Pediatric Epilepsy

Diagnosis and Therapy

Third Edition

Pediatric Epilepsy

Diagnosis and Therapy

Third Edition

EDITORS

JOHN M. PELLOCK, MD
Chairman, Division of Child Neurology
Vice Chair, Department of Neurology
Virginia Commonwealth University
Medical College of Virginia
Richmond, Virginia

BLAISE F.D. BOURGEOIS, MD
Professor of Neurology
Harvard Medical School
Director, Division of Epilepsy and Clinical Neurophysiology
Joseph J. Volpe Chair
Children's Hospital Boston
Boston, Massachusetts

W. EDWIN DODSON, MD
Associate Vice Chancellor and Associate Dean
Professor of Pediatrics and Neurology
Washington University School of Medicine
St. Louis Children's Hopsital
St. Louis, Missouri

ASSOCIATE EDITORS

DOUGLAS R. NORDLI, JR., MD
Director, Children's Memorial Epilepsy Center
Lorna S. and James P. Langdon Chair of Pediatric Epilepsy
Northwestern University's Feinberg School of Medicine
Chicago, Illinois

RAMAN SANKAR, MD, PHD
Professor and Chief, Pediatric Neurology
Rubin Brown Distinguished Chair
David Geffen School of Medicine
Mattel Children's Hospital
University of California, Los Angeles
Los Angeles, California

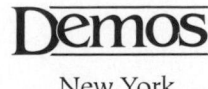

New York

Acquisitions Editor: R. Craig Percy
Cover Designer: Steven Pisano
Compositor and Indexing: Publication Services, Inc.
Printer: Sheridan Books, Inc.

Visit our website at www.demosmedpub.com

Library of Congress Cataloging-in-Publication Data

Pediatric epilepsy: diagnosis and therapy/edited by John M. Pellock, Blaise F.D. Bourgeois, W. Edwin Dodson; associate editors, Douglas R. Nordli Jr., Raman Sankar.—3rd ed.
p.; cm.
Includes bibliographical references and index.
ISBN-13: 978-1-933864-16-7 (hardcover: alk. paper)
ISBN-10: 1-933864-16-8 (hardcover: alk. paper)
1. Epilepsy in children. I. Pellock, John M. II. Bourgeois, Blaise F.D. III. Dodson, W. Edwin
[DNLM: 1. Epilepsy. 2. Child. 3. Epilepsy—therapy. 4. Infant.WL 385 P3795 2008]
RJ496.E6P43 2008
618.92'853—dc22

2007032323

Medicine is an ever-changing science undergoing continual development. Research and clinical experience are continually expanding our knowledge, in particular our knowledge of proper treatment and drug therapy. The authors, editors, and publisher have made every effort to ensure that all information in this book is in accordance with the state of knowledge at the time of production of the book.

Nevertheless, this does not imply or express any guarantee or responsibility on the part of the authors, editors, or publisher with respect to any dosage instructions and forms of application stated in the book. Every reader should examine carefully the package inserts accompanying each drug and check with a physician or specialist whether the dosage schedules mentioned therein or the contraindications stated by the manufacturer differ from the statements made in this book. Such examination is particularly important with drugs that are rarely used or have newly been released on the market. Every dosage schedule or every form of application used is entirely at the reader's own risk and responsibility. The editors and publisher welcome any reader to report to the publisher any discrepancies or inaccuracies noticed.

Special discounts on bulk quantities of Demos Medical Publishing books are available to corporations, professional associations, pharmaceutical companies, health care organizations, and other qualifying groups. For details, please contact:

Special Sales Department
Demos Medical Publishing
386 Park Avenue South, Suite 301
New York, NY 10016
Phone: 800–532–8663 or 212–683–0072
Fax: 212–683–0118
Email: orderdept@demosmedpub.com

Made in the United States of America

07 08 09 10 5 4 3 2 1

Dedication

To our families and to the children and families for whom we care.

Contents

II CLASSIFICATION, EPIDEMIOLOGY, ETIOLOGY, AND DIAGNOSIS

Section Editor: W. Edwin Dodson

III AGE-RELATED SYNDROMES

Section Editors: Blaise F. D. Bourgeois and Douglas R. Nordli, Jr.

NEWBORNS AND EARLY INFANCY

INFANCY

VII PSYCHOSOCIAL ASPECTS

Section Editor: W. Edwin Dodson

Preface

As with the first and second editions, the goal of this third edition of *Pediatric Epilepsy: Diagnosis and Therapy* is to assist all professionals involved in the care of pediatric patients with seizures and epilepsy. Our goal continues to be the perfect result: no seizures, no side effects, and no stigma to limit these children from achieving their full potential.

The scope and depth of coverage of this book remains unique in its field. We have again tried to balance discussions of practical medical management with the scientific basis of epilepsy and its treatment in a clear and concise manner. The book focuses on the special issues of children with epilepsy and is intended as both a practical guide and a reference for clinicians and investigators. With many more options for the treatment of epilepsy—including new antiepileptic drugs (AEDs), vagus nerve stimulation, the reintroduction of the ketogenic diet, increased emphasis on quality of life, as well as improved presurgical evaluation and surgical intervention—hope for a more normal life for all children with epilepsy should continue to grow. To accomplish all the new goals set for this third edition, the previous editors asked Drs. Douglas R. Nordli and Raman Sankar to join them as associate editors.

Since the publication of the second edition, there has been a rapid expansion of basic knowledge, diagnostic techniques, and treatments affecting the management of epilepsy, including advances in basic neurosciences, genetics, definition of syndromes, as well as medical and surgical therapeutic approaches. Because of the increasing familiarity and refinement of knowledge related to the concept of epilepsy syndromes, a new separate section has been added to this third edition. This section consists of an expanded and comprehensive coverage of the syndromes *by age of onset*, taking into account the difficulties that can be encountered in making a fixed diagnosis of a seizure type or epilepsy syndrome in young infants.

Although the precise diagnosis of epilepsy has become more challenging and complex, the enhanced specificity of the final diagnosis will continue to improve therapeutic and prognostic accuracy. The diagnostic process has been further improved by the growing knowledge of metabolic disturbances, disease processes, and genetics of various forms of epilepsy. This has led to an ever-expanding availability of new diagnostic tests, especially those related to DNA analysis. Although the greater choice of diagnostic testing does not always yield an etiology in every patient, those patients without established etiology still have more and better therapeutic options. There has been further growth in the knowledge about clinical pharmacology of AEDs. In particular, experience and comfort have grown with the AEDs that had just been released at the time of the second edition, with recognition of new indications for some of these drugs. Throughout the discussion of individual drugs, available knowledge is discussed regarding their specific use and pharmacokinetics in newborns, infants, older children, and adolescents. Adverse effects are also covered, to include newer aspects as well as age-related, gender-related, and pregnancy-related issues. Epilepsy surgery has become one of the widely applied standard therapeutic approaches to pediatric epilepsy, and it has now truly been incorporated into the treatment paradigms.

In this third edition, every chapter either has been markedly updated or is a newly written chapter that was not included in the second edition. In the initial section on basic mechanisms of epilepsy, a new chapter by Dr. Edward Cooper on the epileptic channelopathies has been added because of the rapid and clinically relevant expansion of knowledge in this area during the past few years. Coverage of epileptogenic cerebral cortical malformations has been enhanced by the contribution of Drs. Christopher Walsh, Ann Poduri, and Bernard Chang. A new section on age-related syndromes has been created. This section is divided into groups of syndromes by age of onset and provides a more comprehensive and detailed coverage by several international authorities in the field, such as Drs. Shunsuke Ohtahara, Richard Hrachovy, Kazuyoshi Watanabe, Pierre Genton, Shlomo Shinnar, Tracy Glauser, Gregory Holmes, Chrysostomos Panayiotopoulos, Prakash Kotagal, and Samuel Berkovic. All of the chapters in this section now follow a unified structure. The section on general principles of therapy now includes a discussion of the emerging evidence-based approach to AED selection by Dr. Tracy Glauser. The issues of fetal effects of epilepsy and fetal effects of AEDs are covered separately by Drs. Mark Yerby and Torbjörn Tomson.

Systematic coverage of individual drugs and other medical treatment modalities was already quite extensive in the second edition but has now been enhanced and expanded to cover the newer drugs not covered previously, as well as updated to include new information on the previously discussed drugs. A chapter on sulthiame by Dr. Dietz Rating has been added, because of the unique role of this drug in the treatment of the common syndrome of benign rolandic epilepsy. Other new chapters cover vitamins, dietary considerations, and alternative therapies (Dr. Orrin Devinsky); immunotherapy (Dr. Raman Sankar); and AEDs in development (Dr. Jacqueline French). The section on surgical treatment contains updated coverage of neurophysiologic evaluation (including magnetoencephalography), advanced imaging, surgical procedures, and outcomes, in addition to an update on vagus nerve stimulation. The section on psychosocial aspects has been expanded and includes chapters on costs of pediatric epilepsy, quality of life, intelligence, co-morbidities, and educational placement, as well as cognitive side effects of AEDs.

We would be remiss in introducing this third edition without acknowledging the contribution of several of the previous authors who have now died. Drs. Kiffin Penry and Fritz Dreifuss, two of the founding fathers of pediatric epilepsy in the United States, have left us to carry on their work. Dr. Eric Lothman died quite prematurely, but his contribution to the understanding of the pathophysiology of seizures and epilepsy remains current even in this edition and will do so for years to come. In honoring these and others who have encouraged and guided our careers, we hope that this book meets the needs of those who care for children with epilepsy as well as the children and families who have to deal with seizures.

For some, epilepsy will be a transient and distant memory, while for others epilepsy is an ever-present burden. Evaluating and treating these children in the most appropriate and efficient fashion while avoiding adverse cognitive and psychosocial effects remains both challenging and rewarding, and it requires state-of-the-art knowledge. We hope that you will find such knowledge in this book, and we hope that this third edition of *Pediatric Epilepsy: Diagnosis and Therapy* will help you and your colleagues provide state-of-the-art care to your patients and their families.

John M. Pellock, MD
Blaise F.D. Bourgeois, MD
W. Edwin Dodson, MD
Douglas R. Nordli, Jr., MD
Raman Sankar, MD, PhD

Contributors

Joan K. Austin, DNS, RN, FAAN
Distinguished Professor and Sally Reahard Chair
Indiana University School of Nursing
Indianapolis, Indiana
Chapter 66: Quality of Life in Children with Epilepsy

Stéphane Auvin, MD, PhD
Department of Pediatric Neurology
Lille University Hospital
Pharmacology Laboratory
Lille Medical School
Lille, France
Chapter 58: Inflammation, Epilepsy, and Anti-Inflammatory Therapies

Caroline E. Bailey, PhD
Assistant Professor
Department of Human Services
California State University
Fullerton, California
Chapter 68: Academic Deficits and Interventions in Pediatric Epilepsy

P. Nina Banerjee, PhD
Gertrude H. Sergievsky Center
College of Physicians and Surgeons
Columbia University
New York, New York
Chapter 9: Epidemiology of Epilepsy in Children

Thomas Bast, MD
Department of Paediatric Neurology
Epilepsy Centre
Children's Hospital
University of Heidelberg
Heidelberg, Germany
Chapter 50: Sulthiame

Dina Battino, MD
Fondazione I.R.C.C.S. Istituto Neurologico "Carlo Besta"
Milan, Italy
Chapter 36: Teratogenic Effects of Antiepileptic Medications

Charles E. Begley
Co-Director, Center for Health Services Research
University of Texas Health Science Center at Houston
Houston, Texas
Chapter 65: Economics of Pediatric Epilepsy

Reza Behrouz, DO
Assistant Professor
Department of Neurology
University of South Florida College of Medicine
Tampa, Florida
Chapter 25: Idiopathic Generalized Epilepsy of Adolescence

Selim R. Benbadis, MD
Professor and Director
Comprehensive Epilepsy Program
Departments of Neurology and Neurosurgery
University of South Florida and Tampa General Hospital
Tampa, Florida
Chapter 25: Idiopathic Generalized Epilepsy of Adolescence

Samuel F. Berkovic, MD, FRS
Director, Epilepsy Research Centre
Department of Medicine
University of Melbourne
West Heidelberg, Victoria, Australia
Chapter 26: Progressive Myoclonus Epilepsies

Blaise F. D. Bourgeois, MD
Professor of Neurology
Harvard Medical School
Director, Division of Epilepsy and Clinical Neurophysiology
Joseph J. Volpe Chair
Children's Hospital Boston
Boston, Massachusetts
Part III: Age-Related Syndromes, Section Editor
Part V: Antiepileptic Drugs and Ketogenic Diet, Section Editor
Chapter 32: Combination Drug Therapy: Monotherapy Versus Polytherapy
Chapter 43: Ethosuximide, Methsuximide, and Trimethadione
Chapter 44: Felbamate
Chapter 53: Valproate

Rochelle Caplan, MD
Professor
David Geffen School of Medicine
University of California, Los Angeles
Los Angeles, California
Chapter 68: Academic Deficits and Interventions in Pediatric Epilepsy

Bernard S. Chang, MD, MMSc
Assistant Professor of Neurology
Harvard Medical School
Comprehensive Epilepsy Center
Beth Israel Deaconess Medical Center
Boston, Massachusetts
Chapter 6: Epileptogenic Cerebral Cortical Malformations

Richard Civil
Vice President, Global Product Safety
Cephalon, Inc.
West Chester, Pennsylvania
Chapter 51: Tiagabine

James C. Cloyd, MD
Professor and Lawrence C. Weaver Endowed Chair–Orphan Drug Development
Director, Center for Orphan Drug Research
College of Pharmacy
University of Minnesota
Minneapolis, Minnesota
Chapter 38: Dosage Form Considerations in the Treatment of Pediatric Epilepsy

Edward C. Cooper, MD, PhD
Assistant Professor
Department of Neurology
University of Pennsylvania
Philadelphia, Pennsylvania
Chapter 3: Channel Mutations in Epilepsy: A Neurodevelopmental Perspective

J. Helen Cross, MB, ChB, PhD, FRCP, FRCPCH
Professor of Pediatric Neurology
Neurosciences Unit
UCL–Institute of Child Health
Great Ormond Street Hospital for Children NHS Trust
London, United Kingdom
Chapter 63: Outcome of Epilepsy Surgery in Childhood

Olivier Delalande
Service de Neurochirurgie Pédiatrique
Fondation Opthalmologique A. de Rothschild
Paris, France
Chapter 62: Surgical Treatment of Therapy-Resistant Epilepsy in Children

Robert J. DeLorenzo, MD, PhD, MPH
George Bliley Professor of Neurology
Professor of Pharmacology and Toxicology
Professor of Molecular Biophysics and Biochemistry
Virginia Commonwealth University
Richmond, Virginia
Chapter 2: Ion Channels, Membranes, and Molecules in Epilepsy and Neuronal Excitability

Laxmikant S. Deshpande, MPharm, PhD
Research Scientist
Department of Neurology
Virginia Commonwealth University
Richmond, Virginia
Chapter 2: Ion Channels, Membranes, and Molecules in Epilepsy and Neuronal Excitability

Orrin Devinsky, MD
Professor of Neurology, Neurosurgery and Psychiatry
New York University School of Medicine
New York, New York
Chapter 55: Vitamins, Herbs, and Other Alternative Therapies

Darryl C. De Vivo, MD
Sidney Carter Professor of Neurology
Professor of Pediatrics
College of Physicians and Surgeons
Columbia University
New York, New York
Chapter 57: The Ketogenic Diet

W. Edwin Dodson, MD
Associate Vice Chancellor and Associate Dean
Professor of Pediatrics and Neurology
Washington University School of Medicine
St. Louis Children's Hospital
St. Louis, Missouri
Part II: Classification, Epidemiology, Etiology, and Diagnosis, Section Editor
Part VII: Psychosocial Aspects, Section Editor
Chapter 37: Pharmacokinetic Principles of Antiepileptic Therapy in Children
Chapter 42: Carbamazepine and Oxcarbazepine
Chapter 49: Phenytoin and Related Drugs
Chapter 67: Epilepsy, Cerebral Palsy, and IQ

Michael Duchowny, MD
Professor of Clinical Neurology
University of Miami School of Medicine
Miami Children's Hospital
Miami, Florida
Chapter 60: Surgical Evaluation

Kevin Farrell, MB, ChB, FRCPC
Professor
Division of Child Neurology
University of British Columbia
British Columbia's Children's Hospital
Vancouver, British Columbia, Canada
Chapter 41: Benzodiazepines

Colin D. Ferrie, MB, ChB, MD, MRCP, FRCPCH
Consultant Paediatric Neurologist
Leeds General Infirmary
Leeds, United Kingdom
Chapter 23: Benign Focal Epilepsies of Childhood

Jacqueline A. French, MD
Professor
Department of Neurology
New York University Medical School
New York, New York
Chapter 59: Antiepileptic Drugs in Development

James D. Frost, Jr., MD
Professor of Neurology and Neuroscience
Peter Kellaway Section of Neurophysiology
Department of Neurology
Baylor College of Medicine
Houston, Texas
Chapter 16: Severe Encephalopathic Epilepsy in Infants: Infantile Spasms (West Syndrome)

William R. Garnett, PharmD
Professor of Pharmacy and Neurology
Department of Pharmacy
Virginia Commonwealth University
Richmond, Virginia
Chapter 38: Dosage Form Considerations in the Treatment of Pediatric Epilepsy

Pierre Genton, MD
Hôpital Henri Gastaut–Centre Saint Paul
Marseille, France
Chapter 17: Myoclonic Epilepsies in Infancy and Early Childhood

Barry E. Gidal, PharmD
Professor
University of Wisconsin
School of Pharmacy and Department of Neurology
Madison, Wisconsin
Chapter 39: Principles of Drug Interactions: Implications for Treatment with Antiepileptic Drugs

Tracy A. Glauser, MD
Director, Comprehensive Epilepsy Program
Cincinnati Children's Hospital Medical Center
Professor of Pediatrics and Neurology
University of Cincinnati College of Medicine
Cincinnati, Ohio
Chapter 19: Febrile Seizures
Chapter 21: Lennox-Gestaut Syndrome
Chapter 31: Evidence-Based Medicine Issues Related to Drug Selection
Chapter 52: Topiramate

Stavros Hadjiloizou, MD
Division of Epilepsy and Clinical Neurophysiology
Department of Neurology
Children's Hospital Boston
Instructor of Neurology
Harvard Medical School
Boston, Massachusetts
Chapter 24: The Landau-Kleffner Syndrome and Epilepsy with Continuous Spike-Waves during Sleep

William Harkness, ChB, FRCS
Consultant Paediatric Neurosurgeon
Department of Neurosurgery
National Hospital for Neurosurgery and Neurology
London, United Kingdom
Chapter 63: Outcome of Epilepsy Surgery in Childhood

W. Allen Hauser, MD
Professor of Neurology and Epidemiology
Gertrude H. Sergievsky Center
College of Physicians and Surgeons and Mailman School of Public Health
Columbia University
New York, New York
Chapter 9: Epidemiology of Epilepsy in Children

Gregory L. Holmes, MD
Professor of Neurology and Pediatrics
Chairman, Department of Neurology
Neuroscience Center at Dartmouth
Dartmouth Medical School
Lebanon, New Hampshire
Chapter 22: Childhood Absence Epilepsies
Chapter 45: Gabapentin and Pregabalin

Carolyn R. Houser, MD
Professor of Neurobiology
David Geffen School of Medicine
University of California, Los Angeles
Los Angeles, California
Chapter 5: Neuropathologic Substrates of Epilepsy

Richard A. Hrachovy, MD
Professor of Neurology
Peter Kellaway Section of Neurophysiology
Department of Neurology
Baylor College of Medicine
Michael E. DeBakey Veterans Affairs Medical Center
Houston, Texas
Chapter 16: Severe Encephalopathic Epilepsies in Infants: Infantile Spasms (West Syndrome)

Sejal V. Jain, MD
Neurophysiology Fellow
Department of Clinical Neurophysiology
Virginia Commonwealth University
Richmond, Virginia
Chapter 11: Evaluating the Child with Seizure

James M. Johnston, MD
Department of Neurosurgery
Washington University–St. Louis
St. Louis, Missouri
Chapter 13: Basics of Neuroimaging in Pediatric Epilepsy

Michael V. Johnston, MD
Chief Medical Officer
Kennedy Krieger Institute
Professor of Neurology, Pediatrics and Physical Medicine and Rehabilitation
The Johns Hopkins School of Medicine
Baltimore, Maryland
Chapter 4: Metabolic and Pharmacologic Consequences of Seizures

John F. Kerrigan, MD
Assistant Professor of Clinical Neurology and Pediatrics
University of Arizona College of Medicine, Phoenix
Director of Pediatric Epilepsy
Barrow Neurological Institute
Phoenix, Arizona
Chapter 56: Zonisamide

Prakash Kotagal, MD
Head, Pediatric Epilepsy Section
Epilepsy Center
Cleveland Clinic Neurological Institute
Cleveland, Ohio
Chapter 27: Localization-Related Epilepsies: Simple Partial Seizures, Complex Partial Seizures, and Rasmussen Syndrome

Günter Krämer, MD
Medical Director
Swiss Epilepsy Center
Zurich, Switzerland
Chapter 54: Vigabatrin

Josiane LaJoie, MD
Assistant Professor of Neurology and Pediatrics
New York University School of Medicine
New York, New York
Chapter 55: Vitamins, Herbs, and Other Alternative Therapies

David J. Leszczyszyn, MD, PhD
Medical Director, Center for Sleep Medicine
Assistant Professor, Division of Child Neurology
Virginia Commonwealth University
Richmond, Virginia
Chapter 34: Status Epilepticus and Acute Seizures

David E. Mandelbaum, MD, PhD
Professor of Clinical Neurosciences and Pediatrics
Warren Alpert Medical School of Brown University
Director of Child Neurology and the Children's Neurodevelopment Center
Hasbro Children's Hospital
Providence, Rhode Island
Chapter 69: Cognitive Side Effects of Antiepileptic Drugs

Gary W. Mathern, MD
Professor
Department of Neurosurgery, The Mental Retardation Research Center, and The Brain Research Institute
David Geffen School of Medicine
University of California, Los Angeles
Los Angeles, California
Chapter 62: Surgical Treatment of Therapy-Resistant Epilepsy in Children

John W. McDonald, MD, PhD
Director, The International Center for Spinal Cord Injury
Kennedy-Krieger Institute
Department of Neurology
The Johns Hopkins School of Medicine
Baltimore, Maryland
Chapter 4: Metabolic and Pharmocologic Consequences of Seizures

Robert C. McKinstry, MD, PhD
Associate Professor of Radiology and Pediatrics
Chief, Pediatric Radiology and Pediatric Neuroradiology
St. Louis Children's Hospital
Washington University
St. Louis, Missouri
Chapter 13: Basics of Neuroimaging in Pediatric Epilepsy

Aspasia Michoulas, BSc Pharm, MD
Neurology Fellow
Division of Child Neurology
University of British Columbia
British Columbia's Children's Hospital
Vancouver, British Columbia, Canada
Chapter 41: Benzodiazepines

Daniel Miles, MD
Assistant Professor of Neurology and Pediatrics
New York University School of Medicine
New York, New York
Chapter 55: Vitamins, Herbs, and Other Alternative Therapies

Eli M. Mizrahi, MD
Head, Peter Kellaway Section of Neurophysiology
Vice Chairman, Department of Neurology
Director, Baylor Comprehensive Epilepsy Center
Professor of Neurology and Pediatrics
Baylor College of Medicine
Houston, Texas
Chapter 14: Neonatal Seizures

Diego A. Morita, MD
Assistant Professor of Pediatrics and Neurology
Division of Neurology
Department of Pediatrics
Cincinnati Children's Hospital Medical Center
University of Cincinnati College of Medicine
Cincinnati, Ohio
Chapter 21: Lennox-Gastaut Syndrome
Chapter 31: Evidence-Based Medicine Issues Related to Drug Selection

Lawrence D. Morton, MD
Medical Director, Clinical Neurophysiology
Associate Professor, Neurology and Pediatrics
Virginia Commonwealth University
Richmond, Virginia
Chapter 11: Evaluating the Child with Seizures
Chapter 28: Selected Disorders Associated with Epilepsy

Solomon L. Moshé, MD
Professor of Neurology, Neuroscience and Pediatrics
Vice Chair, Department of Neurology
Albert Einstein College of Medicine
Bronx, New York
Chapter 1: Pathophysiology of Seizures and Epilepsy in the Immature Brain: Cells, Synapses, and Circuits

Douglas R. Nordli, Jr., MD
Director, Children's Memorial Epilepsy Center
Lorna S. and James P. Langdon Chair of Pediatric Epilepsy
Northwestern University's Feinberg School of Medicine
Chicago, Illinois
Part III: Age-Related Syndromes, Section Editor
Part VI: Epilepsy Surgery and Vagus Nerve Stimulation, Section Editor
Chapter 8: Classification of Epilepsies of Childhood
Chapter 12: The Use of Encephalography in the Diagnosis of Epilepsy in Childhood
Chapter 20: Generalized Epilepsy with Febrile Seizures Plus (GEFS+)
Chapter 23: Benign Focal Epilepsies of Childhood
Chapter 57: The Ketogenic Diet

Christine O'Dell, RN, MSN
Critical Nurse Specialist
Department of Neurology
Montefiore Medical Center
Bronx, New York
Chapter 29: Treatment Decisions in Childhood Seizures

Shunsuke Ohtahara, MD, PhD
Professor of Child Neurology, Emeritus
Department of Child Neurology
Okayama University
Graduate School of Medicine, Dentistry and Pharmaceutical Sciences
Okayama, Japan
Chapter 15: Severe Encephalopathic Epilepsy in Early Infancy

Chrysostomos P. Panayiotopoulos, MD, PhD, FRCP
Consultant Emeritus
Department of Clinical Neurophysiology and Epilepsies
St. Thomas' Hospital
London, United Kingdom
Chapter 23: Benign Focal Epilepsies of Childhood

Shekhar Patil, MD, DM
Epilepsy Fellow
UCL–Institute of Child Health
Great Ormond Street Hospital for Children NHS Trust
London, United Kingdom
Chapter 63: Outcome of Epilepsy Surgery in Childhood

Phillip L. Pearl, MD
Department of Neurology
Children's National Medical Center
George Washington University School of Medicine
Washington, DC
Chapter 22: Childhood Absence Epilepsies
Chapter 45: Gabapentin and Pregabalin

Timothy A. Pedley, MD
Henry and Lucy Moses Professor of Neurology
Chairman, Department of Neurology
Columbia University
New York, New York
Chapter 12: The Use of Encephalography in the Diagnosis of Epilepsy in Childhood

John M. Pellock, MD
Chairman, Division of Child Neurology
Vice Chair, Department of Neurology
Virginia Commonwealth University
Richmond, Virginia
Part VI: General Principles of Therapy, Section Editor
Chapter 20: Generalized Epilepsy with Febrile Seizures Plus (GEFS+)
Chapter 33: Adverse Effects of Antiepileptic Drugs
Chapter 34: Status Epilepticus and Acute Seizures
Chapter 46: Lamotrigine
Chapter 56: Zonisamide

Annapurna Poduri, MD
Assistant in Neurology
Division of Epilepsy and Clinical Neurophysiology
Children's Hospital Boston
Boston, Massachusetts
Chapter 6: Epileptogenic Cerebral Cortical Malformations

John R. Pollard, MD
Assistant Professor
Department of Neurology
University of Pennsylvania
Philadelphia, Pennsylvania
Chapter 59: Antiepileptic Drugs in Development

Asuri N. Prasad, MBBS, MD, FRCPC, FRCPE
Associate Professor
Departments of Pediatrics and Clinical Neurosciences
University of Western Ontario
London, Ontario, Canada
Chapter 7: Genetic Influences on the Risk for Epilepsy

Chitra Prasad, MD, FRCPC, FCCMG, FACMG
Associate Professor
Section of Genetics, Metabolism
Department of Pediatrics
University of Western Ontario
London, Ontario, Canada
Chapter 7: Genetic Influences on the Risk for Epilepsy

Arthur L. Prensky, MD
Professor of Neurology and Pediatrics, Emeritus
Division of Pediatric Neurology
Washington University School of Medicine
St. Louis, Missouri
Chapter 10: An Approach to the Child with Paroxysmal Phenomena with Emphasis on Nonepileptic Disorders

Amir Pshytycky, MD
Neurophysiology and Epilepsy Fellow
Department of Neurology
Children's Hospital of Philadelphia
Philadelphia, Pennsylvania
Chapter 10: An Approach to the Child with Paroxysmal Phenomena with Emphasis on Nonepileptic Disorders

Rajesh RamachandranNair, MD
Assistant Professor
McMaster University
Pediatric Epileptologist
McMaster Children's Hospital
Hamilton, Ontario, Canada
Chapter 40: ACTH and Steroids

Dietz Rating, MD
Professor of Pediatrics
Director, Department of Paediatric Neurology
Epilepsy Centre
Children's Hospital
University of Heidelberg
Heidelberg, Germany
Chapter 50: Sulthiame

James J. Riviello, Jr., MD
George Peterkin Endowed Chair in Pediatrics
Professor of Pediatrics
Department of Pediatrics
Section of Neurology and Developmental Neuroscience
Baylor College of Medicine
The Blue Bird Circle Clinic for Pediatric Neurology
Chief of Neurophysiology
Texas Children's Hospital
Houston, Texas
Chapter 24: The Landau-Kleffner Syndrome and Epilepsy with Continuous Spike-Waves during Sleep

Robert S. Rust, MA, MD
Thomas E. Worrell, Jr., Professor of Epileptology and Neurology
Professor of Pediatrics
The University of Virginia School of Medicine
Co-Director, F. E. Dreifuss Comprehensive Epilepsy and Child Neurology Clinics
Charlottesville, Virginia
Chapter 48: Barbiturates and Related Drugs

Noriko Salamon, MD
Assistant Professor of Radiology
Department of Radiology
David Geffen School of Medicine
University of California, Los Angeles
Los Angeles, California
Chapter 61: Advanced Neuroimaging: PET-MRI Fusion and Diffusion Tensor Imaging

Raman Sankar, MD, PhD
Professor and Chief, Pediatric Neurology
Rubin Brown Distinguished Chair
David Geffen School of Medicine
Mattel Children's Hospital
University of California, Los Angeles
Los Angeles, California
Part I: Basic Mechanisms, Section Editor
Part V: Antiepileptic Drugs and Ketogenic Diet, Section Editor
Chapter 47: Levetiracetam
Chapter 58: Inflammation, Epilepsy, and Anti-Inflammatory Therapies

Nancy Santilli, MSN, PNP, FAAN
Vice President of Commercial Strategy and Portfolio Planning
Endo Pharmaceuticals, Inc.
Chadds Ford, Pennsylvania
Chapter 66: Quality of Life in Children with Epilepsy

W. Donald Shields, MD
Professor of Neurology and Pediatrics
David Geffen School of Medicine
University of California, Los Angeles
Los Angeles, California
Chapter 47: Levetiracetam

Shlomo Shinnar, MD, PhD
Professor of Neurology, Pediatrics and Epidemiology and Population Health
Hyman Climenko Professor of Neuroscience Research
Director, Comprehensive Epilepsy Management Center
Montefiore Medical Center,
Albert Einstein College of Medicine
Bronx, New York
Chapter 19: Febrile Seizures
Chapter 29: Treatment Decisions in Childhood Seizures
Chapter 51: Tiagabine

Matthew D. Smyth, MD, FACS, FAAP
Assistant Professor of Neurosurgery and Pediatrics
Director, Pediatric Epilepsy Surgery Program
St. Louis Children's Hospital
Washington University
St. Louis, Missouri
Chapter 13: Basics of Neuroimaging in Pediatric Epilepsy

O. Carter Snead III, MD
Head, Division Of Neurology
Department Pediatrics
Hospital For Sick Children
University of Toronto
Toronto, Ontario, Canada
Chapter 40: ACTH and Steroids

Kenneth W. Sommerville, MD
Vice President, Area of Neurology
Schwarz Biosciences, Inc.
UCB
Adjunct Assistant Professor of Medicine
Duke University
Raleigh, North Carolina
Chapter 51: Tiagabine

Torbjörn Tomson, MD, PhD
Professor of Neurology
Department of Clinical Neuroscience
Karolinska Institutet
Stockholm, Sweden
Chapter 36: Teratogenic Effects of Antiepileptic Medications

Christine L. Trask, PhD
Clinical Assistant Professor
Department of Psychiatry and Human Behavior
Warren Alpert Medical School of Brown University
Pediatric Neuropsychologist
Rhode Island Hospital
Providence, Rhode Island
Chapter 69: Cognitive Side Effects of Antiepileptic Drugs

Libor Velíšek, MD, PhD
Associate Professor of Neurology and Neuroscience
Albert Einstein College of Medicine
Bronx, New York
Chapter 1: Pathophysiology of Seizures and Epilepsy in the Immature Brain: Cells, Synapses, and Circuits

Harry V. Vinters, MD, FRCP(C), FCAP
Professor of Pathology and Laboratory Medicine and Neurology
Daljit S. and Elaine Sakaria Chair in Diagnostic Medicine
David Geffen School of Medicine
University of California, Los Angeles
Chief, Section of Neuropathology
UCLA Medical Center
Los Angeles, California
Chapter 5: Neuropathologic Substrates of Epilepsy

Christopher A. Walsh, MD, PhD
Chief, Division of Genetics
Children's Hospital Boston
Howard Hughes Medical Institute
Beth Israel Deaconess Medical Center
Bullard Professor of Neurology
Harvard Medical School
Boston, Massachusetts
Chapter 6: Epileptogenic Cerebral Cortical Malformations

Kazuyoshi Watanabe
Faculty of Medical Welfare
Aichi Shukutoku University
Chikusa-ku, Nagoya, Japan
Chapter 18: Partial Epilepsies in Infancy

James W. Wheless, MD
Professor and Chief of Pediatric Neurology
LeBonheur Chair in Pediatric Neurology
University of Tennessee Health Science Center
Director, LeBonheur Comprehensive Epilepsy Program and Neuroscience Institute
LeBonheur Children's Medical Center
Memphis, Tennessee
Chapter 33: Adverse Effects of Antiepileptic Drugs
Chapter 64: Vagus Nerve Stimulation Therapy in Pediatric Patients: Use and Effectiveness

H. Steve White, PhD
Professor and Director
Anticonvulsant Drug Development Program
Department of Pharmacology and Toxicology
University of Utah
Salt Lake City, Utah
Chapter 30: Comparative Anticonvulsant Profile and Proposed Mechanisms of Action of Antiepileptic Drugs

L. James Willmore, MD
Associate Dean and Professor of Neurology and Pharmacology and Physiology
Department of Neurology and Psychiatry
St. Louis University School of Medicine
St. Louis, Missouri
Chapter 33: Adverse Effects of Antiepileptic Drugs

Karen S. Wilcox, PhD
Research Associate Professor
Anticonvulsant Drug Development Program
Department of Pharmacology and Toxicology
University of Utah
Salt Lake City, Utah
Chapter 30: Comparative Anticonvulsant Profile and Proposed Mechanisms of Action of Antiepileptic Drugs

Gabriele Wohlrab, MD
Department of Paediatric Neurology
Epilepsy Centre
Children's Hospital
University of Zurich
Zurich, Switzerland
Chapter 54: Vigabatrin

Nicole Wolf, MD
Department of Paediatric Neurology
Epilepsy Centre
Children's Hospital
University of Heidelberg
Heidelberg, Germany
Chapter 50: Sulthiame

Yasuko Yamatogi, MD, PhD
Professor, Faculty of Health and Welfare Science
Okayama Prefectural University
Soja, Okayama, Japan
Chapter 15: Severe Encephalopathic Epilepsy in Early Infancy

Mark S. Yerby, MD, MPH
Associate Clinical Professor of Neurology
Public Health and Preventive Medicine
Oregon Health and Science University
Portland, Oregon
Chapter 35: The Female Patient and Epilepsy

I

BASIC MECHANISMS

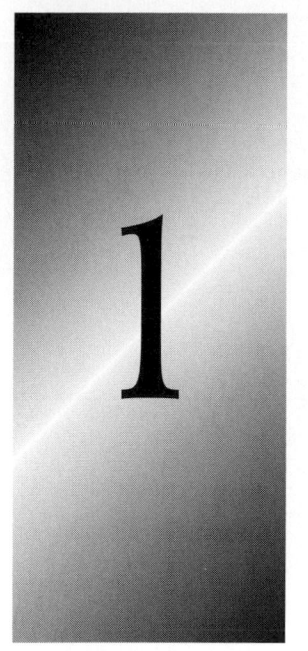

Pathophysiology of Seizures and Epilepsy in the Immature Brain: Cells, Synapses, and Circuits

Libor Velíšek
Solomon L. Moshé

Epidemiological studies show that the propensity of the young brain to develop seizures is much greater than that of the adult brain. These comprehensive studies cover not only the U.S. population (1, 2) but also populations in France, Great Britain, and Scandinavia, and thus the results appear to be geographically independent (3).

There are many more provoked seizures in neonates and infants than in adults. Their causes may involve trauma, hypoxic-ischemic encephalopathy, hypertension, metabolic abnormalities (amino acid disturbances, hypocalcemia, hypoglycemia, and electrolyte imbalance), infections, drug withdrawal, pyridoxine dependency, and toxins (4). Similarly, a genetic predisposition to epilepsy may be expressed in infancy. Genetic factors may involve congenital cerebral malformations and familial seizures such as neurocutaneous syndromes, genetic syndromes, and benign familial epilepsy (4). Additionally, several intractable seizure syndromes occur in early infancy or childhood and not later on (5). In children, focal dysfunction may often produce multifocal seizures and status epilepticus, suggesting less effective barriers for seizure spread and generalization (6).

There are several questions that can be posed. What are the conditions that make a part of the population prone to develop seizures or epilepsy at certain stages of development? Are these conditions acquired or inherited? Are there any seizure-provoking factors in epileptic patients? What are the factors that recruit interictal activity in an epileptic patient to a full seizure? Are these factors intrinsic features of the neurons, glial cells, or extracellular space in the patient's brain or are they extrinsic, environmental factors? How do the seizures propagate? How (why) do they stop? What are the consequences?

Table 1-1 summarizes some important factors that may play a role for these developmental windows of increased susceptibility to seizures and in the development of epilepsy in the immature brain. In this table, factors A1 through A5 are operant in the normal and abnormal brain while factors B1 through B3 may be more specific for abnormal brains. The contribution of these factors in the pathophysiology of childhood seizures can be studied in animal models of seizures and, if available, in models of epilepsy. To study the age-related changes in seizure susceptibility in experimental animals, the investigator has to correlate the brain development of the animal to human brain development. Such correlations are difficult and should be viewed cautiously. Not all parameters studied follow similar developmental curves in animals and humans. This issue is very carefully reviewed in a recent article (7). Nevertheless, based on comparative ontogenetic studies of the rate of brain growth, an 8–10-day-old rat (PN8–10) may be considered equivalent to a full-term

TABLE 1-1
Factors That May Explain the Propensity of the Immature Brain to Develop Frequent Seizures Compared to the Adult Brain

A. In Animals with Normal Brain Development

1. Excitatory processes developing before inhibitory processes
2. Differences in ionic microenvironment
3. Delayed development of circuits that can modify the expression of seizures
4. Seizures begetting seizures as a consequence of frequent seizures early in life
5. High chance of exposure to potentially epileptogenic stimuli (fever, infection, hypoxia)

B. In Animals with Altered Brain Development

1. Genetic predisposition
2. High incidence of structural brain anomalies
3. High probability of seizures begetting seizures as a consequence of frequent seizures early in life

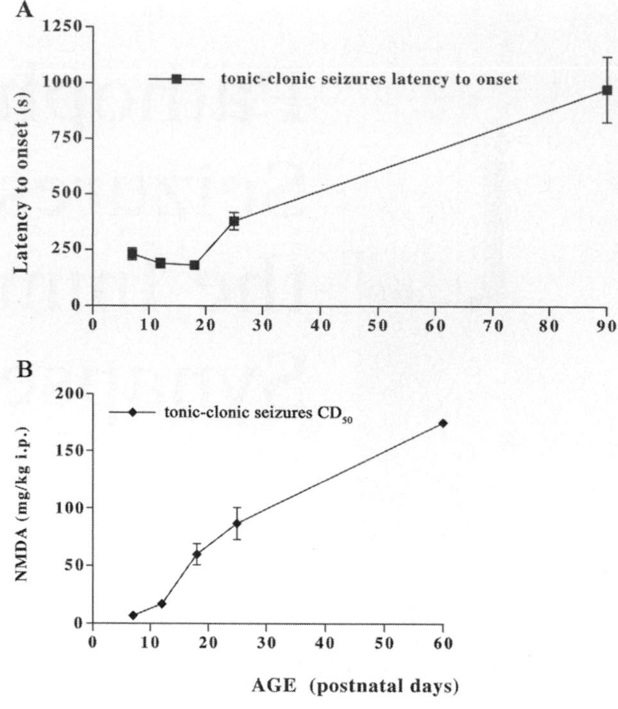

FIGURE 1-1

Increased susceptibility of immature rats to tonic-clonic seizures induced by pentylenetetrazol or NMDA. Increased susceptibility to seizures in immature rats is illustrated using two parameters. (A) Male rats at PN12, 18, 25, and adult rats were injected with 100 mg/kg of pentylenetetrazol subcutaneously. Latency to onset of tonic-clonic seizures, which occur throughout development (20), was determined. A shorter latency to onset of seizures indicates increased susceptibility to seizures. PN12 and PN18 rats have the shortest latencies. (B) Convulsant dose eliciting seizures in 50% of rats (CD_{50}) was calculated from dose responses for NMDA-induced tonic-clonic seizures, which also occur throughout development (21). A lower CD_{50} indicates increased susceptibility to seizures. PN12 rats required lowest doses of NMDA for induction of tonic-clonic seizures. Modified from (21, 22).

human. In this case a rat less than 8–10 days old may be considered as equivalent to a human premature infant (7–10). On the other end, the male rat undergoes puberty from 35–36 to 55 days of age, whereas the female rat is in puberty between days 33 to 45 postnatally (11). Thus, the brain development in the rat at 2–3 weeks postnatally may be equivalent to a human infant/toddler, while at 4–5 weeks it may be considered as equivalent to an older, pre- or peripubescent child (7). Additionally, there may be different developmental dynamics. In a previous review (12), we attempted to calculate the aging rate in developing rat versus developing human. Although our calculations were purely mathematical and did not consider major developmental milestones, we can conclude that the rate of aging in the immature rat compared to that in the child is much higher.

There is ample evidence that seizure susceptibility changes with age in experimental animals as it does in humans. In vitro studies of immature rat cortical neurons (2–3 weeks old) indicate that these neurons are more prone to develop epileptiform discharges following a variety of stimuli, such as low extracellular calcium (13), repetitive stimulation (14), penicillin, bicuculline, picrotoxin (15–18), or high potassium administration (19). In vivo studies indicate that, in 2–3-week-old rats, the susceptibility to seizures is higher, and seizures spread more easily than in any other ages in many seizure models including pentylenetetrazol (Figure 1-1A), bicuculline, allylglycine, kainic acid, N-methyl-D-aspartate (NMDA) (Figure 1-1B), and kindling (Figure 1-2) (20–34). These young, 2–3-week-old rats are also more prone to develop status epilepticus than older rats. Indeed, in many seizure models 2–3-week-old rats are also more prone than younger, 1-week-old rats, to develop seizures, defining thus a specific developmental window for increased seizure susceptibility.

It should be noted that most of the experimentally induced seizures are models of *acute* seizures following the single administration of chemical or electric stimulation (34). There is a *semichronic* model of seizures in the young brain represented by kindling, which is induced by repeated electrical stimulation of susceptible brain sites over 2–3 days in developing rats (29, 35). Until now, there have been only a few successful efforts to develop *chronic* models of seizures in the developing brain that would

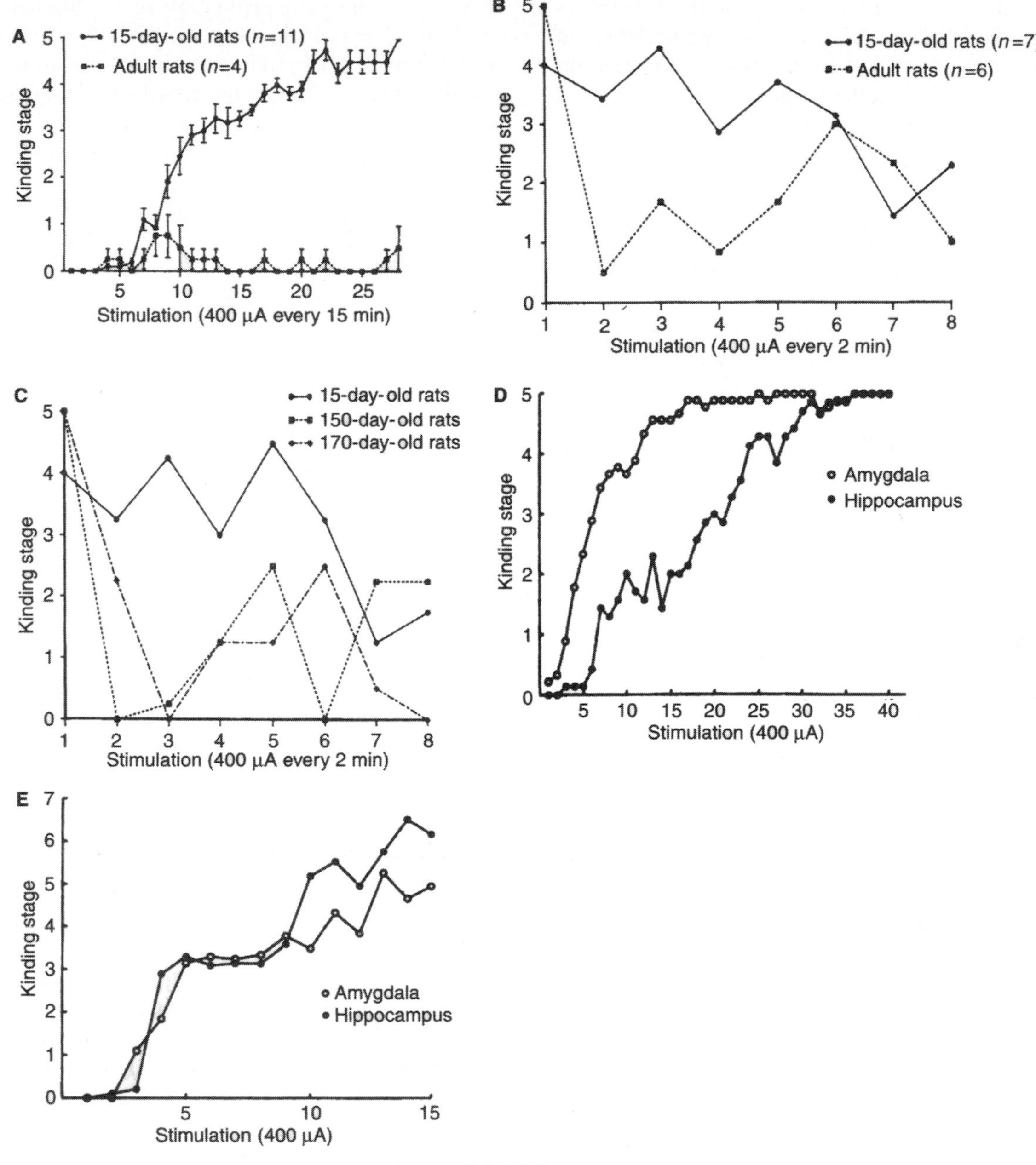

FIGURE 1-2

Increased seizure susceptibility of the immature PN15 brain to kindling-related seizures. Electrodes were implanted in the amygdala in A, B, and C and into the amygdala and hippocampus in D and E. In this composite, the *x*-axis depicts the severity of kindled seizures using the kindling scale of Racine (23) as modified by Moshé (24) and later on by Haas et al. (25). Kindling stages higher than 4 are secondarily generalized convulsions. Each point represents the mean behavioral kindling stage for the particular stimulation. (A) Kindling can be induced in PN15 rats using a 15-minute interstimulus interval; this stimulation paradigm fails to elicit kindling in adult rats. (B) The intensity of postictal depression is decreased in PN15 rats. In this paradigm, PN15 and adult rats that had experienced a generalized seizure received 7 additional stimuli, each delivered at 2-minute intervals. PN15 rats experienced more secondarily generalized seizures than adults, especially during the first 8 minutes. (C) The intensity of postictal refractoriness increases with age. The same rats were tested at 3 different ages: PN15, PN150 and PN170. (D) Kindling antagonism in adult rats. Kindling stimuli were delivered in the amygdala and ipsilateral hippocampus on an alternating basis, and each stimulation is plotted separately. Kindling was induced from the amygdala but not the hippocampus. (E) Lack of kindling antagonism between amygdala and hippocampus in PN16–17 rats under the same experimental conditions that induce antagonism in adults. Modified from (25–27).

better mimic human epilepsy. Examples of such studies include kindling in kittens (36) and the long-term effects of the administration of tetanus toxin in the hippocampus of young rats (37). The epileptic potential of the gamut of either chemically, physically, or genetically experimentally induced brain structural abnormalities has not been adequately explored (38–45). Why do these potentially useful models not attract more research interest? They are very expensive, labor-intensive, and time-consuming, and the data yield is relatively low. Yet this path may be required to establish models for refractory epileptic syndromes in children—catastrophic epilepsies of childhood. Recently, there has been an increase in utilization of these developmental models of pre- or perinatal brain damage, as discussed later.

This review is intended to summarize current information about the differences in the epileptogenicity of young and adult brain and to point out possible future research directions in the field of developmental epilepsy. Since the first publication of this chapter there has been a tremendous increase in the available information about developing cells, synapses, and circuits; we attempt to include all the high points in this edition.

NORMAL IMMATURE BRAIN: EXCITATORY PROCESSES PREDOMINATING

Physiologic, morphologic, biochemical, and molecular biology studies have been performed to determine differences between the young and adult brain that may answer two questions: (1) What are the mechanisms responsible for the enhanced seizure susceptibility of the developing brain? (2) Why is the seizure spread less well controlled in the immature than in the adult brain?

Physiology

In vivo microelectrode studies show no evidence of inhibition in the paired-pulse paradigm in the cornu ammonis 1 (CA1) area of the hippocampus prior to PN18 in rats, after which the intensity of inhibition steadily increases to reach adult levels by PN28. In contrast, already at PN14 the measures of excitation (i.e., excitability and spike width) are at fully mature levels (46). These results indicate that in the rat hippocampus, excitatory processes are well established or fully mature within 2 weeks after birth, whereas the maturation of inhibitory processes to adult levels may not be achieved until several weeks later (46). Two additional features should be discussed here. First, in the hippocampus and other structures in the immature rats, gamma-aminobutyric $acid_A$ ($GABA_A$) receptors have been shown to have depolarizing effects and at times mediate excitatory events (19, 47, 48). Second, in immature animals (kittens, rats, and mice), excitatory NMDA transmission peaks early in development (49–53), with the immature form of the NMDA receptor present in rats until PN14 (54). Both these features may significantly contribute to the increased epileptogenicity of the immature brain.

The available data in seizure models support these findings. The intensity of postictal refractoriness (the period that follows a seizure) may increase with age (Figures 1-2, 1-3). Thus, in rats younger than 2–3 weeks of age, electrical kindling in the amygdala or hippocampus can be induced with stimuli (400 μA, 60 Hz current for 1 s), given at short interstimulus intervals (26, 35, 55, 56). This is not the case in adult rats (57, 58). In younger rats, if two sites are kindled concurrently, both sites develop severe kindled seizures (25, 59). In adults, one of them develops kindling while the other site is suppressed (Figure 1-2) (60). The age-specific failure of both inter- and intrahemispheric mechanisms to suppress the development of multiple kindling foci may explain the high incidence of multifocal seizures in the immature CNS (25, 59). In PN15 rats, additional kindling stimulations easily induce severe seizures classified as stages 6–8 (25). In contrast, in adult rats, severe seizures may occur after approximately 250 kindling stimulations (61).

The increased epileptogenesis may arise from age-specific conditions for excitation and inhibition in the brain (51). Early postnatally, cortical glutamate-mediated excitation utilizes mostly NMDA receptors. This unusual role of NMDA receptors diminishes with increasing age in favor of alpha-amino-3-hydroxy-5-methyl-4-isoxazolepropionic acid (AMPA)-receptor-mediated glutamate transmission (49, 62). Additionally, early postnatally, GABA has excitatory effects through $GABA_A$ receptors in several structures, such as hippocampus, cerebral cortex, cerebellum, and spinal cord, and therefore rather supports than antagonizes glutamate excitatory actions (47, 51, 63). Thus, early in life, GABAergic inhibition may be mediated solely via $GABA_B$ receptors (51), and a fragile balance is maintained between powerful excitatory events mediated by $GABA_A$, NMDA, and AMPA receptors (64) and inhibitory events relying solely on $GABA_B$ transmission (51). Therefore in the developing brain, it seems logical that the $GABA_B$ inhibition may be strengthened; this appears to be the case also in the site critical for control of seizures, the substantia nigra pars reticulata (65), although this enhancement probably cannot compensate for abundant excitation. This indicates that early postnatal arrangement of principal ionotropic receptors favors excitatory processes and that the rearrangement of these receptors is necessary for the decrease of seizure susceptibility in the adolescent and adult brain. It should be noted, however, that the rearrangement of the function of $GABA_A$ receptors is activity dependent and may be altered by significant early postnatal activation, including seizures (66).

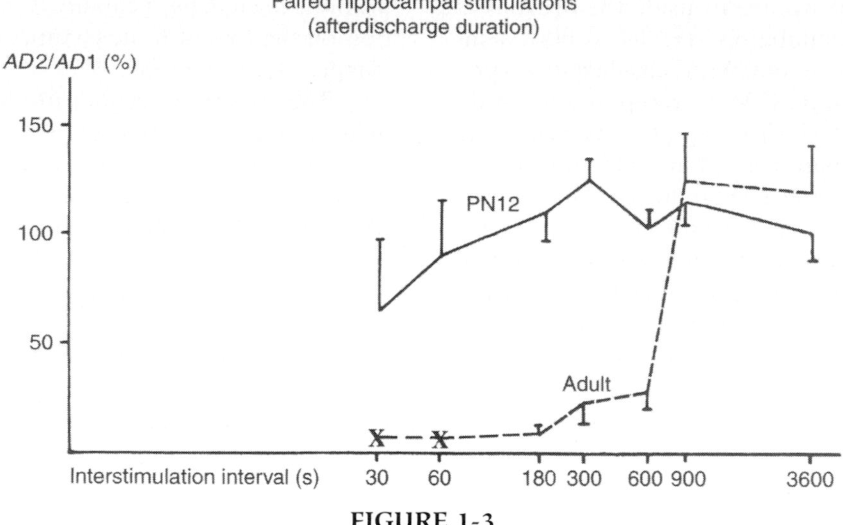

FIGURE 1-3

Insufficient postictal refractory period in the PN12 hippocampus. PN12 and adult rats were implanted with hippocampal stimulating electrodes and cortical recording electrodes. Each of two stimulations consisted of two trains of 121 constant-current rectangular pulses (8 Hz, 1 ms duration; total train length 15 s) with intensity twice as high as necessary to induce a hippocampal-cortical evoked potential using stimulation with a single pulse. Interstimulation intervals (*x*-axis) were in the range from 30 s to 3600 s (1 hour). The duration of the afterdischarge (AD) was recorded after each stimulation, and the results were expressed as AD2/AD1 × 100. The postictal refractory period in PN12 rats was shorter than 30 s because already at this interstimulation interval there was no difference between the duration of the AD1 and AD2. In contrast, in adult rats the postictal refractory period lasted between 600 and 900 s because at 900 s interstimulation interval the duration of AD2 was equal to the AD1.

Morphology

Earlier anatomical studies have suggested that there is a differential development of morphologically distinct types of synapses that can be assigned to "excitatory" and "inhibitory" functions. The classic study of Schwartzkroin showed that the "excitatory type" of the synapse is already present during the first and second postnatal week in the rabbit hippocampal area CA1, whereas the synapses of the "inhibitory type" start to occur during the third postnatal week (67). Thus, net excitation develops in parallel with the "excitatory type" of synapses, while the development of inhibition follows the occurrence of the "inhibitory type" of synapses (68). In the area CA3 of the immature hippocampus, the development of inhibition occurs earlier than in CA1. However, abundant excitatory axonal collaterals in this area form a complex network, which loses its complexity with maturation. Thus, the excessive excitatory wiring in the area CA3 may also contribute to increased epileptogenicity of the immature hippocampus and also to faster, less controlled seizure propagation early in life (69, 70). Finally, faster spread of seizures and recruitment of additional areas in the immature nervous system, compared to the adult, may be due to an extensive direct coupling of the neurons demonstrated in the neocortex of young rats lost with maturation (71). Similar findings have been reported in the PN12–18 rat hippocampus (72).

Biochemistry and Molecular Biology

The developmental hyperexcitability of the all subtypes of glutamate receptors (49, 73) may be a function of their developmentally regulated subunit composition (74). The AMPA subtype of glutamate receptors may change their subunit composition during development from calcium-permeable isoforms in the immature brain to calcium-impermeable isoforms in adulthood (75). In this scenario, it is possible that the enhanced calcium influx into the immature neurons via fast excitatory receptor channels may be a powerful source of depolarization. Similarly, there are significant developmental differences in the expression of $GABA_A$ receptor subunit messenger RNAs (mRNAs), which also suggest age-specific composition of $GABA_A$ receptors (76). The striking correlation between the seizure-specific function and the distribution of certain $GABA_A$ receptor subunit mRNAs in certain brain areas suggests the existence of developmentally regulated $GABA_A$ receptor isoforms that may affect seizures in an opposite way compared to adult $GABA_A$ receptor isoforms (77). Molecular biology studies also indicate that ionic transporter systems such as NKCC1 and KCC2 go through maturational processes, which may affect excitatory and inhibitory features of the neurotransmitter receptors, particularly $GABA_A$ responses (78–80). One of the functional features that may comprise both the differential composition of $GABA_A$ receptors and the ionic (chloride) environment inside the neurons is GABA-mediated tonic inhibition (81). It has been demonstrated that the spillover of GABA outside the synaptic cleft acts on extrasynaptic $GABA_A$ receptors. Addition of bicuculline would block these receptors as well as the chloride currents they control. This tonic inhibition, which may be age-specific, presets excitability of the neuronal plasma membrane and modulates the gain of the transmission (82). These extrasynaptic receptors exhibit a high affinity for GABA (hence low ambient concentrations of GABA are sufficient), and do not inactivate rapidly, thus producing a tonic form of inhibition (83). Unlike the synaptic (phasic) receptors, they do not bind benzodiazepines (84, 85). Recent studies indicate that during this "excitatory GABA" developmental period, tonic and phasic GABA activation in immature neurons may play a critical role in their synaptic integration, which is activity dependent. This process takes place in both the immature brain and newly born neurons in the adult brain (86–88).

The relatively delayed maturation of other neuromodulatory systems may contribute to the increased epileptogenicity of the immature brain. In adult rats, norepinephrine depletion accelerates the rate of kindling, decreases the intensity of postictal refractoriness levels, and permits the development of multiple seizure foci (89–91). In this respect, the norepinephrine-depleted adult rats resemble developing 2-week-old rats in which the norepinephrine transmission has not reached adult levels (29).

NORMAL IMMATURE BRAIN: DIFFERENCES IN IONIC MICROENVIRONMENT AND GLIAL SUPPORT

Setting the Scene

In young children, the brain is more vulnerable to insults from the external environment (92, 93). These insults may be due to epileptogenic features of exogenous or endogenous pyrogens, toxins produced by infectious agents, or reactive metabolic byproducts of the host tissues. The increased vulnerability of the young brain is probably the result of the still developing blood-brain barrier, which, in fact, reflects the development of glial cells (94). Glia have an essential role in maintaining constant extracellular environment of the nervous system (95). In the mature brain, glia contribute to neuronal stability by maintaining ion homeostasis. Almost all ions involved in synaptic transmission undergo age-specific changes, as reflected by the availability of ionic channels and the efficacy of energy-dependent ionic transporters, both in glia and in neurons (96). There is no general rule that the development of ionic channels follows; however, it seems that in the early developmental stages many ionic channels promote calcium permeability (96). For detailed information on the role of ionic channel in epileptogenesis, see Chapter 3, this volume.

The relevant questions are these: Are the developmental changes in ionic environment powerful enough to affect age-specific seizure susceptibility? How does the maturation of transporter systems affect the development of seizures in the immature brain?

Potassium

Potassium has an important role in the regulation of ionic fluxes early in the development of the nervous system. Intracellular concentration of potassium in neurons increases with maturation. This may be due to an increase in Na^+/K^+-ATPase content and probably also activity. Na^+/K^+-ATPase is responsible for the afterhyperpolarization of the neuron following glutamate-induced excitatory postsynaptic potentials (EPSPs) (97). During afterhyperpolarization, it is more difficult to elicit another population spike. In young rats, the afterhyperpolarization is minimal until PN11 and increases during first five postnatal weeks (97). Therefore, young neurons have more favorable conditions to generate repetitive action potentials than adult neurons have, which may further increase the susceptibility of the immature brain to seizures.

Extracellular K^+ efflux accompanies repetitive neuronal discharges (98). The rises in the extracellular K^+ as a consequence to neuronal (and epileptiform) activity are higher in the immature brain (99, 100) and the ceiling for extracellular K^+ concentration ($[K^+]_o$) induced by excessive neuronal activity is much lower in the adult than in the immature rats (10–12 mM versus 1420 mM) (17, 100). In any age group, accumulation of extracellular K^+ causes proportionate moderate depolarization of the neurons and thereby increases neuronal excitability. However, the capability of young CNS to accumulate extracellular K^+ is much larger than that of the adult brain, because of the immature clearance systems in the young (101). Additionally, repetitive discharges in the young brain tend to depolarize the neurons more than similar discharges in the adult brain, because the accumulation of potassium during afterdischarges is higher in the young (P9–11) rats than in older ages (101). In an environment with repeated epileptiform discharges, high $[K^+]_o$ may promote a transition from interictal to ictal state. This situation is more likely to occur in the immature brain (17, 101). This is because there are several extracellular K^+ clearance systems, all of which are immature in the young brain and may contribute to decreased K^+ removal from the extracellular space. The first clearance system is Na^+/K^+-ATPase with a neuronal (97) and a glial (102) pool. The second system is K^+–Cl^- transport into astrocytes (103). The density of astrocytes in the hippocampus during the first postnatal week in the rat is very low, while during the second postnatal week it is sparse only in hippocampal stratum pyramidale (104). The third mechanism of K^+ clearence is spatial redistribution by hiding and diluting K^+ in the remote and narrow processes of the extracellular space. Neurons, astrocytes, and oligodendrocytes share this function; however, the maturation of oligodendrocytes in not finished before four weeks of age (104). Therefore, in the young brain, the extracellular space is wider (105) and spatial redistribution, as measured by extracellular slow potentials (106), is slower, contributing to higher activity–dependent local concentrations of potassium. These findings demonstrate delayed maturation of various glial elements, which increases epileptogenesis of the immature brain and may support the progression of ongoing epileptiform activity (95, 107). Finally, there is a maturational pattern of potassium-chloride cotransporters (KCC), which are less significant for potassium clearance but very significant for chloride distribution (64).

The developmental features of potassium concentration and clearance as well as potassium effects on neuronal membrane excitability make potassium a good ionic candidate responsible in part for the increased seizure susceptibility in the immature brain, especially for the promotion of the transition from interictal to ictal seizure state.

Calcium

Extracellular calcium has age-specific effects on neuronal excitability. Electrophysiological studies have shown that glutamate, and especially NMDA, receptors in the immature hippocampal pyramidal neurons are regulated by extracellular calcium instead of magnesium as in the case of mature neurons (108, 109). Therefore, in the immature brain, activity-dependent changes in extracellular calcium may have a greater influence on ion flow produced by activation of the NMDA receptor. As mentioned previously, enhanced calcium influx into the developing neurons due to the immature form of the AMPA subtype of glutamate receptor channels lacking the GluR2 subunit may be a powerful source of depolarization (75).

The role of intracellular calcium in seizure susceptibility of the immature brain is less obvious and probably indirect. Intracellular calcium affects neuronal maturation through calcium-regulated transcription (110). However, the correlation between this calcium effect and seizure susceptibility of the immature brain has not been yet systematically studied. Further, developmentally regulated intracellular calcium levels (96, 111, 112) may determine the speed by which the axon reaches its synaptic target. Thus, higher intracellular calcium levels early in the development may affect the complexity of the neuronal network and also its excitability by delaying the "plug-in" of the inhibitory elements. Additionally, reciprocal calcium channel (T/R and L type), opening together with voltage-gated sodium channel activity, may contribute to intrinsic bursting, found in CA1 pyramidal cells during the third postnatal week of the rat (113), right after the $GABA_A$ receptor depolarization diminishes, extending effectively the period of increased seizure susceptibility demonstrated in vivo (34).

Chloride

Intracellular chloride can significantly affect features of the neuron and its responses to the neurotransmitter operating via chloride environment (i.e., $GABA_A$) receptors. Intracellular concentration of chloride has powerful effects on chloride fluxes out from and into the neuron (Figure 1-4). If the chloride concentration inside the cell is above electrochemical equilibrium, opening the GABA-operated chloride channel in $GABA_A$ receptors leads to chloride leakage from the cell and consequent depolarization. This is the situation often found in immature neurons. The reason is the developmentally regulated expression of KCC (NKCC1 and KCC2) in the immature neurons, which results in significant intracellular accumulations of chloride (114). NKCC1 pumps all ions, including chloride, into the immature neuron. Its expression (and thus, function) significantly decreases with maturation (64, 80, 115). Therefore, blockade of this cotransporter by the specific antagonist bumetamide significantly suppresses high (8.5 mM) potassium–induced epileptiform activity in brain slices from PN7–12 old rats but is ineffective in PN21–23 rats with already decreased NKCC1 expression; and, of course, bumetamide is also ineffective in slices from NKCC1 knockout mice. Similarly, bumetamide suppresses kainic acid seizures in PN10 rats (80). KCC2 lowers the intraneuronal chloride concentration below its electrochemical equilibrium, and this function increases with maturation (116, 117). If the NKCC1 concentration is high and KCC2 concentration is low, as demonstrated in immature neurons, chloride accumulates in the neurons (78). After $GABA_A$ receptor–operated chloride channels are opened, chloride leaks out, and the cell membrane depolarizes with possible firing of an action potential (64). In mice with disruption of the KCC2-encoding gene (118), electrophysiological recording showed hyperexcitability in the hippocampus, and heterozygotes had increased seizure susceptibility compared to those animals with uninterrupted genes (119). Additional data indicate activity-dependent and also sex-specific expression of KCC2 (79, 120). These findings may contribute to seizure modulation of consequent seizure susceptibility and to sex-differences synaptic events as well as seizure susceptibility (121).

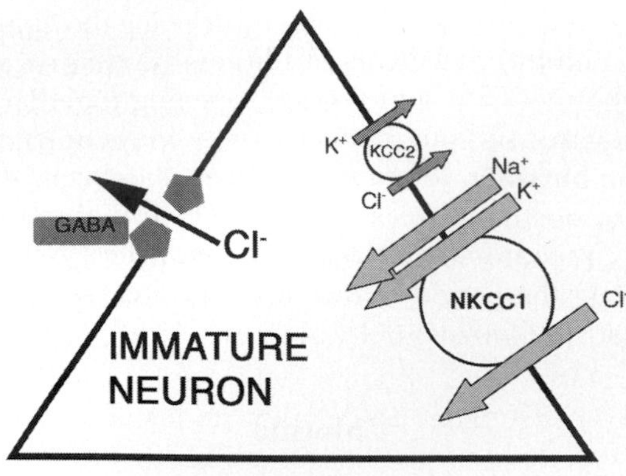

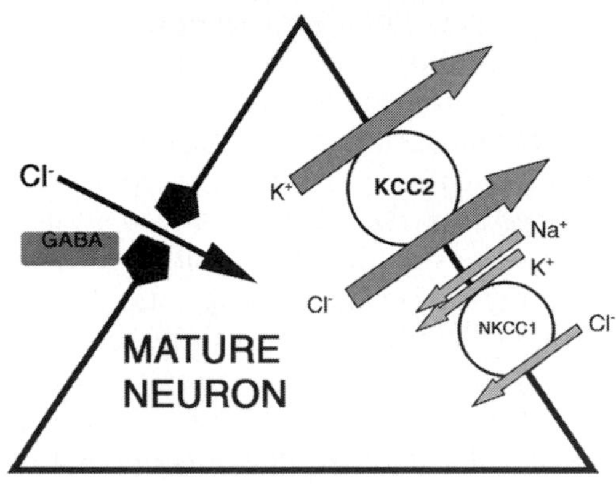

FIGURE 1-4

Main factors affecting chloride concentrations in the immature and mature neurons. In the immature neuron, a sodium-potassium-chloride cotransporter (NKCC1) is expressed in high concentrations. As a result, chloride anions are pumped in and accumulate inside the cell, since the low expression of the potassium-chloride cotransporter (KCC2) cannot extrude them out of the cell. This chloride accumulation shifts chloride reversal potential to a more positive value than the membrane potential. After the $GABA_A$ receptor-operated chloride channel is open after GABA binding, chloride flux is directed from inside the cell outward, carrying negative charge and thus making the inside of the immature neurons more positive—membrane depolarization occurs. This depolarization can generate sodium and calcium action potentials (64).

In the mature neuron, NKCC1 expression is low, while the KCC2 expression is high. This arrangement keeps intracellular chloride concentration low, and the chloride reversal potential is more negative than the membrane potential. After GABA binding to the $GABA_A$ receptor, chloride channels open and chloride anions flow into the cell. This renders the cell more negative inside, and a membrane hyperpolarization occurs. Hyperpolarization makes firing action potentials more difficult.

Sodium

Sodium also plays a significant role in early developmental seizures, as demonstrated by seizures resulting from sodium channel dysfunctions, which occur during infancy or early childhood and often disappear later on (122). The reasons for the developmental occurrence of seizures associated with sodium channel dysfunction are not clear. Although there are age-dependent expression patterns of sodium channel subunits (123), they do not define vulnerability windows. As an alternative, the age specificity of sodium channel defects may be a result of age-specific insults that interact with these channels. For example, increased body temperature (fever) may unmask specific deficits of mutated sodium channels (124). Consistently, sodium channel defects are particularly common in individuals with febrile seizures (125).

NORMAL IMMATURE BRAIN: DELAYED DEVELOPMENT OF CIRCUITS THAT MODIFY THE EXPRESSION OF SEIZURES

Spread of Metabolic Activation during Seizures

Studying the role of brain structures in the initiation and propagation of seizures has, unfortunately, serious limitations. Although several morphological and physiological methods are available, none of them can give a direct answer as to whether the seizure propagates directly from one structure to another via a specific pathway, or whether these additional structures are involved indirectly through relay areas. The best way to approach involvement of different structures is a combination of electrophysiology and imaging that may provide significant correlates of seizure spread. Electrophysiology itself provides limited findings because surface electrodes cover only superficial neocortical regions; depth electrodes record from a restricted area only, and thus many electrodes must be placed to assess the electrical activity of the brain, including the brainstem. Therefore, metabolic imaging studies are more helpful.

Metabolic studies using a radioactive glucose analog 2-deoxyglucose (2-DG) have provided significant information about changes in the metabolic activity of several structures during seizures but also during the immediate postictal period. This information points only to the metabolic activity of the structures; their actual role in seizure generation, propagation, or control, however, can only be estimated. It should be noted that, although 2-DG is an excellent source of qualitative information about brain metabolism changes, 2-DG studies in animals undergoing seizures may not provide absolute quantification because certain assumptions proposed by Sokoloff are applicable only under normal (resting) conditions (126). Additionally, 2-DG uptake informs about the activity of presynaptic elements in the structures but cannot give a simple answer about increases in inhibition or excitation. Further, excessive motor behavior (as during seizures) can change 2-DG uptake pattern and confound the results. Therefore, the 2-DG results should be interpreted with caution.

Several 2-DG metabolic studies demonstrate age-specific metabolic involvement of brain structures in kainic acid-, kindling-, bicuculline-, and pentylenetetrazol-seizures, with somewhat limited data on flurothyl seizures (28, 127–130). The excitotoxin kainic acid, as well as kindling, induces age-specific seizures that originate focally with subsequent generalization. In addition, kainic acid–induced seizures progress into status epilepticus (28, 32, 131, 132). Pentylenetetrazol and flurothyl seizures are believed to be primarily generalized seizures and also have age-specific features; these seizures can lead to status epilepticus (20, 22, 133–138). More recently, the lithium-pilocarpine model of epilepsy has been explored (139).

In young rats until the third week of age, kainic acid–induced status epilepticus produces a rise in metabolism restricted to the hippocampus and lateral septum (28, 130). This is paralleled by paroxysmal discharges observed on electroencephalogram (EEG) that are recorded in the hippocampus, although some studies have proposed that seizures are more prominent in the neocortex (28, 130, 132, 140, 141). Starting from the end of the third week, there is a rise in labeling of other structures that are part of or closely associated with the limbic system: the amygdala complex, the mediodorsal and adjacent thalamic nuclei, the piriform, entorhinal, and rostral limbic cortical regions, and areas of projection of the fornix. These metabolic maps are thus similar to those observed in adults (130, 142). In amygdala kindling in PN15, the metabolic activation during severe seizures is restricted to limbic structures (128, 129), even when the rats experience secondarily generalized seizures. Another interesting seizure-induced difference between the metabolic activation of the young and adult brain is in the involvement of the substantia nigra pars reticulata (SNR). Whereas in the adult rats there is a significant metabolic activation of the SNR during kindling and kainic acid status epilepticus (143–147), neither kindled seizures nor kainic acid status epilepticus induce metabolic activation of the SNR in young rats (28, 148).

A series of studies on pentylenetetrazol-induced status epilepticus have shown an age-specific pattern of metabolic activity and blood flow. In young rats at PN10, there is a uniform increase in the cerebral metabolism and blood flow throughout the brain. At PN21, an age when developmentally specific pentylenetetrazol clonic seizures begin to occur (20, 22), there are significant decreases of local metabolism and blood flow in the cortex and hippocampus as well as in mammillary body, thalamic nuclei, and white matter areas. Moderate metabolic and blood flow increases are restricted to a few structures (134, 137). In the adult rats, there is a rise in metabolism primarily in the neocortex, cerebellum, and vestibular nuclei (136). The data show consistency between metabolic rate and blood flow rate and demonstrate age-specific patterns of brain metabolic activation due to seizures.

Recently, there has been an increased interest in the brain metabolic patterns in the lithium-pilocarpine model of epilepsy. Studies have demonstrated that, in agreement with previous work, spontaneous seizures consistently develop in PN21 and older rats subjected to lithium-pilocarpine status epilepticus (139, 149, 150). No spontaneous seizures were observed in those rats subjected to status epilepticus on PN10 (139), and the spontaneous seizures developed infrequently (23%) in 2-week-old rats exposed to lithium-pilocarpine status epilepticus (150). Similarly, there was no neuronal damage and no metabolic consequences in the youngest group. Older groups than PN10 had neuronal damage in the hippocampal CA1 (2-week-old) (149) and lateral thalamus (PN12) (151). Adult rats additionally had damage in the piriform cortex and basolateral amygdala, whereas the PN21 rats displayed neuronal damage also in the entorhinal cortex.

During the latent period between the status epilepticus and development of spontaneous seizures, in PN21 and adult rats, there were decreases in metabolic activation in forebrain regions corresponding to the damaged areas. At the end of the latent period, metabolic increases in the brainstem occurred (139). Additionally, this model with lithium-pilocarpine status epilepticus induced on PN21 has been used in MRI studies for prediction of epilepsy development (152, 153). Rats with no MRI abnormalities did not develop epilepsy. Spontaneous seizures developed in two groups: with visible MRI abnormalities in one group and without visible abnormalities but with changes in T2 relaxation times in the other. These MRI changes did not correlate with neuronal damage, suggesting that subcellular changes may be responsible for the future development of spontaneous seizures (152, 153).

In flurothyl-induced moderate seizures (20% mortality) in PN15 rats, there is an activation of glucose metabolism in the midbrain and brainstem (excluding the SNR, however) and a decrease of metabolism in the neocortex. Other structures are not affected (EF Sperber, personal communication).

Brain Structures Controlling Seizures

Several brain sites play a critical role in the control or activation of seizures. These sites involve SNR, superior colliculus, subthalamic nucleus, pedunculopontine nucleus, anterior thalamus, and area tempestas (154–163). Unfortunately, developmental data are currently available only for the SNR (77, 164).

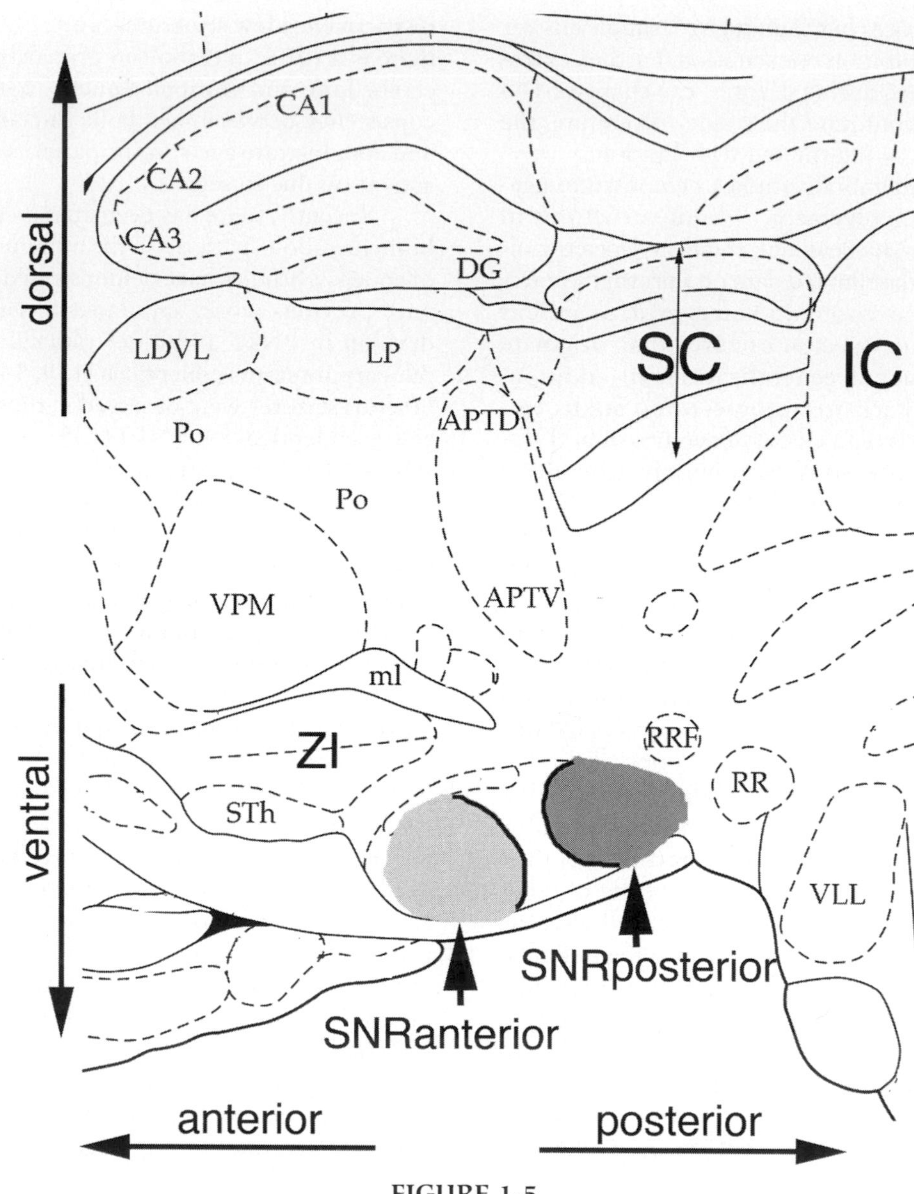

FIGURE 1-5

Two compartments of the substantia nigra pars reticulata (SNR) that in the adult rat brain differentially control seizures. Sagittal section of the rat brain 2.4 mm lateral from midline (168) limited to parts of diencephalon, midbrain, and the brainstem. The diagram illustrates both subregions of the SNR. In the adult male brain, microinfusions of muscimol placed bilaterally and symmetrically in the light gray area ($SNR_{anterior}$) have anticonvulsant effects in flurothyl-induced clonic seizures. In the adult male brain, bilaterally symmetrical microinfusions of muscimol in the dark gray area ($SNR_{posterior}$) have proconvulsant effects. In the adult female brain, symmetrical microinfusions of muscimol into $SNR_{anterior}$ have similar anticonvulsant effects as in the adult males. However, symmetrical muscimol infusions into $SNR_{posterior}$ in adult female rats are without any effect on seizures. Arrows mark the main directions.

Abbreviations: APTD: anterior pretectal nucleus, dorsal. APTV: anterior pretectal nucleus, ventral. CA1, CA2, CA3, CA4: hippocampal cornu ammonis regions 1, 2, 3, and 4. DG: dentate gyrus. IC: inferior colliculus. LDVL: laterodorsal thalamic nucleus, ventrolateral. LP: lateral posterior thalamic nucleus. ml: medial lemniscus. Po: group of posterior thalamic nuclei. RR: retrorubral nucleus. RRF: retrorubral field. SC and the arrow mark the extent of the superior colliculus layers. STh: subthalamic nucleus. VLL: ventral nucleus of lateral lemniscus. VPM: ventral posteromedial thalamic nucleus. ZI: zona incerta.

In the adult male rat SNR, there are two $GABA_A$-sensitive, topographically distinct functional regions localized in the anterior and posterior SNR: $SNR_{anterior}$ and $SNR_{posterior}$, respectively (165–168; Figure 1-5). These two SNR regions mediate differential effects on clonic flurothyl seizures. In the $SNR_{anterior}$, bilateral microinfusions of muscimol have anticonvulsant effects, while in the $SNR_{posterior}$, muscimol microinfusions have proconvulsant effects. Similarly, microinfusions of other GABA receptor–acting drugs (such as bicuculline, ZAPA (Z)-3-[(aminoiminomethyl) thio]prop-z-enoic acid sulfate], and zolpidem) have site-specific effects on seizures in the SNR (Table 1-2) (166, 169, 170). Site-specific effects of the SNR on flurothyl-induced seizures are probably not confined only to GABAergic drugs. Infusions with different pH as an effector have differential actions in the $SNR_{anterior}$ and $SNR_{posterior}$ (171). In situ histochemistry studies have demonstrated that in adult male rats there are two SNR functional regions, which differ in the distribution of the $GABA_A$ receptor alpha-1 subunit mRNA (165). This subunit is the most abundant $GABA_A$ receptor subunit in the adult SNR (172). At the cellular level, there are a few large clusters of labeled cells with high expression of hybridization grains in the $SNR_{anterior}$. In the $SNR_{posterior}$, there is a high density of labeled cells that have moderate expression of the alpha-1 hybridization grains. The two SNR regions use different output pathways for their effects on seizures, as determined by 2-DG studies. In the $SNR_{anterior}$, muscimol infusions decrease glucose utilization in the striatum, sensorimotor cortex, and ventromedial thalamus and increase glucose utilization in superior colliculus (165). In contrast, in the $SNR_{posterior}$, muscimol infusions increase glucose utilization in the dorsal striatum, globus pallidus, and superior colliculus and decrease glucose utilization in thalamus (165). These data support the findings of the topographic and functional segregation of the SNR-mediated systems involved in the control of seizures in adult male rats. An additional study exploring the effects of unilateral SNR muscimol injections on 2-DG uptake revealed that the activation maps in this experimental paradigm have age-, sex-, and SNR region-specific patterns (173).

However, the two regions of the SNR do not develop simultaneously. In PN15 male rats, activation of high-affinity $GABA_A$ receptors (using muscimol or gaboxadol-4, 5, 6, 7-tetrahydroisoxazolo[5, 4-c]pyridin-3-ol(THIP)) mediates only proconvulsant effects (174, 175). Thus, the organization of the SNR into two functional regions, which was described for adult male rats (165, 166), is absent in PN15 male rats (165, 166). In PN15 rats, there is only one functional region within the SNR with respect to the effects of microinfusions of $GABA_A$ergic drug on seizures. These results suggest that the immature, undifferentiated SNR has some similarities with the $SNR_{posterior}$ in terms of the presence of the "proconvulsant" $GABA_A$ receptor subtype. Similarly, in situ hybridization studies have revealed that at the cellular level the silver grains of alpha-1 subunit are clustered over the labeled cells and uniformly distributed throughout the SNR with moderate amounts of the hybridization grains in these clusters. Thus, the distribution and density of these clusters resembles the pattern described in the $SNR_{posterior}$ in adult male rats. In PN15 male rats, muscimol infusions in the SNR also produce specific metabolic changes compared to controls. Irrespective of the site of muscimol infusion, glucose utilization is increased in the ipsilateral dorsal striatum, in the globus pallidus and superior colliculus and not changed in the sensorimotor cortex. In contrast, muscimol infusions decrease glucose utilization in the ipsilateral ventromedial thalamus (165). Thus, the data suggest that in PN15 male rats, there is only one output network, which resembles the one observed in the $SNR_{posterior}$ in adult rats.

TABLE 1-2

Region- and Age-Specific Effects of Nigral GABAergic Drug Microinfusions on Flurothyl Seizures in Male Rats

Drug	PN15 Rats	Adult Rats	
	$SNR_{anterior}$ or $SNR_{posterior}$	$SNR_{anterior}$	$SNR_{posterior}$
Muscimol	Proconvulsant	Anticonvulsant	Proconvulsant
Bicuculline	Proconvulsant	Proconvulsant	No effect
ZAPA	Biphasic effects	Anticonvulsant	Proconvulsant
Zolpidem	Anticonvulsant	Anticonvulsant	No effect
γ-vinyl GABA	Anticonvulsant	Anticonvulsant	Proconvulsant

Muscimol: $GABA_A$ receptor agonist on both low- and high-affinity receptors. Bicuculline: $GABA_A$ receptor antagonist on low-affinity receptors. ZAPA: $GABA_A$ receptor agonist on low-affinity receptors. Zolpidem: agonist of benzodiazepine I binding site of $GABA_A$ receptor. γ-vinyl GABA: irreversible inhibitor of the GABA degradation enzyme, GABA-transaminase.

Based on data in (165, 166, 169, 170).

The question is, When does the differentiation of the two SNR seizure-modifying regions occur? At PN25, the SNR starts to differentiate; infusions of muscimol in the $SNR_{anterior}$ have no effects on flurothyl seizures, while infusions in the $SNR_{posterior}$ have proconvulsant effects. This maturation of the "anticonvulsant" SNR region strikingly coincides with sexual maturation (11). In male rats, there is a sudden drop in plasma testosterone levels (PN20–25) (176–178) just prior to the age when the $SNR_{anteior}$ assumes its "anticonvulsant" characteristics. To test the hypothesis that testosterone may play a role in formation of the "anticonvulsant" $SNR_{anterior}$, male rats were castrated on the day of birth. The rats were exposed to flurothyl at ages PN15 and PN25 following bilateral infusions of muscimol in the $SNR_{anterior}$ or $SNR_{posterior}$. In the $SNR_{anterior}$ in PN15 neonatally castrated male rats, muscimol infusions had no effects on seizures; in PN25, muscimol infusions had anticonvulsant effects compared to saline-infused neonatally castrated controls. Thus, in neonatally castrated male rats the emergence of the "anticonvulsant" $SNR_{anterior}$ shifted to an earlier time point than that observed in intact or sham-operated male rats, suggesting that the depletion of postnatal testosterone may accelerate the appearance of the "anticonvulsant" $SNR_{anterior}$ (170).

In female rats, a proconvulsant muscimol-sensitive SNR region does not develop. In PN15 female rats, there is only one functional region in the SNR. Infusions of muscimol into this region do not change seizure threshold. In adult female rats, the $SNR_{anterior}$ mediates anticonvulsant effects of muscimol similarly to the $SNR_{anterior}$ in adult male rats. In contrast to adult male rats, infusions of muscimol in the $SNR_{posterior}$ in female rats have no effects on seizure threshold. As just mentioned, maturation of the SNR regions is under control of perinatal testosterone or its metabolites. Thus, in females, postnatal administration of testosterone leads to the male SNR phenotype (170, 179). The male–female differences in seizure control seem to be associated with sex-specific differences in the GABAergic system within the SNR as well as in connectivity patterns (173). Further, it appears that the developmental control of seizures in the SNR is affected by sexually dimorphic maturation of KCC2 in this structure (79).

The data demonstrate that the age-specific susceptibility to seizures may be partly due to developmental maturation of structures controlling seizures. This maturation may be under the influence of gonadal hormones and may exert sexually dimorphic features.

ROLE OF STRUCTURAL BRAIN ANOMALIES

Childhood epilepsies are often associated with a variety of brain anomalies. Among epileptic syndromes of childhood, catastrophic epilepsies, including West and Lennox-Gastaut syndromes, are associated with the broadest spectrum of pathoanatomic abnormalities (180), including neuronal migration disorders and small foci of neuronal necrosis. Therefore, pre- and perinatal brain alterations become a condition *sine qua non* for the development of experimental seizures in the immature brain. The long-term goal of these studies is to induce a form of brain injury that would constitute a basis for the development of spontaneous seizures. The model, therefore, should demonstrate structural abnormalities and subsequent increased epileptogenicity in response to environmental stimuli, as well as spontaneous seizures. Until now, only few attempts have been made to approach developmental seizures in the presence of morphologic brain anomalies. How does the presence of brain anomalies or malformations lead to the development of epilepsy? Currently, data exist in four models of experimentally induced malformations: methylazoxymethanol-induced migration disorder, neocortical freezing lesions, neuronal migration disorder induced by irradiation in utero, and the double cortex mutation.

Methylazoxymethanol-Induced Neuronal Migration Disorders

Methylazoxymethanol (MAM) is a powerful alkylating agent (181) acting during the gap 1 (G1) and mitosis (M) phases of the mitotic cell cycle. Administration of MAM on embryonic day 15 in the rat interferes with neuroblastic division and neuronal migration toward cortical layers II–V (182) and is associated with the disruption of radial glia scaffolding with premature astroglia differentiation and thickening of the marginal zone, with redistribution of Cajal-Retzius neurons to deeper layers (183). These actions result in the disruption of the cortical plate and appearance of subventricular zone nodules (183). Consistent brain alterations are present in 100% of cases (Table 1-3; Figure 1-6) (184). Young rats with MAM-induced neuronal migration disorders have indeed a modest increase in seizure susceptibility in several models. In PN14 MAM-exposed rats, hyperthermia induced seizures in 14 of 39 rats, while in age-matched controls only one rat out of 30 had a seizure (39). The higher seizure susceptibility in MAM-exposed rats exposed to hyperthermia was associated with a higher mortality rate. Young MAM rats at PN14 have a lower threshold to kainic-acid–induced seizures, in terms of seizure onset and duration of seizures, than saline-exposed controls (38, 184, 185). These effects may be associated with the alterations in AMPA receptor GluR2 flip and NMDA receptor NR1 subunit distribution in the dysplastic areas of neocortex and hippocampus (186). Additionally, brain slices from rats exposed in utero to MAM display an increased proportion of bursting cells in the hippocampal CA1 pyramidal cells compared to controls (187, 188). Spontaneous seizures have not been observed in this model.

TABLE 1-3
Prenatal Brain Injury

Model	Age of application	Results
MAM	E14, E15	Decreased brain size, decreased cortical thickness, loss of normal lamination in layers II–V of the neocortex with abnormally migrated neurons, bilateral ectopias in the pyramidal layer of the hippocampal CA1, cell loss in the striatum and thalamus (38)
Irradiation	E16, E17	Diffuse cortical dysplasia, periventricular heterotopia, dispersion of hippocampal pyramidal cell layer, corpus callosum agenesis (40)
Double cortex	Mutation	Layers of gray matter placed inside the forebrain white matter; inverted migration pattern (42)

Freezing Lesions

A search for a model of perinatal damage resulting in dysplastic cortex rekindled the interest in the neocortical freezing-induced focus used in adult rats by Escueta (189, 190) and in neonatal rats by Dvořák and Feit (191). In this model, a relatively restricted freezing lesion is produced by a probe (cooled usually by liquid nitrogen) in the neonatal rat neocortex on PN0 or PN1 (41). The treatment results in the loss of normal cortical lamination and results in the creation of a focal microgyrus. Moreover, there are ectopic cell clusters in the layer I of the neocortex and in the white matter (41, 192). There is no significant loss of GABAergic neurons in the hyperexcitable tissue (193), but the GABAtransmission is impaired because of loss of alpha-1, alpha-2, alpha-5, and gamma-2 $GABA_A$ receptor subunits (194). Electrophysiology reveals prominent hyperexcitability of the disorganized neocortical network in the region of focal lesion as early as on PN12 (195). In adult (4–6 months old) rats, electrical stimulation of the neocortical afferents supplying the microgyrus leads to epileptiform discharges that propagate over 4 mm in the horizontal direction, whereas in sham-operated control tissue the horizontal propagation is limited to under 1 mm (41). A metabolic study demonstrated a similar extent of 2-deoxyglucose uptake reduction (196). Although the administration of the NMDA receptor antagonist MK-801 (dizocilpine maleate) prior to the lesion can prevent the development of the discharges, it has little or no effects on an already developed focus and on its propagation (41, 197). Discharges of the already developed focus can be inhibited by the AMPA receptor antagonist 6-nitro-7-sulfamoylbenzo[*f*] quinoxaline-2, 3-dione (NBQX) (41). Optical recordings in brain slices have demonstrated high epileptogenicity of these lesions. In the low-Mg^{2+} model in vitro, epileptiform discharges started in variable locations in control slices. In the dysplastic brains after the freeze lesion, the discharges always emerged from the dysplastic cortex (198). This finding has been confirmed in vivo, since the rats with neonatal (P1) freeze lesions developed hypothermic seizures on P10 earlier (decreased threshold) and the ictal manifestations lasted longer than in control rats (44). However, in the case of freezing lesions in developing rats, spontaneous seizures may develop (43).

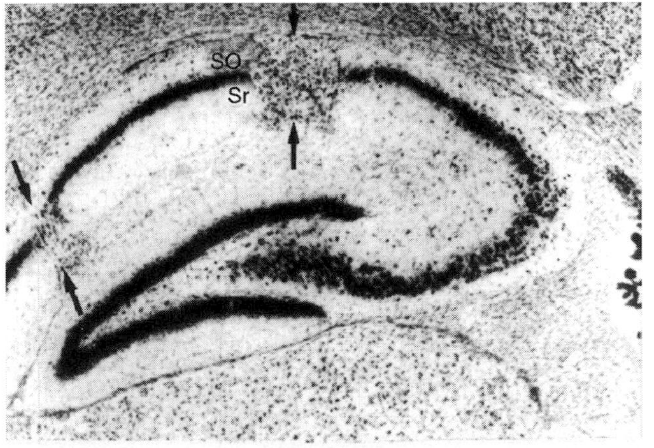

FIGURE 1-6

Brain section from PN15 rat with neuronal migration disorder induced by prenatal treatment with MAM. Coronal section of hippocampus showing areas of neuronal ectopias in the CA1 subfield (arrows). Ectopic neurons are scattered in the stratum oriens (so) and stratum radiatum (sr). Reprinted from Germano IM, Sperber EF. Transplacentally induced neuronal migration disorders: an animal model for the study of the epilepsies. *J Neurosci Res* 1998;51:473–488 (184). Copyright © 1998 Wiley-Liss, Inc., with permission of Wiley-Liss, Inc., a subsidiary of John Wiley & Sons, Inc.

Irradiation Lesions

Exposure of embryonic day 16 (E16) or E17 rat embryos to irradiation disrupts migration patterns, resulting in the creation of numerous dysplastic lesions (40). These rats have a higher susceptibility to the development of electrographic epileptiform discharges after seizure-provoking test with acepromazine or xylazine. Similarly, in vitro neocortical slices from adult rats exposed to irradiation in utero demonstrate more robust epileptiform activity in bicuculline-containing medium than slices from control rats (45). The results suggest that irradiation lesions express their epileptogenic potential in the environment with altered GABAergic transmission. However, spontaneous seizures have not been observed.

Recently this model has been revived. It has been demonstrated that E17 and E19 irradiation is associated with more severe pilocarpine-induced status epilepticus than E13 or E15 irradiation is (199, 200). Similarly, the survival in E13 and E15 groups was higher than in E17 and E19 groups. Interestingly, irradiation on E13 also decreased epileptogenicity of the postnatal mechanical injury inflicted on P30 (201). If the kainic acid status epilepticus model was employed, the profile was opposite to that found in pilocarpine model; that is, irradiation on E13 and E15 produced more severe symptoms than the irradiation on E17 and E19 did (202).

GENETIC PREDISPOSITION TO SEIZURES AND EPILEPSIES

Many forms of human epilepsy are genetically determined (203). The mechanisms by which a multitude of genetic aberrations alter epileptogenicity are unclear. To date, there are several models of genetically determined epilepsy available in baboons, in rats, and many mutant mouse strains with epileptic disorders (42, 204). The major advantage of gene mutation models is the occurrence of spontaneous seizures. The disadvantages may be that there may not be any obvious human correlate, or if there is, the developmental profile may not be similar to that of human epilepsy.

BABOONS

There is a subpopulation of Senegalese baboon with genetically determined photosensitive epilepsy, which was one of the earliest genetic epileptic disturbances studied (205–210). Rhythmic photic stimulation induces progressing myoclonus. The model reflects a quite rare human condition of reflex myoclonus (211). These baboons do not develop their photosensitivity until prepubertal age. The model is now rarely used because of decreased availability of these baboons and the ample availability of mutant mouse models. However, spontaneous myoclonic as well as tonic-clonic seizures have been observed in other baboon subspecies such as *Papio hamadryas anubis* and *cynocephalus/anubis* (212, 213). Photosensitivity is also present in these baboons (213).

RATS

There is a well-established model of generalized tonic-clonic (or brainstem) seizures in the rat induced by intense auditory stimulation. This genetically epilepsy-prone rat (GEPR) is susceptible to environmentally induced seizures that cannot be precipitated in neurologically normal subjects. Drug studies suggest that decrements in monoaminergic transmission may be one of the seizure susceptibility determinants. However, nonmonoaminergic abnormalities may also play an important role in seizure predisposition of the GEPR (214–216).

There are two rat models with spontaneous spike-and-wave discharges akin to human absence seizures: The genetic absence epileptic rat of Strasbourg (GAERS) (217) and WAG/Rij strain with spontaneous absence epilepsy from Nijmegen (218) bring potentially useful information about the mechanisms involved in the generation of absence epilepsy in humans. The age of onset of these seizures is relatively late, so these models cannot be used for study of absence seizures early in life. Thus, spontaneous seizures in GAERS begin to occur well after 4 weeks of age, and their incidence increases till adulthood (219). In the WAG/Rij strain, the seizures occur even later, around PN75 (220). This is in contrast to human absence epilepsy, which begins in childhood and by puberty may even spontaneously remit. On the other hand, the electroclinical correlation between these models and absence seizures is quite good, and thus the models may bring new information on the mechanisms of genesis of spike-and-wave rhythm and the associated behaviors (Table 1-4).

In the flathead mutant rat, the seizures develop in immature animals already during the second postnatal week. The seizure phenotype is related to cortical malformations, including microcephaly, and cellular abnormalities such as cytomegalic neurons and abnormal neuronal death with preferential loss of GABAergic interneuons (221–224). These seizures are myoclonic with loss of posture. Toward the third postnatal week, the seizures become rather tonic and lead to premature death (222).

Mice

A single-locus neurological mutation in mice provides a powerful genetic model system for exploration of the diversity of mechanisms that widely underlie epilepsy.

TABLE 1-4
Pros and Cons of Genetic Absence Models in Rats

Absence Seizure Models in Genetically Prone Rats	
Positive features	Spontaneous seizures Good electroclinical correlation to human absences Good response to antiabsence drugs
Negative features	Developmental discrepancy with the onset of human absence seizures

Many spontaneous as well as engineered gene mutations were identified in mice and are now an important tool to study epilepsy syndromes, with the information well exceeding the extent of this chapter. Recently, several excellent reviews on this topic have been published (225–228); thus, we will not cover this topic in any detail, and only some models will be briefly discussed.

Significant efforts have concentrated on the search for the genes responsible for absence epilepsy. A systematic EEG survey of over 110 mapped mouse mutants revealed 5 mutant genes, located on separate chromosomes, that display a pattern of spontaneous 6–7 Hz spike-and-wave discharges accompanied by behavioral arrest, myoclonic jerks, and uniform responsivity to treatment with ethosuximide (204). These mouse strains have been classified according to the prevalent behavioral feature such as "lethargic" (*lh/lh*), "tottering" (*tg/tg*), "ducky" (*du/du*), "mocha (2J)" (mh^{2J}/mh^{2J}), and "stargazer" (*stg/stg*) and provide a strong evidence for the genetic heterogeneity of the spike-and-wave trait in the mammalian brain. Developmentally, strains *tg* and *stg* show the onset of spontaneous seizures during a 2-day period between PN16 and PN18. Seizure frequency increases with age and reaches adult levels within one week. Seizure severity varies across the strains and is apparently also genetically linked. Thus, the rates for spontaneous seizure are greatest in *stg* and lowest in *du* mice: $stg >> tg >> lh > mh^{2J} > du$ (229). These data show that a defect at a single gene locus is sufficient to produce a spontaneous, generalized spike-and-wave seizure disorder. Additionally, the EEG trait is genetically heterogeneous and can arise from several different recessive mutations. Finally, the background cellular mechanisms responsible for these mutations are not necessarily identical, and each mutation gives rise to a distinct syndrome with a typical seizure frequency, sensitivity to antiepileptic drugs (AEDs), and severity of the associated neurological phenotype (229).

Another mouse strain, with a mutation of the *reeler* gene, has a significant brain anomaly, with layers of gray matter placed inside the forebrain white matter. Similarly, in the *scrambler* mice, mutation of the same gene pathway as in *reeler* mice leads to a disruption of the "inside-out" migration pattern of neocortical neurons during cortical development; instead, an "outside-in" pattern of migration is seen (42). Analogous situations are observed in humans, and the anomaly is termed double cortex. Like the X-linked genetically induced double cortex in humans (230), these large ectopias in mice are associated with seizures (42).

The tottering mouse exhibits intermittent focal myoclonic seizures with ataxia from the fourth postnatal week (231–233). In this model there is an increase in the axonal projections originating from the locus coeruleus, which corresponds to overproduction of norepinephrine in the terminal fields, especially within the cortex (233, 234).

The *Otx1–/–* mouse is characterized by microcephaly, with the reduction expressed especially in the neocortex (235–238). Reduction of neuronal numbers involves mostly GABAergic interneurons. The seizures in these mice start occurring during the fourth postnatal week and are characterized by head nodding and forelimb clonus with rearing and falling.

EXPOSURE TO EPILEPTOGENIC STIMULI (FEVER, INFECTION, HYPOXIA) DURING DEVELOPMENT

Infants are exposed to a high risk of epileptogenic stimuli, represented by greater exposure to infectious agents that lead to fever and sometimes to cerebral infections. Neonates and infants may also often suffer from perinatal hypoxia/ischemia. In susceptible subjects, these stimuli may induce seizures, and because of the higher susceptibility of the young brain to seizures, these seizures occur multiple times a day and may be difficult to control with currently available AEDs (239–245). Several investigators have begun studying the effects of high temperature or hypoxia on seizures in rats with normal and abnormal brain. The pertinent questions are the following: In the experimental models, do the stimuli, such as fever or hypoxia, induce seizures if delivered early in life? If yes, do they increase subsequent seizure susceptibility? Is this change permanent? If the stimuli do not produce acute seizures, do they alter future susceptibility anyway? To date, there are studies using hyperthermia or hypoxia as the seizure-triggering stimuli in the developing brain. So far, there are no reports on infection-induced seizures.

Normal Brain

Hyperthermia-induced seizures can be effectively and reliably induced in developing rats (246–249), and may be a valuable model to assess developmental seizure susceptibility as a result of preexisting alterations, such as hypoxia (250). In PN10–11 rats, hyperthermia can be induced by a stream of heated air, and the seizures are easily determined by both behavioral and electroencephalographic criteria (247). In this model, stereotyped seizures are generated in almost 95% of subjects. EEG correlates of these seizures are not evident in cortical recordings but are present in recordings from the amygdala and hippocampus. There is a low mortality (11%) and long-term survival. This model is suitable for long-term studies and appears to be extremely valuable for studying the mechanisms and sequelae of febrile seizures (247). Although hyperthermic insult produces seizures in infant rats, the question is whether this insult results in spontaneous seizures. A long-term follow-up study indicates that in normal, brief hyperthermic seizures on PN10, there is no spontaneous seizure outcome. However, if prolonged (24-min duration) hyperthermic seizures are inflicted on PN10–11, spontaneous limbic seizures, defined by both motor and EEG patterns, occurred in about 35% of subjects at 3 months of age (251). Interictal discharges were found in 88% of rats in the hyperthermic seizure group. None of these phenomena were recorded in rats subjected to hyperthermia without seizures (blocked by pentobarbital) or in the rats removed from the cage for separation stress control (251). This was elegant experimental evidence that severe hyperthermic seizures early during development may result in development of epilepsy. An additional study demonstrated that there are sex differences in cytogenic response to hyperthermic seizures induced on PN10, determined at PN66 by counts of 5-bromo-2′-deoxyuridine (BrdU)-positive cells after BrdU administration between PN11 and PN16 (252). Male rats had significantly more BrdU-positive cells than controls, while there was no difference in female rats. The model of hyperthermic seizures in normal brain has been further developed by using a neuroimmune challenge with lipopolysaccharide to increase body temperature while concurrently a subconvulsive dose of kainic acid has been administered. This treatment resulted in seizures in about 50% of rats with no neuropathology (253).

Other studies concentrated on compromising the young brain with a hypoxic insult (254–257). In one study, rat pups, exposed to a 3% O_2 on PN10, were either kindled or exposed to corneal electroshock at adulthood PN70. Neither kindled seizure development from the septal nucleus or amygdala nor electroconvulsive shock profiles were significantly altered by hypoxic pretreatment (258). In another study, rat pups were subjected to 6% O_2 hypoxia on PN1 or PN10. In flurothyl-induced seizures and amygdala kindling, there were no differences between hypoxic rats and rats not exposed to hypoxia (255). In contrast, a study that subjected rats on PN5 to hypoxia demonstrated a slight transient increased susceptibility to seizures induced by hippocampal stimulation (256). In the hippocampal kindling model, mild or moderate hypoxia at PN15 did not change seizure susceptibility, while severe hypoxia associated with ischemia delayed the development of kindled seizures (259). Jensen et al. (254) determined the long-term consequences of exposure to hypoxia at PN10 in adult rats. While young rats exposed to hypoxia on PN10 did not perform differently in the water maze, open field, and handling tests compared to nonhypoxic age-matched controls, these rats were more susceptible to flurothyl-induced seizures in adulthood. This effect was enhanced in those PN10 hypoxic rats that had suffered from seizures during hypoxia. A detailed analysis (260) showed that global hypoxia (3–4%) induces acute seizure activity in young rats during a developmental window between PN5 and PN17 with a peak around PN10–12. Animals rendered hypoxic between PN10 and PN12 had long term decreases in seizure threshold. Hypoxia-induced seizures and long-term changes in seizure susceptibility could be prevented by excitatory amino acid antagonists. There was no apparent histological damage in these rats, suggesting that the neuronal changes are only functional (260). Chiba (257) showed that rats suffering from severe 0% O_2 hypoxia on PN10 have increased susceptibility to pentylenetetrazol-induced seizures in adulthood. Moreover, 13 of 20 hypoxic rats developed status epilepticus, while none of the 20 controls experienced status epilepticus. Additionally, the amygdala kindling rate in adult rats subjected to hypoxia on PN10 was twice as fast as in controls. Although none of the hypoxia models induced spontaneous seizures, their value is in showing that hypoxia and hypoxia-induced seizures in young brain may increase (under certain circumstances) seizure susceptibility in adult brain although it may not alter other brain functions. The mechanism for increased seizure susceptibility after neonatal hypoxia may be the plastic calcium-dependent downregulation of GABAergic synaptic transmission (261). In a recent study, a combined hypoxia-ischemia was accomplished by a ligation of the right common carotid artery in PN7 rats together with 2-hour exposure to 8% oxygen. The outcome included development of spontaneous seizures in 40% of rats, along with ipsilateral hippocampal lesions and bilaterally increased Timm stain scores in the inner molecular layer of the dentate gyrus (262).

Thus, the available data suggest that febrile seizures and hypoxia-induced seizures may have model-specific consequences (254, 258). This is in agreement with epidemiological prospective studies in humans, which suggest that the outcome depends on the underlying disease rather than on the seizure itself (239).

Abnormal Brain

There are only few attempts to study the role of elevated temperature or hypoxia in animals with abnormal brain, although this situation may be relatively frequent in neonates and infants with seizures (263, 264).

In one study, where neuronal migration disorders were induced by prenatal administration of the alkylating agent MAM, rat pups at PN14 had a higher incidence of hyperthermia-induced behavioral seizures and mortality rate than controls. Moreover, in rats with the neuronal migration disorder, hyperthermia resulted in hippocampal pyramidal cell loss independent of seizure activity (39). Similarly, neonatal (PN1) freeze lesion enhances susceptibility to hyperthermic seizures on PN10 (44), and in this case, with a long-term observation, spontaneous seizures may occur (43). However, more long-term studies are needed to better understand the long-term effects of developmental seizures.

CONSEQUENCES OF SEIZURES

In human epilepsy as well as in epilepsy models in animals, there are frequent findings of brain anomalies (265).

In temporal lobe epilepsy in adulthood, sclerosis of the cornu ammonis (CA) is frequently found. Detrimental seizure syndromes in childhood (catastrophic epilepsies such as West syndrome and Lennox-Gastaut syndrome) are associated with a broad spectrum of pathoanatomic abnormalities involving dysraphic states, disruption of neuronal migration with pachygyria, neuronal necrosis, and microdysgenesis (180, 266). The principal questions that divide clinicians and researchers are the following: Are repeated seizures or status epilepticus the primary cause for hippocampal damage? Do severe seizures develop as a consequence of previous seizure-induced hippocampal damage? Is seizure-induced hippocampal damage developmentally regulated (267)?

Seizure-Induced Structural Hippocampal Damage

Studies in adult animals have shown that severe or repeated seizures can indeed induce hippocampal damage (268–274). In the adult rats, kainic acid or pilocarpine administration or electric stimulation produce status epilepticus and hippocampal damage. This seizure-induced damage is more pronounced in CA3 and hilar cells than in CA1 (145, 269, 273, 274) and is accompanied by sprouting of the mossy fibers of the granule cells in the dentate gyrus to the supragranular layers (275–281). Later, after 1–2 months, this damage may facilitate the development of spontaneous seizures and may result in serious behavioral deficits (140, 282, 283). Thus, the relationship between seizures and hippocampal damage in the adult brain appears to suggest that repeated prolonged seizures induce hippocampal damage, which further deteriorates brain function and begets further seizures.

The situation in the developing brain is still under investigation. Several studies in developing animals indicate that severe seizures induced by kainic acid, pilocarpine, or flurothyl do not produce extensive damage in the dorsal hippocampus until the end of the third postnatal week (28, 284–289). In PN15 rats, minor hippocampal damage was observed after pilocarpine- (lithium/pilocarpine) induced status epilepticus (289), specific for the CA1 region (150). Similarly in this age group rats, there is no synaptic reorganization following kindling, kainic acid, or flurothyl-induced status epilepticus (284). This is in contrast with the propensity of the immature brain to develop status epilepticus, which is much higher than that of the adult brain (26, 290). However, under certain circumstances in certain models (149), damage may occur even in young rats. Already in PN15 rats, lithium/pilocarpine-induced status epilepticus may induce damage in hippocampal CA1, subiculum, neocortex, amygdala, and thalamus, demonstrating additional involvement of extrahippocampal structures (150). In weanling PN21 rats, this injury is widespread (150, 267, 291), and with time, spontaneous seizures occur in 73% of rats (149, 152). Another study determined neuron-specific enolase as a marker of neuronal damage after lithium/pilocarpine-induced status epilepticus. Interestingly, this enzyme increased in serum already in PN15 rats after status epilepticus; however, the increase was about 50% compared to controls. In contrast, there was a 500% increase in adult rats (292). Taken together, the data suggest that the immature hippocampus is more resistant to the development of seizure-induced hippocampal damage than the adult hippocampus, at least in terms of the classical pathology termed mesial temporal sclerosis (Figure 1-7) (293).

Thus, it seems that the young hippocampus is more resistant to seizure-induced damage and reorganization; however, this feature is seizure model specific. Similarly, the transfer from damage-resistant to damage-sensitive phenotype is not as abrupt as thought previously but follows an age-dependent continuum. The question why the young hippocampus is less sensitive to seizure-induced damage is still unanswered. One possible explanation may be that it is the extracellular calcium influx into adult neurons, due to excessive depolarizations (such as during status epilepticus), that induces neuronal death (294).

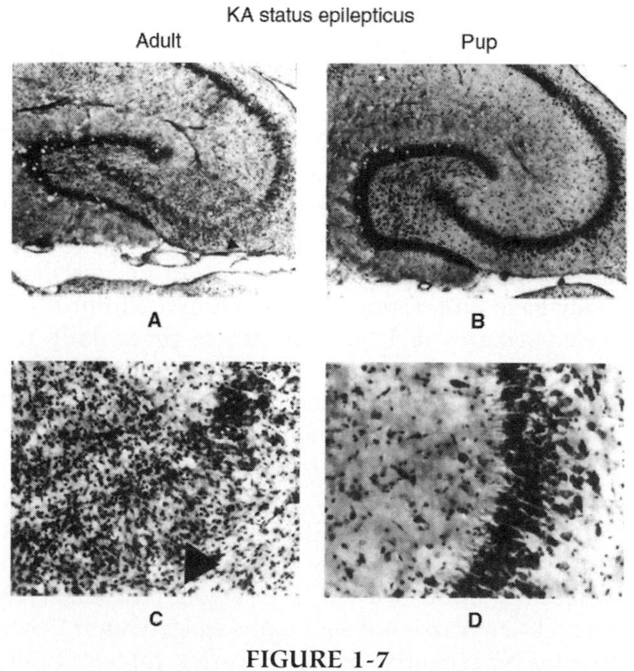

FIGURE 1-7

Kainic acid–induced status epilepticus produces age-related hippocampal damage. Horizontal sections from adult rat (A, C) showing extensive cell loss in the hippocampal CA3 subfield following status epilepticus. In comparison, in PN15 rat, no cell loss is apparent (B, D). It should be noted that the severity of status epilepticus was greater in the PN15 rats than in the adults. Reprinted from Sperber EF, Haas KZ, Moshé SL. Developmental aspects of status epilepticus. *Int Pediatr* 1992;7:213–222 (293) with permission.

Immature neurons receive larger loads of calcium through Ca^{2+}-permeable, GluR2-free AMPA receptors. In contrast to adult neurons, they utilize powerful enzymatic, transport, and storage systems for management of these increased calcium loads, as demonstrated in neocortical neurons (295). After status epilepticus, these systems may clear intracellular excess of calcium rapidly enough either to prevent cell damage completely (296) or to induce only transient metabolic stress (137).

Seizure-Induced Functional Alterations

Are there any functional alterations in the immature brain as a consequence of severe seizures, similarly to those observed in the catastrophic epilepsies in childhood?

In developing rats, there are several studies with follow-up after severe seizures. An interesting difference between kainic acid- and pentylenetetrazol-induced status epilepticus in PN10 and PN25 rats has been demonstrated (297). At PN45, only status epilepticus induced by kainic acid at both juvenile groups elicited deficits in shuttle box conditioned avoidance learning although the other groups experienced pentylenctetrazol-induced status epilepticus of similar duration and intensity. Thus, the learning impairment seems to be specific for kainic acid toxin and not a consequence of status epilepticus. In a different study (140), a correlation between the age, behavioral, and morphological deficits was shown. The rats, which experienced kainic acid–induced status epilepticus on PN5 and PN10, performed normally in behavioral tasks in adulthood. Rats exposed to kainic acid on PN20 demonstrated behavioral alterations in one task, while the rats exposed on PN30 rats were incapable of completing successfully all three tests and already have hippocampal lesions. Repeated flurothyl-induced seizures in PN15 rats (three times daily for 5 days) impaired the performance of these rats in adulthood in the water maze and auditory location but did not induce any gross morphological deficits in the hippocampus (298). Indeed, seizures in immature rats also have long-term metabolic consequences, as shown by several studies (134, 299–301). An interesting insight on long-term effects of status epilepticus in young brain was recently published (134). In young rats subjected to pentylenetetrazol-induced status epilepticus at either PN10 or PN21, neurons in the neocortex, hippocampus, thalamic and hypothalamic nuclei were transiently stained with acid fuchsin, with a peak occurring at 24 hours after the seizures. This staining was accompanied by short-term increase and long term (in adulthood) decrease in the metabolic rate and blood flow rate in the respective structures, but not by cell degeneration. The study demonstrated that immature neurons, in contrast to adult neurons, were only transiently stressed by status epilepticus, without gross morphological damage but with long-term metabolic consequences (134). Several studies have investigated properties of hippocampal neurons after a series of brief flurothyl-induced seizures during neonatal (PN1–5) period. The seizure led to permanent changes in the intrinsic membrane properties of CA1 hippocampal neurons, such as the reduction in spike frequency adaptation and afterhyperpolarizing potential following the spike train (302). Additionally, miniature inhibitory postsynaptic potentials (IPSPs) were reduced in amplitude and frequency in CA3 pyramidal cells, suggesting impairments of $GABA_A$ inhibitory transmission, although there was no change in the $GABA_A$ switch from depolarizing to hyperpolarizing effects (303). An interesting study (304) investigated in cognitive effects of multiple brief seizures, brief seizures combined with preceding status epilepticus, and status epilepticus alone elicited in the immature rats. Only the combination of the status epilepticus and brief seizures caused decrease in performance in the Morris water maze two weeks after the last seizure. Interestingly, there was no histological neuronal injury in any of the groups.

A singe injection of NMDA on PN15, which produced flexion seizures but not tonic-clonic seizures, resulted in significant impairment of spatial navigation in Morris water maze task in adulthood. It should be mentioned that this treatment does not produce any gross morphological deficits (305).

These findings may suggest that although status epilepticus early in life does not produce hippocampal damage, it may impair other behaviors. The effects of seizures may be specific to the seizure type or the agent used to induce the seizures. It appears, however, that at the earlier developmental stages of the brain, the seizures must be very severe to induce at least some long-term functional alterations. It should be noted however that all these studies have been performed in normally developing rats. To better understand the impact of seizures in catastrophic epilepsies, similar studies should be performed in rats with pre- or perinatally compromised brains (39).

Seizure-Induced Alterations in Seizure Susceptibility

Since the nineteenth century, there has been a dictum in human epilepsy that "seizures beget seizures" (306). Animal studies support this theory in adults in many models of seizures. However, the question of whether seizures beget seizures early in life is under investigation.

Prepubescent (PN30) and adult rats subjected to kainic acid–induced status epilepticus demonstrate a high incidence of spontaneous recurrent seizures and an increased susceptibility to seizures induced by kindling and flurothyl. However, kainic acid–induced seizures of similar severity in younger animals (earlier than PN20) have a low rate of spontaneous recurrent seizures in adulthood and do not differ from controls in their susceptibility to kindling- or flurothyl-induced seizures (140, 283,

290). Long-term consequences have also been determined in the pilocarpine model of epilepsy in immature rats. In adult rats, this model is characterized by an acute period of status epilepticus, a silent period, and a chronic period of spontaneous recurrent seizures. However, spontaneous recurrent seizures occurred only in the rats exposed to pilocarpine-induced status epilepticus after PN18 (307).

Kindling in developing rats has demonstrated that rat pups easily kindle beyond stage 5 (25) to severe seizures (stages 6–8) (59, 308). Similarly in kittens, the development of kindling was progressive and permanent (36). These studies demonstrated that in the young brain, kindling is permanent although there are no permanent synaptic changes in the dentate gyrus. Thus, these studies suggest that early in life there may be a dissociation between seizure-induced damage and permanence of seizures. Although permanent, the kindling seizures are still triggered by an external stimulus; however, on rare occasions few spontaneous seizures have been observed (36, 59).

Different results were obtained by unilateral intrahippocampal injection of tetanus toxin in PN9–11 rats (37). Within 24–72 hours the rat pups develop frequent, prolonged behavioral and electrographic seizures in both the injected and contralateral hippocampus and bilaterally in the neocortex with multiple independent spike foci. One week following tetanus toxin injection, the number of seizures decreases; however, interictal spiking persists. In adulthood, some of these rats develop unprovoked behavioral seizures and/or epileptiform EEG activity. Analysis of the hippocampal slices of the seizing rats in adulthood shows burst discharges and paroxysmal depolarizing shifts in CA3 neurons, suggesting long-term changes in neuronal membrane properties (37).

An interesting study investigated the relationship between numbers of hyperthermic seizures early during the development and subsequently to subconvulsant doses of pilocarpine at PN60–70. The study demonstrated that the risk of epilepsy development after the subconvulsant pilocarpine dose was parallel to the number of hyperthermic seizures experienced during the developmental period (309). This finding correlates with a recent study demonstrating that severe hyperthermic seizures on PN10–11 result in development of limbic epilepsy in adulthood (251). These findings indicate that a relatively strong epileptogenic stimulus is required during infantile period for development of seizures in adulthood. The intensity of this stimulus must be sufficient to activate both $GABA_A$ and NMDA transmission, since a collaboration of these two systems has been proposed to result in early developmental epileptogenesis (310).

Thus, the results suggest that in the normal rat, seizures that are triggered prior to the third week of life can on occasion predispose the brain to seizures in adulthood, either triggered (kindling) or spontaneous (tetanus toxin injection). It is interesting that on both occasions seizures early in life altered the subsequent seizure susceptibility if the seizures were multiple. However, a bout of status epilepticus does not appear to beget seizures later on.

COMMENTS ON AGE-SPECIFIC TREATMENTS

Based on clinical experience, it has been accepted that many AEDs that are effective against partial seizures in adults may also be effective against partial seizures in infancy and early childhood (311). However, the developmental neurobiology data discussed in this review suggest that the young brain is not just a small version of the adult brain. There are many age-related features, factors, and functions in the young brain that may specifically affect seizure susceptibility and seizure suppression (312). Therefore, the treatment of seizures should reflect these maturational changes. Additionally, there is the concern about the long-term effects of antiepileptic drug treatment on brain development. Thus, the relevant questions are: What are the best age-specific treatments of seizures for the young brain? How aggressive should this treatment be in terms of total seizure control, if the available drugs produce undesirable (and occasionally long-term) side effects? With this in mind, the consensus conference (311) held on the development of antiepileptic drugs in children proposed that studies for screening putative antiepileptic drugs should be performed in immature animals as well as in adult animals to identify agents that may be age-specific. In addition, the long-term effects of these drugs in the developing brain should be carefully assessed (311).

There are several developmental studies showing age-specific short-term (acute) effects of classic AEDs, GABAergic drugs, and excitatory amino acid antagonists in seizures during development (Table 1-5) (313–320). Unfortunately, for several drugs the beneficiary acute anticonvulsant effects may be associated with long-term toxicity. Some drugs may even have acute toxic effects in the young brain at doses that may be therapeutic in the adult brain.

TABLE 1-5
Age-Specific Effects of Antiepileptic Drugs in Rats

Antiepileptic Drugs		
Effective at All Ages	Highly Effective in Developing Brain, Less Effective or Ineffective in Adult Brain	Effective in Adult Brain, Ineffective or Toxic in Developing Brain
Carbamazepine	Vigabatrin	Phenytoin
Phenobarbital	Baclofen	Pyridoxine
Midazolam	MK-801	
Clonazepam		

Drugs Effective against Seizures at All Ages

Carbamazepine as well as AEDs that enhance $GABA_A$-mediated inhibition, such as phenobarbital and benzodiazepines (i.e., clonazepam and midazolam) are approximately equipotent in both young and adult rats in several seizure models (316, 321–324). However, in PN12 rats in pentylenetetrazol-induced seizures, phenobarbital and carbamazepine can suppress tonic-clonic seizures and at the same time increase the incidence of clonic seizures (322, 323). This suggests that these drugs may have differential effects on various seizure types within a single model. Acute administration of phenobarbital prior to kainic acid inhibits clonic seizures in both PN12 and adult rats (321). However, chronic daily administration of phenobarbital after the kainic acid challenge may have more detrimental effects on memory, learning, and activity level than kainic acid–induced seizures per se (325).

Drugs Effective against Seizures in the Developing Brain but Ineffective or Less Effective in Adults

Systemic administration of vigabatrin (gamma-vinyl GABA; an irreversible inhibitor of the GABA-degrading enzyme GABA-transaminase) 24 hours prior to seizure testing is effective in PN15 but not in adult rats in the flurothyl seizure model (316). Baclofen (a $GABA_B$ receptor agonist) administered systemically is also much more effective in PN15 than in adult rats against flurothyl-, pentylenetetrazol-, and kindling-induced seizures (316, 326, 327).

Most of the excitatory amino acid antagonists, such as MK-801 (dizocilpine; noncompetitive antagonist of NMDA receptors) and 2-amino-7-heptanoic acid (competitive antagonist of NMDA receptors) are more effective in PN12 rats against pentylenetetrazol- and flurothyl-induced seizures than in adult rats (317, 328, 329), an effect that may be associated with blood-brain barrier maturation. In contrast, MK-801 exacerbates kainic acid–induced seizures in neonatal and PN11–12 rats and, in higher doses, induces ictal electrographic and behavioral manifestations (330). Repeated administration of MK-801 in neonatal rats induces a significant decrease in brain size and weight (331, 332). In humans MK-801 has significant behavioral effects, which are the reason for its withdrawal from clinical trials (333).

Drugs Effective against Seizures in Adults but Less Effective or Toxic in Developing Brain

There are drugs with acute toxic effects in the young brain after doses that may be therapeutically effective or even inactive in the adult brain. Phenytoin, which is an effective antiepileptic drug in both adult and young patients (334, 335), may be toxic in high doses (336). Whereas in the pentylenetetrazol model of seizures, phenytoin is anticonvulsant throughout development (337), high doses of phenytoin per se may be toxic and proconvulsant in young rats (319). Similarly, high doses of pyridoxine may be toxic in PN12 and PN18 rats (338).

With certain drugs, such as the NMDA receptor antagonist CGP39551, the anticonvulsant activity is much stronger in adult than in PN12 rats (315). There may be several reasons for this effect, such as the existence of an active metabolite of the drug preferentially synthesized in the adult brain (339) or the delayed maturation of brain uptake mechanisms for the drug. Additionally, an important study revealed that, in fact, some of the anticonvuslant drugs commonly used in children, such as valproate, phenobarbital, phenytoin, and vigabatrin, may significantly increase apoptosis in the therapeutic concentration range (340). The reason for this effect may be a therapy-induced significant decrease in neuronal activity during the developmental period of synaptogenesis, with disruption of the timing and sequence of synaptic connections. This causes nerve cells to receive an internal signal to undergo apoptosis (341).

FUTURE RESEARCH DIRECTIONS

The Need to Create Models of Spectrum of Brain Anomalies and Determine Pathology-Specific Epileptogenicity

Table 1-6 (180, 342) summarizes brain anomalies found in catastrophic epilepsies of childhood. This wide variety of anomalies may have a pre-, peri- or even postnatal

TABLE 1-6
Brain Anomalies Associated with Catastrophic Epilepsies of Childhood

Syndrome	Brain Anomalies
West syndrome	Neuronal migration disruptions, pachygyria, brain weight reduction, neuronal necrosis, dysgenesis, dysraphic states (180)
Lennox-Gastaut syndrome	Small foci of neuronal necrosis in the cortical and subcortical structures of forebrain, also in the cerebellum (342)

origin. Experimentally, there are two models of prenatally induced neuronal migration disorder available: methylazoxymethanol-induced DNA alkylation and prenatal irradiation resulting in severe neuronal migration disorders in the affected offspring (Table 1-3). There is a model of epileptogenic perinatal damage with microgyria induced by neocortical freezing (41) as well as genetically produced models of brain anomalies (42).

There is a need to develop, experimentally, additional severe migration disorders that should involve prenatal and perinatal neuronal alterations, alterations of radial glia, and pre- or perinatal to determine the epileptic potential and consequences of these disorders.

The Need to Create a Model of Chronic Epilepsy/Catastrophic Epilepsy

In the rat, infancy and childhood last a mere 5-week period until the onset of puberty. In cats (36) the process is slower and can be studied for months (with puberty arriving at 7–9 months). Although the developmental models of seizures and progressive epileptic state (kindling) may bear certain similarities to many therapy-responding epileptic seizures in childhood, there are no models of intractable childhood seizures (or catastrophic epilepsies of childhood, such as early infantile epilepsies or West and Lennox-Gastaut syndromes). The available models of severe seizures that eventually express spontaneous seizures have an early developmental limit: they do not occur if the inducing condition (status epilepticus) occurs before PN18 in the rat—that is, later than the age corresponding (7, 9) to the ages of West and Lennox-Gastaut syndrome in infants. Therefore, in the rat, there should be a search for age-specific seizures within the age window between PN10 and PN20 with intractable features that would be similar to catastrophic childhood epilepsies and would provide a model to screen putative AEDs and to determine mechanisms of these therapy-resistant syndromes. In this respect, there may be promise in the tetanus toxin model, which results in the development of spontaneous seizures. NMDA receptor agonists also produce age-specific, intractable flexion seizures with certain features of the West and Lennox-Gastaut syndromes, although without the development of spontaneous seizures (21, 343, 344). These seizures produce long-term cognitive deficits (305). Additional recent data demonstrate that the flexion spasm model induced by systemic injection of NMDA in the brain prenatally exposed to corticosteroids is sensitive to ACTH therapy (345). However, further research in this area is still justified.

The Need for Further Investigations on Gender Differences in Seizure Susceptibility

Historic data from patients suggest that there may be significant gender-related differences in seizure susceptibility (306). These differences have been studied in several animal models of seizures (346–349). The results are mostly in favor of the anticonvulsant action of progesterone and its derivatives and the proconvulsant action of estrogens. However, these conclusions are not supported by all studies. There are many factors involved, including the dose and duration of estrogen effects, estrogen type, and gender of the recipient (Table 1-7). In particular, low doses of beta-estradiol in females may have beneficial effects, especially

TABLE 1-7
Factors Affecting Effects of Estrogens on Seizures and Seizure-Induced Damage

Factors	Anticonvulsant (Neuroprotective) or No Effect	Proconvulsant Effect
Sex	Females	Males
Estrogen dose/level	Low/physiological	High/supraphysiological
Pretreatment	Chronic	Acute
Estrogen type	Beta-estradiol	All other
Brain region/nuclei	Ventral hippocampus Amygdala	Dorsal hippocampus
Seizure model	Flurothyl Pilocarpine Kainic acid NMDA Picrotoxin	Pentylenetetrazol Electroshock
Hormonal status in females	Estrogen replacement Normally cycling	Ovariectomy Aging

It should be emphasized that for the proconvulsant effect to occur, one proconvulsant factor is enough and in a combination of factors, the proconvulsant factor is prevailing.

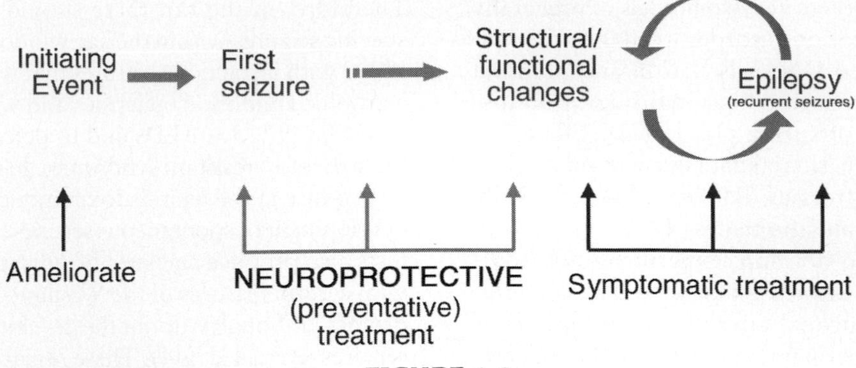

FIGURE 1-8

Simplified scheme of possible treatment interventions during epileptogenesis. The current view is that epileptogenesis proceeds from the initiating (precipitating) event to the first seizure (status epilepticus), which may induce structural and/or functional changes. These changes make the condition permanent and contribute to further generation of recurrent seizures; that is, epilepsy develops. The best treatment opportunity is to ameliorate the initial event; however, this event can be only infrequently diagnosed and rarely predicted, which is a condition for successful amelioration. However, after the first seizure occurs, antiepileptic therapy can be combined with neuroprotection so that the permanent fixation of changes is prevented. This is probably the most promising area for therapy development. Symptomatic (current) treatment, unfortunately, cannot reverse already established morphological changes.

as means of neuroprotection against seizure-induced damage (350–352). Furthermore, Holmes showed that anticonvulsant effects of progesterone in kindling occurred only in developing, but not in adult, rats (353, 354).

Additional studies show that gender differences, as reflected in the control of seizures, may be operant before puberty as a result of sexually dimorphic brain organization (355–358).

The Need to Develop Age-Specific Antiepileptogenic and Neuroprotective Treatments

Though antiepileptic drugs have mostly antiseizure effects, by their mechanisms of action some of these drugs may interfere with both principal mechanisms of neuronal death: necrosis and apoptosis (Figure 1-8). Some of the current AEDs indeed have this potency (359). However, use of phenobarbital with neuroprotective and antiepileptogenic intent in children with febrile seizures may be associated with a decrease in cognition (360). The question is how much this effect is associated with the aforementioned phenobarbital-induced increase in apoptosis (340). Similarly, there are other drugs with neuroprotective potential (such as felbamate) that may be harmful for the developing brain. In this regard, use of those add-on neuroprotective treatments that would not be associated with negative cognitive impacts may be advantageous.

The question remains as to how much this neuroprotective effect of antiepileptic therapy is associated with functional antiepileptogenic effect (361). Here, the data are still controversial. Several authors demonstrate that in animal models, neuroprotective therapy during the window immediately after the status epilepticus reduces the percentage of animals that develop spontaneous seizures (362, 363). On the other hand, recent data indicate that even though several antiepileptic drugs or other compounds (e.g., MK-801) (364) are neuroprotective, none of them are antiepileptogenic in experimental models or in humans (365).

With the rapid expansion of knowledge in basic disciplines such as neurobiology, cell physiology, molecular biology, and neurochemistry, there is hope that appropriate developmental models of epilepsy will be created to deal with epilepsies of infancy and childhood.

ACKNOWLEDGMENTS

Supported by NIH, NINDS grants NS-20253 to S. L. M. and NS-41366 to L. V. S. L. M. is Martin A. and Emily Fisher Fellow.

References

1. Hauser WA, Kurland LT. The epidemiology of epilepsy in Rochester, Minnesota, 1935–1967. *Epilepsia* 1975; 16:1–66.
2. Hauser W. The prevalence and incidence of convulsive disorders in children. *Epilepsia* 1994; 35:1–6.
3. Hauser WA. Incidence and prevalence. In: Engel J Jr, Pedley TA, eds. *Epilepsy: A Comprehensive Textbook*. Philadelphia: Lippincott-Raven Publishers, 1997:47–57.
4. Scher M. Neonatal seizures. In: Wyllie E, ed. *The Treatment of Epilepsy: Principles and Practice*. Baltimore: Williams & Wilkins, 1996:600–621.

5. Shields WD. Investigational antiepileptic drugs for the treatment of childhod seizure disorders: a review of efficacy and safety. *Epilepsia* 1994; 35 Suppl 2:S24–S29.
6. Swann JW, Moshé SL. Developmental issues in animal models. In: Engel J Jr, Pedley TA, eds. *Epilepsy: A Comprehensive Textbook*. Philadelphia: Lippincott-Raven Publishers; 1997:467–479.
7. Avishai-Eliner S, Brunson KL, Sandman CA, Baram TZ. Stressed-out, or in (utero)? *Trends Neurosci* 2002; 25:518–524.
8. Dobbing J, Sands J. Comparative aspects of the brain growth spurt. *Early Hum Dev* 1979; 3:79–83.
9. Gottlieb A, Keydor I, Epstein HT. Rodent brain growth stages. An analytical review. *Biol Neonate* 1977; 32:166–176.
10. Hayakawa K, Konishi Y, Kuriyama M, Matsuda T. Normal brain maturation in MRI. *Eur J Radiol* 1991; 12:208–215.
11. Ojeda, SR, Urbanski, HF. Puberty in the rat. In: Knobil E, ed. *The Physiology of Reproduction*. New York: Raven Press, 1994:363–411.
12. Velíšek L, Moshé SL. Effects of brief seizures during development. In: Sutula T, Pitkanen A, eds. *Do Seizures Damage the Brain?* Amsterdam: Elsevier; 2002:355–364.
13. Hamon B, Heinemann U. Developmental changes in neuronal sensitivity to excitatory amino acids in area CA1 of the rat hippocampus. *Brain Res* 1988; 466:286–290.
14. Schwartzkroin PA. Epileptogenesis in the immature CNS. In: Schwartzkroin PA, Wheal HV, eds. *Electrophysiology of Epilepsy*. London: Academic Press, 1984:389–412.
15. Swann JW, Brady RJ. Penicillin-induced epileptogenesis in immature rats CA3 hippocampal pyramidal cells. *Dev Brain Res* 1984; 12:243–254.
16. Swann JW, Smith KL, Brady RJ. Age-dependent alterations in the operations of hippocampal neural networks. *Ann N Y Acad Sci* 1991; 627:264–276.
17. Hablitz JJ, Heinemann U. Extracellular K^+ and Ca^{2+} changes during epileptiform discharges in the immature rat neocortex. *Brain Res* 1987; 433:299–303.
18. Hablitz JJ, Heinemann U. Alterations in the microenvironment during spreading depression associated with epileptiform activity in the immature neocortex. *Brain Res Dev Brain Res* 1989; 46:243–252.
19. Khazipov R, Khalilov I, Tyzio R, Morozova E, et al. Developmental changes in GABAergic actions and seizure susceptibility in the rat hippocampus. *Eur J Neurosci* 2004; 19:590–600.
20. Vernadakis A, Woodbury DM. The developing animal as a model. *Epilepsia* 1969; 10:163–178.
21. Mareš P, Velíšek L. N-methyl-D-aspartate (NMDA)-induced seizures in developing rats. *Brain Res Dev Brain Res* 1992; 65:185–189.
22. Velíšek L, Kubová H, Pohl M, Staňková L, et al. Pentylenetetrazol-induced seizures in rats: an ontogenetic study. *Naunyn Schmiedebergs Arch Pharmacol* 1992; 346:588–591.
23. Racine RJ. Modification of seizure activity by electrical stimulation: II. Motor seizures. *Electroencephalogr Clin Neurophysiol* 1972; 32:281–294.
24. Moshé SL. The kindling phenomenon and its possible relevance to febrile seizures. In: Nelson, KB, Ellenberg, JH, eds. *Febrile Seizures*. New York: Raven Press, 1981:59–63.
25. Haas K, Sperber EF, Moshé SL. Kindling in developing animals: expression of severe seizures and enhanced development of bilateral foci. *Brain Res Dev Brain Res* 1990; 56: 275–280.
26. Moshé SL, Albala BJ, Ackermann RF, Engel JJ. Increased seizure susceptibility of the immature brain. *Dev Brain Res* 1983; 7:81–85.
27. Moshé SL, Albala BJ. Kindling in developing rats: persistence of seizures into adulthood. *Dev Brain Res* 1982; 4:67–71.
28. Albala BJ, Moshé SL, Okada R. Kainic-acid-induced seizures: a developmental study. *Dev Brain Res* 1984; 13:139–148.
29. Moshé SL, Sharpless NS, Kaplan J. Kindling in developing rats: afterdischarge thresholds. *Brain Res* 1981; 211:190–195.
30. de Feo M, Mecarelli O, Ricci G. Bicuculline-and allylglycine-induced epilepsy in developing rats. *Exp Neurol* 1985; 90:411–421.
31. de Feo MR, Mecarelli O. Ontogenetic models of epilepsy. In: Avanzini G, Fariello R, Heinemann U, Mutani R, eds. *Epileptogenic and Excitotoxic Mechanisms*. London: John Libbey; 1993:89–97.
32. Velíšková J, Velíšek L, Mareš P. Epileptic phenomena produced by kainic acid in laboratory rats during ontogenesis. *Physiol Bohemoslov* 1988; 37:395–405.
33. Zouhar A, Mares P, Lisková-Bernásková K, Mudrochová M. Motor and electrocorticographic epileptic activity induced by bicuculline in developing rats. *Epilepsia* 1989; 30:501–510.
34. Velíšek L. Models of chemically-induced acute seizures. In: Pitkanen A, Schwartzkroin PA, Moshé SL, eds. *Models of Seizures and Epilepsy*. Amsterdam: Elsevier; 2006:127–152.
35. Baram TZ, Hirsch E, Schultz L. Short-interval amygdala kindling in neonatal rats. *Brain Res Dev Brain Res* 1993; 73:79–83.
36. Shouse MN, King A, Langer J, Vreeken T, et al. The ontogeny of feline temporal lobe epilepsy: kindling a spontaneous seizure disorder in kittens. *Brain Res* 1990; 525: 215–224.
37. Lee CL, Hrachovy RA, Smith KL, Frost JD Jr, et al. Tetanus toxin-induced seizures in infant rats and their effects on hippocampal excitability in adulthood. *Brain Res* 1995; 677:97–109.
38. Germano IM, Sperber EF. Increased seizure susceptibility in adult rats with neuronal migration disorders. *Brain Res* 1997; 777:219–222.
39. Germano IM, Zhang YF, Sperber EF, Moshe SL. Neuronal migration disorders increase susceptibility to hyperthermia-induced seizures in developing rats. *Epilepsia* 1996; 37:902–910.
40. Roper SN, Gilmore RL, Houser CR. Experimentally induced disorders of neuronal migration produce an increased propensity for electrographic seizures in rats. *Epilepsy Res* 1995; 21:205–219.
41. Luhmann HJ, Raabe K. Characterization of neuronal migration disorders in neocortical structures: I. Expression of epileptiform activity in an animal model. *Epilepsy Res* 1996; 26:67–74.
42. Gonzalez JL, Russo CJ, Goldowitz D, Sweet HO, et al. Birthdate and cell marker analysis of scrambler: a novel mutation affecting cortical development with a reeler-like phenotype. *J Neurosci* 1997; 17:9204–9211.
43. Scantlebury MH, Gibbs SA, Foadjo B, Lema P, et al. Febrile seizures in the predisposed brain: a new model of temporal lobe epilepsy. *Ann Neurol* 2005; 58:41–49.
44. Scantlebury MH, Ouellet PL, Psarropoulou C, Carmant L. Freeze lesion-induced focal cortical dysplasia predisposes to atypical hyperthermic seizures in the immature rat. *Epilepsia* 2004; 45:592–600.
45. Roper SN, King MA, Abraham LA, Boillot MA. Disinhibited in vitro neocortical slices containing experimentally induced cortical dysplasia demonstrate hyperexcitability. *Epilepsy Res* 1997; 26:443–449.
46. Michelson HB, Lothman EW. An in vivo electrophysiological study of the ontogeny of excitatory and inhibitory processes in the rat hippocampus. *Brain Res Dev Brain Res* 1989; 47:113–122.
47. Michelson HB, Wong RKS. Excitatory synaptic responses mediated by GABA(A) receptors in the hippocampus. *Science* 1991; 253:1420–1423.
48. Cherubini E, Rovira C, Gaiarsa JL, Corradetti R, et al. GABA mediated excitation in immature rat CA3 hippocampal neurons. *Int J Dev Neurosci* 1990; 8:481–490.
49. Tsumoto T, Hagihara H, Sato H, Hata S. NMDA receptors in the visual cortex of young kittens are more effective than those of adult cats. *Nature* 1987; 327:513–514.
50. Brady RJ, Gorter JA, Monroe MT, Swann JW. Developmental alterations in the sensitivity of hippocampal NMDA receptors to AP5. *Brain Res Dev Brain Res* 1994; 83:190–196.
51. Ben-Ari Y, Khazipov R, Leinekugel X, Caillard O, et al. $GABA_A$, NMDA and AMPA receptors: a developmentally regulated "ménage à trois." *Trends Neurosci* 1997; 20:523–529.
52. Luhmann HJ, Prince DA. Transient expression of polysynaptic NMDA receptor-mediated activity during neocortical development. *Neurosci Lett* 1990; 111:109–115.
53. Joshi I, Wang LY. Developmental profiles of glutamate receptors and synaptic transmission at a single synapse in the mouse auditory brainstem. *J Physiol* 2002; 540:861–873.
54. Sircar R. Developmental maturation of the N-methyl-D-aspartic acid receptor channel complex in postnatal rat brain. *Int J Dev Neurosci* 2000; 18:121–131.
55. Velíšek L, Mareš P. Increased epileptogenesis in the immature hippocampus. *Exp Brain Res Series* 1991; 20:183–185.
56. Michelson HB, Williamson JM, Lothman EW. Ontogeny of kindling: The acquisition of kindled responses at different ages with rapidly recurring hippocampal seizures. *Epilepsia* 1989; 30:672.
57. Goddard GV. The kindling model of epilepsy. *Trends Neurosci* 1983; 7:275–279.
58. Racine R. Kindling: the first decade. *Neurosurgery* 1978; 3:234–252.
59. Haas KZ, Sperber EF, Moshé SL. Kindling in developing animals: interactions between ipsilateral foci. *Dev Brain Res* 1992; 68:140–143.
60. Burchfiel JL, Serpa KA, Duffy FH. Further studies of antagonism of seizure development between concurrently developing kindled limbic foci in the rat. *Exp Neurol* 1982; 75:476–489.
61. Pinel JPJ, Rovner LI. Experimental epileptogenesis: kindling induced epilepsy in rats. *Exp Neurol* 1978; 58:190–202.
62. Tremblay E, Roisin MP, Represa A, Charriaut-Marlangue C, et al. Transient increased density of NMDA binding sites in the developing rat hippocampus. *Brain Res* 1988; 461:393–396.
63. Mueller A, Chesnut R, Schwartzkroin P. Actions of GABA in developing rabbit hippocampus: an in vitro study. *Neurosci Lett* 1983; 39:193–198.
64. Ben-Ari Y. Excitatory actions of GABA during development: the nature of the nurture. *Nat Rev Neurosci* 2002; 3:728–739.
65. Garant DS, Sperber EF, Moshé SL. The density of $GABA_B$ binding sites in the substantia nigra is greater in rat pups than in adults. *Eur J Pharmacol* 1992; 214:75–78.
66. Brooks-Kayal AR. Rearranging receptors. *Epilepsia* 2005; 46 Suppl 7:29–38.
67. Schwartzkroin PA, Kunkel DD, Mathers LH. Development of rabbit hippocampus; anatomy. *Dev Brain Res* 1982; 2:452–468.
68. Schwartzkroin PA. Development of rabbit hippocamus; physiology. *Dev Brain Res* 1982; 2:469–486.
69. Swann JW. Synaptogenesis and epileptogenesis in developing neural networks. In: Schwartzkroin PA, Moshé SL, Noebels JL, Swann JW, eds. *Brain Development and Epilepsy*. New York-Oxford: Oxford University Press; 1995:195–233.
70. Swann JW, Smith KL, Gomez CM, Brady RJ. The ontogeny of hippocampal local circuits and focal epileptogenesis. *Epilepsy Res Suppl* 1992; 9:115–125.
71. Peinado A, Yuste R, Katz LC. Extensive dye coupling between rat neocortical neurons during the critical period of circuit formation. *Neuron* 1993; 10:103–114.
72. Venance L, Rozov A, Blatow M, Burnashev et al. Connexin expression in electrically coupled postnatal rat brain neurons. *Proc Natl Acad Sci U S A* 2000; 97:10260–10265.
73. Swann JW, Smith KL, Brady R. Neural networks and synaptic transmissions in immature hippocampus. In: Ben-Ari Y, ed. *Excitatory Amino Acids and Neuronal Plasticity: Advances in Experimental Medicine and Biology*. New York: Putnam Press; 1990:161–171.
74. Pellegrini-Giampietro, D, Bennett, M, Zukin, R. Differential expression of three glutamate receptor genes in developing rat brain: an in situ hybridization study. *Proc Natl Acad Sci U S A* 1991; 88:4157–4161.
75. Pellegrini-Giampietro DE, Gorter JA, Bennett MV, Zukin, RS. The GluR2 (GluR-B) hypothesis: Ca^{2+}-permeable AMPA receptors in neurological disorders. *Trends Neurosci* 1997; 20:464–470.
76. Laurie DJ, Wisden W, Seeburg PH. The distribution of thirteen $GABA_A$ receptor subunit mRNAs in the rat brain. III. Embryonic and postnatal development. *J Neurosci* 1992; 12:4151–4172.

77. Moshé SL, Garant DS, Sperber EF, Velísková J, et al. Ontogeny and topography of seizure regulation by the substantia nigra. *Brain Dev* 1995; 17:61–72.
78. Stein V, Hermans-Borgmeyer I, Jentsch TJ, Hubner CA. Expression of the KCl cotransporter KCC2 parallels neuronal maturation and the emergence of low intracellular chloride. *J Comp Neurol* 2004; 468:57–64.
79. Galanopoulou AS, Kyrozis A, Claudio OI, Stanton PK, et al. Sex-specific KCC2 expression and GABA(A) receptor function in rat substantia nigra. *Exp Neurol* 2003; 183: 628–637.
80. Dzhala VI, Talos DM, Sdrulla DA, Brumback AC, et al. NKCC1 transporter facilitates seizures in the developing brain. *Nat Med* 2005 11:1205–1213.
81. Mody I. Aspects of the homeostaic plasticity of $GABA_A$ receptor-mediated inhibition. *J Physiol* 2005; 562:37–46.
82. Semyanov A, Walker MC, Kullmann DM Silver, RA. Tonically active GABA A receptors: modulating gain and maintaining the tone. *Trends Neurosci* 2004; 27:262–269.
83. Nusser Z, Sieghart W, Somogyi P. Segregation of different $GABA_A$ receptors to synaptic and extrasynaptic membranes of cerebellar granule cells. *J Neurosci* 1998; 18:1693–1703.
84. Yamada J, Furukawa T, Ueno S, Yamamoto S, et al. Molecular basis for the $GABA_A$ receptor-mediated tonic inhibition in rat somatosensory cortex. *Cereb Cortex* 2006.
85. Drasbek KR, Hoestgaard-Jensen K, Jensen K. Modulation of extrasynaptic THIP conductances by $GABA_A$ receptor modulators in mouse neocortex. *J Neurophysiol* 2007.
86. Owens DF, Kriegstein AR. Is there more to GABA than synaptic inhibition? *Nat Rev Neurosci* 2002; 3:715–727.
87. Ge S, Goh EL, Sailor KA, KitabatakeY, et al. GABA regulates synaptic integration of newly generated neurons in the adult brain. *Nature* 2006; 439:589–593.
88. Wadiche LO, Bromberg DA, Bensen AL, Westbrook GL. GABAergic signaling to newborn neurons in dentate gyrus. *J Neurophysiol* 2005; 94:4528–4532.
89. Corcoran ME, Mason ST. Role of forebrain catecholamines in amygdaloid kindling. *Brain Res* 1980; 190:473–484.
90. McIntyre DC, Edson N. Facilitation of amygdala kindling after norepinephrine depletion with 6-hydroxydopamine in rats. *Exp Neurol* 1981; 74:748–757.
91. Burchfiel JL, Applegate CD, Konkol RJ. Kindling antagonism: A role for norepinephrine in seizure suppresion. In: Wada JA, ed. *Kindling 3*. New York: Raven Press; 1986:213–229.
92. Shinnar S, Berg AT, Moshé SL, Petix M, et al. Risk of seizure recurrence following a first unprovoked seizure in childhood. *Pediatrics* 1990; 85:1076–1085.
93. Moshé SL, Shinnar S, Swann JW. Partial (focal) seizures in developing brain. In: Schwartzkroin PA, Moshé SL, Noebels JL, Swann, JW, eds. *Brain Development and Epilepsy*. New York:Oxford University Press, 1995:34–65.
94. Rodier PM. Developing brain as a target of toxicity. *Environ Health Perspect* 1995; 103 Suppl 6:73–76.
95. Nixdorf-Bergweiler BE, Albrecht D, Heinemann U. Developmental changes in the number, size, and orientation of GFAP-positive cells in the CA1 region of rat hippocampus. *Glia* 1994; 12:180–195.
96. Spitzer NC. Regulation of excitability in developing neurons. In: Schwartzkroin PA, Moshé SL, Noebels JL, Swann JW, eds. *Brain Development and Epilepsy*. New York and Oxford: Oxford University Press, 1995:144–170.
97. Fukuda A, Prince DA. Postnatal development of electrogenic sodium pump activity in rat hippocampal pyramidal neurons. *Brain Res Dev Brain Res* 1992; 65:101–114.
98. Kohling R, Lucke A, Nagao T, Speckmann EJ, et al. Extracellular potassium elevations in the hippocampus of rats with long- term pilocarpine seizures. *Neurosci Lett* 1995; 201:87–91.
99. Heinemann U, Lux HD. Ceiling of stimulus-induced rises in extracellular potassium concentration in the cat. *Brain Res* 1977; 120:231–249.
100. Swann JW, Smith KL, Brady RJ. Extracellular K^+ accumulation during penicillin induced epileptogenesis in the CA3 region of immature rat hippocampus. *Dev Brain Res* 1986; 395:243–255.
101. Stringer JL. Regulation of extracellular potassium in the developing hippocampus. *Brain Res Dev Brain Res* 1998; 110:97–103.
102. Grisar T. Glial and neuronal Na-K-pump in epilepsy. *Ann Neurol* 1984; 16:128–134.
103. Ballanyi K, Grafe P, ten Bruggencate G. Ion activities and potassium uptake mechanisms of glial cells in guinea pig olfactory cortex slices. *J Physiol* 1987; 382:159–174.
104. Heinemann U, Albrecht D, Beck H, Ficker E, Nixdorf B, Stabel J, von Haebler D. Potassium homeostasis and epileptogenesis in the immature hippocampus. In: Avanzini G, Fariello R, Heinemann U, Mutani R, eds. *Epileptogenic and Excitotoxic Mechanisms*. London: John Libbey, 1993:99–106.
105. Ransom BR, Carlini WG, Connors BW. Brain extracellular space: developmental studies in rat optic nerve. *Ann N Y Acad Sci* 1986; 481:87–105.
106. Lothman EW, Somjen GG. Extracellular potassium activity, intracellular and extracellular potential responses in the spinal cord. *J Physiol* 1975; 252:115–136.
107. Vernadakis A. Neuronal–glial interactions during development and aging. *Fed Proc* 1975; 34:89–95.
108. Brady RJ, Smith KL, Swann, JW. Calcium modulation of the N-methyl-D-aspartate (NMDA) response and electrographic seizures in immature hippocampus. *Neurosci Lett* 1991; 124:92–96.
109. Mayer ML, Westbrook GL, Guthrie PB. Voltage dependent block by Mg^{2+} of NMDA responses in spinal cord neurons. *Nature* 1984; 309:261–263.
110. Bading H, Ginty DD, Greenberg ME. Regulation of gene expression in hippocampal neurons by distinct calcium signaling pathways. *Science* 1993; 260:181–186.
111. Coulter DA, Huguenard JR, Prince DA. Calcium currents in rat thalamocortical relay neurones: kinetic properties of the transient, low threshold current. *J Physiol* 1989; 414:587–604.
112. Yaari Y, Hamon B, Lux HD. Development of two types of calcium channels in cultured mammalian hippocampal neurons. *Science* 1987; 235:680–682.
113. Chen S, Yue C, Yaari Y. A transitional period of Ca^{2+}-dependent spike after depolarization and bursting in developing rat CA1 pyramidal cells. *J Physiol* 2005; 567:79–93.
114. Payne JA, Rivera C, Voipio J, Kaila K. Cation-chloride co-transporters in neuronal communication; development and trauma. *Trends Neurosci* 2003; 26:199–206.
115. Yamada J, Okabe A, Toyoda H, Kilb W, et al. Cl^- uptake promoting depolarizing GABA actions in immature rat neocortical neurones is mediated by NKCC1. *J Physiol* 2004; 557:829–841.
116. Rivera C, Voipio J, Payne JA, Ruusuvuori E, et al. The K^+/Cl^- cotransporter KCC2 renders GABA hyperpolarizing during neuronal maturation. *Nature* 1999; 397:251–255.
117. Rivera C, Voipio J, Kaila K. Two developmental switches in GABAergic signalling: the K^+/Cl^- cotransporter KCC2 and carbonic anhydrase CAVII. *J Physiol* 2005; 562:27–36.
118. Hubner CA, Stein V, Hermans-Borgmeyer I, Meyer T, et al. Disruption of KCC2 reveals an essential role of K-Cl cotransport already in early synaptic inhibition. *Neuron* 2001; 30:515–524.
119. Woo NS, Lu J, England R, McClellan R, et al. Hyperexcitability and epilepsy associated with disruption of the mouse neuronal-specific K-Cl cotransporter gene. *Hippocampus* 2002; 12:258–268.
120. Ouardouz, M, Sastry, BR. Activity-mediated shift in reversal potential of GABA-ergic synaptic currents in immature neurons. *Brain Res Dev Brain Res* 2005; 160:78–84.
121. Kyrozis A, Chudomel O, Moshé SL, Galanopoulou AS. Sex-dependent maturation of GABA(A) receptor-mediated synaptic events in rat substantia nigra reticulata. *Neurosci Lett* 2006; 398:1–5.
122. Striano P, Bordo L, Lispi ML, Specchio N, et al. A novel SCN2A mutation in family with benign familial infantile seizures. *Epilepsia* 2006; 47:218–220.
123. Gong B, Rhodes, KJ, Bekele-Arcuri, Z, Trimmer JS. Type I and type II Na(+) channel alpha-subunit polypeptides exhibit distinct spatial and temporal patterning, and association with auxiliary subunits in rat brain. *J Comp Neurol* 1999; 412:342–352.
124. Spampanato J, Escayg A, Meisler MH, Goldin AL. Functional effects of two voltage-gated sodium channel mutations that cause generalized epilepsy with febrile seizures plus type 2. *J Neurosci* 2001; 21:7481–7490.
125. Scheffer IE, Berkovic SF. The genetics of human epilepsy. *Trends Pharmacol Sci* 2003; 24:428–433.
126. Sokoloff L, Reivich M, Kennedy C, Des Rosiers MH, et al. The $[^{14}C]$ deoxyglucose method for the measurement of local cerebral glucose utilization: theory, procedures and normal values in the conscious and anesthetized albino rat. *J Neurochem* 1977; 28:897–916.
127. Daval JL, Pereira de Vasconcelos A, el Hamdi G, Werck MC, et al. Quantitative autoradiographic measurements of functional changes induced by generalized seizures in the developing rat brain: central adenosine and benzodiazepine receptors and local cerebral glucose utilization. *Epilepsy Res Suppl* 1992; 9:83–92.
128. Ackermann RF, Moshé SL, Albala BJ. Restriction of enhanced ^{14}C-2-deoxyglucose utilization to rhinencephalic structures in immature amygdala-kindled rats. *Exp Neurol* 1989; 104:73–81.
129. Ackermann RF, Moshé SL, Albala BJ, Engel JJ. Anatomical substrates of amygdala kindling in immature rats demonstrated by 2-deoxyglucose autoradiography. *Epilepsia* 1982; 23:434–435.
130. Tremblay E, Nitecka L, Berger M, Ben-Ari Y. Maturation of kainic acid seizure-brain damage syndrome in the rat. I. Clinical, electrographic and metabolic observations. *Neuroscience* 1984; 13:1051–1072.
131. Cherubini E, DeFeo MR, Mecarelli O, Ricci GF. Behavioral and electrograhic patterns induced by systemic administration of kainic acid in developing rats. *Dev Brain Res* 1983; 9:69–77.
132. Ben-Ari Y, Tremblay E, Berger M, Nitecka L. Kainic acid seizure syndrome and binding sites in developing rats. *Dev Brain Res* 1984; 14:284–288.
133. Nehlig A. Cerebral energy metabolism, glucose transport and blood flow: changes with maturation and adaptation to hypoglycaemia. *Diabetes Metab* 1997; 23:18–29.
134. Nehlig A, Pereira de Vasconcelos A. The model of pentylenetetrazol-induced status epilepticus in the immature rat: short- and long-term effects. *Epilepsy Res* 1996; 26:93–103.
135. Sperber EF, Moshé SL. Age-related differences in seizure susceptibility to flurothyl. *Dev Brain Res* 1988; 39:295–297.
136. Ben-Ari Y, Riche D, Tremblay E, Charton G. Alterations in local glucose consumption following systemic administration of kainic acid, bicuculline or metrazol. *Eur Neurol* 1981; 20:173–175.
137. Pereira de Vasconcelos A, Boyet S, Koziel V, Nehlig A. Effects of pentylenetetrazol-induced status epilepticus on local cerebral blood flow in the developing rat. *J Cereb Blood Flow Metab* 1995; 15:270–283.
138. Pereira de Vasconcelos A, el Hamdi G, Vert P, Nehlig A. An experimental model of generalized seizures for the measurement of local cerebral glucose utilization in the immature rat. II. Mapping of the brain metabolism using quantitative $[^{14}C]$-2-deoxyglucose technique. *Brain Res Dev Brain Res* 1992; 69:243–259.
139. Dube C, da Silva Fernandes MJ, Nehlig A. Age-dependent consequences of seizures and the development of temporal lobe epilepsy in the rat. *Dev Neurosci* 2001; 23:219–223.
140. Stafstrom CE, Chronopoulos A, Thurber S, Thompson JL, et al. Age-dependent cognitive and behavioral deficits after kainic acid seizures. *Epilepsia* 1993; 34:420–432.
141. Stafstrom CE, Holmes GL. Electrophysiologic studies in the newborn. *Semin Neurol* 1993; 13:10–19.
142. Ben-Ari Y. Limbic seizure and brain damage produced by kainic acid: mechanisms and relevance to human temporal lobe epilepsy. *Neuroscience* 1985; 14:375–403.
143. Engel J Jr, Wolfson L, Brown L. Anatomical correlates of electrical and behavioral events related to amygdaloid kindling. *Ann Neurol* 1978; 3:538–544.
144. Campbell KA. Plasticity in the propagation of hippocampal stimulation-induced activity: a $[^{14}C]$2-deoxyglucose mapping study. *Brain Res* 1990; 520:199–207.

145. Lothman EW, Collins RC. Kainic acid induced limbic seizures: metabolic, behavioral, electroencephalographic and neuropathological correlates. *Brain Res* 1981; 218:299–318.
146. Pereira de Vasconcelos A, Vergnes M, Boyet S, Marescaux C, Nehlig A. Forebrain metabolic activation induced by the repetition of audiogenic seizures in Wistar rats. *Brain Res* 1997; 762:114–120.
147. Wooten GF, Collins RC. Regional brain glucose utilization following intrastriatal injections of kainic acid. *Brain Res* 1980; 201:173–184.
148. Sperber EF, Stanton PK, Haas K, Ackermann RF, et al. Developmental differences in the neurobiology of epileptic brain damage. *Epilepsy Res Suppl* 1992; 9:67–80.
149. Sankar R, Shin D, Mazarati AM, Liu H, et al. Epileptogenesis after status epilepticus reflects age- and model- dependent plasticity. *Ann Neurol* 2000; 48:580–589.
150. Sankar R, Shin DH, Liu H, Mazarati A, et al. Patterns of status epilepticus-induced neuronal injury during development and long-term consequences. *J Neurosci* 1998; 18:8382–8393.
151. Kubová H, Druga R, Lukasiuk K, Suchomelová L, et al. Status epilepticus causes necrotic damage in the mediodorsal nucleus of the thalamus in immature rats. *J Neurosci* 2001; 21:3593–3599.
152. Roch C, Leroy C, Nehlig A, Namer IJ. Predictive value of cortical injury for the development of temporal lobe epilepsy in 21-day-old rats: an MRI approach using the lithium-pilocarpine model. *Epilepsia* 2002; 43:1129–1136.
153. Roch C, Leroy C, Nehlig A, Namer IJ. Magnetic resonance imaging in the study of the lithium-pilocarpine model of temporal lobe epilepsy in adult rats. *Epilepsia* 2002; 43:325–335.
154. Gale K. Subcortical structures and pathways involved in convulsive seizure generalization. *J Clin Neurophysiol* 1992; 9:264–277.
155. Gale K. Focal trigger zones and pathways of propagation in seizure generation. In: Schwartzkroin PA, ed. *Epilepsy: Models, Mechanisms and Concepts*. New York: Cambridge University Press, 1993:27–47.
156. Iadarola MJ, Gale K. Substantia nigra: site of anticonvulsant activity mediated by γ-aminobutyric acid. *Science* 1982; 218:1237–1240.
157. Maggio R, Gale K. Seizures evoked from area tempestas are subject to control by GABA and glutamate receptors in substantia nigra. *Exp Neurol* 1989; 105:184–188.
158. Redgrave P, Marrow L, Dean P. Topographical organization of the nigrotectal projection in rat: evidence for segregated channels. *Neuroscience* 1992; 50:571–595.
159. Redgrave P, Marrow L, Dean P. Anticonvulsant role of nigrotectal projection in the maximal electroshock model of epilepsy. II. Pathways from substantia nigra pars lateralis and adjacent peripeduncular area to the dorsal midbrain. *Neuroscience* 1992; 46:391–406.
160. Redgrave P, Simkins M, Overton P, Dean P. Anticonvulsant role of nigrotectal projection in the maximal electroshock model of epilepsy. I. Mapping of dorsal midbrain with bicuculline. *Neuroscience* 1992; 46:379–390.
161. Deransart C, Marescaux C, Depaulis A. Involvement of nigral glutamatergic inputs in the control of seizures in a genetic model of absence epilepsy in the rat. *Neuroscience* 1996; 71:721–728.
162. Velíšková J, Velíšek L, Moshé SL. Subthalamic nucleus: A new anticonvulsant site in the brain. *Neuroreport* 1996; 7:1786–1788.
163. Velíšková J, Miller AM, Nunes ML, Brown LL. Regional neural activity within the substantia nigra during peri-ictal flurothyl generalized seizure stages. *Neurobiol Dis* 2005; 20:752–759.
164. Velíšková J, Liptáková S, Hussain S. The effects of N-methyl-D-aspartate antagonist 2-amino-7-phosphonoheptanoic acid microinfusions into the adult male rat substantia nigra pars reticulata are site-specific. *Neurosci Lett* 2001; 316:108–110.
165. Moshé SL, Brown LL, Kubová H, Velíšková J, et al. Maturation and segregation of brain networks that modify seizures. *Brain Res* 1994; 665:141–146.
166. Velíšková J, Velíšek L, Nunes M, Moshé S. Developmental regulation of regional functionality of substantia nigra $GABA_A$ receptors involved in seizures. *Eur J Pharmacol* 1996; 309:167–173.
167. Shehab S, Simkins M, Dean P, Redgrave P. Regional distribution of the anticonvulsant and behavioural effects of muscimol injected into the substantia nigra of rats. *Eur J Neurosci* 1996; 8:749–757.
168. Paxinos G, Watson C. The rat brain in stereotaxic coordinates. 4th ed. San Diego: Academic Press, 1998.
169. Velíšková J, Löscher W, Moshé SL. Regional and age specific effects of zolpidem microinfusions in the substantia nigra on seizures. *Epilepsy Res* 1998; 30:107–114.
170. Velíšková, J, Moshé, SL. Sexual dimorphism and developmental regulation of substantia nigra function. *Ann Neurol* 2001; 50:596–601.
171. Velíšek L, Velíšková J, Moshé SL. Site-specific effects of local pH changes in the substantia nigra pars reticulata on flurothyl-induced seizures. *Brain Res* 1998; 782:310–313.
172. Wisden W, Laurie DJ, Monyer H, Seeburg PH. The distribution of 13 $GABA_A$ receptor subunit mRNAs in the rat brain. I. Telencephalon, diencephalon, mesencephalon. *J Neurosci* 1992; 12:1040–1062.
173. Velíšek L, Velíšková J, Ravizza T, Giorgi FS, et al. Circling behavior and [^{14}C]2-deoxyglucose mapping in rats: possible implications for autistic repetitive behaviors. *Neurobiol Dis* 2005; 18:346–355.
174. Moshé SL, Albala BJ. Nigral muscimol infusions facilitate the development of seizures in immature rats. *Brain Res* 1984; 315:305–308.
175. Xu SG, Garant DS, Sperber EF, Moshé SL. The proconvulsant effect of nigral infusions of THIP on flurothyl-induced seizures in rat pups. *Brain Res Dev Brain Res* 1992; 68:275–277.
176. Lee VWK, de Kretser DM, Hudson B, Wang C. Variations in serum FSH, LH and testosterone levels in male rats from birth to sexual maturity. *J Reprod Fertil* 1975; 42:121–126.
177. Piacsek BE, Goodspeed MP. Maturation of the pituitary-gonadal system in the male rat. *J Reprod Fertil* 1978; 52:29–35.
178. Döhler KD, Wuttke W. Changes with age in levels of serum gonadotropins, prolactin, and gonadal steroids in prepubertal male and female rats. *Endocrinology* 1975; 97:898–907.
179. Velíšková J, Moshé SL. Update on the role of substantia nigra pars reticulata in the regulation of seizures. *Epilepsy Curr* 2006; 6:83–87.
180. Meencke HJ, Gerhard C. Morphological aspects of aetiology and the course of infantile spasms (West-syndrome). *Neuropediatrics* 1985; 16:59–66.
181. Nagata Y, Matsumoto H. Studies on methylazoxymethanol; methylation of nucleic acids in fetal rat brain. *Proc Soc Exp Biol Med* 1969; 132:383–385.
182. Angerine JB, Sidman RL. Autoradiographic study of cell migration during histogenesis of cerebral cortex of mouse. *Nature* 1961; 1192:766–768.
183. Paredes M, Pleasure SJ, Baraban SC. Embryonic and early postnatal abnormalities contributing to the development of hippocampal malformations in a rodent model of dysplasia. *J Comp Neurol* 2006; 495:133–148.
184. Germano IM, Sperber EF. Transplacentally induced neuronal migration disorders: an animal model for the study of the epilepsies. *J Neurosci Res* 1998; 51:473–488.
185. de Feo MR, Mecarelli O, Ricci GF. Seizure susceptibility in immature rats with microencephaly induced by prenatal exposure to methylazoxymethanol acetate. *Pharmacol Res* 1995; 31:109–114.
186. Rafiki A, Chevassus-au-Louis N, Ben-Ari Y, Khrestchatisky M, et al. Glutamate receptors in dysplasic cortex: an in situ hybridization and immunohistochemistry study in rats with prenatal treatment with methylazoxymethanol. *Brain Res* 1998; 782:147–152.
187. Baraban SC, Schwartzkroin PA. Electrophysiology of CA1 pyramidal neurons in an animal model of neuronal migration disorders: prenatal methylazoxymethanol treatment. *Epilepsy Res* 1995; 22:145–156.
188. Chevassus-au-Louis N, Rafiki A, Jorquera I, Ben-Ari Y, et al. Neocortex in the hippocampus: an anatomical and functional study of CA1 heterotopias after prenatal treatment with methylazoxymethanol in rats. *J Comp Neurol* 1998; 394:520–536.
189. Escueta AV, Davidson D, Hartwig G, Reilly E. The freezing lesion. II. Potassium transport within nerve terminals isolated from epileptogenic foci. *Brain Res* 1974; 78:223–227.
190. Escueta AV, Davidson D, Hartwig G, Reilly E. The freezing lesion. III. The effects of diphenylhydantoin on potassium transport within nerve terminals from the primary foci. *Brain Res* 1975; 86:85–96.
191. Dvořák, K, Feit, J. Migration of neuroblasts through partial necrosis of the cerebral cortex in newborn rats. Contribution of the problems of morphological developmental period of cerebral microgyria. *Acta Neuropathol* 1977; 38:203–212.
192. Rosen GD, Sherman GF, Galaburda AM. Birthdates of neurons in induced microgyria. *Brain Res* 1996; 727:71–78.
193. Schwarz P, Stichel CC, Luhmann HJ. Characterization of neuronal migration disorders in neocortical structures: loss or preservation of inhibitory interneurons? *Epilepsia* 2000; 41:781–787.
194. Redecker C, Luhmann HJ, Hagemann G, Fritschy JM, et al. Differential downregulation of $GABA_A$ receptor subunits in widespread brain regions in the freeze-lesion model of focal cortical malformations. *J Neurosci* 2000; 20:5045–5053.
195. Jacobs KM, Gutnick MJ, Prince DA. Hyperexcitability in a model of cortical maldevelopment. *Cereb Cortex* 1996; 6:514–523.
196. Kraemer M, Roth-Haerer A, Bruehl C, Luhmann HJ, et al. Metabolic and electrophysiological alterations in an animal model of neocortical neuronal migration disorder. *Neuroreport* 2001; 12:2001–2006.
197. Rosen GD, Sigel EA, Sherman GF, Galaburda AM. The neuroprotective effects of MK-801 on the induction of microgyria by freezing injury to the newborn rat neocortex. *Neuroscience* 1995; 69:107–114.
198. Redecker C, Hagemann G, Kohling R, Straub H, et al. Optical imaging of epileptiform activity in experimentally induced cortical malformations. *Exp Neurol* 2005; 192: 288–298.
199. Setkowicz Z, Janeczko K. Long-term changes in susceptibility to pilocarpine-induced status epilepticus following neocortical injuries in the rat at different developmental stages. *Epilepsy Res* 2003; 53:216–224.
200. Setkowicz Z, Klak K, Janeczko K. Long-term changes in postnatal susceptibility to pilocarpine-induced seizures in rats exposed to gamma radiation at different stages of prenatal development. *Epilepsia* 2003; 44:1267–1273.
201. Setkowicz Z, Janeczko K. A strong epileptogenic effect of mechanical injury can be reduced in the dysplastic rat brain. Long-term consequences of early prenatal gamma-irradiation. *Epilepsy Res* 2005; 66:165–172.
202. Setkowicz Z, Janicka D, Kowalczyk A, Turlej A, et al. Congenital brain dysplasias of different genesis can differently affect susceptibility to pilocarpine- or kainic acid-induced seizures in the rat. *Epilepsy Res* 2005; 67:123–131.
203. Pennacchio LA, Lehesjoki AE, Stone NE, Willour VL, et al. Mutations in the gene encoding cystatin B in progressive myoclonus epilepsy (EPM1). *Science* 1996; 271:1731–1734.
204. Noebels JL, Tharp BL. Absence seizures in developing brain. In: Schwartzkroin PA, Moshé SL, Noebels JL, Swann JW, eds. *Brain Development and Epilepsy*. Oxford: Oxford University Press, 1995:66–93.
205. Meldrum B. GABAergic agents as anticonvulsants in baboons with photosensitive epilepsy. *Neurosci Lett* 1984; 47:345–349.
206. Meldrum BS, Croucher MJ, Badman G, Collins JF. Antiepileptic action of excitatory amino acid antagonists in the photosensitive baboon, *Papio papio*. *Neurosci Lett* 1983; 39:101–104.
207. Meldrum BS, Horton RW. Convulsive effects of 4-deoxypyridoxine and of bicuculline in photosensitive baboons (*Papio papio*) and in rhesus monkeys (*Macaca mulatta*). *Brain Res* 1971; 35:419–436.
208. Meldrum BS, Horton RW. Neuronal inhibition mediated by GABA and patterns of convulsions in baboons with photosensitive epilepsy. In: Harris P, Mawdsley C, eds. *Epilepsy*. New York: Churchill-Livingstone, 1974:55–64.

209. Meldrum BS, Horton RW, Brierley JB. Epileptic brain damage in adolescent baboons following seizures induced by allyl-glycine. *Brain* 1974; 97:407–418.
210. Naquet R, Menini C, Riche D, Silva-Barrat C, et al. Photic epilepsy in man and in the baboon, *Papio papio*. In: Meldrum BS, Ferrendelli JA, Wieser HG, eds. *Anatomy of Epileptogenesis*. London-Paris: John Libbey, 1988:107–126.
211. Fisher RS. Animal models of epilepsies. *Brain Res Brain Res Rev* 1989; 14:245–278.
212. Szabo CA, Leland MM, Knape K, Elliott JJ, et al. Clinical and EEG phenotypes of epilepsy in the baboon (*Papio hamadryas* spp.). *Epilepsy Res* 2005; 65:71–80.
213. Szabo CA, Leland MM, Sztonak L, Restrepo S, et al. Scalp EEG for the diagnosis of epilepsy and photosensitivity in the baboon. *Am J Primatol* 2004; 62:95–106.
214. Browning RA, Wang C, Lanker ML, Jobe PC. Electroshock- and pentylenetetrazol-induced seizures in genetically epilepsy-prone rats (GEPRs): differences in threshold and pattern. *Epilepsy Res* 1990; 6:1–11.
215. Browning RA, Wade DR, Marcinczyk M, Long GL, et al. Regional brain abnormalities in norepinephrine uptake and dopamine beta-hydroxylase activity in the genetically epilepsy prone rat. *J Pharmacol Exp Ther* 1989; 249:229–235.
216. Jobe PC, Mishra PK, Ludvig N, Dailey JW. Scope and contribution of genetic models to an understanding of the epilepsies. *Crit Rev Neurobiol* 1991; 6:183–220.
217. Marescaux C, Vergnes M, Depaulis A. Genetic absence epilepsy in rats from Strasbourg—a review. *J Neural Transm Suppl* 1992; 35:37–69.
218. Ramakers GMJ, Peeters BWMM, Vossen JMH, Coenen AML. CNQX, a new non-NMDA receptor antagonist, reduces spike wave discharges in the WAG/Rij rat model of absence epilepsy. *Epilepsy Res* 1991; 9:127–131.
219. Vergnes M, Marescaux C, Depaulis A, Micheletti G, et al. Ontogeny of spontaneous petit mal-like seizures in Wistar rats. *Dev Brain Res* 1986; 30:85–87.
220. Coenen AM, Van Luijtelaar EL. The WAG/Rij rat model for absence epilepsy: age and sex factors. *Epilepsy Res* 1987; 1:297–301.
221. Sarkisian MR. Overview of the current animal models for human seizure and epileptic disorders. *Epilepsy Behav* 2001; 2:201–216.
222. Sarkisian MR, Rattan S, D'Mello SR, LoTurco JJ. Characterization of seizures in the flathead rat: a new genetic model of epilepsy in early postnatal development. *Epilepsia* 1999; 40:394–400.
223. Cogswell CA, Sarkisian MR, Leung V, Patel R, et al. A gene essential to brain growth and development maps to the distal arm of rat chromosome 12. *Neurosci Lett* 1998; 251:5–8.
224. Roberts MR, Bittman K, Li WW, French R, et al. The flathead mutation causes CNS-specific developmental abnormalities and apoptosis. *J Neurosci* 2000; 20:2295–2306.
225. Noebels, JL. The biology of epilepsy genes. *Annu Rev Neurosci* 2003; 26:599–625.
226. Noebels, JL. Exploring new gene discoveries in idiopathic generalized epilepsy. *Epilepsia* 2003; 44 Suppl 2:16–21.
227. Burgess DL. Transgenic and gene replacement models of epilepsy: targeting ion channel and neuroransmission pathways. In: Pitkanen A, Schwartzkroin P, Moshé SL, eds. *Models of Seizures and Epilepsy*. Amsterdam: Elsevier, 2006:199–222.
228. Noebels JL. Spontaneous epileptic mutations in mice. In: Pitkanen A, Schwartzkroin P, Moshé SL, eds. *Models of Seizures and Epilepsy*. Amsterdam: Elsevier, 2006:223–232.
229. Noebels JL. Genetic and phenotypic heterogeneity of inherited spike-and-and wave epilepsies. In Genton, P, Hirsch, E, Marescaux, C, Broglin, D, Bernasconi, R, eds. *Idiopathic Generalized Epilepsies*. London: John Libbey, 1994:215–225.
230. Gleeson JG, Allen KM, Fox JW, Lamperti ED, et al. Doublecortin, a brain-specific gene mutated in human X-linked lissencephaly and double cortex syndrome, encodes a putative signaling protein. *Cell* 1998; 92:63–72.
231. Noebels JL. Analysis of inherited epilepsy using single locus mutations in mice. *Fed Proc* 1979; 38:2405–2410.
232. Noebels JL, Sidman RL. Inherited epilepsy: spike-wave and focal motor seizures in the mutant mouse *tottering*. *Science* 1979; 204:1334–1336.
233. Noebels JL. Mutational analysis of inherited epilepsies. *Adv Neurol* 1986; 44:97–113.
234. Levitt P, Noebels JL. Mutant mouse *tottering*: selective increase of locus ceruleus axons in a defined single-locus mutation. *Proc Natl Acad Sci U S A* 1981; 78:4630–4634.
235. Acampora D, Mazan S, Avantaggiato V, Barone P, et al. Epilepsy and brain abnormalities in mice lacking the Otx1 gene. *Nat Genet* 1996; 14:218–222.
236. Avanzini G, Spreafico R, Cipelletti B, Sancini G, et al. Synaptic properties of neocortical neurons in epileptic mice lacking the *Otx1* gene. *Epilepsia* 2000; 41 Suppl 6:S200–205.
237. Sancini G, Franceschetti S, Lavazza T, Panzica F, et al. Potentially epileptogenic dysfunction of cortical NMDA- and GABA-mediated neurotransmission in *Otx1–/–* mice. *Eur J Neurosci* 2001; 14:1065–1074.
238. Cipelletti B, Avanzini G, Vitellaro-Zuccarello L, Franceschetti S, et al. Morphological organization of somatosensory cortex in *Otx1(–/–)* mice. *Neuroscience* 2002; 115:657667.
239. Verity CM, Ross EM, Golding J. Epilepsy in the first 10 years of life: findings of the Child Health and Education Study. *Br Med J* 1992; 305:857–861.
240. Nelson KB, Ellenberg JH. Predictors of epilepsy in children who have experienced febrile seizures. *N Engl J Med* 1976; 295:1029–1033.
241. Coulter DL. Continuous infantile spasms as a form of status epilepticus. *J Child Neurol* 1986; 1:215–217.
242. Constantinou JE, Gillis J, Ouvrier RA, Rahilly PM. Hypoxic-ischaemic encephalopathy after near miss sudden infant death syndrome. *Arch Dis Child* 1989; 64:703–708.
243. Cowan LD, Bodensteiner JB, Leviton A, Doherty L. Prevalence of the epilepsies in children and adolescents. *Epilepsia* 1989; 30:94–106.
244. Liu CC, Chen JS, Lin CH, Chen YJ, et al. Bacterial meningitis in infants and children in southern Taiwan: emphasis on *Haemophilus influenzae* type B infection. *J Formos Med Assoc* 1993; 92:884–888.
245. Wen DY, Bottini AG, Hall WA, Haines SJ. Infections in neurologic surgery. The intraventricular use of antibiotics. *Neurosurg Clin N Am* 1992; 3:343–354.
246. Morimoto T, Fukuda M, Aibara Y, Nagao H, et al. The influence of blood gas changes on hyperthermia-induced seizures in developing rats. *Brain Res Dev Brain Res* 1996; 92:77–80.
247. Baram TZ, Gerth A, Schultz L. Febrile seizures: an appropriate-aged model suitable for long-term studies. *Brain Res Dev Brain Res* 1997; 98:265–270.
248. Holtzman D, Obana K, Olson J. Hyperthermia-induced seizures in the rat pup: a model for febrile convulsions in children. *Science* 1981; 213:1034–1036.
249. Olson JE, Scher MS, Holtzman D. Effects of anticonvulsants on hyperthermia-induced seizures in the rat pup. *Epilepsia* 1984; 25:96–99.
250. Olson JE, Horne DS, Holtzman D, Miller M. Hyperthermia-induced seizures in rat pups with preexisting ischemic brain injury. *Epilepsia* 1985; 26:360–364.
251. Dube C, Richichi C, Bender RA, Chung G, et al. Temporal lobe epilepsy after experimental prolonged febrile seizures: prospective analysis. *Brain* 2006; 129:911–922.
252. Lemmens EM, Lubbers T, Schijns OE, Beuls EA, et al. Gender differences in febrile seizure–induced proliferation and survival in the rat dentate gyrus. *Epilepsia* 2005; 46:1603–1612.
253. Heida JG, Boisse L, Pittman QJ. Lipopolysaccharide-induced febrile convulsions in the rat: short-term sequelae. *Epilepsia* 2004; 45:1317–1329.
254. Jensen FE, Holmes GL, Lombroso CT, Blume HK, et al. Age-dependent changes in long-term seizure susceptibility and behavior after hypoxia in rats. *Epilepsia* 1992; 33: 971–980.
255. Moshé SL, Albala BJ. Perinatal hypoxia and subsequent development of seizures. *Physiol Behav* 1985; 35:819–823.
256. Marešová D, Mareš P. Effect of hypoxia on hippocampal afterdischarges in young rats. *Exp Brain Res Series* 1991; 20:171–173.
257. Chiba S. Long term effect of postnatal hypoxia on the seizure susceptibility in rats. *Life Sci* 1985; 37:1597–1604.
258. Applegate CD, Jensen F, Burchfiel JL, Lombroso C. The effects of neonatal hypoxia on kindled seizure development and electroconvulsive shock profiles. *Epilepsia* 1996; 37:723–727.
259. Holmes GL, Weber DA. Effects of hypoxic-ischemic encephalopathies on kindling in developing animals. *Exp Neurol* 1985; 90:194–203.
260. Jensen FE. An animal model of hypoxia-induced perinatal seizures. *Ital J Neurol Sci* 1995; 16:59–68.
261. Sanchez RM, Dai W, Levada RE, Lippman JJ, et al. AMPA/kainate receptor-mediated downregulation of GABAergic synaptic transmission by calcineurin after seizures in the developing rat brain. *J Neurosci* 2005; 25:3442–3451.
262. Williams PA, Dou P, Dudek FE. Epilepsy and synaptic reorganization in a perinatal rat model of hypoxia-ischemia. *Epilepsia* 2004; 45:1210–1218.
263. Watanabe K, Hara K, Miyazaki S, Hakamada S. The role of perinatal brain injury in the genesis of childhood epilepsy. *Fol Psychiatr Neurol Jpn* 1980; 34:227–232.
264. Watanabe K, Takeuchi T, Hakamada S, Hayakawa F. Neurophysiological and neuroradiological features preceding infantile spasms. *Brain Dev* 1987; 9:391–398.
265. Haut SR, Velíšková J, Moshé SL. Susceptibility of immature and adult brains to seizure effects. *Lancet Neurol* 2004; 3:608–617.
266. Meencke HJ, Veith G. Hippocampal sclerosis in epilepsy. In: Lüders, HO, ed. *Epilepsy Surgery*. New York: Raven Press, 1991:705–715.
267. Wasterlain CG. Recurrent seizures in the developing brain are harmful. *Epilepsia* 1997; 38:728–734.
268. Bekenstein J, Rempe D, Lothman E. Decreased heterosynaptic and homosynaptic paired pulse inhibition in the rat hippocampus as a chronic sequela to limbic status epilepticus. *Brain Res* 1993; 601:111–120.
269. Nadler JV, Perry BW, Cotman CW. Intraventricular kainic acid preferentially destroys hippocampal pyramidal cells. *Nature* 1978; 271:676–677.
270. Sloviter RS. "Epileptic" brain damage in rats induced by sustained stimulation of the perforant path I. Acute electrophysiological and light microscope studies. *Brain Res Bull* 1983; 10:675–697.
271. Sloviter RS. Decreased hippocampal inhibition and a selective loss of interneurons in experimental epilepsy. *Science* 1987; 235:73–76.
272. Sloviter RS, Dean E, Sollas AL, Goodman JH. Apoptosis and necrosis induced in different hippocampal neuron populations by repetitive perforant path stimulation in the rat. *J Comp Neurol* 1996; 366:516–533.
273. Schmidt-Kastner, R, Heim, C, Sontag, K-H. Damage of substantia nigra pars reticulata during pilocarpine-induced status epilepticus in the rat: immunohistochemical study of neurons, astrocytes and serum-protein extravasation. *Exp Brain Res* 1991; 86: 125–140.
274. Schmidt-Kastner R, Humpel C, Wetmore C, Olson L. Cellular hybridization for BDNF, trkB, and NGF mRNAs and BDNF-immunoreactivity in rat forebrain after pilocarpine-induced status epilepticus. *Exp Brain Res* 1996; 107:331–347.
275. Cronin J, Dudek FE. Chronic seizures and collateral sprouting of dentate mossy fibers after kainic acid treatment in rats. *Brain Res* 1988; 474:181–184.
276. Golarai G, Parada I, Sutula T. Mossy fiber synaptic reorganization induced by repetitive pentylenetetrazol seizures. *Abstr Soc Neurosci* 1988; 14:882.
277. Nadler JV, Perry BW, Cotman CW. Selective reinnervation of hippocampal area CA1 and the fascia dentata after destruction of CA3–CA4 afferents. *Brain Res* 1980; 182:1–9.
278. Sutula T, He X, Cavazos J, Scott G. Synaptic reorganization induced in the hippocampus by abnormal functional activity. *Science* 1988; 239:1147–1150.
279. Sperber EF. The relationship between seizures and damage in the maturing brain. In: Heinemann U, Engel J Jr, Avanzini G, Meldrum BS, et al, eds. *Progressive Nature of Epileptogenesis*. Amsterdam: Elsevier, 1996:365–376.
280. Tauck DL, Nadler JV. Evidence of functional mossy fiber sprouting in hippocampal formation of kainic acid-treated rats. *J Neurosci* 1985; 5:1016–1022.

281. Sperk G, Lassman H, Baran H, Seitelberger F, et al. Kainic acid-induced seizures: dose relationship of behavioural, neurochemical and histopathological changes. *Brain Res* 1985; 338:289–295.
282. Lothman EW, Bertram EH, Kapur J, Stringer JL. Recurrent spontaneous hippocampal seizures in the rat as a chronic sequela to limbic status epilepticus. *Epilepsy Res* 1990; 6:110–118.
283. Holmes, GL. The long-term effects of seizures on the developing brain: clinical and laboratory issues. *Brain Dev* 1991; 13:393–409.
284. Sperber E. The relationship between seizures and damage in the maturing brain. In: Heinemann U, Engel JJ, Avanzini G, Meldrum B, et al, eds. *Progressive Nature of Epileptogenesis*. Amsterdam: Elsevier, 1996:365–376.
285. Holmes GL, Thompson JL. Effects of kainic acid on seizure susceptibility in the developing brain. *Brain Research* 1988; 467:51–59.
286. Holmes GL, Thompson JL. Effects of serial administration of kainic acid on the developing brain. *Neuropharmacology* 1988; 27:209–212.
287. Holmes GL, Thompson JL, Marchi T, Feldman DS. Behavioral effects of kainic acid administration on the immature brain. *Epilepsia* 1988; 29:721–730.
288. Nitecka L, Tremblay E, Charton G, Bouillot JP, et al. Maturation of kainic acid seizure-brain damage syndrome in the rat. II Histopathological sequelae. *Neuroscience* 1984; 13:1073–1094.
289. Cavalheiro EA, Silva DF, Turski WA, Calderazzo-Filho LS, et al. The susceptibility of rats to pilocarpine-induced seizures is age-dependent. *Dev Brain Res* 1987; 465:43–58.
290. Okada R, Moshé SL, Albala BJ. Infantile status epilepticus and future seizure susceptibility in the rat. *Dev Brain Res* 1984; 15:177–183.
291. Sankar R, Shin D, Liu H, Wasterlain C, et al. Epileptogenesis during development: injury, circuit recruitment, and plasticity. *Epilepsia* 2002; 43 Suppl 5:47–53.
292. Sankar R, Shin DH, Wasterlain CG. Serum neuron-specific enolase is a marker for neuronal damage following status epilepticus in the rat. *Epilepsy Res* 1997; 28:129–136.
293. Sperber EF, Haas KZ, Moshé SL. Developmental aspects of status epilepticus. *Int Pediatr* 1992; 7:213–222.
294. Schanne FAX, Kane AB, Young EE, Farber JL. Calcium dependence of toxic cell death: a final common pathway. *Science* 1979; 205:700–702.
295. Alcantara S, de Lecea L, Del Rio JA, Ferrer I, et al. Transient colocalization of parvalbumin and calbindin D28k in the postnatal cerebral cortex: evidence for a phenotypic shift in developing nonpyramidal neurons. *Eur J Neurosci* 1996; 8:1329–1339.
296. Friedman LK, Sperber EF, Moshé SL, Bennett MV, et al. Developmental regulation of glutamate and GABA(A) receptor gene expression in rat hippocampus following kainate-induced status epilepticus. *Dev Neurosci* 1997; 19:529–542.
297. de Feo MR, Mecarelli O, Palladini G, Ricci GF. Long-term effects of early status epilepticus on the acquisition avoidance behavior in rats. *Epilepsia* 1986; 27:476–482.
298. Neill JC, Liu Z, Sarkisian M, Tandon P, et al. Recurrent seizures in immature rats: effect on auditory and visual discrimination. *Brain Res Dev Brain Res* 1996; 95:283–292.
299. Wasterlain CG. Effects of neonatal status epilepticus on rat brain development. *Neurology* 1976; 26:975–986.
300. Wasterlain CG, Dwyer BE. Brain metabolism during prolonged seizures in neonates. In: Delgado-Escueta AV, Wasterlain CG, Treiman, DM, Porter, RJ, eds. *Status Epilepticus*. New York: Raven Press, 1983:241–260.
301. Wasterlain CG, Shirassaka Y. Seizures, brain damage and brain development. *Brain Dev* 1994; 16:279–295.
302. Villeneuve N, Ben-Ari Y, Holmes GL, Gaiarsa JL. Neonatal seizures induced persistent changes in intrinsic properties of CA1 rat hippocampal cells. *Ann Neurol* 2000; 47: 729–738.
303. Isaeva E, Isaev D, Khazipov R, Holmes GL. Selective impairment of GABAergic synaptic transmission in the flurothyl model of neonatal seizures. *Eur J Neurosci* 2006; 23: 1559–1566.
304. Hoffmann AF, Zhao Q, Holmes GL. Cognitive impairment following status epilepticus and recurrent seizures during early development: support for the "two-hit hypothesis." *Epilepsy Behav* 2004; 5:873–877.
305. Stafstrom CE, Sasaki-Adams DM. NMDA-induced seizures in developing rats cause long-term learning impairment and increased seizure susceptibility. *Epilepsy Res* 2003; 53:129–137.
306. Gowers WR. Epilepsy and other chronic convulsive diseases. London: JA Churchill, 1881.
307. Priel MR, dos Santos NF, Cavalheiro EA. Developmental aspects of the pilocarpine model of epilepsy. *Epilepsy Res* 1996; 26:115–121.
308. Sperber EF, Haas KZ, Moshé SL. Mechanisms of kindling in developing animals. In: Wada JA, ed. *Kindling 4*. New York: Plenum Press, 1990:157–168.
309. Gulec G, Noyan B. Do recurrent febrile convulsions decrease the threshold for pilocarpine-induced seizures? Effects of nitric oxide. *Brain Res Dev Brain Res* 2001; 126:223–228.
310. Khalilov I, Le Van Quyen M, Gozlan H, Ben-Ari Y. Epileptogenic actions of GABA and fast oscillations in the developing hippocampus. *Neuron* 2005; 48:787–796.
311. Sheridan PH, Jacobs MP. The development of antiepileptic drugs for children. Report from the NIH workshop, Bethesda, Maryland, February 17–18, 1994. *Epilepsy Res* 1996; 23:87–92.
312. Moshé SL. Sex and the substantia nigra: Administration, teaching, patient care, and research. *J Clin Neurophysiol* 1997; 14:484–494.
313. Velíšek L, Mareš P. Developmental aspects of the anticonvulsant action of MK-801. In: Kamenka J-M, Domino EF, eds. *Multiple Sigma and PCP Receptor Ligands: Mechanisms for Neuromodulation and Neuroprotection?* Ann Arbor, MI: NPP Books, 1992:779–795.
314. Velíšek L, Roztočilová L, Kusá R, Mareš P. Excitatory amino acid antagonists and pentylenetetrazol-induced seizures during ontogenesis: III. The action of kynurenic acid and glutamic acid diethylester. *Brain Res Bull* 1995; 38:525–529.
315. Velíšek L, Vachová D, Mareš P. Excitatory amino acid antagonists and pentylenetetrazol-induced seizures during ontogenesis. IV. Effects of CGP 39551. *Pharmacol Biochem Behav* 1997; 56:493–498.
316. Velíšek L, Velíšková J, Ptachewich Y, Ortíz J, Shinnar S, Moshé SL. Age-dependent effects of gamma-aminobutyric acid agents on flurothyl seizures. *Epilepsia* 1995; 36: 636–643.
317. Velíšek L, Kusá R, Kulovaná M, Mareš P. Excitatory amino acid antagonists and pentylenetetrazol-induced seizures during ontogenesis: I. The effects of 2-amino-7-phosphonoheptanoate. *Life Sci* 1990; 46:1349–1357.
318. Mareš P, Lišková-Bernášková K, Mudrochová M. Convulsant action of diphenylhydantoin overdose in young rats. *Act Nerv Super (Praha)* 1987; 29:30–35.
319. Mareš P, Marešová D, Schickerová R. Effect of antiepileptic drugs on metrazol convulsions during ontogenesis in rats. *Physiol Bohemoslov* 1981; 30:113–121.
320. Mareš P, Velíšek L. Comparison of antiepileptic action of valproate and ethosuximide in adult and immature rats. *Pol J Pharmacol Pharm* 1987; 39:505–512.
321. Velíšek L, Kubová H, Velíšková J, Mareš P, et al. Action of antiepileptic drugs against kainic acid-induced seizures and automatisms during ontogenesis in rats. *Epilepsia* 1992; 33:987–993.
322. Kubová H, Mareš P. Anticonvulsant action of oxcarbazepine, hydroxycarbamazepine, and carbamazepine against metrazol-induced motor seizures in developing rats. *Epilepsia* 1993; 34:188–192.
323. Kubová H, Mareš P. Anticonvulsant effects of phenobarbital and primidone during ontogenesis in rats. *Epilepsy Res* 1991; 10:148–155.
324. Kubová H, Mareš P, Vorlíček J. Stable anticonvulsant action of benzodiazepines during development in rats. *J Pharm Pharmacol* 1993; 45:807–810.
325. Mikati MA, Holmes GL, Chronopoulos A, Hyde P, et al. Phenobarbital modifies seizure-related brain injury in the developing brain. *Ann Neurol* 1994; 36:425–433.
326. Velíšková J, Velíšek L, Moshé SL. Age-specific effects of baclofen on pentylenetetrazol-induced seizures in developing rats. *Epilepsia* 1996; 37:718–722.
327. Wurpel JND, Sperber EF, Moshé SL. Baclofen inhibits amygdala kindling in immature rats. *Epilepsy Res* 1990; 5:1–7.
328. Velíšek L, VelíškováJ, Ptachewich Y, Shinnar S, et al. Effects of MK-801 and phenytoin on flurothyl-induced seizures during development. *Epilepsia* 1995; 36:179–185.
329. Velíšek L, Verešová S, Pobišová H, Mareš, P. Excitatory amino acid antagonists and pentylenetetrazol-induced seizures during ontogenesis: II. The effects of MK-801. *Psychopharmacology* 1991; 104:510–514.
330. Stafstrom CE, Tandon P, Hori A, Liu Z, et al. Acute effects of MK801 on kainic acid-induced seizures in neonatal rats. *Epilepsy Res* 1997; 26:335–344.
331. Facchinetti F, Ciani E, Dall'Olio R, Virgili M, et al. Structural, neurochemical and behavioural consequences of neonatal blockade of NMDA receptor through chronic treatment with CGP 39551 or MK-801. *Brain Res Dev Brain Res* 1993; 74:219–224.
332. Tandon P, Liu Z, Stafstrom CE, Sarkisian M, et al. Long-term effects of excitatory amino acid antagonists NBQX and MK-801 on the developing brain. *Brain Res Dev Brain Res* 1996; 95:256–262.
333. Troupin AS, Mendius JR, Cheng F, Risinger MW. MK-801. In: Meldrum BS, Porter RJ, eds. *New Anticonvulsant Drugs*. London: John Libbey, 1986:191–201.
334. Woodbury DM. Antiepileptic drugs. Phenytoin: introduction and history. In: Glaser GH, Penry JK, Woodbury DM, eds. *Antiepileptic Drugs: Mechanisms of Action*. New York: Raven Press, 1980:305–313.
335. Wyllie E. The treatment of epilepsy: principles and practice. Philadelphia: Lea and Febiger, 1993.
336. Osorio I, Burnstine TH, Remler B, Manon-Espaillat R, et al. Phenytoin-induced seizures: a paradoxical effect at toxic concentrations in epileptic patients. *Epilepsia* 1989; 30: 230–234.
337. Staňková L, Kubová H, Mareš P. Anticonvulsant action of lamotrigine during ontogenesis in rats. *Epilepsy Res* 1992; 13:17–22.
338. Verešová S, Kábová R, Velíšek L. Proconvulsant effects induced by pyridoxine in young rats. *Epilepsy Res* 1998; 29:259–264.
339. Chapman AG, Graham JL, Patel S, Meldrum S. Anticonvulsant activity of two orally active competitive N-methyl-D-aspartate antagonists, CGP 37849 and CGP 39551, against sound-induced seizures in DBA/2 mice and photically induced myoclonus in *Papio papio*. *Epilepsia* 1991; 32:578–587.
340. Bittigau P, Sifringer M, Genz K, Reith E, et al. Antiepileptic drugs and apoptotic neurodegeneration in the developing brain. *Proc Natl Acad Sci U S A* 2002; 99:15089–15094.
341. Olney JW, Young C, Wozniak DF, Jevtovic-Todorovic V, et al. Do pediatric drugs cause developing neurons to commit suicide? *Trends Pharmacol Sci* 2004; 25:135–139.
342. Caviness VSJ, Hatten MF, McConnell SK, Takahashi T. Developmental neuropathology and childhood epilepsies. In: Schwartzkroin PA, Moshé SL, Noebels JL, Swann JW, eds. *Brain Development and Epilepsy*. New York: Oxford University Press,1995:94–121.
343. Velíšek L, Mareš P. Age-dependent anticonvulsant action of clonazepam in the N-methyl-D-aspartate model of seizures. *Pharmacol Biochem Behav* 1995; 52:291–296.
344. Kábová R, Liptáková S, Šlamberová R, Pometlová M, et al. Age-specific N-methyl-D-aspartate-induced seizures: perspectives for the West syndrome model. *Epilepsia* 1999; 40:1357–1369.
345. Velíšek L, Jehle K, Asche S, Velíšková J. Model of infantile spasms induced by NMDA in prenatally impaired brain. *Ann Neurol* 2007; 61:109–119.
346. Woolley DE, Timiras PS. The gonad-brain relationship: effects of female sex hormones on electroshock convulsions in the rat. *Endocrinology* 1962; 70:196–209.
347. Woolley DE, Timiras PS, Woodbury DM. Some effects of sex steroids on brain excitability and metabolism. *Proc West Pharmacol Soc* 1960; 3:11–23.
348. Pericic D, Manev H, Geber J. Sex-related differences in the response of mice, rats and cats to the administration of picrotoxin. *Life Sci* 1986; 38:905–913.

349. Pericic D, Manev H, Lakic N. Sex differences in the response of rats to drugs affecting GABAergic transmission. *Life Sci* 1985; 36:541–547.
350. Velíšková J, Velíšek L, Galanopoulou AS, Sperber EF. Neuroprotective effects of estrogens on hippocampal cells in adult female rats after status epilepticus. *Epilepsia* 2000; 41: S30–35.
351. Velíšek L, Velíšková J. Estrogen treatment protects GABA(B) inhibition in the dentate gyrus of female rats after kainic acid-induced status epilepticus. *Epilepsia* 2002; 43 Suppl 5:146–151.
352. Velíšková J. The role of estrogens in seizures and epilepsy: the bad guys or the good guys? *Neuroscience* 2006; 138:837–844.
353. Chatot CL, Klein NW, Clapper ML, Resor SR, et al. Human serum teratogenicity studied by rat embryo culture: epilepsy, anticonvulsant drugs, and nutrition. *Epilepsia* 1984; 25:205–216.
354. Holmes GL, Weber DA. The effect of progesterone on kindling: a developmental study. *Brain Res* 1984; 318:45–53.
355. Arnold AP, Gorski RA. Gonadal steroid induction of structural sex differences in the central nervous system. *Annu Rev Neurosci* 1984; 7:413–442.
356. Dubrovsky B, Filipini D, Gijsbers K, Birmingham M. Early and late effects of steroid hormones on the central nervous system. *Ciba Foundation Symposium* 1990; 153:240–257.
357. McEwen BS. Non-genomic and genomic effects of steroids on neural activity. *Trends Pharmacol Sci* 1991; 12:141–144.
358. McEwen BS. Steroid hormones: effect on brain development and function. *Horm Res* 1992; 37 (suppl 3):1–10.
359. Pitkanen A, Kubova H. Antiepileptic drugs in neuroprotection. *Expert Opin Pharmacother* 2004; 5:777–798.
360. Sulzbacher S, Farwell JR, Temkin N, Lu AS, et al. Late cognitive effects of early treatment with phenobarbital. *Clin Pediatr (Phila)* 1999; 38:387–394.
361. Pitkanen A. Drug-mediated neuroprotection and antiepileptogenesis: animal data. *Neurology* 2002; 59:S27–33.
362. Pitkanen A, Nissinen J, Nairismagi J, Lukasiuk K, et al. Progression of neuronal damage after status epilepticus and during spontaneous seizures in a rat model of temporal lobe epilepsy. *Prog Brain Res* 2002; 135:67–83.
363. Prasad A, Williamson JM, Bertram EH. Phenobarbital and MK-801, but not phenytoin, improve the long-term outcome of status epilepticus. *Ann Neurol* 2002; 51:175–181.
364. Ebert U, Brandt C, Loscher W. Delayed sclerosis, neuroprotection, and limbic epileptogenesis after status epilepticus in the rat. *Epilepsia* 2002; 43 Suppl 5:86–95.
365. Temkin NR. Antiepileptogenesis and seizure prevention trials with antiepileptic drugs: meta-analysis of controlled trials. *Epilepsia* 2001; 42:515–524.

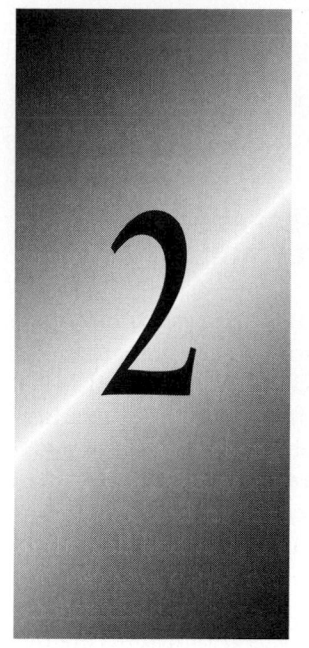

Ion Channels, Membranes, and Molecules in Epilepsy and Neuronal Excitability

Laxmikant S. Deshpande
Robert J. DeLorenzo

Important advances have been made in molecular neurobiology that enhances understanding the regulation of neuronal excitability in epilepsy and other brain functions. This research typically has involved antiepileptic drugs (AEDs) and other pharmacologic probes that have defined different mechanisms affecting neuronal excitability. The investigation of AEDs in these systems has also shed new light on the molecular basis of epilepsy and on the mechanisms of AED action (1–5).

This chapter provides the scientific background to assist the clinician in keeping abreast of several rapidly advancing fields. It highlights issues that influence neuronal excitability and seizures with emphasis on the mechanisms of sustained repetitive firing (SRF), sodium channels, the gamma-aminobutyric acid (GABA)–chloride channel complex, potassium channels, excitatory transmission, regulation of metabotropic receptors, carbonic anhydrase inhibition, neuromodulators, calcium-mediated regulation of neuronal function, and inhibition of epileptogenesis. In considering these quite different mechanisms, this chapter brings together many of the concepts considered in Chapters 4 and 30.

SUSTAINED REPETITIVE FIRING (SRF)

Sustained high-frequency repetitive firing is an important property of vertebrate and invertebrate neurons that correlates with the excitability state of the neuron (6–10). Many central nervous system (CNS) neurons exhibit SRF. Although no direct evidence has demonstrated the link between SRF and epilepsy, information from in vitro studies on isolated neurons may have some bearing on altered neuronal excitability and anticonvulsant action.

Sustained repetitive firing is a nonsynaptic property of neurons. The relevance of limitation of SRF to AED action is strengthened by several important observations. The therapeutic efficacy of each AED in controlling seizures in animals and humans is similar to that for controlling SRF in isolated, cultured neurons. These results indicate (7) that therapeutic levels of AEDs in cerebrospinal fluid (CSF) correlate with the concentrations that are most effective against SRF. The effects of anticonvulsants in limiting SRF have been shown in a variety of neurons from different regions of the mammalian CNS maintained in culture. This argues that this effect is not unique to specific regions or cell types. Anticonvulsants prevent bursting in the epileptic focus and restrict the spread of epileptic activity from the focus to normal surrounding tissue. Thus, suppression of SRF by anticonvulsants may inhibit excitability by inhibiting the spread of seizure activity. Membrane properties of nonepileptic neurons may be important in understanding drug mechanisms of action and may have a special relationship to the properties of SRF. SRF is an important model for studying the excitability of isolated neurons.

SUSTAINED REPETITIVE FIRING AND SODIUM CHANNEL REGULATION

In studying SRF, several properties of neuronal excitability and seizure phenomenon have been recognized. Voltage-gated sodium channels are responsible for the rising phase of neuronal action potentials. Upon neuronal depolarization to action potential threshold, the sodium channel undergoes a conformational change that results in the channel opening for a few milliseconds from its closed (resting), nonconducting state to permit sodium flux. The channel inactivates within a few milliseconds to terminate sodium ion influx. The membrane must repolarize before it can be activated again by a subsequent depolarization. Brain sodium channels can rapidly cycle through the conducting and nonconducting stages, allowing neurons to fire tonic high-frequency action potentials, as is required for both normal brain function and for the expression of epileptic activity characterized by SRF. Several agents block sodium channels to produce an antiepileptic effect. They include phenytoin, lamotrigine, carbamazepine, zonisamide, felbamate, topiramate, and valproate. The AEDs that block SRF have several properties in common. Blocking of SRF is voltage-dependent, and the anticonvulsant effect is use-dependent. Research on the role of the sodium channel in regulating SRF indicates that the drug effects on SRF are mediated through a use-dependent blockage of the sodium channel. Thus the block accumulates with SRF, inhibiting only the pathological high-frequency discharges but not the excitatory or inhibitory synaptic processes essential for normal brain functioning (11). Phenytoin and carbamazepine can reduce the amplitude of the sodium-dependent action potential in a use-dependent fashion (12). Phenytoin is thought to induce a nonconducting state of the sodium channel that is similar to channel inactivation (11, 13). These studies indicate that modulation of sodium channels by anticonvulsants, and possibly endogenous anticonvulsant-like molecules, may play an important role in the regulation of neuronal excitability in seizure discharge. Newer compounds such as safinamide, which is in clinical trials, are thought to produce anticonvulsant effect, at least in part, through inhibition of sodium and calcium channels, stabilizing membrane excitability and inhibiting transmitter release (14). Investigating the heterogeneity of sodium channels and their relationship to altered neuronal excitability is an area of important research.

BENZODIAZEPINE RECEPTORS AND MEMBRANE EXCITABILITY

In the 1970s use of radioactively labeled benzodiazepine derivatives allowed the detection of specific nanomolar benzodiazepine receptor sites in brain membrane (15–17). These sites have a very high affinity for the benzodiazepines, binding in low (nanomolar) concentration ranges. Binding to these receptors is reversible, saturable, and stereospecific. Nanomolar benzodiazepine receptors have now been identified in human brain, where they are widely distributed. The specific membrane protein that accounts for the majority of nanomolar benzodiazepine binding has a molecular weight of approximately 50,000 daltons and has been purified from animal and human brain (18).

High-affinity benzodiazepine binding has also been observed in peripheral, nonneuronal tissue (19). A different class of benzodiazepine receptor molecules causes this binding, because both the potency and the tissue distribution of this binding are different from that at the central-type receptor. This second class of high-affinity benzodiazepine binding sites was designated "peripheral type receptor" (19), but it was subsequently shown that the peripheral-type benzodiazepine receptor is also present in neuronal tissue. Thus, both peripheral and central high-affinity benzodiazepine receptors exist in the brain.

High nanomolar and low micromolar benzodiazepine binding sites have been identified more recently in brain membranes (20, 21). In addition, another benzodiazepine receptor that binds in the high nanomolar range has been identified in brain cytosol (21). These novel benzodiazepine-binding sites are stereospecific and have potencies for benzodiazepine binding that correlate with the ability of these compounds to inhibit maximal electric shock–induced seizures. Benzodiazepine bound to micromolar benzodiazepine receptors is displaced by phenytoin. These results indicate that high nanomolar and low-micromolar-affinity benzodiazepine receptors may represent important anticonvulsant binding sites in brain membrane that mediate some of the effects of benzodiazepines in high concentration in curtailing status epilepticus, generalized tonic-clonic seizures, and maximal electric shock–induced seizures.

Benzodiazepines are effective in nanomolar concentrations in blocking pentylenetetrazol-induced seizures in animals and in treating absence seizures. In addition, benzodiazepines in high nanomolar and low micromolar ranges inhibit maximal electric shock–induced seizures in animals. Furthermore, benzodiazepines are effective in humans in stopping generalized tonic-clonic seizures and status epilepticus when given in intravenous doses that produce low micromolar serum concentrations. The potency of the benzodiazepines in blocking maximal electric shock–induced seizures, however, correlates in neither time nor consequence with their ability to inhibit pentylenetetrazol-induced seizures or bind to the nanomolar central benzodiazepine receptor (20). Thus, other mechanisms appear to underlie this generalized anticonvulsant property of the benzodiazepines in high concentration ranges. Lower-affinity benzodiazepine binding sites in the high nanomolar and low micromolar ranges have also been described (20, 22). These lower-affinity receptor sites come into play in the concentration ranges in which benzodiazepines produce effects on maximal electric shock–induced seizures in animals, on generalized tonic-clonic seizures in man, and on SRF in cultured neurons.

Diazepam and clonazepam reduce SRF in high nanomolar and low micromolar concentrations (7). These concentrations are above therapeutic free-serum concentrations achieved in ambulatory patients treated with benzodiazepines but are within the ranges of free-serum concentrations achieved in patients treated for status epilepticus or acutely for generalized tonic-clonic seizures. In addition to the discrepancy in concentration ranges, the potency of benzodiazepines for suppressing SRF does not correlate with benzodiazepine binding to the nanomolar central receptor or with their ability to inhibit pentylenetetrazol-induced seizures but does correlate with binding to the lower-affinity benzodiazepine binding system.

THE GABA SYSTEM, NEURONAL EXCITABILITY, AND SEIZURE ACTIVITY

Gamma-aminobutyric acid is the major inhibitory neurotransmitter in brain. It has been extensively characterized and plays a major role in regulating neuronal excitability by controlling chloride permeability (23–25). Specific binding sites for GABA molecules have been identified in neuronal membrane. Although not all GABA receptors are linked to the chloride channel, a large proportion of these receptors are directly involved in regulating chloride channel function. The major inhibitory effect of GABA on the nervous system is mediated through its ability to regulate chloride channel permeability. GABA binding to the GABA receptor potentiates the opening of the chloride channel, allowing chloride ions to flow more easily into the cell. This causes cellular hyperpolarization and inhibits neuronal firing, because chloride ions increase the internal electrical negativity of the cell. This is believed to be the major mechanism by which GABA produces its inhibitory effect on neurons.

Functions of GABA in neuronal systems have been closely linked with the effects of the benzodiazepines (23–25). Significant portions of the nanomolar benzodiazepine receptors in the brain are associated with the GABA-binding sites and are thereby functionally linked to the chloride channel in neuronal membranes. The GABA–nanomolar benzodiazepine receptor/chloride ionophore macromolecular complex is an important example of the interrelationship between membrane receptors and neuronal excitability (25). The ability of AEDs and the benzodiazepines to modulate chloride conductances is a major molecular mechanism regulating neuronal excitability.

The GABA–Chloride Channel Complex Regulates Seizure Discharge

The chloride channel is surrounded by a GABA receptor, a nanomolar central benzodiazepine receptor, and a receptor site that binds picrotoxin and related convulsants as well as barbiturates and related depressants. This channel and its properties, related to the benzodiazepines, GABA, and convulsant and barbiturate molecules, have been characterized in detail (26). Picrotoxin binds to the proposed site and modulates benzodiazepine and GABA receptor binding in a way that inhibits chloride channel permeability, therefore making the cell more excitable. Barbiturate binding potentiates benzodiazepine receptor binding and thus indirectly potentiates the GABA effect on opening the chloride channel and enhancing neuronal inhibition. This complex interaction between GABA, benzodiazepines, picrotoxin and related convulsants, and the barbiturates and related depressants is a prime example of how pharmacologic agents modulate the function of ion channels through specific receptor binding.

Benzodiazepines are an important class of compounds that have antianxiety or anxiolytic effects and sedative, muscle relaxant, and anticonvulsant properties (15, 23–25, 27). As anticonvulsants, these compounds are effective in blocking both pentylenetetrazol-induced seizures in animals and, at higher concentrations, maximal electric shock–induced seizures. Benzodiazepines are the most commonly prescribed drugs for the initial treatment of generalized tonic-clonic seizures and status epilepticus in hospital emergency rooms. The anticonvulsant properties of the benzodiazepines, therefore, not only are of academic importance but also have widespread clinical use. The research characterizing this benzodiazepine receptor (16–19, 28, 29) demonstrates AED receptor–mediated regulation of neuronal excitability. Benzodiazepine binding to the nanomolar receptor site potentiates GABA effects on neuronal inhibition, providing one clear mechanism by which these compounds regulate neuronal excitability. Correlative neuropharmacologic studies have indicated that the anxiolytic and anti-pentylenetetrazol-induced anticonvulsant activity of these compounds are mediated through the high-affinity benzodiazepine nanomolar receptors. The effects of benzodiazepines on maximal electric shock–induced seizures and on generalized convulsions, however, cannot be clearly explained by these nanomolar actions.

Stiripentol is a novel antiepileptic compound that is structurally unrelated to any of the other currently marketed antiepileptic drugs (30). Studies in animal models have demonstrated that it produces anticonvulsant effect by increasing GABAergic transmission by enhancing the duration of opening of $GABA_A$ receptor channels (31). However, its clinical development was halted because of its inhibitory effect on cytochrome P450 enzymes. Despite this, it has been found to be beneficial for the treatment of early childhood epilepsy, and clinical trials are under way to further characterize its beneficial effect in pediatric patients (30).

Recently two types of $GABA_A$ receptor–mediated inhibition have come to the forefront: phasic and tonic. Synaptically released GABA, acting on postsynaptic $GABA_A$ receptors, produces "phasic" inhibition, whereas ambient GABA continually present in the extracellular space produces persistent activation of extrasynaptic $GABA_A$ receptors, resulting in "tonic" inhibition (32). Elegant studies by Istvan Mody's group strongly indicate that distinct $GABA_A$ receptor subtypes mediate these tonic and phasic receptor-mediated inhibitions (32–34). They found that the alpha-4 $GABA_A$ receptor subtype were extrasynaptically located and were responsible for tonic inhibition (34). These results suggested that alpha-4/beta/delta and alpha4/beta/gamma subunit–containing $GABA_A$ receptors may be present exclusively extrasynaptically, have a higher affinity for GABA, and not desensitize on the prolonged presence of agonist (35). On the other hand, alpha-1/beta/gamma-2 or alpha-2/beta/gamma-2 receptors are thought to mediate phasic inhibition, since the synaptic currents are known to be sensitive to benzodiazepines (36, 37). These studies provide another mechanism for $GABA_A$ regulation of synaptic activity.

$GABA_A$- and $GABA_B$-Mediated Neuronal Inhibition

As described previously, the best-characterized inhibitory effect of GABA on the nervous system is to open chloride channels and hyperpolarize the membrane, an effect that is mediated through $GABA_A$ receptors. In addition to $GABA_A$ receptors, scientists have characterized $GABA_B$ receptors that primarily open potassium channels in the membrane either pre-or postsynaptically. Opening potassium channels also results in hyperpolarization of the cell. Any alteration or decrease in GABA-mediated inhibition through $GABA_A$ or $GABA_B$ receptors can lead to seizures. Thus $GABA_B$ knockout mice exhibit spontaneous seizures (38). These data clearly indicate that GABA receptors in the regulation of chloride and potassium channels can regulate seizure discharge.

Potassium Channels

Potassium channels play a major role in regulating neuronal excitability. Although more than 20 types of potassium channels have been identified by biophysical studies, there are four major groups: calcium-activated, voltage-gated, sodium-activated, and inwardly rectifying potassium channels. These different types of potassium channels are regulated by neuromodulators, ions, and second messenger systems. The opening of potassium channels has the effect of hyperpolarizing neurons or reversing depolarizing actions that exist during the transmission of the action potential or the neuroexcitatory input. Following depolarization, several calcium-activated potassium channels play a major role in the after-hyperpolarization that occurs to restore the resting potential of a neuron (39). Electrographic studies on hippocampal neurons from patients undergoing temporal lobectomies have demonstrated alterations in potassium channels in epileptic tissue (40). In addition, compounds that can block potassium channels and prevent the effect of these channels on hyperpolarization are potent convulsants. Fluoraminopyridine and dendrotoxin-I are potent convulsants that have been used in numerous animal models to cause seizures (41, 42). In addition, compounds that are currently used as antihypertensive drugs, including chromakalim, minoxidil, diazoxide, and penicidil, act as potassium channel openers in muscle membranes and may have potential for use as anticonvulsant compounds (43, 44). The possibility of developing new classes of compounds that can activate or potentiate potassium channel activity may play an important role in increasing hyperpolarization following excessive excitatory activity and may serve to reverse the decreased levels of some potassium channels observed in patients with epilepsy.

Some anticonvulsant compounds may also play a role as potassium channel openers. Carbamazepine has been found to enhance potassium conductances in neurons (45). Other potential anticonvulsant compounds are being evaluated that may also potentiate potassium channel activation. Investigation of anticonvulsant drugs regulating potassium channels is a major frontier in the development of new anticonvulsant compounds. The small conductance Ca^{2+}-activated K^+ (SK) channels inhibit epileptiform bursting in hippocampal CA3 neurons. Compounds activating or inhibiting voltage-gated potassium channels formed by KCNQ2, KCNQ3, and KCNQ5 assembly (M-channels) are undergoing clinical trials for epilepsy, stroke, and Alzheimer's disease (46). Mutation in KCNQ2/3 causing mild reduction of M-channel activity is thought to enhance neuronal excitability associated with benign neonatal seizures. On the other hand, M-channel openers decrease the hyperexcitability responsible for epileptic seizures and migraine. Indeed, retigabine is thought to produce antiepileptic effect by opening the KNCQ2/3 channels (47, 48). This is a promising area for novel anticonvulsant drug development.

It is only in the recent past that scientists have begun to decipher the role of the hyperpolarization-activated cation (HCN) channel or h-channel (I_h) in regulating neuronal excitability and modulating seizures. The HCN family of genes consists of four subtypes and encodes HCN or I_h (49). HCN1 and HCN2 are the most prevalent subtypes in cortex and hippocampus, and HCN2 and HCN4 predominate in the thalamus. HCN3 is modestly expressed in brain (50). HCN has the unique capacity of being able to produce opposite biophysical effects. Thus, it can be either excitatory or inhibitory with respect to its influence on action potential firing. For example, I_h can diminish the effect of excitatory inputs, or it can set normal resting membrane potential, depolarizing the membrane from the K^+ reversal potential toward the firing threshold, thereby producing an excitatory effect (51). There is a growing body of evidence implicating HCN in epileptogenesis (51–54). For example, I_h- and GABA-mediated inhibition is increased in febrile seizures (55, 56). Moreover, genetic deletion of HCN2 resulted in a mouse phenotype that exhibited spontaneous absence seizures as well as cardiac sinus arrhythmias, indicating that the absence of HCN2 is proconvulsive (57). There is conflicting pharmacologic evidence for the role of HCN in epilepsy (51). Certain AEDs, such as lamotrigine, act beyond their normal target—the Na^+ channels—and upregulate I_h, and they reduce action potential firing that is initiated from dendritic depolarization but not from somatic depolarization (52). On the other hand, other Na^+ channel blockers, such as carbamazepine or phenytoin, did not lower dendritic excitability (52). Thus, the action of lamotrigine on HCN may constitute an important, novel anticonvulsant mechanism. The role of the HCN channel in epilepsy is an important area for further investigation.

EXCITATORY TRANSMISSION

Glutamate is the major excitatory neurotransmitter in the brain. Understanding the role of excitatory transmission and its overactivation in epilepsy is an important area for anticonvulsant drug development. Only since the early 1980s has the role of glutamate, aspartate, and other compounds that serve as excitatory transmitters been clearly identified. Several important receptors have been identified in the brain that respond to glutamate and other excitatory neurotransmitters (58). The major glutamate receptors that regulate ion channels include the N-methyl-D-aspartate (NMDA), quisqualate or alpha-amino-5-methyl-3-hydroxy-4-isoxazolepropionic acid (AMPA), and kainate channels. In addition, there are other, more recently identified subcategories of excitatory amino acid ion channels regulated by glutamate (59).

NMDA receptor–regulated ion channels are an important class of excitatory amino acid coupled channels in the brain that not only play a role in neuronal excitability but also have long-term effects on long-term plasticity changes in the brain. NMDA receptor–activated channels are permeable to sodium, potassium, and calcium. They can be voltage-blocked by magnesium, which indicates that they can be in an operative form only when the cell is partly depolarized by other excitatory receptor activation. This type of modulation allows for complex regulation of NMDA receptor activity. For an NMDA channel to be activated, it is necessary for either the excitatory amino acid transmitter glutamate or aspartate to bind to the NMDA receptor site and for the molecule glycine or D-serine to bind at the neuromodulatory site on the receptor. Antagonists of either glutamate or glycine at their respective recognition sites can block this channel. Regulation of NMDA receptors may play an important role in the development of anticonvulsant drugs. In addition, long-term changes in NMDA channel expression may accompany epileptogenesis. Properties of NMDA receptor channels are altered in neurons from kindled rats (60). Furthermore, NMDA receptor antagonists are anticonvulsants in several models of epilepsy (61). Glutamate (62) and glycine site competitive antagonists (63, 64) also have anticonvulsant activity. Noncompetitive channel blockers that work when the channel is open can also inhibit NMDA channels. These drugs include dizocilpine (MK-801) and phencyclidine. Although both of these compounds are good anticonvulsants, both have major side effects when used in anticonvulsant doses (65). Nevertheless, the possible role of glutamate/NMDA-channel regulation is an important area for the development of anticonvulsant compounds and those that may prevent epileptogenesis. Although there is a plethora of evidence from preclinical in vivo and in vitro models of epilepsy regarding the AED potential for glutamate receptor blockers, use of selective NMDA agents as AEDs has been rather disappointing in the clinical setting. However, there is evidence that some of the clinically used AEDs, such as felbamate, can block NMDA receptor at therapeutic concentrations (66).

AMPA receptors are major excitatory amino acid receptors that play an important role in the fast depolarizing actions of glutamate, contributing to the fast excitatory transmission in the CNS. They are thought to be essential for seizure spread and are thus attractive targets for development of novel AEDs. During epilepsy the AMPA receptors are responsible for the early component of the discharges involved in spike discharges and paroxysmal depolarizing shifts. The later elements of these phenomena are primarily related to NMDA receptor activation. Quinoxalinediones (67) were one of the first AMPA receptor antagonists that were found to have anticonvulsant property in several models of epilepsy (62, 68). Several classes of AMPA channel inhibitors have also been developed that have anticonvulsant activity. Both indirect AMPA antagonists and noncompetitive allosteric inhibitors of AMPA receptors have anticonvulsant property in several animal models (68). The AMPA receptor has several molecular subtypes that are differentially expressed in different neurons (69). Receptors containing the GluR2 subunit have a much lower permeability to calcium and show a component of their activation that has a linear rectifying current–voltage relationship. Receptors lacking the GluR2 subunit are different and show significant calcium permeability and an inwardly rectifying property (70). Evidence indicates that differential expression of the GluR2 subunit may play an important role in epileptogenesis and altered neuronal excitability. Thus, the ability to selectively modify AMPA receptors containing GluR2 subunits may play an important role in the development of anticonvulsant compounds. Selective AMPA receptor antagonists are under intense investigation as potential AEDs, but no currently marketed AEDs act through this mechanism (11).

Kainate channels also play an important role in fast depolarizing actions of glutamate in the CNS. However, only a few drugs have been identified as primary kainate antagonists, although some of the AMPA antagonists also inhibit kainic acid channels (71). At the present time it is not clear whether selective inhibition of kainate channels has any advantage in terms of anticonvulsant development over the development of AMPA channel inhibitors. Sodium ion–permeable kainate receptors not only contribute to the postsynaptic excitation, but the presynaptically located kainate receptors can modulate release of glutamate from excitatory terminals and, interestingly, can also prevent release of GABA from inhibitory interneurons (72). Kainate receptor antagonists have been demonstrated to block seizures in the in vivo and in vitro epilepsy models (73). In fact, among topiramate's multiple actions that contribute toward its being a potent AED, kainate receptor blockade is a participating mechanism of action (74, 75). The possible role of kainate glutamate receptors in modulating seizure discharge and anticonvulsant drug development is an important frontier for further research.

METABOTROPIC RECEPTORS

Metabotropic receptors are glutamate- or excitatory amino acid–activated receptors that are not coupled to ion channels. These excitatory amino acid receptors are coupled to second messenger systems in the membrane that have an important role in regulating cellular metabolism and function (76). Metabotropic receptors are coupled to G proteins and enzymes that regulate adenylate cyclase or guanylate cyclase. Regulating these enzymes by metabotropic receptor activation changes levels of cyclic adenosine monophosphate (cAMP) or cyclic guanasine monophosphate (cGMP). Metabotropic glutamate receptors are classified into eight different types (mGluR1–mGluR8). These mGluRs are further classified according to the second messenger systems to which they are linked. Class I mGluRs consist of mGluR1 and mGluR5, are most potently activated by quisqualate, and are coupled to phospholipase C (PLC) activation. Class II mGluRs, consisting of mGluR2 and mGlur3, are activated by 2R,4R-4-aminopyrrolidine-2-4-dicarboxylate (APDC), and inhibit adenylate cyclase activity. Class III mGluRs (mGluR4 and mGluR6–mGluR8) are most potently activated by l-amino-4-phosphonobutyrate and inhibit adenylate cyclase activity, but to a lesser extent. Metabotropic glutamate receptors are found both on the presynaptic and postsynaptic membranes. Presynaptic mGluRs decrease neurotransmitter release, while mGluRs on the postsynaptic membrane regulate the function of ligand-gated ion channels, including all three subtypes of ionotropic glutamate receptors, as well as inhibit the function of voltage-gated Ca^{2+} channels (VGCCs) and some potassium channels. Thus, metabotropic glutamate receptors can act to modulate synaptic transmission in the CNS (77). Modulating the activation or inhibition of metabotropic receptor activation by excitatory transmission plays an important role in modifying neuronal function over both short- and long-term periods relative to seizure activity. Metabotropic receptors play an important role in producing sustained changes in neuronal excitability that may have implications in epileptogenesis and the development of seizure discharges. In patients with temporal lobe epilepsy (78) or focal cortical dysplasia patients (79), up-regulation of mGluR5 immunoreactivity has been described. In the pilocarpine-induced epilepsy model, mouse strains with differential susceptibility exhibit different expression of mGluR4 receptors, with up-regulation in the dentate gyrus of mice with attenuated seizure phenotype and down-regulation in mice with enhanced seizure susceptibility (80). Evidence has accumulated for a possible role of glutamate metabotropic receptors in the development of epileptogenesis (81). Inhibition of metabotropic receptor activation during epileptogenesis in several models has blocked the development of long-term epilepsy. Competitive antagonists of group I mGluRs have shown efficacy against seizures induced experimentally in several epilepsy models. Metabotropic receptor inhibitors, therefore, are possible future areas for the development of novel AEDs (80, 82, 83).

CARBONIC ANHYDRASE INHIBITION

Carbonic anhydrase (CA) is a major enzyme system that has been found to regulate GABA-mediated inhibitory potentials and therefore has important anticonvulsant or antiepileptic effects (84). GABA receptor ion channels are permeable to both chloride and bicarbonate ions. Bicarbonate ions normally move outward through the GABA receptor, producing a depolarizing effect that is normally smaller than the hyperpolarizing action of the inward movement of chloride ions. The movement of bicarbonate ions out of the neuron following entry of chloride ions can produce a potential depolarizing effect that can be mediated by the GABA-receptor channel. Inhibitors of CA play a role in blocking this effect. Thus, blocking the depolarization effects mediated by the GABA receptor through bicarbonate ion movement may be an important role of CA inhibitors in increasing the hyperpolarizing effect of the GABA receptor in the neuron. There may be other actions of CA inhibitors that go through other mechanisms, but this is another area of research for the development of anticonvulsant drugs. CA inhibitors such as sulthiame and acetazolamide (AZM) have previously been shown to lower neuronal intracellular pH (pHi), which effectively reduced epileptiform activity in epilepsy model systems in vitro (85). Topiramate (86) is shown to produce carbonic anhydrase inhibition that reduces the steady-state pHi of cornu ammonis field 3 (CA3) neurons in slices, thereby inhibiting epileptiform activity.

NEUROMODULATORS

There are many classes of neuromodulators, but two major classes have been widely studied that have significant implications in regulating seizure activity: adenosine and the monoamines. Both adenosine and monoamines influence seizures and epileptogenesis in several models of epilepsy. Adenosine is released during seizure activity and acts as an endogenous anticonvulsant (87, 88). One form of the adenosine receptor (A1 receptor) is coupled to the G protein system in a similar mechanism, as is the metabotropic receptor. Activation of the A1 adenosine receptor stabilizes the resting membrane potential presynaptically and blocks glutamate release but not GABA release (89). Several analogs of adenosine acting at the A1 receptor exhibit good anticonvulsant effects in several models of epilepsy (90, 91). These compounds, however, have significant adverse cardiovascular effects, and their potential role as anticonvulsants needs further investigation. Another major type of adenosine receptor is the A3 receptor. Selected antagonists of the A3 receptor have also been recently shown to have anticonvulsant activity (92).

Regulation of adenosine receptors, both chronically and during seizure activity, may play important roles in developing new anticonvulsant drugs. The major challenge in this area, however, is to develop compounds that do not have complicating side effects, such as cardiovascular alterations or effects on other aspects of the nervous system.

Monoamines are important classes of neurotransmitters that play important roles in modulating both excitatory and inhibitory neurotransmission. Abnormalities in monoaminergic transmission in several animal models and in human epileptic foci taken from patients following epilepsy surgery have indicated that there may a role for monoamine receptor activation in chronic epilepsy. Pharmacologic manipulation of monoaminergic neurotransmission plays a role in the development of several seizure syndromes, such as the reflex epilepsies (93). Noradrenaline agonists, such as alpha$_2$ agonists, are protective against seizure activity, and antagonists act as convulsant compounds. These effects have been well studied in amygdala kindling in rats and kittens (94, 95). Dopamine antagonists have also been shown to be protective in photosensitive epilepsy in animals and humans (96, 97). Monoamine oxidase B inhibitors play a role as anticonvulsants in several seizure models.

There is a growing body of evidence implicating the serotonergic system in the etiology of seizures. For example, depletion of brain 5-hydroxytryptamine (5-HT, serotonin) levels by *p*-chlorophenylalanine (98) and the serotonergic neurotoxin 5,7-dihydroxytrpytamine (99) appears to exacerbate seizures, indicating that experimental manipulations that attenuate serotonergic neurotransmission can induce and/or augment epileptic seizures. In contrast, experimental manipulations that enhance serotonergic function, such as treatment with 5-HTP (100), fluoxetine (101), or stimulation of dorsal raphe nuclei (102–104) has been shown to inhibit seizures. Already there is conflicting evidence regarding the role of selective serotonin reuptake inhibitors (SSRIs) in seizures (105), with fluoxetine reported to elevate hippocampal seizure threshold in rats (106). In light of these findings, the role of 5-HT receptor subtypes is being actively investigated in epilepsy.

Some clinicians consider vagus nerve stimulation (VNS) as an alternative in drug-resistant epilepsy. It is only in the recent past that we have begun to understand the mechanisms underlying VNS-mediated seizure suppression. One of the best indications regarding VNS's mechanisms of action has come from Krahl et al (107). They chemically lesioned the locus coeruleus (LC) to chronically deplete rats of norepinephrine or acutely inactivated LC with lidocaine. Under both circumstances, VNS-induced seizure suppression was attenuated when tested in the maximal electroshock (MES) model. These studies indicate that the LC was necessary for the VNS-mediated anticonvulsant effects. Their studies also suggest that noradrenergic agonists could enhance VNS-induced seizure suppression. Thus, the possible role of monoamines in relation to monoamine receptors in epilepsy is another potential area for development of future anticonvulsants.

CALCIUM REGULATION OF NEURONAL FUNCTION

Calcium plays a major role in modulating normal activity and function of the nervous system (108, 109). One of its most widely recognized roles is modulating synaptic neurotransmission. A host of studies have demonstrated the importance of calcium in stimulus-secretion coupling (110). In addition to its important effects on neurotransmission, calcium plays a major role as a second messenger in neuronal and non-neuronal tissues.

Several lines of evidence indicate calcium's importance in regulating neuronal excitability and producing anticonvulsant effects. Because of calcium's importance as a second messenger, it is reasonable to assume that alterations in the normal function of calcium-regulated processes may underlie some of the abnormalities of neuronal excitability seen in seizure disorders.

Accumulating evidence suggests that abnormalities in major calcium-regulated enzymatic processes or ion channels underlie alterations in neuronal excitability and result in seizure activity (111). The role of calcium in antiepileptic drug action and in regulating seizure excitability has been recently reviewed (111, 112). Certain anticonvulsants have been shown to regulate the entry of calcium into cells through both voltage-regulated and transmitter-regulated calcium channels. In addition, anticonvulsants inhibit important calcium-mediated enzyme systems that play important roles in cell function and neuronal excitability. These mechanisms may also be significant for some anticonvulsant effects.

Calcium Channels and Neuronal Excitability

The entry of calcium into a cell triggers many biochemical and biophysical actions (113, 114). This major second-messenger effect of calcium has been clearly linked to the regulation of neuronal excitability and cell metabolism (109, 114, 115). Thus, controlling calcium entry into the cell is the first major step in regulating the effect of calcium as a second messenger.

Depolarization-dependent action potentials are typically mediated by large sodium currents into the cell. Calcium simultaneously enters the cell during depolarization. Recently, the importance of this calcium entry during action potential generation has been more clearly understood. Accumulation of increased concentrations of calcium within a neuron is related to SRF of neurons, which can occur in vitro or during epileptic activity. Calcium entry is also regulated by specific excitatory amino acid receptors. This type of calcium channel is opened or closed in response to binding of excitatory amino acids (EAA) to specific calcium channel–linked receptors. The ability of these channels to produce tonic, long-lasting excitability changes in hippocampal neurons and in other cortical neurons has implications for long-term potentiation, memory, and excitability.

In conceptualizing the role of calcium in neuronal excitability and anticonvulsant drug action, one must consider both voltage-regulated and excitatory amino acid–modulated calcium channels. The regulation of calcium channels, like the regulation of the chloride channel, by the benzodiazepines, barbiturates, and convulsant drugs may play an important role in modifying neuronal excitability.

Voltage-Gated Calcium Channels

Voltage-regulated or gated calcium channels affect neuronal excitability. As an action potential arrives at a nerve terminal, depolarization of the nerve terminal membrane causes entry of calcium through voltage-gated calcium channels with subsequent release of neurotransmitters. This is the classic paradigm for calcium-mediated neurotransmitter release and was the initial observation that demonstrated the importance of calcium in neuronal excitability, but little was understood about the specific mechanisms of calcium channels in brain.

Early insight into the neuropharmacology of calcium channels came from studies of smooth muscle and cardiac cells during the 1970s. The dihydropyridine type of calcium channel blocker and related molecules were shown to be effective in blocking calcium channels in peripheral tissue (112, 116, 117). These compounds were classified as "organic calcium channel blockers" and represented a major advance in pharmacology. Numerous analogues were developed, and specific binding sites for the dihydropyridines and other analogs were identified and characterized. This led to the first molecular characterization of calcium channels and their regulation by specific receptor sites. A major controversy developed based on the observation that the organic calcium blockers, effective in inhibiting calcium entry into non-neuronal tissue, seemed to be ineffective in blocking voltage-gated calcium entry into neurons (118). Numerous investigators demonstrated that calcium entry as a result of neuronal activity was not significantly inhibited by therapeutic or relevant concentrations of the organic calcium channel blockers (112). Because there was at that time no clear evidence for more than one type of calcium channel, this dichotomy was not well understood and was attributed to unusual properties of the neuronal membrane and to specific differences in drug penetration into the nervous system. More recent studies using benzodiazepines and phenothiazines (119–122) demonstrated that these compounds in fact could significantly block voltage-gated calcium channels in neurons. These results indicated that calcium channels in brain were distinct from calcium channels in peripheral tissue.

With the development of patch and voltage clamp technology, more sophisticated characterization of calcium channels has been possible. It is now clear that there are at least three, and possibly more, types of calcium channels in neurons (118, 123, 124). One type of voltage-gated calcium channel is insensitive to dihydropyridines, while a second type of calcium channel is sensitive to these compounds. A third type of brain membrane calcium channel has also been postulated that is different from the first two types of channels. Although a set terminology has not been developed for these different channels, initial classification by Tsien (124) is currently in use and describes these channels as the T-, N-, and L-type channels, respectively.

The heterogeneity of calcium channels provides a major insight into different mechanisms of regulating calcium excitability in the nervous system. These observations also explain the fact that the major voltage-gated calcium channels in brain that were insensitive to dihydropyridines were a different class of channel from those found in peripheral tissues. In certain regions of the nervous system and at certain sites on the cell body, however, there are calcium channels that are sensitive to dihydropyridines and are similar to those calcium channels in non-neuronal tissue. The different types of calcium channels are distributed in characteristic patterns over the surface of a neuron. Some channels may be localized at the synapse, while others may be present at a higher density at the cell body. The heterogeneity and individual functions of specific types of calcium channels are important areas for further investigation, such as the development of specific drugs to regulate each type of channel.

Several anticonvulsant compounds block or alter calcium entry through voltage-gated calcium channels. Ferrendelli and coworkers (125, 126) described the ability of phenytoin, phenobarbital, carbamazepine, but not ethosuximide, to block voltage-dependent calcium entry into isolated nerve terminal preparations. Subsequent studies have demonstrated that benzodiazepines, as well as phenytoin and barbiturates, can regulate calcium entry into isolated neurons. However, the concentrations of antiepileptic drugs that are required to block calcium entry are in the low micromolar range, concentrations that are approximately one order of magnitude higher than the therapeutic levels of these drugs achieved in spinal fluid. Although these concentrations may be relevant to anticonvulsant actions, they are more likely related to toxic side effects.

Thalamic relay neurons fire in two different modes: burst and tonic. T-type Ca^{2+} channels underlie the burst firings. When activated, T-type channels produce low-threshold Ca^{2+} currents that lead to the generation of a burst of action potentials (127). Burst firing of thalamic neurons have been implicated to play an important role in the pathogenesis of absence epilepsy (128). Ethosuximide, a known antiepileptic drug, is known to block T-type Ca^{2+} channels in thalamic relay neurons (129). Analysis of knockout mouse for the alpha1G gene coding for a subtype of T-type Ca^{2+} channels demonstrated absence of low-threshold, T-type, Ca^{2+} currents and an inability to induce burst firing in the thalamic relay neurons (130, 131). Alpha1G knockout mice were resistant to $GABA_B$ receptor agonists; baclofen and gamma-hydrobutyrate (GHB) induced seizures (132). T-type Ca^{2+} channels represent a novel pharmacologic target for development of drugs for the treatment of epilepsy.

Excitatory Amino Acid Receptors and Calcium Channels

L-glutamate was proposed as an excitatory neurotransmitter over 30 years ago (133). Recently, excitatory amino acids (EAA) have been found to play important roles in epilepsy, neuronal excitability, and learning (133–135). The two main excitatory neurotransmitters currently known are glutamate and aspartate (136). Many pathways in the brain use these neurotransmitters, including hippocampal afferents and major cortical output tracts that are widely activated during convulsions.

Excitatory amino acids bind to specific membrane receptors (58, 137). Currently, four major types of EAA receptors have been characterized. One major EAA receptor is characterized by binding of the EAA analog NMDA. The NMDA receptor has now been well studied and represents a specific type of excitatory amino acid receptor. Three types of non-NMDA receptors that bind other analogs of excitatory amino acids but have different properties from the NMDA receptor have also been identified. The non-NMDA receptors bind EAAs but not NMDA. The non-NMDA receptors include binding sites for kainic acid, quisqualate, and 2-amino-4-phosphonobutyrate (2-APB).

Excitatory transmission regulated by EAA receptors plays a major role in synaptic transmission in the CNS. Excitatory amino acids regulate specific ion channels that allow calcium and sodium to enter the cell when the channel is activated by the EAA receptor (58, 137). These specific channels are actually opened or gated by the EAA. The currents activated by EAA receptors are both rapid and long lasting. The postsynaptic localization of these receptors, as well as their presence over the cell body, have been implicated in explaining how EAAs alter neuronal excitability, causing rapid depolarization in some situations and long-lasting neuronal changes in other cells. Thus, this type of calcium entry is activated by specific EAAs and has been implicated in many neuromodulating effects in the brain. Important convulsants, such as kainic acid, alter neuronal excitability by binding to these receptor sites and activating calcium and sodium channels. Compounds that bind to EAA receptors but do not activate the channel can inhibit EAA effects on these receptors. Several of these compounds have potent anticonvulsant actions and are very effective in maximal electric shock–induced seizure models (58).

Because of their potential importance to epileptogenesis, EAA receptors and the calcium channels that they regulate have been the focus of extensive research (134, 138). These receptor sites are responsible for mediating some of the effects of kainic acid in producing convulsant discharge in the brain. NMDA receptors have been implicated in the phenomenon of long-term potentiation and in long-term alterations of neuronal excitability. The EAA analog 2-amino-7-phosphonoheptanoate (APH, AP7), is a potent anticonvulsant in various seizure models. These and other investigations provide strong evidence that EAA receptors and their regulation of calcium channels are important mechanisms in regulating neuronal excitability and, potentially, in AED actions. It is anticipated that several new anticonvulsant compounds will be developed that act specifically through this mechanism.

Modulating the Calcium Signal in Controlling Neuronal Excitability

The discovery of a calcium-binding protein, calmodulin (CaM), was the first major breakthrough in understanding the molecular mechanisms that mediate calcium second messenger effects (139, 140). Evidence now suggests that many of the effects of calcium on cell function are mediated by calmodulin (120, 121, 141–143). Several important calcium-regulated processes are mediated by calmodulin and by a major calmodulin target enzyme system, calmodulin kinase II (144–146). Evidence from several laboratories has now confirmed the original calmodulin hypothesis of neurotransmission and substantiated the role of calmodulin in mediating some of the effects of calcium on neuronal excitability. Antiepileptic drugs, including phenytoin, carbamazepine, and the benzodiazepines, antagonize calcium-mediated effects and inhibit calmodulin activation of calmodulin kinase II (113, 147). Concentrations required to inhibit CaM kinase II are in the low micromolar concentration ranges for antiepileptic drug effects on the protein kinase. This enzyme plays an important role in mediating calcium-dependent protein phosphorylation of membrane and soluble proteins.

CaM kinase II has been implicated by several investigators to be a major molecular mechanism mediating some of the second-messenger effects of calcium in the cell. Thus, control of this important calcium-mediated event by phenytoin, carbamazepine, and diazepam may be a major action of these drugs. The precise relationship of this particular effect to clinically useful anticonvulsant activity remains to be elucidated.

The importance of calmodulin kinase II in regulating neuronal excitability is widely recognized. Injection of CaM kinase II into invertebrate neurons regulates potassium and calcium currents (148). In addition, CaM kinase II levels in hippocampal neurons are chronically altered during the long-term alteration of neuronal excitability that occurs in kindling (149). CaM kinase II activity is inhibited by specific anticonvulsants (111, 121), and the subunits of CaM kinase II are a major protein component of the postsynaptic density, localizing this important enzyme system directly at the synapse (150, 151). Further understanding the role of CaM kinase II in the pathophysiology of epilepsy and in controlling neuronal excitability is clearly important.

Another major molecular mechanism regulating the effects of calcium on neuronal excitability and cell function is the major enzyme system protein kinase C. Protein kinase C has been implicated in many of the effects of calcium on cell function and has been implicated in some of the effects of calcium in regulating specific ion conductances (108). Although no direct studies have been performed to investigate the effects of anticonvulsant drugs on the C-kinase system, this too is an important area for investigation. Modulation of these calcium target enzyme systems by anticonvulsant drugs is a potential area for new drug development.

Calcium is a ubiquitous signaling molecule with significant regulatory function in neurons (152, 153). As a result even slightest changes in [Ca^{2+}]i could sustain alterations in Ca^{2+}-dependent enzyme systems that could contribute to the generation of epileptiform activity. It has been demonstrated that levels of protein kinase C (alpha) isozyme are decreased after kindling epileptogenesis (154), and the activity of the Ca^{2+}/calmodulin-dependent phosphatase calcineurin is increased after pilocarpine-induced status epilepticus (SE) (155, 156). Further, the activity of CaM kinase II is depressed in human epileptic tissue (157) and in various in vivo models of epilepsy (158–162). Epileptic neurons in culture also manifest some of the biochemical, electrophysiologic, and molecular changes observed in animal models. Thus, decreased CaM kinase II activity and its alpha subunit expression are observed in the low-Mg^{2+} hippocampal neuronal culture model of epilepsy (163). As in epileptogenesis, these changes are dependent on activation of the NMDA receptor (162, 163). Further, mice lacking active CaMKII manifest epileptiform activity after subconvulsive stimulation (164), implicating decreased CaMKII activity in epileptogenesis. In addition, hippocampal neuronal cultures, treated with antisense oligonucleotides to the CaMKII alpha subunit, express decreased levels of CaMKII and exhibit epileptiform discharges similar to the low-Mg^{2+} and glutamate injury-induced epileptogenesis models (165, 166).

Anticonvulsants that Inhibit Vesicular Neurotransmitter Release

SV2A, a synaptic vesicle protein, has recently been identified as a likely target for antiepileptic action. SV2A is a protein component of synaptic vesicles that is structurally similar to 12-transmembrane-domain transporters. SV2A is not essential for synaptic transmission, but mice in which the protein has been deleted by gene targeting exhibit seizures (167). This finding led to a search for compounds acting on SV2A as probable anticonvulsant agents. Levetiracetam (Keppra®) is thought to bind with SV2A and disrupt synaptic release mechanisms to produce an anticonvulsant effect (168). It is also speculated that levetiracetam binding enhances a function of SV2A that inhibits abnormal bursting in epileptic circuits, a function whose loss in the SV2A knockout models results in seizures (168). It is also suggested that a reduction of potassium currents may contribute to the antiepileptic effect(s) of levetiracetam (169). Newer analogs of levetiracetam, such as seleteracetam and brivaracetam, are currently investigated for probable anticonvulsant actions (170). Levetiracetam at clinically relevant concentrations is also reported to inhibit Na^+-dependent Cl^-/HCO_3^- exchange, lower neuronal pH_i, and thereby contribute to its anticonvulsive activity (85).

Anticonvulsants that Target the Endocannabinoid System

Recently the endocannabinoid system—an inhibitory neurotransmitter system—has generated considerable interest as a novel locus of anticonvulsant activity in brain (171–174). This unique system consists of at least two cannabinoid receptors (CB1 and CB2), the endogenous agonists (endocannabinoids: anandamide and 2-Arachidonyl Glycerol (2-AG)), and the protein machinery for their synthesis, transport, and degradation (175). Cannabinoids such as those naturally occurring in marijuana (*Cannabis sativa*) possess anticonvulsant properties (176, 177) and have been used since antiquity for the treatment of seizures (178). Recently synthetic cannabinoids such as WIN 55,212-2 have been demonstrated to produce an anticonvulsant effect in a CB1 receptor–dependent manner (179, 180). Emerging evidences have indicated that the endocannabinoid system controls seizure threshold, duration, and seizure frequency (171, 181).

Endocannabinoids regulate neuronal excitability via depolarization-induced suppression of excitation (DSE) (182) or inhibition (DSI) (183, 184). In response to Ca^{2+}-mediated depolarization of the postsynaptic membrane, endocannabinoids are synthesized "on demand" and then diffuse in a retrograde fashion and activate presynaptic CB1 receptors to inhibit neurotransmitter release and thus modulate neuronal excitability (185). Intense synaptic activity caused by seizure discharges stimulates 2-AG synthesis (171). Such an "on-demand" synthesis of endocannabinoids is thought to produce anticonvulsant effects, ultimately terminate seizures, and regulate seizure duration and frequency in the pilocarpine model of epilepsy. There is also evidence that the endocannabinoids, such as anandamide and 2-AG, dampen epileptiform activity in hippocampal brain slice preparations (186). Cannabinoids and endocannabinoids have also been demonstrated to block seizure spread via a CB1 receptor-dependent mechanism in the MES model of short-term seizure and the rat pilocarpine model of temporal lobe epilepsy (171, 179, 181). This plethora of evidence indicates that an active endogenous cannabinoid tone maintains chronic activation of presynaptic CB1 receptors that play an important role in dampening persistent excitation in epilepsy and may prevent the transition of a single seizure into SE. In the pilocarpine model of acquired epilepsy, inhibiting endogenous cannabinoid tone using a CB1 receptor antagonist caused a marked increase in seizure frequency and duration and produced SE-like activity (171), suggesting that the endocannabinoid system was playing an important role in preventing the development of SE. Thus, the endocannabinoid system appears to be the brain's endogenous mechanism that guards against persistent epileptic neuroexcitation and prevents the transformation of single seizure to SE.

New Frontiers in Epilepsy Treatment: Inhibition of Epileptogenesis

More than half of the epilepsies are described as symptomatic or acquired. These types of epilepsy are acquired through environmental stress or injuries to the nervous system that result in the permanent alteration of neuronal function, resulting in epilepsy (187). Conditions such as stroke, head trauma, metabolic disease, prolonged seizures, tumors, or other neurologic insults can permanently alter the brain and trigger mechanisms of neuronal plasticity that eventually result in the development of epilepsy (188). Because of the diversity of causes of epilepsy, epilepsy is not considered a disease but rather a condition. In addition to the acquired causes as described previously, other idiopathic forms of epilepsy may have a genetic basis (187).

The process of epileptogenesis means the development of spontaneous recurrent seizures in a previously normal brain (188). Symptomatic epilepsy, representing a significant number of patients that develop epilepsy, occurs through the process of epileptogenesis. This is an important area to consider for anticonvulsant drug development. Compounds that prevent the development of epileptogenesis may have important clinical ramifications. If specific antiepileptogenic drugs can be administered following a brain injury, symptomatic epilepsy may be prevented. Although these compounds may not be true anticonvulsant drugs, they would be the ultimate AEDs by preventing the development of epilepsy. This is a new and important area for future research.

Molecular genetics has set the stage for major advances in studying neurologic diseases, and initial advances have been made in understanding specific mutations that are associated with epilepsy and other neurologic conditions (189). In addition to specific mutations, permanent alterations in brain function and diminished expression are associated with epileptogenesis. In symptomatic epilepsy, normal brain tissue is permanently altered and develops spontaneous recurrent seizures. These changes entail long-lasting changes in gene expression at both transcriptional and posttranscriptional levels in association with the induction of epileptogenesis.

Understanding the effects of severe environmental stresses on the multiple sites of transcriptional and posttranscriptional regulation of gene expression is likely to provide important insights into how altered neuronal function develops and point to novel strategies that will prevent epileptogenesis. This important area for future research represents a frontier in the development of AEDs.

References

1. Meldrum BS. Current strategies for designing and identifying new anticonvulsant drugs. In: Engel J, Pedley TA, eds. *Epilepsy: A Comprehensive Textbook*. New York: Raven Press, 1997:1405–1416.
2. Levy, R. H., R. H. Mattson, et al. (1995). Antiepileptic Drugs. New York: Raven Press.
3. Delorenzo, R. J. and L. Dashefsky (1985). Anticonvulsants. *Handbook of Neurochemistry*. A. Lajtha. New York, Plenum Publishing Corp. 9:363–403.
4. Delgado-Escueta, A. V., A. A. Ward, et al. (1986). New wave of research in the epilepsies. New York, Raven Press.
5. Nistico, G., P. Morselli, et al. (1986). Neurotransmitters, Seizures, and Epilepsy III. New York: Raven Press.
6. Macdonald RL, McLean MJ. Cellular bases of barbiturate and phenytoin anticonvulsant drug action. *Epilepsia* 1982; 23 Suppl 1:S7–S18.
7. Macdonald RL, McLean MJ. Anticonvulsant drugs: mechanism of action. *Adv Neurol* 1986; 44:713–736.
8. McLean MJ, Macdonald RL. Multiple actions of phenytoin on mouse spinal cord neurons in cell culture. *J Pharmacol Exp Ther* 1983; 227(3):779–789.
9. McLean MJ, Macdonald RL. Carbamazepine and 10,11-epoxycarbamazepine produce use- and voltage-dependent limitation of rapidly firing action potentials of mouse central neurons in cell culture. *J Pharmacol Exp Ther* 1986; 238(2):727–738.
10. McLean MJ, Macdonald RL. Sodium valproate, but not ethosuximide, produces use- and voltage-dependent limitation of high frequency repetitive firing of action potentials of mouse central neurons in cell culture. *J Pharmacol Exp Ther* 1986; 237(3): 1001–1011.
11. Rogawski MA, Loscher W. The neurobiology of antiepileptic drugs. *Nat Rev Neurosci* 2004; 5(7):553–564.
12. McLean MJ, Macdonald RL. Limitation of high frequency repetitive firing of cultured mouse neurons by anticonvulsants drugs. *Neurology* 1984; 34:288.
13. Kuo CC, and Bean BP. Na^+ channels must deactivate to recover from inactivation. *Neuron* 1994; 12(4):819–829.
14. Salvati P, Maj R, Caccia C, Cervini MA, et al. Biochemical and electrophysiological studies on the mechanism of action of PNU-151774E, a novel antiepileptic compound. *J Pharmacol Exp Ther* 1999; 288(3):1151–9.
15. Killiam EK, Suria A. Benzodiazepine. in Glaser G, Penry JK, and Woodbury DM, eds. *Antiepileptic Drugs: Mechanisms of Action*. New York: Raven Press, p. 1980:597–616.
16. Braestrup C, Squires RF. Pharmacological characterization of benzodiazepine receptors in the brain. Eur J Pharmacol. 1978; 48(3):263–270.
17. Mohler H, Okada T. Properties of ^3H-diazepam binding to benzodiazepine receptors in rat cerebral cortex. *Life Sci* (1977; 20(12):p. 2101–10.
18. Battersby MK, Richards JG, Mohler H. Benzodiazepine receptor: photoaffinity labeling and localization. *Eur J Pharmacol* 1979; 57(2–3):277–278.
19. Mestre M, Carriot T, Belin C, Uzan A, et al. Electrophysiological and pharmacological evidence that peripheral-type benzodiazepine receptors are coupled to calcium channels in the heart. *Life Sci* 1985; 36(4):391–400.
20. Bowling AC, DeLorenzo RJ. Micromolar affinity benzodiazepine receptors: identification and characterization in central nervous system. *Science* 1982; 216(4551):1247–1250.
21. Bowling AC, DeLorenzo RJ. Photoaffinity labeling of a novel benzodiazepine binding protein in rat brain. *Eur J Pharmacol* (1987; 135(1):97–100.
22. Yang J, Johansen J, Kleinhaus AL, DeLorenzo RJ, et al. Effects of medazepam on voltage-gated ion currents of cultured chick sensory neurons. *Eur J Pharmacol* 1987; 143(3):373–381.
23. Tallman JF, Paul SM, Skolnick P, Gallager DW. Receptors for the age of anxiety: pharmacology of the benzodiazepines. *Science* 1980; 207(4428):274–281.
24. Olsen RW, Wong EH, Stauber GB, King RG. Biochemical pharmacology of the gamma-aminobutyric acid receptor/ionophore protein. *Fed Proc* 1984; 43(13):2773–2778.
25. Olsen RW, Wamsley JK, Lee RJ, Lomax P. Benzodiazepine/barbiturate/GABA receptor-chloride ionophore complex in a genetic model for generalized epilepsy. *Adv Neurol* 1986; 44:365–378.
26. Ticku MK, Maksay G. Convulsant/anticonvulsant drugs and GABAergic transmission. In: Nistico G, Morselli P, Lloyd K, Fariello R, et al, eds. *Neurotransmitters, Seizures, and Epilepsy III*. New York: Raven Press, 1986:163–177.
27. Martin IL, Brown CL, Doble A. Multiple benzodiazepine receptors: structures in the brain or structures in the mind? A critical review. *Life Sci* 1983; 32(17):1925–1933.
28. Mohler H, Battersby MK, Richards JG. Benzodiazepine receptor protein identified and visualized in brain tissue by a photoaffinity label. *Proc Natl Acad Sci U S A* 1980; 77(3): 1666–1670.
29. Johansen J, Taft WC, Yang J, Kleinhaus AL, et al. Inhibition of Ca^{2+} conductance in identified leech neurons by benzodiazepines. *Proc Natl Acad Sci U S A* 1985; 82(11): 3935–3939.
30. Chiron C. Stiripentol. *Expert Opin Investig Drugs* 2005; 14(7):905–911.
31. Quilichini PP, Chiron C, Ben-Ari Y, Gozlan H. Stiripentol, a putative antiepileptic drug, enhances the duration of opening of GABA-A receptor channels. *Epilepsia* 2006; 47(4):704–716.
32. Mody I. Aspects of the homeosta[t]ic plasticity of $GABA_A$ receptor-mediated inhibition. *J Physiol* 2005; 562(1):37–46.
33. Stell BM, Mody I. Receptors with different affinities mediate phasic and tonic $GABA_A$ conductances in hippocampal neurons. *J Neurosci* 2002; 22(10):RC223.
34. Nusser Z, Mody I. Selective modulation of tonic and phasic inhibitions in dentate gyrus granule cells. *J Neurophysiol* 2002; 87(5):2624–2628.
35. BencsitsE, Ebert V, Tretter V, Sieghart W. A significant part of native gamma-aminobutyric $acid_A$ receptors containing alpha 4 subunits do not contain gamma or delta subunits. *J Biol Chem* 274(28):19613–19616.
36. Otis TS, Mody I. Modulation of decay kinetics and frequency of $GABA_A$ receptor-mediated spontaneous inhibitory postsynaptic currents in hippocampal neurons. *Neuroscience* 1992; 49(1):13–32.
37. Hajos N, Nusser Z, Rancz EA, Freund TF, et al. Cell type- and synapse-specific variability in synaptic $GABA_A$ receptor occupancy. *Eur J Neurosci* 2000; 12(3):810–818.
38. Schuler V, Luscher C, Blanchet C, Klix N, et al. Epilepsy, hyperalgesia, impaired memory, and loss of pre- and postsynaptic $GABA_B$ responses in mice lacking $GABA_B(1)$. *Neuron* 2001; 31(1):47–58.
39. Sah P. Ca(2+)-activated K+ currents in neurones: types, physiological roles and modulation. *Trends Neurosci* 1996; 19(4):150–154.
40. Beck H, Blumcke I, Kral T, Clusmann H, et al. Properties of a delayed rectifier potassium current in dentate granule cells isolated from the hippocampus of patients with chronic temporal lobe epilepsy. *Epilepsia* 1996; 37(9):892–901.
41. Velluti JC, Caputi A, Macadar O. Limbic epilepsy induced in the rat by dendrotoxin, a polypeptide isolated from the green mamba (*Dendroaspis angusticeps*) venom. *Toxicon* 1987; 25(6):649–657.
42. Rutecki PA, Lebeda FJ, Johnston D. 4-Aminopyridine produces epileptiform activity in hippocampus and enhances synaptic excitation and inhibition. *J Neurophysiol* 1987; 57(6):1911–1924.
43. Weston AH, Edwards G. Recent progress in potassium channel opener pharmacology. *Biochem Pharmacol* 1992; 43(1):47–54.
44. Popoli P, Pezzola A, Sagratella S, Zeng YC, et al. Cromakalim (BRL 34915) counteracts the epileptiform activity elicited by diltiazem and verapamil in rats. *Br J Pharmacol* 1991; 104(4):907–913.

45. Zona C, Tancredi V, Palma E, Pirrone GC, et al. Potassium currents in rat cortical neurons in culture are enhanced by the antiepileptic drug carbamazepine. *Can J Physiol Pharmacol* 1990; 68(4):545–547.
46. Surti TS, Jan LY. A potassium channel, the M-channel, as a therapeutic target. *Curr Opin Investig Drugs* 2005; 6(7):704–711.
47. Blackburn-Munro G, Jensen BS. The anticonvulsant retigabine attenuates nociceptive behaviours in rat models of persistent and neuropathic pain. *Eur J Pharmacol* 2003; 460(2–3):109–116.
48. Blackburn-Munro G, Dalby-Brown W, Mirza NR, Mikkelsen JD, et al. Retigabine: chemical synthesis to clinical application. *CNS Drug Rev* 2005; 11(1):1–20.
49. Santoro B, Liu DT, Yao H, Bartsch D, et al. Identification of a gene encoding a hyperpolarization-activated pacemaker channel of brain. *Cell* 1998; 93(5):717–729.
50. Santoro B, Chen S, Luthi A, Pavlidis P, et al. Molecular and functional heterogeneity of hyperpolarization-activated pacemaker channels in the mouse CNS. *J Neurosci* 2000; 20(14):5264–5275.
51. Poolos NP. The yin and yang of the h-channel and its role in epilepsy. *Epilepsy Curr* 2004; 4(1):3–6.
52. Poolos NP, Migliore M, Johnston D. Pharmacological upregulation of h-channels reduces the excitability of pyramidal neuron dendrites. *Nat Neurosci* 2002; 5(8):767–774.
53. Poolos NP. The h-channel: a potential channelopathy in epilepsy? *Epilepsy Behav* 2005; 7(1):51–56.
54. Poolos NP. H-channel dysfunction in generalized epilepsy: it takes two. *Epilepsy Curr* 2006; 6(3):88–90.
55. Chen K, Baram TZ, Soltesz I. Febrile seizures in the developing brain result in persistent modification of neuronal excitability in limbic circuits. *Nat Med* 1999; 5(8): 888–594.
56. Chen K, Aradi I, Thon N, Eghbal-Ahmadi M, et al. Persistently modified h-channels after complex febrile seizures convert the seizure-induced enhancement of inhibition to hyperexcitability. *Nat Med* 2001; 7(3):331–337.
57. Ludwig A, Budde T, Stieber J, Moosmang S, et al. Absence epilepsy and sinus dysrhythmia in mice lacking the pacemaker channel HCN2. *EMBO J* 2003; 22(2):216–224.
58. Watkins JC, Evans RH, Excitatory amino acid transmitters. *Annu Rev Pharmacol Toxicol* 1981; 21:165–204.
59. Hollmann M, Heinemann S. Cloned glutamate receptors. *Annu Rev Neurosci* 1994; 17:31–108.
60. Kohr G, De Koninck Y, Mody I. Properties of NMDA receptor channels in neurons acutely isolated from epileptic (kindled) rats. *J Neurosci* 1993; 13(8):3612–3627.
61. Croucher MJ, Collins JF, Meldrum BS. Anticonvulsant action of excitatory amino acid antagonists. *Science* 1982; 216(4548):899–901.
62. Swedberg MD, Jacobsen P, Honore T. Anticonvulsant, anxiolytic and discriminative effects of the AMPA antagonist 2,3-dihydroxy-6-nitro-7-sulfamoyl-benzo(*f*) quinoxaline (NBQX). *J Pharmacol Exp Ther* 1995; 274(3):1113–1121.
63. Wlaz P, Loscher W. Weak anticonvulsant effects of two novel glycineB receptor antagonists in the amygdala-kindling model in rats. *Eur J Pharmacol* 1998; 342(1):39–46.
64. Wlaz P, Ebert U, Loscher W. Anticonvulsant effects of eliprodil alone or combined with the $glycine_B$ receptor antagonist L-701,324 or the competitive NMDA antagonist CGP 40116 in the amygdala kindling model in rats. *Neuropharmacology* 1999; 38(2):243–251.
65. Chapman AG, Meldrum BS. Non-competitive N-methyl-D-aspartate antagonists protect against sound-induced seizures in DBA/2 mice. *Eur J Pharmacol* 1989; 166(2): 201–211.
66. Rho JM, Donevan SD, Rogawski MA. Mechanism of action of the anticonvulsant felbamate: opposing effects on N-methyl-D-aspartate and gamma-aminobutyric $acid_A$ receptors. *Ann Neurol* 1994; 35(2):229–234.
67. Honore T, Davies SN, Drejer J, Fletcher EJ, et al. Quinoxalinediones: potent competitive non-NMDA glutamate receptor antagonists. *Science* 1988; 241(4866):701–703.
68. Chapman AG, Smith SE, Meldrum BS. The anticonvulsant effect of the non-NMDA antagonists, NBQX and GYKI 52466, in mice. *Epilepsy Res* 1991; 9(2):92–96.
69. Geiger JR, Melcher T, Koh DS, Sakmann B, et al. Relative abundance of subunit mRNAs determines gating and Ca^{2+} permeability of AMPA receptors in principal neurons and interneurons in rat CNS. *Neuron* 1995; 15(1):193–204.
70. Lomeli H, Mosbacher J, Melcher T, Hoger T, et al. Control of kinetic properties of AMPA receptor channels by nuclear RNA editing. *Science* 1994; 266(5191):1709–1713.
71. Bleakman R, Schoepp DD, Ballyk B, Bufton H, et al. Pharmacological discrimination of GluR5 and GluR6 kainate receptor subtypes by (3S,4aR,6R,8aR)-6-[2-(1(2)H-tetrazole-5-yl)ethyl]decahyd roisdoquinoline[*sic*]-3 carboxylic-acid. *Mol Pharmacol* 1996; 49(4):581–585.
72. Lerma J, Paternain AV, Rodriguez-Moreno A, Lopez-Garcia JC. Molecular physiology of kainate receptors. *Physiol Rev*. 2001; 81(3):971–998.
73. Smolders I, Bortolotto ZA, Clarke VRJ, Warre R, et al. Antagonists of GLUK5-containing kainate receptors prevent pilocarpine-induced limbic seizures. *Nat Neurosci* 2002; 5(8):796–804.
74. Gryder DS, Rogawski MA. Selective antagonism of GluR5 kainate-receptor-mediated synaptic currents by topiramate in rat basolateral amygdala neurons. *J. Neurosci* 2003; 23(18):7069–7074.
75. Kaminski RM, Banerjee M, Rogawski MA. Topiramate selectively protects against seizures induced by ATPA, a GluR5 kainate receptor agonist. *Neuropharmacology* 2004; 46(8):1097–1104.
76. Pin JP, Duvoisin R. The metabotropic glutamate receptors: structure and functions. *Neuropharmacology* 1995; 34(1):1–26.
77. Conn PJ, and Pin JP. Pharmacology and functions of metabotropic glutamate receptors. *Annu Rev Pharmacol Toxicol* 1997; 37:205–237.
78. Notenboom RG, Hampson DR, Jansen GH, van Rijen PC, et al. Up-regulation of hippocampal metabotropic glutamate receptor 5 in temporal lobe epilepsy patients. *Brain* 2006; 129(Pt 1):96–107.
79. Aronica E, Gorter JA, Jansen GH, van Veelen CWM, et al. Expression and cell distribution of group I and group II metabotropic glutamate receptor subtypes in Taylor-type focal cortical dysplasia. *Epilepsia* 2003; 44(6):785–795.
80. Ure J, Baudry M, Perassolo M. Metabotropic glutamate receptors and epilepsy. *J Neurol Sci*. 2006; 247(1):1–9.
81. Akiyama K, Daigen A, Yamada N, Itoh T, et al. Long-lasting enhancement of metabotropic excitatory amino acid receptor-mediated polyphosphoinositide hydrolysis in the amygdala/pyriform cortex of deep prepiriform cortical kindled rats. *Brain Res* 1992; 569(1):71–77.
82. Attwell PJ, Singh KN, Jane DE, Croucher MJ, et al. Anticonvulsant and glutamate release–inhibiting properties of the highly potent metabotropic glutamate receptor agonist (2S,2′R, 3′R)-2-(2′,3′-dicarboxycyclopropyl)glycine (DCG-IV). *Brain Res* 1998; 805(1–2):138–143.
83. Doherty J, Dingledine R. The roles of metabotropic glutamate receptors in seizures and epilepsy. *Curr Drug Targets CNS Neurol Disord* 2002; 1(3):251–260.
84. Staley KJ, Soldo BL, Proctor WR. Ionic mechanisms of neuronal excitation by inhibitory $GABA_A$ receptors. *Science* 1995; 269(5226):977–981.
85. Leniger T, Wiemann M, Bingmann D, Widman G, et al. Carbonic anhydrase inhibitor sulthiame reduces intracellular pH and epileptiform activity of hippocampal CA3 neurons. *Epilepsia* 2002; 43(5):469–474.
86. Shank RP, Gardocki JF, Streeter AJ, Maryanoff BE. An overview of the preclinical aspects of topiramate: pharmacology, pharmacokinetics, and mechanism of action. *Epilepsia* 2000; 41 Suppl 1:S3–S9.
87. Dragunow M. Purinergic mechanisms in epilepsy. *Prog Neurobiol* 1988; 31(2):85–108.
88. During MJ, Spencer DD. Adenosine: a potential mediator of seizure arrest and postictal refractoriness. *Ann Neurol* 1992; 32(5):618–624.
89. Yoon KW, Rothman SM. Adenosine inhibits excitatory but not inhibitory synaptic transmission in the hippocampus. *J Neurosci* 1991; 11(5):1375–1380.
90. Von Lubitz DK, Paul IA, Carter M, Jacobson KA. Effects of N6-cyclopentyl adenosine and 8-cyclopentyl-1,3-dipropylxanthine on N-methyl-D-aspartate induced seizures in mice. *Eur J Pharmacol* 1993; 249(3):p. 265–270.
91. Zhang G, Franklin PH, Murray TF. Activation of adenosine A1 receptors underlies anticonvulsant effect of CGS21680. *Eur J Pharmacol* 1994; 255(1–3):239–243.
92. Von Lubitz DK, Carter MF, Deutsch SI, Lin RC, et al. The effects of adenosine A3 receptor stimulation on seizures in mice. *Eur J Pharmacol* 1995; 275(1):23–29.
93. Horton R, Anlezark G, Meldrum B. Noradrenergic influences on sound-induced seizures. *J Pharmacol Exp Ther*. 1980; 214(2):437–442.
94. Pelletier MR, and Corcoran ME. Infusions of alpha-2 noradrenergic agonists and antagonists into the amygdala: effects on kindling. *Brain Res* 1993; 632(1–2):29–35.
95. Shouse MN, Langer J, Bier M, Farber PR, et al. The alpha 2 adrenoreceptor agonist clonidine suppresses seizures, whereas the alpha 2 adrenoreceptor antagonist idazoxan promotes seizures: pontine microinfusion studies of amygdala-kindled kittens. *Brain Res* 1996; 731(1–2):203–207.
96. Anlezark GM, Blackwood DH, Meldrum BS, Ram VJ, et al. Comparative assessment of dopamine agonist aporphines as anticonvulsants in two models of reflex epilepsy. *Psychopharmacology (Berl)* 1983; 81(2):135–139.
97. Mervaala E, Andermann F, Quesney LF, Krelina M. Common dopaminergic mechanism for epileptic photosensitivity in progressive myoclonus epilepsies. *Neurology* 1990; 40(1):53–56.
98. Racine R, Coscina DV. Effects of midbrain raphe lesions or systemic *p*-chlorophenylalanine on the development of kindled seizures in rats. *Brain Res Bull* 1979; 4(1):1–7.
99. Browning RA, Hoffmann WE, Simonton RL. Changes in seizure susceptibility after intracerebral treatment with 5,7-dihydroxytryptamine: role of serotonergic neurons. *Ann N Y Acad Sci* 1978; 305(1):437–456.
100. De la Torre JC, Kawanaga HM, Mullan S. Seizure susceptibility after manipulation of brain serotonin. *Arch Int Pharmacodyn Ther* 1970; 188(2):298–304.
101. Leander JD. Fluoxetine, a selective serotonin-uptake inhibitor, enhances the anticonvulsant effects of phenytoin, carbamazepine, and ameltolide (LY 201116). *Epilepsia* 1992; 33(3):573–576.
102. Kovacs DA, Zoll JG. Seizure inhibition by median raphe nucleus stimulation in rat. *Brain Res* 1974; 70(1):165–169.
103. Lazarova M, Bendotti C, Samanin R. Studies on the role of serotonin in different regions of the rat central nervous system on pentylenetetrazol-induced seizures and the effect of di-*n*-propylacetate. *Naunyn Schmiedebergs Arch Pharmacol* 1983; 322(2):147–152.
104. Lazarova M, Bendotti C, Samanin R. Evidence that the dorsal raphe area is involved in the effect of clonidine against pentylenetetrazole-induced seizures in rats. *Naunyn Schmiedebergs Arch Pharmacol* 1984; 325(1):12–16.
105. Mazarati AM, Baldwin RA, Shinmei S, Sankar R. In vivo interaction between serotonin and galanin receptors types 1 and 2 in the dorsal raphe: implication for limbic seizures. *J Neurochem* 2005; 95(5):1495–1503.
106. Wada Y, Nakamura M, Hasegawa H, Yamaguchi N. Microinjection of the serotonin uptake inhibitor fluoxetine elevates hippocampal seizure threshold in rats. *Neurosci Res Commun* 1993; 13:143–148.
107. Krahl SE, Clark KB, Smith DC, Browning RA. Locus coeruleus lesions suppress the seizure-attenuating effects of vagus nerve stimulation. *Epilepsia* 1998; 39(7):709–714.
108. Rasmussen H. The calcium messenger system (1). *N Engl J Med* 1986; 314(17):1094–1101.
109. Rasmussen H. The calcium messenger system (2). *N Engl J Med* 1986; 314(18):1164–1170.

110. Katz B, Miledi R. Further study of the role of calcium in synaptic transmission. *J Physiol* 1970; 207(3):789–801.
111. DeLorenzo RJ. A molecular approach to the calcium signal in brain: relationship to synaptic modulation and seizure discharge. *Adv Neurol* 1986; 44:435–464.
112. Taft WC, DeLorenzo RJ. Regulation of calcium channels in brain: implications for the clinical neurosciences. *Yale J Biol Med* 1987; 60(2):99–106.
113. Douglas WW. Stimulus-secretion coupling: the concept and clues from chromaffin and other cells. *Br J Pharmacol* 1968; 34(3):453–474.
114. Rubin RP. The role of calcium in the release of neurotransmitter substances and hormones. *Pharmacol Rev* 1970; 22(3):389–428.
115. Rasmussen H, and Goodman DB. Relationships between calcium and cyclic nucleotides in cell activation. *Physiol Rev* 1977; 57(3):421–509.
116. Bolger GT, Gengo P, Klockowski R, Luchowski E, et al. Characterization of binding of the Ca^{++} channel antagonist, [^{3}H]nitrendipine, to guinea-pig ileal smooth muscle. *J Pharmacol Exp Ther* 1983; 225(2):291–309.
117. Gould RJ, Murphy KM, Snyder SH. [^{3}H]nitrendipine-labeled calcium channels discriminate inorganic calcium agonists and antagonists. *Proc Natl Acad Sci U S A* 1982; 79(11):3656–3660.
118. Miller RJ. Multiple calcium channels and neuronal function. *Science* 1987; 235(4784): 46–52.
119. Leslie SW, Friedman MB, Coleman RR. Effects of chlordiazepoxide on depolarization-induced calcium influx into synaptosomes. *Biochem Pharmacol* 1980; 29(18):2439–2443.
120. DeLorenzo RJ. Role of calmodulin in neurotransmitter release and synaptic function. *Ann N Y Acad Sci* 1980; 356:92–109.
121. DeLorenzo RJ. The calmodulin hypothesis of neurotransmission. *Cell Calcium* 1981; 2(4): 365–385.
122. DeLorenzo RJ, Taft WC, Andrews WT. Regulation of voltage-sensitive calcium channels in brain by micromolar affinity benzodiazepine receptors. In: Katz B, Rahamimoff R, eds. *Calcium, Neuronal Function and Neurotransmitter Release*. Boston: Martinus Nijhoff, 1985:375–394.
123. Nowycky MC, Fox AP, Tsien RW. Three types of neuronal calcium channel with different calcium agonist sensitivity. *Nature* 1985; 316(6027):440–443.
124. Tsien RW. Calcium currents in heart cells and neurons. In Kaczmarek L, Levitan I, eds. *Neuromodulation: The Biochemical Control of Neuronal Excitability*. New York: University Press, 1987; 206–242.
125. Ferrendelli JA, Daniels-McQueen S. Comparative actions of phenytoin and other anticonvulsant drugs on potassium and veratridine-stimulated calcium uptake in synaptosomes. *J Pharmacol Exp Ther* 1982; 220:29–34.
126. Ferrendelli JA, Kinscherf DA. Phenytoin: effects on calcium flux and cyclic nucleotides. *Epilepsia* 1977; 18(3):331–336.
127. Perez-Reyes E. Molecular physiology of low-voltage-activated T-type calcium channels. *Physiol. Rev* 2003; 83(1):117–161.
128. Shin, H-S. T-type Ca^{2+} channels and absence epilepsy. *Cell Calcium* 2006; 40(2): 191–196.
129. Coulter DA, Huguenard JR, Prince DA. Characterization of ethosuximide reduction of low-threshold calcium current in thalamic neurons. *Annals of Neurology* 1989; 25(6):582–593.
130. Talley EM, Cribbs LL, Lee JH, Daud A, et al. Differential distribution of three members of a gene family encoding low voltage-activated (T-type) calcium channels. *J Neurosci* 1999; 19(6):1895–1911.
131. Kim D, Song I, Keum S, Lee T, et al. Lack of the burst firing of thalamocortical relay neurons and resistance to absence seizures in mice lacking [alpha]1G T-Type Ca2+ channels. *Neuron* 2001; 31(1):35–45.
132. Snead OC III, Banerjee PK, Burnham M, Hampson D. Modulation of absence seizures by the $GABA_A$ receptor: a critical role for metabotropic glutamate receptor 4 (mGluR4). *J Neurosci* 2000; 20(16):6218–6224.
133. Rothman SM, Olney JW. Excitotoxicity and the NMDA receptor—still lethal after eight years. *Trends Neurosci* 1995; 18(2):57–58.
134. Turski L, Cavalheiro EA, Turski WA, Meldrum BS. Excitatory neurotransmission within substantia nigra pars reticulata regulates threshold for seizures produced by pilocarpine in rats: effects of intranigral 2-amino-7-phosphonoheptanoate and N-methyl-D-aspartate. *Neuroscience* 1986; 18(1):61–77.
135. Choi DW, Koh JY, Peters S. Pharmacology of glutamate neurotoxicity in cortical cell culture: attenuation by NMDA antagonists. *J Neurosci* 1988; 8(1):185–196.
136. Czuczwar S, Frey H, Loscher W. N-methyl-D,L-aspartic acid-induced convulsions in mice and their blockade by antiepileptic drugs and other agents. In: Nistico G, Morselli P, Lloyd K, Fariello R, et al, eds. *Neurotransmitters, Seizures, and Epilepsy III*. New York: Raven Press, 1986:235–246.
137. Mayer ML, Westbrook GL. The physiology of excitatory amino acids in the vertebrate central nervous system. *Prog Neurobiol* 1987; 28(3):197–276.
138. Meldrum B, Chapman A. Excitatory amino acid antagonists and anticonvulsant agents: receptor subtype involvement in different seizure models, In: Nistico G, Morselli P, Lloyd K, Fariello R, et al, eds. *Neurotransmitters, Seizures, and Epilepsy III*. New York: Raven Press, 1986:223–245.
139. Cheung WY. Calmodulin plays a pivotal role in cellular regulation. *Science* 1980; 207 (4426):19–27.
140. Klee CB, Crouch TH, Richman PG. Calmodulin. *Annu Rev Biochem* 1980; 49:489–515.
141. DeLorenzo RJ, Freedman SD, Yohe WB, Maurer SC. Stimulation of Ca^{2+}-dependent neurotransmitter release and presynaptic nerve terminal protein phosphorylation by calmodulin and a calmodulin-like protein isolated from synaptic vesicles. *Proc Natl Acad Sci U S A* 1979; 76(4):1838–1842.
142. DeLorenzo RJ. Calmodulin in neurotransmitter release and synaptic function. *Fed Proc* 1982; 41(7):2265–2272.
143. DeLorenzo, R. J. (1983). Calcium-calmodulin protein phosphorylation in neuronal transmission: a molecular approach to neuronal excitability and anticonvulsant drug action. *Status Epilepticus*. A. V. Delgado-Escueta, C. G. Wasterlain, L.J. Treiman and R. J. Porter, New York, Raven Press, 34:325–338.
144. Goldenring JR, Gonzalez B, McGuire JS Jr, DeLorenzo RJ. Purification and characterization of a calmodulin-dependent kinase from rat brain cytosol able to phosphorylate tubulin and microtubule-associated proteins. *J Biol Chem* 1983; 258(20):12632–12640.
145. Bennett MK, Erondu NE, Kennedy MB. Purification and characterization of a calmodulin-dependent protein kinase that is highly concentrated in brain. *J Biol Chem* 1983; 258(20): 12735–12744.
146. Schulman H, and Greengard P. Stimulation of brain membrane protein phosphorylation by calcium and an endogenous heat-stable protein. *Nature* 1978; 271(5644):478–479.
147. DeLorenzo RJ, Burdette S, Holderness J. Benzodiazepine inhibition of the calcium–calmodulin protein kinase system in brain membrane. *Science* 1981; 213(4507): 546–549.
148. Sakakibara M, Alkon DL, DeLorenzo R, Goldenring JR, et al. Modulation of calcium-mediated inactivation of ionic currents by Ca^{2+}/calmodulin-dependent protein kinase II. *Biophys J* 1986; 50(2):319–327.
149. Goldenring JR, Wasterlain CG, Oestreicher AB, de Graan PN, et al. Kindling induces a long-lasting change in the activity of a hippocampal membrane calmodulin-dependent protein kinase system. *Brain Res* 1986; 377(1):47–53.
150. Goldenring JR, McGuire JS Jr, DeLorenzo RJ. Identification of the major postsynaptic density protein as homologous with the major calmodulin-binding subunit of a calmodulin-dependent protein kinase. *J Neurochem* 1984; 42(4):1077–1084.
151. Kennedy MB, Bennett MK, Erondu NE. Biochemical and immunochemical evidence that the "major postsynaptic density protein" is a subunit of a calmodulin-dependent protein kinase. *Proc Natl Acad Sci U S A* 1983; 80(23):7357–7361.
152. Ghosh A, and Greenberg ME. Calcium signaling in neurons: molecular mechanisms and cellular consequences. *Science* 1995; 268(5208):239–247.
153. Berridge MJ. Neuronal calcium signaling. *Neuron* 1998; 21(1):13–26.
154. Buzsaki G, Hsu M, Horvath Z, Horsburgh K, et al. Kindling-induced changes of protein kinase C levels in hippocampus and neocortex. *Epilepsy Res Suppl* 1992; 9:279–284.
155. Kurz JE, Sheets D, Parsons JT, Rana A, et al. A significant increase in both basal and maximal calcineurin activity in the rat pilocarpine model of status epilepticus. *J Neurochem* 2001; 78(2):304–315.
156. Kurz JE, Rana A, Parsons JT, Churn SB. Status epilepticus-induced changes in the subcellular distribution and activity of calcineurin in rat forebrain. *Neurobiol Dis* 2003; 14(3):483–493.
157. Battaglia G, Pagliardini S, Ferrario A, Gardoni F, et al. AlphaCaMKII and NMDA-receptor subunit expression in epileptogenic cortex from human periventricular nodular heterotopia. *Epilepsia* 2002; 43 Suppl 5:209–216.
158. Bronstein JM, Farber DB, Micevych PE, Lasher PE, et al. Kindling-induced changes in calmodulin kinase II immunoreactivity. *Brain Res* 1990; 524(1):49–53.
159. Bronstein JM, Micevych P, Popper P, Huez G, et al. Long-lasting decreases of type II calmodulin kinase expression in kindled rat brains. *Brain Res.* 1992; 584(1–2): 257–260.
160. Perlin JB, Churn SB, Lothman EW, DeLorenzo RJ. Loss of type II calcium/calmodulin-dependent kinase activity correlates with stages of development of electrographic seizures in status epilepticus in rat. *Epilepsy Res* 1992; 11(2):111–118.
161. Wasterlain CG, Bronstein JM, Morin AM, Dwyer BE, et al. Translocation and autophosphorylation of brain calmodulin kinase II in status epilepticus. *Epilepsy Res Suppl* 1992; 9:231–238.
162. Kochan LD, Churn SB, Omojokun O, Rice A, et al. Status epilepticus results in an N-methyl-D-aspartate receptor-dependent inhibition of Ca^{2+}/calmodulin-dependent kinase II activity in the rat. *Neuroscience* 2000; 95(3):735–743.
163. Blair RE, Churn SB, Sombati S, Lou JK, et al. Long-lasting decrease in neuronal Ca^{2+}/ calmodulin-dependent protein kinase II activity in a hippocampal neuronal culture model of spontaneous recurrent seizures. *Brain Res.* 1999; 851(1–2):54–65.
164. Butler LS, Silva AJ, Abeliovich A, Watanabe Y, et al. Limbic epilepsy in transgenic mice carrying a Ca^{2+}/calmodulin-dependent kinase II alpha-subunit mutation. *Proc Natl Acad Sci U S A* 1995; 92(15):6852–6855.
165. Churn SB, Kochan LD, DeLorenzo RJ. Chronic inhibition of Ca(2+)/calmodulin kinase II activity in the pilocarpine model of epilepsy. *Brain Res* 2000; 875(1–2):66–77.
166. Churn SB, Sombati S, Jakoi ER, Sievert L, et al. Inhibition of calcium/calmodulin kinase II alpha subunit expression results in epileptiform activity in cultured hippocampal neurons. *Proc Natl Acad Sci U S A* 2000; 97(10):5604–5609.
167. Janz R, Goda Y, Geppert M, Missler M, et al. SV2A and SV2B function as redundant Ca^{2+} regulators in neurotransmitter release. *Neuron* 1999; 24(4):1003–1016.
168. Lynch BA, Lambeng N, Nocka K, Kensel-Hammes P, et al. The synaptic vesicle protein SV2A is the binding site for the antiepileptic drug levetiracetam. *Proc Natl Acad Sci U S A* 2004; 101(26):9861–9866.
169. Madeja M, Margineanu DG, Gorji A, Siep E, et al. Reduction of voltage-operated potassium currents by levetiracetam: a novel antiepileptic mechanism of action? *Neuropharmacology* 2003; 45(5):661–671.
170. Rogawski MA. Diverse mechanisms of antiepileptic drugs in the development pipeline. *Epilepsy Research* 2006; 69(3):273–294.
171. Wallace MJ, Blair RE, Falenski KW, Martin BR, et al. (2003) The endogenous cannabinoid system regulates seizure frequency and duration in a model of temporal lobe epilepsy. *J Pharmacol Exp Ther* 307(1):129–137.

172. Lutz B. On-demand activation of the endocannabinoid system in the control of neuronal excitability and epileptiform seizures. Biochem *Pharmacol*. 2004; 68(9):1691–1698.
173. Smith PF. Cannabinoids as potential anti-epileptic drugs. *Curr Opin Investig Drugs* 2005; 6(7):–6805.
174. Jonsson KO, Holt S, Fowler CJ. The endocannabinoid system: current pharmacological research and therapeutic possibilities. *Basic Clin Pharmacol Toxicol* 2006; 98(2): 124–134.
175. Mackie K. Cannabinoid receptors as therapeutic targets. *Annu Rev Pharmacol Toxicol*. 2006; 46(1):101–122.
176. Karler R, Cely W, Turkanis SA. The anticonvulsant activity of cannabidiol and cannabinol. *Life Sci*. 1973; 13(11):1527–31.
177. Karler R, Cely W, Turkanis SA. Anticonvulsant properties of delta 9-tetrahydrocannabinol and other cannabinoids. *Life Sci* 1974; 15(5):931–47.
178. Adams IB, Martin BR. Cannabis: pharmacology and toxicology in animals and humans. *Addiction* 1996; 91(11):1585–1614.
179. Wallace MJ, Wiley JL, Martin BR, DeLorenzo RJ. Assessment of the role of CB1 receptors in cannabinoid anticonvulsant effects. *Eur J Pharmacol* 2001; 428(1):51–57.
180. Blair RE, Deshpande LS, Sombati S, Falenski KW, et al. Activation of the cannabinoid type-1 receptor mediates the anticonvulsant properties of cannabinoids in the hippocampal neuronal culture models of acquired epilepsy and status epilepticus. *J Pharmacol Exp Ther* 2006; 317(3):1072–1078.
181. Wallace MJ, Martin BR, DeLorenzo RJ. Evidence for a physiological role of endocannabinoids in the modulation of seizure threshold and severity. *Eur J Pharmacol* 2002; 452(3):295–301.
182. Kreitzer AC, Regehr WG. Cerebellar depolarization-induced suppression of inhibition is mediated by endogenous cannabinoids. *J Neurosci* 2001; 21(20):RC174.
183. Wilson RI, Kunos G, Nicoll RA. Presynaptic specificity of endocannabinoid signaling in the hippocampus. *Neuron* 2001; 31(3):453–462.
184. Ohno-Shosaku T, Maejima T, Kano M. Endogenous cannabinoids mediate retrograde signals from depolarized postsynaptic neurons to presynaptic terminals. *Neuron* 2001; 29(3):729–38.
185. Vaughan CW, Christie MJ. Retrograde signalling by endocannabinoids. *Handb Exp Pharmacol* 2005; 168:367–383.
186. Ameri A, Wilhelm A, Simmet T. Effects of the endogeneous cannabinoid, anandamide, on neuronal activity in rat hippocampal slices. *Br J Pharmacol* 1999; 126(8):1831–1839.
187. Hauser WA, Hesdorffer DC. *Epilepsy: frequency, causes and consequences*. New York: Demos, 1990.
188. DeLorenzo RJ, Sun DA, Deshpande LS. Cellular mechanisms underlying acquired epilepsy: the calcium hypothesis of the induction and maintainance of epilepsy. *Pharmacol Ther* 2005; 105(3):229–266.
189. DeLorenzo, R.J., and T. A. Morris (1999). "Long-term modulation of genetic expression in epilepsy and other neurological diseases." *The Neuroscientist* 5(2) 86–99.

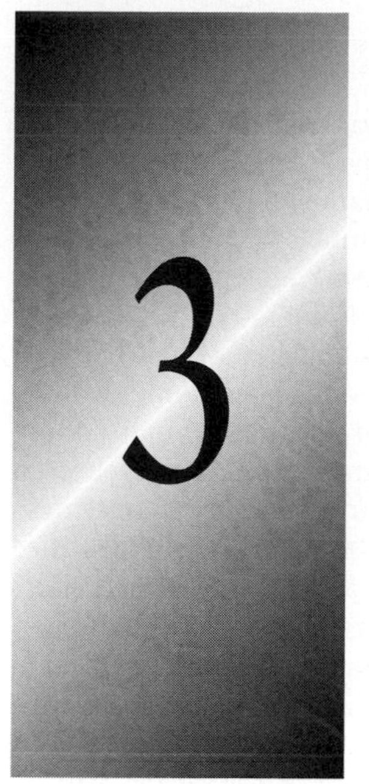

Channel Mutations in Epilepsy: A Neurodevelopmental Perspective

Edward C. Cooper

Searches for genes mutated in several hereditary forms of epilepsy affecting infants and children have resulted in the identification of epileptic channelopathies: that is, epilepsies resulting from mutations in ion channel genes. This is a rapidly evolving field, and reviews of recent progress appear frequently in journals. This chapter attempts to take a broader view and provide background that may serve as an introduction to this ongoing literature for interested pediatricians and pediatric neurologists. In particular, I attempt to make explicit key background, assumptions, and hypotheses underlying this relatively new field and explore (even at the risk of speculation) some of its current directions and promise.

WHY HAVE INVESTIGATORS PURSUED A GENETIC STRATEGY FOCUSED ON RARE MENDELIAN FORMS OF EPILEPSY?

Only a small minority of seizure patients encountered in the clinic have family histories of epilepsy. Why, then, focus on the even smaller group of patients in which pedigree analysis suggests inheritance of epilepsy resulting from effects of mutation in single genes? Investigators have chosen this approach partly out of recognition of the difficult nature of the problem. Seizures and epilepsy are complex phenomena. Seizures emerge suddenly from the brain's interictal activity, often producing elaborate ictal behaviors and myriad consequences for development. During a seizure, normal neuronal firing patterns are replaced by synchronized rhythms that are excessively prominent and widespread. We know that the capacity to seize is latent in normal brain—convulsions can be provoked in any child or adult as a symptom of metabolic disturbances (e.g., hypoglycemia, hypocalcemia, uremia) or acute injury. What is different about the brains of people with epilepsy, who have seizures without such provocations? Furthermore, why do most syndromic forms of epilepsy exhibit distinctive developmental profiles, affecting individuals at particular periods of their lives? These are tough questions.

Genetics is an approach to these questions that has unique advantages. Genetic research can lead to the identification of a responsible gene (or genes), even when no other biologic information about the cause of a disorder is available. So a successful genetic study offers the potential to "think outside the box" by identifying mechanisms previously completely unknown or unsuspected of being involved with a particular disease process (e.g., the nicotinic receptor, KCNQ channel and Lgi1 proteins, discussed subsequently). Genetics is relatively unbiased by preconceptions born from prevailing models and currently available technical approaches. Such an approach is extremely valuable for scientists confronting a process as complex, heterogeneous, and poorly understood as epilepsy. Furthermore, even when the genetic form of a particular disorder is rare, there is a strong possibility that the mechanism revealed may be involved in pathogenesis of more common forms of the disease.

Because of these potential advantages, over the last two decades efforts have been made to identify families in which epilepsy has occurred in patterns suggesting Mendelian inheritance—that is, in patterns suggesting that the epileptic trait resulted from mutations in a single gene. In the last dozen years, with a burst of success aided by tools derived from the Human Genome Project, hundreds of such mutations have now been discovered (Table 3-1). Remarkably, nearly all of the mutations causing idiopathic epilepsy discovered so far lie in genes encoding ion channels, and the exceptions are primarily in genes for proteins that interact directly with channels and regulate their activity. Some types of hereditary epilepsy associated with other features, such as episodic or progressive motor dysfunction and cognitive impairment (i.e., symptomatic or cryptogenic in traditional classification schemes), have also been found to be due to channel mutations. The primary and direct role of ion channels in the pathogenesis of Mendelian forms of idiopathic epilepsy has rapidly gone from hypothesis to irrevocable fact.

The forging of this sturdy conceptual link between epilepsy and channel genes has occurred coincidentally with a period of revolutionary progress in our understanding of channels themselves, coming from basic neuroscience. Very recently, investigators have begun to systematically explore the functions played by the newly identified "epilepsy genes." They have used neurobiologic techniques to analyze with the requisite detail how mutations in particular channels alter the excitability of individual neurons and neural networks, ultimately resulting in epilepsy. These studies of the epileptic channelopathies are revealing important and previously unknown mechanisms controlling brain excitability at particular stages of development that represent novel targets for therapeutic drugs.

TABLE 3.1
Epileptic Channelopathies with Onset in Infancy, Childhood, or Adolescence (Identified as of January 2007)

Syndrome	Gene(s)	Protein	Channel Type
Benign familial neonatal seizures (BFNS)	KCNQ2 (KCNQ3)[1]	Kv7.2 Kv7.3	M-channel; axonal Ks channel; voltage-gated K^+ channel
Benign familial neonatal-infantile seizures (BFNIS)	SCN2A (KCNQ2)	Nav1.2	Axonal voltage-gated Na^+ channel
Generalized epilepsy with febrile seizures plus (GEFS+)	SCN1A (SCN1B)	Nav1.1 Nav beta1	Interneuron voltage-gated Na^+ channel (?);[2] voltage-gated Na^+ channel accessory subunit
	(GABRG2) (GABRD)	$GABA_A$ gamma2 and delta subunits	Ligand-gated (GABA) Cl^- channel subunit
Severe myoclonic epilepsy of infancy (SMEI)	SCN1A	Nav1.1	Interneuron voltage-gated Na^+ channel (?)
Cortical dysplasia-focal epilepsy syndrome (CDFE)	CNTNAP2	Caspr2	Axonal K^+ channel interaction protein
Generalized epilepsy with paroxysmal dyskinesia (GEPD)	KCNMA1	BK subunit	Large conductance Ca-dependent K^+ channel
Childhood absence epilepsy (CAE)	GABRG2	2 $GABA_A$ gamma subunit	Ligand-gated (GABA) Cl^- channel subunit
	CLCN2	CLC-2	Voltage-gated Cl^- channel
Autosomal dominant nocturnal frontal lobe epilepsy (ADNFLE)	CHRNA4 (CHRNA2) (CHRNB2)	$\alpha4$, $\alpha2$, and $\beta2$ subunits of acetyl-choline receptors	Neuronal nicotinic acetylcholine receptor subunits (?inhibitory presynaptic terminals)
Autosomal partial epilepsy with auditory features (ADPEAF)	LGI1	Lgi1	K^+ channel interaction protein (?); glutamate receptor interaction protein (?)
Autosomal dominant juvenile myoclonic epilepsy (ADJME)	GABRA1$\alpha2$	$GABA_A$ subunit	Ligand-gated (GABA) Cl^- channel subunit

[1]Where one gene accounts for most mutations in a disorder, rarely mutated genes are shown enclosed in parentheses.
[2]Where uncertainty exists as to channel function, (?) is shown.

ION CHANNEL FUNCTION, STRUCTURE, DISTRIBUTION, AND DIVERSITY

What are ion channels? Ion channels are membrane proteins, tiny molecular machines about 10 nanometers in size, that allow ions to enter or leave the cell interior at very high rates—usually 10^6 to 10^7 ions per second per channel (1). These ion fluxes through individual channels cause transient, local changes in neuronal membrane potentials that represent the smallest units of brain electrical signaling. All neurons possess different classes of channels that are selectively permeable to the cations sodium (Na^+), potassium (K^+), and calcium (Ca^{2+}) or the anion chloride (Cl^-). Because of the activity of pumps and co-transporters, Na^+, Ca^{2+}, and Cl^- are usually more concentrated extracellularly and K^+ more concentrated intracellularly. To maintain these concentration differences, the pumps consume energy in the form of adenosine triphosphate (ATP). As a result, when channels permeable to Na^+ or Ca^{2+} open, these ions enter the cell, depolarizing the membrane potential. When channels selective for K^+ or Cl^- open, the membrane is made more hyperpolarized as K^+ leaves or Cl^- enters the cell interior. So, at the simplest level, Na^+ or Ca^{2+} channel activity leads to increased excitation, whereas K^+ or Cl^- channel activity reduces excitation.

Although the function of an individual channel type may appear quite simple, groups of such channels can readily underlie complex, dynamic changes in the membrane potential, producing oscillations and rhythmic activity in neurons and neuronal networks. Grouping together even two channels capable of causing opposing changes in the membrane potential in a neuronal membrane creates a mechanism for generating membrane potential oscillations. The propagated action potential, mediated by sequential opening of voltage-gated Na^+ channels (depolarizing phase) and K^+ channels (repolarizing and/or hyperpolarizing phase) grouped along nerve axons, is the best-studied example of such signaling.

We now know, however, that other channel groupings occur everywhere in nervous tissue. Particular channel types are deployed at specific locations, for specialized purposes. Indeed, humans possess several hundred genes encoding ion channel types that differ in key functional properties such as opening and closing rates (kinetics), the types of ions passed (ion selectivity), and the signals that bring about channel opening and closing (gating and modulation) (2). This allows different neurons to express distinct subsets of ion channels and for different channel types expressed by a neuron to be localized at specific sites in the cell membrane with great precision. For example, some channels are expressed at synapses. Some channels are specifically expressed on dendrites, but others are found at particular locations along axons or at presynaptic terminals. Some channels are preferentially expressed on inhibitory or excitatory neurons within a brain region, or on glia. Along with cell shape, cell-specific differences in ion channel expression contribute to each cell's particular electrical "personality," enabling neurons to perform distinctive functions in local networks, and underlying the differences between the network properties of different brain regions. It is important to note that the expression levels of many ion channels are not static during development; instead, ion channel genes exhibit distinctive developmental profiles. One goal of current research is to improve the current fragmentary understanding of how the roles played by different ion channels change in parallel with the achievement of motor, sensory and cognitive development milestones during infancy and childhood.

So, when we learn that an ion channel mutation causes seizures, this leads to functional questions at several levels. At the level of the channel molecule, we seek to learn how the mutation alters intrinsic channel properties such as kinetics, selectivity, gating, and modulation. At the cellular level, we want to know how the mutation affects channel abundance and distribution. At the local network level, we need to know how the mutation alters the rhythmic properties and synchronization of firing occurring in networks of neurons in particular brain regions, since it is at this level that the seizure phenotype is manifest. Finally, we seek understanding of how the channel's roles change during development, seeking clues from the age of onset and natural history of the clinical syndrome.

Ion Channel Structure

Many channel mutations exert their effects by disrupting the normal structure of the encoded channel proteins. Here we introduce some key common aspects of channel structure/function relationships most relevant to the epileptic channelopathies; more detailed reviews are available elsewhere (3–6).

Cellular membranes are bilayers with polar surfaces facing the aqueous cytoplasmic and extracellular spaces and a ~50-angstrom-thick hydrophobic core (Figure 3-1A). Although seemingly thin and fluid, the oily core of biologic membranes represents a formidable barrier for ions, which are even tinier (~1 angstrom) and highly charged. Furthermore, ions in solution attract an admiring "entourage"—a surrounding shell of water molecules that are also repulsed by the hydrophobic core of the membrane. Thus, transport across the membrane requires each ion to be sequentially bound by the channel, dehydrated (stripped of surrounding water molecules), carried across the inhospitable membrane core, rehydrated, and released. These steps must all happen very quickly. It takes the electrical charge from about 10,000 ions to depolarize a 1 μm^2 patch of membrane by

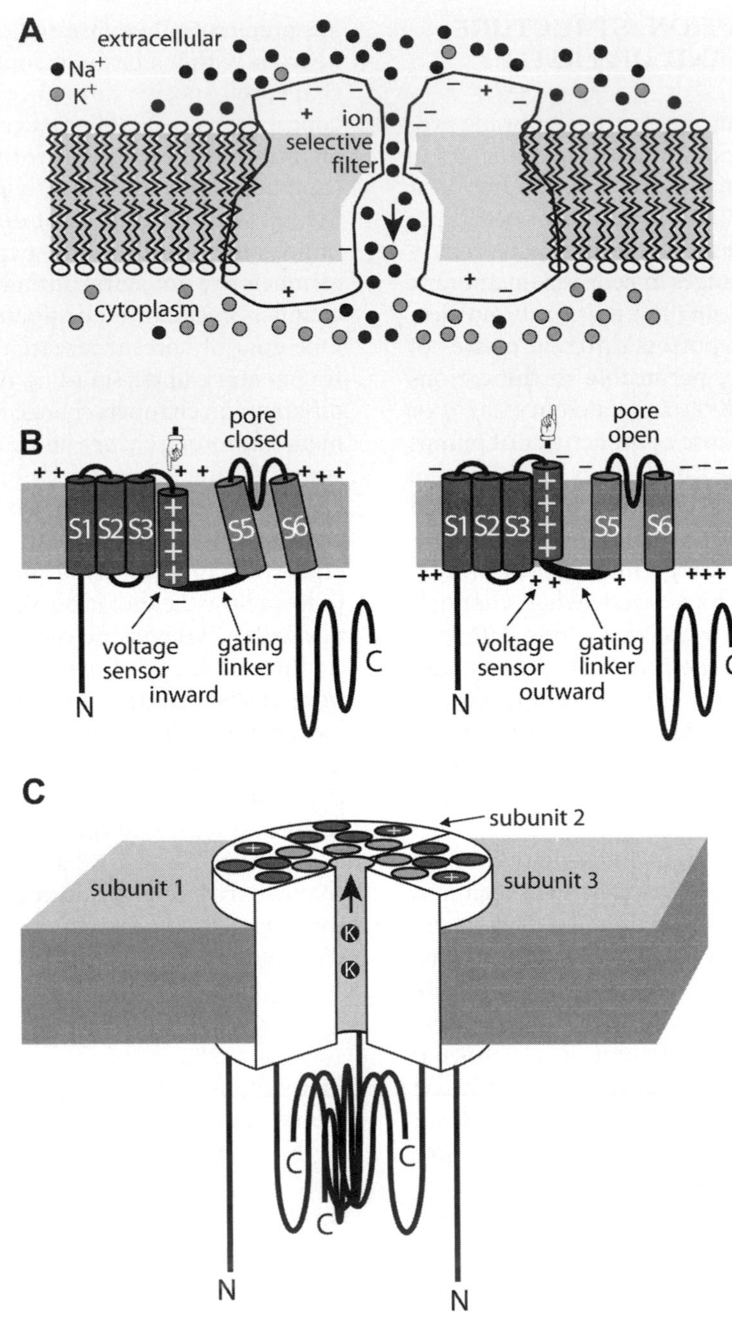

FIGURE 3-1

Structure and gating mechanism of representative ion channels. (A) Cartoon showing a cross-sectional view through the center of a model ion channel. The channel has hydrophobic surfaces facing the membrane lipid core (gray area) and hydrophilic surfaces with charged residues (indicated by +'s and –'s) facing the internal and external solution and lining the centrally located transmembrane ion path. At the narrowest part of the pore, permeant ions bind preferentially to the "ion selective filter." The channel depicted is selectively permeable to Na^+ ions, which are shown moving through the channel from the extracellular solution to the cytoplasm. (B) Transmembrane topology, functional subdomains, and molecular movements of a voltage-gated K^+ channel subunit. The subunit polypeptide has intracellular amino and carboxy terminal domains, and six segments (S1 through S6) that traverse the membrane. S1–S4 form the voltage sensor domain. S5–S6, and the loop that connects them and is folded partly into the membrane, form the pore domain. The S4 domain possesses positively charged residues (indicated by +'s), and as a result, undergoes molecular movements in response to changes in the transmembrane electrical potential, moving outward when the membrane is depolarized (indicated by pointers). Outward movement of the S4 domain pulls the pore at the cytoplasmic end of S5–S6, allowing ion flow (right panel). (C) Cartoon showing K^+ channel subunits arranged around the central pore of an assembled channel—the fourth (front) subunit has been removed to reveal the ion path. Positions of transmembrane segments are indicated as in part B (gray, S5 and S6; dark gray, S1 to S4).

100 mV (the height of a typical action potential). For this to occur within a millisecond, ions must enter this small area of the membrane at a rate approaching 10 million per second. Ion channel routinely achieve this amazing feat, but how?

Ion channel polypeptide chains traverse the membrane several times and assemble into proteins shaped like doughnuts embedded at their midsection in the membrane (Figure 3-1). The surfaces of the channel that face the extracellular and intracellular aqueous solution are hydrophilic and may contain charged residues and sugars that attract ions, whereas the circumferential band touching the oily membrane core is made up of hydrophobic amino acids. Ions traverse the membrane through a centrally located pore (the doughnut's hole). The channel pore is water filled except for a narrow segment known as the selectivity filter. The selectivity filter possesses a row of sites where individual ions are briefly bound and released. The selectivity filter is equally accessible to ions from the intracellular and extracellular sides of the membrane. The net direction of flow is influenced by the fact that randomly moving ions are more likely to access the filter from the side where they are more highly concentrated, and less likely to return once released from the side where they are more dilute. In addition, once ions enter the channel pore, they come under the influence of the electrical potential difference between the two sides of the membrane—Na^+, Ca^{2+}, and K^+ are attracted towards the negative side of the membrane, and Cl^- towards the positive side. The balance between these concentration- and voltage-driven forces determines the direction of net ion flow.

In addition to the pore-forming parts themselves, all ion channels have additional components that control the opening and closing of the ion pathway. Regulatory domains include voltage sensors embedded in the membrane (Figure 3-1B). Alternatively, some channels have parts that bind and respond to intracellular second messengers and metabolites (e.g., Ca^{2+}, ATP, cyclic adenosine monophosphate [cAMP], or polyamines), and extracellular sites for binding neurotransmitters. The best understood regulatory mechanism is that of voltage-gating mechanisms common to Na^+, K^+, and Ca^{2+} channels, which has been revealed through detailed studies combining electrophysiology and X-ray crystallography. A cluster of positive charges on one transmembrane segment (S4) cause it to move inward or outward, depending on which side of the membrane is more negatively charged (Figure 3-1B). In the closed state (inside-negative membrane potential), the S4 is pulled inward, forcing the pore-lining part of the channel into an angled position, so that the inner mouth of the pore is too small for ions to pass (Figure 3-1B, left). When the membrane is depolarized, the voltage sensor moves towards the extracellular space, pulling the pore-lining residues away from the center axis of the pore and opening the inner pore mouth sufficiently to allow ions to flow (Figure 3-1A, C).

Ion Channel Diversity and Nomenclature

Successive waves of technical advance over the last 20 years have left a wake of very confusing nomenclature for ion channel currents, proteins, and genes. First, electrophysiologic methods of improved sensitivity have allowed previously overlooked subtypes in the channel currents to be recorded from neuronal membranes. This led to a new nomenclature subclassifying various voltage- and and ligand-gated channel types based on their kinetics, pharmacology, and other functional properties. Next, the advent of methods for isolating messenger RNAs from neural cells led to the identification of a large number of complementary DNAs (cDNAs) encoding channel subunits. Finally, the sequencing of the genomes of humans and various model organisms led to the identification of many additional channel genes. The process of correlating the channels actually expressed in neurons with specific genes and proteins is slow and painstaking, in part because most native channels are heteromeric—that is, formed by the coassembly of the protein products of two or more different gene. Only rarely do channels appear to be homomeric—that is, formed by multiple copies of the same subunit type. As a result, the exact subunit composition of most of the channels expressed in most brain neurons is not yet known—particularly in humans. The changes in channel composition and expression that occur during normal human development and in disease states are even less understood; with a few exceptions, such developmental changes have not yet been studied.

Although much remains to be learned about the function of particular channel genes, genomics has revealed how ion channel diversity has been generated and, by implication, why. All human channels are derived from a very small number of ancestral genes, already present in the genomes of ancestral prokaryotes over a billion years ago (1, 2, 7). Just as genes are subject to random mutations, it is now known that all genes are subject to random duplication, albeit very rarely, as the result of errors occurring during DNA replication; indeed the rate of such gene duplications is estimated to be one per hundred million years (8, 9). Each gene duplication event creates a "surplus" gene that is relatively free to evolve new functional properties, since the original gene is still present and performing any essential functions. In the vast majority of cases, a duplicate gene does not evolve a novel useful function but instead accumulates inactivating mutations over time and, eventually, disappears from the genome. Rarely, the duplicate gene evolves a new function that provides a survival advantage to the organism—in such cases, both duplicate genes become "fixed" in the genome. The related genes produced by duplication (called "paralogs") can then themselves be subsequently duplicated. The human ion channel families are incredibly large—for example, one such family consists of 80 K^+ channels, 10 voltage-gated Na^+ channels, 11 voltage-gated Ca^{2+} channels, and an additional 42 cation channels of various classes, all derived from the same ancestral K^+ channel (2)! The two other major families of channel genes, encoding voltage-gated Cl^- channels and the ligand-gated channels, were produced by the same process of duplication and subsequent functional divergence (10–12). Because a duplicated neuronal channel gene must provide a survival advantage to first establish itself in its species of origin and remain stably present over the course of evolutionary time, gene survival alone is an indication that a duplicate gene has acquired a needed, novel role. That role may be restricted—for example, to particular neuronal cell types, or to a particular stage of development. Many of these roles remain poorly understood. Indeed, analysis of the phenotypes produced by disease-causing mutations in individual channel genes is an important source for clues regarding these unknown functions.

EPILEPTIC CHANNELOPATHY SYNDROMES

A first expectation, based on earlier studies of channel defects in hyperexcitability disorders of skeletal muscle (e.g., myotonia) and heart (long QT syndrome), would be that channel mutations leading to epilepsy would be associated with increases in Na^+ or Ca^{2+} channel activity (since such activity leads to membrane depolarization) or with reductions in K^+ or Cl^- channel activity (since these currents prevent membrane depolarization) (13, 14). As will be discussed subsequently, we have learned that this expectation is often, but not always, fulfilled. To facilitate further reading, we have provided the listing for each disorder in the National Library of Medicine's Online Mendelian Inheritance in Man (OMIM) database (http://www.ncbi.nlm.nih.gov/omim/), which is frequently updated.

Channel Mutations in Epilepsies with Onset in Neonates and Infants

Benign Familial Neonatal Seizures (BFNS; OMIM 121200). Benign familial neonatal seizures (BFNS, also termed benign familial neonatal convulsions) is a syndrome characterized by recurrent, brief generalized or partial seizures that begin on about the fourth day of life and remit after 1–3 months (15). In the classic syndrome, first described by Rett and Teubel (15), infants otherwise grow and develop normally, without subsequent epilepsy, although affected persons carry a 10–16% risk of experiencing one or more seizures again later in life (16, 17). In 1989, Leppert et al. linked the disease gene to chromosome 20 (18). Later, investigators identified additional families linked to chromosome 8, a first example of genetic heterogeneity in epilepsy (19, 20).

The two BFNS genes on chromosome 20 and 8 encode highly homologous potassium channel subunits, KCNQ2 and KCNQ3 (21–23). These neuronal channel subunits are relatives of a cardiac channel, KCNQ1, which previously was shown to be mutated in both dominantly and recessively inherited forms of the long QT syndrome (24, 25). Four KCNQ1 subunits combine to form the channels in the heart. In neurons, some channels are KCNQ2 tetramers, but many are composed of a combination of KCNQ2 and KCNQ3 subunits (26–31). Some disease-causing missense mutations in KCNQ2 and KCNQ3 are associated with only modest reductions (20–30%) in current magnitude (32). This may imply the critical dependence of neuronal excitability on the absolute magnitude of KCNQ2/KCNQ3 potassium channel activity, especially during the neonatal period. KCNQ channels underlie an extensively studied potassium channel, found in central and autonomic neurons, known as the M-channel (26). The name "M-channel" comes from the fact that these channels are important effectors for acetylcholine acting via muscarinic receptors. Indeed, many neurotransmitters that activate intracellular G proteins increase neuronal excitability by reducing the openings of KCNQ channels (33). These channels open occasionally at the resting membrane potential and are slowly activated by membrane depolarization. Because of their slow kinetics, M-channel activation causes a period of membrane hyperpolarization after a cell receives excitatory input. As a result, neurons expressing M-channels tend to fire one action potential after receiving excitatory input, then become transiently quiescent. Inhibition of the M-channel by neurotransmitter receptors causes these neurons to become slightly depolarized and to fire multiple action potentials rhythmically after receiving excitatory inputs. Thus, M-channels may serve as a general brake on excess neuronal excitation, a brake that can be selectively removed when the cell receives input from neurotransmitters such as acetylcholine.

KCNQ2 subunits are widely expressed in circuits implicated in generation of epileptic seizures (30, 34, 35). Interestingly, one conspicuous localization of KCNQ2 expression is in inhibitory neurons important for synchronization of the firing of excitatory neurons, including the reticular thalamic neurons and several populations of interneurons in the hippocampus and cortex (34). A second important localization of KCNQ2 and KCNQ3 is at spike initiation zones at the beginning of axons, including those of pyramidal cells in the hippocampus and neocortex (30, 36). This localization may allow them to powerfully control the neuronal threshold, since each neuronal action potential originates in the proximal axon (37). In transfection experiments, some BFNS mutations strongly disrupt proper traffic at the axonal initial segment; if this disruption occurs in vivo, it could be the main contributing factor in the BFNS phenotype (38).

Recent studies have identified patients in BFNS pedigrees with KCNQ2 mutations and more severe epilepsy, impaired cognition (39–42) and myokymia (43, 44). KCNQ2 and KCNQ3 have been found at nodes of Ranvier of peripheral nerves and at the axonal initial segments of spinal motor neurons, and loss of their activity likely causes the aberrant impulse initiation in the nerve that is manifest as myokymia (30, 31, 36). It is not clear whether environmental or genetic factors underlie the more severe cognitive, motor, and epileptic phenotypes seen in some BFNS patients.

Retigabine is a novel anticonvulsant, initially identified in the National Institute of Neurological Disease and Stroke (NINDS) antiepileptic (AED) drug screening program, that is effective in preventing seizures induced by electrical shock or by a broad range of chemical convulsants (pentylenetetrazole, N-methyl-D-aspartate [NMDA], 4-aminopyridine, and picrotoxin, but not bicuculline or strychnine) (45). BMS-204352 is another drug initially developed as a potential therapy for acute stroke (46). Remarkably, recent studies have revealed that both these agents are potent activators of neuronal KCNQ channels (47–50). The discover of retigabine's novel mode of action has contributed to new interest in its potential clinical usefulness, and it is currently undergoing stage III trials for adult partial epilepsy (50). Although these agents have not yet been shown to be of clinical usefulness, it is clear that the cloning of the KCNQ channels has revealed an important potential new target for drug screening studies.

Benign Familial Neonatal-infantile Seizures (BFNIS; OMIM 607745). Kaplan and Lacey (51) and Shevell et al. (52) first described families in which nonfebrile seizures, like those seen in BFNS but with a somewhat later onset ranging from the first week of life to 3.5 months, were inherited in an autosomal dominant pattern. This delayed onset led to the suspicion of a distinctive etiology, which was affirmed when the two BFNS loci on chromosomes 8 and 20 were excluded by genetic linkage analysis, and another location on chromosome 2, harboring a cluster of genes encoding several Na^+ channel proteins, was implicated (53–55). Screening of the chromosome 2 genes in BFNIS patients revealed mutations in SCN2A, encoding the Na^+ channel subunit, Nav1.2.

Cell biologic studies using rodents indicate that Nav1.2 channels play an important, transient role on neuronal axons in the developing brain and peripheral nerve (56). In rats and mice, Nav1.2 is at birth the predominant sodium channel at the spike initiation zone in the proximal axon (i.e., the axonal initial segment), but it is largely replaced at this location during the second and third postnatal week. A similar Nav1.2 to Nav1.6 switch occurs at the nodes of Ranvier of many newly myelinating fibers. Based on studies of other proteins, it seems likely that similar subunit switches occur in humans, but over a slower time period of several months (57). The observation that the channels mutated in BFNS and BFNIS are expressed in similar axonal locations during early development is certainly intriguing—but available data do not yet explain why KCNQ2/3 mutations would produce an earlier onset than SCN2A mutations.

Generalized Epilepsy with Febrile Seizures Plus (GEFS+; OMIM 604233), Severe Myoclonic Epilepsy of Infancy (SMEI; OMIM 607208), Intractable Childhood Epilepsy with Generalized Tonic-clonic Seizures (ICEGTCS;OMIM 607208). Febrile seizures occur in 3–5% of all children. When febrile seizures occur in isolation, between age 3 months and 5 years, in children who are otherwise developing normally, the risk of later epilepsy is low (see Chapter 19). For a minority of cases, however, febrile seizures herald epilepsy of a variety of forms and degrees of severity.

In a seminal clinical study, Scheffer and Berkovic (58) described a exceptionally large multigenerational family in which typical febrile seizures of infancy and early childhood were common, but a variety of nonfebrile seizure types also occurred. This spectrum of other seizure types represented in the pedigree included nonfebrile convulsions, absences, myoclonic seizures, atonic seizures, and severe myoclonic-astatic epilepsy with developmental delay. Scheffer and Berkovic argued that this heterogeneity represented variable phenotypes associated with the dominantly inherited trait and introduced the term "generalized epilepsy with febrile seizures plus" (GEFS+) to describe the new seizure syndrome. They further noted that such phenotypic heterogeneity would make this syndrome difficult to detect in smaller families, obscuring its frequency in the clinic. They concluded that molecular studies of large pedigrees such as the one they had analyzed might reveal the underlying genetic mechanism(s). Follow-up studies by the authors and others have confirmed all these predictions.

Mutations in four channel genes have thus far been identified in patients with GEFS+. By far the largest numbers of them are in SCN1A, a close relative of SCN2A, also encoding a voltage-gated Na^+ channel pore-forming subunit. In addition, a few mutations have been found in SCN2A, SCN1B (encoding Nav β1, a voltage-gated Na^+ channel single-transmembrane accessory subunit) and GABRG2 and GABRD (encoding gamma-aminobutyric acid [GABA] receptor subunits).

The single mutation identified in Nav beta1, C121W, has been described in two Anglo-Australian pedigrees (59, 60). C121 is located in the extracellular domain of

Nav beta1, where it forms a disulfide bridge that plays a critical role in the proper assembly of the extracellular domain into an immunoglobulin-like folding pattern (61). Nav beta1 subunits have multiple roles, enhancing surface expression of the pore-forming alpha subunits, participating in protein-protein interactions within the extracellular space that are important for channel clustering at key sites such as the nodes of Ranvier, and enhancing rates of channel inactivation (62). Careful biochemical and electrophysiologic studies using coexpression with neuronal alpha subunits in mammalian cells have revealed two rather subtle effects of C121W (63). The mutation prevents protein-protein interactions mediated by the extracellular domain of Nav beta1 and shifts inactivation to hyperpolarized potentials, thereby increasing the number of channels available for opening.

The discovery of a second GEFS+ locus on chromosome 2q (64, 65), a region that harbors a cluster of three genes encoding sodium channel alpha subunits, led to a search for mutations within these genes in GEFS+ pedigrees. Sequencing of patient DNA revealed many different mutations in SCN1A and a single mutation in SCN2A, all resulting in single amino acid substitutions (missense mutations) in the resulting alpha subunit polypeptides (66–70). Interestingly, these studies have revealed a high frequency of partial seizures in members of some pedigrees that otherwise fit the original GEFS+ profile (60, 69, 70). The electrophysiologic properties of many of the mutant alpha subunits have now been studied fairly intensively in heterologous cells. A subset of the mutations show defective inactivation mechanisms, as observed first in studies of the C121W mutation in beta1 discussed in the preceding paragraph. For example, Lossin et al. found three mutations that exhibited a persistent current during prolonged depolarizations due to an apparent failure of inactivation gating (71). However, other mutations seem to show reduced current amplitudes or changes in gating that are predicted to reduce current flow, without a defect in inactivation (72, 73). Thus, only some GEFS+ mutations appear to be associated with enhanced channel activity similar to the mutations in heart and skeletal muscle Na^+ channels that cause disorders of hyperexcitability and excessive synchrony (myotonia, long QT syndrome) in those tissues (74, 75).

This issue has been further complicated by genetic and clinical evidence that an additional epilepsy syndrome, severe myoclonic epilepsy of infancy (SMEI), represents a severe form of the GEFS+ spectrum (76–78). SMEI, first described by Dravet in 1978, is a progressive syndrome of refractory seizures and cognitive decline. After a normal early infancy, patients present with prolonged generalized or unilateral febrile seizures at 5–12 months of age. Other seizure types, including myoclonic, absence, partial, and atonic seizures, begin between 1 and 4 years of age. Psychomotor slowing becomes apparent during the second year of life, and the patient may also experience obtunded states associated with myoclonus and develop ataxia, pyramidal dysfunction, and refractory generalized tonic-clonic and partial seizures. Intellectual outcome is generally poor. Although a family history of epilepsy had been previously recognized as common in SMEI, the nature of the seizure disorder in family members had not been systematically explored until recently. Singh et al. (76) described 12 SMEI pedigrees within which other family members exhibited forms of epilepsy consistent with the GEFS+ spectrum. Subsequent screening of additional SMEI patients for mutations in SCN1A has identified more than 100 additional mutations. The majority of SMEI mutations are de novo frame-shift, nonsense, or splice-donor mutations predicted to result in markedly aberrant, truncated forms of the channel protein. In contrast to the modest changes in gating seen with GEFS+ mutations that cause single amino acid changes, the SMEI truncations would be expected to produce proteins incapable of conducting ions. Most recently, an additional clinical syndrome, intractable childhood epilepsy with generalized tonic-clonic seizures (ICEGTCS), which is quite similar to SMEI except that patients do not show myoclonic seizures, has also been shown to result from mutations in SCN1A (79).

These clinical and genetic observations are perplexing and lead to many questions concerning genotype-phenotype relations in the GEFS+/SMEI patients. How could gain-of-function mutations (i.e., the impaired inactivation seen in some GEFS+ patients) cause a mild syndrome, if loss-of-function mutations cause a severe phenotype (in SMEI and ICEGTCS). Cell biologic studies are beginning to shed light on this. In early studies, SCN1A was described as widely expressed by excitatory and inhibitory neurons, with Nav1.1 proteins observed on neuronal somata and proximal dendrites (80). Very recent experiments are revising this view, however. In hippocampus, both the protein and mRNA are reportedly much more expressed in inhibitory neurons than in excitatory pyramidal cells, leading to the suggestion that the severe phenotype of null mutations reflects a simple loss of inhibition (81). Furthermore, careful immunohistochemical studies have revealed Nav1.1 channels clustered in the initial segments of some cortical interneurons (82).

In short, the localization and relative importance of various subpopulations of Na^+ channels is incompletely understood but is rapidly being addressed by current studies. Studies using transgenic mouse models that allow mutant channels to be studied in vivo are critical to future success, as are correlative studies of channel distribution in human tissue.

Screening of large clinical populations suggests, however, that amino acid coding mutations in SCN1A, SCN2A, and SCN1B account for only about 20% of familial cases of GEFS+ and a far lower percentage of cases of idiopathic generalized epilepsy (67, 68). This implies that other genes may be involved, and the search has begun. Recently, mutations in the GABRG2 and GABRD genes, which encode the gamma2 and delta subunits of the $GABA_A$ receptor, were also identified as causes of GEFS+ (83, 84). $GABA_A$ receptors are ligand-gated Cl^- channels (85). GABA released at inhibitory synapses binds to sites on the extracellular side of the channel, leading to channel opening and Cl^- influx and generating a fast inhibitory postsynaptic potential (IPSP). There are 16 human genes for subunits of GABA receptors: alpha1–6, beta1–4, gamma1–3, delta, epsilon, and theta. Each GABA receptor is a pentameric complex consisting of two alpha subunits, two beta subunits, and single subunit of class gamma, delta, epsilon, or theta. Although receptors containing a variety of different subunit combinations are represented *in vivo*, the most abundant and widely distributed form of the receptor is formed by alpha1, beta2, and gamma2 subunits. The known gamma2 subunit mutations range widely in the severity of their effects on channel function and the associated clinical phenotype. One mutation (R43N), found in a pedigree with a relatively mild seizure phenotypes (febrile seizures and childhood absence epilepsy), introduces a point mutation in the site for channel modulation by benzodiazepines such as diazepam and lorazepam (86). R43N mutant channels expressed in *Xenopus* oocytes exhibited only 10% reductions in GABA current amplitudes, though responsiveness to benzodiazepines was abolished completely. A second missense mutation (K289M), in an extracellular loop between the M2 and M3 transmembrane segments, was associated with a ~90% reduction in GABA currents and a more severe phenotype of febrile seizures and afebrile generalized tonic-clonic seizures (83). Finally, a truncation mutation in GABRG2 was found in a patient with SMEI within a branch of a large GEFS+ pedigree with bilineal inheritance of epilepsy (87). When expressed in oocytes or cultured mammalian cells, this truncation mutation (Q351X) acted as a potent dominant negative, coassembling with normal GABA receptor subunits and preventing them from leaving the endoplasmic reticulum (87). Beyond these direct effects on GABA receptor functioning, three of the GEFS+ mutations has been shown to impair channel transport to the membrane when expressed in cells maintained at elevated temperature (40°C); by contrast, wild-type channels did not show temperature dependence (88).

Very recently, a fourth GABRG2 mutation was found in a small pedigree with febrile seizures and no other forms of epilepsy (89). The mutation described (R139G) was located in the extracellular portion of the subunit, near the location where benzodiazepines bind and thereby enhance channel openings. R139G had a slight effect on function, speeding the rate of channel closing after an opening elicited by GABA. Although the number of families is very small, so far there is a direct correlation between the severity of epilepsy and the severity of the effects on channel gating observed in the four known GABRG2 mutations.

A single GEFS+ pedigree with four affected patients has been has been linked to a mutation in GABRD. Channels including the delta subunit encoded by GABRD are located at nonsynaptic sites on the soma and dendrites (90). Although delta-containing receptors are present at low density, they make important contributions to regulation of neuronal responsiveness because of their long-lasting openings (91).

Recessive Cortical Dysplasia—Focal Epilepsy Syndrome (CDFE; OMIM 610042). An Amish family was described in which 9 children were affected by a syndrome of cortical dysplasia, focal epilepsy, relative macrocephaly, and diminished deep-tendon reflexes (92). Intractable focal seizures began at 14–20 months of age. Subsequently, autism-like features, including language regression, hyperactivity, impulsive behavior, and mental retardation, developed in all children. Attempts to treat the refractory epilepsy by surgical removal of focal dysplasic cortical regions did not prevent the recurrence of seizures. Pathologic studies of dysplasias showed abnormal neurons, altered neuronal migration, and gliosis. All affected children were found to be homozygous for a mutation in CNTNAP2, encoding the protein contactin-associated protein-like 2 (Caspr2). Caspr2 is a single transmembrane protein possessing a large extracellular domain with multiple protein-protein interaction modules. Remarkably, Caspr2 is localized on axonal membranes at the axon initial segments and the nodes of Ranvier (93, 94). Caspr2 is required for targeting the Kv1 subclass of voltage-gated potassium channels to these important axonal subdomains (95–97).

The Kv1 channel pore-forming subunits are encoded by KCNA genes. Six genes, KCNA1–6, are known to be expressed in the CNS, produced by gene duplication from a single ancient, ancestral gene. Indeed these genes are the homologs of a single fly gene, called *Shaker*. Flies with mutations in *Shaker* are hyperactive when undisturbed and, if exposed to low levels of anesthetic vapors, develop rapid shaking movements of their wings, legs, and abdomen that prevent normal behavior (98). Recordings from *Shaker* flies show failure of action potentials propagated along neuronal axons to repolarize normally (99). In mammals, the role played by Kv1 channels on axons undergoes a developmental switch during myelination (96, 100). Kv1 channels arrive near the node as it begins to form, and they play a key role in axonal action potential repolarization during the early stages of myelination. Once myelination is complete, Kv1 channels have a diminished role at nodes, because they are sequestered beneath the myelin sheath. However, they are also present on unmyelinated portions of the axon both proximally (i.e., the initial segments) and distally (at presynaptic terminals), and in these locations they contribute to control of initiation and neurotransmitter release (93, 101). The basis for epilepsy based on recessive inheritance of Caspr2 mutations is not established, but the connection with axonal excitability is particularly provocative in view of the better-established axonal roles of Nav and KCNQ subunits mutated in neonatal and infantile forms of epilepsy. This family study is also the first human example of recessive inheritance of epilepsy involving channel regulation. A large number of recessive epileptic channelopathies have been identified in inbred stains of laboratory mice (102); the relative lack of such mutations detected in human epilepsy reflects the uncommonness of consanguinity required for the rare pathogenic mutations to become symptomatic, and the difficulty of identifying mutations in small families.

Axonal Hyperexcitability: An Emerging Theme in the Hereditary Epilepsies of Neotates and Infants. From the foregoing discussion, it is clear that recent evidence has linked KCNQ channels, Nav1.2, Nav1.1, and Caspr2 mutations to forms of epilepsy involving neonates and/or infants. In parallel, cell biologic studies have revealed that all of these proteins have major roles in regulation of intrinsic axonal excitability in the developing nervous system. It seems clear that in these early-onset forms of epilepsy, disturbance of the ion channels that mediate the actual initiation and firing of action potentials is centrally important. It is not yet known why, for example, mutations in KCNQ2 should cause onset of seizures at an earlier age than mutations in Nav1.2. Further experiments should help to clarify the specific age-dependent phenotypes associated with various mutations and, in the process, the precise functions played by these channel types.

Channel Mutations in Epilepsies with Onset In Childhood and Adolescence

Autosomal Dominant Nocturnal Frontal Lobe Epilepsy (ADNFLE; OMIM 600513). In 1994, Scheffer et al. described a new epilepsy syndrome characterized by clusters of brief nocturnal motor seizures (103, 104). The attacks began in childhood (median age 8 years) and persisted throughout life, often misdiagnosed as night terrors, nightmares, hysteria, or paroxysmal nocturnal dystonia. Video-EEG recordings revealed that the nocturnal attacks were epileptic seizures heralded by frontally predominant sharp- and slow-wave activity (104), usually arising from stage 2 non-REM sleep. In spite of improved understanding of the disorder, clinical differentiation from parasomnias and other paroxysmal disorders of sleep can be challenging and may require video-EEG monitoring and polysomnography (105, 106).

Initial analysis of ADNFLE pedigrees suggested autosomal dominant inheritance with incomplete (~70%) penetrance. Subsequent molecular genetic studies have revealed mutations in genes for three subunits of neuronal nicotinic acetylcholine receptors (nAchRs) in affected individuals: CHRNA4 on chromosome 20, CNRNB2 on chromosome 1, and CHRNA2 on chromosome 8 (107–111).

Central nAchRs are pentameric cation channels, closely related to the well-studied nAchRs at skeletal muscle endplates, but are composed of alpha and beta subunits expressed only (or at least, primarily) by neurons. Binding of acetylcholine to sites on alpha subunits leads to channel opening and membrane depolarization. Although there are distinct genes for seven neuronal nAchR alpha subunits and three beta subunits, heteromeric channels formed by coassembly of alpha4 and beta2 subunits appear to be the most abundant form expressed in brain. The subunits share a common basic structure, with a large, extracellular amino-terminal domain and four transmembrane alpha-helices. The second (M2) helix lines the transmembrane ion pathway and is believed to undergo a twisting conformational change after acetylcholine binding that allows ions to flow.

The ADNFLE mutations in alpha4 or beta2 described so far all result in single amino acid changes at key positions within the pore-lining helices and might therefore be expected to cause changes in gating or ion conductance properties. Indeed, electrophysiologic experiments using the mutant subunits expressed in experimental cells such as *Xenopus* oocytes or mammalian cultured cells have revealed marked, albeit complex, changes in these properties (108, 112, 113). The α4 S248F mutant AchR responses showed faster desensitization, slower recovery from desensitization, less inward rectification, and virtually no Ca^{2+} permeability as compared with wild-type α4/β2 AChRs (112). Although these effects would all tend to reduce channel activity, this mutation also caused use-dependent up-regulation of activity and was more strongly activated by low levels of agonist, effects that might result in enhanced activity in vivo. Studies of the two known CHRNB2 mutants show differing effects: The V287M mutation shows normal kinetics but 10-fold increased Ach sensitivity (110), whereas the V287L mutation shows normal Ach sensitivity but 30-fold slower kinetics (109). The alpha2 mutation, I279N, is in the first transmembrane segment (M1) that links the extracellular ligand-binding domain to the pore-lining segment (M1). Recordings of transfected cells expressing either the mutant or the wild-type receptor showed that I279N markedly increases the receptor sensitivity to acetylcholine (109).

Immunolocalization studies show that the alpha4 subunit is widely expressed and is localized on neuronal somata and dendrites in cortical and subcortical structures, and it is particularly highly expressed by dopaminergic neurons in the substantia nigra (114). Labarca et al generated CHRNA mutant mice harboring a point mutation in the pore near the position of the ADNFLE mutations (115). This mutation caused 30-fold increased Ach sensitivity and is partially activated by choline at levels that are normally present in cerebrospinal fluid. Mice exhibited early lethality and loss of nigral dopaminergic neurons. More recently, investigators generated two lines of transgenic mice expressing different ADNFLE mutations and found, paradoxically, a 20-fold increase in nicotine-induced GABAergic *inhibitory* postsynaptic currents in cortical neurons, with no change in excitatory currents (116).

How could increased inhibition lead to seizures? Because cortical GABAergic interneurons project widely to large numbers of neighboring pyramidal cells, they are powerful synchronizers of cortical output. Neurons in basal cholinergic nuclei project to the thalamocortical circuits that mediate transitions between sleep and wakefulness; acetylcholine release in these circuits contributes to arousal and alertness (117). Excessive cholinergic responsiveness during a critical stage of desynchronization of this circuit appears to be sufficient to cause seizures. The frontal lobe predominance of the semiology and epileptic discharges in ADNFLE patients is not explained by the distribution patterns of the receptors, which are widespread, but may reflect the inportance of the physiologic contribution made by the frontal lobes to the critical arousal transition that is disrupted in the disorder.

Episodic Ataxia with Myokymia (and Partial Epilepsy) (EA-1; OMIM 160120). EA-1 is a dominantly inherited disorder involving both the brain and peripheral nerves (118–120). Patients experience recurrent attacks of unsteady gait and loss of limb coordination lasting minutes to hours. This phenotype suggests an intermittent derangement of cerebellar function. In some cases, transient cognitive deficits accompany the motor symptoms. Attacks may be provoked by a sudden stress or startle. Myokymia is continuously present in many EA-1 patients. This myokymia is unaffected by pharmacologic block at the proximal portion of peripheral nerves but is reduced by distal nerve block and abolished by inhibition of neuromuscular transmission. This observation suggests that, unlike myotonia or epilepsy, myokymia results from abnormal hyperactivity in the peripheral nerve. However, patients with EA-1 have about a 10-fold greater risk of epileptic seizures compared to the general population (118, 121).

In 1994, Browne et al linked EA-1 to missense mutations in KCNA1 (120). KCNA1, one of the mammalian *Shaker* homologs, encodes voltage-gated potassium Kv1.1 channels that, as discussed previously in connection with the severe CDFE syndrome, are targeted to axons by interaction with Caspr2. Extensive further work, including physiologic studies of the mutant channels, anatomical studies of KCNA channel localization in the central nervous system and peripheral nerve, and studies of knockout and knockin mice, gives useful clues for understanding the basis of the EA-1 phenotype in the brain and peripheral nerve (14). Studies in *Xenopus* oocytes indicate that the mutations causing EA-1 result in reductions in KCNA1 expression and current magnitude (121–123). In some cases, EA-1 mutant channels in heterologous cells exhibit clear "dominant negative" effects, interacting with coexpressed normal channels and preventing them from functioning normally or trafficking to the cell surface. Other EA-1 mutants exhibit simple loss-of-function properties in vitro. As discussed previously, Kv1 family channels have been localized along axons and on presynaptic terminals (101, 124–126). Smart et al. generated knockout mice lacking KCNA1 (127). Interestingly, mice heterozygous for the knockout allele appear normal; this is in contrast to the dominantly inherited effects of EA-1 mutations in humans. Mice that are homozygous for the knockout allele have subtle defects in cerebellar function (128), but the most obvious aspects of their phenotype are very frequent generalized epileptic seizures and associated premature death (127). It has proved difficult to identify the alterations in cellular physiology that cause frequent spontaneous seizures in the Kv1.1 knockout mice; hippocampal slices prepared from the knockouts exhibit remarkably normal intrinsic neuronal and synaptic properties (127). A possible explanations for this was that channels containing the subunit are often localized to small axons and presynaptic termini, which are difficult to study directly using currently available physiologic methods (126). An interesting clue to the pathophysiology of EA-1 is the responsiveness of the condition in some but not all pedigrees to treatment with the carbonic anhydrase inhibitor acetazolamide (129). To further understand the EA-1 phenotype, Herson et al generated knockin mice bearing a human EA-1 point mutation (130). Heterozygous mutant mice exhibited stress-induced loss of coordination that was ameliorated by pretreatment with acetazolamide. Recordings from brain slices suggest that expression of the mutant subunits results in increased neurotransmitter release at presynaptic terminals after invasion by action potentials. Seizures were not reported in the knockin heterozygous mutants, and the homozygous state was lethal early in embryonic development.

As a larger number of patients with EA-1 have been identified, it has become clear that they differ in the severity of their symptoms over a broad spectrum and that more severe forms of the disorder are often associated with epilepsy. Zuberi et al described a family containing five patients with episodic ataxia and myokymia, two of which additionally had partial complex seizures (121). Eunson et al described a second family with this combination of symptoms, as well as families with severe and acetazolamide-resistant ataxia, or isolated myokymia (131). When studied in heterologous cells, the mutations associated with severe ataxia and epilepsy caused severe reductions in channel activity (132). In some cases, the EA-1 plus epilepsy mutant subunits were capable of dominant-negative interactions with wild-type subunits; that is, they were capable of coassembling with the wild-types, but the resulting channels were hypofunctional because of failure of intracellular trafficking or lack of intrinsic channel activity (132). Trafficking defects are likely to be particularly critical in neurons, because the KCNA channel proteins are normally localized to sites along myelinated and nonmyelinated axons and at presynaptic terminals, which are very distant from their sites of translation and assembly in the endoplasmic reticulum (125, 126, 133).

Autosomal Dominant Juvenile Myoclonic Epilepsy (JME; OMIM 606904). JME is characterized by the onset, usually during adolescence, of bilateral single or repetitive myoclonic jerks, occurring most commonly upon morning awakening (134). A majority of patients have at least one generalized tonic-clonic seizure, and about 15% have absences. A characteristic EEG finding is frontally predominant bilateral 4–6 Hz polyspike-wave discharges. JME is not uncommon and represents approximately 4–6% of all patients with epilepsy (134). Nevertheless, identifying genes for JME has been particularly difficult, likely as a result of the genetic heterogeneity and complexity underlying the syndrome. Recently, mutations in genes for a GABA receptor subunit and a subtype of voltage-gated Cl^- channel were identified.

Cossette et al. ascertained a large family in which epilepsy, with characteristic clinical and electroencephalographic features of common JME, was inherited in an autosomal dominant pattern (135). A missense mutation was found in GABRA1, resulting in an A322D change in a conserved site in the third transmembrane helix of the GABA receptor alpha1 subunit. Two alpha subunits are present in each pentameric GABA receptor; each of these subunits contributes both to a binding site for GABA and to the transmembrane pore. Peak currents mediated by receptors that included the A322D GABA alpha1 mutants were only 10% of those of wild-type receptors, and this weak response required 200-fold higher concentrations of GABA. Accordingly, the epileptic phenotype would be expected to be associated with greatly reduced responsiveness to inhibitory neurotransmission. It is unclear why this mutation results in epilepsy of the JME type.

A genomewide linkage analysis of 130 families with idiopathic generalized epilepsy (IGE) identified a susceptibility locus on chromosome 3q (135). The gene CLCN2, encoding a voltage-gated Cl^- channel protein (called ClC-2 or CLC-2), was identified within the linked region and sequenced for mutations in samples from 46 families (137). Three mutations were identified among these families, one in a small family with 5 patients with JME. CLC-2, like other members of the chloride channel family, forms dimeric channel complexes. Heretically, each chloride channel subunit possesses its own transmembrane ion path, and gating of the two pores within each channel is regulated by allosteric interactions within the protein (10). The JME mutation identified in the single family produced a truncated form of the protein that was unable to conduct ions itself or coassemble with wild-type subunits.

Epilepsy with Grand Mal Seizures on Awakening (EGMA, OMIM 607628) and Childhood Absence Epilepsy (CAE; OMIM 600131). JME overlaps with another syndrome, termed "awakening epilepsy" or "epilepsy with grand mal seizures on awakening." Patients with EGMA have difficulty falling asleep, abnormal sleep architecture, and the vast majority of their seizures occur clustered within the first minutes after awakening from sleep (irrespective of the time of day) (138). A CLCN2 mutation encoding a nonfunctional channel was identified in a large family with EGMA (137).

A subset of JME and EGMA patients experience absence spells. A third CLCN2 mutation was found to segregate in a small family in which three children had typical childhood absence epilepsy (CAE) (137). This CAE-linked mutation resulted in a single amino acid change (G715E); mutant channels were reported to be functional but were reported to exhibit altered voltage dependence. This finding has been contradicted by two subsequent investigations showing activity of the mutant indistinguishable from wild type, further weakening the modest genetic evidence provided by the small family studied (10). A more recent survey of 55 families with IGE failed to identify additional CLCN2 mutations (138). At present, the strongest evidence linking CLCN2 to generalized epilepsy is provided by the large EGMA pedigree.

Autosomal Dominant Partial Epilepsy with Auditory Features (ADPEAF, OMIM 600512). In 1995 Ottman et al described a large family in which partial seizures associated with unusual auditory auras were inherited in an autosomal dominant pattern linked to a gene on chromosome 10 (140). Several additional families with this distinctive syndrome were subsequently identified (141, 142). The age of seizure onset was typically at 9 to 12 years of age. Seizures are heralded by a variety of stereotyped, but in nearly all cases nonverbal, auditory hallucinations (141). Mutations were subsequently identified in the gene Lgi1, a gene of unknown function previously shown to be disrupted in some patients with primary brain tumors (143). This set in motion efforts to understand the function of the Lgi1 protein in brain development, auditory processing, and epileptogenesis.

At present, evidence supporting two conflicting models has been described. One set of experiments shows that the Lgi1 protein is physically associated with and enhances the activity of Kv1 family voltage-gated potassium channels whose pore-forming subunits are encoded by the KCNA genes (144). In this model, Lgi1 is a cytosolic protein that binds to the intracellular portion of channels that contain both pore-forming subunits and previously described channel intracellular accessory units, called beta subunits. The beta1 subunit causes Kv1 channels to close after a period of milliseconds of membrane depolarization. This time- and voltage-dependent closing, called inactivation, is similar to the fast inactivation of sodium channels that helps terminate each action potential. However, inactivation of K^+ channels will generally tend to increase neuronal excitability. Wild-type Lgi1 proteins antagonize this inactivation, prolonging channel opening. Mutations derived from ADPEAF patients, which produce truncated proteins, all abolish the ability of the Lgi1 protein to prolong the K^+ channel opening. This model is consistent with previously discussed findings that loss-of-function KCNA1 mutations that cause epilepsy in some patients with EA-1, and mutations in Caspr2 that disrupt Kv1 channel targeting in the recessive focal epilepsy.

The alternative, and very different, model is based on the recent report that Lgi1 protein is packaged in secretory vesicles and released into the synaptic cleft, where it binds tightly to a cluster of proteins linked to postsynaptic glutamate receptors (145, 146). Lgi1 binds directly to ADAM22, and is thereby linked to PSD-95 and stargazin, all of which are components of the excitatory postsynaptic density. Application of soluble Lgi1 proteins to brain slices in vitro results in enhancement of alpha-amino-3-hydroxy-5-methylisoxazole-4-propionic acid (AMPA)-type glutamate receptor currents. Lgi1 applied to neurons grown in dissociated culture increases the number of AMPA receptors at the cell surface. Mutations in stargazin and ADAM22 that are capable of disrupting the protein complex are associated with epilepsy in mice (although human mutations in these genes are unknown) (146–148). Effects of Lgi1 mutations on this complex and the implications for receptor function are incompletely known, but the implication is that mutations would tend to reduce postsynaptic excitatory currents.

How can the two proposed functional roles of Lgi1 be reconciled? Immunoblots of proteins separated by sodium dodecyl sulfate (SDS) gel electrophoresis reveal two forms of Lgi1 that differ by 3–5 kDa, indicating that the protein is either alternatively spliced or post-translationally processed (150). Moreover, the larger form localizes to the cytoplasm, whereas the smaller is found in a microsomal fraction containing secretory vesicles. Although it is not clear which form is most important for epilepsy, hippocampal and cerebellar cortex (areas with particularly high densities of AMPA-type glutamatergic synapses) showed predominantly the smaller, presumed secreted form. The highest percentage of the cytosolic, high-molecular-weight form was present in temporal neocortex (150). This result favors the idea that the cytoplasmic interaction with potassium channel contributes to the auditory auras and seizures in ADPEAF, but additional studies are needed.

Generalized Epilepsy with Paroxysmal Dyskinesias (OMIM 609446). Clinical studies have noted patients, sometimes in familial groups, with a combination of generalized epilepsy and paroxysmal dyskinesia (151, 152). Du et al. described an unusual family with 16 affected individuals in five consecutive generations, strongly indicating dominant inheritance. Seven had paroxysmal nonkinesogenic dyskinesias, four developed epilepsy only, and five exhibited both symptoms. The symptom onset age ranged broadly from 3 to 15 years, with one patient developing seizures before 6 months. After establishing linkage to chromosome 10, the investigators identified a mutation in KCNMA1, which encodes a pore-forming alpha subunit of a type of calcium-activated potassium channel called BK ("Big-K"; also "Maxi-K") because these channels pass ions at higher rates than other K^+ channel types. BK channels are activated synergistically by membrane depolarization and elevated intracellular Ca^{2+} (1). Their opening rates are very fast, enabling them to speed repolarization of action potentials, shortening the sodium channel refractory period and thereby facilitating rapid neuronal bursting. The pathogenic mutation in BK identified increases channel activity (153). Interestingly, a knockout mutation in a BK accessory subunit has also recently been shown to cause epilepsy in transgenic mice (154). Careful electrophysiologic analysis of these mice indicates that this mutation also increases the activity of BK, leading to increased neuronal firing. The detailed biophysical mechanism whereby excitability is increased in the mice is intriguingly indirect. First, the enhanced BK activity and associated shortened action potential duration causes a reduction in Ca^{2+} entry during each spike. This diminishes the activation of a second type of Ca^{2+}-activated K^+channel, known as SK ("small-conductance K^+ channel"). Despite their name, SK channels very potently limit excitability by means of their long-lasting openings. So preventing SK activation (by increasing BK openings) leads to markedly increased cellular excitability. In effect, the cell must balance BK and SK activity precisely to maintain the desired overall level of excitability. This elegant electrophysiologic analysis again illustrates the importance of transgenic mouse models for current studies of the epileptic channelopathies, and it begins to hint at how very indirect the effects of a mutation can be.

CONCLUSIONS AND IMPLICATIONS FOR THERAPEUTICS

Although the first identification of a channel gene mutation in epilepsy occurred only in 1994, many such mutations have now been identified in 15 different channel subunits and channel-associated proteins. What do these efforts reveal about the causes of epilepsy and potential for novel treatments? One remarkable result is that many of the mutations have been found in subunits of voltage-dependent Na^+ channels and GABA receptors, important targets of the majority of currently approved drugs, all developed through in vivo pharmacologic screening. Many (but not all) Na^+ channel mutations in GEFS+, for example, result in increased Na^+ channel activity; by contrast, such drugs as phenytoin, carbamazepine, and lamotrigine act by blocking Na^+ channel activity. Similarly, in autosomal dominant JME and some cases of GEFS+, mutations in GABA receptor subunits that reduce activity are implicated, whereas benzodiazepines and barbiturates potentiate GABA receptor activity. This is satisfying, but is also potentially a cause for concern. If genetics were only to lead us back to the therapeutic targets we know about, it would be informative but of little practical use. In this regard, the stories of the identification of the KCNQ channel mutations in BFNS, nicotinic acetylcholine receptor mutations in ADNFLE, and Lgi1 mutations in ADPEAF are exciting and reassuring counterexamples. The neuronal KCNQ channels and the functions of Lgi1 regulating K^+ channels and glutamate receptors were unknown before these mutations led to the recent mechanistic studies discussed in this chapter. It seems possible that a new class of KCNQ opener drugs may be developed, with patterns of clinical usefulness that are quite different from available agents. The Lgi1-dependent augmentation of K^+ channel activity is another potential target for future drug development. As neurobiologic studies allow us to understand the mechanistic pathways through which individual mutations lead to seizures, additional targets will be revealed beyond the mutated gene itself. An example of this is the unexpected observation that nicotinic receptor mutations in ADNFLE may cause seizures through enhanced inhibition during arousal from deep sleep. Interestingly, low doses of picrotoxin, a GABA antagonist that is strongly convulsant at higher doses, blocked epileptiform EEG activity and spontaneous seizures in transgenic mice bearing ADNFLE mutations (116).

Although many aspects of genotype-phenotype relationships remain poorly understood, recent years have brought considerable progress, encouraging optimism that the pathogenic mechanisms in these disorders can be understood in detail. Examples of such progress are the identification of the role for KCNQ channels in setting thresholds by targeting to the axonal spike initiation zone, the discovery that SCN1A subunits are preferentially expressed on inhibitory interneurons, and the analysis showing how KCNM1 mutations increasing the activity of BK channels can paradoxically increase neuronal excitability (30, 81, 155). However, it remains unclear whether, in GEFS+ families, the variable phenotype seen within pedigrees may reflect differences in genetic background between individuals, environmental exposures, or both. The spectrum of phenotypes associated with SCN1A mutations, ranging from normal gene carriers or patients with only FS in GEFS+ pedigrees to SMEI patients with severe refractory seizures and progressive motor and cognitive decline, is impressive and requires further study. It remains unclear whether the more severe phenotypes in GEFS+ pedigrees and SMEI should be seen as a part of the GEFS+ spectrum, since they are almost certainly associated with secondary changes in brain structure and function (e.g., cell death, network reorganization, changes in the levels of expression of other channels and signaling proteins) that do not occur in mildly affected individuals. Finally, as pathogenic mechanisms in these Mendelian forms of epilepsy become clearer, efforts will focus on understanding to what extent these mechanisms contribute to the common, non-Mendelian forms of epilepsy. Already, the epileptic channelopathies fit poorly with our traditional classification of the epilepsies as idiopathic (i.e., hereditary, with normal function except for seizures) versus symptomatic (associated with cognitive, motor, and other deficits). Not only can different mutations in the same channel cause varying degrees of impairment—the same mutation can have variable effects within a pedigree.

Resolving these and unforeseen questions arising with the identification of novel epilepsy mutations should be extremely fruitful both in terms of a better understanding of basic mechanisms underlying seizures and epileptogenesis and for drug development.

References

1. Hille B. Ionic channels of excitable membranes. 3rd ed. Sunderland, MA.: Sinauer, 2001.
2. Yu FH, Catterall WA. The VGL-chanome: A protein superfamily specialized for electrical signaling and ionic homeostasis. *Sci STKE* 2004;2004:re15. http://stke.sciencemag.org.
3. Tombola F, Pathak MM, Isacoff EY. How far will you go to sense voltage? *Neuron* 2005; 48:719–725.
4. Madden DR. The structure and function of glutamate receptor ion channels. *Nat Rev Neurosci* 2002; 3:91–101.
5. Long SB, Campbell EB, Mackinnon R. Voltage sensor of Kv1.2: structural basis of electromechanical coupling. *Science* 2005; 309:903–908.
6. Jiang Y, Lee A, Chen J, et al. X-ray structure of a voltage-dependent K^+ channel. *Nature* 2003; 423:33–41.

7. Okamura Y, Nishino A, Murata Y, et al. Comprehensive analysis of the ascidian genome reveals novel insights into the molecular evolution of ion channel genes. *Physiol Genomics* 2005; 22:269–282.
8. Zhang J. Evolution by gene duplication: an update. *Trends Ecol Evol* 2003; 18:292–298.
9. Lynch M, Conery JS. The origins of genome complexity. *Science* 2003; 302:1401–1404.
10. Jentsch TJ, Poet M, Fuhrmann JC, et al. Physiological functions of CLC Cl^- channels gleaned from human genetic disease and mouse models. *Annu Rev Physiol* 2005; 67:779–807.
11. Mohler H. GABA(A) receptor diversity and pharmacology. *Cell Tissue Res* 2006; 326: 505–516.
12. Paoletti P, Neyton J. NMDA receptor subunits: function and pharmacology. *Curr Opin Pharmacol* 2007; 7:39–47.
13. Ptacek L. The familial periodic paralyses and nondystrophic myotonias. *Am J Med* 1998; 105:58–70.
14. Cooper EC, Jan LY. Ion channel genes and human neurological disease: Recent progress, prospects, and challenges. *Proc Natl Acad Sci U S A* 1999; 96:4759–4766.
15. Rett A, Teubel R. Neugeborenenkrämpfe im Rahmen einer epileptisch belasteten Familie. *Wien Klin Wochenschr* 1964; 74:609–613.
16. Ronen GM, Rosales TO, Connolly M, et al. Seizure characteristics in chromosome 20 benign familial neonatal convulsions. *Neurology* 1993; 43:1355–1360.
17. Zimprich F, Ronen GM, Stogmann W, et al. Andreas Rett and benign familial neonatal convulsions revisited. *Neurology* 2006; 67:864–866.
18. Leppert M, Anderson VE, Quattlebaum T, et al. Benign familial neonatal convulsions linked to genetic markers on chromosome 20. *Nature* 1989; 337:647–648.
19. Lewis TB, Leach RJ, Ward K, et al. Genetic heterogeneity in benign familial neonatal convulsions: Identification of a new locus on chromosome 8q. *Am J Hum Genet* 1993; 53:670–675.
20. Steinlein O, Schuster V, Fischer C, et al. Benign familial neonatal convulsions: Confirmation of genetic heterogeneity and further evidence for a second locus on chromosome 8q. *Hum Genet* 1995; 95:411–415.
21. Singh NA, Charlier C, Stauffer D, et al. A novel potassium channel gene, KCNQ2, is mutated in an inherited epilepsy of newborns. *Nat Genet* 1998; 18:25–29.
22. Charlier C, Singh NA, Ryan SG, et al. A pore mutation in a novel KQT-like potassium channel gene in an idiopathic epilepsy family. *Nat Genet* 1998; 18:53–55.
23. Biervert C, Schroeder BC, Kubisch C, et al. A potassium channel mutation in neonatal human epilepsy. *Science* 1998; 279:403–406.
24. Neyroud N, Tesson F, Denjoy I, et al. A novel mutation in the potassium channel gene KvLQT1 causes the cardioauditory syndrome. *Nat Genet* 1997; 15:186–189.
25. Wang Q, Curran ME, Splawski I, et al. Positional cloning of a novel potassium channel gene: KvLQT1 mutations cause cardiac arrhythmias. *Nat Genet* 1996; 12:17–23.
26. Wang H-S, Pan Z, Shi W, et al. KCNQ2 and KCNQ3 potassium channel subunits: molecular correlates of the M-channel. *Science* 1998; 282:1890–1893.
27. Hadley JK, Passmore GM, Tatulian L, et al. Stoichiometry of expressed KCNQ2/KCNQ3 potassium channels and subunit composition of native ganglionic M channels deduced from block by tetraethylammonium. *J Neurosci* 2003; 23:5012–5019.
28. Martire M, Castaldo P, D'Amico M, et al. M channels containing KCNQ2 subunits modulate norepinephrine, aspartate, and GABA release from hippocampal nerve terminals. *J Neurosci* 2004; 24:592–597.
29. Shen W, Hamilton SE, Nathanson NM, et al. Cholinergic suppression of KCNQ channel currents enhances excitability of striatal medium spiny neurons. *J Neurosci* 2005; 25:7449–7458.
30. Pan Z, Kao T, Horvath Z, et al. A common ankyrin-G-based mechanism retains KCNQ and NaV channels at electrically active domains of the axon. *J Neurosci* 2006; 26: 2599–2613.
31. Schwarz JR, Glassmeier G, Cooper EC, et al. KCNQ channels mediate Iks, a slow K^+ current regulating excitability in the rat node of Ranvier. *J Physiol* 2006; 573:17–34.
32. Schroeder BC, Kubisch C, Stein V, et al. Moderate loss of function of cyclic-AMP-modulated KCNQ2 KCNQ3 K^+ channels causes epilepsy. *Nature* 1998; 396:687–690.
33. Brown D. M-currents: an update. *Trends Neurosci* 1988; 11:294–299.
34. Cooper EC, Harrington E, Jan YN, et al. M-channel KCNQ2 subunits are localized to key sites for control of neuronal network oscillations and synchronization in mouse brain. *J Neurosci* 2001; 21:9529–9540.
35. Cooper EC, Aldape KD, Abosch A, et al. Colocalization and coassembly of two human brain M-type potassium channel subunits that are mutated in epilepsy. *Proc Natl Acad Sci U S A* 2000; 97:4914–4919.
36. Devaux JJ, Kleopa KA, Cooper EC, et al. KCNQ2 is a nodal K^+ channel. *J Neurosci* 2004; 24:1236–1244.
37. Stuart G, Spruston N, Sakmann B, et al. Action potential initiation and backpropagation in neurons of the mammalian CNS. *Trends Neurosci* 1997; 20:125–131.
38. Chung HJ, Jan YN,Jan LY. Polarized axonal surface expression of neuronal KCNQ channels is mediated by multiple signals in the KCNQ2 and KCNQ3 C-terminal domains. *Proc Natl Acad Sci U S A* 2006; 103:8870–8875.
39. de Haan GJ, Pinto D, Carton D, et al. A novel splicing mutation in KCNQ2 in a multigenerational family with BFNC followed for 25 years. *Epilepsia* 2006; 47:851–859.
40. Dedek K, Fusco L, Teloy N, et al. Neonatal convulsions and epileptic encephalopathy in an Italian family with a missense mutation in the fifth transmembrane region of KCNQ2. *Epilepsy Res* 2003; 54:21–27.
41. Borgatti R, Zucca C, Cavallini A, et al. A novel mutation in KCNQ2 associated with BFNC, drug resistant epilepsy, and mental retardation. *Neurology* 2004; 63:57–65.
42. Pereira S, Roll P, Krizova J, et al. Complete loss of the cytoplasmic carboxyl terminus of the KCNQ2 potassium channel: A novel mutation in a large Czech pedigree with benign neonatal convulsions or other epileptic phenotypes. *Epilepsia* 2004; 45: 384–390.
43. Dedek K, Kunath B, Kananura C, et al. Myokymia and neonatal epilepsy caused by a mutation in the voltage sensor of the KCNQ2 K^+ channel. *Proc Natl Acad Sci U S A* 2001; 98:12272–12277.
44. Zhou X, Ma A, Liu X, et al. Infantile seizures and other epileptic phenotypes in a Chinese family with a missense mutation of KCNQ2. *Eur J Pediatr* 2006; 165:691–695.
45. Rostock A, Tober C, Rundfeldt C, et al. D-23129: A new anticonvulsant with a broad spectrum activity in animal models of epileptic seizures. *Epilepsy Res* 1996; 23:211–223.
46. Gribkoff VK, Starrett JE, Jr., Dworetzky SI, et al. Targeting acute ischemic stroke with a calcium-sensitive opener of maxi-K potassium channels. *Nat Med* 2001; 7:471–477.
47. Schroder RL, Jespersen T, Christophersen P, et al. KCNQ4 channel activation by BMS-204352 and retigabine. *Neuropharmacology* 2001; 40:888–898.
48. Wickenden AD, Yu W, Zou A, et al. Retigabine, a novel anti-convulsant, enhances activation of KCNQ2/Q3 potassium channels. *Molec Pharmacol* 2000; 58:591–600.
49. Main MJ, Cryan JE, Dupere JR, et al. Modulation of KCNQ2/3 potassium channels by the novel anticonvulsant retigabine. *Molec Pharmacol* 2000; 58:253–262.
50. Porter RJ, Nohria V, Rundfeldt C. Retigabine. *Neurotherapeutics* 2007; 4:149–154.
51. Kaplan RE, Lacey DJ. Benign familial neonatal-infantile seizures. *Am J Med Genet* 1983; 16:595–599.
52. Shevell MI, Sinclair DB, Metrakos K. Benign familial neonatal seizures: Clinical and electroencephalographic characteristics. *Pediatr Neurol* 1986; 2:272–275.
53. Lewis TB, Shevell MI, Andermann E, et al. Evidence of a third locus for benign familial convulsions. *J Child Neurol* 1996; 11:211–214.
54. Malacarne M, Gennaro E, Madia F, et al. Benign familial infantile convulsions: Mapping of a novel locus on chromosome 2q24 and evidence for genetic heterogeneity. *Am J Hum Genet* 2001; 68:1521–1526.
55. Leppert M, McMahon WM, Quattlebaum TG, et al. Searching for human epilepsy genes: a progress report. *Brain Pathol* 1993; 3:357–369.
56. Boiko T, Rasband MN, Levinson SR, et al. Compact myelin dictates the differential targeting of two sodium channel isoforms in the same axon. *Neuron* 2001; 30:91–104.
57. Dzhala VI, Talos DM, Sdrulla DA, et al. NKCC1 transporter facilitates seizures in the developing brain. *Nat Med* 2005; 11:1205–1213.
58. Scheffer IE, Berkovic SF. Generalized epilepsy with febrile seizures plus. A genetic disorder with heterogeneous clinical phenotypes. *Brain* 1997; 120:479–490.
59. Wallace RH, Wang DW, Singh R, et al. Febrile seizures and generalized epilepsy associated with a mutation in the Na^+-channel β1 subunit gene SCN1B. *Nat Genet* 1998; 19:366–370.
60. Wallace RH, Scheffer IE, Parasivam G, et al. Generalized epilepsy with febrile seizures plus: Mutation of the sodium channel subunit SCN1B. *Neurology* 2002; 58:1426–1429.
61. McCormick KA, Isom LL, Ragsdale D, et al. Molecular determinants of Na^+ channel function in the extracellular domain of the β1 subunit. *J Biol Chem* 1998; 273:3954–3962.
62. Isom LL. Sodium channel β subunits: anything but auxiliary. *Neuroscientist* 2001; 7: 42–54.
63. Meadows LS, Malhotra J, Loukas A, et al. Functional and biochemical analysis of a sodium channel β1 subunit mutation responsible for generalized epilepsy with febrile seizures plus type 1. *J Neurosci* 2002; 22:10699–10709.
64. Baulac S, Gourfinkel-An I, Picard F, et al. A second locus for familial generalized epilepsy with febrile seizures plus maps to chromosome 2q21–q33. *Am J Hum Genet* 1999; 65:1078–1085.
65. Moulard B, Guipponi M, Chaigne D, et al. Identification of a new locus for generalized epilepsy with febrile seizures plus (GEFS+) on chromosome 2q24–q33. *Am J Hum Genet* 1999; 65:1396–1400.
66. Escayg A, MacDonald BT, Meisler MH, et al. Mutations of SCN1A, encoding a neuronal sodium channel, in two families with GEFS+2. *Nat Genet* 2000; 24:343–345.
67. Wallace RH, Scheffer IE, Barnett S, et al. Neuronal sodium-channel alpha1-subunit mutations in generalized epilepsy with febrile seizures plus. *Am J Hum Genet* 2001; 68:859–865.
68. Escayg A, Heils A, MacDonald BT, et al. A novel SCN1A mutation associated with generalized epilepsy with febrile seizures plus—and prevalence of variants in patients with epilepsy. *Am J Hum Genet* 2001; 68:866–873.
69. Abou-Khalil B, Ge Q, Desai R, et al. Partial and generalized epilepsy with febrile seizures plus and a novel SCN1A mutation. *Neurology* 2001; 57:2265–2272.
70. Sugawara T, Mazaki-Miyazaki E, Ito M, et al. Nav1.1 mutations cause febrile seizures associated with afebrile partial seizures. *Neurology* 2001; 57:703–705.
71. Lossin C, Wang DW, Rhodes TH, et al. Molecular basis of an inherited epilepsy. *Neuron* 2002; 34:877–884.
72. Vanoye CG, Lossin C, Rhodes TH, et al. Single-channel properties of human NaV1.1 and mechanism of channel dysfunction in SCN1A-associated epilepsy. *J Gen Physiol* 2006; 127:1–14.
73. Barela AJ, Waddy SP, Lickfett JG, et al. An epilepsy mutation in the sodium channel SCN1A that decreases channel excitability. *J Neurosci* 2006; 26:2714–2723.
74. Bennett PB, Yazawa K, Makita N, et al. Molecular mechanism for an inherited cardiac arrhythmia. *Nature* 1995; 376:683–685.
75. Cannon SC, Brown RH, Jr.,Corey DP. A sodium channel defect in hyperkalemic periodic paralysis: potassium-induced failure of inactivation. *Neuron* 1991; 6:619–626.
76. Singh R, Andermann E, Whitehouse WP, et al. Severe myoclonic epilepsy of infancy: extended spectrum of GEFS+? *Epilepsia* 2001; 42:837–44.
77. Claes L, Del-Favero J, Ceulemans B, et al. De novo mutations in the sodium-channel gene SCN1A cause severe myoclonic epilepsy of infancy. *Am J Hum Genet* 2001; 68: 1327–1332.
78. Sugawara T, Mazaki-Miyazaki E, Fukushima K, et al. Frequent mutations of SCN1A in severe myoclonic epilepsy in infancy. *Neurology* 2002; 58:1122–1124.

79. Fujiwara T, Sugawara T, Mazaki-Miyazaki E, et al. Mutations of sodium channel alpha subunit type 1 (SCN1A) in intractable childhood epilepsies with frequent generalized tonic-clonic seizures. *Brain* 2003; 126:531–546.
80. Westenbroek RE, Merrick DK,Catterall WA. Differential subcellular localization of the RI and RII Na^+ channel subtypes in central neurons. *Neuron* 1989; 3:695–704.
81. Yu FH, Mantegazza M, Westenbroek RE, et al. Reduced sodium current in GABAergic interneurons in a mouse model of severe myoclonic epilepsy in infancy. *Nat Neurosci* 2006; 9:1142–1149.
82. Ogiwara I, Miyamoto H, Morita N, et al. Nav1.1 localizes to axons of parvalbumin-positive inhibitory interneurons: a circuit basis for epileptic seizures in mice carrying an *SCN1A* gene mutation. *J Neurosci* 2007; 27:5903–14.
83. Baulac S, Huberfeld G, Gourfinkel-An I, et al. First genetic evidence of GABA(A) receptor dysfunction in epilepsy: a mutation in the gamma2-subunit gene. *Nat Genet* 2001; 28:46–48.
84. Dibbens LM, Feng HJ, Richards MC, et al. GABRD encoding a protein for extra- or peri-synaptic GABA(A) receptors is a susceptibility locus for generalized epilepsies. *Hum Mol Genet* 2004; 13:1315–1319.
85. Moss SJ, Smart TG. Constructing inhibitory synapses. *Nat Rev Neurosci* 2001; 2:240–250.
86. Wallace RH, Marini C, Petrou S, et al. Mutant GABA(A) receptor γ2-subunit in childhood absence epilepsy and febrile seizures. *Nat Genet* 2001; 28:49–52.
87. Harkin LA, Bowser DN, Dibbens LM, et al. Truncation of the GABA(A)-receptor γ2 subunit in a family with generalized epilepsy with febrile seizures plus. *Am J Hum Genet* 2002; 70:530–536.
88. Kang JQ, Shen W, Macdonald RL. Why does fever trigger febrile seizures? GABA(A) receptor γ2 subunit mutations associated with idiopathic generalized epilepsies have temperature-dependent trafficking deficiencies. *J Neurosci* 2006; 26:2590–2597.
89. Audenaert D, Schwartz E, Claeys KG, et al. A novel GABRG2 mutation associated with febrile seizures. *Neurology* 2006; 67:687–690.
90. Nusser Z, Sieghart W, Somogyi P. Segregation of different GABA(A) receptors to synaptic and extrasynaptic membranes of cerebellar granule cells. *J Neurosci* 1998; 18:1693–1703.
91. Mortensen M,Smart TG. Extrasynaptic αβ subunit GABA(A) receptors on rat hippocampal pyramidal neurons. *J Physiol* 2006; 577:841–856.
92. Strauss KA, Puffenberger EG, Huentelman MJ, et al. Recessive symptomatic focal epilepsy and mutant contactin-associated protein-like 2. *N Engl J Med* 2006; 354:1370–1377.
93. Inda MC, DeFelipe J,Munoz A. Voltage-gated ion channels in the axon initial segment of human cortical pyramidal cells and their relationship with chandelier cells. *Proc Natl Acad Sci U S A* 2006; 103:2920–2925.
94. Poliak S, Gollan L, Martinez R, et al. Caspr2, a new member of the neurexin superfamily, is localized at the juxtaparanodes of myelinated axons and associates with K^+ channels. *Neuron* 1999; 24:1037–1047.
95. Poliak S, Gollan L, Salomon D, et al. Localization of Caspr2 in myelinated nerves depends on axon-glia interactions and the generation of barriers along the axon. *J Neurosci* 2001; 21:7568–7575.
96. Vabnick I, Trimmer JS, Schwarz TL, et al. Dynamic potassium channel distributions during axonal development prevent aberrant firing patterns. *J Neurosci* 1999; 19:747–758.
97. Rasband MN, Park EW, Zhen D, et al. Clustering of neuronal potassium channels is independent of their interaction with PSD-95. *J Cell Biol* 2002; 159:663–672.
98. Kaplan WD, Trout WE. The behavior of four neurological mutants of *Drosophila*. *Genetics* 1969; 61:399–409.
99. Tanouye MA, Ferrus A, Fujita SC. Abnormal action potentials associated with the *Shaker* complex locus of *Drosophila*. *Proc Natl Acad Sci U S A* 1981; 78:6548–6552.
100. Rasband MN, Shrager P. Ion channel sequestration in central nervous system axons. *J Physiol* 2000; 525 Pt 1:63–73.
101. Geiger JR, Jonas P. Dynamic control of presynaptic Ca^{2+} inflow by fast-inactivating K^+ channels in hippocampal mossy fiber boutons. *Neuron* 2000; 28:927–939.
102. Noebels JL. The biology of epilepsy genes. *Annu Rev Neurosci* 2003; 26:599–625.
103. Scheffer IE, Bhatia KP, Lopes-Cendes I, et al. Autosomal dominant frontal epilepsy misdiagnosed as sleep disorder. *Lancet* 1994; 343:515–517.
104. Scheffer IE, Bhatia KP, Lopes-Cendes I, et al. Autosomal dominant nocturnal frontal lobe epilepsy. A distinctive clinical disorder. *Brain* 1995; 118(Pt 1):61–73.
105. Derry CP, Duncan JS, Berkovic SF. Paroxysmal motor disorders of sleep: the clinical spectrum and differentiation from epilepsy. *Epilepsia* 2006; 47:1775–1791.
106. Provini F, Plazzi G, Tinuper P, et al. Nocturnal frontal lobe epilepsy. A clinical and polygraphic overview of 100 consecutive cases. *Brain* 1999; 122(Pt 6):1017–1031.
107. Steinlein OK, Mulley JC, Propping P, et al. A missense mutation in the neuronal nicotinic acetylcholine receptor alpha 4 subunit is associated with autosomal dominant nocturnal frontal lobe epilepsy. *Nat Genet* 1995; 11:201–203.
108. Steinlein OK, Magnusson A, Stoodt J, et al. An insertion mutation of the CHRNA4 gene in a family with autosomal dominant nocturnal frontal lobe epilepsy. *Hum Mol Genet* 1997; 6:943–947.
109. De Fusco M, Becchetti A, Patrignani A, et al. The nicotinic receptor β2 subunit is mutant in nocturnal frontal lobe epilepsy. *Nat Genet* 2000; 26:275–276.
110. Phillips HA, Favre I, Kirkpatrick M, et al. CHRNB2 is the second acetylcholine receptor subunit associated with autosomal dominant nocturnal frontal lobe epilepsy. *Am J Hum Genet* 2001; 68:225–231.
111. Aridon P, Marini C, Di Resta C, et al. Increased sensitivity of the neuronal nicotinic receptor alpha 2 subunit causes familial epilepsy with nocturnal wandering and ictal fear. *Am J Hum Genet* 2006; 79:342–350.
112. Bertrand S, Weiland S, Berkovic SF, et al. Properties of neuronal nicotinic acetylcholine receptor mutants from humans suffering from autosomal dominant nocturnal frontal lobe epilepsy. *Br J Pharmacol* 1998; 125:751–760.
113. Kuryatov A, Gerzanich V, Nelson M, et al. Mutation causing autosomal dominant nocturnal frontal lobe epilepsy alters Ca^{2+} permeability, conductance, and gating of human α4β2 nicotinic acetylcholine receptors. *J Neurosci* 1997; 17:9035–9047.
114. Arroyo-Jimenez MM, Bourgeois JP, Marubio LM, et al. Ultrastructural localization of the alpha4-subunit of the neuronal acetylcholine nicotinic receptor in the rat substantia nigra. *J Neurosci* 1999; 19:6475–6487.
115. Labarca C, Schwarz J, Deshpande P, et al. Point mutant mice with hypersensitive alpha 4 nicotinic receptors show dopaminergic deficits and increased anxiety. *Proc Natl Acad Sci U S A* 2001; 98:2786–2791.
116. Klaassen A, Glykys J, Maguire J, et al. Seizures and enhanced cortical GABAergic inhibition in two mouse models of human autosomal dominant nocturnal frontal lobe epilepsy. *Proc Natl Acad Sci U S A* 2006; 103:19152–19157.
117. McCormick DA, Bal T. Sleep and arousal: thalamocortical mechanisms. *Annu Rev Neurosci* 1997; 20:185–215.
118. Van Dyke DH, Griggs RC, Murphy MJ, et al. Hereditary myokymia and periodic ataxia. *J Neurol Sci* 1975; 25:109–118.
119. Gancher ST, Nutt JG. Autosomal dominant episodic ataxia: a heterogeneous syndrome. *Mov Disord* 1986; 1:239–253.
120. Browne DL, Gancher ST, Nutt JG, et al. Episodic ataxia/myokymia syndrome is associated with point mutations in the human potassium channel gene, KCNA1. *Nat Genet* 1994; 8:136–140.
121. Zuberi SM, Eunson LH, Spauschus A, et al. A novel mutation in the human voltage-gated potassium channel gene (Kv1.1) associates with episodic ataxia type 1 and sometimes with partial epilepsy. *Brain* 1999; 122:817–825.
122. Adelman JP, Bond CT, Pessia M, et al. Episodic ataxia results from voltage-dependent potassium channels with altered functions. *Neuron* 1995; 15:1449–1454.
123. Zerr P, Adelman JP, Maylie J. Episodic ataxia mutations in Kv1.1 alter potassium channel function by dominant negative effects or haploinsufficiency. *J Neurosci* 1998; 18:2842–2848.
124. Wang H, Kunkel DD, Schwartzkroin PA, et al. Localization of Kv1.1 and Kv1.2, two K channel proteins, to synaptic terminals, somata, and dendrites in the mouse brain. *J Neurosci* 1994; 14:4588–4599.
125. Rhodes KJ, Keilbaugh SA, Barrezueta NX, et al. Association and colocalization of K^+ channel α- and β-subunit polypeptides in rat brain. *J Neurosci* 1995; 15:5360–5371.
126. Cooper EC, Milroy A, Jan YN, et al. Presynaptic localization of Kv1.4-containing A-type potassium channels near excitatory synapses in the hippocampus. *J Neurosci* 1998; 18:965–974.
127. Smart S, Lopantsev V, Zhang CL, et al. Deletion of the Kv1.1 potassium channel causes epilepsy in mice. *Neuron* 1998; 20:809–820.
128. Zhang CL, Messing A,Chiu SY. Specific alteration of spontaneous GABAergic inhibition in cerebellar Purkinje cells in mice lacking the potassium channel Kv1.1. *J Neurosci* 1999; 19:2852–2864.
129. Lubbers WJ, Brunt ER, Scheffer H, et al. Hereditary myokymia and paroxysmal ataxia linked to chromosome 12 is responsive to acetazolamide. *J Neurol Neurosurg Psychiatry* 1995; 59:400–405.
130. Herson PS, Virk M, Rustay NR, et al. A mouse model of episodic ataxia type-1. *Nat Neurosci* 2003; 6:378–383.
131. Eunson LH, Rea R, Zuberi SM, et al. Clinical, genetic, and expression studies of mutations in the potassium channel gene KCNA1 reveal new phenotypic variability. *Ann Neurol* 2000; 48:647–656.
132. Rea R, Spauschus A, Eunson LH, et al. Variable K^+ channel subunit dysfunction in inherited mutations of KCNA1. *J Physiol* 2002; 538:5–23.
133. Laube G, Roper J, Pitt JC, et al. Ultrastructural localization of Shaker-related potassium channel subunits and synapse-associated protein 90 to septate-like junctions in rat cerebellar pinceaux. *Brain Res Mol Brain Res* 1996; 42:51–61.
134. Janz D. Epilepsy with impulsive petit mal (juvenile myoclonic epilepsy). *Acta Neurol Scand* 1985; 72:449–459.
135. Cossette P, Liu L, Brisebois K, et al. Mutation of GABRA1 in an autosomal dominant form of juvenile myoclonic epilepsy. *Nat Genet* 2002; 31:184–189.
136. Sander T, Schulz H, Saar K, et al. Genome search for susceptibility loci of common idiopathic generalised epilepsies. *Hum Mol Genet* 2000; 9:1465–1472.
137. Haug K, Warnstedt M, Alekov AK, et al. Mutations in CLCN2 encoding a voltage-gated chloride channel are associated with idiopathic generalized epilepsies. *Nat Genet* 2003; 33:527–532.
138. Janz D. Epilepsy with grand mal on awakening and sleep-waking cycle. *Clin Neurophysiol* 2000; 111 Suppl 2:S103–S110.
139. Marini C, Scheffer IE, Crossland KM, et al. Genetic architecture of idiopathic generalized epilepsy: clinical genetic analysis of 55 multiplex families. *Epilepsia* 2004; 45:467–478.
140. Ottman R, Risch N, Hauser WA, et al. Localization of a gene for partial epilepsy to chromosome 10q. *Nat Genet* 1995; 10:56–60.
141. Winawer MR, Boneschi FM, Barker-Cummings C, et al. Four new families with autosomal dominant partial epilepsy with auditory features: clinical description and linkage to chromosome 10q24. *Epilepsia* 2002; 43:60–67.
142. Poza JJ, Saenz A, Martinez-Gil A, et al. Autosomal dominant lateral temporal epilepsy: clinical and genetic study of a large Basque pedigree linked to chromosome 10q. *Ann Neurol* 1999; 45:182–188.
143. Kalachikov S, Evgrafov O, Ross B, et al. Mutations in Lgi1 cause autosomal-dominant partial epilepsy with auditory features. *Nat Genet* 2002; 30:335–341.
144. Schulte U, Thumfart JO, Klocker N, et al. The epilepsy-linked Lgi1 protein assembles into presynaptic Kv1 channels and inhibits inactivation by Kvβ1. *Neuron* 2006; 49: 697–706.

145. Fukata Y, Adesnik H, Iwanaga T, et al. Epilepsy-related ligand/receptor complex Lgi1 and Adam22 regulate synaptic transmission. *Science* 2006; 313:1792–1795.
146. Snyder SH. Neuroscience. Adam finds an exciting mate. *Science* 2006; 313: 1744–1745.
147. Letts VA, Felix R, Biddlecome GH, et al. The mouse stargazer gene encodes a neuronal Ca^{2+}-channel gamma subunit. *Nat Genet* 1998; 19:340–347.
148. Chen L, Chetkovich DM, Petralia RS, et al. Stargazin regulates synaptic targeting of AMPA receptors by two distinct mechanisms. *Nature* 2000; 408:936–943.
149. Sagane K, Hayakawa K, Kai J, et al. Ataxia and peripheral nerve hypomyelination in Adam22-deficient mice. *BMC Neurosci* 2005; 6:33.
150. Furlan S, Roncaroli F, Forner F, et al. The Lgi1/epitempin gene encodes two protein isoforms differentially expressed in human brain. *J Neurochem* 2006; 98:985–991.
151. Cuenca-Leon E, Cormand B, Thomson T, et al. Paroxysmal kinesigenic dyskinesia and generalized seizures: clinical and genetic analysis in a Spanish pedigree. *Neuropediatrics* 2002; 33:288–293.
152. Guerrini R, Sanchez-Carpintero R, Deonna T, et al. Early-onset absence epilepsy and paroxysmal dyskinesia. *Epilepsia* 2002; 43:1224–1229.
153. Diez-Sampedro A, Silverman WR, Bautista JF, et al. Mechanism of increased open probability by a mutation of the BK channel. *J Neurophysiol* 2006; 96:1507–1516.
154. Wang B, Rothberg BS, Brenner R. Mechanism of β4 subunit modulation of BK channels. *J Gen Physiol* 2006; 127:449–465.
155. Brenner R, Chen QH, Vilaythong A, et al. BK channel β4 subunit reduces dentate gyrus excitability and protects against temporal lobe seizures. *Nat Neurosci* 2005; 8:1752–1759.

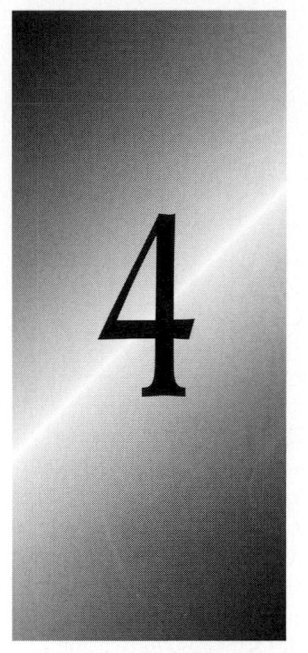

4 Metabolic and Pharmacologic Consequences of Seizures

Michael V. Johnston
John W. McDonald

The electrical discharge of neurons associated with seizure activity stimulates a marked rise in cerebral metabolic activity. Estimates from animal experiments indicate that energy utilization during seizures increases by more than 200 percent, while tissue adenosine triphosphate (ATP) levels remain at more than 95 percent of control, even during prolonged status epilepticus (1, 2). Cerebral metabolic activity can be measured using 2-deoxy-2-[^{18}F]-fluoro-D-glucose positron emission tomography (FDG PET) (3), and magnetic resonance spectroscopy (MRS) can be used to measure the turnover of glutamate, the major excitatory neurotransmitter (4). Comparison of FDG PET and MRS in patients with seizures indicates that glucose metabolism and the turnover of glutamate are tightly coupled (3). This is because the transporters that remove glutamate as well as gamma-aminobutyric acid (GABA), the major inhibitory neurotransmitter, from the synaptic cleft require substantial energy (5). These transporters are located on astroglia that surround synapses, and they remove glutamate and GABA soon after their release from presynaptic nerve terminals to terminate their activity. The transporters are linked to a Na^+/K^+-ATPase, which in turn is powered by anaerobic metabolism of glucose (4). The brain generally withstands the metabolic challenge of seizures quite well because enhanced cerebral blood flow delivers additional oxygen and glucose. Mild to moderate degrees of hypoxemia that commonly accompany seizures are usually harmless. In addition, the immature brain is less vulnerable to injury from seizures than the adult brain (6, 7). However, status epilepticus can sometimes produce an imbalance between metabolic demands and cerebral perfusion, especially if severe hypotension or hypoglycemia is present. Injury can also occur through a direct effect on synapses known as excitotoxicity (8, 9).

Excitotoxicity refers to a process of injury triggered by excessive activation of neuronal receptors for the excitatory amino acid (EAA) neurotransmitters glutamate and aspartate. Under normal circumstances, activation of EAA receptors mediates more than half of the neuronal communication in the brain (10). Seizures initiate release of EAA neurotransmitters from nerve terminals into the synaptic cleft, where they bind to specific neuronal receptors and cause postsynaptic excitation. In the developing brain, EAA receptors serve an additional role as regulators of neuronal development (11). During a prolonged seizure, if the EAA neurotransmitter release continues unabated to raise the synaptic concentration of glutamate, excessive EAA receptor stimulation may damage and eventually kill neurons.

An important component of the excitotoxicity theory holds that EAAs cause intracellular calcium overload, which intoxicates neurons (12–14). Calcium and sodium are allowed to enter neurons through pores or ionophores controlled by EAA receptors. The concentration of calcium within the neuron is normally 10,000 times lower than in the extracellular fluid, and calcium entry is tightly controlled. The neuron has several mechanisms for protecting itself from excessive calcium influx, including sequestration of calcium within mitochondria and endoplasmic reticulum and energy-dependent pumps that move calcium outward across the cell membrane. Continued bombardment of the neuron by EAA neurotransmitters can overwhelm these protective mechanisms, allowing calcium to poison the metabolic machinery of the neuron (15). The EAA theory proposes that excitatory neurotransmitters are a major direct link between excessive seizure activity and neuronal injury; however, metabolic derangements such as hypoxia may play a contributing destructive role by reducing the efficiency of energy-dependent protective mechanisms and hastening EAA-stimulated metabolic exhaustion (16).

PHARMACOLOGY OF EXCITATORY AMINO ACID RECEPTORS

Glutamate is released from presynaptic nerve terminals, but the synaptic concentration is quickly reduced by an active reuptake process mediated by its specific, energy-dependent reuptake pump. Impairment in the activity of the EAA reuptake pump may play an important role in EAA neurotoxicity in disease states. In experimental hypoxia-ischemia, synaptosomal uptake of glutamate is transiently reduced, contributing to marked elevations in extracellular glutamate concentrations, which may reach the micromolar range (17). Metabolic disorders may contribute to EAA neurotoxicity by this mechanism.

The excitatory responses to glutamate are mediated by several receptor subtypes that may be classified into two broad categories as either N-methyl-D-aspartate (NMDA)-type or non-NMDA-type EAA receptors (18, 19) (Figures 4-1 and 4-2). Glutamate is a relatively flexible amino acid molecule that can assume several different conformations, and NMDA is a rigid glutamate analog that represents one of them (20). NMDA maximally activates a glutamate receptor that is linked to an ion channel. Together the receptor and its channel are referred to as the NMDA receptor/channel complex (see Figure 4-1). Molecular cloning of NMDA receptors showed that their diverse characteristics are related to variations in specific combinations of subunits (21). The NMDA channel is permeable to cations such as sodium and calcium, and at normal membrane potential the channel is blocked by magnesium ions (22). Partial depolarization of the membrane potential is necessary for the magnesium block to be removed. As a result, the NMDA receptor/channel complex is not generally involved in ordinary rapid impulse flow.

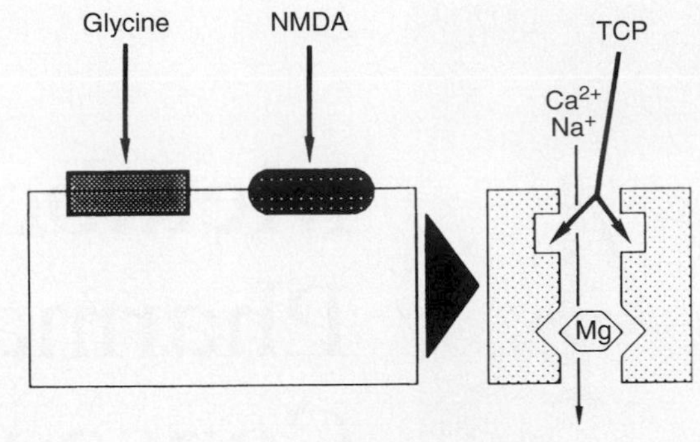

FIGURE 4-1

Current understanding of the components of the NMDA receptor/channel complex, based on biochemical and electrophysiological evidence, is outlined in this schematic diagram. The NMDA recognition site is coupled to a cationic channel that is permeable to Ca^{2+} and Na^+. NMDA receptor activation is modulated by several regulatory sites. Activation of a closely associated glycine recognition site is required for channel activation and markedly enhances responses to NMDA. Physiological concentrations of Mg^{2+} block the NMDA-associated ionophore, and membrane depolarization relieves this blockade. Thus, NMDA receptor/channel activation requires activation of both NMDA and glycine receptors and concurrent membrane depolarization. NMDA-receptor channel activation also can be modulated by Zn^{2+} and polyamines (not illustrated). Noncompetitive NMDA receptor antagonists, such as phencyclidine and its thienyl derivative TCP, block NMDA responses by binding within the NMDA-operated ionophore. Cerebral events that impair the mechanisms that regulate Ca^{2+} homeostasis can produce a prolonged elevation of intracellular Ca^{2+} concentration and cytotoxicity.

Several antagonists of the NMDA receptor/channel complex have been developed, some of which block the NMDA receptor (competitive NMDA antagonists) and others that block the associated cation channel (noncompetitive antagonists). Drugs such as 3-(2-carboxylpiperazin-4-yl)-propyl-1-phosphonic acid (CPP), CGS-19755, and 2-amino-5-phosphonovaleric acid (AP5) are competitive blockers at the NMDA receptor (23). The channel binding site is sometimes referred to as the phencyclidine receptor. Two potent preclinical noncompetitive channel-blocking drugs are MK-801 and phencyclidine (24, 25). The clinically approved anesthetic ketamine (26) and the antitussive dextromethorphan (27), as well as the anticonvulsant felbamate, are also NMDA channel blockers. Memantine, an "un-competitive" NMDA channel blocker, has recently been approved by the Food and Drug Administration for use in Alzheimer disease. It differs from noncompetitive NMDA blockers in that it binds more avidly to open channels, rather than indiscriminately blocking all channel conformations (28). This

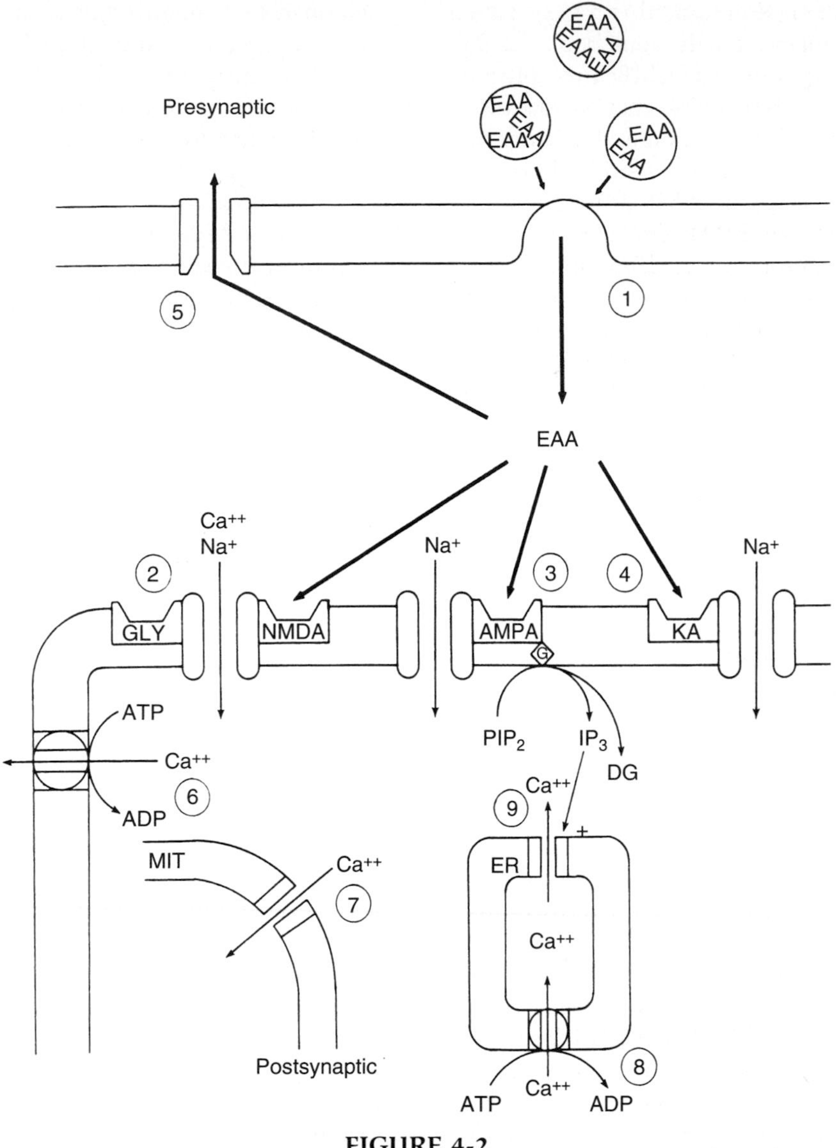

FIGURE 4-2

This schematic diagram outlines the synaptic components that contribute to EAA-mediated synaptic transmission, second-messenger generation, and calcium homeostasis. (1) EAAs such as glutamate are released from presynaptic terminals in a calcium-dependent process by presynaptic depolarization. (2–4) Glutamate in the synaptic cleft depolarizes the postsynaptic membrane by binding to at least three subsets of EAA receptors. Activation of (2) the NMDA receptor/channel complex, (3) AMPA receptors, and (4) kainate receptors, produced calcium (Ca^{2+}) and sodium (Na^+) entry through receptor-associated ionophores. Furthermore, activation of a subset of metabotropic receptors that are linked to phospholipase C produces phosphoinositol hydrolysis and generation of the second messengers inositol triphosphate and diacylglycerol. (5) The excitatory action of synaptically released EAA is terminated by a presynaptic, high-affinity, energy-dependent transport process.

mechanism may be associated with fewer psychotomimetic side effects than are associated with more complete channel blockade.

The NMDA receptor/channel complex also includes several regulatory sites. One receptor is specific for the simple amino acid glycine (29, 30). Unlike the inhibitory glycine site in the spinal cord, this site is not sensitive to strychnine, and activation facilitates opening of the NMDA channel by glutamate. Recognition sites for zinc and polyamines also appear to regulate NMDA receptor/channel complex activity (13). Drugs that block the glycine site on the NMDA receptor are being developed to attempt to avoid the psychotomimetic side effects of noncompetitive NMDA antagonists (31). Non-NMDA receptors were initially identified because they were activated preferentially by the glutamate analogs quisqualic acid and kainic acid (19). Kainic acid is a very potent neurotoxic and convulsant agent in the adult brain (32, 33). Currently, two major types of non-NMDA receptor are recognized: one that is linked to an ion channel that fluxes sodium and to a lesser extent calcium, and another that is linked to stimulation of phosphoinositide (PPI) turnover or downregulation of cyclic-AMP production (20). The so-called ionotropic non-NMDA receptors are now divided into kainate receptors and AMPA (alpha-amino-3-hydroxy-5-methyl-4-isoxazole propionate) receptors. Molecular studies indicate that these two receptors have similar molecular characteristics, with AMPA receptors made up from combinations of GluR1-4 receptor subunits, and kainate receptors made up of GluR5-7 subunits. AMPA receptors mediate most of the fast excitatory activity in the brain, and they include most of the receptors previously referred to as quisqualate receptors (20). The anticonvulsant topiramate is an AMPA receptor blocker. Kainate receptors stimulate presynaptic release of glutamate as well as activating postsynaptic receptors. The glutamate receptors linked to second messengers are called metabotropic receptors. A marked increase in glutamate release, which occurs during a prolonged seizure, is likely to result in the activation of all types of glutamate receptors.

DEVELOPMENT OF EXCITATORY AND INHIBITORY SYNAPTIC MARKERS

Synaptic markers for EAA neurotransmitters undergo marked changes during postnatal development (34–37). Studies of the ontogeny of NMDA and AMPA-sensitive receptor subtypes during postnatal development indicate that NMDA-type and non-NMDA-type glutamate receptors have a unique ontogenetic profile in the hippocampal formation (37). When receptors for NMDA-sensitive ^{3}H-glutamate binding, strychnine-insensitive glycine binding, and ^{3}H-N-(1[2-thienyl]cyclohexyl)3, 4-piperidine (TCP) binding to the channel were examined independently, all were found to be overexpressed in the neonatal period relative to the adult. NMDA-sensitive binding exceeded adult levels by 50 to 120 percent in all regions of the hippocampus examined, with peak densities occurring between postnatal days 10 and 28. The ontogenetic profiles of the glycine modulatory site and the phencyclidine receptor were similar to each other but were delayed with respect to the timing of the NMDA recognition site. The physiologic relevance of overexpression of NMDA recognition sites relative to other components of the NMDA receptor/channel complex is unclear. However, the temporal expression of NMDA recognition sites correlates with the molecular changes in receptor subunits and synaptogenesis (38–40). Studies of NMDA receptors in human cerebral cortex in early life have also demonstrated enhanced levels and different characteristics compared to adults (39, 41).

The ontogeny of NMDA receptor binding also appears to correlate with physiologic changes. Long-term potentiation, a synaptic correlate of memory, is enhanced during the neonatal period in rats, at the same time that NMDA-mediated neurotransmission predominates over AMPA-mediated activity (42). Postsynaptic excitation appears to predominate over inhibition during the first postnatal weeks of hippocampal development, as does enhanced seizure susceptibility (43). In CA3 of the hippocampus, superfusion with NMDA elicits recurrent synchronized burst activity, and the epileptogenic effect of NMDA increases from postnatal days 1 to 10 (44). Also, the susceptibility to epileptiform activity increases from postnatal days 4 to 6 to postnatal day 14 (45). This activity is blocked by specific NMDA receptor antagonists (46). The development of NMDA receptors tends to lag behind the development of sensitivity to NMDA neurotoxicity, which transiently peaks on day seven.

AMPA receptors also undergo developmental changes that make them more calcium permeable and more likely to mediate seizures and excitotoxicity in infancy and childhood (47). AMPA receptors that lack GluR2 subunits are calcium permeable, while AMPA receptors that include GluR2 subunits flux only sodium. Jensen and colleagues have studied the development of AMPA receptor subunits in rats and human postmortem tissue and found a correspondence between the expression of GluR2-lacking receptors and regional susceptibility to brain injury and seizures (48–50). GluR2-lacking AMPA receptors appear first in radial glia and oligodendrocytes in the periventricular white matter at 25–32 weeks gestation in humans (49). Their expression is delayed to around 40 weeks gestation in pyramidal neurons and nonpyramidal neurons of the cerebral cortex, persisting into early infancy and beyond in selected regions (49). These ontogenetic changes in AMPA receptors are consistent with experimental evidence that AMPA-receptor antagonists provide protection against seizures and damage at these stages in development (51).

The development of markers for GABAergic inhibitory synapses also undergoes major changes in the postnatal period and tends to lag behind development of excitatory synapses (52–54). $GABA_A$ receptor antagonists cause prolonged seizure-like discharges in the hippocampus of 2–3-week-old rats (43). However, during early life, extending to the end of the first week postnatal in rats, stimulation of $GABA_A$ receptors paradoxically produces excitation rather than inhibition, as a result of a lag in the development of the chloride KCC2 transporter, which maintains low intracellular Cl^- levels (55–58). Without this transporter, high concentrations of Cl^- accumulate within the dendrite, resulting in depolarization when the

Cl^- channel is opened by GABA. This is consistent with the theme that excitatory neurotransmission is enhanced early in development to support activity-dependent neuronal development and plasticity and becomes more balanced with inhibitory neurotransmission later in life (59). These developmental programs contribute to the higher incidence of seizures in infants and children.

DEVELOPMENTAL CHANGES IN GLUTAMATE NEUROTOXICITY

The immature brain is quite sensitive to neurotoxicity from glutamate and certain of its analogs (33, 60). Olney discovered a number of years ago that feeding monosodium glutamate to neonatal mice produced characteristic lesions in the hypothalamus (33). More recently, it has become clear that the receptors that mediate glutamate neurotoxicity respond differently in the immature brain compared with the adult brain. These observations have important implications for the EAA neurotransmitter hypothesis of epileptic brain injury in children.

In adults, kainic acid is the most potent neurotoxic analog of glutamate, but in neonatal rodents NMDA is the most toxic analog (60–62). Although kainic acid produces seizures in the immature brain, it produces little cytotoxicity (63). In contrast, NMDA injected into the 7-day-old rat brain produces prolonged seizures and extensive neurotoxicity. At 7 days of age, the relative neurotoxicity of several glutamate analogs is NMDA $>>>$ AMPA $>$ kainic $=$ zero, whereas in the adult kainic acid $>>$ NMDA $\geq$ AMPA. The severity of brain injury produced by direct injection of NMDA into the 7-day-old rat brain is approximately 60 times greater than in the adult (60). There is a relatively sharp peak of sensitivity to NMDA neurotoxicity at 7 days of age in the rat, with less sensitivity at times before and after, suggesting a potentially important effect of age on sensitivity to EAA-mediated injury. The shift in sensitivity to NMDA neurotoxicity parallels developmental changes in genetic expression of NMDA subunits that make up the receptor channel complex (40, 64). These changes appear to be programmed to mediate activity-dependent neuronal plasticity during early development (11). NMDA receptor activity is needed to promote normal development, and excessive blockade of these receptors leads to neuronal apoptosis (65). The NMDA receptor is a potential Achilles heel for the developing brain: both overstimulation and blockade can produce damage under certain circumstances (11).

The susceptibility of the developing brain to NMDA-induced brain injury parallels the susceptibility to hypoxic-ischemic brain injury. Olney's studies suggest that the acute neurohistologic picture of NMDA-induced injury in the 7-day-old rat brain is virtually identical to that from a hypoxic-ischemic injury at the same age (66). NMDA may induce metabolic changes similar to hypoxia-ischemia. Studies using ^{31}P MRS in brain slices indicate that NMDA produces a rapid exhaustion of phosphocreatine stores and nucleotide triphosphate levels following its application (67). The noncompetitive antagonist MK-801 protects against hypoxic-ischemic damage in the 7-day-old rat brain (68). These studies suggest that overactivation of NMDA receptors may be a final common pathway for hypoxic-ischemic injury, as well as other types of developmental brain injury.

EVIDENCE THAT EAA NEUROTRANSMITTERS PLAY A ROLE IN SEIZURE-RELATED INJURY

The link between excessive EAA neurotransmitter activity and epileptic brain injury was initially strengthened by Meldrum's pioneering studies in subhuman primates (9). These studies showed that seizures alone could damage the brain and that the EAA analog kainic acid produced sustained seizures and brain injury with a regional histologic pattern resembling epileptic brain injury. Similar studies of selective injury in the hippocampus from kainic acid injection into the brain have been performed in rodents by Nadler and colleagues (69). Two additional models in adult animals have also provided additional, more direct experimental evidence.

In experiments conducted by Sloviter, electrical stimulation of the perforant pathway that projects into the hippocampus from the entorhinal cortex leads to neuronal degeneration in hippocampal zones innervated by perforant pathway fibers (70). The perforant pathway is the major excitatory glutamatergic afferent pathway into the hippocampus (71). The acute neuropathologic changes produced by the persistent stimulation resemble the histopathology seen when glutamate analogues or other convulsant substances are injected into the hippocampus (72).

The pathology replicates the typical "epileptic" pattern of injury with damage to dentate basket cells, hilar cells, and CA3 and CA1 pyramidal cells of the hippocampus. CA2 neurons are typically spared. Electron microscopy shows acutely swollen dendritic segments distributed in a laminar pattern corresponding to the neuronal-receptive fields of EAA pathways in the perforant projection. Somatostatin-containing neurons are especially vulnerable, whereas GABA neurons are relatively spared (73).

In a second model of epileptic brain injury developed by Collins and Olney, persistent focal seizure activity is induced by focal application of the GABA receptor–blocking drug bicuculline onto the cerebral cortex (8). The seizure activity causes acute neurodegenerative changes in specific thalamic regions innervated by the corresponding corticothalamic pathway. This model also produces acute neuropathologic changes that resemble glutamate-like neuronal degeneration. Using this model, Olney's group demonstrated that ketamine and MK-801, two powerful blockers of the action of NMDA-type EAA receptors, completely abolish the thalamic damage caused by the focal seizure activity (74). MK-801 reduced but did not prevent the electrical seizure activity itself, suggesting that the neuroprotective action resulted from blockade of NMDA-type EAA receptor activation rather than from a reduction in neurotransmitter release. The results of these experiments, along with the electrical stimulation studies, support the hypothesis that EAA receptor stimulation plays an important role in seizure-induced neuronal injury. They also suggest that the neurotoxic effects of seizures can be dissociated from effects of excessive electrical activity.

MECHANISMS FOR SEIZURES AND INJURY IN THE IMMATURE BRAIN

The immature brain, especially the seven-day-old rat brain, is quite sensitive to seizures produced by NMDA as well as to NMDA-mediated neurotoxicity, but the relationship between the two is not clear. The models of prolonged direct electrical stimulation of the perforant pathway and of bicuculline-induced focal seizures described for adult animals have not been examined in the infant. However, both perforant pathway stimulation and the lithium-pilocarpine model of status epilepticus have been shown to produce neurotoxicity in the hippocampus of 15-day-old rodents (75). In our experiments, anticonvulsants such as phenytoin, diazepam, and pentobarbital markedly reduced NMDA-induced seizure activity but did not reduce the neurotoxic effects of injected NMDA (76). MK-801 and other NMDA antagonists produce significant levels of neuroprotection at doses that do not block behavioral seizures. Seizures induced by injection of NMDA in immature animals have some similarity to electrographic and behavioral changes seen in infantile spasms, and this is an active area of investigation (77, 78).

Activation of non-NMDA receptors also could contribute to seizure-related injury. A model in which kainic acid is injected into immature rodents has been extensively studied for its effects on brain injury as well as on long-term behavior. This is a useful model for trying to understand subtle effects of seizures themselves, as opposed to direct pathologic effects of neurotoxicity (79). Stimulation of AMPA receptors also produces seizures and brain injury in the immature rat (80). Metabotropic receptor stimulation may also contribute to effects of seizures because seizures stimulate phosphoinositide turnover and release of free fatty acids (81).

EAA mechanisms also could play a role in epileptogenesis and seizure expression (82). In an in vitro model of electrographic seizures in hippocampal slices, NMDA antagonists such as AP4 and MK-801 prevented the progressive development of seizures but did not block previously induced seizures (83). This suggests that the process of establishing a long-lasting seizure-prone state depends on the NMDA receptor/channel complex, whereas the expression of seizures does not. AMPA receptor–mediated mechanisms also appear to play an important role in seizure susceptibility that follows exposure to hypoxia in rodents (84). This suggests an important distinction between antiepileptogenic and anticonvulsant pharmacologic agents (85).

It is also possible that EAA receptors play a role in other more subtle developmental sequelae of seizures (43). In addition to their role in transmembrane signaling, EAA neurotransmitters participate in a variety of neurodevelopmental events. These include promotion of neuronal survival, growth, and differentiation of neurons; regulation of neuronal circuitry and cytoarchitecture; regulation of activity-dependent synaptic plasticity; and certain forms of learning and memory (86). Excitotoxic amino acids may act as neurotrophic factors promoting neuronal survival growth and differentiation during development. The NMDA receptor/channel complex appears to play a critical role in visually determined plasticity in the visual cortex (87). Drugs that block the NMDA receptor/channel complex may block the physiologically determined ocular dominance shifts that normally occur with monocular deprivation. The NMDA receptor/channel complex also appears to play a critical role in the formation of long-term potentiation, an electrical model of learning and memory (88). Disturbances in these normal developmental mechanisms by excessive EAA neurotransmitters released during repeated seizures could potentially be a mechanism for a variety of neurobehavioral disturbances in patients with seizures. Seizure-induced disturbances in EAA mechanisms involved in memory in the hippocampus might be responsible for disturbances in learning and memory in patients with frequent or prolonged seizures. This encephalopathic disturbance might occur in the absence of permanent injury.

Synaptic inhibitory mechanisms also play an important role in both short- and long–term changes that result from seizures. Short-term changes in GABA receptors appear to reduce the efficacy of anticonvulsant drugs that target these receptors after extended periods of status epilepticus (89–93). Injection of tetanus toxin into the hippocampus of immature rats produces selective impairment of GABA neurotransmission and seizures, and this treatment has been shown to induce long-term behavioral and learning deficits as well as changes in the expression of NMDA receptor subunits (43). These experimental results reflect the plastic responses of developing excitatory and inhibitory synaptic mechanisms to seizures.

METABOLIC AND PHARMACOLOGIC CONSEQUENCES OF SEIZURES

Excitatory Amino Acid Mechanisms in the Pathogenesis of Partial Epilepsy

Whether excitotoxic mechanisms play a role in the pathogenesis of childhood temporal lobe epilepsy associated with hippocampal damage is the subject of debate (94, 95). Although laboratory evidence discussed earlier suggests this is likely, human epidemiologic evidence suggest that prolonged seizures are usually harmless in children (7). Although a history of febrile status epilepticus is frequently obtained in patients undergoing temporal lobectomy surgery for partial complex seizures, magnetic resonance imaging (MRI) studies suggest that many patients have hippocampal malformations that predated onset of seizures (96). However, recent serial MRI has identified a few children who acquired hippocampal sclerosis following very prolonged febrile seizures (97). This suggests that EAA pathways may have a role in the pathogenesis of certain forms of chronic epilepsy.

Partial complex seizures following hippocampal injury or malformation are sometimes progressive, suggesting that further seizures lead to progressive injury and synaptic reorganization that promotes more seizures (98). EAA mechanisms could contribute to progressive metabolic disturbances and injury that could perpetuate this process. Studies of epileptogenic hippocampus using intracerebral microdialysis in patients undergoing monitoring prior to surgery showed high basal levels of glutamate, a low glutamate/glutamine ratio, and high lactate levels, which suggest poor glucose utilization (99). This is consistent with the observation that FDG PET commonly shows hypometabolism in epileptogenic hippocampi (100, 101). Interictal energy deficiency could contribute to impaired glutamate reuptake, persistently elevated glutamate, and EAA neurotoxicity. Abnormal recurrent sprouting of excitatory mossy fibers in the hippocampus that have lost their targets in the CA3 region has also been implicated in this process (102). Autoradiography studies of tissue resected from patients with temporal lobe epilepsy shows reduction in binding to the phencyclidine site of the NMDA receptor/channel complex and a relative increase in associated NMDA receptor sites (100). This resembles the ratio of receptor to channel binding found in the immature rat brain (37). Elevations in non-NMDA receptors have also been reported in human hippocampal tissue from patients with partial complex seizures (103). Studies of human hippocampal AMPA and NMDA messenger RNA and protein levels in brain tissue from temporal lobe epilepsy patients also found elevated levels for AMPA GluR1 and NMDA NR2 subunits (104, 105), as well as up-regulation of metabotropic mGluR5 receptors (106). These results suggest that alterations in glutamate receptor levels and subunit composition contribute to neuronal hyperexcitability and seizure generation in temporal lobe epilepsy.

These observations suggest a hypothetical mechanism for progressive epileptic change in certain patients with complex partial seizures (Figure 4-3). In this hypothesis, a severe insult such as prolonged status epilepticus or hypoxia-ischemia leads to EAA release and a glutamate type of injury to neurons in the hippocampus and other susceptible regions. This form of injury causes loss of some pyramidal neurons, but those that remain have stunted dendritic arbors (8, 43, 107). Perhaps in response to a reduced surface area of dendrites, postsynaptic NMDA receptor/channel complexes adjust by up-regulating their NMDA receptors. This would compensate for the reduced dendritic surface area available for excitatory input to the neuron. In addition, a reduction in the number of inhibitory GABA receptors might also serve to increase excitatory tone (100, 108).

An increased ratio of NMDA receptors per channel might sensitize the neuron to enhance excitability and further injury from physiological amounts of synaptic glutamate. Potentially, the seizure threshold might be lower, and further dendritic injury might result from excitatory events that are only mildly superphysiological. This additional injury in turn leads to a cycle of repeated seizures and injury. An important implication of this model is that pharmacological attempts could be made to prevent further EAA-mediated injury and thereby halt the progression of the disorder. Based on studies suggesting that there is a distinction between epileptogenesis and epileptic expression, drugs might be developed that would reduce the progressive epileptic process, although they themselves might not be good antiseizure agents (83, 85, 109).

CONCLUSION

Although seizures dramatically raise the brain's metabolic activity during the ictal event, they generally do not have any long-term damaging effect. However, data from animal models of status epilepticus and supraphysiological stimulation of specific excitatory pathways indicate that neuronal injury in sensitive areas such as the hippocampus can occur through a glutamate-mediated excitotoxic mechanism. Although children appear to be less affected by this mechanism than adults, recent experiments in animals suggest that the effects of prolonged seizures may be more injurious than previously thought (110). Studies in children suggest that hippocampal sclerosis occasionally

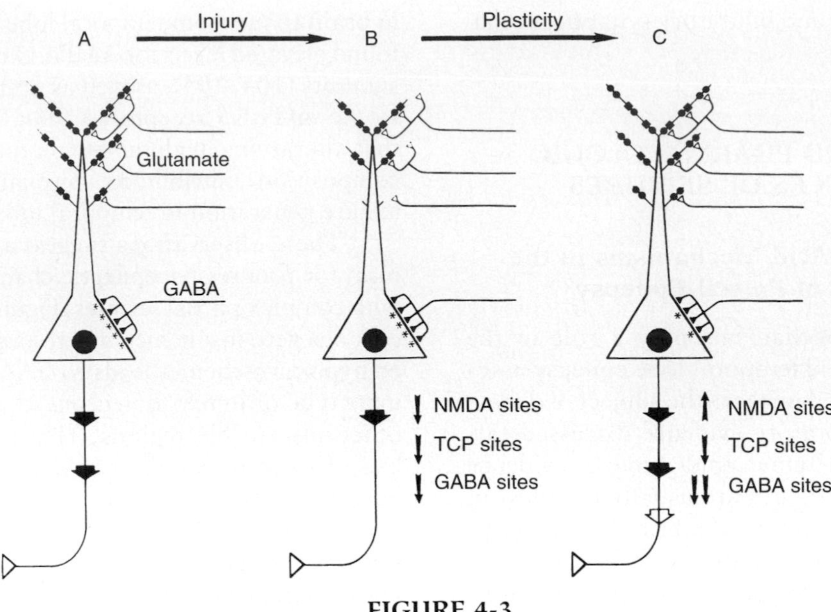

FIGURE 4-3

A speculative proposal of the mechanisms that contribute to the progressive epileptic changes observed in patients with complex partial seizures. (A) Schematic illustration of a typical pyramidal cell from Ca1–3 hippocampal subfields. Glutamatergic input (open triangles) from the perforant path originates in the entorhinal cortex and synapses on distal pyramidal cell dendrites and GABAergic interneurons. A severe focal cerebral insult causes overactivation of EAA receptors and produces excitotoxic injury, localized mainly to dendritic regions of the pyramidal cells. (B) The dendritic regions of surviving pyramidal cells are stunted, and the number of functional NMDA recognition sites (solid circles) and corresponding TCP channels (solid squares) is reduced. Moderate loss of functional $GABA_A$ sites occurs. As a result of impaired EAA synaptic transmission, the level of pyramidal cell excitation is reduced, as depicted by the large arrow of the emerging axon. In response to reduced pyramidal cell excitation, a series of compensatory synaptic alterations take place. (C) Dendritic zones regenerate, EAA neurotransmission is enhanced by up-regulating NMDA recognition sites, and the level of functional inhibition is reduced by down-regulating $GABA_A$ sites. These changes in turn would compensate for the reduced pyramid cell excitation that results from cerebral injury by increasing excitatory tone. However, these compensatory changes could produced enhanced susceptibility to seizure and seizure-related excitotoxicity by lowering the seizure threshold. The compensatory epileptogenic events lead to a cycle of repeated seizures and injury.

may be caused by prolonged febrile status epilepticus. Analysis of hippocampal tissue removed at surgery from patients with temporal lobe epilepsy indicate that levels of specific neuronal glutamate and GABA receptors are altered, which may contribute to epileptogenicity and a progressive cycle of further excitotoxic injury. A better understanding is needed of the factors that contribute to epileptic excitotoxicity.

References

1. Auer RN, Siesjo BK. Biological differences between ischemia, hypoglycemia, and epilepsy. *Ann Neurol* 1988; 24:699–707.
2. Ingvar M, Siesjo BK. Local blood flow and glucose consumption in the rat brain during sustained bicuculline-induced seizures. *Acta Neurol Scand* 1983; 68:129–144.
3. Pfund Z, Chugani DC, Juhasz C, Muzik O, et al. Evidence for coupling between glucose metabolism and glutamate cycling using FDG PET and ^{1}H magnetic resonance spectroscopy in patients with epilepsy. *J Cereb Blood Flow Metab* 2000; 20:871–878.
4. Magistretti PJ, Pellerin L, Rothman DL, Shulman RG. Energy on demand. *Science* 1999; 283:496–497.
5. Magistretti PJ, Pellerin L. Cellular mechanisms of brain energy metabolism. Relevance to functional brain imaging and to neurodegenerative disorders. *Ann N Y Acad Sci* 1996; 777:380–387.
6. Holmes GL, Khazipov R, Ben-Ari Y. Seizure-induced damage in the developing human: relevance of experimental models. *Prog Brain Res* 2002; 135:321–334.
7. Shinnar S, Pellock JM, Berg AT, O'Dell C, et al. Short-term outcomes of children with febrile status epilepticus. *Epilepsia* 2001; 42:47–53.
8. Olney JW, Collins RC, Sloviter RS. Excitotoxic mechanisms of epileptic brain damage. *Adv Neurol* 1986; 44:857–877.
9. Meldrum BS, Brierly JB. Prolonged epileptic seizures in primates. Ischemic cell change and its relationship to ictal physiological events. *Arch Neurol* 1973; 28:10–17.
10. Fonnum F. Glutamate: a neurotransmitter in mammalian brain. *J Neurochem* 1984; 42:1–11.
11. McDonald JW, Johnston MV. Physiological and pathophysiological roles of excitatory amino acids during central nervous system development. *Brain Res Brain Res Rev* 1990; 15:41–70.
12. Siesjo BK. Cell damage in the brain: a speculative synthesis. *J Cereb Blood Flow Metab* 1981; 1:155–185.
13. Choi DW. Ionic dependence of glutamate neurotoxicity. *J Neurosci* 1987; 7:369–379.
14. Rothman SM, Olney JW. Glutamate and the pathophysiology of hypoxic-ischemic brain damage. *Ann Neurol* 1986; 19:105–111.
15. DeLorenzo RJ, Sun DA. Basic mechanisms in status epilepticus: role of calcium in neuronal injury and the induction of epileptogenesis. *Adv Neurol* 2006; 97: 187–197.
16. Novelli A, Reilly JA, Lysko PG, Henneberry RC. Glutamate becomes neurotoxic via the N-methyl-D-aspartate receptor when intracellular energy levels are reduced. *Brain Res* 1988; 451:205–212.

17. Silverstein FS, Buchanan K, Johnston MV. Perinatal hypoxia-ischemia disrupts striatal high-affinity [^{3}H]glutamate uptake into synaptosomes. *J Neurochem* 1986; 47:1614–1619.
18. Watkins JC, Evans RH. Excitatory amino acid transmitters. *Annu Rev Pharmacol Toxicol* 1981; 21:165–204.
19. Monaghan DT, Bridges RJ, Cotman CW. The excitatory amino acid receptors: their classes, pharmacology, and distinct properties in the function of the central nervous system. *Annu Rev Pharmacol Toxicol* 1989; 29:365–402.
20. Watkins JC, Jane DE. The glutamate story. *Br J Pharmacol* 2006; 147 Suppl 1:S100–S108.
21. Moriyoshi K, Masu M, Ishii T, Shigemoto R, et al. Molecular cloning and characterization of the rat NMDA receptor. *Nature* 1991; 354:31–37.
22. Ascher P, Nowak L. The role of divalent cations in the N-methyl-D-aspartate responses of mouse central neurons in culture. *J Physiol* 1988; 399:247–266.
23. Boast CA, Gerhardt SC, Pastor G, Lehmann J, et al. The N-methyl-D-aspartate antagonists CGS 19755 and CPP reduce ischemic brain damage in gerbils. *Brain Res* 1988; 442:345–348.
24. Gill R, Foster AC, Woodruff GN. Systemic administration of MK-801 protects against ischemia-induced hippocampal neurodegeneration in the gerbil. *J Neurosci* 1987; 7:3343–3349.
25. McDonald JW, Silverstein FS, Johnston MV. Neuroprotective effects of MK-801, TCP, PCP and CPP against N-methyl-D-aspartate induced neurotoxicity in an in vivo perinatal rat model. *Brain Res* 1989; 490:33–40.
26. Borris DJ, Bertram EH, Kapur J. Ketamine controls prolonged status epilepticus. *Epilepsy Res* 2000; 42:117–122.
27. Hamosh A, McDonald JW, Valle D, Francomano CA, et al. Dextromethorphan and high-dose benzoate therapy for nonketotic hyperglycinemia in an infant. *J Pediatr* 1992; 121:131–135.
28. Lipton SA. Paradigm shift in neuroprotection by NMDA receptor blockade: memantine and beyond. *Nat Rev Drug Discov* 2006; 5:160–170.
29. Johnson JW, Ascher P. Glycine potentiates the NMDA response in cultured mouse brain neurons. *Nature* 1987; 325:529–531.
30. Slater P, McConnell SE, D'Souza SW, Barson AJ. Postnatal changes in N-methyl-D-aspartate receptor binding and stimulation by glutamate and glycine of [^{3}H]-MK-801 binding in human temporal cortex. *Br J Pharmacol* 1993; 108:1143–1149.
31. Wood PL. The NMDA receptor complex: a long and winding road to therapeutics. *IDrugs* 2005; 8:229–235.
32. Zaczek R, Nelson MF, Coyle JT. Effects of anaesthetics and anticonvulsants on the action of kainic acid in the rat hippocampus. *Eur J Pharmacol* 1978; 52:323–327.
33. Olney JW, Ho OL, Rhee V. Cytotoxic effects of acidic and sulphur containing amino acids on the infant mouse central nervous system. *Exp Brain Res* 1971; 14:61–76.
34. Ritter LM, Vazquez DM, Meador-Woodruff JH. Ontogeny of ionotropic glutamate receptor subunit expression in the rat hippocampus. *Brain Res Dev Brain Res* 2002; 139:227–236.
35. Brennan EM, Martin LJ, Johnston MV, Blue ME. Ontogeny of non-NMDA glutamate receptors in rat barrel field cortex: II. Alpha-AMPA and kainate receptors. *J Comp Neurol* 1997; 386:29–45.
36. Blue ME, Johnston MV. The ontogeny of glutamate receptors in rat barrel field cortex. *Brain Res Dev Brain Res* 1995; 84:11–25.
37. McDonald JW, Johnston MV, Young AB. Differential ontogenic development of three receptors comprising the NMDA receptor/channel complex in the rat hippocampus. *Exp Neurol* 1990; 110:237–247.
38. Harris KM, Jensen FE, Tsao B. Three-dimensional structure of dendritic spines and synapses in rat hippocampus (CA1) at postnatal day 15 and adult ages: implications for the maturation of synaptic physiology and long-term potentiation. *J Neurosci* 1992; 12:2685–2705.
39. Law AJ, Weickert CS, Webster MJ, Herman MM, et al. Expression of NMDA receptor NR1, NR2A and NR2B subunit mRNAs during development of the human hippocampal formation. *Eur J Neurosci* 2003; 18:1197–1205.
40. Sheng M, Cummings J, Roldan LA, Jan YN, et al. Changing subunit composition of heteromeric NMDA receptors during development of rat cortex. *Nature* 1994; 368: 144–147.
41. Slater P, McConnell SE, D'Souza SW, Barson AJ. Postnatal changes in N-methyl-D-aspartate receptor binding and stimulation by glutamate and glycine of [^{3}H]-MK-801 binding in human temporal cortex. *Br J Pharmacol* 1993; 108:1143–1149.
42. Crair MC, Malenka RC. A critical period for long-term potentiation at thalamocortical synapses. *Nature* 1995; 375:325–328.
43. Swann JW. The effects of seizures on the connectivity and circuitry of the developing brain. *Ment Retard Dev Disabil Res Rev* 2004; 33:96–100.
44. King AE, Cherubini E, Ben-Ari Y. N-methyl-D-aspartate induces recurrent synchronized burst activity in immature hippocampal CA3 neurones in vitro. *Brain Res Dev Brain Res* 1989; 46:1–8.
45. Swann JW, Brady RJ. Penicillin-induced epileptogenesis in immature rat CA3 hippocampal pyramidal cells. *Brain Res* 1984; 314:243–254.
46. Brady RJ, Swann JW. Ketamine selectively suppresses synchronized afterdischarges in immature hippocampus. *Neurosci Lett* 1986; 69:143–149.
47. Pellegrini-Giampietro DE, Gorter JA, Bennett MV, Zukin RS. The GluR2 (GluR-B) hypothesis: Ca(2+)-permeable AMPA receptors in neurological disorders. *Trends Neurosci* 1997; 20:464–470.
48. Jensen FE. The role of glutamate receptor maturation in perinatal seizures and brain injury. *Int J Dev Neurosci* 2002; 20:339–347.
49. Talos DM, Follett PL, Folkerth RD, Fishman RE, et al. Developmental regulation of alpha-amino-3-hydroxy-5-methyl-4-isoxazole-propionic acid receptor subunit expression in forebrain and relationship to regional susceptibility to hypoxic/ischemic injury. II. Human cerebral white matter and cortex. *J Comp Neurol* 2006; 497:61–77.
50. Talos DM, Fishman RE, Park H, Folkerth RD, et al. Developmental regulation of alpha-amino-3-hydroxy-5-methyl-4-isoxazole-propionic acid receptor subunit expression in forebrain and relationship to regional susceptibility to hypoxic/ischemic injury. I. Rodent cerebral white matter and cortex. *J Comp Neurol* 2006; 497:42–60.
51. Koh S, Tibayan FD, Simpson JN, Jensen FE. NBQX or topiramate treatment after perinatal hypoxia-induced seizures prevents later increases in seizure-induced neuronal injury. *Epilepsia* 2004; 45:569–575.
52. Brooks-Kayal AR, Pritchett DB. Developmental changes in human gamma-aminobutyric $acid_A$ receptor subunit composition. *Ann Neurol* 1993; 34:687–693.
53. Chandler KE, Princivalle AP, Fabian-Fine R, Bowery NG, et al. Plasticity of GABA(B) receptor-mediated heterosynaptic interactions at mossy fibers after status epilepticus. *J Neurosci* 2003; 23:11382–11391.
54. Johnston MV, Coyle JT. Ontogeny of neurochemical markers for noradrenergic, GABAergic, and cholinergic neurons in neocortex lesioned with methylazoxymethanol acetate. *J Neurochem* 1980; 34:1429–1441.
55. Dzhala VI, Talos DM, Sdrulla DA, Brumback AC, et al. NKCC1 transporter facilitates seizures in the developing brain. *Nat Med* 2005; 11:1205–1213.
56. Ben-Ari Y. Excitatory actions of GABA during development: the nature of the nurture. *Nat Rev Neurosci* 2002; 3:728–739.
57. Leinekugel X, Khalilov I, McLean H, Caillard O, et al. GABA is the principal fast-acting excitatory transmitter in the neonatal brain. *Adv Neurol* 1999; 79:189–201.
58. Chudotvorova I, Ivanov A, Rama S, Hubner CA, et al. Early expression of KCC2 in rat hippocampal cultures augments expression of functional GABA synapses. *J Physiol* 2005; 566:671–679.
59. Ben-Ari Y. Basic developmental rules and their implications for epilepsy in the immature brain. *Epileptic Disord* 2006; 8:91–102.
60. McDonald JW, Silverstein FS, Johnston MV. Neurotoxicity of N-methyl-D-aspartate is markedly enhanced in developing rat central nervous system. *Brain Res* 1988; 459: 200–203.
61. Campochiaro P, Coyle JT. Ontogenetic development of kainate neurotoxicity: correlates with glutamatergic innervation. *Proc Natl Acad Sci U S A* 1978; 75:2025–2029.
62. Ikonomidou C, Price MT, Mosinger JL, Frierdich G, et al. Hypobaric-ischemic conditions produce glutamate-like cytopathology in infant rat brain. *J Neurosci* 1989; 9: 1693–1700.
63. Holmes GL. Seizure-induced neuronal injury: animal data. *Neurology* 2002; 59:S3–S6.
64. Burgard EC, Hablitz JJ. Developmental changes in the voltage-dependence of neocortical NMDA responses. *Brain Res Dev Brain Res* 1994; 80:275–278.
65. Ikonomidou C, Bosch F, Miksa M, Bittigau P, et al. Blockade of NMDA receptors and apoptotic neurodegeneration in the developing brain. *Science* 1999; 283:70–74.
66. Ikonomidou C, Mosinger JL, Salles KS, Labruyere J, et al. Sensitivity of the developing rat brain to hypobaric/ischemic damage parallels sensitivity to N-methyl-aspartate neurotoxicity. *J Neurosci* 1989; 9:2809–2818.
67. Jacquin T, Gillet B, Fortin G, Pasquier C, et al. Metabolic action of N-methyl-D-aspartate in newborn rat brain ex vivo: ^{31}P magnetic resonance spectroscopy. *Brain Res* 1989; 497: 296–304.
68. McDonald JW, Silverstein FS, Johnston MV. MK-801 protects the neonatal brain from hypoxic-ischemic damage. *Eur J Pharmacol* 1987; 140:359–361.
69. Nadler JV, Perry BW, Gentry C, Cotman CW. Fate of the hippocampal mossy fiber projection after destruction of its postsynaptic targets with intraventricular kainic acid. *J Comp Neurol* 1981; 196:549–569.
70. Sloviter RS, Damiano BP. Sustained electrical stimulation of the perforant path duplicates kainate-induced electrophysiological effects and hippocampal damage in rats. *Neurosci Lett* 1981; 24:279–284.
71. Olney JW, deGubareff T, Sloviter RS. "Epileptic" brain damage in rats induced by sustained electrical stimulation of the perforant path. II. Ultrastructural analysis of acute hippocampal pathology. *Brain Res Bull* 1983; 10:699–712.
72. Sloviter RS, Dempster DW. "Epileptic" brain damage is replicated qualitatively in the rat hippocampus by central injection of glutamate or aspartate but not by GABA or acetylcholine. *Brain Res Bull* 1985; 15:39–60.
73. Martin JL, Sloviter RS. Focal inhibitory interneuron loss and principal cell hyperexcitability in the rat hippocampus after microinjection of a neurotoxic conjugate of saporin and a peptidase-resistant analog of Substance P. *J Comp Neurol* 2001; 436:127–152.
74. Clifford DB, Olney JW, Benz AM, Fuller TA, et al. Ketamine, phencyclidine, and MK-801 protect against kainic acid-induced seizure-related brain damage. *Epilepsia* 1990; 31:382–390.
75. Wasterlain CG. Recurrent seizures in the developing brain are harmful. *Epilepsia* 1997; 38: 728–734.
76. McDonald JW, Johnston MV. Excitatory amino acid neurotoxicity in the developing brain. *NIDA Res Monogr* 1993; 133:185–205.
77. Stafstrom CE, Holmes GL. Infantile spasms: criteria for an animal model. *Int Rev Neurobiol* 2002; 49:391–411.
78. Rho JM. Basic science behind the catastrophic epilepsies. *Epilepsia* 2004; 45 Suppl 5:5–11.
79. Stafstrom CE, Chronopoulos A, Thurber S, Thompson JL, et al. Age-dependent cognitive and behavioral deficits after kainic acid seizures. *Epilepsia* 1993; 34:420–432.
80. McDonald JW, Trescher WH, Johnston MV. Susceptibility of brain to AMPA induced excitotoxicity transiently peaks during early postnatal development. *Brain Res* 1992; 583: 54–70.
81. Iadorola MJ, Nicoletti F, Naranjo JR, Putnam F, et al. Kindling enhances the stimulation of inositol phospholipid hydrolysis elicited by ibotenic acid in rat hippocampal slices. *Brain Res* 1986; 374:174–178.

82. Hablitz JJ, Lee WL. NMDA receptor involvement in epileptogenesis in the immature neocortex. *Epilepsy Res Suppl* 1992; 8:139–145.
83. Stasheff SF, Anderson WW, Clark S, Wilson WA. NMDA antagonists differentiate epileptogenesis from seizure expression in an in vitro model. *Science* 1989; 245: 648–651.
84. Jensen FE. The role of glutamate receptor maturation in perinatal seizures and brain injury. *Int J Dev Neurosci* 2002; 20:339–347.
85. Suchomelova L, Baldwin RA, Kubova H, Thompson KW, et al. Treatment of experimental status epilepticus in immature rats: dissociation between anticonvulsant and antiepileptogenic effects. *Pediatr Res* 2006; 59:237–243.
86. Mattson MP. Neurotransmitters in the regulation of neuronal cytoarchitecture. *Brain Res* 1988; 472:179–212.
87. Kleinschmidt A, Bear MF, Singer W. Blockade of "NMDA" receptors disrupts experience-dependent plasticity of kitten striate cortex. *Science* 1987; 238:355–358.
88. Nicoll RA. Expression mechanisms underlying long-term potentiation: a postsynaptic view. *Philos Trans R Soc Lond B Biol Sci* 2003; 358:721–726.
89. Brooks-Kayal AR. Rearranging receptors. *Epilepsia* 2005; 46 Suppl:29–38.
90. Jones-Davis DM, Macdonald RL. GABA(A) receptor function and pharmacology in epilepsy and status epilepticus. *Curr Opin Pharmacol* 2003; 3:12–18.
91. Sankar R, Shin D, Liu H, Wasterlain C, Mazarati A. Epileptogenesis during development: injury, circuit recruitment, and plasticity. *Epilepsia* 2002; 43 Suppl 5:47–53.
92. Nishimura T, Schwarzer C, Gasser E, Kato N, et al. Altered expression of GABA(A) and GABA(B) receptor subunit mRNAs in the hippocampus after kindling and electrically induced status epilepticus. *Neuroscience* 2005; 134:691–704.
93. Naylor DE, Liu H, Wasterlain CG. Trafficking of GABA(A) receptors, loss of inhibition, and a mechanism for pharmacoresistance in status epilepticus. *J Neurosci* 2005; 25: 7724–7733.
94. Lewis DV, Barboriak DP, MacFall JR, Provenzale JM, et al. Do prolonged febrile seizures produce medial temporal sclerosis? Hypotheses, MRI evidence and unanswered questions. *Prog Brain Res* 2002; 135:263–278.
95. Lewis DV. Losing neurons: selective vulnerability and mesial temporal sclerosis. *Epilepsia* 2005; 46 Suppl 7:39–44.
96. Fernandez G, Effenberger O, Vinz B, Steinlein O, et al. Hippocampal malformation as a cause of familial febrile convulsions and subsequent hippocampal sclerosis. 1998. *Neurology* 2001; 57:S13–S21.
97. VanLandingham KE, Heinz ER, Cavazos JE, Lewis DV. Magnetic resonance imaging evidence of hippocampal injury after prolonged focal febrile convulsions. *Ann Neurol* 1998; 43:413–426.
98. Sutula TP, Pitkanen A. More evidence for seizure-induced neuron loss: is hippocampal sclerosis both cause and effect of epilepsy? *Neurology* 2001; 57:169–170.
99. Cavus I, Kasoff WS, Cassaday MP, Jacob R, et al. Extracellular metabolites in the cortex and hippocampus of epileptic patients. *Ann Neurol* 2005 Feb;57:226-235.
100. McDonald JW, Garofalo EA, Hood T, Sackellares JC, et al. Altered excitatory and inhibitory amino acid receptor binding in hippocampus of patients with temporal lobe epilepsy. *Ann Neurol* 1991; 29:529–541.
101. Chassoux F, Semah F, Bouilleret V, Landre E, et al. Metabolic changes and electro-clinical patterns in mesio-temporal lobe epilepsy: a correlative study. *Brain* 2004; 127:164–174.
102. Holmes GL. Epilepsy in the developing brain: lessons from the laboratory and clinic. *Epilepsia* 1997; 38:12–30.
103. Hosford DA, Crain BJ, Cao Z, Bonhaus DW, et al. Increased AMPA-sensitive quisqualate receptor binding and reduced NMDA receptor binding in epileptic human hippocampus. *J Neurosci* 1991; 11:428–434.
104. Mathern GW, Pretorius JK, Kornblum HI, Mendoza D, et al. Human hippocampal AMPA and NMDA mRNA levels in temporal lobe epilepsy patients. *Brain* 1997; 120 (Pt 11):1937–1959.
105. Mathern GW, Pretorius JK, Mendoza D, Lozada A, et al. Increased hippocampal AMPA and NMDA receptor subunit immunoreactivity in temporal lobe epilepsy patients. *J Neuropathol Exp Neurol* 1998 Jun;57:615–634.
106. Notenboom RG, Hampson DR, Jansen GH, van Rijen PC, et al. Up-regulation of hippocampal metabotropic glutamate receptor 5 in temporal lobe epilepsy patients. *Brain* 2006; 129:96–107.
107. Swann JW, Al-Noori S, Jiang M, Lee CL. Spine loss and other dendritic abnormalities in epilepsy. *Hippocampus* 2000; 10:617–625.
108. Loup F, Wieser HG, Yonekawa Y, Aguzzi A, Fritschy JM. Selective alterations in $GABA_A$ receptor subtypes in human temporal lobe epilepsy. *J Neurosci* 2000; 20:5401–5419.
109. McNamara JO, Russell RD, Rigsbee L, Bonhaus DW. Anticonvulsant and antiepileptogenic actions of MK-801 in the kindling and electroshock models. *Neuropharmacology* 1988; 27:563–568.
110. Holmes GL, Ben-Ari Y. Seizures in the developing brain: perhaps not so benign after all. *Neuron* 1998; 21:1231–1234.

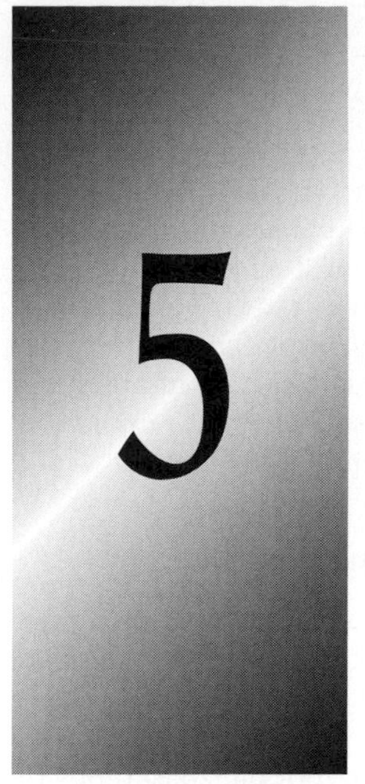

Neuropathologic Substrates of Epilepsy

Carolyn R. Houser
Harry V. Vinters

INTRODUCTION

The purpose of this chapter will be to review selected neuropathologic substrates of intractable epilepsy, including lesions that cause seizures in infants and children, as well as adults. We will not consider the pathologic findings in (usually low-grade) neoplasms that are especially common as a cause of intractable epilepsy.

PATHOLOGY OF TEMPORAL LOBE EPILEPSY

Temporal lobe epilepsy (TLE) is the most common form of epilepsy across all age groups, and hippocampal sclerosis is the most consistent pathology in this disorder. Although TLE is often diagnosed in adolescence or adulthood, the processes leading to epilepsy may have begun earlier and, in many cases, during childhood. In this context, we will consider the patterns of neuronal loss, as well as preservation, in hippocampal sclerosis; evidence for plasticity of remaining neurons, including the reorganization of their axons and synaptic connections; and a disorganization of the granule cells of the dentate gyrus that could be related to alterations in basic developmental programs for neuronal migration.

Neuronal Loss and Resultant Circuitry

Hippocampal sclerosis is characterized by a well-recognized and intriguing pattern of neuronal loss. This typically includes extensive loss of neurons in three major regions of the hippocampal formation—the hilus or polymorph layer of the dentate gyrus, CA3 and CA1 (1–3) (Figure 5-1). In contrast, granule cells of the dentate gyrus and neurons of CA2 and the subiculum are comparatively well preserved (Figure 5-1), even though some cell loss often occurs in these regions also. The cell loss is accompanied by gliosis, and the combined changes lead to a smaller than normal hippocampus (Figure 5-1A, B).

Despite extensive neuronal loss, a functional circuit through the hippocampal formation is likely to remain. Even in the neuron-depleted CA1 and CA3 fields, some neurons are frequently present, either locally, within a hippocampal slice, or at different anterior-posterior levels of the hippocampus. It is presumed that such neurons continue to form a functional hippocampal circuit. Importantly, major input and output regions of the hippocampal formation, the dentate granule cells and subicular neurons, respectively, remain relatively intact. However, the normal inputs to both regions are often severely reduced as a result of cell loss in other hippocampal regions. Loss of both inhibitory gamma-aminobutyric acid (GABA) neurons and

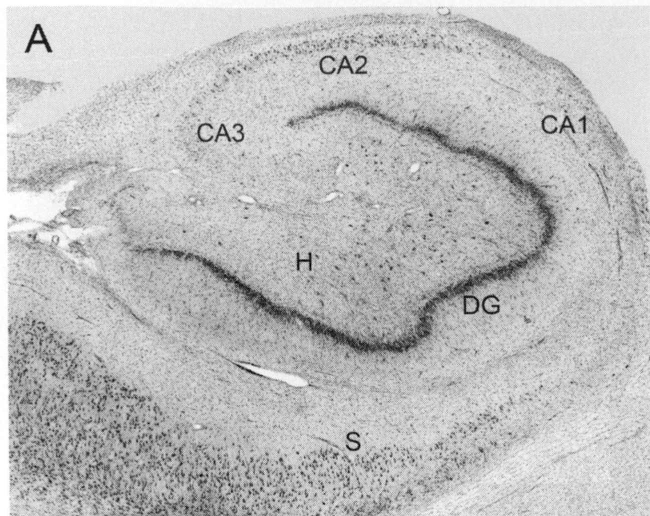

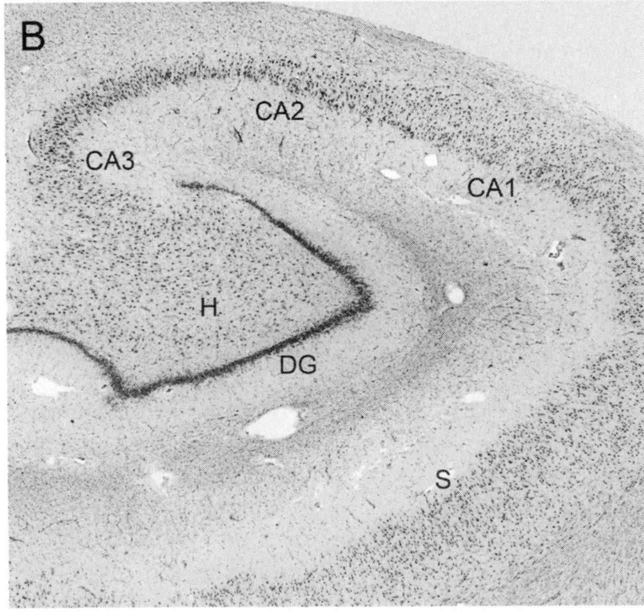

FIGURE 5-1

Hippocampal formation of human temporal lobe epilepsy (A) and normal autopsy (B) specimens that are stained with cresyl violet to demonstrate neuronal cell bodies. (A) The epilepsy specimen exhibits hippocampal sclerosis that is characterized by the smaller size of the hippocampus (compare to control in Panel B) and severe depletion of neurons in the dentate hilus (H), CA3 and CA1. Granule cells of the dentate gyrus (DG) and neurons in CA2 and the subciulum (S) are comparatively well preserved. (B) In a control specimen, neurons are abundant throughout the hilus (H) of the dentate gyrus (DG) and in the pyramidal cell layer of all hippocampal fields (CA3, CA2, CA1) and the subiculum (S). Specimens are shown at the same magnification.

excitatory mossy cells in the hilus reduces their control of the dentate granule cells, and such loss of neurons in the hilus (sometimes referred to as CA4) is one of the most consistent findings in TLE (1, 4, 5). Likewise, the severe depletion of CA1 neurons considerably reduces the normal input to the subiculum. Yet the subiculum remains active and constitutes a major output of the hippocampal formation. Activity from the subiculum can be propagated to the entorhinal cortex and from there to widespread regions of the brain as well as back to the dentate gyrus in a reentrant excitatory path. Thus, despite neuronal loss, a hippocampal circuit persists, and alterations of this remaining basic circuit are likely to form the morphological substrates for the excessive, hypersynchronous activity of epilepsy.

Reorganization of Remaining Neurons

Axonal Reorganization as a Basic Feature of TLE Pathology. Although, for many years, the focus of pathological studies of TLE has been on neuronal loss, it has become increasingly clear that remaining neurons and their connections are a critical part of the "pathology of epilepsy." When the initial cell loss occurs in childhood, remaining neurons are present during a period when the nervous system has the capacity for the greatest developmental plasticity. In particular, processes such as axonal growth and synaptogenesis could be stimulated. Indeed, numerous studies now suggest that reorganization of the synaptic connections of remaining neurons is a central feature of the morphological changes in TLE. This axonal reorganization appears to occur in both principal cells (granule cells of the dentate gyrus and pyramidal cells of the hippocampus) and GABAergic interneurons.

Reorganization of Principal Cells. The reorganization or sprouting of mossy fibers that originate from dentate granule cells is one of the most striking alterations in the hippocampus of humans with TLE. Since the early descriptions of mossy fiber sprouting in human epilepsy (6–8), numerous studies have confirmed the findings in a very high percentage of cases (e.g., 9, 10).

The mossy fibers and their axon collaterals normally innervate neurons in the hilus and CA3, but in many patients with TLE, the mossy fibers are distributed aberrantly in the inner molecular layer, where they form a distinct band above the granule cell layer (Figure 5-2A, C). The inner molecular layer is normally innervated by excitatory mossy cells of the hilus, and these neurons are frequently lost as part of the extensive cell loss in the hilus. Loss of mossy cells may serve as a major stimulus for reorganization of mossy fibers into these regions because, through their loss, many of the normal targets of the granule cells in the hilus are missing (7). Also, synaptic sites on granule cells in the inner molecular layer are vacated as a result of degeneration of mossy cell terminals.

The reorganized mossy fibers in human TLE appear to develop completely and form synaptic contacts in the molecular layer (8, 11, 12). The time course of mossy

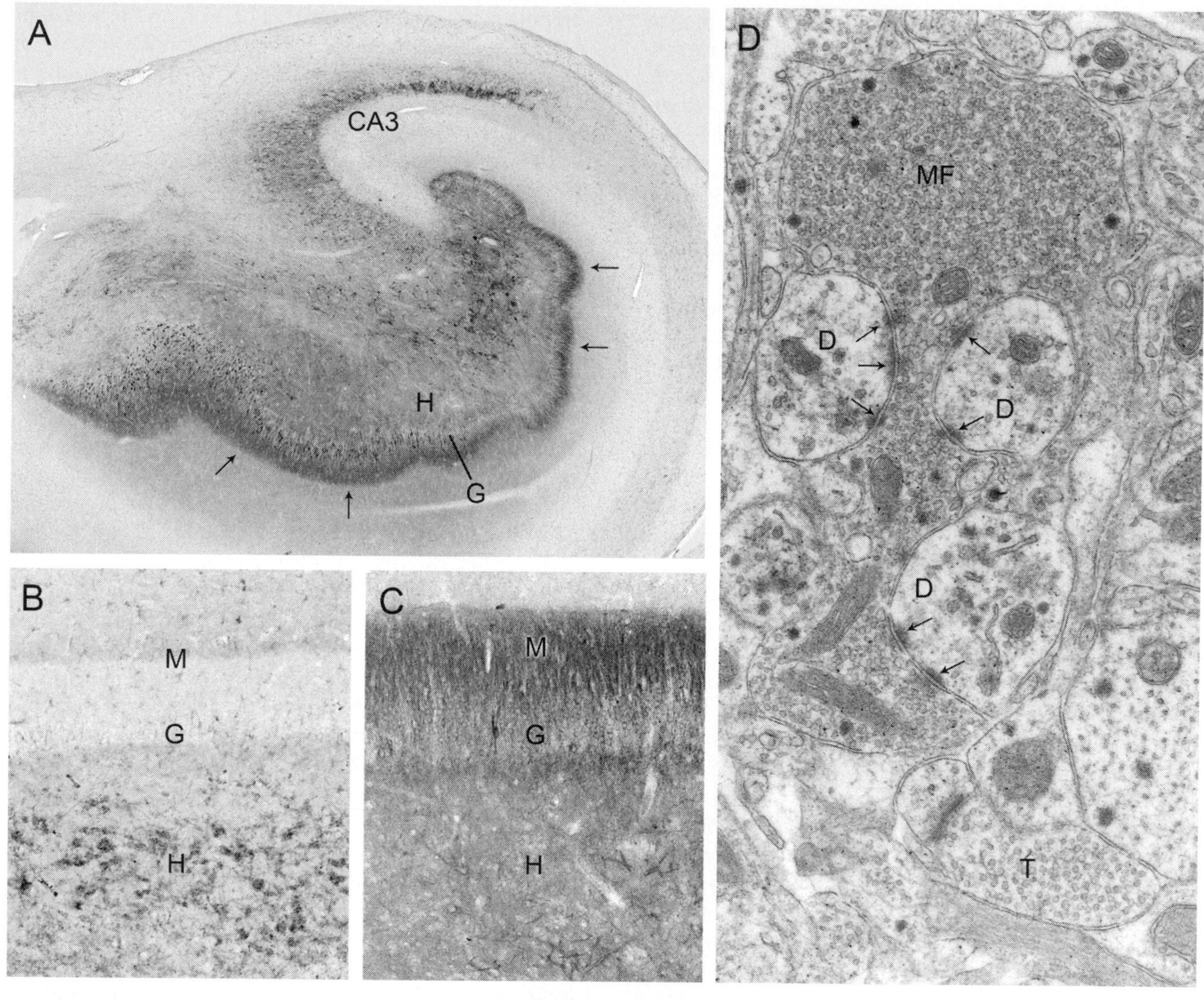

FIGURE 5-2

Dynorphin labeling of mossy fibers in the human hippocampus. (A) In a human temporal lobe epilepsy (TLE) specimen, a dense band of labeled fibers (arrows) is present in the inner molecular layer of the dentate gyrus and indicates an aberrant distribution of mossy fibers from dentate granule cells (G). Normally, such mossy fibers are restricted to the dentate hilus (H) and CA3. (B) In a control autopsy specimen, dynorphin-labeled mossy fibers are concentrated around neurons in the hilus (H) and are not present in the granule cell (G) and molecular (M) layers. (C) In a TLE specimen, dynorphin-labeled mossy fibers are concentrated in the inner molecular layer (M), and the normal labeling around cell bodies in the hilus (H) is reduced due to loss of neurons in this region. (D) In an electron micrograph of a TLE specimen, a dynorphin-containing mossy fiber terminal (MF) in the inner molecular layer contains numerous clear synaptic vesicles as well as several dense core vesicles. The terminal forms distinct, asymmetric synaptic contacts (arrows) with several dendritic profiles (D). The size of the mossy fiber terminal is considerably larger than that of another terminal (T) in the region.

fiber reorganization in humans cannot be determined, but in surgical specimens from patients with chronic epilepsy, the reorganized terminals appear morphologically mature (12). If the mossy fiber terminals had remained in an immature state, they would likely resemble developing mossy fiber terminals in rodents, in which synaptic vesicles are sparse and mitochondrial profiles are few (13). Remarkably, in human TLE, the reorganized mossy fiber terminals are packed with clear synaptic vesicles (Figure 5-2D), presumably containing glutamate, and contain numerous mitochondrial profiles, suggesting that the terminals are functional and capable of strong, excitatory influences. Many of the terminal profiles in humans are relatively large (Figure 5-2D), with a mean major diameter of 2.3 μm, and this exceeds the size of most other axon terminals in the region (12).

Whether the reorganized mossy fibers form synaptic contacts with inhibitory neurons or other granule cells is important for determining their function, and the predominant target of sprouted mossy fibers in animal models continues to be debated (14–16). However, in humans, granule cell dendrites appear to be the most common target, with the vast majority of synaptic contacts being formed with dendritic spines and the remainder with dendritic shafts of granule cells (8, 11, 12).

The morphological features of the reorganized mossy fiber synapses suggest that they could exert strong excitatory influences. The reorganized mossy fiber terminals in humans establish distinct, asymmetric synapses that are characteristic of excitatory synapses, and a single terminal often establishes multiple synaptic contacts (Figure 5-2D). The large aberrant mossy fibers are indented and invaginated by multiple spines (12), and such patterns are characteristic of the final stages of normal mossy fiber development in CA3, when complex spines are formed (13). Thus, reorganized mossy fibers in the human dentate gyrus appear to have progressed through their full development and show synaptic organization that is consistent with a powerful, aberrant, reexcitatory circuit among granule cells.

Reorganized mossy fibers provide the clearest example to date of axonal reorganization and new synapse formation in the human central nervous system (CNS). However, axonal reorganization of other excitatory neurons is also likely to occur in TLE. In the dentate gyrus, the normal projection from the supramammillary region to the inner molecular layer appears to have increased, as indicated by an expanded band of calretinin labeling (17). Thus growth and reorganization of extrinsic as well as intrinsic excitatory projections may occur in the dentate gyrus in TLE and contribute to enhanced excitability in the region.

Axonal reorganization may also occur in CA1 and other regions where there is partial loss of principal neurons. Aberrant collateral sprouting of CA1 pyramidal cell axons into the pyramidal cell layer and stratum radiatum has been described in human TLE following injections of fluorescent tracers in hippocampal slices (18). This network reorganization could contribute to increased excitability and synchrony among the CA1 neurons.

Loss and Reorganization of GABA Neurons. The general histological view of neuronal loss and preservation in TLE emphasizes the principal, excitatory neurons that form the basic circuitry through the hippocampal formation. The fate of GABA neurons that control activity within the circuit has been more difficult to determine. Indeed, early reports appeared to be contradictory, with some studies suggesting that GABA neurons are preserved in the hippocampus of humans with TLE (19) and others demonstrating loss of specific groups of peptide-containing neurons (20, 21) that are known to be subgroups of GABA neurons.

Current findings indicate that the changes in GABA neurons in human TLE are indeed complex but fascinating. First, different classes of GABA neurons appear to have different vulnerabilities, according to whether they innervate dendritic regions or perisomatic sites that include cell bodies and axon initial segments (5, 22). Within the dentate gyrus, neurons that terminate in dendritic regions are among the most vulnerable to damage, and many of these neurons are labeled with somatostatin and neuropeptide Y (NPY). Loss of these neurons was demonstrated initially by de Lanerolle and colleagues and others (20, 23), and their loss has been confirmed in subsequent studies (24). Because many of the cell bodies of somatostatin- and NPY-containing neurons that innervate dentate granule cells are located in the hilus, the loss of hilar neurons in TLE provides additional support for degeneration of these groups of neurons, perhaps as a result of an initial precipitating event (25, 26). This would be consistent with the extreme vulnerability of somatostatin neurons in animal models following status epilepticus, ischemia, and traumatic head injury (27–31). These hilar neurons normally project to the dentate molecular layer, where they help regulate the responses of granule cells to excitatory input from the entorhinal cortex, and loss of these GABA neurons could increase granule cell excitability in response to this input.

Despite the marked loss of hilar neurons, a plexus of somatostatin- and NPY-containing fibers can still be observed in the molecular layer at chronic stages of epilepsy (20). Such findings have suggested that remaining GABA neurons, either within the hilus or other regions of the hippocampus, may have reorganized their axonal connections. This potentially reorganized plexus no longer exhibits a normal laminar pattern in the molecular layer and, instead, is distributed throughout the layer (20, 32). Despite the potential sprouting of these axons, their laminar distribution and associated specificity are altered, and thus it is unlikely that they will compensate fully for loss of the normal GABAergic innervation of the dendritic region.

In contrast to a severe loss of hilar GABA neurons that innervate granule cell dendrites, those that innervate perisomatic regions in the dentate gyrus and hippocampus may be relatively well preserved (33, 34). Many of these neurons normally express the calcium-binding protein parvalbumin, and several studies of human TLE have reported a decrease in parvalbumin labeling (33, 35–37). Although this could reflect a loss of these GABA neurons, electron microscopic studies have found that many GABAergic axon terminals around the cell bodies and axon initial segments, presumed to originate from parvalbumin-containing neurons, are preserved (33, 34, 37). Thus the decreased parvalbumin labeling has been interpreted by some investigators as a decrease in parvalbumin content in persisting interneurons (34). In regions such as the dentate gyrus, the number of terminals and complexity of the innervation around the cell bodies and along the axon initial segments are even increased (33, 38). Such alterations have again suggested sprouting of remaining GABA neurons.

While such changes could be viewed as compensatory, Maglóczky and Freund have suggested that the maintained or increased GABAergic innervation on the cell bodies and axon initial segments of projection neurons could contribute to enhanced, abnormal synchronization of neuronal firing (22). This is consistent with current views of GABAergic function, in which GABAergic innervation at perisomatic locations is considered to be critical for the normal synchronization of ensembles of principal cells (39).

The complexity of changes in GABAergic innervation in TLE has been emphasized in detailed studies of axo-axonic cells by deFelipe (37) and others (38). Despite what appeared to be a general preservation of perisomatic GABAergic innervation in human TLE, a loss of GABAergic terminals along the axon initial segments of some granule cells was identified (38). When a loss was observed, it was often extreme and could be sufficient to severely decrease inhibitory influences at the axon initial segment, which strongly influences the final output of the projection neurons (38). These findings suggest that loss of even a small number of GABA neurons could severely deplete the GABAergic innervation at critical locations on remaining principal cells, and such projection neurons could feasibly become sites of seizure initiation.

Calbindin-containing interneurons are an additional group of GABA neurons that may be preserved in several regions of the hippocampal formation (17, 35). However, these persisting neurons undergo numerous morphological changes that include increased numbers of spines and increased GABAergic innervation (40, 41). Increased inhibitory control of inhibitory interneurons could potentially limit their output and lead to decreased inhibitory control of the principal cells.

Finally, although no loss of GABA neurons and their terminals has been observed in the subiculum (38), functional alterations in GABAergic signaling have recently been described in this region. In a subgroup of pyramidal cells of the subiculum of human TLE specimens, GABA had unexpected depolarizing actions, and the resultant activity contributed to rhythmic interictal discharges (42). These responses are reminiscent of GABA-mediated excitation that occurs during early development and is related to late expression of the potassium-chloride cotransporter (KCC2) that normally extrudes Cl^- from the cell (43). Further studies have demonstrated both down-regulation of the KCC2 transporter mRNA and up-regulation of the Na^+-K^+-$2Cl^-$ (NKCC1) transporter mRNA, a transporter that facilitates accumulation of Cl^- within neurons, in the subiculum in human TLE (44). Interestingly, similar changes were not found in the hippocampus or temporal neocortex. A functional reversion of some neurons in TLE to earlier developmental stages, when GABA has excitatory actions, could substantially alter GABAergic influences and possibly contribute to seizure activity (45–47).

Current findings thus suggest that GABA neurons and their function can be altered in multiple ways in TLE. Clearly some groups of GABA neurons are vulnerable to damage, and their loss could reduce GABAergic control of principal cells at dendritic sites, where they receive their major excitatory input. In contrast, many GABA neurons remain viable, may exhibit substantial axonal reorganization, and could contribute to enhanced neuronal synchronization. Finally, some remaining GABA neurons could exert excitatory influences in specific regions of the hippocampal formation.

Reorganization of the axons and synaptic connections of both principal cells and GABAergic interneurons now appears to be a central component of hippocampal pathology in TLE. Interestingly, the sprouting of excitatory neurons, as well as inhibitory neurons that innervate perisomatic sites, could contribute to enhanced synchrony of the projection neurons of the circuit, although through different mechanisms (22, 48). Determining the "rules" that govern such reorganization and its time course is critical for developing interventions that could limit the formation and maturation of aberrant synaptic connections that are likely to contribute to seizure activity.

Granule Cell Disorganization

Altered Patterns of Dentate Granule Cells. In many patients with TLE and hippocampal sclerosis, the granule cells of the dentate gyrus are one of the most persistent groups of neurons. However, in a subpopulation of these patients, the granule cells have a disorganized appearance that contrasts sharply with the compact, relatively narrow band of granule cells in the normal hippocampus (Figure 5-3A). The most common altered pattern has been described as granule cell dispersion (49) and is characterized by a wider than normal granule cell layer, increased space between many of the granule cells, and poorly defined laminar borders (Figure 5-3B). The granule cells are often aligned in vertical rows that extend into the

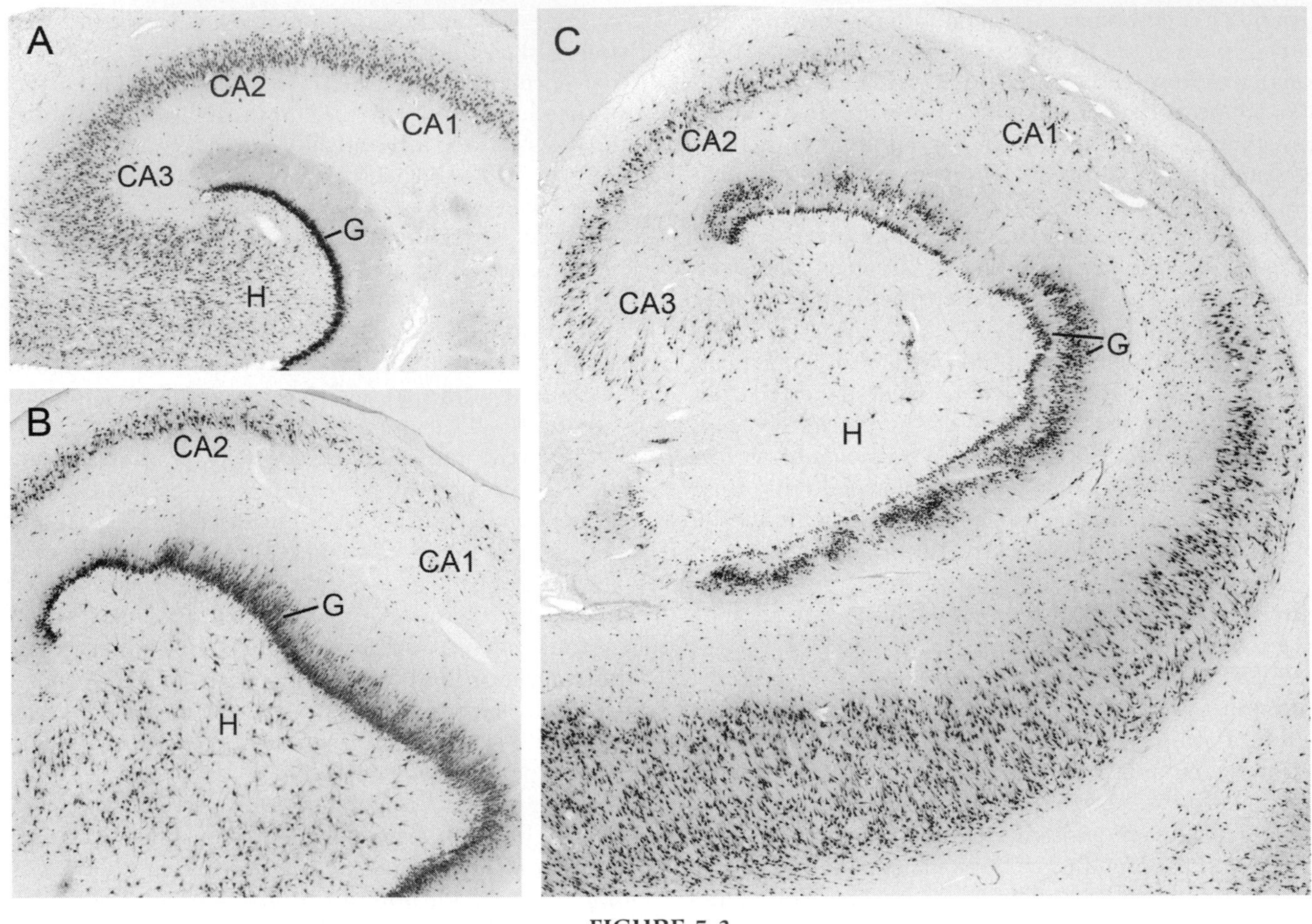

FIGURE 5-3

Granule cell organization in the human hippocampus of control autopsy (A) and temporal lobe epilepsy (TLE) (B, C) specimens as demonstrated by NeuN immunolabling. (A) In control tissue, the granule cells of the dentate gyrus are closely approximated and form a relatively narrow, compact granule cell layer (G). (B) In a TLE specimen, granule cells (G) are dispersed, creating a widened layer with uneven borders. Granule cell somata are more widely separated than normal, particularly in the outer part of the layer. (C) In another TLE specimen, the granule cells (G) form a bilaminar pattern with a relatively cell-free zone between the two layers of neurons. Severe loss of neurons is evident in the hilus (H), CA3 and CA1.

molecular layer to varying extents and create an irregular outer border of the granule cell layer (Figure 5-4A). The vertical alignment of dispersed granule cells and their elongated appearance are remarkably similar to those of developing neurons as they migrate along radial glia (49) (Figure 5-4A). Recent studies have demonstrated a close approximation between dispersed granule cells and radial glia fibers and found that the length of the glial fibers increased with the severity of granule cell dispersion (50).

In several series of TLE patients, granule cell dispersion has been found in approximately 40% of TLE cases (9, 10, 51, 52). Thus, this alteration is not an essential feature of hippocampal sclerosis. However, it is of interest because it suggests alterations in the normal development of the dentate gyrus that could be associated with altered circuitry and contribute to abnormal function of the region.

A second altered pattern is a bilaminar distribution of granule cells in which two layers of granule cells are separated by a clear region that is relatively devoid of neuronal cell bodies (49, 53) (Figure 5-3C) . The bilaminar pattern is observed less frequently than generalized dispersion and has been found in approximately 10% of TLE cases (10). Within dispersed and bilaminar regions, granule cells are numerous, and the laminar alterations do not appear to result primarily from granule cell loss. However, distinct regions of granule cell loss can sometimes be found in the granule cell layer (Figure 5-3C).

Possible Mechanisms of Granule Cell Dispersion. The basic mechanisms responsible for granule cell dispersion in

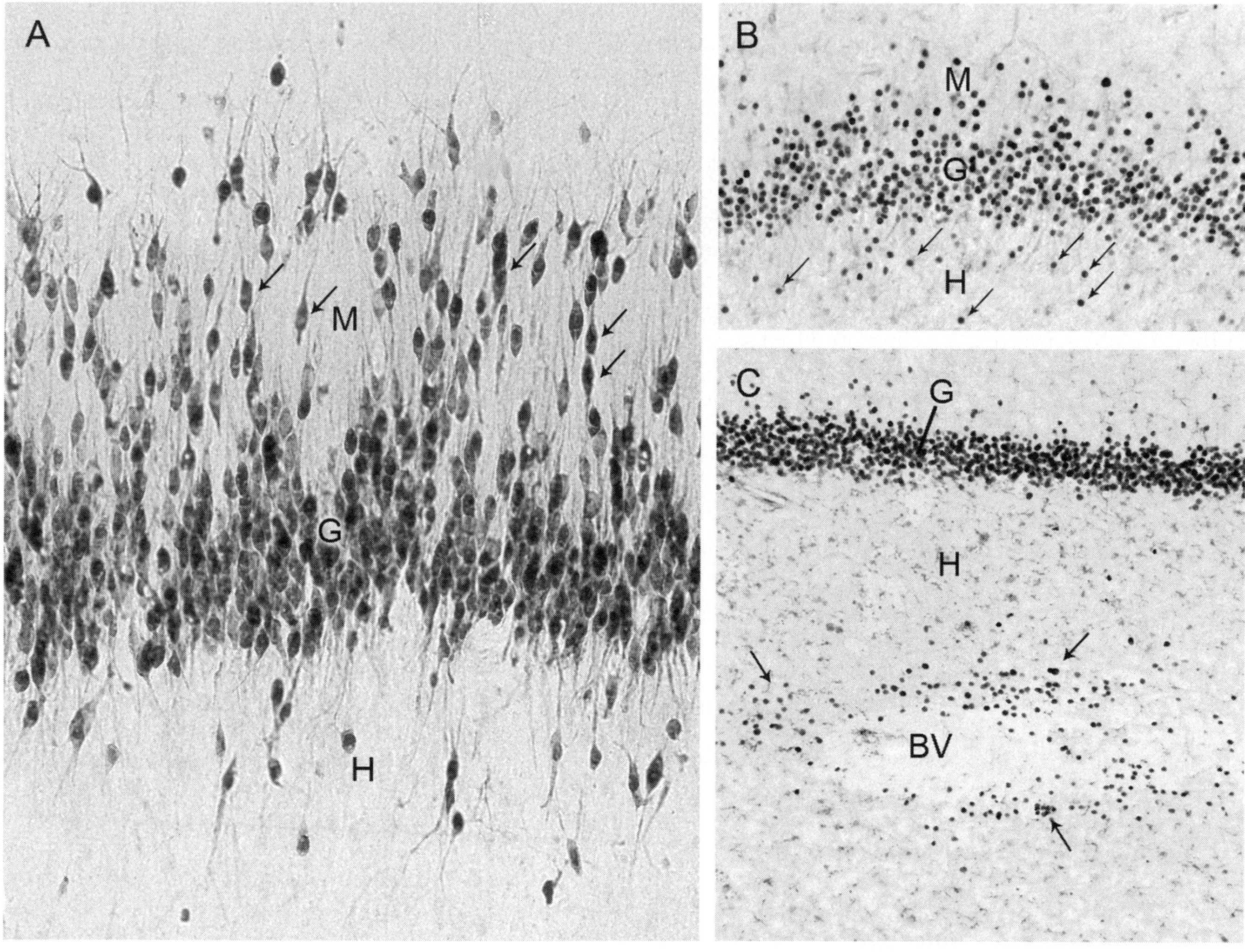

FIGURE 5-4

Granule cell organization in human temporal lobe epilepsy (TLE). (A) In a TLE specimen with granule cell dispersion, many of the NeuN-labeled granule cells have elongated cell bodies (examples at arrows) with vertically oriented processes and often appear to be aligned in columns. Numerous granule cells extend beyond the granule cell layer (G) into the molecular layer (M). Dispersed neurons are also evident in the hilus (H). (B) In a TLE specimen, neurons are identified specifically as granule cells by immunolabeling for Prox1 in their nuclei. Numerous labeled granule cells are evident in the molecular layer (M) as well as in the granule cell layer (G). Some ectopic granule cells (examples at arrows) are also present in the hilus (H). (C) In another TLE specimen, Prox1-labeled neurons in the granule cell layer (G) form a normal, compact layer. However, ectopic granule cells (examples at arrows) are concentrated near a blood vessel (BV) in the hilus (H).

human TLE have not been determined, but recent studies of human tissue and various animal models have suggested several interesting possibilities. Two general hypotheses are being explored. The first is that the alterations reflect an intrinsic, developmental migration disorder. The second is that the altered positioning of the granule cells is acquired as a result of an initial precipitating event such as severe febrile convulsions, status epilepticus, or, possibly, repeated seizure activity. Support can be found for both hypotheses.

The presence of granule cell dispersion has generally been restricted to patients with TLE and has seldom been reported in autopsies of neurologically normal individuals or those with other neurological disorders. However, Harding and Thom (54) recently described bilateral granule cell dispersion in autopsy studies of three pediatric cases. In one case, the child presented with a severe seizure disorder, and bilateral hippocampal sclerosis accompanied the granule cell disorganization. In two other cases, no seizures were documented, and the remainder of the hippocampal formation appeared intact. In all three cases, heterotopias or polymicrogyria were also present. The presence of bilateral granule cell dispersion and other migrational defects suggested that granule cell dispersion could be an independent developmental disorder in at least a small subgroup of cases (54).

Disorganization of dentate granule cells has also been observed in several mouse models with genetic mutations, and these include the Reeler mouse, which lacks the reelin protein, and the p35-deficient mouse. However, some differences exist between the patterns of neuronal lamination in human TLE and those in the mutant mice. In genetic models with altered neuronal migration, multiple groups of cortical and hippocampal neurons are often affected. Yet, in most TLE cases with granule cell dispersion, other regions of the hippocampal formation do not show noticeable laminar disruption (Figure 5-3C). In addition, granule cell dispersion in human TLE is frequently accompanied by severe cell loss in other regions of the hippocampus, and similar patterns of cell loss are not found in the mutant mice.

The association between granule cell dispersion and neuronal loss suggests that either an initial precipitating event or recurrent seizures could have influenced the positions of the granule cells. In several studies of human TLE, a strong association has been found between neuronal loss in the hilar (polymorph) region and the presence of granule cell dispersion (49, 52, 55). Similarly, in a recent study of a large number of TLE cases, Thom and colleagues found that granule cell dispersion correlated more closely with the extent of neuronal loss throughout the hippocampal formation than with any other variables examined (10).

This relationship, when viewed in conjunction with findings from mutant mice with altered granule cell lamination, suggests that the initial precipitating event could have produced specific cellular and molecular changes that, in turn, cause the altered patterns of granule cells. Several potential candidate molecules have recently been identified.

Reelin is an extracellular matrix protein that is important for the proper lamination of the cerebral cortex and hippocampus, and loss of reelin, as occurs in the Reeler mutant mouse, leads to a severely disordered cortex and hippocampus, including nearly complete loss of a compact granule cell layer (56, 57). In the hippocampus, reelin is synthesized and secreted by Cajal-Retzius cells, which are located in the outer molecular layer of the dentate gyrus and are particularly prominent during development (58, 59).

Recent studies by Frotscher and colleagues have found that reelin mRNA expression in Cajal-Retzius neurons of the dentate gyrus is reduced in some patients with TLE (60). Furthermore, the amount of loss of reelin mRNA-labeled cells was correlated with the extent of granule cell dispersion into the molecular layer. These findings are consistent with suggestions that reelin may be providing positional clues for migrating granule cells or controlling their detachment from radial glia and that, following loss of reelin, a compact granule cell layer cannot be established or maintained (50, 60).

The association between neuronal loss and granule cell dispersion suggests further that excitotoxic damage that produces cell loss in the hilus and other regions of the hippocampus could also cause loss of Cajal-Retzius cells and thus reelin. Findings that Cajal-Retzius neurons in rodents are sensitive to damage by glutamate agonists are consistent with this idea (59). While some investigators have found a loss of putative Cajal-Retzius cells (17), others have described a preservation or increase in these neurons, as identified by calretinin labeling, in human TLE (10, 61). Methodological differences may account for some of the discrepancies, or it could be that reelin expression is decreased within persisting neurons.

Granule cell positioning could also be influenced by brain-derived neurotrophic factor (BDNF). In a mouse model of TLE that is produced by the intrahippocampal injection of kainate, granule cells become severely dispersed and enlarged (62). In this model, levels of BDNF are significantly elevated and could have stimulated migration of the granule cells as well as their increased size (63, 64). Injection of BDNF into the hilus in rodents also leads to increased numbers of ectopic granule cells in the region, possibly due to aberrant migration from the subgranular layer (65). Interestingly, increased BDNF mRNA and protein levels also have been found in humans with TLE (66, 67).

The p35 signaling pathway, involved in neuron-specific activation of cyclin-dependent kinase 5 (Cdk5), could also be involved in granule cell dispersion and mossy fiber sprouting. In p35-deficient mice, lamination of the dentate gyrus is altered, and the distribution of granule cells closely resembles that of granule cell dispersion in TLE patients (68). Furthermore, these mice demonstrated spontaneous seizures (69).

Altered migration of granule cells along radial glia or failure of the neurons to leave the scaffold could be a common mechanism underlying granule cell dispersion, through either the reelin or p35 signaling pathway (50, 70). Similarly, immature astrocytes and increased expression of several neural cell adhesion, and related, molecules could contribute to the altered cellular architecture of the dentate gyrus in TLE (71–73).

Finally, evidence for the development of granule cell dispersion following an initial insult, rather than from an intrinsic developmental abnormality, has come from a study of the effects of limbic-like seizures in normal immature monkeys (74). Following a unilateral infusion of bicuculline in the entorhinal cortex and the production of limbic-like seizures, histological changes that resembled hippocampal sclerosis developed, and these included granule cell dispersion, in addition to hippocampal cell loss and mossy fiber sprouting (74). Thus many of the changes observed in humans with TLE can be produced by an initial episode of status epilepticus in a normal, immature primate brain. Although spontaneous seizures were not detected up to 1 year after the initial seizure episode in these animals (74), it seems plausible that a longer postseizure period (years) might be required for such seizures to develop.

Possible Contributions of Neurogenesis. Renewed interest in neurogenesis in the dentate gyrus during postnatal life and evidence that this process can be stimulated by seizure activity (75, 76) have led to speculation about the possible contributions of newborn neurons to granule cell disorganization as well as mossy fiber sprouting. The results of recent studies to determine whether newly generated neurons contribute to granule cell dispersion in patients with TLE have differed. In some studies, immunohistochemical markers of neural stem cells and progenitors, as well as immature glia, have been observed in the dentate gyrus and in regions of dispersion (77, 78). In contrast, other investigators, using similar markers for newly generated neurons in human surgical tissue, have found no evidence for such neurons in regions of dispersion (50) and have concluded that displacement of mature neurons, rather than newly generated neurons, leads to granule cell dispersion in the epileptic hippocampus (50, 79).

The human studies cannot, however, rule out the possibility that increased neurogenesis at earlier times might have contributed to the altered distribution of dentate granule cells. The finding that the number of neurons within regions of dispersion is often greater than that in regions without dispersion is consistent with a contribution of seizure-stimulated neurogenesis to these regions (77). Likewise, in the pilocarpine model of recurrent seizures, some adult-generated granule cells have been identified in ectopic locations in the molecular layer as well as in the hilus (80). Also, in this model, newly generated granule cells in the subgranular zone disperse more rapidly than normal into outer parts of the granule cell layer, but further movement into the molecular layer was not detected (81).

Although observed less frequently than granule cell dispersion in human TLE, clusters of granule cells in the hilus (Figure 5-4C) are consistent with generation of new neurons in a region that is a secondary germinal zone for granule cells during normal development (82). These and other dispersed neurons have been conclusively identified as granule cells by immunohistochemical labeling of Prox1, a homeobox gene that is specific for differentiated granule cells in the dentate gyrus (Figure 5-4B, C) (80). Interestingly, when aberrant clusters of granule cells are found in the hilus in human TLE, they are often located immediately adjacent to blood vessels (Figure 5-4C), and thus these regions have similarities to the vascular niche that has been described in the dentate subgranular zone of rodents and is considered to be a key site for adult neurogenesis (83). More diffusely distributed granule cells in the hilus also could be generated locally or could migrate into the hilus after being generated in the subgranular zone (80).

When considering neurogenesis as well as other types of morphological plasticity in TLE, a distinction between changes that occur at the time of an initial precipitating event and those that may occur as a result of later, spontaneous seizures could be particularly important. The initial event, such as a severe, prolonged seizure, is likely to stimulate neurogenesis acutely, as has been demonstrated in several animal models (76, 84, 85). Although the extent of neurogenesis in humans appears to be considerably less than that in rodents (86), any increased production of granule cells could be significant. The newly generated neurons may then require a period of time to mature and become completely integrated into the hippocampal circuitry, that is, several months in rodents (87, 88) and perhaps longer in humans. Events during this period could be of considerable importance for the functional integration of the newborn neurons (89) and could determine whether granule cells reach normal or abnormal positions, form proper or aberrant connections, and thus compensate for or contribute to an epileptic state.

The effects of spontaneous seizures might differ from those of the acute events. Indeed, several studies have suggested a reduction of neurogenesis in the chronic pilocarpine and intrahippocampal kainate models of recurrent seizures (79, 90, 91), as well as in human pediatric patients with frequent extratemporal seizures (92). Nevertheless, ongoing spontaneous seizures could promote additional changes such as increased production of growth and trophic factors that could continue to influence neuronal migration and circuitry, leading to ectopic positioning of granule cells and the stimulation of axonal sprouting and new synapse formation.

NEOCORTICAL LESIONS ASSOCIATED WITH SEIZURES

Structural lesions (aside from TLE, see previous discussion) associated with epilepsy can be grouped into the following categories: (a) malformative, (b) neoplastic, (c) familial metabolic, (d) vascular/traumatic, and (e) infectious/inflammatory (93, 94). Investigators have suggested that some of these pathologic processes may overlap in epilepsy patients (95, 96) and "dual pathology" (e.g., a cortical resection specimen showing features of *both* a malformative and destructive lesion) is occasionally encountered (97). Some causal lesions—as with TLE, see previous discussion—are amenable to definitive surgical treatment (e.g., low grade neoplasms, malformations of cortical development). This section will focus on developmental malformations and destructive or inflammatory lesions of the neocortex that account for the majority of structural lesions seen in infants and children with intractable epilepsy, especially those with infantile spasms (IS). More subtle malformations are also recognized with increasing frequency in adults with epilepsy; on rare occasions, severe dysplastic lesions may, for unknown reasons, present to a neurologist or epileptologist in adulthood.

MALFORMATIONS OF CORTICAL DEVELOPMENT

Malformations of cortical development (MCDs) have usually been considered to represent disorders of neuronal migration (or vascular formation) and have variously been classified with regard to morphology or putative etiology (98–100). The classification of these lesions is increasingly being modified by (1) the availability of high-resolution multimodality neuroimaging techniques that can be used to predict pathologic abnormalities in a given patient (101–103), and (2) molecular genetic clues to pathogenesis, based upon techniques such as gene expression profiling following laser capture microdissection of surgical specimens (104). The genetic basis of some types of lissencephaly (e.g., Miller-Dieker syndrome, obviously not a surgically treatable lesion) is now well understood (104, 105). They can be categorized as follows: (a) cortical dysplasia (CD), which accounts for the majority of malformations associated with pediatric epilepsy and encompasses the full spectrum of neuronal migration disorders (NMDs), ranging from the most subtle to the most severe; (b) CNS structural lesions associated with tuberous sclerosis complex (TSC); (c) Sturge-Weber-Dimitri syndrome (SWDS), or encephalotrigeminal angiomatosis; (d) neurofibromatosis type II, which may be associated with meningio-angiomatosis; and (e) vascular malformations.

Clinicopathologic Considerations

Seizure disorders have traditionally been subdivided into syndromes based on clinical presentation and electroencephalographic (EEG) findings. However, there is often a marked discrepancy between the clinical phenomenology of a seizure disorder and its neuropathologic substrate(s). Infantile spasms (IS; West syndrome) and Lennox-Gastaut syndrome can be seen with a wide range of cerebral lesions (106–108). The clinical form of epilepsy seen in a given patient appears to depend more on *when* during cerebral development the lesion occurred than on the specific *type* or topographic distribution of lesions (106, 109). It has been suggested that the CNS lesions associated with IS can be functionally categorized into three groups: (a) diffuse, (b) focal or multifocal cerebral lesions, and (c) cases with minimal neuropathologic change (108). Diffuse hemispheric lesions include hemimegalencephaly (HME), agyria/pachygyria-lissencephaly, and Aicardi syndrome (110). Focal and multifocal lesions include CD/MCD and destructive lesions (vascular and infectious), as well as cortical tubers seen in patients with TSC.

MCDs can be viewed as a spectrum of CD resulting from derangement of the normal process of cortical development (111–115). This spectrum consists of a range of morphologic features associated with multiple putative etiologic factors, including genetic and environmental (e.g., destructive) influences. CD encompasses a broad range of neocortical malformations, ranging from the most subtle ("microdysgenesis") to the most severe (HME), and includes such conditions as agyria/pachygyria-lissencephaly, polymicrogyria (PMG), and focal CD. The resultant neuropathologic features may reflect abnormalities that probably occur within well-defined time windows during brain development. Clinically there is an inverse correlation between the size and severity of CD and the age at clinical presentation (102, 111), supporting the notion that there is a predominance of pathologically severe CD in neonates and infants with seizures, including those with IS (116). Although CD accounts for the majority of malformations associated with pediatric epilepsy, other malformative lesions are also capable of producing these epilepsy syndromes, and they frequently show neuropathologic changes that overlap significantly with those seen in patients with CD. Jellinger (106) has noted that the clinical severity of a given seizure disorder appears to be more closely related to the *timing* of the insult (whether genetic or environmental) and its effect on the processes of development than to the nature of the lesion itself. This may explain some of the heterogeneity of neuropathologic lesions seen in children with epilepsy, as the clinical phenotype results not only from the lesion or putative "insult" to the developing CNS but also from the developmental processes it subsequently affects.

A puzzling feature noted in pediatric epilepsy is the finding in cases of IS of *diffuse* and transient suppression of cortical activity in the presence of *focal* or *multifocal* lesions (108). This diffuse cortical suppression has not been linked to particular distributions or types of neuropathologic change. Rather, some have suggested that this feature of IS is associated with neocortical *immaturity*. The pattern of evolution of IS from transient and diffuse suppression of cortical discharge to ultimately focal or generalized seizures may represent a maturation of the malformed cortex (108).

Nosologic Considerations

Understanding of the full clinicopathologic spectrum of CD is currently evolving and reflects a progressive elucidation of the basis of these complex lesions (109–125). Cortical malformations have historically been described largely by their gross characteristics (i.e., agyria/pachygyria-lissencephaly, HME, microgyria). As investigators discovered the range of microscopic cortical malformations that produce epilepsy but show no (or relatively mild) gross abnormalities, additional terms such as microdysgenesis (109, 117, 118), dysplastic cortical architecture (not otherwise specified) (119), focal cortical dysplasia (FCD) (120, 121), and generalized or diffuse cortical dysplasia (122, 123, 124a) came into use. The nomenclature of CD has evolved through several schema of classification, each intended to provide correlations with morphology of seizures or to reflect etiologic mechanisms (98, 99, 111) The term *FCD* was initially used to specify lesions in which cytomegalic neurons were present (121), although its frequent use to describe a localized region of CD renders the term slightly ambiguous. Some investigators prefer to use a traditional classification of migrational disorders into four main groups: (a) agyria/pachygyria-lissencephaly, (b) microgyria-polymicrogyria, (c) dysplastic cortical architecture, and (d) heterotopias (119). Others, to denote the belief that these lesions are related and reflect developmental abnormalities along a continuous spectrum, have chosen to refer to them as neuronal migration disorders (NMDs) (98, 113, 114) or cerebral or synaptic dysgenesis (124, 125). A recent consensus conference resulted in a proposal to subclassify CD or grade its severity (in surgical resection specimens) using simple morphologic criteria identifiable by any experienced neuropathologist, for example, presence or absence of cortical disorganization, enlarged or dysmorphic neuronal cell bodies, and "balloon cells" (see following) (126).

Development of the Neocortex

The neuropathologic changes seen in infants and children with epilepsy frequently represent the end result(s) of insults to a rapidly developing brain. Several reviews have summarized the historical evolution in our understanding of the immensely complex molecular and neurobiologic processes that occur to create a normally functioning cerebral cortex (127–131). Neocortical development after neural tube formation can be roughly considered to be the end result of a series of overlapping processes: (a) cell proliferation in the ventricular and subventricular zones (VZ/SVZ), (b) early differentiation of neuroblasts and glioblasts, (c) programmed cell death of neuronal precursors and neurons, (d) migration of neuroblasts (both radially from the VZ/SVZ and tangentially) to form the mature cortical plate, (e) late neuronal migration, (f) organization and maturation of the cortex, and (g) synaptogenesis/synaptic pruning (98, 110, 119, 132). A discussion of how derangement of these processes contributes to CD is beyond the scope of this review, but can be found elsewhere (133). Most developmental disorders of the brain associated with epilepsy are thought to originate from the perturbation of developmental events after the embryonic period, that is, after 6 weeks' gestation, when cell proliferation starts along the wall of the neural tube. This generates a group of "matrix cells" (134), or precursor cells for all neuroblasts and glioblasts, forming the VZ/SVZ in the pallium, as well as the ganglionic eminence in the subpallium. Programmed cell death (PCD, apoptosis) is also an essential mechanism in normal brain development, determining the cellular constituents of the CNS. In normal brain development, there is a 25% to 50% overproduction of neuroblasts, many of which will undergo physiologic PCD (125). Synapse elimination is intimately intertwined with the remodeling of cortical connections and is a highly dynamic process (135), demonstrated both in vivo and in vitro (136).

As the neocortex develops, the marginal zone, future molecular layer or cortical layer I, is composed largely of Cajal-Retzius cells. As previously discussed, they secrete the extracellular glycoprotein reelin, required for the normal inside-out positioning of neurons as they migrate from the ventricular zone along radial glia. Human Cajal-Retzius cells, characterized by the combined expression of reelin and p73, are transient cells, present from the preplate stage at 8 weeks' gestation, and gradually increase in number (by tangential migration) until they disappear by the end of gestation (137, 138, 138a). In mice carrying mutations in *RELN* (Reeler mice) and in *disabled-1* (*Dab1*), as well as in mice carrying double mutations of both very low-density lipoprotein receptor (*VLDLR*) and apolipoprotein E receptor 2 (*ApoER2*), normal neuroblast migration with an inside-out fashion is inverted (139). This suggests a role for these genes in the control of cell positioning in the developing CNS and predicts a pattern of cytoarchitectural alteration in patients carrying alterations in the reelin/lipoprotein receptor/Dab1 pathway, as well as *RELN* mutations causing lissencephaly (140). LIS1 also appears to have important effects on neuronal migration, and significant interactions with Cajal-Retzius cells (141). The superficial or subpial granular layer (SGL) is a transient cell layer; it appears beneath the pial surface between 13 and 24 weeks' gestation (93, 142). Cells in the SGL originate from the basal periolfactory subventricular zone (142–144) and migrate tangentially beneath the pia to cover the neocortical marginal zone. Cells in this layer express interneuron markers such as calretinin, calbindin, and GABA (145). The biological significance of the SGL, however, remains to be elucidated. PCD may, at least in part, contribute to its elimination (146). The human subplate contains large multipolar neurons. These neurons in the developing cerebrum, though they are transient and most disappear in early postnatal life, are thought to be important in organizing cortical connections in the developing cerebrum and are thought to act as pioneer corticofugal axons (147–150).

Neuropathologic Significance of Cortical Dysplasia

The Pediatric Epilepsy Surgery program at UCLA Center for the Health Sciences, active for over 20 years, has enabled us to examine more than 500 surgically resected specimens from infants and children with intractable seizures, including a spectrum from partial lobectomies to complete and partial (functional) hemispherectomies. The most common morphologic substrate was CD, this being of etiologic importance as a cause of intractable pediatric seizures in more than 80% of children younger than 3 years of age. The extent of CD neuropathology can often be predicted by high-resolution neuroimaging studies. Such neuroimaging allows for stratification of CD cases into those that show hemimegalencephaly (HME), with diffuse enlargement of the gray and white matter, including thickening of the cortical ribbon, within an entire cerebral hemisphere; hemispheric CD, with multifocal CD affecting one cerebral hemisphere (though not causing enlargement of that hemisphere); or multilobar, lobar, or focal CD, the latter affecting as few as one gyrus or two adjacent gyri. The magnetic resonance imaging (MRI) findings of HME include an enlarged cerebral hemisphere and markedly thickened gyri, with loss of sulcation, deformity, and enlargement of the ipsilateral ventricle. Palmini type IIB CD is also easily identified by MRI, with focal thickness of the gyrus (gyri) and associated hyperintense T2-weighted signal changes in the adjacent white matter. It is as yet difficult to visualize Palmini type I CD by MRI; however, combining this with other modalities, such as positron emission tomography (PET) and magnetic source imaging (MSI), it is likely that the detectability of this lesion will increase.

In resection specimens from such patients, macroscopic heterotopia and polymicrogyria (PMG) are occasionally seen. Loss of the normal cortex–white matter junction, best appreciated with a Klüver-Barrera or other myelin stain, is a frequent accompaniment and excellent predictor of severe microscopic CD. Many specimens, however, exhibit no striking gross cortical abnormalities even when severe microscopic lesions are present. CD can be further characterized with regard to specific and easily identifiable microscopic abnormalities, including cortical laminar disorganization, frequent single heterotopic white matter neurons, excess neurons in the neocortical molecular layer, marginal glioneuronal heterotopia, white matter neuronal heterotopia, neuronal cytomegaly with or without associated dysmorphic features of the cytoplasm (the latter often accompanied by cytoskeletal abnormalities and balloon cell change) (111). These microscopic features can be used as the basis for a grading system for CD, for example, one presented recently by Palmini et al (126).

Cortical laminar disorganization is a defining histopathologic feature of CD. As neocortical architecture is the end result of the developmental processes of proliferation of neuronal precursors, migration, terminal differentiation, PCD, and cortical remodeling, abnormalities in any of these processes may result in abnormal cortical architecture. Cortical disorganization (as well as cytologic abnormalities in individual neurons) can be highlighted using immunohistochemistry that incorporates primary antibodies to neurofilament epitopes (104). Although many neurons still reside in the intermediate zone/white matter in the last trimester of pregnancy and even into postnatal life (151, 152), the phenomenon of single heterotopic neurons in the white matter is accentuated in CD (109). It has been demonstrated in other series using morphometric techniques (153). It has been suggested that injury to the radial glial fibers leads to a "stranding" of the migrating neuroblasts within the white matter, where they further differentiate into mature neurons (125). Alternatively, overproduction of neurons late in neurogenesis may lead to crowding of migrating neurons toward the cortical surface (154). Morphometric analysis has demonstrated a statistically significant increase in the number of neurons within the molecular layer of the cortex in epileptic patients (118); this is considered to be evidence of a slight maldevelopment of the neocortex, sometimes described as microdysgenesis (108, 126). Persistence of the superficial granular layer (SGL) has been seen in association with many cortical malformations (111). Marginal glioneuronal heterotopia consists of excrescences of disorganized neuroglial tissue extending from the pial surface into the subarachnoid space. They are often found in association with persistent SGL. These lesions may be associated with a failure of the glia limitans. White matter neuronal heterotopia consists of disorganized masses of neurons in the white matter that usually occur in a periventricular position with a nodular morphology, although rare instances of laminar subcortical bands of heterotopic gray matter have been known to produce the appearance of a double cortex. These lesions may be associated with injury to a group of radial glia, leading to failure of a group of neuroblasts to migrate normally (125). Alternatively, a defect in genes controlling, neuroblast proliferation, neuroglial interactions, and PCD has been suggested as being causal (119).

PMG denotes small, meandering gyri, often with bridging of the sulci by fusion of the molecular layers. It consists of two histologic types. Four-layered PMG is most frequently considered to result from a destructive lesion occurring at approximately 20 to 24 weeks

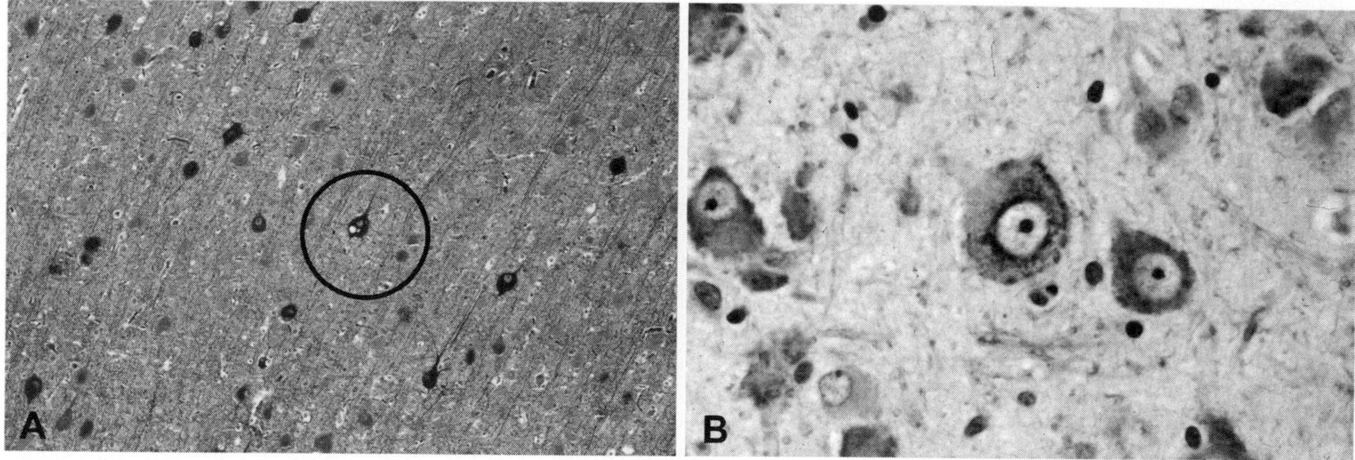

FIGURE 5-5

Cytologic neuronal changes in severe cortical dysplasia (CD). Panel A (stained with the Bielschowsky technique) shows many neurons with cytoskeletal abnormalities, and some with cytoplasmic vacuolization (circled neuron). The neuronal changes resemble neurofibrillary tangles (NFTs) seen in neocortex of patients with Alzheimer disease, although at the ultrastructural level paired helical filaments (typical of Alzheimer NFT) are not present in CD. Nissl techniques (Panel B, stained with Kluver-Barrera) also highlight neuronal disorganization, enlargement of neuronal cell bodies (e.g., neuron in the middle), and clumping of perinuclear Nissl together with clearing of peripheral cytoplasm.

of gestation, and an unlayered form is thought to result from an insult earlier in brain development (at approximately 13–16 weeks) (154).

Neuronal cytomegaly denotes enlarged neurons, some of which may also be dysmorphic (Figure 5-5); these were first described in association with seizure-producing focal cortical malformations by Taylor et al. (121). Nerve cell hypertrophy was convincingly shown using quantitative histochemistry in a case of HME (155). The differentiation of cytomegalic vs. dysmorphic neurons is of importance in assigning a Palmini grade to a given lesion. Neurons that show enlargement of their cell bodies only are, in association with cortical architectural disorganization, typical of Palmini type IB lesions, whereas corticectomies that also contain dysmorphic neurons are characteristic of Palmini type II CD. When balloon cells are absent, the lesion is described as Palmini type IIA; when they are present, it becomes Palmini type IIB. (Palmini IIB CD corresponds to what has been described as Taylor type focal cortical dysplasia, or T-FCD.) Dysmorphic neurons bear an extremely complex dendritic arborization as well as an abundance of perisomatic synapses and a paucity of axosomatic synapses (156, 157). Increased neuronal size has been associated with an increased DNA and RNA content, as well as increased nuclear and nucleolar volume suggestive of heteroploidy (124, 158). Argyrophilic, neurofibrillary-like tangles and cytoplasmic vacuoles have been demonstrated within many such neurons (Figure 5-5) (159), as has the existence of paracrystalline intracytoplasmic structures visible on ultrastructural examination (160). These neurofibrillary-like cytoplasmic inclusions differ from the neurofibrillary tangles of Alzheimer's disease in that they do not contain paired helical filaments (161).

Balloon cells, showing similarity to gemistocytic astrocytes, have eccentric nuclei and ballooned, glassy, or opalescent eosinophilic cytoplasm (Figure 5-6). They often demonstrate binucleation or dysmorphic nuclei, sometimes showing bridges of nucleoplasm between two separate islands of nuclear material within a cell. They may cluster at the cortex–white matter junction or be abundant within subcortical white matter (94, 104). Frequently they are admixed with dysmorphic and enlarged neuronal cell bodies. Ultrastructurally, they are packed with filaments ranging in size from 400 to 600 nm in length and 30 nm in thickness, interspersed with non-membrane-bound, electron-dense, helical structures (162). Vinters et al. (159) and others have demonstrated dual staining of many cells in dysplastic cortex (including some balloon cells) with antibodies to both neuronal and glial markers, implying either a failure of the cells to commit to a specific phenotype or dedifferentiation. The resemblance of balloon cells to cells found within the cortical tubers of TSC has suggested the possibility that cases of CD harboring balloon cell change may represent a forme fruste of TSC (104, 113, 114, 162, 163).

Pathogenesis of Cortical Dysplasia

Although it is accepted that cortical dysplasia involves abnormal cerebral cortical development, it is unclear when this occurs and how it produces seizures. Most MCD classification systems are based on speculating

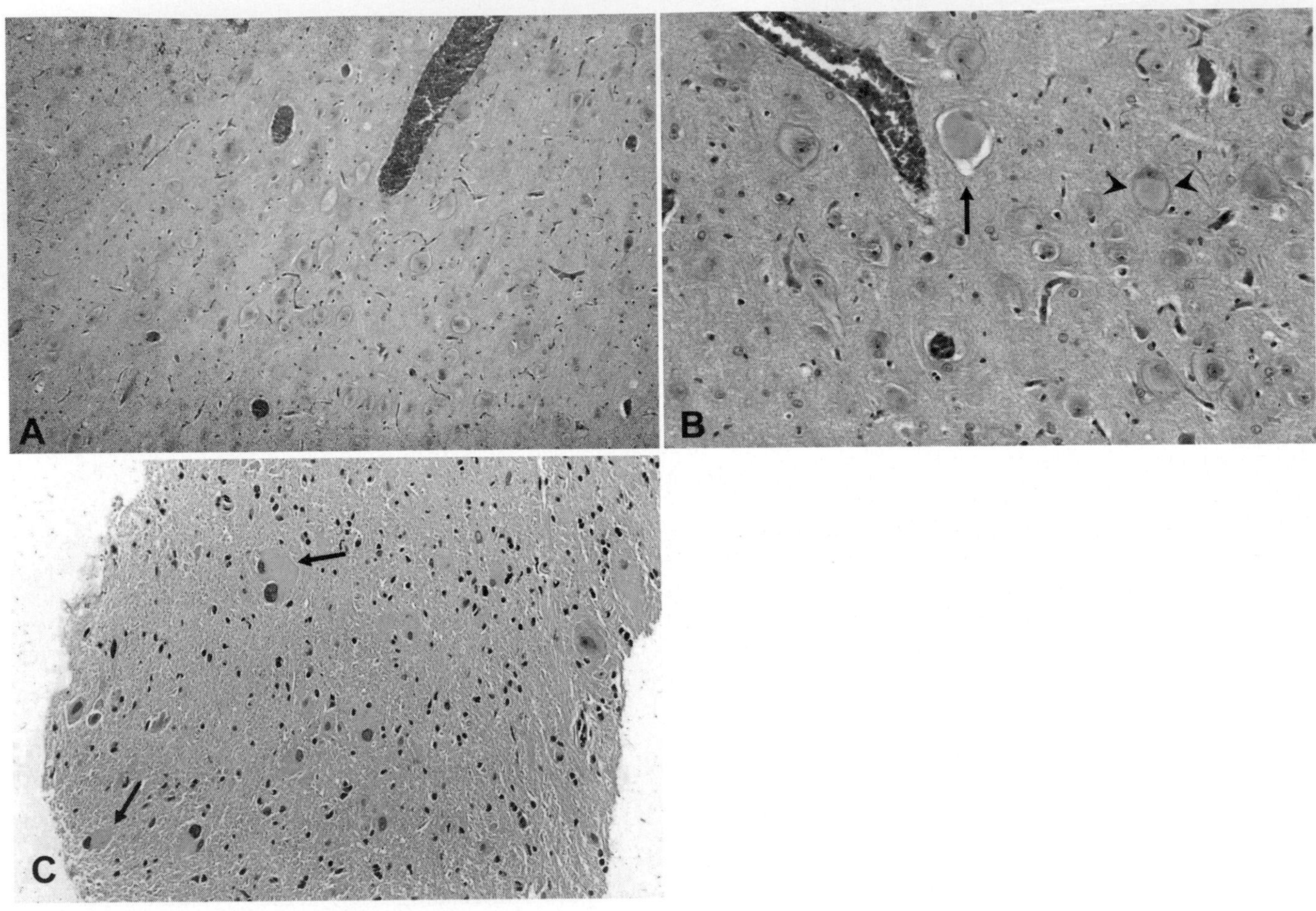

FIGURE 5-6

Changes of CD, Palmini type IIB. All panels are from sections stained with hematoxylin and eosin. Panel A shows marked neuronal disorganization. At higher magnification (Panel B) balloon cells are identified (arrow), as are dysmorphic neurons. Arrowheads highlight a cell with typical neuronal nucleus, but opalescent balloon-like cytoplasm, at the periphery of which Nissl-like substance is seen. Other neurons in this field show changes similar to those in Figure 5-5B. Panel C shows several balloon cells, with glassy eosinophilic cytoplasm (arrows) scattered throughout a surgical resection specimen.

when the first developmental steps involving cell proliferation, neuronal migration, and cortical organization become deranged to produce the malformed cortex. Previously, the presumed mechanisms of CD pathogenesis have been thought to be defects in neuronal migration, as one explanation for subcortical heterotopic neurons, and altered periventricular neuroglial differentiation to account for cytomegalic and dysmorphic neurons and balloon cells (164–166). Although such mechanisms appear to be operant in genetic forms of MCD, clinicopathologic investigations (using corticectomy specimens) have challenged this singular interpretation (98, 101, 102, 167, 168).

In recent studies, the UCLA group has found evidence that surgically treated CD seems to involve retention of cells of the human pre- and subplate, along with an overproliferation of cortical neurons. Prenatal human subplate cells have morphologic similarities to dysmorphic neurons found in postnatal CD tissue (168). Normal human subplate contains large multipolar neurons similar to cytomegalic neurons, and polymorphous and fusiform neurons with thick primary dendrites along with inverted pyramidal-shaped neurons, a feature noted in dysmorphic CD neurons (151). Most human subplate cells degenerate in the 4 to 6 weeks before birth (147, 169), which coincides with increasing definition of the gray-white matter junction and secondary gyral folding (170). Toward the end of normal neurogenesis, periventricular radial glial cells attach themselves to the tailing processes of the last produced cortical pyramidal neurons and migrate toward the cortex, where they detach and eventually transform into protoplasmic astrocytes (171–173). This may explain why balloon cells in CD tissue have some characteristics similar to those of radial glia (174–176).

The UCLA group has proposed that CD pathogenesis probably involves partial failure of the later phases of neocortical formation. As a consequence, subplate and radial glial degeneration and transformation would be reduced or prevented, giving the appearance of abnormal dysmorphic cells in postnatal CD tissue. A failure of late cortical maturation could explain the presence of abnormally thickened gyri with indistinct cortical gray-white matter junctions in the MRI scans of CD patients (101). The precise timing of these events during cortical development would explain the different forms of CD identified by MRI as well as the severity of CD assessed by histopathology. Developmental alterations during the late second or early third trimester would account for severe CD, such as hemimegalencephaly, whereas events occurring closer to birth might explain milder forms of CD. In addition, there appears to be an overproduction of neurons in the later phases of cortical development. Cerebral hemispheric volumes assessed by MRI were normal or increased in the case of hemimegalencephaly, and cortical thickness was the same or slightly increased (103, 154). Furthermore, neuronal densities were increased in the upper gray matter, molecular layer, and subcortical white matter. The location of excess neurons would be consistent with the idea that this process occurred in later periventricular cell cycles (i.e., ones occurring toward the end of neurogenesis). Thus, heterotopic subcortical white matter neurons are likely the result of excessive late generated pyramidal neurons trying to migrate toward the already overly crowded cortical ribbon, in combination with residual prenatal subplate neurons that failed to degenerate before birth.

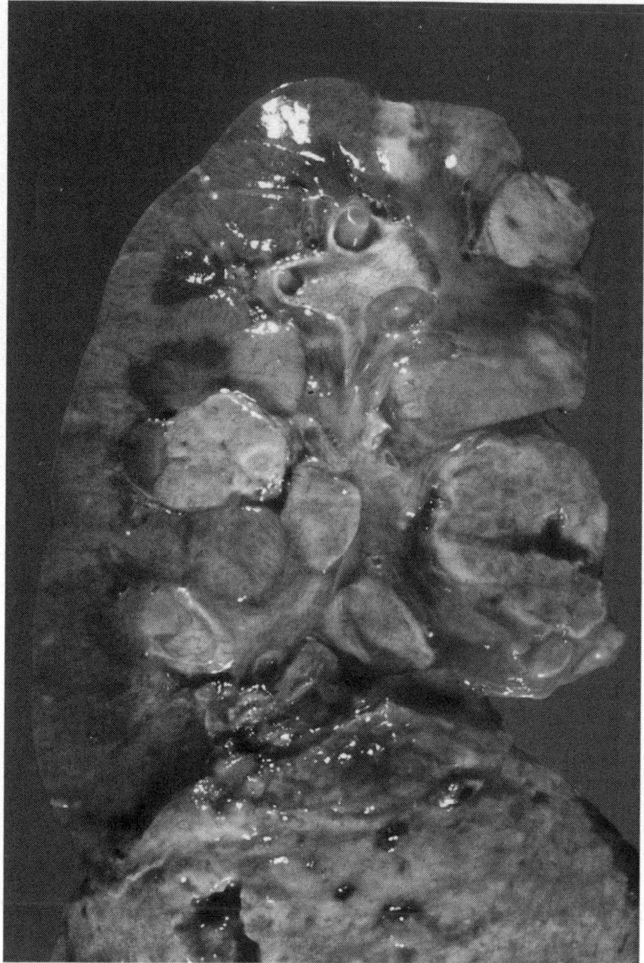

FIGURE 5-7

Angiomyolipoma, a tumor characteristic of TSC, is seen in the sectioned kidney of a patient who came to autopsy.

Cortical Tubers of the Tuberous Sclerosis Complex (TSC)

Tuberous sclerosis complex (TSC) is an autosomal dominant, multisystem disorder in which the CNS, eyes, kidneys (Figure 5-7), skin, and heart are most commonly affected by malformative, hamartomatous, or neoplastic lesions (177–182). It has an incidence of 1:9,400 to 10,000 births (177, 178); however, accurate estimates are difficult to ascertain, and a high rate of spontaneous TSC gene mutations has been described (177, 183). The clinical presentation of an individual with TSC may be with infantile spasms, autism, or mental retardation. Approximately 85% of TSC patients who come to medical attention have experienced a seizure at some time. Because genetic analysis to confirm the diagnosis of TSC remains unavailable to most physicians, diagnostic criteria for TSC have been enunciated (184, 185). In the 1998 criteria, some clinical features previously thought to be pathognomonic for TSC were considered less specific, whereas clinical or radiographic features of the disease were subdivided into major and minor categories, based upon their apparent degree of specificity for TSC. Using these newer revised criteria, a definitive diagnosis of TSC was made by the confirmation of two or more distinct types of lesion in a patient, rather than multiple lesions of the same type (e.g., tubers) in the same organ system. Thus no single lesion defines the disease.

Neuropathology of Cortical Tubers as a Cause of Seizures. Individuals with TSC may rarely present with HME. However, the characteristic brain abnormalities of TSC include neocortical tubers (Figure 5-8), subependymal nodules (SENs), and subependymal giant cell astrocytomas (SEGAs). Cortical tubers are often associated with IS and intractable epilepsy in children. The lesions manifest as enlarged gyri in which the cortex–white matter junction has become blurred, resembling sporadic, severe cortical dysplasia (104, 111). Histologically the lesions show disorganized neocortex, with a variety of dysmorphic, markedly enlarged neurons, and bizarre

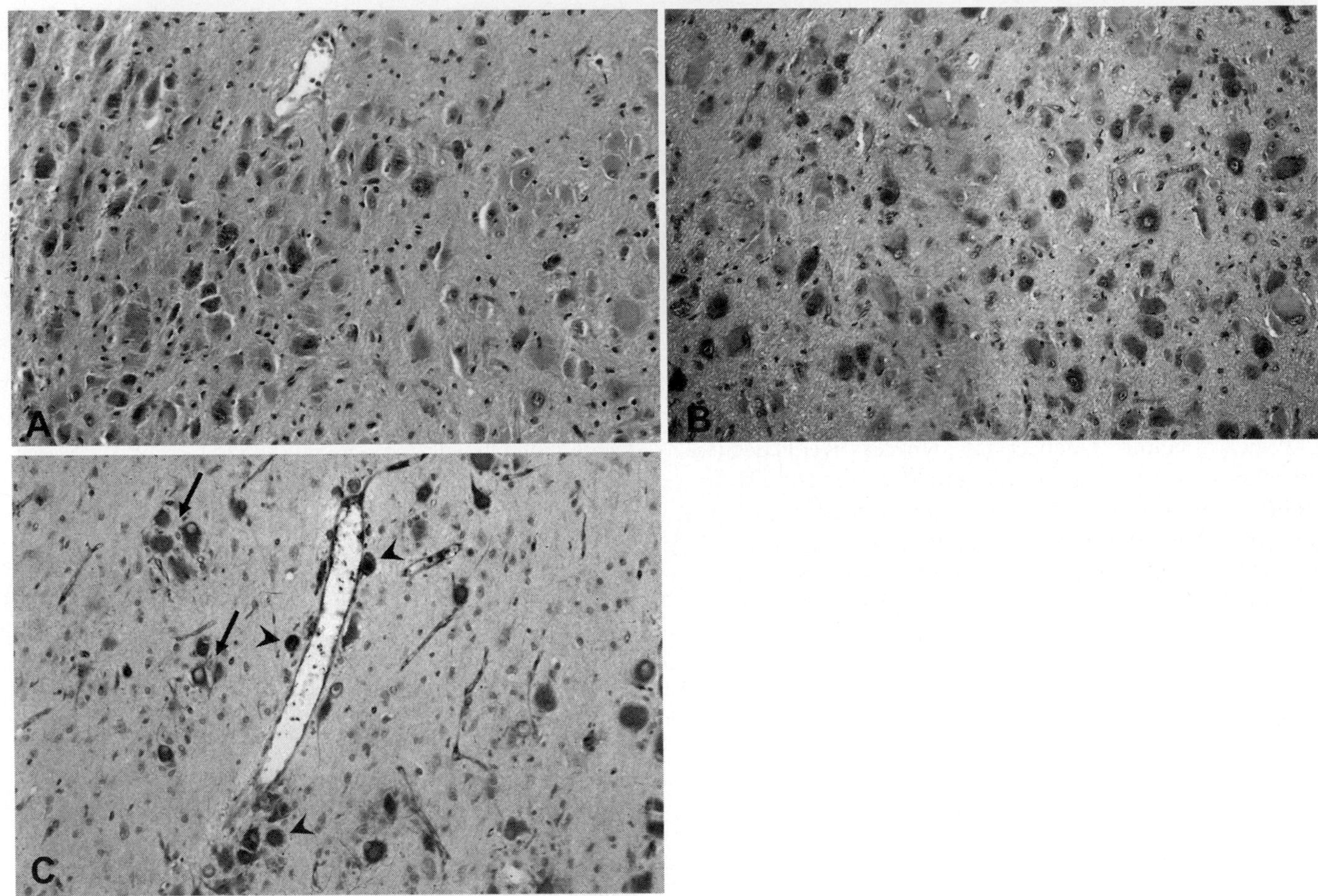

FIGURE 5-8

Tuber of tuberous sclerosis complex. All panels are micrographs from the same specimen, examined using different stains. Panel A (from a hematoxylin and eosin–stained section) shows features akin to those seen in Palmini type IIB cortical dysplasia. Note a markedly disorganized, crowded collection of dysmorphic neurons, and balloon-like cells. Panel B is from a section labeled with a digoxigenin-labeled probe for the *TSC2* gene product. Note differential expression of the gene in various cells, but especially prominent expression within cells of neuronal phenotype. (For details, see M. Menchine, J.k. Emelin, PS Mischel, TA Haag, MG Norman, SH Pepkowitz, CT Welsh, JJ Townsend, HV Vinters. Tissue and cell type specific expression of the tuberous sclerosis-related gene, *TSC2* in human tissues. *Modern Pathology* 1996; 9:1071–1080). Panel C is from a section stained (immunoperoxidase technique) with primary antibodies to the *TSC1* gene product, hamartin. Note prominent immunoreactivity of clusters of cells (with uncertain phenotype, arrows) and perivascular cells (arrowheads). This tuber originated from a patient in whom it was unknown whether a mutation was present in the *TSC1* or *TSC2* gene. (For details of methodology, see MW Johnson J.K. Emelin, S-H Park, H.V. Vinters. Co-localization of TSC1 and TSC2 gene products in tubers of patients with tuberous sclerosis. *Brain Pathology* 1999; 9:45–54.)

gemistocytic astrocyte-like "balloon cells" having eccentric nuclei containing relatively coarse chromatin and glassy, eosinophilic cytoplasm (Figure 5-8). Balloon cells seen in TSC are almost identical to those seen in severe cortical dysplasia (CD). This observation has raised the possibility that cases of CD with balloon cell change represent a forme fruste of TSC (113, 114, 162, 163). Balloon cells, such as those in FCD, show morphological and immunohistochemical features of both neurons and astrocytes, suggesting a failure of commitment in neuroglial differentiation. Tubers may show prominent calcification. Giant cells within TSC tubers show halos of synaptophysin immunoreactivity around neurons, resembling those noted in gangliogliomas, as well as strong immunostaining with antibodies to the microtubule-associated protein 2 (MAP-2) (186). Alpha B-crystallin, a member of the heat shock protein family of peptides, is found within dysgenetic cells of tubers, and within both SEGAs and SENs (187). Dysmorphic cytomegalic neurons express high levels of tuberin, as do individual cells within SEGAs and SENs. Tuberin appears to be present in most neuronal populations of the CNS from at least 20 weeks' gestation, with an apparent up-regulation of its expression after 40 weeks of gestation (181). Hamartin was found, albeit with a weaker signal, in the same cell types during CNS development.

Although architectural disarray is a defining feature of a tuber, cellularity of a lesion may be extremely variable. When high cell density is noted, a tuber may resemble a ganglioglioma (181, 188, 188a). Although the proliferative potential of these lesions appears low, as judged by immunohistochemistry for Ki-67, other markers of cellular proliferation (e.g., collapsin response mediator protein 4/CRMP4, doublecortin/DCX) are expressed within giant cells of cortical tubers and SEGAs, suggesting that they may represent newly generated cells that have migrated into tubers from the SVZ (188).

Our current understanding of the molecular pathogenesis of TSC represents a triumph of multidisciplinary, multicenter collaborations focused on characterizing the complex gene defects that cause this disorder (189–192). TSC results from mutations in one of two nonhomologous tumor suppressor genes, *TSC1* (192) on chromosome 9 (9q34) encoding a 130-kDa protein, hamartin, and *TSC2* (189) on chromosome 16 (16p13.3) encoding a 200-kDa protein, tuberin. About one-half of TSC families show linkage to each of these two genes. *TSC1* mutations, accounting for a minority of mutations identified, are slightly less common in sporadic TSC patients, and are more common in familial cases (13–50%) (193). Putative functions of both *TSC1* and *TSC2* gene products have been studied using mostly *Drosophila* and rodent models of TSC, but also using human tissues. This work initially suggested that both *TSC1* and *TSC2* gene products had growth suppressor properties (194–196). Significant interactions of the TSC gene products with each other, and with intracellular signaling pathways, have been implicated in disease pathogenesis.

Hamartin may also interact with the ERM (ezrin, radixin, and moesin) family of actin-binding proteins to activate small GTPases of the Rho subfamily (Rho GTPases) (197). Rho GTPases are important regulators of the actin cytoskeleton and may be involved in neuronal developmental processes including migration, establishment of polarity, synapse formation, etc. (198). ERM proteins belong to the band-4.1 superfamily of membrane-cytoskeleton linking proteins (199), thought to function in multiple different fashions according to their interaction with various membrane proteins, Ras superfamily GTPases, and the actin cytoskeleton; they may be involved in the formation of microvilli, cell-cell adhesion, maintenance of cell shape, and motility (200). The observation that hamartin binds to ezrin in vivo and can modulate the activity of RhoA (Ras homologous member A) (197), suggests that tuberin and hamartin may be attached to the membrane-cytoskeletal cortex through activated ERM proteins (201, 202). Evidence suggests that ERM proteins function at a position upstream and downstream of Rho GTPases to regulate cellular adhesion and motility (203, 204). ERM proteins (ezrin and moesin) are expressed in germinal matrix cells, migrating cells, and radial glial fibers in the developing human brain (201), correlating with RhoA expression in proliferating and migrating cells in the developing rat brain (205). Dysfunction of tuberin and hamartin may perturb communication between ERM proteins and Rho GTPase to cause abnormal neuronal migration, polarity, and morphology, resulting in the formation of dysplastic cortex. Hamartin and tuberin are coexpressed within a population of abnormal neuroglial cells (206), and both TSC gene products and ERM proteins are also coexpressed within a subpopulation of abnormal neuroglial cells in TSC tubers (201). Abnormalities of radial glia have also been implicated in the pathogenesis of brain lesions of TSC (206a).

Tuberin contains a conserved 163-amino acid carboxy-terminal region that exhibits sequence homology to the catalytic domain of a GTPase-activating protein (GAP) for the small molecular weight GTPase Rap1 (207) and for Rab5 (208). Using in situ hybridization, TSC2 mRNA was found to be widely expressed in various cell types throughout the body, including epithelia, lymphocytes, and endocrine organs; within the CNS, it was prominently and selectively expressed within neurons, especially motor neurons (209). Widespread expression of the *TSC2* gene within developing and adult nervous system was noted in another study using various techniques (210). A study in mice showed that tuberin localized to the perinuclear region of cerebellar Purkinje cells, whereas hamartin was noted to distribute along neuronal or astrocytic processes (211). *TSC2* mRNA and tuberin were found in abundance in many CNS cell types, including neurons and ependymal cells (212).

TSC1 and *TSC2* gene products colocalize within tubers (and sometimes within individual dysmorphic cells) of patients with TSC (206). Tissue culture experiments in various cell types show that both hamartin and tuberin interact with the G2/M cyclin-dependent kinase CDK1 (213). It has also been suggested that hamartin and tuberin have separable and presumably distinct functions in mammalian cell cycle regulation (214); that is, hamartin has the ability to modulate cell proliferation independent of the presence of functional tuberin, and binding to hamartin is not always essential for tuberin to affect cell proliferation. *Tsc1* and *Tsc2*, *Drosophila* homologs of *TSC1* and *TSC2*, function together in vivo to negatively regulate cell size, cell proliferation, and organ size in the insulin signaling pathway (PI3Kinase-Akt/PKB-mTOR-S6K-S6) at a position downstream of *dAkt* (*Drosophila Akt*) and upstream of *dS6k* (*Drosophila S6 kinase*) (215). This has been clearly confirmed in surgically resected TSC tubers by means of quantitative immunohistochemical evaluation using tissue microarray methodology (216); constitutive activation of S6K has been observed in TSC tubers but not in focal cortical dysplasia of Taylor type (T-FCD or CD Palmini type IIB), suggesting one difference between these MCDs (216, 217).

STURGE-WEBER-DIMITRI (SWD) SYNDROME/ENCEPHALOTRIGEMINAL ANGIOMATOSIS

This rare, nonfamilial, neurocutaneous syndrome of unknown etiology (218–220) is encountered in surgical specimens from infants and children with intractable epilepsy, although much less commonly than destructive and malformative/hamartomatous lesions. Its frequency is estimated to be 1 per 50,000 live births (221); 75% to 90% of affected children develop partial seizures by 3 years of age (222). Clinicopathologic reports describe the association of the cerebral lesion, usually localized to the occipital cortex, with facial capillary hemangioma (port-wine stain) in the distribution of the ophthalmic division of the trigeminal nerve (220, 223, 224). Neuroimaging features are highly characteristic. Neuropathologic abnormalities in cortical resection specimens (Figure 5-9) are easily appreciated at low magnification. Soft tissue radiographs of the sliced specimen may show the characteristic "tram-track" pattern of neocortical calcification. Leptomeningeal angiomatosis is a key diagnostic feature of the syndrome (225), characterized by some authors as a venous angioma (224), consisting of dilated and tortuous thin-walled blood vessels within the subarachnoid space and pia, which may extend into the underlying cerebral cortex and subcortical white matter. The cortex itself shows calcifications centered on microvessels, with associated neuronal loss, astrocytic gliosis, and cortical atrophy (218, 219) that is assumed to result from ischemic phenomena secondary, at least in part, to the meningeal angiomatosis. Associated malformations such as polymicrogyria, agyria/pachygyria, heterotopias, and cortical

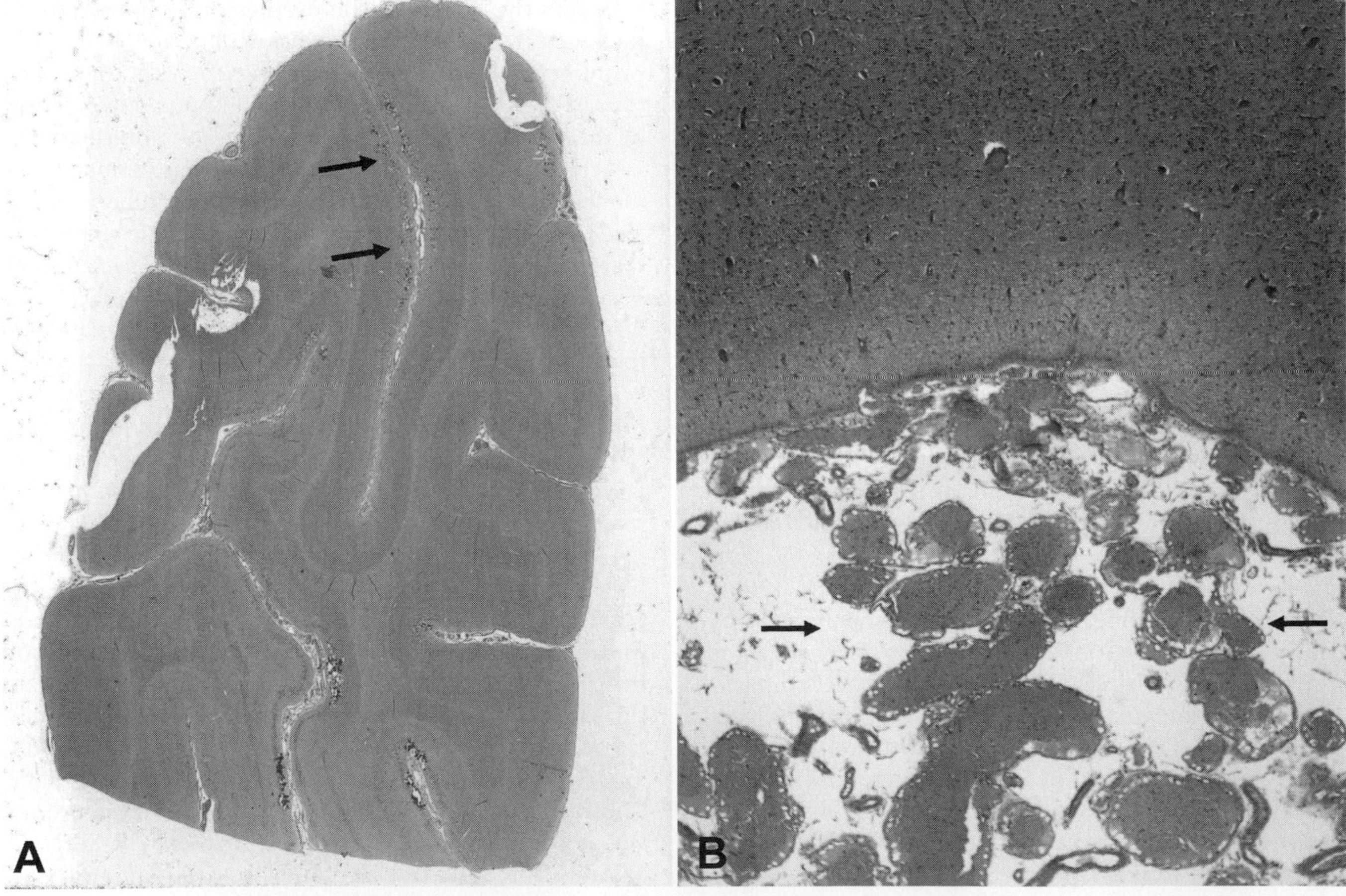

FIGURE 5-9

Sturge-Weber disease (surgical specimens stained with hematoxylin and eosin). (A) A portion of occipital lobe showing barely visible punctate and granular calcification in the superficial cortex (arrows). (B) Venous angioma-like structure in meninges of another case (arrows; cortex is at top of the image).

disorganization may also be seen (220). Ultrastructural studies of the parenchymal calcifications in Sturge-Weber brain have suggested that the earliest calcium deposits occur within perithelial cells (pericytes) of small blood vessels, and that the underlying cause of the calcification may be anoxic injury to endothelial, perithelial, and glial mitochondria (226, 227).

NEUROFIBROMATOSIS AND OTHER NEUROCUTANEOUS SYNDROMES

Central neurofibromatosis (NF-2) is a genetic disorder characterized by neoplastic and dysplastic lesions of Schwann cells, meningeal cells, and glia (182, 228). It is associated with (a) central and peripheral schwannomas, including bilateral acoustic schwannomas, (b) meningiomas, (c) gliomas, and (d) glial hamartomas. It is inherited as autosomal dominant, with a high rate of sporadic mutations. The *NF-2* gene, postulated to be a tumor-suppressor gene, has been localized to chromosome 22q12 and encodes a widely expressed protein, merlin (moesin, ezrin, radixin-like protein) or schwannomin, a new member of the protein 4.1 family of cytoskeleton-associated proteins (228, 229). Although seizures can develop in patients with NF-2, these are usually caused by a primary neoplasm rather than a malformative lesion. The most frequent malformations seen in association with NF-2 are meningio-angiomatosis and glial hamartomas. Meningio-angiomatosis (230, 231) is a rare epilepsy-associated lesion of the cerebral cortex of unknown etiology, with puzzling and rather dramatic vascular, malformative, and neoplastic elements (232, 232a). Rare neurocutaneous syndromes, such as epidermal nevus syndrome and hypomelanosis of Ito (233), have also been associated with pediatric epilepsy. The pathologic changes seen within the cerebral cortex of these patients are virtually identical to those seen in patients with CD.

BRAIN INFLAMMATION AND EPILEPSY

One of the most common inflammatory lesions encountered in corticectomies performed for intractable epilepsy is the chronic inflammatory reaction (often with a giant cell or granulomatous component) that is left by depth electrodes implanted for preoperative monitoring purposes within brain parenchyma. Leaving aside the obvious fact that any inflammatory disorder of the brain (especially viral encephalitides, e.g., caused by *Herpes simplex*) may be accompanied by seizure activity, evidence is emerging of an increasingly important role for brain inflammation in epilepsy. Steroids and adrenocorticotropic hormone (ACTH) have powerful anticonvulsant effects, especially in children with infantile spasms or West syndrome. Seizure activity is regularly associated with a cerebrospinal fluid (CSF) pleocytosis and elevated CSF proinflammatory cytokines. Emerging evidence suggests that patients who develop temporal lobe epilepsy with hippocampal sclerosis (TLE-HS) following febrile convulsions may have been at risk for developing TLE-HS because of polymorphisms in the interleukin (IL)-1β-511T allele (234). Temporal lobes resected from patients with TLE have demonstrated overexpression of NFkappaB, a transcription factor involved in acute inflammation (235). There is indirect evidence that new-onset refractory status epilepticus (NORSE) may have an inflammatory basis in that many patients have an antecedent inflammatory or infectious illness and CSF usually shows a pleocytosis (236).

Rasmussen Syndrome (RS)

Rasmussen syndrome (or Rasmussen encephalitis, RE) is characterized by intractable focal seizures (usually epilepsia partialis continua) with progressive hemiparesis, symptoms attributed to chronic (pathogen-free) inflammation of gray and white matter, with progressive unihemispheric atrophy (237–239). A recent European consensus meeting on RS has formulated diagnostic criteria, which incorporate clinical, EEG, MR, and pathologic findings (240). Although the pathologic appearances of brain tissue affected by RE suggest a chronic viral infection, no virus has ever been consistently isolated from RS brain tissue or discovered within it using modern molecular or microbial culture techniques (241, 242). Circulating anti-glu-R3 antibodies were reported to be of etiologic importance in some patients with RS (243, 244), but subsequently these antibodies were found to occur in other seizure disorders (245, 246). Very recently, autoantibodies against the N-methyl-D-aspartate glutamate receptor (NMDA-type GluR) epsilon2 subunit and its epitopes were reported in RS patients (247). However, although the initial report is highly promising, the diagnostic specificity of GluRepsilon2 for RS remains to be confirmed. Any explanation for RS will ultimately have to account for its unihemispheric topography. Rarely have pathologic studies demonstrated bihemispheric involvement (248).

The neuropathologic findings of RS/RE (Figure 5-10) are said to comprise four merging stages (240, 249, 250), the earliest of which is characterized by inflammation, especially perivascular lymphocytes, and microglial nodule formation within brain parenchyma, but little morphologic evidence of neuronal injury. In stage 2, lymphocytic infiltration increases in density and both astrocytes and microglial cells become more widespread, tending to involve all cortical layers—a "panlaminar" pattern of cortical inflammation and gliosis. Patchy neuronal loss may be present. In stage 3 the neuronal population is depleted in either a patchy or panlaminar pattern, with

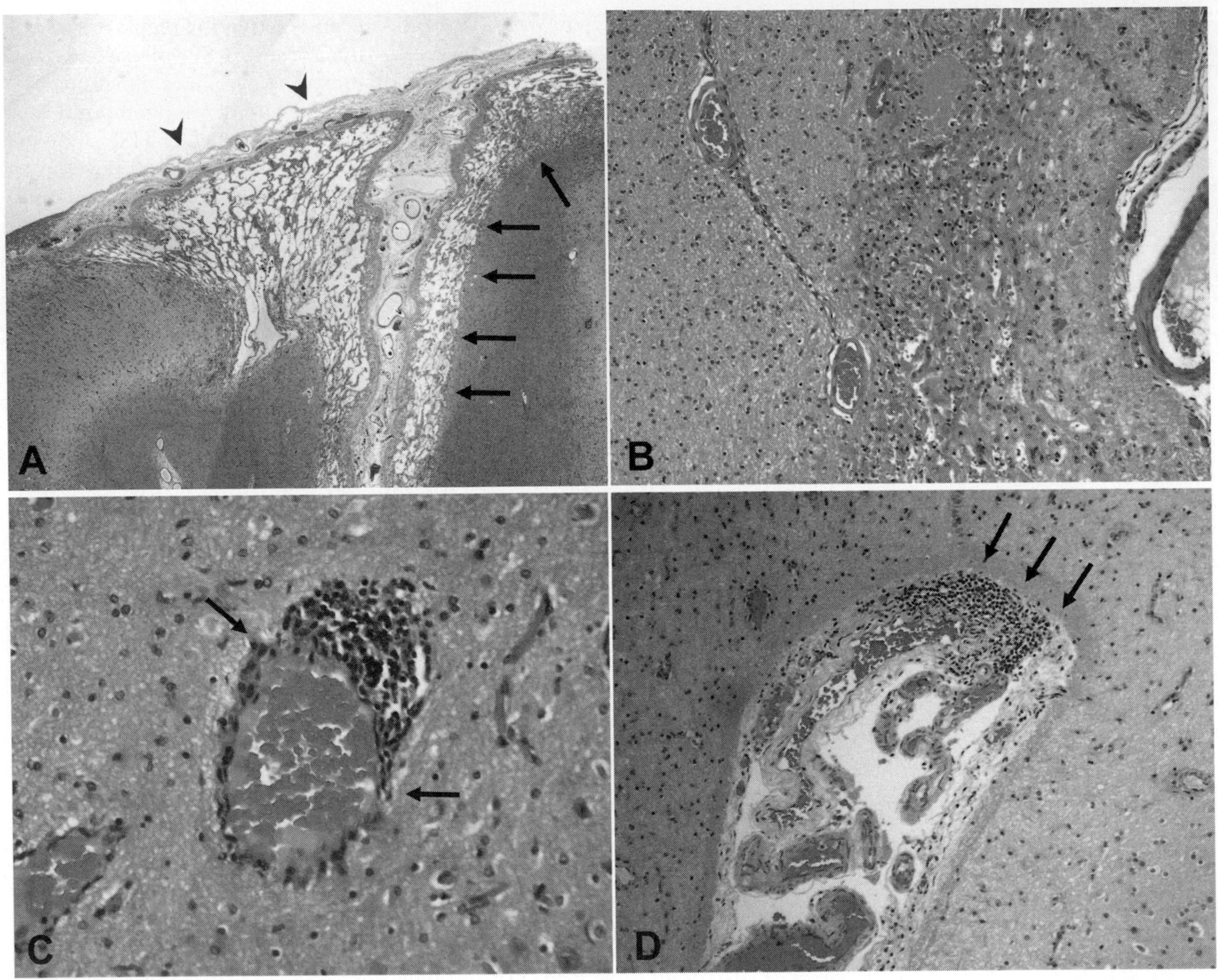

FIGURE 5-10

Histopathology of Rasmussen encephalitis (RE). All panels are from sections stained with hematoxylin and eosin. (A) Extensive cystic cavitation (gyrus at left, arrowheads) and extreme laminar necrosis (gyrus at right, arrows) in a resection specimen from a severely affected child. (B) Large cortical scar, seen in the center of this image, running vertically. (C) Perivascular inflammation by mononuclear inflammatory cells (arrows), accentuated in one part of the vessel wall. (D) Patchy meningeal inflammation (arrows) by mononuclear inflammatory cells.

severe cortical degeneration and gliosis. In stage 4 there is profound cortical atrophy with gliosis and vacuolation of the neuropil, with cystic cavitation in many cases (Figure 5-10). Frequently, areas of relative cortical normality surround zones of badly scarred cortex. This geographically defined severe pathologic change, often seen a few micrometers away from relatively normal brain parenchyma, means that a negative brain biopsy taken with the intent of establishing the diagnosis of RE never truly excludes the diagnosis. Occasionally, dual pathology including malformative elements of cortical dysplasia or vascular malformations and chronic inflammation are seen in a corticectomy originating from an epilepsy patient, suggesting that the two lesions may be etiologically connected (251).

There is some interlobar variation in severity of the neuropathologic change, although usually the occipital cortex is less severely involved than the others. Subcortical white matter may show evidence of axonal injury in the form of neuroaxonal spheroids, although whether this is secondary to Wallerian degeneration or represents a separate cytotoxic attack on axons is uncertain. The

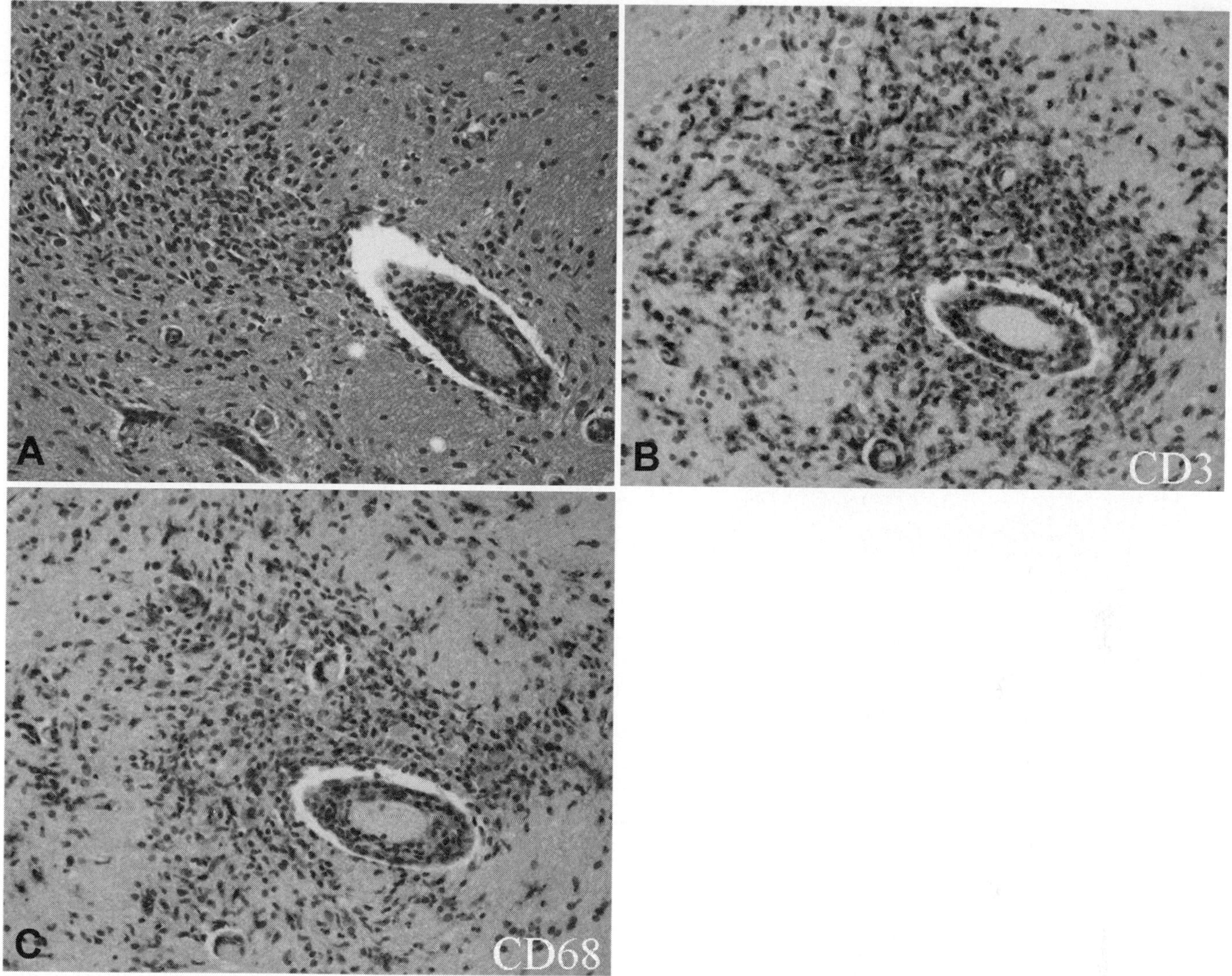

FIGURE 5-11

Immunohistochemical features of Rasmussen encephalitis. The panels represent three parallel fields from a severe case (corticectomy specimen) stained with hematoxylin and eosin (A), or primary antibodies to a T-cell marker (CD3, Panel B) or microglial/macrophage marker (CD68, Panel C), highlighting the heterogeneity of the angiocentric infiltrate. (B lymphocytes are, however, usually few in number.)

inflammation or neuronal destruction varies in its timing and progression from one region to another. Early changes consisting of inflammation only may be located adjacent to areas showing intense neuronal loss and gliosis. The almost unique unilateral nature of RS/RE separates it from all other immune-mediated disorders of the nervous system. Ultrastructural studies of RE/RS have failed to demonstrate viral particles consistently in brain biopsies/resections from affected patients, although rarely measles virus–like particles have been noted; rare cerebral endothelial cells in one case contained tubuloreticular inclusions (252). Gene expression profiling of a brain specimen from an RE patient has shown a dramatic increase in expression of several genes related to inflammation, and a pronounced down-regulation of several GluRs, especially GluR4 (253).

The inflammatory infiltrate in RS brain consists predominantly of CD8-positive T cells (254, 255). The lymphocytes lie adjacent to MHC class I(+)-expressing neurons and contain granzyme B, which has been suggested as the local mediator of T cell–mediated cytotoxic neuronal death in RS (254). There is little evidence to support a humoral

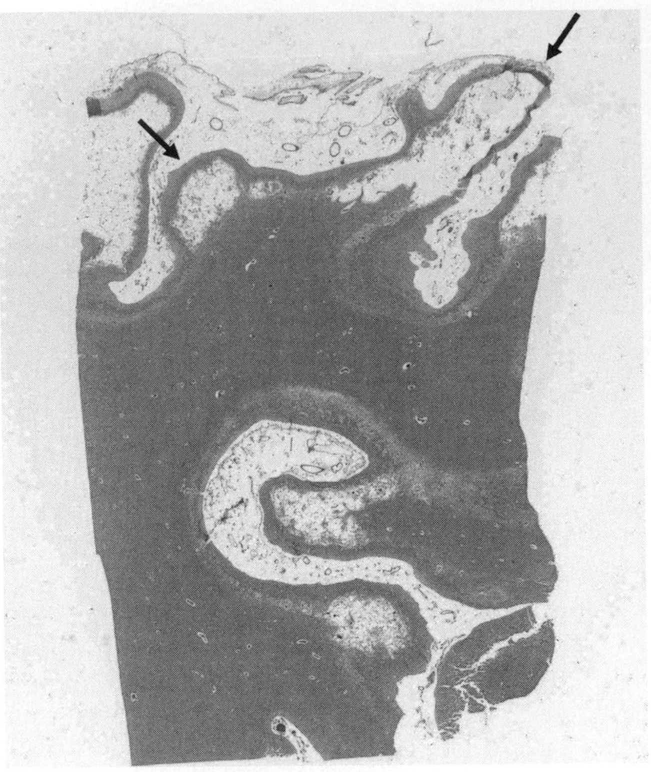

FIGURE 5-12

Severe intrauterine/perinatal brain injury (hematoxylin and eosin–stained section) usually manifests as cystic encephalomalacia, with variably severe involvement of the cortex (arrows) or subcortical white matter (section is from an autopsy rather than a surgical specimen).

process in that B cells, immunoglobulin and complement are rarely found in RS brain tissue. The T cell infiltrate is of relatively restricted clonality (256). Abundant microglia and macrophages may also be present (Figure 5-11).

DESTRUCIVE LESIONS/ ENCEPHALOMALACIA

Destructive lesions, with the neuropathologic appearance of regions of cystic encephalomalacia, are commonly encountered in corticectomies for epilepsy, especially in infants and children (162). They are presumed to represent sequelae of intrauterine, perinatal, or (rarely) postnatal brain infarcts (Figure 5-12) or hemorrhages, the etiology of which is multifactorial, extremely complex, and beyond the scope of this chapter. For excellent recent monographs on pathophysiologic mechanisms important in the evolution of destructive brain lesions in the developing human brain, including ones that may cause seizures, see the works by Kalimo (232) and Golden and Harding (232a).

ACKNOWLEDGMENTS

This work was supported by VA Medical Research Funds and National Institutes of Health Grant NS046524 (CRH), and the Daljit S. & Elaine Sarkaria Chair in Diagnostic Medicine (HVV). Christine Huang and Carol Appleton provided expert assistance with preparation of the figures.

References

1. Margerison JH, Corsellis JAN. Epilepsy and the temporal lobes: a clinical encephalographic and neuropathological study of the brain in epilepsy, with particular reference to the temporal lobes. *Brain* 1966; 89:499–530.
2. Bruton CJ. The neuropathology of temporal lobe epilepsy. London, UK: Oxford, 1988.
3. Wieser HG. ILAE Commission Report. Mesial temporal lobe epilepsy with hippocampal sclerosis. *Epilepsia* 2004; 45:695–714.
4. Sloviter RS. Hippocampal pathology and pathophysiology in temporal lobe epilepsy. *Neurologia* 1996; 11 Suppl 4:29–32.
5. Houser CR. Neuronal loss and synaptic reorganization in temporal lobe epilepsy. In: Delgado-Escueta A, Wilson WA, Olsen RW, Porter RJ, eds. Jasper's *Basic Mechanisms of the Epilepsies*. Philadelphia, PA: Lippincott Williams & Wilkins, 1999:743–761.
6. Sutula T, Xiao-Xian H, Cavazos J, Scott G. Synaptic reorganization in the hippocampus induced by abnormal functional activity. *Science* 1988; 239:1147–1150.
7. Houser CR, Miyashiro JE, Swartz BE, Walsh GO, et al. Altered patterns of dynorphin immunoreactivity suggest mossy fiber reorganization in human hippocampal epilepsy. *J Neurosci* 1990; 10:267–282.
8. Babb TL, Kupfer WR, Pretorius JK, Crandall PH, et al. Synaptic reorganization by mossy fibers in human epileptic fascia dentata. *Neuroscience* 1991; 42:351–363.
9. El Bahh B, Lespinet V, Lurton D, Coussemaq M, et al. Correlations between granule cell dispersion, mossy fiber sprouting, and hippocampal cell loss in temporal lobe epilepsy. *Epilepsia* 1999; 40:1393–1401.
10. Thom M, Sisodiya SM, Beckett A, Martinian L, et al. Cytoarchitectural abnormalities in hippocampal sclerosis. *J Neuropathol Exp Neurol* 2002; 61:510–519.
11. Franck JE, Pokorny J, Kunkel DD, Schwartzkroin PA. Physiologic and morphologic characteristics of granule cell circuitry in human epileptic hippocampus. *Epilepsia* 1995; 36:543–558.
12. Zhang N, Houser CR. Ultrastructural localization of dynorphin in the dentate gyrus in human temporal lobe epilepsy: a study of re-organized mossy fiber synapses. *J Comp Neurol* 1999; 405:472–490.
13. Amaral DG, Dent JA. Development of the mossy fibers of the dentate gyrus: I. A light and electron microscopic study of the mossy fibers and their expansions. *J Comp Neurol* 1981; 195:51–86.
14. Wuarin JP, Dudek FE. Excitatory synaptic input to granule cells increases with time after kainate treatment. *J Neurophysiol* 2001; 85:1067–1077.
15. Buckmaster PS, Zhang GF, Yamawaki R. Axon sprouting in a model of temporal lobe epilepsy creates a predominantly excitatory feedback circuit. *J Neurosci* 2002; 22:6650–6658.
16. Sloviter RS, Zappone CA, Harvey BD, Frotscher M. Kainic acid-induced recurrent mossy fiber innervation of dentate gyrus inhibitory interneurons: possible anatomical substrate of granule cell hyper-inhibition in chronically epileptic rats. *J Comp Neurol* 2006; 494:944–960.
17. Maglóczky Z, Wittner L, Borhegyi Z, Halasz P, et al. Changes in the distribution and connectivity of interneurons in the epileptic human dentate gyrus. *Neuroscience* 2000; 96:7–25.
18. Lehmann TN, Gabriel S, Kovacs R, Eilers A, et al. Alterations of neuronal connectivity in area CA1 of hippocampal slices from temporal lobe epilepsy patients and from pilocarpine-treated epileptic rats. *Epilepsia* 2000; 41 Suppl 6:S190–S194.
19. Babb TL, Pretorius JK, Kupfer WR, Crandall PH. Glutamate decarboxylase-immunoreactive neurons are preserved in human epileptic hippocampus. *J Neurosci* 1989; 9:2562–2574.
20. deLanerolle NC, Kim JH, Robbins RJ, Spencer DD. Hippocampal interneuron loss and plasticity in human temporal lobe epilepsy. *Brain Res* 1989; 495:387–395.
21. Mathern GW, Babb TL, Pretorius JK, Leite JP. Reactive synaptogenesis and neuron densities for neuropeptide Y, somatostatin, and glutamate decarboxylase immunoreactivity in the epileptogenic human fascia dentata. *J Neurosci* 1995; 15:3990–4004.
22. Maglóczky Z, Freund TF. Impaired and repaired inhibitory circuits in the epileptic human hippocampus. *Trends Neurosci* 2005; 28:334–340.
23. Robbins RJ, Brines ML, Kim JH, Adrian T, et al. A selective loss of somatostatin in the hippocampus of patients with temporal lobe epilepsy. *Ann Neurol* 1992; 29:325–332.

24. Sundstrom LE, Brana C, Gatherer M, Mepham J, et al. Somatostatin- and neuropeptide Y-synthesizing neurones in the fascia dentata of humans with temporal lobe epilepsy. *Brain* 2001; 124:688–697.
25. Sagar HJ, Oxbury JM. Hippocampal neuron loss in temporal lobe epilepsy: correlation with early childhood convulsions. *Ann Neurol* 1987; 22:334–340.
26. Mathern GW, Adelson PD, Cahan LD, Leite JP. Hippocampal neuron damage in human epilepsy: Meyer's hypothesis revisited. *Prog Brain Res* 2002; 135:237–251.
27. Sloviter RS. Decreased hippocampal inhibition and a selective loss of interneurons in experimental epilepsy. *Science* 1987; 235:73–76.
28. Lowenstein DH, Thomas MJ, Smith DH, McIntosh TK. Selective vulnerability of dentate hilar neurons following traumatic brain injury: a potential mechanistic link between head trauma and disorders of the hippocampus. *J Neurosci* 1992; 12:4846–4853.
29. Sperk G, Marksteiner J, Gruber B, Bellman R. Functional changes in neuropeptide Y- and somatostatin-containing neurons induced by limbic seizures in the rat. *Neuroscience* 1992; 50:831–846.
30. Matsuyama T, Tsuchiyama M, Nakamura H, Matsumoto M, et al. Hilar somatostatin neurons are more vulnerable to an ischemic insult than CA1 pyramidal neurons. *J Cereb Blood Flow Metab* 1993; 13:229–234.
31. Buckmaster PS, Dudek FE. Neuron loss, granule cell axon reorganization, and functional changes in the dentate gyrus of epileptic kainate-treated rats. *J Comp Neurol* 1997; 385:385–404.
32. de Lanerolle NC. The pathology of the epilepsies: insights from pathology to mechanisms of causation of temporal lobe epilepsy. In: Pellock JM, Dodson WE, Bourgeois BFD, eds. *Pediatric Epilepsy: Diagnosis and Therapy*. New York: Demos Medical Publishing, 2000:45–60.
33. Wittner L, Maglóczky Z, Borhegyi Z, Halász P, et al. Preservation of perisomatic inhibitory input of granule cells in the epileptic human dentate gyrus. *Neuroscience* 2001; 108:587–600.
34. Wittner L, Eröss L, Czirják S, Halasz P, et al. Surviving CA1 pyramidal cells receive intact perisomatic inhibitory input in the human epileptic hippocampus. *Brain* 2005; 128:138–152.
35. Sloviter RS, Sollas AL, Barbaro NM, Laxer KD. Calcium-binding protein (calbindin-D28K) and parvalbumin immunocytochemistry in the normal and epileptic human hippocampus. *J Comp Neurol* 1991; 308:381–396.
36. Zhu ZQ, Armstrong DL, Hamilton WJ, Grossman RG. Disproportionate loss of CA4 parvalbumin-immunoreactive interneurons in patients with Ammon's horn sclerosis. *J Neuropathol Exp Neurol* 1997; 56:988–998.
37. DeFelipe J. Chandelier cells and epilepsy. *Brain* 1999; 122 Pt 10:1807–1822.
38. Arellano JI, Muñoz A, Ballesteros-Yáñez I, Sola RG, et al. Histopathology and reorganization of chandelier cells in the human epileptic sclerotic hippocampus. *Brain* 2004; 127:45–64.
39. Cobb SR, Buhl EH, Halasy K, Paulson O, et al. Synchronization of neuronal activity in hippocampus by individual GABAergic interneurons. *Nature* 1995; 378:75–78.
40. Wittner L, Eröss L, Szabó Z, Toth S, et al. Synaptic reorganization of calbindin-positive neurons in the human hippocampal CA1 region in temporal lobe epilepsy. *Neuroscience* 2002; 115:961–978.
41. Tóth K, Wittner L, Urbán Z, Doyle WK, et al. Morphology and synaptic input of substance P receptor-immunoreactive interneurons in control and epileptic human hippocampus. *Neuroscience* 2007; 144:495–508.
42. Cohen I, Navarro V, Clemenceau S, Baulac M, et al. On the origin of interictal activity in human temporal lobe epilepsy in vitro. *Science* 2002; 298:1418–1421.
43. Rivera C, Voipio J, Payne JA, Ruusuvuori E, et al. The K+/Cl− co-transporter KCC2 renders GABA hyperpolarizing during neuronal maturation. *Nature* 1999; 397:251–255.
44. Palma E, Amici M, Sobrero F, Spinelli G, et al. Anomalous levels of Cl− transporters in the hippocampal subiculum from temporal lobe epilepsy patients make GABA excitatory. *Proc Natl Acad Sci U S A* 2006; 103:8465–8468.
45. Cohen I, Navarro V, Le Duigou C, Miles R. Mesial temporal lobe epilepsy: a pathological replay of developmental mechanisms? *Biol Cell* 2003; 95:329–333.
46. Cossart R, Bernard C, Ben Ari Y. Multiple facets of GABAergic neurons and synapses: multiple fates of GABA signalling in epilepsies. *Trends Neurosci* 2005; 28:108–115.
47. Dzhala VI, Talos DM, Sdrulla DA, Brumback AC, et al. NKCC1 transporter facilitates seizures in the developing brain. *Nat Med* 2005; 11:1205–1213.
48. Nadler JV. The recurrent mossy fiber pathway of the epileptic brain. *Neurochem Res* 2003; 28:1649–1658.
49. Houser CR. Granule cell dispersion in the dentate gyrus of humans with temporal lobe epilepsy. *Brain Res* 1990; 535:195–204.
50. Fahrner A, Kann G, Flubacher A, Heinrich C, et al. Granule cell dispersion is not accompanied by enhanced neurogenesis in temporal lobe epilepsy patients. *Exp Neurol* 2007; 203:320–323.
51. Houser CR, Swartz BE, Walsh GO, Delgado-Escueta AV. Granule cell disorganization in the dentate gyrus: possible alterations of neuronal migration in human temporal lobe epilepsy. *Epilepsy Res Suppl* 1992; 9:41–49.
52. Mathern GW, Kuhlman PA, Mendoza D, Pretorius JK. Human fascia dentata anatomy and hippocampal neuron densities differ depending on the epileptic syndrome and age at first seizure. *J Neuropathol Exp Neurol* 1997; 56:199–212.
53. Armstrong DD. The neuropathology of temporal lobe epilepsy. *J Neuropathol Exp Neurol* 1993; 52:433–443.
54. Harding B, Thom M. Bilateral hippocampal granule cell dispersion: autopsy study of 3 infants. *Neuropathol Appl Neurobiol* 2001; 27:245–251.
55. Suckling J, Roberts H, Walker M, Highley JR, et al. Temporal lobe epilepsy with and without psychosis: exploration of hippocampal pathology including that in subpopulations of neurons defined by their content of immunoreactive calcium-binding proteins. *Acta Neuropathol (Berl)* 2000; 99:547–554.
56. Stanfield BB, Cowan WM. The morphology of the hippocampus and dentate gyrus in normal and reeler mice. *J Comp Neurol* 1979; 185:393–422.
57. D'Arcangelo G, Miao GG, Chen SC, Soares HD, et al. A protein related to extracellular matrix proteins deleted in the mouse mutant reeler. *Nature* 1995; 374:719–723.
58. D'Arcangelo G, Nakajima K, Miyata T, Ogawa M, et al. Reelin is a secreted glycoprotein recognized by the CR-50 monoclonal antibody. *J Neurosci* 1997; 17:23–31.
59. Del Rio JA, Heimrich B, Borrell V, Forster E, et al. A role for Cajal-Retzius cells and reelin in the development of hippocampal connections. *Nature* 1997; 385:70–74.
60. Haas CA, Dudeck O, Kirsch M, Huszka C, et al. Role for reelin in the development of granule cell dispersion in temporal lobe epilepsy. *J Neurosci* 2002; 22:5797–5802.
61. Blümcke I, Beck H, Suter B, Hoffmann D, et al. An increase of hippocampal calretinin-immunoreactive neurons correlates with early febrile seizures in temporal lobe epilepsy. *Acta Neuropathol (Berl)* 1999; 97:31–39.
62. Bouilleret V, Schwaller B, Schurmans S, Celio MR, et al. Neurodegenerative and morphogenic changes in a mouse model of temporal lobe epilepsy do not depend on the expression of the calcium-binding proteins parvalbumin, calbindin, or calretinin. *Neuroscience* 2000; 97:47–58.
63. Suzuki F, Junier M-P, Guilhem D, Sorensen JC, et al. Morphogenetic effect of kainate on adult hippocampal neurons associated with a prolonged expression of brain-derived neurotrophic factor. *Neuroscience* 1995; 64:665–674.
64. Guilhem D, Dreyfus PA, Makiura Y, Suzuki F, et al. Short increase of BDNF messenger RNA triggers kainic acid-induced neuronal hypertrophy in adult mice. *Neuroscience* 1996; 72:923–931.
65. Scharfman H, Goodman J, Macleod A, Phani S, et al. Increased neurogenesis and the ectopic granule cells after intrahippocampal BDNF infusion in adult rats. *Exp Neurol* 2005; 192:348–356.
66. Mathern GW, Babb TL, Micevych PE, Blanco CE, et al. Granule cell mRNA levels for BDNF, NGF, and NT-3 correlate with neuron losses or supragranular mossy fiber sprouting in the chronically damaged and epileptic human hippocampus. *Mol Chem Neuropathol* 1997; 30:53–76.
67. Takahashi M, Hayashi S, Kakita A, Wakabayashi K, et al. Patients with temporal lobe epilepsy show an increase in brain-derived neurotrophic factor protein and its correlation with neuropeptide Y. *Brain Res* 1999; 818:579–582.
68. Wenzel HJ, Robbins CA, Tsai LH, Schwartzkroin PA. Abnormal morphological and functional organization of the hippocampus in a p35 mutant model of cortical dysplasia associated with spontaneous seizures. *J Neurosci* 2001; 21:983–998.
69. Patel LS, Wenzel HJ, Schwartzkroin PA. Physiological and morphological characterization of dentate granule cells in the p35 knock-out mouse hippocampus: evidence for an epileptic circuit. *J Neurosci* 2004; 24:9005–9014.
70. Gupta A, Sanada K, Miyamoto DT, Rovelstad S, et al. Layering defect in p35 deficiency is linked to improper neuronal-glial interaction in radial migration. *Nat Neurosci* 2003; 6:1284–1291.
71. Mikkonen M, Soininen H, Kälviäinen R, Tapiola T, et al. Remodeling of neuronal circuitries in human temporal lobe epilepsy: increased expression of highly polysialylated neural cell adhesion molecule in the hippocampus and the entorhinal cortex. *Ann Neurol* 1998; 44:923–934.
72. Crespel A, Coubes P, Rousset MC, Alonso G, et al. Immature-like astrocytes are associated with dentate granule cell migration in human temporal lobe epilepsy. *Neurosci Lett* 2002; 330:114–118.
73. Pirttilä TJ, Manninen A, Jutila L, Nissinen J, et al. Cystatin C expression is associated with granule cell dispersion in epilepsy. *Ann Neurol* 2005; 58:211–223.
74. Wenzel HJ, Born DE, Dubach MF, Gunderson VM, et al. Morphological plasticity in an infant monkey model of temporal lobe epilepsy. *Epilepsia* 2000; 41 Suppl 6:S70–S75.
75. Lie DC, Song H, Colamarino SA, Ming GL, et al. Neurogenesis in the adult brain: new strategies for central nervous system diseases. *Annu Rev Pharmacol Toxicol* 2004; 44:399–421.
76. Parent JM, Yu TW, Leibowitz RT, Geschwind DH, et al. Dentate granule cell neurogenesis is increased by seizures and contributes to aberrant network reorganization in the adult rat hippocampus. *J Neurosci* 1997; 17:3727–3738.
77. Thom M, Martinian L, Williams G, Stoeber K, et al. Cell proliferation and granule cell dispersion in human hippocampal sclerosis. *J Neuropathol Exp Neurol* 2005; 64:194–201.
78. Crespel A, Rigau V, Coubes P, Rousset MC, et al. Increased number of neural progenitors in human temporal lobe epilepsy. *Neurobiol Dis* 2005; 19:436–450.
79. Heinrich C, Nitta N, Flubacher A, Müller M, et al. Reelin deficiency and displacement of mature neurons, but not neurogenesis, underlie the formation of granule cell dispersion in the epileptic hippocampus. *J Neurosci* 2006; 26:4701–4713.
80. Parent JM, Elliott RC, Pleasure SJ, Barbaro NM, et al. Aberrant seizure-induced neurogenesis in experimental temporal lobe epilepsy. *Ann Neurol* 2006; 59:81–91.
81 Jessberger S, Römer B, Babu H, Kempermann G, et al. Seizures induce proliferation and dispersion of doublecortin-positive hippocampal progenitor cells. *Exp Neurol* 2005; 196:342–351.
82. Altman J, Bayer SA. Migration and distribution of two populations of hippocampal granule cell precursors during the perinatal and postnatal periods. *J Comp Neurol* 1990; 301:365–381.
83. Palmer TD, Willhoite AR, Gage FH. Vascular niche for adult hippocampal neurogenesis. *J Comp Neurol* 2000; 425:479–494.
84. Bengzon J, Kokaia Z, Elmér E, Nanobashvili A, et al. Apoptosis and proliferation of dentate gyrus neurons after single and intermittent limbic seizures. *Proc Natl Acad Sci USA* 1997; 94:10432–10437.
85. Gray WP, Sundstrom LE. Kainic acid increases the proliferation of granule cell progenitors in the dentate gyrus of the adult rat. *Brain Res* 1998; 790:52–59.

86. Kornack DR, Rakic P. Continuation of neurogenesis in the hippocampus of the adult macaque monkey. *Proc Natl Acad Sci U S A* 1999; 96:5768–5773.
87. van Praag H, Schinder AF, Christie BR, Toni N, et al. Functional neurogenesis in the adult hippocampus. *Nature* 2002; 415:1030–1034.
88. Zhao C, Teng EM, Summers RG Jr, Ming GL, et al. Distinct morphological stages of dentate granule neuron maturation in the adult mouse hippocampus. *J Neurosci* 2006; 26:3–11.
89. Overstreet-Wadiche LS, Bromberg DA, Bensen AL, Westbrook GL. Seizures accelerate functional integration of adult-generated granule cells. *J Neurosci* 2006; 26: 4095–4103.
90. Hattiangady B, Rao MS, Shetty AK. Chronic temporal lobe epilepsy is associated with severely declined dentate neurogenesis in the adult hippocampus. *Neurobiol Dis* 2004; 17:473–490.
91. Kralic JE, Ledergerber DA, Fritschy JM. Disruption of the neurogenic potential of the dentate gyrus in a mouse model of temporal lobe epilepsy with focal seizures. *Eur J Neurosci* 2005; 22:1916–1927.
92. Mathern GW, Leiphart JL, De Vera A, Adelson PD, et al. Seizures decrease postnatal neurogenesis and granule cell development in the human fascia dentata. *Epilepsia* 2002; 43 Suppl 5:68–73.
93. Friede RL. *Developmental Neuropathology*. 2nd ed. Berlin: Springer-Verlag, 1989.
94. Vinters HV, Armstrong DL, Babb TL, Daumas-Duport C, et al. The neuropathology of human symptomatic epilepsy. In: Engel J Jr, ed. *Surgical Treatment of the Epilepsies*. 2nd ed. New York: Raven Press, 1993:593–608.
95. Becker AJ, Blümcke I, Urbach H, Hans V, et al. Molecular neuropathology of epilepsy-associated glioneuronal malformations. *J Neuropathol Exp Neurol* 2006; 65:99–108.
96. Blümcke I, Thom M, Wiestler OD. Ammon's horn sclerosis: a maldevelopmental disorder associated with temporal lobe epilepsy. *Brain Pathol* 2002; 12:199–211.
97. Mischel PS, Vinters HV. Destructive lesions associated with cortical dysplasia: analysis of eleven cases. *J Neuropathol Exp Neurol* 1995; 54:413 (abstract).
98. Barkovich AJ, Kuzniecky RI, Jackson GD, Guerrini R, et al. A developmental and genetic classification for malformations of cortical development. *Neurology* 2005; 65:1873–1887.
99. Barth PG. Disorders of neuronal migration. *Can J Neurol Sci* 1987; 14:1–16.
99a. Pilz D, Stoodley N, Golden JA. Neuronal migration, cerebral cortical development, and cerebral cortical anomalies. *J Neuropathol Exp Neurol* 2002; 61:1–11.
100. Prayson RA. Some thoughts on the classification of malformations of cortical development. *Arch Pathol Lab Med* 2006; 130:1101–1102.
101. Cepeda C, André VM, Flores-Hernandez J, Nguyen OK, et al. Pediatric cortical dysplasia: correlations between neuroimaging, electrophysiology and location of cytomegalic neurons and balloon cells and glutamate/GABA synaptic circuits. *Dev Neurosci* 2005; 27:59–76.
102. Cepeda C, André VM, Levine MS, Salamon N, et al. Epileptogenesis in pediatric cortical dysplasia: the dysmature cerebral developmental hypothesis. *Epilepsy Behav* 2006; 9:219–235.
103. Salamon N, Andres M, Chute DJ, Nguyen ST, et al. Contralateral hemimicrencephaly and clinical-pathological correlations in children with hemimegalencephaly. *Brain* 2006; 129:352–65.
104. Crino PB, Miyata H, Vinters HV. Neurodevelopmental disorders as a cause of seizures: neuropathologic, genetic, and mechanistic considerations. *Brain Pathol* 2002; 12:212–233.
105. Reiner O, Carrozzo R, Shen Y, Wehnert M, et al. Isolation of a Miller-Dieker lissencephaly gene containing G protein beta-subunit-like repeats. *Nature* 1993; 364:717–721.
106. Jellinger K. Neuropathological aspects of infantile spasms. *Brain Dev* 1987; 9:349–357.
107. Meencke HJ. Morphological aspects of etiology and the course of infantile spasms (West syndrome). *Neuropediatrics* 1985; 16:59–66.
108. Robain O, Vinters HV. Neuropathological studies. In: Dulac O, Chugani HT, Dalla Bernardina B, eds. *Infantile Spasms and West Syndrome*. London: WB Saunders, 1994:99–117.
109. Meencke HJ, Janz D. Neuropathological findings in primary generalized epilepsy: a study of eight cases. *Epilepsia* 1984; 25:8–21.
110. Aicardi J. Diseases of the nervous system in childhood. Clinics in Developmental Medicine. Nr 115/118. London: MacKeith, 1992.
111. Mischel PS, Nguyen L, Vinters HV. Cerebral cortical dysplasia associated with pediatric epilepsy. Review of neuropathologic features and proposal for a grading system. *J Neuropathol Exp Neurol* 1995; 54:137–153.
112. Morris EB, Parisi JE, Buchhalter JR. Histopathologic findings of malformations of cortical development in an epilepsy surgery cohort. *Arch Pathol Lab Med* 2006; 130:1163–1168.
113. Palmini A, Andermann F, Olivier A, Tampieri D, et al. Focal neuronal migration disorders and intractable partial epilepsy: results of surgical treatment. *Ann Neurol* 1991; 30:750–757.
114. Palmini A, Andermann F, Olivier A, Tampieri D, et al. Focal neuronal migration disorders and intractable partial epilepsy: a study of 30 patients. *Ann Neurol* 1991; 30:741–749.
115. Rakic P. Defects of neuronal migration and the pathogenesis of cortical malformations. *Prog Brain Res* 1988; 73:15–37.
116. Jonas R, Asarnow RF, LoPresti C, Yudovin S, et al. Surgery for symptomatic infant-onset epileptic encephalopathy with and without infantile spasms. *Neurology* 2004; 64:746–750.
117. Hardiman O, Burke T, Phillips J, Murphy S, et al. Microdysgenesis in resected temporal neocortex: incidence and clinical significance in focal epilepsy. *Neurology* 1988; 38:1041–1047.
118. Meencke HJ. Neuron density in the molecular layer of the frontal cortex in primary generalized epilepsy. *Epilepsia* 1985; 26:450–454.
119. Rorke LB. A perspective: the role of disordered genetic control of neurogenesis in the pathogenesis of migration disorders. *J Neuropathol Exp Neurol* 1994; 53:105–117.
120. Moreland DB, Glauser FE, Egnatchik JG, Heffner RR, et al. Focal cortical dysplasia. *J Neurosurg* 1988; 68:487–490.
121. Taylor DC, Falconer MA, Bruton CJ, Corsellis JA. Focal dysplasia of the cerebral cortex in epilepsy. *J Neurol Neursurg Psychiatry* 1971; 34:369–387.
122. Kazee AM, Lapham LW, Torres CF, Wang DD. Generalized cortical dysplasia. Clinical and pathological aspects. *Arch Neurol* 1991; 48:850–853.
123. Kuzniecky R. Familial diffuse cortical dysplasia. *Arch Neurol* 1994; 51:307–310.
124. Becker LE. Synaptic dysgenesis. *Can J Neurol Sci* 1991; 18:170–180.
124a. Marchal G, Andermann F, Tampieri D, Robitaille Y, et al. Generalized cortical dysplasia manifested by diffusely thick cerebral cortex. *Arch Neurol* 1989; 46:430–434.
125. Sarnat HB. Cerebral dysgeneses: embryology and clinical expression. New York: Oxford University Press, 1993.
126. Palmini A, Najm I, Avanzini G, Babb T, et al. Terminology and classification of the cortical dysplasias. *Neurology* 2004; 62 Suppl 3:S2–S8.
127. Chuong CM. Differential roles of multiple adhesion molecules in cell migration: granule cell migration in cerebellum. *Experientia* 1990; 46:893–899.23.
128. Gray GE, Leber SM, Sanes JR. Migratory patterns of clonally related cells in the developing central nervous system. *Experientia* 1990; 46:929–940.
129. Jan YN, Jan LY. Genes required for specifying cell fates in *Drosophila* embryonic sensory nervous system. *Trends Neurosci* 1990; 13:493–498.
130. Rakic P. Specification of cerebral cortical areas. *Science* 1988; 241:170–176.
131. Schmahl W, Knoedlseder M, Favor F, Davidson D. Defects of neuronal migration and the pathogenesis of cortical malformations are associated with Small eye (Sey) in the mouse, a point mutation at the Pax-6 locus. *Acta Neuropathol* 1993; 86:126–135.
132. ten Donkelaar HJ, Lammens M, Hori A. Clinical neuroembryology. Berlin: Springer-Verlag, 2006.
133. Vinters HV, Salamon N, Miyata H, Khanlou N, et al. Neuropathology of developmental disorders associated with epilepsy. In: Engel J Jr, Pedley TA, eds. *Epilepsy. A Comprehensive Textbook*. 2nd ed. Philadelphia-New York: Lippincott-Raven, 2007:in press.
134. Fujita S. The matrix cell and cytogenesis in the developing central nervous system. *J Comp Neurol* 1963; 120:37–42.
135. Purves D, Lichtman JW. Elimination of synapses in the developing nervous system. *Science* 1980; 210:153–157.
136. Van Huizen F, Romijn HJ, Corner MA. Indications for a critical period for synapse elimination in developing rat cerebral cortex cultures. *Brain Res Dev Brain Res* 1987; 31:1–6.
137. Meyer G, Goffinet AM. Prenatal development of reelin-immunoreactive neurons in the human neocortex. *J Comp Neurol* 1998; 397:29–40.
138. Meyer G, Pérez-García CG, Abraham H, Caput D. Expression of p73 and Reelin in the developing human cortex. *J Neurosci* 2002; 22:4973–4986.
138a. Marín-Padilla M. Cajal-Retzius cells and the development of the neocortex. *Trends Neurosci* 1998; 21:64–71.
139. Trommsdorff M, Gotthardt M, Hiesberger T, Shelton J, et al. Reeler/disabled-like disruption of neuronal migration in knockout mice lacking the VLDL receptor and ApoE receptor 2. *Cell* 1999; 97:689–701.
140. Hong SE, Shugart YY, Huang DT, Shahwan SA, et al. Autosomal recessive lissencephaly with cerebellar hypoplasia is associated with human RELN mutations. *Nat Genet* 2000; 26:93–96.
141. Meyer G, Pérez-García CG, Gleeson JG. Selective expression of doublecortin and LIS1 in the developing human cortex suggests unique modes of neuronal movement. *Cereb Cortex* 2002; 12:1225–1236.
142. Brun A. The subpial granular layer of the fetal cerebral cortex in man. *APMIS Suppl* 1965; 179:1–71.
143. Gadisseux J-F, Goffinet AM, Lyon G, Evrard P. The human transient subpial granular layer: an optical, immunohistochemical, and ultrastructual analysis. *J Comp Neurol* 1992; 324:94–114.
144. Meyer G, Wahle P. The paleocortical ventricle is the origin of reelin-expressing neurons in the marginal zone of the foetal human neocortex. *Eur J Neurosci* 1999; 11:3937–3944.
145. Rakic S, Zecevic N. Emerging complexity of layer I in human cerebral cortex. *Cerebral Cortex* 2003; 13:1072–1083.
146. Spreafico R, Arcelli P, Frassoni C, Canetti P, et al. Development of layer I of the human cerebral cortex after midgestation: architectonic findings, immunocytochemical identification of neurons and glia, and in situ labeling of apoptotic cells. *J Comp Neurol* 1999; 410:126–142.
147. Chun JJM, Shatz CJ. Interstitial cells of the adult neocortical white matter are the remnant of the early generated subplate neuron population. *J Comp Neurol* 1989; 282:555–569.
148. Ghosh A, Antonin A, McConnell SK, Shatz CJ. Requirement for subplate neurons in the formation of thalamocortical connections. *Nature* 1990; 347:179–181.
149. Ghosh A, Shatz CJ. Involvement of subplate neurons in the formation of ocular dominance columns. *Science* 1993; 255:1441–1443.
150. McConnell SK, Ghosh A, Shatz CJ. Subplate pioneers and the formation of descending connections from cerebral cortex. *J Neurosci* 1994; 14:1893–1907.
151. Kostovic I, Rakic P. Developmental history of the transient subplate zone in the visual and somatosensory cortex of the macaque monkey and human brain. J Comp Neurol 1990; 297:441–70.
152. Sidman RL, Rakic P. Neuronal migration, with special reference to developing human brain: a review. *Brain Res* 1973; 62:1–35.

153. Meencke HJ. The density of dystopic neurons in the white matter of the gyrus frontalis inferior in epilepsies. *J Neurol* 1983; 30:171–181.
154. Andres M, André VM, Nguyen S, Salamon N, et al. Human cortical dysplasia and epilepsy: An ontogenetic hypothesis based on volumetric MRI and NeuN neuronal density and size measurements. *Cerebral Cortex* 2004; 15:194–210.
155. Bignami A, Palladini G, Zappella M. Unilateral megalencephaly with nerve cell hypertrophy. An anatomical and quantitive histochemical study. *Brain Res* 1968; 9:103–114.
156. Choi BH, Matthias SC. Cortical dysplasia associated with massive ectopia of neurons and glial cells within the subarachnoid space. *Acta Neuropathol* 1987; 73:105–109.
157. Robain O, Chiron C, Dulac O. Electron microscopic and Golgi study in a case of hemimegalencephaly. *Acta Neuropathol* 1989; 77:664–666.
158. Manz HJ, Phillips TM, Rowden G, McCullough DC. Unilateral megalencephaly, cerebral cortical dysplasia, neuronal hypertrophy and heterotopia: cytomorphometric, fluorometric, cytochemical, and biochemical analyses. *Acta Neuropathol* 1979; 45:97–103.
159. Vinters HV, Fisher RS, Cornford ME, Mah V, et al. Morphological substrates of infantile spasms: studies based on surgically resected cerebral tissue. *Childs Nerv Syst* 1993; 8:8–17.
160. DeRosa MJ, Secor DL, Barsom M, Fisher RS, et al. Neuropathologic findings in surgically treated hemimegalencephaly: immunohistochemical, morphometric, and ultrastructural study. *Acta Neuropathol* 1993; 84:250–260.
161. Duong T, DeRosa MJ, Poukens V, Vinters HV, et al. Neuronal cytoskeletal abnormalities in human cerebral cortical dysplasia. *Acta Neuropathol* 1994; 87:493–503.
162. Farrell MA, DeRosa MJ, Curran JG, Secor DL, et al. Neuropathologic findings in cortical resections (including hemispherectomies) performed for the treatment of intractable childhood epilepsy. *Acta Neuropathol* 1993; 83:246–259.
163. Robitaille Y, Rasmussen T, Dubeau F, Tampieri D, et al. Histopathology of non-neoplastic lesions in frontal lobe epilepsy. In: Chauvel P, Delgado-Escueta AV, et al, eds. *Advances in Neurology*. Vol. 57. New York: Raven Press, 1993:499–513.
164. Raymond AA, Fish DR, Sisodiya SM, Alsanjari N, et al. Abnormalities of gyration, heterotopias, tuberous sclerosis, focal cortical dysplasia, microdysgenesis, dysembryoplastic neuroepithelial tumour and dysgenesis of the archicortex in epilepsy. Clinical, EEG and neuroimaging features in 100 adult patients. *Brain* 1995; 118 Pt 3:629–660.
165. Schwartzkroin PA, Walsh CA. Cortical malformations and epilepsy. *Ment Retard Dev Disabil Res Rev* 2000; 6:268–280.
166. Urbach H, Scheffler B, Heinrichsmeier T, von Oertzen J, et al. Focal cortical dysplasia of Taylor's balloon cell type: a clinicopathological entity with characteristic neuroimaging and histopathological features, and favorable postsurgical outcome. *Epilepsia* 2002; 43:33–40.
167. Cepeda C, André VM, Vinters HV, Levine MS, et al. Are cytomegalic neurons and balloon cells generators of epileptic activity in pediatric cortical dysplasia? *Epilepsia* 2005; 46 Suppl 5:82–88.
168. Cepeda C, Hurst RS, Flores-Hernandez J, Hernandez-Echeagaray E, et al. Morphological and electrophysiological characterization of abnormal cell types in pediatric cortical dysplasia. *J Neurosci Res* 2003; 72:472–486. 170.
169. Friauf E, McConnell SK, Shatz CJ. Functional synaptic circuits in the subplate during fetal and early postnatal development of cat visual cortex. *J Neurosci* 1990; 10:2601–2613.
170. Chi JG, Dooling EC, Gilles FH. Gyral development of the human brain. *Ann Neurol* 1977; 1:86–93.
171. Kriegstein AR, Noctor SC. Patterns of neuronal migration in the embryonic cortex. *Trends Neurosci* 2004; 27:392–399.
172. Nadarajah B. Radial glia and somal translocation of radial neurons in the developing cerebral cortex. Glia 2003; 43:33–36.
173. Noctor SC, Martinez-Cerdeno V, Ivic L, Kriegstein AR. Cortical neurons arise in symmetric and asymmetric division zones and migrate through specific phases. *Nat Neurosci* 2004; 7:136–144.
174. Englund C, Folkerth RD, Born D, Lacy JM, et al. Aberrant neuronal-glial differentiation in Taylor-type focal cortical dysplasia (type IIA/B). *Acta Neuropathol* 2005; 109:519–533.
175. Thom M, Martinian L, Sisodiya SM, Cross JH, et al. Mcm2 labelling of balloon cells in focal cortical dysplasia. *Neuropathol Appl Neurobiol* 2005; 31:580–588.
176. Ying Z, Gonzalez-Martinez J, Tilelli C, Bingaman W, et al. Expression of neural stem cell surface marker CD133 in balloon cells of human focal cortical dysplasia. *Epilepsia* 2005; 46:1716–1723.
177. Crino PB, Henske EP. New developments in the neurobiology of the tuberous sclerosis complex. Neurology 1999; 53:1384–1390.
178. Gomez MR, Sampson JR, Whittemore VH, eds. Tuberous sclerosis complex. 3rd ed. New York-Oxford: Oxford University Press, 1999.
179. Kwiatkowski DJ, Short MP. Tuberous sclerosis. *Arch Dermatol* 1994; 130:348–354.
180. Short MP, Richardson EP Jr, Haines JL, Kwiatkowski DJ. Clinical, neuropathological and genetic aspects of the tuberous sclerosis complex. *Brain Pathol* 1995; 5:173–179.
181. Vinters HV, Park SH, Johnson MW, Mischel PS, et al. Cortical dysplasia, genetic abnormalities and neurocutaneous syndromes. *Dev Neurosci* 1999; 21:248–259.
182. McLendon RE, Rosenblum MK, Bigner DD, eds. Russell and Rubinstein's pathology of tumors of the nervous system. 7th ed. London: Hodder Arnold, 2006.
183. Webb DW, Osborne JP. Non-penetrance in tuberous sclerosis. *J Med Genet* 1991; 28:417–419.
184. Roach ES, Gomez MR, Northrup H. Tuberous sclerosis complex consensus conference: revised clinical diagnostic criteria. *J Child Neurol* 1998; 13:624–628.
185. Roach ES, Smith M, Huttenlocher P, Bhat M, et al. Report of the Diagnostic Criteria Committee of the National Tuberous Sclerosis Association. *J Child Neurol* 1992; 7:221–224.
186. Yamanouchi H, Ho M, Jay V, Becker LE. Giant cells in cortical tubers in tuberous sclerosis showing synaptophysin-immunoreactive halos. *Brain Dev* 1997; 19:21–24.
187. Iwaki T, Tateishi J. Immunohistochemical demonstration of alphaB-crystallin in hamartomas of tuberous sclerosis. *Am J Pathol* 1991; 139:1303–1308.
188. Lee A, Maldonado M, Baybis M, Walsh CA, et al. Markers of cellular proliferation are expressed in cortical tubers. *Ann Neurol* 2003; 53:668–673.
188a. Richardson EP Jr. Pathology of tuberous sclerosis. Neuropathologic aspects. *Ann N Y Acad Sci* 1991; 615:128–139.
189. The European Chromosome 16 Tuberous Sclerosis Consortium. Identification and characterization of the tuberous sclerosis gene on chromosome 16. *Cell* 1993; 75:1305–1315.
190. Janssen B, Sampson J, van der Est M, Deelen W, et al. Refined localization of TSC1 by combined analysis of 9q34 and 16p13 data in 14 tuberous sclerosis families. *Hum Genet* 1994; 94:437–440.
191. Povey S, Burley MW, Attwood J, Benham F, et al. Two loci for tuberous sclerosis: one on 9q34 and one on 16p13. *Ann Hum Genet* 1994; 58:107–127.
192. van Slegtenhorst M, de Hoogt R, Hermans C, Nellist M, et al.Identification of the tuberous sclerosis gene TSC1 on chromosome 9q34. *Science* 1997; 277:805–808.
193. MacCollin M, Kwiatkowski D. Molecular genetic aspects of the phakomatoses: tuberous sclerosis complex and neurofibromatosis 1. *Curr Opin Neurol* 2001; 14:163–169.
194. Carbonara C, Longa L, Grosso E, Borrone C, et al. 9q34 loss of heterozygosity in a tuberous sclerosis astrocytoma suggests a growth suppressor-like activity also for the TSC1 gene. *Hum MolGenet* 1994; 3:1829–1832.
195. Green AJ, Johnson PH, Yates JRW. The tuberous sclerosis gene on chromosome 9q34 acts as a growth suppressor. *Hum Mol Genet* 1994; 3:1833–1834.
196. Green AJ, Smith M, Yates JRW. Loss of heterozygosity on chromosome 16p13.3 in hamartomas from tuberous sclerosis patients. *Nat Genet* 1994; 6:193–196.
197. Lamb RF, Roy C, Diefenbach TJ, Vinters HV, et al. The *TSC1* tumour suppressor hamartin regulates cell adhesion through ERM proteins and the GTPase Rho. *Nat Cell Biol* 2000; 2:281–287.
198. Luo L. Rho GTPases in neuronal morphogenesis. *Nat Rev Neurosci* 2000; 1:173–180.
199. Takeuchi K, Kawashima A, Nagafuchi A, Tsukita S. Structural diversity of band 4.1 superfamily members. *J Cell Sci* 1994; 107:1921–1928.
200. Louvet-Vallée S. ERM proteins: from cellular architecture to cell signaling. *Biol Cell* 2000; 92:305–316.
201. Johnson MW, Miyata H, Vinters HV. Ezrin and moesin expression within the developing human cerebrum and tuberous sclerosis-associated cortical tubers. *Acta Neuropathol* 2002; 104:188–196.
202. McKay DJG, Esch F, Furthmayr H, Hall A. Rho- and rac-dependent assembly of focal adhesion complexes and actin filaments in permeabilized fibroblasts: an essential role for ezrin/radixin/moesin proteins. *J Cell Biol* 1997; 138:927–938.
203. Takahashi K, Sasaki T, Mammoto A, Hotta I, et al. Interaction of radixin with Rho small G protein GDP/GTP exchange protein Dbl. *Oncogene* 1998; 16:3279–3284.
204. Takahashi K, Sasaki T, Mammoto A, Takaishi K, et al. Direct interaction of the Rho GDP dissociation inhibitor with ezrin/radixin/moesin initiates the activation of the Rho small G protein. *J Biol Chem* 1997; 272:23371–23375.
205. Olenik C, Aktories K, Meyer DK. Differential expression of the small GTP-binding proteins RhoA, RhoB, Cdc42u and Cdc42b in developing rat neocortex. *Brain Res Mol Brain Res* 1999; 18:9–17.
206. Johnson MW, Emelin JK, Park SH, Vinters HV. Co-localization of *TSC1* and *TSC2* gene products in tubers of patients with tuberous sclerosis. *Brain Pathol* 1999; 9:45–54.
206a. Park SH, Pepkowitz SH, Kerfoot C, De Rosa MJ, et al. Tuberous sclerosis in a 20-week gestation fetus: immunohistochemical study. *Acta Neuropathol* 1997; 94:180–186.
207. Wienecke R, König A, DeClue JE. Identification of tuberin, the tuberous sclerosis-2 product. Tuberin possesses specific Rap1GAP activity. *J Biol Chem* 1995; 270:16409–16414.
208. Xiao GH, Shoarinejad F, Jin F, Golemis EA, et al. The tuberous sclerosis 2 gene product, tuberin, functions as a Rab5 GTPase activating protein (GAP) in modulating endocytosis. *J Biol Chem* 1997; 272:6097–6100.
209. Menchine M, Emelin JK, Mischel PS, Haag TA, et al. Tissue and cell type-specific expression of the tuberous sclerosis-related gene, TSC2, in human tissues. *Mod Pathol* 1996; 9:1071–1080.
210. Geist RT, Gutmann DH. The tuberous sclerosis 2 gene is expressed at high levels in the cerebellum and developing spinal cord. *Cell Growth & Differentiation* 1995; 6:1477–1483.
211. Gutmann DH, Zhang Y, Hasbani J, Goldberg MP, et al. Expression of the tuberous sclerosis complex gene products, hamartin and tuberin, in central nervous system tissues. *Acta Neuropathol* 2000; 99:223–230.
212. Kerfoot C, Wienecke R, Menchine M, Emelin J, et al. Localization of tuberous sclerosis 2 mRNA and its protein product tuberin in normal human brain and in cerebral lesions of patients with tuberous sclerosis. *Brain Pathol* 1996; 6:367–377.
213. Catania MG, Mischel PS, Vinters HV. Hamartin and tuberin interaction with the G2/M cyclin-dependent kinase CDK1 and its regulatory cyclins A and B. *J Neuropathol Exp Neurol* 2001; 60:711–723.
214. Miloloza A, Kubista M, Rosner M, Hengstschläger M. Evidence for separable functions of tuberous sclerosis gene products in mammalian cell cycle regulation. *J Neuropathol Exp Neurol* 2002; 61:154–163.
215. Potter CJ, Huang H, Xu T. *Drosophila Tsc1* functions with *Tsc2* to antagonize insulin signaling in regulating cell growth, cell proliferation, and organ size. *Cell* 2001; 105:357–368.
216. Miyata H, Chiang ACY, Vinters HV. Insulin signaling pathways in cortical dysplasia and TSC-tubers: tissue microarray analysis. *Ann Neurol* 2004; 56:510–519.
217. Baybis M, Yu J, Lee A, Golden JA, et al. mTOR cascade activation distinguishes tubers from focal cortical dysplasia. *Ann Neurol* 2004; 56:478–487.

218. Norman MG, Ludwig SK. Congenital malformations of the nervous system. In: Davis RL, Richardson DM, eds. Textbook of neuropathology. 2nd ed. Baltimore: Williams and Wilkins, 1991:207–280.
219. Norman MG, McGillivray BC, Kalousek DK, Hill A, et al. Congenital malformations of the brain. Pathologic, embryologic, clinical, radiologic and genetic aspects. New York: Oxford University Press, 1995.
220. Venes JL, Linder S. Sturge-Weber-Dimitri syndrome encephalotrigeminal angiomatosis. In: Edwards MSB, Hoffman HJ, eds. Cerebral vascular disease in children and adolescents. Baltimore: Williams and Wilkins, 1989:337–341.
221. Haslam R. Neurocutaneous syndromes. In: Nelson WE, Behrman RE, Kliegman RM, Arvin AM, eds. Nelson textbook of pediatrics. 15th ed. Philadelphia: WB Saunders, 1996:1707–1709.
222. Maria BL, Hoang K, Robertson RL, Barnes PD, et al. Imaging brain structure and functions in Sturge-Weber syndrome. In: Bodensteiner JB, Roach ES, eds. Sturge-Weber syndrome. Mount Freedom, NJ: The Sturge-Weber Foundation, 1999:43–69.
223. Oakes WJ. The natural history of patients with the Sturge-Weber syndrome. *Pediatr Neurosurg* 1992; 18:287–290.
224. Wohlwill FJ, Yakovlev PI. Histopathology of meningo-facial angiomatosis (Sturge-Weber's disease). *J Neuropathol Exp Neurol* 1957; 16:341–364.
225. Thomas-Sohl KA, Vaslow DF, Maria BL. Sturge-Weber syndrome: a review. *Pediatr Neurol* 2004; 30:303–310.
226. Guseo A. Ultrastructure of calcification in Sturge-Weber disease. *Virchows Arch A Pathol Anat Histol* 1975; 366:353–356.
227. Norman MG, Schoene WC. The ultrastructure of Sturge-Weber disease. *Acta Neuropathol* 1977; 37:199–205.
228. Louis DN, Ramesh V, Gusella JF. Neuropathology and molecular genetics of neurofibromatosis 2 and related tumors. *Brain Pathol* 1995; 5:163–172.
229. MacCollin M, Ramesh V, Jacoby LB, Louis DN, et al. Mutational analysis of patients with neurofibromatosis 2. *Am J Hum Genet* 1994; 55:314–320.
230. Kasantikul V, Brown WJ. Meningioangiomatosis in the absence of von Recklinghausen's disease. *Surg Neurol* 1981; 15:71–75.
231. Paulus W, Peiffer J, Roggendorf W. Meningio-angiomatosis. *Pathol Res Pract* 1989; 184:446–452.
232. Kalimo H, ed. Pathology and genetics. Cerebrovascular diseases. Basel: ISN Neuropath Press, 2005.
232a. Golden JA, Harding BN, eds. Pathology and genetics. Developmental neuropathology. ISN Neuropath Press, Basel, 2004:116–191.
233. Kotagal P, Rothner AD. Epilepsy in the setting of neurocutaneous syndromes. *Epilepsia* 1993; 34 Suppl 3:571–578.
234. Kanemoto K, Kawasaki J, Yuasa S, Kumaki T, et al. Increased frequency of interleukin-1beta-511T allele in patients with temporal lobe epilepsy, hippocampal sclerosis, and prolonged febrile convulsion. *Epilepsia* 2003; 44:796–799.
235. Crespel A, Coubes P, Rousset MC, Brana C, et al. Inflammatory reactions in human medial temporal lobe epilepsy with hippocampal sclerosis. *Brain Res* 2002; 952:159–169
236. Wilder-Smith EP, Lim EC, Teoh HL, Sharma VK, et al. The NORSE (new-onset refractory status epilepticus) syndrome: defining a disease entity. *Ann Acad Med Singapore* 2005; 34:417–420.
237. Rasmussen T, Olszewski J, Lloyd-Smith D. Focal seizures due to chronic localized encephalitis. *Neurology* 1958; 8:435–445.
238. Rasmussen T. Further observations on the syndrome of chronic encephalitis and epilepsy. *Appl Neurophysiol* 1978; 41:1–12.
239. Robitaille Y. Neuropathologic aspects of chronic encephalitis. In: Andermann F, ed. Chronic encephalitis and epilepsy. Rasmussen's syndrome. Boston: Butterworth-Heinemann, 1991:79–110.
240. Bien CG, Granata T, Antozzi C, Cross JH, et al. Pathogenesis, diagnosis and treatment of Rasmussen encephalitis: a European consensus statement. *Brain* 2005; 128:454–471.
241. Farrell MA, Cheng L, Cornford ME, Grody WW, et al. Cytomegalovirus and Rasmussen's encephalitis *Lancet* 1991; 337:1551–1552.
242. Vinters HV, Wang R, Wiley CA. Herpesviruses in chronic encephalitis associated with intractable childhood epilepsy. *Hum Pathol* 1993; 24:871–879.
243. Andrews PI, McNamara JO. Rasmussen's encephalitis: an autoimmune disorder? *Curr Opin Neurol* 1996; 6:673–678.
244. Rogers SW, Andrews PI, Gahring LC, Whisenand T, et al. Autoantibodies to glutamate receptor GluR3 in Rasmussen's encephalitis. *Science* 1994; 265:648–651.
245. Mantegazza R, Bernasconi P, Baggi F, Spreafico R, et al. Antibodies against GluR3 peptides are not specific for Rasmussen's encephalitis but are also present in epilepsy patients with severe, early onset disease and intractable seizures. *J Neuroimmunol* 2003; 131:179–185
246. Wiendl H, Bien CG, Bernasconi P, Fleckenstein B, et al. GluR3 antibodies: prevalence in focal epilepsy but no specificity for Rasmussen's encephalitis. *Neurology* 2001; 57:1511–1514.
247. Takahashi Y, Mori H, Mishina M, Watanabe M, et al. Autoantibodies and cell-mediated autoimmunity to NMDA-type GluRepsilon2 in patients with Rasmussen's encephalitis and chronic progressive epilepsia partialis continua. *Epilepsia* 2005; 46 Suppl 5:152–158.
248. Tobias SM, Robitaille Y, Hickey WF, Rhodes CH, et al. Bilateral Rasmussen encephalitis: postmortem documentation in a five-year-old. *Epilepsia* 2003; 44:127–130.
249. Bien CG, Urbach H, Deckert M, Schramm J, et al. Diagnosis and staging of Rasmussen's encephalitis by serial MRI and histopathology. *Neurology* 2002; 58:250–257.
250. Pardo CA, Vining EPG, Guo L, Skolasky RL, et al. The pathology of Rasmussen syndrome: stages of cortical involvement and neuropathological studies in 45 hemispherectomies. *Epilepsia* 2004; 45:516–526.
251. Hart YM, Andermann F, Robitaille Y, Laxer KD, et al. Double pathology in Rasmussen's syndrome. A window on the etiology? *Neurology* 1998; 50:731–735.
252. Park S-H, Vinters HV. Ultrastructural study of Rasmussen encephalitis. *Ultrastruct Pathol* 2002; 26:287–292.
253. Baranzini SE, Laxer K, Bollen A, Oksenberg JR. Gene expression analysis reveals altered brain transcription of glutamate receptors and inflammatory genes in a patient with chronic focal (Rasmussen's) encephalitis. *J Neuroimmunol* 2002; 128:9–15.
254. Bien CG, Bauer J, Deckwerth TL, Wiendl H, et al. Destruction of neurons by cytotoxic T cells: a new pathogenic mechanism in Rasmussen's encephalitis. *Ann Neurol* 2002; 51:311–318.
255. Farrell MA, Droogan O, Secor DL, Poukens V, et al. Chronic encephalitis associated with epilepsy: immunohistochemical and ultrastructural studies. *Acta Neuropathol Berl* 1995; 89:313–321.
256. Li Y, Uccelli A, Laxer KD, Jeong MC, et al. Local-clonal expansion of infiltrating T lymphocytes in chronic encephalitis of Rasmussen. *J Immunol* 1997; 158:1428–1437.

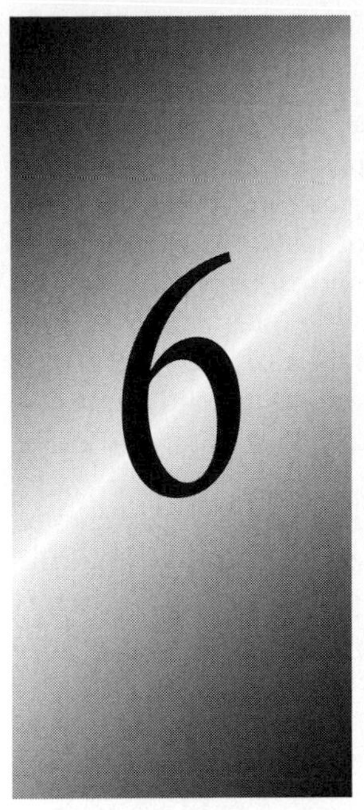

6 Epileptogenic Cerebral Cortical Malformations

Annapurna Poduri
Bernard S. Chang
Christopher A. Walsh

Neuroimaging has become a standard part of the evaluation of patients with localization-related epilepsy or with any type of epilepsy in the setting of abnormal cognitive development. In this setting, malformations of cortical development are recognized more and more frequently as the etiology of epilepsy in children.

The more aggressive pursuit of detailed neuroimaging in children with epilepsy is due in part to the more accepted role of focal resective epilepsy surgery as a treatment option in medically refractory localization-related epilepsy. Neuropathological data from patients undergoing surgical resection of epileptogenic foci have shed further light on the prevalence and histopathological properties of cerebral cortical malformations, even among some patients with normal magnetic resonance imaging (MRI). As such, the role of these malformations is proving to be substantial in the pathogenesis of refractory epilepsy in children.

We use the terms "cerebral cortical malformation" and "malformation of cortical development" interchangeably in this chapter to discuss malformations that represent known or presumed disruptions of brain development. We reserve the term "disorders of neuronal migration" for disorders in which there is radiological, pathological, or other evidence implicating the abnormal migration of cortical neurons during development. In addition, whereas "cortical dysplasia" can refer to the broad range of cerebral cortical malformations (1, 2), we restrict our use of this term to discussions of focal cortical dysplasia (FCD), since to some readers the term may connote a specific, pathologically confirmed entity.

We begin by highlighting the important role of malformations of cortical development in pediatric epilepsy. We discuss mechanisms of epileptogenesis in cerebral cortical malformations, with examples drawn from several types of malformations. In the second half of the chapter we review what has become a well-established framework for the understanding and classification of these disorders, taking into account central nervous system ontogeny and the genes that regulate it.

CEREBRAL CORTICAL MALFORMATIONS IN PEDIATRIC EPILEPSY

Type of Seizures and Epilepsy Associated with Cerebral Cortical Malformations

The majority of patients with malformations of cortical development and epilepsy have symptomatic, localization-related epilepsy. This classification applies to any patient with a cerebral cortical malformation and seizures that originate in a focal region of cortex, regardless of whether the malformation itself is a focal lesion, such as a focal cortical dysplasia, or whether it represents a more widespread abnormality affecting the entire cortex, such as lissencephaly.

An individual with a cerebral cortical malformation may have seizures that appear generalized; such a patient most likely has secondarily generalized localization-related epilepsy, but symptomatic generalized epilepsy is also possible. In these cases, under the most recent semiology-based International League against Epilepsy (ILAE) classification of seizures and epilepsy, the seizure phenomenology is classified as "generalized," and the etiology should be specified as the malformation of cortical development (3).

Epidemiology of Cerebral Cortical Malformations in Pediatric Epilepsy

½ to 1% of children are estimated to have epilepsy (4–6). About one-third of children with epilepsy do not respond to medication and are considered medically refractory (7), and it is in this group that malformations of cortical development are most frequently encountered.

The role of cortical malformations has been widely recognized in cases of refractory localization-related epilepsy in children and adults, with malformations ranging from small heterotopia to large hemispheric malformations such as hemimegalencephaly (8–12). 10% to 20% of patients seen in subspecialty epilepsy centers are estimated to have cerebral cortical malformations by some authors (13). In an observational study of patients aged 15 years or older with localization-related epilepsy, only 70% of whom had any form of imaging performed, 3% of patients were found to have cerebral cortical malformations by MRI (14). In one series of adults with refractory epilepsy, 12% malformations of cortical development on MRI (15).

Epidemiological studies performed in the era preceding the routine use of MRI do not reflect the role of malformations of cortical development in pediatric epilepsy, but there are several reports suggesting that their role is even greater in children than in adults with epilepsy. Kuzniecky and colleagues reported that one-quarter of a series of 44 children who underwent surgical resection for treatment of epilepsy demonstrated cortical malformations (16). Pasquier and colleagues described 230 consecutive children and adults undergoing epilepsy surgery, the majority of whom had childhood-onset epilepsy; nearly one-quarter had some form of cerebral cortical malformation, including FCD, tubers suggesting tuberous sclerosis complex (TSC), and dysembryoplastic neuroepithelial tumor (DNET) (17). Sinclair and colleagues described a series of 42 children undergoing temporal lobectomy, in whom four had pathological evidence of FCD and four had tubers; additionally, of 13 patients who had temporal lobe tumors, eight fell into the spectrum of developmental malformations (seven gangliogliomas and one DNET) (18, 19).

In the subgroup of children undergoing epilepsy surgery for refractory infantile spasms, malformations of cortical development are a leading cause (20–22). Furthermore, there is a growing body of pathological evidence from epilepsy surgery series demonstrating that many adults and children with intractable localization-related epilepsy *without* MRI abnormalities have malformations of cortical development that are currently appreciated only microscopically (12, 23–28) or identified using [^{19}F]2-fluoro-2-deoxy-D-glucose ([^{19}F]2-FDG) (29).

To our knowledge, large population-based studies of children with epilepsy have yet to fully capture the role of cerebral cortical malformations as a common etiology. Nonetheless, the accruing evidence and our personal experience lead us to conclude that malformations of cortical development account for a substantial portion of children with refractory localization-related epilepsy.

EPILEPTOGENESIS OF CEREBRAL CORTICAL MALFORMATIONS

The discussion of the epileptogenesis of malformations of cortical development draws on observations regarding the pathological, electrophysiological, and molecular properties that may underlie their propensity to generate seizures. Many features suggest the persistence of fetal patterns, suggesting a disruption of the early process of neuronal and glial precursor proliferation, which in turn may lead to perturbations of the later processes of neuronal migration, lamination, and later cortical organization. The mechanisms of epileptogenesis may differ among malformations of cortical development according to the stage at which development was disrupted (30). We will consider epileptogenesis as a phenomenon common to all of the malformations together, because specific influences of the timing of disruption have yet to be elucidated.

Pathology of Cerebral Cortical Malformations

Pathological studies provided an initial understanding of developmental malformations of the brain. Despite advances in neuroimaging, there are still patients with relatively subtle disturbances of cortical development that are manifest only as pathological changes; it is only on the basis of accurate neuropathological analysis that these patients' lesions can be appropriately characterized and classified. Even in those patients with malformations evident by neuroimaging, the pathological abnormalities continue to provide insight into the developmental origin of these lesions.

Both neurons and glia may appear abnormal in location and morphology in malformations of cortical development, as described by Taylor and colleagues in focal cortical lesions, now referred to as FCD with balloon cells or Taylor-type FCD (8). They and others since have reported the following abnormalities in neurons in these developmental lesions: (1) neurons may be abnormally large and clustered; (2) many abnormal neurons are located in cortical layer I and sometimes heterotopically in the white matter; (3) the malformations contain bizarrely shaped cells of presumed glial origin; and (4) there is potential for severe disorganization of the cortex in these lesions (8, 31, 32). Similar pathological changes have been described in many other types of cerebral cortical malformations, including hemimegalencephaly (33, 34). Figure 6-1 depicts these abnormal neuronal and glial features from a child with hemimegalencephaly who underwent hemispherectomy for seizure control. Beyond these cellular and architectural findings, Sankar and colleagues described severe dysmyelination underlying regions of pathologically abnormal cortex in cerebral cortical malformations, suggesting a more prominent role of white matter in the pathogenesis as well as epileptogenesis (23).

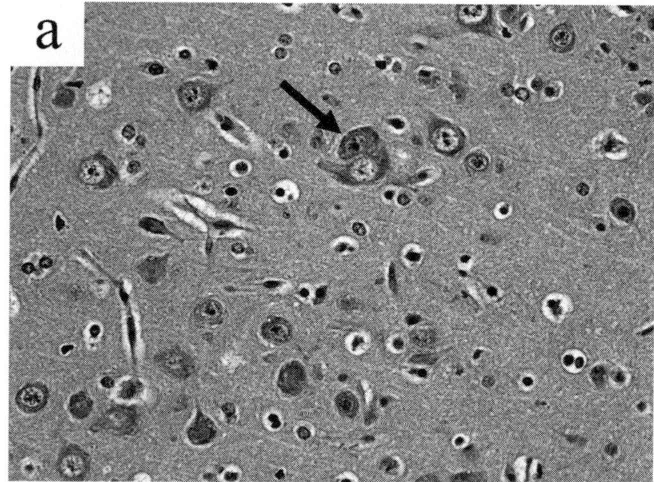

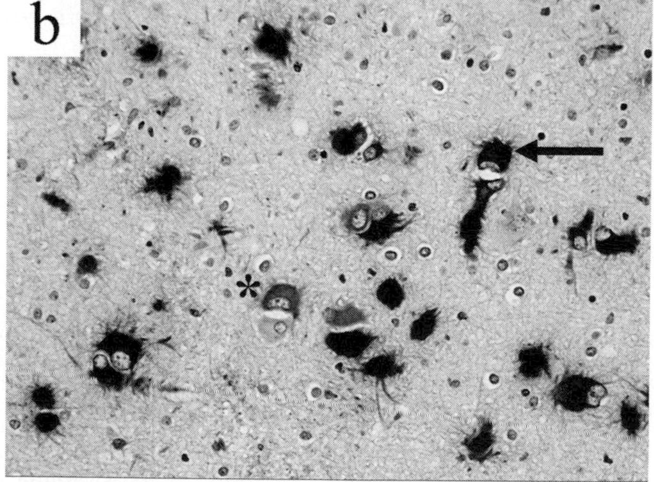

FIGURE 6-1

Abnormal neuronal and glial features from the hemisphere involved in hemimegalencephaly in a child who underwent hemispherectomy for refractory epilepsy. (a) Hematoxylin and eosin staining shows neurons with abnormal morphology, size, and orientation in the gray matter. The arrow indicates two abnormally shaped neurons with abnormal orientation and clustering. (b) Glial fibrillary acidic protein (GFAP) staining depicts abnormal astrocytes in the white matter (arrow) as well as intermediately stained cells with mixed neuronal and glial morphological properties (asterisk).

One feature shared by many malformations of cortical development is disruption of the cortical architecture, which can be profound in such examples as double cortex syndrome and pachygyria, or more subtle in cases with only mild dyslamination. In some cases, the distinction between gray matter and white matter can be difficult to discern (35). Palmini and colleagues grouped the histopathological abnormalities seen in cerebral cortical malformations into four categories, listed by increasing degree of abnormality (36):

1. Isolated architectural abnormalities, including dyslamination and columnar disorganization.
2. Architectural abnormalities with the predominant abnormal cell type of giant neurons (pyramidal-shaped neurons that are larger than normal layer V neurons).
3. Architectural abnormalities with predominant dysmorphic neurons (neurons with abnormal cytoplasmic neurofilament accumulation leading to abnormalities in shape, size, orientation, and processes), along with which giant neurons may also be present.
4. Architectural abnormalities with dysmorphic neurons and balloon cells (large cells that have thin cell membranes and eosinophilic cytoplasm, may be multinucleated, and typically display immunoreactivity to markers of both neurons and glia).

The third and fourth of these categories correspond to what is often termed Taylor-type FCD (36).

An additional feature sometimes seen in malformations of cortical development is the immature neuron, which is neither enlarged nor dysmorphic but has a large, immature-appearing nucleus and relatively sparse cytoplasm (36). From a pathological perspective, the abnormal cells seen in malformations of cortical development can be arranged from least to most severe in the following order: heterotopically placed but morphologically normal neurons, immature and giant neurons, dysmorphic neurons, and balloon cells (listed in Table 6-1). There is some evidence to suggest that pathological severity may reflect the severity of the associated epilepsy (37, 38).

Pathological analysis of malformations of cortical development clearly demonstrates that the neurons and glia within these lesions display unusual morphological properties. One might expect that neurons with abnormal morphological features and cell surface properties would display abnormal connectivity that would give rise to

TABLE 6-1
Range of Abnormal Cells Identified in Cerebral Cortical Malformations, from Least Severe to Most Severe

Type of Neuron	Characteristics
Normal-appearing neurons	Located in abnormal locations (most commonly layer I)
Immature neurons	Normal shape and size, abnormally large nucleus
Giant neurons	Normal shape, abnormal size
Dysmorphic neurons	Abnormal shape, size, orientation, clustering
Balloon cells	Abnormal shape, size, orientation, clustering, neuronal and glial features

epilepsy (39). Some cells seen in malformations of cortical development recall features of neuronal-glial progenitor cells or immature neurons, suggesting the abnormal persistence of a fetal-like state. These and other features may contribute to the proclivity of cerebral cortical malformations to engender seizures. Efforts to understand these malformations on a molecular level should render further insight into the precise means of epileptogenesis, both in and around the malformations and in epileptogenic foci in general.

Persistence of Immature Patterns of Expression in Cerebral Cortical Malformations

Analogous to the pathological features of cerebral cortical malformations, the abnormalities observed at the protein level are also reminiscent of immature patterns. Immunohistochemical study of neurons in malformations of cortical development reveals excessive reactivity to the neurofilament protein SMI311 and the microtubule associated protein MAP2, which are typically expressed early in the immature brain (32, 35). Immunoreactivity to the cell adhesion molecule L1, which usually peaks in expression near the end of normal human gestation, has been found in excess in abnormal neurons from samples of hemimegalencephaly (40). The simultaneous neuronal nuclei (NeuN) and glial fibrillary acidic protein (GFAP) immunoreactivity of some cells corresponds to their morphological ambiguity and suggests absent or aberrant differentiation of neuronal-glial precursors and possible arrest in, or return to, a pre-differentiated state.

The immature and undifferentiated features of many of the cells seen in cerebral cortical malformations certainly suggest a dysregulation of the processes of cell fate determination among neurons and glia. The mechanisms leading to these common features of many malformations of cortical development are not yet known, so it is not possible to state precisely which stage of cortical development is first disrupted. It is conceivable that a disruption during cell proliferation results in a more profound pathological picture, whereas a milder defect influencing neuronal migration may lead to more subtle ultrastructural changes with preserved neuronal maturation and cellular architecture. Until we discover the fundamental inciting events leading to each type of malformation, hypotheses based on the pathology and immunohistochemistry remain speculative.

Abnormal Neurotransmitter Receptor Subunits in Cerebral Cortical Malformations

An imbalance of excitatory and inhibitory synaptic activity can be implicated in any discussion of epileptogenesis. One approach to this issue in the realm of cerebral cortical malformations has been the study of expression of excitatory and inhibitory neurotransmitter receptor subunit proteins in surgical specimens from epilepsy surgery in humans as well as in animal models of malformations of cortical development. A thorough description of the role of excitatory and inhibitory neurotransmission in normal synaptic activity and epileptogenesis is provided elsewhere in this text. We concentrate here on the neurotransmitters for which there are data specific to malformations of cortical development.

Glutamate Receptors

Two classes of excitatory glutamate receptors that have been implicated in the epileptogenesis of malformations of cortical development are the *N*-methyl-D-aspartate (NMDA) and alpha-amino-3-hydroxy-5-methyl-4-isoxazole propionic acid (AMPA) receptors. A functioning NMDA receptor comprises of a four-part complex of NMDAR1 (or NR1) and NMDAR2 (or NR2) subunits, which have eight and four different forms, respectively; although the NMDAR2 subunits do not alone function as ion channels, they potentiate the conductance of NMDAR1 currents when the two subunits are combined (41, 42). Immunohistochemical studies of abnormal neurons from human malformation of cortical development have shown alterations in expression of the NMDAR2 type A and B subunits (43–45). Crino and colleagues evaluated mRNA expression in individual abnormal neurons from regions of focal cortical dysplasia and reported increased expression of NMDAR2 type B and C subunits but decreased expression of NMDAR2 type A subunits in abnormal neurons from FCD (46). The relatively increased NMDAR2 subunit expression correlates with hyperexcitability in neurons in malformations of cortical development; electrocorticography within malformations has revealed abnormal electroencephalographic (EEG) activity in regions subsequently found to have abnormal NMDA receptor profiles (42, 44).

The AMPA receptor complex is formed by four subunits: GluR1 through GluR4. Immunohistochemical studies have shown increases in GluR2 and GluR3 subunit expression in giant neurons and dysplastic neurons from human malformations of cortical development (45). In contrast, mRNA expression studies have shown decreased GluR1 and increased GluR4 expression in abnormal neurons from cerebral cortical malformations, compared to normal neurons from control samples (46). Some authors suggest that the functional implications of any or all of these deviations from normal AMPA receptor subunit expression may involve altered subunit stoichiometry, leading to neuronal hyperexcitability (42), but the precise mechanisms have yet to be worked out.

GABA Receptors

Gamma-aminobutyric acid (GABA) is the chief inhibitory neurotransmitter in the mature central nervous system. Assaying regions of FCD with immunohistochemical markers that identify GABAergic neurons, Ferrer and colleagues reported a decrease in the number of GABAergic neurons (47). In the study mentioned in the preceding section, Crino and colleagues reported a decrease in mRNA expression of the alpha-1, alpha-2, beta-1, and beta-2 subunits of the [GABA-A] receptor (46). During early brain development, there is limited GABA-mediated inhibitory activity (48), and the role of GABA evolves over time from excitatory to inhibitory (49). Abnormalities in GABA receptor expression in malformations of cortical development must therefore be considered against the backdrop of this developmental shift in GABA function (see also Chapter 1). If abnormalities in GABA receptor subunit expression represent yet another recapitulation of an immature state, the persistence of GABA-mediated excitability could contribute to the epileptogenicity of malformations of cortical development (50).

Clearly, in a patient with a cerebral cortical malformation or any predisposition to epilepsy, there are dynamic factors mediating the excitatory-inhibitory balance and establishing an electrophysiological threshold that is intermittently crossed, allowing a seizure to be generated and propagated. While the available data from neurotransmitter receptor subunit expression studies do not provide a complete model for epileptogenesis in malformations of cortical development, the pattern seen in these lesions appears to represent a developmental dysregulation of the balance of excitatory and inhibitory activity. Further study into the unique receptor properties in cerebral cortical malformations may not only shed further light onto the developmental aspects of the malformations but also lead to the targeting of specific pharmacological treatment strategies for patients with malformations of cortical development. Given the important role of glutamate and other neurotransmitters in learning and memory, a more complete understanding of neurotransmitter dysfunction in cerebral cortical malformations may also ultimately provide insight into the cognitive difficulties that often accompany the seizures in patients with malformations of cortical development.

Genomic Study of Focal Cerebral Cortical Malformations

The publication of the human genome, coupled with advances in informatics, allow us to study mRNA expression profiles and to conduct genome-wide studies to assay for deletions, duplications, and chromosomal rearrangements in the malformations of cortical development resected during epilepsy surgery. Kim and colleagues identified upregulation of genes associated with apoptosis and downregulation of other genes associated with apoptosis in tissue from focal malformations of cortical development (51). Immediate early genes have been similarly found to be upregulated in tissue from focal cerebral cortical malformations as well as in epileptic tissue not associated with malformations (52). In such studies, it is difficult to implicate the involvement of the identified genes in the causality of either the malformation or the epilepsy, because the abnormalities seen may represent an effect of electroclinical or electrographic seizures that have occurred. Using evidence from targeted microarrays, Yu and colleagues reported increased expression of genes encoding growth factors and transcription factors in tissue from hemimegalencephaly lesions, pointing to several potential pathways that may be involved in the aberrant growth responsible for these malformations (53). These latter studies may point to the very mechanisms that underlie the formation of malformations of cortical development, and the role of the genes identified in the lesions' epileptogenicity remains to be studied.

In our own study of tissue from epilepsy surgery samples, we have used single-nucleotide polymorphism-based copy number analysis and quantitative polymerase chain reaction to identify three copies of chromosome 1q in two cases of large hemispheric malformation; in one case, there was no evidence of this duplication in the patient's leukocytes, suggesting that a somatic event occurred in the brain (55). Further study is required to determine the implications of chromosomal aneuploidy in the development of focal malformations of cortical development and epilepsy. Although these DNA-based strategies may lead to further understanding of the genetic mechanisms underlying development of cerebral cortical malformations, they may not fully explain their epileptogenic potential.

TABLE 6-2
EEG Characteristics of Cerebral Cortical Malformations

Type of Recording	EEG Characteristics
Scalp EEG	• High-amplitude (>100 μV) rhythmic theta and delta activity (55) • High-amplitude sharp-slow waves, alpha and beta activity (52) • Fluctuating amplitude theta and delta activity, faster than expected for age, possibly asynchronous (55) • High-amplitude or fluctuating amplitude >15 Hz beta activity, in bursts or continuous (55) • Localized slowing and epileptiform spikes (37) • Repetitive or nearly continuous spikes or seizures (60, 61)
Subdural extraoperative EEG	Continuous epileptiform discharges (60)
Intraoperative corticography	• Repetitive bursts of alpha and beta activity (>10 Hz) (61) • "Recruiting/derecruiting pattern" of spikes increasing in rhythmicity and frequency up to 12–16 Hz followed by focal slowing (61) • Continuous or nearly continuous rhythmic spiking (61–63)

Epileptogenic Activity Arising in and around Cerebral Cortical Malformations

Electroencephalographic data from scalp, subdural, and depth electrode recordings suggest intrinsic epileptogenicity of neurons within malformations of cortical development as well as the regions that surround them (9, 55–59). Table 6-2 (60–63) presents electrophysiologic characteristics that have been described in association with various types of cerebral cortical malformations based on routine or prolonged scalp EEG, subdural EEG recorded outside of the operating room with the intent of localizing seizure onset, and intraoperative corticography, the last of which is almost exclusively interictal (37, 55, 60–63). The common theme that emerges from all of these methods of recording is excessive rhythmicity, with higher than expected amplitudes and frequencies for age. Notably, investigators have reported abnormal electrophysiological properties and seizure onset zones in the regions immediately surrounding focal malformations of cortical development (9, 60, 64, 65). These latter findings have important implications for the treatment of cerebral malformations with resective surgery; the epileptogenic capacity of the tissue surrounding the regions of malformation that are visible macroscopically and by MRI suggest that subdural EEG recording may be required to establish seizure onset firmly, since it may not be restricted to the malformation.

CLINICAL PRESENTATION AND CLASSIFICATION OF CEREBRAL CORTICAL MALFORMATIONS BY STAGES OF CORTICAL DEVELOPMENT

The process of brain development, which follows a sequence that is under genetic regulation, provides a framework for understanding the variety of cerebral cortical malformations encountered in patients with pediatric epilepsy. The classification presented by Barkovich and colleagues has evolved to include an ever-expanding list of genetic etiologies for many cerebral malformations (1, 19, 66). The importance of its emphasis on genetic causes cannot be overstated; even when epilepsy is not the presenting symptom of a cerebral malformation, clinicians must address important questions regarding possible genetic etiologies. Table 6-3 presents the major categories of malformations of cortical development according to the stage that is thought to be first or primarily disrupted in brain development.

We begin this section with some general clinical observations regarding patients with epilepsy caused by cerebral cortical malformations. We briefly review the normal sequence of cortical development before discussing representative examples from each major group according to the first stage of brain development known or thought to be disrupted.

General Clinical Observations

The focus of this chapter is the relationship between malformations of cortical development and epilepsy, so we provide estimates of the prevalence of epilepsy among patients with specific malformations when this information is available. In general, though the prevalence of epilepsy in each group is not 100 percent, we recommend advising patients with cerebral cortical malformations and their families that epilepsy is a common symptom of any structural brain malformation.

Apart from the minority of patients with cerebral cortical malformations who are asymptomatic, many patients with malformations of cortical development have what some clinicians term a "chronic static encephalopathy,"

TABLE 6-3
Cortical Malformations Classified by Stages of Cortical Development

STAGE OF DEVELOPMENT	ASSOCIATED MALFORMATIONS
Neuronal and glial proliferation	Net decrease in neurons and glia—primary microcephaly • Normal or simplified gyral pattern • Normal or thin cortex • Microlissencephaly (thick cortex) • With or without polymicrogyria Net increase in neurons and glia—macrocephaly Abnormal proliferation • Cortical tuber • Focal cortical dysplasia with balloon cells, including trans-mantle dysplasia • Hemimegalencephaly Tumors—DNET, ganglioglioma, gangliocytoma
Neuronal migration and cortical lamination	Abnormal radial migration, including arrested migration • Lissencephaly (formerly type I lissencephaly) • Subcortical band heterotopia • Other subcortical heterotopia • Subependymal, periventricular heterotopia Abnormal radial migration, including overmigration • Cobblestone lissencephaly (formerly type II lissencephaly) Abnormal radial and tangential migration • X-linked lissencephaly with abnormal genitalia
Later cortical organization	• Polymicrogyria, bilateral and unilateral • Schizencephaly, bilateral and unilateral • Cortical dysplasia without balloon cells • Lesions with microscopic evidence of abnormal development (not apparent on MRI)

Adapted with permission from Dr. AJ Barkovich.

manifest not only as epilepsy but also varying degrees of developmental delay or mental retardation as well as other neurological problems. It is helpful to frame the individual patient's neurological problems, including the epilepsy, as stemming from the malformation of cortical development and to attribute the malformation itself, along with any associated nonneurological sequelae, to the underlying genetic etiology whenever possible. The likelihood and typical age of onset of epilepsy vary among syndromes, and the most precise characterization of patients' conditions will aid in the prognosis of their epilepsy as well as their neurodevelopmental outcome. In Table 6-4 we present a list of genes known to be associated with specific malformations of cortical development at the time of the writing of this chapter (67–86). Note that most of the conditions described thus far have been associated with autosomal recessive or X-linked patterns of inheritance, which is important when providing counseling to families about recurrence risk in subsequent children.

The treatment of epilepsy caused by malformations of cortical development is beyond the scope of this chapter, and general principles of treatment of epilepsy are covered in depth elsewhere in the text. Patients with refractory epilepsy due to cerebral cortical malformations and well-localized anatomical and seizure foci are often considered candidates for epilepsy surgery, and the outcome has been reported to be favorable in one-third to two-thirds of patients with brain malformations undergoing resective surgery for the treatment of seizures (87–89).

Classification by Stage of Cortical Development Disrupted and Presentations

Normal Cortical Development

The processes underlying normal cortical development in the human continue to be elucidated in increasing detail. The currently accepted paradigm for the formation of the human cortex was outlined elegantly by Sidman and Rakic in 1973 (90) and includes in the following sequence of events: (1) proliferation of progenitor cells in ventricular zone, (2) neuronal migration along a radial glial scaffold, leading to the establishment of the six layers of the neocortex, and (3) further organization, including formation

TABLE 6-4
Genes Responsible for Malformations of Cortical Development and Epilepsy

Malformation of Cortical Development	Identified Gene(s)	Inheritance
Disorders of neuronal and glial proliferation		
Primary microcephaly	*MCPH1, ASPM* (67, 68)	AR
With seizures	*ASPM* (69)	AR
Microcephaly with bilateral periventricular heterotopia	*ARFGEF2* (70)	AR
Disorders with macrocephaly		
Neurofibromatosis type 1	*NF1* (71)	AD or sporadic
Sotos syndrome	*NSD1* (72)	AD or sporadic
Cowden syndrome	*PTEN* (73)	AD
Tuberous sclerosis complex	*TSC1, TSC2* (74, 75)	AD or sporadic
Disorders of neuronal migration and lamination		
Lissencephaly, male or female	*LIS1* (76)	AD or sporadic
Lissencephaly with cerebellar hypoplasia	*RELN* (77)	AR
Lissencephaly, male	*DCX* (76, 78)	X-linked
with abnormal genitalia	*ARX* (79)	X-linked
Double cortex syndrome, female	*DCX* (78, 80)	X-linked
Pachygyria	*DCX, LIS1* (76, 78, 80)	X-linked, AD, or sporadic
Cobblestone lissencephaly	*POMT1* (81) *POMT2* (82) *POMGnT1* (83) others	AR
Bilateral periventricular heterotopia	*FLNA* (84)	X-linked
Disorders of later organization		
Bilateral fronto-parietal polymicrogyria	*GPR56* (85)	AR
Schizencephaly	*EMX2* (86)	AD or sporadic

AR = autosomal recessive, AD = autosomal dominant

of gyri and sulci of the appropriate size and orientation, synaptic organization, and myelination. Figure 6-2 presents a schematic version of cortical development.

This model for cortical development provides an excellent general framework and continues to be refined. Evidence that cortical neurons and the radial glia that guide their migration arise from a common neuronal-glial progenitor pool (91, 92) suggests that there are other elements between steps (1) and (2) in the aforementioned sequence that may be affected to produce malformations of cortical development, including the processes of cell fate determination and formation of the radial glial scaffold, which must occur before migration can begin. There is evidence from studies in *Drosophila* that neuronal differentiation occurs after a progenitor cell undergoes an asymmetric mitotic division, dividing into one "daughter" cell that eventually becomes a neuron and another "daughter" cell that continues to divide, maintaining the pool of progenitor cells; this process is directed and regulated by the action of a number of intrinsic and extrinsic proteins (93–96). Aberrations in these aspects of neuronal differentiation would also result in disorders of proliferation, though they have not yet been identified as such in humans.

Another development that has added complexity to the paradigm of brain development as outlined above is the phenomenon of nonradial neuronal migration (97), characterized as tangential migration from the ventral telencephalon, giving rise predominantly to interneuron populations (98). If they lead to deficiencies of GABAergic interneurons in the cortex, abnormalities of tangential migration may be particularly likely to lead to cortical hyperexcitability and epileptogenesis. Advances in basic neuroscience will continue to shed light on the complex processes that may be disrupted to produce the broad range of known malformations of cortical development, and new clinical syndromes will likely invoke mechanisms that are yet to be described.

Disorders of Neuronal and Glial Proliferation

Disorders of neuronal and glial proliferation most likely result from abnormal proliferation of the undifferentiated progenitor of neurons and glia. These disorders may reflect an imbalance between proliferation of progenitor cells and apoptosis, or programmed cell death. This category includes those conditions thought to be a result of relative underproduction of neurons and glia or, conversely, those with a relative overproduction, as

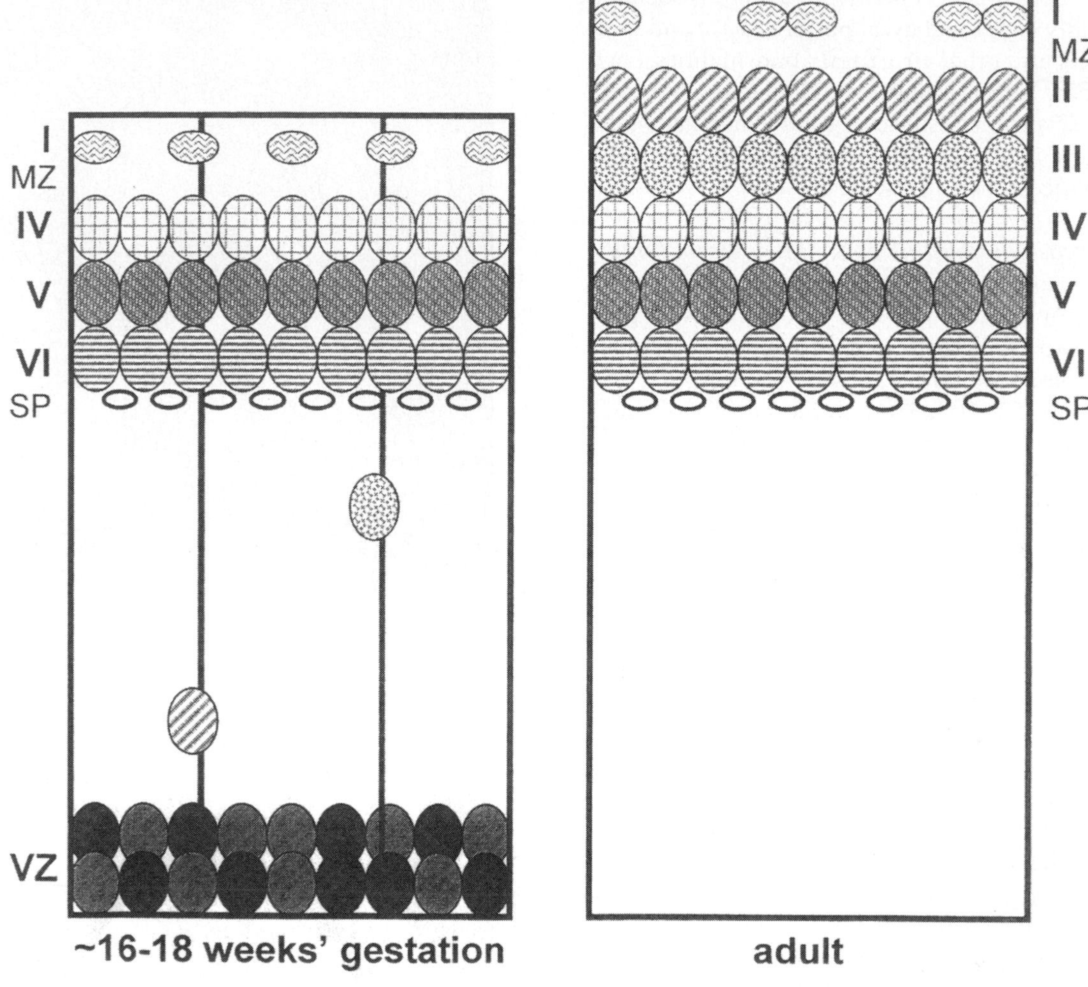

FIGURE 6-2

The formation of the cerebral cortex in humans involves the proliferation of progenitor cells (light gray ovals) in the ventricular zone (VZ); establishment of a radial glial scaffold (vertical lines) following differentiation of some progenitors into glial cells (cell bodies shown as dark gray ovals) and others into neurons (patterned ovals); and (3) neuronal migration along the radial glial scaffold. The panel on the left depicts the stage of approximately 16 to 18 weeks' human gestation, by which time the layer I Cajal-Retzius neurons have migrated to the pial surface (represented by the top of the panel) followed by layer VI, layer V, and layer IV; representative neurons from layers III and II are shown migrating along radial glia. The panel on the right represents the adult six-layer cortex after neuronal migration is complete; note that the cortical plate has expanded with the addition of layers III and II. Not shown are the final stages of further cortical organization, including formation of gyri and sulci of the appropriate size and orientation, synaptic organization, and myelination. (MZ: marginal zone; SP: subplate neurons.)

outlined in Table 6-3. Conditions resulting in the production of abnormal cell types are also included in this group, with both nonneoplastic and low-grade neoplastic subgroups (19). It is important to note that any perturbation at this early stage of development is likely to have downstream effects on the later stage, and it is therefore not surprising that cortical lamination and further organization also appear abnormal in this group of disorders.

Net decrease in neurons and glia—microcephaly. Microcephaly can be the result of a number of etiologies, including hypoxic-ischemic injury and exposure to viral pathogens in utero that result in an underproduction, excessive apoptosis, or abnormal destruction of neurons and glia during gestation. When microcephaly is seen in the absence of such factors, it is considered primary microcephaly. At least seven genetic loci have been associated with autosomal recessive forms of primary microcephaly (99). Nonsense mutations in the gene *ASPM* have been found to be responsible for a particular familial form of microcephaly with seizures (69), reinforcing the connection between this structural brain malformation and epilepsy.

The MRIs of patients with primary microcephaly, as described above, typically have normal or mildly simplified gyral pattern (100). Microcephaly can also be associated with a markedly simplified gyral pattern (101) and with polymicrogyria and other structural abnormalities, such as agenesis of the corpus callosum (102). Generally speaking, the more severe the associated gyral abnormality, the more severe the neurodevelopmental prognosis and the higher the chance of seizures will be (100).

Net increase in neurons and glia—macrocephaly. Macrocephaly, or megalencephaly, is seen in isolation or in association with syndromes associated with general dysregulation of growth in multiple tissues, including neurofibromatosis type 1, Cowden syndrome, and Sotos syndrome (72, 103, 104). Some but not all individuals with these syndromes have epilepsy, but it is a less prominent feature than in those with most of the other malformations described (72, 105, 106). Orstavik and colleagues report a syndrome of macrocephaly, epilepsy, autism, and dysmorphic features in two sisters, the genetic basis of which is not yet known (107). In these cases of primary macrocephaly of known or likely genetic etiology, epilepsy may be one of many clinical manifestations but generally does not dominate the clinical picture.

Abnormal proliferation—TSC, FCD, and hemimegalencephaly. Abnormalities at the time of proliferation of neuronal-glial progenitor cells are thought to be responsible for the formation of cortical tubers in TSC, FCD with balloon cells, and hemimegalencephaly, all of which share many pathological features (31, 33).

Eighty to 90% of individuals with TSC have epilepsy; seizures typically begin during childhood and often are refractory to medical treatment (108). In particular, children with TSC have a particular propensity for developing infantile spasms (109).

FCD with balloon cells is a common pathological finding in epilepsy surgery series, as previously discussed in the section on Epidemiology in this chapter. Subtypes of FCD with balloon cells include transmantle dysplasia (shown in Figure 6-3), extending from the ventricle through the white matter and into the gray matter, and the "bottom of the sulcus" cortical dysplasia (19). MRI features include thickening of the gray matter and blurring of the gray-white matter junction (110). FCDs that have ultimately been found to have balloon cells on pathological analysis have been far more likely than those without balloon cells to be associated with abnormal MRI T2 signal in the white matter underlying the cortical lesion (111). FCD with balloon cells is typically diagnosed by MRI after an individual has presented with epilepsy. Although some such individuals are assessed as cognitively normal, mild to severe mental retardation is also reported, with younger age of onset of epilepsy (particularly under one year) associated with worse cognitive outcome (110).

The other characteristic malformation of cortical development in the category of abnormal proliferation is hemimegalencephaly, an example of which is shown in Figure 6-4. These lesions are large, hemispheric malformations with varying degrees of macroscopically disrupted architecture. As reviewed by Flores-Sarnat and colleagues, the presence of a unilateral malformation, with its characteristic appearance and associated pathological findings, strongly suggests a disruption early in the proliferative stage of brain development (34). Hemimegalencephaly can occur as an isolated entity or as part of a syndrome with somatic components, such as linear sebaceous syndrome, hypomelanosis of Ito, and, rarely but not surprisingly, other neurocutaneous syndromes such as TSC and neurofibromatosis type 1 (112). Why such a profound change occurs primarily unilaterally in the developing brain of patients with hemimegalencephaly is not yet understood. There is a report of microscopic evidence of abnormal development on the side contralateral to the large hemispheric malformation (113), the reason for which is also not known. Epilepsy inevitably occurs in patients with hemimegalencephaly, with a large number of infants presenting with severe neonatal seizures, and hemispherectomy is often a necessary component of seizure management (100).

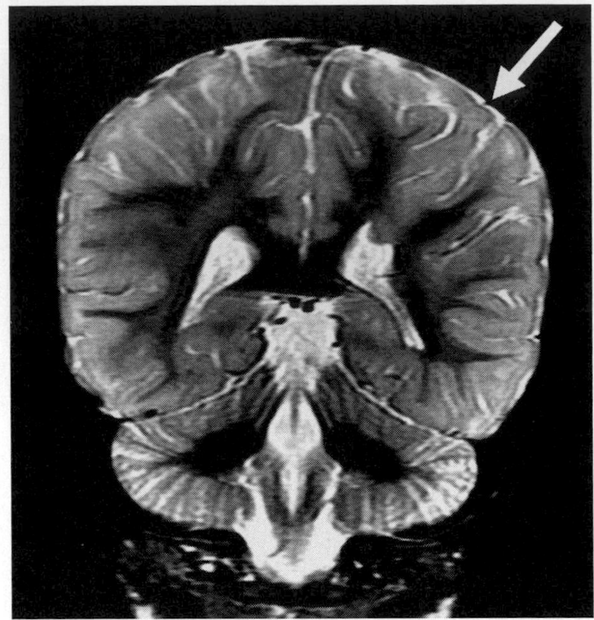

FIGURE 6-3

This coronal T2 fast spin echo inversion recovery (FSEIR) image is from the MRI of a patient with focal seizures due to a transmantle dysplasia, a subtype of focal cortical dysplasia (arrow). This malformation of cortical development likely reflects a focal abnormality at the proliferative stage of brain development.

Abnormal neoplastic proliferation—developmental tumors. As listed in Table 6-3, DNET, ganglioglioma, and gangliocytoma are the developmental tumors associated with abnormal proliferation of progenitor cells and

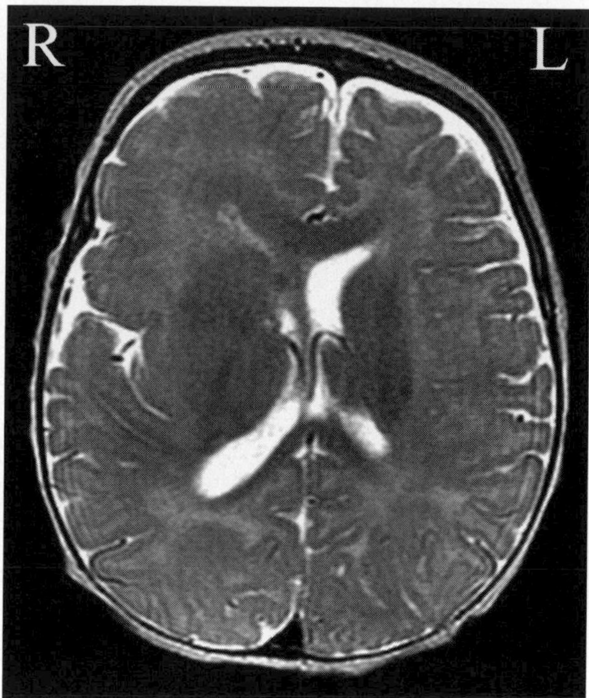

FIGURE 6-4

This axial T2 MR image from a child with intractable localization-related epilepsy shows right-sided hemimegalencephaly. The entire right hemisphere is larger than the left, and there are abnormalities involving the gray and white matter (R: right, L: left).

associated with epilepsy. As previously detailed in the section on Epidemiology, they are reported with varying frequency in series of children undergoing epilepsy surgery (17–19). The line between such nonneoplastic lesions as FCD and this group of neoplastic lesions remains to be better defined by detailed comparative pathological and molecular studies of the two groups.

Disorders of Neuronal Migration and Cortical Lamination

Disorders of neuronal migration include a group of disorders with macroscopic disruptions in cortical architecture, resulting in either absent or profoundly abnormal cortical lamination. Classic examples in this category include lissencephaly as well as the X-linked conditions of double cortex syndrome and periventricular heterotopia, discussed in detail subsequently. In Table 6-3 we have subdivided this category slightly differently from Barkovich and colleagues (19) to highlight that disrupting the two different streams of migration—radial and tangential—can result in different phenotypes.

Theoretically, a disruption at the earlier stage of proliferation could establish an abnormal substrate of neurons and glia, leading to abnormalities in migration and lamination. For the disorders in this group, it is helpful to conceptualize them as those with a dominant defect in migration with possible origin from an earlier defect or with defects at both the proliferation and migration stages. Indeed, molecular evidence from studies of *LIS1*, a gene classically associated with neuronal migration, demonstrates a role for the gene at the stage of progenitor proliferation in the developing mammalian brain (114). That these disorders that are primarily attributed to defects in radial migration are also associated with abnormalities in gyral folding emphasizes that defects in early stages of development will result in disruption of later stages.

Abnormal radial migration—classical lissencephaly and subcortical heterotopia. Classic examples of these malformations of cortical development include the conditions of lissencephaly and double cortex syndrome, representing abnormal radial migration of neurons. Lissencephaly, meaning "smooth brain," affects the entire cortex but can do so variably depending on the underlying genetic etiology. It is helpful to think of classical, or type I, lissencephaly as agyria-pachygyria with either an anterior-posterior or posterior-anterior gradient of smoothness (115). Epilepsy and severe mental retardation are nearly universal features of classical lissencephaly. On the other hand, females with double cortex syndrome, or bilateral subcortical band heterotopia, typically have mild to moderate mental retardation and epilepsy that is generally less severe than in individuals with lissencephaly (116, 117)

Classical lissencephaly occurs in both males and females. When a genetic cause can be identified, it is most often a deletion or mutation in the *LIS1* gene (120). Figure 6-5 presents the MRI from a patient with lissencephaly due to a mutation in the *LIS1* gene and symptomatic generalized epilepsy. The posterior-predominant agyria accompanied by anterior pachygyria is typical of *LIS1*-associated lissencephaly. When there is a deletion of *LIS1* and other genes in the 17p13.3 region, the affected individuals have not only lissencephaly and its consequences but also the dysmorphic features that are characterized as the Miller-Dieker syndrome (119).

Classical lissencephaly in males also occurs as a result of mutations in the *DCX* gene (78, 79). Females with *DCX* mutations typically display double cortex syndrome, and their male offspring have a 50% risk of inheriting a mutated form of *DCX* and presenting with classical lissencephaly. Mutations include single amino acid substitutions as well as protein-truncating mutations, and somatic and germline mosaicism have been observed (120, 121). More recently, Guerrini and colleagues have shown that another phenotype, anteriorly predominant pachygyria and mental retardation, can be associated with *DCX* mutations as well; pharmacoresistant epilepsy occurred in all of the affected boys described (122). Figure 6-6 shows a range of patients with mutations in the *DCX* gene, including classical lissencephaly in a boy, pachygyria in a boy, and double cortex in a girl.

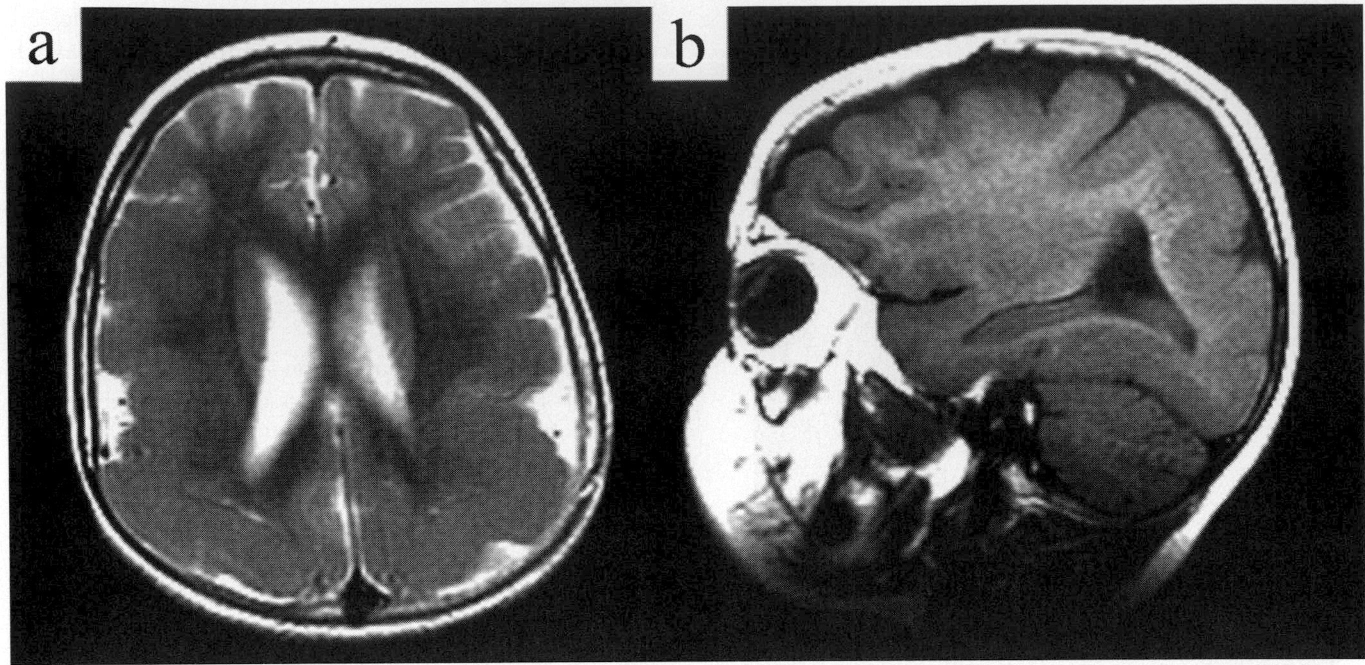

FIGURE 6-5

An example of a disorder predominantly due to a defect in radial neuronal migration is shown in this MRI from a patient with lissencephaly due to a *LIS1* mutation and symptomatic generalized epilepsy. An axial T2 image (a) and a sagittal T1 image (b) are shown.

Focal abnormalities of migration, such as focal subcortical heterotopia, are also seen in association with refractory epilepsy (123). An example is shown in Figure 6-7, which shows an image from the MRI of a patient with subcortical heterotopia, adjacent abnormal cortex, and also focal regions of periventricular heterotopia in the contralateral hemisphere. Genetic causes of subcortical heterotopia have yet to be identified, and the focal nature of these lesions makes them attractive candidates for epilepsy surgery, though long-term outcome data are not available.

Abnormal radial overmigration—cobblestone lissencephaly. Type II lissencephaly, or cobblestone lissencephaly, may resemble classical lissencephaly radiologically

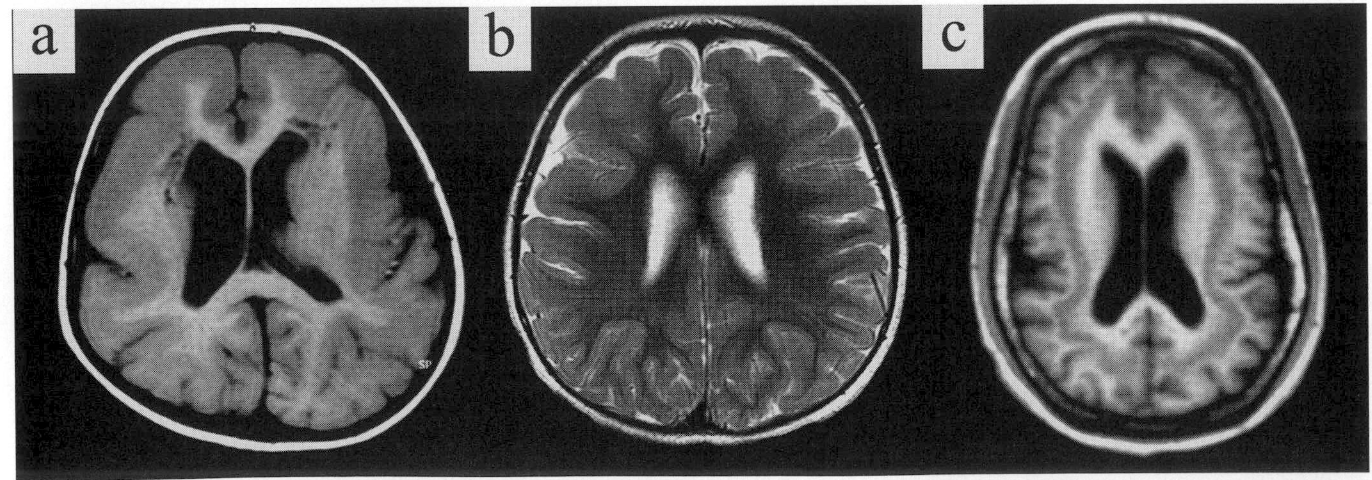

FIGURE 6-6

These axial images show a range of MRI abnormalities in patients with epilepsy and mutations in the *DCX* gene range from (a) lissencephaly in a boy, (b) pachygyria in a boy, and (c) double cortex in a girl. These cases illustrate global disruptions of neuronal migration.

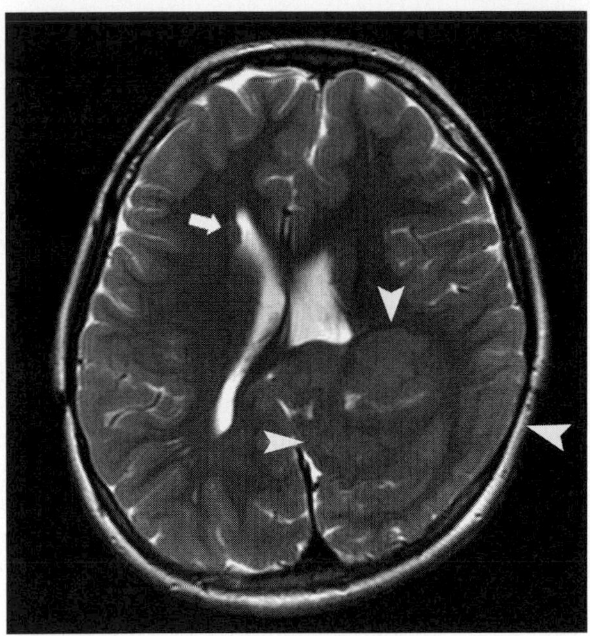

FIGURE 6-7

MRI is shown from a patient with localization-related epilepsy due to a large subcortical heterotopia with abnormal overlying cortex (arrowheads). The patient also had a small contralateral region of heterotopia (arrow), so these lesions appear to represent separate and asymmetric focal disruptions of neuronal migration.

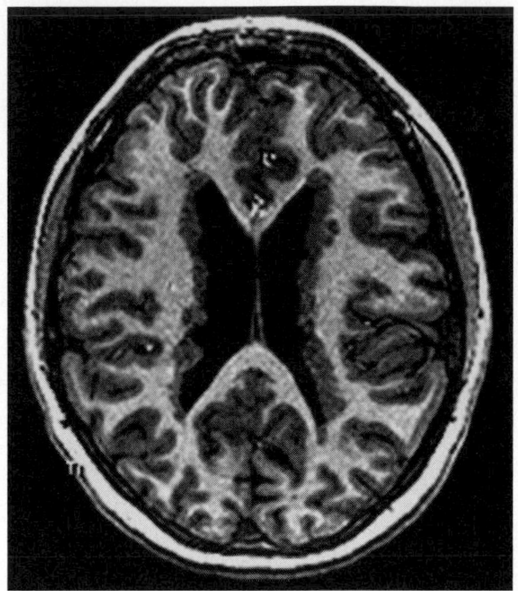

FIGURE 6-8

This axial T1 spoiled gradient recalled (SPGR) MR image shows bilateral periventricular heterotopia in a female with a *FLNA* mutation, representing a disorder of radial neuronal migration.

but represents a different pathophysiological entity that arises from an overmigration of neurons beyond the pial surface. There is a strong clinical association with cobblestone lissencephaly and congenital muscular dystrophy in conditions such as Walker-Warburg syndrome, muscle eye brain disease, and Fukuyama muscular dystrophy (124–126). Epilepsy is often an early component of these syndromes, which are also associated with other MRI abnormalities, varying degrees of mental retardation, and hypotonia. The pathophysiology of this group of disorders involves abnormal glycosylation of alpha-dystroglycan, as described in a recent review by Endo (127).

Abnormal radial migration—periventricular heterotopia. X-linked bilateral periventricular heterotopia (PH) provides another example of abnormal radial neuronal migration, in this case with the appearance of arrested or minimal migration of a subset of neurons from the ventricular zone during cortical development. Figure 6-8 is an MRI from a female patient with this form of malformation due to a mutation in the *FLNA* gene on the X chromosome, the typical genetic abnormality associated with bilateral PH (84, 128). Females with bilateral PH usually have epilepsy, with age of onset in their teens or twenties and milder severity than patients with the other disorders of migration; cognition is often normal, though specific defects in reading ability have been identified (129). Less commonly, this condition can occur in males with a similar overall phenotype (128). Not all females with bilateral PH harbor mutations in FLNA (128); another gene that has been associated with PH is *ARFGEF2*, described in autosomal recessive pedigrees with PH and microcephaly (70) and classified by Barkovich and colleagues as a disorder of neuronal proliferation (19).

Abnormal radial and tangential neuronal migration—XLAG. The last example in this section represents a disorder in which both radial and tangential migration of neurons is affected. X-linked lissencephaly with abnormal genitalia (XLAG) is the most severe phenotype described in association with mutations in the *ARX* gene (79). The lissencephaly is posterior-predominant, similar to classical lissencephaly seen with *LIS1* mutations, and may be accompanied by agenesis of the corpus callosum and basal ganglia abnormalities (130). Also notable are *ARX* mutations in nonsyndromic boys with infantile spasms *without* lissencephaly (131) but presumably with disrupted migration at a microscopic level.

Disorders of Later Cortical Organization

Disorders of later cortical organization chiefly include polymicrogyria (PMG) and schizencephaly. FCD without balloon cells, and lesions that are evident only by

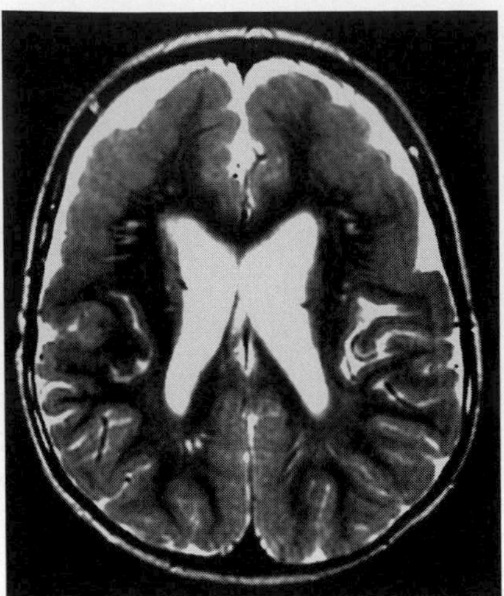

FIGURE 6-9

Bilateral fronto-parietal PMG (BFPP) is often associated with mutations in the gene *GPR56,* as in the patient whose axial T2 MRI is shown here. Note the increased apparent cortical thickness in the regions of polymicrogyria in both frontal and parietal lobes. PMG is classified as a disorder of cortical organization.

microscopic analysis, are included in this category as well. All of these conditions are associated with epilepsy.

PMG can be created experimentally by freeze lesions in rodent cortex (132), suggesting that local disruptions of either genes or the environment during human brain development could produce similar focal lesions in humans. PMG has also been associated with disorders of peroxisome function and with in utero exposure to cytomegalovirus (133, 134). Epilepsy has been a defining feature of the bilateral PMG syndromes, occurring in the vast majority of cases, and these conditions bear further discussion. It is the bilateral PMG syndromes that most strongly suggest a genetic etiology for PMG, and a representative example is shown in Figure 6-9. Bilateral generalized polymicrogyria affects most or all of the cortex and is associated with epilepsy in almost all patients; nearly half of the patients have macrocephaly (135), suggesting a possible disruption as early as the stage of proliferation. The bilateral perisylvian PMG (BPP) syndrome consists of epilepsy and a characteristic oromotor apraxia; epilepsy occurs in nearly 90% of affected individuals (136). Genetic linkage studies of familial BPP suggest a locus on the X chromosome (137), and studies of pedigrees also suggest an autosomal dominant mode of inheritance (138). BPP has also been described in association with deletions of the 22q11 locus (139). Thus, BPP is clearly a genetically heterogeneous syndrome. The bilateral fronto-parietal PMG (BFPP) syndrome—which includes epilepsy, mental retardation, dysconjugate gaze, and pyramidal signs—has been associated with mutations in the gene *GPR56* (85, 140). Interestingly, in a series of 13 patients with a form of bilateral PMG restricted to the frontal regions, only five had epilepsy (141).

Schizencephaly is a cerebral malformation consisting of one or more clefts that span the depth of the cortex, from the lateral ventricle to the pial surface, and that are lined by gray matter (142). Similarly to polymicrogyria, schizencephaly can occur unilaterally or bilaterally and can result from a variety of viral, vascular, or genetic abnormalities (86, 142, 143). About half of the individuals affected are reported to have epilepsy, and as yet there is not a clear correlation between the type of schizencephaly and the occurrence or severity of epilepsy in these patients (144).

CONCLUSIONS

The majority of patients with cerebral cortical malformation will experience clinical epilepsy, often with onset during childhood. The clinical neurologist treating any patient with localization-related epilepsy or treating any child with presumed symptomatic epilepsy, should have a high index of suspicion for a malformation of cortical development as the etiology.

Understanding the mechanisms through which malformations of cortical development occur will continue to teach us about normal brain development and will allow us to provide better explanations of causality to patients and their families. A detailed understanding of the genetic underpinnings of these malformations and the molecular basis of their epileptogenesis should ultimately lead to more refined and individualized approaches to treatment.

ACKNOWLEDGMENTS

A. P. was supported by a Clinical Research Training Fellowship from the American Academy of Neurology. B. S. C. was supported by a K23 award from the NINDS. C. A. W. was supported by grants from the NINDS, the NLM Foundation, and the Marilyn and James Simons Foundation. C. A. W. is an Investigator of the Howard Hughes Medical Institute.

References

1. Barkovich AJ. Congenital malformations of the brain and skull. In: *Pediatric Neuroimaging*. Philadelphia: Lippincott Williams and Wilkins, 2005; 291–439.
2. Guerrini R, Andermann F, Canapicchi R, Roger J, et al., eds. Dysplasias of the cerebral cortex and epilepsy. Philadelphia: Lippincott-Raven, 1996.
3. Engel J; International League Against Epilepsy (ILAE). A proposed diagnostic scheme for people with epileptic seizures and with epilepsy: report of the ILAE Task Force on Classification and Terminology. *Epilepsia* 2001; 42(6):796–803.
4. Cockerell OC, Eckle I, Goodridge DM, Sander JW, et al. Epilepsy in a population of 6000 re-examined: secular trends in first attendance rates, prevalence, and prognosis. *J Neurol Neurosurg Psychiatry* 1995; 58(5):570–576.
5. Cowan LD. The epidemiology of the epilepsies in children. *Mental Retard Dev Disabil Res Rev* 2002; 8(3):171–181.
6. Hauser WA, Annegers JF, Kurland LT. Incidence of epilepsy and unprovoked seizures in Rochester, Minnesota: 1935–1984. *Epilepsia* 1993; 34(3):453–468.

7. Berg AT, Shinnar S, Levy SR, Testa FM, et al. Two-year remission and subsequent relapse in children with newly diagnosed epilepsy. *Epilepsia* 2001; 42(12):1553–1562.
8. Taylor DC, Falconer MA, Bruton CJ, Corsellis JA. Focal dysplasia of the cerebral cortex in epilepsy. *J Neurol Neurosurg Psychiatry* 1971; 34(4):369–387.
9. Palmini A, Andermann F, Olivier A, Tampieri D, et al. Focal neuronal migration disorders and intractable partial epilepsy: a study of 30 patients. *Ann Neurol* 1991; 30(6):741–749.
10. Farrell MA, DeRosa MJ, Curran JG, Secor DL, et al. Neuropathologic findings in cortical resections (including hemispherectomies) performed for the treatment of intractable childhood epilepsy. *Acta Neuropathol (Berl)* 1992; 83(3):246–259.
11. Vinters HV. Histopathology of brain tissue from patients with infantile spasms. *Int Rev Neurobiol* 2002; 49:63–76.
12. Sisodiya SM. Malformations of cortical development: burdens and insights from important causes of epilepsy. *Lancet Neurol* 2004; (3):29–38.
13. Sisodiya SM, Fish DR. Structural neuroimaging in the presurgical evaluation of patients with malformations of cortical development and neurocutaneous syndromes. In: Luders HO, Comair YG, eds. *Epilepsy Surgery*. Philadelphia: Lippincott Williams and Wilkins, 2001; 239–246.
14. Wieshmann UC. Clinical application of neuroimaging in epilepsy. *J Neurol Neurosurg Psychiatry* 2003; 74(4):466–470.
15. Li LM, Fish DR, Sisodiya SM, Shorvon SD, et al. High resolution magnetic resonance imaging in adults with partial or secondary generalised epilepsy attending a tertiary referral unit. *J Neurol Neurosurg Psychiatry* 1995; 59(4):384–387.
16. Kuzniecky R, Murro A, King D, Morawetz R, et al. Magnetic resonance imaging in childhood intractable partial epilepsies: pathologic correlations. *Neurology* 1993; 43(4):681–687.
17. Pasquier B, Peoc'h M, Barnoud R, Pasquier T, et al. Surgical pathology of cortical dysplasia, tuberous sclerosis, and dysembryoplastic neuroepithelial tumours: experience with 55 cases in a recent series of 230 patients with chronic epilepsy. In: Spreafico R, Avanzini G, Andermann F, eds. *Abnormal Cortical Development and Epilepsy: from Basic to Clinical Science*. London: John Libbey, 1999; 227–240.
18. Sinclair DB, Wheatley M, Aronyk K, Hao C, et al. Pathology and neuroimaging in pediatric temporal lobectomy for intractable epilepsy. *Pediatric Neurosurgery* 2001; 35:239–246.
19. Barkovich AJ, Kuzniecky RI, Jackson GD, Guerrini R, et al. A developmental and genetic classification for malformations of cortical development. *Neurology* 2005; 65(12):1873–1887.
20. Vinters HV, De Rosa MJ, Farrell MA. Neuropathologic study of resected cerebral tissue from patients with infantile spasms. *Epilepsia* 1993; 34(4):772–779.
21. Wyllie E, Comair YG, Kotagal P, Raja S, et al. Epilepsy surgery in infants. *Epilepsia* 1996; 37(7):625–637.
22. Vinters HV, Fisher RS, Cornford ME, Mah V, et al. Morphological substrates of infantile spasms: studies based on surgically resected cerebral tissue. *Childs Nerv Syst* 1992; 8(1):8–17.
23. Sankar R, Curran JG, Kevill JW, Rintahaka PJ, et al. Microscopic cortical dysplasia in infantile spasms: evolution of white matter abnormalities. *Am J Neuroradiol* 1995; 16(6):1265–1272.
24. Keene D, Jimenez C, Ventureyra E. Cortical microdysplasia and surgical outcome in refractory epilepsy of childhood. *Pediatr Neurosurg* 1998; 29:69–72.
25. Russo GL, Tassi L, Cossu M, Cardinale F, et al. Focal cortical resection in malformations of cortical development. *Epileptic Disord* 2003; 5 Suppl 2:S115–S123.
26. Porter BE, Judkins AR, Clancy RR, Duhaime A, et al. Dysplasia: a common finding in intractable pediatric temporal lobe epilepsy. *Neurology* 2003; 61(3):365–368.
27. Sinclair DB, Aronyk K, Snyder T, McKean JD, et al. Extratemporal resection for childhood epilepsy. *Pediatr Neurol* 2004; 30(3):177–185.
28. Said RR, Poduri A, Bundock EA, Black PM, et al. Non-lesional focal epilepsy surgery: pathology identifies focal cortical dysplasia, gliosis, and mesial temporal sclerosis. *Ann Neurol* 2004; 58(S8):S112 (abstract).
29. Chugani HT, Shewmon DA, Shields WD, Sankar R, et al. Surgery for intractable infantile spasms: neuroimaging perspectives. *Epilepsia* 1993; 34(4):764–771.
30. Mochida G. Cortical malformation and pediatric epilepsy: a molecular genetic approach. *J Child Neurol* 2005; 20:300–303.
31. Tassi L, Colombo N, Garbelli R, Francione S, et al. Focal cortical dysplasia: neuropathological subtypes, EEG, neuroimaging and surgical outcome. *Brain* 2002; 125(8):1719–1732.
32. Garbelli R, Pasquier B, Minotti L, Tassi L, et al. Immunocytochemical studies in epileptogenic dysplastic tissue. In Spreafico R, Avanzini G, Andermann F, et al, eds. *Abnormal Cortical Development and Epilepsy: From Basic to Clinical Science*. London: John Libbey, 1999; 241–252.
33. Arai Y, Edwards V, Becker LE. A comparison of cell phenotypes in hemimegalencephaly and tuberous sclerosis. *Acta Neuropathol* 1999; 98(4):407–413.
34. Flores-Sarnat L, Sarnat HB, Dávila-Gutiérrez G, Alvarez A. Hemimegalencephaly: part 2. Neuropathology suggests a disorder of cellular lineage. *J Child Neurol* 2003; 18(11):776–785.
35. Yamanouchi H, Zhang W, Jay V, Becker LE. Enhanced expression of microtubule-associated protein 2 in large neurons of cortical dysplasia. *Ann Neurol* 1996; 39(1):57–61.
36. Palmini A, Najm I, Avanzini G, Babb T, et al. Terminology and classification of the cortical dysplasias. *Neurology* 2004; 62(6 Suppl 3):S2–8.
37. Foldvary-Schaefer N, Bautista J, Andermann F, Cascino G, et al. Focal malformations of cortical development. *Neurology* 2004; 62(6 Suppl 3):S14–19.
38. Widdess-Walsh P, Kellinghaus C, Jeha L, Kotagal P, et al. Electro-clinical and imaging characteristics of focal cortical dysplasia: correlation with pathological subtypes. *Epilepsy Res* 2005; 67(1–2):25–33.
39. Chevassus-au-Louis N, Congar P, Represa A, Ben-Ari Y, et al. Neuronal migration disorders: heterotopic neocortical neurons in CA1 provide a bridge between the hippocampus and the neocortex. *Proc Natl Acad Sci U S A* 1998; 95:10263–10268.
40. Tsuru A, Mizuguchi M, Uyemura K, Becker LE, et al. Immunohistochemical expression of cell adhesion molecule L1 in hemimegalencephaly. *Pediatr Neurol* 1997; 16(1):45–49.
41. Nakanishi S. Molecular diversity of glutamate receptors and implications for brain function. *Science* 1992; 258(5082):597–603.
42. Najm I, Ying Z, Babb T, Crino PB, et al. Mechanisms of epileptogenicity in cortical dysplasias. *Neurology* 2004; 62(6 Suppl 3):S9–13.
43. Ying Z, Babb TL, Comair YG, Bingaman W, et al. Induced expression of NMDAR2 proteins and differential expression of NMDAR1 splice variants in dysplastic neurons of human epileptic neocortex. *J Neuropathol Exp Neurol* 1998; 57(1):47-62.
44. Najm IM, Ying Z, Babb T, Bingaman W, et al. Epileptogenicity correlated with increased N-methyl-D-aspartate receptor subunit NR2A/B in human focal cortical dysplasia. *Epilepsia* 2000; 41(8):971–976.
45. André VM, Flores-Hernández J, Cepeda C, Starling AJ, et al. NMDA receptor alterations in neurons from pediatric cortical dysplasia tissue. *Cereb Cortex* 2004; 14:634–646.
46. Crino PB, Duhaime AC, Baltuch G, White R. Differential expression of glutamate and GABA-A receptor subunit mRNA in cortical dysplasia. *Neurology* 2001; 56(7):906–913.
47. Ferrer I, Oliver B, Russi A, Casas R, et al. Parvalbumin and calbindin-D28k immunocytochemistry in human neocortical epileptic foci. *J Neurol Sci* 1994; 123(1–2):18–25.
48. Swann JW. Synaptogenesis and epileptogenesis in developing neural networks. In Schwartzkroin PA, Moshé SL, Noebels JL, Swann JW, eds. *Brain Development and Epilepsy*. New York: Oxford University Press, 1995.
49. Brooks-Kayal AR. Rearranging receptors. *Epilepsia* 2005; 46 Suppl 7:29–38.
50. Jacobs KM, Khazaria VN, Prince DA. Mechanisms underlying epileptogenesis in cortical malformations. *Epilepsy Res* 1999; 36:165–188.
51. Kim SK, Wang KC, Hong SJ, Chung CK, et al. Gene expression profile analyses of cortical dysplasia by cDNA arrays. *Epilepsy Res* 2003; 56(2–3):175–183.
52. Rakhade SN, Yao B, Ahmed S, Asano E, et al. A common pattern of persistent gene activation in human neocortical epileptic foci. *Ann Neurol* 2005; 58(5):736–747.
53. Yu J, Baybis M, Lee A, McKhann G, et al. Targeted gene expression analysis in hemimegalencephaly: activation of beta-catenin signaling. *Brain Pathol* 2005; 15(3):179–186.
54. Poduri A, Beroukhim R, Apse K, Bourgeois BFD, et al. Single nucleotide polymorphism analysis suggests increased allele copy number at chromosome 1q in focal malformations of cortical development. *Epilepsia* 2005; 46(suppl 8):370 (abstract).
55. Dalla Bernardina B, Perez-Jimenez A, Fontan A, et al. Electroencephalographic findings associated with cortical dysplasias. In Guerrini R, Andermann F, Canapicchi R, et al., eds. *Dysplasias of the Cerebral Cortex and Epilepsy*. Philadelphia: Lippincott-Raven, 1996.
56. Gambardella A, Palmini A, Andermann F, Dubeau F, et al. Usefulness of focal rhythmic discharges on scalp EEG of patients with focal cortical dysplasia and intractable epilepsy. *Electroencephalogr Clin Neurophysiol* 1996; 98(4):243–249.
57. Kuzniecky R, Guthrie B, Mountz J, Bebin M, et al. Intrinsic epileptogenesis of hypothalamic hamartomas in gelastic epilepsy. *Ann Neurol* 1997; 42(1):60–67.
58. Kothare SV, VanLandingham K, Armon C, Luther JS, et al. Seizure onset from periventricular nodular heterotopias: depth-electrode study. *Neurology* 1998; 51(6):1723–1727.
59. Tassi L, Colombo N, Cossu M, Mai R, et al. Electroclinical, MRI and neuropathological study of 10 patients with nodular heterotopia, with surgical outcomes. *Brain* 2005; 128(Pt 2):321–37.
60. Chassoux F, Devaux B, Landré E, Turak B, et al. Stereoelectroencephalography in focal cortical dysplasia: a 3D approach to delineating the dysplastic cortex. *Brain* 2000; 123(8):1733–1751.
61. Palmini A, Gambardella A, Andermann F, et al. The human dysplastic cortex is intrinsically epileptogenic. In Guerrini R, Andermann F, Canapicchi R, et al, eds. *Dysplasias of the Cerebral Cortex and Epilepsy*. Philadelphia: Lippincott-Raven, 1996.
62. Andermann F. Cortical dysplasias and epilepsy: a review of the architectonic, clinical, and seizure patterns. *Adv Neurol* 2000; 84:479–496.
63. Rosenow F, Lüders HO, Dinner DS, Prayson RA, et al. Histopathological correlates of epileptogenicity as expressed by electrocorticographic spiking and seizure frequency. *Epilepsia* 1998; 39(8):850–856.
64. Palmini A, Gambardella A, Andermann F, Dubeau F, et al. Intrinsic epileptogenicity of human dysplastic cortex as suggested by corticography and surgical results. *Ann Neurol* 1995; 37(4):476–487.
65. Raymond AA, Fish DR, Sisodiya SM, Alsanjari N, et al. Abnormalities of gyration, heterotopias, tuberous sclerosis, focal cortical dysplasia, microdysgenesis, dysembryoplastic neuroepithelial tumour and dysgenesis of the archicortex in epilepsy. Clinical, EEG and neuroimaging features in 100 adult patients. *Brain* 1995; 118 (Pt 3):629–660.
66. Barkovich AJ, Kuzniecky RI, Dobyns WB, Jackson GD, et al. A classification scheme for malformations of cortical development. *Neuropediatrics* 1996; 27(2):59–63.
67. Jackson AP, Eastwood H, Bell SM, Adu J, et al. Identification of microcephalin, a protein implicated in determining the size of the human brain. *Am J Hum Genet* 2002; 71(1):136–142.
68. Bond J, Scott S, Hampshire DJ, Springell K, et al. Protein-truncating mutations in *ASPM* cause variable reduction in brain size. *Am J Hum Genet* 2003; 73(5):1170–1177.
69. Shen J, Eyaid W, Mochida GH, Al-Moayyad F, et al. *ASPM* mutations identified in patients with primary microcephaly and seizures. *J Med Genet* 2005; 42(9):725–729.
70. Sheen VL, Ganesh VS, Topcu M, Sebire G, et al. Mutations in *ARFGEF2* implicate vesicle trafficking in neural progenitor proliferation and migration in the human cerebral cortex. *Nat Genet* 2004; 36(1):69–76.
71. Viskochil D, Buchberg AM, Xu G, Cawthon RM, et al. Deletions and a translocation interrupt a cloned gene at the neurofibromatosis type 1 locus. *Cell* 1990; 62(1):187–192.
72. Tatton-Brown K, Rahman N. Clinical features of NSD1-positive Sotos syndrome. *Clin Dysmorphol* 2004; 13(4):199–204.
73. Liaw D, Marsh DJ, Li J, Dahia PL, et al. Germline mutations of the *PTEN* gene in Cowden disease, an inherited breast and thyroid cancer syndrome. *Nat Genet* 1997; 16(1):64–67.
74. Haines JL, Short MP, Kwiatkowski DJ, Jewell A, et al. Localization of one gene for tuberous sclerosis within 9q32–9q34, and further evidence for heterogeneity. *Am J Hum Genet* 1991; 49(4):764–772.
75. The European Chromosome 16 Tuberous Sclerosis Consortium. Identification and characterization of the tuberous sclerosis gene on chromosome 16. *Cell* 1993; 75(7): 1305–1315.

76. Reiner O, Carrozzo R, Shen Y, Wehnert M, et al. Isolation of a Miller-Dieker lissencephaly gene containing G protein β-subunit-like repeats. *Nature* 1993; 364:717–721.
77. Hong SE, Shugart YY, Huang DT, Shahwan SA, et al. Autosomal recessive lissencephaly with cerebellar hypoplasia is associated with human RELN mutations. *Nat Genet* 2000; 26(1):93–96.
78. des Portes V, Pinard JM, Billuart P, Vinet MC, et al. A novel CNS gene required for neuronal migration and involved in X-linked subcortical laminar heterotopia and lissencephaly syndrome. *Cell* 1998; 92(1):51–61.
79. Kitamura K, Yanazawa M, Sugiyama N, Miura H, et al. Mutation of *ARX* causes abnormal development of forebrain and testes in mice and X-linked lissencephaly with abnormal genitalia in humans. *Nat Genet* 2002; 32(3):359–369.
80. Gleeson JG, Allen KM, Fox JW, Lamperti ED, et al. Doublecortin, a brain-specific gene mutated in human X-linked lissencephaly and double cortex syndrome, encodes a putative signaling protein. *Cell* 1998; 92(1):63–72.
81. Beltran-Valero de Bernabé D, Currier S, Steinbrecher A, Celli J, et al. Mutations in the O-mannosyltransferase gene *POMT1* give rise to the severe neuronal migration disorder Walker-Warburg syndrome. *Am J Hum Genet* 2002; 71(5):1033–1043.
82. van Reeuwijk J, Janssen M, van den Elzen C, Beltran-Valero de Bernabé D, et al. *POMT2* mutations cause alpha-dystroglycan hypoglycosylation and Walker-Warburg syndrome. *J Med Genet* 2005; 42(12):907–912.
83. Yoshida A, Kobayashi K, Manya H, Taniguchi K, et al. Muscular dystrophy and neuronal migration disorder caused by mutations in a glycosyltransferase, *POMGnT1*. *Dev Cell* 2001; 1(5):717–724.
84. Fox JW, Lamperti ED, Ekşioğlu YZ, Hong SE, et al. Mutations in filamin 1 prevent migration of cerebral cortical neurons in human periventricular heterotopia. *Neuron* 1998; 21(6):1315–1325.
85. Piao X, Hill RS, Bodell A, Chang BS, et al. G protein-coupled receptor-dependent development of human frontal cortex. *Science* 2004; 303(5666):2033–2036.
86. Brunelli S, Faiella A, Capra V, Nigro V, et al. Germline mutations in the homeobox gene EMX2 in patients with severe schizencephaly. *Nat Genet* 1996; 12(1):94–96.
87. Hamiwka L, Jayakar P, Resnick T, Morrison G, et al. Surgery for epilepsy due to cortical malformations: ten-year follow-up. *Epilepsia* 2005; 46(4):556–560.
88. Edwards JC, Wyllie E, Ruggeri PM, Bingaman W, et al. Seizure outcome after surgery for epilepsy due to malformation of cortical development. *Neurology* 2000; 55(8):1110–1114.
89. Fauser S, Schulze-Bonhage A, Honegger J, Carmona H, et al. Focal cortical dysplasias: surgical outcome in 67 patients in relation to histological subtypes and dual pathology. *Brain* 2004; 127(Pt 11):2406–2418.
90. Sidman RL, Rakic P. Neuronal migration, with special reference to developing human brain: a review. *Brain Research* 1973; 62:1–35.
91. Malatesta P, Hartfuss E, Gotz M. Isolation of radial glial cells by fluorescent-activated cell sorting reveals a neuronal lineage. *Development* 2000; 127(24):5253–5263.
92. Noctor SC, Flint AC, Weissman TA, Wong WS, et al. Dividing precursor cells of the embryonic cortical ventricular zone have morphological and molecular characteristics of radial glia. *J Neurosci* 2002; 22(8):3161–3173.
93. Kaltschmidt JA, Davidson CM, Brown NH, Brand AH. Rotation and asymmetry of the mitotic spindle direct asymmetric cell division in the developing central nervous system. *Nat Cell Biol* 2000; 2(1):7–12.
94. Albertson R, Doe CQ. Dlg, Scrib and Lgl regulate neuroblast cell size and mitotic spindle asymmetry. *Nat Cell Biol* 2003; 5(2):166–170.
95. Lee CY, Robinson KJ, Doe CQ. Lgl, Pins and aPKC regulate neuroblast self-renewal versus differentiation. *Nature* 2006; 439(7076):594–598.
96. Siegrist SE, Doe CQ. Extrinsic cues orient the cell division axis in *Drosophila* embryonic neuroblasts. *Development* 2006; 133(3):529–536.
97. Walsh C, Cepko CL. Widespread dispersion of neuronal clones across functional regions of the cerebral cortex. *Science* 1992; 255(5043):434–440.
98. Anderson SA, Kaznowski CE, Horn C, Rubenstein JL, et al. Distinct origins of neocortical projection neurons and interneurons in vivo. *Cereb Cortex* 2002; 12(7):702–709.
99. Woods CG, Bond J, Enard W. Autosomal recessive primary microcephaly (MCPH): a review of clinical, molecular, and evolutionary findings. *Am J Hum Genet* 2005; 76(5):717–728.
100. Gaitanis JN, Walsh CA. Genetics of disorders of cortical development. *Neuroimaging Clin N Am* 2004; 14(2):219–229.
101. Peiffer A, Singh N, Leppert M, Dobyns WB, et al. Microcephaly with simplified gyral pattern in six related children. *Am J Med Genet* 1999; 84(2):137–144.
102. Sztriha L, Dawodu A, Gururaj A, Johansen JG. Microcephaly associated with abnormal gyral pattern. *Neuropediatrics* 2004; 35(6):346–352.
103. Moore BD, Slopis JM, Jackson EF, De Winter AE, et al. Brain volume in children with neurofibromatosis type 1: relation to neuropsychological status. *Neurology* 2000; 54(4):914–920.
104. Nelen MR, Padberg GW, Peeters EA, Lin AY, et al. Localization of the gene for Cowden disease to chromosome 10q22–23. *Nat Genet* 1996; 13(1):114–116.
105. Korf BR, Carrazana E, Holmes GL. Patterns of seizures observed in association with neurofibromatosis 1. *Epilepsia* 1993; 34(4):616–620.
106. Eng C, Murday V, Seal S, Mohammed S, et al. Cowden syndrome and Lhermitte-Duclos disease in a family: a single genetic syndrome with pleiotropy? *J Med Genet* 1994; 31(6):458–461.
107. Orstavik KH, Strømme P, Ek J, Torvik A, et al. Macrocephaly, epilepsy, autism, dysmorphic features, and mental retardation in two sisters: a new autosomal recessive syndrome? *J Med Genet* 1997; 34(10):849–851.
108. Thiele EA. Managing epilepsy in tuberous sclerosis complex. *J Child Neurol* 2004; 19: 680–686.
109. Curatolo P, Seri S, Verdecchia M, Bombardieri R. Infantile spasms in tuberous sclerosis complex. *Brain Dev* 2001; 23(7):502–507.
110. Bast T, Ramantani G, Seitz A, Rating D. Focal cortical dysplasia: prevalence, clinical presentation and epilepsy in children and adults. *Acta Neurol Scand* 2006; 113(2):72–81.
111. Lawson JA, Birchansky S, Pacheco E, Jayakar P, et al. Distinct clinicopathologic subtypes of cortical dysplasia of Taylor. *Neurology* 2005; 64(1):55–61.
112. Gupta A, Carreno M, Wyllie E, Bingaman WE. Hemispheric malformations of cortical development. *Neurology* 2004; 62(6 Suppl 3):S20–26.
113. Jahan R, Mischel PS, Curran JG, Peacock WJ, et al. Bilateral neuropathologic changes in a child with hemimegalencephaly. *Pediatr Neurol* 1997; 17(4):344–349.
114. Tsai JW, Chen Y, Kriegstein AR, Vallee RB. *LIS1* RNA interference blocks neural stem cell division, morphogenesis, and motility at multiple stages. *J Cell Biol* 2005; 170(6):935–945.
115. Dobyns WB, Truwit CL, Ross ME, Matsumoto N, et al. Differences in the gyral pattern distinguish chromosome 17-linked and X-linked lissencephaly. *Neurology* 1999; 53(2):270–277.
116. Palmini A, Andermann F, Aicardi J, Dulac O, et al. Diffuse cortical dysplasia, or the "double cortex" syndrome: the clinical and epileptic spectrum in 10 patients. *Neurology* 1991; 41(10):1656–1662.
117. D'Agostino MD, Bernasconi A, Das S, Bastos A, et al. Subcortical band heterotopia (SBH) in males: clinical, imaging and genetic findings in comparison with females. *Brain* 2002; 125(Pt 11):2507–2522.
118. Pilz DT, Matsumoto N, Minnerath S, Mills P, et al. *LIS1* and *XLIS* (*DCX*) mutations cause most classical lissencephaly, but different patterns of malformation. *Hum Mol Genet* 1998; 7(13):2029–2037.
119. Dobyns WB, Reiner O, Carrozzo R, Ledbetter DH. Lissencephaly. A human brain malformation associated with deletion of the LIS1 gene located at chromosome 17p13. *J Am Med Assoc* 1993; 270(23):2838–2842.
120. Gleeson JG, Minnerath SR, Fox JW, Allen KM, et al. Characterization of mutations in the gene doublecortin in patients with double cortex syndrome. *Ann Neurol* 1999; 45(2):146–153.
121. Gleeson JG, Minnerath S, Kuzniecky RI, Dobyns WB, et al. Somatic and germline mosaic mutations in the doublecortin gene are associated with variable phenotypes. *Am J Hum Genet* 2000; 67(3):574–581.
122. Guerrini R, Moro F, Andermann E, Hughes E, et al. Nonsyndromic mental retardation and cryptogenic epilepsy in women with doublecortin gene mutations. *Ann Neurol* 2003; 54(1):30–37.
123. Barkovich AJ. Subcortical heterotopia: a distinct clinicoradiologic entity. *Am J Neuroradiol* 1996; 17(7):1315–1322.
124. Dobyns WB, Pagon RA, Armstrong D, Curry CJ, et al. Diagnostic criteria for Walker-Warburg syndrome. *Am J Med Genet* 1989; 32(2):195–210.
125. Diesen C, Saarinen A, Pihko H, Rosenlew C, et al. *POMGnT1* mutation and phenotypic spectrum in muscle-eye-brain disease. *J Med Genet* 2004; 41(10):e115(1–5).
126. Yoshioka M, Kuroki S. Clinical spectrum and genetic studies of Fukuyama congenital muscular dystrophy. *Am J Med Genet* 1994; 53(3):245–250.
127. Endo T. Aberrant glycosylation of alpha-dystroglycan and congenital muscular dystrophies. *Acta Myol* 2005; 24(2):64–69.
128. Sheen VL, Dixon PH, Fox JW, Hong SE, et al. Mutations in the X-linked filamin 1 gene cause periventricular nodular heterotopia in males as well as in females. *Hum Mol Genet* 2001; 10(17):1775–1783.
129. Chang BS, Ly J, Appignani B, Bodell A, et al. Reading impairment in the neuronal migration disorder of periventricular nodular heterotopia. *Neurology* 2005; 64(5): 799–803.
130. Kato M, Dobyns WB. X-linked lissencephaly with abnormal genitalia as a tangential migration disorder causing intractable epilepsy: proposal for a new term, "interneuronopathy." *J Child Neurol* 2005; 20(4):392–397.
131. Kato M, Das S, Petras K, Kitamura K, et al. Mutations of *ARX* are associated with striking pleiotropy and consistent genotype-phenotype correlation. *Hum Mutat* 2004; 23(2):147–159.
132. Jacobs KM, Hwang BJ, Prince DA. Focal epileptogenesis in a rat model of polymicrogyria. *J Neurophysiol* 1999; 81(1):159–173.
133. Kaufmann WE, Theda C, Naidu S, Watkins PA, et al. Neuronal migration abnormality in peroxisomal bifunctional enzyme defect. *Ann Neurol* 1996; 39(2):268–271.
134. de Vries LS, Gunardi H, Barth PG, Bok LA, et al. The spectrum of cranial ultrasound and magnetic resonance imaging abnormalities in congenital cytomegalovirus infection. *Neuropediatrics* 2004; 35(2):113–119.
135. Chang BS, Piao X, Giannini C, Cascino GD, et al. Bilateral generalized polymicrogyria (BGP): a distinct syndrome of cortical malformation. *Neurology* 2004; 62(10):1722–1728.
136. Kuzniecky R, Andermann F, Guerrini R. Congenital bilateral perisylvian syndrome: study of 31 patients. The CBPS Multicenter Collaborative Study. *Lancet* 1993; 341(8845):608–612.
137. Villard L, Nguyen K, Cardoso C, Martin CL, et al. A locus for bilateral perisylvian polymicrogyria maps to Xq28. *Am J Hum Genet* 2002; 70(4):1003–1008.
138. Guerreiro MM, Andermann E, Guerrini R, Dobyns WB, et al. Familial perisylvian polymicrogyria: a new familial syndrome of cortical maldevelopment. *Ann Neurol* 2000; 48(1):39–48.
139. Bingham PM, Lynch D, McDonald-McGinn D, Zackai E. Polymicrogyria in chromosome 22 delection syndrome. *Neurology* 1998; 51(5):1500–1502.
140. Chang BS, Piao X, Bodell A, Basel-Vanagaite L, et al. Bilateral frontoparietal polymicrogyria: clinical and radiological features in10 families with linkage to chromosome 16. *Ann Neurol* 2003; 53(5):596–606.
141. Guerrini R, Barkovich AJ, Sztriha L, Dobyns WB. Bilateral frontal polymicrogyria: a newly recognized brain malformation syndrome. *Neurology* 2000; 54(4):909–913.
142. Denis D, Chateil JF, Brun M, Brissaud O, et al. Schizencephaly: clinical and imaging features in 30 infantile cases. *Brain Dev* 2000; 22(8):475–483.
143. Tietjen I, Erdogan F, Currier S, Apse K, et al. EMX2-independent familial schizencephaly: clinical and genetic analyses. *Am J Med Genet* 2005; 135(2):166–170.
144. Granata T, Freri E, Caccia C, Setola V, et al. Schizencephaly: clinical spectrum, epilepsy, and pathogenesis. *J Child Neurol* 2005; 20(4):313–318.

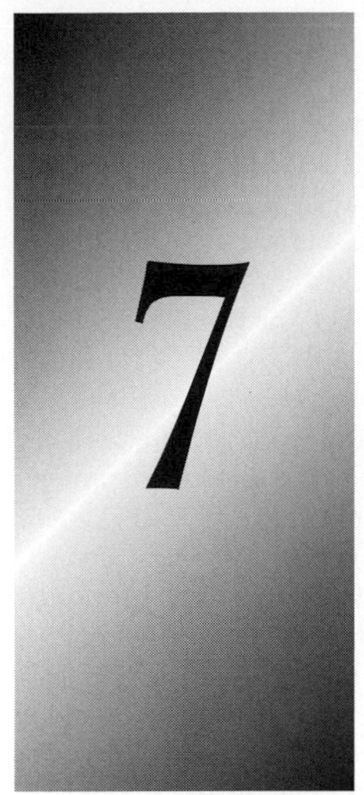

7 Genetic Influences on the Risk for Epilepsy

Asuri N. Prasad
Chitra Prasad

INTRODUCTION

Of the many neurologic disorders affecting humans, epilepsy has been recognized since antiquity, with well-documented references in records dating back to the Mesopotamians. The word *epilepsy* is derived from the Greek verb *epilambanein*, which means "to seize or attack"; that is, a seizure was taken to mean that the patient was being literally seized by gods or demons, and hence the condition was given the status of a "sacred disease" in medical writings that date back to 400 B.C. However, in lay society the diagnosis of epilepsy has spelt fear, hopelessness, social stigma, and isolation.

Epilepsy is a heterogeneous disorder with diverse etiologies, affecting nearly 1% of the world population (1). In the last century, epidemiological studies of families and twins with epilepsy have provided incontrovertible evidence in support of a genetic contribution to the risk of developing certain epilepsies. The discovery of the first single-gene defect underlying idiopathic epilepsy was made in 1995 (mutation in a gene coding for a neuronal nicotinic cholinergic receptor, leading to autosomal dominant nocturnal frontal lobe epilepsy). The subsequent identification of other gene defects has provided added evidence to support the role played by genetic susceptibility in the development of human epilepsy.

The relatively recent breakthroughs in gene-sequencing technologies, accompanied by development of animal models and bioinformatics, have speeded up the identification of new gene defects underlying the many epilepsy syndromes. These have been summarized in several reviews in recent years (2–4). Though a long list of gene defects and mutations associated with human epilepsy is presently known, these are mostly monogenic disorders that are rare; a complete understanding of the genetic basis of the more common epilepsies remains a distant goal. The large majority of individuals affected with epilepsy do not have affected relatives, nor do they have a family pedigree that is consistent with the traditional Mendelian patterns of inheritance. Epileptic disorders such as those currently considered under the umbrella of idiopathic generalized epilepsies (IGE) are now considered as genetically complex as to their inheritance patterns and expression. In this chapter we explore the implications of considering human epilepsy as a complex disorder and how genetic studies can shed light on our understanding of the risk of developing epilepsy in the clinical setting.

MENDELIAN VERSUS COMPLEX INHERITANCE: HISTORICAL BACKGROUND

Before proceeding to a discussion of the genetic influences in human epilepsy, it might be useful to introduce readers to the basic issues on how inheritance plays a role in epilepsy. Mendel in 1866 had worked out inheritance patterns and rules applicable to the segregation of distinct features termed "traits." The traits Mendel studied focused on were qualitative differences (nature of the skin on the seeds, or color of the flowers); it soon became evident that many traits in the general population did not follow these rules of segregation. Galton and Pearson in the 1900s observed that quantitative traits (e.g., growth parameters and IQ scores) followed a Gaussian (normal) distribution among offspring, thus raising contradictions to Mendel's conclusions. The work of Sir Ronald Fisher was instrumental in providing an explanation to this apparent contradiction. His work showed that the observed effects in the case of quantitative traits could be explained through the involvement of multiple genes that carried small effects, which acted in an additive manner (5). The influence of environmental factors was also recognized, and the cumulative additive effects of the combination tended to nudge the resultant effect toward a normative (Gaussian) distribution. This model, called "multifactorial and polygenic," was extended to explain disorders such as epilepsy by Falconer. He postulated a normal distribution of risk in the form of a nonmeasurable quantity termed "liability" that led to people being affected if the liability crossed a particular "threshold." In the case of epilepsy this could be considered as a "seizure threshold" (6). Other factors such as age, sex, puberty, or pregnancy can influence this threshold. Idiopathic epilepsy occurs with higher frequency in relatives of affected individuals; yet the different types do not conform to the expected frequencies for Mendelian traits. In these epilepsies, inheritance is considered to be multifactorial, where intrinsic susceptibility genes interact with environmental factors, producing a particular seizure phenotype (7).

CAUSES OF EPILEPSY

Broadly, epilepsy can be categorized on the basis of etiology (Figure 7-1) as symptomatic (a clear etiology can be demonstrated, such as a tumor, cortical dysplasia, or scarring), cryptogenic (a cause is suspected on the basis of associated neurologic features but remains hidden), or idiopathic (the individual appears to be normal on neurologic assessment, and no cause other than a hereditary predisposition established). Etiologies in the symptomatic category can be attributed to chromosomal aberrations (Angelman syndrome, Wolff-Hirschhorn syndrome) or single-gene defects for conditions such as tuberous sclerosis or lissencephaly. Though the epilepsy phenotypes encountered here are highly variable, these disorders display typical Mendelian inheritance patterns, wherein mutations at a single locus can explain the pattern of segregation of the disease within families. It is possible to list a large number of disorders of this type, but these conditions are uncommon in clinical practice and account for <1% of cases of genetic epilepsies.

At least 40–50% of all epilepsies are considered to belong to the category of idiopathic epilepsy (i.e., with a presumed genetic basis). In the case of idiopathic epilepsies, it is now clear that inheritance patterns can involve a monogenic (single-gene defects), oligogenic (few genes), or polygenic (many genes) models. Even within the monogenic epilepsies the relationship between gene defect and clinical phenotype is susceptible to modification by "epigenetic factors." These factors modify the penetrance of the gene, often resulting in fewer than expected recurrences within families. The disorders displaying polygenic or a complex inheritance pattern display marked phenotypic variability (intrafamilial as well as interfamilial), and recurrence of the trait and its expression within families is much harder to predict.

Genetic inheritance patterns not conforming to classic Mendelian inheritance have also been recognized in the epilepsies. The mechanisms of genetic transmission in these conditions include triplet and dodecamer expansions and mitochondrial inheritance involving nonnuclear (mitochondrial) genome.

GENETIC INFLUENCES IN EPILEPSY

The importance of heredity in epilepsy has been recognized for more than a century. Gowers estimated a figure of around 30% in his case series as having a heritable form of epilepsy in his treatise on *Epilepsy and Other Convulsive Disorders* (8). In the early part of the twentieth century this idea was further explored in family studies using electroencephalography (EEG) in the identification of individuals with an epileptic trait (9). By the end of the twentieth century, different lines of evidence came to strongly support a genetic basis to several forms of common epilepsies. These lines of evidence included (1) linkage analysis and positional cloning of susceptibility genes as well as candidate genes, (2) molecular studies of single-gene defects associated with human epilepsy, and in animal models, (3) aggregation studies in families and twins, and finally (4) association studies (10).

Linkage Analysis

Linkage studies have traditionally provided the lead in the identification of susceptibility genes in monogenic as well as complex phenotypes of epilepsy (11). Typically, classic linkage analysis requires large family sizes, with multiple

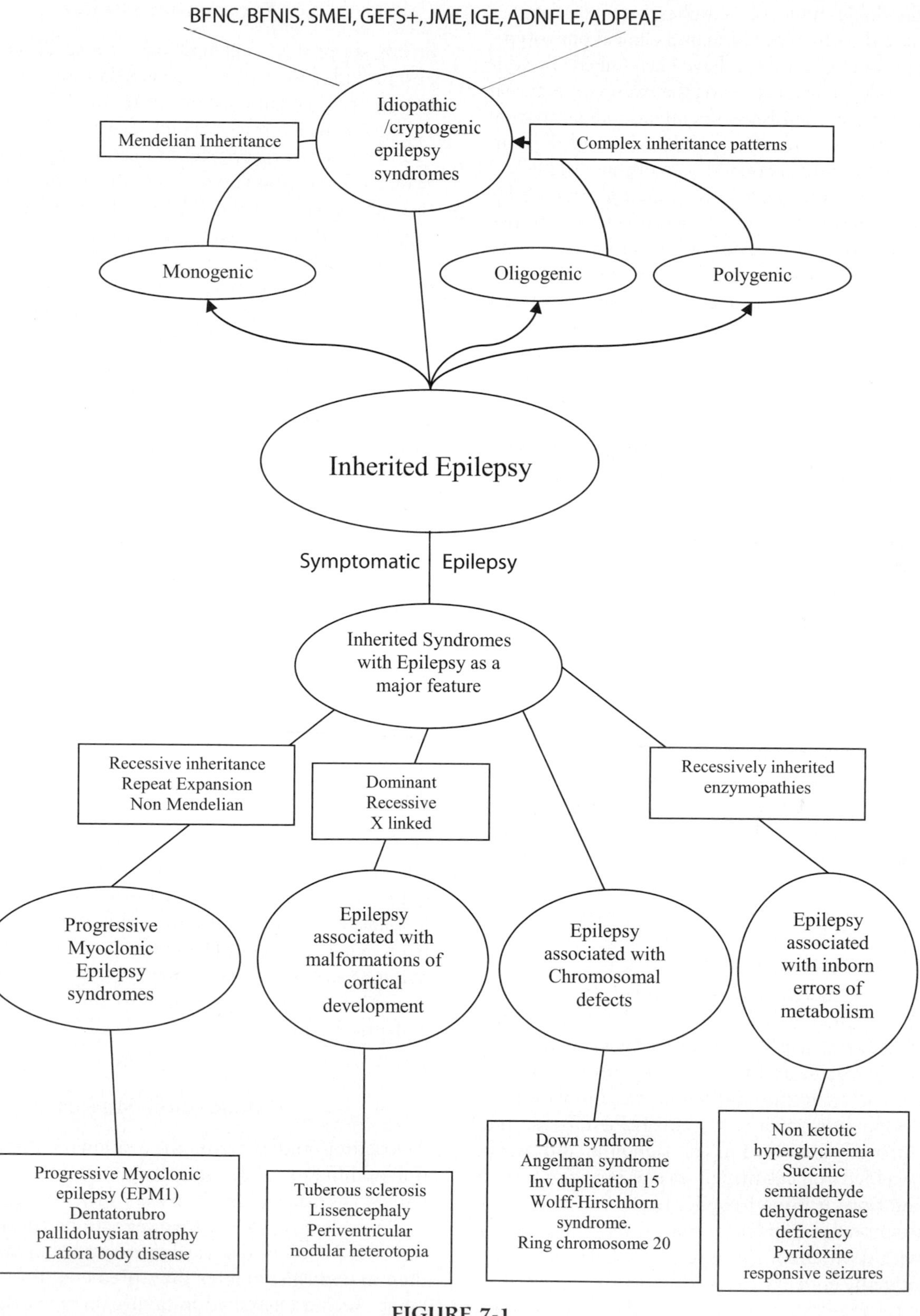

FIGURE 7-1

Genetic influences in human epilepsies; modes of inheritance and examples. BFNC = benign familial neonatal convulsions, BFNIS = Benign Familial Infantile Seizures, SMEI = Severe Myoclonic Epilepsy of Infancy, GEFS+ = Generalized Epilepsy with Febrile Seizures+, JME = Juvenile Myoclonic Epilepsy, IGE = Idiopathic Generalized Epilepsy, ADNFLE = Autosomal Dominant Nocturnal Frontal Lobe Epilepsy, ADPEAF = Autosomal Dominant Partial Epilepsy with Auditory Features.

affected individuals (multiplex families) or many families that may share the same mutation and clinical phenotype. Using this approach several loci have been linked with different partial epilepsy syndromes for, for example, nocturnal frontal lobe epilepsy (NFLE), autosomal dominant partial epilepsy with auditory features (ADPEAF), and the syndrome of benign familial neonatal convulsions (BFNC).

However, this approach seems to work less well for the situations where there may be incomplete penetrance or presence of multiple phenocopies (relatives with epilepsy caused by etiologies other than genetic). Although it is possible to adopt nonparametric approaches, studies carried out lacked sufficient power to detect the weaker susceptibility genes in the complex epilepsies. Thus, success with this approach has been limited.

Single-Gene Defects in Human Epilepsy, Animal Models, and Molecular Studies of Mutations

Single-gene defects are rare as causes of epilepsy and constitute a heterogeneous group of metabolic, degenerative conditions or malformations of cortical development in which epilepsy is often part of a much wider disorder. However, identification of single-gene defects in selected forms of idiopathic epilepsy has provided useful insights into epileptogenesis. The concept of epilepsy as a "channelopathy" was supported by the identification of mutations in voltage- and ligand-gated ion channels underlying BFNC; generalized epilepsy with febrile seizures plus (GEFS+) and severe myoclonic epilepsy of infancy (SMEI) as discussed later in this chapter. Genotype-phenotype correlations in these disorders have led to the conclusion that genetic heterogeneity is considerable, even in single-gene defects leading to inherited epilepsy. Mutations in different genes have been found to cause the same epilepsy syndrome (locus heterogeneity), while mutations in the same gene have been known to be associated with completely different epilepsy phenotypes (allelic heterogeneity) (Figure 7-2).

Additional insight has been gained through studies of the molecular aspects of epileptogenesis in these monogenic disorders, and the study of animal models of epilepsy. The structure and subunit composition of membrane channels, synapses, neurotransmitters, and receptors (proteins involved in cell signaling and transport) have yielded and confirmed several targets affected by gene mutations leading to epilepsy.

Mouse models of epilepsy (both transgenic models and mice with spontaneous seizures) have led to the identification of many epilepsy genes. Broadly these genes are involved in the regulation of (1) neuronal differentiation, migration, and cerebral morphogenesis; (2) membrane excitability (ion- and ligand-gated channels, neurotransmitter biosynthesis, release and reuptake) (3) intracellular pathways of intermediary metabolism, protein synthesis, degradation, and cellular homeostasis) (12).

Aggregation Studies

Strong support for a genetic basis for several epilepsies is also provided by studies of concordant rates of epilepsy in twin pairs. The concordance rate for IGE among monozygotic twins is up to 95% (13). The risk of occurrence of IGE in first-degree relatives of affected individuals is about 8–12%, and shows a significant drop to 1–2% in second-degree relatives. These risk assessments are very suggestive of an oligogenic pattern of inheritance (14).

Whereas monozygotic twins share an identical genotype, dizygotic twins are as different in genotype as siblings. However, both types of twinning share a similar environment in utero. So if two cotwins (in a monozygotic pair) share a given disorder at a greater frequency than two cotwins of a dizygotic pair, the inference drawn supports a strong role for genetic factors in disease causation. Concordance rates for both febrile and afebrile seizures are consistently higher in monozygotic twins as compared to dizygotic twins (13, 15–17) (Table 7-1).

Using the Danish population–based twin registry at the University of Southern Denmark, 34,076 twins were screened for epilepsy. A total of 214 pairs with epileptic seizures (single seizure events, febrile seizures included), and 190 pairs with epilepsy (recurrent unprovoked seizures, 2 or more events) were identified. Higher concordance rates were found in monozygotic over dizygotic twins for epileptic seizures (0.56 vs. 0.21, $p < 0.001$) and for epilepsy (0.49 vs. 0.16, $p < 0.001$). In terms of epilepsy syndromes, concordance rates were higher for monozygotic twins for both generalized epilepsy (0.65 vs. 0.12) and for localization related epilepsy (0.30 vs. 0.10), but significantly more for the former (17, 18). Similar findings of higher concordance rates in monozygotic twins over dizygotic twins for seizure are reported in a larger recent multinational study combining data from twin registries of Denmark, Norway, and the United States (18a). The data from this larger sample is likely to provide even stronger support for a genetic basis for epileptic seizures.

Association Studies

Association studies permit the examination of the association of different alleles at different loci between unrelated individuals using a genetic marker such as single nucleotide polymorphisms (SNPs). An allele can be considered to be associated with the disease if its frequency in cases is higher than in controls, greater than predicted through chance alone. Such an association favors linkage disequilibrium (LD). Association studies have the ease of case collection and enabling greater statistical power. However, there are limitations to this approach, because mere association does not imply causation. The findings have to be replicable and have to fulfill biological plausibility in order to be

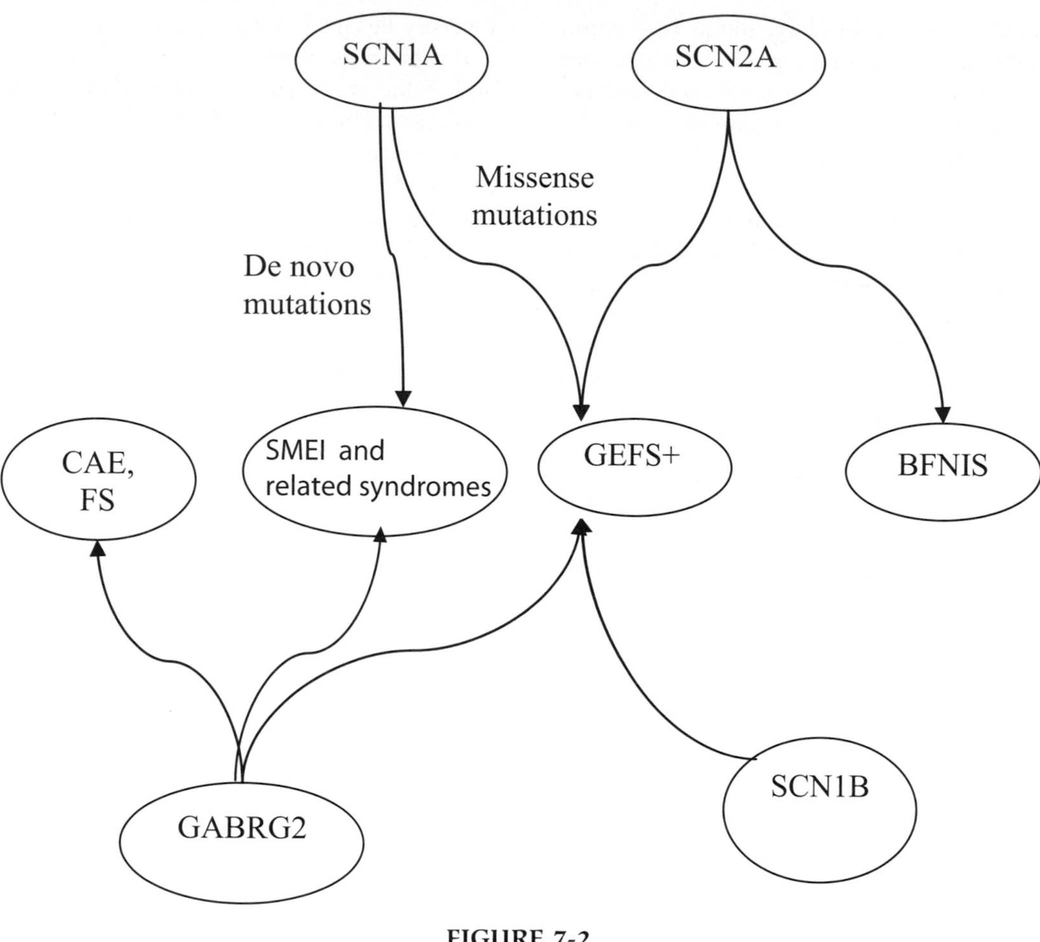

FIGURE 7-2

Locus heterogeneity and allelic heterogeneity in epilepsy phenotypes. SCN1A (Sodium channel, alpha 1 subunit), SCN2A (Sodium channel, alpha 2 subunit), GABRG2 (GABA receptor gamma2 subunit), SCN1B (Sodium channel, beta 1 subunit), CAE (Childhood Absence Epilepsy), SMEI (Severe Myoclonic Epilepsy of Infancy), GEFS+ (Generalized Epilepsy with Febrile Seizures plus), BFNIS (benign familial neonatal-infantile seizures).

TABLE 7-1

Concordance Rate for Epilepsy among Monozygotic and Dizygotic Twin Pairs

Study Authors Nature of Epilepsy in Proband		Population Cohorts	Probandwise Concordance Rates in Twins	
			Monozygotic	Dizygotic
Sillanpaa et al, 1991 (16)	Epilepsy	Finnish	0.10	0.05
Corey et al, 1991 (15)	Epilepsy	Norwegian	0.19	0.07
	Febrile seizures	Virginia	0.33	0.11
Berkovic et al, 1998 (13)	Generalized epilepsy	Australian	0.82	0.26
	Localization related		0.36	0.05
Kjeldsen et al, 2003 (17)	Generalized epilepsy	Danish	0.65	0.12
	Localization related		0.30	0.10

successful. Thus, these limitations have made association studies less popular, and have been regarded with greater skepticism than they once were. More recently there have been efforts to address these deficiencies through population stratification, use of family controls, and the use of two independent datasets of cases and controls as well as using rigorous measures of statistical significance. The results of more than 50 association studies carried out to date have either led to conflicting and nonreplicable findings or have failed to meet the requirement of biologic plausibility.

The availability of a human genome map for SNPs (30,000 of them) will accelerate the use of whole-cell linkage disequilibrium techniques to detect association between a marker and the occurrence of disease (19). Such genomewide association studies are likely to inflate the number of associations reported. Whether the marker locus actually turns out to be the disease locus is dependent on the potential confounding effects of variables such as the presence or absence of linkage disequilibrium and population stratification. Microarray technology will further strengthen and accelerate the process of understanding gene expression regulation, as well as levels and timing of expression, by allowing us to monitor mRNAs of multiple genes in parallel (20).

GENETICS OF EEG ABNORMALITIES

Any consideration of the heritability of epilepsy is incomplete without a brief consideration of the genetics of EEG abnormalities. The same lines of evidence as for epilepsy support the inheritance of EEG abnormalities as a genetic trait. Even normal EEG patterns and variants are known to aggregate within families and co-occur in monozygotic twins. Studies have shown generalized spike wave discharges, photoparoxysmal responses, rolandic spikes, and multifocal spikes to conform to known inheritance patterns (21). However, EEG studies are complicated by problems related to sampling, because the occurrence of EEG abnormalities in a single record is influenced by many factors. Even in those with epilepsy, a single EEG record is likely to show abnormalities only 50% of the time. The association between epileptiform patterns on the EEG and the epilepsy syndromes in which they have been described are not considered to be invariable. In addition, lack of association between the presence of EEG abnormalities and clinically manifest epilepsy, as well as age-dependent penetrance of the trait, also act as confounders (10).

ROLE FOR EPIGENETIC FACTORS?

The enormous diversity of cells and organ systems, their constituent proteins, and their functions all arise from the same genetic code. The biological explanation for this diversity lies in understanding the process of modulation and regulation of gene expression during cell development and proliferation. The rapidly expanding field of epigenetics sheds new light on our understanding of cellular phenomena. Epigenetic processes do not affect the genetic code; however they modulate gene expression through changes in metagenetic information. These processes are stable and are also passed on during mitotic cell division. DNA methylation is one example of an epigenetic control mechanism; other examples include histone hypoacetylation, chromatin modifications, X-inactivation, and imprinting (22).

Through the addition of a methyl group to a CpG dinucleotide, the gene is effectively silenced. Thus, methylation and demethylation processes effectively function as off-on switches for gene expression. Rett syndrome, a neurodegenerative disorder with significant epileptic seizures, results from heterozygous mutations in the X-linked methyl CpG binding protein 2 (MeCP2) gene. The MeCP2 gene product functions as a transcriptional repressor by binding to methylated DNA. The genetic deregulation that follows the occurrence of mutations in the X linked MeCP2 genes has been shown to affect the expression of genes (*UBE3A* and *GABRB3*) at other locations (e.g., 15q11–q13, Angelman syndrome) through possible histone modifications (23, 24). Both Angelman and Rett syndromes share significant features of their clinical phenotype, particularly in the occurrence of epileptic seizures. The reduced expression of *GABRB3*, a GABA receptor gene, is particularly interesting given the epilepsy phenotypes encountered in both Rett and Angelman syndromes. A better understanding of epigenetic factors no doubt will unravel many of the mysteries of variability in human epilepsy. Although the entire genome has been decoded, the information by itself is likely useless without understanding of the cellular processes involved in the timing and translation of this code.

Recent research using advances in genome scanning technology have shed light in characterizing structural variations in human DNA that are ~1 Kb to ~3 Mb in size along the human genome. These copy number variations (CNV) occur at high frequencies when compared to other classes of cytogenetically detected variations. These variants, existing in a heterozygous state, lie between neutral polymorphisms and lethal mutations. Their position may directly interrupt genes or may influence neighboring gene function by virtue of a position effect. These CNVs or copy number polymorphisms (CNPs) are capable of influencing biochemical, morphologic, physiologic, and pathologic processes, thus yielding potentially new mechanisms to explain diversity in human genetic diseases. CNVs and CNPs have been used to identify genetic susceptibility loci and potential candidate genes successfully for complex genetic disorders such as schizophrenia, autism, and severe speech and language disorder (25, 26). It is only a question of time before such an approach will yield new information on the genetically complex epilepsies.

IDENTIFIED GENE DEFECTS IN IDIOPATHIC EPILEPSIES

Broadly these defects fall into two major categories: (1) gene defects expressed in excitatory or inhibitory ion channels (Table 7-2) and (2) non–ion channel genes. It is of interest to note that despite the involvement of many channels, the net effect achieved is an increase in the excitability of the neuronal membrane and its ability to sustain repetitive firing.

Mutations Affecting Ion Channel Genes

Evidence linking channel defects with specific epilepsy phenotype came with discovery of K channel mutations associated with the clinically defined syndromes of BFNC, while Na channel defects have been associated with the recently defined benign familial neonatal-infantile seizures (BFNIS). Voltage-gated potassium channels play a number of crucial roles in neuronal physiology, including regulation of resting membrane potential and action potential duration. By impairing the restoration of ionic balance after neuronal firing, potassium channel dysfunction could lead to repetitive neuronal firing and a state of heightened excitability.

In the BFNIS families, changes have been identified in the alpha2 subunit of the sodium channel (SCN2A). Sodium channels have a single pore-forming alpha subunit, and two beta subunits that modulate the gating effects. Both the mutations (L1330F and L1563V) affect a highly conserved leucine, resulting in an increased sodium current, thus reducing the rate of inactivation and increased excitability. Similarly, a mutation affecting a voltage-gated sodium channel beta subunit (associated with GEFS+ phenotype) renders ineffective the rate of channel inactivation, and thereby increases excitability by permitting greater transmembrane sodium influx. Mutations affecting the alpha 1 subunit of the sodium channel (SCN1A) have come to be established as an important gene defect underlying a wide variety of idiopathic epilepsy syndromes (severe myoclonic epilepsy (SMEI) and other borderline epileptic encephalopathies). Truncation mutations account for nearly 50%, while missense, deletions, and splice site mutations account for the remainder. The spectrum of epileptic syndromes in early life associated with SCN1A mutations appears to be ever widening, further confirming an emerging role for this ion channel as a major contributor to the polygenic model of idiopathic/cryptogenic epilepsy.

In a family with individuals affected only by juvenile myoclonic epilepsy (JME), a novel gene mutation (Ala322Asp) affecting the gene encoding for GABARA1 (alpha subunit of the GABA receptor subtype A) was identified. Voltage clamp recordings from HEK293 whole-cell lines transfected with mutant and wild-type GABA receptors show a reduction in GABA activated currents in the former. This effect is attributed to altered GABA receptor function, and not to reduced expression (27).

GABA receptor dysfunction may also be the consequence of mutations affecting other channels. Three different heterozygous mutations, a premature stop codon (M200fsX231), an atypical splicing site (del74-117), and an amino acid substitution (G715E), have been identified in the voltage-gated chloride channel gene (CLCN2), which co-segregate with other IGE traits in three families of 46 selected for the study (28). Mutations in the CLCN2 gene have been associated with common subtypes of idiopathic generalized epilepsy as well as focal epilepsy (28, 29). Whole-cell patch clamp recordings, after transfecting tsA201 cells with both mutant and wild-type genes, suggest an alteration of human ClCN2 channel function through different mechanisms. The M200fsX231 and the del 174-117 mutation abolish chloride currents, while the G715E mutation alters chloride channel gating to induce a reverse current that affects membrane polarity and electrical stability. The end result is the induction of a hyperexcitable state of GABAergic synapses at a postsynaptic level. Altered GABA-related inhibitory influences underlie the IGE phenotype, despite the differing molecular targets of gene mutations.

In addition to chloride channels, the T-type calcium channel is an obvious target channel, because it plays a critical role in the thalamocortical oscillatory network. Missense mutations in a heterozygous state were identified in a gene coding for a calcium channel (CACN1H) in the 16p13 region in a small group of individuals with absence epilepsy, suggesting a role for calcium channels in the genetic susceptibility to absence epilepsy (30). The described mutations affect highly conserved regions in the T-type calcium channel. Functional studies using site directed mutagenesis have shown a gain of function effect on calcium influx during physiologic activation, leaving the neuron vulnerable to repetitive firing (31).

Several themes appear to be emerging: one, that mutations in different genes may encode for subunits of the same channel, resulting in an epilepsy phenotype that is essentially related to the channel dysfunction in a nonspecific manner (e.g., K channel mutations in BFNC, nAchR mutations in NFLE); on the other hand, mutations affecting different channels may result in the same phenotype (GEFS+ from mutations affecting $GABA_A$ receptor or sodium channel subunits); finally, mutations may affect subunits of the same channel yet result in two entirely different phenotypes. The latter situation is illustrated by mutations in the alpha1 and gamma2 subunits of the $GABA_A$ receptor, resulting in the completely different phenotypes of GEFS+ and autosomal

TABLE 7-2
Ion Channels: Structure and Subunit Composition, Mutations and Mutagenic Effects

Ion Channel	Type	Associated Epilepsy	Composition	Mutations	Effect of Mutations on Channel Function
Nicotinic acetylcholine receptors CHRNA4/ CHRNB2	Ligand gated	NFLE	Pentamers with each subunit containing 4 transmembrane domains. n the human brain there are 10 subunits that can be expressed and may combine in heteromeric or homomeric combinations to form receptors. Relatively nonselective channel	CHRNA4: α4S248F, α4L776ins3, α4S252L	Gain of function resulting in an increase in Ach receptor sensitivity in reconstitution experiments.
				CHRNB2: β2V287L, β2V287M	Mutations appear to affect the constituents around the pore.
Gamma-aminobutyric acid, subtype A (GABRG2/ GABRA1	Ligand gated	GEFSP ADJME	Also shares a pentameric structure with 4 transmembrane domains. Channel shows selective permeability to small anions and allows both chloride and bicarbonate.	GABRG2 γ2K289M GABRA1 α1A322D	Loss of function. Mutations cause reduced amplitude of GABA-activated currents.
Sodium channel SCN1A/SCN2A SCN1B	Voltagegated	GEFSP BFNIS SMEI	Each sodium channel is formed by one pore-forming α-subunit and two α-subunits that serve to modulate channel gating kinetics. Each α-subunit is made from 4 tandem domains, each of which contains 6 transmembrane domains.	SCN1B: β1C121W SCN2A: α2L1330F, α2L1563V SCN1A: Mutations are many and often occur de novo in the gene coding for this channel.	Loss of function. Slower sodium channel inactivation.
Potassium channel KCNQ2/KCNQ3	Voltage gated	BFNC BFNC with myokymia	Each K channel is a tetramer made of 4 homologous subunits that contain 6 trans membrane domains. The 4th transmembrane domain carries amino acids that are positively charged, which effects confor mational change during depolarization. The pore forming loop connects domains 5 and 6.	Multiple mutations described, 6 for KCNQ2	Loss of function. Reduction of the M current. Both KCNQ2 and KCNQ3 form heterometric units that permits the M current K channels form the predominant inhibitory system in the neonatal period.
Chloride channel	Voltage gated	IGE	Chloride channels have two subunits, each with its own pore	3 different mutations: M200fsX231, IVS2-14del11, del 74-117 G715E	The first two mutations caused a loss of function effect, while the third modifies the voltage-dependent gating effect.

dominant juvenile myoclonic epilepsy (ADJME). It is of interest to note that de novo mutations in sodium channel lead to SMEI, while missense mutations in the same channel have been shown to lead to the phenotypically distinct syndrome of GEFS+.

Mutations Affecting Non–Ion Channel Genes

It is important to point out that not all idiopathic epilepsies are turning out to be channelopathies. The identification of mutation in a G protein–coupled receptor underlying a murine audiogenic epilepsy phenotype (Frings mouse) led to a search for mutations in the human ortholog (hMASS1) (32). The gene was mapped to the 5q34 locus, which exhibits linkage to febrile seizures (FEB4). Screening for mutations in the hMASS1 gene in a family with this febrile seizure phenotype led to the identification of a nonsense mutation in one family. Although that mutation did not co-segregate with the febrile seizure phenotype in all families, it was suggested that a loss of function in this gene could lead to febrile and afebrile seizures (33). hMass1 and another gene, VLGR1, appear to be two halves of a single gene now called MASSive G protein–coupled receptor 1 gene (MGR1), which belongs to a family of genes coding for secretin-coupled receptors.

Similarly the identification of a gene mutation in the leucine-rich, glioma-inactivated 1 gene (LGI1) underlying the rare autosomal dominant partial epilepsy with auditory features (ADPEAF) appears to involve non–ion channel genes. However, the structural aspects of the proteins coded by this and other genes (VLGR1 on 5q14.1, and TNEP1 on 21q22.3) share a sevenfold repeated motif in the C terminal region that appears to define a superfamily of related proteins. These tandem repeats have been termed EPTP (34). The mechanisms through which these gene products influence epileptogenesis remain unclear at this stage. Recent studies indicate that even non–ion channel genes may carry an influence in regulating ionic currents across ion channels. Five missense mutations have been identified in unrelated individuals with JME in the EFHC1 gene (6p12-p11 region) that codes for a protein with an EF hand motif (35). This protein has been demonstrated to affect neuronal apoptosis as well as affect R-type calcium currents. It is postulated that individuals with the EFHC1 mutation could carry excess numbers of dystopic neurons that are unstable electrically, giving rise to hypersynchronous neuronal networks (36). Other highly significant associations have been described with non–ion channel genes in families with JME. These include polymorphisms in genes coding for a transcriptional regulator BRD2 (37, 38), and ME2 (malic enzyme 2), a mitochondrial enzyme (39). The functions of the BRD2 gene product remain speculative, while ME2 is involved in GABA biosynthesis/metabolism (40). Whether these polymorphism associations are causal or merely one of the many genes involved in the generation of the complex phenotype in JME remains to be established.

The genes underlying the syndrome of X-linked infantile spasms with mental retardation can also be considered as examples of mutations in non–ion channel genes leading to a specific epilepsy syndrome. The ARX homeobox and cyclin-dependent kinase-like 5 (CDKL-5/STK-9) gene products have functional effects that are not yet well understood (41).

GENETICS OF GENERALIZED EPILEPSIES: THE CLINICAL PHENOTYPES

A genetic basis is widely accepted for the IGEs, which include JME, childhood and juvenile absence epilepsy (CAE, JAE), epilepsy with generalized tonic-clonic seizures (GTCS), and epilepsy with grand mal on awakening. The clinical and EEG characteristics of IGEs overlap considerably. Seizure types include tonic, tonic-clonic, clonic, or myoclonic seizures that are generalized, and the interictal EEG shows bursts of synchronous generalized epileptiform patterns over both cerebral hemispheres. In each syndrome, there is an age-dependent onset of a particular seizure type, while the EEG background is often normal. Affected individuals are of normal intelligence; the neurologic examination is usually normal. While this applies to the idiopathic epilepsies with onset in later years, disorders such as SMEI and related borderline conditions beginning in early life may be associated with epileptic encephalopathy and cognitive decline. Table 7-3 summarizes the chromosomal loci and known gene defects linked to idiopathic generalized epilepsy syndromes.

Childhood Absence Epilepsy (CAE)

There is much overlap in the clinical features between CAE and JAE, within the IGE umbrella. At present, mutations in calcium and chloride channel genes have been reported associated with the CAE phenotype (28, 31).

Juvenile Myoclonic Epilepsy (JME)

JME appears to be a more distinct genetic phenotype in comparison to other forms of IGE (CAE, and JAE) (42). Mutations affecting both ion channel genes (CACNB4) (43) and non–ion channel genes (EFHC1, BRD2) are reported to result in a JME phenotype (35, 37, 38).

Benign Familial Neonatal Convulsions (BFNC)

Mutations affecting the genes coding for a family of voltage-gated potassium channels (KCNQ) that are

TABLE 7-3
Idiopathic Epilepsy and Febrile Seizure Syndromes

Epilepsy Type	Gene Defect	Chromosomal Locus and Mode of Inheritance
Benign familial neonatal convulsions (EBN1), MIM 121200	Potassium channel gene KCNQ2	Autosomal dominant, 20q13.3
Benign familial neonatal convulsion (EBN2), MIM 121201	Potassium channel gene KCNQ3	Autosomal dominant, 8q24
Benign familial neonatal-infantile seizures (BFN-IS), MIM #607745	Sodium channel gene SCN2A	Autosomal dominant, 2q
Benign familial infantile convulsions (BFIC1), MIM %601764	?	Autosomal dominant, 19q11–13 in Italian families
Benign familial infantile convulsions (BFIC2), MIM %605751	?	16p in French kindred
Idiopathic generalized epilepsy (IGE), MIM 600669;		Complex polygenic
childhood absence epilepsy (CAE), MIM 607682;	Calcium channel genes CACNA1A (IGE), CACNB4 (IGE, JME), CACN1H (CAE)	2q22–23
juvenile absence epilepsy (JAE);	GABA receptor genes GABARA1 (JME)	5q34
juvenile myoclonic epilepsy (JME), MIM 606904;	Chloride channel gene CLCN2 (CAE)	3q26
epile psy with grand mal on awakening	Non–ion channel gene EFHC1 (JME), BRD2 (JME), ME2 (IGE)	6p12, 6p21.3
X linked infantile spasms syndrome	Non–ion channel genes Aristaless (ARX), serine-threonine kinase (STK9) gene or cyclin-dependent kinase-like 5 (CDKL5)	X linked, Xp22.13
Generalized epilepsy with febrile seizures plus (GEFS+), MIM #604233: GEFS+1,		Autosomal dominant Genetic heterogeneity Oligogenic in some famiilies
GEFS+2, GEFS+3	Sodium channel genes SCN2A (GEFS+), SCN1B (GEFS+1), SCN1A (GEFS+2)	19q13, 2q24
	GABA receptor gene GABRG2 (GEFS+3), GABARD (GEFS+)	5q31
Familial febrile seizures		Genetic heterogeneity: 8q13 (FEB1), 19p13 (FEB2), 5q14 (FEB4)
Severe myoclonic epilepsy of infancy (SMEI)	Sodium channel gene SCN1A (SMEI)	2q24, 5q31

responsible for the neuronal repolarization appear to underlie this form of epilepsy. Two loci are now recognized: one on chromosome 20q13.3 (EBN1) (44), another on chromosome 8q24 (EBN2) (45). The gene for EBN1, called KCNQ2 (46) codes for one potassium channel component, while the gene for EBN2, termed KCNQ3 (47) codes for another portion of the potassium channel. When expressed in *Xenopus* oocytes, KCNQ2 facilitates the development of potassium currents, whereas expression of the mutant channel shows no such currents (48). The reason why a fixed genetic deficit in potassium channel structure should lead only to intermittent seizures that tend to remit over time in early life may be related to changing levels in the expression of potassium channel genes during brain development (49). It is also possible that the M-current mediated by KCNQ2/3 is less critical as GABA inhibition matures. During early life, GABA plays an excitatory role in the immature hippocampus. Coinciding with this period, KCNQ channels seem to perform predominantly an inhibitory role. The functional switching of GABA's role from excitation to inhibition seems to interact with the KCNQ channels in an intricately time locked sequence that modulates hippocampal excitability to demonstrate an "on" and "off" effect (50, 51).

Benign Familial Neonatal-Infantile Seizures (BFNIS)

Among the families described with benign familial neonatal convulsions, there exist families with an age of onset intermediate between the classic BFNC seizures and the BFIC (i.e., onset predominantly after 1 month). The seizures are partial onset with secondary generalization beginning between 2 to 7 months and carry a good prognosis (52). A mutation in the alpha2 subunit of the voltage-gated sodium channel (SCN2A) has been identified in such individuals in an Australian family and in a family previously described by Lewis et al (53). Thus, the association suggests yet another seizure susceptibility syndrome in early life and has been named benign familial neonatal-infantile seizures (BFNIS).

Infantile Spasms (IS)

Infantile spasms represent a specific syndrome of generalized seizure associated with a characteristic EEG pattern of hypsarrhythmia. Although a variety of etiologies (tuberous sclerosis, inborn errors of metabolism, Down syndrome) are associated with this epilepsy syndrome, mutations in genes underlying X-linked IS and mental retardation have now been identified. These include the Aristaless homeobox gene (ARX) (54, 55) and the serine–threonine kinase (STK-9 or CKL5, cyclin-dependent kinase-like 5) gene (56), both of which are located on the short arm of chromosome X. The ARX gene defect may lead to defects in a putative transcription factor, while the STK-9/CDKL-5 gene may have a pivotal role in synaptic plasticity, thus suggesting divergent mechanisms leading to this specific epilepsy phenotype (41). The phenotypic features of the latter condition clinically overlap with a Hanefeld variant of the Rett syndrome phenotype (57, 58).

Febrile Seizures and Related Syndromes

Table 7-3 summarizes the known gene loci and mutations associated febrile seizures and associated syndromes.

Febrile Seizures (FS). A genetic basis for FS is likely, based on their increased occurrence in families, though the precise mode of inheritance remains uncertain. In particular, twin studies have demonstrated a much higher risk in monozygotic than in dizygotic twins (40% vs. 7%) (13, 15). A complex polygenic rather than simple Mendelian inheritance pattern is currently favored. Several gene loci have been identified for familial febrile seizure; however, no specific gene mutations have so far been identified.

Linkage analysis suggests that a locus on chromosome 8q (FEB1) is involved (60%) (59) with other loci (FEB2 at 19p13, and FEB4 at 5q14) identified so far. The FEB4 locus was also confirmed in nuclear families and may account for 70% of febrile seizure susceptibility. The FEB3 locus at 2q23 was reported in large Utah family, and the seizure descriptions are considered as close to GEFS+, so this may be considered more as a GEFS+ locus rather than as one linked to febrile seizures (60).

Generalized Epilepsy with Febrile Seizures Plus (GEFS+). Scheffer and Berkovic (61) identified an interesting pattern of FS in an Australian family. A variety of dominantly inherited epilepsy phenotypes occurred in these families, and they proposed a syndrome designated as "generalized epilepsy with FS plus" (GEFS+). The most common phenotype, termed "febrile seizures plus" (FSP), consisted of multiple FS in infancy and the continued occurrence of afebrile seizures beyond age 6 years. All seizures remit by adolescence. Other phenotypes identified in this family include FS plus absences, FS plus myoclonic seizures, and FS plus atonic seizures. The mode of inheritance in GEFS+ remains a matter of debate; in some a dominant pattern observed, in others an oligogenic effect, accounting for a wide variation in clinical phenotype.

So far only a single gene defect has been identified in each family with GEFS+ phenotype. Mutations appear to involve subunits of voltage gated sodium channels (62) and subunits of the ligand-gated GABAergic receptors (63). Both types of mutations appear to affect the functional properties of the respective channels and may serve to enhance seizure susceptibility in a nonspecific manner. An overlap is noted between the clinical features and genetic bases of GEFS+ and SMEI (see following paragraph), exemplifying the enormous complexity of genotype-phenotype correlations in the epilepsies.

Severe Myoclonic Epilepsy of Infancy (SMEI, Dravet syndrome). Dravet in 1982 (64) first described the clinical features of this syndrome, where seizures begin in infancy and progress to an epileptic encephalopathy with myoclonic seizures as a prominent feature. Initially the seizures are triggered by febrile events and intercurrent infections, occurring between the second month and the first year of life, after a period of normal development. Seizures are generalized clonic or hemiclonic in character, often prolonged and recurrent. Hemiclonic seizures are thought to be a distinct feature; myoclonic jerks appear later in the course of the disease, accompanied by cognitive and motor decline. Missense and truncating mutations of

TABLE 7–4
Idiopathic Partial Epilepsies

Epilepsy Type	Gene Defect	Chromosomal Locus and Mode of Inheritance
Nocturnal frontal lobe epilepsy (ENFL1, 2, 3) MIM 600513 #605375 (ENFLE3)	Cholinergic receptor gene CHRNA4 (NFL1), CHRNB2 (NFL3)	Autosomal dominant 20q13.2-13.3 15q24 1q
Familial lateral temporal lobe epilepsy with auditory features (ADPEAF), MIM#600512	Non–ion channel gene LGI1	Autosomal dominant Genetic heterogeneity 10q22
Familial Partial Epilepsy with variable foci, MIM %604364	?	Autosomal dominant 22q11–q12
Benign epilepsy of childhood with central temporal spikes	?	Autosomal dominant with incomplete penetrance (EEG trait) 15q13

the SCN1A gene (coding for the alpha1 subunit for the sodium channel) have been identified in many families with SMEI (65–67). As pointed out earlier, a wide spectrum of idiopathic/cryptogenic epilepsy syndromes with both generalized and focal forms of epileptic seizures beginning in early life are being linked with mutations in the SCNA1 gene. SMEI likely represents the more severe end of this spectrum of overlapping conditions that includes both the milder variants of GEFS+ and the severe epileptic encephalopathies (68).

Genetics of Partial Epilepsies

Most partial or focal epilepsies are assumed to not have a genetic basis. However, relatives of probands with partial epilepsy have an increased risk of epilepsy compared to the general population, suggesting a genetic influence in at least some forms of partial epilepsy. A defective gene might cause localized cortical hyperexcitability if it is expressed only in certain vulnerable neuronal regions, or if its effects are modified by local factors (69). The partial epilepsy syndromes and the chromosomal loci to which they are mapped are summarized in Table 7-4.

Benign Epilepsy of Childhood with Central-Temporal Spikes (BECTS). A strong genetic influence in benign rolandic epilepsy has been observed (70). The disorder appears to be inherited in an autosomal dominant manner with age-dependent penetrance, and the EEG trait is inherited similarly (71). There is an increased incidence of both focal and generalized EEG abnormalities among first-degree relatives. (Interestingly, in relatives, generalized abnormalities are even more common than focal ones.) Doose considers typical BECTS to be a special case in a broad spectrum of clinical manifestations due to this genetic excitability defect (72). Linkage to 15q13 locus has been demonstrated in family studies (73).

Autosomal Dominant Nocturnal Frontal Lobe Epilepsy. This type of epilepsy (abbreviated ADNFLE) was first described in an Australian kindred of 27 affected individuals spanning six generations (74–76). ADNFLE is transmitted in an autosomal dominant fashion with incomplete penetrance. Seizures begin in mid-childhood, occurring in clusters during drowsiness or sleep. Affected individuals are of normal intelligence; they experience frequent nocturnal motor seizures (tonic or hyperkinetic), often preceded by an aura; cases are often misdiagnosed as nightmares or sleep disorders. The neurologic examination and the interictal EEG are normal; during the ictus, seizures can be shown to originate from the frontal lobes (77). There is considerable intrafamilial variability in clinical expression. Using exclusion mapping (i.e., by systematic elimination of candidate genes mapping to the same region), the disorder was assigned a chromosomal locus of 20q13.2. A missense mutation (α4S248F) in the alpha4 subunit of the nicotinic acetylcholine receptor (CHRNA4) mapped to this region in all 21 affected members of one ADNFLE family (76). However, there is allelic heterogeneity in this condition, as other families have shown different mutations in the CHRNA4 gene (78).

It appears that mutations that directly affect the ion pore can result in the epilepsy phenotype, as all of the known mutations appear to affect transmembrane domains that form the wall of the ion channel. Differences in the electrophysiologic and pharmacologic profiles among the different receptor mutations have been shown in addition to the common effect of increasing cholinergic sensitivity. In reconstitution experiments carried out in *Xenopus* oocytes, nicotinic cholinergic receptors with mutant alpha4 subunits had faster desensitization kinetics than wild-type receptors; that is, they became rapidly unresponsive to acetylcholine stimulation (79). Reconstituted mutant receptors also show significantly reduced calcium permeability (80). These differences may account for additional specific phenotypic features, such as the occurrence of neuropsychiatric symptoms reported in α4776ins3 carriers (81).

Familial Temporal Lobe Epilepsy. Ottman and colleagues described a single family of 11 affected individuals who presented with partial seizures and nonspecific auditory disturbances with onset during adolescence (82). This syndrome consists of the familial occurrence of mild temporal lobe seizures with age-dependent onset, with seizures originating from the mesial as well as the lateral temporal lobe. The hippocampal pathology seen in typical temporal lobe epilepsy is absent in the familial variety (83, 84). Using linkage analysis, the epilepsy susceptibility gene mapped to chromosome 10q22–24. The condition is now recognized by the phrase "autosomal dominant partial epilepsy with auditory features (ADPEAF)."

When all the 28 genes in the implicated 10q24 locus were sequenced, mutations were identified in the leucine-rich glioma-inactivated 1 gene (LGI1) (85). The implications of this finding have been discussed separately. Other autosomal dominant inheritance patterns for partial epilepsies have been identified in clinical studies of large families: autosomal dominant partial epilepsy with variable foci (83, 86), autosomal dominant rolandic epilepsy with speech dyspraxia (74), and benign familial infantile convulsions (BFIC) (87). Linkage studies have suggested associated loci; however, so far in none of these inherited syndromes has a mutation been identified.

GENE-ENVIRONMENT INTERACTIONS

Environmental factors can strongly influence the expression and risk of developing seizures. The gene-environment connection is challenging to study, and available studies show conflicting results. Although one would intuitively suspect factors such as head trauma to dramatically increase the risk of epilepsy in individuals with a genotype of increased seizure susceptibility, family studies suggest quite the opposite for some factors (identified postnatal insults such as head trauma) (88) but are in agreement for others (alcohol-induced seizures) (89). Alcohol exposure may carry a significant relationship with genetic susceptibility to seizures, a hypothesis that merits further exploration.

Another example of this interaction is operative in the case of pregnant women. Pregnancy exposes the fetus to myriad environmental influences on early development. An increased risk of epilepsy (4–5-fold increase) has been shown in the offspring of women with a history of spontaneous abortions, and such a history may be a marker for increased genetic susceptibility to epilepsy in the mother (90). The molecular basis of this increased susceptibility remains unclear.

In the case of febrile seizures, interesting insights have been provided at a molecular level between mutation effects on $GABA_A$ receptors and temperature effects (91). Impaired gamma2 subunit function has been strongly suspected as a factor in seizure susceptibility in patients with febrile seizures in the GEFS+ spectrum. The gamma2 receptor subunit plays a critical role in receptor trafficking, clustering, and synapse maintenance, and when mutant receptors (with the described mutations in the GEFS+ phenotype) are challenged with temperature elevation, a rapid deterioration in receptor trafficking and increased endocytosis is demonstrable, thus leading to reduced surface expression and increased vulnerability to fever induced seizures (91). The future will likely disclose many more interesting insights at the molecular level of the gene-environment interaction.

PHARMACOGENOMICS IN EPILEPSY

With accelerated-throughput technologies that are increasingly available, the pace of identification of gene mutations has been hastened. With that, opportunities to understand the interactions of gene products and other proteins within the cell have opened up. As the intricate and complex mechanisms underlying epilepsies is unraveled, we have entered into the era of understanding the interaction between drugs and genotype. In the case of epilepsy, the developing branches of proteomics and pharmacogenomics will help us better understand the mechanisms of effectiveness of antiepileptic drugs as well as drug resistance. Variations in genotype will account for differences in drug pharmacokinetics as well as other factors that influence such differences (age, sex, race, etc.) (92).

The effect of genetic polymorphisms on drug metabolism carries with it significant implications for serum drug levels and metabolite concentrations. These in turn can affect the clinical response. Therefore, dosage scheduling by genotype may well come to be an important treatment consideration in the future. End organ targets for antiepileptic drugs may be yet another source of genetically determined pharmacoresistance. Genetic polymorphisms in drug-metabolizing enzymes CYP2C9 and in the SCN1A sodium channel receptor seem to carry significant implications for the prediction of maximal tolerated doses of phenytoin and carbamazepine in one study (93). Further studies are needed to confirm and to extend these observations.

Drug efflux transporters are another area where the relationship of pharmacoresistence to antiepileptic drugs and genotype has been explored. An association between genetic polymorphisms in the ATP-binding cassette binding member 1 (ABCB1) and the phenotype

TABLE 7-5
Risks of Epilepsy in First Degree Relatives and in Offspring

Genetic Counseling Issues	Variables	Risk Estimate Approx %
Risk of developing epilepsy in other family members and relatives	General population risk estimates	1
	Acute symptomatic	
	Febrile seizure	2.3
	Febrile seizure, then epilepsy	6
	Epilepsy age of onset	
	Onset < age 15	4
	Onset > age 25	2.6
	Epilepsy etiology	
	Postnatally acquired	1
	Epilepsy and MR/CP	3
	Epilepsy seizure type	
	Partial epilepsy	2.5
	EEG pattern	
	Epilepsy and GSW	6
	Epilepsy +(GSW+ PPR) or GSW+multifocal spikes	8
	Proband with epilepsy	
	Parent also affected	8
	Parent also affected either with GSW	12
	GSW in probands and sib	15
	Seizure type	
	Myoclonic	4–8
	Absence	5–9
Risk to offspring (% of children with epilepsy by age 20)	Risk of overall epilepsy in children of probands	2–5%
	Mother with epilepsy	2.8–8.7%
	Father with epilepsy	2.4%
	Parent with IGE	3.3%
	Parent with pure absence epilepsy	9%
	Parent with partial epilepsy	4.6%
	Parent age of onset	
	Onset < 20	2.3–6%
	Onset > 20	1.0–3.6%

of drug-resistant epilepsy was suggested by Siddiqui and associates (94). The associated polymorphism is silent, and the haplotype associated with drug resistance was not clearly identified. Subsequently the findings have been replicated in one study (95) but could not be replicated in other studies with a much larger sample size (96, 97). A biologically plausible result may sometimes be a false positive finding (98). Nevertheless the hypothesis of drug resistance mediated by transporters under genetic control remains attractive and merits continued exploration.

Drug reactions are another area where genetic variation can influence the development of such reactions. Serious skin reactions to carbamazepine have been associated with a polymorphism at position 308 in the TNF alpha promoter region (99) as well as variants in HLA gene alleles such as HLA-B*1502 (100, 101). Eventually, genotyping could be used to predict drug reactions prior to initiating treatment with drugs to avoid such serious reactions.

An improved understanding of pharmacogenetic interactions in epilepsy will eventually lead the physician in making correct choices of AEDs in treatment of seizures, improvements in drug design, prediction and avoidance of aberrant drug effects, and better strategies in dealing with pharmacoresistance.

GENETIC COUNSELING ISSUES IN EPILEPSY

The issues relating to genetic counseling center around addressing the heritability of epilepsy, the risk of epilepsy in family members and offspring, and the value of genetic testing in epilepsy (10). We have attempted to summarize the risk estimates in comparison to the general population risk in family relatives (sibship) and offspring (Table 7-5) based on the data from epidemiologic studies in the literature presented in (102).

At the outset, it should be clarified that epilepsy is not a single disorder, but a collection of many disorders with great a deal of variability in phenotype and causation. Therefore no single gene defect could account for the different kinds of epilepsy. The concept of the risk of developing epilepsy being influenced by single, few or many genes will need to be explained. Differences in penetrance could result in people being affected or remaining as asymptomatic carriers. The fact that common epilepsies are influenced by several genes (polygenic) and that inheritance patterns are likely to be complex and difficult to predict will need added emphasis. Finally, it must be pointed out that recurrence risks are likely to be influenced by other environmental factors.

For disorders with single gene defects, which are inherited in true Mendelian fashion, risk estimates for family members are likely straightforward. But for the non-Mendelian disorders (i.e., most common idiopathic epilepsies), estimates of risks are best expressed in terms of absolute risk (%) with a range of values as well as to provide comparison figures for the general population. It may also be possible to express this risk as a ratio rather than a percentage (1 in 25 rather than 4%). It is customary to use data from epidemiologic studies while estimating the risk. The class of relative (in relationship to the probands) should be taken into account. Sibling risks are useful in helping families with one affected child and who are at the stage of planning a pregnancy. Offspring risks are similarly based on information from epidemiologic studies. Risk estimates are influenced by a number of factors, including seizure and syndrome type, type of EEG abnormality, age of onset, parental attributes (sex and affected status), and the number of individuals with epilepsy in the family (Box 7-1).

The role of genetic testing in the routine management of common idiopathic epilepsies is limited. Affected families may undergo genetic testing through participation in numerous research studies and programs such as the gene discovery project of the Epilepsy Foundation of America. This project allows families to link up with researchers working in that area. These disorders are relatively benign, and the complex modes of inheritance and various confounders that can influence the reliability of a result preclude routine use of genetic testing in this group. For the monogenic disorders that are rare, but where the genes and common mutations are identified, direct mutation analysis is possible in disorders such as the progressive myoclonic epilepsies (EPM1, EPM2, MERRF, and the ceroid lipofuscinoses). These are serious disorders with considerable morbidity and mortality, and genetic testing can be justified. Information gleaned can be used for appropriate genetic counseling. Molecular diagnostic tests for BFNC (KCNQ2 DNA sequencing), SMEI, and GEFS+ (SCN1A DNA sequencing), are becoming commercially available (e.g., Athena Diagnostics, http://www.AthenaDiagnostics.com), and the list will, no doubt, grow longer.

BOX 7-1
KEY ISSUES IN GENETIC COUNSELING

Is epilepsy inherited?
The risk to other family members (sibs, offspring, class of relatives)
Seizure etiology
Age of onset of epilepsy
Epilepsy syndrome
Number of affected relatives
Role of genetic testing in epilepsy

SUMMARY

In summary, the modes of inheritance of epilepsy in the light of current understanding suggest diverse mechanisms and both Mendelian and non-Mendelian inheritance (complex oligogenic, polygenic). In essence, gene defects that can lead to the generation of an epilepsy phenotype display a remarkable functional diversity. The pathway from an altered genomic sequence meanders through mRNA, its stability and processing, protein translation defects, stability of the proteome, subcellular localization and expression, and, finally, to a state of electrical instability and a regional or generalized expression of seizures (Figure 7-3). Studies of other areas—for instance, regulatory molecular processes (integrins, growth factors, metabotropic glutamate receptors, GABA transporters) and mechanisms that underlying brain plasticity—will no doubt yield additional genes and their proteins linked with epilepsy. It is recognized that abnormalities of cortical development can lead to epilepsy, but the early occurrence of seizures also carries consequences for the development of neural networks in the developing brain. The genetic and epigenetic factors regulating these complex interactions will no doubt be essential for understanding the genetic-molecular aspects of epileptogenesis (12). Pathologic mutations leading to defects in the function of subcellular organelles (mitochondrial respiratory chain defects, peroxisome biogenesis defects) as well as enzymatic defects in critical metabolic pathways provide additional routes to an epileptogenesis. Ultimately, these numerous pathways seem to converge on the neuron, producing an unstable electrical state that promotes synchronized burst firing in vulnerable neuronal networks.

Thus, the state of present-day understanding of epilepsy is at a crossroads in terms of complexity. In the discussion in this chapter we have highlighted the diversity

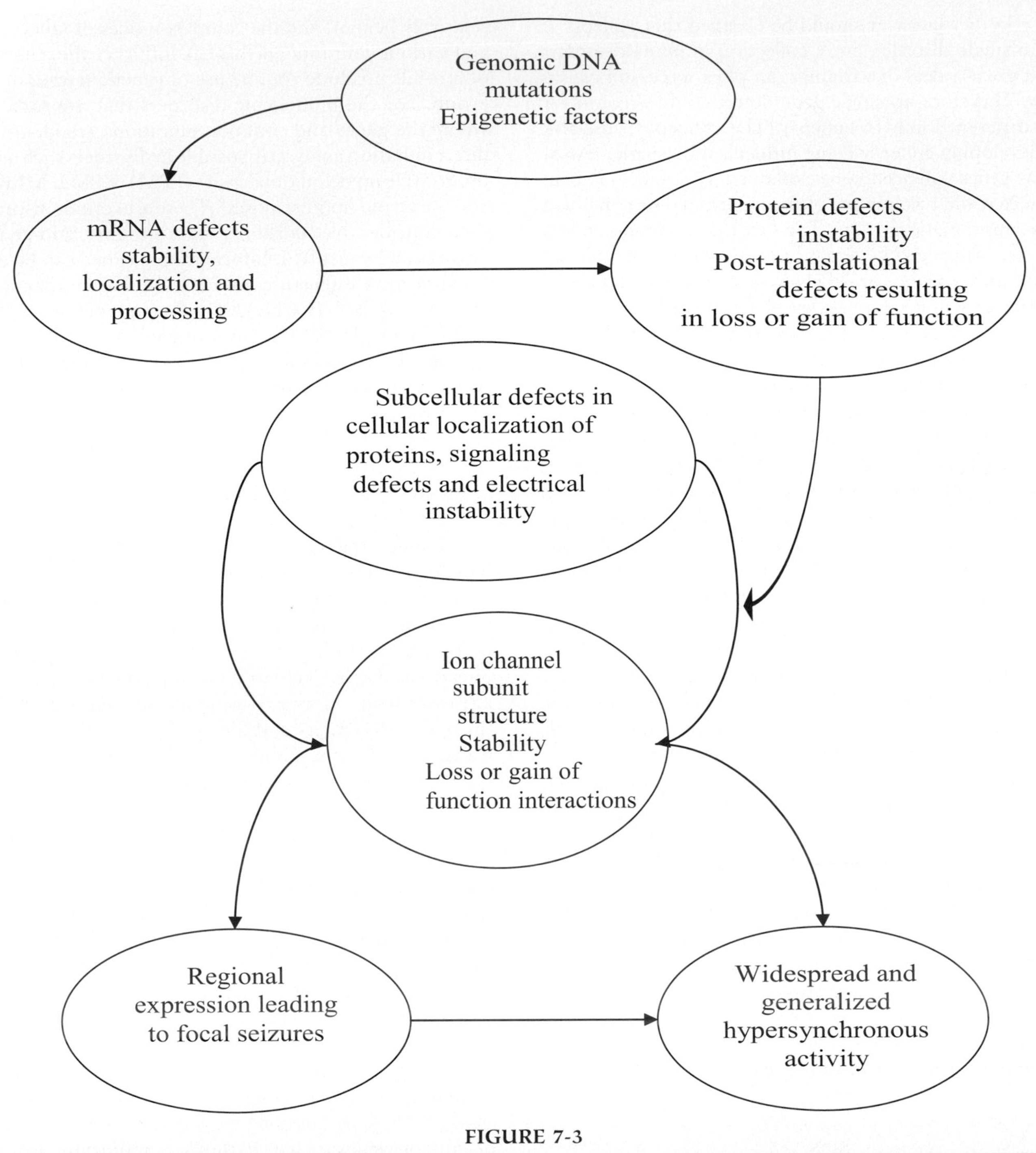

FIGURE 7-3

Genetic and epigenetic processes that can influence epileptogenesis.

of causes and mechanisms and the role of epilepsy genes in the process of epileptogenesis.

Even within the span of a decade, the list of gene defects and mutations has increased at a steady pace each year. Our understanding of the role of these genes and the proteins that they code for is in its infancy, but it underscores the many pathways to epileptogenesis. Does the practicing epileptologist and neurologist have to know all of the numerous gene defects described? We do not think that is necessary. However, we do believe that these discoveries lay the foundation for our understanding human epilepsy and its protean presentations. From genetic defects in ion- and ligand-gated channels and signaling and regulatory molecules, chromosomal aberrations, and defects in intermediary metabolism, the multiplicity of mechanisms underlying the heterogeneity of inherited epilepsy is truly breathtaking. For the clinician, a detailed collection of information on seizure semiology, age of onset, ethnic background, and family history remains critical in recognizing genetic contributions to the individual's epilepsy. In selected instances of single-gene defects mutation analysis will be of help in diagnosis, and even in selecting treatment, where it is or becomes commercially available. In the majority of more common epilepsy syndromes, any form of mutation analysis to determine susceptibility genes is still a long way away. When such technology becomes available, the clinical implications of the findings will have to be carefully examined. These advances hold the promise of improving our understanding of epileptogenesis and will likely lead to methods of early detection and counseling and newer, more effective therapies for affected individuals and their family stricken by this complex disorder.

ACKNOWLEDGMENTS

The authors are indebted to Dr. T Frewen, Dept. of Pediatrics, the Children's Hospital Western Ontario, for their support and encouragement, and Ms. J Carrier (Rathbun Library) for her help with obtaining original articles.

References

1. Hauser WA, Hesdorffer DC, Epilepsy Foundation of America. *Epilepsy: frequency, causes, and consequences*. Landover, MD: Epilepsy Foundation of America, 1990.
2. Prasad AN, Prasad C, Stafstrom CE. Recent advances in the genetics of epilepsy: insights from human and animal studies. *Epilepsia* 1999; 40:1329–1352.
3. Scheffer IE, Berkovic SF. The genetics of human epilepsy. *Trends Pharmacol Sci* 2003; 24:428–433.
4. Robinson R, Gardiner M. Molecular basis of Mendelian idiopathic epilepsies. *Ann Med* 2004; 36:89–97.
5. Hopper JL. Variance components for statistical genetics: applications in medical research to characteristics related to human diseases and health. *Stat Methods Med Res* 1993; 2:199–223.
6. Falconer D. The inheritance of liability to certain diseases, estimated from the incidence among relatives. *Ann Hum Genet* 1965; 29:51–76.
7. Durner M, Keddache MA, Tomasini L, Shinnar S, et al. Genome scan of idiopathic generalized epilepsy: evidence for major susceptibility gene and modifying genes influencing the seizure type. *Annals of Neurology* 2001; 49:328–335.
8. Temkin O. *The falling sickness: a history of epilepsy from the Greeks to the beginings of modern neurology*. Baltimore: The Johns Hopkins University Press; 1994.
9. Metrakos K, Metrakos JD. Genetics of convulsive disorders. II. Genetic and electroencephalographic studies in centrencephalic epilepsy. *Neurology* 1961; 11:474–483.
10. Winawer MR. Epilepsy genetics. *Neurologist* 2002; 8:133–151.
11. Greenberg DA. There is more than one way to collect data for linkage analysis. What a study of epilepsy can tell us about linkage strategy for psychiatric disease. *Arch Gen Psychiatry* 1992; 49:745–750.
12. Noebels J. The inherited epilepsies. In: Scriver CR, Beaudet AL, Sly WS, ValleD, eds. *The Metabolic and Molecular Basis of Inherited Disease*, 8th ed. New York: McGraw-Hill, 2001; 5807–5832.
13. Berkovic SF, Howell RA, Hay DA, Hopper JL. Epilepsies in twins: genetics of the major epilepsy syndromes. *Annals of Neurology* 1998; 43:435–445.
14. Steinlein OK. Genes and mutations in human idiopathic epilepsy. *Brain Dev* 2004; 26:213–218.
15. Corey LA, Berg K, Pellock JM, Solaas MH, et al. The occurrence of epilepsy and febrile seizures in Virginian and Norwegian twins. *Neurology* 1991; 41:1433–1436.
16. Sillanpaa M, Koskenvuo M, Romanov K, Kaprio J. Genetic factors in epileptic seizures: evidence from a large twin population. *Acta Neurol Scand* 1991; 84:523–526.
17. Kjeldsen MJ, Corey LA, Christensen K, Friis ML. Epileptic seizures and syndromes in twins: the importance of genetic factors. *Epilepsy Res* 2003; 55:137–146.
18. Kjeldsen MJ, Kyvik KO, Friis ML, Christensen K. Genetic and environmental factors in febrile seizures: a Danish population-based twin study. *Epilepsy Res* 2002; 51:167–177.

18a. Kjeldsen MJ, Corey LA, Solaas MH, Friis ML, Harris JR, Kyvik KO, Christensen K, Pellock JM. Genetic factors in seizures: a population-based study of 47,626 US, Norwegian, and Danish twin pairs. *Twin Res Hum Genet* 2005; 8(2):138–47.

19. Sachidanandam R, Weissman D, Schmidt SC, Kakol JM, et al. A map of human genome sequence variation containing 1.42 million single nucleotide polymorphisms. *Nature* 2001; 409:928–933.
20. Del Rio JA, Barlow C. Genomics and neurological phenotypes: applications for seizure-induced damage. *Prog Brain Res* 2002; 135:149–160.
21. Niedermeyer E. EEG patterns and genetics. In: Niedermeyer E, Lopes da Silva F, ed. *Electroencephalography: Basic Principles, Clinical Applications, and Related Fields*, 4th ed. Philadelphia: Williams & Wilkins, 1999.
22. Falsenfeld G, Groudine M. Controlling the double helix. *Nature* 2003; 421(6921): 448–53 (review).
23. Makedonski K, Abuhatzira L, Kaufman Y, Razin A, et al. MeCP2 deficiency in Rett syndrome causes epigenetic aberrations at the PWS/AS imprinting center that affects *UBE3A* expression. *Hum Mol Genet* 2005; 14:1049–1058.
24. Samaco RC, Hogart A, LaSalle JM. Epigenetic overlap in autism-spectrum neurodevelopmental disorders: MeCP2 deficiency causes reduced expression of UBE3A and GABRB3. *Hum Mol Genet* 2005; 14:483–492.
25. Feuk L, Carson AR, Scherer SW. Structural variation in the human genome. *Nat Rev* 2006; 7:85–97.
26. Freeman JL, Perry GH, Feuk L, Redon R, et al. Copy number variation: new insights in genome diversity. *Genome Res* 2006; 16:949–961.
27. Cossette P, Liu L, Brisebois K, Dong H. Mutation of GABRA1 in an autosomal dominant form of juvenile myoclonic epilepsy. *Nat Genet* 2002; 31:184–189
28. Haug K, Warnstedt M, Alekov AK, Sander T, et al. Mutations in CLCN2 encoding a voltage-gated chloride channel are associated with idiopathic generalized epilepsies. *Nat Genet* 2003; 33:527–532.
29. D'Agostino D, Bertelli M, Gallo S, Cecchin S, et al. Mutations and polymorphisms of the CLCN2 gene in idiopathic epilepsy. *Neurology* 2004; 63:1500–1502.
30. Chen Y, Lu J, Pan H, Zhang Y, et al. Association between genetic variation of CACNA1H and childhood absence epilepsy. *Ann Neurol* 2003; 54:239–243.
31. Khosravani H, Altier C, Simms B, Hamming KS, et al. Gating effects of mutations in the Cav3.2 T-type calcium channel associated with childhood absence epilepsy. *J Biol Chem* 2004; 279:9681–9684.
32. Skradski SL, Clark AM, Jiang H, White HS, et al. A novel gene causing a mendelian audiogenic mouse epilepsy. *Neuron* 2001; 31:537–544.
33. Nakayama J, Fu YH, Clark AM, Nakahara S, et al. A nonsense mutation of the MASS1 gene in a family with febrile and afebrile seizures. *Ann Neurol* 2002; 52:654–657.
34. Staub E, Pérez-Tur J, Siebert R, Nobile C, et al. The novel EPTP repeat defines a superfamily of proteins implicated in epileptic disorders. *Trends Biochem Sci* 2002; 27:441–444.
35. Suzuki T, Delgado-Escueta AV, Aguan K, Alonso ME, et al. Mutations in EFHC1 cause juvenile myoclonic epilepsy. *Nat Genet* 2004; 36:842–849.
36. Turnbull J, Lohi H, Kearney JA, Rouleau GA, et al. Sacred disease secrets revealed: the genetics of human epilepsy. *Hum Mol Genet* 2005; 14:2491–2500.
37. Lorenz S, Taylor KP, Gehrmann A, Becker T, et al. Association of BRD2 polymorphisms with photoparoxysmal response. *Neurosci Lett* 2006; 400:135–139
38. Pal DK, Evgrafov OV, Tabares P, Zhang F, et al. BRD2 (RING3) is a probable major susceptibility gene for common juvenile myoclonic epilepsy. *Am J Hum Genet* 2003; 73:261–270.
39. Greenberg DA, Cayanis E, Strug L, Marathe S, et al. Malic enzyme 2 may underlie susceptibility to adolescent-onset idiopathic generalized epilepsy. *Am J Hum Genet* 2005; 76:139–146.
40. Gardiner M. Genetics of idiopathic generalized epilepsies. *Epilepsia* 2005; 46 Suppl 9:15–20.
41. Crino PB. New candidate genes for infantile spasms and mental retardation. *Epilepsy Curr* 2004; 4:11–12.
42. Marini C, Scheffer IE, Crossland KM, Grinton BE, et al. Genetic architecture of idiopathic generalized epilepsy: clinical genetic analysis of 55 multiplex families. *Epilepsia* 2004; 45:467–478.
43. Escayg A, De Waard M, Lee DD, Bichet D, et al. Coding and noncoding variation of the human calcium-channel beta4-subunit gene CACNB4 in patients with idiopathic generalized epilepsy and episodic ataxia. *Am J Hum Genet* 2000; 66:1531–1539.
44. Leppert M, Anderson VE, Quattlebaum T, Stauffer D, et al. Benign familial neonatal convulsions linked to genetic markers on chromosome 20. *Nature* 1989; 337:647–648.
45. Lewis TB, Leach RJ, Ward K, O'Connell P, Ryan SG. Genetic heterogeneity in benign familial neonatal convulsions: identification of a new locus on chromosome 8q. *Am J Hum Genet* 1993; 53:670–675.
46. Singh NA, Charlier C, Stauffer D, DuPont BR, et al. A novel potassium channel gene, KCNQ2, is mutated in an inherited epilepsy of newborns. *Nat Genet* 1998; 18:25–29.
47. Charlier C, Singh NA, Ryan SG, Lewis TB, et al. A pore mutation in a novel KQT-like potassium channel gene in an idiopathic epilepsy family. *Nat Genet* 1998; 18:53–55.
48. Biervert C, Schroeder BC, Kubisch C, Berkovic SF, et al. A potassium channel mutation in neonatal human epilepsy. *Science* 1998; 279:403–406.
49. Tinel N, Lauritzen I, Chouabe C, Lazdunski M, et al. The KCNQ2 potassium channel: splice variants, functional and developmental expression. Brain localization and comparison with KCNQ3. *FEBS Lett* 1998; 438:171–176.

50. Okada M, Zhu G, Hirose S, Ito KI, et al. Age-dependent modulation of hippocampal excitability by KCNQ-channels. *Epilepsy Res* 2003; 53:81–94.
51. Sankar R. A time to convulse, a time to stop . . . . *Epilepsy Curr* 2003; 3:82–83.
52. Berkovic SF, Heron SE, Giordano L, Marini C, et al. Benign familial neonatal-infantile seizures: characterization of a new sodium channelopathy. *Ann Neurol* 2004; 55:550–557.
53. Heron SE, Crossland KM, Andermann E, Phillips HA, et al. Sodium-channel defects in benign familial neonatal-infantile seizures. *Lancet* 2002; 360:851–852.
54. Stromme P, Mangelsdorf ME, Scheffer IE, Gecz J. Infantile spasms, dystonia, and other X-linked phenotypes caused by mutations in Aristaless related homeobox gene, ARX. *Brain Dev* 2002; 24:266–268.
55. Stromme P, Mangelsdorf ME, Shaw MA, Lower KM, et al. Mutations in the human ortholog of Aristaless cause X-linked mental retardation and epilepsy. *Nat Genet* 2002; 30:441–445.
56. Kalscheuer VM, Tao J, Donnelly A, Hollway G, et al. Disruption of the serine/threonine kinase 9 gene causes severe X-linked infantile spasms and mental retardation. *Am J Hum Genet* 2003; 72:1401–1411.
57. Hanefeld F. The clinical pattern of the Rett syndrome. *Brain Dev* 1985; 7:320–325.
58. Scala E, Ariani F, Mari F, Caselli R, et al. CDKL5/STK9 is mutated in Rett syndrome variant with infantile spasms. *J Med Genet* 2005; 42:103–107.
59. Wallace RH, Berkovic SF, Howell RA, Sutherland GR, et al. Suggestion of a major gene for familial febrile convulsions mapping to 8q13–21. *J Med Genet* 1996; 33:308–312.
60. Iwasaki N, Nakayama J, Hamano K, Matsui A, et al. Molecular genetics of febrile seizures. *Epilepsia* 2002; 43 Suppl 9:32–35.
61. Scheffer IE, Berkovic SF. Generalized epilepsy with febrile seizures plus. A genetic disorder with heterogeneous clinical phenotypes. *Brain* 1997; 120:479–490.
62. Escayg A, Heils A, MacDonald BT, Haug K, et al. A novel SCN1A mutation associated with generalized epilepsy with febrile seizures plus—and prevalence of variants in patients with epilepsy. *Ame J Hum Genet* 2001; 68:866–873.
63. Harkin LA, Bowser DN, Dibbens LM, Singh R, et al. Truncation of the GABA(A)-receptor gamma2 subunit in a family with generalized epilepsy with febrile seizures plus. *Am J Hum Genet* 2002; 70:530–536.
64. Dravet C, Bureau M, Oguni H, Fukuyama Y, Cokar O. Severe myoclonic epilepsy in infancy (Dravet syndrome). In: Roger J, Bureau M, Dravet C, Genton P, et al, eds: *Epileptic Syndromes in Infancy, Childhood and Adolescence*. 3rd ed. Eastleigh, UK: John Libbey & Co Ltd, 2002:81–103.
65. Claes L, Ceulemans B, Audenaert D, Smets K, et al. De novo SCN1A mutations are a major cause of severe myoclonic epilepsy of infancy. *Hum Mutat* 2003; 21:615–621.
66. Nabbout R, Gennaro E, Dalla Bernardina B, Dulac O, et al. Spectrum of SCN1A mutations in severe myoclonic epilepsy of infancy. *Neurology* 2003; 60:1961–1967.
67. Wallace RH, Hodgson BL, Grinton BE, Gardiner RM, et al. Sodium channel alpha1-subunit mutations in severe myoclonic epilepsy of infancy and infantile spasms. *Neurology* 2003; 61:765–769.
68. Harkin LA, McMahon JM, Iona X, Dibbens L, et al. The spectrum of SCN1A—related infantile epileptic encephalopathies. *Brain* 2007; 130(Pt 3):843–52.
69. Ryan SG. Partial epilepsy: chinks in the armour. *Nat Genet* 1995; 10:4–6.
70. Degen R, Degen HE. Some genetic aspects of rolandic epilepsy: waking and sleep EEGs in siblings. *Epilepsia* 1990; 31:795–801.
71. Heijbel J, Blom S, Rasmuson M. Benign epilepsy of childhood with centrotemporal EEG foci: a genetic study. *Epilepsia* 1975; 16:285–293.
72. Doose H. Genetic EEG traits in the pathogenesis of the epilepsies. *J Epilepsy* 1997; 10:97–110.
73. Neubauer BA. The genetics of rolandic epilepsy. *Epileptic Disord* 2000; 2 Suppl 1: S67–S68.
74. Scheffer IE, Bhatia KP, Lopes-Cendes I, Fish DR, et al. Autosomal dominant frontal epilepsy misdiagnosed as sleep disorder. *Lancet* 1994; 343:515–517.
75. Phillips HA, Scheffer IE, Berkovic SF, Hollway GE, et al. Localization of a gene for autosomal dominant nocturnal frontal lobe epilepsy to chromosome 20q 13.2. *Nat Genet* 1995; 10:117–118.
76. Steinlein OK, Mulley JC, Propping P, Wallace RH, et al. A missense mutation in the neuronal nicotinic acetylcholine receptor alpha 4 subunit is associated with autosomal dominant nocturnal frontal lobe epilepsy. *Nat Genet* 1995; 11:201–203.
77. Oldani A, Zucconi M, Ferini-Strambi L, Bizzozero D, et al. Autosomal dominant nocturnal frontal lobe epilepsy: electroclinical picture. *Epilepsia* 1996; 37:964–976.
78. Steinlein OK, Magnusson A, Stoodt J, Bertrand S, et al. An insertion mutation of the CHRNA4 gene in a family with autosomal dominant nocturnal frontal lobe epilepsy. *Hum Mol Genet* 1997; 6:943–947.
79. Weiland S, Witzemann V, Villarroel A, Propping P, et al. An amino acid exchange in the second transmembrane segment of a neuronal nicotinic receptor causes partial epilepsy by altering its desensitization kinetics. *FEBS Lett* 1996; 398:91–96.
80. Kuryatov A, Gerzanich V, Nelson M, Olale F, et al. Mutation causing autosomal dominant nocturnal frontal lobe epilepsy alters Ca^{2+} permeability, conductance, and gating of human alpha4beta2 nicotinic acetylcholine receptors. *J Neurosci* 1997; 17:9035–9047.
81. Magnusson A, Stordal E, Brodtkorb E, Steinlein O. Schizophrenia, psychotic illness and other psychiatric symptoms in families with autosomal dominant nocturnal frontal lobe epilepsy caused by different mutations. *Psychiatr Genet* 2003; 13:91–95.
82. Ottman R, Risch N, Hauser WA, Pedley TA, et al. Localization of a gene for partial epilepsy to chromosome 10q. *Nat Genet* 1995; 10:56–60.
83. Berkovic SF, Scheffer IE. Genetics of human partial epilepsy. *Curr Opin Neurol* 1997; 10:110–114.
84. Cendes F, Lopes-Cendes I, Andermann E, Andermann F. Familial temporal lobe epilepsy: a clinically heterogeneous syndrome. *Neurology* 1998; 50:554–557.
85. Kalachikov S, Evgrafov O, Ross B, Winawer M, et al. Mutations in LGI1 cause autosomal-dominant partial epilepsy with auditory features. *Nat Genet* 2002; 30:335–341.
86. Berkovic SF. Epilepsy genes and the genetics of epilepsy syndromes: the promise of new therapies based on genetic knowledge. *Epilepsia* 1997; 38:S32–S36.
87. Vigevano F, Fusco L, Di Capua M, Ricci S, et al. Benign infantile familial convulsions. *Eur J Pediatr* 1992; 151:608–612.
88. Ottman R, Annegers JF, Risch N, Hauser WA, et al. Relations of genetic and environmental factors in the etiology of epilepsy. *Ann Neurol* 1996; 39:442–449.
89. Schaumann BA, Annegers JF, Johnson SB, Moore KJ, et al. Family history of seizures in posttraumatic and alcohol-associated seizure disorders. *Epilepsia* 1994; 35:48–52.
90. Schupf N, Ottman R. Risk of epilepsy in offspring of affected women: association with maternal spontaneous abortion. *Neurology* 2001; 57:1642–1649.
91. Kang JQ, Shen W, Macdonald RL. Why does fever trigger febrile seizures? $GABA_A$ receptor gamma2 subunit mutations associated with idiopathic generalized epilepsies have temperature-dependent trafficking deficiencies. *J Neurosci* 2006; 26: 2590–2597.
92. Holmes GL. The interface of preclinical evaluation with clinical testing of antiepileptic drugs: role of pharmacogenomics and pharmacogenetics. *Epilepsy Res* 2002; 50:41–54.
93. Tate SK, Depondt C, Sisodiya SM, Cavalleri GL, et al. Genetic predictors of the maximum doses patients receive during clinical use of the anti-epileptic drugs carbamazepine and phenytoin. *Proc Natl Acad Sci U S A* 2005; 102:5507–5512.
94. Siddiqui A, Kerb R, Weale ME, Brinkmann U, et al. Association of multidrug resistance in epilepsy with a polymorphism in the drug-transporter gene ABCB1. *N Engl J Med* 2003; 348:1442–1448.
95. Zimprich F, Sunder-Plassmann R, Stogmann E, Gleiss A, et al. Association of an ABCB1 gene haplotype with pharmacoresistance in temporal lobe epilepsy. *Neurology* 2004; 63:1087–1089.
96. Sills GJ, Mohanraj R, Butler E, McCrindle S, et al. Lack of association between the C3435T polymorphism in the human multidrug resistance (MDR1) gene and response to antiepileptic drug treatment. *Epilepsia* 2005; 46:643–647.
97. Tan NC, Heron SE, Scheffer IE, Pelekanos JT, et al. Failure to confirm association of a polymorphism in ABCB1 with multidrug-resistant epilepsy. *Neurology* 2004; 63:1090–1092.
98. Ott J. Association of genetic loci: replication or not, that is the question. *Neurology* 2004; 63:955–958.
99. Pirmohamed M, Lin K, Chadwick D, Park BK. TNFalpha promoter region gene polymorphisms in carbamazepine-hypersensitive patients. *Neurology* 2001; 56:890–896.
100. Hung SI, Chung WH, Jee SH, Chen WC, et al. Genetic susceptibility to carbamazepine-induced cutaneous adverse drug reactions. *Pharmacogenet Genomics* 2006; 16:297–306.
101. Hung SI, Chung WH, Liou LB, Chu CC, et al. HLA-B*5801 allele as a genetic marker for severe cutaneous adverse reactions caused by allopurinol. *Proc Natl Acad Sci U S A* 2005; 102:4134–4139.
102. Anderson V, Andermann E, Hauser WA. Genetic counseling. In: Engel JJ, Pedley T, eds. *Epilepsy: A Comprehensive Textbook*. Philadelphia: Lippincott-Raven, 1997:225–230.

II

CLASSIFICATION, EPIDEMIOLOGY, ETIOLOGY, AND DIAGNOSIS

8 Classification of Epilepsies in Childhood

Douglas R. Nordli, Jr.

HISTORICAL BACKGROUND

Early discussions on epilepsy rarely differentiated between epilepsies in childhood and those in adult life. The history of classification of the epilepsies might be defined in three major eras: the philosophical era before the twentieth century, marked by patient observation and, to a large degree, philosophical speculation as to the nature of the disease; the era of the localizationalists and pathologists, spanning roughly the first half of the twentieth century; and the present molecular era, including neurochemistry and particularly receptor pharmacology, the physiology of excitatory and inhibitory systems, and molecular biology.

The Philosophical Era

In 1861 Reynolds (1) described convulsions in children by the name *eclampsia*. So-called eclamptic seizures in those days referred to seizures characteristic of the childhood age group, which encompassed febrile convulsions and convulsions due to specific systemic diseases. Although Poupart had described absence in a young girl in 1705 (2), different seizure types were not particularly related to different age groups until much later. In 1772 Tissot (3) classified epileptic seizures but made a more specific contribution that is often lost and that was further elaborated by Sachs (4) in the first English-language pediatric neurology textbook: that is, the concept that epilepsy is composed of an ongoing predisposing condition or diathesis, but that the individual epileptic seizures, or expression of the epileptic process, is triggered by a concatenation of factors that might be considered as precipitating or triggering factors. The latter are not always recognized, and epilepsy therefore has been defined as a liability to unprovoked seizures, which is probably a procrustean attempt to exclude febrile convulsions from the epilepsy rubric.

Sachs divided childhood epilepsies into the eclamptic and the epileptic. The epileptic seizures were further divided into focal and generalized as well as lesional and idiopathic. He believed that idiopathic seizures on a heritable basis had an ultimately bad prognosis and that symptomatic seizures had an even worse prognosis. He thought that symptomatic epilepsies were the result of neonatal abnormalities, including brain hemorrhage. Freud (5) wrote about epilepsy in his text on the infantile cerebral palsies and related childhood seizures to major brain disturbances leading to the conditions included under the heading of cerebral palsy. Smith (6), in his book on diseases in children published over 100 years ago, stated that eclampsia in children was relatively benign except when severe and protracted, when it might be the cause of certain lesions, and he separated this from epilepsy occurring in older children, which he regarded as symptomatic. Sachs, agreeing with Tissot in defining an underlying predisposition and a precipitating cause, also stated that the prognosis largely depended on the underlying cause of the epilepsy and was otherwise not inherent in the convulsions—a somewhat different conclusion than had been arrived at by Gowers (7), who studied predominantly adults and who believed that the periodicity or repetitiveness of a convulsive disorder carried within it the seeds of a progressive disorder.

The Localizationalist and Pathologist Era

The period of the localizationalists and pathologists began with the experiments of Fritsch and Hitzig and of Ferrier and formed the basis of Hughlings Jackson's localizational endeavors, which in turn inspired the beginning of epilepsy surgery 100 years ago by Victor Horsley. The landmark activities of Penfield, Erickson, and Jasper during the past 50 years more clearly defined the nature of epileptic seizures and their localization in the nervous system. The development of electroencephalography (EEG) and, in more recent times, electroencephalography with simultaneous visualization of epileptic seizure behavior on a split-screen TV (video EEG, vEEG) has contributed to understanding epilepsy. This allowed the elaboration of the 1981 classification of epileptic seizures (8), which represented an advance made possible by objective methods of documenting seizures. The addition of other factors, such as anatomic substrate, cause, and age, based on information other than intensive monitoring, were then incorporated into the definition of individual epileptic syndromes (9).

The Molecular and Genetic Era Modeling of the epilepsies using various animal models; sophisticated neurophysiological, neurochemical, and pharmacological techniques; tissue slice preparations with the application of excitatory and inhibitory neurotransmitters and both extracellular and intracellular recordings; and the individual neuronal culture preparations have advanced the study of the epilepsies immensely. More recent advances in basic science research, oddly enough, could be seen as taking us back hundreds of years to the original postulates of Tissot regarding epileptogenesis. He postulated that certain factors influence the threshold for seizures, and others act in a role of acute provocation. Baraban (10) elegantly summarized the parallels in modern scientific studies: genomic research has identified factors that alter the threshold for seizures, and other factors, including glial activation, may act as the acute provocation. With these studies has come the realization of epilepsy as a system disease with an interplay of factors alluded to by students of epilepsy hundreds of years ago, the details of which are only becoming clear in the current era.

CLASSIFICATION OF EPILEPTIC SEIZURES AND THE EPILEPSIES

Evolution of the Classification Schemes

Classification is an ongoing process that is sequentially refined by addition of new information regarding seizures and the epilepsies. Our predecessors worked hard to lay down the foundations of our currently used classification schemes: the 1981 International League Against Epilepsy (ILAE) classification of seizures and the 1989 ILAE classification of epilepsy syndromes (8, 9). These classifications, intimately familiar to all epileptologists and many neurologists, have stood the test of time—a remarkable feat given the fact that these classifications were devised at a time when video EEG units were just starting to proliferate. Still, some of the terms are clearly outdated (e.g., "partial" is out of vogue and has been replaced by "focal"), new syndromes have been recognized in the interim, and some older syndromes have not held-up under further scrutiny. Modern genetics is challenging some of our assumptions, as in the dialectic of idiopathic versus symptomatic. Some epilepsies with strong genetic predeterminants (e.g., Dravet syndrome) do not phenotypically match the other idiopathic (*sui generis*) epilepsies. Clinical neurophysiological techniques and imaging have shown that seizures previously thought to have been "generalized" are really regional, or even triggered by focal processes. Many have recognized the need, therefore, to change the classification, but the critical question is how. What are the needs of the classification systems? Should they be practical, like a gardener's system, or scientific, like a botanist's (11)? If a scientific system is desired—one that provides insight into the underlying shared mechanisms—how is this done when we have only an incomplete knowledge of the pathogenesis of most epilepsies (12)? Some of the most thoughtful and well-informed people in the epilepsy field actively debate these issues, and we await their sage advice in the form of a newly revised ILAE classification system. Until then, the ILAE has made it clear that the only currently sanctioned classification systems are the ones from the 1980s (13). Accordingly, we will present the 1981 and 1989 classification schemes in this chapter, with modifications that incorporate the most recent published thoughts; however, the reader is encouraged to maintain an open mind and to think creatively of new ways to organize emerging information. Our predecessors never envisioned that the classification systems would remain stagnant; rather, they foresaw the need for further revisions. These will undoubtedly come forth, guided by the many exciting scientific advances in our field, and allow us to better understand and care for people with epilepsy.

Seizure Classification

Seizures have historically been categorized as either focal or generalized (Table 8-1). Focal (or localization-related) seizures arise in specific loci in the cortex, which carry with them identifiable signatures, either subjective or observational. These may range from disorders of sensation or thought to convulsive movement of a part of the body. Originally, simple focal (partial) seizures were defined as those in which consciousness is preserved. The concept was that these arose from the six-layered isocortex and remained localized sufficiently long to allow specific symptoms to be discerned. In contrast, complex focal (partial) seizures were defined as those in which consciousness was impaired. The implication of complex focal (partial) seizures was that they involved elaboration elements of the limbic system, thus leading to early bilateral dysfunction. The most recent work of the ILAE classification core group has moved away from the "simple" and "complex" designations. This is a welcomed change in pediatrics, because accurate determination of alteration of consciousness was often very challenging, particularly in the preverbal infant or the child with impaired ability to communicate (14)

TABLE 8-1
Seizure Categories

I. Focal Seizures (previously known as partial or local seizures)
   - A. Simple focal seizures (consciousness not impaired)
     1. With motor symptoms
     2. With somatosensory or special sensory symptoms
     3. With autonomic symptoms
     4. With psychic symptoms
   - B. Complex focal seizures (with impairment of consciousness)
     1. Beginning as simple focal seizures and progressing to impairment of consciousness
        - a. With no other features
        - b. With features as in A.1-4
        - c. With automatisms
     2. With impairment of consciousness at onset
        - a. With no other features
        - b. With features as in A.1-4
        - c. With automatisms
   - C. Focal seizures secondarily generalized

II. Generalized Seizures (convulsive or nonconvulsive)
   1. Absence seizures
   2. Atypical absence seizures
   3. Myoclonic seizures
   4. Clonic seizures
   5. Tonic seizures
   6. Tonic-clonic seizures
   7. Atonic seizures

III. Unclassified Epileptic Seizures

Generalized seizures involve large volumes of brain from the outset and are usually bilateral in their initial manifestations and associated with early impairment of consciousness. They may range from absence seizures, characterized only by impaired consciousness, to generalized tonic-clonic seizures (GTCS), in which widespread convulsive activity takes place. Myoclonic seizures, tonic seizures, and clonic seizures may also occur as generalized attacks.

The latest report from the ILAE Classification Core Group has divided seizure types into those that are self-limited and status epilepticus. It further divides the self-limited seizures into those that are generalized at onset and those that are focal at onset. It does not do the same for status epilepticus. A simplified version is presented in Table 8-2 (15).

The newly suggested classification scheme for seizures is more complex than the 1981 scheme. As mentioned, the elimination of the simple and complex categories is useful in pediatrics since it is often challenging or impossible to reliably assess alteration of consciousnsess in preverbal children. The current scheme may still be difficult to apply to children, even for experts aided by concurrent vEEG data. Focal seizures in the immature lack declarative focal features that might otherwise point to the type of cortex generating the ictus: contralateral dystonic hand posture, ipsilateral hand automatisms, and contralateral hand and eye version rarely occur (16–18). Automatisms, when expressed, tends to be elementary and to feature simple mouthing movements or swallowing motions. Tonic postures are often nonspecific and may relate to primitive subcortical reflexes that are disinhibited during a seizure (17). Preverbal children, of course, cannot volunteer auras and cannot cooperate with testing to determine alteration of consciousness or amnesia. For all these reasons, accurately diagnosing a focal seizure in an infant, unless there is focal limb clonus, can be very difficult. Reliable differentation of neocortical versus hippocampal seizures is probably next to impossible.

Accordingly, many different seizures in the immature would be left unclassified. This may result in a loss of valuable diagnostic and prognostic information

TABLE 8-2
Seizure Types

I. Self-limited epileptic seizures
- A. Generalized onset
  - 1. Seizures with tonic and/or clonic manifestations
    - a. Tonic-clonic seizures
    - b. Clonic seizures
    - c. Tonic seizures
  - 2. Absences
    - a. Typical absences
    - b. Atypical absences
    - c. Myoclonic absences
  - 3. Myoclonic seizure types
    - a. Myoclonic seizures
    - b. Myoclonic astatic seizures
    - c. Eyelid myoclonia
  - 4. Epileptic spasms
  - 5. Atonic seizures
- B. Focal onset
  - 1. Local
    - a. Neocortical
      - i. Without local spread
      - ii. With local spread
    - b. Hippocampal and parahippocampal
  - 2. With ipsilateral propagation to:
    - a. Neocortical areas
    - b. Limbic areas
  - 3. With contralateral spread to:
    - a. Neocortical areas
    - b. Limbic areas
  - 4. Secondarily generalized
    - a. Tonic-clonic seizures
    - b. Absence seizures
    - c. Epileptic spasms
- C. Neonatal seizures

II. Status epilepticus
- A. Epilepsia partialis continua (EPC)
- B. Supplementary motor area (SMA)
- C. Aura continua
- D. Dyscognitive focal
- E. Tonic-clonic
- F. Absence
- G. Myoclonic
- H. Tonic
- I. Subtle

Modified slightly from Engel et al. (15).

and will undoubtedly thwart the refinement of further classification schemes. Classifying these seizures in semiologically descriptive terms therefore may be more useful. (See Chapter 14 on neonatal seizures for more information.)

The same difficulties apply to the propagation of seizures, even when high quality scalp EEG data is available. Most infantile seizures do not progress in the same orderly sequence that one observes in adults (19). Morever, there is often a mismatch between the scalp EEG and clinical findings. For example, a seizure with overt focal clinical findings may be accompanied by a diffuse attenuation on EEG, suggesting that a deep ictal focus is not spreading to the scalp in an organized fashion. Differentiating between the various types of spread would not possible for the majority of infantile seizures. For these reasons, a semiology-based scheme or a simple description of the fundamental clinical aspects of the seizures may be preferable, especially for the very young (20). Alternatively; one may add some modification to the new classification scheme to allow it to better encompass the full range of pediatric seizures. One such modification for self-limited seizures is listed in Table 8-3.

CLASSIFICATION OF EPILEPSIES AND EPILEPTIC SYNDROMES

In the 1989 ILAE classification scheme epilepsies are classified according to seizure type and EEG findings (for example, either focal or generalized) or according to cause (that is, idiopathic, genetic, or symptomatic). They are classified by anatomic localization (for example, frontal, rolandic, occipital, or temporal lobe epilepsies). Finally, they are sometimes classified according to precipitating factors. Other factors taken into consideration are age of onset and certain diurnal influences. All of these factors (Table 8-4) are taken into account in the 1989 ILAE classification, and this is outlined in Table 8-5.

DEFINITIONS

Benign Childhood Epilepsy with Centrotemporal Spikes

Benign childhood epilepsy with centrotemporal spikes is a syndrome of brief, simple, focal, hemifacial motor seizures, frequently with somatosensory symptoms, which have a tendency to evolve into GTCS (21–26). Both seizure types are often related to sleep. Onset is between 3 and 13 years of age (peak, 9–10), and recovery before ages 15 to 16. Genetic predisposition is frequent, and there is male predominance. The EEG has blunt high-voltage centrotemporal spikes, often followed by slow waves that are activated by sleep.

TABLE 8-3
Self-Limited Seizure Types

I. Generalized onset

A. Seizures with tonic and/or clonic manifestations
1. Tonic-clonic seizures
2. Clonic seizures
3. Tonic seizures

B. Absences
1. Typical absences
2. Atypical absences
3. Myoclonic absences

C. Myoclonic seizure types
1. Myoclonic seizures
2. Myoclonic astatic seizures
3. Eyelid myoclonia

D. Epileptic spasms

E. Atonic seizures

II. Focal (identified by the most prominent feature at onset)

A. Autonomic
B. Asymmetric epileptic spasms
C. Behavioral arrest (with or without version)
D. Clonus
E. Gelastic
F. Hypermotor
G. Jacksonian march
H. Myoclonus
I. Sensory
J. Tonic-clonic
K. Tonic posture-asymmetric
L. Versive

Childhood Epilepsy with Occipital Paroxysms

Two types of epilepsy have been described in this category: early-onset benign childhood occipital epilepsy (Panayiotopoulos type) and late-onset childhood occipital epilepsy (Gastaut type). In the former type, attacks are rare but may be prolonged. The seizures have pronounced autonomic features, often associated with vomiting. The affected child may be listless for a prolonged period with a pale countenance. Early reports highlighted the occpital predominance of the interictal epileptiform discharges, but later reports showed that spikes are multifocal and highly stereotyped so that they have a "cloned-like" appearance. The latter type, described by Gastaut, features brief seizures with variable manifestations, but often including some type of visual phenomena. The EEG shows occipital spikes enhanced by eye closure. The latest work from the ILAE classification commission raised some doubts about the Gastaut variant because of the paucity of recent reports.

TABLE 8-4
Features of Epileptic Syndromes

Seizure type(s)
Age of onset
Etiology
Anatomy
Precipitating factors
Severity
EEG, both ictal and interictal
Duration of epilepsy
Associated clinical features
Chronicity
Diurnal and circadian cycling
Prognosis (occasionally)

Benign Neonatal Familial Convulsions

Benign neonatal familial convulsions are rare, dominantly inherited disorders manifesting mostly on the second and third days of life, with clonic or apneic seizures and no specific EEG criteria (27). History and investigations reveal no etiological factors. Approximately 14 percent of these patients later develop epilepsy.

Benign Neonatal Convulsions

Benign neonatal convulsions are very frequently repeated clonic or apneic seizures occurring around the fifth day of life. They have no known cause or concomitant metabolic disturbance (28). Interictal EEG often shows alternating sharp theta waves (theta pointu alternant). There is no recurrence of seizures, and psychomotor development is not affected.

Benign Myoclonic Epilepsy in Infancy

Benign myoclonic epilepsy in infancy is characterized by brief bursts of generalized myoclonus that occur during the first or second year of life in otherwise normal children who often have a family history of convulsions or epilepsy (29). The EEG shows generalized spike waves occurring in brief bursts during the early stages of sleep. These attacks are easily controlled by appropriate treatment. They are not accompanied by any other types of seizures, although GTCS may occur during adolescence. The epilepsy may be accompanied by a relative delay of intellectual development and minor personality disorders.

TABLE 8-5
International Classification of Epilepsies and Epileptic Syndromes (1989)

1.0 Localization-related (focal, local, focal) epilepsies and syndromes

- 1.1 Idiopathic (with age-related onset)
- 1.2 Symptomatic
- 1.3 Unknown as to whether the syndrome is idiopathic or symptomatic

2.0 Generalized epilepsies and syndromes

- 2.1 Idiopathic (with age-related onset-listed in order of age)
  - Benign neonatal familial convulsions
  - Benign neonatal convulsions
  - Benign myoclonic epilepsy in infancy
  - Childhood absence epilepsy (pyknolepsy)
  - Juvenile absence epilepsy
  - Juvenile myoclonic epilepsy (impulsive petit mal)
  - Epilepsy with grand mal (GTCS) seizures on awakening
  - Other generalized idiopathic epilepsies, if they do not belong to one of the above syndromes, can still be classified as generalized idiopathic epilepsies.
- 2.2 Cryptogenic or symptomatic (in order of age)
  - West syndrome (infantile spasms, Blitz-Nick-Salaam Krampfe)
  - Lennox-Gastaut syndrome
  - Epilepsy with myoclonic-astatic seizures
  - Epilepsy with myoclonic absences
- 2.3 Symptomatic
  - 2.3.1 Nonspecific etiology
    - Early myoclonic encephalopathy
  - 2.3.2 Specific syndromes
    - Epileptic seizures may complicate many disease states. Under this heading are included those diseases in which seizures are a presenting or predominant feature.

3.0 Epilepsies and syndromes undetermined whether focal of generalized

- 3.1 With both generalized and focal seizures
  - Neonatal seizures
  - Severe myoclonic epilepsy in infancy
  - Epilepsy with continuous spike-waves during slow wave sleep
  - Acquired epileptic aphasia (Landau-Kleffner syndrome)
- 3.2 Without unequivocal generalized or focal features

4.0 Special syndromes

- 4.1 Situation-related syndromes (Gelegenheitsanfalle)
  - Febrile convulsions
  - Isolated seizures or isolated status epilepticus
  - Seizures occurring only when there is an acute metabolic or toxic event due to, for example, alcohol, drugs, eclampsia, nonketogenic hyperglycemia, uremia

Childhood Absence Epilepsy (Pyknolepsy)

This syndrome of childhood absence epilepsy (pyknolepsy) occurs in children of school age (peak manifestation, age 6 to 7) with a strong genetic predisposition in otherwise normal children (30–34). It appears more frequently in girls than in boys and is characterized by very frequent (several to many per day) absences. The EEG reveals bilateral, synchronous symmetrical spike waves, usually three per second, on a normal background activity. GTCS often develop during adolescence. Otherwise, absences may remit or, more rarely, persist as the only seizure type.

Juvenile Absence Epilepsy

The absences of this syndrome are the same as in pyknolepsy, but absences with retropulsive movements are less common (35). Age of manifestation is around puberty. Seizure frequency is lower than in pyknolepsy, with absences occurring less frequently than every day, mostly sporadically. Association with GTCS is frequent, and they precede the absence manifestations more often than in childhood absence epilepsy, often occurring on awakening. Not infrequently, the patients also have myoclonic seizures. Sex distribution is equal. The spike wave rate is often faster than 3 per second. Response to therapy is excellent.

Juvenile Myoclonic Epilepsy (Impulsive Petit Mal)

Juvenile myoclonic epilepsy appears around puberty and is characterized by seizures with bilateral, single or repetitive arrhythmic, irregular myoclonic jerks, predominantly in the arms (36–40). Some patients may suddenly fall from a jerk. No disturbance of consciousness is noticeable. The disorder may be inherited, and sex distribution is equal. Often, there are GTCS and, less often, infrequent absences. The seizures usually occur shortly after awakening and are often precipitated by sleep deprivation. Interictal and ictal EEG have rapid, generalized, often irregular spike waves and polyspike waves; there is no close phase correlation between EEG spikes and jerks. Frequently, the patients are photosensitive. Response to appropriate drugs is good.

Epilepsy with GTCS on Awakening

Epilepsy with GTCS on awakening is a syndrome with onset mostly in the second decade of life. The "grand mal" seizures are presumably mainly GTCS and occur exclusively or predominantly (over 90% of the time) shortly after awakening, regardless of the time of day, or in a second seizure peak in the evening period of relaxation. If there are other seizures, they are mostly absences or myoclonic, as in juvenile myoclonic epilepsy. Seizures may be precipitated by sleep deprivation and other external factors. Genetic predisposition is relatively frequent. The EEG shows idiopathic generalized epilepsy. There is a significant correlation with photosensitivity. The most recent work of the ILAE commission has brought into question whether this is a distinct entity (15).

West Syndrome (Infantile Spasms, Blitz-Nick-Salaam Krampfe)

West syndrome usually consists of a characteristic triad: infantile spasms, arrest of psychomotor development, and hypsarhythmia, although one element may be missing (41–45). Spasms may be flexor, extensor, lightning, or nods but most commonly are mixed. Onset peaks between 4 and 7 months and is always before 1 year. Boys are more commonly affected, and the prognosis is generally poor. West syndrome may be separated into two groups. The symptomatic group is characterized by the previous existence of brain damage signs (psychomotor retardation, neurologic signs, radiologic signs, or other types of seizures) or by a known cause. The smaller, idiopathic group is characterized by the absence of previous signs of brain damage and of known cause. The prognosis is dependent upon etiology and response to treatment; a subgroup of infants with no prior brain damage and good response to treatment may have an excellent prognosis with normal development and no recurrence of seizures. Patients with symptomatic etiology and incomplete response to treatment do poorly and often have mental retardation and persistent seizures.

Lennox-Gastaut Syndrome

Lennox-Gastaut syndrome manifests itself in children from 1 to 8 years of age but appears mainly in preschool-age children (46–48). The most common seizure types are tonic-axial, atonic, and absence seizures, but other types such as myoclonic, GTCS, or focal are frequently associated with this syndrome. Seizure frequency is high, and status epilepticus is frequent (stuporous states with myoclonias, tonic, and atonic seizures). The EEG usually has abnormal background activity, slow spike waves of less than 3 per second, and often multifocal abnormalities. During sleep, bursts of fast rhythms (around 10 per second) appear. In general, there is mental retardation. Seizures are difficult to control, and the development is mostly unfavorable. In 60% of cases, the syndrome occurs in children suffering from a previous encephalopathy, but it is primary in other cases.

Epilepsy with Myoclonic-Astatic Seizures

Manifestation begins between the ages of 7 months and 6 years, mostly from 2 to 5 years, with (except if beginning in the first year) twice as many boys affected (49, 50). There is frequently hereditary predisposition and usually a normal developmental background. The seizures are myoclonic, astatic, myoclonic-astatic, absences with clonic and tonic components, and tonic-clonic. Status epilepticus frequently occurs. Tonic seizures develop late in the course of unfavorable cases. The EEG is initially often irregular with fast spike waves or polyspike waves, often occurring in bursts so short that it is difficult to determine the repetition rate precisely. Biparietal rhythmic theta activity has also been noted. Course and outcome are variable.

Epilepsy with Myoclonic Absences

The syndrome of epilepsy with myoclonic absences is clinically characterized by absences accompanied by severe bilateral rhythmical clonic jerks, often associated with a tonic contraction (51). They are always accompanied on the EEG by bilateral, synchronous, and symmetrical discharge of rhythmical spike waves at 3 per second, similar to childhood absence. These seizures occur many times a day. Awareness of the jerks may be maintained. Associated seizures are rare. Age of onset is about seven years, and there is a male preponderance. Prognosis is less favorable than in pyknolepsy because of resistance to therapy for the seizures, mental deterioration, and possible evolution to other types of epilepsy such as Lennox-Gastaut syndrome.

Early Myoclonic Encephalopathy and Early Infantile Epileptogenic Encephalopathy

The principal features of early myoclonic encephalopathy are onset before 3 months of age; initially fragmentary myoclonus, then erratic focal seizures; and massive myoclonias or tonic spasms (52). The EEG is characterized by suppression-burst activity, which may vary in the awake and sleeping states. The course is severe, psychomotor development is arrested, and death may occur in the first year. Familial cases are frequent and suggest the influence of one or several congenital metabolic errors, but there is no constant genetic pattern. Early infantile epileptic encephalopathy with suppression bursts, described by Ohtahara and coworkers (52), presents in a similar fashion, but the predominant seizure type in this disorder is tonic and the EEG shows an invariant burst-suppression pattern with bursts occurring about every 3–5 seconds. It frequently evolves into a syndrome indistinguishable from West syndrome.

Neonatal Seizures

Neonatal seizures differ from those of older children and adults (53). The most frequent neonatal seizures are described as subtle because the clinical manifestations are frequently overlooked. These include tonic, horizontal deviation of the eyes with or without jerking; eyelid blinking or fluttering; sucking, smacking, or other buccal-lingual oral movements; swimming or pedaling movements; and occasionally apneic spells. Other neonatal seizures occur as tonic extension of the limbs, mimicking decerebrate or decorticate posturing. These occur particularly in premature infants. Multifocal clonic seizures characterized by clonic movements of a limb, which may migrate to other body parts or other limbs, or focal clonic seizures, which are much more localized, may occur. In the latter, the infant is usually not unconscious. Rarely, myoclonic seizures may occur, and the EEG pattern is frequently that of suppression-burst activity. The tonic seizures have a poor prognosis because they frequently accompany intraventricular hemorrhage. The myoclonic seizures also carry a poor prognosis because they are frequently a part of the early myoclonic encephalopathy syndrome.

Dravet Syndrome (Severe Myoclonic Epilepsy in Infancy)

Dravet syndrome is now the preferred term for what used to be called severe myoclonic epilepsy in infants, because myoclonus is not seen in all cases (54). Characteristics include a family history of epilepsy or febrile convulsions, normal development before onset, seizures beginning during the first year of life in the form of generalized or unilateral febrile clonic seizures, secondary appearance of myoclonic jerks, and often focal seizures. EEGs show generalized spike waves and polyspike waves, and early photosensitivity and focal abnormalities occur. Psychomotor development is often delayed from the second year of life on. Ataxia, pyramidal signs, and interictal myoclonus often appear. This type of epilepsy is very resistant to many forms of treatment.

Epilepsy with Continuous Spike Waves During Slow Sleep

Epilepsy with continuous spike waves during slow sleep results from the association of various seizure types, focal or generalized, occurring during sleep, and atypical absences when awake (55). Tonic seizures do not occur. The characteristic EEG pattern consists of continuous diffuse spike waves during slow-wave sleep, which occurs after the onset of seizures. Duration varies from months to years. The prognosis is guarded because of the appearance of neuropsychologic disorders despite the usually benign evolution of seizures.

Acquired Epileptic Aphasia (Landau-Kleffner Syndrome)

The Landau-Kleffner syndrome is a childhood disorder associating an acquired aphasia, multifocal spikes, and spike-and-wave discharges (56). Epileptic seizures and behavioral and psychomotor disturbances occur in two-thirds of the patients. There is verbal auditory agnosia and rapid reduction of spontaneous speech. The seizures are mostly generalized convulsive or focal motor, are rare, and remit before the age of 15 years, as do the EEG abnormalities.

Kozhevnikov's Syndrome

Two types of Kozhevnikov's syndrome are now recognized, but only one of these two types is included among the epileptic syndromes of childhood because the other one is not specifically related to this age group (57). The first type represents a particular form of rolandic focal epilepsy in both adults and children and is related to a variable lesion of the motor cortex. Its principal features are motor focal seizures, always well localized; often late appearance of myoclonias in the same site where there are somatomotor seizures; an EEG with normal background activity and focal paroxysmal abnormalities (spikes and slow waves); occurrence at any age in childhood and adulthood; frequently demonstrable cause (tumoral, vascular); and no progressive evolution of the syndrome (clinical, EEG, or psychological) except the evolutive character of the causal lesion. The childhood disorder Rasmussen syndrome (58), which is suspected to be of viral etiology, has onset between 2 and 10 years (peak, 6 years) with seizures that are motor focal seizures but are often associated with other types. Fragmentary motor seizures appear early in the course of the illness and are initially localized but later become erratic and diffuse and persist during sleep. A progressive motor deficit follows, and mental deterioration occurs. The EEG background activity shows asymmetric and slow diffuse delta waves, with numerous ictal and interictal discharges that are not strictly limited to the rolandic area.

References

1. Reynolds JR. Epilepsy: its symptoms, treatment and relation to other chronic convulsive diseases. London: Churchill, 1861.
2. Temkin O. The falling sickness. a history of epilepsy from the greeks to the beginnings of modern neurology. 2nd ed. Baltimore: Johns Hopkins Press, 1971.
3. Tissot SA. Traité de l'epilepsie faisant le tome troisième du traité des nerfs et de leurs maladies. Paris: PF Didot, 1772.
4. Sachs B. A treatise on the nervous system of children for physicians and students. New York: William Wood, 1985.
5. Freud S. Infantile cerebral paralysis. Coral Gables, FL: University of Miami Press, 1968.
6. Smith JL. A treatise on the diseases of infancy and childhood. Philadelphia: Lea Brothers, 1886.
7. Gowers WR. Epilepsy and other chronic convulsive disorders. London: Churchill, 1881.
8. Commission on Classification and Terminology of the International League Against Epilepsy. Proposal for revised clinical and electroencephalographic classification of epileptic seizures. *Epilepsia* 1981; 22:489–501.
9. Commission on Classification and Terminology of the International League Against Epilepsy: Proposal for revised classification of epilepsies and epileptic syndromes. *Epilepsia* 1989; 30:389–399.
10. Baraban SC. Epileptogenesis in the dysplastic brain: a revival of familiar themes. *Epilepsy Curr* 2001; 1(1):6–11.
11. Wolf P. Of cabbages and kings: some considerations on classifications, diagnostic schemes, semiology, and concepts. *Epilepsia* 2003; 44(1):1–4, 13.
12. Berg ATB, N.W. Of cabbages and kings: perspectives on classification from the field of systematics. *Epilepsia* 2003; 44(1):8–12.
13. Engel J Jr. Reply to "Of cabbages and kings: some considerations on classifications, diagnostic schemes, semiology and concepts." *Epilepsia* 2003; 44(1):4–6.
14. Nordli DR Jr, Bazil CW, Scheuer ML, Pedley TA. Recognition and classification of seizures in infants. *Epilepsia* 1997; 38(5):553–560.
15. Engel J Jr. Report of the ILAE classification core group. *Epilepsia* 2006; 47(9):1558–1568.
16. Nordli DR, Bazil CW, Scheuer ML, Pedley TA. Recognition and classifiction of seizures in infants. *Epilepsia* 1997; 38:553–560.
17. Duchowny MS. Complex focal seizures of infancy. *Arch Neurol* 1987; 44:911–914.
18. Wyllie E, Chee M, Granstrom ML, et al. Temporal lobe epilepsy in early childhood. *Epilepsia* 1993; 34:859–868.
19. Korff CM, Nordli DR Jr. The clinical-electrographic expression of infantile seizures. *Epilepsy Res* 2006; 70 Suppl 1:S116–S31.
20. Loddenkemper T, Kellinghaus C, Wyllie E, Najm IM, et al. A proposal for a five-dimensional patient-oriented epilepsy classification. *Epileptic Disord* 2005; 7(4):308–320.
21. Nayrac P, Beaussart M. Les pointe-ondes prerolandique: expression EEG très particulière. *Rev Neurol (Paris)* 1958; 99:201–206.
22. Beaussart M. Benign epilepsy of children with rolandic (centro-temporal) paroxysmal foci. *Epilepsia* 1972; 13:795–811.
23. Beaumanoir A, Ballist T, Varfis G, et al. Benign epilepsy of childhood with rolandic spikes. *Epilepsia* 1974; 15:301–315.
24. Loiseau P, Beaussart M. The seizures of benign childhood epilepsy with rolandic paroxysmal discharges. *Epilepsia* 1973; 14:381–389.
25. Lombroso CT. Sylvian seizures and midtemporal spike foci in children. *Arch Neurol* 1967; 17:52–59.
26. Heijbel J, Blom S, Rasmuson M. Benign epilepsy of childhood with centrotemporal EEG foci: A genetic study. *Epilepsia* 1975; 16:285–293.
27. Bjerre I, Corelius E. Benign familial neonatal convulsions. *Acta Paediatr Scand* 1968; 57:557–561.
28. Brown JK. Convulsions in the newborn period. *Dev Med Child Neuol* 1973; 15:823–846.
29. Dravet C, Bureau M. Roger J. Benign myoclonic epilepsy in infants. In: Roger J, Dravet C, Bureau M, et al, eds. *Epileptic Syndromes in Infancy, Childhood and Adolescence.* London: John Libbey Eurotext, 1985:121–129.
30. Drury I, Dreifuss FE. Pyknoleptic petit mal. *Acta Neurol Scand* 1985; 72:353–362.
31. Loiseau P. Childhood absence epilepsy. In: Roger J, Dravet C, Bureau M, et al, eds. *Epileptic Syndromes in Infancy, Childhood and Adolescence.* London: John Libbey Eurotext, 1985:106–120.
32. Penry JK, Porter RJ, Dreifuss FE. Simultaneous recording of absence seizures with videotape and electroencephalography: a study of 374 seizures in 48 patients. *Brain* 1975; 98:427–440.
33. Currier RD, Kooi KA, Saidman LJ. Prognosis of pure petit mal. A follow-up study. *Neurology* 1963; 13:959–967.
34. Livingston S, Torres I, Pauli LL, et al. Petit mal epilepsy. Results of a prolonged follow-up study of 117 patients. *JAMA* 1965; 194:113–118.
35. Wolf P. Juvenile absence epilepsy. In: Roger J, Dravet C, Bureau M, et al, eds. *Epileptic Syndromes in Infancy, Childhood and Adolescence.* London: John Libbey Eurotext, 1985:242–246.
36. Janz D. Christian W. Impulsive-petit mal. *Dtsch Z Nervenh* 1957; 176:346–386.
37. Delgado-Escueta AV, Enrile-Bascale F: Juvenile myoclonic epilepsy of Janz. *Neurology* 1984; 34:285–294.
38. Tsuboi T. Primary generalized epilepsy with sporadic myoclonias of myoclonic petit mal type. Stuttgart: Theime, 1977.
39. Asconape J, Penry JK. Some clinical and EEG aspects of benign juvenile myoclonic epilepsy. *Epilepsia* 1984; 25:108–114.
40. Dreifuss FE. Juvenile myoclonic epilepsy: characteristics of a primary generalized epilepsy. *Epilepsia* 1989; 30(Suppl 4):S1–S7.
41. West WJ. On a peculiar form of infantile convulsions. *Lancet* 1841; 1:724–725.
42. Jeavons PM, Bower BD. Infantile spasms: a review of the literature and a study of 112 cases. Clinics in Developmental Medicine 15. London: Spastics Society and Heinemann, 1964.
43. Jeavons PM, Bower BD. Infantile spasms. In: Vinken PJ, Bruyn GW, eds. *Handbook of Clinical Neurology,* vol. 15. Amsterdam: North Holland, 1974:219–234.
44. Kellaway P, Hrachovy RA, Frost JD, et al. Precise characteristics and quantification of infantile spasms. *Ann Neurol* 1979; 6:214–218.
45. Lombroso CT. A prospective study of infantile spasms: clinical and therapeutic correlations. *Epilepsia* 1983; 24:135–158.
46. Lennox WG, Davis JP. Clinical correlates of the fast and the slow spike and wave electroencephalogram. *Trans Am Neurol Assoc* 1949; 74:194–197.
47. Lennox WG. The slow-spike-wave EEG and its clinical correlates. In: Lennox WG, ed. *Epilepsy and Related Disorders,* vol. 1. Boston: Little, Brown, 1966:156–170.
48. Gastaut H, Roger J, Soulayrol R, et al. Childhood epileptic encephalopathy with diffuse slow spike-waves (otherwise known as "petit mal variant") or Lennox syndrome. *Epilepsia* 1966; 7:139–179.

49. Doose H, Gerken H, Leonhardt R, et al. Centrencephalic myoclonic-astatic petit mal. *Neuropediatrics* 1970; 2:59–78.
50. Doose H, Gundel A. 4–7 cps rhythms in the childhood EEG. In: Anderson VE, Hauser WA, Penry JK, et al. (eds.). *Genetic Basis of the Epilepsies.* New York: Raven Press, 1982:83–93.
51. Tassinari CA, Bureau M. Epilepsy with myoclonic absences.In: Roger J, Dravet C, Bureau M, et al, eds. *Epileptic Syndromes in Infancy, Childhood and Adolescence.* London: John Libbey Eurotext, 1985:121–129.
52. Ohtahara S, Ishida T, Oka E, et al. On the age-dependent epileptic syndromes: the early infantile encephalopathy with suppression-burst. *Brain Dev* 1976; 8:270–288.
53. Volpe JJ. Neonatal seizures. In: Volpe JJ, ed. *Neurology of the Newborn.* Philadelphia: Saunders, 1981:111–137.
54. Dravet C, Bureau M, Roger J. Severe myoclonic epilepsy in infants. In: Roger J, Bureau M, Dravet C, et al, eds. *Epileptic Syndromes in Infancy, Childhood and Adolescence.* London: John Libbey Eurotext, 1985:58–67.
55. Tassinari CA, Bureau M, Dravet C, et al. Epilepsy with continuous spike and waves during slow sleep. In: Roger J, Dravet C, Bureau M, et al, eds. *Epileptic Syndromes in Infancy, Childhood and Adolescence.* London: John Libbey Eurotext, 1985:194–204.
56. Landau WM, Kleffner FR. Syndrome of acquired aphasia with convulsive disorder in children. *Neurology* 1957; 7:523–550.
57. Kojewnikow L. Eine besondere Form von corticaler Epilepsie. *Neurol Centralb* 1895; 14:47–48.
58. Rasmussen TE, Olszewski J, Lloyd-Smith D. Focal cortical seizures due to chronic localized encephalitides. *Neurology* 1958; 8:435–445.

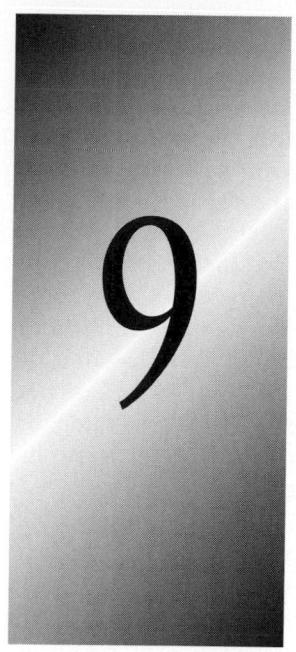

9 Epidemiology of Epilepsy in Children

W. Allen Hauser
P. Nina Banerjee

As a group, the convulsive disorders are among the most frequently occurring neurologic conditions in children. In the United States approximately 5% of children and adolescents experience a seizure of some type by the age of 20 (1). This proportion may be very different in other cultures—higher, for example, in Japanese and lower in Chinese or Asian Indians. The greatest proportion of these children experience convulsions only in association with a febrile illness. Only about a quarter of those experiencing seizures actually meet criteria for "epilepsy"—a condition characterized by *recurrent unprovoked seizures* (2, 3).

Despite efforts of organizations such as the International League Against Epilepsy (ILAE) to develop standardized definitions for the convulsive disorders for epidemiological uses (3), there remain differences in definitions that preclude direct comparison across studies. Population-based studies dealing specifically with children are few and suffer from difficulties with definitions and differences in methodology. Further, total-population studies of the epidemiology of the convulsive disorders or epilepsy seldom provide sufficient detail regarding the specifics of seizure type and etiology in children.

In this chapter we concentrate on studies targeted toward children while integrating data from total population studies. We focus on studies of incidence (newly diagnosed cases), since these are more useful in the assessment of etiology and outcome than prevalence studies. In addition, there is less variation in definitions of seizures and epilepsy in incidence studies than in prevalence studies, allowing some comparison across geographic areas.

DEFINITIONS

Epilepsy

Epilepsy is a condition characterized by recurrent (two or more) unprovoked seizures separated by more than 24 hours. Although epilepsy is the focus of this chapter, only a few of the cited studies here limit cases included to children with epilepsy. Rather, authors include various combinations so the other classes of convulsive disorders, so one must read papers carefully if cross-study comparisons are to be made.

Seizure

A seizure is the clinical manifestation of an abnormal and excessive activity of a set of cortical neurons.

Acute Symptomatic Seizure

Acute symptomatic seizures occur in close temporal association with a systemic or central nervous system (CNS) insult.

About 5% of children with infections of the CNS have acute symptomatic seizures at the time of infection (4). About 10% of children who suffer traumatic brain injury experience seizures early after their injury (5, 6). By age 20, 1% of all children have experienced acute symptomatic seizures (7). Inclusion of children with acute symptomatic seizures as epileptic probably doubles the reported incidence of epilepsy.

Febrile Seizure

A febrile seizure is a convulsive episode occurring in association with an acute febrile illness. This is actually a subcategory of acute symptomatic seizure, differing only in that all children are exposed to the risk factor. Some authors place restrictions for inclusion in this category based on age or clinical symptomatology.

In the United States and in northern European countries, between 2% and 4% of all children can be expected to experience a convulsion during a febrile illness by the age of 5 years (8–10), but there is striking variation in the frequency of occurrence of febrile convulsions worldwide (11–19). The high frequency reported in Japan (9%) has been attributed to recognition of symptoms. It is hypothesized that the typical sleeping arrangement, in which children tend to sleep with or in close proximity to parents, facilitates recognition of symptoms. However, this theory may not explain all geographic difference, because similar sleeping accommodations are common in China and India as well—regions in which incidence is low. It is possible that a selective genetic predisposition for febrile convulsions and the accompanying generalized spike and wave electroencephalograph (EEG) pattern exist in Japanese. The very high frequency of febrile seizures reported in Nigeria may be related to misclassification of children suffering from cerebral malaria, who probably have parasitemia (20). These children have temperature elevation, but probably do not have febrile seizures as defined in Western countries.

Most contemporary studies segregate febrile seizures from epilepsy, but a few series have included selected cases, primarily those with "complex" features. Since such studies comprise 20% to 30% of all febrile convulsion cases, their inclusion may double the apparent incidence or prevalence of unprovoked seizures or epilepsy (21).

Neonatal Seizures

Neonatal seizures are those that occur in the first 28 days of life. This definition, which is derived from concepts of mortality statistics, is conceivably in flux. Infants less than 32 weeks gestational age (a group with improving survivorship) are incapable of developing integrated cerebral electrical activity. In some studies of premature infants, convulsive events occurring between birth and 44 weeks gestational age have been considered a neonatal seizure. From the standpoint of the above classification, most neonatal seizures, particularly those occurring in the first few days of life, would fall into the acute symptomatic category. Epidemiologically, there seems little unique about seizures after the first 7 days of life in full-term infants when compared with seizures identified after the first month of life.

Definitional difficulties are superimposed upon differences in risk within economic groups and geographic areas. Among full-term infants, the reported frequency of neonatal seizures ranges from slightly over 1 per 1,000 live births to 8 per 1,000 live births (22–24). The incidence is lower in developed countries than in developing countries; the incidence may be higher in infants born to mothers of low social-economic class. The frequency is higher among those with low birth weight, and may be higher in children with intracerebral hemorrhage and those who are small for gestational age. There are definite temporal trends in incidence in recent years, with a reduced frequency among full-term infants in most but not all industrialized countries (2, 25, 26). There are also differences in causes over time. Metabolic insults such as hypoglycemia and hypocalcemia were important in the 1950s and 1960s, while in most contemporary studies hypoxic-ischemic insults account for the majority of cases.

Among survivors of neonatal seizures (about 75% of the total), one-third to one-half have adverse neurologic outcomes. Approximately one-third might be expected to experience subsequent unprovoked seizures, mostly in those with neonatal seizures attributable to anoxic insults. Given that the majority of these children experiencing anoxia have associated neurologic disability, their epilepsy may be also be intractable. Children with "benign familial neonatal seizures" (27) and those experiencing "fifth day" seizures (28) have a slightly increased risk for later seizures, but their long-term prognosis in general is quite good. While most epidemiologic studies of epilepsy exclude neonatal seizures unless the patients have subsequent unprovoked seizures, their inclusion would substantially increase the reported incidence of epilepsy, particularly incidence reported in the first year of life.

Unprovoked Seizures

Unprovoked seizures occur in the absence of an identified acute precipitant. In studies in the United States and Iceland, about 25% of newly diagnosed unprovoked seizures in children occur as a single event and never meet criteria for epilepsy (see the following paragraph) (29–31). Half of newly identified unprovoked seizures in childhood in Japan (11) and Spain (32) were isolated events and did not recur.

THE EPIDEMIOLOGY OF EPILEPSY

Incidence cohorts are necessary if one wishes to understand the geographic distribution, causes, and prognosis of epilepsy. A number of recent studies of the incidence have used similar methodology and definition, allowing some comparison. These studies form the basis for most of the following discussion.

Incidence

Information about the incidence of epilepsy in children is derived from studies of total populations that provide age-specific information about incidence (29, 31, 33) and from studies limited to children. Even in studies limited to children, there are difficulties in comparisons across studies because of the inclusion of different age groups as "children," differences in inclusion criteria, and, for the total population studies that provide age specific incidence, different age grouping.

Incidence rates have been estimated from many different populations over the past several years (11, 14, 30, 33, 35–54) and have been found to range from 35 per 100,000 in Finland (34) and Iceland (30) to 124 per 100, 000 in Chile (35) (Table 9-1). Methodological differences in case ascertainment may account for some variation in rate, although the majority of studies have captured information using medical contacts. Some studies conducted in developing countries, however, have relied on door-to-door survey and may have been able to capture cases in the community who may not seek medical attention.

Most recent incidence studies of all unprovoked seizures have been conducted in developed countries (30, 55–59) (Table 9-2). The incidence of "all unprovoked seizures" should be somewhat higher than the incidence of epilepsy. An examination of the studies that have provided rates of all unprovoked seizures shows a reasonable similarity, with the exception of a study in Finland, representing the only outlier. In the most recent studies, the incidence in Tunisia (59) seems substantially higher than the incidences reported by the more recent studies in Iceland and in Sweden.

One of the more intriguing observations from longitudinal studies in children has been a reduction in the incidence of epilepsy over time. In a study in Rochester, Minnesota, incidence of epilepsy fell by about 40% between 1935 and 1975; however, this trend seems to have reversed after 1975 (31) (Table 9-3). On the other hand, among the studies that included all afebrile seizures (60–64) (Table 9-4), a study of a British general practice reported that incidence under age 20 fell from 154 per 100,000 between 1975 to 1984 to 61 per 100,000 from 1985 to 1994 (62). The fall in the middle decades of the past century is largely unexplained, but the increase after 1975 may be related to increased survivorship of very low-birth-weight infants. Interpretation of studies reporting frequency of afebrile seizures is difficult, since there seems to be wide variation. Again, some differences in rate may be due to definition or methodology. For example, the high incidence in Ecuador is likely due to the inclusion of acute symptomatic seizures.

Some studies (12, 65, 66) have used other definitions of "epilepsy" (Table 9-5). In general, these studies seem consistent with studies from the same geographic area, taking into consideration the age structure studied. While there are a number of studies that report global incidence, there are few studies that provide data on gender, age, etiology, or seizure type. The following sections summarize results available from studies that report such data.

Age-Specific Incidence

In all studies providing separate information regarding the incidence by detailed age groups, the incidence is highest in the first year of life. The most recent studies report incidence in the first year of life of about 100 per 100,000 children. Incidence falls after age 1 year, although the rate of the fall varies. In Canada, for example, incidence appears to be stable from ages 1 through 10 years at about 40 per 100,000, and in early adolescence incidence is similar to that reported in adult years of life (20 per 100,000) (45).

In many studies, incidence is typically provided only for 5- or 10-year age groups. In developing countries, incidence may be higher in adolescence than in early childhood, whereas in developed countries, incidence is lower in the second decade of life than in the first decade. The exception is a British study from which one can calculate age-specific incidence: the incidence seems highest in the late teenage years (65). Although this study used an unique definition of "epilepsy," internal comparisons should be consistent, assuming that there is no bias in identification related to age group. As a result these investigators' observations may be valid.

Gender-specific Incidence

For most recent studies that report gender, gender-specific incidence in children is higher in males, although seldom significantly so. This seems to be true regardless of study definition. Only one Swedish study demonstrates a clearly higher incidence in females (58).

TABLE 9-1
Incidence of Epilepsy (Recurrent Unprovoked Seizures per 100,000)

						Etiology (%)		Seizure Type (%)	
Region and Time Period	Reference First Author	Publication Date	Age Group	Incidence	Gender	Idiopathic/ Cryptogenic	Symptomatic	Generalized	Partial
Mariana Islands, Guam 1958–1967	Stanhope (14)	1972	5–10	72					
Sweden 1974	Blom (36)	1978	0–15	82	M>F	81	19	67	33
Connecticut, United States 1960–1970	Shamansky (37)	1979	0–14	56	M=F				
Modena, Italy 1968–1973	Cavazzuti (38)	1980	5–14	82	M>F	71	29	34	66
England 1958 Birth Cohort	Ross (39)	1980	0–4 0–10 0–23	68 41 35		75	25	30	70
Copparo, Italy 1964–1978	Granieri (40)	1983	0–9	97	M>F			80	20
Piedmontese District, Italy 1978	Benna (41)	1984	0–14	83	M>F	60	40		
Faeroe Islands 1970–1980	Joensen (42)	1986	0–20	85	M>F			51	49
Tokyo 1972 Birth Cohort	Tsuboi (11)	1988	0–14	54	M>F			85	15
England 1970 Birth Cohort	Verity (43)	1992	0–10	43		72	30	50	50
Chile 1984–1988	Lavados (35)	1992	0–14	124	M>F		65	35	
Tanzania 1989	Rwiza (33)	1992	0–19	95	M=F				
Minnesota, United States 1935–1984	Hauser (31)	1993	0–14	53					

Sweden 1990–1992	Braathen (44)	1995	0–16	53		70	30	48	52
Nova Scotia, Canada 1977–1985	Camfield (43)	1996	1m–16	41	M=F			47	53
Ethiopia 1990	Tekle-Haimanot (46)	1997	0–9	94					
Yelandur, India 1990	Mani (47)	1998	0–19	62	M>F				
Texas, United States 1995	Annegers (48)	1999	5–14	65					
Minnesota, United States 1980–1984	Zarrelli (49)	1999	0–14	62		74	26	45	55
Estonia 1995–1997	Beilmann (50)	1999	1m–19	45	M>F	63	37	56	44
Spain 1987–1991	Ramirez (51)	1999	1m–11	45				42	58
England 2000	MacDonald (52)	2000	0–4	86					
			5–9	46					
			10–14	94					
Finland 1961–1964	Sillanpaa (53)	2000	0–15	35					
Germany 1999–2000	Freitag (54)	2001	1m–15	61	M>F	62	38	58	42
Iceland 1995–1999	Olafsson (30)	2005	0–14	35	M<F	95	5	23	76

TABLE 9-2
Incidence of All Unprovoked Seizures (per 100,000)

						Etiology (%)		Seizure Type (%)	
Region and Time Period	Reference First Author	Publication Date	Age Group	Incidence	Gender	Idiopathic/ Cryptogenic	Symptomatic	Generalized	Partial
Northern Sweden 1973–1974	Heijbel (55)	1975	0–15	134				45	35
Germany 1957–1966	Doose (56)	1983	1m–9	72	M>F	60	40	80	20
Finland 1966 birth cohort	Wendt (57)	1985	0–14	132	M>F			58	42
Northern Sweden 1985–1987	Sidenvall (58)	1993	0–15	79	F>M	97	3	57	40
Tunisia 1998–1999	Dogui (59)	2003	1m–15	102	M>F	91	9		
Iceland 1995–1999	Olafsson (30)	2005	0–14	63	M>F	85	15	54	46

TABLE 9-3
Incidence of All Unprovoked Seizures in Rochester, Minnesota, by Decade

DECADE	AGE GROUP		
	0–4	*0–9*	*0–14*
1935–44	129	104	91
1945–54	124	101	87
1955–64	85	74	63
1965–74	73	69	59
1975–84	93	79	72

Source: Hauser et al. (31).

Race

One may make broad comparisons across studies of different races, but these are unreliable because of different definitions. In one study of children that used broad definitions of epilepsy, the incidence in African-American children was higher than that in Caucasian children (67). This study did not control for socioeconomic status.

Seizure Type

Most recent studies of epilepsy in developed countries report a slight predominance of partial seizure disorders over generalized seizure disorders. One must consider the age distribution being studied as well as seizures classified, because generalized onset seem to predominate in the first year of life, after which partial seizures seem to predominate. Some studies that seem to find exceptions to this, however, notably those from Tokyo, Japan (11), and Copparo, Italy (40), where 80% to 85% of new cases were considered generalized. Because both areas would be expected to have access to modern diagnostic techniques, the predominance is puzzling. When seizure type is reported, studies in developing countries seem to have a predominance of generalized epilepsy. Whether this represents misclassification related to limited evaluation of incidence cases remains uncertain. An excess of generalized-onset seizures may account for the higher incidence in some countries such as Chile. Studies of "all unprovoked seizures" and studies using more inclusive definitions (e.g., "all afebrile seizures") tend to report a preponderance of generalized seizures. It is likely that in children both single, nonrecurrent, unprovoked seizures and acute symptomatic seizures are predominantly generalized. This should account for the apparent difference in distribution by seizure type based upon study inclusion criteria.

TABLE 9-4
Incidence of All Afebrile Seizures (per 100,000)

REGION AND TIME PERIOD	REFERENCE FIRST AUTHOR	PUBLICATION DATE	AGE GROUP	INCIDENCE	GENDER	SEIZURE TYPE (%)	
						GENERALIZED	PARTIAL
California, United States 1965–1966	Van den Berg (60)	1969	0–6	152	M>F		
England 1970 British birth cohort	Verity (43)	1992	0–10	57		50	50
Ecuador 1984	Placencia (61)	1992	0–19	219	M>F		
England	Cockerell (62)	1995	0–20				
1974–1983				154			
1984–1993				61			
Geneva, Switzerland 1990	Jallon (63)	1997	0–20	69	M>F		
Martinique Islands 1995	Jallon (64)	1999	0–15	82	M>F	60	40
Minnesota, United States 1975–1984	Hauser (31)	1993		90			

TABLE 9-5
Incidence of "Epilepsy" Using Other Definitions (per 100,000)

Region and Time Period	Reference First Author	Publication Date	Age Group	Incidence	Gender	Definition
Japan 1992	Ohtahara (12)	1993	0–10	145	M>F	AUS + some FS
			5–9	63		
England 1995	Wallace (65)	1998	10–14	54		AUS or first AED + some FS
			15–19	101		
England 2001–2003	Reading (66)	2006	0–14	66		

AUS = all unprovoked seizures; FS = febrile seizures.

Etiology

When reported, between 60% and 80% of all new cases in children have no obvious antecedent to explain the condition. This is true even with the use of magnetic resonance imaging. A small proportion of new cases can be attributed to trauma, infection, postnatal vascular lesions, or CNS degenerative conditions. About 20% of cases are associated with neurologic handicaps presumed present from birth, mental retardation (MR), cerebral palsy (CP), or a combination thereof. Whereas most cases of MR or CP in and of themselves usually lack obvious causes, a more appropriate estimate for the proportion with identified cause may be 3%, as reported in a recent study from Sweden (68).

Familial (genetic) predisposition certainly plays a role in the risk for developing epilepsy (69–71). The offspring or sibling of a person with epilepsy has a threefold increase in risk of developing epilepsy. Although familial aggregation consistent with Mendelian inheritance is rare, there are a few childhood-onset syndromes with clear genetic patterns of inheritance. Examples of these include benign familial neonatal seizures, benign infantile epilepsy, and Baltic myoclonic epilepsy. A localization on chromosome 6 and other chromosomal localizations for juvenile-onset epilepsies remains controversial, and the mode of inheritance is not understood. A linkage for the EEG pattern (not the epilepsy) has been reported for rolandic epilepsy with central temporal spikes (72, 73).

It is important to point out factors that are *not* causal for epilepsy. Once cases of CP are accounted for, there has been no evidence of an association between adverse pre- and perinatal factors and the development of epilepsy. The concept of "birth trauma" or of "pregnancy complications" being a cause of epilepsy has not been supported in a variety of studies performed over the past 20 years (74–77). From a similar standpoint, febrile seizures are not "causal" for epilepsy. They are more likely a marker for a preexisting susceptibility—in some cases genetic, and in other cases "structural."

EPILEPSY SYNDROMES

Considerable emphasis has been placed on epilepsy syndromes in recent years (78). The classification to date is most useful in children, but, even in epidemiologic studies in children, a substantial proportion of cases fall into nonspecific categories (30). Syndrome classification has generally not been useful for classification in population-based studies, although its failure may occur primarily in studies of adults (79, 80). Despite limitations in these and other population-based studies, some information regarding the frequency of epilepsy syndromes is available.

Only three population-based incidence studies of all ages classified all cases according to epilepsy syndromes. The incidence of epileptic syndromes for the period between 1980 and 1984 has been investigated for the population of Rochester, Minnesota (49). In this study approximately 20% of childhood cases fell into nonspecific categories, and about one-third were considered localization-related cryptogenic epilepsies without further localization. In the other two studies (conducted in Bordeaux, France, and Iceland), data on the incidence of seizure and epilepsy syndromes were not presented separately for children (30, 80). In France, approximately 1% of the population with newly diagnosed epilepsy had juvenile myoclonic epilepsy, grand mal on awakening, or West syndrome, and 2% had pyknolepsy. The incidence of idiopathic localization-related epilepsy was 1.7 per 100,000 (7% of all cases, adults and children). These proportions correspond to those reported for studies in children alone. In the population-based, prospective study of epilepsy in Iceland, juvenile myoclonic epilepsy, West syndrome, and childhood absence epilepsy again each accounted for 1% of all newly diagnosed cases, with an incidence of 0.7 per 100,000 person years. Benign

TABLE 9-6
Incidence of West Syndrome (Infantile Spasms) per 10,000 Live Births

Region	Reference First Author	Publication Date	Incidence	Gender
California, United States	Van den Berg (60)	1969	1.6	
Denmark	Howitz (81)	1978	3.0	
Finland	Riikonen (82)	1979	4.0	M>F
Texas, United States	Annegers (69)	1982	2.5	
Germany	Doose (56)	1983	4.8	
Finland	Wendt (57)	1985	5.0*	
Faeroe Islands	Joensen (42)	1986	6.0	
Tokyo, Japan	Tsuboi (11)	1988	1.3	
Oklahoma, United States	Cowan (83)	1989	1.9*	
Minnesota, United States	Hauser (84)	1991	2.0	M>F
England	Verity (43)	1992	2.0	M>F
Sweden	Sidenvall (58)	1993	6.0	
Iceland	Ludvigsson (85)	1994	3.0	M>F
Okayama	Oka (86)	1995	3.3	
Finland	Eriksson (87)	1997	3.2*	
Atlanta	Trevathan (88)	1997	7.0*	
Lithuania	Endziniene (89)	1997	7.5*	
Finland	Rantala (90)	1999	4.1	M>F
Iceland	Olafsson (30)	2005	4.3	

*Estimated from prevalence data.

rolandic epilepsy accounted for 20% of new-onset cases in children and 5% of cases in the total population, providing an incidence rate of 2.8 per 100,000 person years. In summary, most population studies show that specific syndromes are rare, with few exceptions.

West Syndrome

The incidence of West syndrome has been evaluated in several geographic areas and seems consistent across studies (11, 30, 42, 43, 56, 57, 69, 81–90). Incidence ranges from 2 to 8 per 10,000 live births (Table 9-6). In all studies reporting gender-specific incidence, there is a male preponderance.

The clinical perception of West syndrome is that the prognosis is poor, but population-based studies in Iceland and Minnesota suggest an excellent prognosis in idiopathic cases (85). These findings underscore the need for more population-based incidence cohorts examining West syndrome.

Lennox-Gastaut Syndrome

The incidence of Lennox-Gastaut syndrome (11, 39, 42, 56, 87, 90) is between 2 and 5 per 10,000 live births (Table 9-7), but there probably is little variation in frequency worldwide. The syndrome typically accounts for 2% to 3% of new cases of epilepsy in children. However,

TABLE 9-7
Incidence of Lennox-Gastaut Syndrome (per 100,000)

Region	Reference First Author	Publication Date	Age Group	Incidence	Gender
England	Ross (39)	1980	0–11	1	
Germany	Doose (56)	1983	0–8	3	
Faeroe Islands	Joensen (42)	1986	0–19	3	
Tokyo, Japan	Tsuboi (11)	1988	0–14	2	
Finland	Eriksson (87)	1997	0–14	2	M>F
Finland	Rantala (90)	1999	1m–2	3	M>F

TABLE 9-8
Incidence of Absence Epilepsy (per 100,000)

Region	Reference First Author	Publication Date	Age Group	Incidence	Percent Total
Germany	Doose (56)	1983	0–8	8	11% AUS
Italy	Granieri (40)	1983	0–14	15	17% RUS
Faeroe Islands	Joensen (42)	1986	0–19	2	2.2% RUS
Tokyo, Japan	Tsuboi (11)	1988	0–14	4	7% RUS
Sweden	Sidenvall (58)	1993	0–15	7	9% AUS
Sweden	Braathen (44)	1995	0–15	4	8% RUS
Nova Scotia, Canada	Camfield (45)	1996	0–14	6	14% RUS
Finland	Eriksson (87)	1997	0–14	2	1.3% AUS
Minnesota, United States	Zarrelli (49)	1999	0–15	5	8% AUS
Tunisia	Dogui (59)	2003	0–15	2	2% AUS
Iceland	Olafsson (30)	2005	0–15	3	1 % AUS

RUS = recurrent unprovoked seizures; AUS = all unprovoked seizures.

in Kiel, Germany, Doose syndrome accounts for about 3 per 100,000 cases age 8 and under.

Severe Myoclonic Epilepsy of Infancy (Dravet Syndrome)

Based upon one case identified in the National Perinatal Collaborative Project (54,000 live births), and on five cases identified from clinics in western Texas, the cumulative risk through age 7 has been suggested to be approximately 1 in 40,000 (91).

Absence Epilepsy: Pyknolepsy and Juvenile Absence Epilepsy

Epilepsies characterized by absence seizures are separated into pyknolepsy and juvenile absence epilepsy. Although these syndromes are considered to be distinct, they are difficult to distinguish clinically and epidemiologically. As a result, they are lumped together in most epidemiologic studies (11, 30, 40, 42, 44, 45, 49, 56, 59, 58, 87). In Sweden, Finland, and Rochester, Minnesota, absence epilepsy comprised approximately 8% of all childhood-onset epilepsy, and the incidence was about 7 per 100,000 (Table 9-8). Incidence was somewhat lower in the Faeroes and another Finnish study (less than 2 per 100,000) and highest in Copporo, Italy (15 per 100,000). Overall, there seems to be considerable consistency for this combined epilepsy syndrome category.

Juvenile Myoclonic Epilepsy

Juvenile myoclonic epilepsy (JME) has received a considerable amount of attention and is perceived as a frequent epilepsy syndrome in children. Most of the studies reporting this syndrome in children (24, 30, 42, 44, 49, 54, 58) have been performed in Scandinavian countries (Table 9-9).

TABLE 9-9
Incidence of Juvenile Myoclonic Epilepsy (per 100,000)

Region	Reference First Author	Publication Date	Age Group	Incidence	Percent Total
Faeroes	Joensen (42)	1986	0–19	3.2	3.8% RUS
Finland	Tudehope (24)	1988	0–14	2.0	1.3% AUS
Sweden	Sidenvall (58)	1993	0–15	5.9	8% AUS
Sweden	Braathen (44)	1995	0–15	0.5	1% RUS
Minnesota, United States	Zarrelli (49)	1999	0–14	1.0	0.75% RUS
Germany	Freitag (54)	2001	0–15	1.7	3% RUS
Iceland	Olafsson (30)	2005	0–25	1.7	1% AUS

TABLE 9-10
Incidence of Benign Rolandic Epilepsy (per 100,000)

Region	Reference First Author	Publication Date	Age Group	Incidence	Percent Total
Italy	Cavazzuti (38)	1980	4–15	20	25% AUS
Germany	Doose (56)	1983	0–8	8	11% AUS
Sweden	Sidenvall (58)	1993	0–15	11	14% AUS
Sweden	Braathen (44)	1995	0–15	5	11% RUS
Minnesota, United States	Zarrelli (49)	1999	0–14	3	5% RUS
Tunisia	Dogui (59)	2003	0–15	8	8% AUS
Iceland	Olafsson (30)	2005	0–15	12	5% AUS

RUS = recurrent unprovoked seizures; AUS = all unprovoked seizures.

In Sweden, five children under the age of 15 had a diagnosis of JME with an incidence of 6 per 100,000. In the studies in Iceland and Rochester, Minnesota, most cases were identified between the ages of 15 and 24. If these age groups are included, the incidence under age 25 is approximately 6 per 100,000. In both Rochester and Iceland, between 5% and 10% of newly diagnosed epilepsy in children may meet criteria for this syndrome. This contrasts with the study in Bordeaux, France, in which 30% of cases were diagnosed at age 5.

Benign Rolandic Epilepsy

Benign rolandic epilepsy is among the more common childhood epilepsy syndromes as based on studies (30, 38, 44, 49, 56, 58, 59) from Scandinavia, Italy, and other countries (Table 9-10). In Italy and Iceland this syndrome accounts for approximately 25% of incidence cases of epilepsy in children from birth through age 15 (38, 90). In Sweden the incidence in those under age 15 is 10.7 per 100,000, and this syndrome accounts for about 14% of childhood epilepsy. Benign rolandic epilepsy accounted for less than 5% of childhood-onset epilepsy in Rochester, Minnesota.

PREVALENCE OF CHILDHOOD EPILEPSY

Tables 9-11–9-13 summarize numerous studies of the prevalence of epilepsy worldwide (11, 14, 19, 32–34, 39, 40–43, 47, 56, 61, 62, 65, 83, 84, 86, 92–124). As mentioned earlier, prevalence provides little information beyond that required for health service needs. Prevalence data are virtually useless for prognosis or etiology. Furthermore, differences in methodology and definitions frequently preclude the ability to make comparisons across studies. Nonetheless, a presentation regarding the epidemiology of epilepsy would not be complete without some discussion of prevalence.

The definitions of prevalence vary as extensively as the definitions of incidence. Prevalence rates in various studies worldwide are usually confound by a dizzying array of definitions. In Tables 9-11–9-13 we have attempted to stratify studies according to definition. When definitions are comparable, there seems little variation in the prevalence of epilepsy (12, 17, 32, 84, 103, 122), except for a moderately higher prevalence in developing countries such as Tanzania (32), Ecuador (90), Thailand (101), Zambia (102), and South Africa (99). Compared with the studies in the United States and Europe, the prevalence of epilepsy may be higher in South America (125–127), and lower in some parts of Asia.

In studies that have defined prevalence as seizures or medication in the past 5 years, estimates remain between 3 and 7 per 1,000 in developed countries and in the range of 9–22 per 1,000 in developing countries. It is hypothesized that the increased prevalence in these regions is a result of parasitic infections. In some studies, prevalence rates seem to increase with age (40, 114, 117, 120). Studies that have measured lifetime prevalence (Table 9-13) within the same population at different points in time show that prevalence of epilepsy has decreased (62).

Prevalence by Seizure Type

Most prevalence studies find a preponderance of generalized-onset seizures. This appears to be true regardless of study site, although the proportion with partial seizures is higher in studies from developed countries.

Etiology

When etiology is reported in incidence studies, between 60% and 80% of cases are of unknown cause. Even fewer prevalence studies report etiology in children. Epilepsy associated with neurologic handicap present from birth

TABLE 9-11

Prevalence of Epilepsy (per 1000) Defined as Seizures or Medication in the Past 1–3 Years

						Etiology (%)		Seizure Type (%)	
Region	Reference First Author	Publication Date	Age Group	Prevalence	Gender	Idiopathic/ Cryptogenic	Symptomatic	Generalized	Partial
Mississippi, United States	Haerer (92)	1986	0–19	5.9	M>F				
Nigeria	Osuntokun (93)	1987	0–19	6.0	M>F				
Spain	Ochoa (32)	1991	6–14	3.7	M>F				
England	Verity (43)	1992	10	2. 8			50	50	
Tanzania	Rwiza (33)	1992	0–9	3.5	M>F				
			10–19	11.1					
Ecuador	Placencia (61)	1992	0–20	6.2 **	M>F				
Tunisia	Attia-Rhomdhane (94)	1993	0–9	4.8	M>F		93	7	
			10–19	5.7					
Kenya	Snow (95)	1994	6–9	2.9	M>F		100		
			10–19	5.5					
England	Cockerell (62)	1995		4.8**					
India	Pal (96)	1998	2–18	2.6					
Serbia	Pavlovic (97)	1998	0–6	4.2	M>F		35	70	30
England	Wallace (65)	1998	5–9	3.2**					
			10–14	4.1**					
			15–19	5.2**					
Iceland	Olafsson (98)	1999	0–14	3.4	M>F	80	20		
South Africa	Christianson (99)	2000	2–9	6.7					
Saudi Arabia	Al Rajeh (100)	2001	0–19	8.1	M>F				
Thailand	Asawavichienjinda (101)	2002	0–14	7.3	F>M				
Zambia	Birbeck (102)	2004	0–4	6.9	M>F				
			5–15	26.2					

*AU = all unprovoked seizures; **AS = acute symptomatic seizures.

TABLE 9-12

Prevalence of Epilepsy (per 1000) Defined as Seizures or Medication in the Past 5 Years

Region	Reference First Author	Publication Date	Age Group	Prevalence	Idiopathic/ Gender	Etiology		Seizure Type	
						Cryptogenic	Symptomatic	Generalized	Partial
Guam	Stanhope (14)	1972	0–19	4.2	M>F				
Finland	Ross (39)	1980	0–15	3.9	M>F				
Copparo, Italy	Granieri (40)	1983	0–9	4.7	M>F				
			10–19	13.9					
Germany	Doose (56)	1983	0–8	4.3*					
Faeroe Islands	Joensen (42)	1986	0–19	6.5	M>F		49	51	
Mississippi, United States	Haerer (92)	1986	0–19	8.3	M>F				
Italy	Pisani (103)	1987	3–14	4.3	M>F		94	6	
Nigeria	Osuntokun (93)	1987	0–19	6.0	M>F				
Tokyo, Japan	Tsuboi ([11])	1988	9–14	3.4	M>F				
Mumbai, India	Bharucha (19)	1988	0–5	4.6	M>F		26	54	
			10–19	3.4					
Kashmir, India	Koul (104)	1988	<14	3.2	M>F				
Oklahoma, United States	Cowan (83)	1989	0–19	4.7	M>F	69	25	38	22
Minnesota, United States	Hauser (84)	1991	0–14	3.9	M>F	80	20		
			0–14	7.1*	M>F	85	15		
Chile	Lavados (35)	1992	0–14	17	F>M				
Pakistan	Aziz (105)	1994	0–9	9.3					
			10–19	9.9					
Turkey	Okan (106)	1995	0–5	9.5	M>F				
Sicily	Reggio (107)	1996	0–9	3.5	M>F	54	46		
Guatemala	Mendizabal (108)	1996	0–9	7.7*					
			10–19	4.6					
Sweden	Sidenvall (109)	1996	0–16	4.2	F<M	57	43	43	52
Lithuania	Endziniene (89)	1997	0–15	4.3	M>F	60	40	30	50
Anatolia, Turkey	Aziz (110)	1997	0–9	10.7	M>F				
			10–19	7.3					
Kerala, India	Hackett (111)	1997	8–12	22	M>F				
Yelandur, India	Mani (47)	1998	0–20	4.6	M>F				
Estonia	Beilmann (112)	1999	1m–19	3.6	M>F	60	40	58	42
Norway	Waaler (113)	2000	6–12	5.1	M>F	54	46		
Kerala, India	Radhakrishnan (114)	2000	0–9	4.0	M>F				
			10–19	6.5					
Turkey	Karabiber (115)	2001	7–12	.8	M>F			83	10
Italy	Rocca (116)	2001	0–19	3.5	M>F				
Brazil	Borges (117)	2002	0–4	4.9					
			5–14	11.7					
Istanbul, Turkey	Onal (118)	2002	0–19	8.9	M=F				
Argentina	Somoza (119)	2005	6–16	2.7	M>F			57	43
Honduras	Medina (120)	2005	0–9	9.5	F>M	41	59		
			10–19	18.4		22	78		

*AUS = all unprovoked seizures; **AAS = atypical absence seizures.

TABLE 9-13
Prevalence of Epilepsy (per 1000) in Lifetime

Region	Reference First Author	Publication Date	Age Group	Prevalence	Gender	Etiology: Idiopathic/Cryptogenic	Etiology: Symptomatic	Seizure Type: Generalized	Seizure Type: Partial
Italy	Pazzaglia (121)	1976	6–14	3.0		74	26	42	58
Kentucky	Baumann (122)	1978	6–16	9.3					
				11.0*					
England	Ross (39)	1980	11	4.1	M>F				
Italy	Cavazzuti (38)	1980	5–9	4.6	M>F	59	41	58	42
			10–14	4.5					
Germany	Doose (56)	1983	0–8	6.3 *	M>F				
Sudan	Younis (123)	1983	6–19	0.9	M>F				
Italy	Benna (41)	1984	0–14	4.5	M=F				
Nigeria	Osuntokun (93)	1987	0–19	6.0	M>F				
Japan	Tsuboi (11)	1988	9–14	8.2	M>F				
Minnesota, United States	Hauser (84)	1991	0–14	4.0	M>F	80	20		
Spain	Ochoa (32)	1991	6–14	5.7	M>F				
England	Verity (43)	1992	0–10	5.7	M=F				
Finland	Sillanpaa (34)	1992	4–15	6.8		60	40	45	55
Ecuador	Placencia (61)	1992	0–9	7.4**	M>F		52	46	
			10–19	13.9					
			0–20	10.5					
England (1983)	Cockerell (62)	1995	0–9	8.1**	F>M				
			10–19	20.7					
			0–20	14.9					
England- (1993)	Cockerell (62)	1995	0–9	5.1**	F>M				
			10–19	14.7					
			0–20	10.2					
Japan	Oka (86)	1995	0–10	8.3	M>F	70	30	31	44
Georgia, United States	Murphy (67)	1995	10	6.0	M>F	60	40	42	58
Yelandur, India	Mani (47)	1998	0–20	4.9	M>F				
Singapore	Kun (124)	1999	18	4.9	Males only	73	27	65	35

*AUS = all unprovoked seizures; **AAS = acute symptomatic seizures.

TABLE 9-14
Cumulative Incidence of Epilepsy

Region	Reference First Author	Publication Date	Age Group	Cumulative Incidence (%)	Definition	Gender	Etiology (%)		Seizure Type (%)	
							Idiopathic/ Cryptogenic	Symptomatic	Generalized	Partial
Finland 1960 Birth Cohort	Hagberg (128)	1976	0–14	1.5	AUS			58	42	
United States NCPP	Ellenberg (129)	1984	0–7	1.0	AS					
Finland 1966 Birth Cohort	Wendt (57)	1985	0–13	1.7	AUS	M>F	65	35	63	37
Tokyo, Japan	Tsuboi (11)	1988	0–15	1.6	AUS					
				0.8	RUS					
Minnesota, United States 1965–84	Hauser (31)	1993	0–15	0.7	RUS					
				0.8	AUS					
				1.1	AS					
England	Cockerell (62)	1995	0–20	1.0	AS					
Serbia	Pavlovic (130)	1999	0–6	0.7	RUS		65	35	70	30
Finland 1987 Birth Cohort	Gissler (131)	1999	0–7	0.7	AUS	Male				
				0.6		Female				

RUS = recurrent unprovoked seizures; AUS = all unprovoked seizures; AS = acute symptomatic seizures.

(e.g., MR or CP) is the most common antecedent, but few studies provide quantitative data. Several studies report the frequency of developmental delay (independent of MR) and other handicap that occurs in up to 25% of cases.

Gender

Except for the British general practice study (62), which used broad definitions of epilepsy, there is a male excess in all studies, although it seldom reaches statistical significance. When age or gender breakdown is provided, females have a higher prevalence in the teenage years in some studies (109, 120).

Race

Prevalence by racial subgroups can be compared in some studies in the United States. Prevalence is higher in African Americans than in Caucasians. These studies do not address whether this difference is attributable to racial or socioeconomic factors.

Cumulative Incidence

A concept more useful than prevalence in terms of epidemiologic measurements is "cumulative incidence," which is the risk of developing a convulsive disorder through to a specific age. It is the cumulative incidence, not prevalence, that is important for comparisons of risk for epilepsy.

Cumulative incidence alone is reported from several studies (11, 31, 57, 62, 128–131) (Table 9-14) and has been reported in or may be calculated from data provided in many papers reporting incidence. If there is no mortality attributable to epilepsy (mortality is negligible in children without handicap), cumulative incidence of epilepsy and lifetime prevalence of epilepsy at age 20 should be similar. The cumulative incidence for all convulsive disorders through age 20 was slightly more than 4% in Rochester, Minnesota; that for epilepsy was slightly more than 1%; and that for all afebrile seizures was about 2%. These proportions should be similar to the lifetime prevalence for these same definitions.

SUMMARY

Epilepsy contributes to a substantial amount of neurologic disease morbidity in children. Recent studies report incidence rates of 35 to 94 per 100,000 and, despite differences in methods and definitions, prevalence rates of 3 to 11 per 1,000, depending on children's ages. There are definite time trends, largely unexplained, that indicate that the incidence of epilepsy in certain populations is declining.

With regard to the burden of epilepsy, it seems greater in males. Developing countries also seem to have a higher burden of disease. Some of the difference between developing and developed countries may be explained by methodological differences. Other factors include misclassification of cases or cases due to parasitic infections, which account for a large proportion of additional epilepsy cases in developing countries.

More studies investigating the etiology of epilepsy are needed, since the large majority of convulsive disorders—more than 60%—have no known cause. Particularly useful would be population-based data on the natural history of untreated and treated epilepsies.

It is difficult to compare seizure type between studies, since not all studies have used the same classification system. In addition, some individuals may have more than one seizure type, and different studies may report this information differently. Regardless of variations by study, generalized-onset seizures are reported to predominate in the first year of life, but later in life partial seizures are more common, at least in developed countries.

The well-defined epilepsy syndromes are important but are less frequent than presumed, even in children. Because of the rarity of epileptic syndromes, information on etiology and classification is limited.

Although no study answers all questions and there is still much to learn, descriptive epidemiological studies of epilepsy provide insights into the frequency of the burden of epilepsy and other convulsive disorders in childhood. This information serves to assist in generating hypotheses regarding the risk factors of epilepsy. Still, more research needs to be done to further our knowledge of the etiology and prevention of epilepsy.

References

1. Hauser WA, Annegers JF, Rocca WA. Descriptive epidemiology of epilepsy: contributions of population-based studies from Rochester, Minnesota. *Mayo Clin Proc* 1996; 71(6):576–586.
2. Hauser WA, Lee JR, Annegers JF, Anderson VE. Risk of recurrent seizures after two unprovoked seizures. *N Engl J Med* 1998; 338(7):429–34.
3. Commission on Epidemiology and Prognosis, International League Against Epilepsy. Guidelines for epidemiologic studies on epilepsy. *Epilepsia* 1993; 34(4):592–596.
4. Annegers JF, Hauser WA, Beghi E, Nicolosi A, et al. The risk of unprovoked seizures after encephalitis and meningitis. *Neurology* 1988; 38(9):1407–1410.
5. Hauser WA, Tabaddor K, Factor PR, Finer C. Seizures and head injury in an urban community. *Neurology* 1984; 34(6):746–751.
6. Annegers JF, Grabow JD, Groover RV, Laws ER, et al. Seizures after head trauma: a population study. *Neurology* 1980; 30(7 Pt 1):683–689.
7. Annegers JF, Hauser WA, Lee JR, Rocca WA. Incidence of acute symptomatic seizures in Rochester, Minnesota, 1935–1984. *Epilepsia* 1995.36(4):327–333.
8. Forsgren L, Sidenvall R, Blomquist HK, Heijbel J. A prospective incidence study of febrile convulsions. *Acta Paediatr Scand* 1990; 79(5):550–557.
9. Verburgh, ME, Bruijnzeels MA, van der Wouden JC, van Suijlekom-Smit LW. et al. Incidence of febrile seizures in The Netherlands. *Neuroepidemiology* 1992; 11(4–6): 169–172.
10. Verity CM, Golding J. Risk of epilepsy after febrile convulsions: a national cohort study. *Br Med J* 1991; 303(6814):1373–1376.
11. Tsuboi T. Prevalence and incidence of epilepsy in Tokyo. *Epilepsia* 1988; 29(2):103–110.
12. Ohtahara S, Oka E, Ohtasuka Y, et al. An investigation on the epidemiology of epilepsy. In: *Frequency, Causes and Prevention of Neurological, Psychiatric and Muscular Disorders*. Ministry of Health and Welfare, Japan 1993:55–60.

13. Hauser WA. The natural history of febrile seizures. In: Nelson KB, Ellenberg J, editors. *Febrile Seizures*, New York: Raven Press, 1982:5–18.
14. Stanhope JM, Brody JA, and Brink E, Convulsions among the Chamorro people of Guam, Mariana islands. I. Seizure disorders. *Am J Epidemiol* 1972; 95(3):292–8.
15. Fukuyama Y, Kagawa K, Tanaka K. A genetic study of febrile seizures. *Eur Neurology* 1978; 18:166–182.
16. Fu Z, Lavine L, Wang Z, et al. Prevalence and incidence of febrile seizures (FBS) in China. *Neurology* 1987.37(Suppl 1):149.
17. Hauser WA, Ortega R, Zarrelli M. The prevalence of epilepsy in a rural Mexican village. *Epilepsia* 1990; 31:604.
18. Gracia F, de Lao SL, Castillo L, Larreategui M, et al. Epidemiology of epilepsy in Guaymi Indians from Bocas del Toro Province, Republic of Panama. *Epilepsia* 1990; 31(6): 718–723.
19. Bharucha NE, Bharucha AE, Bhise AV, Schoenberg BS. Prevalence of epilepsy in the Parsi community of Bombay. *Epilepsia* 1988.29(2):p. 111–1115.
20. Akpede GO, Sykes RM, Abiodum PO. Convulsions with malaria: febrile or indicative of cerebral involvement? *J Trop Pediatr* 1993; 39:350–355.
21. Annegers JF, Hauser WA, Shirts SB, Kurland LT. Factors prognostic of unprovoked seizures after febrile convulsions. *N Engl J Med* 1987; 316(9):493–498.
22. Aireda KI. Neonatal seizures and a 2 year neurological outcome. *J Trop Pediatr* 1991; 37:3313–3317.
23. Eriksson M, Zetterstrom R. Neonatal convulsions. Incidence and causes in the Stockholm area. *Acta Paediatr Scand* 1979; 68:807–811.
24. Tudehope DI, Harris A, Hawes D, Hawes M. Clinical spectrum and outcome of neonatal convulsions. *Austral Paediatr J* 1988; 24:249–253.
25. Kawakami T, Yoda H, Shima Y, Akamatsu H. Incidence and causes of neonatal seizures in the last 10 years (1981–1990). No To Hattatsu 1992; 24:525–529.
26. Goldberg HJ. Neonatal convulsions—a 10 year review. *Arch Dis Child* 1983; 58:976–978.
27. Leppert M, Singh N. Benign familial neonatal epilepsy with mutations in two potassium and channel genes. *Curr Opin Neurol* 1999; 12:143–147.
28. Pryor DS, Don N, Macourt DC. Fifth day fits: a syndrome of neonatal convulsions. *Arch Dis Child* 1981; 56:753–758.
29. Olafsson E, Hauser WA, Ludvigsson P, Gudmundsson G. Incidence of epilepsy in rural Iceland: a population-based study. *Epilepsia* 1996; 37(10):951–955.
30. Olafsson E, Ludvigsson P, Gudmundsson G, Hesdorffer D, et al. Incidence of unprovoked seizures and epilepsy in Iceland and assessment of the epilepsy syndrome classification: a prospective study. *Lancet Neurol* 2005; 4(10):627–634.
31. Hauser WA, Annegers JF, Kurland LT. Incidence of epilepsy and unprovoked seizures in Rochester, Minnesota: 1935–1984. *Epilepsia* 1993; 34(3):453–468.
32. Ochoa Sangrador C, Palencia Luaces R. Study of the prevalence of epilepsy among schoolchildren in Valladolid, Spain. *Epilepsia* 1991; 32(6):791–797.
33. Rwiza HT, Kilonzo GP, Haule J, Matuja WB, et al. Prevalence and incidence of epilepsy in Ulanga, a rural Tanzanian district: a community-based study. *Epilepsia* 1992; 33(6):1051–1056.
34. Sillanpaa M. Epilepsy in children: prevalence, disability, and handicap. *Epilepsia* 1992; 33(3):444–449.
35. Lavados J, Germain L, Morales A, Campero M, et al. A descriptive study of epilepsy in the district of El Salvador, Chile, 1984–1988. *Acta Neurol Scand* 1992; 85(4):249–56.
36. Blom S, Heijbel J, Bergfors PG. Incidence of epilepsy in children: a follow-up study three years after the first seizure. *Epilepsia* 1978; 19(4):343–350.
37. Shamansky SL, Glaser GH. Socioeconomic characteristics of childhood seizure disorders in the New Haven area: an epidemiologic study. *Epilepsia* 1979; 20(5): 457–474.
38. Cavazzuti GB. Epidemiology of different types of epilepsy in school age children of Modena, Italy. *Epilepsia* 1980; 21(1):57–62.
39. Ross EM, Peckham CS, West PB, Butler NR. Epilepsy in childhood: findings from the National Child Development Study. *Br Med J* 1980; 280(6209):207–210.
40. Granieri E, Rosati G, Tola R, Pavoni M, et al. A descriptive study of epilepsy in the district of Copparo, Italy, 1964–1978. *Epilepsia* 1983; 24(4):502–514.
41. Benna P, Ferrero P, Bianco C, Asteggiano G, et al. Epidemiological aspects of epilepsy in the children of a Piedmontese district (Alba-Bra). *Panminerva Med* 1984; 26(2): 113–118.
42. Joensen P. Prevalence, incidence, and classification of epilepsy in the Faroes. *Acta Neurol Scand* 1986; 74(2):150–155.
43. Verity CM, Ross EM, Golding J. Epilepsy in the first 10 years of life: findings of the child health and education study. *Br Med J* 1992; 305(6858):857–861.
44. Braathen G, Theorell K. A general hospital population of childhood epilepsy. *Acta Paediatr* 1995; 84(10):1143–1146.
45. Camfield CS, Camfield PR, Gordon K, Wirrell E, et al. Incidence of epilepsy in childhood and adolescence: a population-based study in Nova Scotia from 1977 to 1985. *Epilepsia* 1996; 37(1):19–23.
46. Tekle-Haimanot R, Forsgren L, Ekstedt J. Incidence of epilepsy in rural central Ethiopia. *Epilepsia* 1997; 38(5):541–546.
47. Mani KS, Rangan G, Srinivas HV, Kalyanasundaram S, et al. The Yelandur study: a community-based approach to epilepsy in rural South India—epidemiological aspects. *Seizure* 1998; 7(4):281–288.
48. Annegers JF, Dubinsky S, Coan SP, Newmark ME, et al. The incidence of epilepsy and unprovoked seizures in multiethnic, urban health maintenance organizations. *Epilepsia* 1999; 40(4):502–506.
49. Zarrelli MM, Beghi E, Rocca WA, Hauser WA. Incidence of epileptic syndromes in Rochester, Minnesota: 1980–1984. *Epilepsia* 1999; 40(12):1708–1714.
50. Beilmann A, Napa A, Hamanik M, Soot A, et al. Incidence of childhood epilepsy in Estonia. *Brain Dev* 1999; 21(3):166–174.
51. Ramirez IO, Rodriguez MH, Aparicio Meix JM, Romero CC. Incidencia de las epilepsias y sindromes epilepticos de la infancia en la provincia de Albacete. *An Esp Pediatr* 1999; 51(2):154–158.
52. MacDonald BK, Cockerell OC, Sander JW, Shorvon SD. The incidence and lifetime prevalence of neurological disorders in a prospective community-based study in the UK. *Brain* 2000; 123 (Pt 4):665–676.
53. Sillanpaa M. Long-term outcome of epilepsy. *Epileptic Disord* 2000; 2:79–88.
54. Freitag CM, May TW, Pfafflin M, Konig S, et al. Incidence of epilepsies and epileptic syndromes in children and adolescents: a population-based prospective study in Germany. *Epilepsia* 2001; 42(8):979–985.
55. Heijbel J, Bohman M. Benign epilepsy of children with centrotemporal EEG foci: intelligence, behavior, and school adjustment. *Epilepsia* 1975; 16(5):679–687.
56. Doose H, Sitepu B. Childhood epilepsy in a German city. *Neuropediatrics* 1983; 14(4): 220–224.
57. Wendt L, Rantakallio P, Saukkonen AL, Maikinen H. Epilepsy and associated handicaps in a year birth cohort in Northern Finland. *Eur J Pediatr* 1985; 144:149–151.
58. Sidenvall R, Forsgren L, Blomquist HK, Heijbel J. A community-based prospective incidence study of epileptic seizures in children. *Acta Paediatr* 1993; 82(1):60–65.
59. Dogui M, Jallon P, Tamallah JB, Sakly G, et al. EPISOUSSE: incidence of newly presenting seizures in children in the region of Sousse, Tunisia. *Epilepsia* 2003; 44(11):1441–1444.
60. Van den Berg BJ, Yerushalamy J. Studies on convulsive disorders in young children. Incidence of febrile and nonfebrile convulsions by age and other factors. *Pediatr Res* 1969; 3:298–304.
61. Placencia M, Shorvon S, Paredes V, Bimos C, et al. Epileptic seizures in an Andean region of Ecuador. Incidence and prevalence and regional variation. *Brain* 1992; 115 (Pt 3):771–782.
62. Cockerell OC, Eckle I, Goodridge DM, Sander JW, et al. Epilepsy in a population of 6000 re-examined: secular trends in first attendance rates, prevalence, and prognosis. *J Neurol Neurosurg Psychiatry* 1995; 58(5):570–576.
63. Jallon P, Goumaz M, Haenggeli C, Morabia A. Incidence of first epileptic seizures in the canton of Geneva, Switzerland. *Epilepsia* 1997; 38(5):547–552.
64. Jallon P, Smadja D, Cabre P, Le Mab G, et al. EPIMART: prospective incidence study of epileptic seizures in newly referred patients in a French Carribean island (Martinique). *Epilepsia* 1999; 40(8):1103–1109.
65. Wallace H, Shorvon S, Tallis R. Age-specific incidence and prevalence rates of treated epilepsy in an unselected population of 2,052,922 and age-specific fertility rates of women with epilepsy. *Lancet* 1998; 352(9145):1970–1973.
66. Reading R, Haynes R, Beach R. Deprivation and incidence of epilepsy in children. *Seizure* 2006; 15(3):190–193.
67. Murphy CC, Trevathan E, Yeargin-Allsopp M. Prevalence of epilepsy and epileptic seizures in 10-year-old children: results from the Metropolitan Atlanta Developmental Disabilities Study. *Epilepsia* 1995; 36(9): 866–872.
68. Forsgren L, Bucht G, Eriksson S, Bergmark L. Incidence and clinical characterization of unprovoked seizures in adults: a prospective population-based study. *Epilepsia* 1996; 37(3):224–229.
69. Annegers JF, Hauser WA, Anderson VE, Kurland LT. The risks of seizure disorders among relatives of patients with childhood onset epilepsy. *Neurology* 1982; 32(2):174–179.
70. Beck-Mannagetta G, Janz D, Hoffmeister U, Behl I, et al. Morbidity risk for seizures and epilepsy in offspring of patients with epilepsy. In: Beck-Mannagetta G, Anderson VE, Doose H, Janz D, eds. *Genetics of the Epilepsies*. Berlin: Springer-Verlag, 1989:119.
71. Anderson E, Hauser WA. Genetics. In: Laidlow R, Richens A, Chadwick D, eds. *Textbook of Epilepsy.* Edinburgh: Churchill-Livingstone, 1993:47–75.
72. Vadlamudi L, Kjeldsen MJ, Corey LA, Solaas MH, et al. Analyzing the etiology of benign rolandic epilepsy: a multicenter twin collaboration. *Epilepsia* 2006; 47(3):550–555.
73. Neubauer BA, Fiedler B, Himmelein B, Kampfer F, et al. Centrotemporal spikes in families with rolandic epilepsy: linkage to chromosome 15q14. *Neurology* 1998; 51(6):1608–1612.
74. Rocca WA, Sharbrough FW, Hauser WA, Annegers JF, et al. Risk factors for complex partial seizures: a population-based case-control study. *Ann Neurol* 1987; 21:22–31.
75. Rocca WA, Sharbrough FW, Hauser WA, Annegers JF, et al. Risk factors for absence seizures: a population-based case-control study in Rochester, Minnesota. *Neurology* 1987; 37:1309–1314.
76. Rocca WA, Sharbrough FW, Hauser WA, Annegers JF, et al. Risk factors for generalized tonic-clonic seizures: a population-based case-control study in Rochester, Minnesota. *Neurology* 1987; 37:1315–1322.
77. Nelson K, Ellenberg JH. Antecedents of seizure disorders in early childhood. *Am J Dis Child* 1986; 40:1053–1061.
78. Commission on Classification and Terminology of the International League Against Epilepsy. Proposal for revised classification of epilepsies and epileptic syndromes. *Epilepsia* 1989; 30(4):389–399.
79. Manford M, Hart YM, Sander JW, Shorvon SD. The National General Practice Study of Epilepsy: the syndromic classification of the International League Against Epilepsy applied to epilepsy in a general population. *Arch Neurol* 1992; 49(8):801–808.
80. Loiseau J, Loiseau P, Guyot M, Duche B, et al. Survey of seizure disorders in the French southwest. I. Incidence of epileptic syndromes. *Epilepsia* 1990; 31(4):391–396.
81. Howitz P, Platz P. Infantile spasms and HLA antigens. *Arch Dis Child* 1978; 53(8): 680–682.
82. Riikonen R, Donner M. Incidence and aetiology of infantile spasms from 1960 to 1976: a population study in Finland. *Dev Med Child Neurol* 1979; 21(3):333–343.
83. Cowan LD, Bodensteiner JB, Leviton A, Doherty L. Prevalence of the epilepsies in children and adolescents. *Epilepsia* 1989; 30(1):94–106.
84. Hauser WA, Annegers JF, Kurland LT. Prevalence of epilepsy in Rochester, Minnesota: 1940–1980. *Epilepsia* 1991; 32(4):429–445.

85. Ludvigsson P, Olafsson E, Sigurdardottir S, Hauser WA. Epidemiological features of infantile spasms in Iceland. *Epilepsia* 1994; 35:802–805.
86. Oka E, Ishida S, Ohtsuka Y, Ohtahara S. Neuroepidemiological study of childhood epilepsy by application of international classification of epilepsies and epileptic syndromes (ILAE, 1989). *Epilepsia* 1995; 36(7):658–661.
87. Eriksson KJ, Koivikko MJ. Prevalence, classification, and severity of epilepsy and epileptic syndromes in children. *Epilepsia* 1997; 38(12):1275–1282.
88. Trevathan E, Murphy CC, Yeargin-Allsopp M. Prevalence and descriptive epidemiology of Lennox-Gastaut syndrome among Atlanta children. *Epilepsia* 1997; 38(12):1283–1288.
89. Endziniene M, Pauza V, Miseviciene I. Prevalence of childhood epilepsy in Kaunas, Lithuania. *Brain Dev* 1997; 19(6):379–387.
90. Rantala H, Ingalsuo H. Occurrence and outcome of epilepsy in children younger than 2 years. *J Pediatr* 1999; 135(6):761–764.
91. Hurst DL, Epidemiology of severe myoclonic epilepsy of infancy. *Epilepsia* 1990; 31(4):397–400.
92. Haerer AF, Anderson DW, Schoenberg B.S. Prevalence and clinical features of epilepsy in a biracial United States population. *Epilepsia* 1986; 27(1):66–75.
93. Osuntokun BO, Adeuja AO, Nottidge VA, Bademosi O, et al. Prevalence of the epilepsies in Nigerian Africans: a community-based study. *Epilepsia* 1987; 28(3):272–279.
94. Attia-Romdhane N, Mrabet A, Ben Hamida M. Prevalence of epilepsy in Kelibia, Tunisia. *Epilepsia* 1993; 34(6):1028–1032.
95. Snow RW, Williams RE, Rogers JE, Mung'ala VO, et al. The prevalence of epilepsy among a rural Kenyan population. Its association with premature mortality. *Trop Geogr Med* 1994; 46(3):175–179.
96. Pal DK, Das T, Sengupta S. Comparison of key informant and survey methods for ascertainment of childhood epilepsy in West Bengal, India. *Int J Epidemiol* 1998; 27(4):672–676.
97. Pavlovic M, Jarebinski M, Pekmezovic T, Levic Z. Seizure disorders in preschool children in a Serbian district. *Neuroepidemiology* 1998; 17(2):105–110.
98. Olafsson E, Hauser WA. Prevalence of epilepsy in rural Iceland: a population-based study. *Epilepsia* 1999; 40(11):1529–1534.
99. Christianson AL, Zwane ME, Manga P, Rosen E, et al. Epilepsy in rural South African children—prevalence, associated disability and management. *S Afr Med J* 2000; 90(3):262–266.
100. Al Rajeh S, Awada A, Bademosi O, Ogunniyi A. The prevalence of epilepsy and other seizure disorders in an Arab population: a community-based study. *Seizure* 2001; 10(6):410–414.
101. Asawavichienjinda T, Sitthi-Amorn C, Tanyanont W. Prevalence of epilepsy in rural Thailand: a population-based study. *J Med Assoc Thai* 2002; 85(10):1066–1073.
102. Birbeck GL, Kalichi EM. Epilepsy prevalence in rural Zambia: a door-to-door survey. *Trop Med Int Health* 2004; 9(1):92–95.
103. Pisani F, Trunfio C, Oteri G, Primerano G, et al. Prevalence of epilepsy in children of Reggio Calabria, southern Italy. *Acta Neurol (Napoli)* 1987; 9(1):40–43.
104. Koul R, Razdan S, Motta A. Prevalence and pattern of epilepsy (Lath/Mirgi/Laran) in rural Kashmir, India. *Epilepsia* 1988; 29(2):116–122.
105. Aziz H, Ali SM, Frances P, Khan MI, et al. Epilepsy in Pakistan: a population-based epidemiologic study. *Epilepsia* 1994; 35(5):950–958.
106. Okan N, Okan M, Eralp O, Aytekin AH. The prevalence of neurological disorders among children in Gemlik (Turkey). *Dev Med Child Neurol* 1995; 37(7):597–603.
107. Reggio A, Failla G, Patti F, Nicoletti A, et al. Prevalence of epilepsy. A door-to-door survey in the Sicilian community of Riposto. *Ital J Neurol Sci* 1996; 17(2):147–151.
108. Mendizabal JE, Salguero LF. Prevalence of epilepsy in a rural community of Guatemala. *Epilepsia* 1996; 37(4):373–376.
109. Sidenvall R, Forsgren L, Heijbel J. Prevalence and characteristics of epilepsy in children in northern Sweden. *Seizure* 1996; 5(2):139–146.
110. Aziz H, Guvener A, Akhtar SW, Hasan KZ. Comparative epidemiology of epilepsy in Pakistan and Turkey: population-based studies using identical protocols. *Epilepsia* 1997; 38(6):716–722.
111. Hackett RJ, Hackett L, Bhakta P. The prevalence and associated factors of epilepsy in children in Calicut District, Kerala, India. *Acta Paediatr* 1997; 86(11):1257–1260.
112. Beilmann A, Napa A, Soot A, Talvik T. Prevalence of childhood epilepsy in Estonia. *Epilepsia* 1999; 40(7):1011–1019.
113. Waaler PE, Blom BH, Skeidsvoll H, Mykletun A. Prevalence, classification, and severity of epilepsy in children in western Norway. *Epilepsia* 2000; 41(7):802–810.
114. Radhakrishnan K, Pandian JD, Santhoshkumar T, Thomas SV, et al. Prevalence, knowledge, attitude, and practice of epilepsy in Kerala, South India. *Epilepsia* 2000; 41(8):1027–1035.
115. Karabiber H, Yakinci C, Durmaz Y, Kutlu O, et al. Prevalence of epilepsy in 3637 children of primary school age in the Province of Malatya, Turkey. *J Trop Pediatr* 2001; 47(5):317–318.
116. Rocca WA, Savettieri G, Anderson DW, Meneghini F, et al. Door-to-door prevalence survey of epilepsy in three Sicilian municipalities. *Neuroepidemiology* 2001; 20(4):237–241.
117. Borges MA, Barros EP, Zanetta DM, Borges AP. [Prevalence of epilepsy in Bakairi Indians from Mato Grosso State, Brazil]. *Arq Neuropsiquiatr* 2002; 60(1):80–85.
118. Onal AE, Tumerdem Y, Ozturk MK, Gurses C, et al. Epilepsy prevalence in a rural area in Istanbul. *Seizure* 2002; 11(6):397–401.
119. Somoza MJ, Forlenza RH, Brussino M, Licciardi L. Epidemiological survey of epilepsy in the primary school population in Buenos Aires. *Neuroepidemiology* 2005; 25(2):62–68.
120. Medina MT, Duron RM, Martinez L, Osorio JR, et al. Prevalence, incidence, and etiology of epilepsies in rural Honduras: the Salama Study. *Epilepsia* 2005; 46(1):124–131.
121. Pazzaglia P, Frank-Pazzaglia L. Record in grade school of pupils with epilepsy: an epidemiological study. *Epilepsia* 1976; 17(4):361–366.
122. Baumann RJ, Marx MB, Leonidakis MG. Epilepsy in rural Kentucky: prevalence in a population of school age children. *Epilepsia* 1978; 19(1):75–80.
123. Younis YO. Epidemiology of epilepsy among school populations in Khartoum Province, Sudan. *J Trop Med Hyg* 1983; 86(6):213–216.
124. Kun LN, Ling LW, Wah YW, Lian TT. Epidemiologic study of epilepsy in young Singaporean men. *Epilepsia* 1999; 40(10):1384–1387.
125. Gomez JG, Arciniegas E, Torres J. Prevalence of epilepsy in Bogota, Colombia. *Neurology* 1978; 28(1):90–94.
126. Chiofalo N, Kirschbaum A, Fuentes A, Cordero ML, et al. Prevalence of epilepsy in children of Melipilla, Chile. *Epilepsia* 1979; 20(3):261–266.
127. Garcia-Pedroza F, Rubio-Donnadieu F, Garcia-Ramos F, Escobedo-Rios, F, et al. Prevalence of epilepsy in children: Tlalpan, Mexico City, Mexico. *Neuroepidemiology* 1983; 2:16–23.
128. Hagberg G, Hansson O. Childhood seizures. *Lancet* 1976; 2(7978):208.
129. Ellenberg JH, Hirtz DG, Nelson KB. Age at onset of seizures in young children. *Ann Neurol* 1984; 15(2):127–134.
130. Pavlovic MV, Jarebinski MS, Pekmezovic TD, Marjanovic BD, et al. Febrile convulsions in a Serbian region: a 10-year epidemiological study. *Eur J Neurol* 1999; 6(1):39–42.
131. Gissler M, Jarvelin MR, Louhiala P, Hemminki E. Boys have more health problems in childhood than girls: follow-up of the 1987 Finnish birth cohort. *Acta Paediatr* 1999; 88(3):310–314.

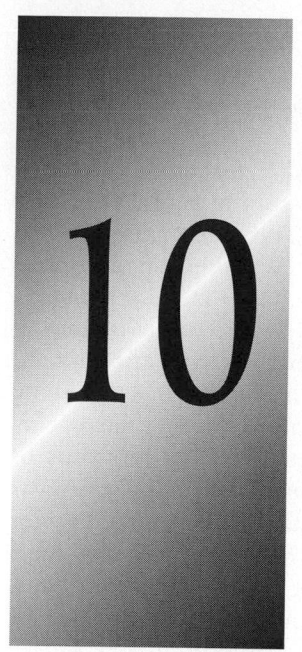

An Approach to the Child with Paroxysmal Phenomena with Emphasis on Nonepileptic Disorders

Arthur L. Prensky
Amir Pshytycky

Seizures are symptoms of abnormal brain function that occur due to excessive electrical discharge of cerebral neurons. Any acute or chronic insult to the brain can produce seizures. During infancy and childhood, seizures may assume many different clinical forms (1). When a child presents with what may be his first seizure, the physician is obligated to define the nature of the event and, if necessary, to search for a specific cause. The most common type of seizure in children is associated with moderate to high fever (2). These seizures rarely result in epilepsy (recurrent unprovoked seizures) or cause neurologic damage (see Chapter 19). Unless there is reason to suspect sepsis or an infection of the central nervous system (CNS), the child does not require an extensive evaluation if prior development has been normal. Even if an initial seizure occurs in the absence of fever, a search for a specific cause is often not fruitful, as many occur in patients in whom there is no detectable evidence of brain damage or systemic illness. Some of these children have family members who have been diagnosed with epilepsy. This suggests a genetic predisposition for the patient's seizure.

EVALUATION OF THE FIRST SEIZURE

There are two populations of children whose seizures are more likely to be associated with an identifiable insult to the brain: those who have other neurologic signs or a history of abnormal development and those who have partial seizures that arise from a specific region of the cerebral cortex. However, in infants and young children, in particular, it is not unusual for a generalized seizure to be the first sign of an acute or chronic metabolic disorder or an infection of the brain or meninges. All children who have had their first seizure, with or without fever, should be evaluated with a complete history and physical examination to determine whether prior development is suspicious, whether there are focal neurologic signs or evidence of increased intracranial pressure, and whether there is indication of other organ involvement. It is the history and physical examination, along with the age of the child at the time of the initial seizure, that determine the extent of the subsequent laboratory evaluations.

The incidence of seizures in the neonatal period is greater than at any other time of life. Most of these seizures occur during the first week of life (3). Neonatal seizures are rarely idiopathic and often have multiple etiologies (4, 5); therefore, an extensive diagnostic evaluation is required. Prognosis often depends upon etiology (6). The most common etiologies are hypoxic-ischemic encephalopathy (HIE), intracranial hemorrhage, or infection and developmental defects. The timing of these seizures may suggest the etiology. Seizures due to HIE or hypoglycemia often begin in the first day of life. Infections, congenital malformations, and other metabolic derangements usually cause seizures after 48 hours of life.

The evaluation of neonatal seizures is based upon the history and physical examination. It includes an electroencephalogram (EEG) to confirm or support seizure activity, neuroimaging, and laboratory studies aimed at identifying a treatable etiology. This includes serum chemistries: pH, electrolytes, glucose, calcium, magnesium, lactate, and pyruvate. Spinal fluid should also be obtained for routine analysis as well as lactate, pyruvate, and amino acids if seizures are repeated. If the cause of the seizures is still obscure, ancillary studies include titers for toxoplasmosis, syphilis, rubella, cytomegalovirus, and herpes simplex virus (TORCH), human immunodeficiency virus (HIV) testing, a drug screen, genetic studies, very-long-chain fatty acids, and lysosomal enzymes. Intractable seizures in a neonate can result from pyridoxine dependency (7). In this treatable autosomal recessive disorder, seizures can begin shortly after a normal birth. Seizures caused by hypoglycemia require evaluation of causes of limited sugar production or hyperinsulinism, including disorders involving organic acid, amino acid, and fatty acid metabolism.

Neuroimaging can identify intracranial hemorrhage, congenital malformations, and other brain injuries. Cranial ultrasound (US) can detect intraventricular hemorrhage and many parenchymal hemorrhages but has limitations detecting convexity hemorrhages, developmental abnormalities, and infarcts (8). Once the neonate is stable, magnetic resonance imaging (MRI) should be performed because it is superior to ultrasound and computerized tomography (CT) scans in identifying these lesions. As timing of the insult is important, the MRI should include diffusion-weighted images (9).

Older children and adolescents who are otherwise normal when they present with their first generalized seizure constitute a different situation (10). If the history is benign and the examination is normal, an EEG is the only test that is indicated. Even the EEG is helpful only in a minority of instances. A normal EEG would not exclude the diagnosis of a seizure if the history was sufficiently clear. An abnormal interictal EEG helps if the diagnosis made by history was uncertain. Many children who have had a seizure have a normal EEG in the interictal period or they show nonspecific abnormalities such as diffuse slowing. Just as the EEG does not always assist in the diagnosis of a seizure disorder, it also is not entirely reliable in predicting whether there will be further episodes (see Chapter 12); however, the initial EEG may define a focus of abnormal brain activity or occasionally show a specific pattern that has some predictive value and helps to plan the child's treatment. The history is always the most critical part of making the diagnosis of a seizure unless the episode itself is observed by the doctor. It is very important to obtain a history from adolescents in the absence of their parents. This may help to determine whether they are at risk for a sexually transmitted disease or whether they have a drug history that could have resulted in a convulsion.

The evaluation of the initial seizure should be much more extensive if the child's history or physical examination is not entirely normal. The following questions must be answered in the history: Was the event a seizure? Was the seizure focal or generalized? Is there a history of neurologic illness? Has the seizure occurred during the course of an acute or subacute systemic or neurologic illness—that is, were there prior or continuing symptoms such as fever, diarrhea, vomiting, headache, or change in level of consciousness or alterations of comprehension, speech, vision, balance, or strength? Does the child have other chronic disorders that might make his seizure more likely to be the result of structural damage to the brain, such as congenital heart disease, hypertension, sickle cell anemia, immunodeficiencies, or collagen vascular disease? A family history is also critical and should emphasize whether other members of the family have had epilepsy, febrile seizures, or other types of neurologic disorders.

The child who presents with a first seizure deserves a thorough neurologic examination and general physical examination with special attention to signs of neuroectodermal diseases, including screening with a Wood's lamp. Emphasis should be placed on whether the child has focal neurologic signs such as visual loss, weakness of one part of the body, reflex changes, or disturbances of balance or coordination that might suggest an area of brain damage that could also be the source of the seizure. Signs of elevated intracranial pressure should also be looked for (a bulging fontanel, split sutures, papilledema, slow pulse, and high blood pressure for age), as should signs of meningeal irritation (a stiff neck, Kernig's signs, Brudzinski's sign). Finally, any recent changes in the child's intellectual capacities or language should be documented. The child with a generalized seizure who has a benign history and physical examination need have little more done than a serum glucose, calcium, and magnesium, and a routine awake and asleep EEG. If the history or physical findings suggest the possibility of focal brain damage or elevated intracranial pressure, CT or MRI is indicated. The latter is more sensitive, especially if one suspects there may be migrational abnormalities that have affected the cortex (11). The CT scan is a better indicator of subependymal deposits of calcium. The ways in which a child's history and physical examination may influence the further evaluation of a child with a first seizure are outlined in Table 10-1.

At times, more sophisticated metabolic studies are indicated to define the cause of an epileptic disorder. For example, infants or children whose seizures are poorly controlled with medication should have their cerebrospinal fluid (CSF) glycine levels determined. Type II hyperglycinemia may result in an intractable

TABLE 10-1
Clinical Basis for Laboratory Investigations

History and Physical Examination	Seizure Type	Type of Evaluation
1. Normal	Generalized	Routine EEG; serum glucose, calcium, magnesium
2. Normal	Partial (focal)	Routine or sleep-deprived EEG; brain scan (CT or MRI); serum glucose, calcium, magnesium
3. Suggests a chronic neurologic insult not previously evaluated with focal physical findings	Generalized or partial	Routine or sleep-deprived EEG; brain imaging (CT or MRI); serum glucose, calcium, magnesium
4. Presence of mental retardation or slow development without focal signs	Generalized or partial	Routine EEG; serum glucose, calcium; serum and urine amino acids; chromosome studies, if otherwise indicated; TORCH titers, if under age 12 months. If seizure is partial, brain imaging is indicated.
5. Normal other than for presence of fever ± vomiting or diarrhea		Brain Imaging
a. Seen acutely	Generalized or partial	Lumber puncture; serum glucose, calcium, electrolytes, BUN; EEG
b. Seen some days later when well	Generalized	Fasting glucose, calcium; EEG
6. Normal other than for a clouded sensorium	Generalized or partial	Brain imaging (CT or MRI). If scan is normal, a lumbar puncture, glucose, calcium, electrolytes. If these are normal, liver chemistries including a serum ammonia, urine ketones, drug screen; EEG; AIDS testing.
7. Presence of increased ICP ± focal signs	Generalized or partial	Brain imaging with contrast enhancement (CT or MRI); calcium, electrolytes, urinalysis; lumbar puncture if scan is normal; EEG. If no cause is found, an MRI may be indicated at a later date.
8. Presence of focal signs of recent onset	Generalized or partial	Contrasted brain scan (CT or MRI); lumbar puncture if scan is normal; EEG; glucose, calcium, electrolytes. If CT scan normal, cardiac evaluation; screen for hemoglobinopathies and coagulation defects, sedimentation rate, antinuclear antibodies, serum cholesterol, triglycerides. Anticardiolipin antibodies if an infarct is seen on imaging.

Abbreviations: EEG, electroencephalogram; CT, computed tomography; MRI, magnetic resonance imaging; MRV, magnetic resonance imaging of venous sinuses and veins; TORCH, toxoplasmosis, other (congenital syphilis and viruses), rubella, cytomegalovirus, and herpes simplex virus; BUN, blood urea nitrogen; AIDS, acquired immune deficiency syndrome; ICP, increased cranial seizures causes by hypoglycemia require evaluation of the causes of limited sugar production or hyperinsulinism including disorders involving organic or fatty acids.

epilepsy, which can be diagnosed only by evaluation of glycine levels in the spinal fluid. Transport defects can affect the entry of glucose and other substrates (such as folate) (12, 13) into the spinal fluid, which can result in repeated seizures when serum levels are normal. Lactate may be more elevated in the CSF than in blood in some mitochondrial disorders. Any infant or young child with poorly controlled seizures should also be tested for partial pyridoxine dependency after by being placed on 25–150 mg of pyridoxine daily for at least 1 month to see whether that affects seizure control. Pyridoxine dependency after infancy cannot always be diagnosed by a single intravenous injection of the vitamin during an EEG.

DISORDERS THAT IMITATE EPILEPSY

Physicians are often asked to distinguish between many forms of epilepsy and other transient disturbances of neurologic function (Table 10-2). Nonepileptic neurologic disorders can produce recurrent, paroxysmal changes of movement, consciousness, or behavior that are similar to those exhibited by a child with epilepsy. Some disorders that mimic seizures are more likely to occur in children who have epilepsy, to be associated with epileptiform EEGs, or to be relieved by antiepileptic drugs. This makes their differentiation from epilepsy even more difficult; however, many of these disorders are benign and do not carry the prognosis or stigma attached to many of the epilepsies. They require no treatment and disappear spontaneously. Others are best treated by medications other than antiepileptic drugs. Thus, it is extremely important to distinguish between repeated paroxysmal events that mimic a seizure and the recurrent seizures that define epilepsy. Epilepsy and the disorders that imitate it present at all ages and in many different forms. There are several excellent reviews of nonepileptic disorders

TABLE 10-2
Imitators of Epilepsy

	Relative Incidence with Age		
Symptoms/Signs	Neonate and Infant 0–2 Years	Early Childhood 2–8 Years	Late Childhood 8–18 Years
A. Unusual movements			
Masturbation	XXX	X	X
Shuddering	XXX	X	X
Benign sleep myoclonus	XXX	X	X
Startle responses	XX	XX	X
Paroxysmal torticollis	X	XX	
Self-stimulating behaviors		XXX	XX
Tics	X	XXX	
Chorea		X	XX
Paroxysmal dyskinesias	XX	X	
Pseudoseizures		X	XX
Unusual eye movements	XXX	XX	X
B. Loss of tone or consciousness			
Syncope		XX	XXX
Drop attacks		X	X
Narcolepsy/cataplexy		X	X
Attention deficits		XXX	XXX
C. Disorders of respiration			
Apneic attacks		XXX	
Breath-holding	XXX	X	
Hyperventilation		X	X
D. Perceptual disturbances			
Dizziness		XXX	XX
Headache		XXX	XXX
Abdominal pain		XXX	X
E. Behavioral disorders			
Head banging	X	XXX	
Night terrors	X	XXX	
Sleepwalking		XXX	X
Nightmares		XX	XX
Hallucinations			
Rage	XXX	XX	
Confusion		X	XXX
Fear	X	XXX	

based on cause (14–17). This discussion considers disorders based on their symptoms and signs and the age at which they are most likely to be confused with seizures, as well as whether they occur when the patient is awake or asleep.

DISORDERS THAT OCCUR DURING SLEEP

Movement Disorders (18)

Benign Nenoatal Sleep Myoclonus. Benign neonatal sleep myoclonus is the most common quasi-epileptic disorder (19, 20). It usually occurs during sleep and begins early in infancy, often in the first weeks or months of life; however, it can be seen in older infants and even in young children. The disorder occurs during non–rapid eye movement (NREM) sleep. Rapid, forceful jerks may occur in the distal extremities, such as the hands or feet, or in the more proximal muscles, moving the entire limb or the trunk. The jerking usually recurs every 2 to 3 seconds, and episodes may last as long as 30 minutes, although most subside in 1 to 3 minutes only to recur repeatedly during the night. The movements migrate from one muscle group to another. Movements occur on both sides of the body. The involvement usually is synchronous, but it need not be. However, prolonged, repetitive involvement of the same muscles or repetitive synchronous involvement of the same muscle groups on the right and left sides of the body are more likely to be a true seizure. The movements of benign neonatal myoclonus are not stimulus sensitive, and the EEGs taken during sleep reveal that epileptiform activity is not present while the events are going on. The source of the myoclonic movements is thought to be in the brainstem. The movements stop if the child is awakened. When alert, the infant is seen to be developing normally and to have a normal neurologic examination.

Benign neonatal myoclonus is extremely disturbing to parents, but the movements rarely interfere with the infant's sleep and normally do not require treatment. If absolutely essential, the movements can generally be reduced by giving a small dose of clonazepam before bed. The prognosis for these infants is a good one. If the movements begin in early infancy, they tend to disappear in 3 to 4 months. Those few children who develop sleep myoclonus later in infancy may continue to exhibit the movements into the second year of life. There is no indication that benign neonatal myoclonus is associated with a higher incidence of epilepsy or abnormal neurologic development later in life.

Head Banging and Other Rhythmic Parasomnias. Repetitive episodes of head banging can occur as an infant is falling asleep and may be mistaken for a seizure because, unlike diurnal episodes of stereotyped movements, they are not associated with emotional disturbances such as anxiety or frustration (21, 22). Other rhythmic movements of the neck and trunk, such as head rolling, body rocking, and leg banging, can occur in children during stage 2 of sleep. These movements are unassociated with EEG abnormalities and can easily be differentiated from seizures by video-EEG or polysomnographic monitoring. If the movements are violent enough to require treatment, they can usually be modified by giving clonazepam before bedtime. Periodic leg movements do not appear to quantitatively alter the quality of sleep in adults (23).

Paroxysmal Hypnogogic Dyskinesia. Hypnogogic paroxysmal dyskinesia or dystonia is a rare disorder in which sleep is interrupted for brief periods of time (usually less than 1 minute) several times each night by severe dystonic, ballistic, or choreic movements sometimes accompanied by screaming (21). The motor patterns are complex with bimanual/bipedal activity, rocking axial and pelvic movements, and sometimes ambulation. Prolonged attacks are believed to be epileptic and arise from the frontal lobe from areas that cannot be accessed by scalp tracings. Thus, the interictal EEG is usually normal as are many ictal EEGs, although carbamazepine often reduces the number of events. Many patients with this disorder go on to develop other forms of diurnal seizures. The disorder indicates how difficult it may be to separate epileptic from nonepileptic events (24, 25).

Disorders of Respiration

Apnea. Disturbances of breathing during sleep are common in infants and children. Periods of apnea without other signs are rarely epileptic when they occur during sleep, but the abrupt cessation of respiration can sometimes be the only sign of a seizure in infants and young children (26, 27). The associated electrical abnormality is usually focal and in the temporal area; however, apnea has been described as the only manifestation of diffuse epileptiform discharges as well.

Usually disorders leading to periods of apnea during sleep are classified as central, obstructive, or mixed (28). Most premature infants and some older infants have apneic events that can be central, secondary to delayed maturation of the centers that control breathing (29), or obstructive, resulting from partial constriction of the upper airway. Polysomnography uses airflow monitors and strain gauges to relate movement of the chest and abdominal musculature to effective rhythmic inspiration and expiration. In obstructive apnea, movements of chest or abdominal musculature continue while the flow of air is markedly decreased or stopped. This is followed by a significant drop in the oxygen saturation of the blood. In central apnea, muscle movements decrease coincident with the drop in airflow. More sophisticated measures of P_{CO_2} and transesophageal pressure may identify more subtle disorders of breathing during sleep (30, 31).

Central apnea has been reported with tumors of the brainstem or compression of the medulla or upper cord by a mass, bony deformities of the upper spine or foramen magnum (32), partial herniation of the brain, or a Chiari malformation. Metabolic or infectious disorders that damage the respiratory center in the medulla may result in loss of automatic control of respiration during sleep (Ondine's curse), producing long periods of apnea sufficient to cause further brain damage or even death.

Obstructive or mixed forms of apnea are frequently seen in young children with cranial-facial deformities that narrow the oropharynx or with adenotonsillar hypertrophy (33, 34). Aspiration may cause similar problems and is more likely to occur in infants or children with significant neurologic damage. However, gastroesophageal reflux can occur in children who are neurologically normal and produce significant repeated periods of apnea in sleep as well as in the waking child.

Studies indicate sleep-disordered breathing is sometimes associated with attention deficit disorders and learning difficulties that may improve with treatment of the sleep disorder (35).

Behavioral Disorders

The behavioral parasomnias noted in children that are often mistaken for epileptic activity include sleepwalking (somnambulism), night terrors (pavor nocturnus), and nightmares (36, 37). The violent behaviors in non-REM sleep in older adults that can result in injury to themselves or to others are rarely seen in children (38).

Sleepwalking. Sleepwalking usually begins between 5 and 10 years of age and can persist into adult life (39). Approximately 15% of all children sleepwalk at least one time. Repeated episodes are much less frequent involving less than 2% of the population. Sleepwalking is often confused with automatisms seen with complex partial seizures. The cause of the disorder is not known, but there is a definite increase in the prevalence of sleepwalking in the family members of children who suffer from the problem. Sleep-disordered breathing is also a predisposing factor. Episodes of sleepwalking usually occur 1 to 3 hours after sleep begins. The child arises and walks about the room or the house in a trance and then walks back to bed. Semipurposeful behavior such as undressing and dressing may occur during the attack. The child's eyes are open and the child rarely walks into objects. The child often mumbles, but there is no purposeful speech. Sleepwalkers can sometimes be directed back to bed, but they often become agitated if restrained. If the child is left alone, physical violence is usually not a part of the attack. The child has no memory of the event the next morning. Attacks sometimes increase with stress.

Usually no treatment is required other than providing for the safety of the child, and the disorder subsides spontaneously over a period of several years. Frequent or prolonged attacks can be treated with benzodiazepines. Polysomnography may reveal a predisposing sleep disorder. Treatment of the underlying problem may also reduce or eliminate episodes of sleepwalking (37).

Night Terrors (Pavor Nocturnus). Night terrors are most commonly seen in children between 5 and 10 years of age. The disorder also occurs in the first 3 hours of sleep in stages 3 or 4 of slow-wave sleep. It may be confused with complex partial seizures. The cause is not known, but there is a familial predisposition. As with sleepwalking, night terrors can be associated with disturbed sleep and a result of disordered breathing or periodic leg movements. Night terrors do not appear to be related to the presence or development of epilepsy or other neurologic or psychiatric disorders. Approximately 3% of all children have this disorder. The child often screams and then sits up. The child continues to scream and appears to be terrified. There are signs of increased sympathetic activity such as excessive sweating and dilated pupils. The attack can last up to 10 minutes, after which the child falls back to sleep. When awakened, the child has no recollection of the event.

Nightmares. Night terrors must be distinguished from nightmares. The latter usually occur later in the night during REM sleep. The EEG is normal. The child may be restless during the dream but usually does not scream. The child often recalls the nightmare and develops a fear of sleeping alone.

Complex partial seizures that occur during sleep are usually associated with automatisms other than walking or with episodes that can be mistaken for night terrors (41). The behaviors are usually abrupt at onset, and if there are movements, they are frequently the same in each attack. The patient may appear anxious, but screaming and sympathetic overactivity are not seen unless someone tries to interrupt the seizure. The child may be incontinent. A video-EEG is sometimes needed to make a diagnosis.

DISORDERS THAT OCCUR WHEN AWAKE

Simple Paroxysmal Movement Disorders

Myoclonus. Rapid, forceful but isolated or nonrhythmic jerks that occur when the infant or child is awake are considered myoclonic. Whether such movements are epileptic may be a matter of semantics. Myoclonus, like other transient, paroxysmal movements, can originate in areas of brain other than the cortex (42) and can occur in the absence of paroxysmal activity in the EEG at the time the movement is seen. The physiologic processes that regulate large groups of subcortical cells, causing them to fire synchronously and repeatedly, may be similar to those seen in the recognized epilepsies involving gamma-aminobutyric acid or glycine-mediated inhibitory mechanisms that control neuronal hyperexcitability (43). However, if the patient has no other neurologic signs, a repeatedly normal EEG, and a benign course in which he fails to develop other seizure types and the movements remain static and eventually disappear, the disorder is usually considered nonepileptic.

Benign waking myoclonic patterns are usually seen in infants in the first year of life and almost always disappear spontaneously within 18 months. The jerks may be limited to head flexion, or there may be bilateral synchronous jerks of the arms (44). At times they can occur repetitively in brief clusters (45). Lombroso and Fejerman (46) described infants who had bursts of flexor or, less often, extensor movements of neck, trunk, and arms resembling those seen in infantile spasms. Their EEG tracings were always normal, and the children continued to develop normally. There was no increased incidence of epilepsy later in childhood.

Spasmodic Torticollis. Benign paroxysmal torticollis (BPT) of infancy is a disorder characterized by recurrent episodes of head tilt. Episodes begin within the first 12 months of life and resolve by 5 years. It presents with torticollis, with or without associated pallor, vomiting, and ataxia, settling spontaneously within hours or days. The torticollis is episodic, may occur to either side, and usually lasts between 4 hours and up to 4 days in duration. This syndrome may include two different situations: one, "periodic," which is more common, that lasts several hours or days; the other, more rare, that is short-lived and "paroxysmal," lasting only minutes and accompanied by ocular signs that are generally lacking in the periodic version (47). Typically the frequency and duration of these episodes decline as the child gets older, and by early to mid childhood they have resolved in their entirety. The etiology of BPT is not known. It has been related to an underlying vestibular disorder such as labyrinthitis or an immaturity of the central nervous system (48) and of the neurotransmitters in a given period of development. Some cases of BPT have evolved into classic migraine. BPT is considered as one of the pediatric migraine equivalent syndromes. Attacks of torticollis can also occur intermittently in the presence of gastroesophageal reflux (Sandifer's syndrome). These episodes are usually not paroxysmal and tend to last longer (49). Inflammatory, developmental, and neoplastic disease of the cervical cord, spine, and neck also tend to produce sustained torticollis, but not a series of brief episodes. If no secondary cause can be discovered, spasmodic torticollis of infancy usually subsides in the first 3 years of life. No treatment is indicated.

Paroxysmal Kinesogenic Dyskinesia (PKD). Children with paroxysmal kinesogenic dyskinesia have abrupt attacks of dystonia, chorea, ballismus, and combinations of different hyperkinesias (50, 51). These episodes are triggered by movement, most commonly whole-body activity such as initiation of standing or walking, and less frequently, by focal movement or a startle. Multiple episodes less lasting less than a minute can occur each day. The EEG is normal during the episode or shows movement artifacts. Paroxysmal kinesogenic dyskinesia most commonly presents between ages 6 and 15 years, although it has been reported in the first year of life. The disorder can be familial or sporadic. It is responsive to carbamazepine and phenytoin. Sporadic cases sometimes follow such insults as hypoxia, hypoglycemia or hyperglycemia, hypocalcemia, cerebral vascular injury, multiple sclerosis, and thyrotoxicosis. Some have postulated it is a form of subcortical epilepsy (52).

Paroxysmal Nonkinesogenic Dyskinesia (PNKD). Paroxysmal nonkinesogenic dyskinesia usually manifests during childhood and early adolescence. Movements may involve trunk, lips, jaw, or tongue. It is rarely generalized. The movement is usually the same from one attack to another (53). The majority of cases are familial with autosomal dominant inheritance, although spontaneous cases do occur. Some cases are linked to chromosome 2q (54). Unlike PKD, the movements and abnormal postures of PNKD generally last longer, from 10 minutes to several hours, and their frequency is often as low as a few episodes per month with only few patients suffering up to three paroxysms per day. PNKD is not triggered by physical activity, but may be primed by fatigue, stress, excitement, alcohol, or caffeine. Paroxysmal nonkinesogenic dyskinesia does not respond to anticonvulsants, and limited success has been achieved with benzodiazepines.

Paroxysmal Exercise-Induced Dyskinesia. Paroxysmal exercise-induced dyskinesia (PED) is the rarest form of paroxysmal dyskinesias. The paroxysms are triggered by prolonged exercise, usually running or walking, and not by exposure to cold or passive joint movements. The distribution of the attacks is either focal dystonia of the foot, hemidystonia, or generalized dyskinesias, involving the legs with and additional involvement of the trunk. The frequency is daily to monthly. Duration of the episodes is extremely variable, from seconds to hours, even in the same patient. Several drugs including antiepileptic drugs, L-DOPA, trihexyphenidyl, and acetazolamide have been reported to be of some benefit in isolated cases (55, 56).

Other Movements

Neurologically impaired children may have many repetitive movements that can be mistaken for seizures. These include head shaking and nodding, staring, tongue thrusting, chewing movements, periodic hyperventilation, tonic postures, tics, and excessive startle reactions. Many have been treated for epilepsy unnecessarily because of these symptoms. In addition, self-stimulatory behaviors (discussed later) such as rhythmic hand shaking and body rocking are seen more often in retarded children.

Jitteriness. Jitteriness occurs in newborns and young infants (57). It can be so severe when a neonate is handled or is irritable or crying that it is sometimes mistaken for a clonic seizure; however, purely clonic generalized seizures are extremely rare in the neonate. Furthermore, the jittery infant is usually alert. The movements of a jittery child have more of an oscillatory quality to them than the clonic jerks seen during a seizure. The tremors seen in jitteriness either occur spontaneously or can be provoked by stimulation (58). They diminish or stop when the extremity is repositioned. However, jittery neonates are much more likely to develop seizures than the normal infant, and they often have abnormal EEGs with epileptiform transients. Jitteriness sometimes has a specific, often treatable cause. The movements are often seen in response to metabolic encephalopathies caused by hypoxia, hypoglycemia, hypocalcemia, and narcotic withdrawal. If possible, the underlying cause of jitteriness should be treated. The movements themselves usually decrease rapidly with time and require no specific therapy. If they are so severe that it is not possible to care for the baby, the baby may have to be sedated for a brief period.

Shuddering. Older infants and children can suffer from paroxysmal bouts of shivering during which spontaneous activity decreases and the upper extremities are adducted and flexed at the elbows or, less often, abducted and extended (59, 60). The head and knees are also frequently flexed. Aside from artifact, there are no EEG abnormalities during the attacks, and the incidence of epilepsy is no higher in these children than in the general population. Antiepileptic medications do not modify the attacks. Shuddering episodes gradually decrease in frequency and intensity in the first decade of life. Many children who have episodes of shuddering come from families in which many members have an essential tremor, and the two disorders may be related.

Rumination. Rumination is a stereotypical behavior beginning with repetitive contractions of the abdominal muscles, diaphragm, and tongue, and culminating in regurgitation of gastric contents into the mouth, where the material is either expectorated or rechewed and reswallowed. During a typical attack the neck is hyperextended, and there are repetitive swallowing movements and tongue thrusts. It can be one of the presentations of gastroesophageal reflux disorder (GERD) in infancy. Because episodes usually occur during or directly following infant feedings, while the infants are alert and often uncomfortable, the event is usually easily distinguished from a seizure. Rumination can occur as voluntary habitual regurgitation of stomach contents into the mouth for self-stimulation in mentally handicapped children or in infants with infant rumination syndrome. This syndrome is rare and has its onset between 3 and 8 months of age (61).

Startle Responses. Startle disease (hyperekplexia) is a rare familial disorder that occurs in major and minor forms in the newborn period. In the minor form the startle response is exaggerated (62–64). In the major form, the infant becomes stiff when handled. Flexor spasms (without habituation) can be elicited by repeated tapping on the infant's nasal bridge. The episodes of hypertonia may be severe, causing apnea, bradycardia, and, rarely, sudden death. Anecdotal reports suggest that forced flexion of the neck or hips interrupts the hypertonic episode. Stiffness decreases during the first year of life and disappears by 2 to 3 years of age. During the same period, the infant develops violent, repetitive jerks upon falling asleep. Many of these children have paroxysmal abnormalities in their EEGs. When they are recorded during a startle response, there are bilateral centroparietal sharp waves followed by a train of slow waves. This complex is considered to be evoked by sensory stimuli and not an epileptiform transient. Older children, juveniles, and adults suddenly stiffen and fall. This is most likely to occur when they are startled, and this is what is usually misinterpreted as an epileptic disorder. The symptoms of hyperekplexia (stiffness, jerking, and falling) respond to antiepileptic drugs such as clonazepam or valproic acid. Despite these features, the disorder is not considered a form of stimulus-sensitive epilepsy. It more likely represents a defect in inhibitory regulation of brainstem centers by the cerebrum. The disorder remains stable or improves with age. Children who have these symptoms do not develop typical seizures more frequently than the average child. Recently, one gene for this disorder has been localized to chromosome 5q33–q35 (65). Mutations that involve the gene that encodes the alpha-1 subunit of the glycine receptor result in exaggerated startle responses (66). The disorder is usually inherited as a dominant but can be recessive. Genetic analysis helps to distinguish difficult cases of hyperekplexia from epilepsy or psychogenic disorders. It should prove most useful in those cases that were considered sporadic.

Chorea. Choreic movements are rapid, purposeless movements that are not repetitive or rhythmic (67). They can involve any muscles but are more prominent in the distal musculature. In most disorders, the abnormal movements are bilateral but not synchronous. Hemichorea is limited to only one side of the body. It is seen, at times, with vascular and inflammatory disorders. In alert children, single movements such as chorea and tics can be confused with myoclonus, although, unlike myoclonic jerks, these movements almost always disappear in sleep (Table 10-3). At times, choreiform movements and multifocal myoclonic jerks are indistinguishable and must be categorized by the diseases with which they

TABLE 10-3
Tics, Chorea, and Myoclonus

	TIC	CHOREA	MYOCLONUS
Common age of onset (years)	(5–10)	(5–15)	Any age
Clinical picture	Stereotyped, repetitive movements of one or more muscle groups most often located in the face, neck or upper trunk. They may be rhythmic for brief periods, but usually are irregular.	Rapid, jerky, arrhythmic movements that randomly migrate from one muscle group to another. May be unilateral. Movements tend to involve the limbs, tongue, and mouth more than other areas. Almost never synchronous.	Focal: repetitive and rhythmic jerks. Multifocal: lightening fast movements that can involve multiple muscle groups and move from one part of the body to another. May be synchronous.
Intent	Purposeless	Purposeless. Patient may consciously integrate the jerk into a willed movement	Purposeless
Voluntary inhibition	Possible for brief periods	Rare	None
Sleep	Improves markedly or disappears	Improves markedly or disappears	Slight or no improvement
Stress or startle	May worsen	No change	May worsen
Level of consciousness		Alert or obtunded	Alert or obtunded or comatose
Associated neurological problems	Compulsive behaviors, Attention deficit, learning disabilities, echolalia, coprolali	Hypotonia, mild, encephalopathic changes	Focal: none or mild encephalopathic changes Multifocal: often evidence of acute or chronic, severe diffuse brain dysfunction
EEG	Normal or background slowing unrelated to the movements	Normal slow or epileptiform but unrelated to the movements	Slow or epileptiform. Spikes can occasionally be linked to the movement.
Brain scan	Normal	Normal or hypodense areas in the corpus striatum or subthalamic region	Often normal. Acute: occasionally evidence of cerebral edema. Chronic: occasional evidence of diffuse atrophy.
Treatment	Haloperodol, clonidine, or other antipychotics such as respiridone	Benzodiazepines, haloperidol	Antiepileptics, especially clonazepam, zonisamide

are associated. Multifocal myoclonus is more likely to occur in patients who have progressive degenerative disease of the brain or who have an acute encephalopathy. Acute chorea can occur with metabolic disorders but is more likely to be seen as the patient recovers from an encephalopathic illness. It also occurs as a sequel to beta-hemolytic streptococcal infections (Sydenham's chorea) (68) and as a result of drug ingestions or head trauma. Lupus erythematosus can be associated with unilateral or bilateral chorea, as can the antiphospholipid syndrome (69). Mass lesions or cerebrovascular accidents are more likely to produce a hemichorea. Usually this form of chorea is easily distinguished clinically from seizures. However, the EEG often fails to distinguish between diffuse chorea and multifocal myoclonus, as it is possible for both to occur in the presence of an EEG with slow background activity without epileptiform transients or with unrelated paroxysmal bursts. The presence of multifocal spikes throughout the record favors the diagnosis of myoclonus, especially when the spike is linked to the jerk. Both types of movements may respond favorably to clonazepam. Chorea may also respond to dopaminergic blockers such as haloperidol or pimozide or drugs that deplete dopamine such as tetrabenazine.

Tics. Tics are rarely mistaken for myoclonus. They usually involve only one or, at most, several muscle groups, and only in the most severe cases are they migratory (70, 71). The movements are usually repetitive and stereotyped. Tics occur sometime during childhood in approximately 20% of the pediatric population, but they are usually "simple" in that they are always characterized by the same movement involving only one or two muscle groups. The face and neck muscles are most commonly involved, but a simple tic can involve muscles of respiration and the extremities. Eye blinking, facial twitches, shrugging of the shoulders, head turning, sniffing, grunting, and repetitive clearing of one's throat are common forms of simple tics. In some children, simple tics may be caused or worsened by anxiety or stress. If left alone, most simple tics subside within weeks to months, although they sometimes recur for another brief period of time. The EEG is usually normal and has no epileptiform activity. Multiple types of tics or tics that involve quite complicated movements of a number of muscle groups are known as complex tics. When they are chronically associated with vocal tics, the diagnosis of Gilles de la Tourette's syndrome can be made. This is an organic brain disorder with a definite genetic component. It is inherited as an autosomal dominant with variable penetrance and variable expression. There is a much higher family incidence of simple and complex tics in relatives of these children when compared with the general population (72). Based on response to therapy, the syndrome may be the result of abnormal metabolism of dopamine in the brain. Although the disorder may stabilize or improve slightly in adolescence or early adult life, it fluctuates in childhood and can be sufficiently severe to modify normal activity. If so, it needs to be treated. The movements usually respond to small amounts of neuroleptics such as respiridone or olanzapine or to alpha blockers such as clonidine (73). Both tics and chorea can be associated with each other and with neuropsychiatric disorders, particularly obsessive compulsive disease. When this is seen following clinically apparent streptococcal infections or with high antistreptolysin-O (ASO titers), it is known as the PANDAS syndrome (74).

Ocular Movements

Paroxysmal Upgaze Deviation. Episodic upgaze is a feature of the oculogyric crisis and is usually part of a dystonic reaction to medications such as phenothiazines, carbamazepine, and lithium (75). Tonic upgaze is sometimes a transient event in neonates. Tonic upward deviation of the eyes has been observed in patients with Chédiak-Higashi disease, Rett's and Tourette's syndromes, and Wilson's disease.

Spasmus Nutans. Classically, spasmus nutans consists of a triad of signs: nystagmus, head nodding, and a head tilt (76). Head nodding and intermittent nystagmus are often the first abnormalities noted by the parents. The nystagmoid movements are often more pronounced in one eye than in the other and frequently lack a quick and slow component. Both symptoms can fluctuate in intensity and may come and go during the course of the day, resulting in some confusion as to whether the infant is having seizures. Infants with spasmus nutans have a somewhat higher incidence of EEG abnormalities than other children their age, but they are alert, in contact with the environment, and no more likely to develop epilepsy than the average child. The pathophysiology of spasmus nutans is not known. A small subgroup of these infants have mass lesions in the area of the optic chiasm or anterior third ventricle. A child who is diagnosed as having spasmus nutans should have an MRI scan. If the scan is normal, no further treatment is necessary. The majority of children with this disorder no longer have signs by 5 years of age; however, some may have nystagmoid eye movements that persist into adult life, and these children cannot be differentiated from those who have congenital nystagmus.

Opsoclonus (77). Opsoclonus-myoclonus syndrome is the presenting sign of 2% of children with neuroblastoma and ganglioneuroblastoma. The majority of patients with opsoclonus-myoclonus have a neuroblastoma. There are also reports of delayed onset opsoclonus-myoclonus syndrome and development of opsoclonus-myoclonus syndrome in the face of recurrent disease. The presence of opsoclonus-myoclonus syndrome is typically associated with a good prognosis for treatment of the tumor and long-term survival. It is believed to be of autoimmune etiology, as supported by identification of antineural protein antibodies in patients who have the disorder (78). It is believed that the precipitation of opsoclonus-myoclonus by certain viruses, such as coxsackie, Epstein-Barr virus, mumps, and rubella, occur as a result of molecular mimicry. Patients with opsoclonus-myoclonus syndrome have responded to immunomodulatory treatments such as steroids and intravenous immunoglobulin or plasmapheresis (79). The majority of children with opsoclonus-myoclonus syndrome have multiple relapses that require prolonged treatment. Developmental sequelae are frequent (80).

TABLE 10-4
Causes of Sudden Loss of Posture

Generalized epilepsy
Syncope
Basilar migraine
Basilar insufficiency
Cataplexy
Compression of the upper cervical cord
Hyperventilation syndrome
Vestibular disorders
Psychogenic illness: hysteria, malingering

Loss of Tone or Consciousness

Attention Deficits and Daydreaming. Children with typical absence seizures have brief episodes in which their activity suddenly ceases and there is a brief loss of contact with the environment. Posture is maintained. Automatisms can occur, but they are unusual. Normal activity is usually resumed immediately. Atypical attacks are more indicative of complex partial seizures, during which the episodes last longer, automatisms are more common, incontinence can occur, and the child may be sleepy at the end of the seizure. Few problems mimic absence or complex partial seizures. The most common is daydreaming (81).

Daydreaming is a common occurrence in children who have attention deficit disorders. They can be unaware of their immediate surroundings for a few seconds or as long as a minute. They may not react to voice or visual stimuli, but generally, they respond to touch. They may have no recollection of what transpired around them during the time their thoughts were elsewhere, but often they say they were thinking of something else at the time. Automatisms are rare, but some children have nervous habits such as picking at their nails or rubbing their hands, and these may continue while they stare ahead. The history can sometimes differentiate between daydreaming and absence seizures. Children who daydream never interrupt their own public recitations to stare ahead and lose track of time. A child who stops speaking in the middle of a sentence and has an episode of absence almost invariably has a seizure disorder. In some instances, video-EEG analysis of the spells is needed to arrive at the correct diagnosis (81).

Drop Attacks. One form of generalized epilepsy only involves sudden loss of tone (82). There may not be a recognizable loss of consciousness. These attacks must be distinguished from other disorders that produce a similar clinical picture. Some of the causes of sudden drop attacks are listed in Table 10-4.

These episodes can occur at any age but are more likely to be confused with epilepsy in later childhood and adolescence. Many disorders in which posture is suddenly lost are much more common in elderly patients. Certainly, this is true of basilar insufficiency and the peculiar vestibular disorders that suddenly throw people to the ground. Cataplexy is also much more likely to occur in adults. Compression of the upper cervical cord that presents with sudden drop attacks is exceedingly rare at any age. Basilar insufficiency and cervical cord compression are often associated with ictal and interictal neurologic signs that point to an insult of the brainstem or the cord. Hyperventilation leading to a loss of tone and consciousness can easily be recognized by observing the attack, and the patient or family often give a history of a period of intense overbreathing preceding the loss of posture and consciousness. An adolescent hysteric has many other symptoms of an emotional disorder that help to make the diagnosis. The malingerer may not fall abruptly and when "unconscious" may resist the limbs or eyelids being moved. The ultimate diagnosis of psychogenic drop attacks may depend on recording the attack with EEG telemetry. The three diagnoses that are most often confused with recurrent postural seizures in children and adolescents are syncope, narcolepsy or cataplexy, and basilar migraine. The latter two problems are relatively rare in the pediatric population, whereas syncope is a common event at all ages.

Syncope. Most syncopal episodes in children are neurally mediated (83) (Table 10-5). There is reflex slowing of the heart producing a sinus bradycardia or a significant drop in systolic and, to a lesser degree, diastolic blood pressure, or both. This may be precipitated by well-defined physical events that overactivate the autonomic nervous

TABLE 10-5
Causes of Syncope

A. Secondary to known precipitating events
  1. Neurocardiogenic
    a. Vasovagal
      1. Fear
      2. Pain
      3. Unpleasant sights (situational)
    b. Reflex
      1. Cough
      2. Micturition
      3. Swallowing
      4. Carotid sinus pressure
  2. Decreased venous return
    a. Orthostatic (with change to an erect position)
    b. Soldier's syncope (standing at attention)
    c. With Valsalva's maneuver
  3. Hypovolemia or severe anemia

B. No clear precipitating event by history
  1. Cardiac
    a. Arrhythmia
    b. Obstructive outflow
  2. Cerebrovascular insufficiency
  3. Psychogenic with or without hyperventilation
  4. No known cause

system, especially the parasympathetic division. Coughing, micturition, swallowing, and carotid sinus pressure are among the more common reflex causes of neurogenic syncope. Vasovagal syncope is also neurogenic, but the physical stimuli are less well defined and include such sensations as heat, pain, and fear. The physiologic basis for neurogenic syncope is yet to be defined completely. Venous pooling may activate cardiac stretch receptors, which leads to reflex bradycardia and a drop in peripheral vascular resistance (84, 85). A second major cause of syncope in children results from decreased blood volume or decreased return of venous blood to the heart.

The majority of syncopal events that are neurogenic in origin or due to decreased blood volume or venous return can be diagnosed by clinical history even if the decrease in blood flow to the brain is sufficiently severe or prolonged to result in seizure activity shortly after the loss of consciousness (86). Most of these children faint in response to one or more limited provocations, that is, micturition, the sight of blood, or a warm, crowded environment, or, in the case of decreased venous return, assumption of upright posture or prolonged standing (87). Many patients realize they are going to faint before losing consciousness. Nausea or vague epigastric sensations are experienced by patients with either syncope or seizures (88). However, other warning signs differ. Patients suffering from syncope are more likely to feel light-headed or dizzy than they are to complain of vertigo. Their visual sensations are also more simple than the visual auras of epileptic children. Vision begins to dim and objects lose their color, becoming gray or brown. Brief syncopal episodes are almost never followed by confusion lasting more than seconds after arousal. Drowsiness is less common after a syncopal episode than a seizure and is almost always less prolonged. After an ictal event, a deep sleep from which the patient can hardly be aroused suggests a seizure. Headache may also follow a brief syncope or a seizure, but it is usually more severe after the latter. Unfortunately, if the syncope is prolonged (lasting minutes) and is severe and the brain is deprived of oxygen for a relatively long period of time, the postictal signs of syncope and seizures may be indistinguishable, or the faint may lead to a seizure.

Of course, the most serious causes of syncope are cardiac, and they often occur without warning and produce significant brain hypoxia, which may result in a confused child after consciousness returns. Disorders of cardiac conduction, particularly the long QT syndrome, are the most common cause of this type of syncope (89, 90). Rarely, lesions of the brainstem or upper cord can cause transient cardiac arrhythmias or arrest. Because cardiogenic syncope can sometimes result in sudden death, it is this group of disorders that must be eliminated as a possible cause of fainting when children repeatedly lose consciousness. One clue to a cardiac cause for syncope is that a child faints while exercising (91). Neurogenic syncope can also occur with exercise, but the proportion of children who have cardiac conduction disorders or reduced cardiac output is greater in the group that faints during exercise than in children who faint at rest.

The physical examination may be of little help in distinguishing syncope from seizures because it is often normal in patients with either symptom, although seizures are more likely to be associated with signs of CNS injury. At the time of the event, pallor, sweating, a slow pulse, and low blood pressure are more suggestive of syncope than a seizure (86). At times, the cause of syncope can be suspected by obtaining supine blood pressure and noting its change when the child rapidly assumes the standing position. In normal children, the blood pressure remains stable (± 5 points) or transiently increases slightly with an increase in the pulse rate of 8 to 20 beats. A drop in blood pressure of 15 or more points or a sinus bradycardia when rapidly standing confirms the history of possible orthostatic hypotension. Auscultation of the heart may also assist in the diagnosis. An irregular rhythm or a murmur may suggest that a cardiac abnormality is the cause of the faint. Provocative office tests such as carotid sinus massage and ocular pressure are not recommended and are rarely informative in children.

The laboratory evaluation of children who faint has become a complicated and argumentative issue regardless of age (92). In the absence of a suspicious history or neurologic findings, an interictal EEG does not differentiate syncope from seizures even if there are paroxysmal transients in the tracing. Neuroimaging is almost always negative unless there are abnormalities on examination. An unexplained episode of fainting mandates an electrocardiogram (ECG). If repeated episodes of fainting have occurred with a typical history, we still obtain a routine 12-channel ECG as the initial study. Further testing may be indicated if the timing of the fainting suggests possible hypoglycemia. If there is no history of a provocative event or an aura, a more extensive cardiac evaluation is indicated if the syncope is repeated. This may include prolonged ambulatory recording of the ECG, stress testing, and possibly an echocardiogram. These are expensive and stressful tests, and their yield, even in high risk patients by history, is probably less than 20% of those tested (93).

Should children suspected of having syncope undergo tilt-table testing, and at what point should such a test be attempted? Studies in pediatric patients and young adults thought to have neurocardiogenic syncope show that they have a statistically significant increase in either bradycardia, systolic hypotension, or asystole with head-up tilting for up to 60 minutes when compared with asymptomatic controls. Drugs such as isoproterenol increase the rate of positive responses and further separate the two groups (94). However, there are still many false positives in the control group and 10% to 15% false negatives in the neurocardiogenic group. Furthermore, positive responses in another group of young adults could only be reproduced 54.5% of the time (95). It is not likely that a head-up tilt test has any more relevance to differentiating syncope from seizures than the EEG. Furthermore, tilt-table testing rarely adds useful information for patients who have a good history to suggest neurocardiogenic syncope (96). This leaves those children who have recurrent syncope without a definable cause, especially if it occurs during exercise. Most of these patients will have neurocardiogenic syncope. In this group a positive response to the head-up tilt test may establish the diagnosis and eliminate the need for further expensive tests. Hence, if a routine ECG and echocardiogram, ambulatory monitoring, and an exercise tolerance test fail to establish the diagnosis, a positive head-up tilt test might suggest appropriate therapy and allow the gradual resumption of full activity by the child. That would be particularly important for children who are interested in resuming competitive sports. A detailed study of the evaluation of syncope, irrespective of age, has been published by the American Heart Association (97).

Narcolepsy and Cataplexy. Children who have cataplexy suddenly drop to the ground with bilateral loss of muscle tone in response to an unexpected touch or emotional stimulus such as laughter. The attacks are brief, and it is not clear if some patients lose consciousness during them, but that is unlikely. Most children with cataplexy also suffer from narcolepsy, a state of excessive daytime drowsiness punctuated by periods during which the patient rapidly falls asleep, frequently under unusual circumstances such as while engaged in conversation (98). This sometimes leads to confusing narcoleptic attacks with episodes of absence, or subliminal status, although the narcoleptic patient appears to be in a state of normal sleep and continues to sleep for many minutes unless aroused by an external stimulus. In addition to cataplexy and narcolepsy, the narcoleptic syndrome includes transient episodes of inability to move when awakening (sleep paralysis) and brief hallucinatory episodes on arousal, which are usually visual. The four components of the syndrome do not appear simultaneously, and some may never occur in a narcoleptic patient. Narcolepsy and cataplexy are the two that are most commonly associated. These four phenomena are consistent with features of REM sleep, in the waking state, probably as a result of yet undescribed defects in the reticular activating system.

The EEG clearly differentiates between cataplexy and narcolepsy and a tonic or absence seizure if recorded during an attack. In the interictal period, a multiple sleep latency test using the EEG can be helpful. The child is allowed to go to sleep on five different occasions during the day. If REM sleep occurs within 10 minutes of the onset of sleep on two of these occasions, the tracing is compatible with the diagnosis of narcolepsy. The HLA-DR2 haplotype has a high degree of association with the syndrome and may be helpful in making a diagnosis. Reduced hypocretin (orexin A) is found in the spinal fluid. The symptoms of narcolepsy can sometimes be ameliorated by the use of stimulant drugs such as modafanil, and cataplexy by antidepressant drugs such as fluoxetine (99) or rarely by an antiepileptic, carbamazepine (100).

Basilar Migraine. The basilar variant of migraine generally begins in adolescence but may occur in children in the first years of life (101, 102). It is more common in females. Some attacks begin with sudden loss of consciousness and posture. Upon recovery, the child often experiences a severe occipital or vertex headache; however, most patients have symptoms of other abnormalities of brainstem function such as dizziness or vertigo or bilateral visual loss. Diplopia, dysarthria, and bilateral paresthesias occur less often. Frequently, there is a family history of migraine. Close relatives may have had similar attacks. Up to one-third of children with basilar migraine have paroxysmal interictal EEGs, some with occipital spike and wave complexes (103). A diagnosis must be made on clinical grounds. Many children with basilar migraine respond to antiepileptic drugs, and others respond to agents that block the transport of calcium into the cell.

Disorders of Respiration

Apnea. Sudden apneic attacks that occur when the infant is awake are even more likely to be thought of as possible seizures, especially if the infant also suddenly develops a fixed stare or begins to flail about (104). However, these kinds of attacks are exactly what one sees with some infants who have gastroesophageal reflux (105). Each of these signs—apnea, staring, and flailing—may occur alone or in combination. Of the three, episodic apnea is the most frequent sign of reflux. The problem is the result of incompetence of the upper and lower esophageal sphincters, which leads to the reflux and sometimes to the aspiration of stomach contents. This occurs most often when infants are in a flat position just after they are fed. The flailing movements are generally thought to be a response to esophageal pain resulting from the acidic refluxed stomach contents. The episodes are not associated with EEG abnormalities. Proof of reflux is often difficult to obtain, although in many infants it can be seen during a barium swallow. Lesser degrees of reflux can, at times, be diagnosed by the use of radioisotopes or the measurement of esophageal pH. The presence of reflux does not necessarily mean that the physician has found the cause of the child's symptoms unless the disorder coincides with the time of reflux. The presence of significant reflux in a symptomatic infant is sufficient reason to start therapy. Treatment usually involves positioning the baby in a more upright posture after feeding, thickening feedings, and finally, in rare instances, fundoplication (106). Video-EEG studies may be needed to prove an apneic attack is a form of epilepsy.

Breath-Holding. Breath-holding also involves attacks of respiratory arrest that can be mistaken for seizures, but the episodes occur in a very different setting (107). There are two forms of breath-holding spells: pallid and cyanotic. Cyanotic spells were the first to be described. They usually peak in the second or third year of life. Almost invariably, the child has been frightened or frustrated or has had a minor injury and begins to cry vigorously. Then the child suddenly stops breathing, often on inspiration. After several seconds, the child turns blue and loses consciousness. The child is often limp at this time. The period of unconsciousness is brief, usually lasting less than 1 minute, although it can be more prolonged. When the child regains consciousness, he or she is alert and frequently resumes normal activities immediately. Pallid breath-holding attacks often follow minor trauma and actually represent vasovagal episodes. Crying is minimal or absent. The child quickly loses consciousness and is limp. The attacks last more than 1 minute and may result in a seizure caused by cerebral ischemia (108).

Both cyanotic and pallid forms of breath-holding result from reflex changes that decrease cerebral blood flow. The exact mechanism may vary from one child to another. If there is a reflex cessation of respiration in inspiration, venous return to the thorax may be decreased, resulting in a decreased cardiac output. Children with pallid spells experience changes in heart rate and rhythm and a decrease in blood pressure.

Neither type of breath-holding attack is accompanied by an epileptic EEG discharge. These attacks are not associated with an increased incidence of epileptic seizures later in life, even if generalized clonic jerks occur secondarily during the attack. The diagnosis is usually made by the history. Breath-holding attacks usually occur less than two to three times a month in susceptible children, and the episodes invariably cease by 5 to 6 years of age. Occasionally children have pallid attacks that occur several times a week or even daily. The frequency of the episodes in these children may sometimes be reduced with the use of atropine-like agents or iron supplementation, but the optimal treatment is behavioral modification directed at reducing the parents' emotional reactions to the episodes. Pallid attacks that are associated with severe bradycardia or asystole have been successfully treated with implantation of a cardiac pacemaker (109). Recently, it has been suggested that severe breath-holding spells may be inherited as an autosomal dominant trait with variable penetrance (110).

Hyperventilation. Hyperventilation is defined as physiologically inappropriate overbreathing (111). Acute hyperventilation is often associated with a feeling of intense anxiety or even panic. Patients may feel they are suffocating or choking during the attack. Other symptoms of acute anxiety may occur, including dry mouth, globus hystericus, chest pain, palpitations, and tachycardia. If the patient becomes severely alkalotic, he may complain of headache, tinnitus, dizziness or vertigo, tingling of the face and hands, or carpopedal spasm. The patient may lose consciousness. This may be followed by a generalized seizure. The diagnosis is usually made by the history of symptoms and signs that precede the loss of consciousness. In the past, the diagnosis was assumed confirmed if (1) the attack were seen and aborted by having the patient rebreathe into a paper bag, and (2) the symptoms could be reproduced by the hyperventilation provocation test. Recently, however, studies have shown that patients' symptoms may have nothing to do with their P_{CO_2}. Hyperventilation may be a consequence and not a cause of these attacks (112).

Perceptual Disturbances

Hallucinations. Hallucinatory episodes can be an aura to an ictus or less frequently or ictal event. However, hallucinatory experiences can be seen with psychoses and with extreme stress in nonpsychotic children (113). They also may result from drugs, particularly antiepileptics (114, 115). Episodes can be visual, auditory or, less often, sensory. The history is essential to the diagnosis. An EEG taken during the event is also helpful.

Headache and Other Pains. Headache is often seen following a generalized motor seizure. Less frequently it occurs as an aura before a complex partial seizure (116). Ictal pain is usually unilateral; it occurs most often in the arm, and it may be the only manifestation of a seizure (117). The focus is often in the contralateral rolandic area. Headache may be the only symptom of a partial seizure, although this is extremely rare. Children who have this type of headache often have signs of cerebral injury, do not get relief from sleep, and do not have a family history of migraine (118).

Paroxysmal recurrent headaches are characteristic of migraine. When children with migraine headaches have an aura, it usually is visual. A migrainous aura is usually made up of loss of part of a visual field or of simple lines or dots that are black and white. Visual phenomena more often associated with epilepsy consist of changes in the size or shape of objects or the intrusion of colored objects. Less common migrainous auras are loss of motor, speech, or sensory function. The headaches are apt to be throbbing and are sometimes unilateral. They are often relieved by a brief period of sleep. They are frequently associated with gastrointestinal disturbances. There is a strong history of migraine in the immediate family in more than half of the patients.

Epilepsy and migraine coexist in many children. Between 3% and 7% of children with migraine have epilepsy. Most have partial seizures. Benign occipital and rolandic seizures are frequently associated with migraine (119). A large percentage of migraineurs (perhaps as high as 20%) have interictal records that are paroxysmal even though they have no seizures. Approximately 60% of children who have migraine headaches obtain significant relief with antiepileptic medication (120). Because migraine occurs in 4% to 12% of children, depending on age, and epilepsy occurs in less than 1%, the most recurrent paroxysmal headaches are likely to be migrainous, even in those children who have complex partial seizures. Furthermore, migraine headaches can be clinically defined by their associated symptoms and family history. The distinction between migraine and epilepsy is made more difficult by the fact that a migrainous aura may not be followed by headache (acephalgic migraine). In addition, several paroxysmal events that occur in children such as recurrent episodes of abdominal pain or vomiting, vertigo, confusion, and alternating hemiplegia may be followed by migraine, not epilepsy, later in life (121).

The criteria for diagnosing an isolated headache as an ictal event should rely heavily on recording a paroxysmal change in the EEG taken at the time of the episode.

Recurrent abdominal pain (122), usually periumbilical, with or without vomiting, pallor, or an idiopathic fever, can be caused by migraine and perhaps, in rare cases, by epilepsy. Most children who have this problem do not have either disorder. Children with recurrent abdominal pain frequently see a physician to rule out epilepsy. The range of interictal paroxysmal EEGs in children with this syndrome is 7% to 76% in different series. Approximately 15% of these children do have epileptic seizures, and more than 40% have recurrent headaches. Approximately 20% have a family history of migraine. Even those children who have other epileptic seizures do not generally have isolated abdominal pain that is epileptic in origin. Children with abdominal pain usually do not respond to antiepileptic drugs, but approximately 20%, in our experience, do respond to antimigrainous drugs such as beta blockers or tricyclic antidepressants. Children with recurrent abdominal pain who do not have other seizures at the time they first present are unlikely to develop epilepsy. However, they are at greater risk for developing migraine later in life (123). In the majority, the attacks recede and are infrequent or have disappeared by the end of puberty. This is another pain syndrome in which the few cases that have been definitely diagnosed as the result of epilepsy have had EEG recordings at the time of the attack. The tracing becomes paroxysmal coincident with the onset of clinical symptoms.

Vertigo and Ataxia

Benign Paroxysmal Vertigo. Sudden or repeated attacks of dysequilibrium in children are sometimes confused with epilepsy. Children with benign paroxysmal vertigo (124) have repeated attacks of vertigo lasting minutes to hours. These episodes can occur as often two or three times a week, but many children have only one attack every 2 to 3 months. The onset is sudden. During the attack, the child is often unable to walk unaided and may be nauseated. Nystagmus need not be present. There is no hearing loss or tinnitus. The child is alert, responsive, and distressed. Interictally, the examination and the EEG are normal. There is no change in the audiogram. Caloric tests of vestibular function are usually normal, but a minority of children have evidence of canal paresis indicating dysfunction of the vestibular end organ in the ear.

Many of these children have a family history of migraine, and some already have migraine headaches. They may have a directional preponderance to their nystagmus on testing. A substantial number develop migraine later in life. The association between these attacks of vertigo in childhood and migraine is so strong that some have defined benign paroxysmal vertigo as a migraine variant. No treatment is indicated. The attacks do not seem to respond to either antiepileptic or antimigrainous medicines. The disorder usually subsides by 6 to 8 years of age. The term benign paroxysmal vertigo is also used to describe positional vertigo in adults. This disorder is associated with positional nystagmus and appears to be labyrinthine in origin (125).

Vestibulocerebellar Ataxia. There are several forms of paroxysmal ataxia that may be mistaken for a seizure. One form is associated with nystagmus, but tests of the semicircular canals are normal. The disorder frequently responds to acetazolamide. It is an autosomal dominant disorder that has been mapped to chromosome 19p (126). In other families, similar symptoms and signs start in adult life and do not localize to chromosome 19p (127). These patients often do not respond to acetazolamide. In both disorders, the patients remain oriented and there is no other history to suggest seizures.

Behavioral Disorders

Stereotyped Movements. Stereotyped movements are patterned repetitive movements that recur frequently, often many times each day, in the same form (128, 129). These movements can be seen in normal children but are much more common in children who are mentally retarded or autistic. Head banging, head rolling, and body rocking often occur when the older infant or child is awake. Head banging is often part of a temper tantrum. Head rolling and body rocking are forms of self-stimulation that seem to result in pleasurable sensations. Flapping the hands or arms is a movement that also seems to relieve anxiety. The normal infant or child may stop these repetitive movements if touched or diverted by other stimuli. None of these behaviors have any direct association with future epileptic attacks, and they occur without a significant change in the EEG (when it is technically possible to record the patient). They are more apt to occur in irritable, excessively active, or retarded children. The movements decline rapidly toward the end of the second year of life. No treatment is necessary unless they persist until the child is 30 to 36 months of age. At that time, the movements may be reduced by behavioral modification techniques. There is no specific drug that is effective in treating these disorders without producing significant sedation, although recently it has been suggested, on the basis of a small series, that clomipramine may reduce the movements (130).

Masturbation. Infants who are masturbating are usually sitting with their legs held tightly together, sometimes straddling the bars of their crib or playpen, rocking back and forth (131, 132). The behavior can almost always be aborted by a distracting stimulus and usually disappears spontaneously in several months. Masturbatory movements in older children are less likely to be confused with seizure activity. They usually lay prone on a flat surface such as a rug or bed and rub their genitals back and forth against the fibers. The children are alert and usually stop on command. Furthermore, they can demonstrate the movements when requested to do so. What the parents usually mistake as the seizure is the detached look and lack of responsiveness that the children get during the period of climax. The history preceding the climax makes the diagnosis. At times, home video or EEG documentation of these events may allow the physician to determine the nature of the behavior (133).

Acute Confusion. Episodic confusion is not usually seen in children unless accompanied by other signs of acute disease such as fever, vomiting, or obtundation. Metabolic disorders that produce recurrent episodes of ketosis, acidosis, hypoglycemia, or hyperammonemia can also be the cause of recurrent confusional states. Children who have this problem should be screened for a metabolic disorder or drug ingestion (see Table 10-1).

Repeated attacks of confusion, usually associated with delirium, may also occur in children with migraine (134, 135). There is often no associated headache, and there is no clinical or laboratory evidence of an infection or a metabolic disturbance. There may be a history of recent trauma. The attack lasts for hours but is almost always over within a day. There is usually a family history of migraine, and the patient may have had typical migraine headaches on other occasions. Confusional migraine is much more likely to occur in adolescence than in the first decade of life. Periods of confusion can be seen with complex parietal and absence seizures without ictal motor behaviors (136). Nonconvulsive status epilepticus may present as an acute confusional state at any age and can only be diagnosed by the EEG (137).

Panic or Fear. Ictal fear is usually a brief event and often precedes or is accompanied by other evidence of a complex partial seizure (138). It is not related to provocation and can be overwhelming. Panic attacks can occur as an acute event during the course of a more chronic anxiety disorder or in patients who are depressed or schizophrenic, but they can also occur in the absence of an underlying emotional disorder. Ictal fear begins in childhood.

Panic attacks last minutes to hours and are accompanied by many symptoms such as palpitations, sweating, dizziness or vertigo, and feelings of unreality or loss of control. The frequency of panic attacks increases in late adolescence and adult life. These symptoms are less prominent with ictal or preictal fear. Ictal fear is also more likely to be associated with repeated, stereotyped behaviors with each attack. Only an EEG at the time of the attack differentiates ictal fear from a nonepileptic panic attack if the history is not clear. Recent studies suggest that individuals who do not have seizures but do suffer from panic disorder may also have excessive neuronal activity in the frontotemporal region. Nonictal panic does not respond to antiepileptic drugs. The underlying disorder must be treated with psychiatric care using cognitive therapy, which can be combined with drugs to modify mood or anxiety (138, 139).

Rage. Rage attacks (intermittent explosive disorder) (140) are not unusual in epileptic children, especially those who have frontal or temporal lobe lesions, but they are usually not part of the ictal event. Rage is also more common in hyperactive children and in others who have conduct, mood, or personality disorders. Ictal rage is unprovoked and not focused on a particular object or individual. Interictal rage or rage reactions without seizures usually occurs in response to frustration, stress, or threatening situations. It is not the only evidence of a behavioral problem. It is often preceded by a period of whining, screaming, and crying. The anger is frequently directed at the source. The child may remember the attack. Behavior can frequently be modified during the episode. The event can rarely be recorded by EEG because of artifact. This type of rage does not respond to antiepileptic drugs, with the possible exception of carbamazepine, and is best treated by behavior modification. Propranolol, antipsychotic, antidepressant, and mood stabilizing drugs may also help.

Pseudoseizures (Nonepileptic Seizures) (141). Pseudoseizures are psychogenic seizures defined as episodes that resemble an epileptic seizure but are unaccompanied by EEG abnormalities (142, 143). Such episodes are felt to be the symptom of a dissociative disorder. Implicit in the definition is the idea that individuals who have pseudoseizures do not consciously produce or control them and thus are not malingerers. The definition of a pseudoseizure has always been an uncomfortable one because a number of unusual symptoms that are presumed to be epileptic can occur without an abnormality on the scalp EEG. Pseudoseizures do not respond to antiepileptic drugs. At least 20% of those who have these nonepileptic seizures are children with true epilepsy that is often poorly controlled, which further complicates the differential diagnosis.

No particular behavior or movement before, during, or after the ictal state differentiates a seizure from a pseudoseizure. The onset of pseudoseizures often builds over minutes; the symptoms at the onset frequently suggest anxiety or a panic attack, that is, dyspnea, paresthesias, light-headedness, and palpitations; the ictal movements are often asymmetric and without rhythm, such as thrashing or flailing arm movements; the patient may scream or weep (144). There can be pelvic thrusting; unfortunately, similar movements and behaviors can be seen with seizures that arise deep in the frontal lobe. However, none of these may occur. A period of absence may still represent a psychologically determined event rather than epilepsy.

The diagnosis of pseudoseizures has been aided considerably in recent years by the development of techniques that allow the EEG to be recorded for long periods of time. EEG telemetry allows the patient's brain waves to be recorded during the episodes in question. The physician can also see and evaluate the clinical event. There are a number of clues that help distinguish seizures from pseudoseizures (Table 10-6), although none allow an absolute diagnosis. Pseudoseizures can sometimes be elicited by suggestion, usually by giving the patient a saline infusion (145). In our experience, this technique is not suitable for younger children or moderately to severely retarded patients. Photic stimulation or hyperventilation are more satisfactory to techniques for these populations. Suggestion may also induce true seizures in patients who have both pseudoseizures and epilepsy.

The separation of epileptic seizures from pseudoseizures is often difficult and expensive, requiring prolonged EEG recordings and possible hospitalization. However, the distinction is extremely important because pseudoseizures can be sometimes be treated effectively as an emotional disturbance, thus avoiding inappropriate antiepileptic drug administration.

SUMMARY

In this chapter we have presented some of the clinical conditions that can be mistaken for epilepsy or an isolated seizure in an infant, young child, or adolescent. The large number of these conditions that encompass motor function, respiration, sensory experience, and behavior, both when awake and asleep in all ages from infancy into adult life, is testimony to the variety of ways in which epilepsy can present. Many families are often perplexed by—or often ignore—unusual behaviors their

TABLE 10-6
Seizures and Pseudoseizures

	Epileptic Seizures	Pseudoseizures
Type of movement	Clonic jerks that are usually flexor, rhythmic, and in all involved extremities. Sudden drops to the ground.	Movements are often lateral, as well as flexor and extensor. Often out of phase in the involved limbs. Some movements have a tremor-like quality. Others are flailing. There are unusual movements such as pelvic thrusts, sudden drops to the ground
Automatisms	Simple, such as lip smacking, picking at clothes. Complex, such as dressing, undressing, walking in circles	Not usually seen or when noted, may not be stereotyped.
Consciousness	Usually out of contact with the environment	May be responsive during the attack
Language	Initial scream, groans, mumbling	Yelling and vulgar language sometimes occur
Incontinence	Frequent	Rare
Self-injury	Rare	Rare
Postictal confusion, headache, drowsiness	Frequent	Rare
Precipitating events	Can be present, specific stressful situations may increase seizure incidence	Incidence can be increased by specific stressful situations
Frequency	Usually single episodes	May occur in clusters
EEG		
Interictal	Often epileptiform transients	Often epileptiform transients
Ictal	Almost always a sudden, paroxysmal discharge, coincident with the attack	No paroxysmal changes
Elevated prolactin after ictus	Yes, but normal levels do not rule out a true seizure (146)	No
Response to antiepileptics	Usually	Rare. There may be a placebo effect.

child is experiencing and postpone seeing a physician because their notion of epilepsy involves a sudden fall to the ground with stiffening and jerking of the limbs. It is important to recognize how many experiences that are out of the normal flow of events during the day or during sleep can be epileptic and how many nonepileptic disorders can mimic those events and confuse the physician.

References

1. Tharp BR. An overview of pediatric seizure disorders and epileptic syndromes. *Epilepsia* 1987; 28 Suppl:36–45.
2. Arnold ST, Dodson WE. Epilepsy in children. *Baillieres Clin Neurol* 1996; 5:783–802.
3. Mizrahi E. Acute and chronic effects of seizures in the developing brain: lessons from clinical experience. *Epilepsia* 1999; 40 Suppl 1:42–50.
4. Arpino C. Prenatal and perinatal determinants of neonatal seizures occurring in the first week of life. *J Child Neurol* 2001; 9:651–656.
5. Lombroso CT. Neonatal seizures: a clinician's overview. *Brain Dev* 1996; 18:1–28.
6. Tekgul H, Gauvreau K, Soul J, et al. The current etiologic profile and neurodevelopmental outcome of seizures in term newborn infants. *Pediatrics* 2006; 7 Suppl 4:1270–1280.
7. Gospe SM Jr. Pyridoxine-dependent seizures: new genetic and biochemical clues to help with diagnosis and treatment. *Curr Opin Neurol* 2006; 2:148–153.
8. Cowan F. Does cranial ultrasound indentify arterial cerebral infarction in term neonates? *Arch Dis Child Fetal Neonatal Ed* 2005; 6:2252–2256.
9. Kieker W. MRI for the management of neonatal cerebral infarction: importance of timing. *Childs Nerv Syst* 2004; 20:742–748.
10. Hirtz D, Ashwal S, Berg D, et al. Practice parameter: evaluating a first nonfebrile seizure in children: report of the quality standards subcommittee of the American Academy of Neurology, the Child Neurology Society, and the American Epilepsy Society. *Neurology* 2000; 55:616–623.

11. Sharma S, Riviello JJ, Harper MB, et al. The role of emergent neuroimaging in children with new-onset afebrile seizures. *Pediatrics* 2003; 111:1–5.
12. Wang D, Pascual JM, Yang H, et al. Glut-1 deficiency syndrome: clinical, genetic, and therapeutic aspects. *Ann Neurol* 2005; 57:111–118.
13. Ramaekers VT, Blau N. Cerebral folate deficiency. *Dev Med Child Neurol* 2004; 46:843–851.
14. Pedley TA. Differential diagnosis of episodic symptoms. *Epilepsia* 1983; 24 Suppl: 31–44.
15. Rothner AD. Not everything that shakes is epilepsy. *Cleve Clin J Med* 1989; 56 Suppl 2:206–213.
16. Williams J, Grant M, Jackson M, et al. Behavioral descriptors that differentiate between seizure and nonseizure events in a pediatric population. *Clin Pediatr* 1996; 35:243–249.
17. Fejerman N. Nonepileptic disorders imitating generalized idiopathic epilepsies. *Epilepsia* 2005; 46 Suppl 9:80–83.
18. Montagna P. Sleep-related non epileptic motor disorders. *J Neurol* 2004; 251:781–794.
19. Turanli G, Senbil N, Altunbasak S, et al. Benign neonatal sleep myoclonus mimicking status epilepticus. *J Child Neurol* 2004; 19:62–63.
20. Ramelli GP, Sozzo AB, Vella S, et al. Benign neonatal sleep myoclonus: an under-recognized, non-epileptic condition. *Acta Paediatr* 2005; 94:962–963.
21. Dyken ME, Rodnitzky RL. Periodic, aperiodic, and rhythmic motor disorders of sleep. *Neurology* 1992; 42 7 Suppl 6:68–74.
22. Dyken ME, Lin-Dyken DC, Yamada T. Diagnosing rhythmic motor movement disorder with video-poly-somnography. *Pediatr Neurol* 1997; 16:37–41.
23. Mendelson WB. Are periodic leg movements associated with clinical sleep disturbance? *Sleep* 1996; 19:219–223.
24. Meierkord H, Fish DR, Smith SJM, et al. Is nocturnal paroxysmal dystonia a form of frontal lobe epilepsy? *Mov Disord* 1992; 7:38–42.
25. Provini F, Plazzi G, Lugaresi E. From nocturnal paroxysmal dystonia to nocturnal frontal lobe epilepsy. *Clin Neurophysiol* 2000; 111 Suppl 2:S2–S8.
26. Watanabe K, Hara K, Hakamada S, et al. Seizures with apnea in children. *Pediatrics* 1982; 79:87–90.
27. Donati F, Schaffler L, Vassella F. Prolonged epileptic apneas in a newborn: a case report with ictal EEG recording. *Neuropediatrics* 1995; 26:223–225.
28. Thach BT. Sleep apnea in infancy and childhood. *Med Clin North Am* 1985; 69: 1289–1315.
29. Katz-Salamon M. Delayed chemoreceptor responses in infants with apnoea. *Arch Dis Child* 2004; 89:261–266.
30. Guilleminault C, Pelayo R, Leger D, et al. Recognition of sleep-disordered breathing in children. *Pediatrics* 1996; 98:871–882.
31. Goldstein NA, Pugazhendhi V, Rao SM, et al. Clinical assessment of pediatric obstructive sleep apnea. *Pediatrics* 2004; 114:33–34.
32. Yglesias A, Narbona J, Vanaclocha V, et al. Chiari type I malformation, glossopharyngeal neuralgia and central sleep apnoea in a child. *Dev Med Child Neurol* 1996; 38:1126–1130.
33. Kahn A, Groswasser J, Sottiaux M, et al. Mechanisms of obstructive sleep apneas in infants. *Biol Neonate* 1994; 65:235–239.
34. Deutsch ES. Tonsillectomy and adenoidectomy. Changing indications. *Pediatr Clin North Am* 1996; 43:1319–1338.
35. Halbower AC, Mahone ME. Neuropsychological morbidity linked to childhood sleep-disordered breathing. *Sleep Med Rev* 2006; 10:97–107.
36. Schenck CH, Mahowald MW. Parasomnias. Managing bizarre sleep-related behavior disorders. *Postgrad Med* 2000; 107:145–156.
37. Guilleminault C, Biol D, Palombini L, et al. Sleepwalking and sleep terrors in prepubertal children: what triggers them? *Pediatrics* 2003; 111:e17–e25.
38. Moldofsky H, Gilbert R, Lue FA, et al. Sleep-related violence. *Sleep* 1995; 18:731–739.
39. Masand P, Popli AP, Weilburg JB. Sleepwalking. *Am Fam Physician* 1995; 51:649–654.
40. Szelenberger W, Niemeewicz S, Dabrowska AJ. Sleepwalking and night terrors: psychopathological and psychophysiological correlates. *Int Rev Psychiatry* 2005; 17:263–270.
41. Scheffer IE, Bhatia KP, Lopes-Cendes I, et al. Autosomal dominant frontal epilepsy misdiagnosed as sleep disorder. *Lancet* 1994; 343:515–517.
42. Rothwell JC. Brainstem myoclonus. *Clin Neurosci* 1995–96; 3:214–218.
43. Caviness JN, Brown P. Myoclonus: current concepts and recent advances. *Lancet Neurol* 2004; 3:598–607.
44. Shuper A, Mimouni M. Problems of differentiation between epilepsy and non-epileptic paroxysmal events in the first year of life. *Arch Dis Child* 1995; 73:342–344.
45. Ricci S, Cusmai R, Fusco L, et al. Reflex myoclonic epilepsy in infancy: a new age-dependent idiopathic epileptic syndrome related to startle reaction. *Epilepsia* 1995; 36:342–348.
46. Lombroso CT, Fejerman N. Benign myoclonus of early infancy. *Ann Neurol* 1977; 1:138–143.
47. Drigo P, Carli G, Laverda AM. Benign paroxysmal torticollis of infancy. *Brain Dev* 2000; 22:169–172.
48. Eviatar L. Benign paroxysmal torticollis. *Pediatr Neurol* 1994; 11:72. (comment).
49. Greco F, Finocchiaro M, Spino M, et al. Sandifer's syndrome: a rare form of torticollis in childhood. A report of a patient. *Pediatr Med Chir* 1997; 19:227–230.
50. Lance JW. Familial paroxysmal dystonic choreoathetosis and its differentiation from related syndromes. *Ann Neurol* 1977; 2:285–293.
51. Bruno MK, Hallett M, Gwinn-Hardy K, et al. Clinical evaluation of idiopathic paroxysmal kinesigenic dyskinesia: new diagnostic criteria. *Neurology* 2004; 63:2280–2287.
52. Lombroso CT. Paroxysmal choreoathetosis: an epileptic or non-epileptic disorder? *Ital J Neurol Sci* 1995; 16:271–277.
53. Bressman SB, Fahn S, Burke RE. Paroxysmal non-kinesi-genic dystonia. *Adv Neurol* 1988; 50:403–413.
54. Fink JK, Hedera P, Mathay JG, et al. Paroxysmal dystonic choreoathetosis linked to chromosome 2q: clinical analysis and proposed pathophysiology. *Neurology* 1997; 49:177–183.
55. Bhatia KP, Soland VL, Bhatt MH, et al. Paroxysmal exercise-induced dystonia: eight new sporadic cases and a review of the literature. *Mov Disord* 1997; 12:1007–1012.
56. Munchau A, Valente EM, Shahidi GA, et al. A new family with paroxysmal exercise induced dystonia and migraine: a clinical and genetic study. *J Neurol Neurosurg Psychiatry* 2000; 68:609–614.
57. Parker S, Zuckerman B, Bauchner H, et al. Jitteriness in full-term neonates: prevalence and correlates. *Pediatrics* 1990; 85:17–23.
58. Uddin MK, Rodnitzky RL. Tremor in children. *Semin Pediatr Neurol* 2003; 10:26–34.
59. Vanasse M, Bedard P, Andermann F. Shuddering attacks in children: an early clinical manifestation of essential tremor. *Neurology* 1976; 26:1027–1030.
60. Holmes GL, Russman BS. Shuddering attacks. *Am J Dis Child* 1986; 140:72–73.
61. Olden KW. Rumination. *Current Treatment Options in Gastroenterology* 2001; 4:351–358.
62. Andermann F, Keene DL, Andermann E, et al. Startle disease or hyperekplexia: further delineation of the syndrome. *Brain* 1980; 103:985–997.
63. Praveen V, Patole SK, Whitehall JS. Hyperekplexia in neonates. *Postgrad Med J* 2001; 77:570–572.
64. Tijssen MA, Vergouwe MN, van Dijk JG, et al. Major and minor form of hereditary hyperekplexia. *Mov Disord* 2002; 17:826–830.
65. Ryan SG, Sherman SL, Terry JC, et al. Startle disease, or hyperekplexia: a response to clonazepam and assignment of the gene (STHE) to chromosome 5q by linkage analysis. *Ann Neurol* 1992; 31:663–668.
66. Eulenburg V, Wencke A, Heinrich B, et al. Glycine transporters: essential regulators of neurotransmission. *Trends Biochem Sci* 2005; 30:325–333.
67. Shannon KM. Chorea. *Curr Opin Neurol* 1996; 9:298–302.
68. Dale RC. Post-streptococcal autoimmune disorders of the central nervous system. *Dev Med Child Neurol* 2005; 47:785–791.
69. Katzav A, Chapman J, Shoenfeld Y. CNS dysfunction in the antiphospholipid syndrome. *Lupus* 2003; 12:903–907.
70. Saccomani L, Fabiana V, Manuela B, et al. Tourette syndrome and chronic tics in a sample of children and adolescents. *Brain Dev* 2005; 27:349–352.
71. Rickards H. Tics and fits. The current status of Gilles de la Tourette syndrome and its relationship with epilepsy. *Seizure* 1995; 4:259–266.
72. Spencer T, Biederman J, Harding M, et al. The relationship between tic disorders and Tourette's syndrome revisited. *J Am Acad Child Adolesc Psychiatry* 1995; 34:1133–1139.
73. Seahill L, Erenberg G, Berlin CM Jr, et al. Contemporary assessment and pharmacotherapy of Tourette syndrome. *NeuroRX* 2006; 3:192–206.
74. Dale RC, Heyman I, Surtees RAH, et al. Dyskinesias and associated psychiatric disorders following streptococcal infections. *Arch Dis Child* 2004; 89:604–610.
75. Ruggieri VL, Yepez II, Fejerman N. Benign paroxysmal tonic upward gaze syndrome. *Rev Neurol* 1998; 27:88–91.
76. King RA, Nelson LB, Wagner RS. Spasmus nutans. *Arch Ophthalmol* 1986; 104:1501–1504.
77. Averbuch-Heller L, Remler B. Opsoclonus. *Semin Neurol* 1996; 16:21–26.
78. Connolly AM, Pestronk A, Mehta S, et al. Serum autoantibodies in childhood opsoclonus-myoclonus syndrome: an analysis of antigenic targets in neural tissues. *J Pediatr* 1997; 130:878–884.
79. Yiu VW, Kovithavongs T, McGonigle LF, et al. Plasmapheresis as an effective treatment for opsoclonus-myoclonus syndrome. *Pediatr Neurol* 2001; 24:72–74.
80. Mitchell WG, Brumm VL, Azen CG, et al. Longitudinal neurodevelopmental evaluation of children with opsoclonus-ataxia. *J Pediatr* 2005; 116:901–907.
81. Carmant L, Kramer U, Holmes GL, et al. Differential diagnosis of staring spells in children: a video-EEG study. *Pediatr Neurol* 1996; 14:199–202.
82. Meissner I, Weibers DO, Swanson JW, et al. The natural history of drop attacks. *Neurology* 1986; 36:1029–1034.
83. McLeod KA. Syncope in childhood. *Arch Dis Child* 2003; 88:350–353.
84. Somers VK, Abboud FM. Neurocardiogenic syncope. *Adv Intern Med* 1996; 41: 399–435.
85. Grubb BP. Neurocardiogenic syncope. *N Engl J Med* 2005; 352:1004–1010.
86. McKeon A, Vaughan C, Delantyn N. Seizure versus syncope. *Lancet Neurol* 2006; 5:171–180.
87. Thomas JE, Schirger A, Fealey RD, et al. Orthostatic hypotension. *Mayo Clin Proc* 1981; 56:117–125.
88. Benke T, Hochleitner M, Bauer G. Aura phenomena during syncope. *Eur Neurol* 1997; 37:28–32.
89. Beder SD, Cohen MH, Riemenschneider TA. Occult arrhythmias as the etiology of unexplained syncope in children with structurally normal hearts. *Am Heart J* 1985; 109:309–313.
90. Lewis DA, Dhala A. Syncope in the pediatric patient. The cardiologist's perspective. *Pediatr Clin North Am* 1999; 46:205–219.
91. Driscoll DJ, Jacobsen SJ, Porter CJ, et al. Syncope in children and adolescents. *J Am Coll Cardiol* 1997; 29:1039–1045.
92. Savvas H, O'Callaghan P, Smith PEM. The investigation of syncope. *Seizure* 2004; 13:537–548.
93. Steinerg LA, Knilans TK. Syncope in children: diagnostic tests have a high cost and low yield. *J Pediatr* 2005; 146:355–358.

94. Carlioz R, Graux P, Haye J, et al. Prospective evaluation of high-dose or low-dose isoproterenol upright tilt protocol for unexplained syncope in young adults. *Am Heart J* 1997; 133:346–352.
95. Ruiz GA, Scaglione J, Gonzalez-Zuelgaray J. Reproducibility of head-up tilt test in patients with syncope. *Clin Cardiol* 1996; 19:215–220.
96. Levine MM. Neurally mediated syncope in children: results of tilt testing, treatment, and long-term follow-up. *Pediatr Cardiol* 1999; 20:331–335.
97. Strickberger SA, Benson DW, Biaggioni I, et al. AHA/ACCF scientific statement on the evaluation of syncope. *Circulation* 2006; 113:316–327.
98. Stores G. The protean manifestations of childhood narcolepsy and their misinterpretation. *Dev Med Child Neurol* 2006; 48:307–310.
99. Frey J, Darbonne C. Fluoxetine suppresses human cataplexy: a pilot study. *Neurology* 1994; 44:707–709.
100. Vaughn BV, D'Cruz OF. Carbamazepine as a treatment for cataplexy. *Sleep* 1996; 19:101–103.
101. Lapkin ML, Golden GS. Basilar artery migraine. A review of 30 cases. *Am J Dis Child* 1978; 132:278–281.
102. Kirchmann M, Thomsen LL, Olesen J. Basilar-type migraine. Clinical epidemiologic, and genetic features. *Neurology* 2006; 66:880–886.
103. De Romanis F, Buzzi MG, Assenza S, et al. Basilar migraine with electroencephalographic findings of occipital spike-wave complexes: a long-term study in seven children. *Cephalalgia* 1993; 13:192–196.
104. Fogarasi A, Janszky J, Tuxhorn I. Autonomic symptoms during childhood partial epileptic seizures. *Epilepsia* 2006; 47:584–588.
105. Mousa H, Woodley FW, Metheney M, Hayes J. Testing the association between gastroesophageal reflux and apnea in infants. *J Pediatr Gastroenterol Nutr* 2005; 41:169–177.
106. Fonkalsrud EW, Ament ME. Gastroesophageal reflux in childhood. *Curr Probl Surg* 1996; 33:1–70.
107. Lombroso CT, Lerman P. Breath-holding spells (cyanotic and pallid infantile syncope). *Pediatrics* 1967; 39:563–581.
108. Gauk EW, Kidd I, Prichard JS. Mechanism of seizures associated with breath-holding spells. *N Engl J Med* 1963; 268:1436–1441.
109. Kelly AM, Porter CJ, McGoon MD, et al. Breath-holding spells associated with significant bradycardia: successful treatment with permanent pacemaker implantation. *Pediatrics* 2001; 108:698–702.
110. DiMario FJ Jr. Prospective study of children with cyanotic and pallid breath-holding spells. *Pediatrics* 2001; 107:265–269.
111. Evans RW. Neurologic aspects of hyperventilation syndrome. *Semin Neurol* 1995; 15:115–125.
112. Hornsveld HK, Garssen B, Dop MJ, et al. Double-blind placebo-controlled study of the hyperventilation provocation test and the validity of the hyperventilation syndrome. *Lancet* 1996; 348:154–158.
113. Whitfield CL, Dube Sr, Felitti VJ, et al. Adverse childhood experiences and hallucinations. *Child Abuse Negl* 2005; 29:797–810.
114. Benatar MG, Sahin M, Davis RG. Antiepileptic drug-induced visual hallucinations in a child. *Pediatr Neurol* 2000; 23:439–441.
115. Akman CI, Goodkin HP, Rogers DP, et al. Visual hallucinations associated with zonisamide. *Pharmacotherapy* 2003; 23:93–96.
116. Yankovsky AE, Andermann F, Mercho S, et al. Preictal headache in partial epilepsy. *Neurology* 2005; 65:1979–1981.
117. Siegel AM, Williamson PD, Roberts DW, et al. Localized pain associated with seizures originating in the parietal lobe. *Epilepsia* 1999; 40:845–855.
118. Haut SR, Bigal ME, Lipton RB. Chronic disorders with episodic manifestations: focus on epilepsy and migraine. *Lancet Neurol* 2006; 5:148–157.
119. Andermann F, Zifkin B. The benign occipital epilepsies of childhood: an overview of the idiopathic syndromes and of the relationship to migraine. *Epilepsia* 1999; 40:1320–1323.
120. Prensky AL, Sommer D. Diagnosis and treatment of migraine in children. *Neurology* 1979; 29:506–510.
121. Al-Twaijri WA, Shevell MI. Pediatric migraine equivalents: occurrence and clinical features in practice. *Pediatr Neurol* 2002; 26:365–368.
122. Abu-Arafeh I, Russell G. Prevalence and clinical features of abdominal migraine compared with those of migraine headache. *Arch Dis Child* 1995; 72:413–417.
123. Hammond J. The late sequelae of recurrent vomiting of childhood. *Dev Med Child Neurol* 1974; 16:15–22.
124. Lanzi G, Balottin U, Fazzi E, et al. Benign paroxysmal vertigo of childhood: a long-term follow-up. *Cephalalgia* 1994; 14:458–460.
125. Hughes CA, Proctor L. Benign paroxysmal positional vertigo. *Laryngoscope* 1997; 107:607–613.
126. Vehedi K, Joutel A, Van Bogart P, et al. A gene for hereditary paroxysmal cerebellar ataxia maps to chromosome 19p. *Ann Neurol* 1995; 37:289–293.
127. Damji KF, Allingham RR, Pollock SC, et al. Periodic vestibulocerebellar ataxia, an autosomal dominant ataxia with defective smooth pursuit, is genetically distinct from other autosomal dominant ataxias. *Arch Neurol* 1996; 53:338–344.
128. Smith EA, Van Houten R. A comparison of the characteristics of self-stimulatory behaviors in "normal" children and children with developmental delays. *Res Dev Disabil* 1996; 17:253–268.
129. Tan A, Salgado M, Fahn S. The characterization and outcome of stereotypical movements in nonautistic children. *Mov Disord* 1997; 12:47–52.
130. Lewis MH, Bodfish JW, Powell SB, et al. Clomipramine treatment for stereotype and related repetitive movement disorders associated with mental retardation. *Am J Ment Retard* 1995; 100:299–312.
131. Finkelstein E, Amichai B, Jaworowski S, et al. Masturbation in prepubescent children: a case report and review of the literature. *Child Care Health Dev* 1996; 22:323–326.
132. Yang ML, Fullwood E, Goldstein J, et al. Masturbation in infancy and early childhood presenting as a movement disorder: 12 cases and a review of the literature. *Pediatrics* 2005; 116:1427–1432.
133. Bye AM, Nunan J. Video EEG analysis of non-ictal events in children. *Clin Exp Neurol* 1992; 29:92–98.
134. Gascon G, Barlow C. Juvenile migraine presenting as an acute confusional state. *J Pediatr* 1970; 45:628–635.
135. Shaabat A. Confusional migraine in childhood. *Pediatr Neurol* 1996; 15:23–25.
136. Gananamuthu C. Confusional states and seizures. When are they related? *Postgrad Med* 1988; 84:149–152.
137. Primavera A, Giberti L, Scotto P, et al. Nonconvulsive status epilepticus as a cause of confusion in later life: a report of 5 cases. *Neuropsychobiology* 1994; 30:148–152.
138. Biraben A, Taussig D, Thomas P, et al. Fear as the main feature of epileptic seizures. *J Neurol Neurosurg Psychiatry* 2001; 70:186–191.
139. Meuret AE, White KS, Ritz T, Roth WT, et al. Panic attack symptom dimensions and their relationship to illness characteristics in panic disorder. *J Psychiatr Res* 2006; 40(6):520–527.
140. McElroy SL, Soutullo CA, Beckman DA, et al. DSM-IV intermittent explosive disorder: a report of 27 cases. *J Clin Psychiatry* 1998; 59:203–210.
141. Wyllie E, Glazer JP, Benbadis S, et al. Psychiatric features of children and adolescents with pseudoseizures. *Arch Pediatr Adolesc Med* 1999; 153:244–248.
142. Stores G. Practitioner review: recognition of pseudoseizures in children and adolescents. *J Child Psychol Psychiatry* 1999; 40:851–857.
143. Bhatia MS, Sapra S. Pseudoseizures in children: a profile of 50 cases. *Clin Pediatr* 2005; 44:617–621.
144. Kotagal P, Costa M, Wyllie E, et al. Paroxysmal nonepileptic events in children and adolescents. *Pediatrics* 2002; 110:e46. (abstract).
145. Walczak TS, Williams DT, Berten W. Utility and reliability of placebo infusion in the evaluation of patients with seizures. *Neurology* 1994; 44:394–399.
146. Chen DK, Yuen TS, Fisher RS. Use of serum prolactin in diagnosing epileptic seizures. Report of the therapeutics and technology assessment. *Neurology* 2005; 65:668–675.

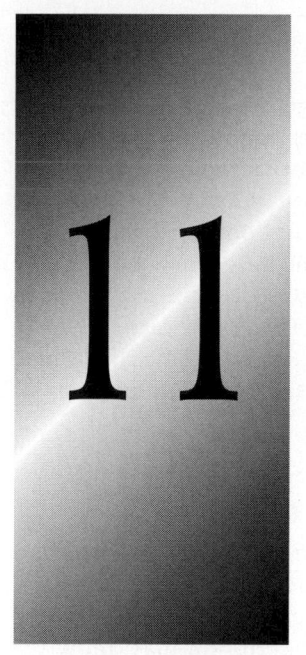

Evaluating the Child with Seizure

Sejal V. Jain
Lawrence D. Morton

Seizures are time-limited paroxysmal events that result from abnormal, involuntary rhythmic neuronal discharges in the brain (1). The term *seizure* appears to arise from a notion that patients were possessed or seized by spirits in old times. Age-adjusted incidence for first diagnosis of unprovoked seizure is 61 per 100,000 person-years (2). Incidence of first nonfebrile seizure in children is 25,000 to 40,000 per year in the United States (3). Although mortality directly related to seizure is low in these children, 45% to 50% will have recurrence (4–6). Therefore it is important to evaluate patients with seizures and events that look like seizures.

Common conditions that are mistaken for seizures are gastroesophageal (GE) reflux, apneic episodes, self-stimulating behavior, breath-holding spells, migraine, attention deficit hyperactivity disorder (ADHD), and sleep disorders (see Chapter 11).

Seizures can be classified based on etiologies and types. Etiologic classification includes provoked and unprovoked seizures. Provoked seizures are defined as seizures occurring in close temporal association with an acute systemic, metabolic, or toxic insult or with an acute central nervous system (CNS) insult (7). Common causes of provoked seizures include metabolic disturbances such as hyponatremia, hypoglycemia and hyperglycemia, hypocalcemia, and acute neurological conditions such as trauma, stroke, meningitis, and recreational drug or alcohol use or withdrawal. Unprovoked seizures can be classified based on etiologies as idiopathic (with particular clinical characteristics and specific electroencephalographic [EEG] findings), symptomatic (due to metabolic, genetic disorders or structural abnormalities), or cryptogenic (unknown etiology) (7). The term cryptogenic suggests a cause may be subsequently discovered. Classification based on seizure types is based on International League Against Epilepsy (ILAE) classification (see Chapter 9).

Epilepsy is defined as occurrence of two or more unprovoked seizures (7). It is important to note that the occurrence of multiple seizures in a 24-hour period is considered as one seizure (7).

When a patient presents with a seizure or seizure-like events, goals are to identify whether the event was a seizure or not; if it was a seizure, to identify the type of seizure based on ILAE criteria, identify the etiology of seizure, and anticipate recurrence and the need for treatment.

Identifying critical elements during the evaluation of a seizure or event that appeared seizure-like is the most important aspect of establishing the diagnosis of epilepsy. This chapter aims to recommend the initial evaluation of a patient presenting with seizure.

PATIENT EVALUATION

History

The following pertinent history should be elicited:

Age

Certain seizure types are age dependent. Examples are infantile spasms, febrile seizures, benign epilepsy with centrotemporal spikes (BECTS), childhood absence seizures, juvenile absence seizures, and juvenile myoclonic epilepsy. Children are most vulnerable to develop epilepsy during the first year of life (2, 8). Etiologies for status epilepticus differ based on age. During the first 2 years of life status epilepticus is more common in neurologically normal children, whereas later on it is more common in neurologically abnormal children (9).

Preceding or Precipitating Events

Knowing the events immediately before a seizure episode is very important. Parents may not perceive that premonitory symptoms or auras are part of a seizure and may not volunteer this information to the physician. Most common manifestations of aura associated with temporal lobe seizures are autonomic. These include "funny feelings," epigastric sensations, flushing, sweating, palpitations, nausea, or dizziness.

The presence of preceding events also helps to differentiate nonepileptic events, such as crying preceding breath-holding spells and feeding preceding reflux. Loud noises and stimuli can lead to hyperekplexia, which may look like seizure.

Certain seizures are provoked by specific stimuli and are called reflex seizures. Well-known precipitating factors are visual stimuli, flickering light, thinking, praxis, reading, somatosensory and proprioceptive stimuli, eating, music, hot water, and startle (10). Other nonspecific factors are also associated with induction of seizure. In a study of 1,677 patients with epilepsy, 53% reported one and 30% reported two or more precipitating factors. Most common factors were emotional stress, sleep deprivation, fatigue, and alcohol consumption. Patients with generalized seizures were more sensitive to sleep deprivation and flickering light than patients with localization-related epilepsy (11).

Timing of Event

Epilepsies associated with awakening seizures are usually primary generalized seizure disorders such as juvenile myoclonic epilepsy and absence seizures. Sleep epilepsies include focal or secondarily generalized seizure disorders such as BECTS, Landau-Kleffner, electrical status epilepticus in sleep (ESES), and frontal lobe seizures. Temporal lobe seizures are also more common during sleep. Complex partial seizures generalize more frequently during sleep. Seizures are more common during stage 1 and 2 sleep and least common during rapid eye movement (REM) sleep. Also nonepileptic seizures do not occur out of sleep (12, 13). Unprovoked seizures occurring out of sleep have a higher risk of recurrence and the sleep state at the time of the first seizure correlates with successive seizures (14). Patients with seizures occurring in sleep have higher chances of having an abnormal EEG (15). Knowing the child's state immediately before and after the event is extremely important and frequently diagnostic.

The Event Itself

Have the parents and family members describe a chronological account of what they witnessed. Caregivers often use diagnostic terms such as "petit mal," drawing conclusions. Often the exact description may allow the physician to determine whether an event was a seizure or not, and if a seizure, what type. Also a majority of the time seizures are described as "shaking." It is not reasonable to speculate that this means clonic activity because it could mean trembling associated with tonic seizure, clonic activity, or simply pelvic thrusting or bicycling motion. Witnesses should be asked to demonstrate the event if they can. A seizure may start in one part of the body and progress to the whole body with loss of consciousness. Therefore, it is important to ascertain how and where it started.

The history of forced eye closure during an event most likely suggests a nonepileptic event. The mouth is usually open during tonic seizure. Forced clenching of the mouth is associated with pseudoseizures (16). Gaze deviation can help determine focal nature of the event and help in localization.

Duration of the event may allow differentiation of seizure from status epilepticus, which is treated differently and has a different prognosis. Status epilepticus is defined as seizure or a series of seizures lasting 30 or more minutes (7). In a study of 407 children presenting with a first unprovoked seizure the authors reported that 50% had seizures lasting 5 minutes or longer, 29% 20 minutes, and 12% 30 minutes. Seizures of partial onset were more likely to be prolonged. 92% of the seizures stopped spontaneously (17). The likelihood of a seizure stopping spontaneously decreases after 5 minutes and reaches a minimum at 15 minutes. Also, the duration of subsequent seizures correlates with the length of the first episode (17). It is not uncommon, however, to overestimate or underestimate the duration of the event.

It is important to ask the patient about what they remember of the event. This may help to identify the exact duration of loss of consciousness or awareness, if any.

After the cessation of the event the patient's condition is important to know. Malingering patients will be back to baseline immediately after a dramatic motor seizure. Others may show confusion, tiredness, sleepiness, or hemiparesis. Continued altered awareness may be due to postictal state or continued subclinical seizure.

Prior history of other paroxysmal events, similar events, other seizures, and febrile seizures is important. Recurrence risk after a second seizure increases to about 70%. High risk was seen if seizure recurred within 6 months of the first seizure (14). In patients with newly diagnosed epilepsy about 17% have seizures of more than one type (18). Such patients have lower a probability of remission of epilepsy (19). A total of 2% to 10% of patients with febrile seizures develop epilepsy. Complex febrile seizures are associated with an increased risk of subsequent development of epilepsy (4, 20).

Associated Events

Common events associated with generalized motor seizures are tongue biting, bowel or bladder incontinence, and respiratory attenuation. Tongue biting can be seen during the clonic phase of a seizure (16).

Irregular respiration and pauses in respirations are seen during clonic and tonic phases of generalized seizures. Cyanosis may be present with a seizure. Often peripheral cyanosis is not associated with central hypoxia. Malingering patients may not be able to demonstrate cyanosis. Respiratory involvement may also make seizures more frightening for the family, and early interventions may be needed in those at risk for prolonged convulsions.

Review of Systems

Fever, lethargy, headache, and photophobia may point toward meningitis and encephalitis as a cause of seizures. Diarrhea and vomiting leading to dehydration and electrolyte imbalance can provoke seizures. It is important to ask about diet, especially in infants and teenage females. In infants who are formula fed, if the formula is improperly mixed, there are chances of electrolyte imbalance leading to seizures. Teenage females should be asked questions regarding bulimia, "dieting" and "diet pills" if suspected. Teenagers should also be asked about recreational drug and alcohol use. History of trauma should be evaluated. Other medical conditions such as diabetes and infections should be considered. Exposure to toxins and heavy metals should be suspected in a younger child.

Medication

It is helpful to know whether the patient is taking medications that are known to decrease seizure threshold. Also, the history of hypoglycemic agents and diuretic use is helpful.

Birth History

Premature newborns who weigh less than 1.5 lb are at higher risk for brain injury leading to acute or remote symptomatic seizures. In-utero exposure to infectious agents, recreational drugs, alcohol, and teratogenic medications can also cause structural brain abnormality. Meningitis, increased bilirubin levels, respiratory problems occurring during the postnatal period are important to know for the same reason. Maternal history of oligohydramnios or polyhydramnios, fetal hiccups, or episodic hammering fetal movements may suggest neurological disorders in the fetus.

Developmental History

History of language, motor or psychosocial delays, and regression and timing of regression should be evaluated. A total of 15% to 30% of patients with childhood-onset epilepsy have cerebral palsy or mental retardation and 11% to 39% of children with autistic spectrum disorders develop epilepsy (8, 21, 22). Patients with severe autism have a higher incidence of epilepsy (23). Developmental delays may be a hallmark of chromosomal disorders and associated epilepsy (24, 25). Language regression and seizures may represent Landau-Kleffner syndrome. Global regression may be seen at the onset of ESES (21) (see Chapter 26). Children with developmental delay or mental retardation have a higher risk of intractable seizure. It is likely that these disorders represent widespread underlying CNS abnormalities (19).

Family History

In a study of patients with seizures about 35% of patients reported seizures in first-degree relatives (26). Inherited epilepsies include autosomal dominant nocturnal frontal lobe epilepsy (ADNFLE), BECTS, juvenile myoclonic epilepsy (JME), generalized epilepsy with febrile seizures plus syndrome, benign familial neonatal convulsions, benign familial infantile convulsions, and other idiopathic generalized epilepsy (27).

In a study looking at risk of epilepsy in adults with seizures, cryptogenic or idiopathic epilepsy with partial onset showed a higher occurrence rate in successive generations, whereas the occurrence rate for generalized epilepsy remained the same in all generations (28). In twin studies there was concordance of occurrence of seizure in monozygotic and dizygotic twins and status epilepticus in monozygotic twins (26, 29).

Physical Examination

General Examination

Head circumference should be measured. Presence of microcephaly could be secondary to congenital infections, hypoxia or maternal diseases, and drug and toxin exposure. Cranial malformations such as lissencephaly, cortical dysplasia, and heterotropia are primary causes of microcephaly (30–32). Macrocephaly is associated with storage disorders and hydrocephalus (31).

Fundoscopic examination may show papilledema suggesting increased intracranial pressure or cherry red spot associated with storage diseases, or findings associated with neurocutaneous syndromes or congenital malformations.

The examiner should look for dysmorphic features. Microcephaly, craniosynostosis, deep-set eyes, hypertelorism, low-set ears, midface hypoplasia, depressed bridge of nose, microstomia or macrostomia, simian crease, and hand and foot abnormalities are some of the features that present in chromosomal disorders associated with seizures (24, 25). Dysmorphic features such as cleft lip and cleft palate are known to be associated with cranial dysplasia. Abnormal hair patterning may suggest abnormalities in brain development before 18 weeks. Microcephaly with abnormal hair patterning may be seen with brain abnormality rather than craniosynostosis (33).

The examination of the skin is important; a number of neurocutaneous syndromes are associated with seizures. Incontentia pigmenti, linear nevus syndrome, hypomelanosis of Ito, tuberous sclerosis, Sturge-Weber syndrome, and neurofibromatosis are examples of these neurocutaneous syndromes (see Chapter 30). Skin examination can also reveal signs of physical abuse.

Nuchal rigidity, positive Kernig's and Brudzinski's signs suggest meningitis. Infants with open fontanel may not present with these signs but will show a bulging or tense fontanel.

Organomegaly may be seen with metabolic storage diseases.

Neurological Examination

Determination of ongoing seizure should be the first step in the evaluation of a patient presenting with a history of seizure. The patient may present with altered sensorium, which could be due to ongoing seizure, postictal phenomena, or medication used. Dysarthria or visual changes may be present postictally. A hemiparesis may suggest Todd's paralysis and a partial seizure. Presence of Todd's paralysis after a first unprovoked seizure is associated with increased risk of recurrence (14).

In patients suspected of having absense seizure hyperventilate for at least 3 minutes as this may precipitate a seizure.

Laboratory Studies

Basic Metabolic Panel

Seizures provoked by metabolic abnormalities in an otherwise normal child are rare. Therefore, basic tests should be done based on clinical judgment per American Academy of Neurology (AAN) guidelines for evaluation of first unprovoked seizure (3).

Lumbar Puncture

If there is clinical suspicion of meningitis or encephalitis, lumbar puncture should be done per AAN guidelines for evaluation of first unprovoked seizure.

Urine Toxicology

Routine urinalysis is not recommended, but if there is clinical suspicion of recreational drug use, a urine drug screen should be obtained.

Liver Function Tests

If there is history suggestive of a potentially degenerative, metabolic or storage disorders or there is anticipation of starting antiepilepsy drugs (AEDs), liver function tests should be performed.

Screening for Inherited Metabolic Disorders

These tests may not be obtained during the initial evaluation, but are very important in seizure evaluation and management and so are mentioned here.

About 200 inherited disorders are associated with seizures (34). There are clues such as certain seizure types, characteristic EEG patterns, and specific epilepsy syndromes that point to some of these disorders. Associated symptoms of mental retardation, developmental delays, hypotonia, macrocephaly and microcephaly, and failure to thrive may also suggest the possibility of a metabolic disorder. In patients with myoclonic seizures, spasms, early-onset tonic seizures, and infantile-onset hypomotor and versive seizures, inherited metabolic disorders should be suspected (34). Other characteristics of seizures associated with inherited disorders include onset in the first month of life, usually partial seizures with migrant nature and successive appearance (35). West syndrome, early myoclonic encephalopathy, and Ohtahara syndrome are known to be associated with metabolic disorders (see Table 11-1).

EEGs showing burst suppression, hypsarhythmia, and diffuse severe depression without obvious cause demand evaluation for inherited disorders (see Table 11-2).

Serum amino acids and urine organic acids can be used as an initial screen in patients with the previously mentioned seizure types and syndromes. Cerebrospinal fluid (CSF) glucose, lactate, and amino acids are recommended for infantile seizures without clear etiology. It is important to obtain samples during the presentation of symptoms before treatment because otherwise samples may be falsely normal or difficult to interpret (36) (see Tables 11-3 and 11-4) (35–37).

Disorders of carnitine and fatty acid oxidation acutely present with a history of decreased oral intake followed by increasing lethargy, obtundation or coma, and seizures. Other features include history of recurrent hypoglycemic, hypoketotic encephalopathy, potential developmental delay, progressive lipid storage myopathy,

TABLE 11-1
Epileptic Syndromes and Inborn Errors of Metabolism

NEONATAL SEIZURES (ILAE 3.1)
Urea cycle defects: argininosuccinic acidemia, ornithine transcarbamylase, carbamylophosphate synthetase
Organic acidurias: maple syrup urine disease
Disorders of biotin metabolism: early-onset multiple carboxylase deficiency (holocarboxylase synthatase deficiency)
Peroxisomal disorders: Zellweger syndrome, acyl-CoA oxidase deficiency
Other: molybdenum cofactor deficiency/sulfite oxidase deficiency, disorders of fructose metabolism, pyridoxine dependency
EARLY MYELOCLONIC ENCEPHALOPATHY/EARLY INFANTILE EPILEPTIC ENCEPHALOPATHY (ILAE 2.3.1)
Nonketotic hyperglycinemia
Propionic acidemia
D-Glyceric academia
Leigh disease
CRYPTOGENIC MYELOCLONIC EPILEPSIES (ILAE 2.2) OTHER THAN INFANTILE SPASMS OR LENNOX-GESTAUT SYNDROME
GM1 gangliosidosis
GM2 gangliosidosis
Infantile neuroaxonal dystrophy
Neuronal ceroid lipofuscinosis
Glucose transporter defect 1 deficiency
Late-onset multiple carboxylase deficiency
Disorders of folate metabolism, methylenetetrahydrofo late reductase deficiency
Arginase deficiency (urea cycle defect)
Tetrahydrobiopterin deficiency (aminoaciduria)
Tyrosinemia type I
WEST SYNDROME, GENERALIZED 2.2
Phenylketonuria/hyperphenylalaninemia
Pyruvate dehydrogenase deficiency
Pyruvate carboxylase deficiency
Carbohydrate-deficient glycoprotein syndrome (type III)
Organic acidurias
Amino acidurias

Abbreviations: ILAE, International League Against Epilepsy; CoA, coenzyme A. Source: Nordli and De Vivo 2002 (34).

recurrent myoglobinuria, hypotonia, neuropathy, and progressive cardiomyopathy. Screening tests should include serum total and free carnitine, acylcarnitines, free fatty acids and ketones and urine organic acids, acylglycines, and acylcarnitines. A serum free-fatty acid to ketone ratio of more than 2:1 suggests a block in fatty acid oxidation. Urine organic acid chain length and type will help to identify the site of block. Confirmations can be obtained by specific cultured skin fibroblast tests (38).

TABLE 11-2
EEG Patterns and Associated Disorders

EEG PATTERN	DISORDER
Comblike rhythm	Maple syrup urine disease Propionic acidemia
Fast central spikes	Tay-Sachs disease
Rhythmic vertex positive spikes	Sialidosis (type I)
Vanishing EEG	Infantile NCL (type I)
High amplitude 16–24 Hz activity	Infantile neuroaxonal dystrophy
Diminished spikes during sleep	PME
Marked photosensitivity	PME and NCL particularly type II
Burst suppression	Neonatal citrullinemia Nonketotic hyperglycinemia Propionic academia Leigh disease D-Glyceric academia Molybdenum cofactor deficiency Menke's syndrome Holocarboxylase synthetase deficiency Neonatal adrenoleukodystrophy
Hypsarrhythmia	Zellweger syndrome Neonatal adrenoleukodystrophy Neuroaxonal dystrophy Nonketotic hyperglycinemia Phenylketonuria Carbohydrate-deficient glycoprotein syndrome (type III)

Abbreviations: EEG, electroencephalogram; NCL, neuronal ceroid lipofuscinosis; PME, progressive myeloclonic epilepsy. Source: Nordli and De Vivo 2002 (34).

A few cases of creatine metabolism defect and epilepsy have been reported. Associated symptoms include hypotonia, mental retardation, neurologic regression, and movement disorders. Initial tests should include serum and urine guanidinoacetic acid and creatine. Magnetic resonance (MR) spectroscopy also helps in the diagnosis (39).

CSF metabolites. Disorders affecting CNS energy metabolism, creatine synthesis, glucose transport, and neurotransmitter metabolism may present with hypotonia,

TABLE 11-3
Metabolic Diseases and Biochemical Abnormalities

SEIZURES AND METABOLIC ACIDOSIS
• Pyruvate dehydrogenase complex deficiency
• Mitochondrial encephalomyopathies
• Multiple carboxylase deficiency disorders
• Intermittent MSUD
• Isovaleric acidemia
• Glutaric aciduria
• Propionic acidemia
• Methylmalonic acidemia
SEIZURES AND HYPOGLYCEMIA
• Glycogen storage disease
• Fructose 1,6-diphosphate deficiency
• Hereditary fructose intolerance
• Organic acidemia
SEIZURES AND HYPERAMMONEMIA
• Biotinidase deficiency
• Carnitine palmitoyl transferase I deficiency
• Hyperammonemic hyperornithinemia with homocitrullinemia
• Urea cycle disorders
• Oxidative metabolism disorders
• Propionic acidemia
• Methylmalonic acidemia

Abbreviation: MSUD, maple syrup urine disease.
Source: Leary LD, Nordli DR, Jr., De Vivo DC 2006 (37).

temperature instability, developmental delay, ptosis, dystonia, and tremors along with seizures. These disorders may not be detected by routine screen for inherited metabolic disorders. If initial metabolic screen and CSF lactate and amino acids are normal in an infant with seizure without clear etiology, profiles of CSF metabolites including biogenic amines should be considered (40).

When gamma-aminobutyric acid (GABA)-related disorders are suspected—that is, GABA transaminase deficiency, succinic semialdehyde dehydrogenase deficiency (SSDD), glutamate decarboxylase or GABA receptor defects—CSF GABA level should be measured. It is increased in patients with SSDD and vigabatrin treatment. SSDD can also be detected in lymphocytes and fibroblasts (41).

In nonketotic hyperglycinemia, CSF glycine is elevated. It is also elevated in patients who are receiving valproate treatment. It is decreased in defective serine synthesis (41).

Guanidinoacetate and creatine measurement can aid in diagnosis of arginine:glycine aminotransferase or guanidinoacetate methyletransferase deficiencies, and creatine transporter defect.

Measurement of tetrahydrobiopterin, neopterin, 7,8-dihydrobiopterin, homovanillic acid, 5-hydroxyindoleacetic acid, and 3-O-methyldopa can help in diagnosis of tetrahydrobiopterin and biogenic amine metabolism.

Pyridoxine-deficient and -responsive seizures are covered in another section (see Chapter 30).

Tests for mitochondrial disorders. Mitochondrial disorders causing epilepsy are rare. It is possible that this rarity is due to our inability to recognize these disorders. A review by DiMauro showed that seizures are associated with MELAS (mitochondrial myopathy, encephalopathy, lactic acidosis, and strokelike episodes), MERRF (myoclonus epilepsy with ragged red fibers), pyruvate dehydrogenase complex deficiencies, cytochrome c oxidase deficiencies, and maternally inherited Leigh's disease (42). All the patients in the review presenting with these disorders and seizure had symptoms such as developmental delay and eventually developed classic symptoms for the disorder. Partial seizures are more common in patients with mitochondrial encephalopathies (43).

Ammonia, serum and CSF lactate, and urine organic acid can be used as an initial screen (36). In cases of intractable seizure and developmental delays, migraine, strokelike episodes, or retinitis pigmentosa, serum testing and muscle biopsy should be considered.

Chromosomal Studies

Chromosomal abnormalities with high association of seizures include 4p– syndrome, Miller-Dieker syndrome, Angelman syndrome, inversion duplication 15 syndrome, terminal deletions of chromosome 1q and 1p, and ring chromosomes 14 and 20. Patients presenting with specific phenotypes and EEG abnormalities should have genetic testing done (24, 25, 44).

EEG

EEG remains the gold standard test for evaluation of seizures, especially when an ictus is captured during the study. It can help to differentiate nonepileptic events from seizure. It can also help to identify an epileptic syndrome, because epilepsy syndromes are classified based on specific patterns of abnormality on EEG. It helps to provide long-term prognosis and identify any need to do further testing. It influences the management by helping to select AEDs. Certain metabolic disorders have classic EEG patterns (see Table 11-2).

In a study of patients with unprovoked seizures, EEG abnormalities were associated with increased recurrence. Abnormal EEGs were more common in patients with partial seizures than with generalized seizures (45). A study by Yoshinaga et al showed that more than 20% of seizures were classified incorrectly or missed when only history was used to identify paroxysmal events (46).

TABLE 11-4
Metabolic Disorders and Diagnostic Laboratory Tests

DIAGNOSIS	LABORATORY TESTS
Amioacidopathies • Urea cycle disorders • HHH syndrome • MSUD • Nonketotic hyperglycinemia • Sulfite oxidase deficiency	Plasma, urine, and CSF amino acids Urine orotic acid
Disorders of carbohydrate metabolism • Glycogen storage disease • Fructose 1,6-diphosphase deficiency • D-Glyceric acidurias	Fasting glucose Blood lactate Fasting urine organic acids
Organic acidurias • Propionic, methylmalonic, glutaric aciduria type I • Multicarboxylase deficiency • Fumarase deficiency	Urine organic acids Plasma acylcarnitine Plasma and urine biotin concentration
Disorders of folic acid and vitamin B_{12} metabolism	Urine organic acids Plasma and urine homocystine and amino acids
Mitochondrial diseases • PDH • Respiratory chain defects • MELAS syndrome • Carnitine transport defects • Defects of beta-oxidation	Plasma acylcarnitine Plasma and CSF lactate Urine organic acids
Peroxisomal disorders	Plasma VLCFA Plasma and urine pipecolic and phytanic acid
CDG syndrome	Isoelectrofocus serum transferrin
Krabbe's disease	High CSF protein concentration
Menkes' syndrome	Serum copper, ceruloplasmin
Pyridoxine dependency	CSF GABA concentration

Abbreviations: HHH, hyperammonemic hyperornithinemia with homocitrullinemia; MSUD, maple syrup urine disease; PKU, phenylketonuria; PDH, pyruvate dehydrogenase deficiency; MELAS, mitochondrial encephalomyopathy, lactic acidosis, and stroke-like episodes; VLCFA, very long chain fatty acids; CDG, carbohydrate-deficient glycoprotein; GABA, gamma-aminobutyric acid. Source: Vigevano and Bartuli 2002 (35).

Recommendations regarding timing for the EEG testing are controversial. In a study by King et al, an EEG performed within the first 24 hours had a higher diagnostic yield (47). In a study done at Virginia Commonwealth University when EEGs were done in the emergency room in patients presenting with a seizure, 80% of patients with an abnormal EEG developed recurrence (48). EEG abnormalities are the best predictors of recurrence in neurologically normal children (3).

Hyperventilation and photic stimulation increase the yield of EEG and are recommended (49). Even though Gilbert et al showed that sleep deprivation did not increase EEG abnormalities (50), a number of other studies have shown that sleep recordings can increase the yield of EEG (3, 13, 45, 49, 51).

Thus EEG is recommended to evaluate paroxysmal events. In patients with altered consciousness and recurrent seizures, emergent EEG is recommended. Hyperventilation and sleep deprivation increase the yield of EEG. When possible, it should be obtained immediately after seizure presentation. A normal or suspicious EEG should be followed by sleep-deprived EEG.

Imaging

In a study by Shinnar et al (52), only 1% of children with a first unprovoked seizure had neuroimaging abnormalities requiring acute intervention. All these children had indications for neuroimaging such as an abnormal neurological examination or prolonged seizure. The most common

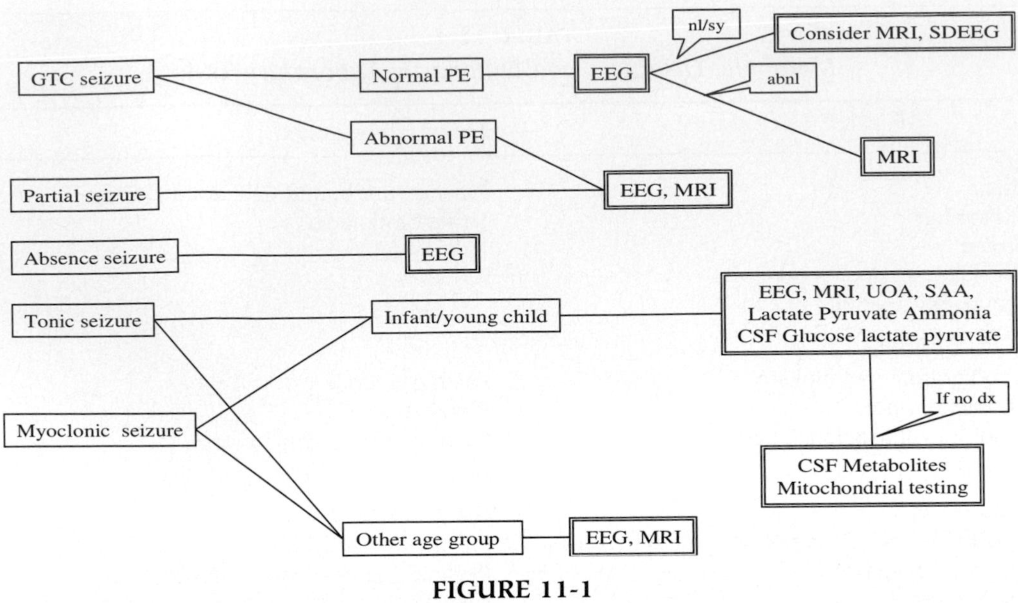

FIGURE 11-1

Recommended algorithm based on seizure types. Abbreviations: GTC, genenralized tonic clonic; PE, physical examination; SDEEG, sleep-deprived EEG; UAO, urine organic acid; SAA, serum amino acid; nl/sy, normal or benign syndromic; abnl, abnormal.

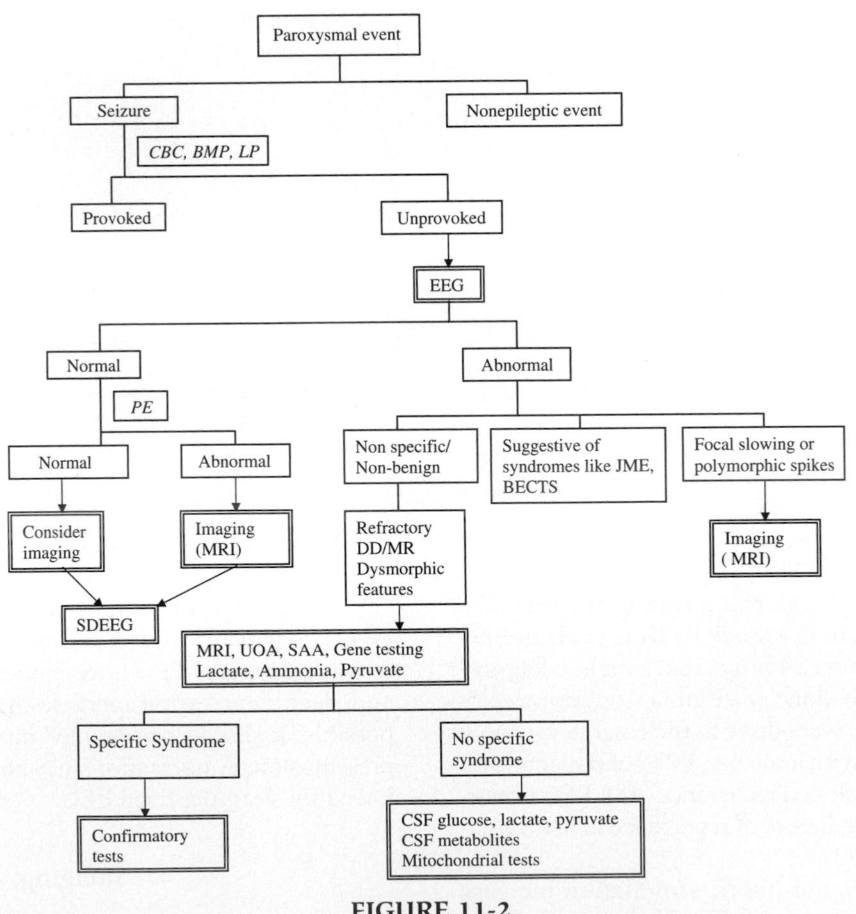

FIGURE 11-2

Recommended algorithm for seizure evaluation. Abbreviations: CBC, complete blood count; BMP, basic metabolic panel; LP, lumbar puncture; PE, physical examination; JME, juvenile myoclonic epilepsy; BECTS, benign epilepsy with centrotemporal spikes; DD, developmental delay; MR, mental retardation; SDEEG, sleep-deprived EEG; UOA, urine organic acid; SAA, serum amino acid.

abnormalities were focal encephalomalacia and cerebral dysgenesis. Suggested risk factors for abnormal imaging were partial seizures, abnormal neurological examination, and abnormal EEG (53). In children with a brief tonic clonic seizure, normal examination, and normal EEG, 10% of imaging studies were abnormal (52).

Imaging is recommended for seizure evaluation (3). Emergent imaging studies are required in case of prolonged seizure, prolonged postictal phase, and postictal hemiparesis to rule out stroke and other structural abnormalities (3). Outside of the acute situation, Magnetic Resonance Imaging is a superior study because it can identify subtle cortical abnormalities (3, 53).

CONCLUSION

Seizures are frightening events for the families and children in whom they occur and require precautions associated with driving, water activities, heights, and work environment. The diagnosis has immense psychosocial impact on both the family and the patient. Thus, the first seizure or similar event should be evaluated carefully to make an accurate diagnosis, the recurrence risk should be explained to the family, and appropriate treatment decisions should be made. Recommended algorithms for seizure evaluation are shown in Figures 11-1 and 11-2.

References

1. Shneker BF, Fountain NB. Epilepsy. *Dis Mon* 2003; 49(7):426–478.
2. Hauser WA, Annegers JF, Kurland LT. Incidence of epilepsy and unprovoked seizures in Rochester, Minnesota: 1935–1984. *Epilepsia* 1993; 34(3):453–468.
3. Hirtz D, Ashwal S, Berg A, Bettis D, et al. Practice parameter: evaluating a first nonfebrile seizure in children: Report of the Quality Standards Subcommittee of the American Academy of Neurology, The Child Neurology Society, and The American Epilepsy Society. *Neurology* 2000; 55(5):616–623.
4. Shinnar S, Berg AT, Moshe SL, O'Dell C, et al. The risk of seizure recurrence after a first unprovoked afebrile seizure in childhood: an extended follow-up. *Pediatrics* 1996; 98 2 Pt 1:216–225.
5. Shinnar S, Berg AT, Moshe SL, Petix M, et al. Risk of seizure recurrence following a first unprovoked seizure in childhood: a prospective study. *Pediatrics* 1990; 85(6):1076–1085.
6. Shinnar S, O'Dell C, Berg AT. Mortality following a first unprovoked seizure in children: a prospective study. *Neurology* 2005; 64(5):880–882.
7. ILAE Commission Report. The epidemiology of the epilepsies: future directions. International League Against Epilepsy. *Epilepsia* 1997; 38(5):614–618.
8. Shinnar S, Pellock JM. Update on the epidemiology and prognosis of pediatric epilepsy. *J Child Neurol* 2002; 17 Suppl 1:S4–S17.
9. Shinnar S, Pellock J, Moshe SL, Maytal J, et al. In whom does status epilepticus occur: age-related differences in children. *Epilepsia* 1997; 38(8):907–914.
10. Ferlazzo E, Zifkia BG, Andermann E, Andermann F. Cortical triggers in generalized reflex seizures and epilepsies. *Brain* 2005; 128 Pt 4:700–710.
11. Nakken KO, Solaas MH, Kjeldsen MJ, Friis ML, et al. Which seizure-precipitating factors do patients with epilepsy most frequently report? *Epilepsy Behav* 2005; 6(1):85–89.
12. Bazil CW, Walczak TS. Effects of sleep and sleep stage on epileptic and nonepileptic seizures. *Epilepsia* 1997; 38(1):56–62.
13. Mendez M, Radtke RA. Interactions between sleep and epilepsy. *J Clin Neurophysiol* 2001; 18(2):106–127.
14. Shinnar S, Berg AT, O'Dell C, Newstein D, et al. Predictors of multiple seizures in a cohort of children prospectively followed from the time of their first unprovoked seizure. *Ann Neurol* 2000; 48(2):140–147.
15. Shinnar S, Berg AT, Ptachewich Y, Alemany M. Sleep state and the risk of seizure recurrence following a first unprovoked seizure in childhood. *Neurology* 1993; 43(4): 701–706.
16. DeToledo JC, Ramsay RE. Patterns of involvement of facial muscles during epileptic and nonepileptic events: review of 654 events. *Neurology* 1996; 47(3):621–625.
17. Shinnar S, Berg AT, Moshe SL, Shinnar R. How long do new-onset seizures in children last? *Ann Neurol* 2001; 49(5):659–664.
18. Berg AT, Shinnar S, Levy SR, Testa FM. Newly diagnosed epilepsy in children: presentation at diagnosis. *Epilepsia* 1999; 40(4):445–452.
19. Oskoui M, Webster RI, Zhang X, Shevell MI. Factors predictive of outcome in childhood epilepsy. *J Child Neurol* 2005; 20(11):898–904.
20. Shinnar S, Glauser TA. Febrile seizures. *J Child Neurol* 2002; 17 Suppl 1:S44–S52.
21. Ballaban-Gil K, Tuchman R. Epilepsy and epileptiform EEG: association with autism and language disorders. *Ment Retard Dev Disabil Res Rev* 2000; 6(4):300–308.
22. Filipek PA, Accardo PJ, Ashwal S, Baranek GT, et al. Practice parameter: screening and diagnosis of autism: report of the Quality Standards Subcommittee of the American Academy of Neurology and the Child Neurology Society. *Neurology* 2000; 55(4):468–479.
23. Danielsson S, Gillberg IC, Billstedt E, Gillberg C, et al. Epilepsy in young adults with autism: a prospective population-based follow-up study of 120 individuals diagnosed in childhood. *Epilepsia* 2005; 46(6):918–923.
24. Kumada T, Ito M, Miyajima T, Fujii T, et al. Multi-institutional study on the correlation between chromosomal abnormalities and epilepsy. *Brain Dev* 2005; 27(2):127–134.
25. Schinzel A, Niedrist D. Chromosome imbalances associated with epilepsy. *Am J Med Genet* 2001; 106(2):119–124.
26. Miller LL, Pellock JM, Boggs JG, DeLorenzo RJ, et al. Epilepsy and seizure occurrence in a population-based sample of Virginian twins and their families. *Epilepsy Res* 1999; 34(2–3):135–143.
27. Callenbach PM, van den Maagdenberg AM, Frants RR, Brouwer OF. Clinical and genetic aspects of idiopathic epilepsies in childhood. *Eur J Paediatr Neurol* 2005; 9(2): 91–103.
28. Ottman R, Lee JH, Risch N, Hauser WA, et al. Clinical indicators of genetic susceptibility to epilepsy. *Epilepsia* 1996; 37(4):353–361.
29. Corey LA, Pellock JM, Boggs JG, Miller LL, et al. Evidence for a genetic predisposition for status epilepticus. *Neurology* 1998; 50(2):558–560.
30. Barkovich AJ, Kuzniecky RI, Jackson GD, Guerrini R, et al. Classification system for malformations of cortical development: update 2001. *Neurology* 2001; 57(12):2168–2178.
31. Glass RB, Fernbach SK, Norton KI, Choi PS, et al. The infant skull: a vault of information. *Radiographics* 2004; 24(2):507–522.
32. Sztrha L, Dawodu A, Gururaj A, Johansen JG. Microcephaly associated with abnormal gyral pattern. *Neuropediatrics* 2004; 35(6):346–352.
33. Smith DW, Gong BT. Scalp-hair patterning: its origin and significance relative to early brain and upper facial development. *Teratology* 1974; 9(1):17–34.
34. Nordli DR Jr, De Vivo DC. Classification of infantile seizures: implications for identification and treatment of inborn errors of metabolism. *J Child Neurol* 2002; 17 Suppl 3:3S3–3S7; discussion 3S8.
35. Vigevano F, Bartuli A. Infantile epileptic syndromes and metabolic etiologies. *J Child Neurol* 2002; 17 Suppl 3:3S9–3S13; discussion 3S14.
36. Buist NR, Dulac O, Bottiglieri T, Gartner J, et al. Metabolic evaluation of infantile epilepsy: summary recommendations of the Amalfi Group. *J Child Neurol* 2002; 17 Suppl 3:3S98–3S102.
37. Leary LD, Nordli DR, Jr., De Vivo DC. Epilepsy in the setting of inherited metabolic and mitochondrial disorders. In: Wyllie E, Gupta A, Lachhwani DK. *The Treatment of Epilepsy: Principles and Practice.* Philadelphia: Lippincott, Williams, & Wilkins, 2006:562.
38. Tein I. Role of carnitine and fatty acid oxidation and its defects in infantile epilepsy. *J Child Neurol* 2002; 17 Suppl 3:3S57–3S82; discussion 3S82–3S83.
39. Leuzzi V. Inborn errors of creatine metabolism and epilepsy: clinical features, diagnosis, and treatment. *J Child Neurol* 2002; 17 Suppl 3:3S89–3S97; discussion 3S97.
40. Hyland K, Arnold LA. Value of lumbar puncture in the diagnosis of infantile epilepsy and folinic acid-responsive seizures. *J Child Neurol* 2002; 17 Suppl 3:3S48–3S55; discussion 3S56.
41. Jaeken J. Genetic disorders of gamma-aminobutyric acid, glycine, and serine as causes of epilepsy. *J Child Neurol* 2002; 17 Suppl 3:3S84–3S87; discussion 3S88.
42. DiMauro S, Andreu AL, De Vivo DC. Mitochondrial disorders. *J Child Neurol* 2002; 17 Suppl 3:3S35–3S45; discussion 3S46–3S47.
43. Canafoglia L, Franceschetti S, Antozzi C, Carrara F, et al. Epileptic phenotypes associated with mitochondrial disorders. *Neurology* 2001; 56(10):1340–1346.
44. Singh R, Gardner RJ, Crossland KM, Scheffer IE, et al. Chromosomal abnormalities and epilepsy: a review for clinicians and gene hunters. *Epilepsia* 2002; 43(2): 127–140.
45. Shinnar S, Kang H, Berg AT, Goldensohn ES, et al. EEG abnormalities in children with a first unprovoked seizure. *Epilepsia* 1994; 35(3):471–476.
46. Yoshinaga H, Hattori J, Ohta H, Asano T, et al. Utility of the scalp-recorded ictal EEG in childhood epilepsy. *Epilepsia* 2001; 42(6):772–777.
47. King MA, Newton MR, Jackson GD, Pitt GJ, et al. Epileptology of the first-seizure presentation: a clinical, electroencephalographic, and magnetic resonance imaging study of 300 consecutive patients. *Lancet* 1998; 352:1007–1011.
48. Alehan FK, Morton LD, Pellock JM. Utility of electroencephalography in the pediatric emergency department. *J Child Neurol* 2001; 16(7):484–487.

49. Jan MM. Assessment of the utility of paediatric electroencephalography. *Seizure* 2002; 11(2):99–103.
50. Gilbert DL, DeRoos S, Bare MA. Does sleep or sleep deprivation increase epileptiform discharges in pediatric electroencephalograms? *Pediatrics* 2004; 114(3):658–662.
51. Flink R, Pederson B, Guekhi AB, Malmgren K, et al. Guidelines for the use of EEG methodology in the diagnosis of epilepsy. International League Against Epilepsy: commission report. Commission on European Affairs: Subcommission on European Guidelines. *Acta Neurol Scand* 2002; 106(1):1–7.
52. Shinnar S, O'Dell C, Mitnick R, Berg AT, et al. Neuroimaging abnormalities in children with an apparent first unprovoked seizure. *Epilepsy Res* 2001; 43(3):261–269.
53. Berg AT, Testa FM, Levy SR, Shinnar S. Neuroimaging in children with newly diagnosed epilepsy: a community-based study. *Pediatrics* 2000; 106(3):527–532.

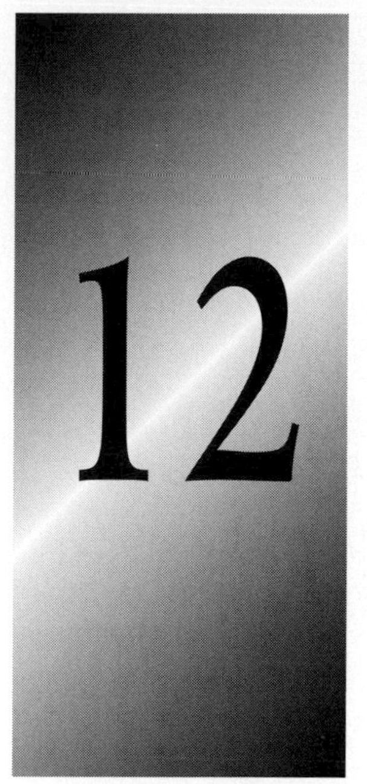

The Use of Electroencephalography in the Diagnosis of Epilepsy in Childhood

Douglas R. Nordli, Jr.
Timothy A. Pedley

The electroencephalogram (EEG) is often the single most informative laboratory test in evaluating children with seizures. At the most rudimentary level, it helps in differentiating epileptic from nonepileptic behavior. Because many conditions, including breathholding spells, movement disorders, syncope, cardiac arrhythmias, sleep disorders, migraine, and various psychiatric syndromes, may mimic epilepsy, EEG findings are often essential in making an accurate diagnosis.

EEG, however, offers much more. More detailed analysis of epileptiform abnormalities assists in distinguishing focal from generalized seizures and in identifying epileptic syndromes, which are indispensable cornerstones of rational therapy. EEG aids in recognizing subclinical and nonconvulsive seizures, in documenting antiepileptic drug (AED) toxicity, and probably in selecting patients for AED withdrawal after remission of seizures. Finally, EEG is critical in evaluating patients with medically refractory seizures for focal resective and other surgical procedures.

EEG TECHNIQUE

To record the EEG, a technician places electrodes, usually gold or silver discs, at standard locations on the scalp using collodion adhesive or a conducting paste. Potential differences between pairs of electrodes are then amplified and the net signal from each amplifier is displayed on a monitor (digital EEG machines) or written on paper (historical EEG machines) to provide a graphic record of EEG voltage changes over time. In practice, modern EEG machines display activity from 20 or more channels (1 pair of electrodes = 1 amplifier channel) simultaneously to provide a comprehensive survey of cerebral electrical activity.

Much of the value of EEG lies in determining the spatial distribution of voltage fields on the scalp. To do this, electrodes are grouped in logical arrangements called *montages*. Montages typically allow comparisons between symmetric areas of the two hemispheres and between parasagittal and temporal areas in the same hemisphere. Most laboratories use as minimum a series of standard montages recommended by the American EEG Society (1). In addition to these, special montages may have to be designed to address issues posed by a particular patient. Creative use of rationally designed montages significantly enhances the utility of the EEG.

A technician typically records spontaneous EEG activity for approximately 30 minutes. However, the yield of positive findings is greatly increased by several activating procedures: hyperventilation, photic stimulation, and sleep. All three are useful in children with suspected seizures or epilepsy.

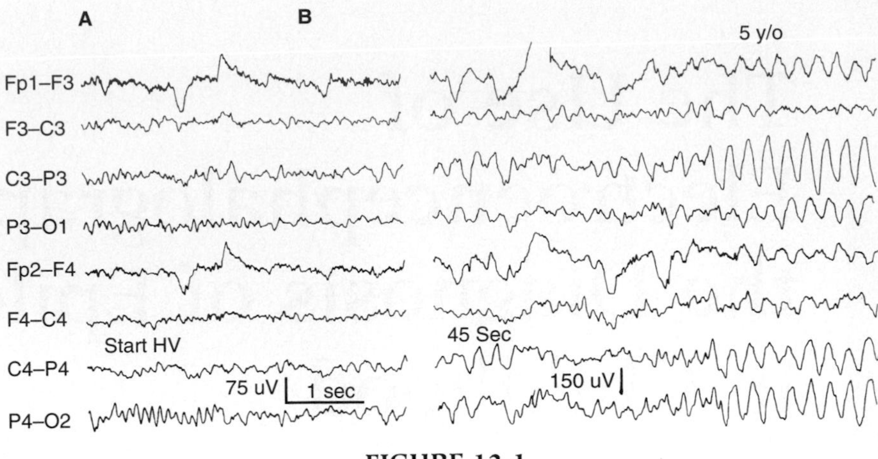

FIGURE 12-1

Effects of hyperventilation in a 5-year-old child. (A) EEG at onset of overbreathing effort; (B) 45 seconds later. There is a moderate buildup of generalized rhythmic slow-wave activity, maximal over the posterior head regions.

Hyperventilation

Hyperventilation for at least 3 minutes, preferably 5 minutes if absence seizures are strongly suspected, should be performed whenever possible. Overbreathing can be achieved even with preschool children if the technician incorporates playful strategies such as blowing a pinwheel or "having a race" to see who can breathe faster. The effect of hyperventilation on EEG activity in children is usually dramatic, with high-voltage, generalized, rhythmic slow waves appearing promptly (Figure 12-1). The mechanisms underlying this age-related normal phenomenon are not known, but changes in cerebral blood flow and the neuronal metabolic milieu are probable factors. What is more important, however, is the empiric observation that a brief period of vigorous overbreathing potently activates generalized epileptiform discharges, especially 3-Hz spike-wave activity. Sometimes focal slow-wave activity associated with structural lesions may appear or be accentuated during hyperventilation. The only responses to hyperventilation that can be unambiguously categorized as abnormal are asymmetric changes and epileptiform discharges.

Photic Stimulation

Photic stimulation is performed using stroboscopic flashes of high-intensity white light at rates of 1 to 30 flashes per second. Stimulation is intermittent, with each frequency delivered for 10 to 20 seconds. A normal physiologic response is entrainment of EEG activity over the occipital lobes at the flash frequency (photic driving) (Figure 12-2A). In some normal children, photic stimulation produces no effect, and in others, the photic driving may be asymmetric. A photoparoxysmal response characterized by generalized bursts of irregular spikes, spike-wave discharges, and multiple spike-wave discharges (Figure 12-2B) occurs in some patients with idiopathic generalized epilepsy. However, it also occurs in a significant percentage of normal children without seizures, presumably as an asymptomatic marker of a genetic trait. Doose and Gerken (2) propose a multifactorial mode of inheritance.

Sleep and Sleep Deprivation

Light sleep substantially increases the percentage of EEGs showing epileptiform activity in patients with epilepsy. The occurrences of both focal and generalized discharges are increased in non-rapid-eye-movement (non-REM) sleep, but rapid eye movement (REM) sleep has a differential effect. Generalized epileptiform activity diminishes markedly or disappears altogether in REM, whereas focal spikes and sharp waves either are unaffected or actually increase in abundance (3).

Sleep deprivation also activates epileptiform activity independent of its sleep-inducing effect (4, 5). Kellaway and Frost (6) have speculated that sleep deprivation and spontaneous or sedated sleep activate abnormalities via different mechanisms.

Scheduling the EEG at the time a child normally naps facilitates sleep recordings. Older children may be partially sleep-deprived with benefit. If children do not sleep spontaneously, they may be given chloral hydrate (30–60 mg/kg) with appropriate guidelines for conscious sedation.

Special Electrodes

Some cortical areas (mesial temporal, orbital frontal, and interhemispheric regions) are relatively inaccessible to

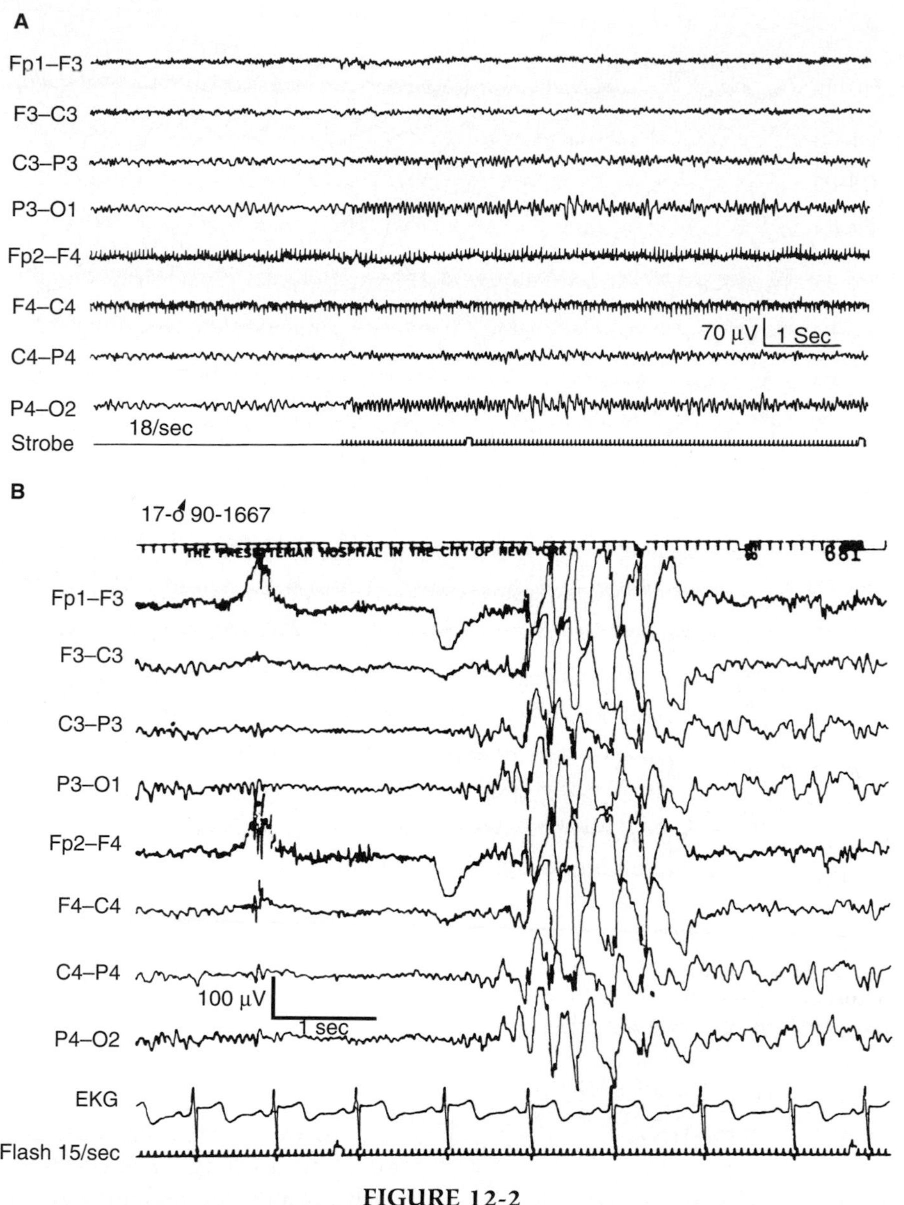

FIGURE 12-2

(A) Normal physiologic response is entrainment of cerebral electrical activity over the occipital regions at the frequency of light stimulation (driving response). (B) Photoparoxysmal response in another child occurring during stroboscopic light stimulation. Bursts of spikes and irregular spike-wave discharges occur during and immediately after the light stimulus. In this case, there were no clinical manifestations during the photoparoxysmal response and no clinical history of photosensitivity.

conventional recording electrodes. If one of these areas is suspected of being the epileptogenic focus, supplemental electrode placements can augment standard ones. Thus, surface placement of anterior temporal, mandibular notch, and supraorbital electrodes are useful in documenting inferior frontal and mesiobasal temporal epileptiform discharges (7).

More invasively, sphenoidal electrodes, which are fine wires inserted transcutaneously through the mandibular notch so that the tips lie near the foramen ovale at the base of the skull, are commonly used in monitoring units evaluating patients for resective surgery (8). Nasopharyngeal electrodes, which are flexible wires that are inserted through the nose to lie in the posterior pharynx, have been widely used in the past, but subsequent studies have cast doubt on their superiority over surface locations, especially anterior and inferior temporal leads, in recording mesial temporal lobe discharges (7, 9, 10).

Invasive electrodes should not be used in children except in special circumstances. Adequate information can usually be obtained using standard scalp electrodes supplemented, as necessary, with additional special placements.

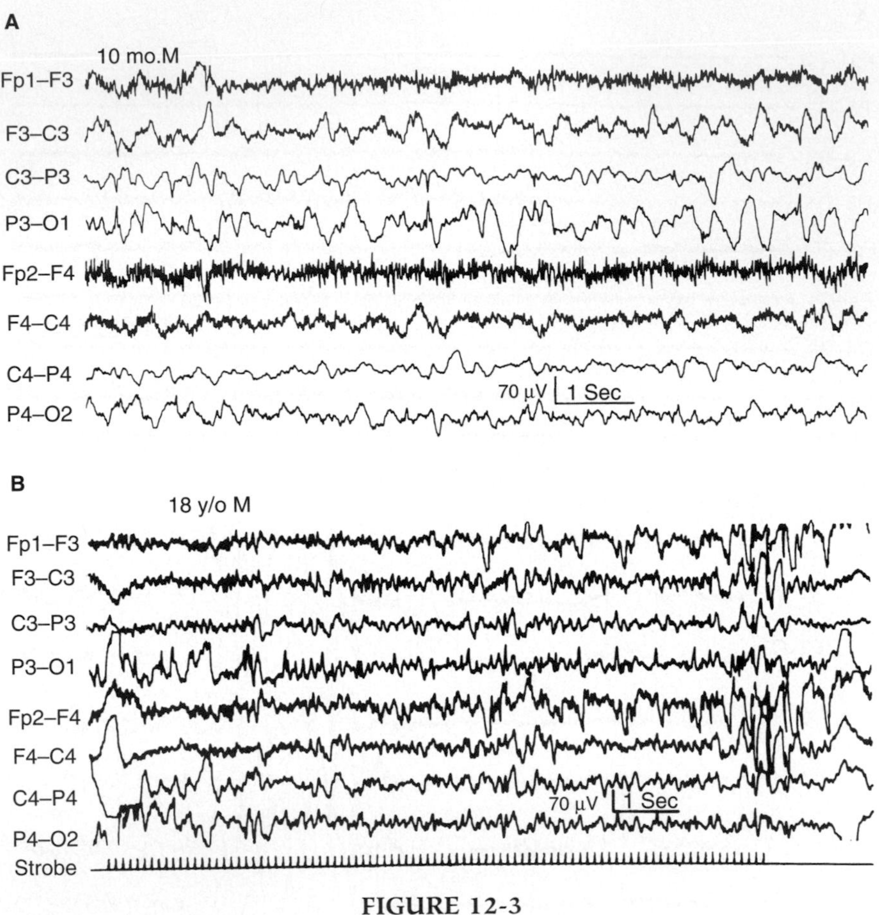

FIGURE 12-3

(A) Focal left parietal spikes (discharge is at P3 in third and fourth channels) in a 10-month-old boy with simple partial seizures involving his right arm and face. (B) Generalized 4- to 5-Hz spike-wave activity in an 18-year-old male with idiopathic generalized tonic-clonic seizures, precipitated by stimluation.

SPECIFIC EEG FINDING

Epileptiform Activity and Epileptogenicity

The only EEG finding that indicates a susceptibility to epileptic seizures is epileptiform activity, that is, spikes, sharp waves, or spike-wave discharges (Figure 12-3).

Although epileptiform discharges indicate an increased risk of seizures, they vary in degree of epileptogenicity, that is, the association with active epilepsy. Epileptogenicity is at least partly age-related. In adults, epileptiform discharges have a high association with seizures and occur only rarely in normal individuals. The situation is more complicated in children, largely because of the occurrence of genetic patterns that may not be associated with clinical seizures. Nonetheless, even in children, epileptiform discharges are uncommon in normal individuals, approximating perhaps 2% in the prevalence studies of Petersen and coworkers (11). From another perspective, Trojaborg (12) found that 83% of children whose EEGs contained focal spikes had seizures.

Another variable that relates to epileptogenicity is location of the discharge. The likelihood of epilepsy is highest when epileptiform discharges are multifocal or when they involve the temporal lobe: 76% and 90%, respectively (13). Risk of epilepsy is considerably lower (approximately 50%) when epileptiform activity involves the central-midtemporal (rolandic) or occipital regions (13).

All epileptiform activity decreases in abundance with age or the passage of time, and less than 10% persists indefinitely (13). In general, there is no useful correlation in individual patients between the amount of epileptiform activity in the EEG and the number and intensity of clinical seizures.

NONSPECIFIC EEG ABNORMALITIES

Abnormalities other than epileptiform discharges are also common in the EEGs of patients with epilepsy. Nonepileptiform abnormalities are termed *nonspecific* because

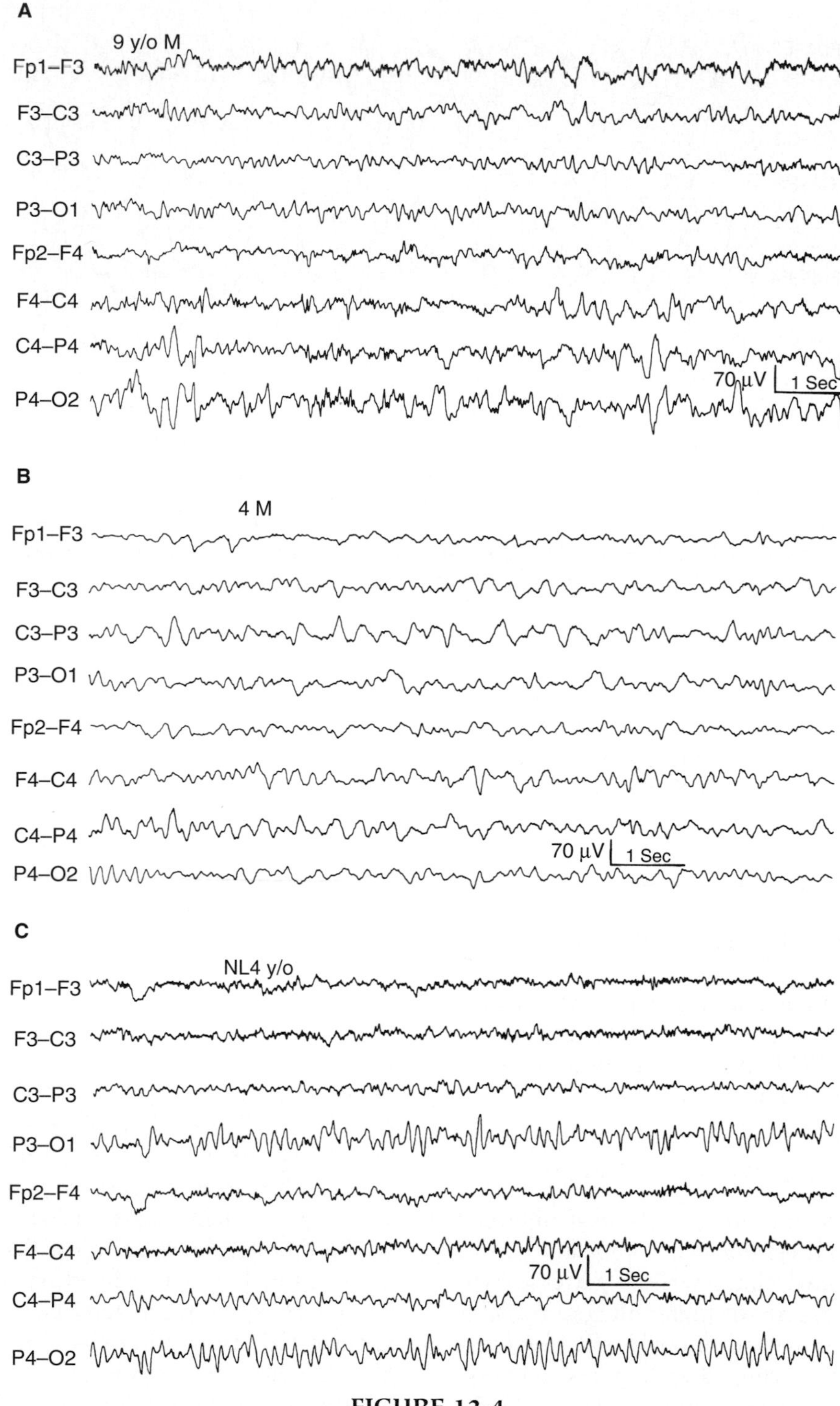

FIGURE 12-4

(A) This EEG sample demonstrates continuous focal arrhythmic slow activity in the right central-parietal region (bottom three channels). (B) In contrast, this EEG sample shows excessive generalized arrhythmic slow activity. The EEG of a normal 4-year-old is shown for comparison (C).

they occur in many other conditions as well, or sometimes even in normal subjects. Examples of nonspecific abnormalities include focal or generalized slow-wave activity (Figure 12-4) or, less often, asymmetries of frequency or voltage. Unlike epileptiform discharges, such findings do not provide support for a diagnosis of epilepsy because of their varied clinical associations and because they do not reflect an epileptogenic disturbance of neuronal function.

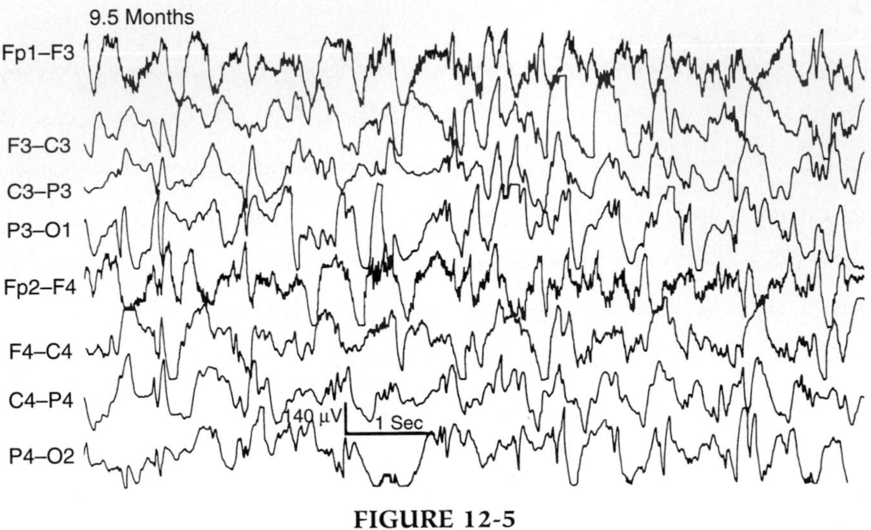

FIGURE 12-5

Hypsarhythmia in a 9.5-month-old infant with infantile spasms. There is extremely high-voltage slow-wave activity diffusely, multifocal spikes, and lack of normal organization and patterns.

Nonspecific findings are important, however, in providing general information about cerebral function. Thus, evaluation of nonspecific EEG abnormalities may help identify associated static or reversible encephalopathies, underlying focal cerebral lesions, or progressive neurologic syndromes.

PEDIATRIC EPILEPTIC SYNDROMES

Electroencephalography is crucial for accurate classification of different forms of epilepsy. The following are brief descriptions of EEG findings in the more common epileptic syndromes encountered in childhood.

Infantile Spasms (West Syndrome)

The EEG is always abnormal, grossly so if obtained when seizures are well established. Gibbs and Gibbs (14) identified the most characteristic pattern, hypsarhythmia, which consists of high-voltage, irregular slow waves occurring asynchronously and randomly over all head regions, intermixed with spikes and polyspikes from multiple independent loci (Figure 12-5). fiVariations of the pattern (modified hypsarhythmia) occur in up to 10% to 15% of children with infantile spasms (15). These other abnormalities, however, are more likely to occur in older infants or if the EEG is performed later in the course of the disorder. Like infantile spasms, hypsarhythmia is age-specific. It is usually most pronounced in slow-wave sleep and may disappear completely in REM. Ictal recordings show various patterns (16), but the most common accompaniment to a spasm is one or more generalized, high-voltage slow or sharp-slow waves followed by abrupt voltage attenuation of background activity lasting from 1 to several seconds, the so-called electrodecremental event (Figure 12-6) (17). Type of spasm does not always correlate well with a particular EEG ictal pattern, and neither do all spasms have EEG correlates. EEG and clinical improvement usually parallel one another, but they may be dissociated.

Childhood Absence Epilepsy

EEGs are rarely normal in untreated children with childhood absence epilepsy (formerly referred to as petit mal epilepsy), and hyperventilation is particularly effective in provoking the characteristic EEG abnormality. In fact, repeated normal EEGs in a child with lapse attacks argue strongly against a diagnosis of childhood absence epilepsy. Each absence seizure is accompanied by generalized, symmetric, stereotyped 3- to 4-Hz spike-wave activity (Figure 12-7A). Background activity is otherwise normal or near normal. Sleep produces striking effects on appearance of the epileptiform activity (Figure 12-7B). Classic features are lost, and instead epileptiform bursts are fragmented, are of shorter duration, and contain more single spikes and multiple spikes.

Spike-wave paroxysms begin abruptly, producing immediate alteration in the child's responsiveness (18). Conversely, when the 3-Hz spike-wave discharge ends, the child's behavior becomes normal at once (18). Detailed analysis of motor and cognitive effects reveals differences in their time course and evolution

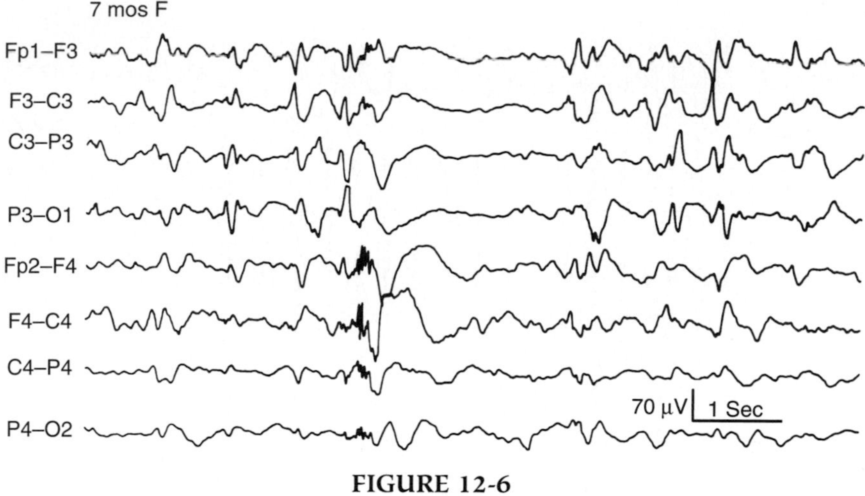

FIGURE 12-6

Electrodecremental event in a 7-month-old child characterized by transient flattening of background activity (middle of figure). Such events frequently accompany the massive spasms of West syndrome.

in relation to the ictal discharge (19). Even short bursts of 3-Hz spike-wave activity produce some functional impairment that may go unrecognized clinically. Thus, childhood absence epilepsy is one instance in which follow-up EEGs are often necessary to gauge how effective treatment is; clinical reports alone may be inadequate.

Lennox-Gastaut Syndrome

The name *Lennox-Gastaut syndrome* (childhood epileptic encephalopathy) has been applied to a heterogeneous group of children with severe seizures, mental retardation, and a characteristic EEG pattern. EEG findings are most typical between 2 and 7 years of age and are remarkably consistent despite widely different underlying causes, including progressive degenerative or metabolic disease, cerebral malformations, perinatal asphyxia, severe head injury, anoxic encephalopathy, and central nervous system infection (20).

EEGs show generalized, bisynchronous sharp- and-slow-wave complexes occurring repetitively, often in extended runs, at 1.5 to 2.5 Hz (Figure 12-8). Within the same record and among patients, the sharp-slow waves vary somewhat in distribution, voltage, and repetition rate. Sleep usually activates epileptiform activity markedly; hyperventilation does so less consistently. Multifocal spikes or sharp waves also occur, especially in older children. Electrodecremental or tonic seizure patterns (Figure 12-9) lasting 2 to 4 seconds occur frequently during sleep, sometimes as often as hundreds of times per night. Clinical correlates of these nocturnal seizure discharges are minimal, most often being slight stiffening of the axial muscles. Background activity is almost always moderately to severely abnormal because of excessive slowing and poor development of normal patterns for age.

A history of West syndrome is present in up to one-third of children with Lennox-Gastaut syndrome (21), suggesting that EEG manifestations of severe encephalopathies reflect, in part, an age-dependent continuum with particular patterns emerging from interaction of maturational and pathologic factors.

Myoclonic-Astatic Epilepsy As Described by Doose

Myoclonic-astatic epilepsy (MAE) as described by Doose is sometimes confused with Lennox-Gastaut syndrome (21b). Children with MAE are usually normal at onset of the epilepsy. The most prominent seizure consists of a sudden drop attack, or myoclonic-astatic seizure, characterized by a combination of sudden myoclonic jerk of the arms and head followed by a brief period of atonia. This results in sudden falls with the potential for injury. This is often accompanied by a brief bursts of generalized spike or repeated spike-wave activity followedy by a diffuse profound attenuation (Figure 12-10). Nocturnal tonic seizures may be seen in some individuals, but more common are clonic-tonic-clonic seizures of intermediate duration ("moyen-mal"). Absence seizures can also occur, and sometimes children develop absence or myoclonic status epilepticus. The interictal EEG may show runs of rhythmic parasagittal slowing (Figure 12-11) and brief generalized spike-wave discharges. These discharges may appears as single spike-wave discharges or as doublets or triplets, so that it may be hard to determine the

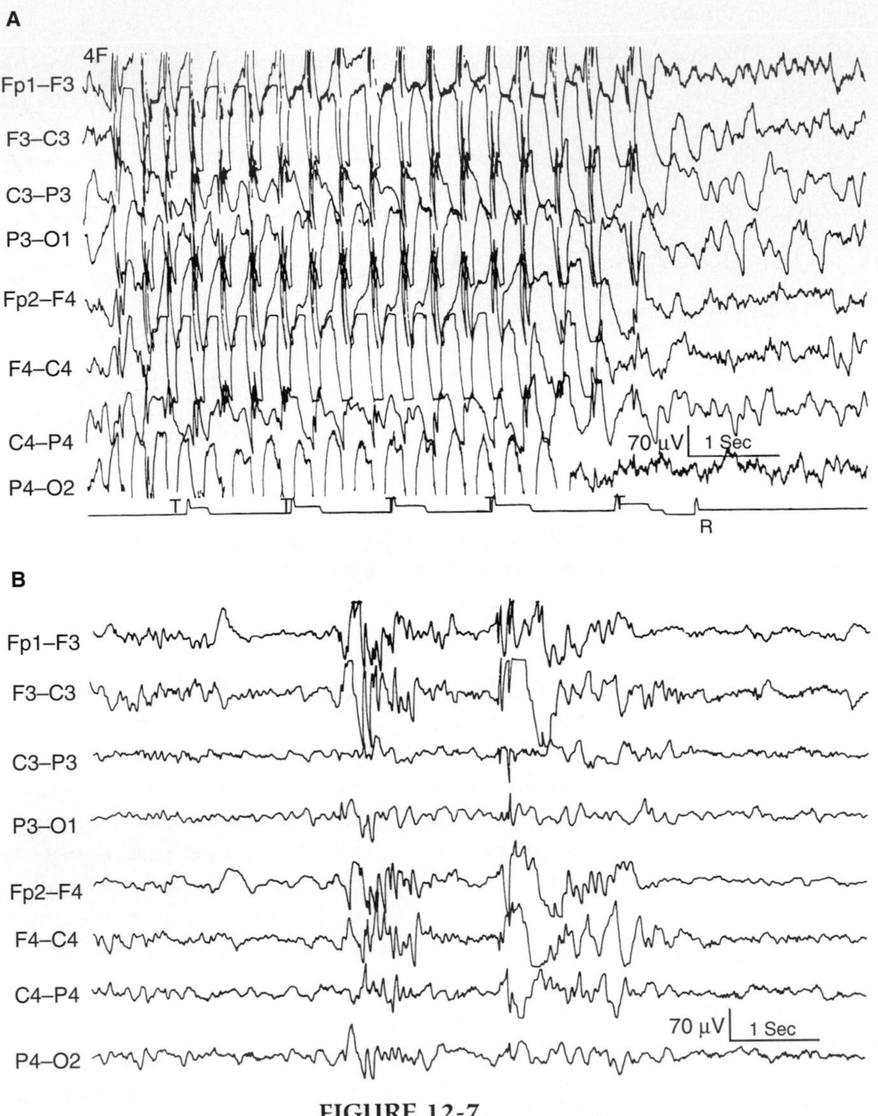

FIGURE 12-7

(A) Stereotyped 3-Hz spike-wave activity in a 4-year-old child with childhood absence epilepsy. The bottom channel records a test tone (T) to which the child has been trained to respond by pressing a button (R). During the generalized spike-wave activity, the child's ability to respond is impaired (absence attack). Normal responsiveness returns immediately upon cessation of the discharge. (B) EEG from same child showing alteration in spike-wave morphology during sleep. The epileptiform activity has become fragmented and contains multiple spikes (polyspikes). The well-formed 3-Hz spike-wave complexes seen during wakefulness no longer occur. Such changes, although varying in degree, are typical of generalized epileptiform abnormalities.

repetition rate accurately. When discernible, repetition rates may be slow (i.e., below 3 Hz) or fast (i.e., above 3 Hz) (Figure 12-12).

Benign Focal Epilepsy with Central-Midtemporal Spikes

The syndrome of benign focal epilepsy with central-midtemporal spikes, which is also referred to as central-temporal epilepsy, sylvian seizures, and rolandic epilepsy, is an idiopathic localization-related epilepsy with highly characteristic EEG and clinical features (22–24).

EEG findings are distinctive and diagnostic. Focal di- or triphasic sharp waves of almost invariant morphology occur in the central and midtemporal regions (Figure 12-13). Epileptiform discharges are usually of high voltage (>100 µV), tend to occur in clusters, and activate dramatically during sleep, when they may seem almost continuous. Discharges may be unilateral in a single EEG, but they are almost always bilaterally present with prolonged or repeated recordings. Lateralization

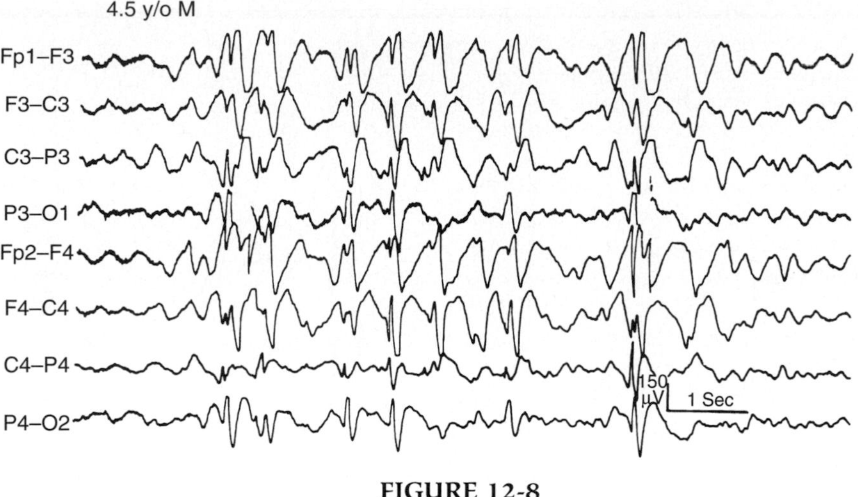

FIGURE 12-8

Generalized sharp- and slow-wave complexes (slow spike-and-wave discharges) occurring repetitively at about 2 Hz in a child with Lennox-Gastaut syndrome.

may switch in serial tracings (22, 23). Generalized spikes and spike-wave activity occasionally occur, usually during sleep (23, 25, 26), and "benign" occipital spikes or multifocal spikes may coexist, especially in younger patients (22, 25).

There is no correlation between EEG findings and seizure occurrence or frequency. As a rule, EEG abnormalities are much more impressive than clinical seizure activity. Indeed, when central-midtemporal spikes are recorded in children without seizures who have EEGs for other reasons, only about half eventually develop typical seizures (13). Furthermore, in symptomatic children, EEG abnormalities persist long after seizures cease. Thus, EEG does not provide assistance in making decisions about when or how long to treat.

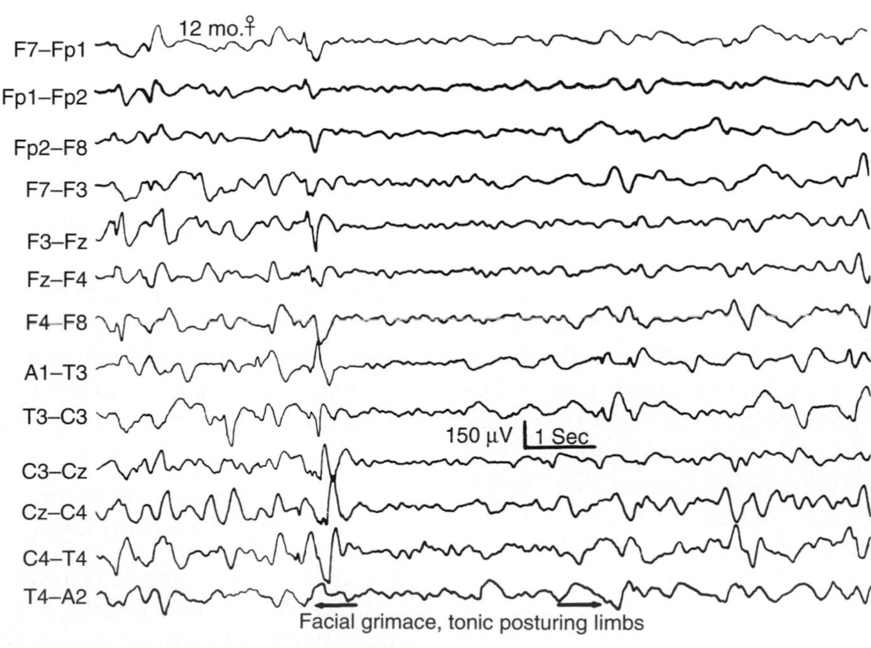

FIGURE 12-9

Tonic seizure during sleep in a child with severe mental retardation and uncontrolled tonic, atonic, and atypical absence seizures. The EEG correlate is an electrodecremental event. Sometimes a low voltage 16- to 25-Hz rhythmic discharge (tonic seizure pattern) occurs during this type of clinical event.

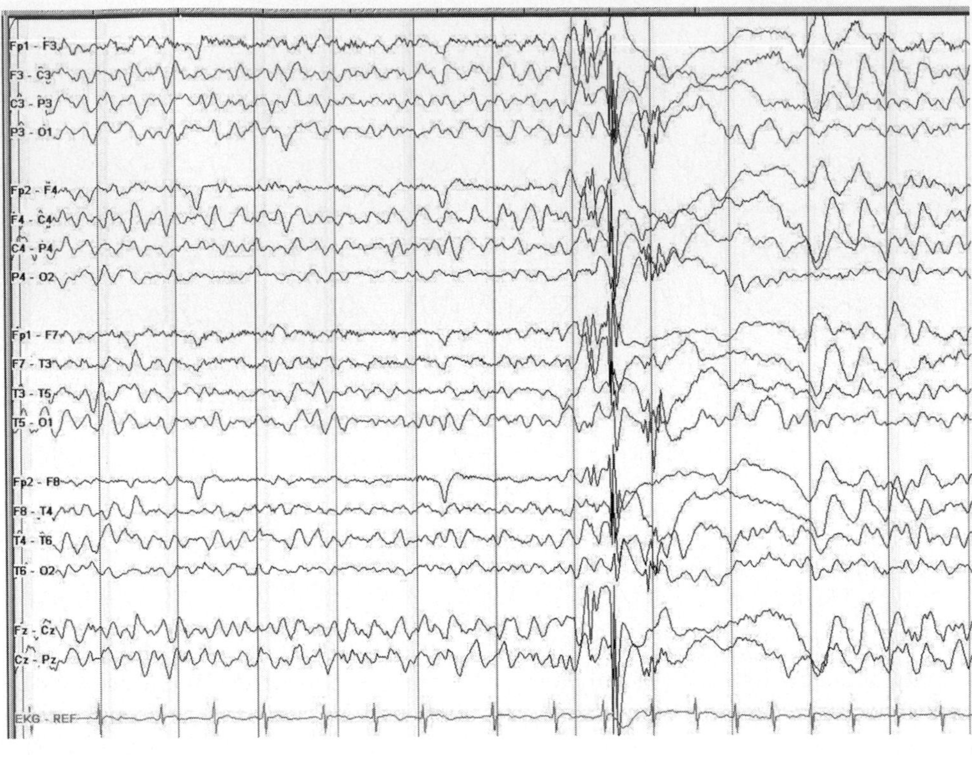

FIGURE 12-10

This patient with myoclonic-astatic epilepsy had a head drop accompanied by a diffuse spike-wave discharge with after-going attenuation.

Genetic studies indicate that the EEG trait is controlled by an autosomal dominant gene with age-dependent penetrance (27, 28).

Benign Focal Epilepsy with Occipital Spikes

Gastaut (29) has described another form of idiopathic localization-related epilepsy in children, in which visual symptoms—either amblyopia or hallucinations—are a common early feature of ictal events. The EEG shows stereotyped, high-voltage (200–300 μV) sharp-wave discharges over one or both occipital regions. Epileptiform activity is attenuated by eye opening and is activated by sleep. Discharge morphology resembles that of central-midtemporal spikes. Background activity is normal. This electroclinical entity is more heterogeneous than benign focal epilepsy with central-midtemporal spikes. Nonetheless, outcome is usually benign in a typical case, with complete resolution of clinical and EEG findings in most children by 18 years of age. Like central-midtemporal spikes, occipital spikes do not correlate with clinical seizure activity or prognosis, and they often persist after seizures cease. Generalized spike-wave discharges and centralmidtemporal spikes may coexist.

A more common benign epilepsy has been described by Panayiotopoulos (29b). Affected children are usually younger than those described by Gastaut and have few clinical attacks. Seizures are, however, often prolonged and have prominent autonomic features. Children characteristically vomit and become listless during the seizures (autonomic status epilepticus). Early descriptions highlighted the importance of stereotyped occipital spikes, but Panayiotopoulos has subsequently showed that "cloned-like" or highly stereotyped interictal epileptiform discharges may be seen in multiple different locations. Spikes may be most prominent in the occipital regions in younger individuals, but they "migrate" to more anterior locations in older individuals (Figure 12-14).

Dravet Syndrome (Severe Myoclonic Epilepsy in Infancy)

Dravet syndrome manifests in the first year of life, often with febrile convulsions (29c). These may be hemiconvulsions and are often prolonged. Later, myoclonic seizures, atypical absences, and focal seizures develop. Not all seizure types are seen in each individual child. The interictal EEG may initially be normal. Some infants will show

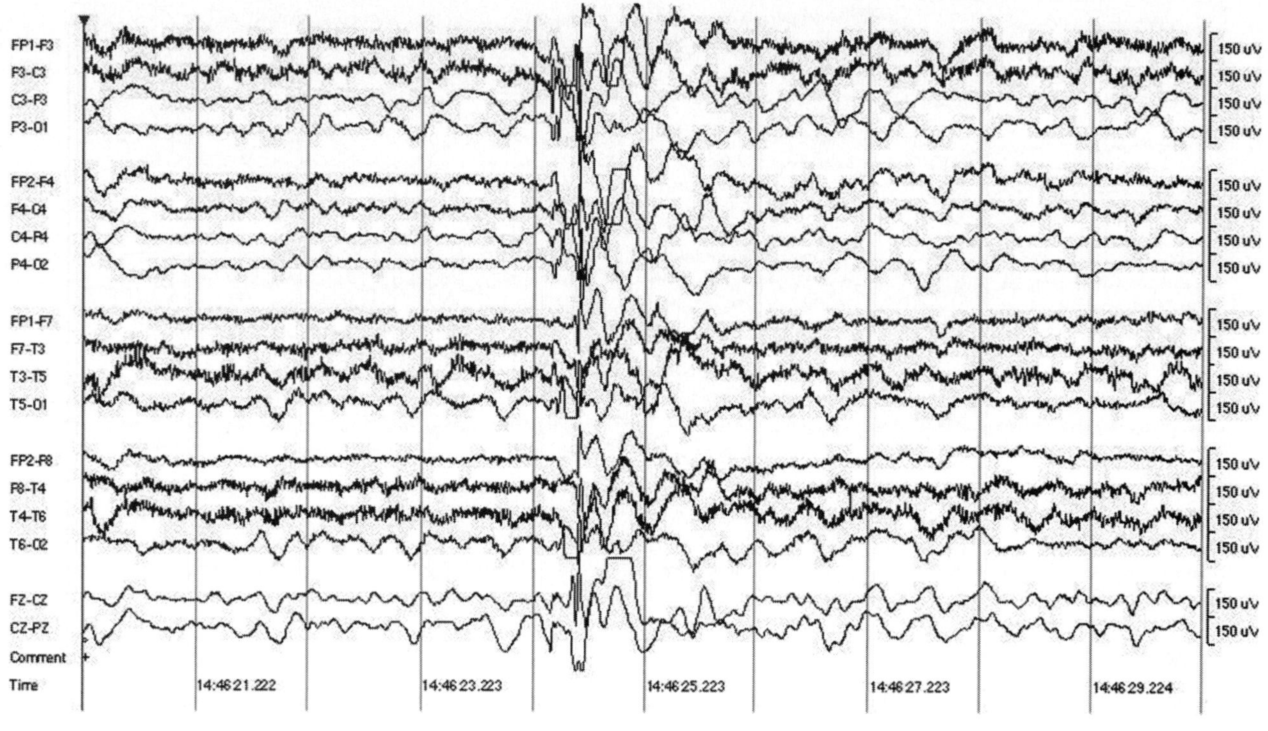

FIGURE 12-11

Children with MAE may have prominent runs of rhythmic biparietal slowing.

photoparoxysmal responses. Usually within one year of onset, the EEG becomes abnormal with background slowing and the appearance of interictal epielptiform discharges. In our experience, these are often most marked in the posterior derivations, and later multifocal spikes and generalized spike-wave discharges are commonly seen. Myoclonic jerks are often accompanied by generalized spike or polyspike-wave discharges. Focal seizures correlate with focal ictal patterns.

Juvenile Myoclonic Epilepsy

Janz and Christian (30) described juvenile myoclonic epilepsy (JME) or "impulsive petit mal" as a subtype of idiopathic generalized epilepsy. Interictal EEGs show generalized 4- to 6-Hz "atypical" spike-wave activity, short bursts of polyspikes, and polyspike-wave discharges (Figure 12-15). An incrementing run of 10- to 16-Hz polyspikes, maximal over the frontal-central areas, followed by a generalized burst of spikes or spike-wave activity accompanies bilateral myoclonic jerks (30, 31). If absence seizures occur, the EEG shows 3.5- to 4-Hz generalized spike-wave paroxysms. Photoparoxysmal responses are common in JME, occurring in approximately one-third of patients (32).

Acquired Epileptic Aphasia

Acquired epileptic aphasia, which is also known as the Landau-Kleffner syndrome, is not primarily an epileptic disorder, although epileptiform activity is part of the diagnostic criteria. Seizures occur in approximately 70 percent of cases but usually are infrequent. EEGs show abundant high-voltage epileptiform activity, which may be temporal, bitemporal, or generalized. Considerable slow activity accompanies epileptiform discharges. In the early stages, EEG abnormalities may occur only during sleep, and throughout the illness slow-wave sleep produces marked activation, sometimes with almost continuous generalized spike-wave activity. Review of the original case (33) and subsequent cases (34–37) of acquired epileptic aphasia does not support any single EEG feature or combination of features as being distinctive of this syndrome. AED treatment does not clearly alter the natural evolution of EEG abnormalities, clinical findings, or outcome.

Epilepsia Partialis Continua

Epilepsia partialis continua manifests as several different subtypes, but one variant—Rasmussen syndrome—occurs primarily in children as a reasonably distinct entity (38).

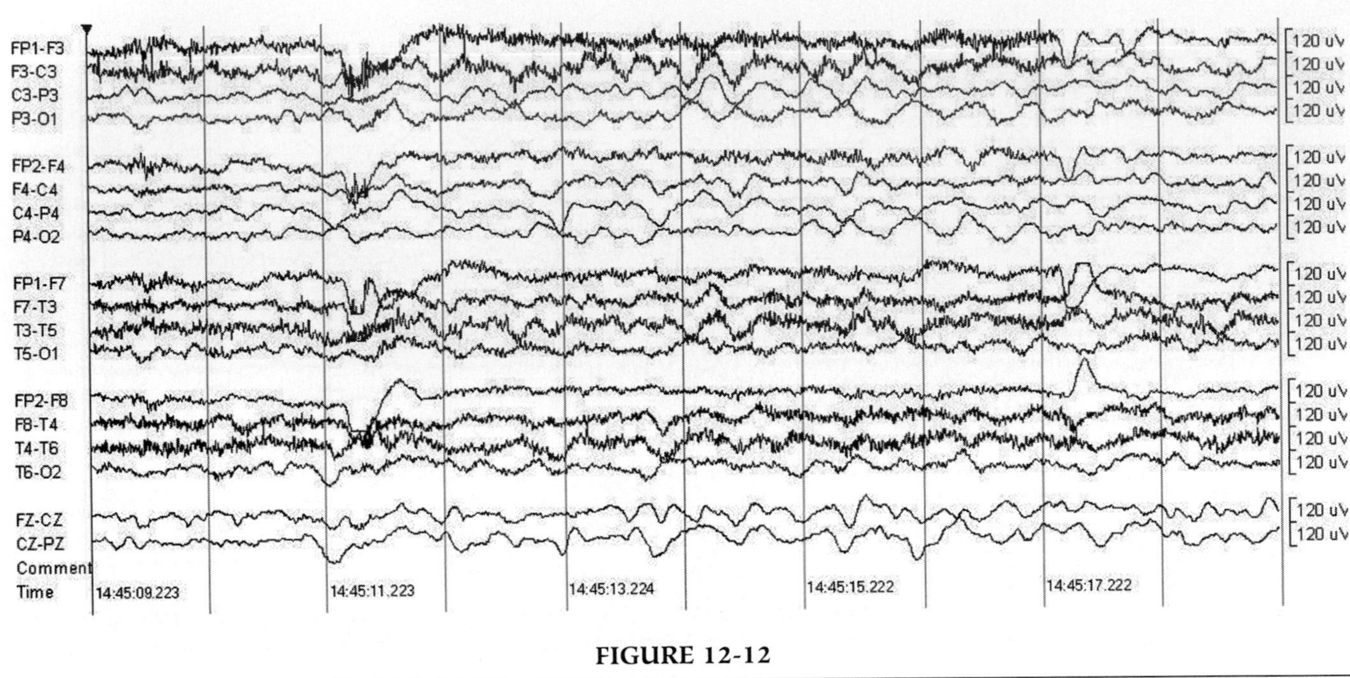

FIGURE 12-12

The interictal epileptiform discharges in MAE are often brief generalized discharges with an irregular repetition rate.

EEG findings are variable, and their topography is often difficult to characterize precisely (38, 39). Most often, interictal EEGs show excessive arrhythmic or rhythmic delta activity that is usually bilateral but accentuated over a large area contralateral to the partial seizures. Epileptiform discharges are rarely well localized and often sporadic, especially early in the illness. As the disease progresses, more abundant pleomorphic spikes and sharp waves appear over an extensive area or bilaterally. It is usually difficult to recognize distinct ictal discharges with scalp recordings; in any event, correlation of EEG changes with muscle jerks is always poor to nonexistent.

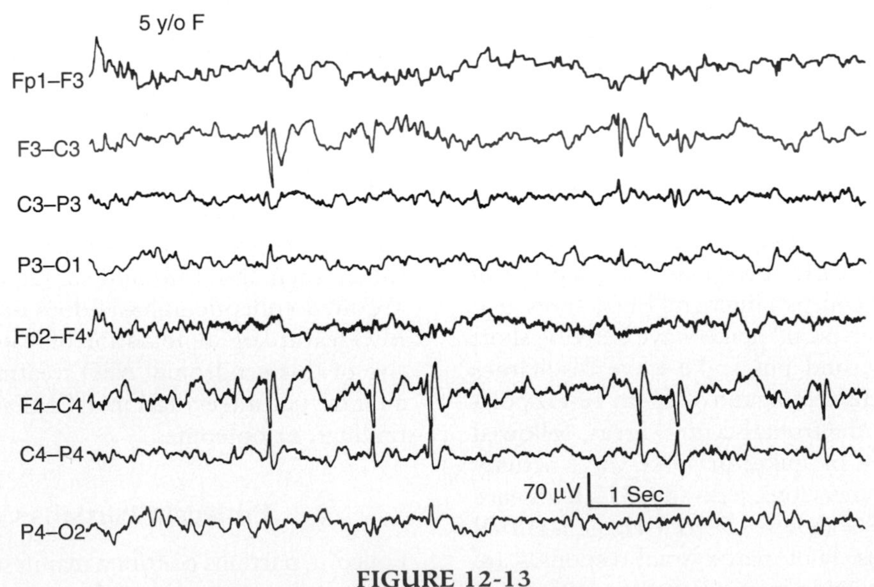

FIGURE 12-13

Stereotyped di- and triphasic sharp wave discharges occur independently in the central regions bilaterally in this child with partial seizures (benign rolandic epilepsy).

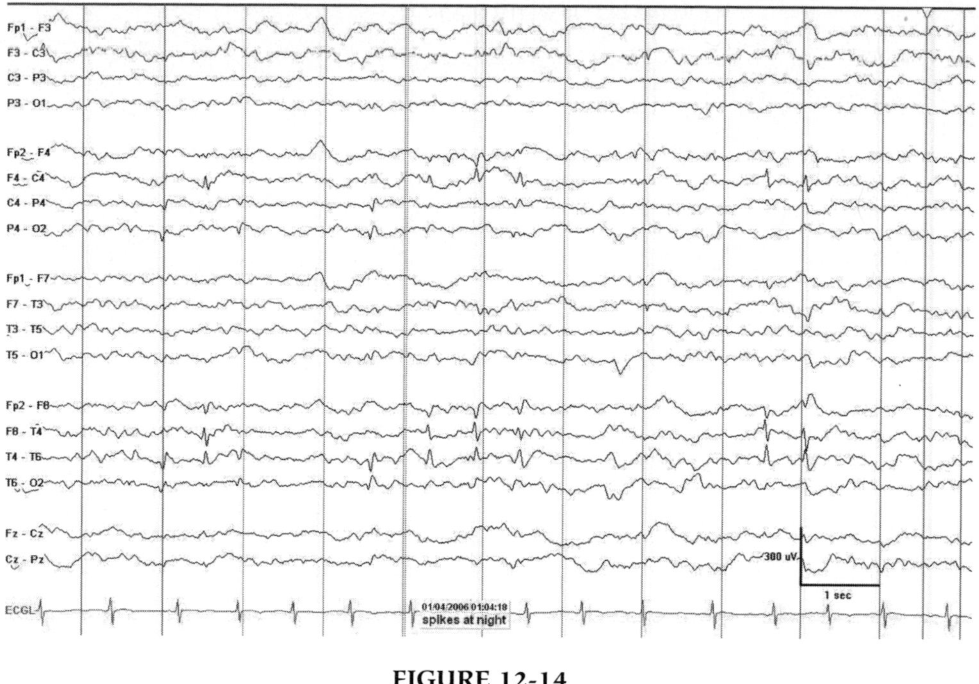

FIGURE 12-14

Highly stereotypsed interical epileptiform discharges are seen in patients with Panayiotopoulos Syndrome.

NEONATAL EEG

EEGs of neonates pose special problems in interpretation. From 26 to 40 weeks of gestation, there are explosive maturational changes in the brain that result in rapid changes in neuronal orientation, alignment, and layering accompanied by substantial dendritic development, extensive synaptogenesis, glial proliferation, and onset of myelination. These biological developments underlie rapid and predictable sequences of EEG changes that are sufficiently consistent as to allow accurate determination of conceptional age in healthy newborns to within 2 weeks.

EEGs in newborns are sufficiently different from those of older children and adults that one must take considerable caution not to overinterpret the significance of certain normal or inconsistent findings, all of which may be only transiently present. Thus, isolated spikes, or sharp transients, are common normal components of the

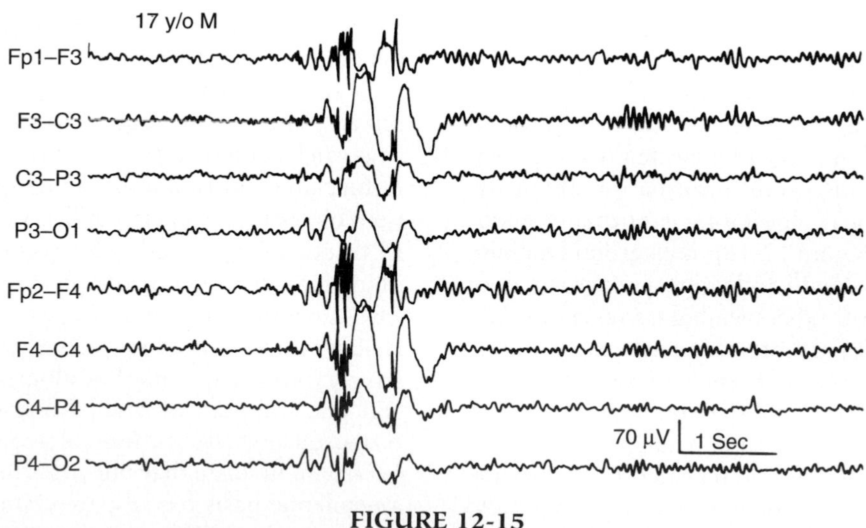

FIGURE 12-15

Generalized multiple spike-wave (polyspike-wave) discharge followed by a single spike-wave complex in a child with juvenile myoclonic epilepsy.

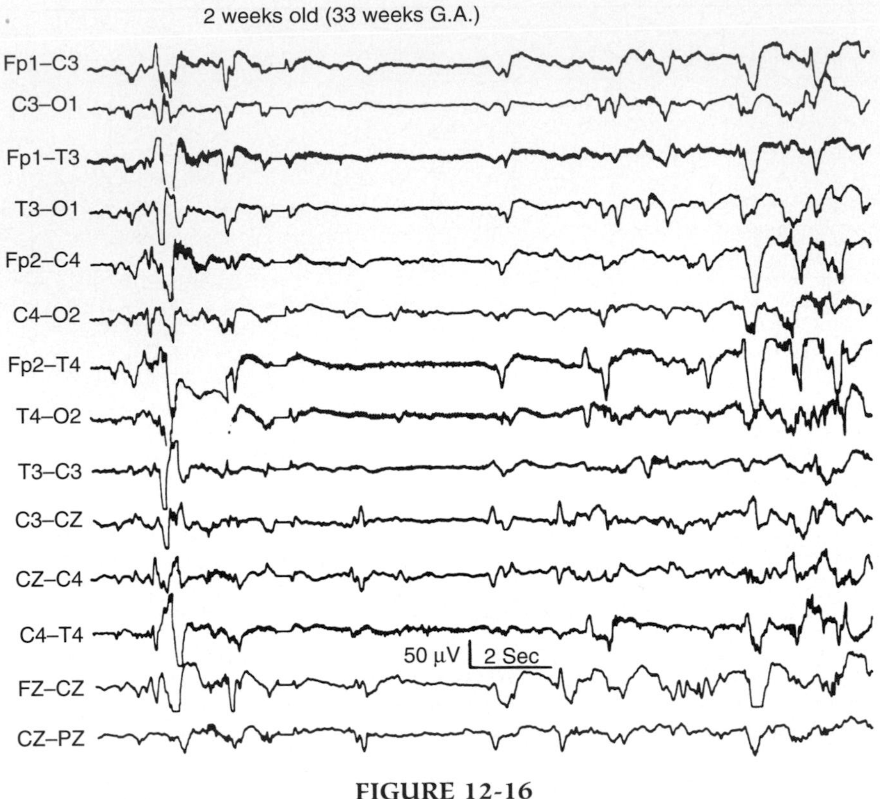

FIGURE 12-16

Severely abnormal EEG in a 2-week-old newborn born at 33 weeks gestational age. EEG activity is depressed and poorly differentiated bilaterally, with intermittent low-voltage activity and random sharp transients punctuated by higher-voltage mixed-frequency burst activity. Note the positive sharp transients occurring at Cz (channels 10–11 and 13–14) (*middle portion of figure*). Such positive rolandic discharges have a high correlation with periventricular leukomalacia.

newborn's EEG, and their significance depends on their location and abundance and the infant's state and conceptional age. Tharp (40), Lombroso (41), and Hrachovy and coworkers (42) give complete discussions of neonatal EEG interpretation.

Just as there are special considerations that relate generally to EEG interpretation in the newborn, some cautionary notes are indicated about using EEG in diagnosing and treating newborns with seizures. EEG background activity characterized in terms of expected developmental features provides important information about the extent to which cortical physiology is normally maintained or disturbed (Figure 12-16). Background activity often deteriorates transiently following a seizure because of associated hypoxia or other metabolic stresses. Interictal background activity, therefore, is extremely variable, reflecting the severity of any encephalopathy underlying or associated with seizures and the timing of the EEG in relation to seizure activity. In some infants, specific patterns or evolution of findings on repeated EEGs provide helpful and reliable prognostic information. When EEG background activity is used to help predict long-term neurologic outcome, interpretation should be based on interictal tracings to avoid problems related to reversible postictal abnormalities. Identifying and visually quantifying spikes is important, but in newborns these results are less an indication of specific susceptibility to seizures (epileptogenicity) than a measure of the underlying encephalopathy. In general, one should be extremely conservative in using interictal spikes or sharp waves to diagnose neonatal seizures.

To establish that an observed behavior is an epileptic seizure, one must record an associated ictal discharge. This can be done using conventional EEG recording if the technician makes copious and temporally accurate notations on the tracing. Better still, however, are simultaneous EEG, polygraphic, and video recordings, which provide objective documentation of the relationship among EEG activity, other physiologic variables, and behavior. Kellaway and colleagues at Baylor College of Medicine have exploited this methodology creatively to identify epileptic and nonepileptic paroxysmal behaviors and to propose a new classification of neonatal seizures (43–45). Such data indicate that one must be cautious in inferring an epileptic basis for all paroxysmal clinical events and that concurrent EEG recordings are usually necessary to distinguish epileptic seizures from similar phenomena caused by different mechanisms (43, 46).

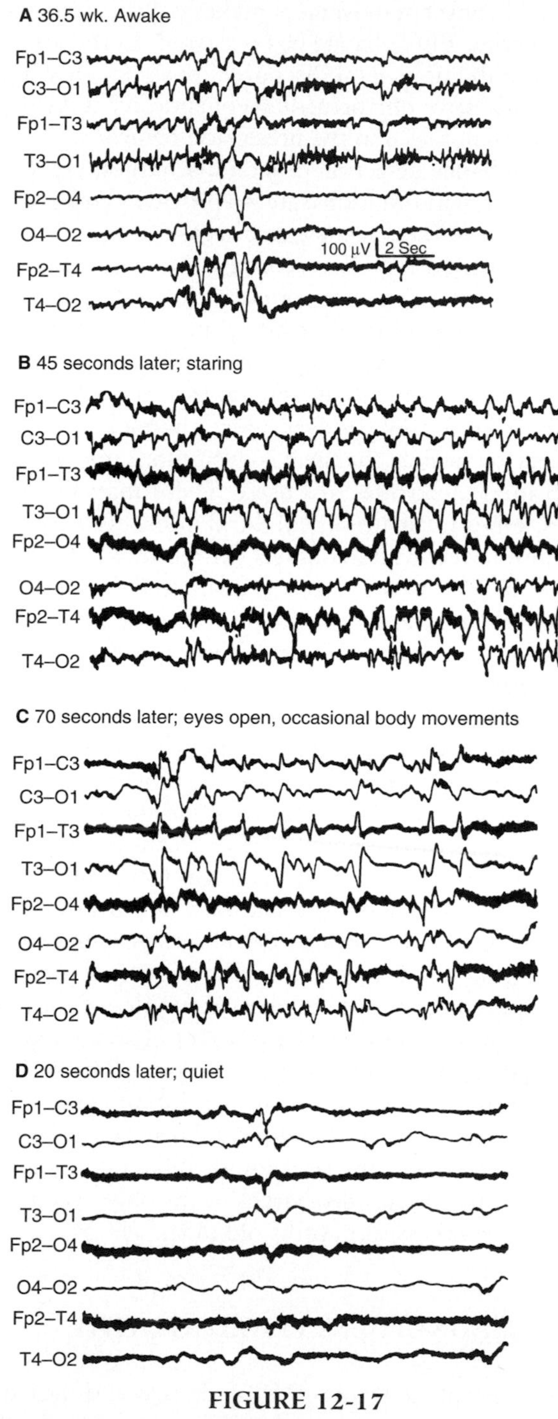

FIGURE 12-17

EEG of a newborn with a postconceptional age of 36.5 weeks demonstrating onset of a repetitive sharp-wave discharge from the left occipital region (A). Forty-five seconds later the discharge involves the entire left hemisphere and is associated with staring (B). Simultaneously, there is a buildup of spiking in the right temporal area that evolves independently from the seizure pattern on the left (B, C). The baby's eyes remain open, and there are occasional irregular body movements (C). Just over 2 minutes after the seizure begins, clinical and EEG seizure activity subside, and EEG background is severely depressed bilaterally (D).

Focal or multifocal clonic seizures, focal tonic seizures, some generalized myoclonic seizures, and ictal apnea are consistently associated with EEG ictal patterns. In contrast, staring, ocular movements, excessive salivation, and various autonomic phenomena occurring in isolation, such as changes in heart rate and blood pressure, may be accompanied by EEG discharges but often are not. Motor automatisms, including various oral-buccal-lingual movements; progression movements such as stepping, pedaling, or swimming; and complex asynchronous motor activities such as thrashing and writhing are not consistently accompanied by EEG seizure patterns. Generalized tonic seizures in the newborn also have no EEG correlate. These latter events presumably arise either from nondetectable (at the scalp) epileptic mechanisms or, more likely, from nonepileptic dysfunction of motor systems at subcortical and brainstem levels (release phenomena) (43).

Ictal discharges are almost always focal or multifocal in newborns, with variable spread to ipsilateral regions and the contralateral hemisphere (Figure 12-17). Repetitive rapid spiking is unusual at this age, especially in premature babies, and most seizure patterns consist of rhythmic sequences at almost any frequency or slowly repetitive (0.5–2 Hz) sharp waves. Seizures may occur simultaneously in the same hemisphere or in different hemispheres and progress independently.

LONG-TERM MONITORING

It is often desirable to record EEG activity for longer periods than conventional EEG recordings allow, so as to increase the likelihood of detecting epileptiform activity or capturing intermittent behavioral events. Two methods of long-term monitoring are now widely available; they have greatly improved diagnostic accuracy and reliability of seizure classification. Both have value in providing continuous recordings through one or more complete wake-sleep cycles and in documenting ictal episodes. Each has additional specific advantages and disadvantages (47–49). Which method one selects depends on the question posed by a particular patient. Gumnit (50) has provided a useful overview.

Ambulatory Monitoring

Multichannel cassette records allow relatively inexpensive continuous EEG recording in the outpatient setting. In terms of EEG information alone, ambulatory cassette recordings are only slightly less accurate in yield of epileptiform abnormalities than recordings made in intensive monitoring units (51). For this purpose, both methods are substantially more useful than routine EEG. Ambulatory EEG is often especially helpful in the pediatric setting, where the young child is often more comfortable in his familiar and unrestricted home environment (52). Limitations include the relatively limited coverage of cortical areas and the absence of video documentation. Thus, ambulatory cassette recordings are inadequate for detailed localization of epileptogenic foci, and very discrete foci may be missed. Furthermore, negative ambulatory EEG recordings are not usually helpful when the question is one of nonepileptic paroxysmal events. Here the video image of the child is frequently indispensable in recognizing and definitively characterizing the event.

Most makers of ambulatory EEG equipment have also converted to digital technology. This technique has all of the advantages of digital technology (described subsequently), allows more channels to be recorded, and offers automated computerized detection of interictal and ictal discharges. These technical advantages have greatly expanded the role of ambulatory monitoring.

Intensive Closed Circuit Television–Video EEG Monitoring

Closed circuit television (CCTV)–Video EEG monitoring in a specialty equipped inpatient unit is the procedure of choice to document pseudoseizures, establish precise electrical–clinical correlations, and localize epileptogenic foci for resective surgery Emphasis in intensive monitoring units usually is on behavioral events, not interictal activity.

Demonstrating that an electrical seizure discharge accompanies undiagnosed disturbances in behavior is unequivocal proof of an epileptic mechanism. Unfortunately, the converse is not true without qualifications. Various physiologic and technical considerations conspire to obscure some ictal discharges and thus lead potentially to false negative results. When the epileptogenic focus lies deep to the surface and the ictal discharge remains localized to this area, scalp recordings may be negative. For example, epileptiform discharges confined to mesiobasal limbic structures may go undetected at the scalp. This means that simple partial seizures manifesting as autonomic, cognitive, affective, or special sensory changes (auras) have EEG correlates in only approximately 15 percent of cases (53). As another confounding variable, consider epileptogenic foci whose physical geometry is such that electrical activity is not ideally oriented for detection by scalp electrodes. Discharges arising from orbital frontal or mesial parasagittal areas may not result in long current loops (dipoles) whose vectors are orthogonal to the surface, the optimal orientation for scalp detection of electrical events. Finally, seizures may be associated with sufficient muscle activity that high-voltage noncerebral electrical activity [electromyography (EMG), movement artifact] prevents detection of low-voltage EEG changes. This is frequently the case with frontal lobe seizures, in which early onset of movement makes it difficult to determine whether EEG change has occurred. In the absence of an unambiguous ictal discharge, postictal slowing is usually indicative of a preceding epileptic event if similar changes are not seen in the preseizure record.

To enhance detection of ictal discharges, especially their earliest manifestations, and to provide a comprehensive analysis of the epileptogenic region, most laboratories supplement usual EEG recording sites with additional placements, including extratemporal electrodes, nasopharyngeal and sphenoidal electrodes, and supraorbital electrodes. Because of the many additional recording sites, it is not unusual for monitoring units to record simultaneously from 32, 64, or even more channels. The need for many recording channels is even more urgent when intracranial electrodes are used. These may be depth probes, subdural strips, or subdural grids, each containing multiple recording contacts. Intracranial electrodes are required in patients being evaluated for resective surgery when extensive surface (including sphenoidal) recordings do not provide definitive localization of the epileptogenic zone (54–57) or when other clinical data conflict with EEG findings (58).

A variety of ictal patterns may be seen in children. For the most part, these are similar to those encountered in adults. Focal ictal discharges are often characterized by sustained runs of rhythmic delta or theta-alpha activity that evolve in frequency and voltage. Generalized convulsive seizures may be characterized by runs of diffuse rhythmic fast activity during tonic phases or runs of spike-wave discharges during clonic phases. Some patterns, however, are peculiar to children. Examples of these are runs of rhythmic positive sharp waves in some infantile focal seizures and electrodecremental events (Figure 12-6) during infantile spasms. Seizures in infants and young children usually are focal and secondarily generalize less often than in adolescents and adults. Bilaterally synchronous generalized ictal discharges occur only very rarely in infants less then 13 months old (59).

MAGNETOENCEPHALOGRAPHY

Magnetoencephalography (MEG) detects and measures magnetic activity of the cortex using superconductive quantum interference devices (SQUIDs). Neuronal aggregates that are current sources of brain electrical activity also generate magnetic fields. Models depicting the head as a homogeneously conducting sphere demonstrate that measurements of magnetic fields can provide three-dimensional localization of a neuronal source. MEG differs from EEG in ways that are potentially very useful. For example, MEG is more accurate than EEG in localizing dipoles of neuronal activity oriented parallel to the surface. Furthermore, MEG is relatively unaffected by overlying tissue and bone, which significantly attenuate volume conduction of electrical potentials between cortex and scalp. Finally, MEG appears to arise solely from intracellular currents in active neurons (60, 61). Thus, for some current sources, MEG may offer greater spatial resolution than EEG.

Several investigators have used MEG to map epileptogenic foci, and results have compared favorably with EEG localization (61–64). Applications are currently limited by the complex technology required to detect the extraordinarily weak magnetic fields of the brain. Until now, most investigators have used only a single SQUID, which is then moved from place to place on the head. Multichannel recording is clearly feasible, however, and reports are appearing of recording devices with 20 or more channels. There is promise, therefore, of using MEG as a complement to EEG to improve source localization in studying epileptiform activity in people with epilepsy.

Digital technology has quickly changed how EEG signals are collected and stored in many laboratories across the country. One difference is that digital signals are not contaminated by sources of noise encountered with analog technologies. The EEG signal is electronically stored and may be reviewed in any desired montage, sensitivity, or filter setting. The digital format also allows for quantitative methods of EEG analysis, including Fourier (spectral cross-correlation) and cross-spectral analysis. In addition, interpolation techniques may be applied to estimate the electric potentials at intermediate scalp positions from known values at each electrode position. Topographic or spatial maps are another way of displaying EEG data that differs from the conventional display by producing maps of electrical potentials that loosely resemble images seen with MR or CT. Finally, source dipole localization has been proposed as a method to find the intracranial sources generating scalp potentials. Most of these techniques are still research tools and have not yet come into common clinical practice.

CONCLUSIONS

In this chapter we have indicated the role of EEG in evaluating children with known or suspected seizures. EEG is an important, perhaps *the* most important, adjunct to history and examination. But, as with any laboratory test, care and judgment must be used in relating EEG findings to other clinical data. Indeed, the full potential of EEG can be realized only when interpretations are placed in the full clinical context.

EEG interpretation in infants and children is complicated by two important considerations. First, many normal potentials are high-voltage, occur paroxysmally, and have spiky waveforms. Unusual benign variants are common. Thus, EEGs of children are easy to overinterpret or misinterpret. The second issue is that the developing brain has unique neuroanatomic, biochemical, and neurophysiologic features. The various EEG abnormalities in childhood epilepsy and the their clinical expression result from the interaction of developmental features with genetic or acquired pathology.

The EEG examination should always be framed to answer a particular question. There is no evidence that routine follow-up EEGs every 6 or 12 months serve any useful purpose. Dialog between the clinician and laboratory is essential, especially if special recording circumstances are necessary to obtain maximal information. Questions that the EEG may help answer include:

1. Does the child have epilepsy?
2. Are seizures of localized or generalized onset?
3. Does the child fit a specific electroclinical syndrome?
4. Is clinical deterioration the result of unrecognized seizures, a progressive neurological syndrome, or drug toxicity?
5. Is the child a candidate for surgery?
6. Can AEDs be safely withdrawn?

References

1. American EEG Society. Guidelines in EEG and evoked potentials. Guideline seven: a proposal for standard montages to be used in clinical EEG. *J Clin Neurophysiol* 1986; 3(Suppl 1):26–33.
2. Doose H, Gerken H. On the genetics of EEG anomalies in childhood. IV. Photoconvulsive reaction. *Neuropädiatrie* 1973; 4:162–171.
3. Dinner DS. Sleep and pediatric epilepsy. *Cleve Clin J Med* 1989; 56(Suppl 2):S234–S239.
4. Ellingson RJ, Wilken V, Bennett DR. Efficacy of sleep deprivation as an activation procedure in epilepsy patients. *J Clin Neurophysiol* 1984; 1:83–101.
5. Rowan AJ, Veldhuizen RJ, Nagelkerke NJD. Comparative evaluation of sleep deprivation and sedated sleep EEGs as diagnostic aids in epilepsy. *Electroencephalogr Clin Neurophysiol* 1982; 54:357–364.
6. Kellaway P, Frost JD. Biorhythmic modulation of epileptic events. In: Pedley TA, Meldrum BS, eds. *Recent Advances in Epilepsy*. Edinburgh: Churchill-Livingstone, 1983:139–154.
7. Sadler RM, Goodwin J. Multiple electrodes for detecting spikes in partial complex seizures. *Can J Neurol Sci* 1989; 16:326–329.
8. Binnie CD, Marston D, Polkey CE, Amin D. Distribution of temporal spikes in relation to the sphenoidal electrode. *Electroencephalogr Clin Neurophysiol* 1989; 73:403–409.
9. Sperling MR, Engel J. Electroencephalographic recording from the temporal lobes: a comparison of ear, anterior temporal, and nasopharyngeal electrodes. *Ann Neurol* 1985; 17:510–513.
10. Sperling MR, Mendius JR, Engel J. Mesial temporal spikes: a simultaneous comparison of sphenoidal, nasopharyngeal, and ear electrodes. *Epilepsia* 1986; 27:81–86.
11. Petersen I, Eeg-Olofsson O, Sellden U. Paroxysmal activity in EEG of normal children. In: Kellaway P, Petersen I, eds. *Clinical Electroencephalography of Children*. Stockholm: Alinquist and Wiksell, 1968:167–188.
12. Trojaborg W. Changes of spike foci in children. In: Kellaway P, Petersen I, eds. *Clinical Electroencephalography of Children*. Stockholm: Almquist and Wiksell, 1968:213–226.
13. Kellaway P. The incidence, significance, and natural history of spike foci in children. In: Henry CE, ed. *Current Clinical Neurophysiology, Update on EEG and Evoked Potentials*. New York: Elsevier North-Holland, 1980:151–175.
14. Gibbs RA, Gibbs EZ. *Atlas of Electroencephalography. Vol 2. Epilepsy*. Cambridge: Addison Wesley, 1952.
15. Hrachovy RA, Frost JD, Kellaway P. Hypsarrhythmia: variations on the theme. *Epilepsia* 1984; 25:317–325.

16. Kellaway P, Hrachovy RA, Frost JD, Zion T. Precise characterization and quantification of infantile spasms. *Ann Neurol* 1979; 6:214–218.
17. Hrachovy R, Frost JD. Infantile spasms. *Cleve Clin J Med* 1989; 56(Suppl 1):S10–S16.
18. Browne TR, Penry JK, Porter RJ, Dreifuss FE. Responsiveness before, during and after spike-wave paroxysms. *Neurology* 1974; 24:659–665.
19. Dalby MA. Epilepsy and 3 per second spike and wave rhythms. A clinical, electrographic and prognostic analysis of 346 patients. *Acta Neurol Scand* 1969; 45(Suppl 40):1–83.
20. Markand ON. Slow spike-wave activity in EEG and associated clinical features often called "Lennox" or "Lennox-Gastaut" syndrome. *Neurology* 1977; 27:746–757.
21. Roger J, Dravet C, Bureau M. The Lennox-Gastaut syndrome. *Cleve Clin J Med* 1989; 56(Suppl 2):S172–S180.
21b. Kaminska A, Ickowicz A, Ploin P, Bru MF, Dellatolas G, Dulac O. Delineation of cryptogenic Lennox-Gastaut syndrome and myclonic epilepsy using multiple correspondence analysis. *Epilepsy Res* 1999; 36:15–29.
22. Lerman P, Kivity S. The benign focal epilepsies of childhood. In: Pedley TA, Meldrum BS, eds. *Recent Advances in Epilepsy*. Vol 3. Edinburgh: Churchill-Livingstone, 1986:137–156.
23. Loiseau P, Duche B. Benign childhood epilepsy with centrotemporal spikes. *Cleve Clin J Med* 1989; 56:S17–S22.
24. Beaumanoir A, Ballis T, Varfis G, Ansari K. Benign epilepsy of childhood with rolandic spikes. *Epilepsia* 1974; 15:301–315.
25. Beaussart M. Benign epilepsy of childhood with rolandic (centrotemporal) paroxysmal foci. *Epilepsia* 1972; 13:795–811.
26. Petersen J, Nielsen CJ, Gulann NC. Atypical EEG abnormalities in children with benign partial (rolandic) epilepsy. *Acta Neurol Scand* 1983; 94(Suppl):57–62.
27. Bray FP, Wiser WC. Hereditary characteristics of familial temporal central focal epilepsy. *Pediatrics* 1965; 36:207–211.
28. Heijbel J, Blom S, Rasmuson M. Benign epilepsy of childhood with centrotemporal EEG foci: a genetic study. *Epilepsia* 1975; 16:285–293.
29. Gastaut H. A new type of epilepsy: benign partial epilepsy of childhood with occipital spike-waves. *Clin Electroencephalogr* 1982; 13:13–22.
29b. Caraballa R, Cersosimo R, Fejerman N. Panayiotopoulos Syndrome: a prospective study of 193 patients. *Epilepsia* 2007; 48:1054–1061.
29c. Korff C, Laux L, Kelley K, Goldstein J, Koh S, Nordli D Jr. Dravet syndrome (severe myoclonic epilepsy in infancy): a retrospective study of 16 patients. *J Child Neurol* 2007; 22:185–194.
30. Janz D, Christian W. Impulsiv-Petit mal. *Dtsch Z Nervenheilkd* 1957; 176:348–386.
31. Delgado-Escueta AV, Enrile-Bascal FE. Juvenile myoclonic epilepsy of Janz. *Neurology* 1984; 34:285–294.
32. Wolf P, Goosses R. Relation of photosensitivity to epileptic syndromes. *J Neurol Neurosurg Psychiatry* 1986; 49:1368–1391.
33. Landau WM, Kleffner F. Syndrome of acquired aphasia with convulsive disorder in children. *Neurology* 1957; 7:523–530.
34. Holmes GL, McKeever M, Saunders Z. Epileptiform activity in aphasia of childhood: an epiphenomenon? *Epilepsia* 1981; 22:631–639.
35. Sato S, Dreifuss FE. Electroencephalographic findings in a patient with developmental expressive aphasia. *Neurology* 1973; 23:181–184.
36. Gascon G, Victor D, Lombroso L, Goodglass H. Language disorder, convulsive disorder and electroencephalographic abnormalities. *Arch Neurol* 1973; 28:156–162.
37. Sawhney INS, Suresh N, Dhand UK, Chopra JS. Acquired aphasia with epilepsy—Landau-Kleffner syndrome. *Epilepsia* 1988; 29:283–287.
38. Rasmussen T, Andermann E. Update on the syndrome of "chronic encephalitis" and epilepsy. *Cleve Clin J Med* 1989; 56(Suppl 2):S181–S184.
39. Bancaud J. Kojewnikow's syndrome (epilepsia partialis continua) in children. In: Roger J, Dravet C, Bureau M, Dreifuss FE, et al, eds. *Epileptic Syndromes in Infancy, Childhood, and Adolescence*. London: John Libbey, 1985:286–298.
40. Tharp BR. Pediatric electroencephalography. In: Aminoff M, ed. *Electrodiagnosis in Clinical Neurology*.New York: Churchill-Livingstone, 1986:67–117.
41. Lombroso CT. Neonatal electroencephalography. In: Niedermeyer E, Lopes da Silva E, eds. *Electroencephalography: Basic Principles: Clinical Applications, and Related Fields*. 2nd ed. Baltimore: Urban & Schwarzenberg, 1987:725–762.
42. Hrachovy RA, Mizrahi EM, Kellaway P. Electroencephalography of the newborn. In: Daly DD, Pedley TA, eds. *Current Practice of Clinical EEG*. 2nd ed. New York: Raven Press, 1990:201–242.
43. Mizrahi EM, Kellaway R. Characterization and classification of neonatal seizures. *Neurology* 1987; 37:1837–1844.
44. Kellaway P, Mizrahi EM. Clinical, electroencephalographic, therapeutic, and pathophysiologic studies of neonatal seizures. In: Wasterlain CG, Vert P, eds. *Neonatal Seizures. Pathophysiology and Pharmacologic Management*. New York: Raven Press, 1989.
45. Mizrahi EM. Clinical and neurophysiologic correlates of neonatal seizures. *Cleve Clin J Med* 1989; 56(Suppl 1):S100–S104.
46. Volpe JJ. Neonatal seizures: current concepts and revised classification. *Pediatrics* 1989; 84:422–428.
47. Binnie CD. Telemetric EEG monitoring in epilepsy In: Pedley TA, Meldrum BS, eds. *Recent Advances in Epilepsy*. Edinburgh: Churchill-Livingstone, 1983:155–178.
48. Binnie CD, Rowan AJ, Overweg, et al. Telemetric EEG and video monitoring in epilepsy. *Neurology* 1981; 31:298–303.
49. Kaplan P, Lesser R. Long-term monitoring. In: Daly DD, Pedley TA, eds. *Current Practice of EEG*. 2nd ed. New York: Raven Press, 1990.
50. Gumnit RJ. Intensive neurodiagnostic monitoring: role in the treatment of seizures. *Neurology* 1986; 36:1340–1346.
51. Bridgers SL, Ebersole JS. The clinical utility of ambulatory cassette EEG monitoring. *Neurology* 1985; 35:166–173.
52. Stores G. Ambulatory diagnostic monitoring of seizures in children. In: Gumnit RJ, ed. *Intensive Neurodiagnostic Monitoring*. Advances in Neurology 46. New York: Raven Press, 1987:157–167.
53. Devinsky O, Kelley K, Porter RJ, Theodore WH. Clinical and electroencephalographic features of simple partial seizures. *Neurology* 1988; 38:1347–1352.
54. Lüders H, Hahn J, Lesser RP, et al. Basal temporal subdural electrodes in the evaluation of patients with intractable epilepsy. *Epilepsia* 1989; 30:131–142.
55. Spencer SS, Spencer DD, Williamson PD, Mattson R. Combined depth and subdural electrode investigation in uncontrolled epilepsy. *Neurology* 1990; 40:74–79.
56. Wyler AR, Richey ET, Hermann BP. Comparison of scalp to subdural recordings for localizing epileptogenic foci. *J Epilepsy* 1989; 2:91–96.
57. Sperling MR, O'Connor MJ. Comparison of depth and subdural electrodes in recording temporal lobe seizures. *Neurology* 1989; 39:1497–1504.
58. Sammaritano M, De Lotbiniere A, Andermann F, et al. False lateralization by surface EEG of seizure onset in patients with temporal lobe epilepsy and gross focal cerebral lesions. *Ann Neurol* 1987; 21:361–369.
59. Nordli DR, Bazil CW, Scheuer ML, Pedley TA. Recognition and classification of seizures in infants. *Epilepsia* 1997; 38:553–560.
60. Williamson SJ, Kaufman L. Analysis of neuromagnetic signals. In: Gevins AS, Rémond A, eds. *Methods of Analysis of Brain Electrical and Magnetic Signals*. Handbook of Electroencephalography and Clinical Neurophysiology, Revised Series, 1. Amsterdam: Elsevier, 1987:405–448.
61. Salustri C, Chapman RM. A simple method for 3-dimensional localization of epileptic activity recorded by simultaneous EEG and MEG. *Electroencephalogr Clin Neurophysiol* 1989; 73:473–478.
62. Wheless JW, Castillo E, Maggio V, Kim HL, Breier JI, Simss PG, Papanicolaou AL. Magnetoencephalography (MEG) and magnetic source imaging (MSI). *Neurologist* 2004; 10:138–153.
63. Barth DS, Baumgartner C, Sutherling WW. Neuromagnetic field modeling of multiple brain regions producing interictal spikes in human epilepsy *Electroencephalogr Clin Neurophysiol* 1989; 73:389–402.
64. Rose DF, Sato S, Smith PD, et al. Localization of magnetic interictal discharges in temporal lobe epilepsy. *Ann Neurol* 1987; 22:348–354.

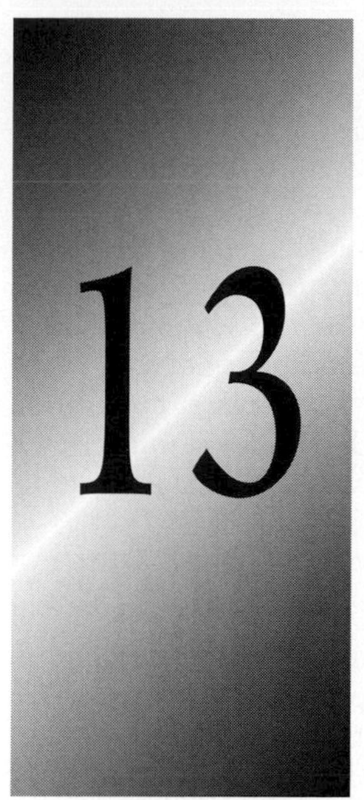

13 Basics of Neuroimaging in Pediatric Epilepsy

James M. Johnston
Matthew D. Smyth
Robert C. McKinstry

Neuroimaging, especially magnetic resonance imaging (MRI), has become a critical tool in the evaluation of the child with epilepsy. The introduction and ongoing refinement of MRI have allowed noninvasive visualization of the many substrates of epileptogenesis. Identification of mesial temporal sclerosis, neoplasms, vascular malformations, and subtle cortical dysplasias converts some cases of heretofore "nonlesional" to "lesional" epilepsy, and thus amenable to surgical intervention and improved outcomes.

Imaging is an essential component of a multidisciplinary evaluation of children with epilepsy. Because imaging is only one of many evaluation tools available to help locate epileptogenic foci, imaging results need to be interpreted in the context of the medical history, physical exam, electroencephalogram (EEG), neuropsychologic testing, and, where indicated, invasive intracranial electrophysiologic monitoring. In this chapter we aim to provide a general overview of the many imaging modalities available to the clinician in furthering our understanding of the pathophysiology of epilepsy. We also briefly review newer technologies aimed at noninvasively localizing epileptogenic cortex.

SEDATION

Movement significantly decreases the resolution and quality of most advanced imaging techniques, especially MRI, making adequate sedation for uncooperative children quite important. Neonates often do not require sedation if they are fed immediately before arrival, kept warm, and provided with ear plugs during the study. Some institutions have installed audiovisual systems in their MR scanners, with subsequent reductions in sedation, motion artifact, and room time. However, most children under 7 years of age will require some form of sedation. When sedation is needed, most institutional protocols call on the expertise of nurse anesthetists, hospitalists, or anesthesiologists to ensure safe and effective sedation.

IMAGING MODALITIES

Head Sonography

Fetal ultrasound is a screening tool that has an established role in the diagnosis of cerebral malformations, congenital anomalies, and complex syndromes. In the postnatal period, ultrasound is often the initial study in a diagnostic workup for seizure activity. It has the benefits of being noninvasive and avoiding radiation exposure.

Neonatal head ultrasound's primary role has traditionally been in the evaluation of the preterm newborn for diagnosis of parenchymal hemorrhage, germinal matrix hemorrhage, and hydrocephalus. Ultrasound may detect changes of hypoxic ischemic injury, vascular anomalies, or brain malformations.

Computed Tomography

Computed tomography (CT) is most helpful in the identification of intracranial hemorrhage, major vascular malformations, and ventriculomegaly. The sensitivity of CT is approximately 30% in the detection of many of the causes of epilepsy (1–5). Given these limitations, as well as the risks of radiation exposure in infants and young children, CT has been replaced by MRI in the elective workup of childhood epilepsy.

In cases of recording in order to localize epileptic foci with electrode grids, CT may also be used to obtain images of electrodes in situ that can later be fused onto preoperative MR images with standard software. This technique allows the use of neuronavigation to guide operative resection of epileptogenic lesions (6).

Magnetic Resonance Imaging

Technical Considerations. The continued development of MRI has improved our ability to visualize the most common causes of epilepsy. Routine sequences should include high-resolution T2-weighted, fluid attenuation inversion recovery (FLAIR), T-2*- weighted gradient echo, 3D high resolution T1W gradient echo, and diffusion-weighted imaging. Imaging after administration of gadolinium contrast agents helps differentiate neoplasia from dysplasia and should be done whenever a structural abnormality is present.

The advent of high-resolution, multichannel coils and higher field strength (⩾ 3 Tesla) has enhanced signal-to-noise ratio and reduced scan times. Phased-array coil imaging has improved cortical lesion detection by 64% compared with standard 1.5-T coils (7). As phased-array technology is adapted for 3-T systems, signal-to-noise ratio and resolution should improve even more (8). Research with 7-T multichannel array technology promises visualization of cortical abnormalities of less than 100 µm in the near future, prompting some authorities to predict an era of "in vivo histology" (9).

Overview of Myelination in the Normal Brain

Any interpretation of magnetic resonance imaging of the developing brain must take into account the dynamic process of myelination and changes in water content, with corresponding signal intensity changes on T1- and T2-weighted imaging. In most basic terms, T1 and T2 relaxation times become shorter as maturation progresses, as a result of increased myelin and decreased water content in imaged tissue. Myelination begins in the dorsal brainstem and cerebellum as early as the fifth fetal month, then involves the pyramidal and somatosensory radiations, and progresses later to the subcortical white matter of the prefrontal and anterior temporal regions over the first two years of life (10). Thus, white-matter maturation is evaluated best with T1-weighted images until 6 to 8 months of age, after which T2-weighted images become more sensitive to white-matter changes.

Quantitative MR Techniques

Detailed manual segmentation of specific brain regions and structures such as hippocampus and amygdala has permitted a more quantitative formulation of standardized growth trajectories and better understanding of both normal and abnormal development (8). For example, mesial temporal sclerosis (MTS) has been studied using quantitative techniques that have excellent sensitivity and specificity for detecting hippocampal asymmetry (11). Quantitative studies of regional brain volume also have found decreases in cerebral and cerebellar size in children with epilepsy (12).

Surface-based and volume-based representations of cortex provide population-averaged "architectonic" maps to permit truer comparisons of functional or structural data between individuals or research cohorts (13). For example, construction of a surface-based atlas has permitted the identification of cortical folding abnormalities in Williams syndrome (14).

Cortical Malformations

A wide spectrum of cortical malformations, due to genetic or environmental insults, can cause pediatric epilepsy. These can be classified in terms of disruption of neuronal production, differentiation, and migration. The most common malformations are well visualized on MRI, especially with the use of high resolution 3-T and modern phased-array technology. The examples that follow illustrate the types of abnormalities that can be identified. For a more extensive review of this topic, see the references by Barkovich and by Raybaud et al (15, 16).

Transmantle Dysplasias

Transmantle dyplasias are disorders of neuronal and glial differentiation with or without abnormal migration. Histologically, these abnormalities contain dysplastic glioneuronal elements that increase signal on T2/FLAIR imaging depending on the child's age and state of myelination of the brain. In many ways these dysplasias represent a one pole of a spectrum that blends into low-grade neoplasia. As a result, it can be difficult to differentiate the two based on imaging alone.

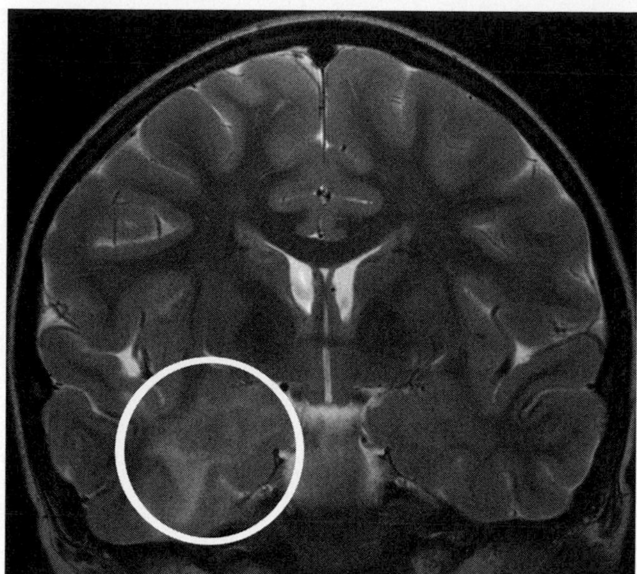

FIGURE 13-1

Cortical dysplasia. Coronal high-resolution T2W image demonstrates extensive abnormal signal hyperintensity in the right inferomedial temporal lobe (within the circle). The cortex has elevated signal, as does the subcortical white matter. The junction between the gray matter and the white matter is indistinct.

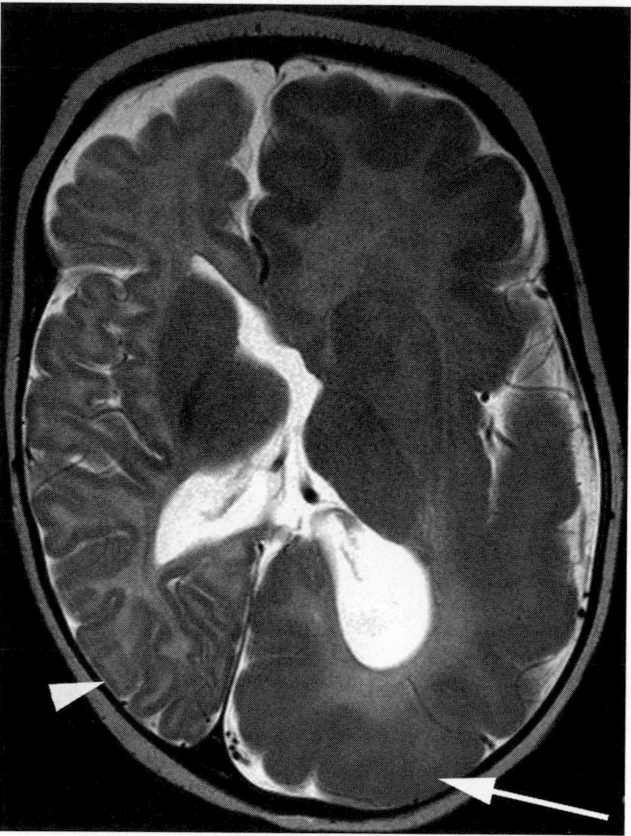

FIGURE 13-2

Hemimegalencephaly. Horizontal T2W image reveals the extensive transmantle dysplasia of left hemimegalencephaly. The right hemisphere is normal. On the left the cortical ribbon is thickened (long white arrow) relative to the normal cortex (white arrow head), the gray-white junction is indistinct, and the left ventricle is dysmorphic and enlarged.

Focal cortical dysplasias of Taylor are the most common of the transmantle dysplasias. Histologically, they are characterized by abnormal dendritic arborization, disorganized neurons, and large dysmorphic astrocytes called "balloon cells." The poorly differentiated glioneuronal cells span the cerebral mantle, with blurring of the gray–white junction. These lesions are best visualized as high signal on T2 and FLAIR images. Classically they have a triangular shape with the apex pointed at the superolateral margin of the ventricle and the base on the cortical surface (Figure 13-1). Imaging after contrast administration helps differentiate this entity from a neoplasm.

Hemimegalencephaly is a highly epileptogenic transmantle dysplasia. It is characterized by an enlarged hemisphere and ipsilateral ventricle, with tilting of the corpus callosum and septum pellucidum towards the involved side (Figure 13-2). There is variable loss of gray–white matter differentiation throughout the abnormal hemisphere. Typically, the white matter has increased T1 and decreased T2 signal, thought to represent hypercellularity or an advanced myelination (17).

In pathologic specimens these hamartomas were described as "candle dripping" (Figure 13-3). Over time, because of increasing myelination and calcification, they are most easily identified on T1-weighted images and variably enhance with contrast. *Cortical hamartomas* (tubers) are characterized histologically by a dense gliosis, disordered myelination, and bizarre giant cells similar to those seen in cortical dysplasia. Sometimes calcified, the MR appearance of tubers changes with advancing age and myelination. In neonates, tubers appear as T1-hyperintense, T2-hypointense to surrounding white matter. With myelination, the lesions slowly become isointense, then T2/FLAIR hyperintense in older infants. Approximately 5–10% of children with TSC will develop a subependymal giant cell astrocytoma. Typically found near the foramen of Monro, these lesions can acutely become symptomatic when they enlarge and obstruct flow of CSF at the foramen. On MRI, they have increased T1 and decreased T2 signal and enhance homogeneously after contrast administration. Degeneration into diffuse astrocytoma is rare but should be suspected when associated with increased T2 signal in the surrounding white matter.

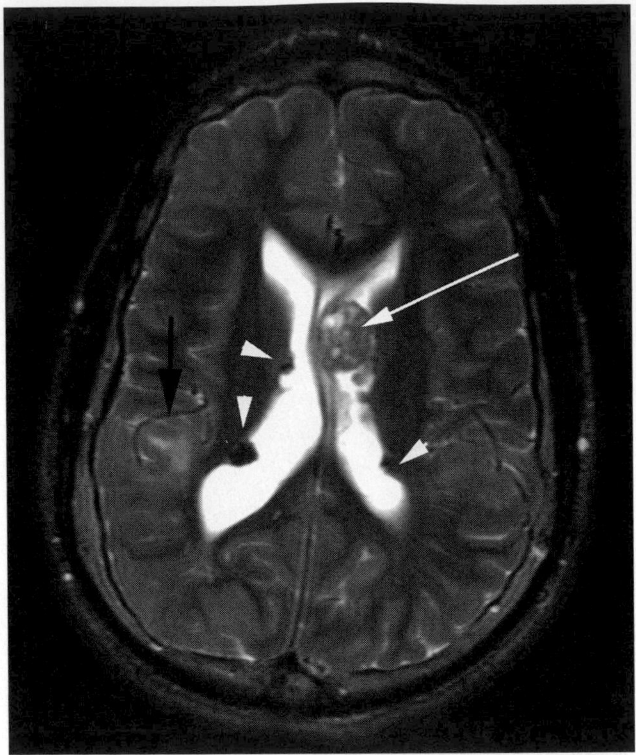

FIGURE 13-3

Tuberous sclerosis. Horizontal T2W image demonstrates three classic features of tuberous sclerosis. The black arrow indicates an area of subcortical flame-like hyperintensity typical of a cortical tuber. The arrow heads illustrate the T2-hypointense subependymal nodules, which are likely calcified. The white arrow identifies an intraventricular heterogeneous mass with bowing of the septum pellucidum due to a subependymal giant cell astrocytoma.

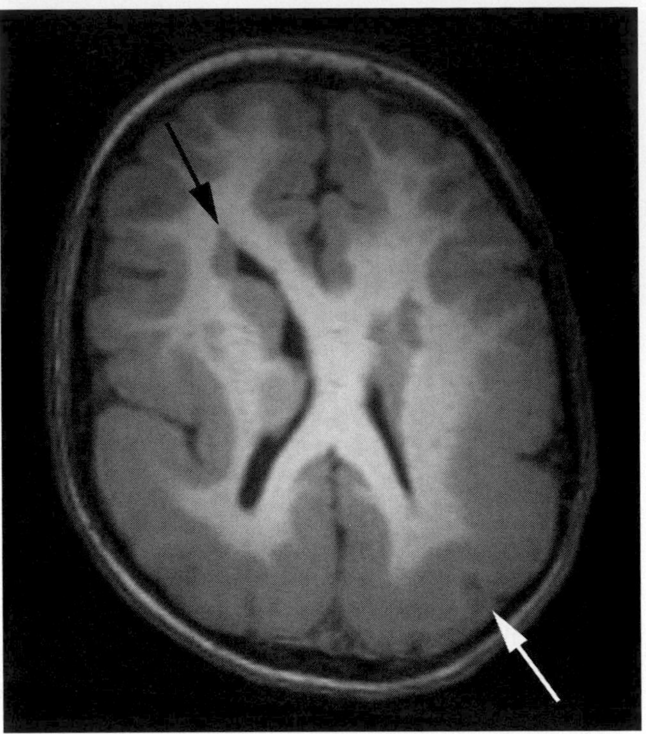

FIGURE 13-4

Periventricular nodular heterotopia and pachygyria. Horizontal T1W image from a child with extensive periventricular nodular heterotopia (black arrow) and bilateral posterior parieto-occipital pachygyria. Note the thickened, broadened, and flattened appearance to the pachygyria relative to normal cortex.

Disorders of Migration. Heterotopias are characterized by groups of neurons in abnormal locations. Unlike the transmantle dysplasias described in the preceding paragraphs, signal characteristics are identical to normal cortex, without T2/FLAIR abnormality. However, the advent of increasingly sensitive MR techniques has allowed visualization of more subtle structural abnormalities.

Nodular heterotopias are either isolated or diffuse clumping of gray matter adjacent to the ventricular wall (subependymal) (Figure 13-4, black arrow) or between the ventricle and cortical mantle (subcortical). The nodules may be unilateral or bilateral and vary greatly in size, and are often associated with commissural agenesis, polymicrogyria, or schizencephaly.

Band heterotopias, also known as laminar heterotopias, are characterized by a duplication of the cortical gray matter extending below and then away from normal cortex. Typically they are bilateral and symmetrical, and they occur almost exclusively in females.

Polymicrogyria (or microgyria) is a disorder of cortical sulcation and lamination with loss of intermediate cortical layers and fusion of the molecular layer. On MRI, the sylvian fissure extends posteriorly beyond its normal confines at the temporoparietal junction, and the remainder of the brain has an "overfolded" appearance (Figure 13-5, white arrows) as compared with normal cortex (Figure 13-5, black arrow). The peri-insular cortex is typically the most severely affected, and variable atrophy of the hemisphere is usually apparent. Often there is increased T2/FLAIR signal in the periventricular and subcortical white matter, suggestive of dysmyelination.

Schizencephaly or split brain refers to the presence of a pia-lined cleft extending from the cortical surface to the ventricle (Figure 13-5, black arrow head). Subclassified as fluid filled ("open-lip") or collapsed ("closed-lip"), it is often associated with adjacent polymicrogyria (Figure 13-5, white arrows), septal agenesis, partial agenesis of the corpus callosum, and cortical heterotopias. This malformation should be differentiated from encephaloclastic porencephaly, in which the cleft is lined with white matter.

Lissencephaly (agyria-pachygyria complex) is a series of brain abnormalities with decreased sulcal and gyral

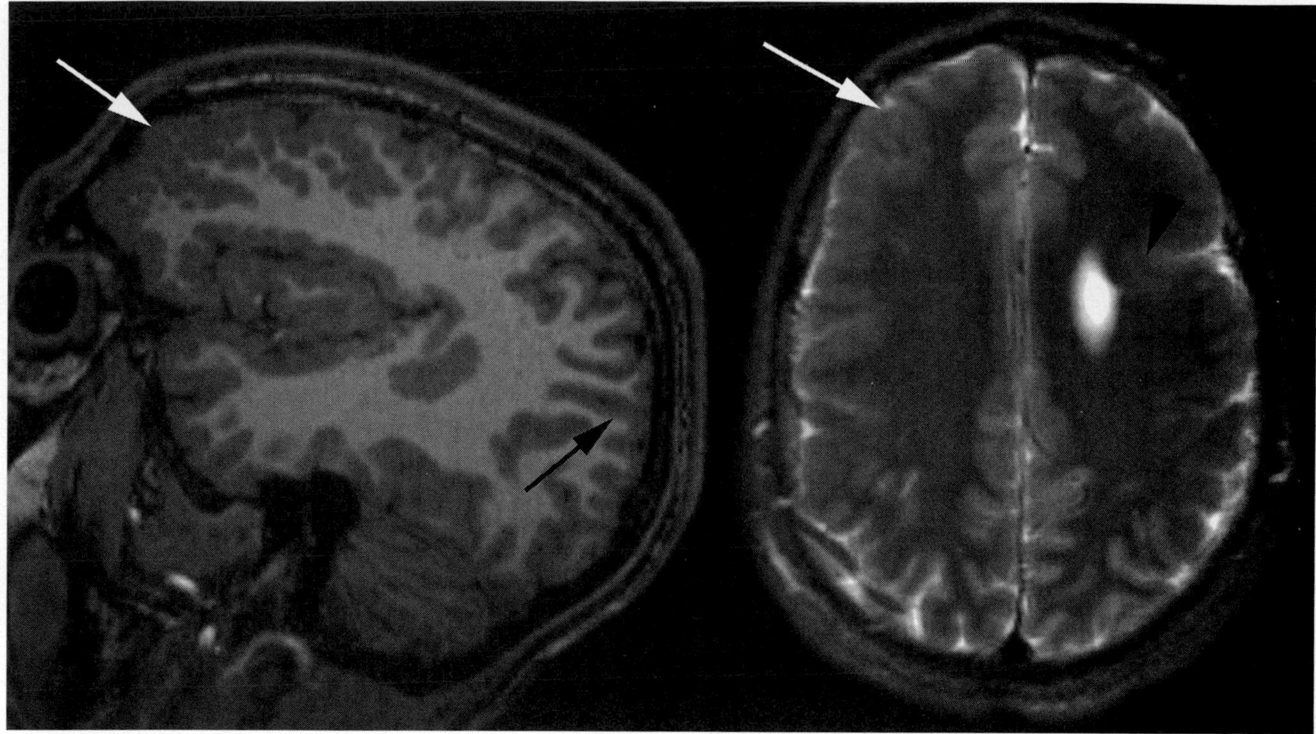

FIGURE 13-5

Polymicrogyria and schizencephaly. Parasagittal T1W image and horizontal T2W image from a child with extensive malformation of cortical development. The white arrows show cobblestone irregularity of the frontal lobe cortex with numerous small gyri compared with the normal cortex (black arrow). The black arrow head points to a closed lip schizencephalic cleft, which is lined by polymicrogyria. The dimple in the lateral wall of the left lateral ventricle is the site of the pial-ependymal seam.

development. "Agyria" refers to an absence of gyri (complete lissencephaly), while "pachygyria" refers to areas of broad, flat gyri (incomplete lissencephaly). Both are characterized by thickened cortex, and result from abnormal neuronal migration (Figure 13-4, white arrow).

Neoplasms

Dysembryoplastic neuroepithelial tumors (DNET or DNT) are benign glioneuronal neoplasms of the cortex associated with partial complex epilepsy, usually without neurologic deficit. Accounting for nearly 20% of the pathology found in pediatric cases of surgically treated epilepsy (18), approximately 60% of these tumors are located in the temporal lobe with 30% in the frontal lobe and the remainder distributed in other brain regions. Imaging findings on MR include decreased T1, increased T2/FLAIR signal without surrounding edema, and enhancement in approximately one-third of cases. Most have cystic or microcystic components and are well demarcated from the surrounding brain parenchyma (Figure 13-6, black arrow).

Gangliogliomas and gangliocytomas are relatively rare. These mixed glioneuronal tumors account for 3% of pediatric brain tumors and usually are seen in older children and young adults with long histories of partial seizures, occasionally with focal neurologic deficits (19). Gangliogliomas are most commonly located in the neocortex and temporal lobe, though they have been described near the hypothalamus and third ventricle. Lesions may be solid or cystic, with or without mural nodule. Solid portions of the tumor demonstrate increased T2 signal with variable enhancement, and calcification is occasionally present (Figure 13-7). Differential diagnosis includes astrocytoma, oligodendroglioma, and DNET. Surgical resection of these tumors usually cures the patient's seizures.

Oligodendrogliomas, though relatively rare (1% of all pediatric brain tumors), commonly cause seizures when they are present. These are most commonly found in the frontal and temporal lobes and are frequently cystic and calcified on CT. MR appearance is nonspecific: They are commonly isointense to surrounding brain on T1 and T2, with areas of T1 hyperintensity (related to calcification) and variable enhancement (Figure 13-8).

Hypothalamic hamartomas are rare, congenital malformations located in the region of the tuber cinereum of the hypothalamus. Clinically, these are associated with precocious puberty, epilepsy, developmental delay, and

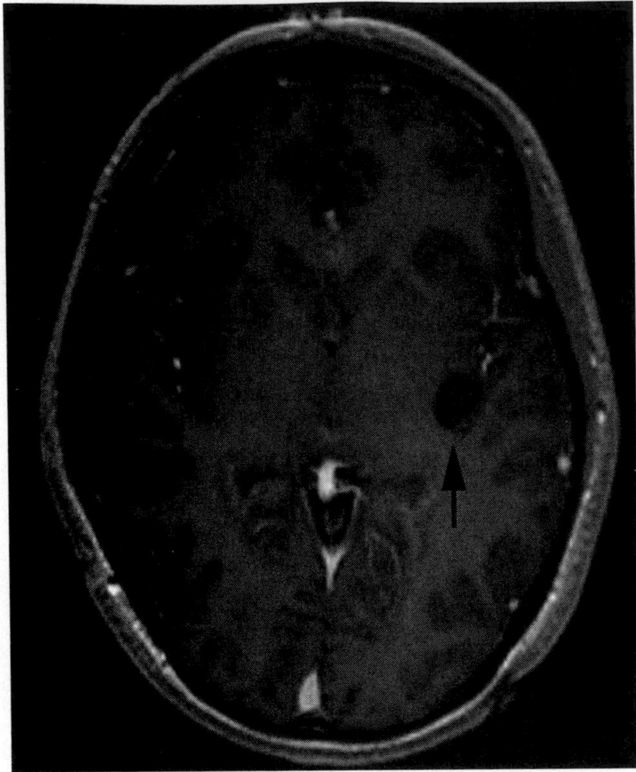

FIGURE 13-6

Dysembryoplastic neuroepithelial tumor (DNET). Horizontal post-contrast T1W image of a child with a DNET. The lesion is based in the cortical and subcortical region of the posterior insula on the left. The lesion has minimal mass effect and a cystlike appearance medially with a posterolateral nodule that follows gray matter signal (black arrow).

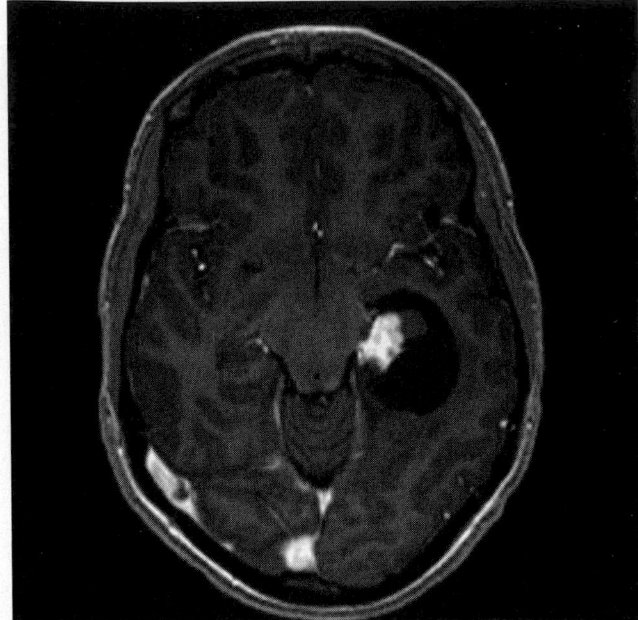

FIGURE 13-7

Ganglioglioma. Horizontal post-contrast T1W image of a left posteriomedial temporal lobe mass. The cystlike lesion with an enhancing mural nodule is a classic appearance for ganglioglioma.

gelastic seizures as well as other types of partial and generalized seizures, including atypical absence and drop attacks (20). Lesions usually are isointense to gray matter on T1 and iso/hyper intense on T2 sequences without enhancement. Large hamartomas (up to 4 cm) may have cystic components extending into the sella or even middle cranial fossa.

Vascular Malformations

Cavernous angioma (or cavernoma) has been associated with epilepsy in children and is frequently associated with a benign venous malformation. Histologically, cavernomas are characterized by sinusoidal vascular spaces with dilated capillary beds filled with blood and breakdown products of varying age. MRI shows a lobulated center ("popcorn") with high T1, T2, and FLAIR signal surrounded by a rim of T2 hypointensity related to hemosiderin and ferritin breakdown products. The rim, related to intermittent small hemorrhages, is best visualized with T2*-weighted gradient echo sequences. Some cavernomas have surrounding gliosis and increased T2 signal (21).

Sturge-Weber (encephalotrigeminal angiomatosis) is a sporadic disorder characterized by angiomatosis involving the eye, face (facial nevus flammus, or port-wine stain), and/or leptomeninges. Intracranially, there is a disorganized angiomatosis of the leptomeninges involving the capillaries, venous channels, and arteries, with characteristic "matting" and fibrosis. There is also typically diffuse calcification of the underlying cortex, most commonly in the temporo-parieto-occipital region secondary to ischemia. Typical findings on MR include weblike enhancement of the subarachnoid space, corresponding to the matted vasculature of the pial angioma (Figure 13-9). Calcification of the underlying cortex is best visualized on CT or MR T2-weighted images and is usually unilateral. The ipsilateral choroid plexus may also be enlarged (22), and may be correlated with the extent of pial angiomatosis (23).

Arteriovenous malformations (AVM) are abnormal, often friable connections between cerebral arteries and veins without intervening capillaries. Thought to be congenital, AVMs may grow over time, resulting in hypoperfusion and the development of aneurysms, and can cause seizures, neurologic deficits, headache, hydrocephalus, or hemorrhage (24). CT is most sensitive in the detection of hemorrhage that presents acutely. CT angiography with 3D reconstructions can help delineate feeding artery and draining vein anatomy (25) (Figure 13-10, long white

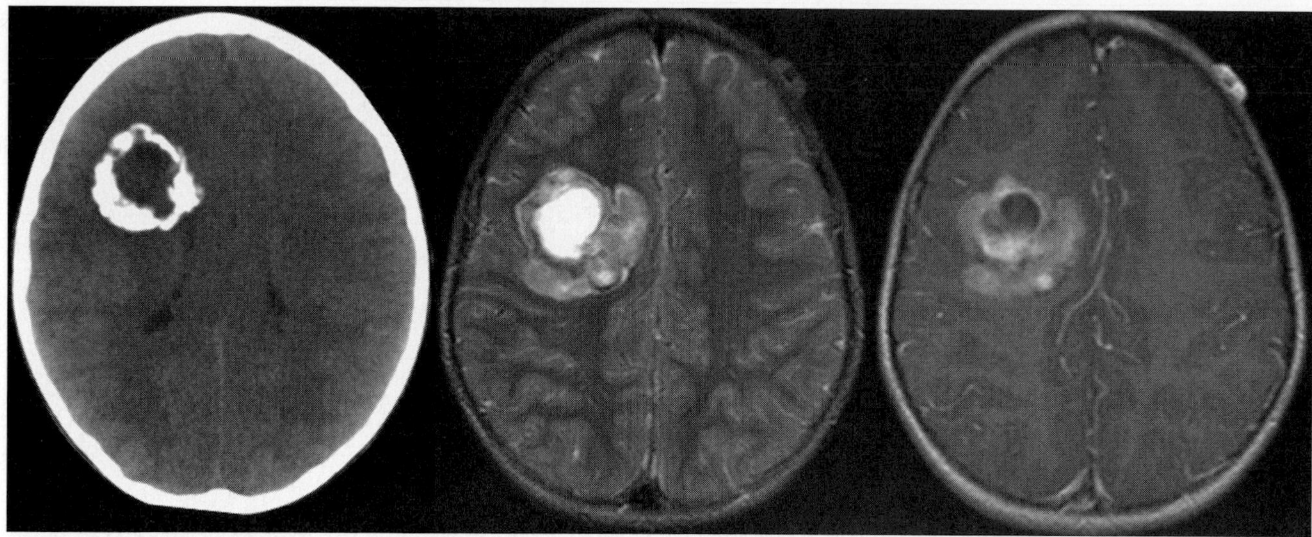

FIGURE 13-8

Oligodendroglioma. Horizontal CT, T2W, and post-contrast T1W images from a right frontal lobe mass. The hyperdensity on the CT peripherally indicates calcification, a common feature of oligodendroglioma. The heterogeneous T2W signal with enhancement are nonspecific but common features in this neoplasm.

arrow). Imaging findings on MR include flow voids on T2 spin echo sequences and low intensity T2* signal in areas of old hemorrhage.

Mesial Temporal Sclerosis

The term *mesial temporal sclerosis* (MTS) refers to hippocampal atrophy, with or without damage to surrounding structures in the mesial temporal lobe. Clinically, MTS is synonymous with temporal lobe epilepsy (TLE) or epilepsy with partial complex seizures. Typically, MTS involves lateral temporal neocortex as well as extratemporal structures, especially the frontal lobe. Histopathologically, hippocampal sclerosis refers to a small, firm hippocampus with neuronal loss in CA1 and CA3, as well as sclerosis in all sectors. As mentioned above, pathologic changes may be discerned in other mesial structures, including the amygdala, fornix, and mammillary body. MTS may be associated with other developmental abnormalities of the brain, especially porencephaly (26, 27). A current area of active investigation includes better delineating the relationship of MTS to complex febrile seizures of childhood as well as status epilepticus.

The classic imaging findings in mesial temporal sclerosis are hippocampal atrophy, increased T2 signal, and loss or distortion of adjacent white matter (Figure 13-11, right image). In addition, quantitative methods have been developed by several groups with excellent results (11, 28). Both automatic and manual segmentation techniques have been applied to high-resolution T1 images in an

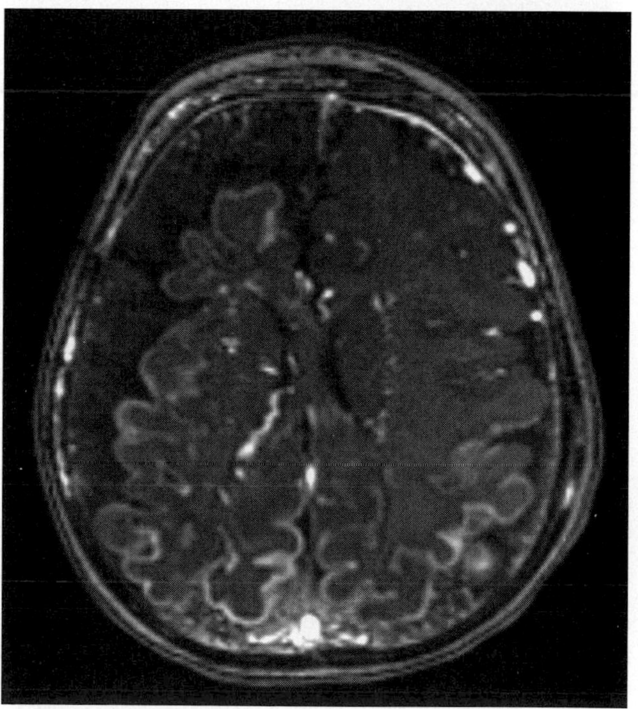

FIGURE 13-9

Sturge-Weber. Horizontal post contrast T1W image demonstrates diffuse, bilateral leptomeningeal enhancement and atrophy of the right hemisphere typical of encephalotrigeminal angiomatosis. The surface of the cortical gyri are enhancing. Bilateral involvement is present in this example, but unilateral involvement is the more typical presentation.

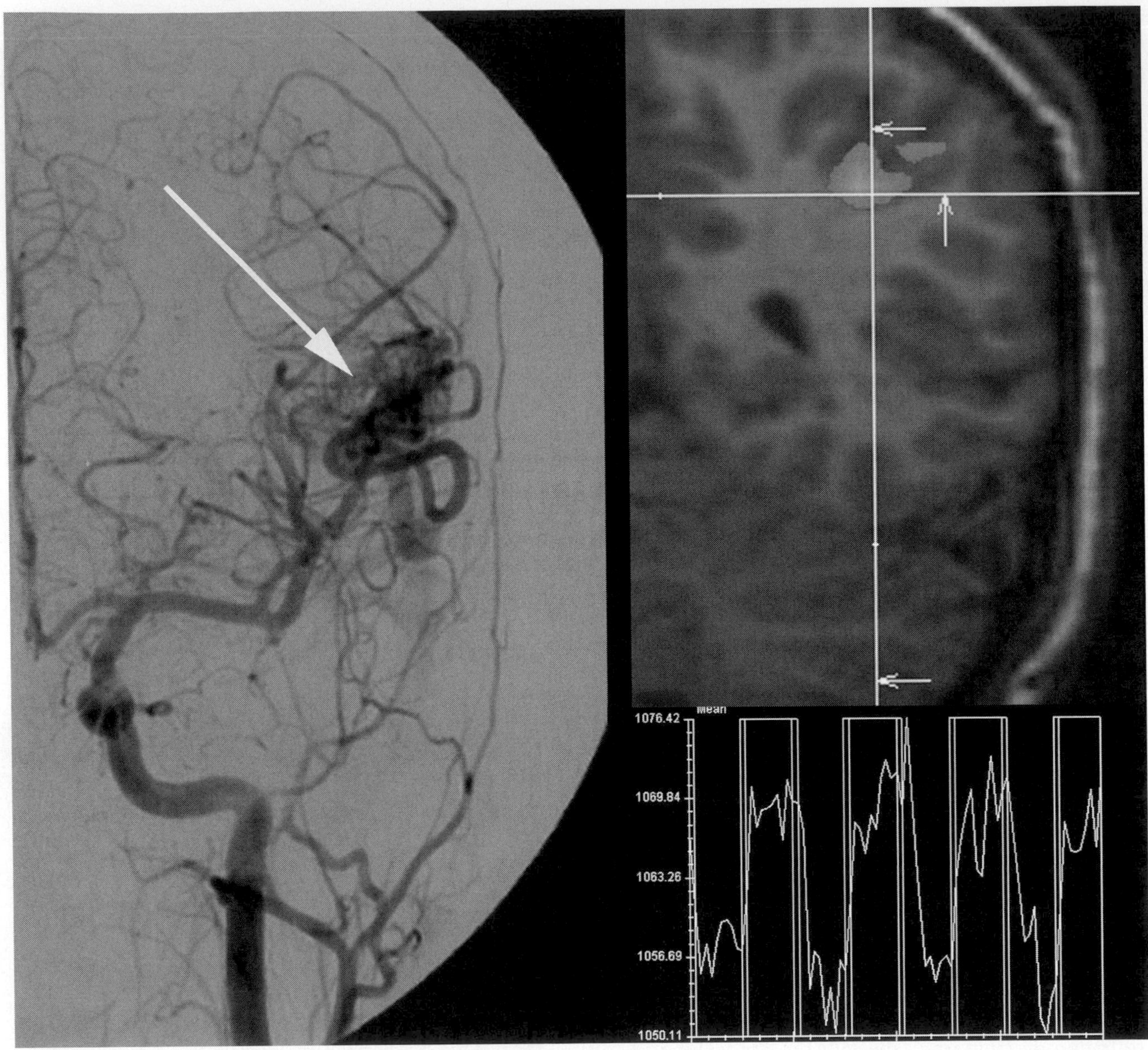

FIGURE 13-10

Arteriovenous malformation. Cerebral angiography (left) of a temporoparietal arteriovenous malformation (AVM). The long white arrow points to a tangle of vessels in the nidus of the AVM. BOLD functional MRI was performed (right) to determine whether the AVM involved eloquent cortex. The circle encloses the AVM. The crossing lines localize activation along the precentral gyrus. The graph confirms that the activation is synchronized with the finger-tapping task paradigm.

oblique coronal plane, perpendicular to the long axes of the hippocampi (Figure 13-11, left image). Volumetric analysis of hippocampi in normal children can provide normative data used for diagnosing hippocampal sclerosis (29). Hippocampal volume has been correlated with prognosis for seizure freedom and neuropathologic findings after surgical resection (30, 31).

Rasmussen's Encephalitis

The term *Rasmussen's encephalitis* describes a syndrome of partial-onset seizures and progressive neurologic deficits that commence between 14 months and 14 years of age. Fluctuating deficits follow seizures, lengthen, and then become permanent in more than half of affected children. Partial and generalized seizures often evolve over time, and progressive deterioration of neurologic status with hemiparesis, focal neurologic deficits, and dementia characterize the most severe cases. Histopathologically, the affected brain shows diffuse lymphocytic infiltration and perivascular cuffing, consistent with chronic viral encephalitis (32). MRI features have been correlated with quantitative histopathology, showing higher numbers of

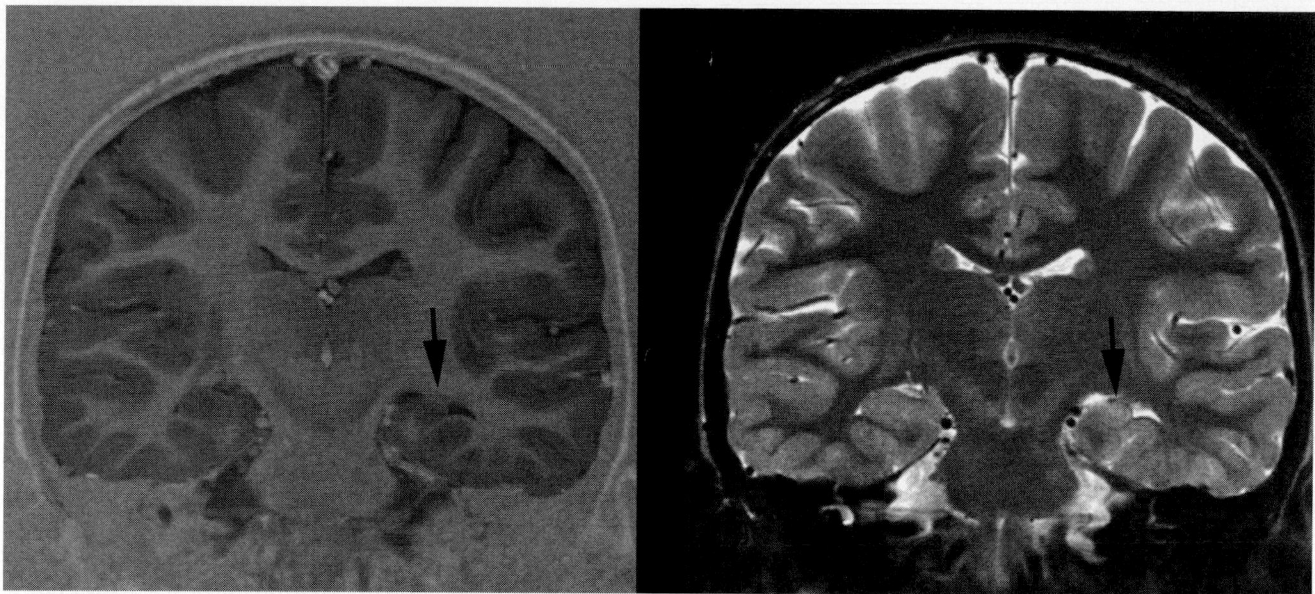

FIGURE 13-11

Mesial temporal sclerosis. Coronal inversion recovery T1W and high resolution T2W images of left hippocampal sclerosis. The black arrows localize a small, T2-hyperintense left hippocampus. The internal architecture of the left hippocampus is indistinct as well.

T cells and reactive astrocytes in the earlier, acute inflammatory stage of the disease (33). Classic imaging findings include progressive brain atrophy, edema of the cortical ribbon with increased T2 and FLAIR signal, and relative enlargement of the ipsilateral ventricle.

Diffusion Tensor Imaging

Diffusion tensor imaging (DTI) has emerged as a powerful tool in the analysis of brain development and myelination of axons, and in visualization of the fine detail of white matter organization in children. Diffusion MR imaging, acquired using single-shot spin echo echo-planar pulse sequence using Stejskal-Tanner pulsed diffusion gradients, is sensitive to the subvoxel movement of water in brain tissue. Signal intensity in DTI is inversely related to the magnitude of water diffusion (hyperintense = decreased movement of water) (10).

The apparent diffusion coefficient (ADC) is a quantitative measure of water diffusion along a given applied gradient. Water diffuses more freely in the direction of white matter bundles structural elements such as the myelin sheath, axolemma, and neurofilaments. The term *fractional anisotropy* (FA) refers to the degree of asymmetric water diffusion (e.g., greater along a fiber tract as opposed to between fiber tracts) within a given location (voxel). Thus, by measuring ADC along multiple diffusion-encoding directions it is possible to obtain information about rate, magnitude, and directionality of water diffusion. This information is then translated into images depicting white matter tract location and directionality.

During normal brain development, there is a general decrease in water diffusivity and increase in anisotropy associated with myelination and tract development. In general, these changes follow both a temporal and spatial sequence that parallels that of myelination noted previously.

Diffusion tensor imaging has proven useful in the study of epilepsy. In MTS, increased diffusivity and decreased fractional anisotropy are present in the epileptogenic zone (34–36). Combining DTI with statistical parametric mapping (SPM) or zonally magnified oblique multi-slice echo planar imaging (ZOOM-EPI) acquisition, some investigators have suggested that increased diffusivity may be an early marker of mesial temporal lobe epilepsy (MTLE), even when the MRI is normal (37, 38). Recent work demonstrates more widespread bilateral changes, including increased diffusivity throughout the ipsilateral hippocampus and mesial temporal lobe, decreased anisotropy in posterior ipsilateral extratemporal regions, as well as decreased anisotropy in the contralateral hippocampus, ipsilateral thalamus (39), and bilateral limbic system (40), suggesting multiple abnormalities over the course of an "epileptogenic network" (41, 42).

Diffusion tensor imaging has also been applied to extratemporal epilepsy with good results. DTI with SPM has demonstrated either reduced anisotropy or increased diffusivity in brain surrounding cortical malformations (43, 44). Paradoxically, dyplastic gray matter demonstrates increased anisotropy in some reports (45). Among children with tuberous sclerosis, DTI studies have identified abnormalities in cortical tubers and in associated white matter lesions (46). Asymmetries in temporal anisotropy have been associated with atypical language lateralization (47). Fractional anisotropy in frontotemporal regions has been correlated with interictal psychosis (48). Generalized decreased fractional anisotropy in injured brain regions may be useful in predicting epileptogenesis in patients with traumatic brain injuries (49). Diffusion tensor imaging tractography is sensitive enough to detect both axonal fragmentation and delayed myelin degradation in patients undergoing corpus callosotomy (50). In combination with functional MRI and MR spectroscopy, DTI provides a noninvasive window on the functional, microstructural, and biochemical characteristics of epileptogenic tissue (51).

DTI has also been utilized for both preoperative and intraoperative applications in the surgical treatment of intractable epilepsy (52). Preoperative DTI visualization of the optic pathways may also be useful for predicting visual field defects after resection of the temporal lobe (53).

Diffusion spectroscopic imaging (DSI) and tractography uses probabilistic map calculation algorithms to better visualize small tracts, as well as the white matter organization outside large tracts, with a spatial resolution of 8 mm^3 (Figure 13-12). Increased resolution of this approach has the potential to allow better definition of the microanatomy of seizures.

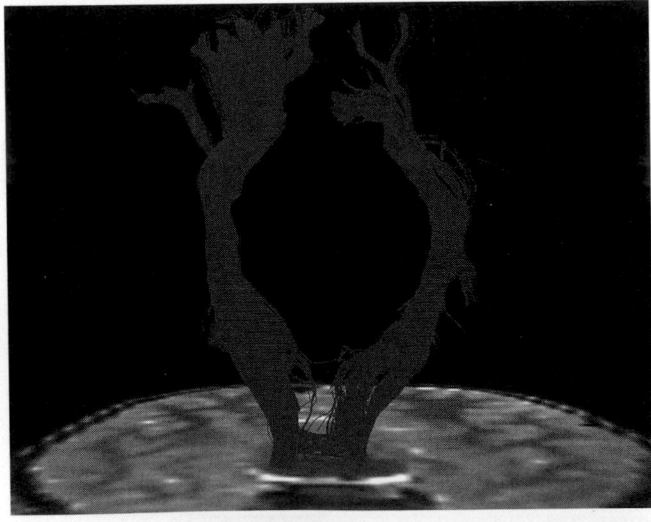

FIGURE 13-12

Diffusion tensor tractography. Diffusion tensor tractography (DTT) of bilateral corticospinal tracts in a 3-year old child. (Figure courtesy of Joshua Shimony, Mallinckrodt Institute of Radiology, Washington University School of Medicine.)

Proton MR Spectroscopic Imaging

Proton magnetic resonance spectroscopy (MRS) is a technique for the assessment of chemical composition and cellular metabolism of the brain in vivo. The most commonly used nuclei are ^{1}H and ^{31}P. Magnetic resonance spectroscopy provides a qualitative and quantitative depiction of metabolites present in brain tissue. In clinical applications ^{1}H-MRS is more commonly used because of its better spatial resolution. The most common metabolites imaged are N-acetyl aspartate (NAA), choline (Cho), glutamate/glutamine (Glx), lactate/lipid (Lac), myo-inositol (mI), and creatine/phosphocreatine (Cr/PCr). In general terms, NAA is a marker of neuronal health, and its concentration probably reflects neuronal density. Cho is thought to be a marker of cell membrane turnover and thus glial health or myelin turnover. Lactate is a marker of anaerobic glycolysis, whereas creatine is a marker of high-energy metabolism. Myo-inositol is an osmolyte and marker of glial health. Glutamate is elevated in ischemia and excitotoxic injury. ^{31}P-MRS is useful in the imaging of phosphate-containing compounds such as adenosine triphosphate (ATP), phosophodiesters, phosphocreatine, and inorganic phosphate. It is also useful in determining tissue acidity/pH (54).

MR spectroscopy has a role in the differentiation of high-grade tumors, in which choline is typically elevated relative to NAA and Cr, as compared to metabolic disorders, ischemia, and glial scarring. Other MR spectroscopy applications include metabolic disorders, stroke, hypoxia and monitoring gene therapy; however, this discussion focuses on its application in the study and localization of epileptogenic cortex.

Studies of children with intractable epilepsy have shown a significantly decreased NAA/(Cho+Cr) ratio (55–59), on the order of 19% in the involved temporal lobe compared with normal controls (56). Postictal ^{1}H-MRS of hippocampi has also shown increased NAA/(Cho+Cr) and lipid/lactate levels if performed within 7–24 hours following a seizure. When the findings were unilateral, they always corresponded to the affected side and were somewhat helpful in the localization of extratemporal foci (60–62). Although ipsilateral apparent diffusion coefficient (ADC) but not NAA/(Cr+Cho) correlated with disease duration, neither ADC nor NAA/(Cr+Cho) correlated with hippocampal volume. Hence these three variables appear to capture different but complementary aspects of hippocampal pathology (35).

Spectroscopy has emerged as a means of locating epileptogenic cortex in children with otherwise normal MRI and hippocampal volumetry (63) and in children with complex febrile convulsions (64). When combined with amygdalo-hippocampal volumetry, the accuracy of ^{1}H spectroscopic imaging (MRSI) maps approaches that of the EEG for lateralizing epileptogenic temporal cortex (65).

Quantitative ^{1}H-MRS has also proven useful in detecting metabolic changes in hippocampi in children with asymptomatic localization-related epilepsy and infrequent seizures (66). Some children with juvenile myoclonic epilepsy have reduced frontal lobe concentrations of NAA (67). In tuberous sclerosis, researchers have found significantly lower NAA/Cr and NAA/(Cho+Cr) in cortical tubers than in normal brain (68).

In summary, proton MR spectroscopy holds great promise for improving our understanding of the metabolic dysfunction that accompanies or predisposes to epilepsy. Future applications will likely allow observation of transport and metabolism of macromolecules in the brain, combination with functional MRI, and assessment of the short-term effects of CNS-targeted pharmacologic interventions (69).

Functional Neuroimaging

Positron Emission Tomography

Functional neuroimaging provides information complementary to structural MR imaging in the diagnosis of epilepsy. Positron emission tomography (PET) allows visualization of brain glucose metabolism with the use of positron-emitting ligands such as 2-deoxy-2-[^{18}F]fluoro-D-glucose (FDG). Other ligands more specific to epilepsy have been developed, including [^{11}C]flumazenil (FMZ), which binds to $GABA_A$ receptors (70), and alpha-[^{21}C]methyl-L-tryptophan (AMT), which measures tryptophan metabolism (71). Research continues regarding the use of radiolabeled ligands to opioid, histamine H1, monoamine oxidase type B enzyme, N-methyl-D-aspartate, peripheral-type benzodiazepine, and serotonin 1A receptors.

Baseline glucose metabolism varies significantly as a function of age, with low values in infants, increasing to a maximum between 4 and 12 years, slowly declining during adolescence (72). Quantitative analysis by statistical parametric mapping (SPM) and statistical probabilistic anatomical mapping improves diagnostic performance (45).

PET has proven useful in the evaluation of many disorders associated with partial-onset seizures. These include infantile spasms, Rasmussen's syndrome(73), as well as partial epilepsies without MRI abnormality (74). Interictal FDG PET imaging of patients with medically refractory temporal lobe epilepsy shows glucose hypometabolism of the involved temporal lobe in about 85% of cases (75). It is important to note that if unrecognized epileptic discharges occur during a PET scan that is thought to be interictal, hypermetabolism may be occurring in the affected cortex. When this occurs, it may lead to false lateralization to the normal side, which appears to be relatively hypometabolic in this setting. Furthermore, the degree of hypometabolism is related to seizure duration and is thus likely to be less sensitive in younger children than in adolescents or adults (76).

PET seems to be most useful in the localization of hypometabolic epileptogenic areas that appear to be normal by MRI (74, 75, 77–82). When areas of hypometabolism are found, they can guide the placement of intracranial electrodes used to further hone in on the epileptogenic region. In children with frontal lobe epilepsy, PET sensitivity of 92% and specificity of 62.5% have been reported (75). Though it is less commonly used than functional magnetic resonance imaging (fMRI), PET may also be useful in functional brain mapping to identify speech and sensory/motor areas (77).

PET has also proven useful in furthering our understanding of certain epileptic syndromes. Heterogeneous metabolic patterns have been correlated with subtypes of Lennox-Gastaut syndrome (82–85). Bilateral abnormalities have been demonstrated in hemimegalencephaly (86). Finally, some authors propose that PET may provide a sensitive measure of the extent of involvement and correlate with clinical course in Sturge-Weber disease (73, 87).

Single-Photon Emission Computed Tomography (SPECT)

Single-photon emission computed tomography (SPECT) noninvasively measures changes in cerebral blood flow (CBF) associated with epileptic discharge. The agents (iodinated radiotracers or technetium-99m methyl cysteinate dimer) that are used in these studies quickly cross the blood-brain barrier and "imprint" the local brain parenchyma, providing a snapshot of CBF. The injection can occur either during seizure activity (ictal), in which case it is associated with an increase in CBF in discharging cortex; just after an event (postictal), when CBF is decreased; or at baseline (interictal) (88–89).

In addition to being aware of the occurrence of seizure activity when SPECT is obtained, SPECT imaging in children must be interpreted with an understanding of the changes in cerebral metabolism and CBF that accompany growth and development. At birth, there is high baseline CBF in the thalamus, central white matter, and cerebellar vermis. By age 3 months, the striatum and occipitoparietal frontal and cerebellar cortex all become relatively hypometabolic. At 12 months of age, the infant brain is very similar to the adult one, but then between 2 and 6 years of age it doubles adult values, finally decreasing to adult levels by age 15 (90).

In adults with temporal lobe epilepsy, ictal and postictal SPECT have sensitivities of 97% and 75%, respectively (91). In extratemporal epilepsy the sensitivity of SPECT is less than 50%, though it may be improved to 80% when subtraction ictal SPECT is coregistered to MRI in the so-called SISCOM (89, 92). Interictal SPECT is most useful as a baseline that can be compared with periictal images, and it has a reported sensitivity of 67% (93). SPECT has also been found to be useful in classification of absence seizures associated with localization-related epilepsies (94).

In pediatric patients, the role of SPECT is less well established. Among children who had a favorable surgical outcome, there was approximately a 70% correlation between areas of increased ictal perfusion and areas of cortical resection, suggesting that SPECT can help optimize the placement of intracranial electrodes (95). However, in a recent meta-analysis, data regarding the use of SPECT failed to support the use of SPECT in extra-temporal epilepsy in children, although ictal combined with immediately post-ictal SPECT scanning might improve results (91). In practical terms, however, performing true peri-ictal SPECT with the subtraction techniques like this requires a highly significant institutional commitment for radioactive tracer acquisition, tracer storage, coordination of peri-ictal injection, and prompt scanning of patients (92).

Functional MRI (fMRI)

Functional MRI allows visualization of active brain regions based on changes in CBF and oxygen metabolism. The most common contrast mechanism used in fMRI is blood oxygenation level-dependent (BOLD). Since neuronal activity drives cerebral metabolism and CBF, fMRI acts as a surrogate marker of cortical activation. Though originally applied to study the localization of movement, language, and memory, fMRI has been applied for the study of epilepsy as well.

Practically speaking, task-related fMRI has been very useful in older children and adults, but can be difficult to impossible to perform in younger children. The most common applications of fMRI include lateralization of language and memory function as well as localization of epileptic phenomena (96). Among many helpful roles, fMRI can help localize eloquent cortex prior to epilepsy surgery (Figure 13-10), help guide the placement of subdural electrode grids, influence the extent of resection, especially in cases of subcortical abnormalities, and generally contribute positively to outcome (97). Recent work shows that fMRI imaging of the amygdala during the fearful face task plus Roland's Hometown Walking Task highly increases the reliability of lateralization in patients with MTLE (98).

Functional MRI data complement EEG data in the elucidating the pathophysiology of epilepsy (99). In approximately 68% of patients with focal epilepsy, BOLD signal and EEG data correlate significantly (100, 101). Atypical language lateralization identified with fMRI has been correlated with duration of epilepsy in pediatric patients (102).

Magneto Encephalography and Magnetic Source Imaging

Magnetoencephalography (MEG) and magnetic source imaging (MSI) are additional noninvasive techniques for localizing epileptogenic cortex. Highly sensitive magnetometers detect faint magnetic fields associated with current flow at postsynaptic membranes of neurons. These data are processed and then superimposed on anatomic MR images to produce MSI (103). Because there is no distortion of magnetic signals by the scalp or skull, MEG has the potential to surpass EEG in the localization of epileptic discharges (104), but this potential has yet to be realized. Compared with invasive monitoring, attempts at localization with MEG have a lower yield in classic temporal lobe epilepsy (105).

Applications for MEG are expanding, with studies describing its use in preoperative evaluation, subdural electrode grid placement, and identification of the central sulcus and somatosensory cortex using evoked somatosensory fields. However, MEG mapping of language, primary motor areas, and memory has been inconsistent. As equipment and mathematical processing of data have improved, MEG is being investigated as a means of reducing the need for invasive subdural electrode monitoring (106–110). MEG may have a role in the localization of epileptogenic tubers in children with TSC (111, 112).

References

1. Duncan R, Patterson J, Hadley DM, et al. CT, MR and SPECT imaging in temporal lobe epilepsy. *J Neurol Neurosurg Psychiatry* 1990; 53:11–15.
2. Heinz ER, Heinz TR, Radtke R, et al. Efficacy of MR vs CT in epilepsy. *AJR Am J Roentgenol* 1989; 152:347–352.
3. Kuzniecky R, Murro A, King D, et al. Magnetic resonance imaging in childhood intractable partial epilepsies: pathologic correlations. *Neurology* 1993; 43:681–687.
4. Schorner W, Meencke HJ, Felix R. Temporal-lobe epilepsy: comparison of CT and MR imaging. *AJR Am J Roentgenol* 1987; 149:1231–1239.
5. Theodore WH, Katz D, Kufta C, et al. Pathology of temporal lobe foci: correlation with CT, MRI, and PET. *Neurology* 1990; 40:797–803.
6. Johnston JM, Smyth MD. CT/MRI image fusion for neuronavigation in grid-based epilepsy surgery. Presented at Annual Meeting of AANS/CNS Section on Pediatric Neurological Surgery, Denver, Colorado, 2006.
7. Grant PE, Barkovich AJ, Wald LL, Dillon WP, et al. High-resolution surface-coil MR of cortical lesions in medically refractory epilepsy: a prospective study. *AJNR Am J Neuroradiol* 1997; 18:291–301.
8. Grant PE. Imaging the developing epileptic brain. *Epilepsia* 2005; 46 Suppl 7:7–14.
9. Bridge H, Clare S. High-resolution MRI: in vivo histology? *Philos Trans R Soc Lond B Biol Sci* 2006; 361:137–146.
10. Mukherjee P, McKinstry RC. Diffusion tensor imaging and tractography of human brain development. *Neuroimaging Clin N Am* 2006; 16:19–43, vii.
11. Lawson JA, Nguyen W, Bleasel AF, et al. ILAE-defined epilepsy syndromes in children: correlation with quantitative MRI. *Epilepsia* 1998; 39:1345–1349.
12. Lawson JA, Vogrin S, Bleasel AF, Cook MJ, et al. Cerebral and cerebellar volume reduction in children with intractable epilepsy. *Epilepsia* 2000; 41:1456–1462.
13. Van Essen DC. A population-average, landmark- and surface-based (PALS) atlas of human cerebral cortex. *Neuroimage* 2005; 28:635–662.
14. Van Essen DC, Dierker D, Snyder AZ, Raichle ME, et al. Symmetry of cortical folding abnormalities in Williams syndrome revealed by surface-based analyses. *J Neurosci* 2006; 26:5470–5483.
15. Barkovich AJ. Pediatric neuroimaging. 4th ed. Philadelphia: Lippincott Williams & Wilkins, 2005.
16. Raybaud C, Shroff M, Rutka JT, Chuang SH. Imaging surgical epilepsy in children. *Childs Nerv Syst* 2006; 22:786–809.

17. Yagishita A, Arai N, Tamagawa K, Oda M. Hemimegalencephaly: signal changes suggesting abnormal myelination on MRI. *Neuroradiology* 1998; 40:734–738.
18. Pasquier B, Peoc HM, Fabre-Bocquentin B, et al. Surgical pathology of drug-resistant partial epilepsy. A 10-year-experience with a series of 327 consecutive resections. *Epileptic Disord* 2002; 4:99–119.
19. Rickert CH, Paulus W. Epidemiology of central nervous system tumors in childhood and adolescence based on the new WHO classification. *Childs Nerv Syst* 2001; 17:503–511.
20. Mullatti N, Selway R, Nashef L, et al. The clinical spectrum of epilepsy in children and adults with hypothalamic hamartoma. *Epilepsia* 2003; 44:1310–1319.
21. Rigamonti D, Drayer BP, Johnson PC, Hadley MN, et al. The MRI appearance of cavernous malformations (angiomas). *J Neurosurg* 1987; 67:518–524.
22. Stimac GK, Solomon MA, Newton TH. CT and MR of angiomatous malformations of the choroid plexus in patients with Sturge-Weber disease. *AJNR Am J Neuroradiol* 1986; 7:623–627.
23. Griffiths PD, Blaser S, Boodram MB, Armstrong D, et al. Choroid plexus size in young children with Sturge-Weber syndrome. *AJNR Am J Neuroradiol* 1996; 17:175–180.
24. Perret G, Nishioka H. Report on the cooperative study of intracranial aneurysms and subarachnoid hemorrhage. Section VI. Arteriovenous malformations. An analysis of 545 cases of cranio-cerebral arteriovenous malformations and fistulae reported to the cooperative study. *J Neurosurg* 1966; 25:467–490.
25. Bittles MA, Sidhu MK, Sze RW, Finn LS, et al. Multidetector CT angiography of pediatric vascular malformations and hemangiomas: utility of 3-D reformatting in differential diagnosis. *Pediatr Radiol* 2005; 35:1100–1106.
26. Ho SS, Kuzniecky RI, Gilliam F, Faught E, et al. Congenital porencephaly and hippocampal sclerosis. Clinical features and epileptic spectrum. *Neurology* 1997; 49:1382–1388.
27. Ho SS, Kuzniecky RI, Gilliam F, Faught E, et al. Congenital porencephaly: MR features and relationship to hippocampal sclerosis. *AJNR Am J Neuroradiol* 1998; 19:135–141.
28. Jack CR, Jr., Sharbrough FW, Twomey CK, et al. Temporal lobe seizures: lateralization with MR volume measurements of the hippocampal formation. *Radiology* 1990; 175:423–429.
29. Mulani SJ, Kothare SV, Patkar DP. Magnetic resonance volumetric analysis of hippocampi in children in the age group of 6 to 12 years: a pilot study. *Neuroradiology* 2005; 47:552–557.
30. Jack CR Jr, Sharbrough FW, Cascino GD, Hirschorn KA, et al. Magnetic resonance image-based hippocampal volumetry: correlation with outcome after temporal lobectomy. *Ann Neurol* 1992; 31:138–146.
31. Cascino GD, Jack CR, Jr., Parisi JE, et al. Magnetic resonance imaging-based volume studies in temporal lobe epilepsy: pathological correlations. *Ann Neurol* 1991; 30:31–36.
32. Raybaud C, Guye M, Mancini J, Girard N. Neuroimaging of epilepsy in children. *Magn Reson Imaging Clin N Am* 2001; 9:121–147, viii.
33. Bien CG, Urbach H, Deckert M, Schramm J, et al. Diagnosis and staging of Rasmussen's encephalitis by serial MRI and histopathology. *Neurology* 2002; 58:250–257.
34. Dumas de la Roque A, Oppenheim C, Chassoux F, Rodrigo S, et al. Diffusion tensor imaging of partial intractable epilepsy. *Eur Radiol* 2005; 15:279–285.
35. Duzel E, Kaufmann J, Guderian S, Szentkuti A, et al. Measures of hippocampal volumes, diffusion and ^{1}H MRS metabolic abnormalities in temporal lobe epilepsy provide partially complementary information. *Eur J Neurol* 2004; 11:195–205.
36. Assaf BA, Mohamed FB, Abou-Khaled KJ, Williams JM, et al. Diffusion tensor imaging of the hippocampal formation in temporal lobe epilepsy. *AJNR Am J Neuroradiol* 2003; 24:1857–1862.
37. Salmenpera TM, Simister RJ, Bartlett P, Symms MR, et al. High-resolution diffusion tensor imaging of the hippocampus in temporal lobe epilepsy. *Epilepsy Res* 2006; 71:102–106.
38. Rugg-Gunn FJ, Eriksson SH, Symms MR, Barker GJ, et al. Diffusion tensor imaging of cryptogenic and acquired partial epilepsies. *Brain* 2001; 124:627–636.
39. Kimiwada T, Juhasz C, Makki M, Muzik O, et al. Hippocampal and thalamic diffusion abnormalities in children with temporal lobe epilepsy. *Epilepsia* 2006; 47:167–175.
40. Concha L, Beaulieu C, Gross DW. Bilateral limbic diffusion abnormalities in unilateral temporal lobe epilepsy. *Ann Neurol* 2005; 57:188–196.
41. Arfanakis K, Hermann BP, Rogers BP, Carew JD, et al. Diffusion tensor MRI in temporal lobe epilepsy. *Magn Reson Imaging* 2002; 20:511–519.
42. Thivard L, Lehericy S, Krainik A, et al. Diffusion tensor imaging in medial temporal lobe epilepsy with hippocampal sclerosis. *Neuroimage* 2005; 28:682–690.
43. Eriksson SH, Rugg-Gunn FJ, Symms MR, Barker GJ, et al. Diffusion tensor imaging in patients with epilepsy and malformations of cortical development. *Brain* 2001; 124:617–626.
44. Okumura A, Fukatsu H, Kato K, Ikuta T, et al. Diffusion tensor imaging in frontal lobe epilepsy. *Pediatr Neurol* 2004; 31:203–206.
45. Lee JJ, Kang WJ, Lee DS, et al. Diagnostic performance of ^{18}F-FDG PET and ictal ^{99m}Tc-HMPAO SPET in pediatric temporal lobe epilepsy: quantitative analysis by statistical parametric mapping, statistical probabilistic anatomical map, and subtraction ictal SPET. *Seizure* 2005; 14:213–220.
46. Karadag D, Mentzel HJ, Gullmar D, Rating T, et al. Diffusion tensor imaging in children and adolescents with tuberous sclerosis. *Pediatr Radiol* 2005; 35:980–983.
47. Briellmann RS, Mitchell LA, Waites AB, et al. Correlation between language organization and diffusion tensor abnormalities in refractory partial epilepsy. *Epilepsia* 2003; 44:1541–1545.
48. Flugel D, Cercignani M, Symms MR, et al. Diffusion tensor imaging findings and their correlation with neuropsychological deficits in patients with temporal lobe epilepsy and interictal psychosis. *Epilepsia* 2006; 47:941–944.
49. Gupta RK, Saksena S, Agarwal A, Hasan KM, et al. Diffusion tensor imaging in late posttraumatic epilepsy. *Epilepsia* 2005; 46:1465–1471.
50. Concha L, Gross DW, Wheatley BM, Beaulieu C. Diffusion tensor imaging of time-dependent axonal and myelin degradation after corpus callosotomy in epilepsy patients. *Neuroimage* 2006; 32:1090–1099.
51. Krakow K, Wieshmann UC, Woermann FG, Symms MR, et al. Multimodal MR imaging: functional, diffusion tensor, and chemical shift imaging in a patient with localization-related epilepsy. *Epilepsia* 1999; 40:1459–1462.
52. Akhtari M, Salamon N, Duncan R, Fried I, et al. Electrical conductivities of the freshly excised cerebral cortex in epilepsy surgery patients; correlation with pathology, seizure duration, and diffusion tensor imaging. *Brain Topogr* 2006; 18:281–290.
53. Powell HW, Parker GJ, Alexander DC, et al. MR tractography predicts visual field defects following temporal lobe resection. *Neurology* 2005; 65:596–599.
54. Hunter JV, Wang ZJ. MR spectroscopy in pediatric neuroradiology. *Magn Reson Imaging Clin N Am* 2001; 9:165–189, ix.
55. Park YD, Allison JD, Weiss KL, Smith JR, et al. Proton magnetic resonance spectroscopic observations of epilepsia partialis continua in children. *J Child Neurol* 2000; 15:729–733.
56. Cross JH, Connelly A, Jackson GD, Johnson CL, et al. Proton magnetic resonance spectroscopy in children with temporal lobe epilepsy. *Ann Neurol* 1996; 39:107–113.
57. Garcia PA, Laxer KD, van der Grond J, Hugg JW, et al. Proton magnetic resonance spectroscopic imaging in patients with frontal lobe epilepsy. *Ann Neurol* 1995; 37:279–281.
58. Kuzniecky R, Hetherington H, Pan J, et al. Proton spectroscopic imaging at 4.1 tesla in patients with malformations of cortical development and epilepsy. *Neurology* 1997; 48:1018–1024.
59. Woermann FG, McLean MA, Bartlett PA, Barker GJ, et al. Quantitative short echo time proton magnetic resonance spectroscopic imaging study of malformations of cortical development causing epilepsy. *Brain* 2001; 124:427–436.
60. Holopainen IE, Lundbom NM, Metsahonkala EL, Komu ME, et al. Temporal lobe pathology in epilepsy: proton magnetic resonance spectroscopy and positron emission tomography study. *Pediatr Neurol* 1997; 16:98–104.
61. Duc CO, Trabesinger AH, Weber OM, Meier D, et al. Quantitative ^{1}H MRS in the evaluation of mesial temporal lobe epilepsy in vivo. *Magn Reson Imaging* 1998; 16:969–979.
62. Castillo M, Smith JK, Kwock L. Proton MR spectroscopy in patients with acute temporal lobe seizures. AJNR Am J Neuroradiol 2001; 22:152-157.
63. Connelly A, Van Paesschen W, Porter DA, Johnson CL, et al. Proton magnetic resonance spectroscopy in MRI-negative temporal lobe epilepsy. *Neurology* 1998; 51:61–66.
64. Holopainen IE, Valtonen ME, Komu ME, Sonninen PH, et al. Proton spectroscopy in children with epilepsy and febrile convulsions. *Pediatr Neurol* 1998; 19:93–99.
65. Cendes F, Caramanos Z, Andermann F, Dubeau F, et al. Proton magnetic resonance spectroscopic imaging and magnetic resonance imaging volumetry in the lateralization of temporal lobe epilepsy: a series of 100 patients. *Ann Neurol* 1997; 42:737–746.
66. Varho T, Komu M, Sonninen P, Lahdetie J, et al. Quantitative HMRS and MRI volumetry indicate neuronal damage in the hippocampus of children with focal epilepsy and infrequent seizures. *Epilepsia* 2005; 46:696–703.
67. Savic I, Lekvall A, Greitz D, Helms G. MR spectroscopy shows reduced frontal lobe concentrations of N-acetyl aspartate in patients with juvenile myoclonic epilepsy. *Epilepsia* 2000; 41:290–296.
68. Mukonoweshuro W, Wilkinson ID, Griffiths PD. Proton MR spectroscopy of cortical tubers in adults with tuberous sclerosis complex. *AJNR Am J Neuroradiol* 2001; 22:1920–1925.
69. Novotny E, Ashwal S, Shevell M. Proton magnetic resonance spectroscopy: an emerging technology in pediatric neurology research. *Pediatr Res* 1998; 44:1–10.
70. Henry TR, Frey KA, Sackellares JC, et al. In vivo cerebral metabolism and central benzodiazepine-receptor binding in temporal lobe epilepsy. *Neurology* 1993; 43:1998–2006.
71. Chugani DC, Chugani HT, Muzik O, Shah JR, et al. Imaging epileptogenic tubers in children with tuberous sclerosis complex using alpha-[^{11}C]methyl-L-tryptophan positron emission tomography. *Ann Neurol* 1998; 44:858–866.
72. Bentourkia M, Michel C, Ferriere G, Bol A, et al. Evolution of brain glucose metabolism with age in epileptic infants, children and adolescents. *Brain Dev* 1998; 20:524–529.
73. Lee JS, Asano E, Muzik O, Chugani DC, et al. Sturge-Weber syndrome: correlation between clinical course and FDG PET findings. *Neurology* 2001; 57:189–195.
74. Juhasz C, Chugani HT. Imaging the epileptic brain with positron emission tomography. *Neuroimaging Clin N Am* 2003; 13:705–716, viii.
75. Sood S, Chugani HT. Functional neuroimaging in the preoperative evaluation of children with drug-resistant epilepsy. *Childs Nerv Syst* 2006; 22:810–820.
76. Gaillard WD, Kopylev L, Weinstein S, Conry J, et al. Low incidence of abnormal (18)FDG-PET in children with new-onset partial epilepsy: a prospective study. *Neurology* 2002; 58:717–722.
77. Mohan KK, Chugani DC, Chugani HT. Positron emission tomography in pediatric neurology. *Semin Pediatr Neurol* 1999; 6:111–119.
78. Zupanc ML. Neuroimaging in the evaluation of children and adolescents with intractable epilepsy: II. Neuroimaging and pediatric epilepsy surgery. *Pediatr Neurol* 1997; 17:111–121.
79. Shulkin BL. PET applications in pediatrics. *Q J Nucl Med* 1997; 41:281–291.
80. Cummings TJ, Chugani DC, Chugani HT. Positron emission tomography in pediatric epilepsy. *Neurosurg Clin N Am* 1995; 6:465–472.
81. Messa C, Grana C, Lucignani G, Fazio F. Functional imaging using PET and SPECT in pediatric neurology. *J Nucl Biol Med* 1994; 38:85–88.
82. Chugani HT. The role of PET in childhood epilepsy. *J Child Neurol* 1994; 9 Suppl 1: S82–S88.
83. Miyauchi T, Nomura Y, Ohno S, Kishimoto H, et al. Positron emission tomography in three cases of Lennox-Gastaut syndrome. *Jpn J Psychiatry Neurol* 1988; 42:795–804.

84. Yanai K, Iinuma K, Matsuzawa T, et al. Cerebral glucose utilization in pediatric neurological disorders determined by positron emission tomography. *Eur J Nucl Med* 1987; 13:292–296.
85. Chugani HT, Mazziotta JC, Engel J Jr, Phelps ME. The Lennox-Gastaut syndrome: metabolic subtypes determined by 2-deoxy-2[^{18}F]fluoro-D-glucose positron emission tomography. *Ann Neurol* 1987; 21:4–13.
86. Rintahaka PJ, Chugani HT, Messa C, Phelps ME. Hemimegalencephaly: evaluation with positron emission tomography. *Pediatr Neurol* 1993; 9:21–28.
87. Pinton F, Chiron C, Enjolras O, Motte J, et al. Early single photon emission computed tomography in Sturge-Weber syndrome. *J Neurol Neurosurg Psychiatry* 1997; 63:616–621.
88. Newton MR, Berkovic SF, Austin MC, Rowe CC, et al. SPECT in the localisation of extratemporal and temporal seizure foci. *J Neurol Neurosurg Psychiatry* 1995; 59:26–30.
89. O'Brien TJ, So EL, Mullan BP, et al. Subtraction SPECT co-registered to MRI improves postictal SPECT localization of seizure foci. *Neurology* 1999; 52:137–146.
90. Chiron C, Raynaud C, Maziere B, Zilbovicius M, et al. Changes in regional cerebral blood flow during brain maturation in children and adolescents. *J Nucl Med* 1992; 33:696–703.
91. Devous MD Sr, Thisted RA, Morgan GF, Leroy RF, et al. SPECT brain imaging in epilepsy: a meta-analysis. *J Nucl Med* 1998; 39:285–293.
92. O'Brien TJ, O'Connor MK, Mullan BP, Brinkmann BH, et al. Subtraction ictal SPET co-registered to MRI in partial epilepsy: description and technical validation of the method with phantom and patient studies. *Nucl Med Commun* 1998; 19:31–45.
93. Spencer SS. The relative contributions of MRI, SPECT, and PET imaging in epilepsy. *Epilepsia* 1994; 35 Suppl 6:S72–S89.
94. Iannetti P, Spalice A, De Luca PF, Boemi S, et al. Ictal single photon emission computed tomography in absence seizures: apparent implication of different neuronal mechanisms. *J Child Neurol* 2001; 16:339–344.
95. Kaminska A, Chiron C, Ville D, Dellatolas G, et al. Ictal SPECT in children with epilepsy: comparison with intracranial EEG and relation to postsurgical outcome. *Brain* 2003; 126:248–260.
96. Detre JA. fMRI: applications in epilepsy. *Epilepsia* 2004; 45 Suppl 4:26–31.
97. Liegeois F, Cross JH, Gadian DG, Connelly A. Role of fMRI in the decision-making process: epilepsy surgery for children. *J Magn Reson Imaging* 2006; 23:933–940.
98. Schacher M, Haemmerle B, Woermann FG, Okujava M, et al. Amygdala fMRI lateralizes temporal lobe epilepsy. *Neurology* 2006; 66:81–87.
99. Gotman J, Kobayashi E, Bagshaw AP, Benar CG, et al. Combining EEG and fMRI: a multimodal tool for epilepsy research. *J Magn Reson Imaging* 2006; 23:906–920.
100. Salek-Haddadi A, Diehl B, Hamandi K, Merschhemke M, et al. Hemodynamic correlates of epileptiform discharges: an EEG-fMRI study of 63 patients with focal epilepsy. *Brain Res* 2006; 1088:148–166.
101. Jokeit H, Okujava M, Woermann FG. Memory fMRI lateralizes temporal lobe epilepsy. *Neurology* 2001; 57:1786-1793.
102. Yuan W, Szaflarski JP, Schmithorst VJ, et al. fMRI shows atypical language lateralization in pediatric epilepsy patients. *Epilepsia* 2006; 47:593–600.
103. Chuang NA, Otsubo H, Pang EW, Chuang SH. Pediatric magnetoencephalography and magnetic source imaging. *Neuroimaging Clin N Am* 2006; 16:193–210, ix–x.
104. Verrotti A, Pizzella V, Trotta D, Madonna L, et al. Magnetoencephalography in pediatric neurology and in epileptic syndromes. *Pediatr Neurol* 2003; 28:253–261.
105. Sperli F, Spinelli L, Seeck M, Kurian M, et al. EEG source imaging in pediatric epilepsy surgery: a new perspective in presurgical workup. *Epilepsia* 2006; 47:981–990.
106. Grondin R, Chuang S, Otsubo H, Holowka S, et al. The role of magnetoencephalography in pediatric epilepsy surgery. *Childs Nerv Syst* 2006; 22:779–785.
107. Knowlton RC, Elgavish R, Howell J, Blount J, et al. Magnetic source imaging versus intracranial electroencephalogram in epilepsy surgery: a prospective study. *Ann Neurol* 2006; 59:835–842.
108. Knowlton RC, Shih J. Magnetoencephalography in epilepsy. *Epilepsia* 2004; 45 Suppl 4:61–71.
109. Otsubo H, Ochi A, Elliott I, et al. MEG predicts epileptic zone in lesional extrahippocampal epilepsy: 12 pediatric surgery cases. *Epilepsia* 2001; 42:1523–1530.
110. Minassian BA, Otsubo H, Weiss S, Elliott I, et al. Magnetoencephalographic localization in pediatric epilepsy surgery: comparison with invasive intracranial electroencephalography. *Ann Neurol* 1999; 46:627–633.
111. Wu JY, Sutherling WW, Koh S, Salamon N, et al. Magnetic source imaging localizes epileptogenic zone in children with tuberous sclerosis complex. *Neurology* 2006; 66:1270–1272.
112. Kamimura T, Tohyama J, Oishi M, et al. Magnetoencephalography in patients with tuberous sclerosis and localization-related epilepsy. *Epilepsia* 2006; 47:991–997.

III

AGE-RELATED SYNDROMES

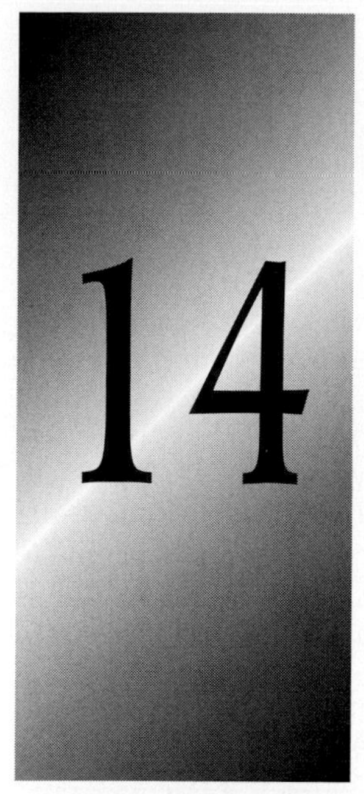

Neonatal Seizures

Eli M. Mizrahi

The first four weeks of life are one of the greatest periods of seizure hazard during childhood. The occurrence of seizures within this neonatal period is associated with significant morbidity and mortality. These seizures are often difficult to recognize clinically and treat effectively and can represent significant diagnostic and management challenges. In addition, despite their clinical importance, there are a number of unresolved issues concerning aspects of pathophysiology, mechanisms of comorbidity, and therapeutic strategies; these issues can complicate the care of affected infants.

Reported incidence rates of neonatal seizures range from 1.5 to 5.5 per 1,000 neonates (1–7). Most have onset within the first week of life with a slow accumulation of incidence over the ensuing three weeks (5). Seizure occurrence may vary with risk factors such as degree of illness, possible etiology, and—according to several investigators—birth weight (5). Scher and colleagues (8, 9) reported that seizures occurred in 3.9% of neonates of less than 30 weeks' conceptional age and 1.5% in neonates older than 30 weeks. Similarly, Kohelet and colleagues (10) found an overall incidence of seizures in a cohort of very low-birth-weight infants to be 5.6/1,000, higher than most reported incidence in full-term infants.

The International League Against Epilepsy (ILAE) has used the terms "acute reactive" or "symptomatic" to classify most neonatal seizures, implying an immediate cause of these events. However, the ILAE has also designated some so-called unprovoked neonatal seizures as the basis of epileptic syndromes. Two are relatively benign and two considered catastrophic (11–13). The benign syndromes are discussed in this chapter and include benign neonatal convulsions and benign familial neonatal convulsions. Two catastrophic syndromes are referred to below, but discussed in more detail in Chapter 15: early myoclonic encephalopathy (EME) and early infantile epileptic encephalopathy (EIEE). Acute reactive or symptomatic seizures are the most frequent; neonatal epileptic syndromes are rare.

CLINICAL FEATURES

Neonatal seizures have clinical features that are unique compared to those of infants and children. Neonatal seizures may be fragmented; be disorganized; exhibit unusual patterns of spread; and may appear in various limbs simultaneously but asynchronously. These features are, for the most part, based on mechanisms of epileptogenesis in the immature. Other differences are based on the relative importance of nonepileptic mechanisms of "seizure" generation in this age group.

Neonatal seizures are classified by various methods: clinical features; the relation between clinical seizures and electrical seizure activity on the electroencephalogram (EEG); seizure pathophysiology; and epileptic syndromes. Each classification can be clinically useful. There have been a number of classification system proposed over the years (14–20). Early classification schemes focused on the differences between neonatal seizures and those of older children; neonatal seizures were reported to be clonic or tonic, not tonic-clonic, and when the seizures were focal, there were characterized as unifocal or multifocal (14). Later classifications included myoclonus (15).

Early investigators also identified clinical events that had less of a traditional organization of motor activity (14, 21, 22). Such seizures were initially characterized as "anarchic" (14) and then later as "subtle" (16) or "minimal" (18). These descriptions included oral-buccal-lingual movements such as sucking and chewing; movements of progression, such as bicycling of the legs and swimming movements of the arms; and random eye movements. While these events were initially considered to be epileptic in origin, others later suggested that they were exaggerated reflex behaviors and referred to them as "brainstem release phenomena" or "motor automatisms" (20).

Tables 14-1 and 14-2 list the clinical characteristics of neonatal seizures according to a current classification scheme (23). This scheme can be applied through clinical observation of the neonate. The basic classifica-

TABLE 14-1

Clinical Characteristics, Classification, and Presumed Pathophysiology of Neonatal Seizures

Classification	Characterization	Pathophysiology
Focal clonic	Repetitive, rhythmic contractions of muscle groups of the limbs, face, or trunk May be unifocal or multifocal May occur synchronously or asynchronously in muscle groups on one side of the body May occur simultaneously, but asynchronously on both sides Cannot be suppressed by restraint or repositioning	Epileptic
Focal tonic	Sustained posturing of single limbs Sustained asymmetrical posturing of the trunk Sustained eye deviation Cannot be provoked by stimulation or suppressed by restraint	Epileptic
Generalized tonic	Sustained symmetrical posturing of limbs, trunk, and neck May be flexor, extensor, or mixed flexor/extensor May be provoked or intensified by stimulation May be suppressed by restraint or repositioning	Presumed nonepileptic
Myoclonic	Random, single, rapid contractions of muscle groups of the limbs, face, or trunk Typically not repetitive or may recur at a slow rate May be generalized, focal, or fragmentary May be provoked by stimulation	May be epileptic or nonepileptic
Spasms	May be flexor, extensor, or mixed flexor/extensor May occur in clusters Cannot be provoked by stimulation or suppressed by restraint	Epileptic
Motor Automatisms		
Ocular signs	Random and roving eye movements or nystagmus (distinct from tonic eye deviation) May be provoked or intensified by tactile stimulation	Presumed nonepileptic
Oral-buccal-lingual movements	Sucking, chewing, tongue protrusions May be provoked or intensified by stimulation	Presumed nonepileptic
Progression movements	Rowing or swimming movements Pedaling or bicycling movements of the legs May be provoked or intensified by stimulation May be suppressed by restraint or repositioning	Presumed nonepileptic

From Mizrahi and Kellaway, 1998 (23).

TABLE 14-2
Classification of Neonatal Seizures with Electroclinical Correlation

Clinical Seizures with a Consistent Electrocortical Signature (Pathophysiology: Epileptic)

Focal clonic
- Unifocal
- Multifocal
- Hemiconvulsive
- Axial

Focal tonic
- Asymmetrical truncal posturing
- Limb posturing
- Sustained eye deviation

Myoclonic
- Generalized
- Focal

Spasms
- Flexor
- Extensor
- Mixed extensor/flexor

Clinical Seizures without a Consistent Electrocortical Signature (Pathophysiology: Presumed Nonepileptic)

Myoclonic
- Generalized
- Focal
- Fragmentary

Generalized tonic
- Flexor
- Extensor
- Mixed extensor/flexor

Motor automatisms
- Oral-buccal-lingual movements
- Ocular signs (aside from sustained eye deviation)
- Progression movements
- Complex purposeless movements

Electrical Seizures without Clinical Seizure Activity

From Mizrahi and Kellaway, 1998 (23).

tion includes seizures characterized as focal clonic, focal tonic, myoclonic, spasms, generalized tonic and motor automatisms (also referred to as "subtle seizures"). Paroxysmal changes in autonomic nervous system measurements have also been reported to be manifestations of seizures, such as alterations in heart rate, respiration, and blood pressure as well as flushing, salivation, and pupillary dilation (19, 24, 25). However, any of these findings occurring as isolated epileptic events are rare, and when they do occur, they do so most consistently in association with other clinical manifestations of seizures (20).

Other classification systems are based upon the temporal relation of clinical events to the occurrence of electrical seizure activity on EEG. An "electroclinical" seizure occurs when the clinical event overlaps in time with electrographic seizure activity. A seizure is referred to as "clinical only" when it occurs in the absence of any EEG seizure activity. A seizure is referred to as electrographic "only" if the electrical seizure occurs without any coincident clinical seizure activity (26).

Seizures may also be classified according to their pathophysiology: epileptic or nonepileptic in character (20). Some seizures may be confidently classified as "epileptic" in nature just by their clinical appearance: focal clonic, focal tonic, some types of myoclonic seizures, and spasms (Table 14-1). These seizure types can be recognized and characterized at the bedside by the visible features of the spontaneous event. In addition, during the event, the clinician can attempt to suppress the motor behavior by holding the affected limb; a continuation of rhythmic muscle contractions indicates the epileptic basis of the event. When EEG is available, these events occur in close association with EEG seizure activity, and the clinical event cannot be provoked by stimulation nor suppressed by restraint of the infant. When EEG is utilized, seizures characterized as electrical-only seizures are also considered, by definition, epileptic in origin.

Other behaviors, previously referred to as "subtle" seizures, are best considered as nonepileptic in origin (4, 20) including some types of myoclonic events, generalized tonic posturing, and motor automatisms such as oral-buccal-lingual movements, movements of progression, and some ocular signs (Table 14-1). These events occur in the absence of electrical seizure activity but, more importantly, have clinical characteristics similar to reflex behaviors. These clinical events can be provoked by stimulation of the infant. Both the provoked and spontaneous events can be suppressed by restraint or by repositioning the infant during the event. In addition, the clinical events may increase in intensity with the increase in the repetition rate of stimulation (temporal summation) or the number of sites of simultaneous stimulation (spatial summation). The response can spread to regions of the body distant from the site of stimulation.

CLINICAL NEUROPHYSIOLOGY

Electroencephalography

The application of the EEG in the evalution of a newborn suspected of seizures differs from its application to older children and adults in terms of the significance of interictal focal abnormalities and the interpretation of the background activity.

Interictal EEG Findings. Although focal sharp waves may be present interictally in the neonatal EEG, they are not considered epileptiform. Some focal sharp waves are normal features of the neonatal EEG, such as frontal sharp transients and some temporal sharp waves (those that occur randomly, are low or moderate in voltage, and present in transitional or light sleep) (27). Other focal sharp waves are abnormal. They are persistent, excessively numerous, and high in amplitude; they are present in wakefulness and sleep; and they have complex morphology. Persistent focal sharp waves may suggest focal injury. When multifocal, such sharp waves may suggest diffuse dysfunction. There may also be focal spikes. These may suggest focal injury, such as localized stroke, or may have uncertain diagnostic significance (28). Despite the interpretation of some interictal focal sharp waves or spikes as abnormal, in the neonate they are are not usually considered direct evidence or confirmation that an individual has had or will have electrographic seizures.

The background EEG activity can provide information concerning degree of associated central nervous system (CNS) dysfunction, potential risk for seizures, and prognosis. The degree of abnormality of the interictal background activity may suggest the extent and type of CNS dysfunction associated with seizures. The nature of the interictal background activity may also indicate the potential risk the individual infants have in experiencing a seizure (29). Infants with initial normal background activity are less likely to eventually experience electrographic seizures than those with persistent diffuse background abnormalities. In addition, the extent, degree, evolution, and rate of resolution (if any) of background EEG abnormalities can suggest prognosis. An EEG with normal background activity recording within the first 24 hours of life may suggest a good outcome (30), while EEG background activity with abnormal features that persist or resolve slowly suggest a poorer outcome (28).

Ictal EEG Findings. Although not clearly defined, it appears that electrical seizure activity in neonates is rare before 34–35 weeks. When recorded, the manifestations of electrical seizures have wide-ranging features (27, 31). Frequency, voltage, and morphology of the seizure discharges may change within an individual seizure, between seizures in an individual infant or among infants. The minimum duration has been designated to be 10 seconds (32), but the duration discharges can vary widely. Electrical events are typically focal and well circumscribed. They frequently arise from the central or centro-temporal region of one hemisphere and less commonly in the occipital, frontal, or midline central regions. Although seizures may arise focally and remain confined to that region, they may also spread to other regions. This spread may appear as a gradual widening of the focal area, by an abrupt change from a small regional focus to involvement of the entire hemisphere (as in a hemiconvulsive seizure) or by migration of the electrical seizure from one area of a hemisphere to another or from one hemisphere to another (23, 27).

There are some relatively unique ictal neonatal patterns that are typically associated with severe encephalopathies and accompanying abnormal background EEG. *Seizure discharges of the depressed brain* are typically low in voltage, long in duration, and highly localized (4). They may be unifocal or multifocal and show little tendency to spread or modulate; typically are not associated with clinical seizures; and occur when the EEG background is depressed and undifferentiated. Their presence suggest a poor prognosis. *Alpha seizure activity* is characterized by a sudden appearance of paroxysmal, rhythmic activity of the alpha frequency (8–12 Hz) typically in the temporal or central region and may evolve from the more typical seizure discharges or may appear *de novo* (33–35). Like seizure discharges of the depressed brain, alpha seizure discharges usually are not accompanied by clinical events and usually indicate the presence of a severe encephalopathy and poor prognosis.

Video-EEG Monitoring

Video-EEG monitoring has proved to be a powerful tool in diagnosis and management of neonatal seizures and as well as in clinical research (20, 36–38). It is now becoming more available at many centers for routine use and more widely employed in neonatal intensive care units (39). Correlation of EEG with video can be very helpful in seizure characterization and classification, although attended EEG can also provide important clinical information, when preformed by a well-trained electroneurodiagnostic technologist who can carefully observe an infant's behavior and characterize the events.

Computer-Assisted EEG Analysis of Neonatal Seizures

Computer-assisted analysis of EEG has been applied to detect and quantify electrical seizure activity in neonates. Such programs have been developed and may provide reliable data, particularly if the recordings are attended by a trained electroneurodiagnostic technician (ENDT) (40, 41). Amplitude integrated EEG (aEEG) or cerebral function monitors (CFM) have experienced a renewed interest (42–44). However, these techniques are limited in terms of their ability to provide data from all brain regions, low resolution, compressed time frame, and reliance on nonexpert health care professionals. One recent study reports that, using CFMs, up to 50% of neonatal seizures were misclassified or unrecognized (45). Shellhaas et al (46) examined 851 electrographic neonatal seizures detected in 125 conventional, full-array EEG recordings. A one-channel EEG (C3 → C4) was digitally created to simulate the contemporary use of single-channel EEGs for seizure detection by CFMs. Although 78% of the seizures were visible in the single-EEG channel, the seizures were briefer and lower in amplitude, and less than half were diagnosed by aEEG based on the C3 → C4 channel. On the other hand, advocates suggest that the ability to monitor specific brain regions with aEEG for long periods may balance the restricted localization and other limitations (47).

ETIOLOGY

Neonatal seizures are typically a correlate of CNS disease. In clinical practice, these seizures prompt a detailed evaluation for etiology. If the etiology is identified, etiologic-specific therapy is initiated. There is a wide range of protential causes of neonatal seizures, and this, in association with the susceptibility of the immature brain to injury, may account for the high incidence of acute neonatal seizures. The list of potential etiologies is extensive (23); however, most can be broadly categorized as hypoxia-ischemia, metabolic disturbances, CNS or systemic infections, and structural brain lesions. Table 14-3 (23) lists the most frequently identified etiologies of neonatal seizures.

TABLE 14-3
Most Frequently Occurring Etiologies of Neonatal Seizures

Hypoxia-ischemia
Intracranial hemorrhage
Intracerebral
Intraventricular
Subarachnoid
Subdural
Infection, CNS
Encephalitis
Intrauterine
Meningitis
Cerebral infarction
Metabolic
Hypocalcemia
Hypoglycemia
Hypomagnesemia
Chromosomal anomalies
Congenital abnormalities of the brain
Neurodegenerative disorders
Inborn errors of metabolism
Benign neonatal convulsions
Benign familial neonatal convulsions
Drug withdrawal or intoxication

Main categories are listed in relative order of frequency (subcategories listed alphabetically). "Unknown" etiology is not listed, although encountered in approximately 10% of cases (although some in this category may be benign neonatal convulsions). From Mizrahi and Kellaway, 1998 (23).

Symptomatic Neonatal Seizures

Hypoxic-ischemic encephalopathy (HIE) is often cited as the most frequent cause of neonatal seizures. The diagnosis may be difficult to establish, because diagnostic criteria have not been uniformly accepted. In addition, some proposed criteria have been so restrictive that infants with encephalopathy may not meet all of them but still carry the diagnosis of "suspected HIE." At other centers, clinical practice is directed towards identification of measures of asphyxia that have predictive value in the occurrence of long-term sequelae (48). This strategy has resulted in less restrictive criteria for HIE. Both approaches, however, include the tabulation of delivery room Apgar scores, blood gases, requirement for resuscitation, recognition of clinical aspects of encephalopathy including seizures, and confirmation of multisystem involvement. There is also an emerging discussion of the use of computer-assisted analysis of EEG, including aEEG, to aid in the staging of the severity of HIE (49), although this is still considered investigational.

Associated metabolic disturbances range from electrolyte imbalances to inborn errors of metabolism. This category is important because of its potentially treatable disorders such as hypocalcemia, hypomagnesemia, and hypoglycemia. Inborn errors of metabolism are much less frequent and include aminoacidurias, urea cycle defects, or organic acidurias. Other rare causes of medically refractory neonatal seizures that are potentially treatable include pyridoxine and biotinidase deficiency.

Bacterial and viral agents are associated with seizures to such an extent that almost all neonates with new-onset seizures are investigated for such infection. Some viral infections, such as herpes simplex encephalitis, may be treated empirically at clinical presentation prior to confirmation of the diagnosis. In addition, prenatal toxoplasmosis, rubella, cytomegalovirus, herpes simplex, or other (so-called TORCH) infections can be risk factors for neonatal seizures.

Associated structural brain lesions include both acquired and congenital conditions, such as stroke or hemorrhage and developmental anomalies of the brain. Congenital brain malformations may range from highly localized focal dysplasias to catastrophic defects such as holoprosencephaly and lissencephaly.

Neonatal Epileptic Syndromes

In its Classification of Epilepsies and Epileptic Syndromes, the ILAE has designated only four syndromes in the neonatal period (11): benign neonatal convulsions, benign neonatal familial convulsions, early myoclonic encephalopathy, and early infantile epileptic encephalopathy. These have been reviewed recently (50). The first two are associated with a relatively good prognosis and are discussed here, while the others suggest a poor outcome, have been included among the catastrophic pediatric epilepsy syndromes (51) and are discussed elsewhere in this volume (Chapter 15) and compared in Table 14-4 (12, 52, 53).

Benign Neonatal Convulsions. The syndrome of benign neonatal convulsions (BNC) has also been referred to as "benign idiopathic neonatal convulsions," because of the lack of an identifiable etiology (54), and "fifth day fits" because of the timing of onset (55), and has been recently extensively reviewed by Plouin and Anderson (56). The features of this syndrome are normal interictal neonate; focal clonic seizures or, rarely, focal tonic seizures; no family history of neonatal seizures; full-term gestational age; and a history of an uncomplicated, normal pregnancy, labor, and delivery. Seizure onset is usually between the fourth and sixth day after birth. The seizures are typically brief (1 to 3 minutes), although, rarely, the seizures can be prolonged. The seizure disorder is self-limited in that seizures may recur only during a 24- to 48-hour period after onset, although this period on rare occasion may also be prolonged. The clinical seizures are usually unifocal clonic and may be associated with apnea. A critical feature for diagnosis is that no etiology for the seizures can be identified. In the past this disorder has been associated with a finding of rotavirus in stool but not in cerebro-

TABLE 14-4
Comparison of Early Myoclonic Encephalopathy (EME) and Early Infantile Epileptic Encephalopathy (EIEE).

	EME	EIEE
Age of onset	Neonatal period	Within first 3 months
Neurologic status at onset	Abnormal at birth or at seizure onset	Always abnormal even prior to seizure onset
Characteristic seizure type	Erratic or fragmentary myoclonus	Tonic spasm
Additional seizure types	Massive myoclonus, simple partial seizures, hemiconvulsions, infantile spasms (tonic)	Focal motor seizures, generalized seizures
Background EEG	Suppression-burst	Suppression-burst
Etiology	Cryptogenic, inborn errors of metabolism, familial	Cerebral dysgenesis, anoxia, cryptogenic
Natural course	Progressive impairment	Static impairment
Incidence of death	Very high, occurring in infancy	High, occurring in infancy, childhood, or adolescence
Status of survivors	Vegetative state	Severe mental retardation. quadriplegic, and bedridden
Long-term seizure evolution	Infantile spasms	West syndrome, Lennox-Gastaut

Based on data from Aicardi, 1997 (52), and Ohtahara et al, 1992 (53). Reprinted from Mizrahi and Clancy, 2000 (12).

spinal fluid (CSF) (57) and with acute zinc deficiency in CSF (25); these findings are now considered of doubtful etiologic relevance.

The ictal EEG is characterized by focal, rhythmic, recurrent sharp wave or spike activity that is closely correlated with the clinical seizures. The background EEG is typically normal, although it has also been reported that in up to 60% of neonates with this syndrome the interictal EEG pattern referred to as "*theta pointu alternant*" may be present (58). The background activity is discontinuous and nonreactive. The bursts include rhythmic (4 to 7 Hz) theta activity, which may be mixed with sharp waves that alternate between hemispheres. Although in this disorder this pattern has not been considered diagnostic for BNC (56). The *theta pointu alternant* EEG pattern may persist for up to 2 weeks after the clinical syndrome resolves.

This syndrome is a diagnosis of exclusion, since the initial clinical presentation may resemble infants with symptomatic focal clonic seizures. Thus, a thorough evaluation for an etiology is conducted in order to identify a potentially treatable cause of seizures, even though the diagnosis of benign neonatal convulsions may be considered at the onset (56). Treatment is controversial, although most frequently the seizures are treated with phenobarbital. Because the seizures tend to be brief and infrequent, it has been argued that antiepileptic drug (AED) therapy may not be needed. If AEDs are used, they are typically discontinued once the seizures subside. The prognosis is considered to be generally good. However, one group of investigators has found either transient or persistent psychomotor delays in affected infants (55). Plouin (59) found neurodevelopmental deficits at 2 years of age in 50% of those with this syndrome and a slightly higher incidence of postneonatal epilepsy (0.5% of those patients) than in the general population.

Benign Neonatal Familial Convulsions. This syndrome is characterized by early-onset focal clonic or focal tonic seizures in a neonate with a family history of neonatal seizures and with no other neurological findings (60–62). There is an autosomal dominant pattern of inheritance with incomplete penetrance with two known chromosomal loci: one on chromosome 20q13 (63) and one on chromosome 8q (64–66). Genes responsible for this disorder are potassium channel genes, referred to as KCNQ2 for the chromosome 20q gene (67, 68) and KCNQ3 for the chromosome 8q gene (66).

The clinical seizures are best characterized as focal clonic or focal tonic. Seizure onset is between the first few days and one week of life (69), although there have been reports of onset as late as the second month of life. These various ages of onset may be developmentally determined, since infants who are born prematurely with this disorder will have seizure onset at an older chronological age than the infants born at term. The seizures may be brief but can recur up to 2–3 months of age, when they will remit spontaneously. The interictal EEG is typically normal, although *theta pointu alternant* pattern has also been reported. While the outcome is generally good, there is a higher incidence of seizures in affected infants later in life; ranging from 11% to 16% (58, 70). Phenobarbital therapy is often used with success, although some investigators use valproate as an alternative (59).

TREATMENT

With seizure onset, basic principles of medical management are initially applied to establish and maintain airway patency and access the circulatory system. Some seizures, as well as the use of some AEDs, may be associated with changes in respiration, heart rate, and blood pressure, and the anticipation and potential treatment of these associated conditions are critical to the overall care of neonates with seizures.

Following clinical stabilization, the assessement of seizure etiology and the initiation of the first phase of AED treatment are typically undertaken concurrently. Etiologic-specific therapy, if appropriate, is directed to treat the underlying cause of seizures and potentially limit associated brain injury. In addition, some seizures may not be controlled effectively with AEDs unless the underlying cause is treated—in particular, seizures associated with metabolic disturbances such as hypocalcemia, hypomagnesemia, and hypoglycemia. Additional etiologic-specific therapies include appropriate antiviral agents, antibiotics, treatments for some in-born errors of metabolism, and, in rare instances, surgery (71).

Initiation of AED Therapy

The decision to initiate AED therapy is based upon seizure type and seizure frequency and severity. Ideally, only seizures of epileptic origin should be treated with AEDs. These include electroclinical seizures when clinical seizures are witnessed during EEG recording. When clinical observation alone is the basis for management, focal clonic seizures and focal tonic seizures are the seizure types most clearly characterized as epileptic in origin. Clinical events considered nonepileptic in origin are generalized tonic and motor automatisms (those provoked by stimulation and suppressed by restraint) and are typically not treated with AEDs. Electrical seizures without clinical events are also treated with AEDs.

An important, although unresolved issues, is whether all neonates with seizures of epileptic origin should be treated with AEDs, since some are brief, infrequent, and self-limited, presenting only as reaction to an acute CNS insult. It has been argued that these brief, reactive events many not warrant AEDs, with potential risks of acute and chronic AED therapy perhaps outweighing the potential risks of the seizures themselves. On the other hand, epileptic seizures that are long in duration, frequent, and not self-limited are treated acutely and aggressively with AEDs. The management of seizures with features that fall between these two extremes represent more of a clinical challenge. In clinical practice, almost all neonatal epileptic seizures within this intermediate category receive AEDs.

Acute AED Therapy

First-line AEDs that are most frequently used and their dosing schedules are listed in Table 14-5 (23, 72–74), although comprehensive clinical trials have not established the most effective regimen (75). The most established strategy is acute treatment with an AED that can be subsequently given as maintenance therapy; most often this is phenobarbital, and less frequently phenytoin or fosphenytoin.

Phenobarbital is given as a loading dose followed by additional boluses titrated to response until the maximum tolerated dose, or serum level in the high therapeutic range, is reached. Boylan and colleagues prospectively assessed the efficacy of phenobarbital utilizing video-EEG monitoring (38) and found that only 4 of 14 infants responded, while the remainder experienced a reduction in electroclinical seizures but an increase in electrical seizures.

After phenobarbital, phenytoin is the AED most often used as a first-line AED, now typically initiated with fosphenytoin because of reports of reduced adverse effects with acute administration (76). Phenytoin administration is increased to maximum tolerated dose or high therapeutic serum levels, and then a maintenance dose is established. Painter and colleagues (77) compared the effectiveness of acute administration of phenobarbital and phenytoin in seizure control and found no significant difference between the two medications. However, neither proved as efficacious as generally believed.

Another strategy for initial AED treatment is acute administration of repeated doses of short-acting benzodiazepines (lorazepam or midazolam) until seizures are controlled. Chronic AED therapy or maintenance doses are avoided if seizures do not recur.

Control of both the clinical and electrical seizures is ideal but often difficult to acheive or, on occasion, unattainable. Typically, the initial response of electroclinical seizures to acute AED therapy is characterized by control of the clinical seizures with the persistence of the electrical seizure activity, referred to as "uncoupling" (20). While additional dosing may eventually control the electrical seizures (78) there are instances in which the EEG seizures cannot be controlled despite increasing doses of the initial AED and addition of other AEDs.

In current practice, if no EEG is available and the clinician relies only on observation, acute AED therapy is given until clinical seizures are controlled. The first AED is given to serum levels in the high therapeutic range or maximum tolerated dose followed by the second. Benzodiazepines are also given as needed. If EEG is utilized, the same AED strategy is followed. The AEDs are given to achieve high therapeutic serum levels even if electrical seizure discharges persist, since most are often resistant to further AED therapy. A second AED may be added to high serum levels, but if electrical seizures continue unabated, additional drugs are typically not given, beyond a second maintenance AED and dosing of benzodiazepines, in order to avoid adverse effects without significant benefit.

The pharmacology of phenobarbital and phenytoin in the neonate is discussed elsewhere in detail (Chapters 48 and 49). However, there it is important to emphasize that some pathologic conditions can alter the availability of active drug given at standard doses in sick neonates (79–82).

TABLE 14-5
Dosages of First-Line and Second-Line AEDs in the Treatment of Neonatal Seizures

Drug	Dose: Loading	Dose: Maintenance	Average Therapeutic Range	Apparent Half-life
Diazepam	0.25 mg/IV (bolus) 0.5 mg/kg (rectal)	May be repeated 1–2 times		31–54 h
Lorazepam	0.05 mg/kg (IV) (over 2–5 min)	May be repeated		31–54 h
Phenobarbital	20 mg/kg IV (up to 40 mg)	3–4 mg/kg in 2 doses	20–40 μg/L	100 h after day 5–7
Phenytoin	20 mg/kg IV (over 30–45 min)	3–4 mg/kg in 2–4 doses	15–25 μg/L	100 h (40–200)

*Based on Fenichel, 1990 (72); Aicardi, 1994 (73); Volpe, 2001 (74). Table originally from Mizrahi and Kellaway, 1998 (23).

Phenobarbital is a weak acid and is protein bound. Infants with acidosis may have less active AED available, and those with hypoalbuminemia may have greater unbound or active drug available. Both conditions may be found in sick neonates. In addition, the drug is eliminated by the liver and kidney. Infants with impaired hepatic or renal function, such as those with hypoxic ischemic encephalopathy, may have a reduced rate of drug elimination and thus a potential for toxicity with standard dosing. In preterm infants, the half-life of phenobarbital is longer than in term infants, and in term infants it is reduced with chronologic age in the first month of life. Thus, in preterm infants there is a potential for higher serum levels with standard doses, and with that the potential for toxicity. With increasing age, there is the potential for established doses to result in lower serum levels over time, creating the potential for breakthrough seizures with no other change in the infant's clinical condition (74, 83–85).

Important pharmacologic characteristics of phenytoin require individualization of dosing after initiation of therapy. These include nonlinear pharmacokinetics; a variable rate of hepatic metabolism; a decrease in elimination rates during the first weeks of life; and a variable bioavailability of the drug with various generic preparations (86, 87). After initial dosing, there is a redistribution of the AED with a relative drop in brain concentrations after the first dose, which may result in breakthrough seizures with established doses.

Alternative and Adjuvant AED Therapy

Alternative or adjuvant AEDs fall into two categories: those administered in attempts to control otherwise medically refractory seizures and those used for control of acute seizures. The latter holds the most promise. Agents in both classes have been utilized either intravenously or orally with variable success. Those given intravenously and primarily as alternatives to acute therapy include: clonazepam (88), lidocaine (89), midazolam (90) and paraldehyde (not available in the United States) (91). One recent study reported success with continuous midazolam infusion in the treatment of otherwise uncontrolled neonatal seizures (92), although infants experienced treatment-related hypotension that was medically managed. Midazolam is given first as a 0.15 mg/kg bolus followed by initial continuous infusion of 1µg/kg/min, titrated by 0.5 to 1 µg/kg/min increments to termination of clinical or electrical seizures or a maximal dose of 18 µg/kg/min. Lidocaine is another medication that has been the topic of renewed interest. Boylan and colleagues (93) reported limited success with lidocaine in refractory neonatal seizures. Others (94) reported that during the use of lidocaine (initial loading dose of 2 mg/kg over 10 minutes followed by a continuous infusion of 6 mg/kg per hour), 4.8% of infants experienced a cardiac arrhythmia (all responding to lidocaine discontinuation).

Other agents have been given orally to control medically refractory seizures after acute AEDs have failed include carbamazepine (95), primidone (96), valproate (97), vigabatrin (98), and lamotrigine (99). The success of this latter group of AEDs is difficult to assess, since they have been used in conjunction with other AEDs and well into the course of the seizure disorder.

Chronic AED Therapy

After acute seizures have been controlled, maintenance therapy is typically initiated. However, there are no well-defined criteria for maintenance AED treatment. When chronic therapy is considered, either phenobarbital or phenytoin is given in maintenance doses of 3 to 5 mg/kg/day and serum levels are monitored. There are also no well-established criteria for discontinuation of maintenance AED therapy. Reported schedules range from 1 week up to 12 months after the last seizure, although a currently utilized and successful schedule is to withdraw AEDs 2 weeks after the infant's last seizure (72). At some centers, an EEG is also performed at the end of this 2-week period to be certain there are no subclinical electrical seizures.

Potential Adverse Effect of AED Therapy

There has been much concern about the potential adverse effects of AEDs on the developing brain. These have included alteration in cell growth and energy substrate utilization, although the applicability of these findings to humans has been called into question. There have been few studies of clinically significant adverse effects of acute AED therapy. However, vigorous acute AED administration can result in CNS depression, hypotension, bradycardia, and respiratory depression. Any of these clinical events represent risk for secondary CNS hypoxia or ischemia. More recently, Ikonomidou and colleagues (100) assessed the effect of phenytoin, phenobarbital, diazepam, clonazepam, vigabatrin, and valproate on apoptotic neurodegeneration in the developing rat brain in plasma concentrations relevant for seizure control in humans. The basis of their study was the consideration that AEDs' mechanisms of action are also those essential for the endogenous neuroprotective system crucial for neuronal survival during development. Thus, they suggested that these vital mechanisms would be blocked by AEDs and have an adverse effect on development. However, it is unclear whether these results can be extrapolated to the human. In addition, recent data from the same group show that another AED, topiramate, lacks the toxicity seen with some of the other drugs mentioned above (101).

PROGNOSIS

In general, the long-term outcome of neonates with seizures is predominantly determined by the etiology underlying seizure onset, although the relative contribution, if any, of adverse effects of seizures and of AEDs on the developing brain has not been definitively determined.

Early investigators suggested that, even though the immature brain was more likely to develop seizures in response to injury than the more mature brain, either the immature brain was more resistant to seizure-induced injury or any seizure-related alterations were either transient or not clinically significant. More recent data suggests otherwise: Seizures in early life may result in permanent anatomical and functional alterations and enhanced epileptogenicity (102–105). A number of mechanisms of seizure-induced injury have been investigated, including direct neuronal injury; the so-called "double-hit" mechanism of enhanced vulnerability to a second injury after seizures; aberrant cell growth or reorganization of circuitry (104, 106); or the interference of fiber tracts projections during development (102, 107).

Recent findings indicate that seizures in immature animals do not, in the immediate postseizure period, result in significant alterations of learning, memory, or activity levels. However, animals exposed to seizures early in life have demonstrated impairments and alterations in learning and behavior later in life in comparison to those exposed to seizures when mature (108–110). Adverse effects of seizures are more apparent when animals exposed to prolonged seizures early in life are then exposed to seizures when mature (111, 112). Holmes and colleagues (102, 113) indicate that prolonged seizures in immature animals result in minimal behavioral consequences when the animals are studied later in life and are associated with minimal morphological changes. However, such early-onset seizures result in changes in the brain that make it more vulnerable to the development of cognitive impairment when animals are exposed to post-neonatal seizure.

Clinical studies describe the outcome of infants with neonatal seizures in terms of survival, neurological disability, developmental delay, and postneonatal epilepsy. Ortibus and colleagues (114) reported that 28% of those with neonatal seizures died, 22% of survivors were neurologically normal at an average of 17 months of age, 14% had mild abnormalities, and 36% had severe abnormalities. In a prospective study of full-term infants 2 years following neonatal seizures, Mizrahi and colleagues (115) found that 28% died, and in survivors 42.7% had abnormal neurological examinations, 55.2% had Bayley Developmental Assessment of Mental Development Index less than 80, 49.6% had a Bayley Developmental Assessment of Psychomotor Developmental Index less that 80, and 26% had postneonatal epilepsy (115). Brunquell and colleagues (116) found that 30% of those with neonatal seizures died and 59% of survivors had abnormal neurological examinations, 40% were mentally retarded, 43% had cerebral palsy, and 21% had postneonatal epilepsy after a follow-up to a mean of 3.5 years. Most recently, Tekgul et al (117), describing a selected population, found that 7% of neonates who had experienced seizures died and, of the survivors, 28% had a poor outcome.

Ellenberg and colleagues (118) studied postneonatal epilepsy in more detail. Postneonatal epilepsy occurred in approximately 20% of survivors of neonatal seizures studied; nearly two thirds of post-neonatal seizures occurred within the first 6 months of life (118). Similar rates of postneonatal epilesy were found by Scher and colleagues (8), 17-30%; Ortibus and colleagues (114), 28%; Bye and colleagues (36), 21%; Mizrahi and colleagues (115), 26%; Brunquell et al (116), 21%; and, most recently Da Silva et al (119), 22% at 12-month follow-up and 33.8% within 48 months. Clancy and Legido (120) found a much higher (56%) rate of postneonatal epilepsy in a population skewed toward severe brain injury.

Some clinical factors that may influence outcome may include seizure duration or severity and seizure type. Some infants who experience brief and infrequent seizures may have relatively good long-term outcomes, while those with prolonged seizures may not do as well. Easily controlled seizures or self-limited seizures may be the result of transient or more benign CNS disorders, whereas medically refractory neonatal seizures may be the result of more sustained, refractory, or more severe brain disorders. On the other hand, a relationship has been shown in infants with perinatal asphyxia between a greater amount of electrographic seizure activity and subsequent relative increased mortality and morbidity (121). Other investigators, utilizing proton magnetic resonance spectroscopy in neonates, found an association between seizure severity and impaired cerebral metabolism measured (122).

However, the dominant variable that predicts neurodevelopmental outcome may be the underlying cause of the seizures rather than the presence, duration or degree of brain involvement of the seizures themselves. Mizrahi and Kellaway (23) analyzed a number of clinical studies indicating that normal outcomes occurred with increasing frequency in association with the following etiologies: HIE, infection, hemorrhage, hypoglycemia and hypocalcemia. In discussing prognosis, Volpe emphasized the clinical factors of gestational age and etiology on outcome and found that mortality increased with the greater degree of prematurity and that specific etiologies were associated with varying degrees of developmental delay. Most recently, Tekgul et al (117) suggested that seizure etiology and background EEG patterns—themselves markers of the degree and distribution of brain injury—remain powerful prognostic factors.

It has been suggested that clinical seizure type may also predict outcome (20), also most likely as a reflection of etiology or the degree of associated brain dysfunction at the onset of seizures. Focal clonic and focal tonic seizures were associated with a relatively good outcome, primarily because these seizure types are typically associated with relatively confined, nondiffuse brain injury and significant spared CNS function. Generalized tonic posturing and motor automatisms where associated with a poor outcome, since they are associated with diffuse CNS dysfunction. Recently Brunquell and colleagues (116) demonstrated similar findings in long-term studies.

In multivariate analyses, predictors of outcome have included features of the interictal EEG from one or serial recordings, the ictal EEG, the neurological examination at the time of seizures, the character or duration of the seizures, etiology, findings on neuroimaging, conceptional age, and birth weight. Multiple rather than single factors appear to be most accurate in predicting outcome. Ortibus and colleagues (114) found that the predicted outcome is less reliable when based solely on EEG variables from a single recording obtained at seizure onset than when based on a combination of imaging findings and clinical and EEG data. Pisani and colleagues (123) also considered several different independent variables and found the character of the EEG background activity is predictive of developmental outcome. However, in these studies all variables related to a single factor—the degree of brain injury at the time of seizure occurrence—and this, in turn, is related to etiology.

ACKNOWLEDGMENTS

This work was, in part, supported by Contract NO 1-01255, National Institutes of Neurological Disorders and Stroke, NIH, Bethesda, MD, and the Peter Kellaway Research Endowment, Baylor College of Medicine, Houston, TX. The Stiftung Michael, Bonn, Germany, is gratefully acknowledged.

References

1. Eriksson M, Zetterström R. Neonatal convulsions. Incidence and causes in the Stockholm area. *Acta Paediatr Scand* 1979; 68:807–811.
2. Bergman I, Painter MJ, Hirsch RP, et al. Outcome in neonates with convulsions treated in an intensive care unit. *Ann Neurol* 1983; 14:642–647.
3. Spellacy WN, Peterson PQ, Winegar A, et al. Neonatal seizures after cesarean delivery: higher risk with labor. *Am J Obstet Gynecol* 1987; 157:377–379.
4. Kellaway P, Hrachovy RA. Status epilepticus in newborns: a perspective on neonatal seizures. In: Delgado-Escueta AV, Wasterlain CG, Treiman DM, et al, eds. *Status Epilepticus*. Advances in Neurology 34. New York: Raven Press, 1983:93–99.
5. Lanska MJ, Lanska DJ, Baumann RJ, et al. A population-based study of neonatal seizures in Fayette County, Kentucky. *Neurology* 1995; 45:724–732.
6. Ronen GM, Penney S. The epidemiology of clinical neonatal seizures in Newfoundland, Canada: a five-year cohort study. *Ann Neurol* 1995; 38:518–519.
7. Saliba RM, Annegers JF, Mizrahi EM. Incidence of clinical neonatal seizures. *Epilepsia* 1996; 37:13.
8. Scher MS, Aso K, Berggarly ME, et al. Electrographic seizures in pre-term and full-term neonates: clinical correlates, associated brain lesions, and risk for neurologic sequelae. *Pediatrics* 1993; 91:128–134.
9. Scher MS, Hamid MY, Steppe DA, et al. Ictal and interictal electrographic seizure durations in preterm and term neonates. *Epilepsia* 1993; 34:284.
10. Kohelet D, Shochat R, Lusky A, Reichman B. Israel Neonatal Network. Risk factors for neonatal seizures is very low birthweight infants: population-based survey. *J Child Neurol* 2004; 19(2):123–128.
11. Commission on Classification and Terminology of the International League Against Epilepsy. Proposal for revised clinical and classification of epilepsies and epileptic syndromes. *Epilepsia* 1989; 30:389–399.
12. Mizrahi EM, Clancy RR. Neonatal seizures: Early-onset seizure syndromes and their consequences for development. *Ment Retard Dev Disabil Res Rev* 2000; 6:229–241.
13. Tharp BR. Neonatal seizures and syndromes. *Epilepsia* 2002; 43:2.
14. Dreyfus-Brisac C, Monod N. Electroclinical studies of status epilepticus and convulsions in the newborn. In: Kellaway P, Petersén I, eds. *Neurological and Electroencephalographic Correlative Studies in Infancy*. New York: Grune & Stratton, 1964:250–272.
15. Rose AL, Lombroso CT. Neonatal seizure states. *Pediatrics* 1970; 45:404–425.
16. Volpe JJ. Neonatal seizures. *N Engl J Med* 1973; 289:413–415.
17. Volpe JJ. Neonatal seizures. *Pediatrics* 1989; 84:422–428.
18. Lombroso CT. Seizures in the newborn. In: Vinken PJ, Bruyn GW, eds. *Handbook of Clinical Neurophysiology*. Vol 15. Amsterdam: North-Holland, 1974:189–218.
19. Watanabe K, Hara K, Miyazaki S, et al. Electroclinical studies of seizures in the newborn. *Folia Psychiatr Neurol Jpn* 1977; 31:383.
20. Mizrahi EM, Kellaway P. Characterization and classification of neonatal seizures. *Neurology* 1987; 37:1837–1844.
21. Sainte-Anne-Dargassies S, Berthault F, Dreyfus-Brisac C, et al. La convulsion du tout jeune nourrisson aspects cephalographiques du probleme. *Presse Med* 1953; 46:965.
22. Minkowski A, Sainte-Anne-Dargassies S, Dreyfus-Brisac C, et al. L'état du mal convulsive du nouveau-né. *Arch Franc de Pediatr* 1955; 12:271–284.
23. Mizrahi EM, Kellaway P. Diagnosis and management of neonatal seizures. Philadelphia, PA: Lippincott-Raven Publishers, 1998:181.
24. Lou HC, Friis-Hansen B. Arterial blood pressure elevations during motor activity and epileptic seizures in the newborn. *Acta Paediatr Scand* 1979; 68:803–806.
25. Goldberg RN, Goldman SL, Ramsay RE, et al. Detection of seizure activity in the paralyzed neonate using continuous monitoring. *Pediatrics* 1982; 69:583–586.
26. Clancy RR, Mizrahi EM. Neonatal seizures. In: Wyllie E, ed. *The Treatment of Epilepsy: Principles & Practice*. Philadelphia, PA: Lippincott Williams & Wilkins, 2006:487–510.
27. Mizrahi EM, Hrachovy RA, Kellaway P. Atlas of neonatal electroencephalography. 3rd ed. Philadelphia, PA: Lippincott Williams & Wilkins, 2003:274.
28. Hrachovy RA, Mizrahi EM, Kellaway P. Electroencephalography of the newborn. In: Daly D, Pedley TA, eds. *Current Practice of Clinical Electroencephalography*. 2nd edition. New York: Raven Press, 1990:201–242.
29. Laroia N, Guillet R, Burchfiel J, et al. EEG background as predictor of electrographic seizures in high-risk neonates. *Epilepsia* 1998; 39:545.
30. Holmes GL, Lombroso CT. Prognostic value of background patterns in the neonatal EEG. *J Clin Neurophysiol* 1993; 10:323.
31. Patrizi S, Holmes GL, Orzalesi M, et al. Neonatal seizures: characteristics of EEG ictal activity in preterm and fullterm infants. *Brain Dev* 2003; 25:427.
32. Clancy RR, Legido A. The exact ictal and interictal duration of electroencephalographic neonatal seizures. *Epilepsia* 1987; 28:537.
33. Knauss TA, Carlson CB. Neonatal paroxysmal monorhythmic alpha activity. *Arch Neurol* 1978; 35:104.
34. Willis J, Gould JB. Periodic alpha seizures with apnea in a newborn. *Dev Med Child Neurol* 1980; 22:214.
35. Watanabe K, Hara K, Miyazaki S, et al. Apneic seizures in the newborn. *Am J Dis Child* 1982; 136:980.
36. Bye AM, Cunningham CA, Chee KY, et al. Outcome of neonates with electrographically identified seizures, or at risk of seizures. *Pediatr Neurol* 1997; 16:225.
37. Clancy RR, McGaurn SA, Wernovsky G, et al. Risk of seizures in survivors of newborn heart surgery using deep hypothermic circulatory arrest. *Pediatric* 2003; 111:592.
38. Boylan GB, Rennie JM, Presler RM, et al. Phenobarbitone, neonatal seizures, and video-EEG. *Arch Dis Child Fetal Neonatal Ed* 2002; 86:F165.
39. Clancy RR. Prolonged electroencephalogram monitoring for seizures and their treatment. *Clin Perinatol* 2006; 33(3):649–665.
40. Gotman J, Flanagan D, Rosenblatt B, et al. Automatic seizure detection in newborns: validation with multicenter data. *Epilepsia* 1996 7(suppl):62.
41. Karayiannis NB, Mukherjee A, Glover JR, Ktonas PY, et al. Detection of pseudosinusoidal epileptic seizure segments in the neonatal EEG by cascading a rule based algorithm with a neural network. *IEEE Trans Biomed Eng* 2006; 53(4):633–641.
42. Toet MC, van der Meij W, de Vries LS, et al. Comparison between simultaneously recorded amplitude integrated electroencephalogram (cerebral function monitor) and standard electroencephalogram in neonates. *Pediatrics* 2003; 109:772.
43. Hellstrom-Westas L, deVries L, Rosen I. An atlas of amplitude-integrated EEGs in the newborn. New York: Parthenon Publishing, 2003:51–66.
44. Shah DK, Lavery S, Doyle LW, Wong C, et al. Use of 2-channel bedside electroencephalogram monitoring in term-born encephalopathic infants related to cerebral injury defined by magnetic resonance imaging. *Pediatrics* 2006; 118(1):47–55.

45. Rennie JM, Chorley G, Boylan GB, et al. Non-expert use of the cerebral function monitor for neonatal seizure detection. *Arch Dis Child Fetal Neonatal Ed* 2004; 89:F37.
46. Shellhaas, Venkat A, Clancy RR. Use of single channel EEG for neonatal seizure detection. *Epilepsia* 2006; 47(suppl 4):13–14.
47. DeVries LS, Toet MC. Amplitude integrated electroencephalography in the full-term newborn. *Clin Perinatol* 2006; 33(3):619–632.
48. Perlman JM. Intrapartum hypoxic-ischemic cerebral injury and subsequent cerebral palsy: medicolegal issues. *Pediatrics* 1997; 99:851.
49. Shalak LF, Laptook AR, Velaphi SC, Perlman JM. Amplitude-integrated electroencephalography coupled with an early neurologic examination enhances prediction of term infants at risk for persistent encephalopathy. *Pediatrics* 2003; 111:351.
50. Mizrahi EM. Neonatal seizures. In: Swaiman KF, Ashwal S, Ferriero D, eds. *Pediatric Neurology: Principles and Practice*. 4th ed. Philadelphia: Mosby-Elsevier, 2006:257–278.
51. LaJoie J, Moshe SL. Neonatal seizures and neonatal epilepsy. In Devinsky O, ed. *Epilepsy and Developmental Disabilities*. Woburn, MA: Butterworth-Heinemann, 1999:.
52. Aicardi J. Overview: neonatal syndromes. In: Engel J Jr, Pedley TA, eds. *Epilepsy: A Comprehensive Textbook*. Philadelphia, PA: Lippincott-Raven Publishers, 1997:2243.
53. Ohtahara S, Ohtsuka Y, Yamatogi Y, et al. Early-infantile epileptic encephalopathy with suppression-bursts. In: Roger J, Bureau M, Dravet Ch, et al, eds. *Epileptic Syndromes in Infancy, Childhood and Adolescence*. 2nd ed. London: John Libbey & Company Ltd., 1992:25.
54. Plouin P. Benign neonatal convulsions. In: Wasterlain CG, Vert P, eds. *Neonatal Seizures*. New York: Raven Press, 1990:51–59.
55. Dehan M, Quilleron D, Navelet Y, et al. Les convulsions du cinquieme jour de vie: un nouveau syndrome? *Arch Fr Pediatr* 1977; 34:730–742.
56. Plouin P, Anderson VE. Benign familial and non-familial neonatal seizures. In: Roger J, Bureau M, Dravet C, et al, eds. *Epileptic Syndromes in Infancy, Childhood and Adolescence*. 4th ed. Montrouge, France: John Libbey & Co., 2005:3–16.
57. Herrmann B, Lawrenz-Wolf B, Seewald C, et al. 5th day convulsions of the newborn infant in rotavirus infections. *Monatsschr Kinderheilkd* 1993; 141 120.
58. Plouin P. Benign idiopathic neonatal convulsions. In: Roger J, Bureau M, Dravet Ch, Dreifuss FE, et al, eds. *Epileptic Syndromes in Infancy, Childhood and Adolescence*. 2nd ed. John Libbey & Company Ltd., 1992:3.
59. Plouin P. Benign familial neonatal convulsions and benign idiopathic neonatal convulsions. In: Engel J Jr, Pedley TA, eds. *Epilepsy: A Comprehensive Textbook*. Philadelphia, PA: Lippincott-Raven, 1997:2247.
60. Pettit RE, Fenichel GM. Benign familial neonatal seizures. *Arch Neurol* 1980; 37:47.
61. Hirsch E, Velez A, Sellal F, et al. Electroclinical signs of benign neonatal familial convulsions. *Ann Neurol* 1993; 34:835.
62. Bye AM. Neonate with benign familial neonatal convulsions. *Pediatr Neurol* 1994; 10:164.
63. Leppert M, Anderson VE, Quattelbaum TG, et al. Benign familial neonatal convulsions linked to genetic markers on chromosome 20. *Nature* 1989; 337:647–648.
64. Ryan SG, Wiznitzer M, Hollman C, et al. Benign familial neonatal convulsions: evidence for clinical and genetic heterogeneity. *Ann Neurol* 1991; 29:469.
65. Lewis TB, Leach RJ, Ward K, et al. Genetic heterogeneity in benign familial neonatal convulsions: identification of a new locus on chromosome-8q. *Am J Hum Genet* 1993; 53:670–675.
66. Steinlein O, Schuster V, Fischer C, et al. Benign familial neonatal convulsions: confirmation of genetic heterogeneity and further evidence for a second locus on chromosome 8q. *Hum Genet* 1995; 95:411.
67. Biervert C, Schroeder BS, Kubisch C, et al. A potassium channel mutation in neonatal human epilepsy. *Science* 1998; 279:403.
68. Singh NA, Charlier C, Stauffer D, et al. A novel potassium channel gene, KCNQ2, is mutated in an inherited epilepsy of newborns. *Nat Genet* 1998; 18:25.
69. Quattlebaum TG. Benign familial convulsions in the neonatal period and early infancy. *J Pediatr* 1979; 95:257–259.
70. Ronen GM, Rosales TO, Connolly M, et al. Seizure characteristics in chromosome 20 benign familial neonatal convulsions. *Neurology* 1993; 43:1355–1360.
71. Lortie A, Plouin P, Chiron C, Delalande O, Dulac O. *Epilepsy Res.* 2002; 51(1–2):133–145.
72. Fenichel GM. Neonatal neurology. 3rd ed. New York: Churchill-Livingstone, 1990.
73. Aicardi J. Neonatal seizures. In: *Epilepsy in Children*. 2nd ed. International Review of Child Neurology Series. New York; Raven Press, 1994:217.
74. Volpe JJ. Neonatal seizures. In: *Neurology of the Newborn*. Philadelphia: WB Saunders, 2001:Chapter 5.
75. Clancy RR, Mizrahi EM. Neonatal seizures. In: Wyllie E, ed. *The Treatment of Epilepsy: Principles and Practice*. 4th ed. Philadelphia: Lippincott, 2006:487–510.
76. Pellock JM. Treatment of seizures and epilepsy in children and adolescents. *Neurology* 1998; 51:S8.
77. Painter MJ, Scher MS, Paneth NS, et al. Randomized trial of phenobarbital v. phenytoin treatment of neonatal seizures. *Pediatr Res* 1994; 35:384.
78. Scher MS. Neonatal seizures. *Pediatr Neurol* 2003; 29:381.
79. DeLorenzo RJ. Phenytoin. Mechanisms of action. In: Levy RH, Mattson RH, Meldrum BS, eds. *Antiepileptic Drugs*. 4th ed. New York: Raven Press, 1995:271.
80. Levy RA, Mattson RH, Meldrum BS, eds. Antiepileptic drugs. 4th ed. New York: Raven Press, 1995.
81. MacDonald RL. Benzodiazepines. In: Levy RH, Mattson RH, Meldrum BS, eds. *Antiepileptic Drugs*. 4th ed. New York: Raven Press, 1995:695–703.
82. Painter MJ, Gaus LM. Phenobarbital: clinical use. In: Levy H, Mattson RH, Meldrum BS, eds. *Antiepileptic Drugs*. 4th ed. New York: Raven Press, 1995:401.
83. Painter MJ, Pippenger C, MacDonald H, et al. Phenobarbital and diphenylhydantoin levels in neonates with seizures. *J Pediatr* 1978; 92:315.
84. Gal P, Toback J, Boer HR, et al. Efficacy of phenobarbital monotherapy in treatment of neonatal seizures—relationship to blood levels. *Neurology* 1982; 32:1401–1404.
85. Donn SM, Grasela TH, Goldstein GW. Safety of a higher loading dose of phenobarbital in the term newborn. *Pediatrics* 1985; 75:1061.
86. Bourgeois BFD, Dodson WE. Phenytoin elimination in newborns. *Neurology* 1983; 33:173.
87. Dodson WE. Antiepileptic drug utilization in pediatric patients. *Epilepsia* 1984; 25:s132.
88. André M, Boutray MJ, Dubruc O, et al. Clonazepam pharmacokinetics and therapeutic efficacy in neonatal seizures. *Eur J Clin Pharmacol* 1986; 305:585.
89. Hellström-Westas L, Westgren U, Rosen I, et al. Lidocaine for treatment of severe seizures in newborn infants. I. Clinical effects and cerebral electrical activity monitoring. *Acta Paediatr Scand* 1988; 77:79.
90. Sheth RD, Buckley DJ, Gutierrez AR, et al. Midazolam in the treatment of refractory neonatal seizures. *Clin Neuropharmacol* 1996; 19:165.
91. Koren G, Warwick B, Rajchgot R, et al. Intravenous paraldehyde for seizure control in newborn infants. *Neurology* 1986; 36:108.
92. Hu KC, Chiu NC, Ho CS, et al. Continuous midazolam infusion in the treatment of uncontrollable neonatal seizures. *Acta Paediatr Taiwan* 2003; 44:279.
93. Boylan GB, Rennie JM, Chorley G, Pressler RM, et al. Second-line anticonvulsant treatment of neonatal seizures: a video-EEG monitoring study. *Neurology* 2004; 62(3):486–488.
94. Van Rooij LGM, Toet MC, Rademaker KMA, et al. Cardiac arrhythmias in neonates receiving lidocaine as anticonvulsive treatment. *Eur J Pediatr* 2004; 163:637.
95. Mackintosh DA, Baird-Lampert J, Buchanan N. Is carbamazepine an alternative maintenance therapy for neonatal seizures? *Dev Pharmacol Ther* 1987; 10:100.
96. Sapin JI, Riviello JJ Jr, Grover WD. Efficacy of primidone for seizure control in neonates and young infants. *Pediatr Neurol* 1988; 4:292.
97. Gal P, Oles KS, Gilman JT, Weaver R. Valproic acid efficacy, toxicity, and pharmacokinetics in neonates with intractable seizures. *Neurology* 1988; 38(3):467–471.
98. Aicardi J, Mumford JP, Dumas C, Wood S. Vigabatrin as initial therapy for infantile spasms: a European retrospective survey. Sabril IS Investigator and Peer Review Groups. *Epilepsia* 1996; 37:638.
99. Mikati MA, Fayad M, Koleilat M, Mounla N, et al. Efficacy, tolerability, and kinetics of lamotrigine in infants. *J Pediatr* 2002; 141(1):31–35.
100. Bittigau P, Sifringer M, Genz K, et al. Antiepileptic drugs and apoptotic neurodegeneration in the developing brain. *Proc Natl Acad Sci U S A* 2002; 99:15089.
101. Glier C, Dzietko M, Bittigau P, et al. Therapeutic doses of topiramate are not toxic to the developing brain. *Exp Neurol* 2004; 187:403.
102. Holmes GL. Effects of early seizures on later behavior and epileptogenicity. *Ment Retard Dev Disabil Res Rev* 2004; 10:101.
103. Holmes GL, Khazipov R, Ben-Ari Y. New concepts in neonatal seizures. *Neuroreport* 2002; 13:A3.
104. Swann JW, Hablitz JJ. Cellular abnormalities and synaptic plasticity in seizure disorders of the immature nervous system. *Ment Retard Dev Disabil Res Rev* 2000; 6:258–267.
105. Volpe JJ. Perinatal brain injury: from pathogenesis to neuroprotection. *Ment Retard Dev Disabil Res Rev* 2001; 7:56.
106. McCabe BK, Silveira DC, Cilio MR, et al. Reduced neurogenesis after neonatal seizures. *J Neurosci* 2001; 21:2094.
107. Schwartzkroin PA. Plasticity and repair in the immature central nervous system. In: Schwartzkroin PA, Moshé SL, Noebels JL, Swann JW, eds. *Brain Development and Epilepsy*. New York: Oxford University Press, 1995:234.
108. Holmes GL, Chronopoulos A, Stafstrom CE, et al. Effects of kindling on subsequent learning, memory, behavior, and seizure susceptibility. *Brain Res Dev Res* 1993; 73:71–77.
109. Ni H, Jiang YW, Bo T, et al. Long-term effects of neonatal seizures on subsequent N-methyl-aspartate receptor-1 and gamma-aminobutyric acid receptor A-alpha 1 receptor expression in hippocampus of the Wistar rat. *Neurosci Lett* 2004; 368:254.
110. Sogawa Y, Monokoshi M, Silveira DC, et al. Timing of cognitive deficits following neonatal seizures: relationship to histological changes in the hippocampus. *Brain Res Dev Brain Res* 2001; 131:73.
111. Koh S, Storey TW, Santos TC, et al. Early-life seizures in rats increase susceptibility to seizure-induced brain injury in adulthood. *Neurology* 1999; 53:915.
112. Sarkisian MR, Tandon P, Liu Z, et al. Multiple kainic acid seizures in the immature and adult brain: Ictal manifestations and long term effects on learning and memory. *Epilepsia* 1997; 38:1157.
113. Hoffman AF, Zhao Q, Holmes GL. Cognitive impairment following status epilepticus and recurrent seizures during early development: support for the "two-hit" hypothesis. *Epilepsy Behav* 2004; 5:873.
114. Ortibus EL, Sum JM, Hahn JS. Predictive value of EEG for outcome and epilepsy following neonatal seizures. *Electroencephalogr Clin Neurophysiol* 1996; 98:175.
115. Mizrahi EM, Clancy RR, Dunn JK, et al. Neurologic impairment, developmental delay and postnatal seizures 2 years after EEG-video documented seizures in near-term and term neonates: report of the clinical research centers for neonatal seizures. *Epilepsia* 2001; 42:102.
116. Brunquell PJ, Glennon CM, DiMario FJ Jr, et al. Prediction of outcome based on clinical seizure type in newborn infants. *J Pediatr* 2002; 140:707.
117. Tekgul H, Gauvreau K, Soul J, et al. The current etiologic profile and neurodevelopmental outcome of seizures in term newborn infants. *Pediatrics* 2006; 117(4):1270–1280.
118. Ellenberg JH, Hirtz DG, Nelson KB. Age at onset of seizures in young children. *Ann Neurol* 1984; 15:127.
119. Da Silva LFG, Nunes ML, Da Costa JC. Risk factors for developing epiliepsy after neonatal seizures. *Pediatr Neurol* 2004; 30:271.
120. Clancy RR, Legido A. Postnatal epilepsy after EEG-confirmed neonatal seizures. *Epilepsia* 1991; 32:69–76.
121. McBride MC, Laroia N, Guillet R. Electrographic seizures in neonates correlate with poor neurodevelopmental outcome. *Neurology* 2000; 55:506.
122. Miller SP, Weiss J, Barnwell A, et al. Seizure-associated brain injury in term newborns with perinatal asphyxia. *Neurology* 2002; 58:542.
123. Pisani F, Leali L, Parmigiani S, et al. Neonatal seizures in preterm infants: clinical outcome and relationship with subsequent epilepsy. *J Matern Fetal Neonatal Med* 2004 16(suppl 2):51.

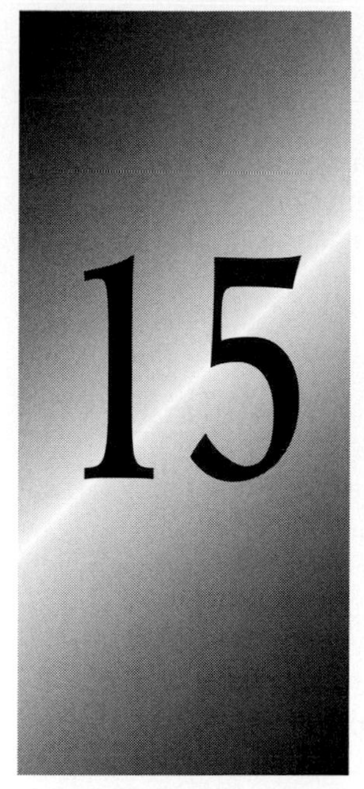

Severe Encephalopathic Epilepsy in Early Infancy

Shunsuke Ohtahara
Yasuko Yamatogi

From the neonatal to the early infantile periods, seizures are relatively rare, compared with other periods of childhood, because of the structural and biochemical immaturity of the brain, which may regulate the seizure susceptibility or threshold. Only a few epileptic syndromes have their onset during these periods, and most of them are severe epilepsies (1). Peculiar representatives are early-infantile epileptic encephalopathy with suppression bursts or Ohtahara syndrome (OS) (2) and early myoclonic encephalopathy (EME) (2, 3). Both syndromes are classified as symptomatic generalized epilepsies with nonspecific etiology according to the present international classification (1), and are designated as epileptic encephalopathies in a newly proposed diagnostic scheme of International League Against Epilepsy (ILAE) classification (4). They could be inclusively called "early infantile epileptic syndromes with suppression-burst" or "severe neonatal epilepsies with suppression-burst pattern" (3) because of shared common characteristics: very early onset with frequent minor seizures and suppression-burst (S-B) pattern on the electroencephalogram (EEG).

EARLY-INFANTILE EPILEPTIC ENCEPHALOPATHY WITH SUPPRESSION BURSTS OR OHTAHARA SYNDROME

Ohtahara syndrome was first described by Ohtahara and coworkers in 1976 (5) as the earliest form of an age-dependent epileptic encephalopathy, and it is characterized by frequent tonic spasms of early onset within the first few months of life and a S-B EEG pattern (6–8). Its evolutional change with age is specific (2, 3, 6, 9–12). The seizures are refractory to medications and the prognosis for neurological development is very poor.

The age-dependent epileptic encephalopathy includes OS, West syndrome (WS), and Lennox-Gastaut syndrome (LGS). Although each of these syndromes is an independent electroclinical entity with its own special features, they have the following common characteristics (5–9, 12, 13):

1. Onset during a specific period of life
2. Peculiar types of frequent, minor generalized seizures
3. Severe and continuous massive epileptic EEG abnormality

4. Heterogeneous cause
5. Frequent association with mental defect
6. Therapy resistance and grave prognosis

Furthermore, transition is often observed over time among patients with these syndromes. A considerable number of OS cases evolve into West syndrome and from West to Lennox-Gastaut syndrome in their clinical course (9–12). Because of these common characteristics and mutual transition with age, the inclusive term *age-dependent epileptic encephalopathy* has been applied to this group of syndromes (7, 13). "Epileptic encephalopathy" was applied to them according to the following four characteristics: (1) the presence of serious underlying disorders, (2) extremely frequent seizures, (3) continuously and diffusely appearing marked epileptic abnormality on EEG, and (4) mental deterioration often manifesting with the persistence of seizures.

As the electroclinical features specific to each syndrome appear on the basis of many causes commonly observed in the three syndromes, the age factor should be considered as the determinant for the manifestation of their individual characteristics. These syndromes, therefore, may be the age-specific epileptic reaction, at a special developmental stage, to various nonspecific exogenous brain insults.

Epidemiology

Several dozens of cases of OS have been reported, but its incidence is rare compared with those of West and Lennox-Gastaut syndromes. An epidemiological study on childhood epilepsy carried out in Okayama, Japan, in 1980, detected one case of OS (0.04%) and four cases of EME (0.17%) among 2,378 epileptic children younger than 10 years of age (14). Compared to the 40 cases (1.68%) of WS observed in the same study, the prevalence of OS and EME is low. Similarly, Kramer et al (15) described one case of OS (0.2%) and 40 cases of WS (9.1%) in a cohort of 440 consecutive children with epilepsy under 15 years of age in Tel Aviv, Israel. Thus, the relative prevalences of OS and EME to WS may be 1:40 or less and 1:10 or less, respectively.

No obvious sex difference has been observed in either syndrome.

Clinical Manifestations

The onset of seizures is very early and is confined to the first 2 or 3 months after birth, mainly the first month. The main seizure type is tonic spasms with or without clustering. The duration of each tonic spasm is up to 10 seconds. One cluster consists of 10 to 40 spasms, at intervals of 5 to 15 seconds. These epileptic spasms occur not only in waking states but also during sleep states in most cases. Daily seizure frequency is very high, ranging from 100 to 300 isolated spasms or 10 to 20 series in those with clustering spasms. In addition to tonic spasms, partial seizures such as erratic focal motor seizures and hemiconvulsions are observed in about one-third of the cases. In contrast to EME, myoclonic seizures or myoclonia are rarely observed (2, 6).

EEG Findings

The most characteristic feature is the S-B pattern, which is persistently observed regardless of the circadian cycle (Figure 15-1). This is a diagnostically most important and indispensable finding. The S-B pattern is characterized by high-voltage bursts alternating with nearly flat patterns at an approximately regular rate. Bursts of 1 to 3 seconds' duration comprise 150 to 350 μV high-voltage slow waves intermixed with multifocal spikes. Duration of the suppression phase is 3 to 5 seconds. The burst-burst interval, measured from onset to onset of the bursts, ranges from 5 to 10 seconds. Presumably reflecting the underlying organic brain lesion, some asymmetry in S-B occurs in about two-thirds of cases, but no remarkable asynchrony is found except for the case of Aicardi syndrome (16).

The ictal EEG of tonic spasms shows principally a desynchronization with or without evident, sometimes remarkable, initial rapid activity (6, 11). A low-voltage fast activity is also often observed. Tonic spasms appear concomitant with bursts. Partial seizures usually originate in some fixed foci and are followed by tonic spasms in series, or sometimes they follow them.

Other Investigations

Brain imaging such as computed tomography (CT) and magnetic resonance imaging (MRI) reveal structural abnormalities, notably asymmetric lesions even at the early stage of seizure onset in most cases. Progressive brain atrophy is often suspected with seizure persistence, particularly in infancy. No abnormalities are found in routine laboratory examinations of blood, urine, cerebrospinal fluid, bone marrow, and liver functions, or in metabolic studies including amino acids, lysosomal enzymes, pyruvate and lactate, and organic acids, or in immunological and virological examinations.

Etiology

Although the causes of OS are heterogeneous, obvious brain lesions including brain malformations are often found. Porencephaly, Aicardi syndrome (3, 16), hemimegalencephaly (17–19), olivary-dentate dysplasia (20, 21), lissencephaly, linear sebaceous nevus (22), Leigh encephalopathy (23), and subacute diffuse encephalopathy (3) have all been associated with the syndrome. In a few cases no cause has been identified, and these are labeled cryptogenic (3). But cryptogenic cases may have undetectable

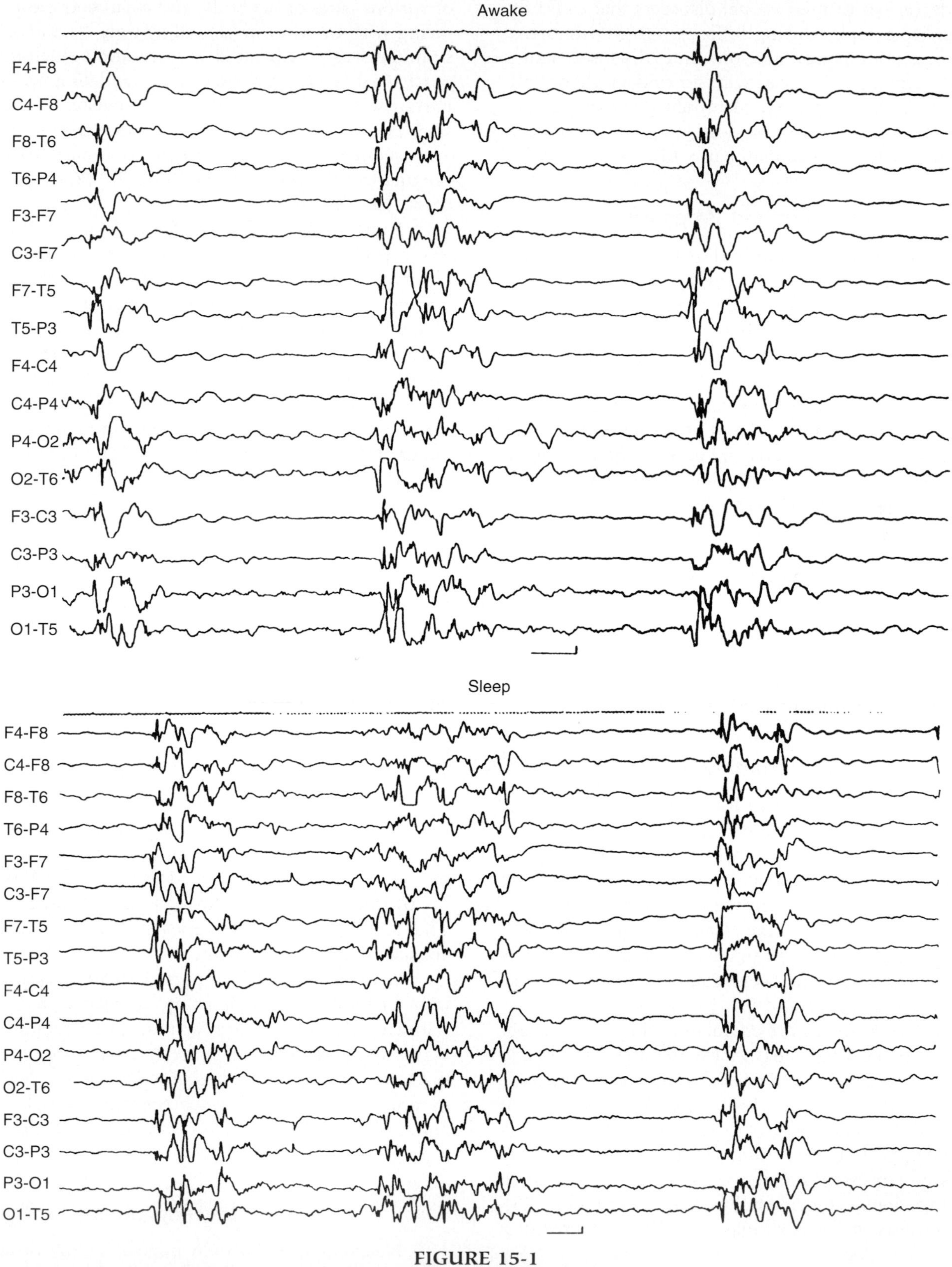

FIGURE 15-1

Interictal EEG (Ohtahara syndrome). Two-month-old boy. High-voltage bursts and almost flat suppressions alternately repeat continuously and consistently throughout the waking (upper) and sleeping (lower) states. The horizontal calibration mark, 1 second; the vertical one, 50 μV.

microdysgenesis or migrational disorders that cause the progressive atrophy during follow-up (6). Postmortem pathologic examination has sometimes disclosed significant abnormalities in cases with no evident abnormalities on neuroimaging (18). Metabolic disorder was not reported except in rare cases of cytochrome c oxidase deficiency or Leigh encephalopathy (3).

Treatment and Prognosis

Seizures are intractable. Natural or synthetic adrenocorticotropic hormone (ACTH) therapy is partially effective in only a few cases (6). Clobazam, acetazolamide, vitamin B_6, valproate, vigabatrin, and zonisamide are recommended to be tried (6). Successful resection of focal cortical dysplasia is reported (24, 25). Although seizures possibly subside by school age in about half of the cases, developmental and life prognoses are very poor. All those who survive are severely handicapped, both mentally and physically. Mortality is high, especially in the early stage of the disease (6).

EARLY MYOCLONIC ENCEPHALOPATHY

Early myoclonic encephalopathy is a rare epileptic syndrome of very early onset with frequent myoclonias and partial seizures, and S-B in the EEG. It was first described by Aicardi and Goutières (26) in 1978.

Clinical Manifestations

The onset of seizures is in the first 3 months of life, mostly during the neonatal period. The cardinal seizures are myoclonias, which are mostly fragmentary. Frequent erratic partial seizures, massive myoclonias, and tonic spasms are also seen. Among these types of seizures, fragmentary myoclonias are the essential symptom in EME and the initial seizure type in most cases (2–3, 26). They may occur within the first several hours of life or perhaps even prenatally (27).

Such myoclonias are characterized by only a slight twitching of the distal ends of the extremities, eyelids, and corners of the mouth, and are sometimes too subtle to be detected without careful observation. The frequency of these myoclonias varies greatly from several times a day to several dozen times a minute. The ictal EEG usually shows no consistent change with myoclonia, although some myoclonias coincidentally occur with bursts (2, 28). This suggests that myoclonias in EME are mainly of a nonepileptic type.

Throughout the course of the syndrome, the main seizure types are partial seizures; those include complex partial seizures with eye deviation or autonomic symptoms such as apnea and facial flushing, clonic seizures of various parts of the body, and asymmetric tonic posturing with or without generalization. Partial seizures simultaneously associated with erratic myoclonias are particularly characteristic of this syndrome (2, 3, 29). Partial seizures have a tendency to cluster in the early stage. They are seen during both waking and sleep states. The frequency of partial seizures is remarkably high, ranging from 7 to 8 times to 30 to 100 times a day, but decreases with age.

Tonic spasms are also often observed, but massive myoclonias and tonic spasms are not necessarily observed in all cases. Cases with tonic spasms are considered WS when tonic spasms appear at 3 to 4 months of age. The period of WS is, however, transient, and the EME state recurs and persists for a long period thereafter (28, 30). Tonic spasms are usually seen during both waking and sleeping states and appear either in series or in isolation. Tonic spasms in series sometime appear following a partial seizure, but a partial seizure may appear just after tonic spasms in other occasions or infants.

EEG Findings

Interictal EEG of EME is also characterized by a S-B pattern with bursts lasting 1 to 5 seconds and nearly flat periods of 3 to 10 seconds. This pattern becomes more distinct during sleep and more pronounced as sleep deepens (28, 29) (Figure 15–2).

The S-B pattern tends to be replaced by atypical hypsarrhythmia or by multifocal paroxysms after 3 to 5 months of age. In most cases, however, the appearance of atypical hypsarrhythmia is transient, lasting up to 2 years 6 months of age at the latest (28, 30), after which the S-B pattern returns again and persists for a long period thereafter (28, 30). In addition to the S-B pattern, multifocal spikes persist throughout the clinical course. The location of spike foci varies in every case and is not consistent in a given patient.

With the ictal EEG of partial seizures, various patterns of focal onset, such as fast activity, alpha or theta patterns, rhythmic sharp waves, and irregular spike waves, are observed, usually from two or more sites with migration in each individual case (2, 28–31). Ictal EEG of tonic spasms shows desynchronization, which appears concomitant with bursts. Myoclonic seizures also occur during bursts (31, 32).

Other Investigations

Neuroimaging is often normal at the onset, but progressive cortical and periventricular atrophies are observed in some cases (2–3, 29). Abnormalities are often detected from 3 to 10 months of age, that is, 3 to 8 months after the onset. Diffuse cortical atrophy is noted

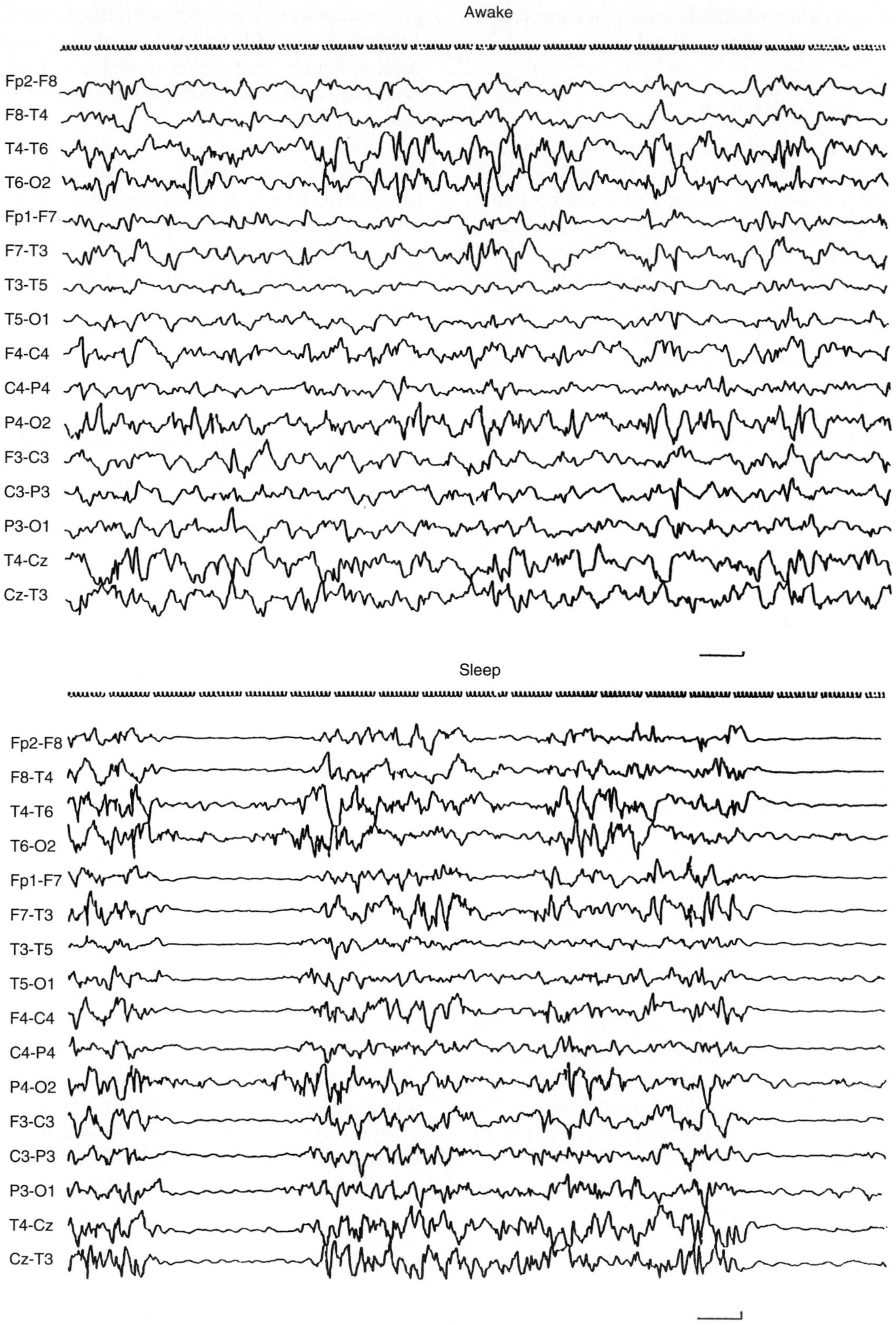

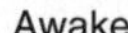

FIGURE 15–2

Intterictal EEG (early myoclonic encephalopathy). Six-month-old girl. Mutifocal spikes are noted frequently in the disorganized background activity in the waking record (upper), but suppression-burst pattern is apparent in the sleeping record (lower).

in all, with associated ventricular dilatation in some cases, but focal abnormalities are exceptional.

Etiology

The most striking feature of this disorder is the high incidence of familial cases as found in 4 of 12 families in the series of Aicardi and Ohtahara (3) and 2 of 8 families in the series of Dalla Bernardina et al (29). This suggests the etiologic participation of some kinds of genetic and congenital metabolic errors in many cases. Nonketotic hyperglycinemia (32–34), propionic acidemia, methylmalonic acidemia, and D-glyceric acidemia, carbamyl-phosphate synthetase deficiency (34), pyridoxine-dependency, molybdenum cofactor deficiency, Menkes disease (3, 35), and Zellweger syndrome (36) have been reported to be associated with EME. In many cases; however, the cause remains unknown.

Treatment and Prognoses

None of the conventional antiepileptic drugs, ACTH, corticosteroids, or pyridoxine has been effective, excepting pyridoxine-dependency (3). Both partial seizures and myoclonias, however, decrease gradually with age. EME has an extremely poor prognosis including a high mortality, with death usually occurring before 2 years of age. Survivors have persistent partial seizures and progressive psychomotor deterioration to a vegetative state (3, 29).

DEVELOPMENTAL ASPECTS

Compared to EME, the remarkable characteristic of OS is its age-dependent evolutional change. It develops from OS to WS in middle infancy, particularly during 3 to 6 months of age, in many cases, and further from WS to LGS in early childhood, at 1 to 3 years of age, in some cases (12, 30).

The EEG also evolves from the S-B pattern to hypsarrhythmia in many cases at around 3 to 6 months of age, and further from hypsarrhythmia to diffuse slow spike-waves in some cases at around 1 year of age (9,12). Some cases evolve further to the severe epilepsy with multiple independent spike foci (37).

Concerning the changing process of S-B pattern in OS, its transition to hypsarrhythmia starts with a gradual increase in the amplitude of the suppression phase. Disappearance of the S-B pattern in waking precedes that in sleep, and S-B remains in the sleeping EEG even after the waking EEG has already transformed to hypsarrhythmia. In the course of evolution from hypsarrhythmia to diffuse slow spike-waves, the change in the waking EEG is followed by the change in the sleep EEG. Thus, the evolution from a S-B pattern to hypsarrhythmia and further to diffuse slow spike-waves proceeds in a close relation with the waking and sleeping cycle (2, 9, 12, 30). The timing of transition among the three epileptic syndromes and EEG patterns is specific; evolving syndromes and EEG patterns appear at characteristic ages.

EME, however, manifests no fundamental change in the electroclinical feature throughout its course, except for the EEG change from suppression-burst or burst-suppression pattern to a disorganized pattern with frequent multifocal spikes that occur within several months of life (3, 26, 29) and transient manifestation of WS and hypsarrhythmia in some cases (28, 30).

DIFFERENTIAL DIAGNOSIS

Differential Diagnosis between OS and WS

The age of onset of the two syndromes is different: OS appears from the neonatal to early infantile periods and WS in middle infancy. Although the main seizure type is tonic spasms in both syndromes, tonic spasms in OS appear not only while awake but also during sleep, and not only in clusters. Partial seizures also occur in some OS cases but are rare in WS. Most cases with OS have severe cortical pathology, often displaying asymmetric lesions on neuroimaging.

The EEG discriminates the S-B pattern in OS from hypsarrhythmia in WS. The S-B pattern differs from the periodic type of hypsarrhythmia in which periodicity becomes evident only during sleep.

Seizures are more intractable in OS, and ACTH therapy is usually not effective. Furthermore, children with OS have less favorable prognoses than those with WS.

Differential Diagnosis between EME and OS

As EME and OS have common clinical and electrical characteristics such as early onset within a few months of life and the S-B pattern on EEG, differentiation may be difficult (28, 30). The main seizure type is tonic spasms, and myoclonias are rarely seen in OS. In contrast, myoclonias, especially erratic myoclonias, and frequent partial seizures predominate in EME (28, 30).

Electroencephalographically, the S-B pattern is a common feature of both syndromes, but its relation to the circadian cycle and age of its appearance and disappearance differ considerably. The S-B pattern in OS is characterized by consistent appearance during both waking and sleeping states, whereas in EME it is enhanced by sleep and often not manifest in the waking state. Concerning the duration of appearance, the S-B pattern appears at the beginning of the disease and disappears within the first 6 months of life in OS, whereas in EME, it becomes distinct at 1 to 5 months of age in some cases and characteristically persists for a long period (28, 30).

The evolution of the EEG abnormalities during the clinical course is a characteristic feature of OS: from the S-B pattern to hypsarrhythmia in many cases and further from hypsarrhythmia to diffuse slow spike-waves in some cases (2, 11, 12, 30). In EME, the S-B pattern persists for a long time, although atypical hypsarrhythmia appears transiently in some cases. Therefore, the age-related evolutional pattern differs considerably between OS and EME (30).

Regarding epileptic syndromes, OS shows a characteristic evolution as the earliest form of the age-dependent epileptic encephalopathy, whereas EME has no specific evolution with age (28, 30).

Etiologically, OS is usually based on evident organic brain lesions including brain malformations. Neuroimaging demonstrates abnormal findings even at the early stage. No familial cases have been reported in OS. In contrast, the frequent incidence of familial cases suggests some undetermined inborn metabolic disorders as the cause in many cases of EME.

The differences between OS and EME indicate that they are independent electroclinical entities (30). Efficiency of the developmental study should be stressed to clearly delineate both syndromes.

References

1. Commission on Classification and Terminology of the International League Against Epilepsy. Proposal for revised classification of epilepsies and epileptic syndromes. *Epilepsia* 1989; 30:389–399.
2. Ohtahara S, Yamatogi Y. Epileptic encephalopathies in early infancy with suppression-burst. *J. Clin Neurophysiol* 2003; 20:398–407.
3. Aicardi J, Ohtahara S. Severe neonatal epilepsies with suppression-burst pattern. In: Roger J, Bureau M, Dravet Ch, et al, eds. *Epileptic Syndromes in Infancy, Childhood and Adolescence* 4th ed. Montrogue: John Libbey Eurotext, 2005:39–50.
4. Engel Jr J. ILAE Commission Report. A proposed diagnostic scheme for people with epileptic seizures and with epilepsy: Report of the ILAE Task Force on Classification and Terminology. *Epilepsia* 2001; 42:796–803.
5. Ohtahara S, Ishida T, Oka E, et al. On the specific age dependent epileptic syndrome: the early-infantile epileptic encephalopathy with suppression-burst. *No To Hattatsu* (Tokyo) 1976; 8:270–280 (in Japanese).
6. Yamatogi Y, Ohtahara S. Early-infantile epileptic encephalopathy with suppression-bursts, Ohtahara syndrome; its overview referring to our 16 cases. *Brain Dev* 2002; 24:13–23.
7. Ohtahara S. A study on the age-dependent epileptic encephalopathy. *No To Hattatsu* (Tokyo) 1977; 9:2–21 (in Japanese).
8. Ohtahara S. Clinico-electrical delineation of epileptic encephalopathies in childhood. *Asian Med J* 1978; 21:499–509.
9. Ohtahara S,Yamatogi Y. Evolution of seizures and EEG abnormalities in childhood onset epilepsy. In: Wada JA, Ellingson RJ, eds. *Clinical Neurophysiology of Epilepsy, Handbook of Electroencephalography and Clinical Neurophysiology.* Revised Series, Vol. 4. Amsterdam: Elsevier, 1990:457–477.
10. Ohtsuka Y, Ogino T, Murakami N, et al. Developmental aspects of epilepsy with special reference to age-dependent epileptic encephalopathy. *Jpn J Psychiatry Neurol* 1986; 40:307–313.
11. Yamatogi Y, Ohtahara S. Age-dependent epileptic encephalopathy: a longitudinal study. *Folia Psychiatr Neurol Jpn* 1981; 35:321–331.
12. Ohtahara S, Ohtsuka Y, Yamatogi Y, et al. The early-infantile epileptic encephalopathy with suppression-burst: developmental aspects. *Brain Dev* 1987; 9:371–376.
13. Donat JF. The age-dependent epileptic encephalopathies, *J Child Neurol* 1992; 7:7–21.
14. Oka E, Ishida S, Ohtsuka Y, Ohtahara S. Neuroepidemiological study of childhood epilepsy by application of international classification of epilepsies and epileptic syndromes (ILAE, 1989). *Epilepsia* 1995; 36:658–661.
15. Kramer U, Nevo Y, Neufeld MY, et al. Epidemiology of epilepsy in childhood: a cohort of 440 consecutive patients. *Pediatr Neurol* 1998; 18:46–50.
16. Ohtsuka Y, Oka E, Terasaki T, et al. Aicardi syndrome: a longitudinal clinical and electroencephalographic study. *Epileplsia* 1993; 34:627–634.
17. Bermejo AM, Martin VL, Arcas J, et al. Early infantile epileptic encephalopathy: a case associated with hemimegalencephaly, *Brain Dev* 1992; 14:425–428.
18. Miller SP, Dilenge M-E, Meagher-Villemure K, et al. Infantile epileptic encephalopathy (Ohtahara syndrome) and migrational disorder. *Pediatr Neurol* 1998; 19:50–54.
19. Ohtsuka Y, Ohno S, Oka E. Electroclinical characteristics of hemimegalencephaly. *Pediatr Neurol* 1999; 20:390–393.
20. Robain O, Dulac O. Early epileptic encephalopathy with suppression bursts and olivary-dentate dysplasia. *Neuropediatrics* 1992; 23:162–164.
21. Harding BN, Boyd SG. Intractable seizures from infancy can be associated with dentato-olivary dysplasia. *J Neurol Sci* 1991; 104:157–165.
22. Hirata Y, Ishikawa A, Somiya K. A case of linear nevus sebaceous syndrome associated with early-infantile epileptic encephalopathy with suppression burst (EIEE). *No To Hattatsu* (Tokyo) 1985; 17:577–582 (in Japanese).
23. Tatsuno M, Hayashi M, Iwamoto H, et al. Leigh's encephalopathy with wide lesions and early infantile epileptic encephalopathy with burst-suppression; an autopsy case. *No To Hattatsu* 1984; 16:68–75 (in Japanese).
24. Pedespan JM, Loiseau H, Vita A, et al. Surgical treatment of an early epileptic encephalopathy with suppression-bursts and focal cortical dysplasia. *Epilepsia* 1995; 36:37–40.
25. Komaki H, Sugai K, Sasaki M et al. Surgical treatment of a case of early infantile epileptic encephalopathy with suppression-bursts associated with focal cortical dysplasia. *Epilepsia* 1999; 40:365–369.
26. Aicardi J, Goutières F. Encéphalopathie myoclonique néonatale. *Rev EEG Neurophysiol* 1978; 8:99–101.
27. Du Plessis AJ, Kaufmann WE, Kupsky WJ. Intrauterine-onset myoclonic encephalopathy associated with cerebral cortical dysgenesis, *J Child Neurol* 1993; 8:164–170.
28. Murakami N, Ohtsuka Y, Ohtahara S. Early infantile epileptic syndromes with suppression-bursts: early myoclonic encephalopathy vs. Ohtahara syndome. *Jpn J Psychiatry Neurol* 1993; 47:197–200.
29. Dalla Bernardina B, Dulac O, Fejerman N, et al. Early myoclonic epileptic encephalopathy (EMEE). *Eur J Pediatr* 1983; 140:248–252.
30. Ohtahara S, Yamatogi Y. Ohtahara syndrome: with special reference to its developmental aspects for differentiating from early myoclonic encephalopathy. *Epilepsy Res* 2006; 705:s58–67.
31. Otani K, Abe J, Futagi Y, et al. Clinical and electroencephalographical follow-up study of early myoclonic encephalopathy. *Brain Dev* 1989; 11:332–337.
32. Dalla Bernardina B, Aicardi J, Goutières F, et al. Glycine encephalopathy. *Neuropädiatrie* 1979; 10:209–225.
33. Terasaki T, Yamatogi Y, Ohtahara S, et al. A long-term follow-up study on a case with glycine encephalopathy. *No To Hattatsu* (Tokyo) 1988; 20:15–22 (in Japanese).
34. Lombroso CT. Early myoclonic encephalopathy, early infantile epileptic encephalopathy, and benign and severe infantile myoclonic epilepsies: a critical review and personal contributions. *J Clin Neurophysiol* 1990; 7:380–408.
35. Vigevano F, Bartuli A. Infantile epileptic syndromes and metabolic etiologies. *J Child Neurol* 2002; 17(suppl 3):359–14.
36. Spreafico R, Angelini L, Binelli S et al. Burst suppression and impairment of neocortical ontogenesis: electroclinical and neuropathologic findings in two infants with early myoclonic encephalopathy. *Epileplsia* 1993; 34:800–808.
37. Yamatogi Y, Ohtahara S. Severe epilepsy with multiple independent spike foci. *J Clin Neurophysiol* 2003; 20:442–448.

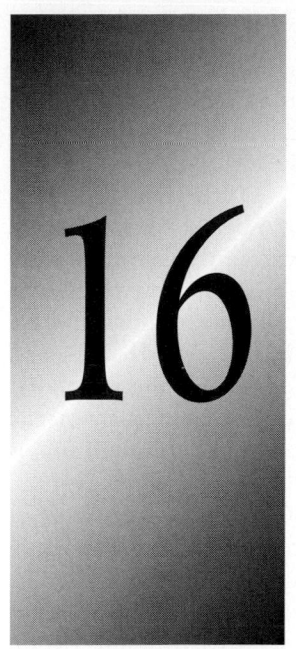

16 Severe Encephalopathic Epilepsy in Infants: Infantile Spasms (West Syndrome)

Richard A. Hrachovy
James D. Frost Jr.

INTRODUCTION AND DEFINITION

Infantile spasms (West syndrome) is a unique disorder that is peculiar to infancy and early childhood. More than 75 different names have been applied to the disorder (1), including massive spasms, flexion spasms, jackknife seizures, infantile myoclonic seizures, and the like, and they have been recognized as an epileptic phenomenon since they were first described by William West in 1841 (2). Approximately 100 years later, Gibbs and Gibbs (3) described the interictal electroencephalogram (EEG) pattern, hypsarrhythmia, which was noted to occur in a large number of patients with infantile spasms. Most patients with infantile spasms have some degree of mental and developmental retardation. In 1958, the first therapeutic breakthrough was reported by Sorel and Dusaucy-Bauloye (4), who observed improvement in EEGs and amelioration of spasms in patients treated with adrenocorticotropic hormone (ACTH).

A considerable amount of literature pertaining to this disorder has accumulated over the past several decades. However, classifications and clinical descriptions of the seizures, based largely on routine bedside observations, have been highly variable, and this lack of uniformity has led to considerable confusion and controversy. Our understanding of the clinical manifestations of this disorder was greatly increased by the development of long-term polygraphic-video monitoring techniques in the 1970s (5). These techniques also provided objective means of evaluating the acute effects of therapy on seizure frequency and the EEG. The introduction of computed tomography (CT), magnetic resonance imaging (MRI), and positron emission tomography (PET) scanning in the 1970s and 1980s greatly increased our understanding of associated brain abnormalities seen in these patients. Such information has not only been helpful in the classification of patients (symptomatic versus cryptogenic) but has also aided our understanding of the possible pathophysiological mechanism(s) underlying this condition.

In this chapter, we briefly describe the clinical and EEG features of infantile spasms and review some of the more controversial and as yet unresolved issues, including therapy and pathophysiology.

EPIDEMIOLOGY

Although the reported incidence of infantile spasms has ranged from 0.05 to 0.60 per 1,000 live births, the average incidence of this disorder is approximately 0.31 per 1,000 live births (1 in 3,225 live births) (1, 6). Spasm onset is usually within the first 4 to 8 months of life with a peak at 6 months. Most cases occur before 3 years of age. Although several studies have reported that infantile spasms occur more commonly in males, there is no clear evidence of a preponderance of one sex over the other (1).

The information concerning the familial occurrence of infantile spasms is limited. The percentage of patients who have a family member with infantile spasms has ranged from none to 7% (7–9). The percentage of cases having a positive family history for any type of epilepsy has ranged from none to 33% (7, 10–14). A major problem with most of these studies is that the authors do not provide comparable data for normal subjects.

CLINICAL MANIFESTATIONS

Description of Spasms

The motor spasm typically consists of a brief, bilaterally symmetrical contraction of the muscles of the neck, trunk, and extremities. This muscle activity is typically characterized by an initial phasic contraction lasting less than 2 seconds, which may be followed by a less intense, but more sustained, tonic contraction lasting up to 10 seconds in duration. The exact character of the seizure depends on whether the flexor or extensor muscles are predominantly affected and on the distribution of the muscle groups involved (5, 15). The position of the body (e.g., supine versus sitting) usually influences the type of spasm. The intensity of the spasm may vary from a massive contraction of all flexor muscles, resulting in a jackknife at the waist, to a minimal contraction of muscles such as the abdominal recti.

Three main types of motor spasm have been identified: flexor, extensor, and mixed flexor-extensor. In our polygraphic-video monitoring experience, mixed spasms were the most frequent (approximately 42%), followed by flexor spasms (approximately 34%), and extensor spasms were the least common (approximately 25%). Asymmetrical spasms were rare (less than 1%). Periods of attenuated responsiveness, which have been termed *arrest phenomena*, may occur following a motor spasm or may occur independently. Most infants with this disorder have more than one type of spasm (15, 16).

A variety of clinical phenomena have been reported to occur in association with the motor spasms. These include autonomic changes (heart rate alterations, cyanosis, pallor, sweating, and flushing), respiratory rate changes, vocalizations (crying, laughter, and grunting sounds), hiccups, smiling, grimacing, tongue and mouth movements, and ocular events (eye deviation, nystagmus, eye opening or closing, pupillary dilation, and tearing).

Monitoring studies have shown that there is little variation in the number of spasms recorded from the same patient in consecutive 24-hour monitoring periods; however, there is a marked variation in spasm frequency when patients are monitored at 2-week intervals (17). The number of spasms recorded during 24-hour periods has ranged from a handful to several hundred in different patients (15, 16).

Approximately the same number of spasms occurs during the day as at night; however, the spasms rarely occur when the infant is actually asleep (less than 3%) (18–20). Instead, they frequently occur immediately upon, or soon after, arousal (10, 12, 15, 16, 21, 22). The spasms are not precipitated by feeding or photic stimulation but may occasionally be elicited by tactile stimulation or unexpected loud noises, although this is uncommon (15).

Although spasms may occur in an isolated fashion, they frequently occur in clusters, with clusters being reported in 47% to 84% of cases (13, 15, 16, 20, 23). In the series reported by Kellaway et al (15), the number of spasms per cluster varied from 2 to 138. Succession rates of up to 15 spasms per minute were recorded, and the intensity of the motor spasms within a cluster would usually wax and then wane.

Spontaneous Remission

The phenomenon of spontaneous remission of infantile spasms is poorly understood. Published data concerning the duration of this disorder have been infrequent and imprecise. In 1973, Jeavons and coworkers (24) reported that 28% of patients were free of spasms by 1 year of age, 49% before age 2, 65% before age 3, and 74% by age 4. Unfortunately, some of their patients had been treated with steroids, and EEG findings were not presented. To further investigate spontaneous remission in this disorder, we retrospectively studied 44 patients who had not been treated with hormonal drugs (25). Our results indicated that spontaneous remission of spasms and disappearance of the hypsarrhythmic EEG pattern can begin within 1 month of the onset of this disorder and that 25% of patients with infantile spasms experience spontaneous remission within 1 year.

Spontaneous remission in two consecutively identified patients with infantile spasms being evaluated for possible admission to a trial of ACTH therapy is illustrated in Figures 16-1 and 16-2. This phenomenon must always be remembered when interpreting results of any therapeutic trial in this disorder and must also be considered in discussing possible pathophysiological mechanisms underlying infantile spasms.

Coupling of Spasms with Other Seizures

The coexistence of partial seizures and spasms in patients with infantile spasms has been recognized for many years (10, 12, 14, 26–28). Partial seizures may appear before the onset of spasms, concurrently with spasms, or after

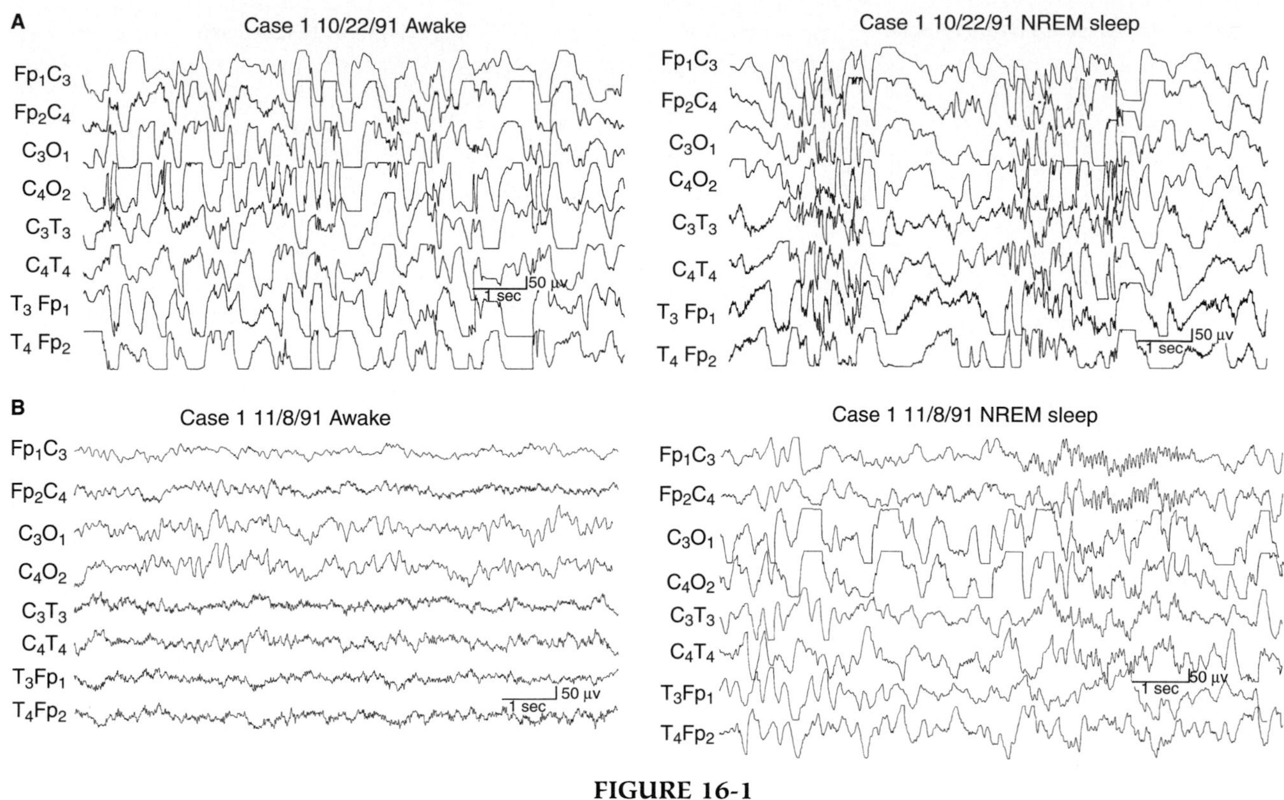

FIGURE 16-1

Spontaneous remission in a 7-month-old girl with cryptogenic infantile spasms. ACTH was not initiated in this patient because of a concurrent infection. Representative samples of the awake and NREM-sleep EEG selected from 18-channel-24-hour polygraphic-video monitoring records. (A) Recording at the time of diagnosis shows hypsarrhythmia. Spasms were recorded. (B) Repeat study 3 weeks later showing normal activity awake and during NREM sleep. Awake sample shown was taken with the patient's eyes open (eyes-closed recording revealed a well-defined occipital rhythm of 5–5.5 Hz). No spasms were recorded during the 24-hour monitoring study.

spasms have ceased, either spontaneously or following treatment. Recently, there has been increased interest in the observation that in some patients with infantile spasms focal electrical seizure discharges (FS) may be tightly coupled with spasms. Our group first described this association in 1984 (29), and since that time several additional reports of this phenomenon in small groups of patients have appeared (30–35). Although this is an interesting phenomenon, its significance remains uncertain. These observations have been used by some investigators to support the hypothesis that infantile spasms occur as a result of an interaction between a primary cortical generator and subcortical structures (see subsequent section). To further investigate the significance of the temporal coupling of FS and spasms, we analyzed the video-EEG studies performed on 96 consecutive patients newly diagnosed with infantile spasms and hypsarrhythmic EEGs (36). Ten of these patients also demonstrated FS; however, in only five patients was there an apparent coupling of FS with spasms. More importantly, in only three patients (3% of the entire population) was the observed coupling statistically significant. Three different couplings were documented: FS could precede a cluster of spasms, could occur during a cluster of spasms, or could follow a cluster of spasms. FS always arose independently from various sites in a given patient, and in some patients coupling of spasms and FS always occurred on arousal from sleep.

Our conclusion from this study is that coupling of FS and spasms at the time of diagnosis of infantile spasms occurs only rarely. We believe there are several possible explanations for this coupling phenomenon. In some instances, apparent coupling may best be explained by random coincidence. A second possibility is that FS may facilitate or induce the appearance of spasms (or vice versa), as has been the major explanation suggested by others. Finally, the coupling of spasms and FS may result from the effect of some "critical factor" that simultaneously affects the seizure thresholds of the neuronal systems involved in the generation of both seizure types. This final hypothesis assumes that in the presence of the critical factor, the seizure thresholds for FS and epileptic spasms are concurrently altered, resulting in the simultaneous or

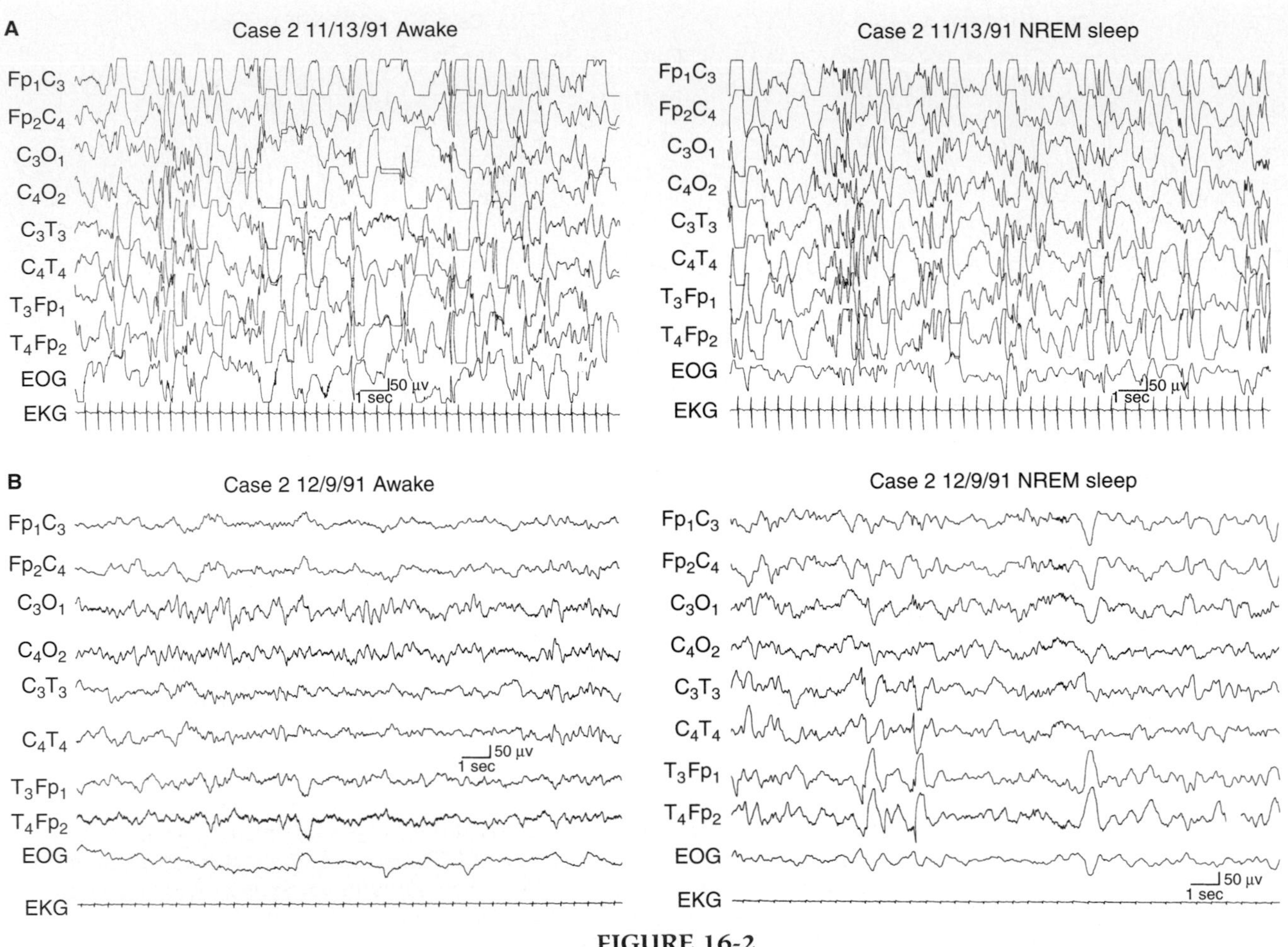

FIGURE 16-2

Spontaneous remission in a 5-month-old boy with symptomatic infantile spasms. The parents refused to give permission for treatment. Representative samples of the awake and NREM-sleep EEG selected from 18-channel 24-hour polygraphic-video monitoring records. (A) Recording at the time of initial diagnosis shows hypsarrhythmia. Spasms were recorded. (B) Repeat study 3 weeks later, showing normal background for age. NREM-sleep sample shows right temporal spikes. Left temporal spikes (not shown) were also present in the sleep tracing. No spasms were recorded during the 24-houir monitoring study.

near simultaneous occurrence of both seizure types. In some of our patients the critical factor appeared to be the arousal mechanism, a known potent activator of spasms and other seizures.

Tonic seizures may also be coupled with spasms, and these two seizure types may be difficult to differentiate because the clinical and EEG features are very similar. The major distinguishing features between the two are that tonic seizures usually are more prolonged and lack the intense initial phasic component seen with most spasms. An interesting observation is that tonic seizures may rarely immediately precede a cluster of spasms. A review of video-EEG monitoring studies of 57 consecutive patients with infantile spasms revealed coupling of tonic seizures with spasms in three (5%) cases (personal observations). Because of the similarities between tonic seizures and spasms, it is likely that these two seizure types are generated by a similar mechanism and arise from the same region of the brain, possibly the brainstem.

ELECTROENCEPHALOGRAPHIC FEATURES

Interictal Patterns

The interictal pattern most commonly associated with infantile spasms is hypsarrhythmia (Fig 16-3), which was originally defined by Gibbs and Gibbs (3) as follows:

> . . . random high voltage slow waves and spikes. These spikes vary from moment to moment, both in duration and in location. At times they appear to be focal, and a few seconds later they seem to originate from multiple foci. Occasionally the spike discharge becomes generalized, but it never appears as a rhythmically

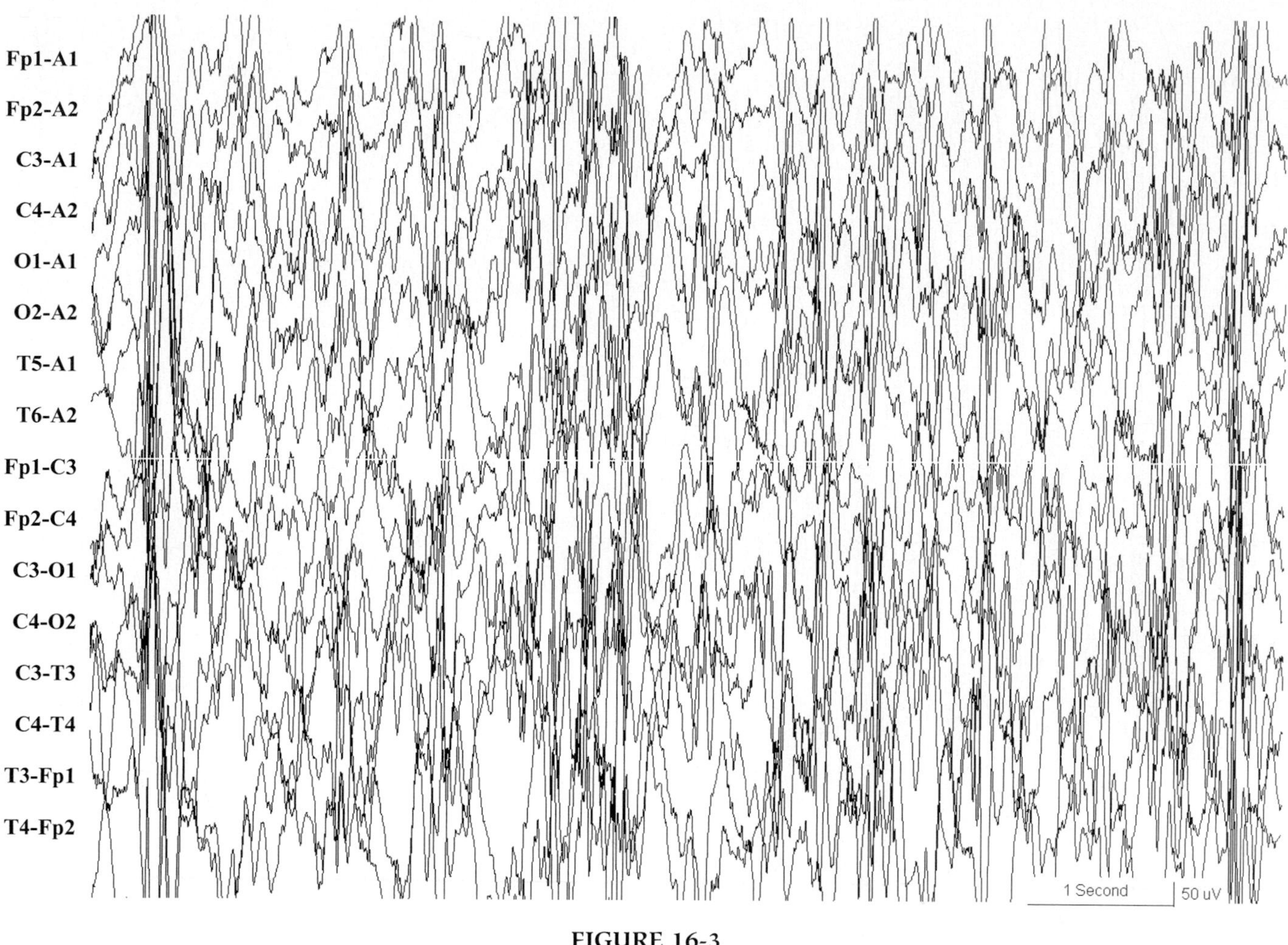

FIGURE 16-3

Hypsarrhythmia. Digital recording from a 6-month-old male.

> repetitive and highly organized pattern that could be confused with a discharge of the petit mal or petit mal variant type. The abnormality is almost continuous, and in most cases it shows as clearly in the waking as in the sleeping record.

This prototypic pattern is usually seen in the early stages of the disorder and most often in younger infants (younger than 1 year of age). The pattern has been reported in 7% to 75% of patients with infantile spasms (10, 12, 37–41). In addition, variations or modifications of this pattern may be seen in many patients. In 1984, we identified five variations of the originally described pattern after reviewing the 24-hour EEG-video monitoring studies in 67 infants with infantile spasms (29). These variations include hypsarrhythmia with a consistent focus of abnormal discharge, hypsarrhythmia with increased interhemispheric synchronization, hypsarrhythmia comprising primarily high-voltage, slow-wave activity with very little spike or sharp wave activity, asymmetrical or unilateral hypsarrhythmia, and hypsarrhythmia with episodes of generalized, regional, or localized voltage attenuation, which, in its maximal expression, is referred to as the "suppression-burst variant." These variations were subsequently confirmed by Alva-Moncayo et al (37) in 100 cases.

In addition to demonstrating these basic variations, 24-hour EEG-video monitoring studies have shown that hypsarrhythmia is a highly dynamic pattern, with transient alterations in the pattern occurring throughout the day. The hypsarrhythmic activity tends to be most pronounced and to persist to the latest age in slow-wave (non-rapid-eye movement [NREM]) sleep. During NREM sleep there is a tendency for grouping of the multifocal spike and sharp wave discharges resulting in a quasi-periodic appearance of the background activity (29, 42, 43). Also during NREM sleep, attenuation episodes frequently occur. The hypsarrythmic pattern is least evident or completely absent during REM sleep, when the background activity may

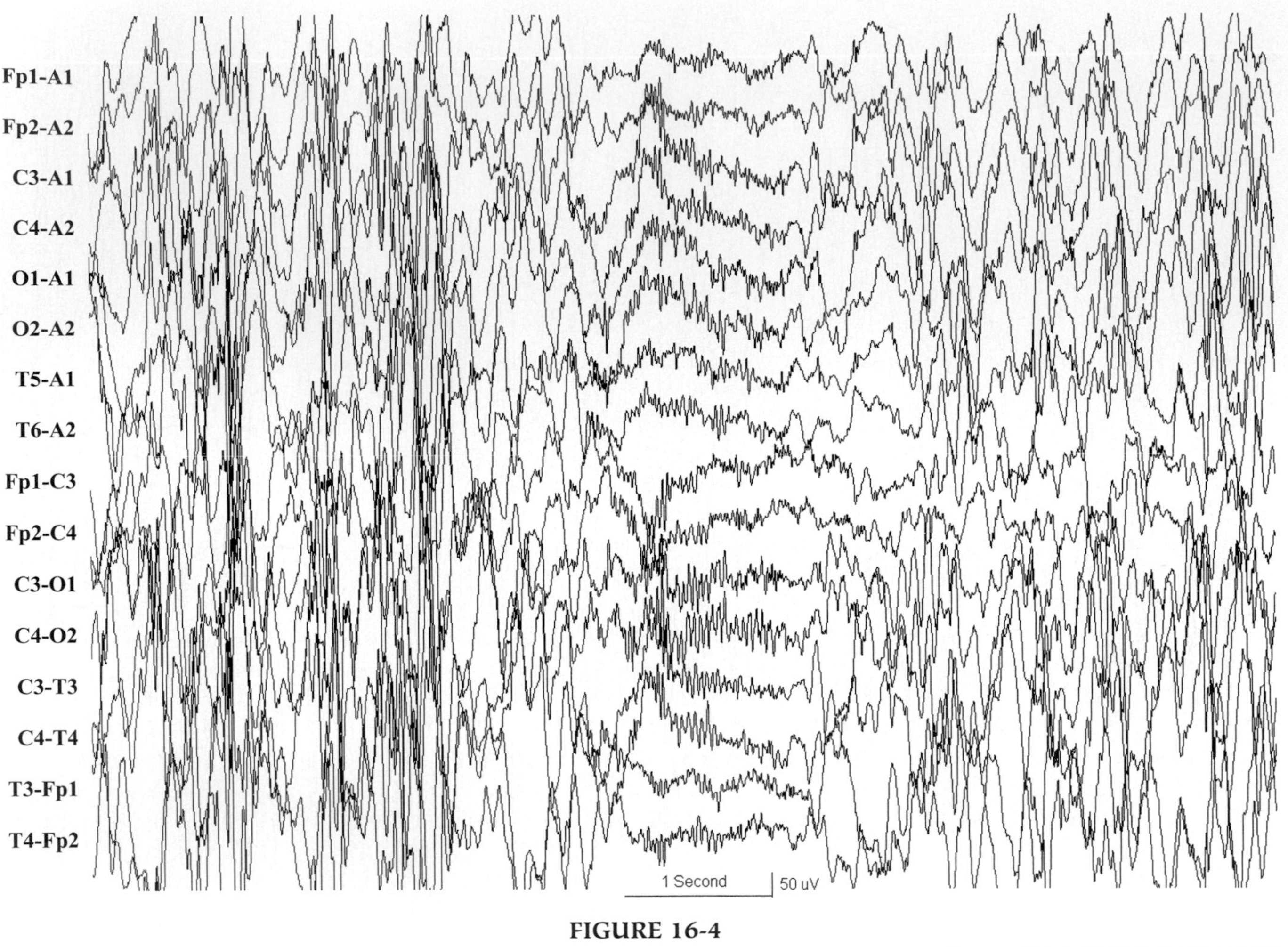

FIGURE 16-4

Digital recording from a 6-month old male showing ictal EEG change associated with infantile spasms. Note the period of voltage attenuation associated with superimposed fast activity.

appear normal (42). Transient disappearance or reduction of the hypsarrhythmic activity is usually seen on arousal from sleep; this normalization may last from a few seconds to many minutes. In addition, there is usually a reduction or disappearance of the hypsarrhythmic pattern during a cluster of spasms, with the pattern returning immediately following cessation of the spasms (15).

Although hypsarrythmia or one of its variants is most commonly seen in patients with infantile spasms, several other interictal patterns may occur (1, 26). These include diffuse slowing of the background activity, focal slowing, focal or multifocal spikes and sharp waves, generalized slow-spike-and-slow-wave activity, focal depression, paroxysmal slow or fast bursts, or continuous spindling. These patterns may occur in isolation or in various combinations. In a small number of infants, the background activity may appear normal.

Ictal Patterns

A variety of ictal EEG patterns have been identified (15). These include generalized slow-wave transients, sharp-and-slow-wave transients, and attenuation episodes, occurring alone or with superimposed faster frequencies. These patterns occur singly or in various combinations. However, the most common ictal EEG change is a generalized slow-wave transient, followed by an abrupt attenuation of background activity in all regions (Fig 16-4). The duration of the ictal EEG event may range from less than 1 second to more than 1 minute, with the longer episodes being associated with arrest phenomena. Also, episodes of generalized voltage attenuation may occur in the absence of clinical spasms. These observations have been confirmed by many authors (16, 33, 44–55). There is no close correlation between the character of the ictal EEG event and the type of spasm, with the exception that an asymmetric ictal pattern usually correlates with focal or lateralized brain lesions (47, 56).

PATHOPHYSIOLOGY

The pathophysiological mechanism underlying infantile spasms is not known, and a suitable animal model exhibiting the major clinical and electroencephalographic features of this disorder has yet to be developed. At present, it is not even known whether the disorder occurs in any species other than humans. For those interested in a thorough discussion of the proposed pathophysiological mechanisms underlying this disorder, it is suggested that the reader review our recently published study on this topic (1). Here, we will provide only a brief overview of some of the hypotheses that have been proposed.

Considerable evidence implicates the brainstem as the area in which epileptic spasms and the hypsarrhythmic EEG pattern originate (42, 57–61). We previously described a pathophysiological model of infantile spasms, based on our long-term polygraphic-video monitoring experience (42, 62), which suggested that dysfunction of certain monoaminergic or cholinergic regions of the brainstem involved in the control of sleep cycling may be responsible for the generation of the spasms and the EEG changes seen in this disorder (62). According to this model, the clinical spasms would result from phasic interference of descending brainstem pathways that control spinal reflex activity, whereas the hypsarrhythmic EEG pattern, and perhaps the cognitive dysfunction seen in these patients, would result from activity occurring in ascending pathways projecting from these brainstem regions to the cerebral cortex. Various other investigators have also suggested that dysfunction of monoaminergic neurotransmitter systems may be responsible for the generation of epileptic spasms (63–68). It has also been reported that corticosteroids (65) and ACTH (69) suppress central serotonergic activity, a finding consistent with this brainstem hypothesis. However, this model did not exclude the possibility that these critical brainstem region(s) might be affected by distant sites, because the brainstem sleep system receives input from many other areas (62). Several years later, Chugani and coworkers (60, 70) expanded our hypothesis. Primarily on the basis of PET scan studies, these authors suggested that the brainstem dysfunction causing infantile spasms was produced by an abnormal functional interaction between the brainstem (raphe nuclei) and a focal or diffuse cortical abnormality. According to this hypothesis, the cortical abnormality exerts a noxious influence over the brainstem from where the discharges spread caudally and rostrally to produce spasms and the hypsarrhythmic EEG pattern. The association of partial seizures with infantile spasms (described previously) was further evidence used to support the hypothesis that a primary cortical generator interacts with subcortical structures, resulting in infantile spasms. This model provides for the observation that a subset of infantile spasms patients with localized lesions in the cortex may have cessation of seizures and improved EEGs after resection of focal cortical lesions (70–73). A similar model proposing that spasms arise from subcortical structures was provided by Dulac et al (74). This group hypothesized that the epileptic spasms result from a functional deafferentation of subcortical structures such as the basal ganglia caused by abnormal cortical activity, but the hypsarrhythmic EEG pattern directly reflects the cortical dysfunction. A cortical-subcortical interaction was also postulated by Avanzini et al (75) and Lado and Moshe (76).

Another major hypothesis is that infantile spasms is the result of a defect in the immunological system (62, 77, 78). Supportive evidence for this hypothesis includes the presence of antibodies to extracts of normal brain tissue in the sera of patients with infantile spasms (79, 80), the presence of increased numbers of activated B cells and T cells in the peripheral blood of patients with infantile spasms (81), and abnormal leukocyte antigen studies in patients with infantile spasms compared with control subjects (82–84). Although these findings indicate abnormal immune function in patients with infantile spasms, there is no direct evidence that an immunologic defect causes this disorder.

Another hypothesis is that corticotropin-releasing hormone (CRH) may play a mechanistic role in infantile spasms (85–87). According to this model, stress or injury during early infancy results in the release of excess amounts of CRH, which in the presence of an abundance of CRH receptors, produces epileptogenic alterations in the brainstem pathways that result in spasms. The therapeutic benefit of corticosteroids and ACTH in this disorder would be secondary to the suppression of CRH synthesis by these hormones. However, although injection of CRH into the brains of infant rodents does produce seizures, the ictal behaviors and EEG features are not typical of those seen in the human condition (88). In addition, CRH levels are not elevated in the cerebrospinal fluid (CSF) of patients with infantile spasms (86). Furthermore, treatment of patients with infantile spasms with a competitive antagonist of CRH did not alter spasm frequency or significantly change the EEG pattern (89).

Several additional pathophysiological mechanisms underlying this disorder have also been proposed. It has been suggested that infantile spasm results from a failure or delay of normal developmental processes (90). This theory is based largely on the assumption that ACTH and corticosteroids accelerate certain normal developmental processes in immature animals (91–95).

Also, several biochemical and metabolic disturbances have been reported in patients with infantile spasms. These include dysfunction of metabolic pathways for neuropeptides, pyridoxine, and amino acids, such as aspirate, glutamate, and gamma-aminobutyric acid (1).

Finally, there are 13 genetically based conditions associated with infantile spasms (1), some of which involve the same region of the X chromosome. For example, Aicardi syndrome has been associated with X chromosome abnormalities near Xp22 (96). Patients with incontinentia pigmenti type I have abnormalities in the same region, with evidence of X/autosomal translocation at Xp11 (97). Patients with X-linked infantile spasms have mutations involving the ARX gene located on the X chromosome at Xp22 (98–102) and the CDKL5 (STK9) gene (103–109). Pyruvate dehydrogenase complex deficiency, a metabolic defect associated with infantile spasms, has been localized to Xp22.1–Xp22.2, a region similar to that associated with X-linked infantile spasms (110). These findings suggest that defects in the involved region of the X chromosome and products of the involved gene (or genes) may play a role in the pathophysiology of this disorder (1, 101, 111).

Recently, we proposed a new model concerning the pathophysiology of this disorder based on developmental desynchronization (112). According to this model, infantile spasms results from a particular temporal desynchronization of two or more developmental processes, resulting in a specific disturbance of brain function. As shown in Figure 16-5, the developmental desynchronization could be produced by (1) a mutation or inherited abnormality affecting the primary genes governing ontogenesis, (2) a mutation or inherited abnormality affecting the genes specifying transcription factors (or other genetic modulators), or (3) an injurious external environmental factor affecting the maturational processes of brain tissues, neurochemical systems, or both. Each mechanism (or combination of mechanisms) could be manifested at different locations and at different points of development. As a

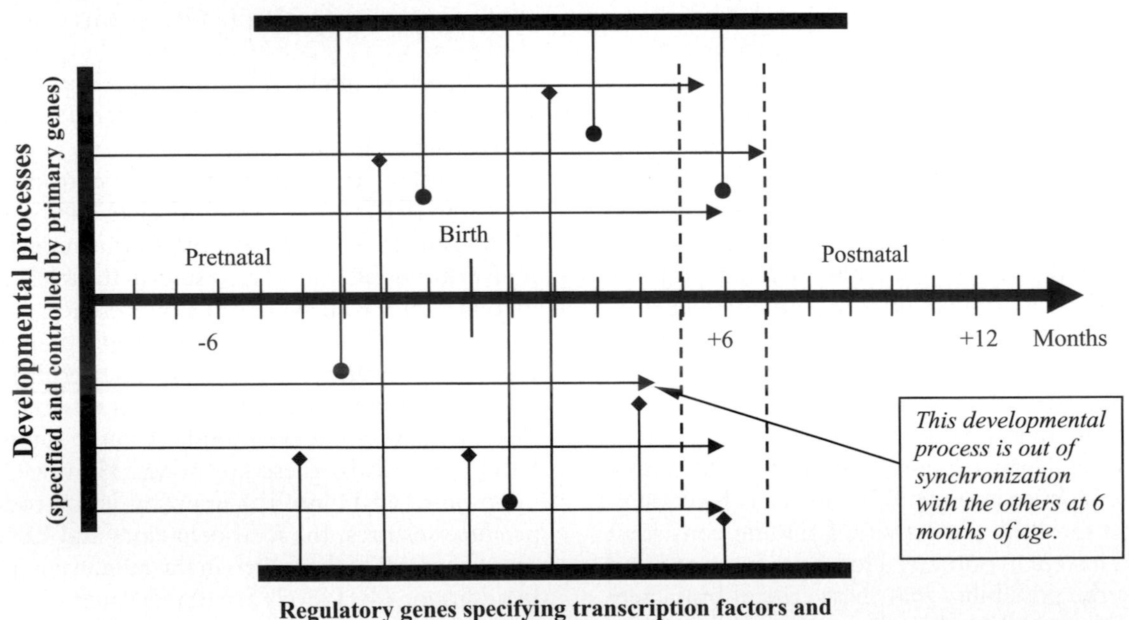

FIGURE 16-5

Developmental desynchronization model of infantile spasms pathogenesis showing schematically the interaction of developmental processes controlled by primary genes (e.g., neurogenesis, myelination, synaptogenesis, apoptosis, neurotransmitter systems) (horizontal lines) with regulatory gene effects (vertical lines from bottom) and environmental factors (vertical lines from top). Vertical dashed lines indicate hypothetical maximal extent of desynchronization consistent with normal function at 6 months. Reprinted from J.D. Frost, Jr. and R.A. Hrachovy, Pathogenesis of infantile spasms: A model based on developmental desynchronization, *J. Clin Neurophysiol.* 22:25–36, Figure 1, page 28; copyright 2005, with kind permission from Wolters Kluwer/Lippincott Williams & Wilkins.

result, at least one developmental process would lag behind other processes, resulting in a loss of integration of brain function. This model would allow for the observation that multiple, seemingly unrelated, conditions and insults occurring at different points of development (prenatal, perinatal, or postnatal) could result in the same functional deficit. Also, this hypothetical model would be consistent with the response of patients with infantile spasms to a diverse group of therapeutic agents with different modes of action. All agents would not be effective in all patients because of the different fundamental impairments responsible for the common functional deficit resulting in spasms. Also, the phenomenon of spontaneous remission could result from internal control mechanisms detecting the developmental desynchronization that caused spasms and responding to it by the activation or modulation of other gene regulatory systems.

DIAGNOSTIC EVALUATION AND TREATMENT

Diagnostic Evaluation

The diagnosis of infantile spasms is suggested on the basis of a good clinical history. Thorough general physical and neurological examinations must be performed. This should include a careful ophthalmic evaluation and close examination of the skin using a Wood's lamp to rule out such conditions as tuberous sclerosis. A routine EEG, recorded with the infant awake and asleep, is then obtained, which helps confirm the diagnosis. If the routine EEG does not reveal hypsarrhythmia and if the typical ictal EEG patterns (described previously) or spasms are not recorded, a prolonged video-EEG monitoring study should be performed to establish the presence of the disorder. Neuroimaging studies, preferably MRI, should be obtained to search for structural brain abnormalities. If ACTH or corticosteroids are to be started, the neuroimaging studies should be obtained before institution of such therapy, because these agents produce enlargement of CSF spaces that cannot be easily distinguished from preexisting cerebral atrophy. Routine laboratory studies including complete blood count with differential, renal panel with electrolytes and glucose, liver panel, serum calcium, magnesium, and phosphorus, and urinalysis should be obtained in all cases before institution of therapy. If an associated etiology is not identified on the basis of the previous information, a metabolic workup including serum lactate and pyruvate, plasma ammonia, urine organic acids, serum and urine amino acids, and serum biotinidase should be obtained. Chromosomal analysis should be performed. The CSF should be evaluated for cell count, glucose, protein, viral and bacterial culture, lactate and pyruvate, and amino acids.

Associated Etiological and Clinical Factors

In approximately 40% of patients, no associated etiological factor can be clearly identified. In the other 60%, various prenatal, perinatal, and postnatal factors have been implicated. In our recent review of the more than 400 published reports concerning etiology (1) more than 200 associated conditions were identified. These include such prenatal conditions as cerebral dysgenesis (e.g., lissencephaly), intrauterine infection, hypoxia-ischemia, prematurity, and genetic disorders (e.g., tuberous sclerosis), perinatal conditions such as traumatic delivery and hypoxia-ischemia, and postnatal conditions such as inborn errors of metabolism (e.g., nonketotic hyperglycinemia), head injury, central nervous system (CNS) infection, hypoxia-ischemia, and intracranial hemorrhage.

Approximately 80% of patients with infantile spasms show some degree of mental and developmental retardation, and approximately the same percentage of patients have neurologic deficits (1).

Diffuse and focal abnormalities on MRI and CT scans may be seen in (70–80%) of cases. In addition, MRI may also reveal evidence of delayed myelination (113–115). PET reportedly detects focal or diffuse hypometabolic changes in up to 97% of patients with infantile spasms (116). However, these changes do not necessarily persist over time, suggesting that cortical hypometabolism in some patients with infantile spasms does not represent a structural lesion, but only a functional change (115, 117, 118).

Immunization

During the last several decades, there has been a major disagreement as to whether immunization is an etiological factor for infantile spasms. This is an important issue, not only from a medical standpoint but also from a legal point of view, as evidenced by the large number of lawsuits against manufacturers of vaccines. Of the various vaccines that have been reported to be associated with infantile spasms, the one most frequently implicated is the diphtheria-pertussis-tetanus (DPT) vaccine. The pertussis agent has generated the most concern, and a number of publications have reported its apparent relationship to the development of infantile spasms (119–125). The major problem in determining whether there is a causal relationship between DPT immunization and infantile spasms is that the vaccine is given at the same age as the usual onset of infantile spasms. Therefore, if a large population were studied, an association between infantile spasms and DPT immunization would be expected on the basis of coincidence alone. Few studies have approached this problem in a manner amenable to statistical analysis; however, those that have done so have demonstrated that the apparent association between DPT immunization and infantile spasms is coincidental and that no causal relationship exists (126–129).

Patient Classification

In the past, the classification of infantile spasm patients was variable and inconsistent (1, 26). Currently, patients are best classified on the basis of medical history, developmental history, neurologic examination, and neuroimaging studies (MRI, CT, and perhaps PET). Based on these criteria, patients can be divided into two main groups: cryptogenic or symptomatic. Those with no abnormality on neurologic examination, no known associated etiological factor, normal development before onset of the spasms, and normal neuroimaging studies are categorized as cryptogenic. Currently, approximately 20% of patients with infantile spasms are classified as cryptogenic (1), with the remaining 80% classified as symptomatic. This classification scheme can be helpful in the management of these patients because patients in the cryptogenic category have the best prognosis for spasm control and long-term developmental outcome (see following discussion).

Differential Diagnosis

The diagnosis of infantile spasms is often delayed for weeks or months because parents, and even physicians, do not recognize the motor phenomena as seizures. Colic, Moro reflexes, and startle responses are diagnoses frequently made by pediatricians. Parents also may confuse infantile spasms with hypnagogic jerks occurring during sleep, head banging, transient flexor-extensor posturing of trunk and extremities of nonepileptic origin, and other types of myoclonic activity.

Infants with benign myoclonic epilepsy in infancy (BMEI) may have repetitive jerks, but the seizures are much briefer than spasms, and the EEG during the seizures reveals 3-Hz spike-and-wave or polyspike-and-wave activity. The background EEG activity is usually normal. These myoclonic seizures are treated with standard anticonvulsants, and the long-term prognosis in these patients is favorable. Another type of myoclonic movement that has been reported to be confused with infantile spasms is so-called benign myoclonus of early infancy (130). Infants with this disorder reportedly have tonic and myoclonic movements involving either the axial or limb musculature, which, like infantile spasms, may occur in clusters. The age at onset of this disorder (3 to 8.5 months) coincides with the age at onset of infantile spasms. In none of the reported cases did these movements persist beyond the age of 2 years. Unlike patients with infantile spasm, infants with benign myoclonus of early infancy have normal development, normal neurologic examinations, and normal EEGs. The motor movements are not accompanied by EEG changes, thus suggesting a nonepileptiform basis for the events. Patients with severe myoclonic epilepsy in infancy (SMEI), a disorder that may be confused with infantile spasms, usually have a family history of seizures and the disorder often begins following a prolonged febrile seizure. Unilateral clonic seizures, generalized tonic-clonic seizures, and myoclonic seizures, but not epileptic spasms, typically occur in these patients. The EEG reveals generalized spike-and-wave or polyspike-and-wave activity (131–133). The seizures are typically refractory to anticonvulsants and mental retardation and neurological deficits are common. Epilepsy with myoclonic-astatic seizures (EMAS) may also be confused with infantile spasms. However, these patients experience brief myoclonic seizures, not epileptic spasms. The EEG typically shows spike-and-wave or polyspike-and-wave activity (134). Most patients are developmentally normal before onset of this disorder, which tends to be at a later age (7 months to 10 years) than infantile spasms.

Related Syndromes

Three different epilepsy syndromes—early myoclonic encephalopathy (EME), early infantile myoclonic epilepsy (EIEE) and Lennox-Gastaut syndrome—may be difficult to differentiate from infantile spasms. They may share a common pathophysiological basis, with each disorder being expressed at a different age. A comparison of the important ictal and interictal features of these disorders, as well as the other myoclonic epilepsies described previously, is provided in Table 16-1.

Ohtahara (135) proposed that the syndrome of infantile spasms, suppression-burst activity in the EEG, and developmental retardation, when seen in the first few months of life, represents a disorder different from that seen in older infants, and he termed this disorder early infantile epileptic encephalopathy (EIEE). This disorder, which has been reported by many authors (133, 136–143), has a high mortality rate. The major reported difference between EIEE and infantile spasms is that the suppression-burst pattern seen with EIEE is continuous during wakefulness and sleep, whereas infantile spasms are associated with hypsarrhythmia. However, as discussed previously, a suppression-burst variant of hypsarrhythmia may be seen in patients with infantile spasms. Without knowing the age and clinical history of the patient, it is not possible to differentiate between these two suppression-burst patterns. Another reported difference between EIEE and infantile spasms is that in infantile spasms the spasms occur almost entirely while the patient is awake, whereas the spasms associated with EIEE reportedly occur both during wakefulness and sleep (138, 142).

A similar syndrome, early myoclonic encephalopathy (EME), has an onset within the first few weeks of life (132, 133, 144). This syndrome differs from EIEE and infantile spasms chiefly by the main type of clinical seizure observed. EME patients reportedly have fragmentary myoclonus, whereas patients with infantile spasms and EIEE have epileptic spasms. However, EME patients reportedly begin to experience epileptic spasms as they grow older. Also, the EEG in EME shows a suppression-burst pattern, but it is

TABLE 16-1
Comparison of Childhood Epileptic Syndromes: Typical or Most Common Features

	Early Infantile Epileptic Encephalopathy	Early Myoclonic Encephalopathy	Infantile Spasms	Lennox-Gastaut Syndrome	Benign Myoclonic Epilepsy in Infancy	Severe Myoclonic Epilepsy in Infancy	Epilepsy with Myoclonic Astatic Seizures
Age of onset	0–3 m	0–3 m	3–8 m	1–8 y	1–2 y	3 m–7 y	7 m–10 y
Ictal events							
Epileptic (tonic) spasms	+++	+	+++	+	–	–	–
Tonic seizures	–	–	+	+++	–	+	+
Clonic seizures	–	–	+	+	–	+++	+
Tonic-clonic seizures	–	–	+	++	+	+	+
Myoclonic seizures	–	+++	+	+	+++	++	+++
Atonic seizures	–	–	–	+++	–	–	–
Absence seizures	–	–	–	+++	–	+	+
Partial seizures	++	++	++	++	–	++	–
Interictal EEG pattern							
Hypsarrhythmia	–	–	+++	–	–	–	–
Suppression-burst	+++	+++	+	–	–	–	–
Slow spike-wave	–	–	–	+++	–	–	–
Other abnormality	–	–	+	+	+	+++	+++
Normal	–	–	–	–	+++	–	–

+++ very common; ++ common; + occasional; – rare or never.
Reprinted from Frost JD Jr, Hrachovy RA, *Infantile Spasms*, Table 7.2, page 91, copyright © 2003 Kluwer Academic Publishers, with kind permission from Springer Science and Business Media.

reportedly less persistent than the suppression-burst pattern seen in EIEE. The various etiologies associated with these three disorders overlap, although EME has been reported to be associated primarily with metabolic disorders, whereas EIEE is more likely to be associated with structural brain abnormalities (133, 137, 142, 144–146).

It is usually not difficult to differentiate Lennox-Gastaut syndrome from infantile spasms in the infant younger than 1 year of age. However, in older patients, the myoclonic, brief tonic and atonic seizures seen in the patient with Lennox-Gastaut syndrome may be confused with infantile spasms, particularly on the basis of clinical description alone.

The fact that these syndromes transition from one to the other also complicates the issue. For example, an average of 71% of patients with EIEE transition to infantile spasms. Some of these patients then transition to Lennox-Gastaut syndrome. Some cases of EME reportedly transition to EIEE, and some cases of EIEE may evolve directly to Lennox-Gastaut (1, 136, 138, 147). In addition, an average of 17% of patients with infantile spasms will evolve to Lennox-Gastaut syndrome. If these disorders do share a common pathophysiological mechanism, with the stage of brain maturation being the only factor affecting the appearance of each disorder, it is difficult to explain why the following evolution is not seen in all or most patients: EME → EIEE → infantile spasms → Lennox-Gastaut syndrome. From this brief discussion, it is clear that much additional work is needed to clarify the relationship of these disorders.

Differentiation of infantile spasms from nonepileptic events, other types of myoclonic activity, and the three syndromes just described frequently requires that video-EEG monitoring studies be performed to capture the questionable episodes and thus provide a definitive diagnosis.

TREATMENT

No aspect of this disorder has created as much confusion and controversy as the area of therapy. During the past four decades, numerous studies on the treatment of infantile spasms have been published; however, the results of these studies are so diverse that no consensus exists, and no true "standard of care" has been established. In this section, we briefly review the prevailing attitudes and opinions on the treatment of this disorder and make recommendations for the most appropriate therapy based on the best available data.

Medical Therapy

Since 1958, when Sorel and Dusaucy-Bauloye (4) reported that treatment of patients with infantile spasms using ACTH resulted in cessation or amelioration of spasms and disappearance of the hypsarrhythmic EEG pattern, many reports have appeared on the treatment of this disorder with ACTH and corticosteroids and more traditional anticonvulsants (1, 148, 149). To date, most of these studies have been plagued with methodological shortcomings that hamper interpretation and comparison of results. Some of the problems encountered are the following:

1. The natural history of the disorder is not completely understood—particularly the phenomenon of spontaneous remission. As noted previously, we reported in a retrospective study (25) that spontaneous remission could begin within 1 month of onset of the disorder, and within 12 months of onset, one quarter of patients had disappearance of the hypsarrhythmic pattern and cessation of spasms. More recently, Appleton et al. (150) performed a comparative trial of vigabatrin and placebo and reported that 2 of 20 patients (10%) responded to placebo. In addition, there are several case reports documenting the spontaneous remission of infantile spasms (1, 151–153).
2. There have been marked variations in dosages of medications used and durations of treatment.
3. Usually, an objective method of determining treatment response (video-EEG monitoring) has not been used. Instead, most studies have relied on parental observation to determine spasm frequency, which, as we have shown in previous studies, is unreliable. As shown in Figure 16-6, parents often underestimate spasm frequency to such an extent that they might

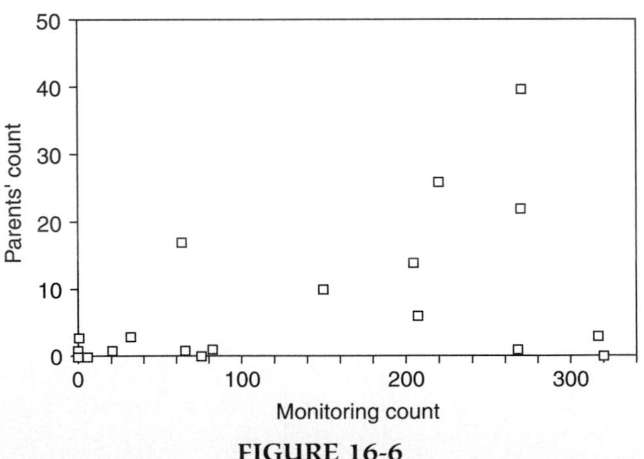

FIGURE 16-6

Spasm frequency after institution of ACTH or prednisone therapy: comparison of parents' estimates with results of 24-hour polygraphic-video monitoring. The coefficient of determination (r^2) between the parents' and video monitoring counts was 0.26. The 24-hour monitoring studies were performed 2 to 4 weeks after institution of ACTH or prednisone therapy. Patients who failed to respond to ACTH were treated with prednisone and vice versa. Sixteen patients eventually responded to hormonal therapy.

report that no spasms occurred in a child who, in fact, is experiencing many spasms per day. In 8 of 24 patients, parents reported complete cessation of spasms during ACTH or prednisone therapy; however, in 3 of these patients, the presence of spasms was documented by long-term polygraphic-video monitoring. Conversely, parents may report that spasms did occur in a child who, in reality, does not have spasms. These discrepancies are probably related to the fact that spasms often occur in clusters shortly after arousal from sleep; they occur relatively equally during the nighttime and daytime; they are relatively brief in duration and may be subtle in appearance, and they are easily confused with other types of infant behavior (see previous discussion).

4. In most studies, response to therapy has been defined in a graded fashion. However, there is no reliable evidence that spasms respond to any form of therapy in such a manner. Our long-term monitoring of patients with infantile spasms treated with ACTH and prednisone indicates that the response to therapy is an all-or-none phenomenon—complete control or no control (154–157). This point is emphasized in the Guidelines to Antileptic Drug Trials in Children (Commission, 1994 [158]).
5. Almost all reported studies were inadequately powered because of small study populations and so do not provide meaningful statistical data.
6. Few well-controlled, prospective studies have been performed. Most studies have been case reports or retrospective studies that are uncontrolled and unblinded (1, 26, 148, 149). In our initial analysis of the various therapeutic agents used to treat this disorder, we categorized 214 treatment studies into six different groups (1) (Table 16-2). The most rigorously designed studies are listed in the first column of the table. The remaining studies meeting progressively less stringent criteria are listed in the remaining columns. Only six studies (150, 156, 157, 159–161) were prospective, using blinded and randomized protocols. Furthermore, only eight studies (154–157, 159, 162, 163) used serial 24-hour video-EEG monitoring to determine response to therapy objectively. Of the 15 agents shown in the table, 8 have never been evaluated using prospective, blinded, and randomized protocols, or with 24-hour EEG/video monitoring.

In addition, Table 16-2 lists the response rates to the various agents used to treat these patients. The dosages and durations of treatment, side effects, formulations, proposed mechanisms of action, and response characteristics of each of these agents may be found in our review of the topic (1). Between 2003 and 2006, more than 30 additional studies reporting the effectiveness of various treatment modalities have been published. Review of these studies reveals that almost all of these studies suffer from the same methodological shortcomings described previously, with the exception of two randomized, controlled studies (164, 165).

Because of these methodological problems, several opinions have been published regarding the treatment of infantile spasms. After their review of the subject, Hancock and Osborne (148) concluded that no single treatment could be proven to be more efficacious than any other in terms of long-term psychomotor development or subsequent epilepsy rates. Vigabatrin may be more efficacious than placebo, and ACTH may be more efficacious than low doses of prednisone in stopping spasms. Vigabatrin may be more efficacious than hydrocortisone in stopping spasms in the group of patients with tuberous sclerosis. However, they found no treatment to be more efficacious than any other with regard to reduction in number of spasms, relapse rates, or resolution of hypsarrhythmia. Mackay et al (149) published a best practice parameter for the treatment of infantile spasms for the American Academy of Neurology and the Child Neurology Society. This group concluded that ACTH is probably effective in the short-term treatment of infantile spasms, but the evidence was insufficient to recommend the optimal dosage or duration of treatment. Vigabatrin is possibly effective in the short-term treatment of infantile spasms and possibly effective in children with tuberous sclerosis. However, there was insufficient evidence to recommend any other treatment for this disorder. Also, there was insufficient evidence to conclude that successful treatment of infantile spasms improves long-term prognosis.

On the basis of our analysis of the available data, we believe that it is reasonable to conclude that:

1. All agents listed in Table 16-2 have shown some efficacy in the treatment of infantile spasms.
2. As concerns treatment of this disorder with corti costeroids and ACTH, most investigators believe ACTH to be more effective.
3. There is no convincing evidence that higher doses of ACTH are more effective than lower doses of the drug.
4. Vigabatrin appears to be particularly effective in stopping the spasms in patients with tuberous sclerosis.
5. Response to any form of therapy usually occurs relatively quickly (within 1–2 weeks).
6. About 25% to 33% of patients will relapse after initial response to an agent.
7. There are no factors (e.g., treatment lag or patient classification) that can definitely be used to predict response to therapy.

TABLE 16-2

Summary of 214 Therapeutic Trials (1958–2002)

Therapy	Type of Trial											
	24h Mon.[a] Pros.[c] Rand.[d] Blinded		Subj.[b] Pros.[c] Rand.[d] Blinded		24h Mon.[a] Pros.[c] Open[e]		Subj.[b] Pros.[c] Open[e]		Retro.[f]		Case reports[g]	
	N[h]	%[i]	N[h]	%[i]	N[h]	%[i]	N[h]	%[i]	N[h]	%[i]	N[h]	%[i]
ACTH	3	42–58			1	74	11	20–94	27	7–93	25	0–100
ACTH (High dose)	2	50–87					1	93	4	54–100	6	50–100
Corticosteroid	2	29–33			1	25	3	33– 67	9	14–77	9	0–100
Vigabatrin			1	35	1	48	13	23–100	7	47–100	8	0–100
Nitrazepam	1						2	25	5	20–82	3	0–30
Valproate			1				2	22–50	4	18–43	5	0–50
Pyridoxine (vitamin B_6)							5	3–29	3	0–27	4	0–100
Surgery							1	61			16	0–100
Clonazepam							2	12	2	25–26	5	0–40
Immunoglobulin							2	26–82			4	33–43
TRH							2	47–54	1	31	1	
Zonisamide							3	20–36	2	38	2	33
Topiramate					1	45	2	33–50	1	15	2	20–57
Lamotrigine							4	15–29			1	100
Felbamate							1				2	75

[a]24h Mon. = 24-hour video-EEG monitoring.
[b]Subj. = Subjective observation by parent/caregiver and/or short-term video-EEG monitoring (< 24 hours).
[c]Pros. = Prospective design.
[d]Rand. = Randomized study.
[e]Open = Open-label design.
[f]Retro. = Retrospective design.
[g]Case reports = Case reports or trials with fewer than 11 subjects.
[h]N = Number of trials in category.
[i]% = Range of reported initial response to therapy is expressed as the percentage of patients exhibiting complete cessation of spasms.
Reprinted from Frost JD Jr, Hrachovy RA, *Infantile Spasms*, Table 11.1, page 168, copyright © 2003 Kluwer Academic Publishers, with kind permission from Springer Science and Business Media.

Surgical Therapy

Over the decades, several anecdotal reports have appeared reporting the beneficial effects of the surgical removal of anatomical lesions such as tumors and cysts (11, 72, 166–170). In recent years, there has been a greater emphasis on the surgical treatment of infantile spasms in patients with focal abnormalities on EEG, CT, MRI, or PET. In one of the largest series, Chugani and coworkers (171) reported that 9 of 23 patients with either focal or lateralized hypometabolism (18 patients) or focal hypermetabolism (5 patients) on PET also had focal abnormalities on MRI, CT, or both. All 23 patients had focal EEG findings that matched focal areas of abnormality on PET; 15 patients underwent focal cortical resection and 8 underwent hemispherectomy. At an average follow-up of 28 months, 14 (64%) were reported to be seizure-free. Others (172, 173) have reported similar results. The most common pathological finding of the resected tissue was cortical dysplasia.

There are several problems in interpreting the results of these surgical studies.

1. Not all of the patients identified in these reports actually had infantile spasms at the time of surgery. Many of the patients had a prior history of infantile spasms, but at the time of surgery were actually experiencing other seizure types (e.g., partial seizures).
2. The time required for cessation of infantile spasms following surgical treatment is usually not provided. In most instances, it is not possible to determine whether spasms stopped immediately following surgery or weeks to months later. This point is extremely important when one considers the phenomenon of spontaneous remission.
3. Most patients who were treated surgically continued to receive medical therapy after surgical resections were performed.
4. In most cases, video-EEG monitoring was not used to document the presence of spasms immediately before surgery or the cessation of spasms following surgery.

The problem in determining the effect of surgical treatment on spasm frequency can be further demonstrated by comparing studies of the long-term outcome in a group of patients with surgically treated infantile spasms and in a group of patients who failed to respond to hormonal therapy but were not treated surgically. Of the 17 patients reportedly experiencing infantile spasms at the time of surgery in Chugani's series (171), 10 (59%) were reportedly seizure free at follow-up. In a study of 26 patients who failed to respond to hormonal therapy but were not treated surgically (174), 12 (46%) were seizure free at follow-up. Therefore, it is difficult to determine whether cessation of spasms in all of the surgically treated patients was secondary to the surgical procedure itself or to some other factor (i.e., spontaneous remission). Of equal importance is the question whether surgical treatment of patients with infantile spasms affects long-term development. Although some authors report that patients with infantile spasm treated surgically show some improvement in developmental skills following surgery (171), the degree of improvement is difficult to assess because of the limited developmental information provided and the lack of control subjects.

Despite these shortcomings, focal cortical resection and hemispherectomy may contribute significantly to the treatment of a select group of patients with infantile spasms with focal cortical abnormalities who have failed medical treatment.

Recommended Treatment Approach

Based on critical analysis of the data (1, 148, 149), no single drug demonstrates superior efficacy, and several different treatment modalities appear to exert an effect on this disorder. Also, as indicated previously, focal cortical resection or hemispherectomy may benefit a small number of patients who have failed medical therapy. Because it is not possible to predict which patient will respond to a particular medical treatment or surgical approach, the following systematic approach is recommended (Fig 16-7). The primary goal is to obtain a therapeutic response (cessation of spasms and EEG improvement) as soon as possible and to avoid prolonged treatment with ineffective drugs. If the patient fails to respond to one modality, it should be immediately stopped, and another agent immediately initiated. The specific implementation guidelines for each modality are shown in Table 16-3.

As discussed previously, prolonged video-EEG monitoring is the best method to use to determine if a response to treatment has occurred. However, if long-term video-EEG monitoring is not available, or if such monitoring is not reimbursed by third-party payors, the physician will have to rely on the observations of parents and the results of routine EEG studies to evaluate treatment response. In this situation, if the caregiver has not observed spasms during close observation for at least five consecutive days, and if a repeat EEG, including a sleep recording, reveals disappearance of the hypsarrhythmic pattern, it can be assumed that a response has occurred. If a relapse occurs, the treatment protocol should be restarted, beginning with the agent that previously produced a response.

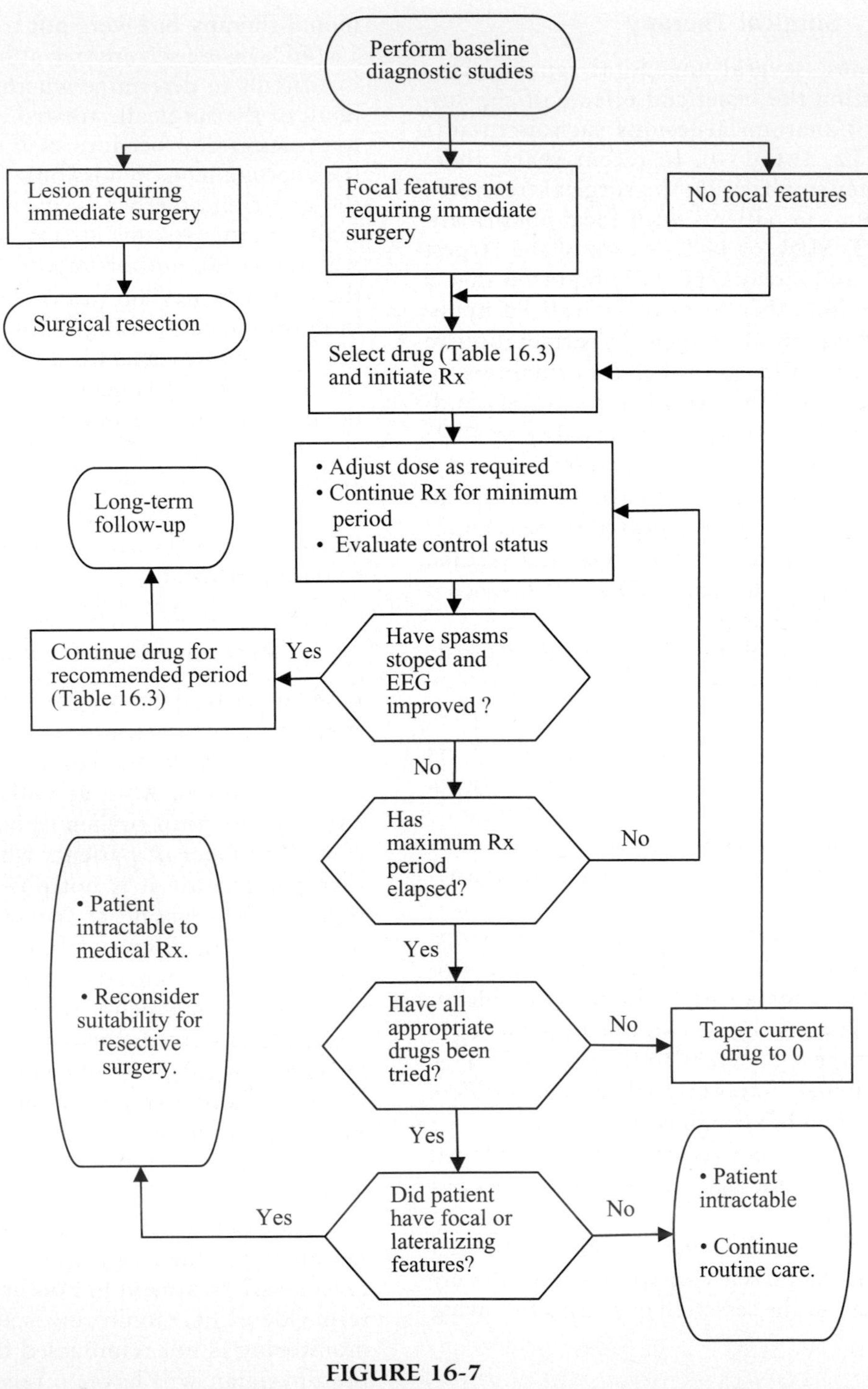

FIGURE 16-7

Flowchart summarizing recommended approach to the treatment of infantile spasms. Reprinted from J.D. Frost Jr. and R.A. Hrachovy, *Infantile Spasms*, Fig. 11.4, page 197; copyright 2003, Kluwer Academic Publishers, with kind permission from Springer Science and Business Media.

COURSE AND PROGNOSIS

Unique to medical treatment of infantile spasms has been the belief that treatment with various modalities not only improves the EEG and stops the spasms but also improves the outlook for mental and motor development. However, there is no conclusive evidence that such treatment alters the developmental or mental outcome in these patients. This is because the designs of most studies concerned with long-term outcome do not permit definitive

TABLE 16-3
Therapeutic Modalities with Demonstrated Efficacy in Infantile Spasms and Suggested Parameters for Implementation

Therapy	Initial Dose	Maximum Maintenance Dose	Minimum Duration of Therapy	Maximum Duration of Therapy if No Response	Continue Therapy if Response Occurs?
ACTH	20 u/day	30 u/day	2 weeks (plus 1 week taper)	6 weeks (plus 1 week taper)	No
Corticosteroid (prednisone)	2 mg/kg/day	2 mg/kg/day	2 weeks (plus 1 week taper)	6 weeks (plus 1 week taper	No
Vigabatrin[a]	50 mg/kg/day	200 mg/kg/day	N/A[b]	8 weeks	Yes[c]
Nitrazepam[a]	1 mg/kg/day	10 mg/kg/day	N/A[b]	12 weeks	Yes[c]
Valproate	40 mg/kg/day	100 mg/kg/day	N/A[b]	8 weeks	Yes[c]
Pyridoxine (vitamin B_6)	100 mg/day or 20 mg/kg/day	400 mg/day or 50 mg/kg/day	1 week	2 weeks	Yes[c]
Topiramate	12 mg/kg/day	24 mg/kg/day	N/A[b]	8 weeks	Yes[c]
Zonisamide	3 mg/kg/day	13 mg/kg/day	N/A[b]	6 weeks	Yes[c]
Immunoglobulin	100–400 mg/kg/day × 1–5 days	400 mg/kg/day × 5 days every 6 weeks	5 days	8 weeks	Yes, up to 6 months
TRH	0.05–0.5 mg/kg/day	1.0 mg/kg/day	2 weeks	4 weeks	No
Surgery	N/A[b]	N/A[b]	N/A[b]	N/A[b]	N/A[b]

[a]These drugs are not approved for general use in the United States.
[b]N/A = Not applicable to this form of therapy.
[c]An attempt at discontinuation is suggested after several months.
Reprinted from Frost JD Jr, Hrachovy RA, *Infantile Spasms*, Table 11.4, page 195, copyright © 2003 Kluwer Academic Publishers, with kind permission from Springer Science and Business Media.

conclusions to be reached. Past studies of long-term prognosis have typically been retrospective, and older studies did not use such diagnostic tests as CT and MRI scans to aid in classifying patients as symptomatic or cryptogenic. Various treatment protocols have been used, and many patients were treated with multiple agents. No placebo-treated groups were included for analysis, and times for follow-up were not standardized. Also, in most studies, standardized tests of developmental and mental status were not utilized (1, 148, 149).

In our review of long-term outcome, we analyzed 67 studies (1). We included studies (minimum of 25 patients per study) for which populations were not preselected. The average duration of follow-up was 31 months in 52 studies that provided data concerning length of follow-up. Only 16% of the patients in these studies had normal development at follow-up, and approximately 47% continued to experience seizures. Symptomatic patients experienced a higher rate of seizure occurrence (54%) compared to cryptogenic patients (23%). The most common seizures observed were tonic, generalized tonic-clonic, and simple partial seizures. Lennox-Gastaut syndrome developed in an average of 17% of patients. Abnormal EEG findings were seen in 61% of patients and 44% had persistent neurologic deficits. The average mortality rate was 12% (mortality has declined slightly over the decades, and this is probably related to better medical care).

Many factors have been reported to be predictive of a good outcome. In our analysis, the most favorable predictive factor was classification into the cryptogenic category. The percentage of cryptogenic patients with normal development (51%) was significantly higher than that of symptomatic patients (6%). Each of the criteria defining the cryptogenic category (normal neuroimaging, normal development before onset of spasms, and absence of associated etiological factors) may also be good prognostic indicators, but additional information is needed to confirm these observations. A sustained response to therapy (no relapse) and the absence of other seizure types are also factors predicting a favorable outcome. The evidence that other factors frequently mentioned in the literature (e.g., a classic hypsarrhythmic pattern, older age at onset, and short treatment lag) are associated with a good outcome is less convincing.

References

1. Frost JD Jr, Hrachovy RA. Infantile spasms. Boston, MA: Kluwer Academic Publishers, 2003.
2. West WJ. On a peculiar form of infantile convulsions. *Lancet* 1841; 1:724–725.
3. Gibbs FA, Gibbs EL. Atlas of electroencephalography. Vol. 2. Epilepsy. Cambridge: Addison-Wesley, 1952.
4. Sorel L, Dusaucy-Bauloye A. A propos de 21 cas d'hyp-sarythmie de Gibbs. Son traitement spectaculaire par l'A. C. T. H. *Acta Neurol Psychiatr Belg* 1958; 58:130–141.
5. Frost JD Jr, Hrachovy RA, Kellaway P, Zion T. Quantitative analysis and characterization of infantile spasms. *Epilepsia* 1978; 19:273–282.
6. van den Berg BJ, Yerushalmy J. Studies on convulsive disorders in young children. I. Incidence of febrile and nonfebrile convulsions by age and other factors. *Pediatr Res* 1969; 3:298–304.
7. Liou HH, Oon PC, Lin HC, Wang PJ, et al. Risk factors associated with infantile spasms: a hospital-based case-control study in Taiwan. *Epilepsy Res* 2001; 47:91–98.
8. Sidenvall R, Eeg-Olofsson O. Epidemiology of infantile spasms in Sweden. *Epilepsia* 1995; 36:572–574.
9. Trojaborg W, Plum P. Treatment of "hypsarrhythmia" with ACTH. *Acta Paediatr Scand* 1960; 49:572–582.
10. Druckman R, Chao D. Massive spasms in infancy and childhood. *Epilepsia* 1955; 4:61–72.
11. Gibbs EL, Fleming MM, Gibbs FA. Diagnosis and prognosis of hypsarrythmia and infantile spasms. *Pediatrics* 1954; 33:66–72.
12. Jeavons PM, Bower BD. Infantile spasms: a review of the literature and a study of 112 cases. Clinics in Developmental Medicine, No. 15. London: Spastics Society and Heinemann, 1964.
13. Kurokawa T, Goya N, Fukuyama Y, et al. West syndrome and Lennox-Gastaut syndrome: a survey of natural history. *Pediatrics* 1980; 65:81–88.
14. Lombroso CT. A prospective study of infantile spasms. *Epilepsia* 1983; 24:135–158.
15. Kellaway P, Hrachovy RA, Frost JD Jr, Zion T. Precise characterization and quantification of infantile spasms. *Ann Neurol* 1979; 6:214–218.
16. King DW, Dyken PR, Spinks IL Jr, Murvin AJ. Infantile spasms: ictal phenomena. *Pediatr Neurol* 1985; 1:213–218.
17. Hrachovy RA, Frost JD Jr. Intensive monitoring of infantile spasms. In: Schmidt D, Morselli PL, eds. *Intractable Epilepsy: Experimental and Clinical Aspects*. New York: Raven Press, 1986:87–97.
18. Horita H. Epileptic seizures and sleep-wake rhythm. *Psychiatr Clin Neurosci* 2001; 55:171–172.
19. Ohtsuka Y, Oka E, Terasaki T, Ohtahara S. Aicardi syndrome: a longitudinal clinical and electroencephalographic study. *Epilepsia* 1993; 34:627–634.
20. Plouin P, Jalin C, Dulac O, Chiron C. [Ambulatory 24-hour EEG recording in epileptic infantile spasms]. *Rev Electroencephalogr Neurophysiol Clin* 1987; 17:309–318.
21. Baird HW. Convulsions in infancy and childhood. *Conn Med* 1959; 23:149–151.
22. Taylor FM. Myoclonic seizures in infancy and childhood. *Tex Med* 1952; 46:647–649.
23. Gaily E, Liukkonen E, Paetau R, Rekola R, Granstrom ML. Infantile spasms: diagnosis and assessment of treatment response by video-EEG. *Dev Med Child Neurol* 2001; 43:658–667.
24. Jeavons PM, Bower BD, Dimitrakoudi M. Long-term prognosis of 150 cases of "West syndrome." *Epilepsia* 1973; 14:153–164.
25. Hrachovy RA, Glaze DG, Frost JD Jr. A retrospective study of spontaneous remission and long-term outcome in patients with infantile spasms. *Epilepsia* 1991; 32:212–214.
26. Lacy JR, Penry JK. *Infantile Spasms*. New York: Raven Press, 1976.
27. Kellaway P. Neurologic status of patients with hypsarrhythmia. In: Gibbs FA, ed. *Molecules and Mental Health*. Philadelphia, PA: Lippincott, 1959:134–149.
28. Fukuyama Y. Studies on the etiology and pathogenesis of flexor spasms. *Adv Neurol Sci (Tokyo)* 1960; 4:861–867.
29. Hrachovy RA, Frost JD Jr, Kellaway P. Hypsarrhythmia: variations on the theme. *Epilepsia* 1984; 25:317–325.
30. Bour F, Chiron C, Dulac O, Plouin P. Caract´electro-eres ´cliniques des crises dans le syndrome d'Aicardi. *EEG Neurophysiol Clin* 1986; 16:341–353.
31. Carrazana EJ, Barlow JK, Holmes GL. Infantile spasms provoked by partial seizures. *J Epilepsy* 1990; 3:97–100.
32. Carrazana EJ, Lombroso CT, Mikati M, Helmers S, et al. Facilitation of infantile spasms by partial seizures. *Epilepsia* 1993; 34:97–109.
33. Donat JF, Wright FS. Simultaneous infantile spasms and partial seizures. *J Child Neurol* 1991; 6:246–250.
34. Plouin P, Jalin C, Dulac O, Chiron C. Enregistrement ambulatoire de l'EEG pendant 24 heures dans les spasmes infantiles epileptiques. *Rev EEG Neurophysiol Clin* 1987; 17:309–318.
35. Yamamoto N, Watanabe K, Negoro I, et al. Partial seizures evolving to infantile spasms. *Epilepsia* 1988; 29:34–40.
36. Hrachovy RA, Frost JD Jr, Glaze DG. Coupling of focal electrical seizure discharges with infantile spasms: incidence during long-term monitoring in newly diagnosed patients. *J Clin Neurophysiol* 1994; 11:461–464.
37. Alva-Moncayo E, Diaz-Leal MC, Olmos-Garcia de Alba G. [Electroencephalographic discoveries in children with infantile massive spasms in Mexico]. *Rev Neurol* 2002; 34:928–932.
38. Anandam R. Clinical and electroencephalographic study of infantile spasms. *Indian J Pediatr* 1983; 50:515–518.
39. Jacobi G, Neirich U. Symptomatology and electroencephalography of the "genuine" type of the West syndrome and its differential diagnosis from the other benign generalized epilepsies of infancy. *Epilepsy Res Suppl* 1992; 6:145–151.
40. Kholin AA, Mukhin K, Petrukhin AS, Il'ina ES. Electroencephalographic characteristics of West syndrome. *Zh Nevrol Psikhiatr Im S S Korsakova* 2002; 102:40–44.
41. Vacca G, de Falco FA, Natale S, et al. EEG findings in West syndrome: a follow-up of 20 patients. *Acta Neurol (Napoli)* 1992; 14:297–303.
42. Hrachovy RA, Frost JD Jr, Kellaway P. Sleep characteristics in infantile spasms. *Neurology* 1981; 31:688–694.
43. Watanabe K, Negoro T, Aso K, Matsumoto A. Reappraisal of interictal electroencephalograms in infantile spasms. *Epilepsia* 1993; 34:679–685.
44. Acharya JN, Wyllie E, Luders HO, et al. Seizure symptomatology in infants with localization-related epilepsy. *Neurology* 1997; 48:189–196.
45. Donat JF, Wright FS. Unusual variants of infantile spasms. *J Child Neurol* 1991; 6:313–318.
46. Fusco L, Vigevano F. Ictal clinical electroencephalographic findings of spasms in West syndrome. *Epilepsia* 1993; 34:671–678.
47. Gaily EK, Shewmon DA, Chugani HT, Curran JG. Asymmetric and asynchronous infantile spasms. *Epilepsia* 1995; 36:873–882.
48. Haga Y, Watanabe K, Negoro T, et al. Do ictal, clinical, and electroencephalographic features predict outcome in West syndrome? *Pediatr Neurol* 1995; 13:226–229.
49. Haga Y, Watanabe K, Negoro T, et al. Ictal electroencephalographic findings of spasms in West syndrome. *Psychiatr Clin Neurosci* 1995; 49:S233–234.
50. Panzica F, Franceschetti S, Binelli S, et al. Spectral properties of EEG fast activity ictal discharges associated with infantile spasms. *Clin Neurophysiol* 1999; 110:593–603.
51. Silva ML, Cieuta C, Guerrini R, et al. Early clinical and EEG features of infantile spasms in Down syndrome. *Epilepsia* 1996; 37:977–982.
52. Viani F, Romeo A, Mastrangelo M, Viri M. Infantile spasms combined with partial seizures: electroclinical study of eleven cases. *Ital J Neurol Sci* 1994; 15:463–471.
53. Vigevano F, Fusco L, Pachatz C. Neurophysiology of spasms. *Brain Dev* 2001; 23:467–472.
54. Wong M, Trevathan E. Infantile spasms. *Pediatr Neurol* 2001; 24:89–98.
55. Yamatogi Y, Ohtahara S. Age-dependent epileptic encephalopathy: a longitudinal study. *Folia Psychiatr Neurol Jpn* 1981; 35:321–332.
56. Donat JF, Lo WD. Asymmetric hypsarrhythmia and infantile spasms in west syndrome. *J Child Neurol* 1994; 9:290–296.
57. Morimatsu Y, Murofushi K, Handa T, Shinohara T, Shiraki H. Pathology in severe physical and mental disabilities in children—with special reference to four cases of nodding spasms. *Adv Neurol Sci (Tokyo)* 1972; 16:465–470.
58. Satoh J, Mizutani T, Morimatsu Y, et al. Neuropathology of infantile spasms. *Brain Dev* 1984; 6:196 (abstract).
59. Chugani HT, Mazziotta JC, Engel J Jr, Phelps ME. Positron emission tomography with 18F-2-fluorodeoxyglucose in infantile spasms. *Ann Neurol* 1984; 16:376–377.
60. Chugani HT, Shewmon DA, Sankar R, Chen BC, et al. Infantile spasms: II. Lenticular nuclei and brain stem activation on positron emission tomography. *Ann Neurol* 1992; 31:212–219.
61. Neville BG. The origin of infantile spasms: evidence from a case of hydranencephaly. *Dev Med Child Neurol* 1972; 14:644–647.
62. Hrachovy RA, Frost JD Jr. Infantile spasms: a disorder of the developing nervous system. In: Kellaway P, Noebels JL, eds. *Problems and Concepts in Developmental Neurophysiology*. Baltimore. MD: Johns Hopkins University Press, 1989:131–147.
63. Coleman M. Infantile spasms associated with 5-hydro-xytryptophan administration in patients with Down's syndrome. *Neurology* 1971; 21:911–919.
64. Klawans HL Jr, Goetz C, Weiner WJ. 5-Hydroxytrypto-phan-induced myoclonus in guinea pigs and the possible role of serotonin in infantile myoclonus. *Neurology* 1973; 23:1234–1240.
65. Nausieda PA, Carvey PM, Braun A. Long-term suppression of central serotonergic activity by corticosteroids: a possible model of steroid-responsive myoclonic disorder. *Neurology* 1982; 32:772–775.

66. Ross DL, Anderson G, Shaywitz B. Changes in monoamine metabolites in CSF during ACTH treatment of infantile spasms. *Neurology* 1983; 33 Suppl 2:75 (abstract).
67. Silverstein F, Johnston MV. Cerebrospinal fluid monoamine metabolites in patients with infantile spasms. *Neurology* 1984; 34:102–104.
68. Yamamoto H, Egawa B, Horiguchi K, Kaku A, et al. [Changes in CSF tryptophan metabolite levels in infantile spasms]. *No To Hattatsu* 1992; 24:530–535.
69. Pranzatelli MR. In vivo and in vitro effects of adrenocorticotrophic hormone on serotonin receptors in neonatal rat brain. *Dev Pharmacol Ther* 1989; 12:49–56.
70. Chugani HT, Shields WD, Shewmon DA, et al. Infantile spasms: I. PET identifies focal cortical dysgenesis in cryptogenic cases for surgical treatment. *Ann Neurol* 1990; 27:406–413.
71. Uthman BM, Reid SA, Wilder BJ, Andriola MR, Beydoun AA. Outcome for West syndrome following surgical treatment. *Epilepsia* 1991; 32:668–671.
72. Wyllie E, Comair YG, Kotagal P, Raja S, et al. Epilepsy surgery in infants. *Epilepsia* 1996; 37:625–637.
73. Wyllie E, Comair Y, Ruggieri P, Raja S, et al. Epilepsy surgery in the setting of periventricular leukomalacia and focal cortical dysplasia. *Neurology* 1996; 46:839–841.
74. Dulac O, Chiron C, Robain O, et al. Infantile spasms: a pathophysiological hypothesis. *Semin Pediatr Neurol* 1994; 1:83–89.
75. Avanzini G, Panzica F, Franceschetti S. Brain maturational aspects relevant to pathophysiology of infantile spasms. *Int Rev Neurobiol* 2002; 49:353–365.
76. Lado FA, Moshe SL. Role of subcortical structures in the pathogenesis of infantile spasms: what are possible subcortical mediators? *Int Rev Neurobiol* 2002; 49:115–140.
77. Mandel P, Schneider J. Sur le mode d'action de l'A. C. T. H. dans l'E. M. I. H. In: Gastaut H, Roger J, Soulayrol R, Pinsard N, eds. *L'encephalopathie myoclonique infantile avec hypsarythmie*. Paris: Masson & Cie, 1964:177–189.
78. Martin F. Physiopathog´enie. In: Gastaut H,Roger J, Soulayrol R, Pinsard N, eds. *L'enc´ephalopathie myoclonique infantile avec hypsarythmie*. Paris: Masson & Cie, 1964:169–176.
79. Reinskov T. Demonstration of precipitating antibody to extract of brain tissue in patients with hypsarrhythmia. *Acta Paediatr Scand* 1963; 140 (Suppl). 73.
80. Mota NGS, Rezkallah-Iwasso MT, Peracoli MTS, Montelli TCB. Demonstration of antibody and cellular immune response to brain extract in West and Lennox-Gastaut syndromes. *Arq Neuropsiquiatr* 1984; 42:126–131.
81. Hrachovy RA, Frost JD Jr, Shearer WT, et al. Immunological evaluation of patients with infantile spasms. *Ann Neurol* 1985; 18:414 (abstract).
82. Hrachovy RA, Frost JD Jr, Pollack M, Glaze DG. Serologic HLA typing in infantile spasms. *Epilepsia* 1988; 29:817–819.
83. Howitz P, Platz P. Infantile spasms and HLA antigens. *Arch Dis Child* 1978; 53:680–682.
84. Suastegui RA, de la Rosa G, Carranza JM, Gonzalez-Astiazaran A, et al. Contribution of the MHC class II antigens to the etiology of infantile spasm in Mexican Mestizos. *Epilepsia* 2001; 42:210–215.
85. Baram TZ. Pathophysiology of massive infantile spasms (MIS): perspective on the role of the brain adrenal axis. *Ann Neurol* 1993; 33:231–237.
86. Baram TZ, Mitchell WG, Snead OC III, Horton EJ, et al. Brain-adrenal axis hormones are altered in the CSF of infants with massive infantile spasms. *Neurology* 1992; 42:1171–1175.
87. Brunson KL, Avishai-Eliner S, Baram TL. ACTH treatment of infantile spasms: mechanisms of its effects in modulation of neuronal excitability. *Int Rev Neurobiol* 2002; 49:185–197.
88. Baram TZ, Hirsch E, Snead OC III, Schultz L. Corticotropin-releasing hormone-induced seizures in infant rats originate in the amygdala. *Ann Neurol* 1992; 31:488–494.
89. Baram TZ, Mitchell WG, Brunson K, Haden E. Infantile spasms: hypothesis-driven therapy and pilot human infant experiments using corticotropin-releasing hormone receptor antagonists. *Dev Neurosci* 1999; 21:281–289.
90. Riikonen R. Infantile spasms: some new theoretical aspects. Epilepsia 1983; 24:159–168.
91. Palo J, Savolainen H. The effect of high doses of synthetic ACTH on rat brain. *Brain Res* 1974; 70:313–320.
92. Ardeleanu A, Sterescu N. RNA and DNA synthesis in developing rat brain: hormonal influences. *Psychoneuroendocrinology* 1978; 3:93–101.
93. Huttenlocher PR, Amemiya IM. Effects of adrenocortical steroids and of adrenocorticotrophic hormone on (Na+-K+)-ATPase in immature cerebral cortex. *Pediatr Res* 1978; 12:104–107.
94. Doupe AJ, Patterson PH. Glucocorticoids and the developing nervous system. In: Ganton D, Pfatt D, eds. *Current Topics in Neuroendocrinology: Adrenal Actions on Brain*. Berlin: Springer-Verlag, 1982:23–43.
95. Pranzatelli MR. On the molecular mechanism of adrenocorticotrophic hormone in the CNS: neurotransmitters and receptors. *Exp Neurol* 1994; 125:142–161.
96. Ropers HH, Zuffardi O, Bianchi E, Tiepolo L. Agenesis of corpus callosum, ocular, and skeletal anomalies (X-linked dominant Aicardi's syndrome) in a girl with balanced X/3 translocation. *Hum Genet* 1982; 61:64–68.
97. Hodgson SV, Neville B, Jones RW, Fear C, et al. Two cases of X/autosome translocation in females with incontinentia pigmenti. *Hum Genet* 1985; 71:231–234.
98. Stromme P, Sundet K, Mork C, et al. X linked mental retardation and infantile spasms in a family: new clinical data and linkage to Xp11.4–Xp22.11. *J Med Genet* 1999; 36:374–378.
99. Strømme P, Mangelsdorf MMS, Lower K, et al. Mutations in the human ortholog of Aristaless cause X-linked mental retardation and epilepsy. *Nat Genet* 2002; 30:441–445.
100. Bienvenu T, Poirier K, Friocourt, et al. ARX, a novel Prd-class-homeobox gene highly expressed in the telencephalon, is mutated in X-linked mental retardation. *Hum Mol Genet* 2002; 11:981–991.
101. Kato M, Dobyns WB. X-linked lissencephaly with abnormal genitalia as a tangential migration disorder causing intractable epilepsy: proposal for a new term, "interneuronopathy." *J Child Neurol* 2005; 63:392–397.
102. OMIM: National Center for Biotechnology Information (NCBI) online Human Genome Resources databases (http://www.ncbi.nlm.nih.gov/genome/guide/ human/), including Online Mendelian Inheritance in Man, (OMIM) [McKusick-Nathans Institute for Genetic Medicine, Johns Hopkins University, Baltimore, MD], MIM No. 300382.
103. Buoni S, Zannolli R, Colamaria V, et al. Myoclonic encephalopathy in the CDKL5 gene mutation. *Clin Neurophysiol* 2006; 117:223–227.
104. Evans JC, Archer HL, Colley JP, et al. Early onset seizures and Rett-like features associated with mutations in CDKL5. *Eur J Hum Genet* 2005; 25:1113–1120.
105. Kalscheuer VM, Tao J, Donnelly A, et al. Disruption of the serine/threonine kinase 9 gene causes severe X-linked infantile spasms and mental retardation. *Am J Hum Genet* 2003; 72:1401–1411.
106. OMIM: National Center for Biotechnology Information (NCBI) online Human Genome Resources databases (http://www.ncbi.nlm.nih.gov/genome/guide/ human/), including Online Mendelian Inheritance in Man, (OMIM) [McKusick-Nathans Institute for Genetic Medicine, Johns Hopkins University, Baltimore, MD], MIM No. 300203.
107. Scala E, Ariani F, Mari F, et al. CDLK5/STK9 is mutated in Rett syndrome variant with infantile spasms. *J Med Genet* 2005; 80:103–107.
108. Tao J, Van Esch H, Hagedorn-Greiwe M, et al. Mutations in the X-linked cyclin-dependent kinase-like (CDLK5/STK9) gene are associated with severe neurodevelopmental retardation. *Am J Hum Genet* 2004; 90:1149–1154.
109. Weaving LS, Christodoulou J, Williamson SL, et al. Mutations of CDLK5 cause a severe neurodevelopmental disorder with infantile spasms and mental retardation. *Am J Hum Genet* 2004; 91:1079–1093.
110. Borglum AD, Flint T, Hansen LL, Kruse TA. Refined localization of the pyruvate dehydrogenase E1 alpha gene (PDHA1) by linkage analysis. *Hum Genet* 1997; 99:80–82.
111. Partington MW, Turner G, Boyle J, Gecz J. Three new families with x-linked mental retardation caused by the 428-451 dup(24bp) mutation in ARX. *Clin Genet* 2004; 114:39–45.
112. Frost JD Jr, Hrachovy RA. Pathogenesis of infantile spasms: a model based on developmental desynchronization. *J Clin Neurophysiol* 2005; 22:25–36.
113. Schropp C, Staudt M, Staudt F, et al. Delayed myelination in children with West syndrome: an MRI-study. *Neuropediatrics* 1994; 25:116–120.
114. Kasai K, Watanabe K, Negoro T, et al. Delayed myelination in West syndrome. *Psychiatr Clin Neurosci* 1995; 49:S265–S266.
115. Natsume J, Watanabe K, Maeda N, et al. Cortical hypometabolism and delayed myelination in West syndrome. *Epilepsia* 1996; 37:1180–1184.
116. Chugani H, Conti J. Classification of infantile spasms in 139 cases: the role of positron emission tomography. *Epilepsia* 1994; 35 Suppl 8:19 (abstract).
117. Maeda N, Watanabe K, Negoro T, et al. Transient focal cortical hypometabolism in idiopathic West syndrome. *Pediatr Neurol* 1993; 9:430–434.
118. Maeda N, Watanabe K, Negoro T, et al. Evolutional change of cortical hypometabolism in West's syndrome. *Lancet* 1994; 343:1620–1623.
119. Baird HW, Borofsky LG. Infantile myoclonic seizures. *J Pediatr* 1957; 50:332–339.
120. Jeavons PM, Bower BD. Infantile spasms: a review of the literature and a study of 112 cases. Clinics in Developmental Medicine, No. 15. London: Spastics Society and Heinemann, 1964.
121. Kulenkampff M, Schwartzman JS, Wilson J. Neurological complications of pertussis inoculation. *Arch Dis Child* 1974; 49:46–49.
122. Miller DL, Ross EM, Alderslade R, Bellman MH, et al. Pertussis immunization and serious acute neurologic illness in children. *Br Med J (Clin Res)* 1981; 282:1595–1599.
123. Millichap JG, Bickford RG, Klass DW, Backus RE. Infantile spasms, hypsarrhythmia, and mental retardation. A study of etiologic factors in 61 patients. *Epilepsia* 1962; 3:188–197.
124. Strom J. Further experience of reactions, especially of a cerebral nature, in conjunction with triple vaccination: a study based on vaccinations in Sweden 1959–65. *Br Med J* 1967; 4:320–323.
125. Wilson J. Neurological complications of DPT inoculation in infancy. *Arch Dis Child* 1973; 48:829–830.
126. Bellman MH, Ross EM, Miller DL. Infantile spasms and pertussis immunization. *Lancet* 1983; 1:1031–1034.
127. Cody CL, Baraff LJ, Cherry JD, Marcy SM, et al. Nature and rates of adverse reactions associated with DPT and DT immunizations in infants and children. *Pediatrics* 1981; 68:650–660.
128. Fukuyama Y, Tomori N, Sugitate M. Critical evaluation of the role of immunization as an etiological factor of infantile spasms. *Neuropaediatrie* 1977; 8:224–237.
129. Melchior JC. Infantile spasms and early immunization against whooping cough. Danish survey from 1970 to 1975. *Arch Dis Child* 1977; 52:134–137.
130. Lombroso CT, Fejerman N. Benign myoclonus of early infancy. *Ann Neurol* 1977; 1:138–143.
131. Ogino T, Ohtsuka Y, Amano R, Yamatogi Y, et al. An investigation on the borderland of severe myoclonic epilepsy in infancy. *Jpn J Psychiatry Neurol* 1988; 42:554–555.
132. Commission on classification and terminology of the International League Against Epilepsy. Proposal for revised classification of epilepsies and epileptic syndromes. *Epilepsia* 1989; 30:389–399.
133. Lombroso CT. Early myoclonic encephalopathy, early infantile epileptic encephalopathy, and benign and severe infantile myoclonic epilepsies: a critical review and personal contributions. *J Clin Neurophysiol* 1990; 7:380–408.
134. Fejerman N. Differential diagnosis. In: Dulac O, Chugani H, Dalla Bernardina B, eds. *Infantile Spasms and West syndrome*. Philadelphia, PA: WB Saunders, 1994:88–98.

135. Ohtahara S. Clinico-electrical delineation of epileptic encephalopathies in childhood. *Asian Med* J 1978; 21:499–509.
136. Chakova L. On a rare form of epilepsy in infants—Ohtahara syndrome. *Folia Med (Plovdiv)* 1996; 38:69–73.
137. Chen PT, Young C, Lee WT, et al. Early epileptic encephalopathy with suppression burst electroencephalographic pattern—an analysis of eight Taiwanese patients. *Brain Dev* 2001; 23:715–720.
138. Clarke M, Gill J, Noronha M, McKinlay I. Early infantile epileptic encephalopathy with suppression burst: Ohtahara syndrome. *Dev Med Child Neurol* 1987; 29:520–528.
139. Itoh M, Hanaoka S, Sasaki M, Ohama E, et al. Neuropathology of early-infantile epileptic encephalopathy with suppression-bursts; comparison with those of early myoclonic encephalopathy and West syndrome. *Brain Dev* 2001; 23:721–726.
140. Martinez Bermejo A, Roche C, Lopez Martin V, Pascual Castroviejo I. Early infantile epileptic encephalopathy. *Rev Neurol* 1995; 23:297–300.
141. Trinka E, Rauscher C, Nagler M, et al. A case of Ohtahara syndrome with olivary-dentate dysplasia and agenesis of mamillary bodies. *Epilepsia* 2001; 42:950–953.
142. Wang PJ, Lee WT, Hwu WL, Young C, et al. The controversy regarding diagnostic criteria for early myoclonic encephalopathy. *Brain Dev* 1998; 20:530–535.
143. Ohtahara S, Ohtsuka Y, Yamatogi Y, Oka E. The early-infantile epileptic encephalopathy with suppression-burst: developmental aspects. *Brain Dev* 1987; 9:371–376.
144. Aicardi J. *Epilepsy in Children*. New York: Raven Press, 1986.
145. Ohtahara S, Ohtsuka Y, Oka E. Epileptic encephalopathies in early infancy. *Indian J Pediatr* 1997; 64:603–612.
146. Otani K, Abe J, Futagi Y, et al. Clinical and electroencephalographical follow-up study of early myoclonic encephalopathy. *Brain Dev* 1989; 11:332–337.
147. Ohtahara S, Ohtsuka Y, Yamatogi Y. The West syndrome: developmental aspects. *Acta Paediatr Jpn* 1987; 29:61–69.
148. Hancock E, Osborne J. Treatment of infantile spasms. *The Cochrane Database of Systematic Reviews* 2003:(3):CD001770. doi: 10.1002/14651858.CD001770.
149. Mackay MT, Weiss SK, Adams-Webber T, et al. Practice parameter: medical treatment of infantile spasms: Report of the American Academy of Neurology and the Child Neurology Society. *Neurology* 2004; 62:1668–1681.
150. Appleton RE, Peters AC, Mumford JP, Shaw DE. Randomised, placebo-controlled study of vigabatrin as first-line treatment of infantile spasms. *Epilepsia* 1999; 40:1627–1633.
151. Bachman DS. Spontaneous remission of infantile spasms with hypsarrhythmia. *Arch Neurol* 1981; 38:785 (abstract).
152. Hattori H. Spontaneous remission of spasms in West syndrome—implications of viral infection. *Brain Dev* 2001; 23:705–707.
153. Nalin A, Facchinetti F, Galli V, et al. Reduced ACTH content in cerebrospinal fluid of children affected by cryptogenic infantile spasms with hypsarrhythmia. *Epilepsia* 1985; 26:446–449.
154. Hrachovy RA, Frost JD Jr, Kellaway P, Zion T. A controlled study of prednisone therapy in infantile spasms. *Epilepsia* 1979; 20:403–407.
155. Hrachovy RA, Frost JD Jr, Kellaway P, Zion T. A controlled study of ACTH therapy in infantile spasms. *Epilepsia* 1980; 21:631–636.
156. Hrachovy RA, Frost JD Jr, Kellaway P, Zion TE. Double-blind study of ACTH vs prednisone therapy in infantile spasms. *J Pediatr* 1983; 103:641–645.
157. Hrachovy RA, Frost JD Jr, Glaze DG. High dose/long duration vs. low dose/short duration corticotropin therapy for infantile spasms: a single blind study. *J Pediatr* 1994; 124:803–806.
158. Commission. Guidelines for Antiepileptic Drug Trials in Children. Commission on Antiepileptic Drugs of the International League Against Epilepsy. *Epilepsia* 1994; 35:94–100.
159. Baram T, Mitchell WG, Tournay A, et al. High-dose corticotropin (ACTH) versus prednisone for infantile spasms: a prospective, randomized, blinded study. *Pediatrics* 1996; 97:375–379.
160. Dreifuss F, Farwell J, Holmes G, et al. Infantile spasms: comparative trial of nitrazepam and corticotropin. *Arch Neurol* 1986; 43:1107–1110.
161. Dyken PR, DuRant RH, Minden DB, King DW. Short-term effects of valproate on infantile spasms. *Pediatr Neurol* 1985; 1:34–37.
162. Glauser TA, Clark PO, Strawsburg R. A pilot study of topiramate in the treatment of infantile spasms. *Epilepsia* 1998; 39:1324–1328.
163. Vigevano F, Cilio MR. Vigabatrin versus ACTH as first-line treatment for infantile spasms: a randomized, prospective study. *Epilepsia* 1997; 38: 1270–1274.
164. Debus OM, Kurlemann G; for the study group. Sulthiame in the primary therapy of West syndrome: a randomized double-blind placebo-controlled add-on trial on baseline pyridoxine medication. *Epilepsia* 2004; 45:103–108.
165. Lux, AL, Edwards, SW, Hancock, E, et al. The United Kingdom Infantile Spasms Study comparing vigabatrin with prednisolone or tetracosactide at 14 days: a multicentre, randomized controlled trial. *Lancet* 2004; 364:1773–1778.
166. Branch CE, Dyken PR. Choroid plexus papilloma and infantile spasms. *Ann Neurol* 1979; 5:302–304.
167. Dolman CL, Crichton JU, Jones EA, Lapointe J. Fibromatosis of dura presenting as infantile spasms. *J Neurol Sci* 1981; 49:31–39.
168. Mimaki T, Ono J, Yabuuchi H. Temporal lobe astrocytoma with infantile spasms. *Ann Neurol* 1983; 14:695–696.
169. Palm DG, Brandt M, Korinthenberg R. West syndrome and Lennox-Gastaut syndrome in children with porencephalic cysts: long-term follow-up after neurosurgical treatment. In: Niedermeyer E, Degen R, eds. *The Lennox-Gastaut Syndrome*. New York: Alan R. Liss, 1988:491–526.
170. Ruggieri V, Caraballo R, Fejerman N. Intracranial tumors and West syndrome. *Pediatr Neurol* 1989; 5:327–329.
171. Chugani HT, Shewmon A, Shields D, et al. Surgery for intractable infantile spasms: neuroimaging perspectives. *Epilepsia* 1993; 34:764–771.
172. Adelson PD, Peacock WJ, Chugani HT, et al. Temporal and extended temporal resections for the treatment of intractable seizures in early childhood. *Pediatr Neurosurg* 1992; 18:169–178.
173. Hoffman HJ. Surgery for West's syndrome. *Adv Exp Med Biol* 2001; 497:57–59.
174. Glaze DG, Hrachovy RA, Frost JD Jr, Kellaway P, et al. Prospective study of outcome of infants with infantile spasms treated during controlled studies of ACTH and prednisone. *J Pediatr* 1988; 112:389–396.

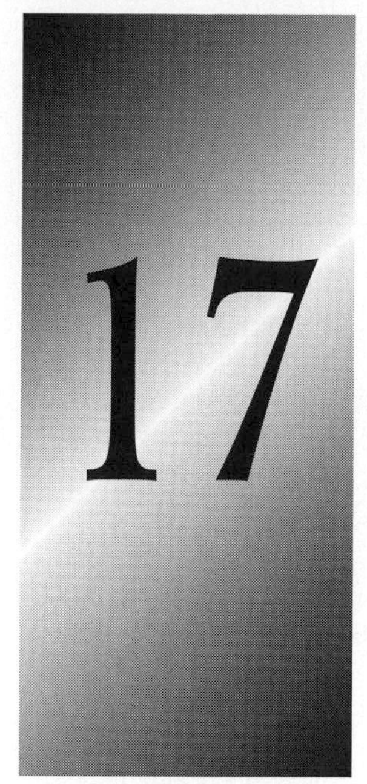

17 Myoclonic Epilepsies in Infancy and Early Childhood

Pierre Genton

It is still common to use the concept of "myoclonic epilepsy" as a diagnosis in epilepsy, although the past decades have led to the individualization of numerous and highly different epileptic syndromes in this category. More important, perhaps, is the fact that myoclonias can be found in the most benign and in the most severe forms of epilepsy, particularly in young children. The clinician's job is to provide patient and family with the best possible treatment, and with a prognosis; diagnosis of a "myoclonic" epilepsy may help narrow the range of possible diagnoses and may also help avoid the risk of using inappropriate therapies. Indeed, myoclonias and myoclonic seizures are (with absences) those that are most likely to be aggravated by a whole range of anticonvulsants (1).

In this paper, we shall review some of the best-established early childhood epilepsy syndromes associated with the word "myoclonic," and this review is based on recent reference textbooks on this subject (2, 3). However, we must acknowledge from the very start that many individual cases fall between the lines that separate syndromes and that diagnoses may remain tentative in some patients until a long-term follow-up has enabled the clinician to confirm (or change) the initial diagnosis.

The traits of the three major myoclonic epilepsy syndromes found in infants and young children and treated in this chapter have been summarized in Table 17-1; we have included "differential diagnoses." Indeed, many patients with myoclonias and myoclonic seizures cannot be diagnosed as having one of the typical syndromes. Several points should be made in this respect:

- Lennox-Gastaut syndrome (LGS) is not typically a myoclonic epilepsy. Myoclonic jerks and seizures have been reported, historically, in some patients who would still be categorized as LGS, whereas most others would now be considered to have Dravet syndrome or Doose syndrome. Important clinical and neurophysiological differences exist between these entities, as shown by a recent neurophysiological study of myoclonic jerks comparing patients with LGS and patients with Doose syndrome: this work underlines the difference between truly generalized myoclonus (as in Doose syndrome) and secondary bilateral synchrony (as in LGS) (4).
- Although epilepsy with myoclonic absences is a well-defined syndrome (5), there are, particularly among the cases with early-onset typical absences before the age of 2 or 3 years, many cases with prominent, nonrhythmic or stereotyped myoclonias. There are also typical childhood absence epilepsy cases with marked myoclonic (eyelid, perioral) features.

TABLE 17-1
Distinctive Features of the Main Types of Myoclonic Epilepsies Occurring in Younger Children

Syndrome	Age at Onset	Seizure Types	Associated Conditions/ Etiology	EEG Features	Prognosis/ Outcome
Benign myoclonic epilepsy in infancy	4 m–3 y (later onset uncommon)	Bilateral jerks; spontaneous or reflex	Idiopathic	Normal background; fast, irregular SW associated with bilateral myoclonic jerks	Excellent in most; self-limited condition; treatment may not be necessary
Severe myoclonic epilepsy in infancy (Dravet syndrome)	3 m–2 y	Febrile, convulsive, unilateral, sleep-related; falsely generalized; myoclonic, atypical absence, polymorphous seizures	Progressive mental decline; Na channelopathy in most	Normal background at onset, progressive deterioration; polymorphic interictal and ictal changes	Poor to very severe; mental handicap; high risk of SUDEP; sensitivity to fever may persist; most severe seizures sleep-related
Myoclonic-astatic epilepsy (Doose syndrome)	1–4 y	Myoclonic; astatic; myoclonic-astatic; absence status; GTCS	Idiopathic; progressive mental deterioration in some; ion channel disorder demonstrated in some	Normal background with some theta slowing; blateral SW, atypical absences and absence states, polymorphous changes during sleep that may include tonic discharges	Excellent to poor; self-limited in some with offset in childhood; chronic in others, with severe seizure and cognitive handicap
Differential Diagnosis					
Lennox-Gastaut syndrome	2–7 y	Tonic, absence, astatic; very rarely myoclonic	Multiple etiologies; no genetic factors	Slow spike-waves; fast activities in sleep	Poor to very severe
Myoclonic absences	1–10 y	Typical absences with rhythmic myoclonias	Usually idiopathic	3-Hz spike-waves with axial hypertonia	Not necessarily poor in all
Early onset absences	6 m–3 y	Typical absences with myoclonus, GTCS	Heterogenous	Typical absences, various interictal changes	Highly variable
Specific conditions with myoclonus	All ages	Various presentations	Various metabolic and genetic disorders	Abnormal background, specific features according to etiology	Usually poor, depending on etiology

However, such cases should be discussed with the absence epilepsy syndromes.

- Numerous specific, metabolic, and/or genetically determined conditions are associated with epileptic seizures and with myoclonias. Such conditions are beyond the sco pe of this chapter and are dealt with in other chapters of this volume.

BENIGN MYOCLONIC EPILEPSY IN INFANCY

Introduction and Definition

Benign myoclonic epilepsy in infancy (BMEI) was individualized among the early-onset myoclonic epilepsies nearly 30 years ago (6). BMEI stands out as the earliest form of idiopathic generalized epilepsy (7, 8). It is easily recognizable, with solid clinical and electroencephalogram (EEG) features. Extensive experience with this syndrome has led to the description of clinical variants, which share its excellent overall prognosis. Its diagnostic criteria can be summarized as follows:

- Onset in a normal infant aged 4 months to 3 years
- Bilateral myoclonic jerks, isolated or in brief series, occurring spontaneously or, less commonly, after unexpected sensory stimulations
- Myoclonic jerks always associated with fast, generalized, irregular spike-wave or polyspike-wave discharges
- EEG showing normal background and few interictal changes
- Favorable neurological and cognitive outcome in most with or without treatment, although some patients may experience infrequent generalized tonic-clonic seizures (GTCS), or rarely other forms of epilepsy, later in life

Epidemiology

In our experience, BMEI is uncommon, and boys clearly outnumber girls (M/F ratio close to 2). BMEI represents less than 1% of all epilepsies and less than 2% of all idiopathic generalized epilepsies (9). This was confirmed by other studies, BMEI representing around 2% of all epilepsies with onset in the first 3 years of life (10), or 1–2% of all epilepsies with onset in the first year of life (11, 12).

Clinical Manifestations

Myoclonic jerks begin usually between the ages of 4 months and 3 years. At the onset, the clinical manifestations are usually rare (seen less often than once/day) and barely noticeable. After some weeks or months, they become more frequent and more obvious. They involve prominently the upper limbs, with a sudden upward extension, but are usually generalized and may be associated with a head drop and a quick upward rolling of the eyes. They may cause falls, drops of objects, or crying. If a short cluster occurs, it does not last more than 2–3 seconds. Sudden brief vocalization (13), or longer myoclonic attacks lasting up to 5 seconds (14), have also been reported, but are uncommon. There are usually no specific triggering factors, and attacks occur unexpectedly (although a slight increase of occurrence may be noted during drowsiness in some children).

A significant clinical variant, now accepted as *reflex* BMEI (15, 16), is characterized by the triggering of myoclonic jerks by sudden tactile or acoustic stimuli. Its prognosis does not differ from the usual type, and it may even be more benign. Some authors have also stressed the possibility of a later age at onset, but such patients still experience the self-limited course of the usual type of BMEI, and there is apparently no overlap with juvenile myoclonic epilepsy (JME) (17).

There are no significant associated features. Cognitive development and behavior remain normal, but some patients may experience various problems in this respect. A recent study showed that attention deficit or slightly below normal IQ can be found in single cases (18), but the significance of such findings is disputable (9).

EEG Features

As an idiopathic type of generalized epilepsy, BMEI is not associated with global changes of the waking or sleeping EEG (Figure 17-1). The interictal EEG is normal, with the exception of rare generalized discharges not associated with myoclonias, especially during sleep. Most importantly, all myoclonias occur in association with EEG discharges. The EEG may remain fully normal if no myoclonic attacks are recorded, and long-term waking video-EEGs should be obtained until the ictal event is well documented. Sleep EEGs are useful in terms of differential diagnosis, because most other syndromes that may be suspected in the early diagnostic phases will be associated with significant global EEG changes during sleep or at awakening. However, drowsiness may in some cases increase the incidence of jerks, and it is recommended that a daytime sleep recording (easy to obtain in infants or very young children) be added to the clinical workup of these patients.

The typical EEG feature is a brief discharge of irregular, often fast spike-waves or polyspike-waves, that is very often associated with myoclonic jerks (Figure 9-1). This discharge can predominate anteriorly. Myoclonic jerks occur as an isolated event, or in very brief rhythmic or near-rhythmic clusters of 2–4 jerks, and may be associated with brief loss of tone in axial muscles (neck). There is no EEG or polygraphic particularity in

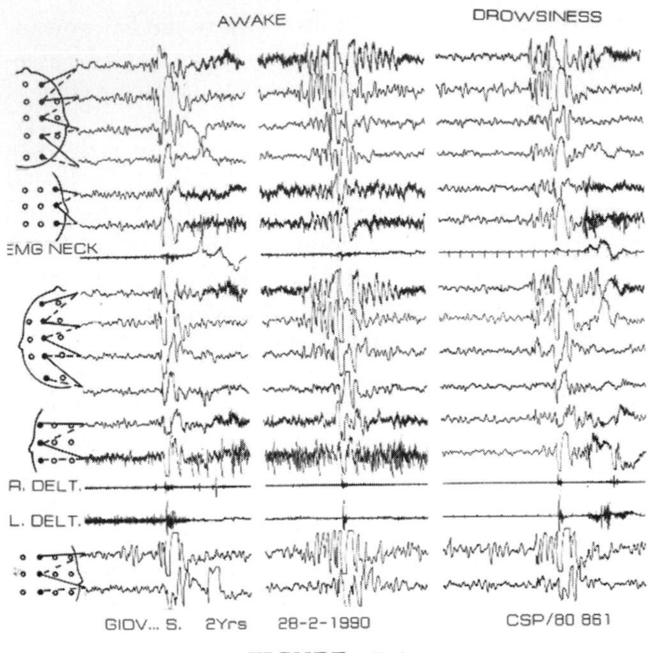

FIGURE 17-1

Benign myoclonic epilepsy in infancy (BMEI). Two-year old female infant with onset before age 1 of myoclonic jerks, who remained untreated until this polygraphic-EEG evaluation at age 2, showing waking and drowsiness. Note the correlation between generalized, irregular spike wave discharges on the EEG and myoclonic jerks shown on the deltoid EMG leads.

the reflex forms, or in patients with slightly later onset, after infancy. The jerks may begin at the eyelids, but they predominate clinically in the arms in most patients (15). A photoparoxysmal response following intermittent light stimulation (ILS) may be found in ca. 10% of patients, sometimes inducing myoclonic jerks (9, 17, 19). Focal changes, mostly in the form of frontal or temporal spike-waves, can be found transiently in rare cases, often only in sleep recordings (9, 19).

Pathophysiology

There is no significant personal history in patients with BMEI, which has all the characteristics of idiopathic epilepsy. The only significant history is the occurrence of simple febrile seizures, which precede (or coexist with) BMEI in up to 26% of cases (9). The main physiopathological discussions surrounding BMEI concern the genetic context. Indeed, family histories of epilepsy (mostly of idiopathic forms) and/or febrile seizures are present in up to 44% of cases. There is no report of familial cases of BMEI, but this condition may occur in association with other forms of epilepsy in some families. One patient had a sibling with myoclonic-astatic epilepsy (20), but other family histories have not been reported in detail. There is, at present, no data to formally link BMEI with other myoclonic epilepsies or to a larger grouping of idiopathic epilepsies. Nor is there data to exclude such linkage.

Diagnostic Evaluation and Differential Diagnosis

The diagnosis of BMEI should immediately come to mind when myoclonic jerks occur in an infant who is progressing normally. The only major differential diagnosis in this age class is with benign infantile spasms (21), a comparatively frequent, likewise benign condition in which the clinical manifestations occur in clusters and in which the EEG remains normal. A familial infantile myoclonic epilepsy was reported in a large kindred, with benign outcome and autosomal recessive inheritance and clinical and EEG characteristics that differ from both BMEI and SMEI (22). These patients had often long-lasting myoclonic attacks preceding GTCS, the GTCS were the initial seizure type in most, and seizures tended to persist into adulthood. Febrile myoclonus is clearly a different entity (23). The diagnosis of SMEI and of myoclonic-astatic epilepsy, which may be confused with BMEI at their very early stages, will be discussed subsequently.

The diagnosis of BMEI can be easily confirmed by video-EEG monitoring, coupled with clinical monitoring. Video documentation of the attacks by the family may be of help at the first consultation and should be requested whenever possible. The frequency of myoclonic jerks is usually such that video-EEG monitoring, coupled with polygraphic recording of the jerks by surface EMG, is productive (Figure 9-1). However, several hours of recording, or repeated recordings, may be necessary in some cases. In the absence of clear video-polygraphic data, or in the presence of atypical findings, the diagnosis and prognosis should remain open; long-term follow-up is necessary to bring about a better established diagnosis in such patients. Neuroimaging procedures are seldom performed and do not reveal significant findings (9). Cognitive and behavioral assessment may be useful for the management of cases with problems in these areas.

Treatment

Myoclonic jerks are easily controlled by valproate (VPA) (9). Untreated patients continue to experience myoclonic attacks, and this may contribute to difficulties in terms of psychomotor development and behavior. Thus the classically recommended attitude is to treat patients with VPA and discontinue treatment after several years of seizure freedom.

In their review of the current literature, Dravet and Bureau (9) have stressed the major efficacy of VPA in BMEI. Out of 87 patients treated in monotherapy, 73/82 became seizure free on VPA, 2/2 on phenobarbital (PB), 2/2 on clonazepam (CZP). Addition of PB, CZP, or clobazam (CLB) resulted in seizure freedom in half of those who had not responded to VPA. Overall, 94% of the patients become seizure free on therapy. Resistance to VPA may be overcome using high initial doses (30 to 40 mg/kg) (13). There are also patients with a very benign course who remained untreated, and the necessity of drug treatment may be discussed in individual cases.

Course and Prognosis

BMEI is a self-limited condition, with an active period lasting seldom more than a few years, and spontaneous remission during childhood. Myoclonic jerks disappear after a period of active epilepsy that may be shortened by anticonvulsant treatment; intellectual development progresses normally, and the EEG normalizes. However, this rule does not apply to all patients. The overall outcome may depend on an early diagnosis and treatment. Persistence of myoclonic attacks may lead to impaired psychomotor development and behavioral disturbances (9, 24). The cases with reflex triggering of myoclonic jerks appear to be more benign than average among BMEI patients, and often do not necessitate treatment.

No other seizure types are usually seen in the course of BMEI, except simple febrile seizures, and afebrile GTCS: the latter occur very late, usually during adolescence, and are often ascribed to drug withdrawal at that age. VPA may still be withdrawn without recurrence of GTCS in some, but has to be maintained in others, for example, because of persisting photosensitivity. Photosensitivity can indeed appear after the cessation of myoclonic jerks and persist into adulthood (13, 25, 26). Some patients may present with other seizure types: two patients had typical absences at age 10 and 11 years, after several years of seizure freedom off VPA (14). A multicentric study reported that, among 34 BMEI cases diagnosed between 1981 and 2002, there were two who later developed JME (27), but such findings need confirmation.

The cognitive outcome is favorable (9). In patients with long-term follow-up, 81.6% are normal, while 14.47% have mild retardation and attend a specialized school, none being institutionalized. Associated conditions may account for some of these unfavorable courses; one of our patients had Down syndrome. In other cases, the myoclonic seizures had remained untreated for many years. Mangano et al. (18) reported the cognitive and behavioral outcome in seven patients. Five were normal, one had a slight and one a moderate mental retardation, and all but one also had attention deficit disorder. The pathogenesis of such unfavorable outcomes is probably multifactorial. In addition to the existence of co-pathologies, it appears that treatment delay (in patients with frequent attacks), familial anxiety, and inappropriate educational attitudes, as well as a putative underlying biological factor, may contribute to a less than fully benign prognosis in some patients.

SEVERE MYOCLONIC EPILEPSY IN INFANCY (DRAVET SYNDROME)

Introduction and Definition

Severe myoclonic epilepsy in infancy (SMEI) was described in the late 1970s (28) as a condition with severe epilepsy and progressive mental impairment, distinct from Lennox-Gastaut syndrome. It was included among the undetermined (as to whether focal or generalized) epilepsies in the 1989 International League Against Epilepsy (ILAE) classification (7) and ranked among the epileptic encephalopathies by the more recent classification scheme proposal (8). Following the increasing description of less typical forms, in which myoclonic jerks seem to play a lesser part, the eponym "Dravet syndrome" is now widely accepted, which puts less emphasis on its myoclonic components.

SMEI has gained a major importance in recent years as a result of the realization that it is a fairly common syndrome, with many cases reported from all continents, and that many cases are related to a specific abnormality of sodium channel receptors (29). SMEI is nowadays considered an archetypical form of an ion channel disorder–related epilepsy.

Although it is fairly easy to diagnose after a certain duration of follow-up, SMEI still poses multiple diagnostic and therapeutic problems. Its diagnostic criteria can be summarized as follows:

- Onset in a normal infant aged 3 months to 2 years
- Repeated simple febrile seizures, becoming progressively longer and afebrile, unilateral, sleep-related, and increasing in duration
- Occurrence of myoclonias, both bilateral and erratic, in the second year of life or thereafter
- Progressive occurrence of multiple seizure types, including falsely generalized seizures, various forms of status epilepticus, atypical absences, myoclonic seizures, and focal seizures, with increased incidence during febrile episodes
- Progressive mental decline after the second-third year of life
- EEG normal at onset, with progressive deterioration of background, frequent and early photosensitivity, and multiple interictal and ictal abnormal patterns
- Poor prognosis, with progressive mental decline during the first years and a fairly stable residual state with marked to severe mental impairment, persisting seizures, and high mortality

Epidemiology

In spite of its major rank among epileptic encephalopathies, SMEI remains uncommon, but far from rare, and increasing numbers of cases are diagnosed nowadays. The incidence was estimated at less than 1 per 40,000 (30). Among epilepsies with onset in the first year of life, SMEI represents 3% (11) or 5% (31). Among epilepsies with onset in the first three years of life, the prevalence has been estimated at 6.1% (29) or 7% (10). Males are more often affected, with a sex ratio of 2 (30, 31).

Clinical Manifestations

SMEI is characterized by a stereotyped clinical course, beginning with simple convulsive febrile seizures, which become frequent and predominantly nocturnal, increase in duration, and are progressively associated with afebrile events, multiple seizure types, myoclonias, and mental decline as well as neurological symptoms and behavioral disturbances.

The first febrile seizures may not be particularly disquieting. In most cases they are associated with intercurrent ear, nose, and throat (ENT) infections, or they follow vaccinations, but Japanese authors have stressed that they can also be triggered by hot baths producing a rise in body temperature (32). Early characteristic features occur in some patients, with long febrile seizures, or clusters (33), or afebrile seizures in 28 to 48% of cases (29). Febrile seizures tend to recur within weeks, and the first afebrile seizures occur within 2 to 14 months (33). The diagnosis of SMEI becomes more apparent when other seizure types appear, and when cognitive problems start manifesting, between 1 and 4 years of age.

There are several types of convulsive seizures in SMEI (29), which can all last 30 minutes or more, or recur after short interruptions:

- GTCS are uncommon, usually short, with a tonic phase often already intermixed with clonias.
- Hemiclonic seizures are seen in the very young, before age 3.
- "Falsely generalized" seizures are complicated, with discrepancies between the EEG onset (which may precede the clinical phenomena) and offset (EEG discharges persisting after the clinical offset). They consist in bilateral, asymmetric, asynchronous tonic contraction and clonias, leading to variable postures during the seizure, and each component may transiently predominate on one side or one one limb. They last up to 2–3 minutes.
- "Unstable" seizures are characterized by shifting EEG predominance, while their clinical appearance resembles the falsely generalized seizures.

Myoclonias appear after age 1 year, usually before age 5. Generalized myoclonic jerks, sometimes with falls, may be prominent upon awakening, disappear during sleep, and be provoked by intermittent light stimulation in the EEG laboratory. Fragmentary, asynchronous myoclonias are also seen (in up to 85% of the patients) in association with the former or, very often, as interictal manifestations, involving the limbs or facial muscles.

Atypical absences, often associated with increased myoclonias, may appear at any age during childhood and are found in 40 to >90% of patients. The clouding of consciousness is incomplete, with some staring and slowing. The EEG correlates range from 3-Hz spike-wave discharges to diffuse slowing interspersed with multifocal spike-waves. Eyelid myoclonias and head drops may also occur during absences. They can culminate in states of obtundation, which occur in close to 50% of SMEI patients, and are characterized by fluctuating contact, slowing, and erratic myoclonias (Figure 9-2). Convulsive seizures may trigger, accompany, or terminate such states, which may last hours to days. The EEG shows diffuse slowing with focal and generalized spikes and spike-waves.

Focal seizures occur early in the course of SMEI, as simple motor seizures or as complex focal seizures with autonomic symptoms, often as soon as 4 months after the first febrile events. They may follow a myoclonic seizure. Complex focal seizures are with drooling, pallor, automatisms, and erratic myoclonias. Simple motor focal seizures are usually versive, or clonic, limited to one side or one limb. The EEG changes are clearly focal, originating in the occipital, temporal, or frontal region.

Tonic seizures are extremely uncommon but have been reported by several authors (29).

Motor milestones are normal at the beginning, with walking at the normal age, but unsteady gait is often noticed. Slight ataxia is noted in 60%, and mild pyramidal signs in 20%, during early childhood. Language also starts at the normal age but progresses slowly. Cognitive delay occurs often in the second year of life, sometimes only later. The children often become hyperkinetic. Twenty patients aged 11 months to 16 years 7 months were investigated with neuropsychological tests (34): motor, linguistic, and visual abilities were strikingly affected. Children with an initial high frequency of convulsive seizures showed earlier cognitive slowing. The number and duration of convulsive seizures correlated with the degree of mental deterioration. Better development correlated with milder epilepsy. In children with marked photosensitivity, self-stimulation (using light sources or geometric patterns) may become prominent (35).

EEG Features

The EEG changes found in SMEI (Figure 17-2) are highly polymorphic and not specific. At the onset the EEG is normal and may remain so after repeated, simple febrile

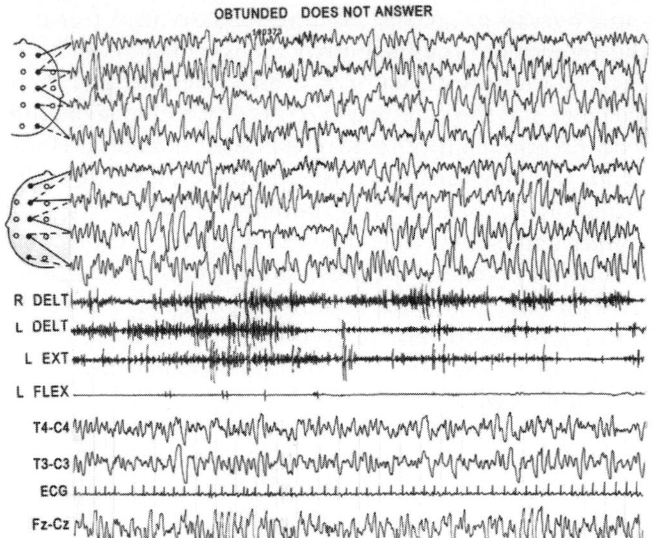

FIGURE 17-2

Dravet syndrome (severe myoclonic epilepsy in infancy, SMEI). This child had a typical history, with early-onset simple febrile seizures. This plate illustrate one of the multiple aspects of clinical manifestations of SMEI. During a state of obtundation, the patient has both segmental, asynchronous, and diffuse myoclonias, as shown on the polygraphic EMG leads. The EEG shows global slowing, and predominantly multifocal sharp waves.

seizures. Later, the background activity is variable, partly in relation to the delay since the last convulsive seizure, showing diffuse slowing in the wake of major seizures. Sharp activities consist in spikes, spike-waves, and polyspike-waves, often predominating over the frontal and central areas, together with multifocal slow activities. Brief generalized discharges are associated with massive jerks, but there are no evident EEG correlates, or only focal spikes, in association with erratic or segmental myoclonias. Sleep patterns are conserved unless sleep-related seizures are frequent. Photoparoxysmal responses can be elicited by intermittent photic stimulation or by geometric patterns, but this EEG laboratory finding is not always correlated with clinical photosensitivity.

The ictal patterns are also highly variable and depend on the seizure type. Some have been summarized in the previous section. The multifocal aspect of changes, both slow and sharp, is highlighted by the recording of a state of obtundation (Figure 17-2).

The EEG changes progress during childhood, with diffuse, but moderate overall slowing, while the sharp changes tend to decrease over time.

Pathophysiology

The genetic context in which SMEI occurs has been stressed repeatedly, with a family history of febrile seizures in up to 71% of cases (34). A new light was shed on the nosology of SMEI after the description of the GEFS+ syndrome (generalized epilepsy with febrile seizures "plus") (36). Probands with SMEI may belong to GEFS+ families, with other members having more benign phenotypes (such as simple febrile seizures, febrile seizures+, but also myoclonic-astatic epilepsy or focal epilepsy) (37). Indeed, although familial occurrence of SMEI remains rare (29), two GEFS+ families, each with two siblings with SMEI, have been reported (38). SMEI was thus related to a group of epilepsies with sensitivity to fever.

The next step in the discovery of pathophysiological mechanisms underlying SMEI occurred in 2001, when mutations in the SCN1A sodium-channel gene were found in all seven SMEI probands studied by Claes et al (39). These mutations occurred *de novo*, and were confirmed by numerous other studies. Mutations are predominantly frameshift and nonsense, but missense and other types have been reported. Most mutations were confirmed to occur *de novo*, but some, all missense, were inherited (40, 41). SCN1A mutations were thus found in most, but not all, patients with SMEI, with a lesser prevalence in borderline or atypical cases (29). Among 11 mutation-negative patients with typical or atypical SMEI, a recent study found that three had microdeletions in the SCN1A gene (42). Other candidate genes, including those implied in some families with GEFS+, were consistently negative, with one exception: a patient with a GABRG2 gene mutation was reported by Harkin et al. (43).

Genotype-phenotype correlations were extensively studied (29). There is a higher frequency of truncating mutations in the patients with SMEI. Some authors emphasize the localization of missense mutations and found that those situated around the pore-forming region and around the voltage-sensor region were more likely to produce the more severe phenotypes (44). Most mutations result in loss of function of the SCN1A channel (45), while others can lead to increased function (46). In spite of marked and rapid progress in the understanding of the cellular mechanisms producing SMEI, there is thus still ample room for further research.

Diagnostic Evaluation and Differential Diagnosis

The diagnosis of SMEI can be suspected on clinical grounds in a context of repeated febrile seizures with a progressive tendency to occur at lower temperatures, to last longer, and to have an apparently unilateral or shifting aspect. It will be confirmed during follow-up, with the onset of myoclonias and multiple seizure types, and of progressive mental alteration. Waking and sleeping polygraphic video-EEG recordings are useful, because the children progressively fulfill the diagnostic criteria of

SMEI. Molecular biology can, nowadays, help characterize a defect in sodium channel receptors in most cases, and positive findings in this field may constitute a diagnostic criterion in the future.

CT scan and MRI are usually normal, or show slight diffuse atrophy, without hippocampal sclerosis, a strange fact given the occurrence of numerous prolonged febrile seizures in these patients (29). However, recent works have shown some significant findings. Ictal single-photon emission computed tomography (SPECT) may show lateralized or bilateral hypoperfusion (47, 48), and interictal positron emission tomography (PET) may show lateralized cortical hypometabolism (49). Contrary to previous studies, unilateral or bilateral hippocampal sclerosis was found in 10 of 14 patients at various stages of SMEI (50), and 6 of these 10 patients had an initially normal MRI. The real incidence and significance of acquired, progressive lesions in SMEI thus remain to be defined. A high-resolution MRI is thus recommended, whenever possible, at the early stages of this condition.

Many differential diagnoses are usually discussed before a consensus can be reached on the diagnosis of SMEI. Simple febrile seizures and BMEI can be easily eliminated after some follow-up. Lennox-Gastaut syndrome (LGS) may begin in infancy, but usually in children with brain lesions, who present with another type of symptomatic epilepsy, such as infantile spasms; moreover, the EEG is much more specific in the LGS, showing fast discharges during sleep, with or without overt tonic seizures. Myoclonic-astatic epilepsy (discussed subsequently) may be more difficult to differentiate in the first or second year of life. Major differential diagnoses are represented by the following:

- Some metabolic disorders, such as mitochondrial encephalomyopathies or neuronal ceroid lipofuscinosis, resemble SMEI; one patient with a condition mimicking SMEI had biological signs of mitochondrial dysfunction (51).
- Severe cryptogenic frontal lobe epilepsy with onset in infancy may be discussed in some patients also but is not associated with the polymorphic association of seizures or the alternating character of unilateral seizures seen in SMEI.
- Recurrent febrile seizures may raise the possibility of SMEI, which remains unlikely if seizure types and febrile threshold do not change over time. Recurrent febrile seizures can occur in a context of GEFS+ and may also be associated with Na channel functional defects.

A major diagnostic problem is raised by the existence of atypical, or « borderline » cases of SMEI, that only partially fulfill the diagnostic criteria, but share the same overall prognosis. Among such atypical features: the absence of prominent myoclonus, which, if all other criteria are present, will not change the practical management and the outcome (12, 31, 48); a clinical picture with predominant refractory GTCS or unilateral clonic or tonic-clonic seizures, onset in infancy, and an evolution similar to SMEI (52). In both cases, recent molecular studies have shown that an SCN1A gene mutation could be demonstrated in patients with borderline SME (53) or with only refractory GTCS seizures (41). Thus the borders of SMEI remain controversial, and the actual weight of molecular biology in its diagnosis has yet to be established.

Treatment

SMEI is characterized by marked drug resistance, and there is no report of full seizure control over a long period with any single drug or drug combination. In spite of this, a rational approach of pharmacological management can be proposed in SMEI.

Some anticonvulsants have a clearly deleterious effect, which has been noted by clinicians and has not received satisfactory explanations. Lamotrigine was shown to aggravate at least 80% of SMEI patients, at any stage of the condition (54). The same phenomenon has been noted for carbamazepine (55), and both drugs (with the likely addition of oxcarbazepine, which is closely related to CBZ) should not be used in SMEI.

Most other anticonvulsants have been used with some benefit in SMEI. Phenobarbital (PB), VPA, and benzodiazepines may decrease the frequency and duration of convulsive seizures. Phenytoin (PHT) can be useful in critical situations. Zonisamide is a potent antimyoclonic agent and has been used with success (56). Other drugs merit special attention:

- Bromides brought major improvement of convulsive seizures in 8 of 22 patientswith SMEI, but did not influence absences or myoclonias (57).
- Topiramate caused a 50–100%, long-term reduction in convulsive seizures (up to 36 months) in 23 patients out of 27 in our experience (Villeneuve, personal communication), and good results have been published by other groups (58, 59).
- Felbamate, in our experience, also proved efficient in several patients with SMEI, reducing all seizure types; there is, however, no published study to confirm this interesting effect in SMEI.
- Stiripentol was efficient in association with VPA and CLB on convulsive seizures in SMEI (60). In this randomized, placebo-controlled, add-on trial, 15 of 21 children (71%) had more than 50% reduction in seizure frequency (nine were seizure free), compared to 1 of 20 (not seizure free) under placebo (5%).

The ketogenic diet is also an option: Of seventeen patients, seven achieved a 75–100%, and two a 50–74% seizure reduction (61). Seizures remained well controlled for more than one year. Steroids may be used in case of repeated status but do not have long-term efficacy. In some patients, immunoglobulins gave satisfactory results (Dravet, personal communication). In case of convulsive status, intravenous benzodiazepines, clonazepam, and midazolam can be used (62), in association with chloral hydrate or barbiturates.

Course and Prognosis

SMEI stands out as a particularly severe epilepsy, with a very poor overall prognosis, confirmed by all published studies. Seizures tend to persist, all patients have cognitive dysfunction, and mortality is high, especially when patients reach adolescence and adulthood (30). The diagnosis of SMEI is comparatively easy in adults, because it is based on a fairly typical clinical evolution. A recent assessment of 14 adult patients with SMEI showed that predominantly nocturnal convulsive seizures persisted and that all patients were mentally disabled and had various degrees of neurological dysfunction (63).

Seizures are drug-resistant at all ages but tend to become less frequent in early adolescence, persisting as nocturnal convulsive attacks, often triggered by intercurrent febrile conditions. In the Tokyo cohort (30), one patient has been seizure free for more than one year, 20 (51%) had weekly seizures, 14 (36%) monthly seizures, 3 (8%) one seizure in 1 to 6 months, and 3 (7%) one seizure in 6 months to 1 year. Febrile status still happens during adolescence, but febrile episodes are less frequent than in young children.

Neurological impairment may appear insidiously during childhood, with poor coordination, tremor, or slight action myoclonus (64). Some patients may necessitate wheelchairs as a result of ataxia, spastic paresis, and kyphoscoliosis. The cognitive outcome is poor, but deficits tend to stabilize in older children. Among the patients followed at our institution (30), all those aged more than 10 years needed institutional care, and half had an IQ below 50. Behavior tended to become less hyperkinetic and rather marked by slowness and perseverations.

Mortality is a major problem in SMEI at any age. Among 128 patients who died in a department of child neurology, there were 4 of 8 patients with SMEI, including three during status epilepticus (65). The experience from our center notes that by 1992, 15.9% of our patients had died during follow-up, with the following causes (30): sudden unexpected death in epilepsy (SUDEP) (2 cases, aged 7 and 13 years), drowning (3 cases, aged 4, 10 and 14 years), status epilepticus during respiratory infection (1 case, age 3years 3 months), accident (1 case, age 15 years), malignant measles under steroids (1 case, age 3 years 4 months), unknown (1 case). Over the past 15 years, several adolescent and adult patients have died in their sleep, with indirect evidence of seizures in some. We now recommend that adolescent and adult patients with SMEI sleep without soft cushions, and we also recommend that febrile episodes be treated as early as possible.

MYOCLONIC-ASTATIC EPILEPSY (DOOSE SYNDROME)

Introduction and Definition

Myoclonic-astatic epilepsy (MAE) is one of the few epileptic syndromes named after a particular seizure type (66), but it is also known under the name of Doose syndrome, a tribute to the German author who first described "centroencephalic myoclonic-astatic petit mal" (67), without, however, separating it clearly from Lennox-Gastaut syndrome (LGS), which had been characterized in the same period, or from SMEI, which was described later. It was classified among the cryptogenic or symptomatic generalized epilepsies in the 1989 international classification of epilepsies (7), but rightly moved to the idiopathic forms in the 2001 proposal (8). Recent studies have stressed the relationship between MAE and other idiopathic epilepsies, including the GEFS+ syndrome. There are still debates about the precise syndromic classification of patients diagnosed with MAE, "cryptogenic" LGS, and some cases with BMEI or SMEI.

The diagnostic criteria of MAE can be summarized in the following manner:

- Onset in a normal child, between age 1 and 5 years
- Absence of structural brain anomalies
- Strong genetic context, with high incidence of idiopathic epilepsy in the family
- Myoclonic-astatic seizures resulting in drops and falls, associated with multiple generalized seizure types: myoclonic, atonic, absence, GTC, less commonly tonic seizures, as well as nonconvulsive status epilepticus
- Variable response to medication, with high efficacy of the valproate + lamotrigine combination
- Possible progressive cognitive impairment in some patients
- Variable prognosis for epilepsy and cognition, ranging from excellent to poor

Epidemiology

The sex ratio is strongly in favor of males (2.7–3:1) (68). Incidence data vary according to the precise definition used, but overall MAE represents 1–2% of all childhood epilepsies (69), or 2.2% of children with seizure onset between age 1 and 10 years in a hospital-based study (70).

Clinical Manifestations

MAE occurs in neurologically normal young children. Seizure onset is between 18 and 60 months, and 94% of the children start their seizures before age 5 years. Onset in children older than 7 has not been reported. MAE may be preceded by (or associated with) simple febrile seizures in 11 to 28% of children in the usual age range (age 17 to 40 months) (70, 71), or 90% if MAE occurs in GEFS+ families (72).

The first seizures are usually generalized tonic-clonic, and soon after, they become myoclonic. They increase in frequence over a few months (73). Up to one-third of the patients can experience within 1–3 months a "stormy" evolution with multiple convulsive seizures per day, episodes of nonconvulsive status, or multiple daily falls due to myoclonic-astatic seizures (68). Such patients do not necessarily have a worse outcome than do those with a more gradual onset.

The characteristic presentation of MAE is as a multiple seizure disorder. Myoclonic and myoclonic-astatic seizures are present in all, as are generalized jerks occurring isolated or in clusters of 2 to 3. A prominent feature consists of sudden falls that may be related to myoclonic jerks or to atonias, usually to the characteristic combination of both. This can be documented by polygraphic video-EEG recording (74). Injuries are common. Minor episodes are limited to head drops.

The following are other seizure types that may occur in MAE (68, 70, 71):

- GTCS are found in 75–95% of patients and may occur during waking, but mostly during sleep after the first months.
- Pure atonic seizures were documented in 11 of 30 patients and associated with sudden falls and immediate recovery (74).
- Atypical absences are found in 62–89% of patients, often associated with lowered muscle tone.
- Stupor, or nonconvulsive status, has been reported in up to 95% of patients. Such episodes may occur upon awakening from sleep or from a nap and last up to one hour or more, or occur as true status, lasting up to several days, often longer in children with unfavorable outcome. Discrete, arrhythmic myoclonias of the face and extremities usually accompany these episodes (Figure 17-3).
- Tonic seizures may occur during sleep.

EEG Features

At first appearance of seizures, the EEG (Figure 17-3) has a normal background and may show brief bursts of 2–3 Hz generalized spike-wave or polyspike-wave discharges, which increase during sleep. The presence of a regular, rhythmic theta activity at 4–7 Hz predominating over the vertex and central areas is considered fairly specific of MAE, but it is not present in all patients and may become less prominent during follow-up. Myoclonic and myoclonic-astatic seizures are characterized by a single generalized (poly)spike-wave complex or by a cluster of sharp elements at 3–4 Hz lasting 2–6 seconds (74). Closer analysis of myoclonic seizures with back-averaging techniques have demonstrated the generalized nature of the ictal phenomenon, with a 2–4 ms latency between sides, which contrasts with the findings in Lennox-Gastaut syndrome, in which the interside latency is much higher and in favor of bilateral synchrony (4). Atonias correlate with a 200–400-ms silent period on the EMG and polyspike discharges on the EEG (73, 74). Tonic seizures are characterized by 10–15 Hz polyspike discharges.

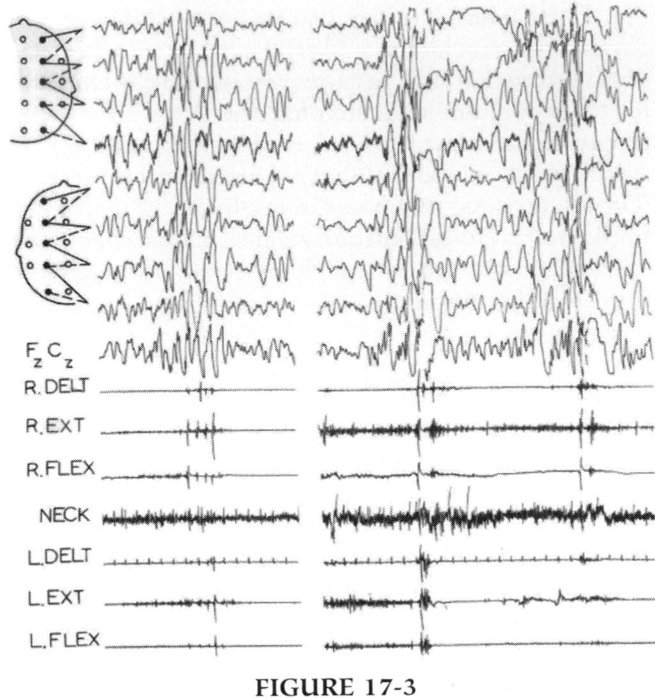

FIGURE 17-3

Doose syndrome (myoclonic-astatic epilepsy, MAE). A typical aspect of the EEG in a patient with MAE. Both segments: generalized or diffuse EEG changes with irregular spike waves. Right segment: a myoclonic-astatic episode, with myoclonias and atonia (as shown on the polygraphic EMG leads).

Stuporous states are associated with mixed, slow and sharp activities, and when they are accompanied by prominent myoclonias, these can be associated, using back-averaging techniques, with cortical events (75).

Pathophysiology

The "idiopathic" character of the Doose syndrome is based on the lack of acquired pathology and on the presence of significant genetic backgrounds. Very rarely, MAE can coexist with brain lesions, as recently shown in a patient with Sturge-Weber syndrome, in whom MAE developed and kept its peculiar pharmacological sensitivity (76). Although the "generalized" nature of MAE remains uncontroversial, magnetoencephalographic findings have pointed to a frontal, premotor generation of myoclonic-astatic attacks (77).

Most studies pointed to a high incidence of positive family histories of epilepsy, found in 15–32% of cases (70, 71). Recent studies have stressed the existence of MAE patients in large GEFS+ pedigrees (36, 37, 72). However, none of the known three genes associated with GEFS+ was found to be mutated in a series of sporadic MAE cases (78), and only three out of 20 patients with sporadic MAE demonstrated SCN1A mutations (79). Other genetic factors may play a major part, and the precise genetic etiology or etiologies of MAE is (are) thus still unknown.

Diagnostic Evaluation and Differential Diagnosis

The diagnosis of MAE can be suspected from the onset but, in most cases, requires a certain amount and duration of follow-up with clinical and EEG monitoring before it can be accepted as likely; as with other epileptic syndromes that lack a clear biological marker, it will never be definitive and can change during the course of the condition. The clinical evaluation ascertains normal development prior to the onset of epilepsy, a family history of idiopathic epilepsy, onset in early childhood, absence of brain pathology, multiple seizure types, as well as fairly characteristic EEG changes awake and asleep; pharmacological sensitivity (discussed subsequently) may also constitute a major diagnostic criterion. Diagnosis of MAE may remain tentative over a prolonged period, especially if atypical features are present in the patient's history or clinical presentation.

Thus, various diagnoses may be considered during the early phases of MAE: BMEI (discussed earlier in this chapter), which may belong to the same spectrum of "idiopathic myoclonic epilepsies," has a different, simpler presentation, but a cryptogenic form of Lennox-Gastaut syndrome may pose difficult problems, as several major clinical features overlap with those of MAE (70). A precise neurophysiological assessment of myoclonic jerks may help differentiate the truly "generalized" features of MAE from those of LGS, which are more likely to be associated with secondary bilateral synchrony (4). Other forms of "encephalopathic" early childhood epilepsies can be diagnosed in this context:

- Atypical benign partial epilepsy (80), or the syndrome of continuous spike-waves during slow-wave sleep (81), may also occur in normal children who present with multiple seizure types, including drop attacks, but the EEG is different, showing focal and diffuse spike-wave discharges with major activation during sleep.
- The late infantile form of ceroid lipofuscinosis, or other specific progressive disorders, may resemble MAE at the onset, especially if there is a "stormy" onset of MAE, or during periods of worsening, but clinical and EEG traits (e.g., visual impairment, single-flash responses on ILS, and rapid cognitive decline) quickly change the diagnostic context.

Treatment

In recent years the treatment of MAE has changed for the better, but it remains difficult, and the multiplicity of therapeutic proposals is a clear witness to this unsatisfactory situation. Valproate (VPA) is still considered the drug of first choice, as it may be effective against the multiple seizure types. Ethosuximide (ESM) can be considered to treat prominent absences and myoclonic attacks. When the initial phase of MAE is "explosive," phenobarbital (PB) may be a reasonable option, as it has proven efficacy in convulsive attacks, but its use should not be continued beyond this initial stage (68). Steroids can help in the management of periods with multiple astatic seizures and frequent prolonged episodes of nonconvulsive status in MAE (73). Others have reported a positive effect of high-dose intravenous gamma-globulins (82) or intravenous lidocaine (83) in the treatment of minor motor status in MAE. The ketogenic diet may also be proposed in the most severe cases (84, 85).

Conversely, such drugs as carbamazepine (CBZ) and vigabatrin (VGB), and probably phenytoin, oxcarbazepine, tiagabine, gabapentin, or pregabalin, should be used with utmost care in MAE, as in other myoclonic epilepsies, as they may be responsible for paradoxical aggravation of seizures, resulting at times in myoclonic status (75, 86).

Newer anticonvulsants may help control MAE. Lamotrigine (LTG) has achieved a major role in the treatment regimen of patients with MAE (87), especially in association with VPA: This synergic combination, recommended in focal epilepsies (88), may have found a major application in MAE. Other newer anticonvulsants such as zonisamide, topiramate, and levetiracetam (LEV) may also be appropriate. However, a case of MAE with paradoxical aggravation (leading to myoclonic status) has been reported with LEV monotherapy (89). Topiramate may have some lasting beneficial effect on seizure control in some patients (90). Felbamate has been used with positive effect in selected cases (91).

Course and Prognosis

MAE stands out as a syndrome with a very variable, difficult-to-predict outcome that ranges from benign (with total remission without sequelae) to very poor (with severe persisting epilepsy and mental impairment). MAE appears to follow a natural course that cannot be accurately predicted on the basis of its characteristics at onset. In spite of frequent seizures and initial apparent resistance to drugs, the condition is self-limited in many patients, with abatement of seizures after an active period of 1–3 years and good cognitive evolution. The proportion of "favorable" cases with total remission of epilepsy has apparently grown in recent years, from around 50% to up to 68% (70, 71, 84). Some patients may experience infrequent, easy-to-control GTCS, while myoclonic-astatic seizures remit in 89% (84). Behavioral problems occur in some patients. The cognitive outcome was considered poor in 18% and was mostly associated with persisting minor motor states (84). Various factors of poor outcome have been proposed: repeated prolonged episodes of nonconvulsive status and positive family histories (71); occurrence of numerous falls, of atypical absences, and of frequent GTCS (17); frequent minor motor attacks and presence of a family history of epilepsy (84). The occurrence of tonic seizures during sleep is often but not always associated with a poorer prognosis (70, 92). In patients with long-term EEG recordings that include nocturnal sleep, they occur in only one-third of patients with favorable outcome but up to 95% of those with poor outcome (70).

For all practical purposes, there are no solid hints at severity or benignity at the onset of the condition, no matter how "stormy" it is. Clinicians in charge of such patients should closely follow the evolution, use adequate drug regimens that avoid toxicity and paradoxical aggravation, and apply less common treatment procedures, together with educational support, when seizures become disabling and cognitive development deteriorates. If the epilepsy has not markedly abated three years after the onset, a poor prognosis is likely.

References

1. Genton P. When antiepileptic drugs aggravate epilepsy. *Brain Dev* 2000; 22:75–80.
2. Roger J, Bureau M, Dravet C, Genton P, et al, eds. Epileptic syndromes in infancy, childhood and adolescence. 4th ed. London: John Libbey; 2005.
3. Delgado-Escueta A, Guerrini R, Medina M, Genton P, et al, eds. Idiopathic myoclonic epilepsies. *Adv Neurology* 2005; 95.
4. Bonanni P, Parmeggiani L, Guerrini R. Different neurophysiologic patterns of myoclonus characterize Lennox-Gastaut syndrome and myoclonic astatic epilepsy. *Epilepsia* 2002; 43:609–615.
5. Genton P, Bureau M. Epilepsy with myoclonic absences. *CNS Drugs* 2006; 20: 911–916.
6. Dravet C, Bureau M. L'épilepsie myoclonique bénigne du nourrisson. *Rev EEG Neurophysiol* 1981; 11:438–444.
7. Commission on Classification and Terminology of the International League Against Epilepsy. Proposal for revised classification of epilepsies and epileptic syndromes. *Epilepsia* 1989; 30:289–299.
8. Engel J. A proposed diagnostic scheme for people with epileptic seizures and with epilepsy: report of the ILAE Task Force on Classification and Terminology. *Epilepsia* 2001; 42:796–803.
9. Dravet C, Bureau M. Benign myoclonic epilepsy in infancy. In: Roger J, Bureau M, Dravet Ch, Genton P., Tassinari CA, Wolf P, eds. *Epileptic Syndromes in Infancy, Childhood and Adolescence.* 4th ed. London: John Libbey Eurotext Ltd, 2005:77–88.
10. Dalla Bernardina B, Colamaria V, Capovilla G, Bondavalli S. Nosological classification of epilepsies in the first three years of life. In: Nistico G, Di Perri R, Meinardi H, eds. *Epilepsy: An Update on Research and Therapy.* New York: Alan Liss, 1983:165–183.
11. Caraballo R, Cersósimo R, Galicchio S, Fejerman N. Epilepsies during the first year of life. *Rev Neurol* 1997; 25:1521–1524.
12. Sarisjulis N, Gamboni B, Plouin P, Kaminska A, et al. Diagnosing idiopathic/cryptogenic epilepsy syndromes in infancy. *Arch Dis Child* 2000; 82:226–230.
13. Lin YP, Itomi K, Takada H, Kuboda T, et al. Benign myoclonic epilepsy in infants: video-EEG features and long-term follow-up. *Neuropediatrics* 1998; 29:268–271.
14. Prats-Vinas JM, Garaizar C, Ruiz-Espinosa C. Benign myoclonic epilepsy in infants. *Rev Neurol* 2002; 34:201–204.
15. Ricci S, Cusmai R, Fusco L, Vigevano F. Reflex myoclonic epilepsy: a new age-dependent idiopathic epileptic syndrome related to startle reaction. *Epilepsia* 1995; 36:342–348.
16. Caraballo R, Cassar L, Monges S, Yepez I, et al. Reflex myoclonic epilepsy in infancy: a new reflex epilepsy syndrome or a variant of benign myoclonic epilepsy in infancy. *Rev Neurol* 2003; 36:429–432.
17. Guerrini R, Dravet Ch, Gobbi G, Ricci S, et al. Idiopathic generalized epilepsies with myoclonus in infancy and childhood. In: Malafosse A, Genton P, Hirsch E, Marescaux C, et al, eds. *Idiopathic Generalized Epilepsies: Clinical, Experimental, and Genetic Aspects.* London, Paris: John Libbey Eurotext Ltd, 1994:267–280.
18. Mangano S, Fontana A, Cusumano L. Benign myoclonic epilepsy in infancy: neuropsychological and behavioural outcome. *Brain Dev* 2005; 27:218–223.
19. Giovanardi Rossi P, Parmeggiani A, Posar A, Santi A, et al. Benign myoclonic epilepsy: long-term follow-up of 11 new cases. *Brain Dev* 1997; 19:473–479.
20. Arzimanoglou A, Prudent M, Salefranque F. Epilepsie myoclono-astatique et épilepsie myoclonique bénigne du nourrisson dans une même famille: quelques réflexions sur la classification des épilepsies. *Epilepsies* 1996; 8:307–315.
21. Lombroso CT, Fejerman N. Benign myoclonus of early infancy. *Ann Neurol* 1977; 1: 138–143.
22. De Falco FA, Majello L, Santangelo R, Stabile M, et al. Familial infantile myoclonic epilepsy: clinical features in a large kindred with autosomal recessive inheritance. *Epilepsia* 2001; 42:1541–1548.
23. Dooley JM, Hayden JD. Benign febrile myoclonus in childhood. *Can J Neurol Sci* 2004; 31:504–505.
24. Zuberi SM, O'Regan ME. Developmental outcome in benign myoclonic epilepsy in infancy and reflex myoclonic epilepsy in infancy: a literature review and six new cases. *Epilepsy Res* 2006; 70 Suppl 1:S110–115.
25. Ribacoba Montero R, Salas Puig J. Benign myoclonic epilepsy in childhood. A case report. *Rev Neurol* 1997; 25:1210–1212.
26. Todt H, Müller D. The therapy of benign myoclonic epilepsy in infants. In: Degen R, Dreifuss FE, eds. *The Benign Localized and Generalized Epilepsies in Early Childhood. Epilepsy Research* Suppl 6. Amsterdam: Elsevier Science, 1992:137–139.
27. Auvin S, Pandit F, De Bellecize J, Badinand N, et al. Benign myoclonic epilepsy in infants: electroclinical features and long-term follow-up of 34 patients. *Epilepsia* 2006; 47: 387–393.
28. Dravet C. Les épilepsies graves de l'enfant. *Vie Med* 1978; 8:543–548.
29. Dravet C, Bureau M, Oguni H, Fukuyama Y, et al. Severe myoclonic epilepsy in infancy (Dravet syndrome). In: Roger J, Bureau M, Dravet C, Genton P, et al, eds. *Epileptic Syndromes in Infancy, Childhood and Adolescence.* 4th ed. London: John Libbey Eurotext Ltd, 2005:89–113.
30. Hurst DL. Epidemiology of severe myoclonic epilepsy of infancy. *Epilepsia* 1990; 31: 397–400.
31. Yakoub M, Dulac O, Jambaque I, Plouin P. Early diagnosis of severe myoclonic epilepsy in infancy. *Brain Dev* 1992; 14: 299–303.
32. Ogino T. Severe myoclonic epilepsy in infancy—a clinical and electroencephalographic study. *J Jpn Epil Soc* 1986; 4:114–126.
33. Ohki T, Watanabe K, Negoro K, Aso K, et al. Severe myoclonic epilepsy in infancy: evolution of seizures. *Seizure* 1997; 6:219–224.
34. Wolff M, Casse-Perrot C, Dravet C. Severe myoclonic epilepsy of infants (Dravet syndrome): natural history and neuropsychological findings. *Epilepsia* 2006; 47:Suppl 2:45–48.
35. Dalla Bernardina B, Capovilla G, Chiamenti C, Trevisan E, et al. Cryptogenic myoclonic epilepsies of infancy and early childhood: nosological and prognostic approach. In: Wolf P, Dam M, Janz D, Dreifuss FE, eds. Advances in Epileptology 16. New-York: Raven Press, 1987:175–180.
36. Scheffer IE, Berkovic SF. Generalized epilepsy with febrile seizures plus: a genetic disorder with heterogeneous clinical phenotypes. *Brain* 1997; 120: 479–490.
37. Singh R, Andermann E, Whitehouse WP, Harvey AS, et al. Severe myoclonic epilepsy of infancy: extended spectrum of GEFS+? *Epilepsia* 2001; 42:837–844.
38. Veggiotti P, Cardinali S, Montalenti E, Gatti A, et al. Generalized epilepsy with febrile seizures plus and severe myoclonic epilepsy in infancy: a case report of two Italian families. *Epil Disord* 2001; 3:29–32.
39. Claes L, Del-Favero J, Ceulemans B, Lagae L, et al. *De novo* mutations in the sodium-channel gene *SCN1A* cause severe myoclonic epilepsy of infancy. *Am J Hum Genet* 2001; 68:1327–1332.

40. Nabbout R, Gennaro E, Dalla Bernardina B, et al. Spectrum of *SCN1A* mutations in severe myoclonic epilepsy of infancy. *Neurology* 2003; 60:1961–1967.
41. Fujiwara T, Sugawara T, Mazaki-Miyazaki E, Takahashi Y, et al. Mutations of sodium channel α subunit type 1 (*SCN1A*) in intractable childhood epilepsies with frequent generalized tonic clonic seizures. *Brain* 2003; 126:531–546.
42. Suls A, Claeys KG, Goossens D, et al. Microdeletions involving the SCN1A gene may be common in SCN1A-mutation-negative SMEI patients. *Hum Mutat* 2006; 27: 914–920.
43. Harkin LA, Bowser DN, Dibbens LM, Singh R, et al. Truncation of the $GABA_A$-receptor γ 2 subunit in a family with generalized epilepsy with febrile seizures plus. *Am J Hum Genet* 2002; 70:530–536.
44. Ceulemans BP, Claes LR, Lagae LG. Clinical correlations of mutations in the *SCN1A* gene: from febrile seizures to severe myoclonic epilepsy in infancy. *Pediatr Neurol* 2004; 30:236–243.
45. Sugawara T, Mazaki-Miyazaki E, Fukushima K, Shimomura J, et al. Frequent mutations of *SCN1A* in severe myoclonic epilepsy in infancy. *Neurology* 2002; 58:1122–1124.
46. Rhodes TH, Lossin C, Vanoye CG, Wang DW, et al. Noninactivating voltage-gated sodium channels in severe myoclonic epilepsy of infancy. *Proc Natl Acad Sci U S A* 2004; 101:11147–11152.
47. Lambarri San Martin I, Garaizar Axpe C, Zuazo Zamalloa E, Prats Vinas JM. Epilepsia polimorfa de la infancia. Revision de 12 casos. *An Esp Pediatr* 1997; 46:571–575.
48. Nieto-Barrera M, Lillo MM, Rodriguez-Collado C, Candau R, et al. Epilepsia mioclonica severa de la infancia. Estudio epidemiologico analitico. *Rev Neurol* 2000; 30:620–624.
49. Ferrie CD, Maisey M, Cox T, et al. Focal abnormalities detected by ^{18}FDG PET in epileptic encephalopathies. *Arch Dis Child* 1996; 75:102–107.
50. Siegler Z, Barsi P, Neuwirth M, Jerney J, et al. Hippocampal sclerosis in severe myoclonic epilepsy in infancy: a retrospective MRI study. *Epilepsia* 2005; 46(5):704–708.
51. Castro-Gago M, Martinon Sanchez JM, Rodriguez-Nunez A, Herranz Fernandez JL, et al. Severe myoclonic epilepsy and mitochondrial cytopathy. *Childs Nerv Syst* 1997; 13 (11–12):570–571.
52. Seino M, Higashi T. A group of patients with infant onset secondary generalized epilepsy characterized by refractory grand mal seizures. (in Japanese). In: Kimura M, ed. *Mental and Physical Disability Research Group Sponsored by Ministry of Health and Welfare. Report of Research Group of Children's Health and Environment (1978)*. 1979: 79–80.
53. Fukuma G, Oguni H, Shirasaka Y, et al. Mutations of neuronal voltage-gated Na+ channel γ 1 subunit gene *SCN1A* in core: severe myoclonic epilepsy in infancy (SMEI) and in borderline SMEI (SMEB). *Epilepsia* 2004; 45:140–148.
54. Guerrini R, Dravet C, Genton P, Belmonte A, et al. Lamotrigine and seizure aggravation in severe myoclonic epilepsy. *Epilepsia* 1998; 39:508–512.
55. Wakai S, Ikehata M, Nihira H, Ito N, et al. Obtundation status caused by complex partial status epilepticus in a patient with severe myoclonic epilepsy in infancy. *Epilepsia* 1996; 37:1020–1022.
56. Kanazawa O, Shirane S. Can early zonizamide medication improve the prognosis in the core and peripheral types of severe myoclonic epilepsy in infants? *Brain Dev* 1999; 21:503.
57. Oguni H, Hayashi K, Oguni M, et al. Treatment of severe myoclonic epilepsy in infants with bromide and its borderline variant. *Epilepsia* 1994; 35:1140–1145.
58. Nieto Barrera M, Candau R, Nieto-Jimenez M, Correra A, et al. Topiramate in the treatment of severe myoclonic epilepsy in infancy. *Seizure* 2000; 9:590–594.
59. Coppola G, Capovilla G, Montagnini A, Romeo A, et al. Topiramate as add-on drug in severe myoclonic epilepsy in infancy: an Italian multicenter open trial. *Epilepsy Res* 2002; 49:45–48.
60. Chiron C, Marchand MC, Tran A, Rey E, et al. Stiripentol in severe myoclonic epilepsy in infancy: a randomised placebo-controlled syndrome-dedicated trial. STICLO study group. *Lancet* 2000; 356:1638–1642.
61. Fejerman N, Caraballo R, Cersosimo R. Ketogenic diet in patients with Dravet syndrome and myoclonic epilepsies in infancy and early childhood. *Adv Neurol* 2005; 95:299–305.
62. Minakawa K. Effectiveness of intravenous midazolam for the treatment of status epilepticus in a child with severe myoclonic epilepsy in infancy. *No To Hattatsu* 1995; 27:498–500.
63. Jansen FE, Sadleir LG, Harkin LA, Vadlamudi L, et al. Severe myoclonic epilepsy of infancy (Dravet syndrome): recognition and diagnosis in adults. *Neurology* 2006; 67: 2224–2226.
64. Guerrini R, Dravet Ch. Severe epileptic encephalopathies of infancy, other than West syndrome. In: Engel J, Pedley TA eds. *Epilepsy. A Comprehensive Textbook*. Vol. 3. Philadelphia, New York: Lippincott-Raven 1998:2285–2302.
65. Miyake S, Tanaka M, Matsui M, Miyagawa T, et al. Mortality patterns of children with epilepsies in a children's medical center. *No To Hattatsu* 1991; 23:329–335.
66. Genton P, Roger J, Guerrini R, Medina MT, et al. History and classification of "myoclonic" epilepsies: from seizures to syndromes to diseases. *Adv Neurol* 2005; 95:1–14.
67. Doose H, Gerken H, Leonhardt R, Voelzke E, et al. Centroencephalic myoclonic-astatic petit mal. Clinical and genetic investigations. *Neuropädiatrie* 1970; 2:59–78.
68. Guerrini R, Parmeggiani L, Bonanni P, Kaminska A, et al. Myoclonic astatic epilepsy. In: Roger J, Bureau M, Dravet Ch, Genton P, et al, eds. *Epileptic Syndromes in Infancy, Childhood and Adolescence*. 4th ed. London: John Libbey Eurotext Ltd, 2005:115–124.
69. Doose H, Sitepu B. Childhood epilepsy in a German city. *Neuropediatrics* 1983; 14: 220–224.
70. Kaminska A, Ickowicz A, Plouin P, Bru MF, et al. Delineation of cryptogenic Lennox-Gastaut syndrome and myoclonic astatic epilepsy using multiple correspondence analysis. *Epilepsy Res* 1999; 36:15–29.
71. Doose H. Myoclonic astatic epilepsy of early childhood. In: Roger J, Bureau M, Dravet Ch, Dreifuss FE, et al, eds. *Epileptic Syndromes in Infancy, Childhood and Adolescence*. London: John Libbey, 1992:103–114.
72. Singh R., Scheffer IE, Crossland K, Berkovic SF. Generalised epilepsy with febrile seizures plus: a common childhood-onset genetic epilepsy syndrome. *Ann Neurol* 1999; 45:75–81.
73. Oguni H, Hayashi K, Imai K, Funatsuka M, et al. Idiopathic myoclonic-astatic epilepsy of early childhood—nosology based on electrophysiologic and long-term follow-up study of patients. *Adv Neurol* 2005; 95:157–174.
74. Oguni H, Fukuyama Y, Imaizumi Y, Uehara T. Video-EEG analysis of drop seizures in myoclonic astatic epilepsy of early childhood (Doose syndrome). *Epilepsia* 1992; 33: 805–813.
75. Guerrini R, Bonanni P, Rothwell J, Hallett M. Myoclonus and epilepsy. In: Guerrini R, Aicardi J, Andermann F, Hallett M, eds. *Epilepsy and Movement Disorder*. Cambridge, UK: Cambridge University Press, 2002:165–210.
76. Ewen JB, Comi AM, Kossoff EH. Myoclonic-astatic epilepsy in a child with Sturge-Weber syndrome. *Pediatr Neurol* 2007; 36:115–117.
77. Kubota M, Ozawa H, Kaneko K, Sakakihara Y. A magnetoencephalographic study of astatic seizure in myoclonic astatic epilepsy. *Pediatr Neurol* 2004; 31:207–210.
78. Nabbout R, Kozlovski A, Gennaro E, Bahi-Buisson N, et al. Absence of mutations in major GEFS+ genes in myoclonic astatic epilepsy. *Epilepsy Res* 2003; 56:127–133.
79. Ebach K, Joos H, Doose H, Stephani U, et al. SCN1A mutation analysis in myoclonic astatic epilepsy and severe idiopathic generalized epilepsy of infancy with generalized tonic-clonic seizures. *Neuropediatrics* 2005; 36:210–213.
80. Aicardi J, Chevrie JJ. Atypical benign partial epilepsy of childhood. *Dev Med Child Neurol* 2002; 24:281–292.
81. Tassinari CA, Rubboli G, Billard C, Bureau M. Electrical status epilepticus during slow sleep (ESES or CSWS) and acquired epileptic aphasia (Landau-Kleffner syndrome). In: Roger J, Bureau M, Dravet Ch, Genton P, et al, eds. *Epileptic Syndromes in Infancy, Childhood and Adolescence*. 4th ed. London: John Libbey Eurotext Ltd, 2005:295–314.
82. Sasagawa M, Kioi Y. A successful treatment with a continuous intravenous lidocaine for a cluster of minor seizures in a patient with Doose syndrome. *No To Hattatsu* 1997; 29: 261–263.
83. Kanemura H, Aihara M, Sata Y, Hatakeyama K, et al. A successful treatment with a continuous intravenous lidocaine for a cluster of minor seizures in a patient with Doose syndrome. *No To Hattatsu* 1996; 28:325–331.
84. Oguni H, Tanaka T, Hayashi K, Funatsuka M, et al. Treatment and long-term prognosis of myoclonic-astatic epilepsy of early childhood. *Neuropediatrics* 2002; 33:122–132.
85. Caraballo RH, Cersosimo RO, Sakr D, Cresta A, et al. Ketogenic diet in patients with myoclonic-astatic epilepsy. *Epileptic Disord* 2006; 8:151–155.
86. Lortie A, Chiron C, Mumford J, Dulac O. The potential for increasing seizure frequency, relapse, and appearance of new seizure types with vigabatrin. *Neurology* 1993; 43 (Suppl 5):S24–S27.
87. Dulac O, Kaminska A. Use of lamotrigine in Lennox-Gastaut and related epilepsy syndromes. *J Child Neurol* 1997; 12(suppl 1):S23–S28.
88. Pisani F, Oteri G, Russo MF, Di Perri R, et al. The efficacy of valproate-lamotrigine comedication in refractory complex partial seizures: evidence for a pharmacodynamic interaction. *Epilepsia* 1999; 40:1141–1146.
89. Kroll-Seger J, Mothersill IW, Novak S, Salke-Kellermann RA, et al. Levetiracetam-induced myoclonic status epilepticus in myoclonic-astatic epilepsy: a case report. *Epileptic Disord* 2006; 8:213–218.
90. Jayawant S, Libretto SE. Topiramate in the treatment of myoclonic-astatic epilepsy in children: a retrospective hospital audit. *J Postgrad Med* 2003; 49:202–205.
91. Szczepanik E, Pakszys M, Rusek G. [Positive effect of felbamate therapy in a boy with refractory epilepsy] (in Polish). *Neurol Neurochir Pol* 2000; 34 Suppl 1:195–201.
92. Hoffmann-Riem M, Diener W, Beninger C, Rating D, et al. Nonconvulsive status epilepticus: a possible cause of mental retardation in patients with Lennox-Gastaut syndrome. *Neuropediatrics* 2000; 31:169–174.

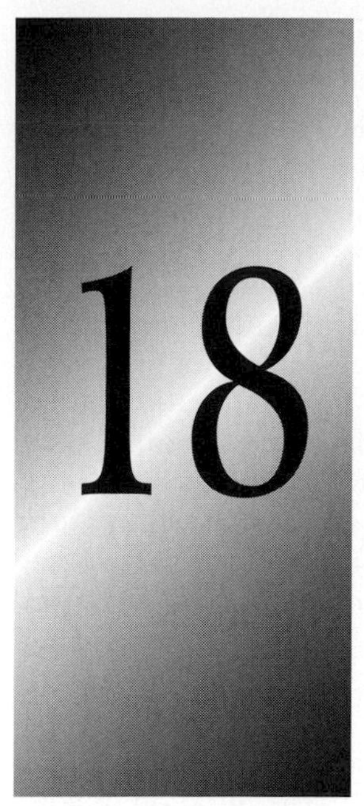

18 Partial Epilepsies in Infancy

Kazuyoshi Watanabe

Partial epilepsies had been considered infrequent in infancy (1–3), but this may be because partial seizure manifestations in infants are subtle and often difficult to identify unless they show definite focal motor phenomena. It is often difficult to distinguish partial from generalized seizures on the basis of clinical observations and interictal encephalograms (EEGs) (4). In a previous study of seizures in the first year of life (2), partial seizures comprised only 12%, whereas infantile spasms accounted for 41% and generalized motor seizures for 35%. Generalized motor seizures, however, may represent partial seizures that are secondarily generalized. Generalized tonic-clonic seizures are very rare in infants, if present, and ictal EEGs of such seizures usually display partial seizure patterns evolving to secondarily generalized tonic-clonic seizures (5, 6). In another study, partial epilepsy comprised 12%, whereas West syndrome represented 69% of the cases (7). Later studies of epilepsies in the first years of life revealed an increased incidence of partial epilepsies, although West syndrome remained the most common syndrome: 17–36% for partial epilepsies vs. 39–48% for West syndrome (8–10). Recent studies have reported a higher incidence of partial epilepsies in the first 2 years of life: 43% for partial epilepsies vs. 28% for infantile spasms at a tertiary center (11), and 60% vs. 35% in the first 2 years of life in a regional general hospital (12). This increased incidence is probably due to an increased recognition of partial seizures with or without secondary generalization in infants.

The prognosis of partial epilepsy in infancy had been considered poor, and benign partial epilepsy was reported to be extremely rare or nonexistent in infancy (13, 14). Complex partial seizures of infancy were reported to be medically intractable and often associated with mental handicap, necessitating aggressive treatment (15). However, Watanabe et al (16) first reported the presence of partial epilepsy in infancy with complex partial seizures in 1987, and, subsequently, of benign partial epilepsy with secondarily generalized seizures (17).

This chapter reviews symptomatic, cryptogenic, and idiopathic benign partial epilepsies and related syndromes in the first 2 years of life, excluding neonatal seizures.

ICTAL CLINICAL MANIFESTATIONS

The repertoire of ictal manifestation of epilepsy in infants is limited. Seizures often begin with a change in facial expression or behavior, but the most striking feature is an arrest or marked reduction of behavioral motor activity, which was formerly called a hypomotor seizure (18). Some authors consider seizures complex partial if nonconvulsive ictal phenomena are associated with disturbance of contact or unresponsiveness and focal or nongeneralized paroxysmal EEG discharges (15, 19), but others avoid the term because of difficulty in determining impairment of consciousness (18). The most ordinary sequence of infantile complex partial seizures consists mainly of motion arrest, decreased responsiveness, staring or blank eyes, or simple gestural automatisms followed by mild convulsive movements and subsequent alimentary automatisms (16, 19). Convulsive movements consist of eye deviation or head rotation; mild clonic movements involving face, eyelids, or limbs; and increased limb tone. These tonic or clonic movements are qualitatively not as intense as those in generalized tonic-clonic seizures. They are more frequent in younger children and may be widespread, covering a wide area of the body, often leading to an erroneous diagnosis of generalized tonic-clonic seizures. Constant focal or unilateral motor seizures are characteristic of symptomatic partial epilepsy. Symmetric motor phenomena of the limbs and head nodding are characteristic of seizures in younger children with temporal lobe seizures (20). Bilaterally synchronous motor seizures (21), or bilateral tonic stiffening and extension of all limbs with or without evolution to a bilateral asymmetric clonic phase, tonic seizures with a sustained fencer posture, epileptic spasms in cluster, or brief loss of muscle tone on one side of the body may also be seen in infants (18). Automatisms consist of simple head, arm, or leg movements, and alimentary automatisms such as chewing, lip and tongue smacking, swallowing, or licking one's lips (19). Alimentary automatisms are the most common form, and no complex, semipurposeful gestural automatisms are present in infants. Eye deviation or head rotation occurs early in the attack, whereas oral automatisms occur later, or postictally. Some authors feel these subtle limb or oral movements difficult to distinguish from background behavior (18). Autonomic changes such as flushing, mydriasis, pallor, cyanosis, apnea, or tachypnea may be seen (22). All focal motor seizures and most versive seizures are associated with focal EEG seizure patterns in the contralateral hemisphere. Generalized motor seizures display focal EEG discharges in 37%, while hypomotor seizures do so in 70% (23). Hypomotor seizures originate from temporal, temporoparietal, or parietooccipital regions. Seizures with localized or bilateral clonic, tonic, or atonic motor phenomena arise predominantly from frontal, frontocentral, central, or frontoparietal areas. Temporal or temporoparietal foci are associated with diminution of behavioral activity, whereas frontal or central foci are associated with localized or generalized motor phenomena (18). Frontal lobe seizures are often initiated by psychomotor arrest followed either by limb hypertonia or tonic posturing and complex global motor behavior, or by simple gestural automatisms and eyelid myoclonias (24). Hypermotor seizures and complex motor automatisms are not seen in young children with frontal lobe seizures (25). Rolandic seizures often begin by uni- or bilateral hypertonia of the limbs, followed by uni- or more frequently bilateral clonic activity. Eye opening or psychomotor arrest mainly occur at the onset of temporal lobe seizures, during which oroalimentary automatisms are observed, often associated with eyelid myoclonias (24). Younger children with temporal lobe seizures show convulsive movements more often than older children (19, 26). The first clinical signs of occipital seizures frequently consist of eye deviation, or more rarely eye opening, frequently followed by oculoclonias and eyelid myoclonias (24, 27). Ictal smile, flush, head nod, and behavioral changes are typical in infants and young children with posterior cortex seizures (28). Focal clonic activity, predominantly unilateral spasms, focal tonic activity, ictal nystagmus, and postictal paresis are good lateralizing signs occurring contralateral to the hemisphere of seizure onset, whereas tonic eye deviation is not a good lateralizing sign (29). The duration of complex partial seizures, timed from the first clinical or EEG change until the end of paroxysmal discharges, excluding postictal polymorphous delta waves, ranges from 40 to 250 seconds in infants, longer than that of older children, ranging from 10 to 110 seconds (19). Partial seizures may evolve into secondarily generalized tonic-clonic seizures. In such cases, initial partial seizures last 5–33 seconds, and the following generalized tonic-clonic seizures 40–120 sec (17). Convulsive movements may be extensive, but secondary generalization is infrequent in symptomatic partial epilepsies (19, 25, 28). In contrast, secondarily generalized seizures are more frequent in idiopathic benign partial epilepsy (11). Epilepsia partialis continua may occur in hemimegalencephaly or focal cortical dysplasia (30, 31). Epileptic spasms are usually considered a seizure manifestation of generalized epilepsy, but they may be seen in partial epilepsy if it is defined by localized ictal EEG or localized lesion on neuroimaging with seizure-free surgical outcome (18, 23). Epileptic spasms are often the initial manifestation or seen transiently during the course of symptomatic partial epilepsy due to focal cortical dysplasia (25, 27, 32–34). About one-third of infants with partial epilepsies beginning in the first 2 years of life presented initially with infantile spasms (12).

EEG FEATURES

In infants with partial epilepsies, interictal EEGs demonstrate paroxysmal discharges infrequently (19). In idiopathic benign partial epilepsy in infancy with complex partial seizures or secondarily generalized seizures, interictal EEGs are normal and do not show paroxysmal discharges, although small vertex spikes with larger bell-shaped slow waves are seen in benign partial epilepsy with vertex spikes and waves during sleep (35). Paroxysmal discharges may be absent even in symptomatic partial epilepsies in infancy. In symptomatic partial epilepsies, interictal background EEG rhythms are usually slow and poorly organized, and regional posterior frequencies are not observed (15). Sleep EEGs display abnormal organization, often without stage II features, and persistent voltage and frequency asymmetry may be observed. Interictal EEGs often show paroxysmal discharges such as spikes, spike and waves, and sharp waves that may be unilateral, bilateral, or multifocal (36).

Ictal EEGs usually display focal discharges of low-voltage fast waves or rhythmic or repetitive sharp alpha or theta waves of increasing amplitude and decreasing frequency, which are followed by theta and delta waves mixed with spikes or sharp waves with gradual or rapid spread to other regions (16, 19). In secondarily generalized seizures, ictal EEGs show focal discharges of low-voltage fast waves or rhythmic or repetitive sharp waves or spikes of increasing amplitude and decreasing frequency, which transmit to the contralateral and adjacent regions, then to all areas. These waves or spikes resemble epileptic recruiting rhythm, which then become mixed with slow waves of decreasing frequency, giving rise to spike, polyspike, or sharp- and slow-wave complexes. Bilateral synchrony of these discharges and associated clonic seizures is poorer in comparison with those observed in older children and adults (17).

IDIOPATHIC PARTIAL EPILEPSIES

Benign Partial Epilepsy in Infancy with Complex Partial Seizures

This syndrome is characterized by complex partial seizures (CPS) occurring in clusters, age at onset mostly during the first year of life, a family history of benign infantile seizures in many cases, normal development prior to onset, no underlying disorders or neurological abnormalities, normal cranial computed tomography (CT) and magnetic resonance imaging (MRI) findings, normal interictal EEGs, excellent response to drug treatment, and normal developmental outcome (11, 16, 37–40). Seizures occur mostly during wakefulness in clusters 1–10 times a day for 1–3 days. They may recur within a few months even on drug treatment. The most frequent site of origin of ictal discharges is the temporal area, but other foci or even dual foci can be seen. We previously proposed to combine this syndrome with benign partial epilepsy with secondarily generalized seizures, described subsequently, and call them benign partial epilepsy in infancy (17). But CPS may be misdiagnosed as generalized tonic-clonic seizures because of concomitant convulsive movements (19). The unique characteristics of this syndrome with CPS as the sole type of seizures should be emphasized, because it may be difficult to diagnose it unless we know its presence. It is important to recognize this subtype, because it may be too subtle or atypical to diagnose it as an epileptic seizure. In fact, gastroesophageal reflux disease was initially thought to be the etiology of symptoms in a substantial number of patients, delaying referral to the pediatric neurologist by as much as 3 months (11).

Benign Partial Epilepsy in Infancy with Secondarily Generalized Seizures (SGS)

The main clinical features are similar to those of the aforementioned subtype with CPS in regard to family history, age of onset, neurodevelopmental normality, absence of underlying disorders, and normal interictal EEGs (17). This subtype presents only with SGS. Seizures occur more frequently during wakefulness than during sleep, but more frequently during sleep than in the subtype with CPS. Partial seizures lasting 5–35 seconds, manifested by motion arrest with staring or blank eyes during wakefulness, or opening of eyes with staring during sleep, are followed by generalized tonic-clonic seizures of 40–150 seconds' duration. Seizures occur in clusters 2–5 times a day for 1–3 days. They may recur within a few months after treatment, but they can be easily controlled with an adjustment of the dosage. The site of initial paroxysmal discharges is usually in the central, occipital, or parietal area (38). Different foci (occipital and central) were disclosed at the onset and recurrence in an infant (17). SGS are easily mistaken for primarily generalized seizures, because it is not always easy to recognize the presence of preceding partial seizures. For their accurate diagnosis, the initial partial seizure manifestation should be specially sought, or an ictal EEG recording should be done.

Diagnosis and Long-Term Follow-up of Benign Partial Epilepsy in Infancy

It is not always easy to make an accurate diagnosis of benign partial epilepsy in infancy (BPEI) at the onset of seizures (41), as the diagnostic criteria include seizure freedom and normal developmental outcome. A positive family history of similar disorders is helpful, but it is absent in many cases. Okumura et al (42) defined *possible BPEI* as partial epilepsy with CPS and/or SGS meeting the aforementioned criteria excluding outcome items, and made the final diagnosis of *definite BPEI* at age 5 years, when there was no seizure beyond age 2 years and normal psychomotor development beyond 5 years. *Definite BPEI* accounted for 76% of the patients diagnosed as having *possible BPEI* at the first presentation and 90% of those who met the conditions on reevaluation at age 2 years. Thus, recognition of BPEI is possible, to some extent, at the first presentation, and reevaluation at age 2 years is useful for a more precise diagnosis. A recent long-term follow-up study revealed that most of patients with *possible BPEI* at age 2 years and almost all of the patients who met the criteria of *definite BPEI* at age 5 years did not have seizure recurrence or mental problems beyond 8 years of age (43). Thus, the diagnosis of BPEI can be made reliably at age 5 years. During the follow-up period in this study, 9% of patients with definite BPEI at age 8 years or older had convulsions with mild gastroenteritis at age 18–22 months after an antiepileptic drug (AED) was discontinued. In view of the long interval between the two types of seizures and the different age of onset of two syndromes, it is reasonable to consider that these patients had two different syndromes rather than a relapse of BPEI. Another 9% of the patients developed paroxysmal kinesigenic choreoathetosis (PKC) at age 6–8 years. The association of PKC with benign infantile convulsions has been recently recognized (see the following section). No patients developed other types of idiopathic epilepsy.

Benign Infantile Convulsions/Seizures

The presence of infantile convulsions with benign outcome was first described by Fukuyama in 1963 (44), who defined them as having the following features: onset before 2 years of age; generalized, symmetrical convulsion, mainly tonic-clonic, lasting 1–2 minutes; no family history of epilepsy; no remarkable past history; normal psychomotor development; no etiology; (EEG normal); and benign course. This type of infantile convulsions has been the subject of many subsequent studies in Japan and has been called benign infantile convulsions (BIC) (38). As generalized, symmetrical convulsions are one of the criteria of BIC, none of the studies considered BIC partial seizures. We pointed out, however, that ictal EEGs of such patients usually display partial seizures evolving to secondarily generalized tonic-clonic seizures (5). Tsurui et al (45) made a similar observation in patients with BIC meeting the criteria of Fukuyama except for a family history. The absence of a family history of epilepsy was another criterion of BIC described by Fukuyama, but a family history of benign convulsions was often elicited in BIC (38). Vigevano et al (46) reported an autosomal dominant disorder, benign infantile familial convulsions (BIFC), characterized by a family history of benign seizures in infancy and secondarily generalized partial seizures confirmed by ictal EEG recordings. The site of origin of ictal discharges was in the parieto-occipital area. Since the description by Vigevano et al (46), there have been reports on BFIC from many different parts of the world (47, 48). This syndrome corresponds to the familial type of BIC described by Fukuyama (44) and to benign partial epilepsy with SGS described by Watanabe et al (17). Later reports recognized the presence of simple or complex partial seizures without secondarily generalization in a number of patients (49–51). These cases may correspond to BPEI with CPS described by Watanabe et al (16). BFIC show an autosomal dominant mode of inheritance. So far, three loci for BFIC have been mapped on chromosomes 19q12–q13.11 (52), 2q24 (53), and 16p12–q12 (51, 54). The last region is the same locus as that for familial infantile convulsions and paroxysmal choreoathetosis (49). Recently, Striano et al (55) have reported a pedigree with BFIC in which genetic analysis revealed a novel SCN2A gene mutation on chromosome 2q24. Mutations in the same gene has been identified in families affected by benign familial neonatal-infantile seizures (BFNIS) (56, 57), suggesting these two benign familial seizures may share the same genetic abnormality. Both share many clinical features except for the age of onset.

Benign Familial Neonatal-Infantile Seizures

This is an autosomal dominant benign seizure disorder, presenting in early infancy, in which mutations of SCN2A gene have been detected (56, 57). The age of onset ranges from day 2 to 7 months (mean, 11.2 weeks). Seizures are characterized by secondarily generalized partial seizures; neonatal seizures were not seen in all families. The frequency of seizures varied; some individuals had only a few attacks without treatment, whereas others had clusters of many per day. Febrile seizures were rare. All cases remitted by 12 months. Ictal recordings showed a focal onset in the posterior quadrants.

Benign Familial Infantile Convulsions and Paroxysmal Choreoathetosis

The association of paroxysmal choreoathetosis with BFIC was first reported by Szepetowski et al (49) and subsequently described by several authors (58–63). This disorder is inherited as an autosomal dominant trait and linked to chromosome 16p12–q12. The clinical expression is variable, and affected individuals may display infantile seizures, paroxysmal dyskinesia, or both. The paroxysmal dyskinesia starts at age 5–28 years and occurs spontaneously at rest or is induced by sudden movements, anxiety, or prolonged exercise. Some patients exhibited recurrence of epileptic seizures at a much later age (59). Two families with this disorder in which one of the members developed temporal lobe seizures in adolescence and adulthood, respectively, were reported (64, 65). Carbamazepine is usually effective against dyskinesia, although the condition may not be so disabling as to make individuals seek medical advice.

Benign Familial Infantile Convulsions and Familial Hemiplegic Migraine

Vanmolkot et al (66) reported novel missense mutations in the ATP1A2 Na^+, K^+-ATPase pump gene on chromosome 1q23 in two families with familial hemiplegic migraine (FHM). The M731T mutation was found in a family with pure FHM, whereas the R689Q mutation was identified in a family in which FHM and benign familial infantile convulsions (BFIC) partially cosegregate. In this family, all available affected family members with FHM, BFIC, or both carry the ATP1A2 mutation. Like FHM linked to 19p13, FHM linked to 1q23 also involves dysfunction of ion transport, and epilepsy is part of its phenotypic spectrum.

Benign Partial Epilepsy in Infancy and Early Childhood with Vertex Spikes and Waves During Sleep

This syndrome is a form of benign partial epilepsy in infancy characterized by the presence of typical focal interictal EEG abnormalities in the vertex regions only during sleep (35, 67). Spikes and waves have a particular morphology consisting of a low-voltage fast spike followed by a higher-voltage bell-shaped slow wave, appearing isolated or grouped in short sequences with spread from vertex to central regions. A family history of febrile or afebrile benign seizures is relatively common (30–50%). The age of onset ranges from 13 to 30 months with a peak between 16 and 20 months, but an earlier onset before age 1 year was reported later (68). Seizures occur infrequently, varying from one episode to three to four per year, mostly in wakefulness, and are characterized by staring and motion arrest, followed by stiffening of the arms, cyanosis, and loss of consciousness, lasting 1–5 minutes. They never occurred in clusters or in the form of status (67). Seizure remission occurred between 2 years 3 months and 3 years 7 months, whereas spike and waves remitted between 3 and 5 years. Antiepileptic treatment is considered unnecessary because of low seizure frequency and short duration (69).

Benign Convulsions with Mild Gastroenteritis

Benign convulsions with mild gastroenteritis (CwG) are situation-related seizures associated with gastroenteritis. They were first described by Morooka in Japan (70) and have been studied by many Japanese and a few Taiwanese investigators (71) but rarely reported from other countries (72–74). Uemura et al (71) studied clinical features of this disorder in 114 episodes of 105 patients. CwG are defined as having the following features: seizures associated with gastroenteritis without signs of dehydration or electrolyte derangement; the body temperature less than 38°C before and after the seizures; patients with bacterial or aseptic meningitis, encephalitis/encephalopathy associated with viral infection, or a history of epilepsy are excluded. The age of onset ranged from 8 to 52 months (average 21.1 months). A family history of febrile or afebrile seizures is infrequent (7%, 6% respectively). A pair of identical twins had CwG on the same day (75). Sakai et al (76) reported a family with CwG and BIC. Only 5% had febrile seizures on occasions unrelated to CwG. Seizures occurred in clusters in 75% of the episodes, presented as generalized convulsions in 87% of patients and complex partial seizures in 13%, and lasted from 30 seconds to 3 minutes. They were induced by pain and/or crying in 43% of episodes, although no patients had convulsions associated with crying on any occasions before and after the episode of CwG. These seizures were clearly different from breath-holding spells. In patients with multiple seizures, the interval between the first and last seizure was 0.5–48 hours (mean 8.6 hours), and seizures ceased within 6 hours in 59% of episodes. None of the patients developed epilepsy, and all patients exhibited normal psychomotor development. Interictal EEGs are normal. Ictal EEGs were recorded in a few cases and showed complex partial seizures evolving to secondarily generalized tonic-clonic seizures (75, 77, 78). The site of origin of ictal discharges was occipital in 5, parietal in one, and centroparietotemporal in one of 7 episodes recorded from 5 patients. One of the patients showed three different foci in three episodes (77). Rotavirus is the most common etiologic agent of gastroenteritis, but other viruses, such as small round structured virus, may also be responsible (79, 80). It is not always easy to distinguish patients with CwG from those with encephalitis/encephalopathy. Hongou et al (81) reported a patient with rotavirus encephalitis mimicking CwG who showed slowing of the background EEG.

Treatment of Benign Partial Epilepsies and Other Benign Infantile Seizure Disorders

Although benign partial epilepsies and other benign infantile seizures have a tendency to spontaneous remission, the seizures often occur in clusters, and the benignity of the condition can not usually be ascertained at the very beginning of the disease, so an AED may be administered for a certain period. However, there is no consensus as to the choice of an AED and the period of administration. Various AEDs have been tried, but the efficacy of each drug is difficult to assess because of the tendency toward spontaneous remission. Breakthrough seizure rates while on AED treatment were 11–37% and highest in the population where phenobarbital was mainly used (11). Recently, a once-daily dose of 5 mg/kg of carbamazepine has been reported to be highly effective for the treatment of benign infantile convulsions (82) or convulsions with mild gastroenteritis (83). In contrast, diazepam is generally ineffective against clusters of seizures in benign infantile convulsions or convulsions with mild gastroenteritis (82, 84). Phenobarbital is considered effective against convulsions with mild gastroenteritis if used in a large dose, but its effect is not usually satisfactory (84).

Lidocaine in drip infusion or in the form of skin tape is reported to be more effective against CwG than diazepam or phenobarbital (85). For the treatment of BIC, it is recommended to administer the aforementioned dose of carbamazepine as quickly as possible, orally or through a nasogastric tube if oral administration is not possible. For BPEI, we previously recommended to administer an AED for one year or until the child reaches 3 years of age, as no seizures occurred after this age (38). But a shorter treatment period may be feasible in view of the short period of seizure persistence in BPEI (average 3 months, range 0–12 months) (39). Nelson et al (11) suggested weaning from AED 6 months after seizure onset in BPEI.

SYMPTOMATIC AND CRYPTOGENIC PARTIAL EPILEPSIES IN INFANCY

Etiology

Etiologies of symptomatic partial epilepsies in infants include focal cortical dysplasia (FCD), pachygyria, polymicrogyria, low-grade dysplastic changes, heterotopic gray matter, schizencephaly, Sturge-Weber syndrome, tuberous sclerosis, hemimegalencephaly, with or without various neurocutaneous syndromes, dysembryoplastic neuroepithelial tumor, ganglioglioma, gangliocytoma, glialneuronal hamartoma, perinatal/postnatal insult, and hippocampal sclerosis with or without cortical dysplasia (18, 86–89). FCD is one of the most frequent causes of symptomatic partial epilepsy in infancy (27). Diffuse or bilateral cortical dysplasia is more often associated with generalized epilepsy, but not infrequently associated with partial epilepsies (90). Inborn errors of metabolism or chromosomal disorders may also induce partial seizures (91–93). Neonatal hypoglycemia may cause posterior cerebral lesions and symptomatic epilepsy, most frequently occipital lobe epilepsy (94). The syndrome of celiac disease, epilepsy, and cerebral calcifications is a rare clinical condition characterized by occipital seizures (95).

Surgical Treatment

The prognosis of symptomatic or cryptogenic partial epilepsies of patients with onset under age 3 years is less favorable than for patients with onset at 3 years or more (96). The probability of seizure control steadily increased until 15 years of treatment, but the cumulative probability of seizure control was small after 5 years of treatment. But epilepsy surgery should be considered in infants with refractory partial epilepsy as early as possible, because partial seizures in early infancy may be catastrophic and associated with poor long-term outcome. Repeated uncontrolled partial seizures in the first months of life may result in cognitive deterioration (97). Cortical resection or hemispherectomy can produce cessation or a dramatic reduction of seizures for highly selected infants with severe, intractable epilepsy and developmental delay (98). Identification of infants for surgery is often challenging, because seizure semiology may yield few clues to the partial nature of the epilepsy in infants. The interictal EEG is often nonlocalizing, and ictal EEG may not be helpful. Neuroimaging with high-resolution MRI, interictal and ictal single-photon emission computed tomography (SPECT), and interictal positron emission tomography (PET) plays an important role in identifying an epileptic lesion. In infants as well as older patients, the location of a potentially resectable epileptogenic zone must be defined by convergence of results from video-EEG, anatomic and functional neuroimaging, and clinical examination (98). Diagnosis of focal cortical dysplasia may be especially difficult during infancy, when myelination is incomplete and MRI does not reveal the abnormality. Sometimes neuroimaging abnormalities are evident only in early life or for a limited period (99–101).

Seizure-free outcome has been reported to be about 50–80% in infants who had cortical resection or hemispherectomy for catastrophic partial epilepsy due to FCD, infantile spasms with focal or hemispheric lesions, Sturge-Weber syndrome, ganglioglioma, or hemimegalencephaly (88, 98, 102–108). Catch-up developmental progress may be expected after surgery in some infants (98). A better developmental outcome is associated with early surgical intervention (109). The presence of a discrete lesion on preoperative neuroimaging correlated with a favorable surgical outcome (88). Seizure outcomes after surgery were less favorable in infants with FCD than for Sturge-Weber syndrome or low-grade glioma, and patients with hemispherectomies had a better outcome than those with focal cortical resections (105–107).

Epilepsy with Periodic Spasms

This is a peculiar type of partial epilepsy in infants and children, characterized by an initial focal clinical manifestation or ictal focal discharges followed by a series of bilateral and asymmetrical spasms in periodic sequence (110). The interictal EEG showed focal or multifocal epileptiform discharges but never hypsarrhythmia. The ictal EEG demonstrated a slow wave with superimposed fast rhythm at 15–25 Hz. This disorder is resistant to treatment and is found only in patients affected by a brain disease consisting of a fixed or progressive encephalopathy.

Partial Epilepsy with Transient West Syndrome

Partial seizures may be combined with epileptic spasms in patients with West syndrome (111–119). In contrast to epilepsy with periodic spasms, the interictal EEG shows hypsarrhythmia. Epilepsy with such combinations often starts with partial epilepsy in the neonatal period or early infancy and evolves into West syndrome, and it often will end up again in partial epilepsy, although it may evolve into Lennox-Gastaut syndrome (120).

Malignant Epilepsy with Migrating Partial Seizures in Infancy

This syndrome was first described by Coppola et al (121) and subsequently reported by several authors (122–126) and is characterized by onset between 1 day and 7 months of frequent or nearly continuous multifocal partial seizures, intractability to conventional AEDs, lack of identifiable etiology, and progressive decline in psychomotor function. Interictal EEGs show diffuse slowing of the background activity with multifocal epileptiform discharges, which may be rare in the early stage of the disorder. Ictal EEGs display paroxysmal discharges occurring in various regions in consecutive seizures in a given patient. They start in one region and progressively involve the adjacent areas. The area of ictal onset shifts from one region to another and from one hemisphere to the other, with occasional overlapping of consecutive seizures. The migratory feature of ictal discharges is not pathognomonic of the disorder and may be seen in BPEI with complex partial seizures (37). Most conventional AEDs have failed to control seizures, although bromides have been reported to be effective (122). The prognosis, although poor, is not uniformly grim as previously reported (126).

Symptomatic Partial Epilepsy with Subcortical Lesions

Gelastic Seizures due to Hypothalamic Hamartoma: Early-onset gelastic seizures, in association with hypothalamic hamartoma and occasionally precocious puberty, are a rare but well-recognized epileptic syndrome (127, 128). Gelastic seizures most commonly begin in infancy, even in the neonatal period, and are brief, frequent, and mechanical in nature (127). Seizures may either evolve toward a catastrophic encephalopathy or be transiently severe and progressively settle down. Intermediate situations also exist, as well as cases presenting with a mild epilepsy (129). Cognitive deterioration occurs, and severe behavior problems are frequent. The interictal EEG shows focal frontal or temporal spikes or generalized spike-waves. The ictal EEG demonstrates generalized fast rhythmic activity, generalized suppression of background activity, or both, sometimes preceded by single or multiple generalized spike-waves (127, 130). The variable expression of the epileptic syndrome renders difficult any dogmatic position on early surgery, but recent data suggest that a surgical solution must be sought early (129).

Hemifacial Seizures of Cerebellar Origin. Harvey et al (131) reported a 6-month old infant with daily episodes of left hemifacial contraction, head and eye deviation to the right, nystagmoid jerks to the right, autonomic dysfunction, and retained conscouness. The episodes began on day 1 of life and were unresponsive to antiepileptic medication. Interictal and ictal scalp recordings were unremarkable. MRI revealed a mass in the left cerebellar hemisphere and middle cerebellar peduncle. Ictal SPECT revealed focal hyperperfusion in the region of the cerebellar mass. Ictal EEG recordings with implanted cerebellar electrodes demonstrated focal seizure discharges in the region of the mass. Resection of the mass resulted in remission of seizures, and histopathology revealed a ganglioglioma. They concluded that this patient constituted a rare but important clinicopathological syndrome of infancy characterized by epileptic seizures of cerebellar origin.

References

1. Oller-Daurella L, Oller LF. Partial epilepsy with seizures appearing in the first three years of life. *Epilepsia* 1989; 30:820–826.
2. Matsumoto A, Watanabe K, Sugiura M, et al. Long-term prognosis of convulsive disorders in the first year of life: mental and physical development and seizure persistence. *Epilepsia* 1983; 24:321–329.
3. Chakova, L. Studies on the frequency and clinical manifestations of epilepsy in infancy and early childhood. *Folia Medica (Plovdiv)* 1996; 38:75–80.
4. Nordli DR Jr, Bazil CW, Scheuer ML, Pedley TA. Recognition and classification of seizures in infants. *Epilepsia* 1997; 38:553–560.
5. Watanabe K, Negoro T, Sugiura T, et al. Ictal EEGs of generalized tonic-clonic seizures in infancy (in Japanese). *Rinsho Noha (Osaka)* 1981; 23:445–447.
6. Korff C, Nordli DR Jr. Do generalized tonic-clonic seizures in infancy exist? *Neurology* 2005; 65:1750–1753.
7. Czochanska J, Langner-Tyszka B, Losiowski Z, Schmidt-Sidor B. Children who develop epilepsy in the first year of life: a prospective study. *Dev Med Child Neurol* 1994; 36:344–350.
8. Kramer U, Phatal A, Neufeld MY, Leitner Y, et al. Outcome of seizures in the first year of life. *Eur J Paediatr Neurol* 1997; 1:165–171.
9. Caraballo R, Cersosimo R, Galicchio S, Fejerman N. Epilepsies during the first year of life (in Spanish). *Revista de Neurologia* 1997; 25:1521–1524.
10. Battaglia D, Rando T, Deodato F, et al. Epileptic disorders with onset in the first year of life:neurological and cognitive outcome. *Eur J Paediatr Neurol* 1999; 3:95–103.
11. Nelson GB, Olson DM, Hahn JS. Short duration of benign partial epilepsy in infancy. *J Child Neurol* 2002; 17:440–445.
12. Okumura A, Hayakawa F, Kato T, et al. Five-year follow-up of patients with partial epilepsies in infancy. *Pediatr Neurol* 2001; 24:290–296.
13. Dulac O, Cusmai R, de Oliveira K. Is there a partial benign epilepsy in infancy? *Epilepsia* 1989; 30:798–801.
14. Dravet C, Catani C, Bureau M, Roger J. Partial epilepsies in infancy: a study of 40 cases. *Epilepsia* 1989; 30:807–812.
15. Duchowny MS, Resnick TJ, Alvarez L. Complex partial seizures of infancy. *Arch Neurol* 1987; 44:911–914.
16. Watanabe K, Yamamoto N, Negoro T, et al. Benign complex partial epilepsies in infancy. *Pediatr Neurol* 1987; 3:208–211.
17. Watanabe, K Negoro T, Aso K. Benign partial epilepsy with secondarily generalized seizures in infancy. *Epilepsia* 1993; 34:635–638.
18. Acharya JN, Wyllie E, Lüders HO, et al. Seizure symptomatology in infants with localization-related epilepsy. *Neurology* 1997; 48:189–196.
19. Yamamoto N, Watanabe K, Negoro T, et al. Partial seizures evolving to infantile spasms. *Epilepsia* 1988; 29:34–40.
20. Brockhaus A, Elger CE. Complex partial seizures of temporal lobe origin in children of different agegroups. *Epilepsia* 1995; 36:1173–1181.
21. Blume, WT. Clinical profile of partial seizures beginning at less than four years of age. *Epilepsia* 1989; 30:813–819.
22. Luna D, Dulac O, Plouin P. Ictal characteristics of cryptogenic partial epilepsies in infancy. *Epilepsia* 1989; 30:827–832.
23. Hamer HM, Wyllie E, Lüders HO, et al. Symptomatology of epileptic seizures in the first three years of life. *Epilepsia* 1999; 40:837–844.

24. Rathgeb JP, Plouin P, Soufflet C, et al. Les cas particuliers des crises partielles du nourrisson: semiologie electroclinique. In: Bureau M, Kahane P, Munari C, eds. *Epilepsies partielles graves pharmaco-resistantes de l'enfant: strategies diagnostiques et traitments chirurgicaux*. Paris: John Libbey Eurotext, 1998:122–134.
25. Fogarasi A, Janszky J, Faveret E, Pieper T, et al. A detailed analysis of frontal lobe seizure semiology in children younger than 7 years. *Epilepsia* 2001; 42:80–85.
26. Fogarasi A, Jokeit H, Faveret E, Janszky J, et al. The effect of age on seizure semiology in childhood temporal lobe epilepsy. *Epilepsia* 2002; 43:638–643.
27. Lortie A, Plouin P, Chiron C, Delalande O, et al. Characteristics of epilepsy in focal cortical dysplasia in infancy. *Epilepsy Res* 2002; 51(1–2):133–45.
28. Fogarasi A, Boesebeck F, Tuxhorn I. A detailed analysis of symptomatic posterior cortex seizure semiology in children younger than seven years. *Epilepsia* 2003; 44:89–96.
29. Loddenkemper T, Wyllie E, Neme S, Kotagal P, et al. Lateralizing signs during seizures in infants. *J Neurol* 2004; 251:1075–1079.
30. Fusco L, Bertini E, Vigevano F. Epilepsia partialis continua and neuronal migration anomalies. *Brain Dev* 1992; 14:323–328.
31. Desbiens R, Berkovic SF, Dubeau F, et al. Life-thestening focal atatus epilepticus due to occult cortical dysplasia. *Arch Neurol* 1993; 50:695–700.
32. Watanabe K, Negoro T, Aso K, et al. Childhood-onset epilepsy due to focal cortical dysplasia. In: Guerrini, R, Andermann, F, Canapicchi, R, et al., eds. *Dysplasias of Cerebral Cortex and Epilepsy*. Philadelphia: Lippincott-Raven Publishers, 1996:227–234.
33. Ohtsuka Y, Sato M, Sanada S, Yoshinaga H, et al. Suppression-burst patterns in intractable epilepsy with focal cortical dysplasia. *Brain Dev* 2000; 22:135–138.
34. D'Agostino MD, Bastos A, Piras C, et al. Posterior quadrantic dysplasia or hemi-hemimegalencephaly: a characteristic brain malformation. *Neurology* 2004; 62: 2214–2220.
35. Capovilla G, Beccaria F. Benign partial epilepsy in infancy and early childhood with vertex spikes and waves during sleep: a new epileptic form. *Brain Dev* 2000; 22:93–98.
36. Ohmori, I, Ohtsuka, Y, Oka, E, Akiyama, T, et al. Electroclinical study of localization-related epilepsies in early infancy. *Pediatr Neurol* 1997; 16:131–136.
37. Watanabe K, Yamamoto N, Negoro T, et al. Benign infantile epilepsy with complex partial seizures. *J Clin Neurophysiol* 1990; 7:409–416.
38. Watanabe K, Okumura A. Benign partial epilepsies in infancy. *Brain Dev* 2000; 22: 296–300.
39. Okumura A, Hayakawa F, Kuno K, Watanabe K. Benign partial epilepsy in infancy. *Arch Dis Child* 1996; 74:19–21.
40. Capovilla G, Giordano L, Tiberti S, Valseriati D, et al. Benign partial epilepsy in infancy with complex partial seizures (Watanabe's syndrome): 12 non-Japanese new cases. *Brain Dev* 1998; 20:105–111.
41. Takeuchi Y, Matsushita H, Yamazoe I, et al. Clinical study on localization-related epilepsy in infancy without underlying disorders. *Pediatr Neurol* 1998; 19:26–30.
42. Okumura A, Hayakawa F, Kato T, Kuno K, et al. Early recognition of benign partial epilepsy in infancy. *Epilepsia* 2000; 41:714–717.
43. Okumura A, Watanabe K, Negoro T, et al. Long-term follow-up of patients with benign partial epilepsy in infancy. *Epilepsia* 2006; 47:181–185.
44. Fukuyama Y. Borderland of epilepsy with special reference to febrile convulsions and so called infantile convulsions (in Japanese). *Seishin Igaku (Tokyo)* 1963; 5:211–223.
45. Tsurui S, Oguni H, Fukuyama Y. Analysis of ictal EEG in benign infantile convulsions (in Japanese). *Tenkan Kenkyu (Tokyo)* 1989; 7:160–168.
46. Vigevano F, Fusco L, Di Capua M, et al. Benign infantile familial convulsions. *Eur J Pediatr* 1992; 151:608–612.
47. Gautier A, Pouplard F, Bednarek N, et al. Benign infantile convulsions. French collaborative study (in French). *Arch Pediatr* 1999; 6:32–39.
48. Vigevano F. Benign familial infantile seizures. *Brain Dev* 2005; 27:172–177.
49. Szepetowski P, Rochette J, Berquin P, et al. Familial infantile convulsions and paroxysmal choreoathetosis: a new neurological syndrome linked to the pericentromeric region of human chromosome 16. *Am J Hum Genet* 1997; 61:889–898.
50. Caraballo RH, Cersosimo RO, Espeche A, Fejerman N. Benign familial and non-familial infantile seizures: a study of 64 patients. *Epileptic Disord* 2003; 5:45–49.
51. Weber YG, Berger A, Bebek N, et al. Benign familial infantile convulsions: linkage to chromosome 16p12–q12 in 14 families. *Epilepsia* 2004; 45:601–609.
52. Guipponi M, Rivier F, Vigevano F, et al. Linkage mapping of benign familial infantile convulsions (BFIC) to chromosome 19q. *Hum Mol Genet* 1997; 6:473–477.
53. Malacarne M, Gennaro E, Madia F, et al. Benign familial infantile convulsions: mapping of a novel locus on chromosome 2q24 and evidence for genetic heterogeneity. *Am J Hum Genet* 2001; 68:1521–1526.
54. Caraballo R, Pavek S, Lemainque A, et al. Linkage of benign familial infantile convulsions to chromosome 16p12–q12 suggests allelism to the infantile convulsions and choreoathetosis syndrome. *Am J Hum Genet* 2001; 68:788–794.
55. Striano P, Bordo L, Lispi ML, et al. A novel SCN2A mutation in family with benign familial infantile seizures. *Epilepsia* 2006; 47:218–220.
56. Heron SE, Crossland KM, Andermann E, et al. Sodium-channel defects in benign familial neonatal-infantile seizures. *Lancet* 2002; 360(9336):851–852. Erratum in: *Lancet* 2002; 360(9344):1520.
57. Berkovic SF, Heron SE, Giordano L, et al. Benign familial neonatal-infantile seizures: characterization of a new sodium channelopathy. *Ann Neurol* 2004; 55:550–557.
58. Hamada Y, Hattori H, Okuno T. Eleven cases of paroxysmal kinesigenic choreoathetosis; correlation with benign infantile convulsions (in Japanese) *No To Hattatsu* 1998; 30:483–488.
59. Lee WL, Tay A, Ong HT, et al. Association of infantile convulsions with paroxysmal dyskinesias (ICCA syndrome): confirmation of linkage to human chromosome 16p12–q12 in a Chinese family. *Hum Genet* 1998; 103:608–612.
60. Hattori H, Fujii T, Nigami H, et al. Co-segregation of benign infantile convulsions and paroxysmal kinesigenic choreoathetosis. *Brain Dev* 2000; 22:432–435.
61. Swoboda KJ, Soong B, McKenna C, et al. Paroxysmal kinesigenic dyskinesia and infantile convulsions: clinical and linkage studies. *Neurology* 2000; 55:224–230.
62. Thiriaux A, de St Martin A, Vercueil L, et al. Co-occurrence of infantile epileptic seizures and childhood paroxysmal choreoathetosis in one family: clinical, EEG, and SPECT characterization of episodic events. *Mov Disord* 2002; 17:98–104.
63. Demir E, Prud'homme JF, Topcu M. Infantile convulsions and paroxysmal choreoathetosis in a consanguineous family. *Pediatr Neurol* 2004; 30:349–353.
64. Kurahashi H, Okumura A, Okada J, Watanabe K. Benign infantile convulsions, paroxysmal kinesgenic choreoathetosis and temporal lobe epilepsy in a family. In *Proceedings of International Symposium on Epileptic Syndromes in Infancy and Early Childhood. Tokyo, April 29–May 1, 2005*:63.
65. Demir E, Turanii G, Yalntzoglu D, Topcu M. Benign familial infantile convulsions: phenotypic variability in a family. *J Child Neurol* 2005; 20:535–538.
66. Vanmolkot KR, Kors EE, Hottenga JJ, et al. Novel mutations in the Na^+, K^+-ATPase pump gene ATP1A2 associated with familial hemiplegic migraine and benign familial infantile convulsions. *Ann Neurol* 2003; 54:360–366.
67. Bureau M, Cokar O, Maton B, Genton P, et al. Sleep-related, low voltage rolandic and vertex spikes: an EEG marker of benignity in infancy-onset focal epilepsies. *Epileptic Disord* 2002; 4:15–22.
68. Capovilla G, Beccaria F, Montagnini A. "Benign focal epilepsy in infancy with vertex spikes and waves during sleep." Delineation of the syndrome and recalling as "benign infantile focal epilepsy with midline spikes and waves during sleep" (BIMSE). *Brain Dev* 2006; 28:85–91.
69. Capovilla G, Vigevano F. Benign idiopathic partial epilepsies in infancy. *J Child Neurol* 2001; 16:874–881.
70. Morooka K. Convulsions and mild diarrhea (in Japanese). *Shonika (Tokyo)* 1982; 23: 131–137.
71. Uemura N, Okumura A, Negoro T, Watanabe K. Clinical features of benign convulsions with mild gastroenteritis. *Brain Dev* 2002; 24:745–749.
72. Contino MF, Lebby T, Arcinue EL. Rotaviral gastrointestinal infection causing afebrile seizures in infancy and childhood. *Am J Emerg Med* 1994; 12:94–95.
73. Gomez-Lado C, Garcia-Reboredo M, Monasterio-Corral L, et al. Benign seizures associated with mild gastroenteritis: apropos of two cases (in Spanish). *An Pediatr (Barc)* 2005; 63:558–560.
74. Chalouhi C, Barnerias C, Abadie V. Afebrile seizures in gastroenteritis: a Japanese peculiarity (in French). *Arch Pediatr* 2006; 13:266–268.
75. Okumura A, Kato T, Hayakawa F, Kuno K, et al. Convulsion associated with mild gastroenteritis: occurrence in identical twins on the same day (in Japanese). *No To Hattatsu* 1999; 31:59–62.
76. Sakai Y, Kira R, Torisu H, Yasumoto S, et al. Benign convulsion with mild gastroenteritis and benign familial infantile seizure. *Epilepsy Res* 2006; 68:269–271.
77. Imai K, Otani K, Yanagihara K, et al. Ictal video-EEG recording of three partial seizures in a patient with the benign infantile convulsions associated with mild gastroenteritis. *Epilepsia* 1999; 40:1455–1458.
78. Maruyama K, Okumura A, Kubota T. Ictal EEG of convulsions with mild gastroenteritis: Report of three cases. *Proceedings of International Symposium on Epileptic Syndromes in Infancy and Early Childhood. Tokyo, April 29–May 1, 2005*:65.
79. Komori H, Wada M, Eto M,et al. Benign convulsions with mild gastroenteritis: a report of 10 recent cases detailing clinical varieties. *Brain Dev* 1995; 17:334–337.
80. Abe T, Kobayashi M, Araki K, et al. Infantile convulsions with mild gastroenteritis. *Brain Dev* 2000; 22:301–306.
81. Hongou K, Konishi T, Yagi S, Araki K, et al. Rotavirus encephalitis mimicking afebrile benign convulsions in infants. *Pediatr Neurol* 1998; 18:354–357.
82. Matsufuji H, Ichiyama T, Isumi H, Furukawa S. Low-dose carbamazepine therapy for benign infantile convulsions. *Brain Dev* 2005; 27:554–557.
83. Ichiyama T, Matsufuji H, Suenaga N, et al. Low-dose therapy with carbamazepine for convulsions associated with mild gastroenteritis (in Japanese) *No To Hattatsu* 2005; 37: 493–497.
84. Okumura A, Uemura N, Negoro T, Watanabe K. Efficacy of antiepileptic drugs in patients with benign convulsions with mild gastroenteritis. *Brain Dev* 2004; 26:164–167.
85. Okumura A, Tanabe T, Kato T, Hayakawa F, et al. A pilot study on lidocaine tape therapy for convulsions with mild gastroenteritis. *Brain Dev* 2004; 26:525–529.
86. Wyllie E, Comair YG, Kotagal P, Raja S, et al. Epilepsy surgery in infants. *Epilepsia* 1996; 37:625–637.
87. Vigevano F, Fusco L, Granata T, et al. Hemimegalencephaly: clinical and EEG characteristics. In: Guerrini R, Andermann F, Canapicchi R, eds. *Dysplasias of Cerebral Cortex and Epilepsy*. Philadelphia: Lippincott-Raven Publishers, 1996:285–294.
88. Duchowny M, Jayakar P, Resnick T., et al. Epilepsy surgery in the first three years of life. *Epilepsia* 1998; 39:737–743.
89. Okumura A, Watanabe K, Negoro T, et al. MRI findings in patients with symptomatic partial epilepsies beginning in infancy and early childhood. *Seizure* 2000; 9:566–571.
90. Guerrini R, Dravet C, Bureau J, et al. Diffuse and localized dysplasias of cerebral cortex: clinical presentation, outcome, and proposal for a morphologic MRI classification based on a study of 90 patients. In: Guerrini R, Andermann F, Canapicchi R, eds. *Dysplasias of Cerebral Cortex and Epilepsy*. Philadelphia: Lippincott-Raven Publishers, 1996:255–269.
91. Ishii K, Oguni H, Hayashi K, et al. Clinical study of catastrophic infantile epilepsy with focal seizures. *Pediatr Neurol* 2002; 27:369–377.
92. Nordli DR Jr, De Vivo DC. Classification of infantile seizures: implications for identification and treatment of inborn errors of metabolism. *J Child Neurol* 2002; 17 Suppl 3:3S3–3S8.

93. Battaglia A, Guerrini R. Chromosomal disorders associated with epilepsy. *Epileptic Disord* 2005; 7:181–192.
94. Caraballo RH, Sakr D, Mozzi M, et al. Symptomatic occipital lobe epilepsy following neonatal hypoglycemia. *Pediatr Neurol* 2004; 31:24–29.
95. Gobbi G. Coeliac disease, epilepsy and cerebral calcifications. *Brain Dev* 2005; 27: 189–200.
96. Aso K, Watanabe K. Limitations in the medical treatment of cryptogenic or symptomatic localization-related epilepsies of childhood onset. *Epilepsia* 2000:41(Suppl 9):18–20.
97. Kramer U, Fattal A, Nevo Y, Leitner Y, et al. Mental retardation subsequent to refractory partial seizures in infancy. *Brain Dev* 2000; 22:31–34.
98. Wyllie E. Surgery for catastrophic localization-related epilepsy in infants. *Epilepsia* 1996; 37(Suppl 1):S22–S25.
99. Kasai K, Watanabe K, Negoro T. Delayed myelination in West syndrome. *Psychiatr Clin Neurosci* 1995; 49:S265–S266.
100. Furusho J, Kato T, Tazaki I, Iikura Y, et al. MRI lesions masked by brain development: a case of infant-onset focal epilepsy. *Pediatr Neurol* 1998; 19:377–381.
101. Eltze CM, Chong WK, Bhate S, et al. Taylor-type focal cortical dysplasia in infants: some MRI lesions almost disappear with maturation of myelination. *Epilepsia* 2005; 46:1988–1992.
102. Vigevano F, Di Rocco C. Effectiveness of hemispherectomy in hemimegalencephaly with intractable seizures. *Neuropediatrics* 1990; 21:222–223.
103. Chugani HT, Shewmon DA, Shields WD, et al. Surgery for intractable infantile spasms: neuroimaging perspectives. *Epilepsia* 1993; 34:764–771.
104. Humbertclaude VT, Coubes PA, Robain O, Echenne BB. Early hemispherectomy in a case of hemimegalencephaly. *Pediatr Neurosurg* 1997; 27:268–271.
105. Sugimoto T, Otsubo H, Hwang PA, et al. Outcome of epilepsy surgery in the first three years of life. *Epilepsia* 1999; 40:560–565.
106. Kossoff EH, Buck C, Freeman JM. Outcomes of 32 hemispherectomies for Sturge-Weber syndrome worldwide. *Neurology* 2002; 59:1735–1738.
107. Gonzalez-Martinez JA, Gupta A, Kotagal P, et al. Hemispherectomy for catastrophic epilepsy in infants. *Epilepsia* 2005; 46:1518–1525.
108. Kang HC, Hwang YS, Park JC, et al. Clinical and electroencephalographic features of infantile spasms associated with malformations of cortical development. *Pediatr Neurosurg* 2006; 42:20–27.
109. Jonas R, Asarnow RF, LoPresti C. Surgery for symptomatic infant-onset epileptic encephalopathy with and without infantile spasms. *Neurology* 2005; 64:746–750.
110. Gobbi G, Bruno L, Pini A, et al. Periodic spasms: an unclassified type of epileptic seizures in childhood. *Dev Med Child Neurol* 1987; 29:766–775.
111. Yamamoto N, Watanabe K, Negoro T, et al. Partial seizures evolving to infantile spasms. *Epilepsia* 1988; 29:34–40.
112. Donat JF, Wright FS. Simultaneous infantile spasms and partial seizures. *J Child Neurol* 1991; 6:246–250.
113. Carrazana EJ, Lombroso CT, Mikati M, Helmers S, et al. Facilitation of infantile spasms by partial seizures. 1993; *Epilepsia* 34:97–109.
114. Plouin P, Dulac O, Jalin C, Chiron C. Twenty-four-hour ambulatory EEG monitoring in infantile spasms. *Epilepsia* 1993; 34:686–691.
115. Hrachovy RA, Frost JD Jr, Glaze DG. Coupling of focal electrical seizure discharges with infantile spasms: incidence during long-term monitoring in newly diagnosed patients. *Epilepsia* 1994; 11:461–464.
116. Viani F, Romeo A, Mastrangelo M, Viri M. Infantile spasms combined with partial seizures: electroclinical study of eleven cases. *Ital J Neurol Sci* 1994; 15:463–471.
117. Kubota T, Aso K, Negoro T, Natsume J, et al. Epileptic spasms preceded by partical seizures with a close temporal association. *Epilepsia* 1999; 40:1572–1579.
118. Pachatz C, Fusco L, Vigevano F. Epileptic spasms and partial seizures as a single ictal event. *Epilepsia* 2003; 44:693–700.
119. Ramachandrannair R, Ochi A, Akiyama T, et al. Partial seizures triggering infantile spasms in the presence of a basal ganglia glioma. *Epileptic Disord* 2005; 7:378–382.
120. Watanabe K, Miura K, Natsume J, et al. Epilepsies of neonatal onset: seizure type and evolution. *Dev Med Child Neurol* 1999; 41:318–322.
121. Coppola G, Plouin P, Chiron C, Robain O, et al. Migrating partial seizures in infancy: a malignant disorder with developmental arrest. *Epilepsia* 1995; 36:1017–1024.
122. Okuda K, Yasuhara A, Kamei A, et al. Successful control with bromide of two patients with malignant migrating partial seizures in infancy. *Brain Dev* 2000; 22:56–59.
123. Wilmshurst JM, Appleton DB, Grattan-Smith PJ. Migrating partial seizures in infancy: two new cases. *J Child Neurol* 2000; 15:717–722.
124. Veneselli E, Perrone MV, Di Rocco M, Gaggero R, et al. Malignant migrating partial seizures in infancy. *Epilepsy Res* 2001; 46:27–32.
125. Gross-Tsur V, Ben-Zeev B, Shalev RS. Malignant migrating partial seizures in infancy. *Pediatr Neurol* 2004; 31:287–290.
126. Marsh E, Melamed SE, Barron T, Clancy RR. Migrating partial seizures in infancy: expanding the phenotype of a rare seizure syndrome. *Epilepsia* 2005; 46:568–572.
127. Berkovic SF, Andermann F, Melanson D, et al. Hypothalamic hamartomas and ictal laughter: evolution of a characteristic epileptic syndrome and diagnostic value of magnetic resonance imaging. *Ann Neurol* 1988; 23:429–439.
128. Striano S, Meo R, Bilo L, et al. Gelastic epilepsy: symptomatic and cryptogenic cases. *Epilepsia* 1999; 40:294–302.
129. Arzimanoglou AA, Hirsch E, Aicardi J. Hypothalamic hamartoma and epilepsy in children: illustrative cases of possible evolutions. *Epileptic Disord* 2003; 5:187–199.
130. Iannetti P, Spalice A, Raucci U, Atzei G, et al. Gelastic epilepsy: video-EEG, MRI and SPECT characteristics. *Brain Dev* 1997; 19:418–421.
131. Harvey AS, Jayakar P, Duchowny M, et al. Hemifacial seizures and cerebellar ganglioglioma: an epilepsy syndrome of infancy with seizures of cerebellar origin. *Ann Neurol* 1996; 40:91–98.

19 Febrile Seizures

Shlomo Shinnar
Tracy A. Glauser

The International League Against Epilepsy (ILAE) defined a febrile seizure as "a seizure in association with a febrile illness in the absence of a CNS infection or acute electrolyte imbalance in children older than 1 month of age without prior afebrile seizures" (1) The temperature associated with the febrile illness must be greater than 38.4°C, although the temperature may not be evident until after the seizure. Prior epidemiological studies have used either one month (2–8) or 3 months (9,10) as the youngest age of occurrence, while no specific upper age limit was employed. Febrile seizures have a peak incidence at about 18 months of age, are most common between 6 months and 5 years of age, and onset above age 7 is rare, although it does occur. The child may be neurologically normal or abnormal.

Febrile seizures can be classified as either simple or complex. A simple febrile seizure is isolated, brief, and generalized. Conversely, a complex febrile seizure is focal, multiple (more than one seizure during the febrile illness), or prolonged, lasting either more than 10 (2–6, 11) or 15 (9–11) minutes. The child's prior neurological condition is not used as part of the classification criteria (1, 12).

EPIDEMIOLOGY

Febrile seizures are the most common form of childhood seizures, affecting between 2% and 4% of children in the United States and Western Europe (4, 8, 9, 13–15), 9% to 10% of children in Japan (16), and up to 14% of children in Guam (17). The peak incidence of febrile seizures is at approximately 18 months of age.

Most febrile seizures are simple. In a study of 428 children with a first febrile seizure (11), at least one complex feature was noted in 35% of children, including focality (16%), multiple seizures (14%), and prolonged duration (>10 minutes, 13%). Five percent of the total group experienced a seizure lasting more than 30 minutes (i.e., febrile status epilepticus) (11). Despite febrile status epilepticus representing only 5% of febrile seizures, it accounts for approximately one quarter of all episodes of childhood status epilepticus (18–23), and more than two thirds of status epilepticus cases in the second year of life (23). The majority of febrile seizures do not occur at the onset of the fever. In the study of Berg et al, only 21% of the children experienced seizures either prior to or within one hour of the onset of fever; 57% had a seizure after 1 to

Substantial portions of this chapter are reprinted with permission from Shinnar S, Glauser TA. Febrile seizures. *J Child Neurol* 2002;17:S44–S52.
Supported in part by grant NS 43209 from NINDS.

24 hours of fever, and 22% experienced their febrile seizure more than 24 hours after the onset of fever (5, 6).

Risk Factors for First Febrile Seizure

Two studies (24, 25) have examined risk factors associated with experiencing a febrile seizure (Table 19-1). In a 1993 case control population-based study, four factors were associated with an increased risk of febrile seizures: (1) a first- or second-degree relative with a history of febrile seizures, (2) a neonatal nursery stay of >30 days, (3) developmental delay, or (4) attendance at day care. There was a 28% chance of experiencing at least one febrile seizure for children with two of these factors (24). A second case control study examined the issue of which children with a febrile illness were most likely to experience a febrile seizure, using febrile controls matched for age, site of routine pediatric care, and date of visit (25). Significant independent risk factors, on a multivariable analysis, were the peak temperature and a history of febrile seizures in a first- or higher-degree relative. Gastroenteritis as the underlying illness appeared to have a significant inverse (i.e., protective) association with febrile seizures.

Risk Factors for Recurrent Febrile Seizures

Overall, approximately one-third of children with a first febrile seizure will experience a recurrence; 10% will have three or more febrile seizures (4–10, 14, 26–29). An assessment of various factors potentially associated with the recurrence of febrile seizures is shown in Table 19-2. The most consistent risk factors reported are a family history of febrile seizures and onset of first febrile seizure at <18 months of age (4–7, 9, 10, 14, 26–29). This relationship is not due to a greater tendency to experience seizures with each specific illness, but rather to the longer period during which a child with a younger age of onset will be in the age group at risk for febrile seizures (27, 28, 30).

Two other definite risk factors for recurrence of febrile seizures are peak temperature (3–5, 27, 28, 31) and the duration of the fever prior to the seizure (3, 4). In general, the higher the peak temperature, the lower the chance of recurrence. In one study, those with peak temperatures of 101°F (38.3°C) had a 42% recurrence risk at one year, compared with 29% for those with peak temperature of 103°F (39.4°C) and only 12% for those with a peak temperature ≥ 105°F (40.6°C) (3, 4). Note that the risk factor is the peak temperature during the illness, not the temperature at the time of the seizure or at the time of presentation to the emergency department. The other risk factor related to the acute illness is duration of recognized fever, with a shorter duration of recognized fever associated with a higher risk of recurrence. The recurrence risk at one year was 46% for those with a febrile seizure within an hour of recognized onset of fever, compared with 25% for those with prior fever lasting 1 to 24 hours, and 15% for those having more than 24 hours of recognized fever prior to the febrile seizure.

Children with multiple risk factors have the highest risk of recurrence (3, 27). A child with two or more risk factors has a greater than 30% recurrence risk at 2 years; a child with three or more risk factors has a greater than 60% recurrence risk (3). In contrast, the 2-year recurrence risk is less than 15% for a child with no risk factors (e.g., older than 18 months with no family history of febrile seizures, who experiences a first febrile seizure associated with a peak temperature > 40°C [104°F] after a

TABLE 19-1
Risk Factors for First Febrile Seizure

In Population (24)
– First- or second-degree relative with history of FS
– Neonatal nursery stay of >30 days
– Developmental delay
– Attendance at day care
– 2 of these factors ⇒ 28% chance of at least 1 FS
In Children with a Febrile Illness (25)
– First- or second-degree relative with history of FS
– High peak temperature

TABLE 19-2
Risk Factors for Recurrent Febrile Seizures

Definite Risk Factor
– Family history of FS
– Age <18 months
– Low peak temperature
– Duration of fever
Possible Risk Factor
– Family history of epilepsy
Not a Risk Factor
– Neurodevelopmental abnormality
– Complex FS
– >1 complex feature
– Sex
– Ethnicity

recognized fever of more than one hour) (3, 27). A recurrent febrile seizure is also more likely to be prolonged if the initial febrile seizure was prolonged (11, 27).

The relationship between a family history of unprovoked seizures or epilepsy and the overall risk of febrile seizure recurrence appears to be doubtful. Some studies report a modest increase in the risk of febrile seizure recurrence in children with a family history of unprovoked seizures, but a large study in Rochester, Minnesota, found no difference in recurrence risk between children with a family history of epilepsy (25%) and those with no such family history (23%) (4). Other studies have found equivocal results (5, 6, 27, 28).

The presence of a neurodevelopmental abnormality in the child, or a history of complex febrile seizures, have not been shown to be significantly associated with an increased risk of subsequent febrile seizures (4-7, 9, 11, 27, 28). Ethnicity and sex have also not been associated with a clear increased risk of recurrent febrile seizures.

Risk Factors for Subsequent Epilepsy

The risk factors for developing epilepsy after febrile seizures are summarized in Table 19-3. Following a single simple febrile seizure, the risk of developing epilepsy is not substantially different from the risk in the general population (2, 3, 9, 13, 32, 33).

Data from five large cohorts of children with febrile seizures indicate that 2% to 10% of children who have febrile seizures will subsequently develop epilepsy (2, 3, 9, 13, 32, 33). In each of these five large studies, the occurrence of a family history of epilepsy and the occurrence of a complex febrile seizure were associated with an increased risk of subsequent epilepsy (2, 3, 9, 13, 32, 33). The occurrence of multiple febrile seizures was associated with a slight, but statistically significant, increased risk of subsequent epilepsy in two studies (2, 33). One study found that children with a febrile seizure that occurred within one hour of a recognized fever (i.e., at onset) had a higher risk for subsequent epilepsy than those children with a febrile seizure associated with longer fever duration (33). Two studies have found that very prolonged febrile seizures (i.e., febrile status epilepticus) were associated with an increased risk of subsequent epilepsy above that of a complex febrile seizure that was less prolonged (2, 33).

TABLE 19-3
Risk Factors for Subsequent Epilepsy

Definite Risk Factor

- Neurodevelopmental abnormality
- Complex FS
- Family history of epilepsy
- Duration of fever

Possible Risk Factor

- >1 complex feature

Not a Risk Factor

- Family history of FS
- Age at first FS
- Peak temperature
- Sex
- Ethnicity

The number of complex features in a febrile seizure may possibly affect the risk of recurrence. Although one study found that patients with two complex features (e.g., prolonged and focal) had further increased risk of subsequent epilepsy (2), another study did not detect this association (33). A family history of febrile seizures, age at first febrile seizure, and the height of fever at first seizure are not associated with a differential risk of developing epilepsy (2, 3, 9, 32, 33). The only common risk factor for both recurrent febrile seizures and for subsequent epilepsy was duration of fever prior to the febrile seizure (5, 6, 33); this may be a marker for overall seizure susceptibility.

In general, the types of epilepsy that occur in children with prior febrile seizures are varied and are not very different from those that occur in children without such a history (2, 34–36). Febrile seizures can also be the initial manifestation of specific epilepsy syndromes, such as severe myoclonic epilepsy of infancy (37).

It is controversial whether febrile seizures are simply an age-specific marker of future seizure susceptibility or have a causal relationship with the subsequent epilepsy (38, 39). Two factors support the former, and not the latter, interpretation. There is not an increased incidence of epilepsy in populations with a high cumulative incidence of febrile seizures (e.g., 10% in Tokyo, Japan) (16). Secondly, no evidence exists that treatment of febrile seizures alters the risk of subsequent epilepsy (5, 40–43). However, newer data suggest that, while in most cases the link is not causal, there is a causal link between very prolonged febrile seizures, or febrile status epilepticus, and subsequent hippocampal injury, mesial temporal sclerosis, and temporal lobe epilepsy (44, 45).

MORBIDITY AND MORTALITY

The morbidity and mortality associated with febrile seizures are extremely low. Multiple studies have demonstrated no evidence of permanent motor deficits following febrile seizures or febrile status epilepticus (8–10, 19, 21, 22, 46–49). No reports of acute deterioration of cognitive abilities have been noted following febrile seizures, even in series limited to status epilepticus (21, 22, 47, 48, 50–52). Three large studies have shown that cognitive abilities and school performance of children with febrile seizures were similar to those of controls (46, 47, 50, 53). Even prolonged febrile seizures do not appear to be associated with adverse cognitive outcomes (47, 48, 50, 52).

No deaths were reported from the National Collaborative Perinatal Project (9, 10) or the British cohort study (8, 46, 47). The mortality of febrile status epilepticus in recent series is extremely low (19–22, 47–49, 51).

GENETICS

Genetic influences are evident in multiple studies. A positive family history of febrile seizures is a definite risk factor for both a first febrile seizure (24, 25) and recurrent febrile seizures (4–7, 9, 27, 28). Tsuboi reported a febrile seizure concordance rate of 56% in monozygotic and 14% in dizygotic twins in a study of 32 twin pairs and 673 sibship cases (54). Correlation of clinical symptoms, including age of onset and degree of fever, was larger in the twin pairs than in the sibship cases. A separate data set from Rochester, Minnesota, demonstrated similar results (55). Most likely, all children have some increased susceptibility to seizures from fever at the specific age window. Genetic influences are therefore likely to account for some, but not all, of the cases.

Overall, there appears to be a multifactorial mode of inheritance for febrile convulsions, but there may be a subset of children with an autosomal dominant mode of inheritance (55–57). To date, no definitive gene or locus for febrile seizure has been established. Some cases of febrile seizures in large families have been linked to genes on chromosomes 8 and 19 (56–58). A discussion of the relationship of febrile seizures and specific syndromes such as GEFS+ is found in Chapter (20).

INITIAL EVALUATION

Meningitis, encephalitis, serious electrolyte imbalance, and other acute neurological illnesses must be excluded in order to make the diagnosis of a febrile seizure. A detailed history and physical and neurological examinations are essential and can eliminate many of those neurological conditions. Routine serum electrolytes, calcium, phosphorus, magnesium, complete blood count (CBC), and blood glucose are of limited value in the evaluation of a child above 6 months of age with a febrile seizure in the absence of a suspicious history (e.g., vomiting, diarrhea) or physical findings (14, 59–62).

The most common evaluation issue is whether a lumbar puncture is necessary to exclude meningitis. The incidence of meningitis in children who present with an apparent febrile seizure is between 2% and 5% (14, 60–67). In each of these series, the majority had identifiable risk factors. In one series, four features were noted in children with meningitis: a visit for medical care within the previous 48 hours; seizures on arrival to the emergency room; focal seizure; or suspicious findings on physical or neurological examination (63). In the absence of risk factors, other authors have found a low yield for routine lumbar puncture (14, 64, 65, 67).

The American Academy of Pediatrics issued guidelines for the neurodiagnostic evaluation of a child with a simple febrile seizure between 6 months and 5 years of age (14). A lumbar puncture should be strongly considered in infants less than 12 months of age. Children between 12 and 18 months of age need careful assessment, because the signs of meningitis may be subtle. In the absence of suspicious findings on history or examination, a lumbar puncture is not necessary in children above 18 months of age. A lumbar puncture is still recommended in children with a first complex febrile seizure, as well as in any child with persistent lethargy. It should also be strongly considered in a child who has already received prior antibiotic therapy. A recent practice parameter of the American Academy of Neurology also recommends that a lumbar puncture be done in children with status epilepticus and fever (68). Any CSF pleocytosis is of concern, because, even in children with febrile status epilepticus,more than 4 or 5 white blood cells (WBCs) per mm^3 are very uncommon (69).

Skull X-rays are of no value. Computed tomography (CT) scans are also of limited benefit in this clinical setting and are used when there is concern about increased intracranial pressure or when trauma is suspected. Magnetic resonance imaging (MRI) scans are not indicated in children with a simple febrile seizure (14). It is unclear whether or not an MRI study is indicated in the evaluation of a child with a prolonged or focal febrile seizure (39, 70). Recent data do indicate that a number of children with prolonged febrile seizures will have acute changes in the hippocampus seen on MRIs done within a few days of the episode (44, 45, 70), but at this point such imaging has not yet become routine practice.

Electroencephalograms (EEG) are of limited value in the evaluation of the child with febrile seizures (14, 71–74). EEGs are more likely to be abnormal in older children, children with preexisting neurodevelopmental abnormalities, children with a family history of febrile seizures, or children with a complex febrile seizure (36, 71, 73, 75–78). Even if present, the clinical significance of these EEG abnormalities is unclear. There is no evidence so far that EEG abnormalities help predict either recurrence of febrile seizures or the development of subsequent epilepsy (14, 36, 71, 73, 75–79), though preliminary data from an ongoing study suggest a high rate of significant EEG abnormalities in children with very prolonged febrile seizures (80).

PATHOPHYSIOLOGY

In general, febrile seizures appear to be an age-specific occurrence, where increased susceptibility to seizures is induced by fever. However, the detailed pathophysiology remains unclear. Decades ago, the key factor was thought to be the rate of rise of the fever (81); recent data suggest that the key factor is the actual peak temperature (25, 82). Gastroenteritis is associated with a lower incidence of febrile seizures (25), whereas herpesvirus-6 infections have had a high reported association with febrile seizures (83–85).

Animal models of febrile seizures also show an age-dependent effect (86–89). In addition, in vitro preparations show induction of epileptiform activity by temperature elevation in hippocampal slices in young rats (90). Recent animal data from Baram and colleagues suggest that prolonged febrile seizures may lead to long-lasting changes in the hippocampal circuits. In a rat model of prolonged febrile seizures, cytoskeletal changes in neurons were evident within 24 hours and persisted for several weeks without leading to cell loss (91). However, altered functional properties of these injured neurons were evident (92, 93). Nevertheless, even in this model, which has produced convincing data for functional changes, a seizure duration of 20 minutes or more was required. Seizures lasting 10 minutes or less were not associated with any anatomic or functional changes.

As may be the case in humans, animals with preexisting neurological abnormalities are more susceptible to seizures and to their consequences. Young rats with neuronal migration disorders appear more susceptible to hyperthermia-induced seizures (87) and are also more susceptible to hippocampal damage. Interestingly, in this model, hippocampal damage occurs with hyperthermia even in the absence of seizures. The availability of animal models provides a new means of studying the pathophysiology of febrile seizures and their consequences.

FEBRILE SEIZURES AND MESIAL TEMPORAL SCLEROSIS

It remains controversial whether prolonged febrile seizures cause mesial temporal sclerosis (MTS) (39, 52). Retrospective studies (from tertiary epilepsy centers) report that many adults with intractable mesial temporal lobe epilepsy had a history of prolonged or atypical febrile seizures in childhood (94–100). However, both population-based studies and prospective studies of children with febrile seizures have failed to find this association (2, 8, 9, 13, 33, 38, 47).

In those studies that reported an association between prolonged febrile seizures and MTS, the duration of the febrile seizures was extremely prolonged. Maher and McLachlan (101) reported on a large family with a high rate of both febrile convulsions and temporal lobe epilepsy. The mean duration of the febrile seizures in those who subsequently developed temporal lobe epilepsy was 100 minutes. Van Landingham et al (70) reported that few children with very prolonged (mean of >90 minutes) focal febrile seizures had acute changes on an MRI, which, in some cases, was followed by later chronic changes (70). However, these MRI changes only occurred in a small minority of patients. Furthermore, all cases of MTS in this study occurred in patients who had focal seizures, some of whom also had focal lesions, which raises the question of preexisting focal pathology.

Overall, febrile seizures are not likely to account for the majority of cases of MTS. Febrile seizures lasting more than 90 minutes are very rare and are uncommon even in series of febrile status epilepticus (9, 11, 15, 21, 22, 33, 47, 48, 50, 51, 70, 102). Very prolonged febrile seizures are also usually focal (70, 102). In cases of febrile status epilepticus, imaging abnormalities are relatively uncommon (70). MTS can also be found in many patients who have no prior history of febrile seizures (103–108). Recent clinico-pathological studies have also provided evidence for multiple etiologies for MTS, as well as the frequent presence of dual pathology, such as subtle migration defects (105–108).

More recent studies do suggest that prolonged febrile seizures can cause acute hippocampal injury in 20–30% of cases and that these may lead to hippocampal volume loss and MTS (44, 45, 109). An ongoing multicenter study currently in progress should eventually provide the answers to the relationship between prolonged febrile seizures and subsequent MTS and temporal lobe epilepsy (109).

TREATMENT

Overview

Two distinct approaches to the treatment of febrile seizures have developed based on the perceived immediate and long-term risks of febrile seizures. One approach is based on the old idea that febrile seizures are harmful and may lead to the development of epilepsy; this approach is aimed at preventing febrile seizures by using either intermittent or chronic treatment with medications (72, 110, 111). The second approach is based on the epidemiological data that febrile seizures are benign; the only concern focuses on aborting febrile seizures to prevent status epilepticus.

Stopping a Febrile Seizure

In Hospital

Ongoing seizure upon arrival in the emergency department is an indication for initiating therapy. Intravenous diazepam is effective in most cases (20, 112). Rectal diazepam or diazepam gel would also be appropriate for use in a prehospital setting, such as an ambulance, and in cases where intravenous access is difficult (20, 113–115). Other benzodiazepines, such as lorazepam, may also be effective but have not been adequately studied (20, 112). If the seizure continues after an adequate dose of a benzodiazepine, a full status epilepticus treatment protocol should be initiated (20, 112).

At Home

The majority of febrile seizures are brief, lasting less than 10 minutes, and no intervention is necessary. Rectal diazepam or diazepam gel has been shown to be effective in terminating febrile seizures and is the therapy of choice for intervention outside the hospital (113–115). It should be used with caution, and only by reliable caregivers who have been trained in its use. Families with children at high risk for, or with a history of, prolonged or multiple febrile seizures (11), and those who live far from medical care, are excellent candidates to have rectal diazepam or diazepam gel readily available in their homes. For many families, the availability of a rectal diazepam formulation will relieve anxiety, even after a single febrile seizure, even though they will most likely never have to use it (116–118).

Preventing a Febrile Seizure

Intermittent Medications at Time of Fever

Antipyretics. Despite the logical assumption that aggressive treatment with antipyretic medication would reduce the risk of having a febrile seizure, and the finding of case control studies that the risk of a febrile seizure is directly related to the height of the fever (25, 82), there is little evidence to suggest that antipyretics reduce the risk of a recurrent febrile seizure (66, 119). It should be recalled that the children in whom the febrile seizure occurs at the onset of the fever have the highest risk of recurrent febrile seizures (5, 6). Any recommendations for antipyretic therapy should take into account its limitations and avoid creating undue anxiety and guilt in the parents.

Benzodiazepines. Diazepam, given orally or rectally at the time of onset of a febrile illness, has demonstrated a statistically significant, yet clinically modest, ability to reduce the probability of a febrile seizure (26, 120–124). In one large, randomized trial comparing placebo with oral diazepam (0.33 mg/kg/dose every 8 hours with fever), 22% of the diazepam-treated group had seizure recurrence by 36 months, compared with 31% of the placebo-treated group (124). One must weigh this modest reduction in seizure recurrence with the side effects of sedating children every time they have a febrile illness.

Barbiturates. Intermittent therapy with phenobarbital at the onset of fever is ineffective in reducing the risk of recurrent febrile seizures (125, 126). Surprisingly, it is still fairly widely used for this purpose (72, 110, 111).

Daily Medications

Barbiturates. Phenobarbital, given daily at doses that achieve a serum concentration of 15 µg/mL or higher, has been shown to be effective in reducing the risk of recurrent febrile seizures in several well-controlled trials (119, 122, 123, 127–130). However, in these studies, a substantial portion of the children had adverse effects, primarily hyperactivity, which required discontinuation of therapy (131–133). More recent studies have cast some doubt on the efficacy of the drug and, more importantly, have raised concerns about potential long-term adverse effects on cognition and behavior (131, 134). Chronic phenobarbital therapy is rarely indicated, as the risks seem to outweigh the benefits in most cases.

Valproate. Daily treatment with valproic acid is effective in reducing the risk of recurrent febrile seizures in both human and animal studies (89, 123, 129, 130). However, it is very rarely used, because children considered most often for prophylaxis (young and/or neurologically abnormal) are also the ones at highest risk for fatal idiosyncratic hepatotoxicity (135, 136).

Other AEDs. Despite evidence of effectiveness when used in intermittent therapy, there is no experience with chronic use of benzodiazepines for treatment of febrile seizures. Even if effective, benzodiazepines' toxicity and adverse effect profile would likely preclude their widespread use in this setting. Phenytoin and carbamazepine are ineffective in preventing recurrent febrile seizures in humans and in animal models of hyperthermia-induced seizures (89, 127, 128, 137). There are no published data on the efficacy of the newer AEDs, such as gabapentin, lamotrigine, topiramate, tiagabine, or vigabatrin, in the treatment of febrile seizures.

Preventing Epilepsy

There is no evidence that preventing febrile seizures will reduce the risk of subsequent epilepsy. One rationale for starting chronic antiepilepsy therapy in children with febrile seizures was to prevent the development of future epilepsy (72, 110, 111). In three studies comparing placebo with treatment (either with daily phenobarbital or with diazepam administered at the onset of fever), treatment significantly and substantially reduced the risk of febrile seizure recurrence, but the risk of later developing epilepsy was no lower in the treated groups than in the controls (26, 40–43, 126). No difference in the occurrence of epilepsy, or in school performance or other cognitive outcomes, was seen between the treated group and control group in two of these studies with more than 10 years of follow-up (40, 41).

Therapy Recommendations

A recent practice parameter by the American Academy of Pediatrics suggests that the best treatment for simple febrile seizures is reassurance of the parents regarding their benign though frightening nature (138). The authors wholeheartedly agree that treatment is only rarely indicated for a simple febrile seizure. In fact, no treatment is needed in most children with complex febrile seizures. Because the data suggest that only prolonged febrile seizures are associated with hippocampal injury and may be causally linked to subsequent epilepsy (39, 44), a rational goal of therapy would be to prevent very prolonged febrile seizures. When treatment is indicated, particularly in those at risk for prolonged or multiple febrile seizures (11) or those who live far away from medical care, rectal diazepam or diazepam gel used at the time of seizure as an abortive agent would seem the most logical choice (20, 112–115). Daily medications or benzodiazepines at the time of fever are rarely used in the management of febrile seizures.

Counseling and Education

Counseling and education will be the sole treatment for the majority of children with febrile seizures. Education is key to empowering the parents, who have just experienced a very frightening and traumatic event (139). Many parents, even of children with a simple febrile seizure, are afraid that their child could have died (140). Parents need to be reassured that the child will not die during a seizure and that keeping the child safe during the seizure is generally the only action that needs to be taken.

The basic facts about febrile seizures should be presented to the family. The amount of information and the level of content will depend largely on the medical sophistication of the parents and their ability to attend to the information given to them at that particular time. The parents' perception of their child's disorder will be an important factor in their later coping and will ultimately impact on their perception of quality of life (139).

Parents will usually be interested in information that will help them manage the illness or specific problems; lengthy explanations are usually not helpful. Information should be provided about how to manage further seizures should they occur. This should include what to do during a seizure, when it may be necessary to call the physician, and when the child should be taken to the emergency department.

In those cases where rectal diazepam or diazepam gel is being recommended for the next seizure, explicit instructions regarding its use should be given. As it is difficult to absorb all this information in an emergency department setting, it is usually advisable to see the family again a few weeks later to review the information and answer any additional questions they may have.

CONCLUSION

Febrile seizures are the most common of childhood seizures and are usually benign. There is accumulating evidence that prolonged febrile seizures lasting more than 30 minutes may have long-term consequences. An understanding of the natural history and prognosis will enable the physician to reassure the families and provide appropriate counseling and management while avoiding unnecessary diagnostic and therapeutic interventions.

References

1. Commission on Epidemiology and Prognosis, International League Against Epilepsy. Guidelines for epidemiologic studies on epilepsy. *Epilepsia* 1993; 34:592–596.
2. Annegers JF, Hauser WA, Shirts SB, et al. Factors prognostic of unprovoked seizures after febrile convulsions. *N Engl J Med* 1987; 316:493–498.
3. Annegers JF, Hauser WA, Elveback LR, Kurland LT. The risk of epilepsy following febrile convulsions. *Neurology* 1979; 29:297–303.
4. Annegers JF, Blakely SA, Hauser WA, Kurland LT. Recurrence of febrile convulsions in a population-based cohort. *Epilepsy Res* 1990; 66:1009–1012.
5. Berg AT, Shinnar S, Darefsky AS, et al. Predictors of recurrent febrile seizures. *Arch Ped Adolesc Med* 1997; 151:371–378.
6. Berg AT, Shinnar S, Hauser WA, et al. Predictors of recurrent febrile seizures: a prospective study of the circumstances surrounding the initial febrile seizure. *N Engl J Med* 1992; 327:1122–1127.
7. Berg AT, Shinnar S, Hauser WA, Leventhal JM. Predictors of recurrent febrile seizures: a metaanalytic review. *J Pediatr* 1990; 116:329–337.
8. Verity CM, Butler NR, Golding J. Febrile convulsions in a national cohort followed up from birth. I. Prevalence and recurrence in the first 5 years of life. *Br Med J* 1985; 290:1307–1315.
9. Nelson KB, Ellenberg JH. Prognosis in children with febrile seizures. *Pediatrics* 1978; 61:720–727.
10. Nelson KB, Ellenberg JH. Predictors of epilepsy in children who have experienced febrile seizures. *N Engl J Med* 1976; 295:1029–1033.
11. Berg AT, Shinnar S. Complex febrile seizures. *Epilepsia* 1996; 37:126–133.
12. National Institutes of Health. Febrile seizures: consensus development conference summary. Vol. 3, No. 2. Bethesda, MD: National Institute of Health, 1980.
13. Van den Berg BJ, Yerushalmi J. Studies on convulsive disorders in young children, I. Incidence of febrile and nonfebrile convulsions by age and other factors. *Pediatr Res* 1969; 3:298–304.
14. American Academy of Pediatrics: Provisional Committee on Quality Improvement. Practice parameter: the neurodiagnostic evaluation of the child with a simple febrile seizure. *Pediatrics* 1996; 97:769–775.
15. Berg AT. The epidemiology of seizures and epilepsy in children. In: Shinnar S, Amir N, Branski D, eds. *Childhood Seizures*. Basel, Switzerland: S Karger, 1995:1–10.
16. Tsuboi T. Epidemiology of febrile and afebrile convulsions in children in Japan. *Neurology* 1984; 34:175–181.

17. Stanhope JM, Brody JA, Brink E, Morris CE. Convulsions among the Chamorro people of Guam, Mariana Islands. II. Febrile convulsions. *Am J Epidemiol* 1972; 95:299–304.
18. Aicardi J, Chevrie JJ. Convulsive status epilepticus in infants and in children. A study of 239 cases. *Epilepsia* 1970; 11:187–197.
19. DeLorenzo RJ, Hauser WA, Towne AR, et al. A prospective population-based epidemiological study of status epilepticus in Richmond, Virginia. *Neurology* 1996; 46:1029–1035.
20. Dodson WE, DeLorenzo RJ, Pedley TA, et al. The treatment of convulsive status epilepticus: recommendations of the Epilepsy Foundation of America's working group on status epilepticus. *JAMA* 1993; 270:854–859.
21. Dunn WD. Status epilepticus in children: etiology, clinical features and outcome. *J Child Neurol* 1988; 3:167–173.
22. Maytal J, Shinnar S, Moshe SL, Alvarez LA. Low morbidity and mortality of status epilepticus in children. *Pediatrics* 1989; 83:323–331.
23. Shinnar S, Pellock JM, Moshe SL, et al. In whom does status epilepticus occur: age related differences in children. *Epilepsia* 1997; 38:907–914.
24. Bethune P, Gordon KG, Dooley JM, et al. Which child will have a febrile seizure? *Am J Dis Child* 1993; 147; 35–39.
25. Berg AT, Shinnar S, Shapiro ED, et al. Risk factors for a first febrile seizure: a matched case-control study. *Epilepsia* 1995; 36:334–341.
26. Knudsen FU. Recurrence risk after first febrile seizure and effect of short-term diazepam prophylaxis. *Arch Dis Child* 1985b; 60:1045–1049.
27. Offringa M, Bossuyt PMM, Lubsen J, et al. Risk factors for seizure recurrence in children with febrile seizures: a pooled analysis of individual patient data from five studies. *J Pediatr* 1994; 124:574–584.
28. Offringa M, Derksen-Lubsen G, Bossuyt, Lubsen J. Seizure recurrence after a first febrile seizure: a multivariate approach. *Dev Med Child Neurol* 1992; 34:15–24.
29. Van den Berg BJ. Studies on convulsive disorders in young children. III. Recurrence of febrile convulsions. *Epilepsia* 1974; 15:177–190.
30. Shirts SB, Annegers JF, Hauser WA. The relation of age at first febrile seizure to recurrence of febrile seizures. *Epilepsia* 1987; 28:625 (abstract).
31. El-Rahdi AS, Banajeh S. Effect of fever on recurrence rate of febrile convulsions. *Arch Dis Child* 1989; 64:869–870.
32. Verity CM, Golding J. Risk of epilepsy after febrile convulsions: a national cohort study. *Br Med J* 1991; 303:1373–1376.
33. Berg AT, Shinnar S. Unprovoked seizures in children with febrile seizures: short term outcome. *Neurology* 1996; 47:562–568.
34. Berg AT, Shinnar S, Levy SR, et al. Characteristics of newly diagnosed epilepsy in children with and without prior febrile seizures. *Epilepsia* 1996; 37(Suppl 5):100.
35. Camfield CS, Camfield PR, Dooley JM, Gordon, K. What type of afebrile seizures are preceded by febrile seizures? A population-based study of children. *Dev Med Child Neurol* 1994; 36; 887–892.
36. Sofianov N, Sadikario A, Dukovski M, Kuturec M. Febrile convulsions and later development of epilepsy. *Am J Dis Child* 1983; 137:123–126.
37. Dravet C, Bureau M, Guerrini R, et al. Severe myoclonic epilepsy in infants. In: Roger J, Bureau M, Dravet C, et al, eds. *Epileptic Syndromes in Infancy, Childhood and Adolescence*. 2nd ed. London: John Libbey, 1992:75–88.
38. Berg AT, Shinnar S. Do seizures beget seizures? An assessment of the clinical evidence in humans. *J Clin Neurophysiol* 1997; 14:102–110.
39. Shinnar S. Prolonged febrile seizures and mesial temporal sclerosis. *Ann Neurol* 1998; 43:411–412.
40. Knudsen FU, Paerregaard A, Andersen R, Andresen J. Long term outcome of prophylaxis for febrile convulsions. *Arch Dis Child* 1996; 74:13–18.
41. Wolf SM, Forsythe A. Epilepsy and mental retardation following febrile seizures in childhood. *Acta Paediatr Scand* 1989; 78:291–295.
42. Rosman NP, Labazzo JL, Colton T. Factors predisposing to afebrile seizures after febrile convulsions and preventive treatment. *Ann Neurol* 1993; 34:452.
43. Shinnar S, Berg AT. Does antiepileptic drug therapy prevent the development of "chronic" epilepsy? *Epilepsia* 1996; 37:701–708.
44. Shinnar S. Febrile seizures and mesial temporal sclerosis. *Epilepsy Curr* 2003; 3:115–118.
45. Lewis DV, Barboriak DP, MacFall JR, Provenzale JM, et al. Do prolonged febrile seizures produce medial temporal sclerosis? Hypothesis, MRI evidence and unanswered questions. *Prog Brain Res* 2002; 135:263–278.
46. Verity CM, Butler NR, Golding J. Febrile convulsions in a national cohort followed up from birth. II. Medical history and intellectual ability at 5 years of age. *Br Med J* 1985; 290:1311.
47. Verity CM, Ross EM, Golding J. Outcome of childhood status epilepticus and lengthy febrile convulsions: findings of national cohort study. *Br Med J* 1993; 307:225–228.
48. Shinnar S, Pellock JM, Berg AT, O'Dell C, et al. Short-term outcomes of children with febrile status epilepticus. *Epilepsia* 2001; 42:47–53.
49. Towne AR, Pellock JM, Ko D, DeLorenzo RJ. Determinants of mortality in status epilepticus. *Epilepsia* 1994; 35:27–34.
50. Ellenberg JH, Nelson KB. Febrile seizures and later intellectual performance. *Arch Neurol* 1978; 35(1):17–21.
51. Maytal J, Shinnar S. Febrile status epilepticus. *Pediatrics* 1990; 86:611–616.
52. Shinnar S, Babb TL. Long term sequelae of status epilepticus. In: Engel J Jr, Pedley TA, eds. *Epilepsy: A Comprehensive Text*. Philadelphia: Lippincot-Raven, 1997:755–763.
53. Ross EM, Peckham CS, West PB, et al. Epilepsy in childhood: findings from the National Child Development Study. *Br Med J* 1980; 1:207.
54. Tsuboi T. Genetic analysis of febrile convulsions: twin and family studies. *Hum Genet* 1987; 75:7–14.
55. Rich SS, Annegers JF, Hauser WA, Anderson VE. Complex segregation analysis of febrile convulsions. *Am J Hum Genet* 1987; 41:249–257.
56. Johnson EW, Dubovsky J, Rich SS, et al. Evidence for a novel gene for familial febrile convulsions, FEB2, linked to chromosome 19p in an extended family from the Midwest. *Hum Mol Genet* 1998; 7:63–67.
57. Wallace RH, Wang DW, Singh R, et al. Febrile seizures and generalized epilepsy associated with a mutation in the Na^+-channel betal subunit gene SCN1B. *Nat Genet* 1998; 19:366–370.
58. Wallace RH, Berkovic SF, Howell RA, et al. Suggestion of a major gene for familial febrile convulsions mapping to 8q13–21. *J Med Genet* 1996; 33:308–312.
59. Gerber MA, Berliner BC. The child with a "simple" febrile seizure: appropriate diagnostic evaluation. *Am J Dis Child* 1981; 135:431–433.
60. Heijbel J, Blom S, Bergfors PG: Simple febrile convulsions: a prospective incidence study and an evaluation of investigations initially needed. *Neuropediatrie* 1980; 11:45–56.
61. Jaffe M, Bar-Joseph G, Tirosh E. Fever and convulsions—indications for laboratory investigations. *Pediatrics* 1981; 57:729–731.
62. Rutter N, Smales ORC: Role of routine investigations in children presenting with their first febrile convulsion. *Arch Dis Child* 1977; 52:188-191.
63. Joffe A, McMcormick M, DeAngelis C. Which children with febrile seizures need lumbar puncture? A decision analysis approach. *Am J Dis Child* 1983; 137:1153–1156.
64. Lorber J, Sunderland R. Lumbar puncture in children with convulsions associated with fever. *Lancet* 1980; 1:785–786.
65. McIntyre PB, Gray SV, Vance JC. Unsuspected bacterial infections in febrile convulsions. *Med J Aust* 1990; 152:183–186.
66. Rutter N, Metcalf DH. Febrile convulsions: What do parents do? *Br Med J* 1978; 2:1345–1346.
67. Wears RL, Luten RC, Lyons RG. Which laboratory tests should be performed on children with apparent febrile convulsions? An analysis and review of the literature. *Pediatric Emer Care* 1986; 2:191–196.
68. Riviello JJ Jr, Ashwal S, et al, American Academy of Neurology Subcommittee, Practice Committee of the Child Neurology Society. Practice parameter: diagnostic assessment of the child with status epilepticus (an evidence-based review): report of the Quality Standards Subcommittee of the American Academy of Neurology and the Practice Committee of the Child Neurology Society. *Neurology* 2006; 67(9):1542–1550.
69. Frank LM, Hesdorffer DC, O'Dell C, et al, FEBSTAT Study Team. Febrile status epilepticus does not cause CSF pleocytosis: results of the FEBSTAT Multicenter Trial. *Epilepsia* 2006; 47(Suppl 4).
70. Van Landingham KE, Heinz ER, Cavazos JE, Lewis DV. MRI evidence of hippocampal injury following prolonged, focal febrile convulsions. *Ann Neurol* 1998; 43:413–426.
71. Koyama A, Matsui T, Sugisawa T. Febrile convulsions in northern Japan. A quantitative and qualitative analysis of EEG and clinical findings. *Acta Neurol Scand* 1991; 83: 411–417.
72. Millichap JG, Colliver JA. Management of febrile seizures: survey of current practice and phenobarbital usage. *Pediatr Neurol* 1991; 7:243–248.
73. Sofianov N, Emoto S, Kuturec M, et al: Febrile seizures: clinical characteristics and initial EEG. *Epilepsia* 1992; 33:52–57.
74. Stores G. When does an EEG contribute to the management of febrile seizures? *Arch Dis Child* 1991; 66:554–557.
75. Doose H, Ritter K, Volzke E. EEG longitudinal studies in febrile convulsions. Genetic aspects. *Neuropediatrics* 1983; 14:81–87.
76. Frantzen E, Lennox-Buchthal M, Nygaard A, Stene J. Longitudinal EEG and clinical study of children with febrile convulsions. *Electroencephalogr Clin Neurophysiol* 1968; 24:197–212.
77. Millichap JG, Madsen JA, Aledort LM. Studies in febrile seizures. V. Clinical and electroencephalographic study in unselected patients. *Neurology* 1960; 10:643–653.
78. Tsuboi T. Correlation between EEG abnormality and age in childhood. *Neuropediatrics* 1978; 9:229–238.
79. Kuturec M, Emoto SE, Sofianov N, et al. Febrile seizures: is the EEG a useful predictor of recurrences? *Clin Pediatr* 1997; 36:31–36.
80. Nordli DR, Moshe SL, Frank LM, et al, FEBSTAT study team. Acute EEG findings in children with febrile status epilepticus. *Epilepsia* 2005; 46(suppl 8):266.
81. Livingston S, Bridge EM, Kajdi L. Febrile convulsions: a clinical study with special reference to heredity and prognosis. *J Pediatr* 1947; 31:509–512.
82. Rantala H, Uhari M, Hietala J. Factors triggering the first febrile seizure. *Acta Paediatr* 1995; 84:407–410.
83. Barone SR, Kaplan MH, Krilov LR. Human herpesvirus-6 infection in children with first febrile seizures. *J Pediatr* 1995; 127:95–97.
84. Hall CB, Long CE, Schnabel KC, et al. Human herpesvirus-6 infection in children: a prospective study of complications and reactivation. *N Engl J Med* 1994; 331:432–438.
85. Kondo K, Nagafuji H, Hata A, et al. Association of human herpesvirus-6 infection of the central nervous system with recurrence of febrile convulsions. *J Infect Dis* 1993; 167:1197–1200.
86. Baram TZ, Gerth A, Schultz L. Febrile seizures: an appropriate-aged model suitable for long-term studies. *Brain Res Dev Brain Res* 1997; 98:265–270.
87. Germano IM, Zhang YF, Sperber EF, Moshe SL. Neuronal migration disorders increase susceptibility to hyperthermia-induced seizures in developing rats. *Epilepsia* 1996; 37:902–910.
88. Holtzman D, Obana K, Olson J. Hyperthermia-induced seizures in the rat pup: a model for febrile convulsions in children. *Science* 1981; 213:1034–1036.
89. Olson JE, Scher MS, Holtzman D. Effects of anticonvulsants on hyperthermia-induced seizures in the rat pup. *Epilepsia* 1984; 25:96–99.

90. Tancredi V, D'Arcangelo G, Zona C, et al. Induction of epileptiform activity by temperature elevation in hippocampal slices from young rats: an in vitro model for febrile seizures? *Epilepsia* 1992; 33:228–234.
91. Toth Z, Yan XX, Haftoglou S, et al. Seizure-induced neuronal injury: vulnerability to febrile seizures in immature rat model. *J Neurosci* 1998; 18:4285–4294.
92. Chen K, Baram TZ, Soltesz I. Febrile seizures in the developing brain result in persistent modification of neuronal excitability in limbic circuits. *Nat Med* 1999; 5:888–894.
93. Dube C, Chen K, Eghbal-Ahmadi M, et al. Prolonged febrile seizures in the immature rat model enhance hippocampal excitability long term. *Ann Neurol* 2000; 47:336–344.
94. Abou-Khalil B, Andermann E, Andermann F, et al. Temporal lobe epilepsy after prolonged febrile convulsions: excellent outcome after surgical treatment. *Epilepsia* 1993; 34:878–883.
95. Bruton CJ. The neuropathology of temporal lobe epilepsy. New York: Oxford University Press, 1988.
96. Cendes F, Andermann F, Dubeau F, et al. Early childhood prolonged febrile convulsions, atrophy and sclerosis of mesial structures, and temporal lobe epilepsy: an MRI volumetric study. *Neurology* 1993; 43:1083–1087.
97. Cendes F, Andermann F, Gloor P, et al. Atrophy of mesial structures in patients with temporal lobe epilepsy: cause or consequence of repeated seizures. *Ann Neurol* 1993; 34: 795–801.
98. French JA, Williamson PD, Thadani M, et al. Characteristics of medial temporal lobe epilepsy: I. Results of history and physical examination. *Ann Neurol* 1993:34:774–780.
99. Sagar HJ, Oxbury JM. Hippocampal neuron loss in temporal lobe epilepsy: correlation with early childhood convulsions. *Ann Neurol* 1987; 22:334–340.
100. Taylor DC, Ounsted C. Biological mechanisms influencing the outcome of seizures in response to fever. *Epilepsia* 1971; 12:33–45.
101. Maher J, McLachlan RS. Febrile convulsions. Is seizure duration the most important predictor of temporal lobe epilepsy? *Brain* 1995; 118:1521–1528.
102. Chevrie JJ, Aicardi J. Duration and lateralization of febrile convulsions. Etiological factors. *Epilepsia* 1975; 16:781–789.
103. Falconer M. Genetic and related etiological factors in temporal lobe epilepsy: a review. *Epilepsia* 1971; 12:13–31.
104. Falconer MA, Serafetinides EA, Corsellis JAN. Etiology and pathogenesis of temporal lobe epilepsy. *Arch Neurol* 1964; 10:233–248.
105. Mathern GW, Babb TL, Mischel PS, et al. Childhood generalized and mesial temporal epilepsies demonstrate different amounts and patterns of hippocampal neuron loss and mossy fibre synaptic reorganization. *Brain* 1996; 119:965–987.
106. Mathern GW, Babb TL, Vickrey BG, et al. The clinical-pathologic mechanisms of hippocampal neuronal loss and surgical outcomes in temporal lobe epilepsy. *Brain* 1995; 118:105–118.
107. Mathern GW, Pretorius JK, Babb TL. Influence of the type of initial precipitating injury and at what age it occurs on course and outcome in patients with temporal lobe seizures. *J Neurosurg* 1995; 82:220–227.
108. Mathern GW, Babb TL, Pretorius JK, et al. The pathophysiologic relationships between lesion pathology, intracranial ictal EEG onsets, and hippocampal neuron losses in temporal lobe epilepsy. *Epilepsy Res* 1995; 21:133–147.
109. Lewis DV, Bello JA, Chan S, FEBSTAT study team. Hippocampal abnormalities subsequent to febrile status epilepticus: Findings on early postictal imaging. Epilepsia 2005; 46(Suppl 8):52–53.
110. Hirtz DG, Lee YJ, Ellenberg J, Nelson KB. Survey on the management of febrile seizures. *Am J Dis Child* 1986; 140:909–914.
111. Millichap JG. Management of febrile seizures: current concepts and recommendations for phenobarbital and the electroencephalogram. *Clin Electroencephalogr* 1991; 22:5–12.
112. Maytal J, Shinnar S. Status epilepticus in children. In: Shinnar S, Amir N, Branski D, eds. *Childhood Seizures*. Basel, Switzerland: S Karger, 1995:111–122.
113. Camfield CS, Camfield PR, Smith E, Dooley, JM. Home use of rectal diazepam to prevent status epilepticus in children with convulsive disorders. *J Child Neurol* 1989; 4: 125–126.
114. Knudsen FU. Rectal administration of diazepam in solution in the acute treatment of convulsions in infants and children. *Arch Dis Child* 1979; 54:855–857.
115. Morton LD, Rizkallah E, Pellock JM. New drug therapy for acute seizure management. *Semin Pediatr Neurol* 1997; 4:51–63.
116. Knudsen FU. Practical management approaches to simple and complex febrile seizures. In: Baram TZ, Shinnar S, eds. *Febrile Seizures*. San Diego, CA: Academic Press, 2002:274–304.
117. O'Dell C. What do we tell the parent of a child with simple or complex febrile seizures? In: Baram TZ, Shinnar S, eds. *Febrile Seizures*. San Diego, CA: Academic Press, 2002:305–316.
118. O'Dell C, Shinnar S, Ballaban-Gil K, et al: Home use of rectal diazepam gel (Diastat). *Epilepsia* 2000; 41(suppl 7):246.
119. Camfield PR, Camfield CS, Shapiro S, et al. The first febrile seizure—antipyretic instruction plus either phenobarbital or placebo to prevent a recurrence. *J Pediatr* 1980; 97:16–21.
120. Autret E, Billard C, Bertrand, et al. Double-blind randomized trial of diazepam versus placebo for prevention of recurrence of febrile seizures. *J Pediatr* 1990; 117:490–495.
121. Knudsen FU. Effective short-term diazepam prophylaxis in febrile convulsions. *J Pediatr* 1985; 106:487–490.
122. Knudsen FU, Vestermark S. Prophylactic diazepam or phenobarbitone in febrile convulsions: a prospective, controlled study. *Arch Dis Child* 1978; 53:660–663.
123. McKinlay I, Newton R. Intention to treat febrile convulsions with rectal diazepam, valproate or phenobarbitone. *Dev Med Child Neurol* 1989; 31:617–625.
124. Rosman NP, Colton T, Labazzo J, et al. A controlled trial of diazepam administered during febrile illnesses to prevent recurrence of febrile seizures. *N Engl J Med* 1993; 329:79–84.
125. Pearce JL, Sharman JR, Forster RM. Phenobarbital in the acute management of febrile seizures. *Pediatrics* 1977; 60:569–572.
126. Wolf SM, Carr A, Davis DC, et al. The value of phenobarbital in the child who has had a single febrile seizure: a controlled prospective study. *Pediatrics* 1977; 59:378–385.
127. Anthony J, Hawke S. Phenobarbital compared with carbamazepine in prevention of recurrent febrile convulsions. *Am J Dis Child* 1983; 137:892–895.
128. Bacon C, Mucklow J, Rawlins M, et al. Placebo-controlled study of phenobarbital and phenytoin in the prophylaxis of febrile convulsions. *Lancet* 1981; 11:600–603.
129. Herranz JL, Armijo JA, Arteaga R. Effectiveness and toxicity of phenobarbital, primidone, and sodium valproate in the prevention of febrile convulsions, controlled by plasma levels. *Epilepsia* 1984; 25:89–95.
130. Newton RW. Randomized controlled trials of phenobarbitone and valproate in febrile convulsions. *Arch Dis Child* 1988; 63:1189–1192.
131. American Academy of Pediatrics: Committee on Drugs. Behavioral and cognitive effects of anticonvulsant therapy. *Pediatrics* 1995; 96:538–540.
132. Camfield CS, Chaplin S, Doyle AB, et al. Side effects of phenobarbital in toddlers: behavioral and cognitive aspects. *J Pediatr* 1979; 95:361–365.
133. Wolf SM, Forsythe A. Behavior disturbance, phenobarbital and febrile seizures. *Pediatrics* 1978; 61:728–731.
134. Farwell J, Lee YJ, Hirtz DG, et al. Phenobarbital for febrile seizures-effects on intelligence and on seizure recurrence. *N Engl J Med* 1990; 322:364–369.
135. Dreifuss FE, Langer DH, Moline KA, et al. Valproic acid hepatic fatalities. II. U.S. experience since 1984. *Neurology* 1989; 39:201–207.
136. Dreifuss FE, Santilli N, Langer DH, et al. Valproic acid hepatic fatalities: a retrospective review. *Neurology* 1987; 37:379–385.
137. Camfield PR, Camfield CS, Tibbles JA. Carbamazepine does not prevent febrile seizures in phenobarbital failures. *Neurology* 1982; 32:288–289.
138. American Academy of Pediatrics. Practice parameter: long-term treatment of the child with simple febrile seizures. *Pediatrics* 1999; 103:1307–1309.
139. Shinnar S, O'Dell C. Treating childhood seizures: when and for how long. In: Shinnar S, Amir N, Branski D, eds. *Childhood Seizures*. Basel: S Karger, 1995:100–110.
140. Baumer JH, David TJ, Valentine SJ, et al. Many parents think their child is dying when having a first febrile convulsion. *Dev Med Child Neurol* 1981; 23:462–464.

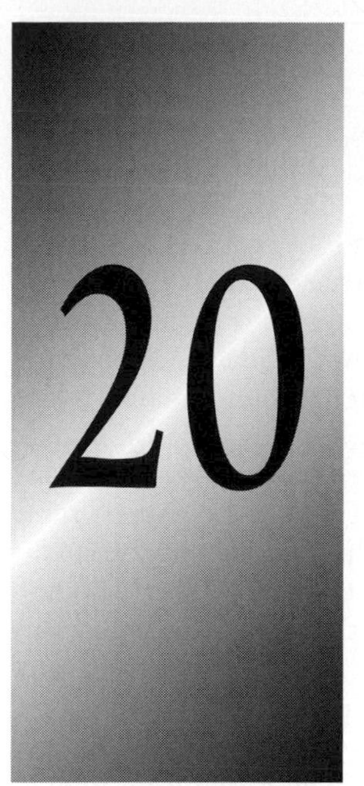

Generalized Epilepsy with Febrile Seizures Plus (GEFS+)

Douglas R. Nordli, Jr.
John M. Pellock

Generalized epilepsy with febrile seizures plus (GEFS+) was defined by Scheffer and colleagues in 1997 and was based upon a very careful and extensive examination of large families with multiple affected individuals (1). Family members had febrile seizures alone (FS); febrile seizures "plus," meaning febrile seizures beyond the typical age limit of 6 years, or a history of febrile seizures along with afebrile generalized seizures; or afebrile seizures. Early descriptions of the afebrile seizures in these individuals highlighted generalized seizures including absence, convulsions, myoclonus, and atonic seizures. Later descriptions included a richer variety of seizures and epilepsy syndromes. Perhaps the most startling revelation was the fact that some families contained children with severe epilepsies, including myoclonic-astatic epilepsy (MAE) as described by Doose, Dravet syndrome, temporal lobe epilepsy, and infantile spasms. It was quickly recognized that this was a very important contribution to our understanding of the genetic contributions to epilepsy. Some characteristics appeared to be inherited in an autosomal dominant fashion, but the extremely broad clinical spectrum of affected individuals in some families strongly suggested polygenic contributions. These genetic influences may involve complex interactions among susceptibility genes, modifier genes, and the environment.

EPIDEMIOLOGY

The discovery of GEFS+ postdates many of the classic and extensive epidemiological studies of childhood epilepsy. The original patients were described in large family kindreds, which are undoubtedly quite rare. GEFS+ more commonly presents in small families, or perhaps with spontaneous mutations where the genetic contributions are probably not appreciated by the physicians caring for the patients, unless the individual presents with a severe phenotype, such as Dravet syndrome, and undergoes SCN1A testing. These facts, coupled with the large and diverse clinical spectrum of the disorder, make it difficult to establish the precise incidence and prevalence. It is nevertheless clear that families with GEFS+ have been confirmed in many different regions of the world with diverse racial backgrounds and that the phenomenon is not isolated to a restricted gene pool. There is no clear gender preponderance.

CLINICAL MANIFESTATIONS

The clinical manifestation of GEFS+ are diverse (1, 2). The commonest phenotype is typical febrile seizures, defined as convulsions in the setting of fever (above 38°C) in children between the ages of 3 months and 6 years. The second most common phenotype is febrile seizures plus, which indicates that febrile seizures continued beyond 6 years of age or that there were afebrile convulsions in addition to the febrile seizures. The least common phenotype was isolated afebrile convulsions in childhood. Generalized seizure types seen include absence, atonic, and myoclonic seizures. Focal seizures arising from the temporal or frontal regions have also been reported (3).

Two of the most severe phenotypes reported in families with GEFS+ include MAE, as described by Doose and colleagues, and Dravet syndrome. About one third of children with myoclonic-astatic epilepsy have a history of febrile seizures. Boys are more commonly affected. Myoclonic-astatic seizures are the commonest manifestation, but myoclonic, atonic, absence, and generalized clonic-tonic-clonic seizures are also observed. Tonic seizures may be present, particularly during the night, and nonconvulsive status epilepticus is also seen. Generalized spike-wave discharges are common, as are rhythmic bursts of biparietal theta activity. Many patients will go into remission with several years of onset, but the outcome is variable, and some patients will be left with substantial cognitive disabilities (4).

Children with Dravet syndrome typically present in the first year of life with febrile hemiclonic seizures or generalized convulsions (5). Children then develop a variety of afebrile seizures including absence, atonic, myoclonic, or focal seizures. The electroencephalogram (EEG) may initially show focal spikes in the posterior derivations, but later, generalized spike-wave discharges develop in most individuals, and a photoparoxysmal response may be seen in some.

EEG FEATURES

EEG backgrounds are usually normal. Interictal features appear to vary according to the clinical phenotype. Those individuals with febrile seizures alone often have normal EEGs (1). Those with febrile seizures and generalized afebrile seizures may have generalized spike-wave discharges. Patients with the MAE or Dravet phenotype have the corresponding EEG features. Patients with focal seizures may have focal spikes, or focal slowing (3).

PATHOPHYSIOLOGY

The pathophysiology of GEFS+ has been well studied. Mutations involving three different genes have been shown to be relevant, but these genes alone cannot explain the large phenotypic variety seen in the families of affected individuals. It is likely that other genes yet to be discovered, the environment, or both play additional roles in determining the phenotype. It has been speculated that a fuller knowledge of these interactions may illuminate important pathophysiological mechanisms in other forms of epilepsy.

These genes involved in GEFS+ encode the gamma-aminobutyric acid A ($GABA_A$) receptor and the neuronal sodium channel. The gene encoding the alpha1 subunit of the sodium channel, SCN1A, is the most frequently mutated in GEFS+. This subunit has four domains, which create the pore of the channel, a voltage sensor, and an anchor to the axonal membrane. Missense mutations are found at may different loci and may cause gain of function, loss of function, or no discernable change in the channel properties (6–8). Mutations of the beta subunit, SCN1B, have also been found, but these are less common (9). The mutations effect an extracellular portion of the protein that is important in altering properties of the channel. Finally, mutations of the gene that encodes the $GABA_A$ receptor are reported in GEFS+. These mutations involve the gamma2 subunit, GABRG2, and the delta subunit, GABRD (10, 11). These mutations are the most rare in GEFS+ but may be of particular importance because of their association with idiopathic generalized epilepsies.

DIAGNOSTIC EVALUATION AND DIFFERENTIAL DIAGNOSIS

Patients with febrile seizures are common, and as many as 15–20% of all patients with epilepsy have had febrile seizures. The main features suggesting GEFS+ are a positive family history, the persistence of seizures beyond 6 years of age, and the coexistence of other, afebrile seizures (see Table 20-1). The evolution to severe forms of epilepsy

TABLE 20-1
Features of GEFS+

Positive Family History

Febrile Seizures +
- Starting earlier than typical febrile seizures (before 6 months)
- Continuing longer than usual (above age 6 years)

Generalized Epilepsy (from early to mid-childhood)
- Brief nonfebrile generalized convulsions
- Absences
- Myoclonic jerks
- Tonic seizures

Focal Seizures
- May be seen, mostly of frontal or temporal origin

Severe Epilepsies (May Be Associated)
- Dravet syndrome
- Myoclonic-astatic epilepsy
- West syndrome

is most likely to be phenotypically consistent with Dravet syndrome or MAE. Genetic testing for SCN1A gene mutations (targeted at identification of individuals with the severe or Dravet phenotype) is now commercially available in the United States.

TREATMENT

The large amount of emerging information regarding the pathogenesis of the seizures in GEFS+ should ultimately direct the development of rational therapies for patients with GEFS+. So far, though, such recommendations are lacking (12). Patients at risk for prolonged or repeated febrile seizures may be prescribed rectal diazepam to be used as needed for these circumstances. There are no formal guidelines for determining when, if ever, one should initiate prophylactic treatment in children with repeated febrile seizures, particularly those whose febrile seizures are persisting beyond the expected age cutoff of 6 years. Treatment of patients with repeated afebrile seizures would depend upon the seizure type. Treatment of Dravet syndrome and MAE is described in Chapter 17.

COURSE AND PROGNOSIS

The course is generally favorable. The majority of patients do not have refractory epilepsies, and their epilepsy, if it develops, usually spontaneously remits, often by mid-childhood (2). Patients with a clinical phenotype consistent with Dravet syndrome have a severe prognosis, and those with MAE must be considered to have a guarded prognosis.

References

1. Scheffer IE, Berkovic SF. Generalized epilepsy with febrile seizures plus. A genetic disorder with heterogeneous clinical phenotypes. *Brain* 1997; 120(Pt 3):479–490.
2. Singh R, Scheffer IE, Crossland K, Berkovic SF. Generalized epilepsy with febrile seizures plus: a common childhood-onset genetic epilepsy syndrome. *Ann Neurol* 1999; 45(1):75–81.
3. Abou-Khalil B, Ge Q, Desai R, Ryther R, et al. Partial and generalized epilepsy with febrile seizures plus and a novel SCN1A mutation. *Neurology* 2001; 57(12):2265–2272.
4. Guerrini R, Aicardi J. Epileptic encephalopathies with myoclonic seizures in infants and children (severe myoclonic epilepsy and myoclonic-astatic epilepsy). *J Clin Neurophysiol* 2003; 20(6):449–461.
5. Dravet C, Bureau M, Oguni H, Fukuyama Y, et al. Severe myoclonic epilepsy in infancy: Dravet syndrome. *Adv Neurol* 2005; 95:71–102.
6. Mulley JC, Scheffer IE, Petrou S, Dibbens LM, et al. SCN1A mutations and epilepsy. *Hum Mutat* 2005; 25(6):535–542.
7. Lossin C, Rhodes TH, Desai RR, Vanoye CG, et al. Epilepsy-associated dysfunction in the voltage-gated neuronal sodium channel SCN1A. *J Neurosci* 2003; 23(36): 11289–11295.
8. Spampanato J, Aradi I, Soltesz I, Goldin AL. Increased neuronal firing in computer simulations of sodium channel mutations that cause generalized epilepsy with febrile seizures plus. *J Neurophysiol* 2004; 91(5):2040–2050.
9. Audenaert D, Claes L, Ceulemans B, Lofgren A, et al. A deletion in SCN1B is associated with febrile seizures and early-onset absence epilepsy. *Neurology* 2003; 61(6):854–856.
10. Baulac S, Huberfeld G, Gourfinkel-An I, Mitropoulou G, et al. First genetic evidence of GABA(A) receptor dysfunction in epilepsy: a mutation in the gamma2-subunit gene. *Nat Genet* 2001; 28(1):46–48.
11. Dibbens LM, Feng HJ, Richards MC, Harkin LA, et al. GABRD encoding a protein for extra- or peri-synaptic $GABA^A$ receptors is a susceptibility locus for generalized epilepsies. *Hum Mol Genet* 2004; 13(13):1315–1319.
12. Burgess DL. Neonatal epilepsy syndromes and GEFS+: mechanistic considerations. *Epilepsia* 2005; 46 Suppl 10:51–58.

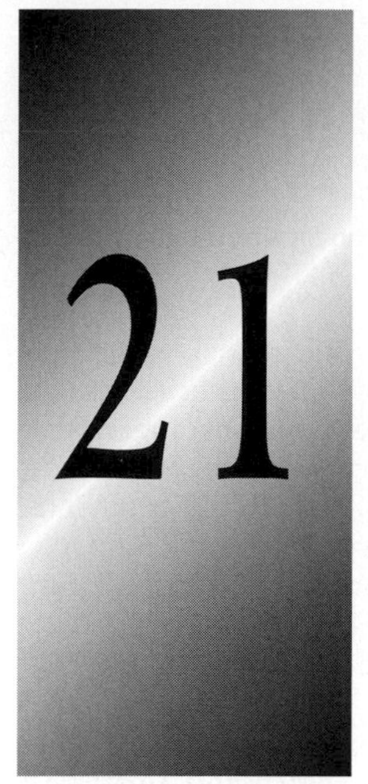

21 Lennox-Gastaut Syndrome

Diego A. Morita
Tracy A. Glauser

Among the numerous epileptic syndromes occurring during childhood, a subset is characterized by severe, treatment-resistant seizures, usually associated with progressive loss of higher intellectual functions and characteristic electroencephalogram (EEG) abnormalities. These age-dependent epileptic syndromes are often called encephalopathic epilepsies or epileptic encephalopathies, a descriptive terminology that does not shed light on their underlying pathophysiologies or specific etiologies. It has been proposed that these syndromes are age-specific epileptic reactions to nonspecific and diverse exogenous insults (1). This subgroup of pediatric epilepsy syndromes includes early infantile epileptic encephalopathy with suppression-burst (EIEE, Ohtahara syndrome) and infantile spasms (West syndrome), both of which are discussed in detail elsewhere in this book (Chapters 15 and 16). The focus of this chapter is on childhood epileptic encephalopathy with diffuse slow spike-and-waves (Lennox-Gastaut syndrome, or LGS).

HISTORY

The clinical manifestations of the Lennox-Gaustat syndrome have been recognized for more than two centuries. In 1772, Tissot described a mentally retarded boy who had multiple daily brief motor seizures with drop attacks (2). In 1886, Jackson reported a young child who had been having stiffening spells (with subsequent falling and facial injury), occurring 20 to 50 times a day, since the age of 2 years (2). In the early twentieth century, Hunt reported more than 10 patients suffering abrupt loss of postural tone, resulting in falls with subsequent significant facial and knee injuries (2).

With the advent of the EEG, neurologists began to look at clinical-electrographic correlates (both ictal and interictal) in patients with epilepsy. In 1935, the 3-Hz spike-and-wave discharge associated with "petit mal" seizures was first described by Gibbs, Davis, and Lennox (3). Subsequently, in 1939, Gibbs, Gibbs, and Lennox identified a similar, yet slower pattern (approximately 2 per second) and proposed to call it a "petit mal variant" to distinguish it from the classic 3-Hz spike and wave (4).

In 1945, Lennox assembled the clinical manifestations and the EEG manifestations into the first semblance of the electroclinical syndrome (5) that we now call childhood epileptic encephalopathy with diffuse slow spike-and-waves, or the Lennox-Gastaut syndrome. Lennox's triad consisted of the slow spike-and-wave interictal EEG pattern, mental retardation, and three types of seizures considered characteristic: myoclonic jerks, atypical absence, and "drop attacks" (also known as akinetic seizures or astatic seizures) (2, 5–7).

This constellation of symptoms initially was not given a formal syndrome name. Renewed interest in this syndrome began in 1964, when Sorel and Doose each described about 20 cases (8, 9). Three meetings held in Marseille (the 13th, 14th, and 16th Symposia of Marseille in 1964, 1966, and 1968, respectively) examined the syndrome in depth (2). After the first meeting ended with divergent views on the subject, multiple investigators sought to better define the electroclinical manifestations of this syndrome (2). Dravet, in her doctoral thesis in 1965 and two subsequent papers in 1966, reported the results of these intensive studies (10–12). The 1966 Marseille meeting culminated in the proposal to name the syndrome the Lennox-Gastaut syndrome, acknowledging the significant contributions of both the United States and French groups to the understanding of the syndrome (2). The 1968 meeting in Marseille reinforced the existence of this syndrome in each of the participants' countries and solidified its position in the pantheon of epileptic syndromes (2).

The importance of recognizing patients with LGS increased in the early 1990s, when this population was identified as a target group to participate in trials of investigational antiepileptic drugs (AEDs). The factors contributing to the targeting of this group for study with investigational AEDs include their high daily seizure frequency, the lack of very effective therapy, and the desire to examine safety and efficacy issues for investigational AEDs in pediatric populations before general release.

The current definition of LGS by the International League Against Epilepsy (ILAE) classification is as follows (13):

> LGS manifests itself in children aged 1–8 years, but appears mainly in preschool-age children. The most common seizure types are tonic-axial, atonic, and absence seizures, but other types such as myoclonic, generalized tonic-clonic seizures (GTCS), or partial seizures are frequently associated with this syndrome. Seizure frequency is high, and status epilepticus is frequent (stuporous states with myoclonias, tonic and atonic seizures). The EEG usually has abnormal background activity, slow spike-and-waves <3Hz and, often, multifocal abnormalities. During sleep, bursts of fast rhythms (10 Hz) appear. In general, there is mental retardation. Seizures are difficult to control, and the development is unfavorable. In 60 percent of cases, the syndrome occurs in children suffering from a previous encephalopathy, but is primary in other cases.

A triad of basic elements needed to make a diagnosis of LGS is usually stated based on this definition, coupled with clinical experience and research:

1. Multiple types of seizures including tonic seizures, atypical absences, and atonic seizures;
2. An EEG pattern consisting of interictal diffuse slow spike-and-wave discharges occurring at a 1.5- to 2-Hz frequency
3. Diffuse cognitive dysfunction and/or mental retardation (2, 13–18)

There is abundant discussion among epileptologists about the minimal necessary and sufficient criteria to diagnose a patient with LGS. Some investigators do not consider cognitive dysfunction or mental retardation indispensable for diagnosis, especially at onset, if the seizures and EEG pattern are typical (15, 19–21). Other authors use a stricter EEG criterion, requiring that the diagnostic EEG pattern include bursts of generalized fast spikes (10 Hz) during non-rapid-eye movement (NREM) sleep (22).

Ohtahara proposed a more comprehensive set of diagnostic criteria consisting of indispensable, supportive, and suggestive criteria (19). The indispensable criteria are the combination of tonic seizures, atypical absences, atonic seizures, myoclonic seizures, and astatic seizures, with an interictal EEG pattern of diffuse slow spike-and-waves. Mental retardation, bursts of generalized fast spikes (10 Hz) during NREM sleep, onset in early childhood, and treatment-resistant seizures are among the supportive features (19).

In the 2001 ILAE proposal for classification and terminology of seizures and epilepsy, LGS was classified as an epileptic encephalopathy in which the epileptiform abnormalities may contribute to progressive dysfunction (23).

EPIDEMIOLOGY

Overall, LGS accounts for 1% to 4% of all cases of childhood epilepsy, but 10% of cases that start in the first 5 years of life (20, 21, 24–30). Epidemiological studies in the Western or industrialized world (Israel, Spain, Estonia, Italy, and the United States) demonstrated that the proportion of LGS seems relatively consistent across various populations (21, 25–28). The annual incidence of LGS in childhood is 2 per 100,000 children (30, 31). The prevalence of LGS ranges from 0.1 to 0.28 per 1,000 in Europe and the United States (21, 31–33).

The prevalence and percentage of LGS in mentally retarded children were reported as 0.06 per 1,000 and 7%, respectively (29). The proportion of LGS in institutionalized patients with mental retardation is as high as 16.3% (34).

Males are affected more often than females. Most studies do not report this gender difference to be statistically significant, but in an epidemiological study in Atlanta, Georgia, the difference between males and females was significant ($P < 0.005$) (21, 30, 35, 36). The relative risk of occurrence of LGS is significantly higher in boys (prevalence rate, 0.1 per 100 for boys, 0.02 per 1,000 for girls; rate ratios 5.31; 95% confidence interval, 1.16–49.35) (32). There are no racial differences in the occurrence of LGS (21). The mean age at epilepsy onset is 26 to 28 months (range, 1 day–14 years) (20, 36). The peak age at epilepsy onset is older in the symptomatic LGS group, but the difference in age of onset between the group with a history of West syndrome compared with the group without such a history was not significant. The average age at diagnosis of LGS in Japan was 6 years (range, 2–15 years) (20). Compared with other patients with less severe epilepsies, patients with LGS have a younger age of onset of epilepsy (30).

Lennox-Gastaut syndrome can be classified according to its suspected etiology as either idiopathic or symptomatic. Patients may be considered to have idiopathic LGS if there is normal psychomotor development before the onset of symptoms, if there are no underlying disorders or definite presumptive causes, and if there are no neurologic or neuroradiologic abnormalities (19). In contrast, patients have symptomatic LGS if there is an identifiable cause for the syndrome.

Population-based studies found that 22% to 30% of patients have idiopathic LGS, and 70% to 78% have symptomatic LGS (19, 20, 35, 37). Examples of underlying pathologies responsible for symptomatic LGS include encephalitis/meningitis, tuberous sclerosis, brain malformations (e.g., cortical dysplasias), birth injury, hypoxic-ischemic injury, frontal lobe lesions, and trauma (18, 19, 38). Infantile spasms precede the development of LGS in 9% to 41% of cases (14, 21, 38).

Some investigators add "cryptogenic" as a different etiological category, in which there is no identified cause when a cause is suspected and the epilepsy is presumed to be symptomatic. In an epidemiological study in Atlanta, Georgia, 44% of all LGS patients were classified in the cryptogenic group (21). Reports of a family history of epilepsy and febrile seizures for patients with LGS range from 2.5% to 47.8% (noted in a series of 23 patients with cryptogenic LGS) (35, 36).

CLINICAL MANIFESTATIONS

Before onset, 20% to 30% of children with LGS are free from neurologic and neuropsychologic deficits. These problems inevitably appear during the evolution of LGS. Factors associated with mental retardation are symptomatic LGS, a previous history of West syndrome, onset of symptoms before 12 to 24 months of age, and higher seizure frequency (18, 35, 37, 39).

The average intelligence quotient (IQ) in a series of 72 patients with LGS followed up for more than 10 years was significantly lower in the symptomatic group than in the cryptogenic group (20, 40). At the time of the first examination, the IQ showed a variable degree of mental retardation in 66% of the cryptogenic group and in 76% of the symptomatic group. At the last examination, mental retardation was found in 95% of the cryptogenic group and in 100% of the symptomatic group (20). A significant correlation exists between age of onset of seizures and mental deterioration, with a favorable cognitive outcome more likely to occur in patients with a later age of LGS onset (40). In one study, almost 98% of the patients who had the onset of seizures before age 2 years, and 63% of those with onset after the age of 2 years, had definite cognitive impairment (39). In some patients with LGS, mental retardation could be a result of nonconvulsive status epilepticus (41).

Psychiatric symptoms in young children consist of mood instability and personality disturbances, whereas slowing or arrest of psychomotor development and educational progress characterize the neuropsychological symptoms. Character problems predominate in older children, and acute psychotic episodes or chronic forms of psychosis with aggressiveness, irritability, or social isolation may occur (35). Prolonged reaction time and information processing are the most impaired of the cognitive functions (18). Kaminska et al found that the main characteristics of mental deterioration were apathy, memory disorders, impaired visuomotor speed, and perseveration (42). The major electrographic abnormalities associated with LGS may account for some of the abnormalities found in higher intellectual functions. Commonly, the epileptiform discharges are frequent and may affect the ability of the patient to engage with the surroundings (43).

Several types of seizures occur in LGS including tonic, atonic, myoclonic, and atypical absences, often associated with other less common types.

Tonic Seizures

Tonic seizures are said to be the most characteristic type of seizure and occur in 17% to 95% of children with LGS (16, 38). Tonic seizures are more frequent during NREM sleep; therefore, researchers who have systematically obtained sleep tracings reported higher prevalences. These seizures can occur during wakefulness or sleep, but if they occur only during sleep they may go unnoticed (35).

Tonic seizures may be (1) axial tonic, involving the head and the trunk, with head and neck flexion, contraction of masticatory muscles, and eventual vocalizations; (2) axorhizomelic tonic, in which there is tonic involvement of the proximal upper limbs, with elevation of the shoulders and abduction of the arm; or (3) global tonic, with contraction of the distal part of the extremities, sometimes leading to a sudden fall and other times mimicking infantile spasms (18, 22, 35).

Tonic seizures can be asymmetric, and some patients may show gestural automatisms after the tonic phase. Duration is from a few seconds to a minute, and, if prolonged, they can end in a vibratory component. In some seizures, the activity may be limited to upward deviation of the eyes ("sursum vergens") and a slowing of respiration (18, 35), which may be mistaken for physiologic phenomena.

Atypical Absences

The reported frequency ranges from 17% to 100% (16, 22). In most studies, the frequency of the different types of seizures reported is based on parental counting of seizures, reviews from charts, or not specifically stated. Unfortunately, parental ability to recognize and identify atypical absences correctly is poor. In one study using video-EEG monitoring in a cohort of children with LGS, parental recognition was 27% for atypical absences, but the sensitivity was as high as 80% for myoclonic seizures and 100% for tonic, atonic, tonic-clonic, clonic, and complex partial seizures (44).

Atypical absences may be difficult to diagnose because the onset may be gradual (18, 22, 35) and there may be an incomplete loss of consciousness that allows the patient to continue activities to some degree. They may be associated with eyelid myoclonias, not as rhythmic as in typical absences, but often associated with perioral myoclonias or progressive flexion of the head secondary to a loss of tone (35). Automatisms may be observed (18). The seizure end may be gradual in some cases or abrupt in others (18, 22, 35).

Atonic Seizures, Massive Myoclonic Seizures, and Myoclonic-Atonic Seizures

Atonic seizures, massive myoclonic seizures, and myoclonic-atonic seizures can be difficult to differentiate by clinical observation alone, and there are considerable discrepancies in how these terms are used. The reported frequency ranges from 10% to 56% (16, 18, 20, 21, 36, 37). They produce sudden fall, producing injuries ("drop attacks," "Sturzanfalle"), sometimes limited to the head, resulting in the head falling on the chest ("head drop," "head nod," "nictatio capitis") (2, 35, 45). Ikeno et al found that pure atonic seizures are exceptional and that most so-called atonic seizures had a tonic or myoclonic component (45).

Other Types of Seizures

Generalized tonic-clonic seizures are reported in 15% of patients with LGS, whereas complex partial seizures occur in 5% (18). Status epilepticus of different types (absence status epilepticus, tonic status epilepticus, nonconvulsive status epilepticus) can occur (16, 18) and is characterized by a long duration and resistance to treatment.

Donat and Wright reported in patients with LGS, infantile spasms–like seizures with clinical characteristics and ictal EEG changes similar to those typically seen in West syndrome. These seizures consisted of brief myoclonic jerks and brief stiffening or flexion of the upper body at the waist (46).

EEG FEATURES

Interictal Manifestations

The interictal EEG is characterized by a slow background that can be constant or transient. Permanent slowing of the background is associated with poor cognitive prognosis (35). The hallmark of the awake interictal EEG is the diffuse slow spike-and-waves. This pattern consist of bursts of irregular, generalized spikes or sharp waves followed by a sinusoidal 35–400-millisecond slow wave (18), with an amplitude that ranges from 200 to 800 μV (39), which can be symmetrical or asymmetrical. The amplitude is very often higher in the anterior region and in the frontal or frontocentral areas, but in some cases the activity may dominate in the posterior regions of the head (39). The frequency of the slow spike-and-wave activity is commonly found between 1.5 and 2.5 Hz (39) (Figure 21-1).

Slow spike-and-waves are usually not activated by photic stimulation. In one series of 83 patients with LGS, activation of slow spike-and-waves with photic stimulation occurred in 2 patients (3 tracings), and decrease in slow spike-and-wave activity was noted in 9% of the tracings (39). Hyperventilation rarely induces slow spike-and-waves (18), although in many patients mental retardation prevents an adequate cooperation (39). During NREM sleep, discharges are more generalized, occur more frequently, and consist of polyspikes and slow waves. In rapid eye movement (REM) sleep there is a decrease in spike-and-waves (18). There is a reduction in the total duration of REM sleep during periods of frequent seizures (18).

Ictal Manifestations

Several types of seizures occur in LGS, including tonic, atonic, myoclonic, and atypical absences, often associated with other less common types.

Tonic Seizures

The tonic seizure EEG is characterized by a diffuse, rapid (10–13 Hz), low-amplitude activity, mainly in the anterior and vertex areas ("recruiting rhythm"), that progressively decreases in frequency and increases in amplitude (Figure 21-2). When the seizure is limited to brief upward

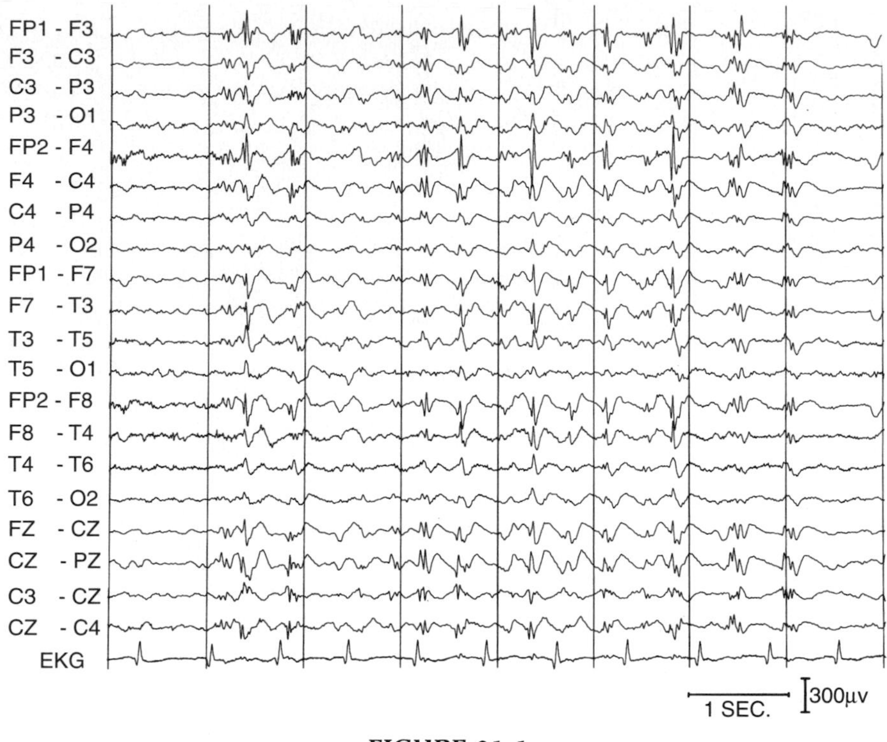

FIGURE 21-1

Slow spike-wave pattern in a 24-year-old awake male with Lennox-Gastaut syndrome. The slow posterior background rhythm has frequent periods of 2–2.5 Hz discharges maximal in the bifrontocentral areas occurring in trains up to 8 seconds without any clinical accompaniment.

deviation of the eyes, the EEG activity may be accentuated in the posterior regions (22). A brief generalized discharge of slow spike-and-waves or flattening of the recording may precede this pattern. Diffuse slow waves and slow spike-and-waves may follow it. These fast discharges are common during NREM sleep. Unlike tonic-clonic seizures, no postictal flattening occurs. Clinical manifestations appear 0.5 to 1 seconds after the onset of EEG manifestations and last several seconds longer than the discharge (18, 35). Yaqub also reported synchronous 3-Hz spike-and-waves associated with tonic seizures (22).

Atypical Absences

The atypical absence seizure EEG is characterized by diffuse, slow (2–2.5 Hz) and irregular spike-and-waves, which may be difficult to differentiate from interictal bursts (18). Discharges of rapid rhythms may be seen preceded by flattening of the record for 1 to 2 seconds, followed by a progressive development of irregular fast rhythm in the anterior and central regions, ending with brief spike-and-waves (22, 35).

Atonic Seizures, Massive Myoclonic Seizures, and Myoclonic-atonic Seizures

The EEG in these seizures is characterized by slow spike-and-waves, polyspike-and-waves, or rapid diffuse rhythms (26, 35). Simultaneous video-EEG recording and polygraphy is necessary for precise diagnosis. In 95% of affected patients, all three types of seizures occur in the same patient (35). Myoclonic seizures in LGS show different neurophysiologic patterns compared to other specific epileptic syndromes such as myoclonic astatic epilepsy (MAE). Epileptic myoclonus in MAE appears to be a primary generalized epileptic phenomenon. In contrast, epileptic myoclonus in LGS seems to be secondarily generalized, originating from a stable generator in the frontal cortex, with interhemispheric spread, likely through transcallosal pathways (47).

Other Types of Seizures

The EEG during absence status epilepticus reveals continuous spike-and-wave discharges, usually at a lower frequency than at baseline, and rapid rhythms during tonic status epilepticus (35). Donat and Wright reported in patients with LGS, infantile spasms–like seizures with clinical characteristics, and ictal EEG changes similar to those typically seen in West syndrome. The interictal EEG showed generalized slow spike-wave discharges (1–2.5 Hz) with occasional multifocal spike waves. The ictal changes consisted of generalized decrement in cerebral activity, identical to the pattern that can be observed with infantile spasms (46).

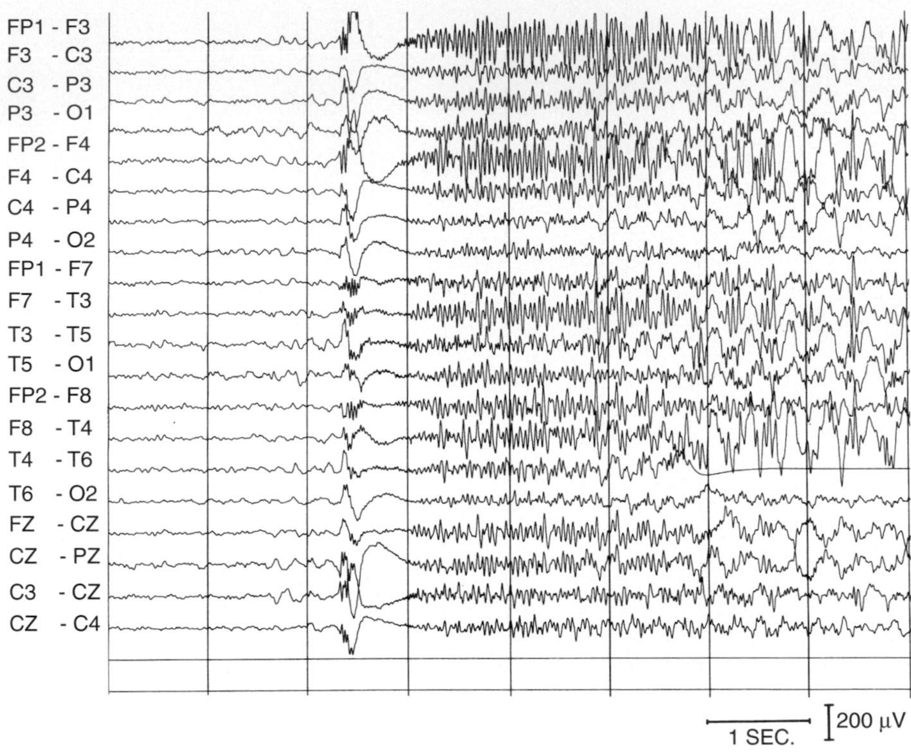

FIGURE 21-2

Tonic seizure with arm extension in a 24-year old male with Lennox-Gastaut syndrome. Before the seizure, the patient is watching television and then has a sudden body jerk, leans forward with arms extended and fixed at shoulder level. The EEG shows a diffuse burst of high-voltage polyspike and slow wave activity followed by 1 second of relative attenuation and then paroxysmal fast activity maximal in the bifrontocentral regions of the head.

PATHOPHYSIOLOGY

The pathophysiology of LGS is not well known (14), and there are no animal models (18). A variety of possible pathophysiologies have been proposed including developmental, immunologic, and metabolic. One hypothesis is that there is excessive permeability in the excitatory interhemispheric pathways in the frontal areas at the time the anterior parts of the brain mature. This maturation commonly occurs around the age of onset of LGS and would allow for synchronization of both frontal lobes (18).

Immunogenetic mechanisms are hypothesized to play a role in triggering or maintaining some cases of LGS. A strong association between LGS and the HLA class I antigen B7 (48) was found in one study, but another group found no statistical difference in the presence of HLA class I antigens, including the antigen B7 (49). This latter study found an increased frequency of HLA class II antigen DR5 and a decrease in DR4 antigen (49).

Two hypotheses have been proposed to explain the cognitive outcome of patients with LGS. It has been suggested that the key LGS electrographic feature of slow spike-and-wave discharges and the paroxysmal fast activity reflect excessive neocortical excitability and subsequent abnormal patterns of central nervous system activity and connectivity. These processes would successfully compete with normal developmental mechanisms, leading to cognitive impairment (50, 51). Another hypothesis postulates a genetic predisposition that is responsible for both the clinical manifestations and the mental retardation (51).

No clear-cut or homogeneous metabolic pattern was noted in six positron emission tomography (PET) studies done in a total of 50 patients with LGS (52–57). Although most studies suggested a focal abnormality, a few others showed diffuse changes or normal findings. Gur et al found temporal lobe unilateral hypometabolism in 2 patients (52). Theodore studied 10 patients with LGS and did not find a region of persistent focal hypometabolism. One of the patients showed hypermetabolism in association with increased epileptiform discharges in EEG (55). Chugani's findings showed four predominant metabolic patterns in 15 children with LGS: unilateral focal hypometabolism, unilateral diffuse hypometabolism, bilateral diffuse hypometabolism, and normal metabolism (56). Iinuma et al reported unilateral hypometabolism in 4 of 5 patients with LGS, particularly in the inferior frontal gyrus or in the posterior portion of the superior temporal gyrus (53). Miyauchi et al found hemispheric metabolic differences in 3 patients with LGS, with hypometabolism in the frontal to the temporal regions (57). Ferrie et al studied 15 patients with LGS and found no areas of hypometabolism in 5 typical cases of LGS, whereas he found them in 3 of 4 atypical cases and in 5 of 6 patients with previous history of West syndrome (54).

Single-photon emission computed tomography (SPECT) in 3 children with LGS showed multiple hypoperfused areas, which contrasted with single areas of hypoperfusion in 11 children with partial secondary generalized epilepsy (58).

DIAGNOSTIC EVALUATION AND DIFFERENTIAL DIAGNOSIS

The diagnosis of LGS is based on the criteria previously defined, which include multiple types of seizures, in particular tonic seizures; an EEG pattern consisting of interictal diffuse slow spike-and-wave discharges occurring at a 1.5–2-Hz frequency, with or without bursts of generalized fast spikes (10 Hz) during NREM sleep; and diffuse cognitive dysfunction, mental retardation, or both.

Because of the nonspecific nature of multiple seizure types and cognitive dysfunction, multiple other pediatric epilepsy syndromes may be confused with LGS. A useful approach to understanding and differentiating these syndromes is to first consider LGS and similar epilepsy syndromes as part of a continuum and then to try to identify characteristics that separate the syndromes. Two scenarios have been proposed. In both scenarios, LGS is at one end of the spectrum. In one scenario, the other end of the continuum is placed in the broad term *myoclonic epilepsies* (16), and another scenario places the end at MAE (42). In both scenarios, the epilepsy syndromes encountered when moving from one end of the spectrum to the other are in the same order: LGS, the "myoclonic variant" of LGS, MAE, and then the lumped "myoclonic epilepsies" (e.g., benign myoclonic epilepsy of infancy, severe myoclonic epilepsy of infancy, and progressive myoclonic epilepsy) (17).

Compared with classic LGS, the "myoclonic variant" of LGS has less frequent and less severe mental retardation; rarer tonic seizures, usually of late onset and almost exclusively nocturnal; an "unusually marked myoclonic component"; a less unfavorable outcome; and frequently faster (>2.5 Hz) spike-and-wave complexes on EEG (16, 38).

Myoclonic astatic epilepsy and LGS have in common myoclonic seizures, atonic seizures, and atypical absences. However, there are major differences: MAE is predominantly idiopathic, is genetically determined, usually has a favorable outcome, and does not follow West syndrome, whereas LGS is mainly symptomatic, is not genetically determined, usually has an unfavorable outcome, and can follow West syndrome (18, 42). Kaminska and coworkers differentiate LGS and MAE using a sophisticated statistical approach called multiple correspondence analysis to study different clinical and EEG parameters. They recognized a group of children with LGS characterized by later onset of epilepsy, atypical absences, tonic and partial seizures, no myoclonus or vibratory tonic seizures, mental retardation, and an EEG pattern with slow spike-and-waves that were, as a group, different from those in the group with MAE features (42). In addition, myoclonic seizures in LGS and MAE show different neurophysiologic patterns, as shown by Bonanni et al using video-EEG, simultaneous surface electromyography, and, when necessary, burst-locked EEG averaging techniques (47).

Compared with patients with LGS, patients with myoclonic epilepsies (in the broadest sense) have myoclonic seizures as the clearly predominant seizure type, only occasionally have tonic seizures, only occasionally have slow spike-and-waves on EEG, almost always have fast (>2.5 Hz) spike-and-wave complexes on EEG, and have variable frequency and levels of mental retardation (16, 17).

Multiple etiologies have been associated with LGS. Knowledge of the cause may affect prognosis and, at times, selection of the best therapy. Neuroimaging is an important part of the search for an underlying etiology in a patient with LGS. Abnormalities revealed by neuroimaging associated with LGS include tuberous sclerosis, brain malformations (e.g., cortical dysplasias), hypoxic-ischemic injury, or frontal lobe lesions. In general, magnetic resonance imaging (MRI) is the preferred neuroimaging study for a patient with LGS rather than a computed tomography (CT) scan. CT scans may be preferred in selected situations (e.g., evaluation of suspected intracranial injury, hematoma, or both in a patient with head trauma resulting from an atonic or tonic seizure). No current indication exists for routine PET or SPECT scanning in patients with LGS. However, PET and SPECT scans may be useful when patients are undergoing evaluation for potential epilepsy surgery.

An EEG in patients with suspected LGS is critical, because the diagnosis depends on the presence of specific electrographic findings. Recording of a prolonged EEG is desirable, because a routine 30-minute EEG may not capture the patient's electrographic activity both awake and asleep and thus may miss crucial specific EEG findings. It is important to capture and classify each of the patient's multiple seizure types. Video-EEG telemetry should be strongly considered because it may also help to educate the parents on which of the patient's events are seizures and which are nonepileptic behavioral events (44).

When assessing learning disability, it is important to differentiate "permanent learning disability" and "state-dependent learning disability." The former refers to the learning disability as a result of an underlying brain damage that leads to both epilepsy and learning disability, or to the epilepsy that leads to brain damage, which in turn results in learning disability (e.g., prolonged status epilepticus). The latter depends on factors affecting the patient, such as adverse medication effects or increased seizures (ictal and postictal effects), both of which are not necessarily permanent and are potentially treatable and reversible (43). Review of the ongoing treatment and recording of a prolonged video-EEG may be of help.

TREATMENT

Overview

The goals of treatment for patients with LGS are the same as for all patients with epilepsy: the best quality of life with the fewest seizures (hopefully none), the fewest treatment side effects, and the least number of medications.

The various treatment options for patients with LGS can be divided into the following three major groups (Table 21-1):

1. First-line treatments based on clinical experience or conventional wisdom
2. Suspected effective treatments based on open-label uncontrolled studies
3. Effective treatments based on double-blind placebo-controlled studies

TABLE 21-1
Treatments for Children with Lennox-Gastaut Syndrome

First-line treatments based on clinical experience or conventional wisdom
Valproic acid
Benzodiazepines
Pyridoxine
Suspected effective treatments based on open-label uncontrolled studies
Adrenocorticotropic hormone–corticosteroids
Intravenous immunoglobulin
Vigabatrin
Zonisamide
Ketogenic diet
Corpus callosotomy
Vagus nerve stimulation
Effective treatments based on double-blind, placebo-controlled studies
Felbamate
Lamotrigine
Topiramate
Rufinamide

In the first and second groups, the efficacy and safety of individual treatment options have not been formally tested. Only options in the third group have been rigorously and scientifically evaluated and found to be effective and safe for specific seizure types in LGS patients. Each treatment group can be subdivided into medical, dietary, and surgical therapies. Unfortunately, no treatment by itself in any of the three groups gives satisfactory relief for all or even a majority of patients with LGS. Combination of treatment modalities is frequently needed (59).

First-Line Treatments Based on Clinical Experience or Conventional Wisdom

Medications

Over the past two decades, valproic acid (VPA) has been considered as a first-line treatment option for children with LGS (24, 52, 53). From a practical viewpoint, by the time a clinician makes a diagnosis of LGS, the patient has already been diagnosed with epilepsy and treatment has been initiated. Because these children have multiple types of generalized seizures and at times coexisting partial seizures, clinicians may initially select a broad-spectrum AED such as VPA. Valproic acid has been reported to be more effective in cryptogenic LGS than in symptomatic LGS (60).

Benzodiazepines, specifically clonazepam, nitrazepam, and clobazam, are also first-line AED therapy options (38, 61, 62). All are considered effective against seizures associated with LGS, but side effects and the development of tolerance limit their usefulness over time (38). Side effects of clonazepam include hyperactivity, sedation, drooling, and incoordination, which can significantly affect the quality of life for patients with LGS (38). The efficacy and tolerability profile of nitrazepam is similar to that of clonazepam (38). Clobazam is considered the least sedating benzodiazepine, with the longest time to the development of tolerance (62). Some recommendations to slow the development of tolerance include dosing on an every-other-day schedule or alternate two different benzodiazepines on an alternate-day basis (63, 64). Unfortunately, not all benzodiazepines are beneficial: intravenous diazepam and lorazepam have been reported to induce tonic status epilepticus in some patients (65, 66). Based on clinical experience, some authors believe a combination of valproic acid and a benzodiazepine may be better than either drug alone, but no data exist to confirm this impression (38).

Although carbamazepine, phenobarbital, phenytoin, and ethosuximide may be first-line therapy for a variety of seizure types or other epilepsy syndromes, none is considered first-line therapy for LGS. Carbamazepine may exacerbate atypical absence seizures despite reducing generalized tonic-clonic seizures (67, 68). Phenobarbital may be effective against a variety of seizures but can exacerbate hyperactivity and aggressiveness or produce sedation and drowsiness (which may exacerbate tonic seizures) (38, 60). Phenytoin can be effective for tonic seizures and tonic status epilepticus but not for atypical absence seizures (69). In contrast, ethosuximide may be useful in atypical absence seizures but is ineffective in other seizure types (59).

Because patients with pyridoxine (vitamin B_6) dependency may have seizures and a slow spike-and-wave pattern on EEG, some clinician investigators have suggested trials of vitamin B_6 in all children with treatment-resistant epilepsy who are younger than 5 years old (61). One study examined the efficacy of high-dose vitamin B_6 in five patients with LGS and found mixed results; three of the five patients with LGS had no response, whereas the others had a more noticeable response (70). Given the lack of serious side effects and the ease of performing a therapeutic vitamin B_6 trial, it is reasonable and appropriate to conduct a vitamin B_6 trial early in treatment of a child with LGS (71). Doses and duration of vitamin B_6 therapy vary widely. In the aforementioned clinical trial, vitamin B_6 was given at 50 to 100 mg/day fifiintramuscularly for the first 5 days, and then 200 to 300 mg/day orally (70). Some clinicians (mainly in Japan) administer high doses of pyridoxal phosphate (30–40 mg/kg/day) (61). Wheless and Constantinou prescribe 100 mg of vitamin B_6 three times daily for 2 weeks, discontinuing vitamin B_6 if there is no response to therapy after 2 weeks (61).

Dietary Treatment

At this time, the ketogenic diet is not a first-line therapy for the seizures associated with LGS.

Surgical Treatment

At this time, neither corpus callosotomy nor the vagus nerve stimulator are first-line therapies for the seizures associated with LGS.

Suspected Effective Treatments Based on Open-Label Uncontrolled Studies

Medications

Medications suspected to have some effectiveness against seizures associated with LGS based on open-label uncontrolled trials include (in alphabetical order): adrenocorticotropic hormone (ACTH) (72, 73), corticosteroids (35, 61, 74), intravenous immunoglobulin (IVIG) (75, 76), vigabatrin (77), and zonisamide (ZNS) (78).

Both ACTH and corticosteroid therapy are proposed to be effective against the seizures associated with LGS. Roger et al propose that prolonged corticosteroid therapy initiated at the onset of cryptogenic LGS can yield "excellent" results (35). Despite this effectiveness, there are multiple potentially significant side effects associated with therapy, and relapse frequently occurs when the drugs are withdrawn (38, 61, 71–74).

The efficacy of adjunctive high-dose IVIG in patients with LGS has been investigated in at least seven open-label trials (75). The results of these trials were very encouraging because 30% to 92% of LGS patients receiving IVIG experienced at least 50% seizure reduction during treatment (75). Dosing schedules varied between studies. Later well-controlled trials (detailed in following discussion) did not confirm the effectiveness of IVIG against seizures associated with LGS (79, 80).

Six studies involving 78 patients treated with vigabatrin showed that 15% of these patients became completely seizure free and 44% of the patients had at least 50% reduction in their seizure frequency (77, 81–85). The best results were noted in an open-label, dose-ranging, adjunctive therapy study of vigabatrin in 20 children with LGS in which monotherapy with VPA did not control their seizures. Seventeen children (85%) experienced at least 50% reduction in their seizure frequency, and eight children (40%) were seizure free at doses ranging from 1 to 3 g/day at study end (77). The authors concluded that vigabatrin and VPA duotherapy was effective and well tolerated in children with LGS (77).

The most common adverse effects of vigabatrin are generally central nervous system related and include hyperactivity, agitation, weight gain, drowsiness, insomnia, facial edema, ataxia, stupor, and somnolence (83, 86–88). Not only can vigabatrin exacerbate myoclonic seizures and even absence seizures in some patients, but it can also cause visual field constriction in children (82, 83, 86, 89, 90). The aforementioned side effects limit significantly the consideration of vigabatrin as long-term therapy for patients with LGS (87).

The effectiveness of ZNS in LGS has been investigated in three small studies. Although Sakamoto et al reported that ZNS was "effective" in 39% of patients with LGS, the definition of effectiveness was not clear (78). In 1991 Yamatogi and Ohtahara reported 50% (10 of 20) of Lennox-Gastaut patients treated with ZNS had at least 50% reduction in seizure frequency (91). Iinuma and Haginoya found that 26% (10 of 39) of patients with LGS treated with ZNS responded with a 50% or greater reduction in seizure frequency (92).

There have been no formal published open-label studies investigating the effectiveness and safety of gabapentin, tiagabine, levetiracetam, or oxcarbazepine in the treatment of seizures associated with LGS. Single reports have suggested that L-tryptophan (transient improvement), amantadine, thyrotropin-releasing hormone, and its analog, DN-1417, may reduce seizure frequency in patients with LGS (93–96).

Dietary Teatment

A number of studies have shown the ketogenic diet to be useful for patients with LGS (71, 72, 97, 98). Response to the diet usually is evident within 1 month of starting the diet (61). Freeman and Vining reported that atonic or myoclonic seizures in 17 consecutively treated patients with LGS at The Johns Hopkins Hospital decreased "by more than 50% immediately," after being started on the ketogenic diet (99). Overall, the benefits of the diet can include fewer seizures along with less drowsiness, better behavior, and fewer concomitant AEDs (61).

Surgical Treatment

Surgical procedures that have been reported to be beneficial for patients with LGS include corpus callosotomy, focal resection (rarely), and electrical stimulation, in particular vagus nerve stimulation (VNS) and the electrical stimulation of the centromedian thalamic nuclei (100, 101).

Corpus callosotomy is effective in reducing drop attacks but typically does not appear to be helpful for other seizure types (38, 102, 103). A recent study from Taiwan reported that anterior corpus callosotomy was effective for "all kinds of medically intractable seizures, especially generalized" in a cohort of 74 patients (80% had LGS) (104). In general, callosotomy is considered palliative rather than curative, and seizure freedom is rare, although it can occur (60, 104).

In six studies, VNS appears effective for patients with LGS (105–110) The three earlier studies reported that a total of 13 of 18 (72%) patients with LGS experienced at least 50% reduction in seizure frequency with follow-up as long as 5 years (105–107). Hosain et al (108) reported on the use of VNS in 13 patients with LGS (age range, 4–44 years; mean, 16.7 years). During the first 6 months of treatment the median seizure rate reduction was 52% (range, 0–93%; $P = 0.04$). At 6 months of follow-up, three patients had >90% reduction in seizure frequency, two patients had >75% reduction, one patient had >50% reduction, six had >25% reduction, and one patient did not improve. The main reported side effects were hoarseness, coughing, and pain in throat. These results suggest VNS could be an effective and safe adjunct therapy for the treatment of LGS (108). Aldenkamp and collaborators in the Netherlands studied the long-term effects of 24 months of treatment with VNS on cognition in 19 patients with LGS or LGS-like syndromes (13 patients with LGS). The average reduction of seizure frequency was 20.6% after 24 months. No deterioration on cognition was seen when baseline was compared to follow-up measurements. The authors concluded that VNS does not have long-term, higher-order functions adverse effects (109). A previous report from the same group reported on the cost-effectiveness of VNS in 16 children with LGS at the 6-month follow-up. There was a significant reduction in direct non-health-care costs and the number of days of suboptimal functioning of the child. Comparing the costs pre and post VNS placement, the payback period was 2.3 years (110). In the largest cohort of LGS patients treated with VNS, Frost et al reported the effectiveness, tolerability, and safety of VNS therapy in 50 patients (median age, 13 years) with LGS. At 6 months after VNS implantation, 58% median reduction in seizure frequency was seen. Quality of life was improved in some patients and the most common adverse effects were voice change and coughing during stimulation (111).

In rare cases, resection of a localized lesion (e.g., vascular lesion or tumor) can improve seizure control in patients with LGS (38, 112).

Effective Treatments Based on Double-Blind Placebo-Controlled Studies

Medications

The gold standard for evaluation of the safety and efficacy of an anticonvulsant medication is the randomized, double-blind, placebo-controlled clinical trial. Six drugs have undergone this rigorous testing to determine safety and efficacy in patients with LGS: cinromide, IVIG, felbamate, lamotrigine, topiramate, and rufinamide. The latter four AEDs successfully demonstrated efficacy against seizures in patients with LGS, whereas the former two did not. Despite the lack of proven efficacy for cinromide and immunoglobulins in double-blind studies, both therapies had open-label trials suggesting efficacy in patients with LGS, reinforcing the need for randomized double-blind controlled trials to definitively establish the efficacy of any proposed therapy.

Cinromide. In 1980 cinromide was reported to be effective for seizures associated with LGS in an open-label uncontrolled trial (113). These results prompted a subsequent double-blind, placebo-controlled adjunctive therapy trial of cinromide in patients with LGS (114). Overall, 73 patients enrolled, but "sufficient data for analysis" were available only for 56 patients (26 receiving cinromide, 30 receiving placebo). There was no difference between cinromide adjunctive therapy and placebo adjunctive therapy in terms of seizure reduction or global evaluations (114). The development of cinromide was halted in 1981 (114).

Immunoglobulins. Two blinded placebo-controlled studies have been published examining the efficacy of IVIG in children with LGS (79, 80). The first study enrolled 10 children, aged 4 to 14 years, in an add-on, placebo-controlled, single-blind study design. Only 2 children showed a response to IVIG (42% and 100% decrease in seizure frequency), and the remaining 8 children were "unaffected" (79). Sixty-one patients with various forms of refractory epilepsy (including LGS and West syndrome) participated in a randomized, double-blind, placebo-controlled, dose-ranging (three different doses) trial of IVIG. Despite 52.5% of the IVIG group having a greater than 50% reduction in seizure frequency, compared with 27.8% in the placebo group, this difference did not reach statistical significance (80).

Felbamate. Felbamate (FBM) was found to be safe and effective in patients with LGS in a randomized, double-blind, placebo-controlled adjunctive therapy trial (115). Seventy-three patients with LGS aged 4 to 36 years enrolled. The FBM dose in the double-blind portion was 45 mg/kg/day (maximum 3,600 mg/day). The FBM treatment group experienced a 34% reduction in atonic seizures compared with 9% in the placebo group ($P < 0.01$). Total seizure frequency dropped 19% in the FBM group compared with a 4% increase in the placebo group ($P < 0.002$). The percentage of patients experiencing at least 50% reduction in atonic seizures was 57% for the FBM group compared with 9% in the placebo group ($P < 0.001$). The percentage of patients experiencing at least 50% reduction in total seizure frequency was 50% for the FBM group compared with 11% in the placebo group ($P < 0.001$) (Table 21-2). FBM was significantly better than placebo in improving global evaluation scores. The types and frequency of side effects were similar in the two treatment groups (107). A 12-month follow-up in patients who completed the controlled part of the study confirmed long-term efficacy (116).

Unfortunately, FBM is associated with dangerous idiosyncratic reactions involving the blood and liver. The most common severe FBM-associated idiosyncratic reaction is aplastic anemia, which has been seen to date in 34 patients receiving FBM (117, 118). The incidence of FBM-associated aplastic anemia is approximately 127 cases per million treated with FBM (approximately 1 in 4,000 to 8,000 FBM-treated patients) versus 2 to 6 per million people in the general population (87, 117, 119, 120). Another report estimates the risk of aplastic anemia in patients receiving FBM to be 1:3,000, with a death rate of 1 in 10,000 FBM-treated patients (87, 121). In perspective, this estimated risk is approximately 20 times greater than that for carbamazepine-associated aplastic anemia (117). Risk factors for FBM-associated aplastic anemia are Caucasian, adult, female, history of autoimmune disorder, a positive antinuclear antibody titer, history of prior AED toxicity or allergy, prior cytopenia, and treatment with FBM for less than 1 year (117, 118, 122).

The second most common severe FBM-associated idiosyncratic reaction is hepatotoxicity. Reported in 18 patients receiving FBM, its estimated incidence is between 64 and 164 per million (approximately 1 in 18,500–25,000 FBM-treated patients) (117). This suggests that the frequency of FBM-associated hepatotoxicity and VPA-associated hepatotoxicity are approximately the same (117). Based on the reported 5 felbamate-related liver failure fatalities, which occurred in approximately 130,000 to 170,000 exposed persons, the estimated incidence would be between 1 per 26,000 to 1 per 34,000 exposures (103). In perspective, the risk of hepatic-related fatalities in the population taking VPA is between 1 in 10,000 and 1 in 49,000, with the risk in high-risk pediatric patients younger than 2 years being 1 in 500 (118). There is no evidence that laboratory monitoring of blood counts and liver function during FBM therapy anticipates these severe idiosyncratic reactions

TABLE 21-2

Responder Rates (at Least 50% Reduction in Seizure Frequency) for Four Antiepileptic Medications Tested in Double-Blind, Placebo-Controlled Trials in Lennox-Gastaut Syndrome

Seizure Type	Felbamate vs. Placebo	Lamotrigine vs. Placebo	Topiramate vs. Placebo	Rufinamide vs. Placebo
Total seizures	50% vs. 11%*			
All major seizures (drop attacks plus tonic-clonic)		33% vs.16%*	33% vs. 8%*	
Drop attack or atonic seizures	57% vs. 9%*	37 vs. 22%*	28% vs. 14%	42% vs. 17%*
Tonic-clonic seizures	60% vs. 23%*	43% vs. 20%*		

*$P < 0.05$.

(117). A suggested management strategy is to use careful clinical monitoring, perform routine laboratory testing, and discontinue the drug if no substantial clinical benefit is observed after 3 to 6 months of therapy.

Although effective, there are significant risks associated with FBM use. In general, it is regarded as a good third-line or fourth-line drug for LGS.

Lamotrigine. The efficacy of lamotrigine (LTG) against seizures associated with LGS has been examined in multiple open-label studies and two controlled trials. In five open-label trials of LTG in patients with LGS, 58% (31 of 53) experienced at least 50% reduction in seizure frequency (123–127). A double-blind, placebo-controlled, crossover study of LTG as adjunctive therapy in 30 patients with treatment-resistant generalized epilepsy was reported in 1998. Twenty study patients had LGS. Seven of the 20 children with LGS responded to LTG therapy with a greater than 50% reduction in seizure frequency. Two patients became seizure-free (128).

Lamotrigine was found to be safe and effective in patients with LGS in a randomized, double-blind, placebo-controlled, adjunctive therapy trial (129). A total of 169 patients enrolled and were randomized to either LTG ($n = 79$) or placebo ($n = 90$) adjunctive therapy. Patients receiving the LTG treatment arm had a greater median percent reduction from baseline in weekly seizure counts (for drop attacks, tonic-clonic seizures, and all major seizures —defined as drop attacks plus tonic clonic seizures) compared with patients on the placebo treatment arm. The responder rate (percentage of patients experiencing at least 50% reduction in seizures) for major seizures (drop attacks and tonic-clonic seizures) was greater in the LTG group (33%) than in the placebo group (16%, $P < 0.01$). For drop attacks, 37% of LTG-treated patients responded, compared with 22% of the placebo-treated patients ($P < 0.04$). Finally, for tonic-clonic seizures, 43% of the LTG-treated patients responded, compared with 20% of patients receiving placebo ($P < 0.007$) (129) (Table 21-2).

Unfortunately, LTG can be associated with idiosyncratic reactions, predominantly involving the skin. The most common skin manifestation is a rash affecting 10% to 12% of LTG patients (130–132). The rash rapidly resolves following LTG withdrawal; sometimes the rash may even resolve without changing LTG dosage (133). However, this dermatologic reaction can progress in some patients to erythema multiforme, Stevens-Johnson syndrome, or even toxic epidermal necrolysis (87, 130, 133). Stevens-Johnson syndrome and toxic epidermal necrolysis are related severe mucocutaneous disorders with mortality rates of 5% and 30%, respectively (130). The risk of a potentially life-threatening rash (based on clinical trials and postmarketing reports) in adults is 0.3% and approximately 1% in children 16 years old and younger (133).

Risk factors for LTG-associated severe dermatologic reactions include younger age (children more than adults), comedication with VPA, a rapid rate of LTG titration, and a high LTG starting dose (87, 133, 134). Careful attention should be given to initial LTG starting dose, titration rate, and comedications. The prompt evaluation of any rash is prudent.

Despite the risk of idiosyncratic reactions, LTG is a very valuable medication for patients with LGS and should be considered for use as soon as the diagnosis of LGS is made. Proper attention to concomitant medications, a low starting dose, and a very slow titration can minimize the risk of dermatologic idiosyncratic reactions.

Topiramate. Topiramate (TPM) was found to be safe and effective as adjunctive therapy for patients with LGS in a multicenter, double-blind, placebo-controlled trial (135). Ninety-eight patients with LGS (older than 1 year and younger than 30 years) were randomized to either TPM adjunctive therapy (target dose, 6 mg/kg/day) or placebo adjunctive therapy. The median percent reduction from baseline in average monthly seizure rate for drop attacks was 14.8% for the TPM group and 5.1% (an increase) for the placebo group ($P < 0.041$). Using parental global evaluations, TPM-treated patients demonstrated greater improvement in seizure severity than did placebo-treated patients ($P < 0.037$). The responder rate for major seizures (drop attacks and tonic-clonic seizures) was greater in the TPM group (15 of 46, or 33%) than in the control group (4 of 50, or 8%; $P < 0.002$). The responder rate for drop attacks in the TPM group was higher than in the placebo group (28% vs. 14%) but did not reach statistical significance (135) (Table 21-2).

In the long-term, open-label extension portion of the above trial, 97 patients were followed up and had their TPM dose adjusted as clinically indicated (136). The mean TPM dose in those patients who had completed 6 months of therapy was 10 mg/kg/day. For those patients who had completed 6 months of TPM therapy, drop attacks were reduced at least 50% in 55% of patients; 15% of patients were free of drop attacks for at least 6 months at the last visit. The median percent reduction in drop attacks was 56%. The median percent reduction in overall seizure frequency was 44%, with 45% of the patients having at least 50% reduction in all seizure types and 2% being seizure-free for the previous 6 months. Long-term TPM therapy was well tolerated. The most common adverse events were somnolence, injury, and anorexia. Behavioral problems during the last 6 months of long-term TPM therapy were reported in only 5% of the patients. During long-term therapy, TPM is effective and well tolerated in controlling drop attacks and seizures associated with LGS (136).

Rufinamide. The efficacy and tolerability of rufinamide adjunctive therapy for patients with LGS was examined in a multicenter, double-blind, placebo-controlled, randomized, parallel-group study (137, 138). A 28-day baseline phase was followed by an 84-day double-blind phase (14-day titration phase followed by a 70-day maintenance phase). Eligible patients were between 4 and 30 years old, had 90 seizures in the month prior to the baseline phase, and were taking one to three concomitant AEDs. The rufinamide target dose was 45 mg/kg/day. Overall, 138 patients with a mean age of 14.1 years (range, 4 to 37 years) were randomized to either rufinamide ($n = 74$) or placebo ($n = 64$). The median dose in both groups was 1,800 mg/day (42–45 mg/kg/day) (137, 138).

The median percent reduction in total seizure frequency per 28 days, relative to the baseline phase, in the rufinamide group was significantly higher than in the placebo group (32.7% vs. 11.7%, $P = 0.0015$). In the rufinamide group, the median percent reduction in tonic-atonic seizure frequency per 28 days, relative to the baseline phase, was significantly higher compared with the placebo group (42.5% vs. 1.4%, $P < 0.0001$). The tonic-atonic seizure responder rate was significantly higher in the rufinamide group compared with the placebo group (42.5% vs. 16.7%, $P = 0.0020$) (137, 138).

The most common adverse events experienced included somnolence (24.3% rufinamide, 12.5% placebo), vomiting (21.6% rufinamide, 6.3% placebo), pyrexia (13.5% rufinamide, 17.2% placebo), and diarrhea (5.4% rufinamide, 10.9% placebo). A lower percentage of patients in the rufinamide group (17.6%) experienced cognitive/psychiatric adverse events of interest, such as psychomotor hyperactivity and lethargy, compared with the placebo group (23.4%). Rufinamide was efficacious and well tolerated as an adjunctive therapy for the treatment of resistant seizures in patients with LGS (137, 138).

Dietary Treatment

In a recent study, Freeman and collaborators reported in abstract form their findings of a blinded, crossover, placebo-controlled trial. Twenty children with LGS were fasted for 36 hours and introduced to the ketogenic diet. Glucose or saccharin was randomly used in a blinded fashion to negate or sustain the effect of the diet. Although the initial fasting to start the ketogenic diet resulted in a significant reduction in median seizures (30 to 10 seizures per day, $P < 0.0001$), the randomized part of the study failed to show a significant effect of ketogenic diet on seizure frequency (139). In a preliminary study, these investigators were able to negate urinary ketosis in patients on the ketogenic diet by giving a drink containing glucose (85). However, in the more recent study, none of the patients in the placebo arm, the ones who received glucose, was completely ketone free (139).

Surgical Treatment

There are no double-blind trials examining the efficacy of surgical intervention in patients with LGS, completed or under way, at this time.

PROGNOSIS

The long-term prognosis is variable, but overall it is unfavorable. Several studies have followed cohorts of children with LGS over time and illustrate this unevenness. Beaumanoir found that 47% of the patients with LGS still had typical characteristics after 10 years of follow-up (33). Roger et al followed 338 patients with LGS until adulthood. In 46.9% of patients, the clinical characteristics and EEG findings persisted into adulthood. In 15.5% of patients, mainly symptomatic cases, the syndrome disappeared, but a severe, multifocal epilepsy persisted. About 17% of patients in which LGS followed another type of epilepsy seemed to have been cured (140). Ohtahara et al reported persistent seizures in 76.4% of patients, and mental retardation present in 91% of patients with LGS in a long-term follow-up study (141). Yagi examined a cohort of 102 patients with LGS, followed up for an average of 16 years; 11.8% of them worked normally, 35.3% worked part-time or at a sheltered workshop, and the remaining 52.9% were under home care or institutionalized (142). The characteristic clinical symptoms and EEG pattern remained in one-third of the patients at the end of the study. In the remaining patients, seizures decreased in type and frequency with treatment (142). In another long-term follow-up of patients with LGS over 42 years, the disappearance of the characteristic slow spike-waves pattern was followed by focal discharges, and focal and diffuse slow waves, which were seen in the majority of patients. Complex partial seizures also became more frequent in this population (143). Hoffman-Riem et al identified by multivariate analysis four independent risk factors for severe mental retardation in patients with LGS: nonconvulsive status epilepticus, odds ratio (OR) 25.2, previous history of West syndrome (OR 11.6), a symptomatic etiology (OR 9.5), and an early age (before age 3 years) at onset of epilepsy (OR 4.7) (41). Long-term follow-up of patients with LGS reveals that only few of them will become seizure free (20, 123). Many authors consider that early and effective seizure treatment might prevent some of the long-term impairments and improve global prognosis (43, 144). However, patients that achieve seizure control and are seizure free for several years may continue to have severe cognitive impairments (51). One hypothesis proposes that this could be due to a genetic predisposition responsible for the mental retardation. Another theory suggests that the treatment may come too late in the course of the disease, at a time when the damage has already occurred.

A worse prognosis is associated with symptomatic LGS, particularly those with a prior history of West syndrome (37), early onset of seizures (37), higher frequency of seizures (18), or constant slow EEG background activity (35). In one report, tonic seizures became more difficult to control over time and persisted (97.8% of the patients), whereas myoclonic and atypical absences appeared easier to control, persisting in 22.5% and 39.3% of the patients, respectively (145). The characteristic diffuse slow spike-and-wave pattern of LGS gradually disappears with age and is replaced by focal epileptic discharges, especially multiple independent spikes. This may reflect that subcortical epileptic discharges are suppressed and focal cortical discharges gain preponderance with brain maturation (37). Mortality has been reported to range from 3% (mean follow-up of 8.5 years) to 7% (mean follow-up of 9.7 years) (35).

The severity of the seizures, frequent injuries, developmental delays, and behavioral problems take a large toll on even the strongest parents and family structures. Attention must be paid to the psychosocial needs of the family (especially siblings). The proper educational setting is also important to help the patients with LGS reach their maximal potential. Because of the high rate of injuries associated with atonic/tonic seizures, some patients with LGS may need to wear a protective helmet. Helmets need to have a faceguard to maximize protection of the patient's forehead, nose, and teeth. Unfortunately, some patients will not tolerate a helmet with a faceguard, and even if tolerated, helmets are often uncomfortable and rarely "cosmetically acceptable" (38).

References

1. Ohtahara S, Ohtsuka Y, Yamatogi Y, Oka E, et al. Prenatal etiologies of West syndrome. *Epilepsia* 1993; 34(4):716–722.
2. Gastaut H. The Lennox-Gastaut syndrome: comments on the syndrome's terminology and nosological position amongst the secondary generalized epilepsies of childhood. *Electroencephalography and Clinical Neurophysiology Supplement* 1982; 35:71–84.
3. Gibbs FA, Davis H, Lennox WG. Electroencephalogram in epilepsy and in conditions of impaired consciousness. *Archives of Neurological Psychiatry* 1935; 34:1133–48.
4. Gibbs F, Gibbs E, Lennox W. Influence of blood sugar level on wave and spike formation in petit mal epilepsy. *AMA Archives of Neurology and Psychiatry* 1939; 41:1111.
5. Lennox W. The petit mal epilepsies: their treatment with tridione. *JAMA* 1945; 129: 1069–1074.
6. Lennox WG, Davis JP. Clinical correlates of the fast and the slow spike-wave electroencephalogram. *Pediatrics* 1950; 5:626–644.
7. Lennox W. Epilepsy and related disorders. Boston, Toronto: Little, Brown, 1960.
8. Doose H. Das akinetische Petit Mal. *Arch Psychiatr Nervenkr* 1964; 205:625–654.
9. Sorel L. L'epilepsie myokinetique grave de la premiere enfance avec pointe-onde lente (petit mal variant) et son traitement. *Rev Neurol* 1964; 110:215–33.
10. Dravet C. Encephalopathie epileptique de l'enfant avec pointe-onde lente diffuse. Marseille: Thèse, 1965.
11. Bernard R, Pinsard N, Draver C, Gastaut H, et al. Aspets diagnostiquest et evolutifs d'ume encephalopathie epileptique de l'enfant avec pointe-ondes lents diffues. *Pediatrie* 1966; 21:712–30.
12. Gastaut H, Roger J, Soulayrol R, Tassinari C, et al. Childhood epileptic encephalopathy with diffuse slow spike-waves (otherwise known as "petit mal variant") or Lennox syndrome. *Epilepsia* 1966; 7(2):139–179.
13. Commission on Classification and Terminology of the International League Against Epilepsy. Proposal for revised classification of epilepsies and epileptic syndromes. *Epilepsia* 1989; 30(4):389–399.
14. Beaumanoir A, Blume W. The Lennox-Gastaut syndrome. In: Roger J, Bureau M, Dravet C, Genton P, et al, eds. *Epileptic Syndromes in Infancy, Childhood and Adolescence*. 4th ed. Montrouge, France: John Libbey Eurotext, 2005:125–148.
15. Farrell K. Classifying epileptic syndromes: problems and a neurobiologic solution. *Neurology* 1993; 43 11 Suppl 5:S8–S11.
16. Aicardi J. Epileptic syndromes in childhood. *Epilepsia* 1988; 29 Suppl 3:S1–S5.
17. Livingston JH. The Lennox-Gastaut syndrome. *Dev Med Child Neurol* 1988; 30(4): 536–540.
18. Dulac O, N'Guyen T. The Lennox-Gastaut syndrome. *Epilepsia* 1993; 34 Suppl 7: S7–S17.
19. Ohtahara S. Lennox-Gastaut syndrome. Considerations in its concept and categorization. *Jpn J Psychiatry Neurol* 1988; 42(3):535–542.
20. Oguni H, Hayashi K, Osawa M. Long-term prognosis of Lennox-Gastaut syndrome. *Epilepsia* 1996; 37 Suppl 3:44–47.
21. Trevathan E, Murphy CC, Yeargin-Allsopp M. Prevalence and descriptive epidemiology of Lennox-Gastaut syndrome among Atlanta children. *Epilepsia* 1997; 38(12): 1283–1288.
22. Yaqub BA. Electroclinical seizures in Lennox-Gastaut syndrome. *Epilepsia* 1993; 34(1):120–127.
23. Engel J Jr. A proposed diagnostic scheme for people with epileptic seizures and with epilepsy: report of the ILAE Task Force on Classification and Terminology. *Epilepsia* 2001; 42(6):796–803.
24. Hauser WA. The prevalence and incidence of convulsive disorders in children. *Epilepsia* 1994; 35 Suppl 2:S1–S6.
25. Kramer U, Nevo Y, Neufeld MY, Fatal A, et al. Epidemiology of epilepsy in childhood: a cohort of 440 consecutive patients. *Pediatr Neurol* 1998; 18(1):46–50.
26. Prats JM, Garaizar C. [Etiology of epilepsy in adolescents]. *Rev Neurol* 1999; 28(1):32–35.
27. Beilmann A, Talvik T. Is the International League against Epilepsy classification of epileptic syndromes applicable to children in Estonia? [In Process Citation]. *Eur J Paediatr Neurol* 1999; 3(6):265–272.
28. Cavazzuti GB. Epidemiology of different types of epilepsy in school age children of Modena, Italy. *Epilepsia* 1980; 21(1):57–62.
29. Steffenburg U, Hedstrom A, Lindroth A, Wiklund LM, et al. Intractable epilepsy in a population-based series of mentally retarded children. *Epilepsia* 1998; 39(7): 767–775.
30. Heiskala H. Community-based study of Lennox-Gastaut syndrome. *Epilepsia* 1997; 38(5):526–531.
31. Rantala H, Putkonen T. Occurrence, outcome, and prognostic factors of infantile spasms and Lennox-Gastaut syndrome. *Epilepsia* 1999; 40(3):286–289.
32. Beilmann A, Napa A, Soot A, Talvik I, et al. Prevalence of childhood epilepsy in Estonia. *Epilepsia* 1999; 40(7):1011–1019.
33. Beaumanoir A. The Lennox-Gastaut syndrome: a personal study. *Electroencephalography and Clinical Neurophysiology Supplement* 1982; 35:85–99.
34. Mariani E, Ferini-Strambi L, Sala M, Erminio C, et al. Epilepsy in institutionalized patients with encephalopathy: clinical aspects and nosological considerations. *Am J Ment Retard* 1993; 98 Suppl:27–33.
35. Roger J, Dravet C, Bureau M. The Lennox-Gastaut syndrome. *Cleve Clin J Med* 1989; 56 Suppl Pt 2:S172–S180.
36. Chevrie JJ, Aicardi J. Childhood epileptic encephalopathy with slow spike-wave. A statistical study of 80 cases. *Epilepsia* 1972; 13(2):259–271.
37. Ohtsuka Y, Amano R, Mizukawa M, Ohtahara S. Long-term prognosis of the Lennox-Gastaut syndrome. *Jpn J Psychiatry Neurol* 1990; 44(2):257–264.
38. Aicardi J. Epilepsy in children. 2nd ed. New York: Raven Press, 1994.
39. Markand ON. Slow spike-wave activity in EEG and associated clinical features: often called "Lennox" or "Lennox-Gastaut" syndrome. *Neurology* 1977; 27(8): 746–757.
40. Goldsmith IL, Zupanc ML, Buchhalter JR. Long-term seizure outcome in 74 patients with Lennox-Gastaut syndrome: effects of incorporating MRI head imaging in defining the cryptogenic subgroup. *Epilepsia* 2000; 41(4):395–399.
41. Hoffmann-Riem M, Diener W, Benninger C, Rating D, et al. Nonconvulsive status epilepticus—a possible cause of mental retardation in patients with Lennox-Gastaut syndrome. *Neuropediatrics* 2000; 31(4):169–174.
42. Kaminska A, Ickowicz A, Plouin P, Bru MF, et al. Delineation of cryptogenic Lennox-Gastaut syndrome and myoclonic astatic epilepsy using multiple correspondence analysis. *Epilepsy Res* 1999; 36(1):15–29.
43. Besag FM. Cognitive and behavioral outcomes of epileptic syndromes: implications for education and clinical practice. *Epilepsia* 2006; 47 Suppl 2:119–125.
44. Bare MA, Glauser TA, Strawsburg RH. Need for electroencephalogram video confirmation of atypical absence seizures in children with Lennox-Gastaut syndrome. *J Child Neurol* 1998; 13(10):498–500.
45. Ikeno T, Shigematsu H, Miyakoshi M, Ohba A, et al. An analytic study of epileptic falls. *Epilepsia* 1985; 26(6):612–621.

46. Donat JF, Wright FS. Seizures in series: similarities between seizures of the West and Lennox-Gastaut syndromes. *Epilepsia* 1991; 32(4):504–509.
47. Bonanni P, Parmeggiani L, Guerrini R. Different neurophysiologic patterns of myoclonus characterize Lennox-Gastaut syndrome and myoclonic astatic epilepsy. *Epilepsia* 2002; 43(6):609–615.
48. Smeraldi E, Scorza Smeraldi R, Cazzullo CL, Guareschi Cazzullo A, et al. Immunogenetics of the Lennox-Gastaut syndrome: frequency of HL-A antigens and haplotypes in patients and first-degree relatives. *Epilepsia* 1975; 16(5):699–703.
49. van Engelen BG, de Waal LP, Weemaes CM, Renier WO. Serologic HLA typing in cryptogenic Lennox-Gastaut syndrome. *Epilepsy Res.* 1994; 17(1):43–47.
50. Blume WT. Lennox-Gastaut syndrome: potential mechanisms of cognitive regression. *Ment Retard Dev Disabil Res Rev* 2004; 10(2):150–153.
51. Filippini M, Boni A, Dazzani G, Guerra A, et al. Neuropsychological findings: myoclonic astatic epilepsy (MAE) and Lennox-Gastaut syndrome (LGS). *Epilepsia* 2006; 47 Suppl 2:56–59.
52. Gur RC, Sussman NM, Alavi A, Gur RE, et al. Positron emission tomography in two cases of childhood epileptic encephalopathy (Lennox-Gastaut syndrome). *Neurology* 1982; 32(10):1191–1194.
53. Iinuma K, Yanai K, Yanagisawa T, Fueki N, et al. Cerebral glucose metabolism in five patients with Lennox-Gastaut syndrome. *Pediatr Neurol* 1987; 3(1):12–18.
54. Ferrie CD, Maisey M, Cox T, Polkey C, et al. Focal abnormalities detected by 18FDG PET in epileptic encephalopathies. *Arch Dis Child* 1996; 75(2):102–107.
55. Theodore WH, Rose D, Patronas N, Sato S, et al. Cerebral glucose metabolism in the Lennox-Gastaut syndrome. *Ann Neurol* 1987; 21(1):14–21.
56. Chugani HT, Mazziotta JC, Engel J Jr, Phelps ME. The Lennox-Gastaut syndrome: metabolic subtypes determined by 2-deoxy- 2[^{18}F]fluoro-D-glucose positron emission tomography. *Ann Neurol* 1987; 21(1):4–13.
57. Miyauchi T, Nomura Y, Ohno S, Kishimoto H, et al. Positron emission tomography in three cases of Lennox-Gastaut syndrome. *Jpn J Psychiatry Neurol* 1988; 42(4): 795-804.
58. Heiskala H, Launes J, Pihko H, Nikkinen P, et al. Brain perfusion SPECT in children with frequent fits. *Brain Dev* 1993; 15(3):214–218.
59. Mattson RH. Efficacy and adverse effects of established and new antiepileptic drugs. *Epilepsia* 1995; 36 Suppl 2:S13–S26.
60. Farrell K, Tatum W. Encephalopathic generalized epilepsy and Lennox-Gastaut syndrome. In: Wyllie E, ed. *The Treatment of Epilepsy: Principles and Practice.* Philadelphia, PA: Lippincott Wilkins & Williams, 2006:429–440.
61. Wheless JW, Constantinou JEC. Lennox-Gastaut syndrome. *Pediatr Neurol* 1997; 17(3):203–211.
62. Gastaut H, Lowe M. Antiepileptic properties of clobazam, a 1.5 benzodiazepine, in man. *Epilepsia* 1979; 20:437–446.
63. Snead OC, Saito M. Encephalopathic epilepsy after infancy. In: Dodson WE, Pellock JM, eds. *Pediatric Epilepsy: Diagnosis and Therapy*. New York: Demos Publications, 1993:147–156.
64. Sher P. Alternate day clonazepam treatment of intractable seizures. *Arch Neurol* 1985; 42:787–788.
65. Bittencourt PR, Richens A. Anticonvulsant-induced status epilepticus in Lennox-Gastaut syndrome. *Epilepsia* 1981; 22(1):129–134.
66. DiMario FJ Jr, Clancy RR. Paradoxical precipitation of tonic seizures by lorazepam in a child with atypical absence seizures. *Pediatr Neurol* 1988; 4(4):249–251.
67. Snead O. Exacerbation of seizures in children by carbamazepine. *N Engl J Med* 1985; 323:916–921.
68. Horn CS, Ater SB, Hurst DL. Carbamazepine-exacerbated epilepsy in children and adolescents. *Pediatr Neurol* 1986; 2(6):340–345.
69. Erba G, Browne T. Atypical absence, myoclonic, atonic and tonic seizures and the "Lennox-Gastaut syndrome." In: Browne T, Feldman R, eds. *Epilepsy, Diagnosis and Management*. Boston: Little, Brown, 1983:75–94.
70. Zouhar A, Slapal R. [Administration of high doses of B6 in age-related epileptic encephalopathies]. *Cesk Neurol Neurochir* 1989; 52(1):28–31.
71. Bourgeois BFD. Antiepileptic drugs in pediatric practice. *Epilepsia* 1995; 36(2): S34–S45.
72. Brett E. The Lennox-Gastaut syndrome: therapeutic aspects. In: Niedermeyer E, Degen R, eds. *The Lennox-Gastaut Syndrome*. New York: Alan Liss, 1988:317–339.
73. Yamatogi Y, Ohtsuka Y, Ishida T, Ichiba N, et al. Treatment of the Lennox syndrome with ACTH: a clinical and electroencephalographic study. *Brain Dev* 1979; 1:267–276.
74. Snead O, Benton J, Myers C. ACTH and prednisone in childhood seizure disorders. *Neurology* 1983; 33:966–970.
75. Duse M, Notarangelo LD, Tiberti S, Menegati E, et al. Intravenous immune globulin in the treatment of intractable childhood epilepsy. *Clin Exp Immunol* 1996; 104 Suppl 1:71–76.
76. van Engelen BG, Renier WO, Weemaes CM, Strengers PF, et al. High-dose intravenous immunoglobulin treatment in cryptogenic West and Lennox-Gastaut syndrome; an add-on study. *Eur J Pediatr* 1994; 153(10):762–769.
77. Feucht M, Brantner-Inthaler S. Gamma-vinyl-GABA (vigabatrin) in the therapy of Lennox-Gastaut syndrome: an open study. *Epilepsia* 1994; 35(5):993–998.
78. Sakamoto K, Kurokawa T, Tomita S, Kitamoto I, et al. Effects of zonisamide on children with epilepsy. *Curr Ther Res* 1988; 43(3):378–383.
79. Illum N, Taudorf K, Heilmann C, Smith T, et al. Intravenous immunoglobulin: a single-blind trial in children with Lennox-Gastaut syndrome. *Neuropediatrics* 1990; 21(2):87–90.
80. van Rijckevorsel-Harmant K, Delire M, Schmitz-Moorman W, Wieser HG. Treatment of refractory epilepsy with intravenous immunoglobulins. Results of the first double-blind/dose finding clinical study. *Int J Clin Lab Res* 1994; 24(3):162–166.
81. Livingston J, Beaumont D, Arzimanoglou A. Vigabatrin in the treatment of epilepsy in children. *Br J Clin Pharmacol* 1989; 27:109S–112S.
82. Gibbs J, Appleton R, Rosenbloom L. Vigabatrin in intractable childhood epilepsy: a restrospective study. *Pediatr Neurol* 1992; 8:338–340.
83. Luna D, Dulac O, Pajot N. Vigabatrin in the treatment of childhood epilepsies. A single-blind placebo-controlled study. *Epilepsia* 1989; 30:430–437.
84. Fois A, Buoni S, Bartolo RD. Vigabatrin treatment in children. *Childs Nerv Syst* 1994; 10:244–248.
85. Maldonado C, Castello J, Fuentes E. Vigabatrin in the management of Lennox-Gastaut syndrome [abstract]. *Epilepsia* 1995; 36:S102.
86. Dulac O, Chiron C, Luna D, Cusmai R, et al. Vigabatrin in childhood epilepsy. *J Child Neurol* 1991; 2 Suppl:S30–S37.
87. Pellock JM. New antiepileptic drugs in pediatric epilepsy syndromes. *Pediatrics* 1999; 104 5 Pt 1:1106–1116.
88. Shields WD, Sankar R. Vigabatrin. *Semin Pediatr Neurol* 1997; 4(1):43–50.
89. Appleton RE. Vigabatrin in the management of generalized seizures in children. *Seizure* 1995; 4(1):45–48.
90. Sankar R, Wasterlain CG. Is the devil we know the lesser of two evils? Vigabatrin and visual fields. *Neurology* 1999; 52(8):1537–1538.
91. Yamatogi Y, Ohtahara S. Current topics of treatment. In: Ohtahara S, Roger J, eds. *Proceedings of the International Symposium, New Trends in Pediatric Epileptology.* Okayama, Japan: 1991:136–148.
92. Iinuma K, Haginoya K. Clinical efficacy of zonisamide in childhood epilepsy after long-term treatment: a postmarketing, multi-institutional survey. *Seizure* 2004; 13 Suppl 1: S34–S39; discussion S40.
93. Prusinski A, Stepien-Barcikowska A. A trial of using tryptophane in the treatment of Lennox-Gastaut syndrome. *Neurochir Polska* 1984; 18:287–289.
94. Slapal R, Zouhar A. [Therapeutic effect of dopaminergic substances in drug-resistant Lennox- Gastaut syndrome]. *Cesk Neurol Neurochir* 1989; 52(1):32–35.
95. Inanaga K, Kumashiro H, Fukuyama Y, Ohtahara S, et al. Clinical study of oral administration of DN-1417, a TRH analog, in patients with intractable epilepsy. *Epilepsia* 1989; 30(4):438–445.
96. Takeuchi Y, Takano T, Abe J, Takikita S, et al. Thyrotropin-releasing hormone: role in the treatment of West syndrome and related epileptic encephalopathies. *Brain Dev* 2001; 23(7):662–667.
97. Ros Perez P, Zamarron Cuesta I, Aparicio Meix M, Sastre Gallego A. [Evaluation of the effectiveness of the ketogenic diet with medium-chain triglycerides, in the treatment of refractory epilepsy in children. Apropos of a series of cases]. *An Esp Pediatr.* 1989; 30(3):155–158.
98. Wheless JW. The ketogenic diet: Fa(c)t or fiction. *J Child Neurol* 1995; 10(6):419–423.
99. Freeman JM, Vining EP. Seizures decrease rapidly after fasting: preliminary studies of the ketogenic diet. *Arch Pediatr Adolesc Med* 1999; 153(9):946–949.
100. Arzimanoglou A, Guerrini R, Aicardi J, eds. Epilepsy In Children. Third Edition ed. Philadelphia: Lippincott Wilkins & Williams; 2004. p. 38–50.
101. Velasco AL, Velasco F, Jimenez F, Velasco M, et al. Neuromodulation of the centromedian thalamic nuclei in the treatment of generalized seizures and the improvement of the quality of life in patients with Lennox-Gastaut syndrome. *Epilepsia* 2006; 47(7): 1203–1212.
102. Wheless J. Evaluation of children for epilepsy surgery. *Pediatr Ann* 1991; 20:41–49.
103. Baumgartner J, Clifton G, Wheless J. Corpus callostomy. *Tech Neurosurg* 1995; 1:45–51.
104. Kwan SY, Wong TT, Chang KP, Chi CS, et al. Seizure outcome after corpus callosotomy: the Taiwan experience. *Childs Nerv Syst* 2000; 16(2):87–92.
105. Hornig GW, Murphy JV, Schallert G, Tilton C. Left vagus nerve stimulation in children with refractory epilepsy: an update. *South Med J* 1997; 90(5):484–488.
106. Ben-Menachem E, Hellstrom K, Waldton C, Augustinsson LE. Evaluation of refractory epilepsy treated with vagus nerve stimulation for up to 5 years [see comments]. *Neurology* 1999; 52(6):1265–1267.
107. Lundgren J, Amark P, Blennow G, Stromblad LG, et al. Vagus nerve stimulation in 16 children with refractory epilepsy. *Epilepsia* 1998; 39(8):809–813.
108. Hosain S, Nikalov B, Harden C, Li M, et al. Vagus nerve stimulation treatment for Lennox-Gastaut syndrome. *J Child Neurol* 2000; 15(8):509–512.
109. Aldenkamp AP, Majoie HJ, Berfelo MW, Evers SM, et al. Long-term effects of 24-month treatment with vagus nerve stimulation on behaviour in children with Lennox-Gastaut syndrome. *Epilepsy Behav* 2002 Oct; 3(5):475–479.
110. Majoie HJ, Berfelo MW, Aldenkamp AP, Evers SM, et al. Vagus nerve stimulation in children with therapy-resistant epilepsy diagnosed as Lennox-Gastaut syndrome: clinical results, neuropsychological effects, and cost-effectiveness. *J Clin Neurophysiol* 2001; 18(5):419–428 (abstract).
111. Frost M, Gates J, Helmers SL, Wheless JW, et al. Vagus nerve stimulation in children with refractory seizures associated with Lennox-Gastaut syndrome. *Epilepsia* 2001; 42(9):1148–1152.
112. Angelini L, Broggi G, Riva D, Lazzaro Solero C. A case of Lennox-Gastaut syndrome successfully treated by removal of a parietotemporal astrocytoma. *Epilepsia* 1979; 20(6):665–669.
113. Lockman L, Rothner A, Erenberg G, Wright F, et al. Cinromide in the treatment of seizures in the Lennox-Gastaut syndrome. *Epilepsia* 1980; 22:241 (abstract).
114. Group for the Evaluation of Cinromide in the Lennox-Gastaut Syndrome. Double-blind, placebo-controlled evaluation of cinromide in patients with the Lennox-Gastaut syndrome. *Epilepsia* 1989; 30(4):422–429.
115. Ritter FJ. Efficacy of felbamate in childhood epileptic encephalopathy (Lennox-Gastaut syndrome). *N Engl J Med* 1993; 328:29–33.

116. Jensen PK. Felbamate in the treatment of Lennox-Gastaut syndrome. *Epilepsia* 1994; 35 Suppl 5:S54–S57.
117. Pellock JM. Felbamate. *Epilepsia* 1999; 40 Suppl 5:S57–S62.
118. Pellock JM, Faught E, Leppik IE, Shinnar S, et al. Felbamate: consensus of current clinical experience. *Epilepsy Res* 2006; 71(2–3):89–101.
119. Patton W, Duffull S. Idiosyncratic drug-induced haematological abnormalities. Incidence, pathogenesis, management and avoidance. *Drug Saf* 1994; 11(6): 445–462.
120. Kaufman DW, Kelly JP, Anderson T, Harmon DC, et al. Evaluation of case reports of aplastic anemia among patients treated with felbamate. *Epilepsia* 1997; 38(12):1265–1269.
121. Bourgeois BF. Felbamate [published erratum appears in *Semin Pediatr Neurol* 1998; 5(1):76]. *Semin Pediatr Neurol* 1997; 4(1):3–8.
122. Pellock JM, Brodie MJ. Felbamate: 1997 update. *Epilepsia* 1997; 38(12):1261–1264.
123. Donaldson JA, Glauser TA, Olberding LS. Lamotrigine adjunctive therapy in childhood epileptic encephalopathy (the Lennox Gastaut syndrome). *Epilepsia* 1997; 38(1):68–73.
124. Timmings PL, Richens A. Lamotrigine as an add-on drug in the management of Lennox-Gastaut syndrome. *Eur Neurol* 1992; 32(6):305–307.
125. Schlumberger E, Chavez F, Palacios L, Rey E, et al. Lamotrigine in treatment of 120 children with epilepsy. *Epilepsia* 1994; 35(2):359–367.
126. Uvebrant P, Bauziene R. Intractable epilepsy in children. The efficacy of lamotrigine treatment, including non-seizure related benefits. *Neuropediatrics* 1994; 25:284–289.
127. Buchanan N. Lamotrigine: Clinical experience in 93 patients with epilepsy. *Acta Neurol Scand* 1995; 92:28–32.
128. Eriksson AS, Nergardh A, Hoppu K. The efficacy of lamotrigine in children and adolescents with refractory generalized epilepsy: a randomized, double-blind, crossover study. *Epilepsia* 1998; 39(5):495–501.
129. Motte J, Trevathan E, Arvidsson JF, Barrera MN, et al. Lamotrigine for generalized seizures associated with the Lennox-Gastaut syndrome. *N Engl J Med* 1997; 337(25):1807–1812.
130. Pellock JM. Overview of lamotrigine and the new antiepileptic drugs: the challenge. *J Child Neurol* 1997; 12 Suppl 1:S48–S52.
131. Schlienger RG, Shapiro LE, Shear NH. Lamotrigine-induced severe cutaneous adverse reactions. *Epilepsia* 1998; 39 Suppl 7:S22–S26.
132. Pellock JM, Watemberg N. New antiepileptic drugs in children: present and future. *Semin Pediatr Neurol* 1997; 4(1):9–18.
133. Matsuo F. Lamotrigine. *Epilepsia* 1999; 40 Suppl 5:S30–36.
134. Pellock J. Overview of lamotrigine and the new antiepileptic drugs: the challenge. *J Child Neurol* 1997; 12:S48–S52.
135. Sachdeo RC, Glauser TA, Ritter F, Reife R, et al. A double-blind, randomized trial of topiramate in Lennox-Gastaut syndrome. *Neurology* 1999; 52(9):1882–1887.
136. Glauser TA, Levisohn PM, Ritter F, Sachdeo RC. Topiramate in Lennox-Gastaut syndrome: open-label treatment of patients completing a randomized controlled trial. Topiramate YL Study Group. *Epilepsia* 2000; 41 Suppl 1:S86–S90.
137. Glauser T, Kluger G, Krauss GL, Perdomo C, et al. Short term and long term efficacy and safety of rufinamide as adjunctive therapy in patients with inadequately controlled Lennox Gastaut syndrome. *Neurology* 2006; 66 Suppl 2:A36.
138. Glauser T, Kluger G, Sachdeo RC, Krauss GL, et al. Efficacy and safety of rufinamide adjunctive therapy in patients with Lennox–Gastaut Syndrome (LGS): a multicenter, randomized, double-blind, placebo-controlled, parallel trial. *Neurology* 2005; 64:1826 (abstract).
139. Freeman J, Vining E, Goodman S, Kossoff E,, et al. A blinded, crossover, placebo-controlled study of the effectiveness of the ketogenic diet (KJD). *Ann Neurol* 2006; 60 Suppl 10:S139 (abstract).
140. Roger J, Remy C, Bureau M, Oller-Daurella L, et al. [Lennox-Gastaut syndrome in the adult]. *Rev Neurol* 1987; 143(5):401–405.
141. Ohtahara S, Ohtsuka Y, Kobayashi K. Lennox-Gastaut syndrome: a new vista. *Psychiatry Clin Neurosci* 1995; 49(3):S179–S183.
142. Yagi K. Evolution of Lennox-Gastaut syndrome: a long-term longitudinal study. *Epilepsia* 1996; 37 Suppl 3:48–51.
143. Hughes JR, Patil VK. Long-term electro-clinical changes in the Lennox-Gastaut syndrome before, during, and after the slow spike-wave pattern. *Clin Electroencephalogr* 2002; 33(1):1–7.
144. van Rijckevorsel K. Cognitive problems related to epilepsy syndromes, especially malignant epilepsies. *Seizure* 2006; 15(4):227–234.
145. Ohtsuka Y, Ohmori I, Oka E. Long-term follow-up of childhood epilepsy associated with tuberous sclerosis. *Epilepsia* 1998; 39(11):1158–1163.

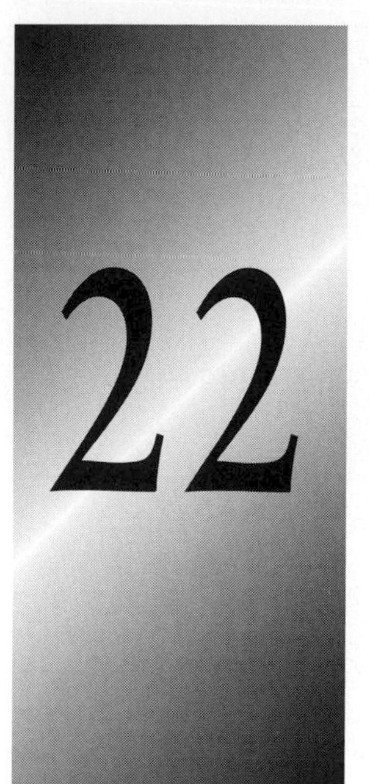

22 Childhood Absence Epilepsies

Phillip L. Pearl
Gregory L. Holmes

The absence seizure is characterized by sudden discontinuation of activity with loss of awareness, responsiveness, and memory, and an equally abrupt recovery. The first description of such an event was by Poupart in 1705 (1). The use of the term *petit mal* to describe all nonconvulsive seizures, proposed by Esquirol in 1815, has contributed to confusion that persists today. "Petit mal" was used to imply the severity of a seizure, more or less, before the electroencephalographic (EEG) description of 3-Hz spike-and-wave by Gibbs, Davis, and Lennox in 1935 (2). Clarification and delineation of absence seizure types was advanced by systematic neurophysiological studies using video-EEG monitoring techniques, which led to the description of protean manifestations and clinical syndromes associated with absence seizures.

Absence seizures are classified by the International League Against Epilepsy (ILAE) as generalized seizures among the self-limited seizure types. Those seizure types that conform to the absence seizure include several entities: typical absence seizures, atypical absence seizures, myoclonic absence seizures, and eyelid myoclonia with absences (Table 22–1). In addition, absence status epilepticus is classified as a type of generalized status epilepticus among the continuous seizure types.

The conceptualization of the epilepsy syndrome, comprising the predominant and associated seizure types associated with other clinical and electroencephalographic characteristics, was a major advance in understanding the patient's underlying condition and, further, to allow for optimal management. Most physicians use the term "petit mal epilepsy" or "childhood absence epilepsy" to describe a syndrome of simple absence seizures in school-age children who are otherwise neurologically and intellectually normal. Of the ILAE epilepsy syndromes, absence seizures are an important component in several entities that would fit the original operational definition of the idiopathic generalized epilepsies (IGE) (Table 22–2) (3): childhood absence epilepsy, epilepsy with myoclonic absences, epilepsy with myoclonic-astatic seizures, juvenile absence epilepsy, and juvenile myoclonic epilepsy (JME). Other proposed syndromes that feature absence seizures include Jeavons syndrome, perioral myoclonia with absences, and phantom absences. The latter two entities are lifelong and associated with absence status epilepticus. "Phantom absences" refers to a type of mild absence occurring before a first generalized tonic-clonic seizure that usually occurs in adulthood. Jeavons syndrome refers to a purely reflex IGE with eyelid myoclonia and EEG abnormalities on eye closure (4). The scope of this chapter encompasses childhood absence epilepsy,

TABLE 22–1
Classification of Absence Seizures (ILAE)

Self-limited seizure types
Generalized seizures
  Typical absence seizures
  Atypical absence seizures
  Myoclonic absence seizures
  Eyelid myoclonia with absences
Continuous seizure types
Generalized status epilepticus
  Absence status epilepticus

TABLE 22–2
Epilepsy Syndromes (ILAE) Featuring Absence Seizures

A. Childhood absence epilepsy
B. Epilepsy with myoclonic absences
C. Epilepsy with myoclonic-astatic seizures
D. Juvenile absence epilepsy
E. Juvenile myoclonic epilepsy

epilepsy with myoclonic absences, and eyelid myoclonia with absences.

EPIDEMIOLOGY

Absence seizures comprise 2% to 11% of seizure types in all ages (5–10). The prevalence is highest in the first decade (11, 12). The incidence is 9.6 per 100,000 in the age group 0 to 15 years (11). Sato and coworkers (13), in a study of 83 patients with absence seizures, reported the age of onset was most commonly in the 5- to 9-year-old group (versus 4 years or younger, or 10 years or older), whereas Wirrell and colleagues (14) found an average age of onset of 5.7 years in 72 children. Occasional cases begin during infancy (15). A population-based case control study found that only a history of febrile seizures was a significant risk factor for the development of absence seizures ($P < 0.01$) (16). None of the other factors studied were significant, including those that were historically suggested such as twin pregnancy, breech presentation, being firstborn, and perinatal asphyxia. A recent population based study in Sweden determined that the syndrome childhood absence epilepsy was diagnosed in 5.9% of children aged 1 month to 16 years with active epilepsy (17).

CLINICAL MANIFESTATIONS

The terms *typical absence seizure* (TAS) and *atypical absence seizure* (AAS) were used by the International Classification of Epileptic Seizures to delineate these two distinct types of absences (18). The simple typical absence seizure consists of the sudden onset of impaired consciousness, usually associated with a blank facial appearance without other motor or behavioral phenomena. This subtype is actually relatively rare and comprised only 9% of 374 absence seizures video recorded from 48 patients by Penry and associates (19). The complex typical absence seizure, alternatively, is accompanied by other motor, behavioral, or autonomic phenomena.

Clonic components may be quite subtle and most frequently consist of eye blinking. Clonic activity may range from nystagmus (20) to rapid jerking of the arms. Changes in tone may include a tonic postural contraction, leading to flexion or extension of the trunk (21). Decreases in tone leading to head nodding or dropping objects may also occur, although they rarely cause a fall.

In a study of 476 typical absence seizures monitored by simultaneous video-EEG telemetry, automatisms were the most common clinical accompaniment, occurring in 44% of 27 patients (22). Automatisms are semipurposeful behaviors of which the patient is unaware and which the patient subsequently cannot recall. They may be either perseverative, reflecting continuation of preictal activities, or de novo. Simple behaviors, such as rubbing the face or hands, licking the lips, chewing, grimacing, scratching, or fumbling with clothes tend to be de novo automatisms. Complex activity such as dealing cards, playing pattycake, or handling a toy are generally perseverative. If it occurs, speech is usually perseverative and often slowed and dysarthric, but it may be totally normal and include both expressive and receptive abilities (23).

Autonomic phenomena associated with absence seizures include pupil dilatation, pallor, flushing, sweating, salivation, piloerection, and even urinary incontinence (21, 24). Neither the autonomic changes nor the automatisms allow one to distinguish absence seizures from other seizure types.

Atypical absence seizures have traditionally been characterized as having less abrupt onset or cessation, more pronounced changes in tone, and longer duration than typical absence (18). They usually begin before 5 years of age and are associated with other generalized seizure types and mental retardation. The ictal EEG is more heterogeneous, showing 1.5- to 2.5-Hz slow spike-and-wave or multiple spike-and-wave discharges that may be irregular or asymmetrical (5, 6). The interictal EEG is usually abnormal, with slowing and multifocal epileptiform features (25).

Using the aforementioned ictal EEG criteria to differentiate atypical from typical absence seizures operationally, Holmes and coworkers (22) compared 426 typical and 500 atypical absence seizures in 54 children. The average duration of the AAS, 10.24 seconds, was longer than that of the TAS, 8.69 seconds ($P < 0.01$). A change in facial expression or appearance of a blank stare was the most common initial clinical manifestation in either type. A pause or slowing of motor activity was also frequently noted as the initial finding in either seizure type. Either diminished postural tone or tonic or myoclonic activity was significantly more likely to be the initial clinical feature in AAS than in TAS. A blank stare or change in facial expression was the sole clinical finding in only 16% of TAS and 28% of AAS. Automatisms, eye blinking, and lip smacking occurred more commonly in TAS. A change in postural tone, either an increase or a decrease, was more commonly seen in AAS. Automatisms were more common in TAS than in AAS and are usually perseverative, such as often playing with a toy or game. De novo automatisms were associated with longer spells and most commonly consisted of rubbing the face or hands in TAS and smiling in AAS.

In the study by Holmes and coworkers (22), the authors found that both TAS and AAS started abruptly without an aura, lasted from a few seconds to half a minute, and ended abruptly. Both were frequently associated with eye blinking, lip smacking, decrease in tone, and automatisms. Although statistically significant differences can be identified between TAS and AAS, there is considerable overlap between the two seizure types, and they more likely represent a clinical continuum. This overlap pertains to the EEG as well as the proposed pathophysiology.

Most patients with typical absence seizures have normal neurologic examinations. In two large studies, abnormalities were found in 23% of patients by Sato and associates (13) and 16% by Dalby (8). Neurologic abnormalities tend to be mild and nonprogressive.

Intelligence scores are more variable, largely attributable to the diverse patient populations. In patients with typical 3-Hz spike-and-wave discharges, Dalby (8) found 17% of patients had IQs below 90, whereas Sato and coworkers (13) found 52% had IQs below 90. Holmes et al (22) found 22% of 27 patients with typical absence seizures to be mentally retarded, whereas 93% of 27 patients with atypical absence were retarded.

Between 40% and 60% of patients with typical absence seizures have generalized tonic-clonic seizures (8, 11, 13, 26–29). The time from the first absence to the first generalized tonic-clonic seizure may range from 1 to 16 years (mean, 6.6 years) (29). Nearly all patients with atypical absence seizures have generalized tonic-clonic seizures, and many also have myoclonic, tonic, and atonic seizures. There appears to be a spectrum of clinical conditions associated with atypical absence seizures, so that children with exclusively atypical absence have a less severe educational disability than children with atypical absence seizures plus other seizure types (30).

The syndrome of childhood absence epilepsy, named pyknolepsy for the frequent clustering of seizures in a day (*pyknos* = "cluster" in Greek), is defined as a disorder of typical absence seizures with occurrence in school age, having peak manifestations during ages 6 to 7 years, with a strong genetic predisposition in otherwise normal children. It is seen more frequently in girls than in boys. The EEG demonstrates bilateral, synchronous, and symmetrical 3-Hz spike-wave paroxysms on a normal background. More recent attempts to fine-tune this definition, especially for research purposes, have provided stricter inclusion criteria (onset between 4 and 10 years, normal neurologic state and development, brief duration [4 to 20 seconds, exceptionally longer], and EEG ictal discharges with generalized high-amplitude spike) and exclusion criteria (other seizure types including generalized tonic-clonic seizures or myoclonic, eyelid myoclonia, perioral myoclonia, rhythmic massive limb jerking, single or arrhythmic myoclonic jerks, mild or no impairment of consciousness during the ictal discharge, brief EEG paroxysms < 4 seconds duration, multiple spikes [more than 3], and visual [i.e., photic] and other sensory precipitation of clinical seizures) (31). Such criteria remain under debate. For example, photosensitivity is well accepted by other authors in childhood absence epilepsy with typical absence seizures (32, 33). Eyelid myoclonia with absences (EMA) is characterized by eyelid myoclonia and absences provoked by eye closure and photosensitivity. This may be seen in idiopathic or symptomatic epilepsies (34).

EEG FEATURES

The EEG signature of a typical absence seizure is the sudden onset of 3-Hz generalized symmetrical spike- or multiple spike-and-slow-wave complexes (Figure 22–1). The voltage of the discharges is often maximal in the frontocentral regions. The frequency tends to be faster, about 4 Hz, at the onset and slows to 2 Hz toward the end of discharges longer than 10 seconds. The ictal discharges during an atypical absence seizure are more variable. They occur at frequencies between 1.5 and 2.5 Hz or may be faster than 2.5 Hz but are irregular or asymmetrical in voltage.

The interictal EEG background is generally normal in TAS and abnormal in AAS. Using the aforementioned ictal EEG criteria to classify absence seizures, Holmes and colleagues (22) found that only 44% of 27 patients with TAS had normal EEG backgrounds. Diffuse slowing was seen in 22%, paroxysmal spikes or sharp waves in 37%, and posterior rhythmic delta (less than 4 Hz) slowing in 15%. Conversely, only 11% of 27 patients with AAS had a normal interictal EEG. Diffuse slowing and focal or multifocal spikes or sharp waves were seen in 85%.

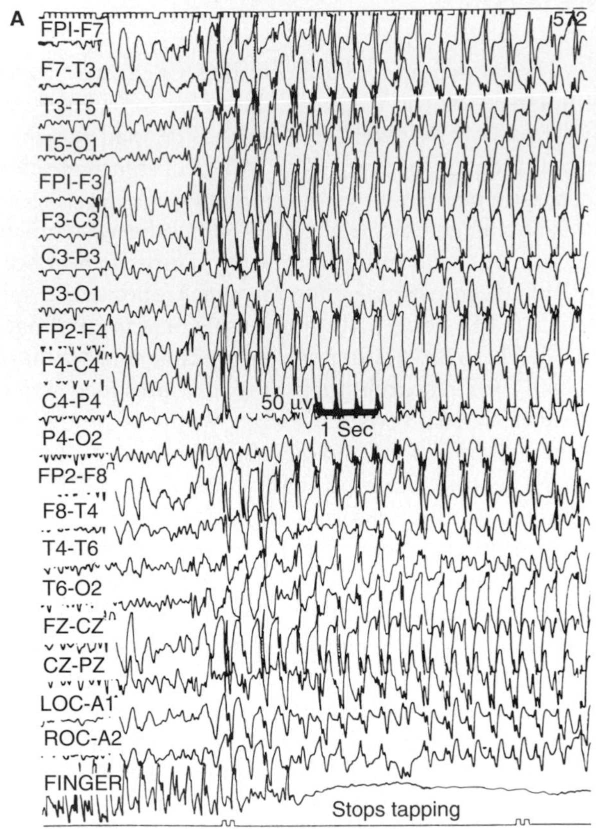

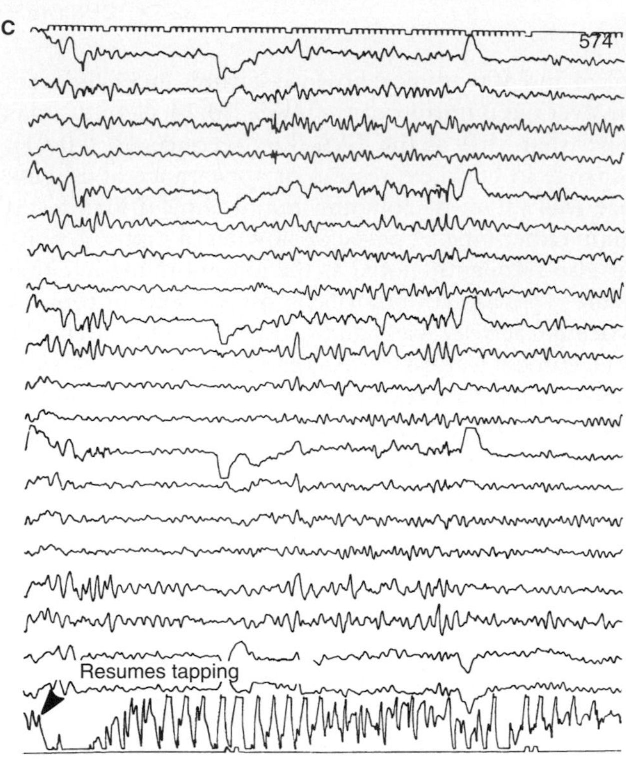

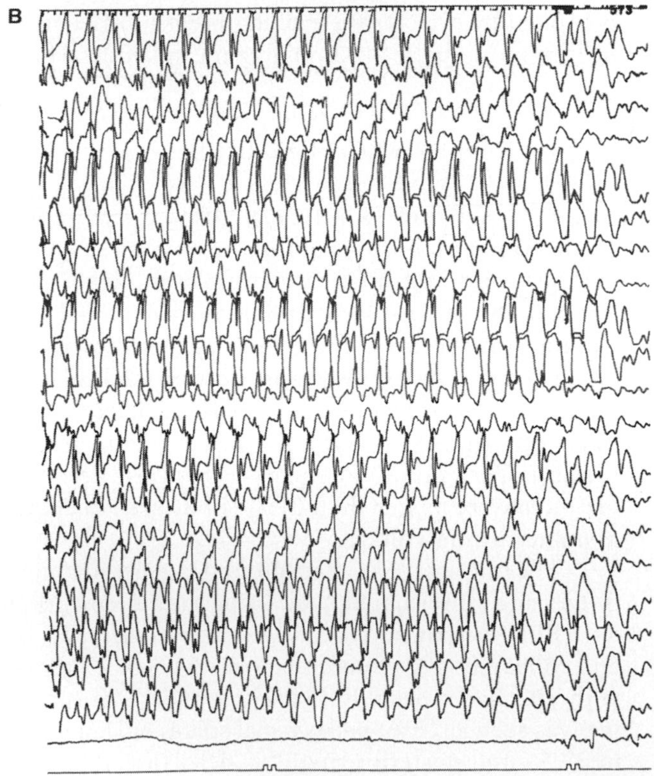

FIGURE 22–1

Typical 3-Hz generalized synchronous and symmetrical spike-and-wave EEG discharge during hyperventilation in an 8-year-old girl with pyknolepsy. Note the drop out of finger tapping 2 seconds into the paroxysm and return on cessation of the discharge.

The discharges are more numerous during all sleep states except rapid eye movement (REM) (35–37). The bursts have a modified appearance in sleep, as they may be briefer, less regular, and slower with a 1.5- to 2.5-Hz frequency range. Hyperventilation, photic stimulation, and hypoglycemia activate typical absence seizures, but hyperventilation is the most effective procedure (8, 38).

Clinical effects are generally perceived accompanying discharges lasting longer than 3 seconds. Detailed neuropsychological investigations have demonstrated functional impairment from a spike-and-wave burst of any duration. Auditory reaction times were delayed 56% of the time when a stimulus was presented at the onset of the EEG paroxysm (39). They were abnormal in 80% when the stimulus was delayed 0.5 second. Responsiveness may improve as the paroxysm continues (40).

ETIOLOGY

Both acquired and inherited factors are implicated in the etiology of absence seizures, reflecting the heterogeneity of the patient population. Genetic factors predominate in children who match the syndromes of idiopathic generalized epilepsy. Alternatively, acquired disorders are frequently found in retarded children with abnormal neurologic findings, abnormal interictal EEGs, and atypical absence seizures. Typical absence seizures, both clinically and electrographically, have been rarely seen in patients with mesial frontal lesions, with diencephalic lesions, and after withdrawal from sedatives (41–44). Nonconvulsive status epilepticus of frontal lobe origin can mimic absence status epilepticus once it has progressed to a full-blown phase (45). A 6-year-old girl with typical (albeit intractable) absence seizures and diffuse 3-Hz spike-and-wave EEG discharges induced by hyperventilation was diagnosed with Moyamoya disease (46). The epilepsy remitted after bilateral revascularization procedures were performed.

The lack of structural pathology and the age-specific window observed in most patients with typical absence seizures implicate a hereditary etiology. Metrakos and Metrakos (47) showed that absence seizures and generalized spike-and-wave EEG discharges are both inherited traits. Generalized spike-and-wave activity was seen in 37% of siblings of patients with generalized spike-and-wave activity on EEG and absence or generalized tonic-clonic seizures compared with 9% of controls. Only 25% of the family members with the EEG trait actually had seizures. They theorized that the inheritance of generalized spike-and-wave discharges is autosomal dominant with age-dependent penetrance, regardless of whether seizures occur. Doose and associates (48) suggested a multigenic inheritance, with both independent and interactive genetic factors. In general, the idiopathic generalized epilepsies are considered genetic in origin, and usually represented by familial but complex, non-Mendelian traits. It has become increasingly clear that a variety of gene defects can result in absence seizures (49). Familial clustering of absence, myoclonic, and generalized tonic-clonic seizures has been demonstrated in the idiopathic generalized epilepsies, providing evidence for distinct genetic effects vis-à-vis seizure type (50). There are also patients with concomitant childhood absence epilepsy (CAE) and localization-related epilepsy, suggesting gene effects that transcend the traditional epilepsy syndrome classification (51).

More recent investigations of the pathophysiology of absence seizures, pointing to altered thalamocortical circuitry with key roles for T-type calcium channels and GABAergic mechanisms (vide infra), have spurred a new generation of molecular studies. The Cav3.2 T-type calcium channel gene has been linked to childhood absence epilepsy with mutations associated with altered channel gating properties (52). Mutations in GABA receptor genes have been invoked in CAE (53, 54). A significant association between a polymorphism in GABARB 3 in chromosome 15q11 was found in 50 families with CAE. Mutations of the $GABA_A$ receptor gamma-1 subunit gene (GABRG2) on chromosome 5 were identified in a large family with CAE and febrile seizures. Multiple mutations and polymorphisms in the calcium channel CACNA1H gene were found in the highly conserved residues of the T-type calcium channel gene (55). Linkage analysis of a five-generation family with childhood absences plus generalized tonic-clonic seizures identified a locus on chromosome 8q24, designated as ECA 1, although the gene remains to be identified (56). Yet another study found no evidence that genes encoding $GABA_A$ and $GABA_B$ receptors, voltage-dependent calcium channels, and the ECA region on chromosome 8q account independently for the childhood absence trait in a majority of families (57). The precise mode of inheritance and the genes involved in CAE remain largely unidentified (58).

PATHOPHYSIOLOGY

The observation that 3-Hz spike-and-wave discharges in absence seizures appear simultaneously and synchronously in all electrode locations led early investigators to speculate that the pathophysiologic mechanisms must involve "deep" structures with widespread connections between the two hemispheres (59–61). The term "centrencephalon" was coined to describe this unknown structure. Although this term was historically useful in emphasizing the fundamental differences between partial seizures and generalized seizures, later investigations have led to a better understanding of the basic mechanism of this disorder.

In the generalized penicillin epilepsy model, parenteral injections of penicillin—a weak $GABA_A$ receptor agonist—produce behavioral unresponsiveness associated with bilateral synchronous slow waves on EEG. Thalamic and cortical cells become synchronized during this event through reciprocal thalamocortical connections. Although it is not clear whether activity in the cortex precedes that in the thalamus in primary generalized seizures, recordings from cortical neurons show an increase in the number of action potentials during a depolarizing burst. This is followed by powerful GABAergic feedback inhibition that hyperpolarizes the cell for approximately 200 milliseconds after each burst. The summated activity of the bursts produces the "spike," which is dependent on alpha-amino-3-hydroxy-5-methylisoxazole-4-propionic acid (AMPA) receptors and T-type calcium channels, and the summated inhibition produces the "wave," due to GABA-mediated inhibition as well as voltage- and calcium-dependent potassium conductances (62).

A number of studies have demonstrated that the basic underlying mechanism in generalized absence epilepsies involves thalamocortical circuitry and the generation of abnormal oscillatory rhythms in this neuronal network (63–66). Studies using both in vivo and in vitro models have demonstrated the neuronal circuit responsible for the generation of the oscillatory thalamocortical burst firing observed during absence seizures. The key role of the thalamus is corroborated by a selective increase in blood flow during absence seizures using positron emission tomography (PET) imaging and functional magnetic resonance imaging (fMRI) technology (67–69).

This circuit includes cortical pyramidal neurons, thalamic relay neurons, and the nucleus reticularis thalami (NRT) (66, 70). The principal synaptic connections of the thalamocortical circuit include glutamatergic fibers between neocortical pyramidal cells and the NRT, and GABAergic fibers from NRT neurons that activate $GABA_A$ and $GABA_B$ receptors on thalamic relay neurons. In addition, recurrent collateral GABAergic fibers from the NRT activate $GABA_A$ receptors on adjacent NRT neurons. As can be seen in Figure 22–2, the NRT is in a position to influence the flow of information between the thalamus and cerebral cortex (71). The NRT cells have rhythmic burst firing (oscillatory firing) during periods of sleep (critical for sleep spindle formation) and continuous single-spike firing (tonic firing) during wakefulness.

The cellular events that underlie the ability of NRT neurons to shift between an oscillatory and tonic firing mode are the low-threshold Ca^{2+} spikes that are present in thalamocortical and NRT neurons (71). Low-threshold, transient Ca^{2+} channels (T-channels) are a key membrane property involved in burst firing excitation and are associated with rhythmic discharges in thalamocortical cells during absence seizures (64, 65, 72, 73). Mild depolarization of these neurons is sufficient to activate these channels and to allow the influx of extracellular Ca^{2+}. Further depolarization produced by Ca^{2+} inflow exceeds the threshold for firing a burst of action potentials. After T-channels are activated, they become inactivated rather quickly, hence the name "transient." Deinactivation of T-channels requires a relatively lengthy hyperpolarization. $GABA_B$ receptor–mediated hyperpolarization is able to deinactivate T-channels.

There is considerable evidence that the pathophysiological basis of absence seizures is the generation of excessive abnormal oscillatory rhythms (74). These abnormal oscillatory rhythms could be caused by abnormalities of the T-channels or enhanced $GABA_B$ function (59, 75). In some animal models of absence seizures T-channel activation in the NRT is significantly different from that in control animals (76). These aberrant T-channels may be one basis for absence seizures. In other models, there has been an increase in $GABA_B$ receptors in thalamic and neocortical neuronal populations compared with controls (74). As would be predicted from the thalamocortical circuits involved in absence seizures, in animal models of absences $GABA_B$ agonists produce an increase in seizure frequency, whereas $GABA_B$ antagonists reduce absence seizure frequency (77–79).

As demonstrated in Figure 22–2, recurrent collateral GABAergic fibers from the NRT neurons activate $GABA_A$ receptors on adjacent NRT neurons. Activating $GABA_A$ receptors in the NRT therefore results in inhibition of output to the thalamic relay neurons and serves to reduce hyperpolarization and delay deinactivation of the T-channels. In animal studies, injection of the $GABA_A$ agonists bilaterally into the NRT reduces absence seizure frequency. This occurs because the GABA output to the thalamic relay neurons is reduced. Because of the decreased $GABA_B$ activation, there would be a reduced likelihood that the Ca^{2+} deinactivation would occur. This would result in decreased oscillatory firing. However, direct $GABA_A$ and $GABA_B$ activation of thalamic relay neurons would be expected to have detrimental effects, increasing depolarization and deinactivation of the T-channels.

As would be expected from these animal findings are the clinical observations that three drugs that are effective in the treatment of absence seizures—valproate, ethosuximide, and trimethadione—all suppress T-currents. In addition, there is some clinical evidence that vigabatrin, which increases endogenous GABA levels and thereby increases the activation of $GABA_B$ receptors, worsens absence seizures in patients. However, clonazepam, which preferentially activates $GABA_A$ receptors in the NRT, can be a highly effective antiabsence drug (80). Hosford and Wang (74) evaluated the effects of a number of antiepileptic drugs (AEDs) on seizure frequency in the *lethargic* (*lh/lh*) mouse model of absence seizures. Previous studies

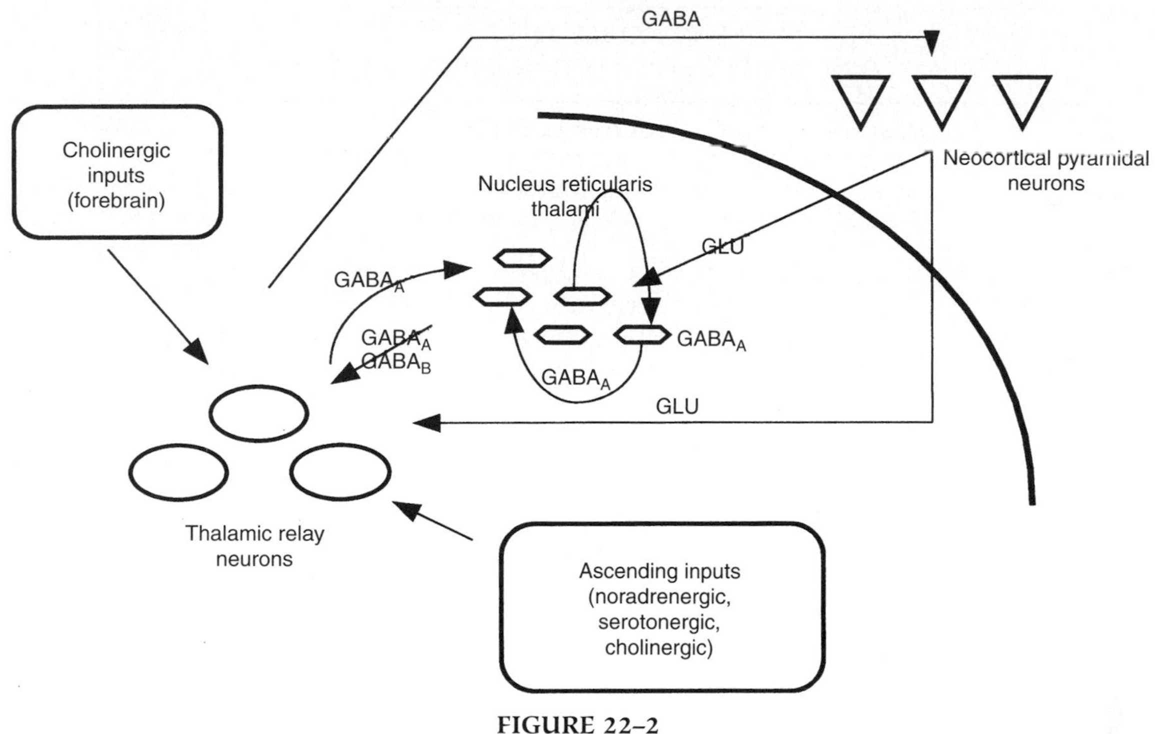

FIGURE 22–2

Thalamocortical circuits and neuronal networks implicated in the genesis of absence seizures. For discussion, see text.

had demonstrated the efficacy of ethosuximide, clonazepam, and valproate in this model. The authors found that lamotrigine significantly reduced seizure frequency, whereas vigabatrin and tiagabine increased seizure frequency and duration. Gabapentin and topiramate had no significant effects on seizure frequency.

The molecular characterization of T-type Ca^{2+} channels identified a family of genes that encode ion channels, alpha1G, alpha1H, and alpha1I, with characteristics similar to T-type Ca^{2+} channels in neurons (81). Thalamic relay neurons express mainly the alpha1G form. A transgenic mouse model with lack of expression of the alpha1G protein fails to exhibit spike-and-wave discharges in response to $GABA_B$ receptor activation (82). The human analogs to these genes have been designated CACNA1G, CACNA1H, and CACNA1I. This provides further support for the critical role of T-type Ca^{2+} channels in absence seizures.

Other neurotransmitter systems (i.e., serotonergic, noradrenergic, and cholinergic) can influence the thalamocortical circuits and therefore influence absence seizure frequency. Diffuse monoamine projections from the locus coeruleus (noradrenergic), raphe magnus (serotoninergic), and ventral tegmentum (dopaminergic) are implicated. For example, the mutant *tottering* mouse model has suggested a role for diffuse noradrenergic hyperinnervation of the cortex from the locus coeruleus in the genesis of paroxysmal spike wave discharge and the phenotype of behavioral arrest (83).

DIAGNOSTIC EVALUATION AND DIFFERENTIAL DIAGNOSIS

The primary diagnostic considerations to be differentiated from absence seizures are complex partial seizures and daydreaming (Table 22–3). Complex partial seizures are more common than absence seizures and are also manifested by an alteration in consciousness with staring, automatisms, changes in tone, and autonomic symptoms (84). The complex partial seizure tends to be longer and less frequent, but clinically there maybe no absolute distinguishing factor. The presence of an aura or postictal impairment is strongly suggestive of a complex partial seizure. When positive, the EEG is the best confirmation of either seizure type.

Daydreaming is associated with boredom, can be "broken" with stimulation, and is not associated with motor activity. Absence seizures, however, may sometimes be terminated with stimulation and tend to increase during periods of relaxation and tiredness. Tics and pseudoseizures may need to be considered as well. A normal EEG that includes several trials of 3 to 5 minutes of hyperventilation, however, virtually rules out absence seizures. Repeated studies or prolonged monitoring occasionally are necessary when diagnostic confusion persists (85).

Childhood absence epilepsy describes typical absence seizures (i.e., both simple and complex) in children between the ages of 3 to 5 years and puberty who are otherwise normal. There is a strong genetic predisposition, and girls

TABLE 22-3
Differential Diagnosis of Typical Absence Seizures

Clinical Data	Absence	Complex Partial	Daydreaming
Frequency/day	Multiple	Rarely over 1–2	Multiple; situation-dependent
Duration	Frequently <10 sec	Average duration over 1 min, 10 sec	Seconds to minutes; rarely more, rarely less
Aura	Never	Frequently	No
Eye blinking	Common	Occasionally	No
Automatisms	Common	Frequently	No
Postictal impairment	None	Frequently	No
Seizures activated by:			
HV	Very frequently	Occasionally	No
Photic	Frequently	Rarely	No
EEG			
Ictal	Generalized spike and wave	Usually unilateral or bilateral temporal frontal discharges	Normal
Interictal	Usually normal	Variable; may be spikes or sharp waves in frontal or temporal lobes	Normal

Source: With permission from publisher and author, Holmes GL. *Diagnosis and Management of Seizures in Children*. Philadelphia: W.B. Saunders Company, 1987:177.

are more frequently affected. The absences are very frequent, occurring at least several times daily, and tend to cluster. The EEG reveals the classic bilateral, synchronous symmetrical 3-Hz spike-and-wave discharge with normal interictal background activity. The absences may remit during adolescence.

The syndrome of epilepsy with myoclonic absences, as recognized by Tassinari and Bureau (86), is characterized by absence seizures accompanied by severe bilateral rhythmical clonic, and sometimes tonic, activity. Age of onset averages 7 years, and boys are more often affected. The ictal EEG discharges are similar to those of pyknolepsy. Seizures are frequent and less responsive to medication than those of CAE. The episodes of myoclonic absence last 10 to 60 seconds' duration and are precipitated by hyperventilation, awakening, and occasionally intermittent light. About half of affected children are normal and half have mental retardation before seizure onset. The majority of cases develop other seizure types, including generalized tonic-clonic seizures, pure absence without myoclonias, and drops. Mental deterioration and evolution to Lennox-Gastaut syndrome may occur (87).

Eyelid myoclonia with (and without) absences is a form of epileptic seizures manifest by myoclonic eyelid jerks and brief absences. These are precipitated by eye closure and lights. The syndrome has genetic underpinnings, is age related, and affects neurologically normal children with a female predominance. The semiology involves an initial and prominent eyelid myoclonia, which may or may not progress to a mild absence. The duration is typically brief, between 3 and 5 seconds. Head deviation or jerking of the hands may occur. The eyelid jerking becomes less violent as the absence component proceeds. Impairment of consciousness is mild and may appear incomplete. Some patients will self-induce the events, with some reports of an associated pleasurable feeling. The events are precipitated by eye closure (in a lit, not dark, environment), whether voluntary, involuntary, or reflex. They may only appear during photic stimulation. The accompanying EEG reveals generalized polyspike and polyspike-slow wave discharges of 3- to 6-Hz frequency and typically duration of 3 to 5 seconds. The symptoms require differentiation from ocular tics, with which they are often confused, and occipital seizures because forced eyelid closure and eyelid blinking are also described in occipital epilepsy. There also appears to be a group of patients having photosensitive epilepsy and concomitant nonepileptic paroxysmal eyelid movements (88). Lifelong treatment is recommended in eyelid myoclonia with absences, as remission is not anticipated (89).

TREATMENT

The extent of diagnostic evaluation required in patients with absence seizures is variable and depends somewhat on which epileptic syndrome might best "fit" the patient. A patient who meets the criteria for one of the idiopathic generalized syndromes by clinical and EEG criteria requires no further studies. Not every patient, however, fits these descriptions. The presence of typical absence seizures with consistent EEG ictal and interictal features and normal intelligence and neurologic examinations is reassuring that further tests are not necessary. Atypical features or history of developmental delay warrant cranial MRI and possibly more specific tests such as lumbar puncture, metabolic studies, and tissue examinations.

AED therapy is recommended for all children with adequate documentation of absence seizures. Although they are not life-threatening, they may lead to poor school performance, ridicule, and accidents. Because even a 1-second generalized spike-and-wave discharge sometimes affects cognitive function (39), it is prudent to try to control the seizures as well as possible with minimal drug toxicity.

Injury prevention counseling should not be underestimated. Accidental injury is common in patients with absence epilepsy and indeed usually occurs after anticonvulsant medication is already started (90). Specific recommendations, including mandatory use of bicycle helmets and avoidance of unsupervised swimming or climbing without protection, are common-sense precautions for any child.

The primary drugs of choice are ethosuximide, valproic acid or disodium valproate, and lamotrigine (91, 92). For the reader's convenience, in this chapter valproic acid and disodium valproate will both be called valproate. Comparative studies of the older AEDs have indicated equivalence in efficacy for ethosuximide and valproate (93–97). A Cochrane Database review indicated that randomized treatment trials possessing good methodological quality or sufficient power to detect a difference in efficacy when these agents are compared to each other or placebo are lacking, and concluded there is insufficient evidence to inform clinical practice (98). A multicenter trial addressing this question, coupled with neuropsychological testing of patients, is in progress at the time of this writing.

In standard clinical practice, a single agent is chosen and, after appropriate laboratory studies, initiated at a low dose and gradually increased. AED levels may be helpful, but dose changes in either direction should follow clinical indications. Upon dosage modifications, drug levels should be obtained only after sufficient time has elapsed to reach steady-state serum concentrations. Some clinicians will begin therapy with ethosuximide, primarily because of the rare but severe hepatotoxicity and pancreatitis associated with valproate (45, 99–101). Valproate is generally considered the drug of choice in the patient who has both absence seizures and generalized tonic-clonic seizures (20, 76). Published expert consensus opinion indicates that if initial monotherapy with ethosuximide, valproate, or lamotrigine is ineffective, other appropriate options are zonisamide or topiramate (91).

The combination of ethosuximide and valproate may be more effective than either drug alone (96, 102), although drug interactions do occur, requiring monitoring of clinical toxicity and serum drug levels (103). Clonazepam has been used in refractory cases, although it is limited because of its side effects of sedation and tachyphylaxis. The combination of valproate and clonazepam has been associated with precipitation of absence status (104), but this is rare.

Lamotrigine appears to be a promising drug in the treatment of absence seizures, with a number of studies demonstrating efficacy (105–108). Lamotrigine has demonstrated some efficacy in the treatment of myoclonic absence seizures (109). In a small, open-label extension study Biton found that four of five patients with absence seizures had a 50% or greater reduction in seizure frequency with topiramate (110). Based on animal studies and limited clinical experience, it does not appear that vigabatrin is effective in the treatment of absence seizures (111). Felbamate may sometimes be useful in the treatment of absence seizures, although the drug is rarely used for this indication because of the associated aplastic anemia (112). Gabapentin also does not appear to be effective in the treatment of absences (113, 114). Small open-label studies suggest potential efficacy for levetiracetam (115). Although trimethadione is rarely used because of its side effect profile and significant teratogenic potential, it is an effective compound, to be considered only in truly refractory absence seizures (116). Aggravation of idiopathic generalized epilepsy syndromes has been increasingly recognized as an iatrogenic complication of AEDs, and carbamazepine, phenytoin, gabapentin, tiagabine, and vigabatrin should be avoided (117).

The cellular mechanisms of action of the antiabsence drugs remain unclear. Valproate increases GABA levels through several possible pathways, but the relevance of this mechanism to its clinical effect has not been demonstrated (118). Valproate has been shown to limit sustained high-frequency repetitive firing of action potentials at therapeutic levels using mouse neurons in cell culture (119). Clonazepam, along with other benzodiazepines and phenobarbital, augments postsynaptic GABA responses (119). The active metabolite of trimethadione, dimathadione, blocks the low threshold, transient (T-type) calcium current in thalamic neurons, an effect shared by ethosuximide but not phenytoin or carbamazepine (116).

As discussed in the section on pathophysiology, the *lh/lh* genetic mouse model has contributed extensively to the investigation of the cellular and molecular mechanisms underlying absence seizures. The model has correctly predicted the therapeutic effects of ethosuximide, clonazepam, and valproate, in contrast to phenobarbital, phenytoin, and carbamazepine, against absence seizures. This same model demonstrated antiabsence efficacy of lamotrigine, proabsence effects of vigabatrin and tiagabine, and lack of effects by gabapentin and topiramate (74).

The duration of therapy is variable, although gradual taper from medication is recommended in general in patients who are seizure free for 2 years. The EEG is indicated in this situation, because even a 1-second generalized spike-and-wave discharge can result in subtle functional impairment (39). A brief discharge in sleep, however, would not preclude drug withdrawal. Hyperventilation should be performed during the EEG for 3 to 5 minutes, and the presence of discharges indicates a high recurrence risk.

Withdrawal seizures may occur with ethosuximide and valproic acid but are more likely to be precipitated by rapid reduction of clonazepam (120). Clonazepam should not be tapered faster than 0.25 mg per week (121). Withdrawal seizures may be delayed weeks after stopping valproate.

Absence status epilepticus is a unique form of nonconvulsive status epilepticus manifested by sustained impairment of consciousness associated with generalized, irregular, approximately 3-Hz spike-and-wave EEG discharges. Most patients are dull and confused but partially responsive and able to carry out tasks of daily living (122). They often exhibit facial twitching, eye blinking, staring, or automatisms (41, 123–125). Absence status may present as periods of stupor in adolescents or adults with a history of childhood absences after a relatively long seizure-free interval. The EEG may also show polyspike-and-wave discharges or prolonged generalized bursts of spike activity or irregular slow spike-and-wave discharges (122). Treatment is usually with intravenous diazepam (125), although intravenous acetazolamide (500 mg, or 250 mg for children weighing less than 35 kg) has been advocated (126). Intravenous valproate is likely to be useful for treatment of absence status.

COURSE AND PROGNOSIS

The average age of cessation of absence seizures is 10.5 years (12); however, some children continue to have absence seizures beyond puberty. Typical absence seizures generally have a favorable prognosis, with remission rates of approximately 80% (7, 127–129). An analysis of 52 patients with childhood absence by Loiseau and coworkers (130) demonstrated complete control in 95% of patients with absence seizures only and in 77% of patients with absence plus generalized tonic-clonic seizures. In contrast, of 62 patients with juvenile absence epilepsy, control was achieved in 77% of patients with absence seizures only and in 37% of patients with absence plus generalized tonic-clonic seizures (130).

Patients with CAE have a favorable response to medication and good prognosis for remission when taken off medication. Sato and colleagues (25) identified favorable prognostic signs for "outgrowing" both absence seizures and other seizure types as a negative family history of epilepsy, normal EEG background activity, and normal intelligence. A subsequent long-term follow-up study of 72 patients having mean seizure onset at 5.7 years (range, 1–14 years) and studied at a mean age of 20.4 years (range, 12–31 years) determined only a 65% remission rate, and furthermore that 15% of the total cohort developed JME. Adverse prognostic factors were cognitive impairment at diagnosis, history of absence status, presence of generalized tonic-clonic or myoclonic seizures during AED treatment, abnormal EEG background, and family history of generalized seizures in first-degree relatives (14). Also troubling is the observation of psychosocial difficulties, in the areas of academic-personal and behavioral categories, in a recent report on 56 young adults having a history of typical childhood absence epilepsy. Remission occurred in 32 (57%) of the patients, and the least favorable outcomes correlated with persistence of seizures (131).

In a study of treatment outcome in 86 children with childhood and juvenile absence epilepsy, initial drug treatment was successful in 52 (60%). Adverse prognostic factors were coexistence of generalized tonic-clonic or myoclonic seizures. As with other epilepsies, ultimate remission was more likely if the initial drug was successful than if it was not (69% vs. 41%, $P < 0.02$) (132). More recent studies of the evolution and prognosis of childhood absence epilepsy have identified that strict ILAE classification criteria impact the ability of a clinician to impart an accurate prognosis. In patients fulfilling strict criteria for CAE compared to children with absence seizures who did not fulfill syndromic criteria, there were significantly better rates of seizure control (95% vs. 77%), terminal remission (82% vs. 51%), fewer generalized tonic-clonic seizures (8% vs. 30%), and shorter mean treatment duration (2.2 vs. 3.8 years) (133). Unfavorable prognostic factors were the presence of generalized tonic-clonic seizures in the active stage of absences, myoclonias, eyelid or perioral myoclonia, and atypical EEG features.

References

1. Temkin O. The falling sickness: A history of epilepsy from the Greeks to the beginnings of modern neurology. 2nd ed. Baltimore: Johns Hopkins University Press, 1971:250.
2. Ajmone Marsan C, Lewis WR. Pathologic findings in patients with "centrencephalic" electroencephalographic patterns. *Neurology* 1960; 10:922–930.
3. Commission on Classification and Terminology of the International League Against Epilepsy. Proposal for revised classification of epilepsies and epileptic syndromes. *Epilepsia* 1989; 30(4):389–399.
4. Panayiotopoulos CP. Syndromes of idiopathic generalized epilepsies not recognized by the International League Against Epilepsy. *Epilepsia* 2005; 46 Suppl 9:57–66.
5. Blom S, Heijbel J, Bergfors PG. Incidence of epilepsy in children: a follow-up study three years after the first seizure. *Epilepsia* 1978; 19(4):343–350.
6. Blume WT, David RB, Gomez MR. Generalized sharp and slow wave complexes. Associated clinical features and long-term follow-up. *Brain* 1973; 96(2):289–306.
7. Cavazzuti GB. Epidemiology of different types of epilepsy in school age children of Modena, Italy. *Epilepsia* 1980; 21(1):57–62.
8. Dalby MA. Epilepsy and 3 per second spike and wave rhythms. A clinical, electroencephalographic and prognostic analysis of 346 patients. *Acta Neurol Scand* 1969; Suppl 40:1–183.
9. Livingston S, Torres I, Pauli LL, Rider RV. Petit mal epilepsy. Results of a prolonged follow-up study of 117 patients. *JAMA* 1965; 194(3):227–232.
10. Okuma T, Kumashiro H. Natural history and prognosis of epilepsy: report of a multi-institutional study in Japan. The group for the study of prognosis of epilepsy in Japan. *Epilepsia* 1981; 22(1):35–53.

11. Hauser WA, Kurland LT. The epidemiology of epilepsy in Rochester, Minnesota, 1935 through 1967. *Epilepsia* 1975; 16(1):1–66.
12. Blume W. Abnormal EEG: epileptiform potentials. In: Blume WT, ed. *Atlas of Pediatric EEG*. New York: Raven Press, 1982.
13. Sato S, Dreifuss Fe, Penry JK, Kirby DD, et al. Long-term follow-up of absence seizures. *Neurology* 1983; 33(12):1590–1595.
14. Wirrell EC, Camfield CS, Camfield PR, Gordon KE, et al. Long-term prognosis of typical childhood absence epilepsy: remission or progression to juvenile myoclonic epilepsy. *Neurology* 1996; 47(4):912–918.
15. Fernandez-Torre JL, Herranz JL, Martiniez-Martinez M, Maestro I, et al. Early-onset absence epilepsy: clinical and electroencephalographic features in three children. *Brain Dev* 2006; 28(5):311–314.
16. Rocca WA, Sharbrough FW, Hauser WA, Annegers JF, et al. Risk factors for absence seizures: a population-based case-control study in Rochester, Minnesota. *Neurology* 1987; 37(8):1309–1314.
17. Larsson K, Eeg-Olofsson O. A population based study of epilepsy in children from a Swedish county. *Eur J Paediatr Neurol* 2006; 10(3):107–113.
18. Commission on Classification and Terminology of the International League Against Epilepsy. Proposal for revised clinical and electroencephalographic classification of epileptic seizures. *Epilepsia* 1981; 22(4):489–501.
19. Penry JK, Porter RJ, Dreifuss RE. Simultaneous recording of absence seizures with video tape and electroencephalography. A study of 374 seizures in 48 patients. *Brain* 1975; 98(3):427–440.
20. Watanabe K, Negoro T, Matsumoto A, Inokuma K, et al. Epileptic nystagmus associated with typical absence seizures. *Epilepsia* 1984; 25(1):22–24.
21. Sato S. Generalized seizures: absence. In: Dreifuss FE, ed. *Pediatric Epileptology*. Littleton, MA: John Wright, 1983:65–91.
22. Holmes GL, McKeever M, Adamson M. Absence seizures in children: clinical and electroencephalographic features. *Ann Neurol* 1987; 21(3):268–273.
23. McKeever M, Holmes GL, Russman BS. Speech abnormalities in seizures: a comparison of absence and partial complex seizures. *Brain Lang* 1983; 19(1):25–32.
24. Mirsky AF, Vanburen JM. On the nature of the "absence" in centrencephalic epilepsy: a study of some behavioral, electroencephalographic and autonomic factors. *Electroencephalogr Clin Neurophysiol* 1965; 18:334–348.
25. Sato S, Dreifuss FE, Penry JK. Prognostic factors in absence seizures. *Neurology* 1976; 26(8):788–796.
26. Charlton MH, Yahr MD. Long-term follow-up of patients with petit mal. *Arch Neurol* 1967; 16(6):595–598.
27. Gibberd FB. The clinical features of petit mal. *Acta Neurol Scand* 1966; 42(2): 176–190.
28. Gibberd FB. The prognosis of petit mal. *Brain* 1966; 89(3):531–538.
29. Loiseau P, Pestre M, Dartigues JF, Commenges D, et al. Long-term prognosis in two forms of childhood epilepsy: typical absence seizures and epilepsy with rolandic (centrotemporal) EEG foci. *Ann Neurol* 1983; 13(6):642–648.
30. Nolan M, Bergazar M, Chu B, Cortez MA, et al. Clinical and neurophysiologic spectrum associated with atypical absence seizures in children with intractable epilepsy. *J Child Neurol* 2005; 20(5):404–410.
31. Panayiotopoulos C. Idiopathic generalized epilepsies. In: Panayiotopoulos CP, ed. *The Epilepsies: Seizures, Syndromes and Management*. Oxford: Bladon Medical Publishing, 2005:271–348.
32. Hirsch E, Blanc-Platier A, Marescaux C. What are the relevant criteria for a better classification of epileptic syndromes with typical absences? In: Malafosse A, Genton P, Hirsch E, Marescaux C, et al, eds. *Idiopathic Generalized Epilepsies: Clinical, Experimental and Genetic Aspects*. London: John Libbey, 1994:87–93.
33. Wolf P, Goosses R. Relation of photosensitivity to epileptic syndromes. *J Neurol Neurosurg Psychiatry* 1986; 49(12):1386–1391.
34. Sevgi Demirci EB, Saygi S. Unusual features in eyelid myoclonia with absences: a patient with mild mental retardation and background slowing on electroencephalography. *Epilepsy Behav* 2006; 8(2):442–445.
35. Niedermeyer E. Sleep electroencephalograms in petit mal. *Arch Neurol* 1965; 12:625–630.
36. Ross JJ, Johnson LC, Walter RD. Spike and wave discharges during stages of sleep. *Arch Neurol* 1966; 14(4):399–407.
37. Sato S, Dreifuss FE, Penry JK. The effect of sleep on spike-wave discharges in absence seizures. *Neurology* 1973; 23(12):1335–1345.
38. Adams DJ, Lueders H. Hyperventilation and 6-hour EEG recording in evaluation of absence seizures. *Neurology* 1981; 31(9):1175–1177.
39. Porter R, Penry JK, Dreifuss FE. Responsiveness at the onset of spike-wave bursts. *Electroencephalogr Clin Neurophysiol* 1973; 34:239–245.
40. Browne TR, Penry JK, Porter RJ, Dreifuss FE. Responsiveness before, during, and after spike-wave paroxysms. *Neurology* 1974; 24(7):659–665.
41. Andermann F, Robb JP. Absence status. A reappraisal following review of thirty-eight patients. *Epilepsia* 1972; 13(1):177–187.
42. Farwell JR, Stuntz JT. Frontoparietal astrocytoma causing absence seizures and bilaterally synchronous epileptiform discharges. *Epilepsia* 1984; 25(6):695–698.
43. Madsen JA, Bray PF. The coincidence of diffuse electroencephalographic spike-wave paroxysms and brain tumors. *Neurology* 1966; 16(6):546–555.
44. Stevens J. Focal abnormality in petit mal epilepsy. *Neurology* 1970; 20:1069–1076.
45. Kudo T, Sato K, Yagi K, Seino M. Can absence status epilepticus be of frontal lobe origin? *Acta Neurol Scand* 1995; 92(6):472–477.
46. Kikuta K, et al. Absence epilepsy associated with Moyamoya disease. Case report. *J Neurosurg* 2006; 104 Suppl 4:265–268.
47. Metrakos K, Metrakos JD. Genetics of convulsive disorders. II. Genetic and electroencephalographic studies in centrencephalic epilepsy. *Neurology* 1961; 11:474–483.
48. Doose H, Gerken H, Horstmann T, Volzke E. Genetic factors in spike-wave absences. *Epilepsia* 1973; 14(1):57–75.
49. Holmes GL. Models for generalized seizures. *Suppl Clin Neurophysiol* 2004; 57: 415–424.
50. Winawer MR, Marini C, Grinton BE, Rabinowitz D, et al. Familial clustering of seizure types within the idiopathic generalized epilepsies. *Neurology* 2005; 65(4):523–528.
51. Grosso S, Galimberti D, Gobbi G, Farnetani M, et al. Typical absence seizures associated with localization-related epilepsy: a clinical and electroencephalographic characterization. *Epilepsy Res* 2005; 66(1–3):13–21.
52. Peloquin JB, Khosravani H, Barr W, Bladen C, et al. Functional analysis of Ca3.2 T-type calcium channel mutations linked to childhood absence epilepsy. *Epilepsia* 2006; 47(3):655–658.
53. Feucht M, Fuchs K, Pichlbauer E, Hornik K, et al. Possible association between childhood absence epilepsy and the gene encoding GABRB3. *Biol Psychiatry* 1999; 46(7):997–1002.
54. Marini C, Harkin LA, Wallace RH, Mulley JC, et al. Childhood absence epilepsy and febrile seizures: a family with a GABA(A) receptor mutation. *Brain* 2003; 126 Pt 1:230–240.
55. Chan Y, Lu J, Pan H, Zhang Y, et al. Association between genetic variation of CACNA1H and childhood absence epilepsy. *Ann Neurol* 2003; 54(2):239–243.
56. Fong GC, Shah PU, Gee MN, Serratosa JM, et al. Childhood absence epilepsy with tonic-clonic seizures and electroencephalogram 3-4-Hz spike and multispike-slow wave complexes: linkage to chromosome 8q24. *Am J Hum Genet* 1998; 63(4):1117–1129.
57. Robinson R, Taske N, Sander T, Heils A, et al. Linkage analysis between childhood absence epilepsy and genes encoding GABAA and GABAB receptors, voltage-dependent calcium channels, and the ECA1 region on chromosome 8q. *Epilepsy Res* 2002; 48(3):169–179.
58. Crunelli V, Leresche N. Childhood absence epilepsy: genes, channels, neurons and networks. *Nat Rev Neurosci* 2002; 3(5):371–382.
59. Gloor P. Generalized spike and wave discharges: a consideration of cortical and subcortical mechanisms of their genesis and synchronization. In: Petsche H, Brazier MAB, eds. *Synchronization of EEG Activities in Epilepsies*. New York and Vienna: Springer Verlag, 1972:382–402.
60. Gloor P. Generalized cortico-reticular epilepsies. Some considerations on the pathophysiology of generalized bilaterally synchronous spike and wave discharge. *Epilepsia* 1968; 9(3):249–263.
61. Gloor P. Neurophysiological bases of generalized seizures termed "centrencephalic." In: Gastaut H, Jasper H, Bancaud J, et al, eds. *The Physiopathogenesis of the Epilepsies*. Springfield, IL: Charles C Thomas, 1969:209–246.
62. Lothman E. The neurobiology of epileptiform discharges. *Am J EEG Technol* 1993; 33:93–112.
63. Coulter D, Zhang Y. Thalamocortical rhythm generation in vitro: physiological mechanisms, pharmacological control, and relevance to generalized absence epilepsy. In: Malafosse A, Genton P, Hirsch E, et al, eds. *Idiopathic Generalized Epilepsies: Clinical, Experimental, and Genetic Aspects*. London: John Libbey, 1994:123–131.
64. Crunelli V, Leresche N. A role for GABAB receptors in excitation and inhibition of thalamocortical cells. *Trends Neurosci* 1991; 14(1):16–21.
65. Huguenard JR, Prince DA. Intrathalamic rhythmicity studied in vitro: nominal T-current modulation causes robust antioscillatory effects. *J Neurosci* 1994; 14(9):5485–5502.
66. Steriade M, McCormick DA, Sejnowski TJ. Thalamocortical oscillations in the sleeping and aroused brain. *Science* 1993; 262(5134):679–685.
67. Prevett MC, Duncan JS, Jones T, Fish DR, et al. Demonstration of thalamic activation during typical absence seizures using H2(15)O and PET. *Neurology* 1995; 45(7):1396–1402.
68. Hamandi K, Salek-Haddadi A, Laufs H, Liston A, et al. EEG-fMRI of idiopathic and secondarily generalized epilepsies. Neuroimage 2006; 31(4):1700–1710.
69. Lebate A, Briellmann RS, Abbott DF, Waites AB, et al. Typical childhood absence seizures are associated with thalamic activation. *Epileptic Disord* 2005; 7(4):373–377.
70. Steriade M, Llinas RR. The functional states of the thalamus and the associated neuronal interplay. *Physiol Rev* 1988; 68(3):649–742.
71. Snead OC 3rd. Basic mechanisms of generalized absence seizures. *Ann Neurol* 1995; 37(2):146–157.
72. Coulter DA, Huguenard JR, Prince DA. Specific petit mal anticonvulsants reduce calcium currents in thalamic neurons. *Neurosci Lett* 1989; 98(1):74–78.
73. Coulter DA, Huguenard JR, Prince DA. Characterization of ethosuximide reduction of low-threshold calcium current in thalamic neurons. *Ann Neurol* 1989; 25(6): 582–593.
74. Hosford DA, Wang Y. Utility of the lethargic (lh/lh) mouse model of absence seizures in predicting the effects of lamotrigine, vigabatrin, tiagabine, gabapentin, and topiramate against human absence seizures. *Epilepsia* 1997; 38(4):408–414.
75. Liu Z, Vergnes M, Depaulis A, Marescaux C. Involvement of intrathalamic GABAB neurotransmission in the control of absence seizures in the rat. *Neuroscience* 1992; 48(1):87–93.
76. Tsakiridou E, Bertollini L, de Curtis M, Avanzini G, et al. Selective increase in T-type calcium conductance of reticular thalamic neurons in a rat model of absence epilepsy. *J Neurosci* 1995; 15(4):3110–3117.
77. Hosford DA, Clark S, Cao Z, Wilson WA, et al. The role of GABAB receptor activation in absence seizures of lethargic (lh/lh) mice. *Science* 1992; 257(5068):398–401.
78. Marescaux C, Vergnes M, Bernasconi R. GABAB receptor antagonists: potential new anti-absence drugs. *J Neural Transm Suppl* 1992; 35:179–188.

79. Marescaux C, Vergnes M, Depaulis A. Genetic absence epilepsy in rats from Strasbourg—a review. *J Neural Transm Suppl* 1992; 35:37–69.
80. Huguenard JR, Prince DA. Clonazepam suppresses GABAB-mediated inhibition in thalamic relay neurons through effects in nucleus reticularis. *J Neurophysiol* 1994; 71(6):2576–2581.
81. Perez-Reyes E. Molecular physiology of low-voltage-activated t-type calcium channels. *Physiol Rev* 2003; 83(1):117–161.
82. Kim D, Song I, Keum S, Lee T, et al. Lack of the burst firing of thalamocortical relay neurons and resistance to absence seizures in mice lacking alpha(1G) T-type Ca(2+) channels. *Neuron* 2001; 31(1):35–45.
83. Noebels JL. Mutational analysis of spike-wave epilepsy phenotypes. *Epilepsy Res Suppl* 1991; 4:201–212.
84. So EL, King DW, Murvin AJ. Misdiagnosis of complex absence seizures. *Arch Neurol* 1984; 41(6):640–641.
85. Duchowny MS, Resnick TJ, Deray MJ, Alvarez LA. Video EEG diagnosis of repetitive behavior in early childhood and its relationship to seizures. *Pediatr Neurol* 1988; 4(3):162–164.
86. Tassinari C, Bureau M, Epilepsy with myoclonic absence. In: Roger J, Dravet C, Bureau M, Dreifuss FE, et al, eds. *Epileptic Syndromes in Infancy, Childhood and Adolescence.* 1985, London: John Libbey; 121–129.
87. Tassinari C, Bureau M, Thomas P. Epilepsy with myoclonic absences. In: Roger J, Bureau M, Dravet C, Dreifuss FE, et al, eds. *Epileptic Syndromes in Infancy, Childhood and Adolescence*. London: John Libbey, 1992:151–160.
88. Camfield CS, Camfield PR, Sadler M, Rahey S, et al. Paroxysmal eyelid movements: a confusing feature of generalized photosensitive epilepsy. *Neurology* 2004; 63(1):40–42.
89. Panayiotopoulos C. Jeavons syndrome (eyelid myoclonia with absences). In: Panayiotopoulos CP, ed. *The Epilepsies: Seizures, Syndromes and Management*. Oxford: Bladon Medical Publishing, 2005:475–480.
90. Wirrel EC, Camfield PR, Camfield CS, Dooley JM, et al. Accidental injury is a serious risk in children with typical absence epilepsy. *Arch Neurol* 1996; 53(9):929–932.
91. Wheless JW, Clarke DF, Carpenter D. Treatment of pediatric epilepsy: expert opinion, 2005. *J Child Neurol* 2005; 20 Suppl 1:S1–S56; quiz S59–S60.
92. French JA, Kanner AM, Bautista J, Abou-Khalil B, et al. Efficacy and tolerability of the new antiepileptic drugs. I: Treatment of new onset epilepsy: report of the Therapeutics and Technology Assessment Subcommittee and Quality Standards Subcommittee of the American Academy of Neurology and the American Epilepsy Society. *Neurology* 2004; 62(8):1252–1260.
93. Callaghan N, O'Hare J, O'Driscoll D, O'Neill B, et al. Comparative study of ethosuximide and sodium valproate in the treatment of typical absence seizures (petit mal). *Dev Med Child Neurol* 1982; 24(6):830–836.
94. Santavuori P. Absence seizures: valproate or ethosuximide? *Acta Neurol Scand Suppl* 1983; 97:41–48.
95. Sato S, White BG, Penry JK, Dreifuss FE, et al. Valproic acid versus ethosuximide in the treatment of absence seizures. *Neurology* 1982; 32(2):157–163.
96. Suzuki M, Maruyama H, Ishibashi Y, et al. A double-blind comparative trial of sodium dipropylacetate and ethosuximide in epilepsy in children with special emphasis on pure petit mal seizures. *Med Prog* 1972; 82:470–488.
97. Hitiris N, Brodie MJ. Evidence-based treatment of idiopathic generalized epilepsies with older antiepileptic drugs. *Epilepsia* 2005; 46 Suppl 9:149–153.
98. Posner EB, Mohamed K, Marson AG. Ethosuximide, sodium valproate or lamotrigine for absence seizures in children and adolescents. *Cochrane Database Syst Rev* 2003(3): CD003032.
99. American Academy of Pediatrics Committee on Drugs. Valproic acid: benefits and risks. *Pediatrics* 1982; 70(2):316–319.
100. Dreifuss F. How to use valproate. In: Morselli PL, Pippenger CE, Penry JK, eds. *Antiepileptic Drug Therapy in Pediatrics*. New York: Raven Press, 1983:219–227.
101. Schmidt D. Adverse effects of valproate. *Epilepsia* 1984; 25 Suppl 1:S44–S49.
102. Rowan AJ, Binnie CD, de Beer-Pawlikowski NKB, Goedhart DM, et al. Sodium valproate: serial monitoring of EEG and serum levels. *Neurology* 1979; 29(11):1450–1459.
103. Mattson RH, Cramer JA. Valproic acid and ethosuximide interaction. *Ann Neurol* 1980; 7(6):583–584.
104. Jeavons PM. Non-dose-related side effects of valproate. *Epilepsia* 1984; 25 Suppl 1: S50–S55.
105. Besag FM, Wallace SJ, Dulac O, Alving J, et al. Lamotrigine for the treatment of epilepsy in childhood. *J Pediatr* 1995; 127(6):991–997.
106. Frank LM, Enlow T, Holmes GL, Manasco P, et al. Lamictal (lamotrigine) monotherapy for typical absence seizures in children. *Epilepsia* 1999; 40(7):973–979.
107. Fitton A, Goa KL. Lamotrigine. An update of its pharmacology and therapeutic use in epilepsy. *Drugs* 1995; 50(4):691–713.
108. Schlumberger E, Chavez F, Palacios L, Rey E, et al. Lamotrigine in treatment of 120 children with epilepsy. *Epilepsia* 1994; 35(2):359–367.
109. Manonmani V, Wallace SJ. Epilepsy with myoclonic absences. *Arch Dis Child* 1994; 70(4):288–290.
110. Biton V. Preliminary open-label experience with topiramate in primary generalized seizures. *Epilepsia* 1997; 38 Suppl 1:S42–S44.
111. Michelucci R, CA. Tassinari, Response to vigabatrin in relation to seizure type. *Br J Clin Pharmacol* 1989; 27 Suppl 1:119S–124S.
112. Theodore W, Jensen PK, Kwan RMF. Felbamate. Clinical use. In: Levy RH, Mattson SN, Meldrum BS, eds. *Antiepileptic Drugs*. 4th ed. New York: Raven Press, 1995: 817–822.
113. Chadwick, D, Leiderman DB, Sauermann W, Alexander J, et al. Gabapentin in generalized seizures. *Epilepsy Res* 1996; 25(3):191–197.
114. Trudeau V, Myers S, LaMoreaux L, Anhut H, et al. Gabapentin in naive childhood absence epilepsy: results from two double-blind, placebo-controlled, multicenter studies. *J Child Neurol* 1996; 11(6):470–475.
115. Di Bonaventura C, Fattouch J, Mari F, Egeo G, et al. Clinical experience with levetiracetam in idiopathic generalized epilepsy according to different syndrome subtypes. *Epileptic Disord* 2005; 7(3):231–235.
116. Pellock J, Coulter DA. Oxazolidinedione: Trimethodione. In: Levy RH, Mattson RH, Meldrum BS, eds. *Antiepileptic Drugs*. 4th ed. New York: Raven Press, 1995:689–694.
117. Thomas P, Valton L, Genton P. Absence and myoclonic status epilepticus precipitated by antiepileptic drugs in idiopathic generalized epilepsy. *Brain* 2006; 129 Pt 5:1281–1292.
118. Fariello R, Smith MC. Valproate: mechanisms of action. In: Levy R, Mattson R, Meldrum B, Penry JK, et al, eds. *Antiepileptic Drugs*. 3rd ed. New York: Raven Press, 1989: 567–575.
119. Macdonald RL, McLean MJ. Mechanisms of anticonvulsant drug action. *Electroencephalogr Clin Neurophysiol Suppl* 1987; 39:200–208.
120. Lund M, Trolle E. Clonazepam in the treatment of epilepsy. *Acta Neurol Scand Suppl* 1973; 53:82–90.
121. Schmidt D. How to use benzodiazepines. In: Morselli PL, Pippenger CE, Penry JK, eds. *Antiepileptic Drug Therapy in Pediatrics*. New York: Raven Press, 1983.
122. Porter RJ, Penry JK. Petit mal status. *Adv Neurol* 1983; 34:61–67.
123. Belafsky Ma, Carwille S, Miller P, Waddell G, et al. Proglonged epileptic twilight states: continuous recordings with nasopharyngeal electrodes and videotape analysis. *Neurology* 1978; 28(3):239–245.
124. Geier S. Prolonged psychic epileptic seizures: a study of the absence status. *Epilepsia* 1978; 19(5):431–445.
125. Moe PG. Spike-wave stupor. Petit mal status. *Am J Dis Child* 1971; 121(4):307–313.
126. Browne T. Status epilepticus. In: Browne TR, Feldman RG, eds. *Epilepsy: Diagnosis and Management*. Boston: Little, Brown, 1983:341–354.
127. Annegers JF, Hauser WA, Elveback LR. Remission of seizures and relapse in patients with epilepsy. *Epilepsia* 1979; 20(6):729–737.
128. Sofijanov NG. Clinical evolution and prognosis of childhood epilepsies. *Epilepsia* 1982; 23(1):61–69.
129. Turnbull DM, Rawlins MD, Weightman D, Chadwick DW. A comparison of phenytoin and valproate in previously untreated adult epileptic patients. *J Neurol Neurosurg Psychiatry* 1982; 45(1):55–59.
130. Loiseau P, Duche B, Pedespan JM. Absence epilepsies. *Epilepsia* 1995; 36(12): 1182–1186.
131. Wilder BJ, Ramsay RE, Murphy JV, Karas BJ, et al. Comparison of valproic acid and phenytoin in newly diagnosed tonic-clonic seizures. *Neurology* 1983; 33(11): 1474–1476.
132. Wirrell E, Camfield C, Camfield P, Dooley J. Prognostic significance of failure of the initial antiepileptic drug in children with absence epilepsy. *Epilepsia* 2001; 42(6):760–763.
133. Grosso C, Galimberti D, Vezzosi P, Farnetani M, et al. Childhood absence epilepsy: evolution and prognostic factors. *Epilepsia* 2005; 46(11):1796–1801.

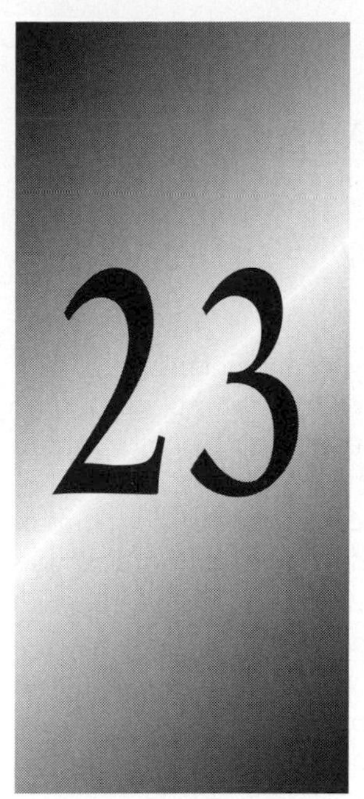

23 Benign Focal Epilepsies of Childhood

Colin D. Ferrie
Douglas R. Nordli, Jr.
Chrysostomos P. Panayiotopoulos

The International League Against Epilepsy's (ILAE's) definition of a benign epilepsy (syndrome) is "A syndrome characterized by epileptic seizures that are easily treated, or require no treatment, and remit without sequelae" (1). In approximately 60% of children with epilepsy seizures will cease, antiepileptic drugs (AEDs) can be withdrawn, and seizures will not recur (2). This indicates that a majority of children with epilepsy have benign conditions.

In its 2001 diagnostic scheme, the ILAE listed around 40 epilepsy syndromes and conditions with recurrent epileptic seizures (3). Only a small number of them satisfy the ILAE criteria for the diagnosis of benign epilepsy. These are (in order of the age at which they characteristically begin):

- Benign familial neonatal seizures
- Benign nonfamilial neonatal seizures
- Benign familial and nonfamilial infantile seizures
- Benign childhood epilepsy with centrotemporal spikes
- Early onset benign childhood occipital epilepsy (Panayiotopoulos type)

If a less rigorous definition is used, the following conditions could reasonably be added:

- Benign myoclonic epilepsy in infancy
- Childhood absence epilepsy
- Late onset childhood occipital epilepsy (Gastaut type)
- Idiopathic photosensitive occipital lobe epilepsy

Although some of these disorders are common, together they still account for well under half of all children with epilepsy. This emphasizes two important points when considering benign childhood epilepsy syndromes. First, among the many children with epilepsy who do not fit within any of the currently recognized syndromes, there are many whose epilepsy follows a benign course. Second, many children who have epilepsy syndromes that are not usually considered benign, nevertheless, have a good outcome. This is perhaps best illustrated by children with congenital hemiplegia who develop focal seizures. Many such children have only a few seizures, respond well to medication, and eventually successfully discontinue treatment. However, even with syndromes usually considered anything but benign (or even "malignant") significant numbers of individuals have a good outcome. For example, this is so in 12% to 25% of children diagnosed with West syndrome (4). This chapter will therefore consider only a fraction of those children with benign forms of focal epilepsy. Idiopathic generalized epilepsies, including those whose courses are usually benign, are considered elsewhere, as are the benign focal epilepsies that occur in the neonatal and infantile periods. The "core group" of benign focal epilepsies left to consider in this chapter (with their official ILAE names in brackets) are

- Rolandic epilepsy (benign childhood epilepsy with centrotemporal spikes)
- Panayiotopoulos syndrome (early onset benign childhood occipital epilepsy—Panayiotopoulos type)
- Idiopathic childhood occipital epilepsy (late onset childhood occipital epilepsy—Gastaut type and idiopathic photosensitive occipital lobe epilepsy)

The main features of these disorders are compared in Table 23-1.

A NOTE ON TERMINOLOGY

We prefer "rolandic epilepsy" to "benign childhood epilepsy with centrotemporal spikes" for the following reasons:

- The term is widely used by pediatricians.
- Centrotemporal spikes are located mainly in the central (rolandic) fissure; they are rarely located in the temporal electrodes.
- Rolandic epilepsy may occur without centrotemporal spikes and conversely centrotemporal spikes occur in children without seizures and in children with other benign focal epilepsies.
- The term "temporal" may suggest the occurrence of temporal lobe symptoms during seizures despite these not being a feature of the condition.

TABLE 23-1
Comparison of the Clinical and EEG Features of the Three Idiopathic Childhood Focal Epilepsies of Childhood

	Panayiotopoulos Syndrome	Rolandic Epilepsy	Idiopathic Childhood Occipital Epilepsy
Prevalence among children 1–15 years with afebrile seizures, %	6	15	1-2
Mean age at onset (range), years	4–5 (1–14)	8–9 (1–15)	8-9 (3-16)
Sex prevalence,%	54 males	60 males	50 males
Seizure characteristics			
Main type of seizures	Autonomic and often with emesis	Focal sensory-motor	Focal visual
Duration	Long (usually 9 minutes or longer)	Moderate (usually 2–4 minutes)	Brief (seconds to 1–2 minute)
Focal nonconvulsive status epilepticus (>30 min), %	44	Rare	Exceptional
Frequency of seizures	Infrequent	Infrequent	Many, sometimes daily
Single seizures only, %	30	10–20	Exceptional
Circadian distribution, %	Mainly in sleep (64)	Mainly in sleep (70)	Mainly when awake (>90)
Reflex provocation of clinical seizures	Probably none	Probably none	10–20% photosensitivity
Interictal EEG	Multifocal spikes	Centrotemporal spikes	Occipital spikes
Reflex provocation of spikes, %	Fixation-off sensitivity (10) and less often somatosensory stimulation (<5)	Somatosensory stimulation (20–25)	Fixation-off sensitivity and 20% occipital photosensitivity
Prophylactic continuous treatment	Often not needed	Often not needed	Needed
Prognosis	Excellent	Excellent	Uncertain
Risk of epilepsy as an adult, %	2?	3	20?
Remission within 1–3 years from first seizure	Common	Common	Uncommon
Similar seizures after remission	None	Only one case is reported	Common
Developmental and social prognosis	Normal	Normal	Usually good

Modified from Ferrie et al (54), with the permission of the Editor of *Developmental Medicine and Child Neurology*.

We prefer "Panayiotopoulos syndrome" to "early onset benign childhood occipital epilepsy (Panayiotopoulos type)," because evidence now suggests that it is a form of multifocal epilepsy with autonomic ictal symptoms rather than an occipital lobe epilepsy.

We use the term "idiopathic childhood occipital epilepsy" to include both late onset childhood occipital epilepsy—Gastaut type and idiopathic photosensitive occipital lobe epilepsy. This is because both conditions share many common features and it is not clear that they merit separation into two distinct syndromes.

CONSIDERATIONS REGARDING THE ETIOLOGY, INCLUDING THE GENETIC BASIS, OF THE BENIGN FOCAL EPILEPSIES OF CHILDHOOD

The benign focal epilepsies of childhood are all idiopathic epilepsies, the ILAE's definition of which is "A syndrome that is only epilepsy, with no underlying structural brain lesion or other neurologic signs or symptoms. These are presumed to be genetic and are usually age-dependent" (3). In keeping with their presumed genetic origin, there is an increased risk of epileptic seizure disorders in the family members of children with benign focal epilepsies, although it is rare to find family members with the same benign focal seizure disorder. Febrile seizures are common both in probands and family members (5). However, to date the likely genetic basis of these disorders has eluded us. Panayiotopoulos has suggested that they (and possibly also febrile seizures) share a common age-related origin and all might be considered as manifestations of a "benign childhood seizure susceptibility syndrome" (5, 6). This is a common, genetically determined, mild and reversible, functional derangement of the brain cortical maturational process. Benign childhood seizure susceptibility is often clinically silent and manifests in more than 90% with electroencephalographic (EEG) sharp and slow waves with an age-related localisation. The remaining 10% have infrequent focal seizures with symptoms that are also localization—and age related—and dependent. It is possible that a few of these children, with or without seizures, also have usually minor and fully reversible neuropsychologic symptoms that are rarely clinically overt and that can only be detected by formal neuropsychologic testing. Finally, there may be a very small number of patients (<1%) in whom this derangement of the brain maturation process may be further derailed in a more aggressive condition with seizures, neuropsychologic manifestations, and EEG abnormalities of various combinations and various degrees of severity, such as in Landau-Kleffner syndrome, and epilepsy with continuous spikes and slow waves during sleep (5, 6).

The benign focal epilepsies of childhood do not, as a whole, follow simple Mendelian inheritance. Vadlamudi et al found strong concordance for idiopathic generalized epilepsies in 26 monozygotic twins, but no concordance for rolandic epilepsy in 6 monozygotic twins (7). Of course, this does not exclude Mendelian inheritance in individual families with forms of benign focal epilepsy. Moreover, the EEG trait characterizing these disorders may show Mendelian inheritance, even if the seizure phenotype does not (8–10). If this is so, by implication, other genetic, environmental factors, or both must also be involved in producing the clinical seizure disorder (7). So far, the only genetic linkage reported for any of the benign focal epilepsies of childhood is to 15q14 for rolandic epilepsy (10, 11).

One of the most significant developments in epileptology in the last decade has been the demonstration that many seizure disorders, albeit to date rare ones, arise as a consequence of mutations in genes encoding neuronal ion channels (12–14). Benign familial neonatal seizures, which are autosomal dominant with high penetrance, is caused by mutations in the voltage-gated potassium channel subunit gene KCNQ2 on chromosome 20q13.3 and KCNQ3 on chromosome 8q.13.3 (12–15). Similarly, benign familial neonatal-infantile seizures, also an autosomal dominant condition, is caused by mutations in the sodium channel subunit gene SCN2A (16). Given this evidence, the likelihood that the benign focal epilepsies of childhood also result from mutations on genes encoding channel ions is high, although other mechanisms are not precluded (94).

Further fascinating clues regarding the pathogenesis of these disorders are descriptions linking them with nonepileptic paroxysmal disorders. Families are described in which benign infantile seizures and paroxysmal choreoathetosis or dystonia occur (17). In some subjects one or other of these disorders is recognized, whereas in others both occur together, or else the benign infantile seizures subside but later the movement disorder begins. A pedigree has also been described with three members in the same generation who had rolandic epilepsy, paroxysmal dystonia, and writer's cramp (18).

Rolandic Epilepsy

Introduction and Definition. This disorder (19, 20), also called benign epilepsy of childhood with centrotemporal spikes (BECTS), was, in 1958, the first of the benign focal epilepsies to be recognized (by Beaussart et al [21]). Later its recognition in the United States was established by Lombroso (22). It is probably the single most common epilepsy syndrome after febrile seizures.

Rolandic epilepsy can be defined as an idiopathic benign focal seizure disorder of childhood manifested with seizures, which are usually infrequent and often single, and whose semiology reflects onset in the lower part of the pre- and postcentral gyri. They are characterized by unilateral facial sensorimotor symptoms, oropharyngolaryngeal manifestations, speech arrest, and hypersalivation. Secondary generalization is frequent. Interictal EEG shows high amplitude sharp and slow wave foci, which are usually localized to the central or centrotemporal electrodes.

Epidemiology. Rolandic epilepsy can start as early as 1 year of age or as late as 15 years of age (23). However, three-quarters of cases have onset of seizure between 7 and 10 years. Boys are more often affected, with a ratio of 3:2. Overall around 15% of children with seizures aged 1 to 15 years of age are considered to have rolandic epilepsy. The EEG trait characteristic of rolandic epilepsy is considered to be inherited in an autosomal dominant manner.

Clinical Manifestations. Rolandic epilepsy, being idiopathic, is expected to occur in children who are otherwise normal. Three-quarters of seizures occur in non-rapid-eye movement (non-REM) sleep, usually shortly after sleep commences or before wakening. The most recognizable seizure manifestations involve oropharyngolaryngeal symptoms and hemifacial motor, sensory, or more usually sensorimotor symptoms. Oropharyngolaryngeal symptoms occur in just over one-half of seizures, with hemifacial sensorimotor manifestations occurring in around one-third of seizures.

Oropharyngolaryngeal symptoms consist of unilateral sensory (numbness and parasthesia) and motor manifestations affecting the structures inside the mouth (i.e., tongue, inner cheeks, teeth, and gums) and the pharynx and larynx. The motor manifestations are responsible for gurgling, grunting, and guttural noises, sometimes producing a so-called death rattle.

The motor manifestations of the hemifacial seizures consist of sudden, continuous, or bursts of clonic contractions usually localized to the lower lip and often accompanied by ipsilateral tonic deviation of the mouth. In a minority of cases the motor manifestations are more widespread with hemifacial clonic activity, sometimes with spread to the ipsilateral upper limb. The sensory manifestations of the hemifacial seizures are usually described as numbness or tingling in the corner of the mouth.

Speech arrest is very common in rolandic seizures, occurring in about 40% of patients. The cause is disputed. Some refer to it as aphemia (implying a motor aphasia), others as aphonia (implying an inability to produce sound as a consequence of laryngeal dysfunction). Panayiotopoulos has argued that it is an anarthria or dysarthria (implying an articulatory disturbance) (19). In support of this, it appears to occur equally in left- and right-sided seizures. The child with speech arrest will often try to communicate using other means, such as gestures.

Hypersalivation is reported to occur in around one-third of rolandic seizures, and recently ictal syncope (described in detail later) has also been reported as a rare feature of rolandic seizures (5).

In more than one-half of rolandic seizures consciousness is retained throughout the seizure, such that the child can often give a vivid description of his or her experiences after the seizure. However, spread of rolandic seizures is common, leading to impairment of consciousness and secondarily generalized tonic-clonic seizures (GTCS). Such spread is much more likely with seizures occurring in sleep; rolandic epilepsy is one of the commonest causes of nocturnal GTCS in children, whereas it is said to be only exceptionally associated with GTCS when awake.

Seizures in rolandic epilepsy are usually brief, mostly lasting 1–2 minutes. However, they may be longer if they progress to GTCS. Focal motor status epilepticus and hemiconvulsive status epilepticus, although rare, are well described. The latter is probably more common when the syndrome occurs in younger children. It may be followed by Todd's paresis, usually sparing the face. Opercular status is encountered as part of the atypical evolution sometimes encountered in the syndrome (24). Convulsive status epilepticus is exceptional.

EEG Features. The interictal EEG in children with rolandic epilepsy usually shows a normal background but with the hallmark centrotemporal (or rolandic) spikes (Figure 23-1). Despite their name, these are usually high amplitude sharp and slow wave complexes localized to the central (C3/C4) electrodes or midway between the central and temporal electrodes (C5/C6). They may be unilateral or bilateral, synchronous or asynchronous.

Centrotemporal spikes have been studied with EEG single- or multiple-dipole modeling computerized techniques. The consensus is that their main negative spike component can usually be modeled by a single and stable tangential dipole source along the central (rolandic) region, with the negative pole maximal in the centrotemporal and the positive pole maximal in the frontal regions (25, 26).

Centrotemporal spikes are highly activated by sleep; normal sleep architecture is preserved.

The interictal EEG (especially if there is no sleep recording) may rarely be normal. Mild background slowing may be a postical effect, reflect antiepileptic drug medication, or may be seen if centrotemporal spikes are particularly abundant. Rarely small inconspicuous spikes may be seen, rather than those with the more characteristic morphology. Sharp- and slow-wave complexes in areas outside the centrotemporal regions, such as occipital, parietal, frontal, and midline regions, may occur concurrently with centrotemporal spikes. They are of similar

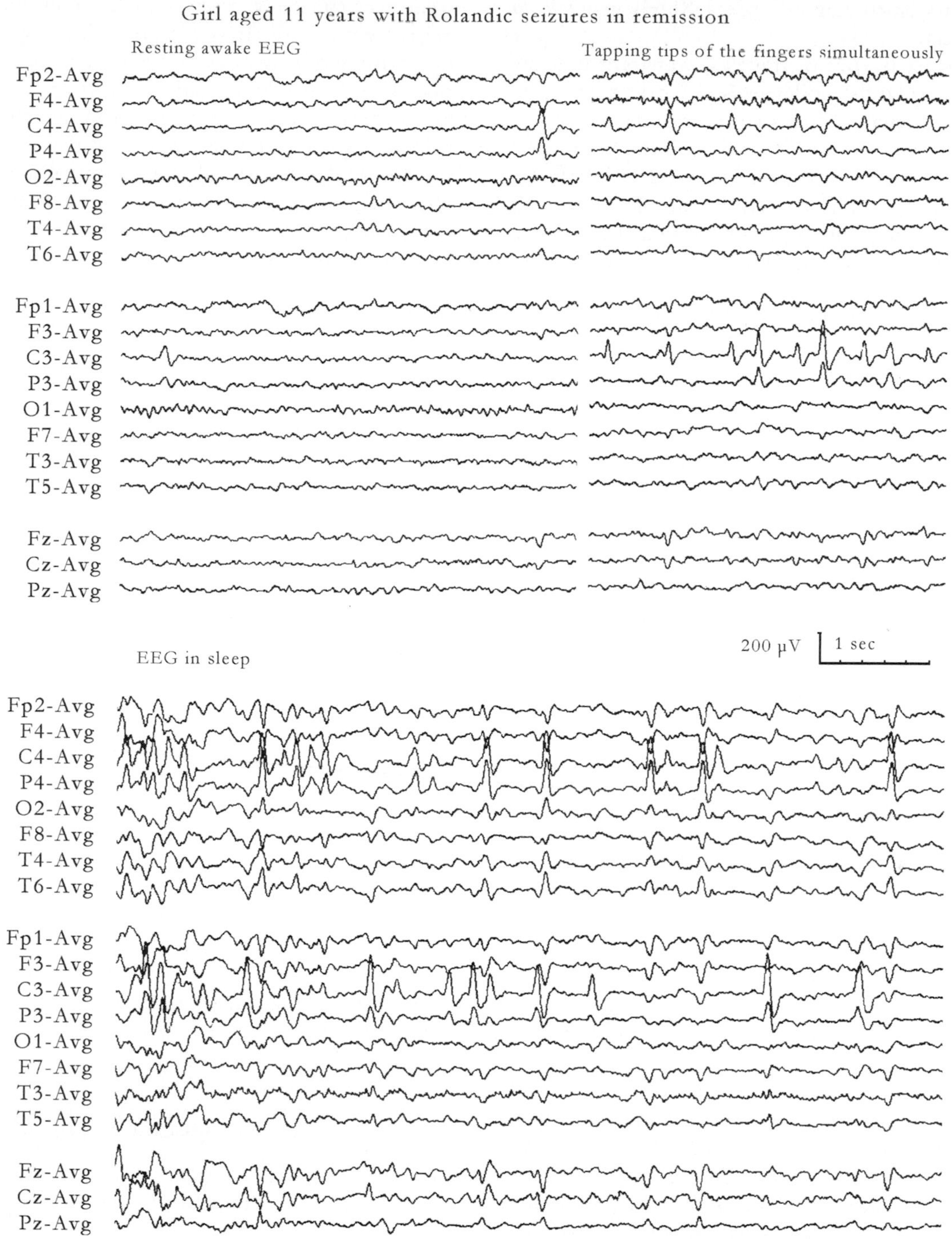

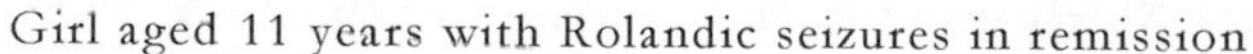

FIGURE 23-1

Centrotemporal spikes recorded from an 11-year-old girl with rolandic seizures that had been in remission for the last 3 years. Note that the spikes have their maximal amplitude in the central rather than temporal electrodes. (Top) EEG in wakefulness. (Top, left) Infrequent spikes occur independently in the right or left central electrodes (C4 or C3). (Top, right) Stimulation of the tips of the fingers elicited high amplitude central spikes, which were contralateral to the side of stimulation. Self-stimulation of the fingers elicited simultaneous bilateral central spikes. In clinical EEG practice, asking the child to tap together the palmar surface of the tips of his or her fingers of both hands is an easy method of testing for evoked spikes. The child should be instructed to strike them with sufficient strength and at random intervals. This may elicit either bilateral or unilateral central spikes. (Bottom) Frequency and amplitude of central spikes is markedly increased in sleep. In previous EEGs their abundance approached that of electrical status epilepticus in sleep. Despite marked EEG abnormalities over many years, the child was otherwise normal, did well in school, and had no linguistic or neuropsychologic deficits.

morphology to centrotemporal spikes. Rarely, generalized discharges occur.

An unusual feature of the EEG apparent in some children with rolandic epilepsy is the provocation by tapping of the fingers or toes of extreme somatosensory evoked spikes (giant somatosensory evoked potentials) in the contralateral hemisphere (5, 27, 28). These are of identical morphology to centrotemporal spikes. It should be noted that although most often encountered in rolandic epilepsy, the phenomenon is not confined to this syndrome.

Centrotemporal spikes, the EEG hallmark of rolandic epilepsy, peak at 8–9 years of age and occur in 2% to 3% of normal children; they are also common in children with neurologic deficits who do not have epileptic seizures (29–31).

The frequency, location, and persistence of centrotemporal spikes do not determine the clinical manifestations, severity, and frequency of seizures or the prognosis (5).

There are very few ictal EEG recordings of rolandic seizures. Before the onset of the ictal discharge, centrotemporal spikes become sparse. The ictal discharge then appears and consists of unilateral slow waves intermixed with fast rhythms and spikes located in the central regions (19, 20, 32). The ictal EEG features of rolandic epilepsy are shown in Figure 23-2 and compared to those of Panayiotopoulos syndrome.

Magnetoencephalography (MEG) studies have shown that the dipoles of the prominent negative sharp waves of rolandic discharges appear as tangential dipoles in the central (rolandic) region, with positive poles being situated anteriorly (32, 33). MEG findings in children with rolandic epilepsy are shown in Figure 23-3 and compared with those in Panayiotopoulos syndrome.

Diagnostic Evaluation and Differential Diagnosis. There is controversy as to the extent to which children with suspected rolandic epilepsy require investigation. Investigations, other than EEG, are expected to be normal. Many, but not all authorities, consider that neuroimaging is not required if the clinical picture, taking into account age, the absence of any comorbidities, seizure semiology, and EEG features, are typical. Neuroimaging, preferably magnetic resonance imaging (MRI), is certainly indicated if atypical features are present or if the evolution is not as expected. Structural lesions in the rolandic regions may occasionally be found (34). If neuroimaging is routinely performed it may detect coincidental abnormalities (35). The significance of reports of hippocampal abnormalities in a minority of children with rolandic epilepsy remains to be determined (36–38).

Treatment. The ultimate prognosis in rolandic epilepsy is almost certainly not influenced by regular AED treatment. Many authorities do not recommend such treatment routinely, reserving it for children whose seizures are unusually frequent or unpleasant (for example, occurring while awake). Some are concerned about the risk of sudden unexpected death in epilepsy (SUDEP), although there is no strong evidence that this is a risk in rolandic epilepsy. If it is decided to treat, it is generally considered that seizures are easily controlled in most cases. However, a recent study suggested that only secondary GTCS, not focal seizures, were significantly reduced by such treatment (38). The evidence base for choosing a particular medication is poor; carbamazepine is probably used most often.

Course and Prognosis. Most children with rolandic epilepsy will have fewer than 10 seizures; indeed, single seizures are common (an argument for considering this as a benign seizure disorder rather than an epilepsy (23, 39). However, perhaps up to one-fifth of subjects will have frequent seizures, especially at the start of the disorder. The prognosis, however, remains excellent, with remission usually occurring within 1–2 years of onset and certainly before the age of 16 years (23). The risk of GTCS in adult life is less than 2% (similar to the normal population). There is probably a higher risk, however, of developing absence seizures (5).

The term "benign" should not be used to imply "trivial" or to suggest that rolandic epilepsy has no neurodevelopmental effects. Transient cognitive impairment has been demonstrated as a consequence of centrotemporal spikes, raising interesting questions concerning the boundary between interictal and ictal EEG abnormalities (40–46). Some children with rolandic epilepsy develop mild, but not insignificant, speech, reading, and behavioral problems (40–46). It is not established whether AED treatment is useful in the management of such problems; the potential adverse cognitive and behavioral effects of such drugs should certainly be borne in mind.

Panayiotopoulos Syndrome

Introduction and Definition. This condition (47–54) was first described by Panayiotopoulos in a 30-year prospective study starting in 1973 (47, 50, 51, 53, 55–57). After rolandic epilepsy, it is the most common of the benign focal epilepsies of childhood and is typically manifested with autonomic seizures and autonomic status epilepticus. Autonomic seizures can be defined as epileptic seizures characterized by altered autonomic function occurring at the onset of the seizure or as the sole manifestation of the seizure. Autonomic status epilepticus is an autonomic seizure that lasts for more than 30 minutes (50, 51, 58).

Panayiotopoulos syndrome, because of its unusual ictal manifestations, is especially likely to be misdiagnosed as a nonepileptic disorder.

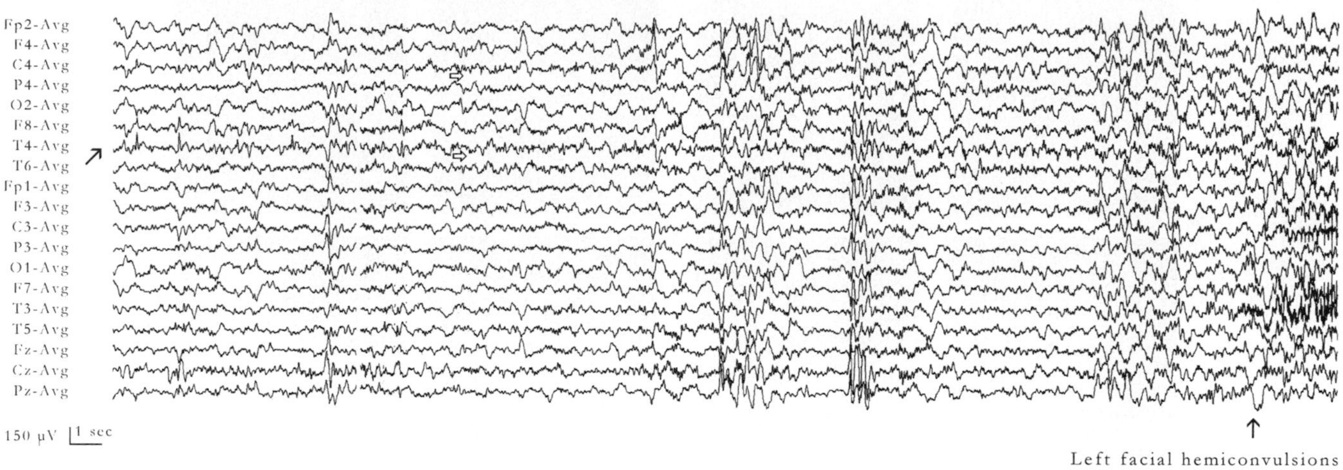

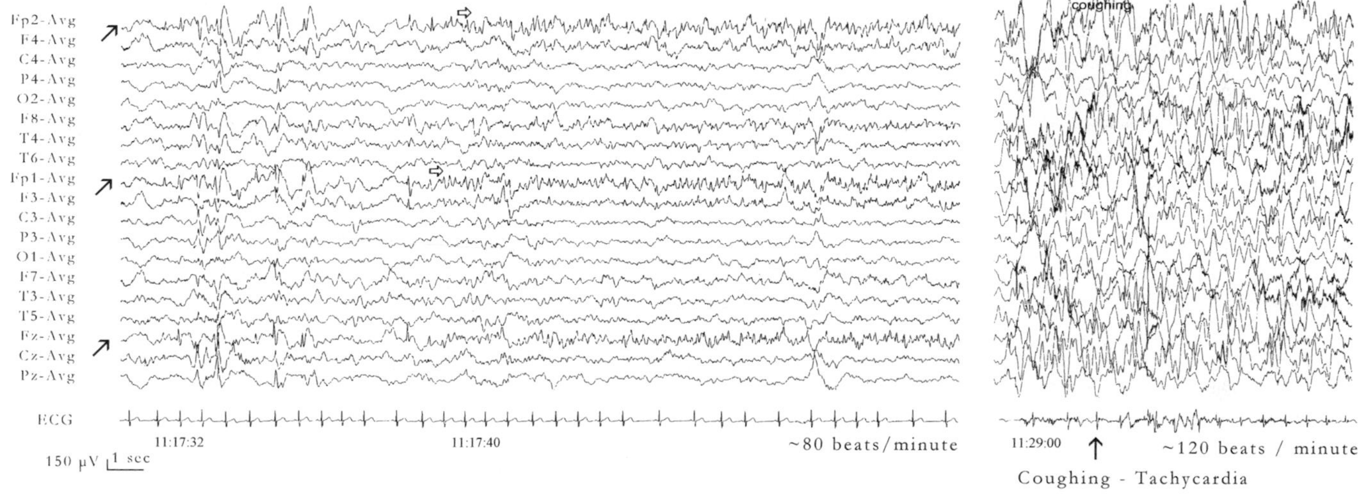

FIGURE 23-2

Samples from video-EEG recorded seizures of rolandic epilepsy and Panayiotopoulos syndrome. (Top) Onset of a rolandic seizure captured during routine sleep video-EEG of a 9-year-old girl. Right-sided centrotemporal spikes (oblique arrows) and brief (2 to 4 seconds) generalized discharges of sharp slow waves intermixed with small spikes occurred in the interictal EEG only during during sleep. The exact onset of the electrical ictal event is not clear but started in the right centrotemporal regions (open horizontal arrows) with 2- to 3-Hz slow waves and irregular, random, and monophasic medium-voltage spikes intermixed and superimposed on the slow waves. This activity tended to spread, and the amplitude of the spikes rapidly increased before the first clinical symptoms of left hemifacial convulsions, which occurred approximate 30 seconds from the onset of the EEG ictal changes (black vertical arrow). At age 18 years, she is entirely normal and is not taking medication. Modified from Reference 5 with the permission of the publisher. (Bottom) Onset of autonomic status epilepticus captured during routine video-EEG of a 4-year-old boy with Panayiotopoulos syndrome. High amplitude spikes and slow waves are recorded from the bifrontal regions (oblique arrows) before the onset of the electrical discharge, which is also purely bifrontal (open horizontal arrows). The first clinical symptoms (black vertical arrow) with three or four coughs and marked tachycardia appeared 13 minutes (see time at the bottom of the figure) after the onset of the electrical discharge, when this had become bilaterally diffuse. Subsequent clinical symptoms were tachycardia, ictus emeticus (without vomiting), and impairment of consciousness. No other ictal manifestations occurred until termination of the seizure with benzodiazepines 70 minutes after onset. Another lengthy autonomic seizure was recorded on video EEG 1 year later. The onset of symptoms was different with mainly tachycardia and agitation despite similar EEG manifestations. Modified from Reference 71 with the permission of the authors and the editor of *Epilepsy & Behavior*.

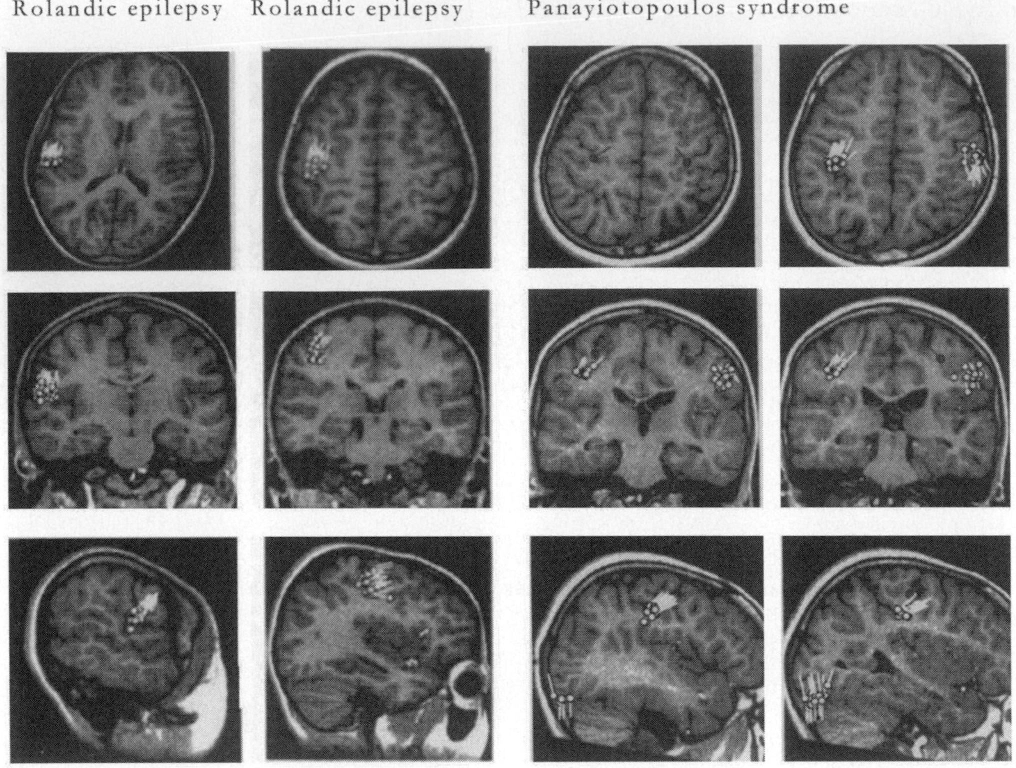

FIGURE 23-3

Magnetoencephalography (MEG) studies from two patients with rolandic epilepsy (left two columns) and a patient with Panayiotopoulos syndrome (right two columns). In rolandic epilepsy, equivalent current dipoles of spikes are located and concentrated in the rolandic regions and have regular directions. In Panayiotopoulos syndrome, equivalent current dipoles of spikes are located and concentrated bilaterally in the rolandic regions and right occipital area. The directions of each equivalent current dipole in each area are quite regular as if three small round toothbrushes are placed in each of the three areas. Small yellow circles represent locations and yellow arrows represent directions of equivalent current dipoles. Blue circles and arrows represent bilateral somatosensory evoked magnetic field. Figure courtesy of Dr. Osamu Kanazawa.

Panayiotopoulos syndrome can be defined as an idiopathic benign focal seizure disorder of childhood manifested with autonomic seizures, which are usually infrequent and often single. Characteristically, seizure semiology includes emetic symptoms, which may be combined with other autonomic features. Syncopal-like episodes may occur. Seizures are often prolonged (autonomic status epilepticus). Interictal EEG shows focal high amplitude sharp and slow wave complexes that, in serial EEGs, shift between various EEG electrodes.

Epidemiology (47, 50, 54, 59). Panayiotopoulos syndrome can start as early as 1 year of age or as late as 14 years of age. However, 76% of cases begin between 3 and 6 years of age and onset peaks at 4 to 5 years of age. It affects boys and girls equally. In those children with epilepsy who are 1–15 years old, prevalence is estimated to be 6%, rising to 13% in those 3–6 years old. Therefore, a clinician might expect to see at least one case of Panayiotopoulos syndrome for every three cases of rolandic epilepsy.

Clinical Manifestations (47, 50, 54, 56, 57, 59–65). Panayiotopoulos syndrome, being idiopathic, is expected to occur in children who are otherwise normal. Two-thirds of seizures occur during sleep, including daytime naps. No precipitants can be identified, although it has been noted that seizures appear to be particularly likely while traveling.

Seizures usually begin with emetic symptoms. These include one or more of nausea, retching, and vomiting. If asleep at seizure onset, the child may be found in bed retching or vomiting. However, many will first waken and complain of nausea. Seizures that occur when awake usually begin with a complaint of nausea often accompanied by behavioral changes, particularly agitation. During the seizure the child commonly vomits a few times; but occasionally vomiting may be repeated many times, sometimes over hours. Seizures in Panayiotopoulos syndrome without at least one feature of the "emetic triad" are rare but do occur.

Other autonomic features may occur concurrently with or follow the emetic features. Pallor is very common; cyanosis and flushing are less common (50). Pupillary abnormalities, especially mydriasis but also miosis, are frequently noticed by eyewitnesses, but will usually require prompting to obtain a report of them. Urinary and occasionally fecal incontinence may occur. A raised temperature may be suspected or measured during or immediately after a seizure and may represent a true ictal symptom, rather than being a precipitant of the seizure. Rarer ictal symptoms that have been reported include headache and other "cephalic sensations," hypersalivation, and coughing (50, 59).

Once it was realized that autonomic features dominated the seizures of Panayiotopoulos syndrome, it was natural to ask whether respiratory and cardiovascular irregularities might occur and, if so, whether these might be dangerous. Breathing changes are sometimes reported, particularly before convulsions (50). Tachycardia is certainly a feature of seizures recorded on EEG with simultaneous ECG recording (50, 66). Cardiorespiratory arrest during a typical seizure of Panayiotopoulos syndrome has been reported (67), and three other children with a diagnosis of Panayiotopoulos syndrome are also suspected to have had cardiorespiratory arrest (50).

When seizures occur in the awake state (or if the child awakens at the start of the seizure), the initial seizure symptoms usually occur in full consciousness (simple focal seizure). However, and after a variable time, consciousness usually becomes impaired (complex focal seizure), although some awareness and ability to respond is often retained. Some observers report behavioral changes such as restlessness, agitation, and terror, apparently in full consciousness (50, 59).

Some seizures in Panayiotopoulos syndrome include features suggestive of syncope, with the child becoming pale, flaccid, and unresponsive (50). Often these features occur along with more typical ones, but can occasionally occur in isolation. The term "ictal syncope" or "ictal syncopal-like episodes" have been used to denote these (50, 51, 53). It is not known if they are a result of transient hypoperfusion of the brain as in a true syncope.

When Panayiotopoulos syndrome was first described, ictal deviation of the eyes and often also the head were reported as prominent features. Reevaluation of the data has confirmed that such versive features are common. However, they usually occur around the time consciousness is becoming impaired, rather than at the start of the seizure.

Seizures in Panayiotopoulos syndrome often end in hemiconvulsions (around one-fifth of seizures) or GTCS (also around one-fifth of seizures).

An important feature of the seizures is that they are generally prolonged. Of those reported in the literature, 44% lasted for 30 minutes or more (maximum reported is 7 hours). These episodes, therefore, represent a form of nonconvulsive status epilepticus and might reasonably be classified as autonomic status epilepticus. They may end spontaneously or as short hemiconvulsions or GTCS. The child is expected to have returned to normal within a few hours of such episodes. Convulsive status epilepticus is exceptional. The mean duration of nonstatus seizures in Panayiotopoulos syndrome is around 9 minutes.

EEG Features (47, 50, 54–57, 59–65). The interictal EEG of Panayiotopoulos usually shows a normal background with high amplitude sharp and sharp and slow wave foci (functional spikes), similar in morphology if not location to those seen in rolandic epilepsy. Previously the occipital location of these was emphasized, along with their occurrence in long trains (occipital paroxysms) and abolition by central fixation (fixation-off sensitivity). It now appears that these features were overemphasized, and in Panayiotopoulos syndrome the characteristic functional spikes can occur in multiple locations, albeit with a posterior predominance. Multifocal spike foci are now considered a characteristic finding in Panayiotopoulos syndrome. These sometimes take the form of cloned-like, repetitive, mulifocal spike wave complexes in which repetitive spike or sharp and slow wave complexes appear concurrently in different brain locations of one or both hemispheres. The EEG abnormalities in Panayiotopoulos syndrome are accentuated in sleep. Figure 23-4 illustrates the variability of the interictal EEG in Panayiotopoulos syndrome.

Rarer EEG findings in Panayiotopoulos syndrome include small, sometimes inconspicuous, spikes, slow waves intermixed with small spikes and brief generalized discharges. Focal or diffuse slowing may be seen postictally. Occasionally, repeated EEGs can all be normal. Although fixation-off sensitivity is common, photosensitivity is exceptional.

The frequency, location, and persistence of spikes do not determine the clinical manifestations, severity, and frequency of seizures or the prognosis of Panayiotopoulos syndrome (53, 54).

A number of ictal EEGs in Panayiotopoulos syndrome have been reported showing focal discharges of rhythmic theta or delta, often with spikes. Onset is usually posterior (61, 66, 68–70), but may be anterior as shown in Figure 23-2 (61, 71).

In MEG combined with MRI, equivalent current dipoles cluster preferentially in cortical locations along the parietal-occipital, the calcarine, or the central fissure. The equivalent current dipole clustering may be unilateral or bilateral, monofocal or multifocal (33, 72, 73). These findings are in keeping with

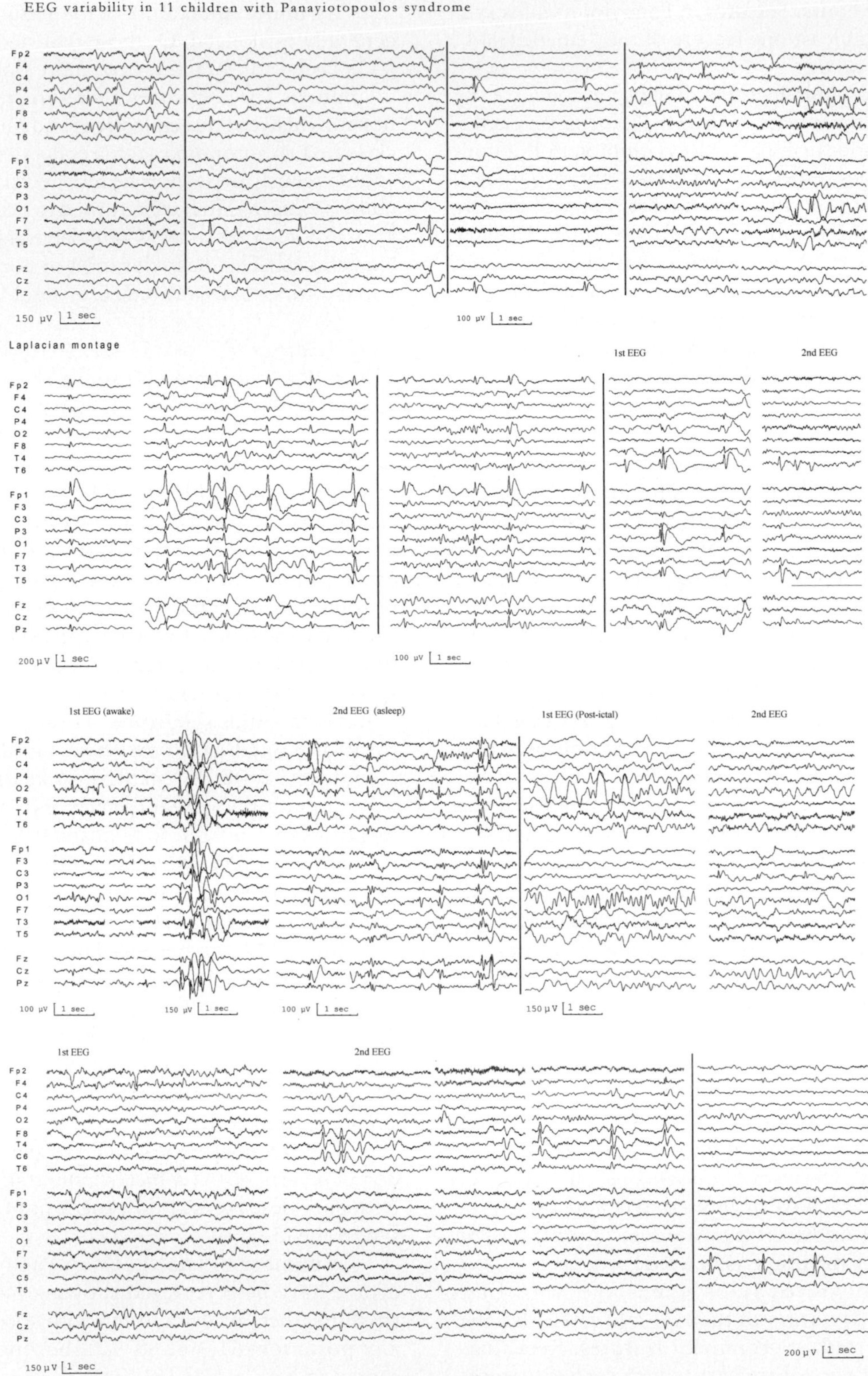

FIGURE 23-4

Interictal EEG variability in 11 children with Panayiotopoulos syndrome. Despite similar clinical features, EEG spikes are often located in different, often shifting, brain locations. EEG may show a single focus, but multifocal locations are more usual. Some interictal EEGs are similar to those seen in rolandic or idiopathic childhood occipital epilepsy. Brief generalized discharges may occur. Of particular interest are the clonedlike, repetitive, multifocal spike wave complexes; these are as common in children with single seizures as in those with multiple seizures. Vertical bars separate the EEGs of an individual patient.

the condition being a multifocal rather than a purely occipital epilepsy.

Diagnostic Evaluation and Differential Diagnosis. Panayiotopoulos syndrome is frequently mistaken for nonepileptic disorders and occasionally for other types of epilepsy. This reflects its unusual ictal clinical features and, for a benign epilepsy, its somewhat unusual interictal EEG features.

Because of the prolonged nature of seizures in Panayiotopoulos syndrome, many children present with it to emergency departments while they are still in an ictal state. However, if the main features of this are impaired consciousness and vomiting, an epileptic state may not even come into the differential diagnosis. Conditions such as encephalitis and meningitis are often considered. If the ictus terminates in a hemi- or generalized convulsion, this may merely strengthen the presumptive (but erroneous) diagnosis. Many such children end up intubated and treated in pediatric intensive care units with antibiotics and antiviral agents. The prolonged seizures of Panayiotopoulos syndrome may also be confused with acute confusional migraine and, if vomiting is particularly prominent, with cyclical vomiting syndrome or gastroenteritis. Some seizures may simply be dismissed as travel sickness.

The EEG of Panayiotopoulos syndrome may be similar or identical to that of idiopathic childhood occipital epilepsy or rolandic epilepsy, and these conditions may be mistakenly diagnosed if the clinical history is ignored (74). More importantly, multifocal spike discharges and cloned-like repetitive multifocal spike wave complexes may suggest more malignant epilepsies such as the Lennox-Gastaut syndrome, although clinically these conditions are completely different.

Unlike the other conditions described in this chapter, children with Panayiotopoulos syndrome commonly present to emergency departments while still seizing or in the immediate postictal period. Panayiotopoulos syndrome should be considered in the differential diagnosis of all previously well young children, especially those between the ages of 3 and 6 years, who have rapid onset of emetic symptoms followed by impaired (often fluctuating) consciousness. Eye or head deviation may be a useful finding. However, it may still be appropriate to manage the child for a suspected encephalopathy.

In the office setting, if Panayiotopoulos syndrome is suspected from the history, the most useful investigation is likely to be the EEG (including sleep if necessary). Symptomatic epilepsies may mimic Panayiotopoulos syndrome, so even if the history is typical, most authorities recommend neuroimaging. However, if MRI will require sedation or general anesthetic, CT may be appropriate. No other investigations are required.

Treatment. A recent consensus statement concluded that regular prophylactic AED medication was probably best reserved for children whose seizures were unusually frequent, distressing, or otherwise significantly interfering with the child's life (54). There are no high quality studies of what treatment is most appropriate. Carbamazepine and sodium valproate appear equally efficacious. Given the benign nature of the condition, it is particularly important to avoid adverse effects. Withdrawal of treatment after 1 or 2 seizure-free years is appropriate. The EEG is not helpful in deciding when to withdraw medication. Whether these recommendations will stand if it is confirmed that seizures in Panayiotopoulos syndrome can be associated with cardiorespiratory arrest remains to be seen.

Course and Prognosis. Total seizure count in Panayiotopoulos syndrome is usually low. Around one-third of patients have a single seizure and only 5% to 10% will have more than 10; sometimes seizures are very frequent. The duration of active seizures is short; remission usually occurring within 1 to 2 years from onset. About one-fifth of subjects with Panayiotopoulos syndrome will have one or more seizures typical of one of the other benign focal epilepsies of childhood, especially rolandic epilepsy (50, 53). However, the likelihood of seizures in adult life is probably no greater than in the general population.

Idiopathic Childhood Occipital Epilepsy (Late-Onset Childhood Occipital Epilepsy—Gastaut Type and Idiopathic Photosensitive Occipital Lobe Epilepsy)

Introduction and Definition. Idiopathic childhood occipital epilepsy (5, 52, 75–80) with and without photosensitivity was first established as an epileptic syndrome by Gastaut (75, 76). Recently, such subjects have generally been classified separately by the ILAE Task Force as late-onset childhood occipital epilepsy—Gastaut type and idiopathic photosensitive occipital lobe epilepsy (3). The likelihood of remission in these syndromes is considerably less than it is for rolandic epilepsy and Panayiotopoulos syndrome. Their inclusion in this chapter could reasonably be questioned. However, it is convenient to consider them here because undoubtedly some children with these conditions remit completely.

Idiopathic childhood occipital epilepsy can be defined as an idiopathic focal seizure disorder of childhood manifested mainly by elementary visual seizures and ictal blindness, which are often frequent and usually occur without impairment of consciousness. EEG shows occipital epileptiform abnormalities, particularly so-called occipital paroxysms. Idiopathic photosensitive occipital epilepsy is an idiopathic focal seizure disorder mainly of childhood manifested mainly by elementary visual seizures provoked by various forms of environmental light stimulation. EEG shows occipital or generalized photoparoxysmal responses to intermittent photic stimulation and often spontaneous, mainly occipital, epileptiform abnormalities.

Epidemiology. Idiopathic childhood occipital epilepsy is reported as starting in children as young as 3 years of age and as old as 15 years of age. Peak age of onset is around 8 years. Boys and girls are equally affected. Idiopathic photosensitive occipital epilepsy may start as early as the second year of life or as late as young adult life. However, it peaks at around 12 years of age. There is probably a slight female preponderance, but nowhere near as great as for photosensitivity per se. Both these epilepsies are rare. Panayiotopoulos estimated that idiopathic childhood occipital epilepsy accounted for about 2–7% of all benign focal epilepsies of childhood (78).

Clinical Manifestations. In both these syndromes the seizures are most characteristically manifested with elementary visual hallucinations. These usually consist of small multicolored circular patterns (79). Often they are reported as arising unilaterally in the periphery of a visual field, becoming larger and multiplying as the seizure progresses. They may move horizontally across the visual field, and other more complex movements are described. In some subjects normal vision is obscured by the hallucinations; in others it is retained. More complex visual hallucinations, such as of formed shapes and faces, and visual illusions may also occur but are much less common. Visual illusions include distortions of shape and distance.

After elementary visual hallucinations, ictal blindness is the second most common visual manifestation of seizures in these syndromes. It usually involves both visual fields but may be unilateral or involve only part of a hemifield. The subject usually reports everything as black, but occasionally everything goes white. Ictal blindness is usually an initial manifestation of the seizure but may follow visual hallucinations.

Other ictal ocular symptoms are relatively common. Some subjects report sensations of their eyes being tugged or of ocular pain. Eye deviation, often with simultaneous head deviation, is also common, possibly occurring in about 70% of cases. It usually follows after the hallucinations begin, although the latter may persist. Forced eye closure and eyelid blinking are other reported phenomena.

Most seizures are short lived, many lasting only a few seconds. However, some last a matter of minutes. Seizures with ictal blindness often last longer. Occasionally, seizures (including those with blindness) can last for hours (status amauroticus).

There is a particularly strong association between seizures in these epilepsies and headache. This can be an ictal or postictal phenomenon, although the latter is more common. It often has a migrainous character. Indeed, it is likely that in many cases the seizure provokes a true migraine. In idiopathic photosensitive occipital lobe epilepsy, seizure symptomatology may also include autonomic features, including emesis, which characterizes Panayiotopoulos syndrome (77, 81).

Consciousness is preserved during most seizures but occasionally may become impaired. This often precedes secondary generalization with GTCS. In exceptional cases spread to cause temporal lobe type symptoms is reported.

In idiopathic childhood occipital lobe epilepsy seizures are mainly diurnal and are usually quite frequent (often several each day or week). Occasional nocturnal seizures, often with hemiconvulsions or GTCS, are not infrequent.

In idiopathic photosensitive occipital lobe epilepsy, seizures are provoked by light factors. Video-game playing appears to be the most provocative, followed by watching TV. Some subjects are very photosensitive, and this is likely to be reflected in a high seizure frequency. Other subjects are less photosensitive and may have very few seizures. However, spontaneous seizures may also occur. It is also reported that some subjects with this epilepsy have other seizure types such as absences and myoclonic jerks provoked by photic factors.

EEG Features (5, 52, 75–82). The interictal EEG in both idiopathic childhood occipital epilepsy and idiopathic photosensitive occipital epilepsy is expected to have a normal background. In the former, occipital paroxysms are characteristic. However, in some subjects only isolated occipital spikes may be seen. Extraoccipital paroxysmal abnormalities may occur, but are much less common than in Panayiotopoulos syndrome. In some subjects EEG abnormalities may only be seen in sleep; occasionally both awake and sleep EEGs may be consistently normal. Figure 23-5 illustrates occipital paroxysms and fixation-off sensitivity.

The ictal EEG is expected to show attenuation of occipital paroxysms followed by appearance of an occipital discharge of fast rhythms, fast spikes, or both.

In idiopathic occipital lobe epilepsy there may be no spontaneous epileptiform abnormalities or else there may be occipital spikes or paroxysms. Extraoccipital epileptiform abnormalities may also be seen. Intermittent photic stimulation will, in all subjects, show occipital or generalized photoparoxysmal responses.

Diagnostic Evaluation and Differential Diagnosis. These syndromes, like all occipital epilepsies, are very prone to misdiagnosis as migraine. In part, this is understandable, because headache, often migrainous, as previously described, is common both ictally and postictally. However, the elementary visual hallucinations are unlike those of migraine. In the latter they tend to be black and white, rather than colored, and have jagged or sharp contours rather than being predominantly rounded.

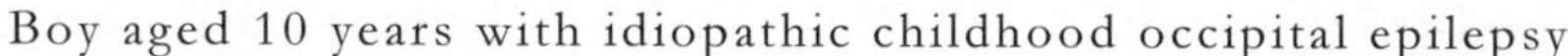

Boy aged 10 years with idiopathic childhood occipital epilepsy

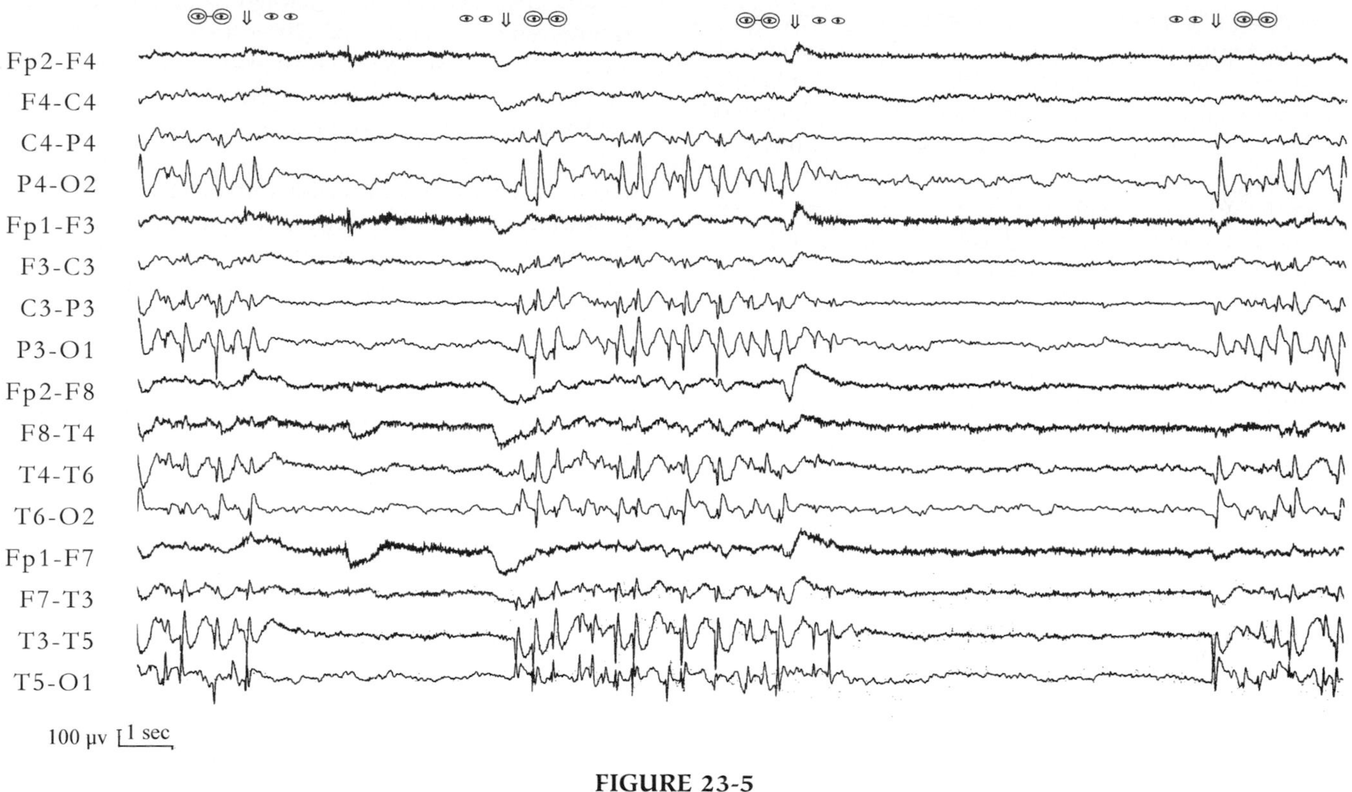

FIGURE 23-5

Occipital paroxysms with fixation off sensitivity of an 11-year-old boy with idiopathic childhood occipital epilepsy. Occipital paroxysms occur immediately after and as long as fixation and central vision are eliminated by any means (eyes closed, darkness, plus 10 spherical lenses, Ganzfeld stimulation). Under these conditions, even in the presence of light, eye opening does not inhibit the occipital paroxysms. Conversely, occipital paroxysms are totally inhibited by fixation and central vision. Symbols of eyes open without glasses indicate conditions in which fixation is possible. Symbols of eyes with glasses indicate conditions in which central vision and fixation are eliminated. At age 18 years, he is entirely normal and is not receiving medication.

These syndromes may mimic symptomatic occipital lobe epilepsies, and neuroimaging, preferably MRI, is indicated. No other investigations, except EEG, are routinely required.

Treatment. Given the frequency of seizures in idiopathic childhood occipital epilepsy, including the likelihood of occasional GTCS, regular AED treatment is considered necessary in most if not all subjects. There are no controlled studies comparing alternatives, although carbamazepine appears to be most often used in subjects who are not photosensitive. It is appropriate to attempt withdrawal after two seizure-free years, although there is a significant risk of relapse.

Some subjects with idiopathic photosensitive occipital lobe epilepsy who are only mildly photosensitive and who do not have spontaneous seizures can remain seizure free by avoiding precipitants. Others will require AED treatment. Broad spectrum agents, such as sodium valproate and levetiracetam, active against focal and generalized seizures and photosensitivity, would appear to be reasonable choices. However, it appears that carbamazepine, not usually considered a useful drug for photosensitivity, may sometimes be effective.

Course and Prognosis. The prognosis for both idiopathic childhood occipital epilepsy and idiopathic photosensitive occipital lobe epilepsy is variable. A majority of the former, perhaps 50% to 60%, have remission of seizures within 2–4 years of them starting. However, in a significant minority seizures will continue into adulthood. In those with idiopathic photosensitive occipital lobe epilepsy who are only mildly photosensitive and can control their exposure to relevant provoking factors, freedom from seizures may be easy. For others, particularly those who are highly photosensitive, the likelihood of seizures continuing into adult life is high.

Atypical Evolutions of the Benign Focal Epilepsies of Childhood

Less than 1% of children with rolandic epilepsy have so-called atypical evolutions (24, 32, 83). These include the development of severe linguistic, cognitive, or behavioral problems. If such problems develop in a child with rolandic epilepsy, a sleep EEG should be obtained, because continuous spike-and-wave during slow-wave sleep (CSWS) may be present. The Landau-Kleffner syndrome is sometimes said to develop from rolandic epilepsy. CSWS may also be seen in children with opercular status characterized by continuous positive or negative myoclonias around the mouth or elsewhere in the face and pseudobulbar problems. Atypical focal epilepsy of childhood in which other seizure types, including tonic and atypical absence seizures, occur may also develop in children with otherwise typical rolandic epilepsy.

There are also case reports of atypical evolutions in Panayiotopoulos syndrome, including the development of absences and drop attacks (32, 84, 85) and in idiopathic childhood occipital epilepsy with cognitive deterioration and CSWS (86).

Carbamazepine is sometimes implicated in precipitating such atypical evolutions (87, 88).

Other Described Benign Focal Epilepsies of Childhood

The syndromes discussed previously are the only benign focal epilepsies of childhood currently recognized by the ILAE. However, others have been proposed and are more or less well characterized. They include the following.

Benign Childhood Seizures with Affective Symptoms (89). This is reported to have its onset between 2 and 9 years of age and is characterized by multiple, usually short, daytime and nighttime seizures in which the predominant symptom appears to be fear or terror, accompanied by autonomic disturbances (pallor, sweating, abdominal pain, and salivation), arrest of speech, and mild impairment of consciousness with automatisms. Interictal EEG shows sharp and slow wave complexes similar to those in rolandic epilepsy but located in the frontotemporal and parietotemporal electrodes. Remission in 1 to 2 years from onset is expected. This is likely to be an intermediate phenotype between Panayiotopoulos syndrome and rolandic epilepsy.

Benign Childhood Epilepsy with Parietal Spikes and Frequent Giant Somatosensory Evoked Potentials (28, 90). This putative disorder is mainly defined by its interictal EEG features reflected in its name. These features are, however, said to often be associated with a phenotype characterized by mainly daytime versive seizures, which are infrequent and have an excellent prognosis.

Benign Childhood Focal Seizures Associated with Frontal or Midline Spikes (5). Again this putative disorder is mainly defined by its interictal EEG features. These EEG features can be seen in children with febrile seizures, rolandic epilepsy, Panayiotopoulos syndrome, and idiopathic childhood occipital epilepsy.

Benign Focal Epilepsy in Infants with Central and Vertex Spikes and Waves During Sleep (91, 92). Benign focal epilepsy in infants with central and vertex spikes and waves during sleep has been recently described as a new benign syndrome. In terms of age of onset, it is on the borderline between benign infantile seizures and Panayiotopoulos syndrome. Age at onset is in the first 2 years of life with both sexes equally affected. Infants are normal and all tests other than EEG are normal. Seizures consist mainly of staring, motor arrest, facial cyanosis, loss of consciousness, and stiffening of the arms. Clonic convulsions and automatisms are rare. Duration is from 1 to 5 minutes. Seizures are mainly diurnal (but may also occur during sleep) and may occur in clusters, but are generally infrequent (1–3 per year). Interictal EEG abnormalities are seen only in non-REM sleep and consist of small, mostly singular, spikes and waves localized at the vertex and central electrodes.

There is a strong family history of epilepsy with benign epilepsies prevailing. The prognosis is excellent with remission of seizures, normal development, and normalization of the EEG before the age of 4 years.

Benign Focal Seizures of Adolescence (5, 93). This syndrome of the second decade, and predominantly occurring in males, features a single seizure or a single cluster of seizures over a period of up to 36 hours. The seizures are mainly diurnal, with consciousness initially preserved. The main manifestations are focal clonic jerking, usually without a Jacksonian march, and somatosensory symptoms. Secondary GTCS occur in about 50% of cases. EEG and brain neuroimaging are normal. The prognosis is excellent and treatment is not required.

References

1. Commission on Classification and Terminology of the International League Against Epilepsy. Proposal for revised classification of epilepsies and epileptic syndromes. *Epilepsia* 1989; 30:389–399.
2. Geelhoed M, Boerrigter AO, Camfield P, Geerts AT, et al. The accuracy of outcome prediction models for childhood-onset epilepsy. *Epilepsia* 2005; 46:1526–1532.
3. Engel J Jr. A proposed diagnostic scheme for people with epileptic seizures and with epilepsy: Report of the ILAE Task Force on Classification and Terminology. *Epilepsia* 2001; 42:796–803.
4. Riikonen R. Long-term outcome of patients with West syndrome. *Brain Dev* 2001; 23:683–687.

5. Panayiotopoulos CP. Benign childhood focal seizures and related epileptic syndromes. In: Panayiotopoulos CP, ed. *The Epilepsies: Seizures, Syndromes and Management*. Oxford: Bladon Medical Publishing, 2005:223–269.
6. Panayiotopoulos CP. Benign childhood partial epilepsies: benign childhood seizure susceptibility syndromes [editorial]. *J Neurol Neurosurg Psychiatry* 1993; 56:2–5.
7. Vadlamudi L, Harvey AS, Connellan MM, Milne RL, et al. Is benign rolandic epilepsy genetically determined? *Ann.Neurol* 2004; 56:129–132.
8. Bray PF,.Wiser WC. Evidence for a genetic etiology of temporal-central abnormalities in focal epilepsy. *N Engl J Med* 1964; 271:926–933.
9. Heijbel J, Blom S, Rasmuson M. Benign epilepsy of childhood with centrotemporal EEG foci: a genetic study. *Epilepsia* 1975; 16:285–293.
10. Neubauer BA, Hahn A, Stephani U, Doose H. Clinical spectrum and genetics of Rolandic epilepsy. *Adv Neurol* 2002; 89:475–479.
11. Neubauer BA, Fiedler B, Himmelein B, Kampfer F, et al. Centrotemporal spikes in families with rolandic epilepsy: linkage to chromosome 15q14. *Neurology* 1998; 51:1608–1612.
12. Scheffer IE, Berkovic SF. The genetics of human epilepsy. *Trends Pharmacol Sci* 2003; 24:428–433.
13. Gutierrez-Delicado E, Serratosa JM. Genetics of the epilepsies. *Curr Opin Neurol* 2004; 17:147–153.
14. Hirose S, Mitsudome A, Okada M, Kaneko S. Genetics of idiopathic epilepsies. *Epilepsia* 2005; 46 Suppl 1:38–43.
15. Coppola G, Castaldo P, Miraglia DG, Bellini G, et al. A novel KCNQ2 K+ channel mutation in benign neonatal convulsions and centrotemporal spikes. *Neurology* 2003; 61:131–134.
16. Berkovic SF, Heron SE, Giordano L, Marini C, et al. Benign familial neonatal-infantile seizures: characterization of a new sodium channelopathy. *Ann Neurol* 2004; 55:550–557.
17. Roll P, Massacrier A, Pereira S, Robaglia-Schlupp A, et al. New human sodium/glucose cotransporter gene (KST1): identification, characterization, and mutation analysis in ICCA (infantile convulsions and choreoathetosis) and BFIC (benign familial infantile convulsions) families. *Gene* 2002; 285:141–148.
18. Guerrini R, Bonanni P, Nardocci N, Parmeggiani L, et al. Autosomal recessive rolandic epilepsy with paroxysmal exercise-induced dystonia and writer's cramp: delineation of the syndrome and gene mapping to chromosome 16p12-11.2. *Ann Neurol* 1999; 45:344–352.
19. Panayiotopoulos CP. Benign childhood epilepsy with centrotemporal spikes or Rolandic seizures. In: Panayiotopoulos CP, ed. *Benign Childhood Partial Seizures and Related Epileptic Syndromes*. London: John Libbey & Company, 1999:33–100.
20. Dalla Bernardina B, Sgro M, Fejerman N. Epilepsy with centro-temporal spikes and related syndromes. In: Roger J, Bureau M, Dravet C, Genton P, et al, eds. *Epileptic Syndromes in Infancy, Childhood and Adolescence*. 4th ed. Montrouge, France: John Libbey Eurotext, 2005:203–225.
21. Beaussart M, Loiseau P, Roger H. The discovery of "benign rolandic epilepsy." In: Berkovic SF, Genton P, Hirsch E, Picard F, eds. *Genetics of Focal Epilepsies*. London: John Libbey & Company, 1999:3–6.
22. Lombroso CT. Sylvian seizures and midtemporal spike foci in children. *Arch Neurol* 1967; 17:52–59.
23. Bouma PA, Bovenkerk AC, Westendorp RG, Brouwer OF. The course of benign partial epilepsy of childhood with centrotemporal spikes: a meta-analysis. *Neurology* 1997; 48:430–437.
24. Fejerman N, Caraballo R, Tenembaum SN. Atypical evolutions of benign localization-related epilepsies in children: are they predictable? *Epilepsia* 2000; 41:380–390.
25. Gregory DL,.Wong PK. Clinical relevance of a dipole field in rolandic spikes. *Epilepsia* 1992; 33:36–44.
26. Yoshinaga H, Amano R, Oka E, Ohtahara S. Dipole tracing in childhood epilepsy with special reference to rolandic epilepsy. *Brain Topogr* 1992; 4:193–199.
27. De Marco P, Tassinari CA. Extreme somatosensory evoked potential (ESEP): an EEG sign forecasting the possible occurrence of seizures in children. Epilepsia 1981; 22:569–575.
28. Fonseca LC, Tedrus GM. Somatosensory evoked spikes and epileptic seizures: a study of 385 cases. *Clin Electroencephalogr* 2000; 31:71–75.
29. Gibbs F A, Gibbs EL. Atlas of electroencephalography. Vol 2: Epilepsy. Reading, MA: Addison-Wesley, 1952:214–290.
30. Smith JMB, Kellaway P. Central (Rolandic) foci in children: an analysis of 200 cases. *Electroencephalogr Clin Neurophysiol* 1964; 17:460–461.
31. Eeg-Olofsson O. The development of the electroencephalogram in normal children and adolescents from the age of 1 through 21 years. *Acta Paediatr Scand Suppl* 1970; 208.
32. Kanazawa O. Benign rolandic epilepsy and related epileptic syndromes: electrophysiological studies including magnetoencephalography in ictal and interictal phenomena. In: Benjamin SM, ed. *Trends in Epilepsy Research*. New York: Nova Science Publishers,Inc., 2005. pp 19–54.
33. Minami T, Gondo K, Yamamoto T, Yanai S, et al. Magnetoencephalographic analysis of rolandic discharges in benign childhood epilepsy. *Ann Neurol* 1996; 39:326–334.
34. Gelisse P, Corda D, Raybaud C, Dravet C, et al. Abnormal neuroimaging in patients with benign epilepsy with centrotemporal spikes. *Epilepsia* 2003; 44:372–378.
35. Gelisse P, Genton P, Raybaud C, Thiry A, et al. Benign childhood epilepsy with centrotemporal spikes and hippocampal atrophy. *Epilepsia* 1999; 40:1312–1315.
36. Lundberg S, Eeg-Olofsson O, Raininko R, Eeg-Olofsson KE. Hippocampal asymmetries and white matter abnormalities on MRI in benign childhood epilepsy with centrotemporal spikes. *Epilepsia* 1999; 40:1808–1815.
37. Lundberg S, Weis J, Eeg-Olofsson O, Raininko R. Hippocampal region asymmetry assessed by 1H-MRS in rolandic epilepsy. *Epilepsia* 2003; 44:205–210.
38. Peters JM, Camfield CS, Camfield PR. Population study of benign rolandic epilepsy: Is treatment needed? *Neurology* 2001; 57:537–539.
39. Loiseau P, Pestre M, Dartigues JF, Commenges D, et al. Long-term prognosis in two forms of childhood epilepsy: typical absence seizures and epilepsy with rolandic (centrotemporal) EEG foci. *Ann Neurol* 1983; 13:642–648.
40. Deonna T, Zesiger P, Davidoff V, Maeder M, et al. Benign partial epilepsy of childhood: a longitudinal neuropsychological and EEG study of cognitive function. *Dev Med Child Neurol* 2000; 42:595–603.
41. Papavasiliou A, Mattheou D, Bazigou H, Kotsalis C, et al. Written language skills in children with benign childhood epilepsy with centrotemporal spikes. *Epilepsy Behav* 2005; 6:50–58.
42. Vinayan KP, Biji V, Thomas SV. Educational problems with underlying neuropsychological impairment are common in children with benign epilepsy of childhood with centrotemporal spikes (BECTS). *Seizure* 2005; 14:207–212.
43. Fonseca LC, Tedrus GM, Tonelotto JM, Antunes TDA, Chiodi MG. [School performance in children with benign childhood epilepsy with centrotemporal spikes]. *Arq Neuropsiquiatr* 2004; 62:459–462.
44. Baglietto MG, Battaglia FM, Nobili L, Tortorelli S, et al. Neuropsychological disorders related to interictal epileptic discharges during sleep in benign epilepsy of childhood with centrotemporal or Rolandic spikes. *Dev Med Child Neurol* 2001; 43:407–412.
45. Yung AW, Park YD, Cohen MJ, Garrison TN. Cognitive and behavioral problems in children with centrotemporal spikes. *Pediatr Neurol* 2000; 23:391–395.
46. Croona C, Kihlgren M, Lundberg S, Eeg-Olofsson O, et al. Neuropsychological findings in children with benign childhood epilepsy with centrotemporal spikes. *Dev Med Child Neurol* 1999; 41:813–818.
47. Panayiotopoulos CP. Vomiting as an ictal manifestation of epileptic seizures and syndromes. *J Neurol Neurosurg Psychiatr* 1988; 51:1448–1451.
48. Ferrie CD, Grunewald RA. Panayiotopoulos syndrome: a common and benign childhood epilepsy [commentary]. *Lancet* 2001; 357:821–823.
49. Koutroumanidis M. Panayiotopoulos syndrome: a common benign but underdiagnosed and unexplored early childhood seizure syndrome [editorial]. *BMJ* 2002; 324:1228–1229.
50. Panayiotopoulos CP. Panayiotopoulos syndrome: a common and benign childhood epileptic syndrome. London: John Libbey & Company, 2002.
51. Panayiotopoulos CP. Autonomic seizures and autonomic status epilepticus peculiar to childhood: diagnosis and management. *Epilepsy Behav* 2004; 5:286–295.
52. Covanis A, Ferrie CD, Koutroumanidis M, Oguni H, et al. Panayiotopoulos syndrome and Gastaut type idiopathic childhood occipital epilepsy. In: Roger J, Bureau M, Dravet C, Genton P, et al, eds. *Epileptic Syndromes in Infancy, Childhood and Adolescence*. 4th ed, with video. Montrouge, France: John Libbey Eurotext, 2005:227–253.
53. Panayiotopoulos CP. Panayiotopoulos syndrome. In: Panayiotopoulos CP, ed. *The Epilepsies: Seizures, Syndromes and Management*. Oxford: Bladon Medical Publishing, 2005:235–248.
54. Ferrie C, Caraballo R, Covanis A, Demirbilek V, et al. Panayiotopoulos syndrome: a consensus view. *Dev Med Child Neurol* 2006; 48:236–240.
55. Panayiotopoulos CP. Inhibitory effect of central vision on occipital lobe seizures. *Neurology* 1981; 31:1330–1333.
56. Panayiotopoulos CP. Benign childhood epilepsy with occipital paroxysms: a 15-year prospective study. *Ann Neurol* 1989; 26:51–56.
57. Panayiotopoulos CP. Extraoccipital benign childhood partial seizures with ictal vomiting and excellent prognosis. *J Neurol Neurosurg Psychiatry* 1999; 66:82–85.
58. Ferrie CD. Nonconvulsive status epilepticus in the benign focal epilepsies of childhood with particular reference to autonomic status epilepticus in Panayiotopoulos syndrome. *Epileptic Disord* 2005; 7:291–293.
59. Sanders S, Rowlinson S, Manidakis I, Ferrie CD, et al. The contribution of the EEG technologists in the diagnosis of Panayiotopoulos syndrome (susceptibility to early onset benign childhood autonomic seizures). *Seizure* 2004; 13:565–573.
60. Ferrie CD, Beaumanoir A, Guerrini R, Kivity S, et al. Early-onset benign occipital seizure susceptibility syndrome. *Epilepsia* 1997; 38:285–293.
61. Oguni H, Hayashi K, Imai K, Hirano Y, et al. Study on the early-onset variant of benign childhood epilepsy with occipital paroxysms otherwise described as early-onset benign occipital seizure susceptibility syndrome. *Epilepsia* 1999; 40:1020–1030.
62. Caraballo R, Cersosimo R, Medina C, Fejerman N. Panayiotopoulos-type benign childhood occipital epilepsy: a prospective study. *Neurology* 2000; 55:1096–1100.
63. Kivity S, Ephraim T, Weitz R, Tamir A. Childhood epilepsy with occipital paroxysms: clinical variants in 134 patients. *Epilepsia* 2000; 41:1522–1523.
64. Lada C, Skiadas K, Theodorou V, Covanis A. A study of 43 patients with Panayiotopoulos syndrome: a common and benign childhood seizure suceptibility. *Epilepsia* 2003; 44:81–88.
65. Ohtsu M, Oguni H, Hayashi K, Funatsuka M, et al. EEG in children with early-onset benign occipital seizure susceptibility syndrome: Panayiotopoulos syndrome. *Epilepsia* 2003; 44:435–442.
66. Parisi P, Ferri R, Pagani J, Cecili M, et al. Ictal video-polysomnography and EEG spectral analysis in a child with severe Panayiotopoulos syndrome. *Epileptic.Disord* 2005; 7:333–339.
67. Verrotti A, Salladini C, Trotta D, di Corcia G, et al. Ictal cardiorespiratory arrest in Panayiotopoulos syndrome. *Neurology* 2005; 64:1816–1817.
68. Beaumanoir A. Semiology of occipital seizures in infants and children. In: Andermann F, Beaumanoir A, Mira L, Roger J, et al, eds. *Occipital Seizures and Epilepsies in Children*. London: John Libbey and Company, 1993:71–86.
69. Vigevano F, Lispi ML, Ricci S. Early onset benign occipital susceptibility syndrome: video-EEG documentation of an illustrative case. *Clin Neurophysiol* 2000; 111 Suppl 2:S81–S86.
70. Demirbilek V, Dervent A. Panayiotopoulos syndrome: video-EEG illustration of a typical seizure. *Epileptic.Disord* 2004; 6:121–124.

71. Koutroumanidis M, Rowlinson S, Sanders S. Recurrent autonomic status epilepticus in Panayiotopoulos syndrome: video/EEG studies. *Epilepsy Behav* 2005; 7:543–547.
72. Kanazawa O, Tohyama J, Akasaka N, Kamimura T. A magnetoencephalographic study of patients with Panayiotopoulos syndrome. *Epilepsia* 2005; 46:1106–1113.
73. Sugita K, Kato Y, Sugita K, Kato M, Tanaka Y. Magnetoencephalographic analysis in children with Panayiotopoulos syndrome. *J Child Neurol* 2005; 20:616–618.
74. Covanis A, Lada C, Skiadas K. Children with rolandic spikes and ictus emeticus: Rolandic epilepsy or Panayiotopoulos syndrome? *Epileptic Disord* 2003; 5:139–143.
75. Gastaut H. A new type of epilepsy: benign partial epilepsy of childhood with occipital spike-waves. *Clin Electroencephalogr* 1982; 13:13–22.
76. Gastaut H, Zifkin BG. Benign epilepsy of childhood with occipital spike and wave complexes. In: Andermann F, Lugaresi E, eds. *Migraine and Epilepsy*. Boston: Butterworths, 1987:47–81.
77. Guerrini R, Dravet C, Genton P, Bureau M, et al. Idiopathic photosensitive occipital lobe epilepsy. *Epilepsia* 1995; 36:883–891.
78. Panayiotopoulos CP. Occipital seizures and related epileptic syndromes. In: Panayiotopoulos CP, ed. *Benign Childhood Partial Seizures and Related Epileptic Syndromes*. London: John Libbey & Company, 1999:101–228.
79. Panayiotopoulos CP. Elementary visual hallucinations, blindness, and headache in idiopathic occipital epilepsy: differentiation from migraine. *J Neurol Neurosurg Psychiatry* 1999; 66:536–540.
80. Panayiotopoulos CP. Idiopathic photosensitive occipital lobe epilepsy. In: Panayiotopoulos CP, ed. *The Epilepsies: Seizures, Syndromes and Management*. Oxford: Bladon Medical Publishing, 2005:469–474.
81. Guerrini R, Bonanni P, Parmeggiani A. Idiopathic photosensitive occipital lobe epilepsy. In: Gilman S, ed. *Medlink Neurology*. San Diego: Arbor Publishing, 2005.
82. Panayiotopoulos CP. Fixation-off, scotosensitive, and other visual-related epilepsies. *Adv Neurol* 1998; 75:139–157.
83. Fejerman N. Atypical evolutions of benign partial epilepsies in children. *Int Pediatr* 1996; 11:351–356.
84. Caraballo RH, Astorino F, Cersosimo R, Soprano AM, et al. Atypical evolution in childhood epilepsy with occipital paroxysms (Panayiotopoulos type). *Epileptic Disord* 2001; 3:157–162.
85. Ferrie CD, Koutroumanidis M, Rowlinson S, Sanders S, et al. Atypical evolution of Panayiotopoulos syndrome: a case report [published with video- sequences]. *Epileptic Disord* 2002; 4:35–42.
86. Tenembaum S, Deonna T, Fejerman N, Medina C, et al. Continuous spike-waves and dementia in childhood epilepsy with occipital paroxysms. *J Epilepsy* 1997; 10:139–145.
87. Corda D, Gelisse P, Genton P, Dravet C, et al. Incidence of drug-induced aggravation in benign epilepsy with centrotemporal spikes. *Epilepsia* 2001; 42:754–759.
88. Kikumoto K, Yoshinaga H, Oka M, Ito M, et al. EEG and seizure exacerbation induced by carbamazepine in Panayiotopoulos syndrome. *Epileptic Disord* 2006; 8:53–56.
89. Dalla Bernardina B, Colamaria V, Chiamenti C, Capovilla G, et al. Benign partial epilepsy with affective symptoms ("benign psychomotor epilepsy"). In: Roger J, Bureau M, Dravet C, Dreifuss FE, et al, eds. *Epileptic Syndromes in Infancy, Childhood and Adolescence*. London: John Libbey & Company, 1992: 219–223.
90. Tassinari CA, De Marco P. Benign partial epilepsy with extreme somato-sensory evoked potentials. In: Roger J, Bureau M, Dravet C, Dreifuss FE, et al, eds. *Epileptic Syndromes in Infancy, Childhood and Adolescence*. London: John Libbey & Company, 1992:225–229.
91. Bureau M, Cokar O, Maton B, Genton P, Dravet C. Sleep-related, low voltage Rolandic and vertex spikes: an EEG marker of benignity in infancy-onset focal epilepsies. *Epileptic Disord* 2002; 4:15–22.
92. Capovilla G, Beccaria F, Montagnini A. "Benign focal epilepsy in infancy with vertex spikes and waves during sleep." Delineation of the syndrome and recalling as "benign infantile focal epilepsy with midline spikes and waves during sleep" (BIMSE). *Brain Dev* 2006; 28:85–91.
93. Loiseau P, Jallon P, Wolf P. Isolated partial seizures of adolescence. In: Roger J, Bureau M, Dravet C, Genton P, et al, eds. *Epileptic Syndromes in Infancy, Childhood and Adolescence*. 4th ed. Montrouge: John Libbey Eurotext, 2005:359–362.
94. Grosso S, Orrica A, Galli L, Di Bartolo R, Sorrentio V, Balestri P. SCN1A mutations associated with a typical Panayiotopoulos syndrome. *Neurology* 2007; 69:609–611.

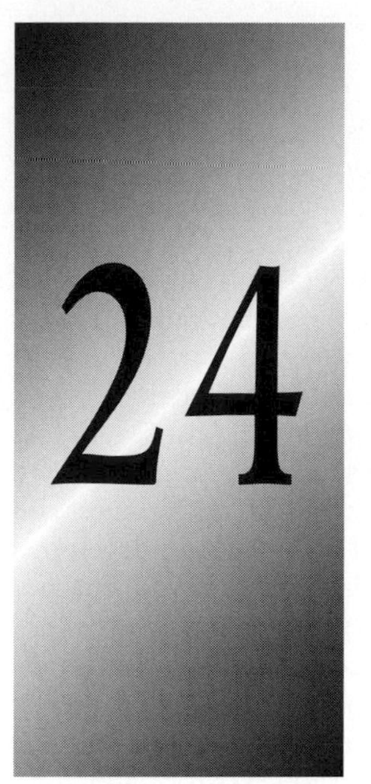

24 The Landau-Kleffner Syndrome and Epilepsy with Continuous Spike-Waves during Sleep

James J. Riviello, Jr.
Stavros Hadjiloizou

The Landau-Kleffner syndrome (LKS) and epilepsy with continuous spikewaves during slow-wave sleep (CSWS) are recognized as specific epilepsy syndromes by the International League Against Epilepsy (ILAE) (1–3). They were first classified as epilepsies and syndromes undetermined as to whether they are focal or generalized (2). They are now classified as an epileptic encephalopathy, defined as disorders in which the epileptiform abnormalities may contribute to progressive dysfunction (3). Other epileptic encephalopathies are early myoclonic encephalopathy, Ohtahara syndrome, West syndrome, Dravet syndrome, myoclonic status in nonprogressive encephalopathies, and the Lennox-Gastaut syndrome (3). LKS and CSWS are also considered special syndromes of status epilepticus (4).

Overt clinical seizures are not present in all children with LKS or CSWS. Both syndromes typically present with regression in cognitive abilities, either a language regression, predominantly in LKS (1, 5), or a more global neuropsychiatric regression in CSWS (5–7), with each demonstrating marked sleep-activated epileptiform activity on electroencepahlogram (EEG). Patry et al defined the term "electrical status epilepticus of sleep" (ESES) (6) before the identification of CSWS by the ILAE. However, ESES and CSWS are synonymous terms, and "status epilepticus during sleep" (SES) is also used (8). The strict definition of ESES requires the presence of sleep-activated epileptiform activity in greater than 85% of slow-wave sleep (6, 7). Veggiotti and colleagues emphasized the difference between the EEG pattern of CSWS and the epileptic syndrome of CSWS (9). Not all patients with a sleep-activated pattern consistent with ESES have the age-related epileptic syndrome of CSWS. We prefer using the term ESES to describe the EEG, and CSWS to describe the epileptic syndrome.

Regression in intellectual or cognitive abilities, associated with behavioral problems, is the hallmark of these syndromes, and regression may even be the presenting manifestation. In general, cognitive regression should always raise the suspicion of a sleep-activated epileptic encephalopathy, especially in those with underlying developmental or neurological disorders. LKS and CSWS may respond to treatment with the standard antiepileptic drugs (AEDs) but often require other therapies, such as corticosteroids (10–15), high dose benzodiazepine (16, 17), and other immune-modulating therapies such as intravenous immunoglobulin (IVIG) (18–21), or the ketogenic diet (22, 23).

EPIDEMIOLOGY

LKS and CSWS are rare syndromes among the pediatric epilepsy syndromes. In a recent 20-year epidemiologic study of childhood epilepsy, Kramer and colleagues reported LKS and CSWS in 0.2% each, compared with West syndrome in 9%, myoclonic seizures in 2.2%, and Lennox-Gastaut syndrome in 1.5% (24). Ohtahara syndrome and myoclonic astatic epilepsy also occurred in 0.2% each.

In a review of LKS, Smith and Hoeppner (25) noted that only 81 cases had been reported between 1956 and 1980, whereas 117 cases were reported between 1980 and 1990. For ESES, 19 cases had been reported between 1971 and 1984 by Tassinari et al and another 25 were reported in the medical literature (7).

CLINICAL MANIFESTATIONS

The onset of LKS usually occurs in children older than 4 years (26), with a range of 3 to 10 years (27). LKS may first manifest as an apparent word deafness or a verbal auditory agnosia. Seizures and behavior disturbances, particularly attention deficits and hyperactivity, each occur in approximately two-thirds of children with LKS (5). The majority of cases are classified as idiopathic, although any pathologic process affecting the auditory cortex may cause LKS. Symptomatic cases have been described (see the section on differential diagnosis), and we have seen symptomatic LKS caused by a left temporal oligodendroglioma, with clinical improvement noted after resection.

The classical features of LKS are a verbal auditory agnosia (word deafness) followed by language regression, seizures, or both in a previously normal child who has an epileptiform EEG. An important corollary is normal hearing, because a central disorder cannot be diagnosed in the presence of peripheral dysfunction. Children with sleep-activated epileptiform activity without the classic features of LKS have been referred to as children with LKS variant (28). These variants include children with involvement of more anterior language areas with dysfunction characterized by oral-motor apraxia, sialorhea, seizures, and an abnormal EEG (29), referred to as anterior LKS; children with pervasive developmental disorder (PDD, autism) with language regression and abnormal EEGs (30–32); and children with congenital aphasias (33), also called developmental language disorders, with or without clinical regression but with epileptiform EEGs, also referred to as developmental LKS.

The evaluation of LKS should include a baseline history, physical examination, sleep-deprived EEG, a formal neuropsychological evaluation, neuroimaging, with magnetic resonance imaging (MRI) preferred, long-term video-EEG monitoring (LTM), and if needed, dipole analysis, functional neuroimaging with single-photon emission computed tomography (SPECT), positron emission tomography (PET), or magnetoencephalography (MEG), and the frequency-modulated auditory evoked response (FM-AER). The FM-AER is an evoked response that tests receptive language function and is usually absent with a verbal auditory agnosia (34).

The hallmark of CSWS is regression in cognitive functioning and behavior, but not primarily language, as occurs in LKS. Although children with CSWS commonly have seizures, these may not be frequent. Tassinari et al reported 29 children with CSWS (7); all except 1 child had seizures, 1 had a single seizure, and 1 had only three seizures. Eighteen of these children had normal, and 11 had abnormal, psychomotor development before onset. In the 18 with normal development, all had severe loss of IQ and behavioral disturbances, including decreased attention span, hyperactivity; aggression, difficulties with interaction and inhibition, and two children developed a psychotic state. In the 11 with abnormal psychomotor development, mental deterioration occurred in all, 3 developed a marked hyperactivity, and 1 showed "massive regression" including language and a loss of interest in all activities. Intellectual regression occurs in virtually all children, although we have seen several in which no regression has been seen. Attention deficits and hyperactivity occur in the majority, and language disturbances, aggression, disinhibition, emotional lability, anxiety, and psychotic behavior may also occur. An expressive aphasia occurs, in contrast to LKS, which is characterized by verbal auditory agnosia (35).

The presence of ESES alone does not diagnose these specific epileptic syndromes. These are identified by the combination of the clinical manifestations and EEG findings. Both LKS and CSWS may have the EEG pattern of ESES; LKS clinically consists predominantly of a language regression, with a more focal ESES pattern, whereas CSWS is characterized clinically by a more global neurobehavioral disorder with a more generalized EEG pattern (36, 37). LKS and ESES have been classified as benign epileptic syndromes; that term refers only to the evolution of the actual seizures and EEG patterns over time. Given the devastating neuropsychological deficits that occur, we prefer to consider these malignant epileptic syndromes.

EEG FEATURES (INTERICTAL, ICTAL)

The EEG pattern of ESES may be seen with both syndromes, but not all children with the ESES pattern may have these specific syndromes. Veggiotti et al emphasized the difference between the EEG pattern of CSWS and the epileptic syndrome of CSWS (9). In their series of 32 patients with CSWS, only 10 (34%) had features of the CSWS syndrome, whereas in the remainder, 4 had LKS, 3 had the acquired opercular syndrome, and 15 had symptomatic epilepsy. Van Hirtum-Das and colleagues identified 102 children with ESES, using a spike-wave index greater than 25% (38). In this group, only 18% had LKS. Although CSWS was named for sleep activation during slow-wave sleep, this term is misleading because EEG activation occurs in non-rapid-eye movement (NREM) sleep, typically starting in drowsiness (8). This is our experience as well. The spike-waves become fragmented during REM sleep, when focality may bc seen, and the spike-wave index usually decreases below 25% (8). Upon awakening, the spike-wave frequency dramatically decreases again.

The EEG in LKS shows bilateral, multifocal spikes and spike-and-wave discharges, occurring usually in the posterior regions, especially the more posterior regions, with a marked activation during NREM sleep (Figure 24-1). However, discharges occur in many locations and may even be generalized. The strict definition of ESES (spike-wave index greater than 85%) is not absolutely necessary to diagnose LKS, because the spike-wave index may reach only 50% (25). The EEG may improve over time, either spontaneously or with treatment (39, 40).

There is speculation that EEG abnormalities are more likely present during the actual period of language regression, with subsequent EEG improvement. This may have been more likely in the past, before the recognition of LKS and CSWS. In the first 20 patients diagnosed with LKS or LKS variant at Children's Hospital, Boston, reviewed by Bolanos et al, the EEG became normal in 4 patients within a year (39).

Guilhoto and Morrell reported that when the ESES pattern was more focal, the LKS with language regression was the most prominent symptom, whereas when the ESES pattern was more generalized, the CSWS syndrome with generalized neurobehavioral dysfunction was the predominant symptoms (36). Guilhoto and colleagues subsequently reported 17 children with ESES. Five had LKS and the EEG showed diffuse activity with accentuation in the centrotemporal region, whereas the others had widespread discharges (37). Therefore, LKS and CSWS may have similar clinical and electrographic features. The EEG abnormalities in LKS may be an epiphenomenon (41).

PATHOPHYSIOLOGY

The underlying mechanisms of LKS and CSWS are complex and not yet specifically identified. However, it is

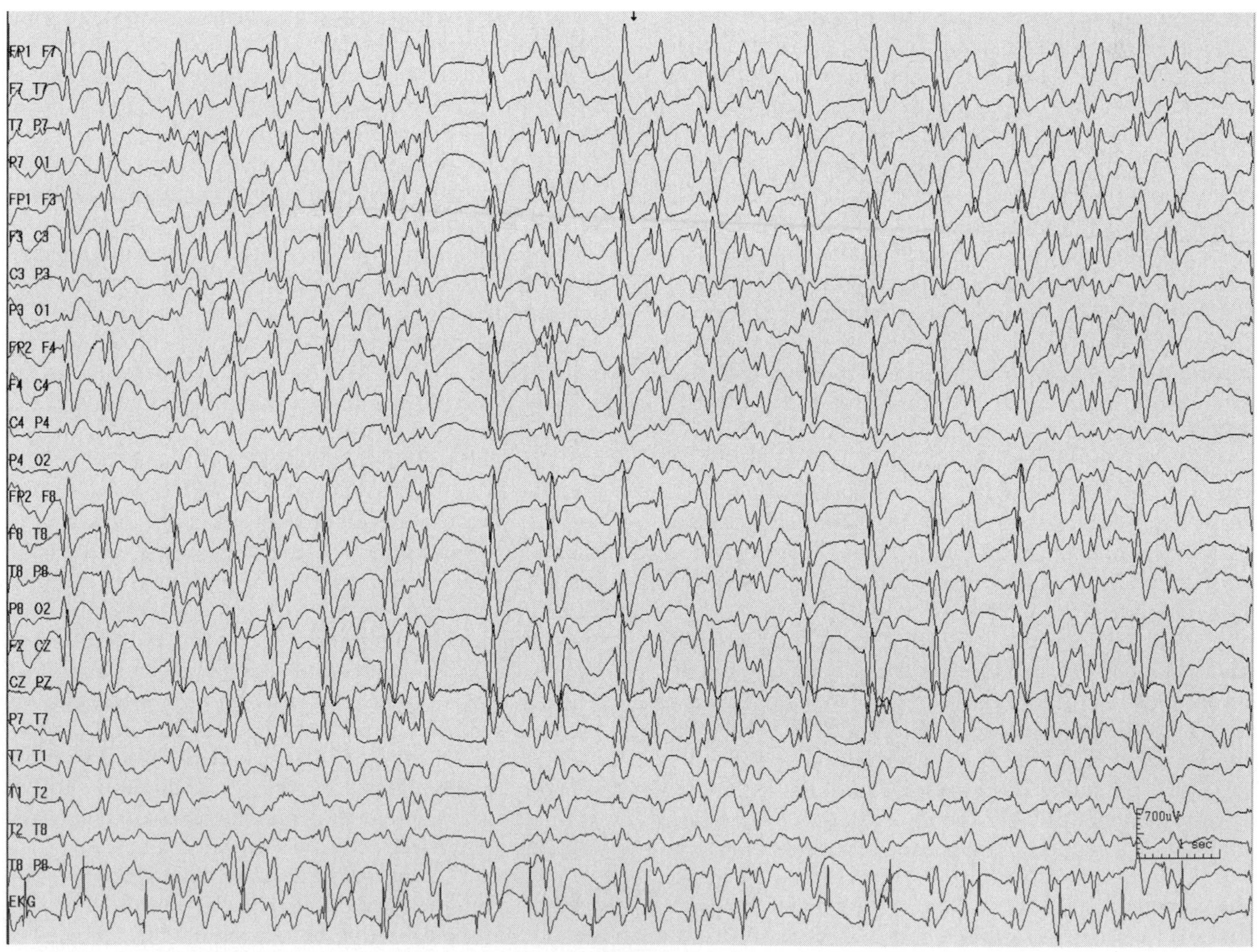

FIGURE 24-1

Electrical status epilepticus of sleep (ESES) electroencephalogram in a child with Landau-Kleffner syndrome.

presumed that the neuropsychological deficits are, at least partially, the result of the epileptiform activity. Landau and Kleffner (1) suggested that "persistent convulsive discharges in brain tissue largely concerned with language communication result in the functional ablation of these areas." Hirsch and colleagues agree with the hypothesis of a functional ablation (27). Poor daytime alertness due to sleep fragmentation may contribute to the neuropsychological deficits (42). Alternatively, the previous potential interrelations are a hypothesis, and a causal relation between abnormal interictal discharges and neuropsychological deficits is still controversial (43). A valid argument is that the dysfunction may represent different manifestations of the same unknown, possibly genetically determined, underlying pathogenic mechanism. An argument against this hypothesis is that the suppression of discharges with medical or surgical therapy may, at least partly, reverse these cognitive deficits (44, 45).

Despite the controversy regarding the underlying pathophysiology of epileptic encephalopathies, the following three crucial questions await answers: (1) what are the mechanisms involved in the generation of such a significant, interictal, sleep activation; (2) what are the mechanisms involved in the cognitive or developmental regression that accompanies these conditions; and (3) what is the interrelation between the two, if any?

Although a genetic predisposition was questioned, there is no strong evidence to support such predilection (46). The response of the epileptiform discharges to corticosteroids raised the question of an autoimmune pathogenesis at least in a subset of patients including central nervous system (CNS) vasculitis or demyelination. IgG and IgM antibodies to brain endothelial cells have been identified in these disorders (28, 47), with higher levels in the patients than in controls. Brain-derived neurotrophic factor (BDNF), BDNF autoantibodies, and IgM and IgG antibodies were elevated in some children with autism and childhood disintegrative disorder (CDD). The authors concluded that these findings suggest a previously unrecognized interaction between the immune system and BDNF (47). Autoantibodies to rat brain auditory cortex, brainstem, and cerebellum have been identified in children with LKS (48).

There is increasing evidence that interictal EEG abnormalities can produce transient cognitive impairment (49–55). Furthermore, benign rolandic epilepsy may be not so benign, because the interictal discharges may have a substantial effect on cognitive function (56, 57), at least for a subset of patients. Additionally, the presence of continuously abnormal discharges during sleep may cause disruption of hippocampal function and interfere with the consolidation of memory (58–60). Hence, the potential impact of the persistent interictal discharges on brain plasticity is proposed as a mechanism for the resulting neuropsychological impairment in these children. More specifically, the occurrence of epileptiform discharges during a critical time of brain development may result in defective synaptogenesis and thalamocortical circuit formation. Secondary bilateral synchrony, facilitated by the corpus callosum with involvement of thalamocortical connections, was hypothesized as a possible mechanism for the generation of the epileptiform discharges (61–64).

DIAGNOSTIC EVALUATION AND DIFFERENTIAL DIAGNOSIS

The diagnosis starts by establishing an epileptic disturbance in the child with regression, usually first with a routine EEG. All pediatric epilepsy syndromes are classified as symptomatic, cryptogenic, or idiopathic. Symptomatic cases exist for both LKS and CSWS, although symptomatic cases are more frequent with CSWS. We have seen only one case of a symptomatic LKS, in a child with a left temporal oligodendroglioma. However, other categories reported include infectious disorders, such as cysticercosis and toxoplasmosis; inflammatory disorders, such as CNS vasculitis; demyelinating disease and acute disseminated encephalomyelitis (ADEM); congenital brain malformations, such as polymicrogyria; and tumors, including temporal lobe astrocytomas and dysembryoplastic neuroepithelial tumors (DNET) (4, 5). Therefore, neuroimaging is warranted.

Typically in the idiopathic cases, no structural abnormalities are seen with routine neuroimaging, although bilateral volume reduction using an MRI cortical parcellation technique has been reported in the superior temporal gyrus (65) and perisylvian polymicrogyria has been reported in a single case (66). Functional neuroimaging has demonstrated temporal dysfunction with SPECT (67, 68), PET (69, 70), or MEG scans (71). These studies are usually done when a patient has failed treatment and epilepsy surgery is considered.

The differential diagnosis of a sleep-activated EEG includes (3): LKS, CSWS, and PDD with regression, congenital aphasia or developmental language disorders, or the epilepsy syndromes benign focal epilepsy with centrotemporal discharges, benign focal epilepsy with occipital discharges, atypical benign partial epilepsy of childhood, the Lennox-Gastaut syndrome, and myoclonic-astatic epilepsy (Doose syndrome). Language or intellectual regression associated with behavioral problems in any of these syndromes may make the differential diagnosis difficult and not all pediatric epilepsy syndromes are readily classified. In our experience, children with PDD with regression and an epileptiform EEG are the largest numbers of children referred for evaluation.

Clinical symptoms other than language regression have been reported with ESES. Hirsch and colleagues suggested that the definition of LKS should be expanded to include the acquired deterioration of any higher cortical function in association with sleep-activated paroxysmal features (72) and not limited just to language regression. Clinical manifestations include epileptic dysgraphia (73), visual agnosia (74), and an acquired frontal syndrome (75). We have seen one child with blindness (Figure 24-2) and another child with a prosopagnosia, with both demonstrating a more posterior ESES on EEG.

TREATMENT

All children with LKS and CSWS should have a formal neuropsychological evaluation to guide their educational program and track developmental changes. Children with LKS will, especially, require intensive speech and language therapy. These two syndromes are associated with significant neuropsychiatric comorbidities, and treatment for hyperactivity, attention deficit disorder, mood instability, behavior problems, and even an autistic picture may require referral to a psychopharmacologist and psychologist. Despite control of seizures and EEG abnormalities, these children may have significant residual neurologic, psychological, and psychiatric dysfunction.

LKS and ESES have similar treatment but the specifics are debated. Smith and Hoeppner recommend that the treatment goal is the complete elimination of epileptiform activity within 2 years (25). Treatment options include standard AEDs, corticosteroids (adrenocorticotropic hormone [ACTH] or prednisone), high-dose benzodiazepines, intravenous immunoglobulins, or multiple subpial transections (MST). Although AEDs may control seizures, the language dysfunction may not improve, whereas corticosteroid treatment may control seizures and decrease the epileptiform activity and improve language (10–12). Early corticosteroid treatment has been considered the treatment of choice for LKS (12). Because relapse may occur, LKS often requires long-term corticosteroid treatment, which increases the risk of side effects (15). Despite either AED or corticosteroid treatment, many children continue with language dysfunction. Regardless of treatment, 50% to 80% of children have long-term language or neurobehavioral abnormalities (76–78).

Landau and Kleffner reported a positive relationship between AED treatment and aphasia improvement (1). In 1967, Deuel and Lenn reported a case with a clear relationship between AED treatment and language improvement (79), and there have been subsequent reports of improvement with various AEDs. However, the conventional wisdom is that the AEDs control the actual clinical seizures but not the aphasia (11, 12). McKinney and McGreal reported a better response with steroids (10). Some children who had not responded to AEDs improved after steroid therapy (11, 12). They also thought that the rapidity of the response and the sequelae depend on the duration and severity of symptoms before treatment, that initial high doses are more effective, and that brief treatment is ineffective or leads to a high relapse rate. Both ACTH and prednisone have been used.

Both carbamazepine and valproatc have been widely used, but there are no data suggesting that any one AED is better than others. We have seen several cases of children treated with carbamazepine for seizures with focal epileptiform abnormalities on EEG who subsequently developed language regression with ESES. We prefer using AEDs with antiepileptogenic properties as first-line AEDs. The term *anticonvulsant* refers to suppression of seizures, whereas *antiepileptogenic* refers to suppression of the development of epilepsy or the underlying process that leads to epilepsy (80). We have historically preferred valproic acid (VPA) because it has both anticonvulsant and antiepileptogenic properties, and it may normalize EEGs. It is well known that carbamazepine may worsen the generalized epilepsies and may even worsen focal spike-and-wave discharges and activate the EEG (81–83). For ESES, VPA, benzodiazepines, and ethosuximide have been the most successful AEDs (7), and lamotrigine and levetiracetam have also been used. However, we have seen seizures worsen with every AED used. In general, for either LKS or ESES, if AEDs do not work, then high-dose corticosteroids are used. These may work through GABAergic effects rather than immune mediation (84).

De Negri and colleagues introduced a high-dose diazepam protocol for electrical status epilepticus (ESE) (85). They gave a rectal dose of 1 mg/kg with EEG monitoring and continued a dose of 0.5 mg/kg orally for several weeks in those that responded. They found that those on chronic benzodiazepine treatment did not respond as well to this treatment. When a clinical relapse occurred, this dosing schedule was repeated. In the group of De Negri and colleagues with ESE, only 1 child had LKS and 1 had ESES. We modified this high-dose diazepam protocol, using 1 mg/kg either orally or rectally under EEG guidance, but then treated all children with a dose of 0.5 mg/kg, orally for 3 to 4 weeks (17). If EEG showed no improvement, we rapidly tapered the diazepam. If EEG showed an improvement, we tapered then by 2.5 mg/month. In our series, every child who initially responded and then had a rapid diazepam taper had either a clinical or electrographic regression. We now continue a maintenance diazepam dose, usually at a dose of 2.5 to 5 mg, for 2 years. The best responders to high-dose diazepam have been children with idiopathic LKS.

Tassinari et al recommend trials with several different drugs, and they report that a long-lasting effect has been achieved with VPA along with clobazam, lorazepam, and clonazepam (8). Smith and Hoeppner recommend initial treatment with high-dose VPA, with or without a benzodiazepine, and, in the absence of response, then several months of corticosteroid therapy (25). Inutsuka and colleagues (86) reported their treatment results in 15 children, using the following protocol: (1) VPA at

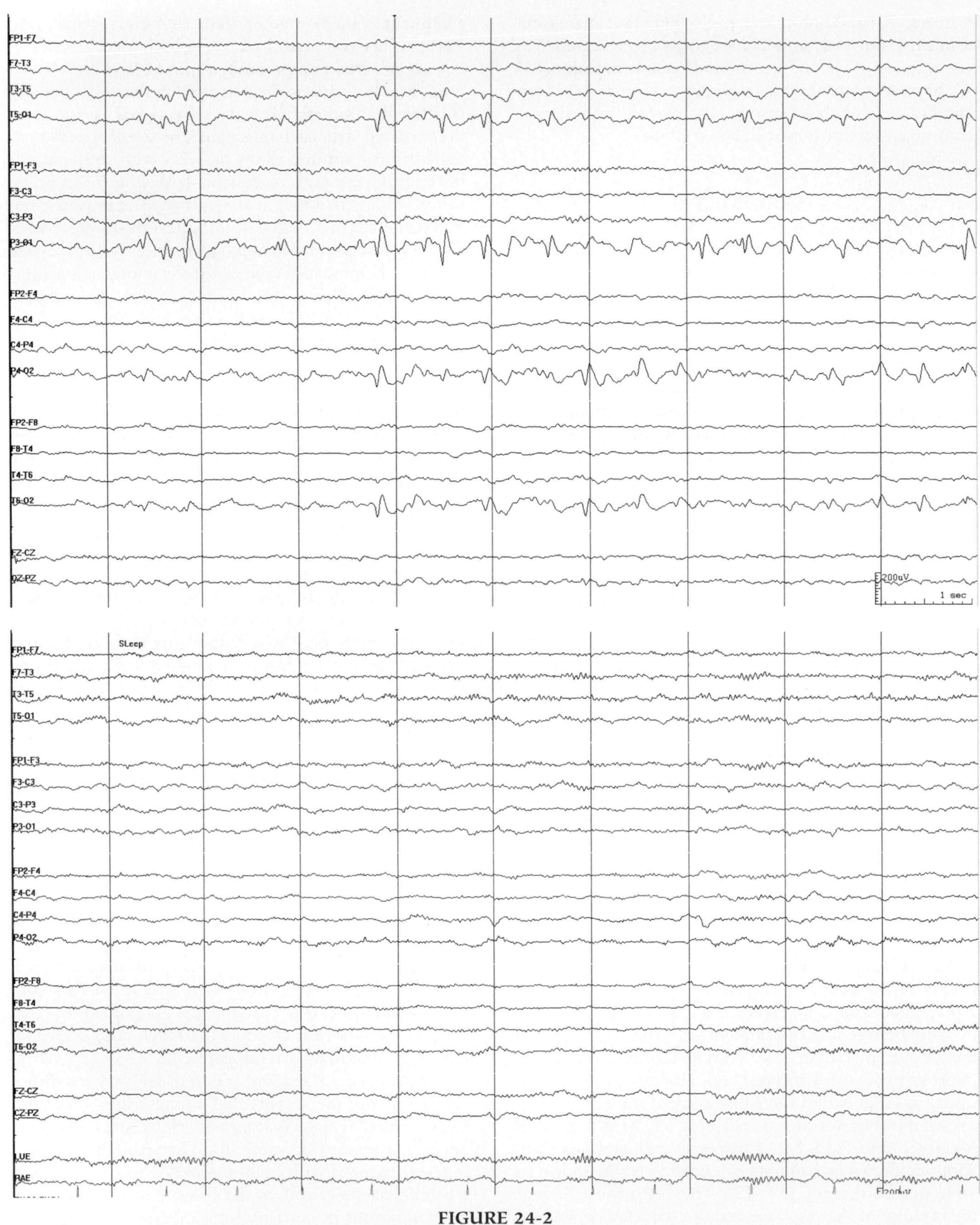

FIGURE 24-2

(A) Electroencephalogram (EEG) in child with blindness and posterior electrical status epilepticus of sleep (ESES). (B) EEG after high dose diazepam treatment; vision has recovered.

levels greater than 100 mg/L, (2) combination of VPA plus ethosuximide, (3) short cycles of high-dose diazepam, (4) or intramuscular ACTH. Treatment with short cycles of ACTH (duration 11 to 43 days) or diazepam (DZP) (duration for 6 to 7 days) did not achieve long-term remission, whereas either high-dose VPA alone ($n = 7$) or in combination with ethosuximide ($n = 3$) achieved remission in 10 children (67%). We retrospectively analyzed our experience with ESES treatment in 12 children (87). Only 1 of 12 responded to initial short-term therapy with VPA. We used prednisone for 6 months in 6 children with the dose schedule outlined in Table 24-1 (88); 5 of 6 had a positive response, but 4 of 5 (80%) relapsed and required another course. Before the elective use of corticosteroids, immunizations should be up to date.

Alternate treatments including immunoglobulins and the ketogenic diet have been tried, with case reports documenting efficacy, but long-term follow-up data are limited (18–22). MST has been performed in selected children who failed medical therapy, and it may provide benefit (62, 89).

TABLE 24-1
Six-Month Dosing Schedule for Oral Prednisone

2 mg/kg/day for 1 month (maximum dose 60 mg)
1.5 mg/kg/day for 1 month
1 mg/kg/day for 1 month
1 mg/kg every other day for 1 month
0.75 mg/kg every other day for 1 month
0.5 mg/kg/day every other day for 1 month

Note: Immunizations should be up to date before the elective use of corticosteroids.

COURSE AND PROGNOSIS

In general, the outcome of epilepsy is favorable in both LKS and CSWS (90), whereas cognitive dysfunction occurs in the majority (25). The prognosis for LKS has varied, depending on the series. Mantovani and Landau conducted a long-term follow-up of the original children reported by Mantovani and Landau (91). In nine patients, with follow-up that varied from 10 to 28 years, four patients had full recovery, one had a mild language disability, and four had moderate disability. Later studies have not reported as positive an outcome. Bishop did a literature review of 45 children with LKS. The age of onset was related to the outcome, which was less favorable if onset occurred before 4 years of age (26). Shinnar and colleagues reported residual language dysfunction in 88% of children who had language regression, and most had autism or autistic features (76). Deonna et al reported that only one of seven adult patients had normal language, with the six others demonstrating varying degrees of language deficits, some with complete absence of language (75). In a recent article on the neuropsychological follow-up of 12 patients, Soprano et al reported that 9 of 12 had a variable degree of persistent language deficit (78). Only 50% have been able to lead a normal life (62, 69).

The prognosis is poor in CSWS (92). In an adult follow-up study of seven patients, only one had active epilepsy, but only two had been in a normal school setting (93). The two patients with LKS had a normal IQ, but had language deficits, whereas the five patients with ESES had global mental deficiency. Scholtes et al (94) performed a long-term follow-up of 10 children with ESES, with a good recovery in only 1 child and a partial recovery in only 4. There are more residual deficits in CSWS, because this syndrome is more likely to be symptomatic, compared to LKS, which is more likely to be idiopathic.

References

1. Landau W, Kleffner FR. Syndrome of acquired aphasia with convulsive disorder in children. *Neurology* 1957; 7:523–530.
2. Commission on Classification and Terminology of the International League Against Epilepsy. Proposal for revised classification of epilepsies and epileptic syndromes. *Epilepsia* 1989; 30:389–399.
3. Engel J Jr. A proposed diagnostic scheme for people with epileptic seizures and with epilepsy: report of the ILAE Task Force on Classification and Terminology. *Epilepsia* 2001; 42:796–803.
4. Riviello JJ. Drislane F, eds. Status epilepticus in children. Status epilepticus: a clinical perspective. Totowa, NJ: Humana Press, 2005:313–338.
5. Hadjiloizou S, Riviello JJ. Epileptic and epileptiform encephalopathies. Neurology. Omaha, NE: eMedicine.com, Inc., 2006.
6. Patry G, Lyagoubi S, Tassinari A. Subclinical "electrical status epilepticus" induced by sleep in children. A clinical and electroencephalographic study of six cases. *Arch Neurol* 1971; 24:242–252.
7. Tassinari CA, Bureau M, Dravet C, Dalla Bernardina B, et al. Epilepsy with continuous spikes and waves during slow sleep-otherwise described as ESES (epilepsy with electrical status epilepticus during slow sleep. In: Roger J, Bureau M, Dravet Ch, Dreifuss FE, et al, eds. *Epileptic Syndromes in Infancy, Childhood, and Adolescencence*. 2nd ed. London: John Libbey, 1992:245–256.
8. Tassinari CA, Rubboli G, Volpi L, Meletti S, et al. Encephalopathy with electrical status epilepticus during slow sleep or ESES syndrome including the acquired aphasia. *Clin Neurophsyiol* 2000; 111 Suppl 2:S94–S102.
9. Veggiotti P, Beccaria F, Guerrini R, Capovilla G, et al. Continuous spike-and-wave activity during slow-wave sleep: syndrome or EEG pattern? *Epilepsia* 1999; 40:1593–1601.
10. McKinney W, McGreal DA. An aphasic syndrome in children. *Can Med J* 1974; 110:637–639.
11. Marescaux C, Finck S, Maquet P, Schlumberger E, et al. Landau-Kleffner syndrome: a pharmacologic study of five cases. *Epilepsia* 1990; 31:768–777.
12. Lerman P, Lerman-Sagie T, Kivity S. Effect of early corticosteroid therapy for Landau-Kleffner syndrome. *Dev Med Child Neurol* 1991; 33:257–260.
13. Tsuru T, Mori M, Mizuguchi M, Momoi MY. Effects of high-dose intravenous corticosteroid therapy in Landau-Kleffner syndrome. *Pediatr Neurol* 2000; 22:145–147.
14. Sinclair DB, Snyder TJ. Corticosteroids for the treatment of Landau-Kleffner syndrome and continuous spike-wave discharge during sleep. *Pediatr Neurol* 2005; 32:300–306.
15. Verhelst H, Boon P, Buyse G, Ceulemans B, et al. Steroids in intractable childhood epilepsy: clinical experience and review of the literature. *Seizure* 2005; 14:412–421.
16. De Negri M, Baglietto MG, Battaglia FM. Treatment of electrical status epilepticus by short diazepam (DZP) cycles after DZP rectal bolus test. *Brain Dev* 1995; 17:330–333.
17. Riviello JJ, Holder DL, Thiele E, Bourgeois BFD, et al. Treatment of continuous spikes and waves during slow wave sleep with high dose diazepam. *Epilepsia* 2001; 42 Suppl 7:56.
18. Fayad MN, Choueiri R, Mikati M. Landau-Kleffner syndrome: consistent response to repeated intravenous gamma-globulin doses: a case report. *Epilepsia* 1997; 38:489–494.
19. Mikati MA, Saab R. Successful use of intravenous immunoglobulin as initial monotherapy in Landau-Kleffner syndrome. *Epilepsia* 2000; 41:880–886.
20. Mikati MA, Saab R, Fayad MN, Choueiri RN. Efficacy of intravenous immunoglobulin in Landau-Kleffner syndrome. *Pediatr Neurol* 2002; 26:298–300.
21. Lagae LG, Silberstein J, Gillis PL, Casaer PJ. Successful use of intravenous immunoglobulins in Landau-Kleffner syndrome. *Pediatr Neurol* 1998; 18:165–168.

22. Prasad AN, Stafstrom CF, Holmes GL. Alternative epilepsy therapies: the ketogenic diet, immunoglobulins, and steroids. *Epilepsia* 1996; 37 Suppl 1:S81–S95.
23. Bergqvist AG, Chee CM, Lutchka LM, Brooks-Kayal AR. Treatment of acquired epileptic aphasia with the ketogenic diet. *J Child Neurol* 1999; 14:696–701.
24. Kramer U, Nevo Y, Neufeld MY, Fatal A, et al. Epidemiology of epilepsy in childhood: a cohort of 440 consecutive patients. *Pediatr Neurol* 1998; 18:46–50.
25. Smith MC, Hoeppner TJ. Epileptic encephalopathy of late childhood: Landau-Kleffner syndrome and the syndrome of continuous spikes and waves during slow sleep. *J Clin Neurophysiol* 2003; 20:462–472.
26. Bishop DVM. Age of onset and outcome in acquired aphasia with convulsive disorder (Landau-Kleffner syndrome). *Dev Med Child Neurol* 1985; 27:705–712.
27. Hirsch E, Valenti MP, Rudolf G, Seegmuller C, et al. Landau-Kleffner syndrome is not an eponymic badge of ignorance. *Epilepsy Res* 2006; 70 Suppl 1:S239–S247.
28. Connolly AM, Chez MG, Pestronk A, Arnold ST, et al. Serum autoantibodies to brain in Landau-Kleffner variant, autism, and other neurologic disorders. *J Pediatr* 1999; 134:607–613.
29. Shafrir Y, Prensky AL. Acquired epileptiform opercular syndrome: a second case report, review of the literature, and comparison to the Landau-Kleffner syndrome. *Epilepsia* 1995; 36:1050–1057.
30. Tuchman RF, Rapin I. Regression in pervasive developmental disorders: seizures and epileptiform electroencephalogram correlates. *Pediatrics* 1997; 99:560–566.
31. Tuchman RF, Rapin I, Shinnar S. Autistic and dysphasic children. I: Clinical characteristics. *Pediatrics* 1991; 88:1211–1218.
32. Tuchman RF, Rapin I, Shinnar S. Autistic and dysphasic children. II: Epilepsy. *Pediatrics* 1991; 88:1219–1225.
33. Echenne B, Cheminal R, Rivier F, Negre C, et al. Epileptic electroencephalographic abnormalities and developmental dysphasias: a study of 32 patients. *Brain Dev* 1992; 14:216–225.
34. Stefanatos GA, Foley C, Grover W, Doherty B. Steady-state auditory evoked responses to pulsed frequency modulations in children. *EEG Clin Neurophysiol* 1997; 104:31–42.
35. Galanopoulou AS, Bojko A, Lado F, Moshe SL. The spectrum of neuropsychiatric abnormalities associated with electrical status epilepticus in sleep. *Brain Dev* 2000; 22:279–295.
36. Guilhoto LMFF, Morrell F. Electrophysiological differences bewteen Landau-Kleffner syndrome and other conditions showing the CSWS electrical pattern. *Epilepsia* 1994; 35 Suppl 8:126.
37. Guilhoto LM, Machado-Haertel LR, Manreza ML, Diament AJ. Continuous spike wave activity during sleep. Electroencephalographic and clinical features. *Arq Neuropsiquiatr* 1997; 55:762–770.
38. Van Hirtum-Das M, Licht EA, Koh S, Wu JY, et al. Children with ESES: Variability in the syndrome. *Epilepsy Res* 2006; 7S; S248–S258.
39. Bolanos A, Mikati M, Holmes G, Helmers S, et al. Landau-Kleffner syndrome: clinical and EEG features. *Neurology* 1995; 45 Suppl 4:A180.
40. Bolanos A, Urion DK, Helmers SL, Lombroso CT, et al. Serial electroencephalographic changes in children with Landau-Kleffner syndrome. *Epilepsia* 1997; 38 Suppl 3:27.pl4:A180.
41. Holmes GL, McKeever M, Saunders Z. Epileptiform activity in aphasia of childhood: an epiphenomenon? *Epilepsia* 1981; 22:631–639.
42. Kohrman MH, Carney PR. Sleep-related disorders in neurologic disease during childhood. *Pediatr Neurol* 2000; 23:107–113.
43. Ben-Ari Y, Holmes GL. Effects of seizures on developmental processes in the immature brain. *Lancet Neurol* 2006; 5:1055–1063.
44. Matsuzaka T, Baba H, Matsuo A, Tsuru A, et al. Developmental assessment-based surgical intervention for intractable epilepsies in infants and young children. *Epilepsia* 2001; 42 Suppl 6:9–12.
45. Holmes GL, Lenck-Santini PP. Role of interictal epileptiform abnormalities in cognitive impairment. *Epilepsy Behav* 2006; 8:504–515. Epub 2006.
46. Landau WM. Landau-Kleffner syndrome. An eponymic badge of ignorance. *Arch Neurol* 1992; 49:353.
47. Connolly 2005.
48. Boscolo S, Baldas V, Gobbi G, Giordano L, et al. Anti-brain but not celiac disease antibodies in Landau-Kleffner syndrome and related epilepsies. *J Neuroimmunol* 2005; 160:228–232. Epub 2004.
49. Shewmon DA, Erwin RJ. The effect of focal interictal spikes on perception and reaction time. II. Neuroanatomic specificity. *Electroencephalogr Clin Neurophysiol* 1988; 69:338–352.
50. Shewmon DA, Erwin RJ. Transient impairment of visual perception induced by single interictal occipital spikes. *J Clin Exp Neuropsychol* 1989; 11:675–691.
51. Kasteleijn-Nolst Trenite DG, Bakker DJ, Binnie CD. Psychological effects of subclinical epileptiform EEG discharges. I. Scholastic skills. *Epilepsy Res* 1988; 2:111–116.
52. Aarts JH, Binnie CD, Smit AM, Wilkins AJ. Selective cognitive impairment during focal and generalized epileptiform EEG activity. *Brain* 1984; 107 Pt 1:293–308.
53. Binnie CD, Kasteleijn-Nolst Trenite DG, Smit AM, et al. Interactions of epileptiform EEG discharges and cognition. *Epilepsy Res* 1987; 1:239–245.
54. Binnie CD. Significance and management of transitory cognitive impairment due to subclinical EEG discharges in children. *Brain Dev* 1993; 15:23–30.
55. Binnie CD. Cognitive impairment during epileptiform discharges: is it ever justifiable to treat the EEG? *Lancet Neurol* 2003; 2:725–730.
56. Massa R, de Saint-Martin A, Carcangiu R, Rudolf G, et al. EEG criteria predictive of complicated evolution in idiopathic rolandic epilepsy. *Neurology* 2001; 57:1071–1079.
57. Nolan MA, Redoblado MA, Lah S, Sabaz M, et al. Memory function in childhood epilepsy syndromes. *J Paediatr Child Health* 2004; 40:20–27.
58. Moruzzi G, Magoun HW. Brain stem reticular formation and activation of the EEG. *J Neuropsychiatry Clin Neurosci* 1995; 7:251–267.
59. Lorincz A, Buzsaki G. Two-phase computational model training long-term memories in the entorhinal-hippocampal region. *Ann N Y Acad Sci* 2000; 911:83–111.
60. Louie K, Wilson MA. Temporally structured replay of awake hippocampal ensemble activity during rapid eye movement sleep. *Neuron* 2001; 29:145–156.
61. Morrell F. Secondary epileptogenesis in man. *Arch Neurol* 1985; 42:318–335.
62. Morrell F, Whisler WW, Smith MC, Hoeppner TJ, et al. Landau-Kleffner syndrome. Treatment with subpial intracortical transection. *Brain* 1995; 118:1529–1546.
63. Kobayashi K, Murakami N, Yoshinaga H, Enoki H, et al. Nonconvulsive status epilepticus with continuous diffuse spike-and-wave discharges during sleep in childhood. *Jpn J Psychiatry Neurol* 1988; 42:509–514.
64. Monteiro JP, Roulet-Perez E, Davidoff V, Deonna T. Primary neonatal thalamic haemorrhage and epilepsy with continuous spike-wave during sleep: a longitudinal follow-up of a possible significant relation. *Eur J Paediatr Neurol* 2001; 5(1):41–47.
65. Takeoka M, Riviello JJ Jr, Duffy FH, Kim F, et al. Bilateral volume reduction of the superior temporal areas in Landau-Kleffner syndrome. *Neurology* 2004; 63:1289–1292.
66. Huppke P, Kallenberg K, Gartner J. Perisylvian polymicrogyria in Landau-Kleffner syndrome. *Neurology* 2005; 64:1660.
67. O'Tuama LA, Urion DK, Janicek MJ, Treves ST, et al. Regional cerebral perfusion in Landau-Kleffner syndrome and related childhood aphasias. *J Nucl Med* 1992; 33: 1758–1765.
68. Guerreiro MM, Camargo EE, Kato M, Menezes Netto JR, et al. Brain single photon emission computed tomography imaging in Landau-Kleffner syndrome. *Epilepsia* 1996; 37:60–67.
69. Maquet P, Hirsch E, Dive D, Salmon E, et al. Cerebral glucose utilization during sleep in Landau-Kleffner syndrome: a PET study. *Epilepsia* 1990; 31:778–783.
70. da Silva EA, Chugani DC, Muzik O, Chugani HT. Landau-Kleffner syndrome: metabolic abnormalities in temporal lobe are a common feature. *J Child Neurol* 1997; 12:489–495.
71. Paetau R, Granstrom M-L, Blomstedt G, Jousmaki V, et al. Magnetoencephalography in presurgical evaluation of Landau-Kleffner syndrome. *Epilepsia* 1999; 40:326–335.
72. Hirsch E, Maquet P, Metz-Lutz M-N, Motte J, et al. The eponym "Landau-Kleffner Syndrome" should not be restricted to childhood-acquired aphasia with epilepsy. In: Beaumanoir A, Bureau M, Deonna T, Mira L, et al, eds. *Continuous Spikes and Slow Waves During Slow Sleep Electrical Status Epilepticus During Slow Sleep: Acquired Epileptic Aphasia and Related Conditions.* London: John Libbey, 1995:57–62.
73. DuBois CM, Zesiger P, Perez ER, Ingvar MM, Deonna T. Acquired epileptic dysgraphia: a longitudinal study. *Dev Med Child Neurol* 2003; 45:807–812.
74. Eriksson K, Kylliainen A, Hirvonen K, Nieminen P, et al. Visual agnosia in a child with non-lesional occipito-temporal CSWS. *Brain Dev* 2003; 25:262–267.
75. Deonna T, Davidoff V, Maeder-Ingvar M, Zesiger P, et al. The spectrum of acquired cognitive disturbances in children with partial epilepsy and continuous spike-waves during sleep. A 4-year follow-up case study with prolonged reversible learning arrest and dysfluency. *Eur J Paediatr Neurol* 1997; 1:19–2916.
76. Shinnar S, Rapin I, Arnold S, Tuchman RF, et al. Language regression in childhood. *Pediatr Neurol* 2001; 24:183–189.
77. Mantovani JF. Autistic regression and Landau-Kleffner syndrome: progress or confusion? *Dev Med Child Neurol* 2000; 42:349–353.
78. Soprano AM, Garcia EF, Caraballo R, Fejerman N. Acquired epileptic aphasia: neuropsychologic follow-up of 12 patients. *Pediatr Neurol* 1994; 11:230–235.
79. Deuel RK, Lenn NJ. Treatment of acquired epileptic aphasia. *J Pediatr* 1977; 90:959–961.
80. Silver JM, Shin C, McNamara JO. Antiepileptogenic effects of conventional anticonvulsants in the kindling model of epilepsy. *Ann Neurol* 1991; 29:356–363.
81. Snead OC 3rd, Hosey LC. Exacerbation of seizures in children by carbamazepine. *N Engl J Med* 1985; 313:916–921.
82. Kochen S, Giagante B, Oddo S. Spike-and-wave complexes and seizure exacerbation caused by carbamazepine. *Eur J Neurol* 2002; 9:41–47.
83. Gansaeuer M, Alsaadi TM. Carbamazepine-induced seizures: a case report and review of the literature. *Clin Electroencephalogr* 2002; 33:174–177.
84. Mtchedlishvili Z, Kapur J. A presynaptic action of the neurosteroid pregnenolone sulfate on GABAergic synaptic transmission. *Mol Pharmacol* 2003; 64:857–864.
85. De Negri M, Baglietto MG, Battaglia FM. Treatment of electrical status epilepticus by short diazepam (DZP) cycles after DZP rectal bolus test. *Brain Dev* 1995; 17:330–333.
86. Inutsuka M, Kobayashi K, Oka M, Hattori J, Ohtsuka Y. Treatment of epilesy with electrical status epilepticus of sleep and its related disorders. *Epilepsy Behav* 2006; 28:281–286.
87. Albaradie RS, Bourgeois BFD, Thiele E, Duffy FH, et al. Treatment of continuous spike and wave during slow wave sleep. *Epilepsia* 2001; 42 Suppl 7:46–47.
88. Stefanatos GA, Grover W, Geller E. Case study: corticosteroid treatment of language regression in pervasive developmental disorder. *J Am Acad Child Adolesc Psychiatry* 1995; 34:1107–1111.
89. Irwin K, Birch V, Lees J, Polkey C, et al. Multiple subpial transection in Landau-Kleffner syndrome. *Dev Med Child Neurol* 2001; 43:248–252.
90. Bureau M. Outstanding cases of CSWS and LKS: analysis of the data sheets provided by the participants. In: Beaumanoir A, Bureau M, Deonna T, Mira L, et al, eds. *Continuous Spikes and Slow Waves During Slow Sleep Electrical Status Epilepticus During Slow Sleep: Acquired Epileptic Aphasia and Related Conditions.* London: John Libbey, 1995:213–216.
91. Mantovani JF, Landau WM. Acquired aphasia with convulsive disorder: course and prognosis. *Neurology* 1980; 30:524–529.
92. Morikawa T, Seino M, Watanabe M. Long-term outcome of CSWS syndrome. In: Beaumanoir A, Bureau M, Deonna T, Mira L, et al, eds. *Continuous Spikes and Slow Waves During Slow Sleep Electrical Status Epilepticus During Slow Sleep: Acquired Epileptic Aphasia and Related Conditions.* London: John Libbey, 1995:27–36.
93. Praline J, Hommet C, Barthez M-A, Brault F, et al. Outcome at adulthood of continuous spike waves of slow sleep and Landau-Kleffner syndrome. *Epilepsia* 2003; 44:1434–1440.
94. Scholtes FB, Hendriks MP, Renier WO. Cognitive detrioration and electrical status epilepticus during slow sleep. *Brain Dev* 2005; 6:167–173.

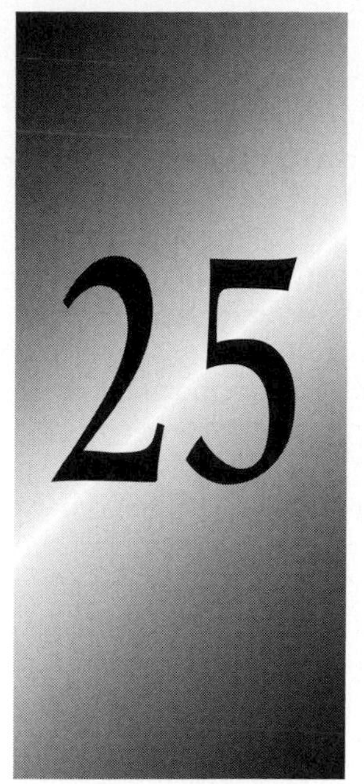

25 Idiopathic Generalized Epilepsy of Adolescence

Reza Behrouz
Selim R. Benbadis

Idiopathic generalized epilepsies (IGEs) are a distinct group of epilepsies, clearly defined in the 1989 International Classification of Epileptic Syndromes and Epilepsies. This classification established an important dichotomy between the idiopathic epilepsies on the one hand, and the symptomatic or cryptogenic epilepsies on the other (1). In prior versions of this classification, IGEs were referred to as primary generalized epilepsies, and symptomatic/cryptogenic generalized epilepsies were categorized under secondary generalized epilepsies. This nomenclature was revised because the term "secondary generalized" was confusing when applied to epilepsy, where it meant that the epilepsy was secondary to some other cause, whereas when applied to seizures, it means that the generalization is secondary from an originally focal seizure.

Unfortunately, the term "idiopathic" in the current classification is also confusing in the context of current medical terminology, because in every other area of medicine "idiopathic" means "of an unknown cause." It is now clearly understood that IGEs are primarily of genetic origin.

IGEs are age-dependent, meaning that a given genotype may express itself differently at different ages. This chapter will focus on the IGE seen in adolescence.

GENETICS & PATHOPHYSIOLOGY

IGEs represent a group of epilepsies best described as a genetically determined low threshold for generalized seizures, as opposed to symptomatic or cryptogenic generalized epilepsies, where there is an underlying anatomic (pathologic) abnormality. Investigations for microscopic lesions (e.g., microdysgenesis) in IGE, using structural imaging, have yielded inconsistent results (2). Functional imaging, not surprisingly, can show evidence for diffuse dysfunction. Proton magnetic resonance spectroscopy (MRS) has revealed frontal lobe (3) or thalamic (4) abnormalities.

Because they have "overlapping" genetic origins, it is appropriate and practical to view IGEs as a continuum of genetic conditions exhibiting variable phenotypes. Recent advances have identified IGEs linked to defects in genes encoding the subunits for voltage- or ligand-gated ion channels including sodium, potassium, calcium, or chloride channels affecting the gamma-aminobutyric acid $(GABA)_A$ receptors. Hence, they are categorically referred to as "ion channelopathies" (5). For the classic and well-defined forms of IGE—juvenile myoclonic epilepsy (JME) or childhood absence epilepsy (CAE), a few mutations, including the KCNQ potassium channels and the ClC-2 chloride channel, have been implicated (6).

The pathophysiology (e.g., the concept of channelopathies) and genetics of IGE are gradually being elucidated. Fundamentally, IGEs appear to be "phenotypes of many, often individually rare, gene defects" (7, 8).

The inheritance of IGEs is complex in the sense that it does not follow a well-defined Mendelian pattern. Moreover, phenotypic expression influencing semiology and frequency of a specific genotype may be quite variable from one individual to another. This is likely due to different degrees of alteration of neuronal excitability induced by gene errors. At least for JME, a maternal inheritance has been proposed and confirmed by some (9). Nevertheless, it is reasonable to state that the genetic complexity of IGEs necessitates additional investigation in order to reach a conclusion regarding their precise mechanism of inheritance.

EPIDEMIOLOGY AND NATURAL HISTORY

IGEs constitute approximately 15–20% of all epilepsies (10). They affect all races equally and may have a slight predilection for women (11). Seizures usually, but not always, have an onset early in life, from childhood to early adulthood. In fact, IGEs are the most frequent group of epilepsies with an adolescent onset (12). IGEs are generally associated with low mortality and favorable response rate to treatment. The morbidity from IGE is primarily a function of how well the condition is treated. As it will be mentioned further in this chapter, the response rate to antiepileptic drugs (AEDs) is good. Additionally, 50% of patients with IGE can outgrow them. A recent intriguing finding is the association between IGE and type 1 diabetes (13).

CLINICAL FEATURES (OF IGE IN GENERAL)

Overall, there are much more similarities than there are differences among the various types of IGE. These epilepsies manifest themselves by the same three seizure types, have similar electroencephalographic (EEG) findings, are said to "evolve" into one another, and have overlapping genetic origins (family members may express different IGE syndromes). In all, IGEs are best viewed as a spectrum of conditions, and many of them may indeed represent a single entity with slightly different clinical phenotypes (14–19). Thus, there are good reasons to study them as a group. In addition, as will be discussed subsequently, making a diagnosis of IGE as a group (as opposed to localization-related epilepsy or a symptomatic/cryptogenic generalized epilepsy) has critical implications for patient care, whereas differentiating among the specific syndromes is relatively less important. The IGEs are genetically determined and have no structural or anatomic cause, and seizures are the only manifestation of the condition. Age of onset is very important, since IGE usually (but not always) begin early in life, from childhood to early adulthood. Neurologic examination is normal, intelligence is normal, imaging studies are normal, and EEG is normal other than for the epileptiform abnormalities (i.e., there is no abnormal slow activity or evidence for diffuse encephalopathy).

Seizure types in IGE include a combination of generalized tonic-clonic (GTC), absence, and myoclonic seizures.

- *Absence seizures* are clinically characterized by a brief (5–15 sec) impairment of consciousness, with few or no other symptoms. More specifically, patients with IGE have *typical* absence seizures, characterized by an abrupt onset and termination and the classic monomorphic 3-Hz spike-wave complexes (ictally and interictally) with no other EEG abnormality. By contrast, atypical absence seizures occur in symptomatic generalized epilepsy of the Lennox-Gastaut type and are less discrete in time, longer, and with slower and more polymorphic spike-wave complexes on EEG. Absence seizures are the defining and predominant seizure type in CAE and juvenile absence epilepsy, but they do occur in the other IGEs.
- *Myoclonic seizures* consist of sporadic jerks, usually appendicular and symmetrical, associated electrically with generalized epileptiform discharges, typically polyspikes (Figure 25-1). Patients sometimes report them as an electric shock sensation. Myoclonic seizures are the defining and predominant seizure type in JME, but they do occur in the other IGEs.
- *Generalized tonic-clonic (GTC) seizures* are of course the most common type of seizures. GTC seizures in the IGEs are by definition "primarily generalized" GTC seizures. They are typically characterized by a tonic phase that which is gradually interrupted by quiescence, thus giving rise to the clonic phase, with rhythmic spikes and spike-wave complexes decreasing in frequency. Often, primarily generalized GTC seizures begin with clonic or myoclonic jerks before the tonic phase, thus in reality being clonic-tonic-clonic rather than tonic-clonic.

The *morning predominance* of convulsive seizures is a general feature in IGE that must be specifically asked about during history taking.

EEG FEATURES (OF IGE IN GENERAL)

The EEG findings of IGEs are characteristic, and consist of generalized epileptiform discharges with normal background activity (i.e., no abnormally slow background and no superimposed slow activity). Epileptiform discharges

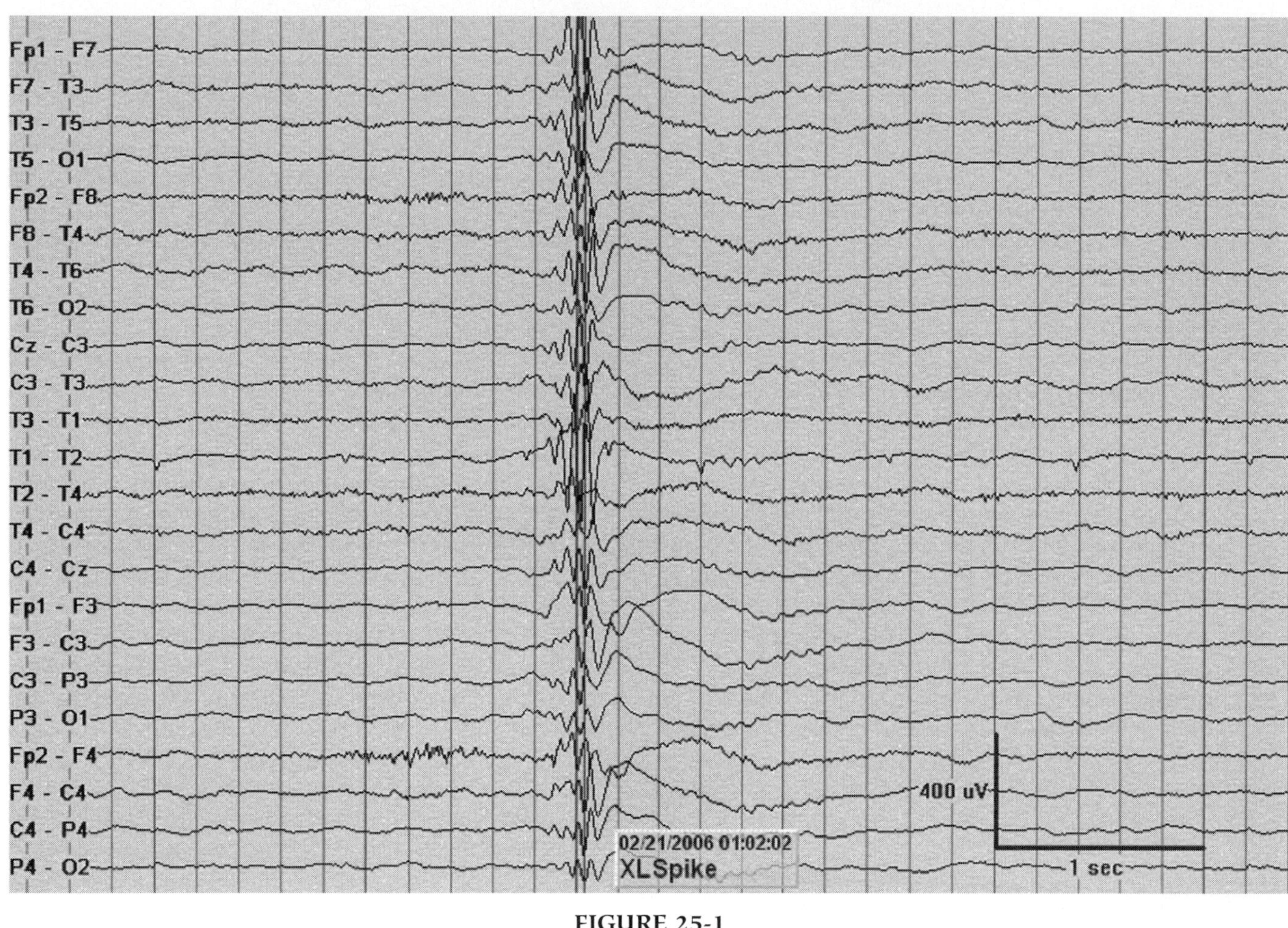

FIGURE 25-1

Typical generalized polyspike during drowsiness in a 17-year-old adolescent with typical juvenile myoclonic epilepsy. Note the high amplitude (see scale) and the aftergoing slow wave and suppression. This discharge was asymptomatic.

can take the form of spikes, sharp waves, spike-wave complexes and polyspikes. Spike-wave complexes can be viewed as the EEG correlate of absence seizures, and polyspikes as the EEG correlate of myoclonic seizures. Just as patients with IGE have various combinations of the three seizure types described in the preceding section, they also have various combinations of generalized epileptiform abnormalities. Although epileptiform discharges are typically generalized and symmetric, minor EEG asymmetries may occasionally be present (20–23) and should not lead to a diagnosis of partial seizures (24).

- *Spikes and sharp waves* are of high amplitude, with aftergoing slow waves disrupting the ongoing background. Those seen in IGE are generalized and typically maximal frontally (F3/F4 or Fp1/Fp2).
- *The spike-wave complexes* seen in IGE are very monomorphic and have the classic frequency of 3 Hz, but this may vary between 2.5 and 3.5 Hz and is often faster at the onset of the discharges (3.5 to 4.5 Hz). The near perfect monomorphism of the spike-wave complexes is as important as the 3-Hz frequency in distinguishing this pattern from the "slow" spike-wave complexes seen in the *symptomatic* generalized epilepsies of the Lennox-Gastaut type. They are generalized and symmetric with a maximum negativity frontally, almost always at F3 and F4. The onset and offset are abrupt. The 3-Hz spike-wave complexes are both an interictal and ictal pattern. The border between the two is imprecise because the clinical impairment may be difficult to detect during short discharges. It is generally stated that a discharge of about 3 seconds or more is associated with detectable impairment of awareness, but this depends of how well short impairments can be detected. The use of a clicker to test responsiveness can be very useful to document very brief impairments in awareness. Clinical seizures and the 3-Hz spike-wave complexes discharges are often precipitated by hyperventilation. The 3-Hz

frequency, and also the striking monomorphism of the spike-wave discharges, distinguish absence epilepsy from other syndromes. Spike-wave complexes can be faster (i.e., 4–6 Hz), especially in patients with IGE of adolescence, as opposed to those with typical CAE.

- *Polyspikes* (Figure 25-1) are also of high amplitude, generalized, bilateral, and grossly symmetric, and followed by significant slowing. Polyspikes are the electrical correlate of myoclonic seizures, and as such they are typically seen in IGE syndromes that include this seizure type, most characteristically JME. Polyspikes can be repetitive and described as polyspike-wave complexes.
- *Photosensitivity* is particularly frequent and, in fact, quite typical of IGE (25). Photosensitivity can be purely an EEG phenomenon, where photic stimulation elicits a photoparoxysmal response (Figure 25-2). It can also be a clinical phenomenon, where photic stimulation triggers a clinical seizure as well (typically motor seizures, i.e., myoclonic and GTC seizures).

Just as convulsive seizures tend to predominate in the morning in IGE, epileptiform discharges on awakening appear to be typical of IGE (26).

TREATMENT

Fortunately, IGEs respond well to therapy if the correct AED is administered. In general, 80-90% will become fully controlled. As mentioned earlier, some (such as typical childhood absence epilepsy) have a tendency to be outgrown.

Correct diagnosis of IGEs (at least as a group) is critical, as the choice of pharmacologic treatment matters. There is good evidence that not all AEDs are optimal choices for IGEs, and some may potentially worsen the condition (27–36, see Table 25-1). In fact, up to 70% of patients with IGE initially receive an ill-advised AED, which causes the seizures to increase in frequency or appear intractable (pseudo-intractability) (37). The use of inadequate AEDs in IGE can also result in absence or myoclonic status epilepticus (36). In general, sodium channel blockers, including phenytoin, carbamazepine, and oxcarbazepine, and GABAergic molecules, such as gabapentin, viagabatrin, and tiagabine, are not advisable in patients with IGE. The exact mechanism for these agents' lack of therapeutic effect and occasional harmful effect has not been established.

Valproic acid is the classic drug of choice for the treatment of IGEs. Both ethosuximide and valproic acid are very effective against absence seizures. In patients

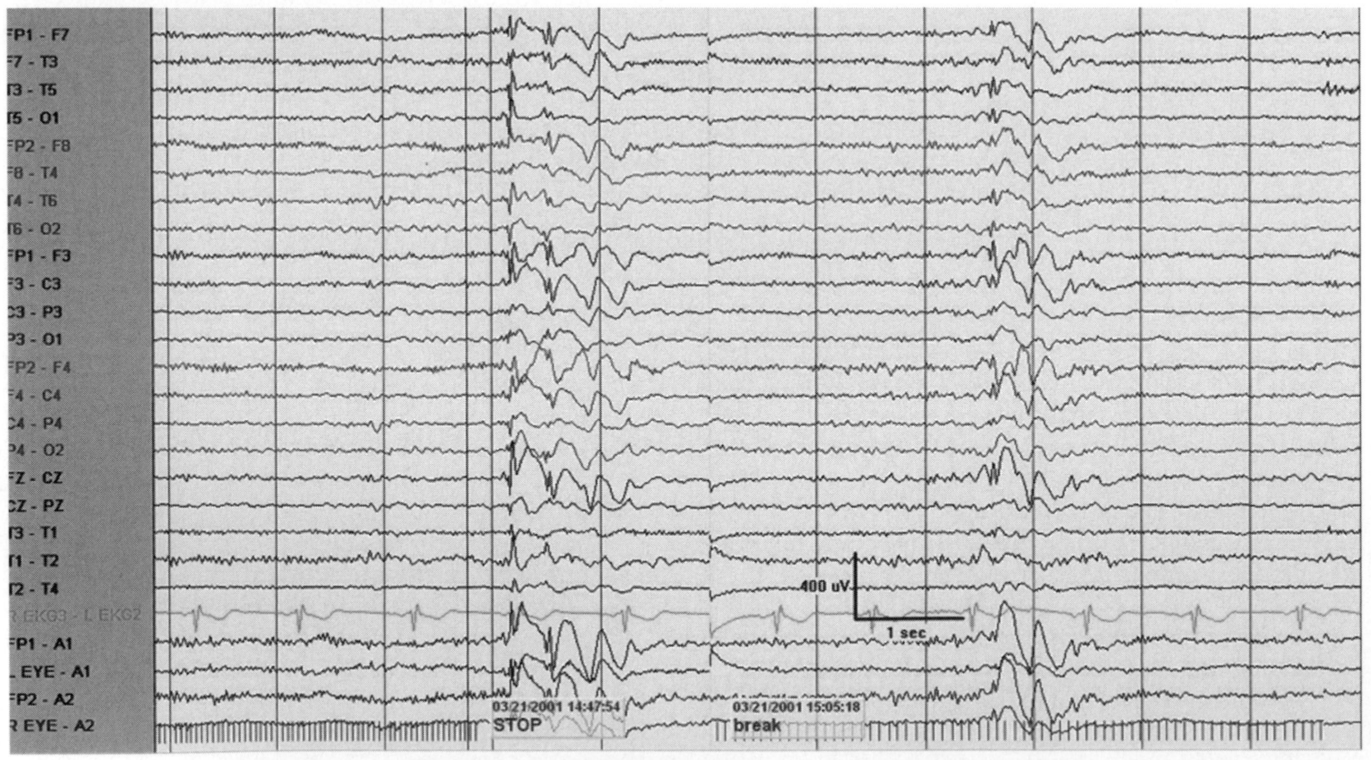

FIGURE 25-2

Photoparoxysmal response in an 18-year-old girl with generalized tonic clonic seizures. Photic stimulation (bottom channel) on 2 occasions triggers a brief but clear burst of spike-wave complexes. This discharge was asymptomatic. The patient also had similar discharges of spike-wave complexes without photic stimulation.

TABLE 25-1
Published Evidence That Some AEDs Are Not Effective in IGEs and May Exacerbate Some Seizure Types

AED	Seizure or Epilepsy Type Studied	Reference
CBZ	IGE	Snead and Hosey, 1985 (27)
CBZ, PHT	JME	Genton et al, 2000 (28)
GBP	CAE	Trudeau et al, 1996 (29)
TGB	IGE	Knake et al, 1999 (30)
CBZ	Unclear	Shields and Saslow, 1983 (31)
CBZ	Mixed	Horn et al, 1986 (32)
CBZ	Unclear	Liporace et al, 1994 (33)
CBZ	Unclear	Talwar et al, 1994 (34)
PHT, CBZ	JME	Panayiotopoulos et al, 1994 (35)
Multiple	IGE	Thomas et al, 2006 (36)

IGE: idiopathic generalized epilepsy; JME: juvenile myoclonic epilepsy; CAE: childhood absence epilepsy. CBZ: carbamazepine, GBP: gabapentin, PHT: phenytoin, TGB: tiagabine.

with both absence and generalized tonic-clonic (GTC) seizures, valproic acid is the medication of choice. A good argument can be made to select valproic acid over ethosuximide even in absence epilepsy, since 50% of patients with absence will develop GTC seizures. However, since children with typical (pure) childhood absence epilepsy rarely develop GTC seizures until the second decade, ethosuximide can be the drug of choice in young children. The limiting factors in the use of valproic acid are its potential long-term side effects, including weight gain, hair loss, tremor, teratogenicity, and polycystic ovarian disease. Ethosuximide is generally associated with a favorable side effect profile. It should be used cautiously with patients who have blood dyscrasias or abnormal renal function.

The newer AEDs are promising based upon growing evidence (38), and their place in the treatment of IGE is evolving. Newer AEDs are typically approved initially as adjunct for partial epilepsies, and only later are some of them tested for and approved for IGE. Thus, their use in IGE may be "off-label" (39–53, Table 25-2). In this regard, however, it should be pointed out that no AED, even standard ones like VPA, has specific indications for epilepsy syndromes, so that the "off-label" terminology in this context is a little artificial. In the recent years, topiramate, levetiracetam, and lamotrigine have received specific approval for IGE (Table 25-2). Lastly, levetiracetam has also recently (August 2006) received specific approval as "adjunctive therapy in the treatment of myoclonic seizures in JME," which in practice means JME (with both GTC and myoclonic seizures), and probably implies efficacy in the IGEs as a group. As usual newer AEDs first obtain approval as adjunctive therapy. However, no AED has ever been found to work as adjunctive therapy and not in monotherapy, and there is no doubt that these newer AEDs will work in monotherapy.

TABLE 25-2
Published Evidence of the Efficacy of New AEDs in the IGEs

AED	Seizure or Epilepsy Type Studied	*N*	Reference
LTG	Absence	45	Frank et al, 1999 (39)
LTG	IGE	26	Beran et al, 1998 (40)
TPM	GTC	8	Biton et al, 1999 (41)
LEV	Photosensitive	12	Kasteleijn-Nolst-Trenite et al, 1996 (42)
LEV	IGE	3	Cohen, 2003 (43)
LTG, ZNS	IGE	3	Wallace, 1998 (44)
TPM	Absence	5	Cross 2002 (45)
LTG	JME	63	Morris et al, 2004 (46)
ZNS	JME	15	Kothare et al, 2004 (47)
LEV	JME	35	Labate et al, 2006 (48)
LEV	IGE	19	Di Bonaventura et al, 2005 (49)
LEV	IGE	55	Krauss et al, 2003 (50)
LEV	IGE	25	Kumar and Smith, 2004 (51)
LEV	IGE	8	Rocamora et al, 2006 (52)
TPM	JME	22	Biton et al, 2005 (53)
LTG[1]	GTCS	117	Biton et al. 2005 (74)
LEV[1]	GTCS	80	Berkovic et al. 2007 (75)

LEV: levetiracetam; LTG: lamotrigine; TPM: topiramate; ZNS: zonisamide.
[1]Double-blind placebo-controlled studies.

INDIVIDUAL SYNDROMES

Juvenile myoclonic epilepsy, juvenile absence epilepsy, and epilepsy with generalized tonic-clonic seizures (GTCS) on awakening are the three syndromes of idiopathic generalized epilepsy of adolescent onset currently included in the ILAE classification. Childhood absence epilepsy is discussed in Chapter 22.

Juvenile Myoclonic Epilepsy (JME)

JME is one of the most common forms of epilepsy seen in the adolescent population, and is one of the best-defined syndromes. Although there is some controversy, JME appears to represent a unique phenotype among IGEs (54). The genetic abnormality in JME has been linked to a gene locus on chromosome 6 (55). In about 80% of cases, it has an age onset of between 12 and 18 years (mean 14.6 years) (56). Seizures occur predominantly in the morning, just upon awakening, in a cluster fashion, and are highly sensitive to sleep deprivation, stress, fatigue, or alcohol. Clusters of myoclonic seizures typically herald a GTC seizure. In fact, this pattern of clonic-tonic-clonic rather than tonic-clonic seizures is quite typical of JME, or at least IGE. Because JME begins as sporadic myoclonic seizures before the patient develops GTC seizures, it is often underdiagnosed and requires careful history taking, specifically inquiring about morning jerks.

Photosensitivity is very common in JME and is found in 30% of patients, the highest rate of all epilepsies (25). The characteristic EEG pattern in JME consists of discharges of high-amplitude generalized symmetric and synchronous 4–6 Hz polyspike-wave complexes.

Probably the most unique feature of JME among IGEs is that it is not outgrown and requires lifelong treatment, as the rate of recurrence is very high after discontinuation of medication, even after a long remission.

Juvenile Absence Epilepsy (JAE)

The individualization of JAE as a separate syndrome is relatively recent (1, 57, 58), because the clinical boundaries of JAE are rather imprecise. JAE falls somewhere in-between childhood absence epilepsy and JME on the spectrum of IGE, and it can have features of both. Most cases begin near or after puberty, typically between 10 and 17 years of age (59).

Absence seizures are similar though, less "pure" than those of CAE. They are clinically characterized by a brief (5–15 seconds) impairment of consciousness with abrupt onset and termination represented electrographically with a classic pattern of 3-Hz spike-wave complexes. During these episodes, the patient often displays automatisms manifesting as lip-smacking, eye blinks, or repetitive head movements. The spells have an abrupt onset (without warning) and termination, a feature distinguishing them from complex partial seizures. In general, these seizures can be reliably provoked by having the child hyperventilate for 3 to 5 minutes.

"Other" IGE or IGE "NOS" or Adult-Onset IGE

In addition to the preceding well-defined syndromes, many patients with IGE, perhaps the majority (37), either have features that do not meet criteria for a specific syndrome or have hybrid features. Seizures typically begin in young adulthood, and neurologic examination is normal. A positive family history is not uncommon. Seizures may predominate in the morning, may be photosensitive, and are sensitive to sleep deprivation. The 1989 ILAE epilepsy classification individualized "epilepsy with grand-mal seizures on awakening" and "epilepsies with specific modes of precipitation," but these entities are less well defined and too restrictive. In that scheme, most adults with IGE would not fit into any syndrome. Thus the evolving classification of IGEs uses more inclusive terms such as "IGE with GTC seizures only" (60). Other terms for the same condition include the "adult-onset IGE" (61) and IGE with pure grand mal (62). This common syndrome is typically characterized by GTC only, and likely the same as GTC "on awakening" in which seizures are not limited to the morning. When other seizure types exist in these IGEs, the seizures can clinically include mixed features, giving rise to confusing names. For example, seizures with features of both absence and myoclonic jerks can be referred to as "myoclonic absence." Examples of questionable syndromes include some reflex epilepsies, such as photosensitive GTC seizures (63), epilepsy with GTC seizures on awakening (1), epilepsy induced by thinking and spatial tasks (64, 65), or adult myoclonic epilepsy (66). In fact, many such variants can be described as, or hypothetized to be, individual syndromes, but it is more practical to view them as variations within the continuum of IGE (60).

Similarly, the EEG patterns can show mixtures of generalized epileptiform discharges of any type (spikes, sharp waves, spike-wave complexes, and polyspikes) and photosensitivity, but can vary to become a hybrid of spike-wave complexes, polyspikes, polyspike-wave complexes, and spikes (21).

Thus, in many patients (especially adolescents and young adults), pigeonholing the IGE syndrome is not necessary and may be futile, but it is critical to diagnose the patient correctly as having an IGE rather then a localization-related epilepsy, since this has crucial therapeutic and prognostic implications.

MEDICALLY INTRACTABLE IGE

The entity of "medically intractable" IGE is not well recognized and has received little attention because the vast majority of patients with IGE are fully controlled with AEDs. In addition, most patients with IGE that are not controlled are not truly intractable but instead have been treated with inadequate AEDs (37, 67, 68). Nevertheless, epilepsy centers encounter patients with clear IGE who are refractory to medications. For these patients, there is some preliminary evidence that vagus nerve stimulation (VNS) is a good option. VNS may have comparable efficacy against IGE as it does in localization-related epilepsy (69, 70), but this (like newer AEDs) is off-label use. One study in an animal model of absence epilepsy found no benefit of VNS (71). Another option in truly intractable IGE may the ketogenic diet, but no data are available to support this.

Secondary bilateral synchrony, in which frontal lobe epilepsy masquerades as IGE, should be considered when seizures appear refractory, but in the absence of a structural lesion or other clear evidence for focality, this should not be pursued surgically (24).

CONCLUSION: THE IMPORTANCE OF MAKING THE DIAGNOSIS OF IGE

Making a diagnosis of IGE is a critical step in the management of patients with seizures. Making a diagnosis of the specific type of IGE is often not possible, usually controversial, and is not necessarily important, but a diagnosis of IGE (as a group) is critical. First, the cause is not "unknown." Rather, it is a genetically determined low threshold for seizures. This is easier for patients and families to accept. Second, not all AEDs are equal for IGE. Missing the diagnosis of IGE results in inadequate drug treatment and poor seizure control (37). Third, a diagnosis of IGE has important (usually optimistic) prognostic implications.

Unfortunately, it is often taught that adults with epilepsy should be assumed to have partial (focal) epilepsy. Staring spells are loosely labeled "complex partial" seizures, and GTCs are assumed to be secondarily generalized (61). This assumption should be avoided, as it will be wrong at least 25% of the time in adults, and even more so in adolescents. A significant proportion of IGEs begin beyond childhood and adolescence: 28% after age 20 (61), and 35% after age 18 (72). And in a study of 300 patients with new-onset seizures (a mean age of 31), a quarter turned out to have an IGE (73). The EEG, when abnormal, is extremely helpful and clearly points to IGE. Occasionally the diagnosis will require video-EEG monitoring. In practice, young adults with rare GTCs often have normal EEGs, and it may be difficult to determine whether they have IGE or a focal (e.g., frontal lobe) epilepsy. In this situation, one should keep an open mind and not assume partial epilepsy. In a patient with infrequent GTC seizures and a normal (not helpful) EEG, the diagnosis should not be assumed to be localization-related epilepsy. Instead, it is prudent to keep an open mind, using a diagnosis such as "epilepsy with GTC seizures, type (IGE vs focal) uncertain," and to use broad-spectrum AEDs.

References

1. Commission on Classification and Terminology of the International League Against Epilepsy: Proposal for revised classification of epilepsy and epileptic syndromes. *Epilepsia* 1989; 30:389–399.
2. Opeskin K, Kalnins RM, Halliday G, Cartwright H, et al. Idiopathic generalized epilepsy: lack of significant microdysgenesis. *Neurology* 2000; 55:1101–1106.
3. Simister RJ, McLean MA, Barker GJ, Duncan JS. Proton MRS reveals frontal lobe metabolite abnormalities in idiopathic generalized epilepsy. *Neurology* 2003; 61:897–902.
4. Bernasconi A, Bernasconi N, Natsume J, Antel SB, et al. Magnetic resonance spectroscopy and imaging of the thalamus in idiopathic generalized epilepsy. *Brain* 2003; 126 (Pt 11):2447–2454.
5. Hirose S, Mitsudome A, Okada M, et al. Genetics of idiopathic epilepsies. *Epilepsia* 2005; 46(Suppl 1):38–43.
6. Lerche H, Weber YG, Jurkat-Rott K, et al. Ion channel defects in idiopathic epilepsies. *Curr Pharm Des* 2005; 11(21):2737–2752.
7. Noebels JL. Exploring new gene discoveries in idiopathic generalized epilepsy. *Epilepsia* 2003; 44 Suppl 2:16–21.
8. Anderson E, Berkovic S, Dulac O, et al. ILAE Genetics Commission conference report: molecular analysis of complex genetic epilepsies. *Epilepsia* 2002; 43:1262–1267. Erratum: *Epilepsia* 2002; 43:1600–1602.
9. Pal DK, Durner M, Klotz I, Dicker E, et al. Complex inheritance and parent-of-origin effect in juvenile myoclonic epilepsy. *Brain Dev* 2006; 28(2):92–98.
10. Jallon P, Latour P. Epidemiology of idiopathic generalized epilepsies. *Epilepsia* 2005; 46(Suppl 9):10–14.
11. Christensen J, Kjeldsen MJ, Andersen H, et al. Gender differences in epilepsy. *Epilepsia* 2005; 46:956–960.
12. Wheless JW, Kim HL. Adolescent seizures and epilepsy syndromes. *Epilepsia* 2002; 43(Suppl 3):33–52.
13. McCorry D, Nicolson A, Smith D, Marson A, et al. An association between type 1 diabetes and idiopathic generalized epilepsy. *Ann Neurol* 2006; 59:204–206.
14. Benbadis SR, Lüders HO. Generalized epilepsies. *Neurology* 1996; 46:1194–1195.
15. Berkovic SF, Andermann F, Andermann E, et al. Concepts of absence epilepsies: discrete syndromes or biological continuum. *Neurology* 1987; 37:993–1000.
16. Janz D. Juvenile myoclonic epilepsy. *Cleve Clin J Med* 1989; 56 (Suppl 1):S23–S33.
17. Reutens DC, Berkovic SF. Idiopathic generalized epilepsy of adolescence: are the syndromes clinically distinct? *Neurology* 1995; 45:1469–1476.
18. Briellmann RS, Torn-Broers Y, Berkovic SF. Idiopathic generalized epilepsies: do sporadic and familial cases differ? *Epilepsia* 2001; 42:1399–1402.
19. Loiseau P, Duché B, Pedespan JM. Absence epilepsies. *Epilepsia* 1995; 36:1182–1187.
20. Lancman ME, Asconapé JJ, Penry JK. Clinical and EEG asymmetries in juvenile myoclonic epilepsy. *Epilepsia* 1994; 35:302–306.
21. Yenjun S, Harvey AS, Marini C, Newton MR, et al. EEG in adult-onset idiopathic generalized epilepsy. *Epilepsia* 2003; 44:252–256.
22. Lombroso CT. Consistent EEG focalities detected in subjects with primary generalized epilepsies monitored for two decades. *Epilepsia* 1997; 38:797–812.
23. Usui N, Kotagal P, Matsumoto R, Kellinghaus C, et al. Focal semiologic and electroencephalographic features in patients with juvenile myoclonic epilepsy. *Epilepsia* 2005; 46:1668–1676.
24. Benbadis SR. Observations on the misdiagnosis of generalized epilepsy as partial epilepsy: causes and consequences. *Seizure* 1999; 8:140–145.
25. Wolf D, Goosses R. Relationship of photosensitivity to epileptic syndromes. *J Neurol Neurosurg Psychiatry* 1986; 49:1386–1391.
26. Fittipaldi F, Curra A, Fusco L, Ruggieri S, et al. EEG discharges on awakening: a marker of idiopathic generalized epilepsy. *Neurology* 2001; 56:123–126.
27. Snead OC 3rd, Hosey LC. Exacerbation of seizures in children by carbamazepine. *N Engl J Med* 1985; 313(15):916–921.
28. Genton P, Gelisse P, Thomas P, Dravet C. Do carbamazepine and phenytoin aggravate juvenile myoclonic epilepsy? *Neurology* 2000; 55(8):1106–1109.
29. Trudeau V, Myers S, LaMoreaux L, Anhut H, et al. Gabapentin in naive childhood absence epilepsy: results from two double-blind, placebo-controlled, multicenter studies. *J Child Neurol* 1996; 11(6):470–475.
30. Knake S, Hamer HM, Schomburg U, Oertel WH, et al. Tiagabine-induced absence status in idiopathic generalized epilepsy. *Seizure* 1999; 8:314–317.
31. Shields WD, Saslow E. Myoclonic, atonic, and absence seizures following institution of carbamazepine therapy in children. *Neurology* 1983; 33:1487–1489.
32. Horn CS, Ater SB, Hurst DL. Carbamazepine-exacerbated epilepsy in children and adolescents. *Pediatr Neurol* 1986; 2:340–345.

33. Liporace JD, Sperling MR, Dichter MA. Absence seizures and carbamazepine in adults. *Epilepsia* 1994; 35:1026–1028.
34. Talwar D, Arora MS, Sher PK. EEG changes and seizure exacerbation in young children treated with carbamazepine. *Epilepsia* 1994; 35:1154–1159.
35. Panayiotopoulos CP, Obeid T, Tahan AR. Juvenile myoclonic epilepsy: a 5-year prospective study. *Epilepsia* 1994; 35:285–296.
36. Thomas P, Valton L, Genton P. Absence and myoclonic status epilepticus precipitated by antiepileptic drugs in idiopathic generalized epilepsy. *Brain* 2006; 129(Pt 5):1281–1292.
37. Benbadis SR, Tatum WO, Gieron M. Idiopathic generalized epilepsy and choice of antiepileptic drugs. *Neurology* 2003; 61:1793–1795.
38. Bergey GK. Evidence-based treatment of idiopathic generalized epilepsies with new antiepileptic drugs. *Epilepsia* 2005; 46 Suppl 9:161–168.
39. Frank LM, Enlow T, Holmes GL, et al. Lamictal (lamotrigine) monotherapy for typical absence seizures in children. *Epilepsia* 1999; 40:973–979.
40. Beran RG, Berkovic SF, Dunagan FM, et al. Double-blind, placebo-controlled, crossover study of lamotrigine in treatment-resistant generalised epilepsy. *Epilepsia* 1998; 39:1329–1333.
41. Biton V, Montouris GD, Ritter F, et al. A randomized, placebo-controlled study of topiramate in primary generalized tonic-clonic seizures. Topiramate YTC Study Group. *Neurology* 1999; 52:1330–1337. Erratum: 1999; 53:1162.
42. Kasteleijn-Nolst Trenite DG, Marescaux C, Stodieck S, Edelbroek PM, et al. Photosensitive epilepsy: a model to study the effects of antiepileptic drugs. Evaluation of the piracetam analogue, levetiracetam. *Epilepsy Res* 1996; 25:225–230.
43. Cohen J. Levetiracetam monotherapy for primary generalised epilepsy. *Seizure* 2003; 12:150–153.
44. Wallace SJ. Myoclonus and epilepsy in childhood: a review of treatment with valproate, ethosuximide, lamotrigine and zonisamide. *Epilepsy Res* 1998; 29:147–154.
45. Cross JH. Topiramate monotherapy for childhood absence seizures: an open label pilot study. *Seizure* 2002; 11:406–410.
46. Morris GL, Hammer AE, Kustra RP, Messenheimer JA. Lamotrigine for patients with juvenile myoclonic epilepsy following prior treatment with valproate: results of an open-label study. *Epilepsy Behav* 2004; 5:509–512.
47. Kothare SV, Valencia I, Khurana DS, Hardison H, et al. Efficacy and tolerability of zonisamide in juvenile myoclonic epilepsy. *Epileptic Disord* 2004; 6:267–270.
48. Labate A, Colosimo E, Gambardella A, Leggio U, et al. Levetiracetam in patients with generalised epilepsy and myoclonic seizures: an open label study. *Seizure* 2006; 15: 214–218.
49. Di Bonaventura C, Fattouch J, Mari F, Egeo G, et al. Clinical experience with levetiracetam in idiopathic generalized epilepsy according to different syndrome subtypes. *Epileptic Disord* 2005; 7:231–235.
50. Krauss GL, Betts T, Abou-Khalil B, et al. Levetiracetam treatment of idiopathic generalised epilepsy. *Seizure* 2003; 12:617–620.
51. Kumar SP, Smith PE. Levetiracetam as add-on therapy in generalised epilepsies. *Seizure* 2004; 13:475–477.
52. Rocamora R, Wagner K, Schulze-Bonhage A. Levetiracetam reduces frequency and duration of epileptic activity in patients with refractory primary generalized epilepsy. *Seizure* 2006; 15:428–433.
53. Biton V, Bourgeois BF, YTC/YTCE Study Investigators. Topiramate in patients with juvenile myoclonic epilepsy. *Arch Neurol* 2005; 62:1705–1708.
54. Martinez-Juarez IE, Alonso ME, Medina MT, et al. Juvenile myoclonic epilepsy subsyndromes: family studies and long-term follow up. *Brain* 2006; 129:1269–1280.
55. Greenberg DA, Durner M, Resor S, Rosenbaum D, et al. The genetics of idiopathic generalized epilepsies of adolescent onset: differences between juvenile myoclonic epilepsy and epilepsy with random grand mal and with awakening grand mal. *Neurology* 1995; 45:942–946.
56. Panayiotopoulos CP, Obeid T, Tahan AR. Juvenile myoclonic epilepsy: a 5-year prospective study. *Epilepsia* 1994; 35:258–296.
57. Obeid T. Clinical and genetic aspects of juvenile absence epilepsy. *J Neurol* 1994; 241: 487–491.
58. Wolf P, Inoue Y. Therapeutic response of absence seizures in patients of an epilepsy clinic for adolescents and adults. *J Neurol* 1984; 231:225–229.
59. Wolf P. Juvenile absence epilepsy. In: Roger J, Bureau M, Dravet C, et al, eds. *Epileptic Syndromes in Infancy, Childhood and Adolescents*. 2nd ed. London: John Libbey, 1992:307–312.
60. Engel J. A proposed diagnostic scheme for people with epileptic seizures and with epilepsy: report of the ILAE Task Force on Classification and Terminology. *Epilepsia* 2001; 42:796–803.
61. Marini C, King MA, Archer JS, et al. Idiopathic generalised epilepsy of adult onset: clinical syndromes and genetics. *J Neurol Neurosurg Psychiatry* 2003; 74:192–196.
62. Unterberger I, Trinka E, Luef G, et al. Idiopathic generalized epilepsies with pure grand mal: clinical data and genetics. *Epilepsy Res* 2001; 44:19–25.
63. Zifkin BG, Kasteleijn-Nolst Trenite D. Reflex epilepsy and reflex seizures of the visual system: a clinical review. *Epileptic Disord* 2002:129–36.
64. Andermann F, Zifkin B, Andermann E. Epilepsy induced by thinking and spatial tasks. *Adv Neurol* 1998; 75:263–272.
65. Goossens LAZ, Andermann F, Andermann E, et al. Reflex seizures induced by calculation, card or board games, and spatial tasks: a review of 25 patients and delineation of the epileptic syndrome. *Neurology* 1990; 40:1171–1176.
66. Gilliam F, Steinhoff BJ, Bittermann HJ, Kuzniecky R, et al. Adult myoclonic epilepsy: a distinct syndrome of idiopathic generalized epilepsy. *Neurology* 2000; 55: 1030–1033.
67. Genton P, Gelisse P, Thomas P, Dravet C. Do carbamazepine and phenytoin aggravate juvenile myoclonic epilepsy? *Neurology* 2000; 55:1106–1109.
68. Perucca E. The management of refractory idiopathic epilepsies. *Epilepsia* 2001; 42(Suppl 3): 31–35.
69. Holmes MD, Silbergeld DL, Drouhard D, Wilensky AJ, et al. Effect of vagus nerve stimulation on adults with pharmacoresistant generalized epilepsy syndromes. *Seizure* 2004; 13:340–345.
70. Ng M, Devinsky O. Vagus nerve stimulation for refractory idiopathic generalised epilepsy. *Seizure* 2004; 13:176–178.
71. Dedeurwaerdere S, Vonck K, Van Hese P, Wadman W, et al. The acute and chronic effect of vagus nerve stimulation in genetic absence epilepsy rats from Strasbourg (GAERS). *Epilepsia* 2005; 46 Suppl 5:94–97.
72. Gastaut H. Individualisation des épilepsies dites "bénignes" ou "fonctionnelles" aux différents âges de la vie. Appréciation des variations correspondantes de la prédisposition épileptiques à ces âges. *Rev EEG Neurophysiol* 1981; 11:346–366.
73. King MA, Newton MR, Jackson GD, et al. Epileptology of the first-seizure presentation: a clinical, electroencephalographic, and magnetic resonance imaging study of 30 consecutive patients. *Lancet* 1998; 352(9133):1007–1011.
74. Biton V, Sackellares JC, Vuong A, Hammer AE, Barrett PS, Messenheimer JA. Double-blind, placebo controlled study of lamotrigine in primary generalized tonic-clonic seizures. *Neurology* 2005; 65:1737–43.
75. Berkovic SF, Knowlton RC, Leroy RF, Schiemann J, Falter U; on behalf of the Levetiracetam N01057 Study Group. Placebo-controlled study of levetiracetam in idiopathic generalized epilepsy. *Neurology* 2007 Jul 11; (*Neurology*, doi:10.1212/01.wnl.0000268699.34614.d3).

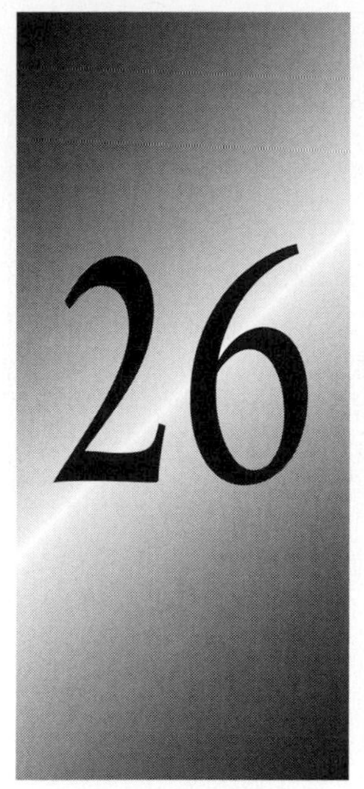

Progressive Myoclonus Epilepsies

Samuel F. Berkovic

The syndrome of progressive myoclonus epilepsy (PME) consists of myoclonic seizures, tonic-clonic seizures, and progressive neurologic dysfunction, particularly ataxia and dementia. Onset may be at any age but is usually in late childhood or adolescence. Myoclonus in PME is typically fragmentary and multifocal and often is precipitated by posture, action, or external stimuli such as light, sound, or touch. It is particularly apparent in facial and distal limb musculature. Bilateral massive myoclonic jerks, which tend to involve proximal limb muscles, may also occur (1, 2).

In its fully developed form with florid, unremitting myoclonic seizures and progressive neurologic deterioration, diagnosis of the PME syndrome can hardly be missed. Diagnosis may be more difficult in the early stages, and confusion with more benign epilepsies is common. There are a large number of causes of the PME syndrome; most are due to specific genetic disorders, which can now be accurately diagnosed in life. Spectacular advances in the molecular genetics of these disorders have occurred in the last few years (Table 26-1).

Diagnosis of the specific type of PME is challenging, as most individual clinicians have limited experience with these rare disorders. The main causes of PME are described in this chapter, which is largely derived from another publication (3). Description of the rarer forms can be found elsewhere (1–3).

UNVERRICHT-LUNDBORG DISEASE

Unverricht-Lundborg disease is the prototypic cause of PME (4, 5). No storage material is present, but there is neuronal loss and gliosis, particularly affecting the cerebellum, medial thalamus, and spinal cord (6).

Clinical Features

Clinical onset is with myoclonus or tonic-clonic seizures between the ages of 8 and 13 years (mean 10, range 6–16).

The myoclonus usually is quite severe and may be precipitated by movement, stress, or sensory stimuli. Repetitive morning myoclonus is also typical, frequently building up and culminating in a major tonic-clonic seizure (7, 8). Seizures may be difficult to control, but progression in terms of ataxia and dementia is mild and late. The clinical course is variable, and there may be considerable intrafamily variation in the severity of the seizures. Some patients are relatively mildly affected and survive to old age. Others have a more fulminant course, with death within a few years of onset; this outcome seems

TABLE 26-1
Molecular Genetics of Major Progressive Myoclonus Epilepsies

Specific Disorder		Linkage	Gene Product
Unverricht-Lundborg disease		21q22	Cystatin B
Myoclonus epilepsy with ragged red fibers		mtDNA	$tRNA^{Lys}$
Lafora disease		6q24	EPM2A (Laforin)
		6p22	EPM2B (NHLRC1)
Neuronal ceroid lipofuscinoses			
	Late infantile	11p15	Tripeptidyl peptidase I (CLN2)
	Finnish late infantile	13q	CLN 5
	Late-infantile variant	15q21	CLN6
	Turkish late infantile	8p23	CLN8
	Juvenile	16p12	CLN3
	Adult	?	?
Sialidosis type I	6p21	Neuraminidase	
Sialidosis type II	20q13	Protective protein/ cathepsin A	

to be rare now and may have been due to unrecognized deleterious effects of phenytoin (9, 10).

The electroencephalogram (EEG) background may show some diffuse theta that increases over years as well as some frontal beta activity. Epileptic activity consists of 3–5 Hz spike-wave or multiple spike-wave activity with the maximum field being anterior. Sporadic focal spikes, particularly in the occipital region, may be seen but are usually not prominent. Photosensitivity typically is marked. The spike-wave activity is diminished during non–rapid-eye-movement (non-REM) sleep (8, 11).

Genetics

Unverricht-Lundborg disease is an autosomal recessive condition (12) initially recognized as a geographic cluster in Finland and eastern Sweden (hence the name "Baltic myoclonus"). An erroneous but frequently held view is that this disorder is confined to the Baltic region. Clusters of a phenotypically identical disorder, the so-called "Mediterranean myoclonus," occur in southern Europe and North Africa (13). It is also found sporadically worldwide in Caucasians, blacks, and Japanese (9, 14, 15).

The disorder was linked to the long arm of chromosome 21 in Finnish cases in 1991 (16), and the gene for cystatin B was identified as the responsible gene in 1996 (17). The clinical prediction that similar cases seen outside the Baltic region have the same condition was confirmed by showing the identification of mutations in the cystatin B gene (CSTB) in families from around the world. The commonest mutation, responsible for about 90% of abnormal alleles, is an unstable expansion of a dodecamer repeat in the 5′ untranslated promoter region. The remaining mutations are missense mutations (18–21).

Diagnosis

Unverricht-Lundborg disease is recognized clinically by its characteristic age of onset and clinical pattern, with an absence of other clinical or pathologic features. Diagnosis is confirmed by molecular genetic study of the cystatin B gene.

MYOCLONUS EPILEPSY WITH RAGGED RED FIBERS

The syndrome of myoclonus epilepsy with ragged red fibers (MERRF) has emerged as one of the most common causes of PME. It may be familial or sporadic, and its clinical features and severity are extremely variable.

Clinical Features

Myoclonus epilepsy with ragged red fibers was first described in cases with a florid clinical myopathy and myoclonus epilepsy (22, 23). It is now clear that the clinical spectrum of MERRF is extremely broad. It should be suspected in a wide variety of situations, even when clinical and pathologic evidence of myopathy are absent (24). Symptoms may begin at any age, and there may be marked intrafamily variation in the age of onset and clinical severity (24, 25). The clinical features include myoclonus, tonic-clonic seizures, dementia, and ataxia, with less common findings of myopathy, neuropathy, deafness, and optic atrophy. Some cases show striking axial lipomas. Occasional patients or families have focal neurologic events, and there is an overlap with the syndrome of mitochondrial encephalomyopathy, lactic acidosis, and strokelike episodes (MELAS), in which strokelike episodes, frequently preceded by migrainous headaches with vomiting, are characteristic.

The EEG shows slowly progressive background slowing, paralleling the degree of clinical deterioration. There are generalized spike-and-wave discharges at 2–5 Hz or multiple spike-and-wave discharges. Sporadic occipital spikes and sharp waves may be seen. Prominent photosensitivity may occur. Non-REM sleep is disorganized, and spike-and-wave discharges are diminished (11, 26).

Genetics

Virtually all familial cases of MERRF are transmitted through the maternal line and are examples of mitochondrial inheritance (25). The peculiarities of mitochondrial inheritance provide an explanation for the wide phenotypic variability in patients with MERRF and the extraordinary intrafamily variation.

A single base substitution at nucleotide pair 8344 of mitochondrial DNA, causing an A-to-G substitution in the $tRNA^{Lys}$ gene, occurs in many familial cases of MERRF (27). The fact that this mutation affects tRNA rather than a gene for a respiratory enzyme probably explains the heterogeneous results for respiratory enzyme assays reported in MERRF. This $tRNA^{Lys}$ mutation has been confirmed in numerous laboratories around the world and appears to underlie most but not all familial cases and some sporadic examples of MERRF. Other rare identified molecular causes of MERRF are mutations at nucleotides 8356 and 8363 in the same $tRNA^{Lys}$ (28, 29) and mutations in $tRNA^{Ser}$ (30), but in some cases no molecular defect has been found. Recently, autosomal recessive mutations in the nuclear encoded mitochondrial gene polymerase gamma (POLG) have been identified in some MERRF cases (31).

Diagnosis

Diagnosis can usually be suspected clinically but may be difficult to confirm with laboratory markers. The clinical clues to the diagnosis include deafness, optic atrophy, myopathy, lipomas, intrafamily variation in age of onset and severity, and a pattern of inheritance compatible with maternal transmission. Serum lactate, ragged red fibers, and respiratory enzyme activities in muscle can all be normal in patients known to be affected (e.g., family members of proven cases). Magnetic resonance spectroscopy (MRS) of muscle may show elevated levels of inorganic phosphate and a decrease of the phosphocreatine:inorganic phosphate concentration ratio (32). When present, molecular defects in mitochondrial DNA can be detected in peripheral blood or muscle (33, 34).

LAFORA DISEASE

Lafora disease is characterized by the presence of Lafora bodies, which are polyglucosan inclusions found in neurons and in a variety of other sites, including the heart, skeletal muscle, liver, and sweat gland duct cells (35, 36).

Clinical Features

Onset of Lafora disease is between the ages of 10 and 18 years, with a mean age of onset of 14 years. Clinical features are myoclonus, tonic-clonic seizures, and relentless cognitive decline. Focal seizures, particularly that arise from the occipital regions, occur in approximately half the patients. Recognition of Lafora disease in its fully developed form is not difficult. At the onset, however, the disorder may resemble a typical benign adolescent generalized epilepsy with no evidence of cognitive decline. It also may present as a dementing illness with relatively infrequent seizures, or it may mimic a nonspecific secondary generalized epilepsy because myoclonus is not obvious (37, 38). The prognosis of Lafora disease is dismal, with death occurring 2 to 10 years after onset and the mean age of death being 20 years.

The clinical picture, including the relatively narrow age range of onset and relentlessly progressive course to death within 2 to 10 years of onset, is constant in all reports with the exception of a few cases. These cases, sometimes erroneously labeled "type Lundborg," had symptoms beginning in late adolescence or early adult life with a milder protracted course. They may represent a genetic subtype of Lafora disease separate from the classic form (39, 40).

At onset the EEG background is well organized, and there are multiple spike-and-wave discharges that are increased by intermittent photic stimulation. Erratic myoclonus is seen without EEG correlation. Spike-and-wave discharges are not accentuated during sleep. Over the next few months to years, the background deteriorates, the physiologic elements of sleep become disrupted, and only REM sleep can be identified. Multifocal, particularly posterior, epileptiform abnormalities appear in addition to the generalized bursts, and in the terminal phase of the illness the EEG is quite disorganized (41).

Genetics

Lafora disease is an autosomal recessive condition. The largest series have been reported from southern Europe (41), but it is found worldwide, apparently without a marked racial or ethnic predilection. Approximately 90% of cases have mutations in the gene EPM2A, which encodes a dual phosphatase known as laforin (42, 43), or in EPM2B (also called NHLRC1), which codes for an E3 ubiquitin ligase known as malin (44, 45). There is evidence for a third, as yet unknown, locus (46).

Diagnosis

The age of onset, eventual inexorable dementia, and frequent occurrence of focal occipital seizures are clinical clues to the diagnosis (38). Lafora bodies can be demonstrated in many tissues, but diagnosis is most simply made by examination of eccrine sweat gland ducts by a simple skin biopsy (36) and can now be confirmed in most cases by molecular study of EPM2A and EPM2B (47).

NEURONAL CEROID LIPOFUSCINOSES

The neuronal ceroid lipofuscinoses (NCL) are characterized by the accumulation of abnormal amounts of lipopigment in lysosomes. Seven types—late infantile (Jansky-Bielschowsky, CLN2), late infantile variants (CLN5, CLN6, CLN7, CLN8), juvenile (Spielmeyer-Vogt-Sjögren, CLN3), and adult NCL (Kufs, CLN4)—may cause the PME syndrome (48). The infantile form (CLN1) presents differently, with regression, hypotonia, and impaired vision, and it is not considered here. The childhood forms are sometimes collectively referred to as Batten's disease.

Clinical Features

The late infantile form has an onset between 2.5 and 4 years. Seizures usually are the first manifestation, with myoclonic seizures, tonic-clonic seizures, atonic seizures, and atypical absences. Ataxia and psychomotor regression are seen within a few months of onset, with visual failure generally developing late.

Examination of the optic fundi reveals attenuated retinal vessels and macular degeneration. The seizures are usually intractable, dementia is relentless, and there is progressive spasticity, with death approximately 5 years after onset (37). The EEG shows background slowing and disorganization with generalized epileptiform discharges. Photosensitivity is marked, and single flashes may provoke giant posterior evoked responses. Visual evoked potentials (VEPs) are abnormally broad and of high amplitude, and sensory evoked potentials (SEPs) are enlarged. The electroretinogram (ERG) becomes progressively attenuated (37, 49).

The late infantile variant form, described in Finland, differs in that onset is later, between 5 and 7 years; psychomotor regression and visual failure occur earlier; myoclonic and tonic-clonic seizures generally appear at approximately age 8 years; and progression is somewhat slower (50). Electrophysiologic findings are similar to those of the late infantile form except that the marked response to photic stimulation develops at approximately age 7–8 years and disappears by age 10–11 years, and the visual evoked response (VER), which initially is large, progressively attenuates (50). Other variants of the late infantile form have been described in other geographic regions (48).

Juvenile NCL begins between the ages of 4 and 10 years. The majority of patients present with visual failure and have gradual development of dementia and extrapyramidal features, with seizures being a relatively minor manifestation. Other patients present with myoclonus and tonic-clonic seizures with visual, cognitive, and motor signs developing later. This is sometimes called the early juvenile variant. Fundoscopy reveals optic atrophy, macular degeneration, and attenuated vessels. Inheritance is autosomal recessive. The course is variable, with death approximately 8 years after onset (37, 51). The EEG shows background slowing and generalized epileptiform discharges that often are of the slow-spike-and-wave type. Sleep activates the epileptic abnormality, but photic stimulation does not. VEPs are of low amplitude and sometimes cannot be elicited. The ERG is flat (37, 49).

The adult form is considerably rarer. It can present as a PME syndrome around the age of 30, although other patients present with a picture of dementia and extrapyramidal or cerebellar disturbance. Visual auras may occur before some seizures. Blindness is notably absent, and the optic fundi are normal. The clinical course from onset to death is approximately 12 years (52). The EEG shows generalized fast spike-and-wave discharges with marked photosensitivity. Single flashes may evoke paroxysmal discharges. The background activity may be normal in the early stages, and ERGs are normal (11, 52).

Genetics

The various forms are genetically distinct and occur worldwide, but with peculiar patterns of geographic clustering. In Finland there are large numbers of infantile and juvenile cases, whereas in Newfoundland late infantile and juvenile cases occur with increased frequency (53, 54). All forms are autosomal recessive disorders. Kufs' disease, however, also occurs in families with dominant inheritance (55).

The storage material(s) in the NCLs has been extremely difficult to characterize and for many years was thought to be lipid. Subunit c of mitochondrial ATP synthase, a very hydrophobic protein, subsequently was identified as the major storage protein in an ovine model (56) and in human late infantile, juvenile, and adult cases (56, 57).

Considerable progress in the molecular genetics of this complex group of disorders has recently occurred. The causative gene has been identified for five of the currently identified seven variants causing PME. The classical late infantile form is due to mutations in the gene CLN2, which encodes a lysosomal enzyme tripetidyl peptidase (TPP1) (48). CLN3, CLN5, CLN6, and CLN8 encode various lysosomal or intracellular membrane proteins whose functions remain to be elucidated (48).

Diagnosis

Diagnosis may often be suspected clinically, particularly if there are visual changes. The electrophysiologic findings previously described may be helpful. Vacuolated lymphocytes may occur in the juvenile form. Neuroradiologic studies show cerebral atrophy and particularly cerebellar atrophy. Definitive diagnosis presently requires the demonstration of characteristic inclusions by electron microscopy. These can be found most simply in eccrine secretory cells. The inclusions take various forms, with curvilinear profiles being characteristic of a late infantile NCL, fingerprint profiles being usual in the juvenile and adult forms, and granular osmiophilic deposits occurring in the infantile form. Considerable expertise may be required in the pathologic interpretation of the electron micrographs (58). In the case of suspected CLN2, enzymatic assays for TPP1 are available, and molecular testing can be performed for CLN2, CLN3, CLN5, CLN6, and CLN8 (48).

SIALIDOSES

The sialidoses are the least common of the major forms of PME. They are autosomal recessive disorders associated with deficiencies of alpha-N-acetyl-neuraminidase.

Clinical Features

In sialidosis type I ("cherry-red spot-myoclonus syndrome"), there is onset in adolescence with myoclonus, gradual visual failure, tonic-clonic seizures, ataxia, and a characteristic cherry-red spot in the fundus. The myoclonus is usually very severe. Lens opacities and a mild peripheral neuropathy with burning feet may occur. Dementia is absent (37, 59).

Juvenile sialidosis type II presents as a PME with features similar to those of sialidosis type I except that onset is sometimes a little later. There may be additional features of coarse facies, corneal clouding, dysostosis multiplex, hearing loss, and low intellect, which may be present from early life (59, 60).

The EEG background shows low-voltage fast activity, but some slowing can be seen in demented patients. Generalized spike-and-wave bursts are absent or infrequent; rather massive myoclonus is associated with trains of 10- to 20-Hz small vertex positive spikes preceding the electromyogram (EMG) artifact. Non-REM sleep is disorganized, and although myoclonus diminishes, the vertex spikes persist and become very frequent in deep sleep (37).

Genetics

Sialidosis type 1 is due to mutations in the alpha-N-acetylneuraminidase gene (NEU1) on chromosome 6 (61). Many of the published cases were of Italian origin (59).

Sialidosis type II comprises a complex group of phenotypes. The juvenile form presents as a PME and occurs predominantly in Japan. In addition to the neuraminidase deficiency, a partial deficiency of beta-galactosidase is also found in most if not all cases (58, 59). The combination of neuraminidase and beta-galactosidase deficiency (galactosialidosis) is due to a lack of protein that is required to protect galactosidase from degradation and is essential for the catalytic action of neuraminidase (62). Missense mutations in the gene that encodes lysosomal protective protein/cathepsin A (PPCA) on chromosome 20 cause the juvenile form with PME (63–65).

Diagnosis

Sialidoses should be identified clinically because of the characteristic optic fundus. Periodic acid-Schiff-positive inclusions may be seen in lymphocytes, bone marrow cells, neurons, and Kupfer cells. Diagnosis is confirmed by grossly elevated urinary sialyloligosaccharides and by a deficiency of cryolabile alpha-N-acetylneuraminidase in leukocytes or cultured fibroblasts (59).

DISTINGUISHING PME FROM OTHER EPILEPSIES AND MYOCLONIC SYNDROMES

It usually is not difficult to diagnose the syndrome of PME some years after onset with the distinctive diagnostic triad of myoclonic seizures, tonic-clonic seizures, and progressive neurologic decline. At the beginning of the illness, however, the clinical and EEG features may be similar to those of benign idiopathic generalized epilepsies, particularly mimicking juvenile myoclonic epilepsy. Initial response to therapy may be relatively favorable. However, seizures may become more frequent with the passage of time, and progressive neurologic decline occurs. Failure to respond to therapy and progressive neurologic signs should lead to consideration of the presence of a PME. Conversely, the clinical picture of patients with idiopathic generalized epilepsies may mimic that of PME if they are inappropriately treated and intoxicated with antiepileptic drugs (AEDs), leading to ataxia, impaired cognitive function, and poorly controlled seizures.

Myoclonus in PMEs is usually quite severe, but in some patients it may be relatively obscure, with convulsive seizures and intellectual decline dominating the clinical picture, leading to a misdiagnosis of a nonspecific symptomatic (secondary) generalized epilepsy or Lennox-Gastaut syndrome. In such cases, a careful search for myoclonus should lead to consideration of the PME syndrome.

Neurophysiologic assessment may also provide clues to the presence of a PME. The EEG background rhythm may be relatively well preserved in the early phases, but generalized slow activity appears as the condition progresses. This is particularly so in those forms of PME associated with relentless dementia, such as Lafora disease and NCL. Generalized epileptiform abnormalities are seen during the resting record, usually in the form of fast spike-and-wave, multiple spike-and-wave, or multiple spike discharges. Photosensitivity is common and may be marked. Focal, particularly posterior, epileptiform abnormalities are common in Lafora disease but also may occur in other forms (11). Somatosensory evoked potentials (SEPs) frequently show giant responses (66).

PMEs should be distinguished from degenerative disorders in which seizures and/or myoclonus can occur but do not form part of the clinical core or usual initial presentation of the disorder. The causes of such progressive encephalopathies with seizures are numerous and include GM2 gangliosidosis, nonketotic hyperglycinemia, Niemann-Pick type C, juvenile Huntington's disease, Alzheimer's disease, and so forth. The distinction between this diverse group of disorders and the PMEs, while not absolute, is clinically useful and provides a practical framework on which to begin specific differential diagnosis. For example, typical Alzheimer's disease may have myoclonus as a relatively late feature and would not be confused with a PME. Rare early-onset cases may, however, present as a PME in early adult life (67). Myoclonus is also prominent in certain static encephalopathies, of which postanoxic myoclonus (Lance-Adams syndrome) is the best known. The absence of progression and the usual clear history of the causative encephalopathy enable clear distinction from PME.

The PME syndrome should also be distinguished from the progressive myoclonic ataxias. The latter term was introduced to denote a group of patients, usually adults, with progressive ataxia and myoclonus but with few, if any, tonic-clonic seizures and little or no evidence of dementia (14). Previously, some authors used the term "Ramsay Hunt syndrome" for these patients' condition, although others used this term for quite different clinical groups, which led to considerable confusion in the literature. The causes of progressive myoclonic ataxia partially overlap with those of PME but also include spinocerebellar degeneration, celiac disease, and Whipple's disease. Although it is now possible to specifically diagnose most patients with the PME syndrome in life (see next section), a larger proportion of carefully studied cases with progressive myoclonic ataxia remain without a known specific cause (14, 68).

Japanese authors have highlighted a condition of benign myoclonic epilepsy of adulthood. In this autosomal dominant disorder, onset is usually between 20 and 40 years, with myoclonus and rare tonic-clonic seizures. Generalized epileptiform EEG abnormalities and giant SEPs are present, but there is little or no evidence of progression (69, 70). This condition may be the same as or similar to that previously described in the German literature as myoclonus epilepsy of Hartung type (39).

Finally, the condition of benign familial myoclonus should be distinguished. In this autosomal dominant disorder, nonepileptic myoclonus begins in the first three decades of life but is not associated with major seizures, epileptiform EEG abnormalities, or neurologic deterioration (71).

DIAGNOSING THE SPECIFIC TYPE OF PME

Once the clinician is convinced that a patient has the PME syndrome, the critical question is to determine which specific disorder is present. This is essential for proper clinical and genetic counseling of the family (see "Treatment" section).

It is now possible to provide a specific diagnosis in life for the majority of patients with PME using clinical methods and minimally invasive investigations. An approach to this problem has been described previously. The clinician should first consider the five major disorders causing PME. Once these conditions are excluded, the rarer disorders should be considered (1–3).

Clinical Features

Although patients with the PME syndrome superficially may appear to have similar clinical features, knowledge of the specific clinical patterns of the common causes of PME often allows the differential diagnosis to be narrowed. Age at onset of symptoms provides some guidance in making the diagnosis, although MERRF may begin at any age. Certain seizure patterns are helpful; very prominent myoclonus suggests Unverricht-Lundborg disease, MERRF, or sialidosis. Partial seizures, particularly of occipital origin, can occur in a variety of the disorders but are often noted in Lafora disease. Characteristic fundal changes are almost invariable in sialidosis and are frequent in the NCLs. Dementia is a constant feature of Lafora disease and NCLs, whereas it is characteristically absent or mild in Unverricht-Lundborg disease and sialidosis type I. The presence of deafness, lipomas, optic atrophy, myopathy, or neuropathy are clinical pointers to MERRF. Neuropathy may also occur in sialidosis. Dysmorphic features are usual in sialidosis type II and may occur in MERRF.

Family History

A detailed family history, including examination of relatives, is essential. Recessive inheritance is usual, and the finding of parental consanguinity or early clinical signs in asymptomatic siblings would support this pattern. Maternal transmission is characteristic of MERRF. In MERRF and the autosomal dominant disorders, older relatives may be found to have mild, incomplete forms of the condition.

Neurophysiology

Findings that may be useful in specific diagnosis include vertex spikes as the main epileptiform abnormality in sialidosis, activation of epileptiform abnormalities in non-REM sleep in the sialidoses and the late-infantile and juvenile forms of NCL, photosensitivity to single flashes in late infantile and adult NCL, and absent ERG in late infantile and juvenile NCL (11).

Laboratory Findings

Hematologic examination may reveal lymphocyte vacuolation in sialidosis and in certain cases of NCL. Routine biochemical tests are not helpful, with the exception of elevated lactate levels in blood and cerebrospinal fluid in some cases of MERRF.

Pathologic Studies

A tissue diagnosis is essential for a number of these disorders. Skin biopsy with or without skeletal-muscle biopsy is the initial procedure. Lafora disease can be reliably diagnosed by examining eccrine sweat gland duct cells with stains for polysaccharides (36). The diagnosis of NCL may be suggested by an acid phosphatase stain, but electron microscopy of the skin biopsy specimen is essential for the definitive identification of inclusions. These inclusions are detectable in many cell types in the late infantile form of the disease, but diagnostic inclusions may be limited to eccrine secretory cells in the juvenile and adult varieties (58). False negative skin biopsies in Lafora disease and in late infantile and juvenile NCL are due to failure to examine the appropriate cell type properly. In suspected Lafora disease, sweat gland ducts must be included in the biopsy and properly examined. Where doubt remains, skin biopsy should be repeated because of the serious prognostic implications of the diagnosis of Lafora disease. The reliability of diagnosis of Kufs' disease from skin biopsy is not yet clear.

Study of muscle biopsy specimens with modified Gomori's trichrome and oxidative enzyme reactions may demonstrate ragged red fibers in MERRF. Abnormal mitochondria may be identified in muscle or skin using electron microscopy. Normal light and electron microscopic studies of muscle do not rule out the diagnosis of MERRF, and a second biopsy may be indicated in clinically suspicious cases.

Molecular Biological Studies

Molecular biological studies are playing an increasing role in the diagnosis of the PMEs. Simple DNA tests for the dodecamer repeat in Unverricht-Lundborg disease and mitochondrial DNA mutations in MERRF are readily available. Testing for mutations associated with Lafora disease, neuronal ceroid lipofuscinososes, and sialidoses is available from more specialized or research-oriented laboratories (see http://www.genetests.org).

TREATMENT

Treatment of these disorders may be distressingly difficult. Accurate diagnosis is the first step, as informed genetic counseling must be given. It is very important to distinguish MERRF, which may show maternal inheritance, from autosomal recessive disorders, such as Unverricht-Lundborg disease, Lafora disease, sialidoses, and the NCLs, and from rare dominant families with Kufs' disease. Genetic counseling may now be extended to prenatal diagnosis in some cases. Specific diagnosis also allows an accurate prognosis to be given, including a realistic appraisal of the educational and vocational goals of the patient.

Valproate and/or clonazepam should be used for symptomatic control of myoclonus. Phenytoin has a clear deleterious effect in Unverricht-Lundborg disease (9, 10), and neither should it be used in the other PMEs. Small doses of barbiturates may be helpful, but sedation should be avoided. Piracetam may be useful in certain cases (72, 73). Care must be taken not to intoxicate the patient with drugs, although there is some evidence that carefully monitored polytherapy may be more effective in some patients than the usual practice of aiming for monotherapy (74). Zonisamide (75, 76) and levetiracetam (77–79) may be quite effective. Programs of physical therapy may be of benefit, and attempts should be made to search for strategies that allow movement without precipitating myoclonus in individual patients. Alcohol may provide symptomatic benefit in some patients, but must be used judiciously (80).

Strategies for replacing enzymes in the storage disorders and augmenting mitochondrial function in the mitochondrial disorders are being developed, but presently they remain in the experimental phase, and results to date have been disappointing.

References

1. Berkovic SF, Andermann F, Carpenter S, Wolfe LS. Progressive myoclonus epilepsies: specific causes and diagnosis. *N Engl J Med* 1986; 315:296–305.
2. Genton P, Malafosse A, Moulard B, Rogel-Ortiz, et al. Progressive myoclonic epilepsies. In: Roger J, Bureau M, Dravet C, Genton P, et al, editors. *Epileptic Syndromes in Infancy, Childhood and Adolescence*. 4th ed. London: John Libbey; 2005:441–465.
3. Berkovic SF. Progressive myoclonus epilepsies. In: Engel JJ, Pedley TA, eds. *Epilepsy: A Comprehensive Textbook*. Philadelphia: Lippincott-Raven; 2007 (in press).
4. Unverricht H. Die Myoclonie. Leipzig: Franz Deuticke, 1891.
5. Koskiniemi M. Baltic myoclonus. *Adv Neurol* 1986; 43:57-64.
6. Haltia M, Kristensson K, Sourander P. Neuropathological studies in three Scandinavian cases of progressive myoclonus epilepsy. *Acta Neurol Scand* 1969; 45:63–77.

7. Koskiniemi M, Donner M, Majuri H, Haltia M, et al. Progressive myoclonus epilepsy. A clinical and histopathological study. *Acta Neurol Scand* 1974; 50:307–332.
8. Koskiniemi M, Toivakka E, Donner M. Progressive myoclonus epilepsy. Electroencephalographical findings. *Acta Neurol Scand* 1974; 50:333–359.
9. Eldridge R, Iivanainen M, Stern R, Koerber T, et al. "Baltic" myoclonus epilepsy: hereditary disorder of childhood made worse by phenytoin. *Lancet* 1983; 2:838–42.
10. Iivanainen M, Himberg JJ. Valproate and clonazepam in the treatment of severe progressive myoclonus epilepsy. *Arch Neurol* 1982; 39:236–238.
11. Berkovic SF, So NK, Andermann F. Progressive myoclonus epilepsies: clinical and neurophysiological diagnosis. *J Clin Neurophysiol* 1991; 8:261–274.
12. Norio R, Koskiniemi M. Progressive myoclonus epilepsy: genetic and nosological aspects with special reference to 107 Finnish patients. *Clin Genet* 1979; 15:382–398.
13. Genton P, Michelucci R, Tassinari CA, Roger J. The Ramsay Hunt syndrome revisited: Mediterranean myoclonus versus mitochondrial encephalomyopathy with ragged-red fibers and Baltic myoclonus. *Acta Neurol Scand* 1990; 81:8–15.
14. Marseille Consensus Group. Classification of progressive myoclonus epilepsies and related disorders. *Ann Neurol* 1990; 28:113–116.
15. Cochius JI, Figlewicz DA, Kalviainen R, Nousiainen U, et al. Unverricht-Lundborg disease: absence of nonallelic genetic heterogeneity. *Ann Neurol* 1993; 34:739–741.
16. Lehesjoki A-E, Koskiniemi M, Sistonen P, Miao J, et al. Localization of a gene for progressive myoclonus epilepsy to chromosome 21q22. *Proc Natl Acad Sci U S A* 1991; 88:3696–3699.
17. Pennacchio LA, Lehesjoki A-E, Stone NE, Willour VL, et al. Mutations in the gene encoding cystatin B in progressive myoclonus epilepsy (*EPM1*). *Science* 1996; 271:1731–1734.
18. Lafreniere RG, Rochefort DL, Chretien N, Rommens JM, et al. Unstable insertion in the 5′ flanking region of the cystatin B gene is the most common mutation in progressive myoclonus epilepsy type 1, EPM1. *Nat Genet* 1997; 15:298–302.
19. Lalioti MD, Scott HS, Antonarakis SE. What is expanded in progressive myoclonus epilepsy? *Nat Genet* 1997; 17:17.
20. Lehesjoki AE. Molecular background of progressive myoclonus epilepsy. *EMBO J* 2003; 22:3473–3478.
21. Virtaneva K, D'Amato E, Miao J, Koskiniemi M, et al. Unstable minisatellite expansion causing recessively inherited myoclonus epilepsy, EPM1. *Nat Genet* 1997; 15:393–396.
22. Tsairis P, Engel WK, Kark P. Familial myoclonic epilepsy syndrome associated with skeletal-muscle mitochondrial abnormalities. *Neurology* 1973; 23:408 (abstract).
23. Fukuhara N, Tokiguchi S, Shirakawa K, Tsubaki T. Myoclonus epilepsy associated with ragged-red fibres (mitochondrial abnormalities): disease entity or a syndrome? Light-and electron- microscopic studies of two cases and review of literature. *J Neurol Sci* 1980; 47:117–133.
24. Berkovic SF, Carpenter S, Evans A, Karpati G, et al. Myoclonus epilepsy and ragged-red fibres (MERRF). 1. A clinical, pathological, biochemical, magnetic resonance spectrographic and positron emission tomographic study. *Brain* 1989; 112:1231–1260.
25. Rosing HS, Hopkins LC, Wallace DC, Epstein CM, et al. Maternally inherited mitochondrial myopathy and myoclonic epilepsy. *Ann Neurol* 1985; 17:228–237.
26. So N, Berkovic S, Andermann F, Kuzniecky R, et al. Myoclonus epilepsy and ragged-red fibres (MERRF). 2. Electrophysiological studies and comparison with other progressive myoclonus epilepsies. *Brain* 1989; 112:1261–1276.
27. Shoffner JM, Lott MT, Lezza AMS, Seibel P, et al. Myoclonic epilepsy and ragged-red fiber disease (MERRF) is associated with a mitochondrial DNA $tRNA^{Lys}$ mutation. *Cell* 1990; 61:931–937.
28. Silvestri G, Moraes CT, Shanske S, Oh SJ, et al. A new mtDNA mutation in the tRNA(Lys) gene associated with myoclonic epilepsy and ragged-red fibers (MERRF). *Am J Hum Genet* 1992; 51:1213–1217.
29. Ozawa M, Nishino I, Horai S, Nonaka I, et al. Myoclonus epilepsy associated with ragged-red fibers: a G-to-A mutation at nucleotide pair 8363 in mitochondrial tRNA(Lys) in two families. *Muscle Nerve* 1997; 20:271–278.
30. Jaksch M, Klopstock T, Kurlemann G, Dorner M, et al. Progressive myoclonus epilepsy and mitochondrial myopathy associated with mutations in the tRNA(Ser(UCN)) gene. *Ann Neurol* 1998; 44:635–640.
31. Tzoulis C, Engelsen BA, Telstad W, Aasly J, et al. The spectrum of clinical disease caused by the A467T and W748S POLG mutations: a study of 26 cases. *Brain* 2006; 129:1685–1692.
32. Matthews PM, Berkovic SF, Shoubridge EA, Andermann F, et al. In vivo magnetic resonance spectroscopy of brain and muscle in a type of mitochondrial encephalomyopathy (MERRF). *Ann Neurol* 1991; 29:435–438.
33. Hammans SR, Sweeney MG, Brockington M, Morgan-Hughes JA, et al. Mitochondrial encephalopathies: molecular genetic diagnosis from blood samples. Lancet 1991; 337:1311–1313.
34. Zeviani M, Amati P, Bresolin N, Antozzi C, et al. Rapid detection of the A—G(8344) mutation of mtDNA in Italian families with myoclonus epilepsy and ragged-red fibers (MERRF). *Am J Hum Genet* 1991; 48:203–211.
35. Lafora G, Glueck B. Beitrag zur Histopathologie der myoklonischen Epilepsie. *Z Gesamte Neurol Psychiatr* 1911; 6:1–14.
36. Carpenter S, Karpati G. Sweat gland duct cells in Lafora disease: diagnosis by skin biopsy. *Neurology* 1981; 31:1564–1568.
37. Rapin I. Myoclonus in neuronal storage and Lafora diseases. In: Fahn S, Marsden CD, Van Woert MH, editors. *Myoclonus*. New York: Raven Press; 1986:65–85.
38. Roger J, Pellissier JF, Bureau M, Dravet C, et al. Early diagnosis of Lafora disease. Significance of paroxysmal visual manifestations and contribution of skin biopsy. *Rev Neurol (Paris)* 1983; 139:115–124.
39. Diebold K. Four genetic and clinical types of progressive myoclonus epilepsies. *Arch Psychiatr Nervenkr* 1972; 215:362–375.
40. Footitt DR, Quinn N, Kocen RS, Oz B, et al. Familial Lafora body disease of late onset: report of four cases in one family and a review of the literature. *J Neurol* 1997; 244:40–44.
41. Tassinari CA, Bureau-Paillas M, Dalla Bernardina B, Picornell-Darder I, et al. Lafora disease (author's transl). *Rev Electroencephalogr Neurophysiol Clin* 1978; 8:107–122.
42. Minassian BA, Lee JR, Herbrick JA, Huizenga J, et al. Mutations in a gene encoding a novel protein tyrosine phosphatase cause progressive myoclonus epilepsy. *Nat Genet* 1998; 20:171–174.
43. Serratosa J, Gomez-Garre P, Gallardo M, Anta B, et al. A novel protein tyrosine phosphatase gene is mutated in progressive myoclonus epilepsy of the Lafora type (EPM2). *Hum Mol Genet* 1999; 8:345–352.
44. Chan EM, Young EJ, Ianzano L, Munteanu I, et al. Mutations in NHLRC1 cause progressive myoclonus epilepsy. *Nat Genet* 2003; 35:125–127.
45. Gentry MS, Worby CA, Dixon JE. Insights into Lafora disease: malin is an E3 ubiquitin ligase that ubiquitinates and promotes the degradation of laforin. *Proc Natl Acad Sci U S A* 2005; 102:8501–8506.
46. Chan EM, Omer S, Ahmed M, Bridges LR, et al. Progressive myoclonus epilepsy with polyglucosans (Lafora disease): evidence for a third locus. *Neurology* 2004; 63:565–567.
47. Ianzano L, Zhang J, Chan EM, Zhao XC, et al. Lafora progressive myoclonus epilepsy mutation database—EPM2A and NHLRC1 (EPM2B) genes. *Hum Mutat* 2005; 26:397.
48. Mole SE, Williams RE, Goebel HH. Correlations between genotype, ultrastructural morphology and clinical phenotype in the neuronal ceroid lipofuscinoses. *Neurogenetics* 2005; 6:107–126.
49. Pampiglione G, Harden A. So-called neuronal ceroid lipofuscinosis. Neurophysiological studies in 60 children. *J Neurol Neurosurg Psychiatry* 1977; 40:323–330.
50. Santavuori P, Rapola J, Sainio K, Raitta C. A variant of Jansky-Bielschowsky disease. *Neuropediatrics* 1982; 13:135–141.
51. Lake BD, Cavanagh NP. Early-juvenile Batten's disease—a recognisable sub-group distinct from other forms of Batten's disease. Analysis of 5 patients. *J Neurol Sci* 1978; 36:265–271.
52. Berkovic SF, Carpenter S, Andermann F, Andermann E, et al. Kufs' disease: a critical reappraisal. *Brain* 1988; 111(Pt 1):27–62.
53. Rapola J, Santavuori P, Savilahti E. Suction biopsy of rectal mucosa in the diagnosis of infantile and juvenile types of neuronal ceroid lipofuscinoses. *Hum Pathol* 1984; 15:352–360.
54. Andermann E, Jacob JC, Andermann F, Carpenter S, et al. The Newfoundland aggregate of neuronal ceroid-lipofuscinosis. *Am J Med Genet Suppl* 1988; 5:111–116.
55. Boehme DH, Cottrell JC, Leonberg SC, Zeman W. A dominant form of neuronal ceroid-lipofuscinosis. *Brain* 1971; 94:745–760.
56. Palmer DN, Fearnley IM, Medd SM, Walker JE, et al. Lysosomal storage of the DCCD reactive proteolipid subunit of mitochondrial ATP synthase in human and ovine ceroid lipofuscinoses. *Adv Exp Med Biol* 1989; 266:211–222; discussion 223.
57. Hall NA, Lake BD, Dewji NN, Patrick AD. Lysosomal storage of subunit c of mitochondrial ATP synthase in Batten's disease (ceroid-lipofuscinosis). *Biochem J* 1991; 275(Pt 1):269–272.
58. Carpenter S, Karpati G, Andermann F, Jacob JC, et al. The ultrastructural characteristics of the abnormal cytosomes in Batten-Kufs' disease. *Brain* 1977; 100 Pt 1:137–156.
59. Lowden JA, O'Brien JS. Sialidosis: a review of human neuraminidase deficiency. *Am J Hum Genet* 1979; 31:1–18.
60. Matsuo T, Egawa I, Okada S, Suetsugu M, et al. Sialidosis type 2 in Japan. Clinical study in two siblings' cases and review of literature. *J Neurol Sci* 1983; 58:45–55.
61. Seyrantepe V, Poupetova H, Froissart R, Zabot MT, et al. Molecular pathology of NEU1 gene in sialidosis. *Hum Mutat* 2003; 22:343–352.
62. D'Azzo A, Hoogeveen A, Reuser AJ, Robinson D, et al. Molecular defect in combined beta-galactosidase and neuraminidase deficiency in man. *Proc Natl Acad Sci U S A* 1982; 79:4535–4539.
63. Mueller OT, Henry WM, Haley LL, Byers MG, et al. Sialidosis and galactosialidosis: chromosomal assignment of two genes associated with neuraminidase-deficiency disorders. *Proc Natl Acad Sci U S A* 1986; 83:1817–1821.
64. Zhou XY, van der Spoel A, Rottier R, Hale G, et al. Molecular and biochemical analysis of protective protein/cathepsin A mutations: correlation with clinical severity in galactosialidosis. *Hum Mol Genet* 1996; 5:1977–1987.
65. Palmeri S, Hoogeveen AT, Verheijen FW, Galjaard H. Galactosialidosis: molecular heterogeneity among distinct clinical phenotypes. *Am J Hum Genet* 1986; 38:137–148.
66. Shibasaki H, Yamashita Y, Neshige R, Tobimatsu S, et al. Pathogenesis of giant somatosensory evoked potentials in progressive myoclonic epilepsy. *Brain* 1985; 108(Pt 1):225–240.
67. Melanson M, Nalbantoglu J, Berkovic S, Melmed C, et al. Progressive myoclonus epilepsy in young adults with neuropathologic features of Alzheimer's disease. *Neurology* 1997; 49:1732–1733.
68. Marsden CD, Harding AE, Obeso JA, Lu CS. Progressive myoclonic ataxia (the Ramsay Hunt syndrome). *Arch Neurol* 1990; 47:1121–1125.
69. Kuwano A, Takakubo F, Morimoto Y, Uyama E, et al. Benign adult familial myoclonus epilepsy (BAFME): an autosomal dominant form not linked to the dentatorubral pallidoluysian atrophy (DRPLA) gene. *J Med Genet* 1996; 33:80–81.
70. Okino S. Familial benign myoclonus epilepsy of adult onset: a previously unrecognized myoclonic disorder. *J Neurol Sci* 1997; 145:113–118.
71. Daube JR, Peters HA. Hereditary essential myoclonus. *Arch Neurol* 1966; 15:587–594.
72. Obeso JA, Artieda J, Luquin MR, Vaamonde J, et al. Antimyoclonic action of piracetam. *Clin Neuropharmacol* 1986; 9:58–64.
73. Koskiniemi M, Van Vleymen B, Hakamies L, Lamusuo S, et al. Piracetam relieves symptoms in progressive myoclonus epilepsy: a multicentre, randomised, double blind, crossover study comparing the efficacy and safety of three dosages of oral piracetam with placebo. *J Neurol Neurosurg Psychiatry* 1998; 64:344–348.
74. Obeso JA, Artieda J, Rothwell JC, Day B, et al. The treatment of severe action myoclonus. *Brain* 1989; 112(Pt 3):765–777.

75. Henry TR, Leppik IE, Gumnit RJ, Jacobs M. Progressive myoclonus epilepsy treated with zonisamide. *Neurology* 1988; 38:928–931.
76. Kyllerman M, Ben-Menachem E. Zonisamide for progressive myoclonus epilepsy: long-term observations in seven patients. *Epilepsy Res* 1998; 29:109–114.
77. Crest C, Dupont S, Leguern E, Adam C, et al. Levetiracetam in progressive myoclonic epilepsy: an exploratory study in 9 patients. *Neurology* 2004; 62:640–643.
78. Magaudda A, Gelisse P, Genton P. Antimyoclonic effect of levetiracetam in 13 patients with Unverricht-Lundborg disease: clinical observations. *Epilepsia* 2004; 45:678–681.
79. Mancuso M, Galli R, Pizzanelli C, Filosto M, et al. Antimyoclonic effect of levetiracetam in MERRF syndrome. *J Neurol Sci* 2006; 243:97–99.
80. Genton P, Guerrini R. Antimyoclonic effects of alcohol in progressive myoclonus epilepsy. *Neurology* 1990; 40:1412–1416.

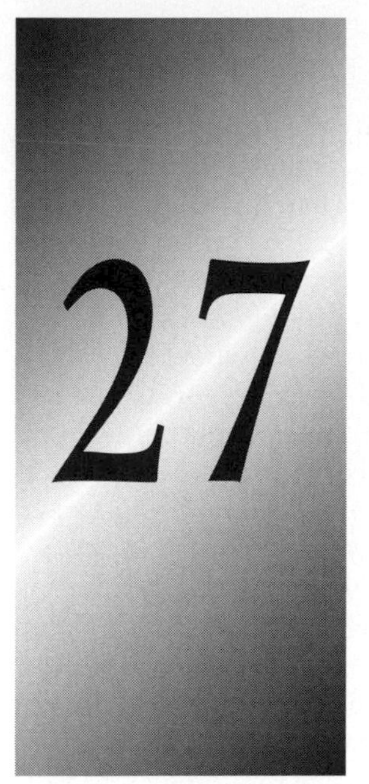

27 Localization-Related Epilepsies: Simple Partial Seizures, Complex Partial Seizures, and Rasmussen Syndrome

Prakash Kotagal

The International Classification of Epilepsies and Epileptic Syndromes (1) divides epilepsy, first, on the basis of whether the seizures are partial (localization-related epilepsies) or generalized (generalized epilepsies) and, second, by etiology (idiopathic, symptomatic, or cryptogenic epilepsy). Idiopathic epilepsies are defined by age-related onset, clinical and electroencephalographic characteristics, and a presumed genetic etiology. Symptomatic epilepsies comprise syndromes based on anatomic localization and are considered to be the consequence of a known or suspected disorder of the central nervous system. Cryptogenic epilepsies are presumed to be symptomatic, but the etiology is not known. Localization-related epilepsies include the following types of seizures:

1. Simple partial seizures
2. Complex partial seizures
   a. With impairment of consciousness at onset
   b. Simple partial onset followed by impairment of consciousness
3. Partial seizures evolving to generalized tonic-clonic (GTC) convulsions
   a. Simple partial evolving into GTC
   b. Complex partial evolving into GTC including those with simple partial onset

DEFINITIONS

A simple partial seizure is one that arises from a localized area within one hemisphere without impairment of consciousness. A complex partial seizure is a partial-onset seizure that is characterized by impaired consciousness, unresponsiveness, and automatic behavior often followed by postictal confusion. Impaired consciousness is defined as the inability to respond normally to exogenous stimuli by virtue of altered awareness or responsiveness (2). *Awareness* refers to the patient's contact with events during the period in question and its recall (2), whereas *responsiveness* is the ability of the patient to carry out simple commands or willed movements.

ETIOLOGY

By definition, partial seizures imply the presence of a focal abnormality in one cerebral hemisphere. A definite etiological factor can be identified by magnetic resonance imaging (MRI) in approximately 75% to 90% of patients with partial seizures (3–5). These include birth asphyxia, intrauterine infections (toxoplasmosis, cytomegalovirus, rubella, or syphilis), congenital anomalies, head trauma, meningitis, viral encephalitis, parasitic infections (cysticercosis and echinococcosis), neoplasms, arteriovenous malformations, cerebral embolization from congenital heart disease, or disorders affecting the intracranial vessels, as in fibromuscular dysplasia and moyamoya disease. Head injury and viral encephalitis have a predilection for the temporal lobe (6, 7). Approximately 30% of patients who undergo surgical treatment for intractable partial seizures have a foreign tissue lesion detected on pathologic examination (8). Mesial temporal sclerosis (MTS) has been established as a causative factor in 50% to 60% of adolescents and adults with temporal lobe epilepsy (TLE) (9–11). Hippocampal pathology shows neuronal loss and gliosis in the Sommer sector, end folium, and dentate gyrus in 50% of cases (12). However, other etiologies predominate in children below the age of 12 years. Duchowny and coworkers found that in their surgical series of 16 patients with TLE, only 2 had MTS, 7 had abnormalities of neuroblast migration, and 3 had ganglioglioma (13). The common tumors associated with intractable partial epilepsy include low-grade gliomas, gangliogliomas, and dysembryoplastic neuroepitheliomas (DNT) (14, 15). Neuronal migration disorders have been increasingly recognized as a cause of epilepsy. Focal cortical dysplasia (16–18), lissencephaly (19), band heterotopia (20), nodular heterotopia (21), the bilateral perisylvian syndrome (22, 23), and schizencephaly (24) often present with seizures. In a study correlating pathology and MRI findings in children with intractable partial seizures, Kuzniecky and coworkers (25) described the presence of cortical lesions in 23% of patients. Tuberous sclerosis, Sturge-Weber syndrome, neurofibromatosis, epidermal nevus syndrome, and hypomelanosis of Ito are neurocutaneous disorders associated with early-onset seizures (26). Coexistence of certain tumors such as ganglioglioma and DNT with cortical dysplasia, most frequently observed in the pediatric population, may suggest a hamartomatous nature of the neoplasms (27, 28). The association of hippocampal sclerosis with cortical dysplasia remote from the mesial structures is well established in patients with TLE (29, 30).

SEIZURE PHENOMENA

The symptomatology of partial seizures depends greatly on the location of the seizure focus within the cerebral cortex. Although a given symptom may occur with seizures arising from different locations, the combined information from seizure symptomatology and electroencephalogram (EEG) findings enables one to determine the location of seizure focus. Simple partial seizures with motor manifestations may result from ictal onset within or propagation to the precentral and postcentral gyri of the contralateral hemisphere or the supplementary motor area (31). The ictal symptomatology of epileptic seizures in general is a reflection of activation of symptomatogenic zones. This activation is usually the result of spreading of the epileptiform discharges from the epileptogenic zone to adjacent cortex, which when activated produces the ictal semiology. Auras consist exclusively of subjective warning symptoms and usually occur at the beginning of a seizure; depending on methodology and selection of patients, auras have been reported anywhere from 20% to 90% of those with partial-onset seizures (32–34). Complex partial seizures (CPS) arise from the temporal lobes in the majority of cases. However, in 15% to 20% of CPS an extratemporal focus in the mesial frontal, opercular insular region, cingulate gyrus, orbitofrontal cortex is seen (35). Postictal dysfunction has localizing value but does not reliably identify the site of ictal onset. The International Classification of Epileptic Seizures provides a useful approach to understanding the symptomatology of partial seizures (2). This classification is electroclinical—in other words, based on both seizure semiology and EEG findings—whereas a recently proposed semiological seizure classification by Lüders is independent of EEG or imaging findings (36).

Simple Partial Seizures with Motor Signs

Simple partial seizures with motor signs are the most common form of simple partial seizures because of the prominent representation of the motor cortex and high epileptogenicity of the frontal cortex. These symptoms are contralateral (at least at onset) and usually consist of positive (irritative) symptoms, less often negative (inhibitory) symptoms, or a combination of the two.

Focal Motor Seizures with and without March

Motor seizures can be clonic or tonic, involving any portion of the body, depending on the site of origin of the ictal discharge. Focal motor seizures may remain strictly focal, or they may spread to contiguous cortical areas, producing a sequential involvement of body parts in an epileptic march. This pattern is often referred to as a Jacksonian march. Postictally, a temporary weakness, Todd's paralysis, may be seen, especially if the seizure is severe or prolonged (7). Focal clonic seizures can occur with ictal discharges in any cortical region. The name *epilepsia partialis continua* (EPC) is given to continuous focal motor seizure activity.

Versive Seizures

Seizures beginning in or spreading to area 8, the frontal eye field, and the supplementary motor area or mesial part of premotor area 6 produce contralateral conjugate deviation of the eyes and turning of the head. When this movement is unquestionably forced and involuntary, the seizures are termed versive seizures and lateralize seizure onset to the contralateral hemisphere (37). Forced and sustained head and eye version, continuing through generalization or occurring within 10 seconds before generalization, was the best lateralizing sign, identifying a contralateral seizure focus in more than 90 percent of seizures (38).

Supplementary Sensorimotor Area Seizures

The supplementary sensorimotor area (SSMA) may be activated during seizures arising in patients with an epileptogenic zone in the posterior mesial or superior frontal area of one hemisphere. Seizures are frequent, brief, and usually out of sleep with abrupt bilateral asymmetric tonic posturing of the extremities. The posturing predominantly affects the proximal musculature with stiffening and gross flailing movements (15, 16, 39, 40). Speech arrest and vocalization are common, but consciousness is often preserved. Ictal contraversive head and eye version may serve as a lateralizing feature if they precede secondary generalization. SSMA seizures may be confused with psychogenic seizures and parasomnias such as night terrors or confusional arousals.

Aphasic Seizures

Ictal language disturbances during epileptic seizures include speech arrest, aphasia, or vocalization. Seizures that begin with aphasic speech arrest, without altered consciousness, are generally considered to originate in the dominant posterolateral temporal region (41, 42). Lüders and coworkers (43) demonstrated the presence of a basal temporal language area (BTLA) by electrical stimulation with subdural electrodes (43, 44). Speech arrest has been demonstrated in seizures originating in the dominant BTLA (45, 46). Seizures arising in the frontal operculum of the dominant hemisphere can give rise to epileptic aphasia (47). Vocalizations, sounds of no speech quality, may be seen with simple partial seizures affecting the suprasylvian area of the frontal lobe as well as complex partial seizures. They have no lateralizing value (48). Following the end of a simple or complex partial seizure, postictal aphasia may be detected by asking the patient to name items or read and is 80–90% reliable in lateralizing seizure onset to the language-dominant hemisphere (49, 50).

Simple Partial Seizures with Somatosensory or Special Sensory Signs

Sensory or motor phenomena are often the initial symptom of seizures starting in or near the postcentral area. Sensory phenomena include tingling, numbness, or paresthesias contralateral to the epileptogenic focus. The sensory phenomena may march to adjacent sensory or motor areas. The frequency of motor phenomena is due to intimate connections between the sensory and motor areas (6), as shown by motor phenomena observed in 25% of cases during electrical stimulation of the postcentral gyrus. Sensory symptoms that are ipsilateral or bilateral in distribution and identical to those occurring only contralaterally are believed to originate in the second sensory area at the base of the motor strip in the frontoparietal operculum (51). Benign rolandic epilepsy often manifests with focal motor seizures with preserved consciousness or as partial-onset, secondarily generalized tonic-clonic seizures. They usually involve the face, oropharyngeal muscles, or arm on one side, and less commonly the leg. Sometimes they are associated with sensory phenomena such as tingling or numbness.

Visual seizures are simple partial seizures involving the visual cortex in the region of the calcarine fissure. They usually consist of flashes of light or colors in the contralateral hemifield. Visual seizures should be distinguished from migraine, which usually produces negative phenomena such as scotomas or hemianopsia. More elaborate visual phenomena (i.e., formed visual hallucinations) are seen with seizures starting in the posterior temporal regions. Seizures starting from the occipital cortex may spread to the temporal lobes producing complex partial seizures (52).

Auditory seizures are seen with onset from the auditory cortex in the superior temporal gyrus. They usually manifest with sounds such as humming, buzzing, roaring, or whistling. More elaborate hallucinations (music, voices, etc.) result from involvement of the auditory association areas (6).

Olfactory and gustatory seizures present with an aura of an unpleasant odor or a bad taste in the mouth. They are usually observed with seizures arising from the anterior temporal lobe or insular region.

Vertiginous phenomena are sometimes reported by patients as the aura preceding their complex partial seizures. This may be a light-headed feeling or actual vertigo. Vertiginous phenomena are encountered with CPS of posterior temporal lobe onset (53, 54).

Simple Partial Seizures with Autonomic Symptoms or Signs

Autonomic symptoms in the form of flushing, pallor, sweating, pupillary dilation, nausea, vomiting, borborygmi, piloerection, or epigastric sensations are often seen in CPS, especially those starting in the anterior temporal lobe, opercular-insular region, and orbitofrontal cortex (54–56). Ictal gastrointestinal symptoms that are limited to visceral sensations are more common in children; they include painful cramping, periumbilical pain, bloating, nausea, vomiting, and diarrhea. Pallor and cold sweating may accompany the abdominal symptoms in children and may be misdiagnosed as psychogenic pain (57). Sinus tachycardia, the most frequent cardiac concomitant of seizures, has been reported in several case studies (58, 59). Sinus bradycardia, sinus arrest, atrioventricular block, and prolonged asystole occur much less frequently. Sudden unexplained death has been postulated to be a result of autonomically mediated fatal cardiac arrhythmia or sudden "neurogenic" pulmonary edema associated with seizures (62–64).

Simple Partial Seizures with Psychic Symptoms

Simple partial seizures with psychic symptoms refer to alterations of higher cerebral function—dysphasia, dysmnesia (déjà vu or jamais vu), affective (fear, anger), cognition (distortion of time sense, dreamy states), illusions (micropsia or macropsia), or hallucinations (voices, music, or scenes). They are usually followed by a complex partial phase; only rarely do they occur in isolation.

As mentioned previously, simple partial seizures may evolve to secondarily generalized tonic-clonic seizures directly or after a complex partial phase. Likewise, CPS may give rise to secondarily generalized tonic-clonic seizures (2). The ictal discharge may spread from the focus to contiguous areas or to distant regions by way of specific pathways or callosal fibers connecting homologous areas of the cortex in the opposite hemisphere.

Complex Partial Seizures

Approximately 50% of patients with CPS report a warning symptom or aura. An aura is, by definition, a simple partial seizure. It may take different forms depending on the location of the seizure focus, as described previously. CPS of mesial temporal onset are most commonly preceded by a rising epigastric sensation. Young children sometimes run to their mother and cling to her fearfully (63). The aura is more clearly expressed as the child gets older. The aura is followed by the complex partial phase with partial or complete loss of consciousness, unresponsiveness often with a vacant stare, behavioral arrest, and some stiffening of the body. Duchowny and coworkers (64) noted that CPS in infants under 2 years of age frequently consisted of behavioral arrest with forced lateralized deviation of the head and eyes and tonic upper extremity extensor stiffening. Automatisms defined as more or less coordinated, involuntary movements occurring during a period of altered awareness are frequently seen in CPS. These invariably take place during the ictus, less commonly in the postictal period. They may consist of stereotyped movements of the mouth and lips, oroalimentary automatisms such as lip smacking or swallowing, fumbling or grasping movements of the hands, blinking, grimacing, bicycling movements of the legs, walking or running about, laughing, crying, or complex motor activity. Automatisms tend to be simpler in the younger children, whereas highly organized behavioral sequences and complex gestural automatisms are observed in the older children and adults (64–66). The motor phenomena in preschool children may consist of symmetric tonic or clonic movements of the limbs and atonic phenomenon such as head nodding resembling infantile spasms or hyper-motor turning movements and postures similar to frontal lobe seizures in adults. Unilateral dystonic posturing is more often seen in CPS of temporal lobe origin and has good lateralizing value (67–68). Posturing in frontal lobe CPS tends to be more often tonic, and bilaterally asymmetric. Temporal lobe CPS usually last 60 to 90 seconds and are followed by a postictal period lasting several minutes or hours (69). The child is often lethargic during the postictal period and may complain of headache. Postictal dysphasia may also be seen. The patient is usually confused postictally and may engage in automatic behavior. Attempts to restrain the patient may result in aggressive behavior, which is usually nondirected (70). One-third to one-half of patients with CPS may go on to have a secondarily generalized tonic-clonic seizure, more often out of sleep. Version may occur during such a seizure and is of lateralizing significance (37). It tends to occur earlier in frontal lobe seizures, probably as a result of rapid propagation (71, 72). During the tonic phase of a partial seizure with secondarily generalization, the contralateral arm may be extended while the other arm is flexed, resembling a figure 4, which has lateralizing value (73).

Occasionally, patients may develop complex partial status epilepticus, which may present as a prolonged confusional state, similar to absence status. This may last several hours or even days. The patient appears to be in a daze, is slow to respond, frequently is unable to talk, and often is restless and disoriented. The diagnosis is established by the finding of a continuous focal ictal pattern on the EEG (76).

Frontal Lobe Seizures

Frontal lobe seizures represent the largest subgroup of extratemporal epilepsy, accounting for 30% of partial epilepsy (75, 76). The most recent epilepsy classification scheme (42) suggests seven different types of frontal lobe seizures related to specific regions of seizure origin (Table 27-1). In practice, large epileptogenic zones, high speed and pattern of seizure propagation, and extensive overlap among different types make it difficult to subclassify CPS of frontal lobe origin accurately into distinct anatomic subregions based on clinical characteristics. Frontal lobe CPS (72, 77–80) can usually be distinguished from CPS arising from the temporal lobes and other regions (Table 27-2). These seizures often have a bizarre clinical presentation, have minimal or absent interictal and

TABLE 27-1
Summary of International League Against Epilepsy (ILAE) Classification of Frontal Lobe Epilepsies

Region	Clinical Features
Primary motor cortex	Contralateral tonic or clonic movements according to somatotopy, speech arrest and swallowing with frequent secondary generalization
SMA	Simple focal tonic seizures with vocalization, speech arrest, fencing postures, and complex focal motor activity
Cingulate	Complex focal motor activity with initial automatisms, sexual features, vegetative signs, changes in mood and affect, and urinary incontinence
Frontopolar	Early loss of consciousness, "pseudo absence," adversive and subsequent contraversive movements of head and eyes, axial clonic jerks, falls, autonomic signs with frequent generalization
Orbitofrontal	Complex focal motor seizures with initial automatisms or olfactory hallucinations, autonomic signs, and urinary incontinence
Dorsolateral (premotor)	Simple focal tonic with versive movements and aphasia and complex focal motor activity with initial automatisms
Opercular	Mastication, salivation, swallowing and speech arrest with epigastric aura, fear, and autonomic phenomena. Partial clonic facial seizures may be ipsilateral, and gustatory hallucination is common

ictal EEG abnormalities, and sometimes are mistaken for psychogenic seizures.

Autosomal Dominant Nocturnal Frontal Lobe Epilepsy

Autosomal dominant nocturnal frontal lobe epilepsy (ADNFLE) was first described as a distinct clinical syndrome in six families in 1994 (81, 82). Mutations have been found in two genes, CHRNA4 and CHRNB2, which code for the neuronal nicotinic acid receptor subunits (83). Seizures begin in childhood (mean age 11.7 years, range 2 months–52 years) and usually persist through adult life. Individuals frequently have an aura followed by a gasp, grunt, or vocalization, and thrashing hyperkinetic activity or tonic stiffening with or without superimposed clonic activity (84). Seizures typically occur in clusters during sleep, and awareness is usually retained. Patients are of normal intellect with normal neurologic examination and neuroimaging tests. Interictal EEG is usually normal. When

TABLE 27-2
Differentiating Features of Frontal versus Temporal Lobe CPS

	Frontal	Temporal
Duration	Brief < 30 seconds	60–90 seconds
Time of day	Night > day	Day > night
Clusters	Common	Uncommon
Aura	General body sensation; cephalic aura	Epigastric, psychic
Automatisms	Proximal and coarse; bicycling movements, pelvic thrusting	Distal and discrete, oroalimentary, manual, gestural, mimetic, ictal speech, perseverative, ictal vomiting
Motor posturing	Bilateral, asymmetric tonic	Contralateral dystonic posturing, often with automatisms on the opposite side
Vocalizations	Prominent	Less common
Partial loss of consciousness	Noted earlier in the seizure	Noted later in the seizure
Version	Ipsilateral head deviation followed by contralateral version before secondary generalization; is usually < 18 seconds after onset	Contralateral version precedes generalization, usually occurs after 18 seconds

not obscured by movement artifact, ictal EEG may show bifrontal epileptiform discharges. Seizures are often misdiagnosed as parasomnias, paroxysmal nocturnal dystonia (which may in actuality be ADNFLE), familial dyskinesia, or a psychiatric disorder. The seizures frequently respond to carbamazepine or oxcarbazepine monotherapy.

RASMUSSEN SYNDROME

Rasmussen syndrome (RS) is characterized by intractable focal motor seizures, declining cognitive function, progressive hemiparesis, visual field abnormality, and contralateral focal, predominantly perisylvian cortical atrophy. Changes in signal intensity may also be seen in the deep gray and white matter. The onset of the disease occurs at 10 years or younger in 85% of patients (85). Epilepsia partialis continua or focal motor status occurs in one-half of patients at some point in their course (86). The etiology is not known, but an autoimmune process is important in the pathogenesis of RS, and it is believed that the glutamate receptor subunit, GluR3 may be an important autoantigen (87–89). Neuropathology characteristically shows perivascular lymphocytic cuffing and proliferation of microglial nodules in the cortex of the affected hemisphere (90–92). In-situ hybridization techniques were reported to show most Rasmussen patients to have neurons with cytomegalic inclusion virus (93); this, however, has not been confirmed by others. T-cell-mediated cytotoxicity may also play a role (94). Following cleavage of the GluR3 protein by Granzyme B, the immunogenic section of the GluR3 protein becomes exposed to the immune system (95).

The EEG may show background slowing, disruption of sleep architecture, and frequent epileptiform discharges over the affected hemisphere; with progression of the disease, the spikes may become bilaterally synchronous and appear in the contralateral hemisphere (96–98). Computed tomography (CT) and MRI scans may show diffuse atrophy of the involved hemisphere (99). Proton MR-spectroscopy may reveal decreased *N*-acetylaspartate (NAA) concentration in patients with RS (100). This finding correlates well with brain atrophy and neuronal loss. For reasons that are not yet clear, Rasmussen encephalitis is essentially a unilateral disease.

Rasmussen syndrome is notoriously difficult to treat and does not show the same dramatic response to IV medications as do other forms of status. IV immunoglobulin, high-dose steroids, or both may produce some reduction of seizure frequency in the short term in a few cases (101), but surgical removal of the affected hemisphere is the standard therapy (102). A trial of tacrolimus was found to slow the rate of neurologic deterioration, but it did not improve seizure frequency (103).

In the Johns Hopkins experience, 88% of children who underwent hemispherectomy became seizure free or have occasional, nondisabling seizures (102, 104, 105). Early hemispherectomy, although increasing the hemiparesis, reduces the overall burden of the illness because of a marked decrease in both frequency and severity of seizures. Because hemiplegia is inevitable with or without surgery, early surgery may allow the child to return to a more normal life by preventing the cognitive decline that is the result of constant seizures.

DIFFERENTIAL DIAGNOSIS

Pseudoseizures are in the differential diagnosis of any seizure, especially if presenting with bizarre and unusual patterns or prolonged generalized seizures with intact memory for the event. There usually is no postictal confusion. Pseudoseizures often can be terminated abruptly with suggestion (108, 109). The frequency of pseudoseizures may be unrelated to antiepileptic drug (AED) levels. Video-EEG monitoring reveals no seizure pattern during the episode. Psychogenic unresponsiveness (that is, unresponsiveness during the presence of a preserved alpha background rhythm) is also very helpful. Pseudoseizures occasionally coexist with true seizures, and the monitoring must document all the seizure types reported by the family. Migrainous phenomena (108) may be difficult to distinguish from CPS, especially if they are associated with visual hallucinations or confusion. Migraine and partial seizures may coexist, or at times migraine may be followed by a partial seizure. The prodrome of the migraine attack usually develops more slowly than the epileptic aura. The frequent occurrence of vomiting and family history make this diagnosis more likely. The recording of a typical episode in the laboratory with EEG and video monitoring is helpful.

Radiologic Findings

MRI is the imaging modality of choice in a child with partial or localization-related epilepsy because of its inherent advantages in soft tissue contrast, spatial resolution, multiplanar capabilities, and lack of bone artifact. Kuzniecky and coworkers correlated the MRI imaging results with pathology in 44 children with intractable epilepsy and showed a potential epileptogenic abnormality in 86% of patients (109). CT scanning is inferior in detecting lesions that may be seen only on MRI, with the exception of revealing intracranial calcification in Sturge-Weber syndrome, congenital brain infections such as toxoplasmosis, or cytomegalovirus. MRI reliably demonstrates hippocampal atrophy in 70% to 90% of patients with mesial TLE (110, 111). Accurate assessment of hippocampal size by volumetric studies has been shown to correlate with severity of neuronal loss in the hippocampus (112) and seizure outcome following resection (113). MRI has led to increased recognition, better characterization, and improved understanding of malformations of cortical development (MCD). The generalized MCDs include lissencephaly, pachygyria, band or laminar heterotopia, and subependymal heterotopias. Localized forms of MCDs include focal cortical dysplasia, polymicrogyria, focal subependymal heterotopias, and schizencephaly (114, 115). The identification of a focal MCD and complete removal of the lesion is followed by good seizure control in 77% of the patients (116). MRI is very sensitive in detection of tumors; vascular malformations such as cavernous hemangiomas, arteriovenous malformations, and subependymal nodules; and cortical tubers in tuberous sclerosis. Positron emission tomography (PET) scans may show an area of hypometabolism interictally and a focus of hypermetabolism on ictal scans (98, 99). Unilateral temporal lobe hypometabolism is present in 70% to 80% of patients with TLE (117) and corresponds pathologically and anatomically to the depth electrode localization of the epileptic zone (118). Focal cortical dysplasia (FCD) may be difficult to visualize in very young children because of incomplete myelination. Interictal PET is useful in demonstrating areas of hypometabolism corresponding to FCD in infants and children with catastrophic epilepsy. In the early stages of Rasmussen encephalitis, the MRI may be normal, but the PET scan may show focal or diffuse hemispheric hypometabolism. Flumazenil PET reveals a reduction in benzodiazepine receptor binding in the epileptic focus of partial epilepsy (119). Carfentanil PET studies of TLE have revealed increased mu-opiate receptor binding in the neocortex of the epileptogenic temporal lobe, correlating directly with a decrease of glucose metabolism seen on FDG-PET (120). Single-photon emission computed tomography (SPECT) has been used in patients with refractory seizures considered for epilepsy surgery. Interictal SPECT demonstrates hypoperfusion in 40% to 70% of patients with focal epilepsy (121). Ictal SPECT has been reported to have a localization accuracy of 70% to 100% in TLE (122) and in up to 90% of selected patients with frontal lobe epilepsy (123, 124).

Interictal EEG

The interictal EEG may be normal in 30% to 40% of patients with clinically documented partial seizures. A normal EEG, however, does not rule out the diagnosis of epilepsy. The chance of finding an abnormality is increased by performing repeated or prolonged EEGs, sleep recordings, additional closely spaced electrodes, appropriate montages, and hyperventilation. With these techniques, the yield may be increased up to 90% (125–127). A unilateral temporal lobe focus is found in most cases of CPS. Bitemporal sharp wave foci are seen in 25% to 33% of patients (118). An extratemporal focus is seen in 15% to 20% of patients, usually in the frontal lobe (13). Focal intermittent rhythmic slowing may be seen intermittently in approximately half the patients with focal seizures (125–128) and has the same significance as focal spikes. One may also find focal slowing that is nonrhythmic with suppression of the normal background rhythms in 75 percent of patients (125). It is important to exclude nonepileptiform sharp transients such as small sharp spikes, psychomotor variant, or 14- and 6-Hz spikes. Additionally, benign focal epileptiform discharges of childhood may occur in asymptomatic children (129). These usually are found in the central or midtemporal location, have a characteristic stereotyped waveform, and are markedly activated during sleep.

Ictal EEG

According to Gastaut (130), the ictal EEG is abnormal in more than 95% of cases. In 75% of patients, the interictal spikes or sharp waves show an abrupt cessation or decrease just before ictal onset. This is then followed by rhythmic activity that shows a progressive buildup of amplitude and frequency (most often in the 13- to 30-Hz range, but possibly in the theta or delta range). This may be well localized to the area of the focus, or it may be more widespread over that hemisphere (125). Focal beta activity at seizure onset seen in scalp recordings occurs in 25% of patients with FLE and is felt to be predictive of good outcome after focal resection (131). Postictally, one may find slowing or flattening, which, if focal, may be helpful in lateralization (132). Sometimes it is difficult to localize or lateralize the seizure onset from scalp recordings. Invasive recordings with subdural or depth electrodes may be indicated in such cases (132–138).

PROGNOSIS

Contrary to previous reports that stated that up to one-third of patients with CPS became seizure-free (139), our experience and that of others indicates that although some patients do become seizure free on medication, spontaneous remission (that is, seizure free off medications) is rare (140). Pazzaglia and coworkers reported that good seizure control was achieved in 31% of patients with simple partial seizures, 37% of those with complex partial seizures, and 61% of those with secondarily generalized epilepsy (141). Loiseau and coworkers found that seizure control could be predicted after 1 year of treatment (142). Thus, it should be possible to document medical intractability within a couple of years after seizure onset. Such patients should undergo prolonged video-EEG monitoring, high-resolution MRI, nuclear imaging (PET, ictal SPECT), and functional assessment. If found to be suitable candidates, epilepsy surgery should be performed sooner rather than later to minimize compromise of psychosocial and intellectual function.

References

1. Dreifuss FE. Proposal for classification of epilepsies and epileptic syndromes. *Epilepsia* 1985; 26:268–278.
2. Dreifuss FE. Proposal for a revised clinical and electrographic classification of epileptic seizures. *Epilepsia* 1981; 22:489–501.
3. Jackson GD. New techniques in magnetic resonance and epilepsy. *Epilepsia* 1994; 35:S2–S13.
4. Li LM, Fish DR, Sisodiya SM, et al. High-resolution resonance imaging in adults with partial or secondarily generalized epilepsy attending a tertiary referral unit. *J Neurol Neurosurg Psychiatry* 1995; 59:384–387.
5. Kuzniecky R, Murro A, King D, Morawetz R, et al. Magnetic resonance imaging in childhood intractable partial epilepsies: pathologic correlations. *Neurology* 1993; 43:681–687.
6. Scarpa P, Carassini B. Partial epilepsy in childhood: clinical and EEG study of 261 cases. *Epilepsia* 1982; 23:333–341.
7. Ounsted C, Lindsay J, Norman R. Biological factors in temporal lobe epilepsy. *Clin Dev Med* 1966; 22.
8. Babb TL, Brown WJ. Pathological findings in epilepsy. In: Engel J Jr, ed. *Surgical Treatment of the Epilepsies*. New York: Raven Press; 1987:511–540.
9. Falconer MA, Taylor DC. TLE: clinical features, pathology, diagnosis and treatment. In: Price JH, ed. *Modern Trends in Psychological Medicine*. London: Butterworths, 1970:346–373.
10. Brown WJ. Structural substrate of seizure foci in the temporal lobe. In: Brazier MAB, ed. *Epilepsy: Its Phenomena in Man*. New York: Academic Press, 1973:339–374.
11. Brown WJ, Babb TL. Central pathological considerations of complex partial seizures. In: Hopkins A, ed. *Epilepsy*. London: Chapman and Hall, 1987.
12. Falconer MA, Taylor DC. Surgical treatment of drug resistant epilepsy due to mesial temporal sclerosis. *Arch Neurol* 1968; 19:353–361.
13. Duchowny M, Levin B, Jayakar P, et al. Temporal lobectomy in early childhood. *Epilepsia* 1992; 33:298–303.
14. Mercuri S, Russo A, Palma L. Hemispheric supratentorial astrocytomas in children: long term results in 29 cases. *J Neurosurgery* 1981; 55:170–173.
15. Gol A. Cerebral astrocytomas in childhood. *J Neurosurgery* 1962; 19:577–582.
16. Taylor DC, Falconer MA, Bruton CJ, Corsellis JAN. FD of the cerebral cortex in epilepsy. *J Neurol Neurosurg Psychiatry* 1971; 34:369–387.
17. Palmini A, Andermann F, Oliver A, Tampieri D, et al. Neuronal migration disorder and intractable partial epilepsy. Results of surgical treatment. *Ann Neurol* 1991; 30:750–757.
18. Guerrini R, Dravet C, Raybaud C, Roger J, et al. Epilepsy and focal gyral abnormalities detected by MRI: electroclinico-morphological correlations and follow-up. *Dev Med Child Neurol* 1992; 34:706–718.
19. Dieker H, Edwards RH, Zukhein G, et al. The lissencephaly syndrome. *Birth Defects* 1969; 5:53–64.
20. Palmini A, Andermann F, Aicardi J, et al. Diffuse cortical dysplasia, "the double cortex" syndrome: the clinical and epileptic syndrome in 10 patients. *Neurology* 1991; 41: 1656–1662.
21. Barkovitch AJ, Kjos B. Grey matter heterotopias: MR characteristics and correlation with developmental and neurologic manifestations. *Radiology* 1992; 182:493–499.
22. Kuzniecky R, Andermann F, Guerrini R, and the CBPS Collaborative Study. Congenital perisylvian syndrome: a study of 31 patients. *Lancet* 1993; 341:608–612.
23. Kuzniecky R, Andermann F, Tampieri D, et al. Bilateral central microgyria: epilepsy, pseudobulbar palsy and mental retardation: a recognizable neuronal migration disorder. *Ann Neurol* 1989; 25:547–554.
24. Liblan CR, Tampieri D, Robitaille Y, Feindel W, et al. Surgical treatment of intractable epilepsy associated with schizencephaly. *Neurosurgery* 1991; 29:421–429.
25. Kuzniecky R, Murro A, King D, et al. MRI in childhood intractable partial epilepsy: pathological correlations. *Neurology* 1993; 43:681–687.
26. Kotagal P, Rothner AD. Epilepsy in the setting of neurocutaneous syndrome. *Epilepsia* 1993; 34(Suppl 3):S71–S78.
27. Prayson R, Estes M, Morris H. Coexistence of neoplasia and cortical dysplasia in patients presenting with seizures: *Epilepsia* 1993; 34:609–615.
28. Prayson RA, Estes ME. Dysembryoplastic neuroepithelial tumor. *Am J Clin Pathol* 1992; 97:398–401.
29. Raymond AA, Fish DR, Stevens JM, et al. Association of hippocampal sclerosis with cortical dysgenesis in patients with epilepsy. *Neurology* 1994; 44:1841–1845.
30. Rush E, Morrell MJ. Cortical dysplasia with mesial temporal sclerosis: evidence for kindling in humans. *Epilepsia* 1993; 34(Suppl 6):15 (abstract).
31. Penfield W, Jasper H. Epilepsy and the functional anatomy of the brain. Boston: Little, Brown, 1954.
32. Quesney LF, Constain M, Fish DR, Rasmussen T. The clinical differentiation of seizures arising in the para-sagittal and anterolateral dorsal frontal convexities. *Arch Neurol* 1990; 47:677–684.
33. Quesney LF. Clinical and EEG features of complex partial seizures of temporal lobe origin. *Epilepsia* 1986; 27(Suppl 2):S27–S45.
34. Kotagal P, Lüders H, Williams G, et al. Temporal lobe complex partial seizures: analysis of symptom clusters and sequences. *Epilepsy Res* 1995; 20:49–67.
35. Jovanovic UJ. Psychomotor epilepsy: a polydimensional study. Springfield, IL: Charles C Thomas, 1974.
36. Lüders H, Acharya J, Baumgartner C, et al. Semiological seizure classification. *Epilepsia* 1998; 39:1006–1013.
37. Wyllie E, Lüders H, Morris HH, Dinner DS. The lateralizing significance of versive head and eye movements during epileptic seizures. *Neurology* 1986; 36:606–611.
38. Kernan JC, Devinsky O, Luciano DJ, Vasquez B, et al. Lateralizing significance of head and eye deviation in secondary generalized tonic clonic seizures. *Neurology* 1993; 43:1308–1310.
39. Morris HH, Dinner DS, Lüders H, Wyllie E, et al. Supplementary motor seizures: clinical and electroencephalographic findings. *Neurology* 1988; 38:1075–1082.
40. Kanner A, Morris HH, Dinner DS, et al. Supplementary motor seizures mimicking pseudoseizures: how to distinguish one from the other. *Neurology* 1988; 38 (Supp 1):347.
41. Commission on Classification and Terminology of the ILAE. Proposal for classification of epilepsies and epileptic syndromes. *Epilepsia* 1985; 26:268–278.
42. Commission on Classification and Terminology of the ILAE. Proposal for classification of epilepsies and epileptic syndromes. *Epilepsia* 1989; 30:389–399.
43. Lüders H, Lesser RP. Hahn J, et al. Basal temporal language area demonstrated by electrical stimulation. *Neurology* 1986; 36:505–510.
44. Lüders H, Lesser RP, Hahn J, et al. Basal temporal language area. *Brain* 1991; 114: 743–754.
45. Suzuki I, Shimizu H, Ishijima B, et al. Aphasic seizures caused by focal epilepsy in the left fusiform gyrus. *Neurology* 1992; 42:2207–2210.
46. Abou-Khalil B, Wilch L, Blumenkopf B, Newman K, et al. Global aphasia with seizure onset in the dominant basal temporal region. *Epilepsia* 1994; 35:1097–1084.
47. Sakai K, Hidari M, Fukai M, et al. A chance SPECT study of ictal aphasia during simple partial seizures. *Epilepsia* 1997; 38:374–376.
48. Gabr M, Lüders H, Dinner DS, Morris H, et al. Speech manifestations in lateralization of temporal lobe seizures. *Ann Neurol* 1980; 25:82–87.
49. Fakhoury T, Abou-Khalil B, Peguero E. Differentiating clinical features of right and left temporal lobe seizures. *Epilepsia* 1994; 35:1038–1044.
50. Privitera MD, Morris GL, Gilliam F. Postictal language assessment and lateralization of complex partial seizures. *Ann Neurol* 1991; 30:391–396.
51. Penfield W, Jasper H. *Epilepsy and the Functional Anatomy of the Human Brain*. Boston: Little, Brown, 1954:517–518.
52. Williamson PD, et al. Complex partial seizures with occipital lobe onset. *Epilepsia* 1981; 22:247–255.
53. Smith BH. Vestibular disturbances in epilepsy. *Neurology* 1960; 10:465.
54. King DW, Ajmone-Marsan C. Clinical features and ictal patterns in epileptic patients with EEG temporal lobe foci. *Ann Neurol* 1977; 2:138–147.
55. Tharp BR. Orbital frontal seizures: a unique electroencephalographic and clinical syndrome. *Epilepsia* 1972; 627–642.
56. Kramer RE, Lüders H, Goldstick LP, et al. Ictus emeticus: an electroclinical analysis. *Neurology* 1988; 48:1048–1052.
57. Singhi PD, Kaur S. Abdominal epilepsy misdiagnosed as psychogenic pain. *Postgrad Med J* 1988; 64:281–282.
58. Marshall DW, Westmoreland BF, Sharbrough FW. Ictal tachycardia during temporal lobe seizures. *Mayo Clin Proc* 1983; 58:443–446.
59. Devinsky O, Price BH, Cohen SI. Cardiac manifestations of complex partial seizures. *Am J Med* 1986; 80:195–202.
60. Neuspiel DR, Kuller LH. Sudden and unexpected natural death in childhood and adolescence. *JAMA* 1985; 254:1321–1325.
61. Leestma JE, Kelkar MB, Teas SS, et al. Sudden unexpected death associated with seizures: analysis of 66 cases. *Epilepsia* 1984; 25:84–88.
62. Terrence CF, Rao GR, Perper JA. Neurogenic pulmonary edema in unexpected death of epileptic patients. *Ann Neurol* 1981; 9:458–464.
63. Blume WT. Temporal lobe seizures in childhood. Medical aspects. In: Blaw ME, Rapin I, Kinsbourne M, eds. *Topics in Child Neurology*. New York: Spectrum, 1977:105–125.
64. Duchowny MS. Complex partial seizures of infancy. *Arch Neurol* 1987; 44:911–914.
65. Brockhaus A, Elger CE. Complex partial seizures of temporal lobe origin in children of different age groups. *Epilepsia* 1995; 36:1173–1181.
66. Bye AME, Foo S. Complex partial seizures in young children. *Epilepsia* 35; 1994: 482–488.
67. Kotagal P, Lüders H, Morris HH, et al. Dystonic posturing in complex partial seizures of temporal lobe onset: a new lateralizing sign. *Neurology* 1989; 39:196–201.
68. Varelas M, Wada JA. Lateralizing significance of unilateral upper limb dystonic posturing in temporal/frontal lobe seizures. *Neurology* 1988; 38(Suppl 1):107.
69. Delgado-Escueta AV, Mattson R, King L, et al. The nature of aggression during epileptic seizures. *N Engl J Med* 1981; 305:711–716.
70. Delgado-Escueta AV, Bascal FE, Treiman DM. Complex partial seizures on closed-circuit television and EEG. A study of 691 attacks in 79 patients. *Ann Neurol* 1982; 11:292–600.
71. Chee M, Kotagal P, Van Ness P, et al. Lateralizing signs in intractable partial epilepsy: blinded multiple-observer analysis. *Neurology* 1993; 43:2519–2525.
72. Kotagal P, Arunkumar G, Hammel J, Mascha E. Complex partial seizures of frontal lobe onset: Statistical analysis of ictal semiology. *Seizure* 2003; 12:268–281.
73. Kotagal P, Bleasel AF, Geller E, Kanirawatana P, et al. Lateralizing value of asymmetric tonic limb posturing (figure 4 sign) observed in secondarily generalized tonic-clonic seizures. *Epilepsia* 2000; 41:457–462.
74. Mayeux R, Lüders H. Complex partial status epilepticus. A case report and proposal for diagnostic criteria. *Neurology* 1978; 28:957.
75. Wieser HG, Hajek M. Frontal lobe epilepsy: compartmentalization, presurgical evaluation, and operative results. In: Jasper HH, Riggio S, Goldman-Rakic PS, eds. *Epilepsy and the Functional Anatomy of the Frontal Lobe*. New York: Raven Press, 1995: 297–319.

76. Manford M, Hart YM, Sander JW, Shorvon SD. National General Practice Study of Epilepsy (NGPSE): partial seizure patterns in a general population. *Neurology* 1992; 42:1911–1917.
77. Williamson PD, Spencer DD, Spencer SS, Novelly R, et al. Complex partial seizures of frontal lobe origin. *Ann Neurol* 1985; 18:497–504.
78. Williamson PD. Frontal lobe epilepsy: some clinical characteristics. In: Jasper HH, Riggio S, Goldman-Rakic PS, eds. *Epilepsy and the Functional Anatomy of the Frontal Lobe*. New York: Raven Press, 1995:297–319.
79. Salanova V, Morris HH, Van Ness P, et al. Frontal lobe seizures: electroclinical syndromes. *Epilepsia* 1995; 36:16–24.
80. Manford M, Fish DR, Shorvon SD. An analysis of clinical seizure patterns and their localizing value in frontal and temporal lobe epilepsies. *Brain* 1996; 119:17–40.
81. Scheffer I, Bhatia K, Lopes-Cendes I, et al. Autosomal dominant frontal epilepsy misdiagnosed as sleep disorder. *Lancet* 1994; 343:515–517.
82. Phillips H, Scheffer I, Berkovic S, et al. Localization of a gene for autosomal dominant nocturnal frontal lobe epilepsy to chromosome 20q13.2. *Nat Genet* 1995; 10:117–118.
83. Combi R, Dalpra L, Luisa-Tenchini ML, Ferini-Strambi L. Autosomal dominant nocturnal frontal lobe epilepsy. A critical overview. *J Neurol* 2004; 251:923–934.
84. Scheffer I, Bhatia K, Lopes-Cendes I, et al. Autosomal dominant nocturnal frontal lobe epilepsy. A distinctive clinical disorder. *Brain* 1995; 118:61–73.
85. Rasmussen T, Andermann F. Update on the syndrome of "chronic encephalitis" and epilepsy. *Cleve Clin J Med* 1989; 56(Suppl):181–184.
86. Oguni H, Andermann F, Rasmussen TB. The natural history of the syndrome of chronic encephalitis and epilepsy: a study of the MNI series of 48 cases. In: Andermann F, ed. *Chronic Encephalitis and Epilepsy: Rasmussen Syndrome*. Boston: Butterworth-Heinemann, 1991:7–25.
87. Rogers SW, Andrews PI, Gahring LC, et al. Autoantibody to glutamate receptor Glu R3 in Rasmussen's encephalitis. *Science* 1994; 265:648–651.
88. Pardo CA, Arroyo S, Ringing EPG, Freeman JM. Neuronal injury in Rasmussen's chronic encephalitis is mediated by cytotoxic T-cells. *Epilepsia* 1994; 35(Suppl 8):89.
89. Andrews PI, Dichter MA, Berkovic SF, McNamara JO. Plasmapheresis in Rasmussen's encephalitis. *Neurology* 1996; 46:242–246.
90. Aguilar MJ, Rasmussen T. Role of encephalitis in the pathogenesis of epilepsy. *Arch Neurol* 1960; 2:663–676.
91. Verhagen WI, Renier WO, Ter Laak H, Jaspar HH, et al. Anomalies of the cerebral cortex in a case of epilepsia partialis continua. *Epilepsia* 1988; 29:57–62.
92. Robitaille Y. Neuropathological aspects of chronic encephalitis. In: Andermann F, ed. *Chronic Encephalitis and Epilepsy: Rasmussen Syndrome*. Boston: Butterworth-Heinemann, 1991:79–110.
93. Power C, Poland SD, Blume WT, Girvin JP, et al. Cytomegalovirus and Rasmussen's encephalitis. *Lancet* 1990; 336:1282–1284.
94. Farrell MA, Droogan O, Secor DL, Poukens V, et al. Chronic encephalitis associated with epilepsy: Immunohistochemical and ultrastructural studies. *Acta Nedur̄opathol Berl* 1995; 89:313–321.
95. Gahring LC, Carlson NG, Meyer EL, Rogers SW. Cutting edge: Granzyme B proteolysis of a neuronal glutamate receptor generates an autoantigen and is modulated by glycosylation. *J Immunol* 2001; 166:1433–1438.
96. Andrews PI, McNamara JO, Lewis DV. Clinical and electroencephalographic correlates in Rasmussen's encephalitis. *Epilepsia* 1997; 38:189–194.
97. Vining EPG, Freeman JM, Brandt J, Carson BS. Progressive unilateral encephalopathy of childhood (RS): a reappraisal. *Epilepsia* 1993; 34:639–650.
98. So NK, Gloor P. Electroencephalographic and electrocorticographic findings in chronic encephalitis of the Rasmussen type. In: Andermann F, ed. *Chronic Encephalitis and Epilepsy: Rasmussen Syndrome*. Boston: Butterworth-Heinemann, 1991:37–46.
99. Tien RD, Ashdown BC, Lewis DV, Atkins MR, et al. Rasmussen's encephalitis: neuroimaging findings in 4 patients. *AJR Am J Roentgenol* 1992; 158:1329–1332.
100. Matthews PM, Andermann F, Arnold DL. A proton magnetic resonance spectroscopic study of focal epilepsy in humans. *Neurology* 1990; 40:985–989.
101. Hart YM, Cortez M, Andermann F, et al. Medical treatment of Rasmussen's syndrome (chronic encephalitis and epilepsy): effect of high dose steroids or immunoglobulins in 19 patients. *Neurology* 1994; 44:1030–1036.
102. Vining PG, Freeman JM, Pillas DJ, Uematsu S, et al. Why would you remove half a brain? The outcome of 58 children after hemispherectomy. *Pediatrics* 1997; 100:163–171.
103. Bien CG, Gleissner U, Sassen R, Widman G, et al. An open study of tacrolimus therapy in Rasmussen encephalıtis. *Neurology* 2004; 62:2106 2109.
104. Villemure JG, Andermann F, Rasmussen T. Hemispherectomy for the treatment of epilepsy due to chronic encephalitis. In: Andermann F, ed. *Chronic Encephalitis and Epilepsy: Rasmussen Syndrome*. Boston: Butterworth-Heinemann, 1991:235–241.
105. Vining PG, Carson B, Brandt J. Hemispherectomy for Rasmussen syndrome: report of 24 cases. *Epilepsia* 1995; 36:S241 (abstract).
106. Theodore WH, Porter RJ, Penry JK. Complex partial seizures: clinical characteristics and differential diagnosis. *Neurology* 1983; 33:1115–1221.
107. Wyllie E, Friedman D, Rothner AD, et al. Psychogenic seizures in children and adolescents: outcome after diagnosis by ictal video and electroencephalographic recording. *Pediatrics* 1990; 85(Suppl 4):480–484.
108. Rothner AD. The migraine syndrome in children and adolescents. *Pediatr Neurol* 1986; 2:121–126.
109. Kuzniecky R, Murro A, King D, et al. Magnetic resonance imaging in childhood intractable partial epilepsies: pathologic correlation. *Neurology* 1993; 43:681–687.
110. Berkovic SF, Andermann F, Olivier A, et al. Hippocampal sclerosis in temporal lobe epilepsy demonstrated by magnetic resonance imaging. *Ann Neurol* 1991; 29:175–182.
111. Jackson GD, Berkovic SF, Duncan JS, Connelly A. Optimizing the diagnosis of hippocampal sclerosis using MRI. *Am J Nucl Radiol* 1993; 14(3):753–762.
112. Cascino GD, Jack CR, Parsi JE, et al. Magnetic resonance imaging based volume studies in temporal lobe epilepsy: pathological correlation. *Ann Neurol* 1991; 30:31–36.
113. Jack C, Sharbrough FW, Cascino GD, Hirschorn KA, et al. Magnetic resonance image-based hippocampal volumetry: correlation with outcome after temporal lobectomy. *Ann Neurol* 1992; 31:138–146.
114. Kuzniecky R, Cascino G, Palmini A, et al. Structural neuroimaging. In: Engel JE, ed. *Surgical Treatment of Epilepsies*. New York: Raven Press, 1993:197.
115. Palmini A, Andermann F, Olivier A, et al. Focal neuronal migrational disorder and intractable partial epilepsy: a study of 30 patients. *Ann Neurol* 1991; 30:741–749.
116. Palmini A, Andermann F, Olivier A, et al. Neuronal migration disorders. A contribution of modern neuroimaging to the etiological diagnosis of epilepsy. *Can J Neurol Sci* 1991; 18:580–587.
117. Theodore WH. Neuroimaging in the evaluation of patients for focal resection. In: Wyllie E, ed. *The Treatment of Epilepsy: Principles and Practice*. Philadelphia: Lea & Febiger, 1993:1039–1050.
118. Henry TR, Chugani HT, Abou-Khalil BW, et al. Positron emission tomography. In: Engel J Jr, ed. *Surgical Treatment of Epilepsies*. 2nd ed. New York: Raven Press, 1993:211–243.
119. Savic I, Persson A, Roland P, et al. In vivo demonstration of BZ receptor binding in human epileptic foci. *Lancet* 1988; 2:863–866.
120. Frost JJ, Mayberg HS, Fisher RS, et al. Mu-opiate receptors measured by positron emission tomography are increased in temporal lobe epilepsy. *Ann Neurol* 1988; 23:231–237.
121. Adams C, Hwang P, Gilday DL, et al. Comparison of SPECT, EEG, CT, MRI and pathology in partial epilepsy. *Pediatr Neurol* 1992; 8:97–103.
122. Markand ON, Shen W, Park HM, Siddiqui AR, et al. Single photon imaging computed tomography (SPECT) for localization of epileptogenic focus in patients with intractable complex partial seizures. *Epilepsy Res Suppl* 1992; 5:121–126.
123. Harvey A, Hopkins I, Bowe J, et al. Frontal lobe epilepsy: clinical seizure characteristics and localization with ictal ^{99m}Tc-HMPAO SPECT. *Neurology* 1993; 43:1966–1980.
124. Marks DA, Katz A, Hoffer P, et al. Localization of extratemporal epileptic foci during ictal single-photon emission computed tomography. *Ann Neurol* 1992; 31:250–255.
125. Geiger LR, Harner RN. EEG seizure patterns at the time of focal seizure onset. *Arch Neurol* 1978; 35:276–286.
126. Gibbs FA, Gibbs EL. Atlas of electroencephalography. In: *Epilepsy*. Vol III. Reading, MA: Addison-Wesley, 1960.
127. Klass DW, Fischer-Williams M. Activation and provocation methods in clinical neurophysiology. I. Sensory stimulation. Sleep and sleep deprivation. In: Remond A, ed. *Handbook of Electroencephalography and Clinical Neurophysiology*. Amsterdam: Elsevier, 1975:5–73.
128. Harner RN. The significance of focal hypersynchrony in clinical EEG. *Electroencephalogr Clin Neurophysiol* 1971; 31:293.
129. Eeg-Olofson O, Peterson I, Seliden U. The development of the electroencephalogram in normal children from the age of 1 through 15 years: paroxysmal activity. *Neuropädiatrie* 1971; 2:375–404.
130. Gastaut H, Broughton R. *Epileptic Seizures*. Springfield, IL: Charles C Thomas, 1972.
131. Worrell GA, So EL, Kazemi J, O'Brien TJ, et al. Focal ictal β discharge on scalp EEG predicts excellent outcome of frontal lobe epilepsy surgery. *Epilepsia* 2002; 43:277–282.
132. Gastaut H, Vigoroux M. Electroclinical correlation in 500 cases of psychomotor seizures. In: Baldwin E, and Bailey P, eds. *Temporal Lobe Epilepsy*. Springfield, IL: Charles C Thomas, 1958:118–128.
133. Wyllie E, Lüders H, Morris HH, et al. Subdural electrodes in the evaluation for epilepsy surgery in children and adults. *Neuropediatrics* 1988; 19:80–86.
134. Lüders H, Lesser RP, Dinner DS, et al. Commentary: chronic intracranial recording and stimulation with subdural electrodes. In: Engel J, ed. *Surgical Treatment of the Epilepsies*. New York: Raven Press, 1987:297–321.
135. Munari C, Bancaud J. The role of stereo-electroencephalography in the evaluation of partial epileptic seizures. In: Porter RJ, Morselli PL, eds. *Epilepsies*. London, Butterworths, 1985:267–306.
136. Engel J, Rausch R, Lieb JP, Kuhl DE, et al. Correlation of criteria used for localizing epileptic foci considered for surgical therapy of epilepsy. *Ann Neurol* 1981; 9:215–224.
137. Spencer SS, Spencer DD, Williamson PD, Mattson R. The localizing value of depth electroencephalography in 32 patients with refractory epilepsy. *Ann Neurol* 1982; 12:248–253.
138. Oliver A, Gloor P, Andermann F, Ives J. Occipitotemporal epilepsy studied with stereotaxically implanted depth electrodes and successfully treated by temporal resection. *Ann Neurol* 1982; 11:428–432.
139. Kotagal P, Rothner AD, Erenberg G, Cruse RP, et al. Complex partial seizures of childhood-onset: a five-year follow-up study. *Arch Neurol* 1987; 44:1177–1180.
140. Lindsay J, Ounsted C, Richards P. Long-term outcome in children with temporal lobe epilepsy: I. Social outcome and childhood factors. *Dev Med Child Neurol* 1979; 21: 285–298.
141. Pazzaglia P, D'Alessandro R, Lozito A, Lugaresi E. Classification of partial epilepsies according to the symptomatology of seizures: Practical value and prognostic implications. *Epilepsia* 1982; 23:343–350.
142. Loiseau P, Dartigues JF, Pestre M. Prognosis of partial epileptic seizures in the adolescent. *Epilepsia* 1983; 24:472–481.

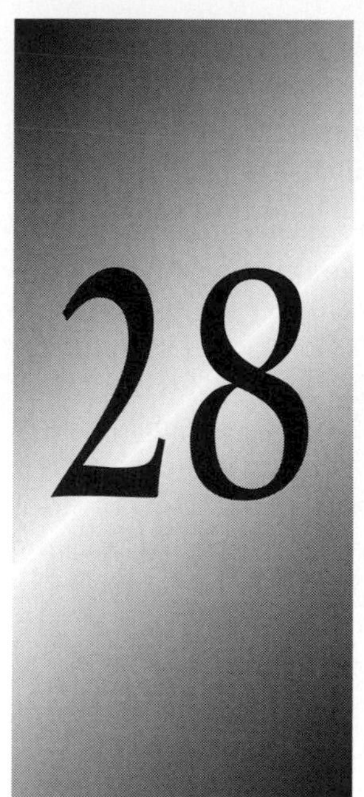

Selected Disorders Associated with Epilepsy

Lawrence D. Morton

Certain diseases and clinical syndromes should be suspected by their presentation with particular types of epilepsy, seizures, or EEG characteristics. A case in point would be the infant who presents with infantile spasms and is found to have hypsarrhythmia on the electroencephalogram (EEG). The clinical evaluation should include an ultraviolet light (Wood's lamp) examination of the skin for hypomelanotic macules (1, 2). The diagnosis of tuberous sclerosis may be confirmed by neurologic evaluation and brain imaging with either computed tomography (CT) or magnetic resonance imaging (MRI). In a similar manner a variety of uncommon diseases in which epilepsy is a prominent symptom can be suspected by recognizing distinctive forms of epilepsy. Additionally, seizures may arise in disorders that otherwise do not have prominent neurologic features. In this context, seizures are important "red flags" that may indicate a cerebral insult and the potential for serious neurologic complications or may be an important prognostic marker. This chapter discusses important examples of childhood disorders in which epilepsy plays a major role.

NEUROCUTANEOUS DISORDERS

Tuberous Sclerosis

Tuberous sclerosis complex is a congenital neurocutaneous disease of autosomal-dominant inheritance and variable expressivity (2). However, only one-third of cases are inherited. Two different mutations have been described that cause the tuberous sclerosis complex: TSC1 (9q34.3) and TSC2 (16p13.3) (3, 4). A mutation in one of these genes can be seen in up to 85% of patients fulfilling clinical criteria for tuberous sclerosis (5). TSC1 encodes a protein called hamartin. Hamartin forms a complex with the tuberin protein, which is encoded by the TSC2 gene, and the complex is thought to function in part as a negative regulator of the cell cycle (6). These proteins appears to participate in normal brain development (7).

Hamartomas, or benign growths, may affect almost any organ but notably the skin, central nervous system (CNS), retina, heart, and kidney. The incidence of tuberous sclerosis varies in different studies from 1 in 10,000 to 1 in 170,000, but with increased evaluation, the disease appears to be more prevalent and not rare (2).

Tuberous sclerosis most often presents with seizures. In all, 80% to 90% of patients develop seizures at some point in their lifetime. Generalized seizures are the most frequent. Infantile spasms occur in 68% of cases presenting in infancy. Tonic, atonic, and atypical absences are also seen, especially in patients who have slow spike-wave EEG patterns and thus conform to the Lennox-Gastaut syndrome. Tonic-clonic seizures usually occur after 1 year of age, replacing other seizure types (8). Complex partial seizures also occur frequently.

Various EEG abnormalities have been documented, depending on the clinical seizure type. Infantile spasms are associated with a hypsarrhythmia, which may progress to multifocal EEG abnormalities including, most frequently, sharp-and-slow-wave discharges and spike-and-wave discharges. In general, the EEG abnormalities relate to the age of onset of the seizures (9, 10).

The neurologic examination is frequently nonfocal; however, focal or diffuse signs occur with increasing size of subependymal or cortical lesions. These include hydrocephalus, movement disorders, visual disturbances, mental retardation, and rare focal motor deficits. The prognosis depends on the number and location of intracerebral lesions. The presence of numerous multifocal lesions correlates with an early onset of difficult-to-control seizures and mental retardation. Approximately 37% of patients with tuberous sclerosis have average intelligence; 50% to 60% are mentally retarded. Seizure-free children usually have normal intelligence. Involvement of other organ systems, especially the heart and kidneys, may affect longevity. Aberrant behavior frequently becomes the most difficult management issue in these children as they become older.

Seizures are surprisingly refractory to treatment. Patients with infantile spasms and myoclonic seizures need to be treated immediately. The treatment of choice for each patient depends on their seizure type, age, and comorbidity (2, 11, 12). Infantile spasms are treated with adrenocorticotropic hormone (ACTH), valproate, vigabatrin, zonisamide, or topiramate (13, 14). Vigabatrin has been reported to be efficacious in the treatment of refractory infantile spasms.

Surgical treatment for focal abnormalities, or tubers, primarily correlated by EEG evidence of partial seizures, has been quite successful (12) (see Chapters 62 and 63). Traditionally, patients with tuberous sclerosis were considered poor surgical candidates. Recently, centers have been performing more epilepsy surgery in these patients and with good results (15). Agreement between EEG, imaging of tubers, and clinical seizures allows this group to compare favorably with other lesional epilepsy surgery outcomes, and seizure-free rates of over 80% have been reported (16).

Neurofibromatosis (von Recklinghausen's Disease)

Neurofibromatosis is inherited as an autosomal-dominant disorder. There are two main types: NF1 (also known as Von Recklinghausen's disease or peripheral neurofibromatosis) and NF2 (also known as bilateral acoustic neurofibromatosis). NF1 is by far the more common and the classic form. NF1 has an incidence of 1 in 4,000 births. Central or acoustic neurofibromatosis, NF2, causes acoustic neuromas, not cutaneous or bony abnormalities. NF1 has been mapped to 17q11.2 and NF2 to the long arm of chromosome 22 (17, 18).

Classic neurofibromatosis is characterized by pigmentary abnormalities and neurofibromas (17, 19). Skin lesions include café-au-lait spots (6 or more > 0.5 cm in prepubertal children and > 1.5 cm in postpubertal children) and intertriginous freckles. Lisch nodules in the iris are present in a minority of affected young children but increase with age. Neurologic features include seizures in 3% to 6% (20, 21), though an incidence as high as 10% has been reported (22); occasional mental retardation, learning disorders, and a heightened risk of developing glial CNS tumors, with visual path glioma being most common in NF1. Although cortical heterotopias are found in rare cases, most often the pathogenesis of epilepsy and learning problems is unclear. Other features include growth disturbances, osseous aplasia or hyperplasia, macrocephaly, scoliosis, precocious puberty, and cerebrovascular lesions causing stroke. There is an increased risk of malignancies, which can limit longevity.

The treatment of seizures associated with neurofibromatosis is dependent on seizure type and whether a specific intracranial mass lesion is present. Most patients are treated with chronic antiepileptic drug (AED) therapy, with very few having spontaneous remission of their epilepsy.

Sturge-Weber Syndrome

Sturge-Weber syndrome is characterized by a portwine stain unilaterally over the upper face, superior eyelid, or supraorbital region, corresponding to the sensory component of the ophthalmic branch of the trigeminal nerve. Buphthalmos or glaucoma is the most characteristic and constant ocular lesion (23). Intracranial calcification occurs in 90% of cases. Seizures are often the presenting symptom and usually in early childhood. The percentage of patients manifesting partial or secondarily generalized seizures increases steadily with age, so that by age 5 years nearly 95% of patients have seizures (24). Seizures are more common with bilateral cutaneous manifestations (87–93%) than unilateral (71%) (24, 25). EEG reveals decreased amplitude and frequency over the affected hemisphere with diffuse multiple and independent spikes (26).

Surgical removal of the affected lobe or hemisphere should be considered when seizures are refractory. Significant improvement in seizure control with no disabling deficit is often seen. Seizure freedom has been seen in up to 81% (27). Results of limited cortical resection were not as dramatic, though there was also relief of seizure activity (28). Tuxhorn and Pannek reported two children with bilateral Sturge-Weber syndrome who benefited from hemispherectomy, suggesting that removal of the dominant epileptogenic focus can be considered in some patients with bilateral disease (29).

Hypomelanosis of Ito

Hypomelanosis of Ito is characterized by macular cutaneous hypopigmentation in patterns of whorls, streaks, and patches, as well as generalized abnormalities. Associated neurologic abnormalities, seen in 61% to 100% of patients, include developmental delay and refractory seizures, sometimes manifesting as infantile spasms (30, 31). Cortical atrophy is seen on imaging studies. The EEG abnormality shows no consistent pattern (32). Seizures occur in 53% (33). No specific antiepileptic drug treatments tailored to the underlying etiology have been recommended; instead, medications are usually selected to treat the seizure type. Surgery has been used successfully but with very few patients (34).

Incontinentia Pigmenti

The skin lesion of incontinentia pigmenti, which is seen mostly in girls, has three stages. Initially, one sees macular papular vesicular and even bullous lesions occurring in the first 2 weeks of life and located primarily over the limbs or trunk. This stage is followed by a keratotic verrucous lesion over the limbs, followed by hypopigmentation or skin atrophy. Subsequent pigmentation then occurs. The CNS is commonly involved, with generalized and focal seizures in 9 percent to 13 percent of patients, typically satisfactory control is often achieved (35). Retardation, spasticity, and microcephaly occur in 5% to 16%. Ocular abnormalities occur in one third of the patients (36).

Epidermal Nevus Syndrome

Epidermal nevi may be present at birth or may develop later, usually around the time of puberty. The skin lesions are slightly raised, ovoid, or linear plaques. As the patient approaches puberty, the lesions may change from skin-colored to an orange-brown and become verrucous (37). Epilepsy, mental retardation, and focal motor deficits are the most commonly encountered neurologic manifestations. Seizures are present in the majority of patients with linear sebaceous nevus (38). A variety of congenital malformations of the CNS have been described including hemimegalencephaly, heterotopias, and schizencephaly (39). A wide variety of seizure disorders may be seen in this disorder.

METABOLIC DISORDERS

Various diseases with underlying inborn metabolic abnormalities may cause epilepsy characterized by a particular EEG abnormality (40). Early identification and appropriate treatment of these specific disorders frequently leads to the best treatment of seizures and optimal developmental outcome. AEDs, however, are sometimes necessary adjuncts.

Urea Cycle Disorders

Urea cycle disorders occur in 1 in 30,000 births. Seizure activity may be the presenting symptom associated with hyperammonemia, which can be precipitated or worsened by valproate therapy in unrecognized ornithine transcarbamylase deficiency (41). Deficiencies of ornithine transcarbamylase and arginosuccinic acid lyase have resulted in abnormal EEG activity characterized mainly by multiple spikes, spike waves, or slow-and-sharp-wave activity. The EEG normalizes with successful treatment of the metabolic disorder (42). Citrullinemia also has presented with seizure activity and an EEG with multifocal spikes (43). However, there is a lag in EEG normalization after treatment (peritoneal dialysis) in this condition. Neurologic deficits persist in reported cases (44).

Phenylketonuria

Phenylketonuria, when untreated, may be associated with infantile spasms and hypsarrhythmia. Phenylketonuria is caused by a deficiency in hepatic phenylalanine hydroxylase, whose gene is located at 12.q24.1 (45). In treated phenylketonuria there is an increased prevalence of EEG abnormalities manifesting as generalized slowing with or without spikes (46). With advancing age, the EEG abnormalities increase but lack any relationship to IQ or dietary treatment (47).

Menkes Disease

Menkes kinky hair disease, a sex-linked disorder with its gene located on the long arm of the X chromosome, causes a marked reduction of serum copper and serum ceruloplasmin levels. Patients typically present at 2–3 months of age. The clinical findings consist of mental retardation, poorly pigmented fragile hair, hypotonia, and generalized seizure activity, frequently infantile spasms (48). Milder forms have been described with less or minimal neurologic sequelae; the mildest Menkes variant is known as occipital horn syndrome, in reference to the pathognomonic wedge-shaped calcification that forms within the trapezius and sternocleidomastoid muscles at their attachment to the occipital bone in affected individuals (49). Parenteral copper benefits some patients with Menkes disease. This may reflect preservation of some activity of certain copper ATPase alleles (50).

Glycine Encephalopathy

Glycine encephalopathy, also known as nonketotic hyperglycinemia, is an autosomal recessive disorder caused by defective function of the multimeric glycine cleavage enzymes. The most common defect, affecting the P protein, is encoded by a gene localized to 9p22. Glycine is elevated in the plasma, urine, and cerebrospinal fluid (CSF). The lack of ketones helps differentiate between nonketotic hyperglycinemia and organic acidurias such as methylmalonic acidemia and propionic acidemia. Infants with the classic form of the disease present in the first week after birth with apnea, lethargy, and hypotonia (51). Intractable seizures develop; the EEG demonstrates burst-suppression or hypsarrhythmia (52). Brain imaging in nearly one half of patients with glycine encephalopathy shows congenital abnormalities including atrophy and agenesis of the corpus callosum (41C). Valproate is contraindicated, because it induces hyperglycinemia (53).

GM2 Gangliosidoses

GM2 gangliosidoses (Tay-Sachs and Sandhoff diseases) have seizures as a frequent complication, particularly in the infantile form. The first symptom is an excessive startle in response to noise, tactile stimuli, or light flashes. This startle response in patients with Tay-Sachs disease, which differs from the Moro response of normal infants, consists of a quick extension of the arms and legs, frequently with clonic movements. There is arrest in development, and axial hypotonia ensues. During the second year after birth, macrocephaly develops, and seizures become more prominent. These may be myoclonic or gelastic and can be induced by auditory or tactile stimulation (54). Later, blindness develops and patients become increasingly less responsive. Autonomic dysfunction is a frequent finding including apnea. In Sandhoff disease the only clinical differences compared to Tay Sach's disease are mild hepatosplenomegaly, secondary to storage of globoside, and bony deformities (54).

Pyridoxine-Dependent Seizures

Seizures beginning in the first week after birth may have pyridoxine dependency. Associated symptoms may include episodes of restlessness, irritability, and feeding difficulties. The seizures are refractory to standard anticonvulsant medications but respond well to pyridoxine administration (55). Atypical forms are common and may outnumber the classical form. Features include late onset after the first week but typically in the first months after birth, transient response to standard therapy, and atypical seizures (56). Very late forms have been described (57), as well as response following failed trials during infancy (58). Some cases have localized to the gene at chromosome 5q31.2–q31.3 (59).

Porphyria

Although porphyria does not become symptomatic until after puberty, it occasionally affects older adolescents. Seizures commonly occur in 15 percent of patients with porphyria, usually during an acute attack. Seizures may be partial or generalized. Therapy of chronic seizures in these patients must avoid drugs that increase porphyria precursors and induce attacks. This includes all commonly used AEDs (60), although gabapentin and levetiracetam should be safe and effective.

Biotinidase Deficiency

Skin rashes and striking neurologic symptoms with seizures are prominent signs of biotinidase deficiency. Hypotonia, developmental delay, and seizures are presenting features in the neonatal form. In the late-onset type, 1 week to 2 years onset, the most common presenting feature is seizures. The most common seizure type is myoclonus, although generalized tonic-clonic and focal clonic seizures have been described (61). Ataxia and hypotonia are present, as are rash and alopecia. Hearing loss may occur. Treatment is oral biotin with rapid response within 24 hours (61, 62).

Other Inborn Errors of Metabolism

Other inborn errors of metabolism may be associated with generalized seizure activity. These include maple syrup urine disease, galactosemia, organic acidurias, hyperammonemia, and peroxisomal disorders, to mention only a few.

INFECTIONS

Infants with prenatal intracranial infections often present with postnatal seizures. A common infection is cytomegalovirus (63). In particular, infants with neonatal herpes simplex encephalitis may have specific EEG patterns consisting of periodic or quasiperiodic patterns. Thus, a periodic pattern in a young infant with partial motor seizures and lymphocytic CSF pleocytosis is highly suggestive of herpes virus encephalitis (64), cytomegalovirus, or toxoplasmosis (65).

Human Immunodeficiency Virus

HIV has emerged as a major prenatal infection with significant neurologic morbidity. Approximately 90 percent of prepubertal cases reflect intrauterine or intrapartum infection. The predominant clinical finding is a triad of impaired brain growth, progressive motor dysfunction, and plateau or loss of developmental milestones (66, 67). In children, CNS effects usually result from direct HIV-1 infection, not from tumors or opportunistic infections, in contrast to adults (66). Seizures occur at only a slightly higher incidence in the pediatric HIV-1 population (68) than in the uninfected population. Seizures may be the presenting symptom in children with new stroke as a complication of HIV (69, 70). The incidence of new-onset seizures in HIV patients has been found to be between 4% and 11%, with most having advanced AIDS (71). The presence of a seizure leads to a workup, including neuroimaging, to look for coexisting focal pathology (72) or opportunistic infection.

Subacute Sclerosing Panencephalitis

This condition was first reported in 1993 as an inclusion body encephalitis. Measles virus is the causal agent and persists in the CNS. Virus persistence appears to be a result of a defect in replication. The progression of the illness has been broken into four stages, with stage I including mild behavioral and intellectual changes and stage IV including flexor posture, mutism, and autonomic instability. Seizures typically develop in stage II. Myoclonus is the best known and typically is periodic and stereotypic. The EEG demonstrates periodic complexes of high-amplitude delta waves occurring every 4 to 12 seconds and are synchronous with the myoclonic jerks (73). Other seizure types include akinetic, atypical absence, generalized tonic-clonic, and focal clonic (74). The prognosis is grave even with treatment, with a median survival of 1 year. Although this condition had become quite rare, an outbreak due to overall low vaccination rates in 1989 to 1991 caused a 10-fold increase in biopsy-proven cases from 1992 through 2003 (75).

Acute CNS Infections

Any acute infection of the CNS may lead to seizures, including bacterial meningitis, viral encephalitis, focal cerebritides, and parasitic infections. Bacterial meningitis should be suspected and excluded by lumbar puncture in any child with seizures in the setting of headache, fever, and meningeal signs. The causal agent typically varies with patient age.

Acute viral encephalitis may produce seizures. Herpes simplex is the most common infectious encephalitis associated with seizures (76). In herpes simplex encephalitis, patients may have a prodrome of malaise, fever, headache, and nausea. This is followed by acute or subacute onset of an encephalopathy whose symptoms include lethargy, confusion, and delirium. Headaches, seizures, aphasia, and other focal deficits may follow. Even with modern treatment, mortality in children may be as high as 20%, and an even larger percentage suffer permanent neurologic sequelae (77). Other viral encephalitides associated with seizures include California, Japanese, and St. Louis encephalitides as well as Eastern and Western encephalitides.

Parasitic infections of the central nervous system may lead to seizures. Although this is more common in the immunosuppressed, some infections may occur in immunocompetent patients. Cysticercosis is caused by the metacestode, or larval stage, of *Taenia solium*, the pork tapeworm. Cysticerci that enter the CSF are initially viable but do not cause much inflammation in surrounding tissues; this phase of infection is usually asymptomatic. The host develops a state of immune tolerance to the parasite, and cysticerci can remain in this stage for many years. Most patients remain in this stage for life. Cysticerci do not produce clinical symptomatology until the cysts begin to degenerate. The leaking cyst leads to a surrounding inflammatory reaction. The most common neurologic manifestation is seizures, occurring in about 75% (78). Trichinosis results from ingesting the nematode parasite *Trichinella* from contaminated pork. Trichinosis has two stages: an intestinal stage and a muscle stage, during the latter of which neurologic symptoms may occur. Involvement of the CNS occurs in 10% to 20% of patients. The mortality rates may be as high as 50% (79). Neurologic disease may develop early or late, and can be diffuse or focal in nature and may include seizures.

Systemic Infections

Systemic infections may lead to seizures, mostly by alterations in electrolytes or other effects such as hypoxia, such as in pneumonia. *Shigella*, however is associated with a high frequency of seizures in young children, occurring in one series at 5% (80). This large study also suggested that factors other than *Shigella* toxin were the cause of the seizures.

CHROMOSOMAL ABNORMALITIES AND CONGENITAL BRAIN ABNORMALITIES

Chromosomal abnormalities, including trisomy 13 and 21, may result in infants and children with seizure activity. Approximately 20 percent of patients with fragile X syndrome have seizures (generalized or partial) with spikes similar to rolandic spikes, which are noted during sleep tracings (81, 82). Five percent to 6% of children with

Down syndrome (trisomy 21) have seizures (83). Infantile spasms may occur but are fairly responsive to therapy.

Congenital malformations with neurologic deficits can cause infantile spasms and hypsarrhythmia as well as other seizure types. The Aicardi syndrome, an X-linked dominant syndrome limited to females, is marked by agenesis of the corpus callosum, mental retardation, vertebral anomalies, and chorioretinal lacunae. In patients with seizures, 97% have had infantile spasms, with many having other seizure types (84). Patients with septo-optic dysplasia, with absence of septum pellucidum, optic nerve hypoplasia, and hypothalamic-pituitary dysfunction, can also present with infantile spasms (85). Various brain gyral malformations such as lissencephaly, agyria-pachygyria, and others may cause infantile spasms or other seizure types (86–88).

Angelman Syndrome

Angelman syndrome occurs in children with a history of nonprogressive delayed development from infancy. Jerky limb movements, stiff ataxic-like gait, paroxysms of inappropriate laughter, and lack of speech are characteristic. Distinctive facial features with a prominent lower jaw, wide mouth, frequent tongue thrusting, and a thin upper lip are consistent. A chromosomal abnormality of maternal origin 15q11–13 has been detected in patients with Angelman syndrome (89).

Seizure activity is a frequent presenting symptom and is found in 86 percent of patients (90). Seizures commence at an early age, appearing by age 11 months at the earliest but often by 2 years of age. Myoclonic, atypical absence, generalized tonic-clonic, and unilateral clonic seizures are the typical clinical patterns, whereas infantile spasms are rare (91–93). In one series almost all patients had nonconvulsive seizures (94). The EEG demonstrates large-amplitude generalized spike-wave activity that may precede the clinical manifestation of seizures. Runs of rhythmic delta may be seen with either a frontal or an occipital predominance. There are often admixed spikes which have an inconsistent relationship to the slow waves, sometimes occurring on the descending portion of the slow wave and giving a "notched" appearance. This large rhythmic activity persists in sleep. The spike-wave activity also tends to be accentuated with eye closure. Thus, this facilitation of the EEG pattern with eye closure and the general pattern present from 1 year of age is suggestive of Angelman syndrome (95). This EEG pattern appears to persist, is not modified by AEDs, and may not be consistently correlated with clinical features. Other EEG findings include high-amplitude 4–6-Hz activity and posterior spike and sharp waves (96). Brain imaging shows variable results, with brain atrophy in perhaps 50 percent of patients. Correlation exists between epilepsy phenotypes and genotypes (97).

Prader-Willi Syndrome

Prader-Willi syndrome consists of short stature, small hands and feet, obesity, and mental retardation preceded in infancy by hypotonia and feeding difficulty. Boys have hypoplastic, flat scrotums with inguinal or abdominal testes. Seizures occur in 15% to 20% (98–100). It is rare to find the distinct EEG features of Angelman syndrome in Prader-Willi syndrome, though some cases exist (100). Although most cases are sporadic, concordance in monozygotic twins has been reported (101).

The disorder results from the specific deletion of 15q11–13 of paternal origin (102). The same region is deleted in Angelman syndrome; the different syndromes result from genetic imprinting (103).

Miller-Dieker Syndrome

Miller-Dieker syndrome includes microcephaly and lissencephaly, epilepsy, profound mental retardation, and occasional anomalies of the heart and genitalia (104, 105). Characteristic features include flat midface, prominent forehead, protuberant upper lip, and small jaw. It results from a deletion of the terminal end of the long arm of chromosome 17p13.3. Smaller deletions in chromosome 17 have also resulted in lissencephaly but without the typical facial features (106, 108). Overall, about 25 syndromes of different genetic basis and varying associated symptoms have been described (108). Infantile spasms are found in almost all Miller-Dieker and isolated lissencephaly syndrome patients. The infantile spasms usually respond to corticotropin. The other seizure types may respond to any seizure medicine. Corpus callosotomy has been used to treat an 11-month-old with bilateral lissencephaly and intractable tonic seizures (109).

MITOCHONDRIAL ENCEPHALOMYOPATHIES

The mitochondrial encephalomyopathies consist of a heterogeneous group of multisystem disorders. Seizures are a common finding in this class of disease. Seizures are a defining symptom in myoclonic epilepsy with ragged red fibers (MERRF) and are a common feature in mitochondrial encephalomyopathy, lactic acidosis, and strokelike episodes (MELAS). Seizures are uncommon in Kearns-Sayre syndrome.

Myoclonic Epilepsy with Ragged Red Fibers

Ataxia, intention and action myoclonus, and progressive mental deterioration have been reported in MERRF. Associated with these features, aggregates of mitochondria in skeletal muscle, known as ragged red fibers, are demonstrated by muscle biopsy. A specific mutation in mitochondrial DNA was discovered,a missense mutation in the gene for transfer RNA for lysine that accounts for 80% to 90% of MERRF cases (110). Generalized tonic-clonic seizures that are photosensitive are a feature and may be a presenting symptom. Spike-wave complexes occurring spontaneously and coinciding with myoclonic activity occur (111).

Mitochondrial myopathies associated with myoclonic epilepsy have been described occurring in families. Recently, mitochondrial abnormalities have been reported in Rett syndrome (112), discussed in a later section. In most reported mitochondrial myopathies, EEGs typically show generalized spike-wave activity. Seizure control is difficult in severe cases (113). The seizures of MERRF have been treated with typical antiseizure agents. Levetiracetam has shown encouraging results in a small number of patients (114).

Mitochondrial Encephalomyopathy with Lactic Acidosis and Strokelike Episodes

MELAS has among its defining features strokelike episodes, typically before age 40; encephalopathy characterized by dementia, seizures, or both; and evidence of a mitochondrial myopathy with ragged red fibers, lactic acidosis, or both. A variety of point mutations have been described that are causal, though one mutation accounts for about 80% of cases (115). Patients with MELAS frequently have seizures. In one group, seizures were the initial clinical symptom in 28%. They were sometimes associated with a strokelike episode. Seizures were both generalized and partial (116). Partial seizures were most typically motor. Seizures typically respond to conventional antiseizure agents, though valproate may exacerbate the disorder (117).

AUTISM AND AUTISTIC SPECTRUM DISORDERS

Autism is a heterogeneous, pervasive developmental disorder (118). Markedly abnormal or impaired development in social interaction and communication skills are evident in the first 3 years. Patients are often described as either passive or overly irritable as infants, and they fail to anticipate being picked up. Dysfunctional behaviors may start to appear, such as self-stimulatory behaviors (i.e., repetitive, non-goal-directed behavior such as rocking or hand flapping), self-injury, sleeping and eating problems, poor eye contact, insensitivity to pain, hyperactivity, and attention deficits (119, 120). More than a third, 41.9%, fall in the severe to profound range of mental retardation (121). However, cognitive skills in individuals with autism may show uneven development.

Underlying disorders include congenital infections (rubella, cytomegalovirus), phenylketonuria, tuberous sclerosis, fragile X, and Rett syndrome, though an etiology is not determined in up to 90% (122). Researchers have located several brain abnormalities in individuals with autism; however, the reasons for these abnormalities is not known, nor is the influence they have on behavior. Selective hypoplasia of the neocerebellar vermis has been reported on midsagittal MRI of autistic patients (123), while in another study, total cerebellar volume has been increased (124). Recent studies show that the cerebellum may have a modulatory role in a wide array of neurobehavioral functions including learning (125), communication, attention, and socialization in addition to motor behavior. Abnormalities have been seen in the amygdala and hippocampus; damage to this region in monkeys has led to autistic-like behavior (126). Dysregulation in serotonin has also been found in some patients with autism (127), while others have implicated dopamine, norepinephrine, or neuropeptide function. There is some indication of a genetic influence in autism. A 60% concordance for autism was found in monozygotic twin pairs versus 0% in dizygotic twins, with an estimated heritability of over 90% in one study (128).

Electrencephalographic abnormalities are present in 27% to 77% of individuals (129, 130). However, many individuals have abnormal EEGs but not clinical epilepsy. Incidence of clinical epilepsy has been observed to be as high as 40% with higher rates in children in the more impaired range of autism (131).

Treatment has focused primarily on the behavioral aspects. In addition to medications, behavioral, educational, and language training have been employed. Commonly used medications include selective serotonin reuptake inhibitors (SSRIs) as well as classic and newer neuroleptics; stimulants are also commonly used. Many of the antiseizure medications, particularly valproate, have been used to treat behavior problems in a variety of patients with different medical and psychiatric problems. This has been true in autism as well. Many experts have found antiseizure medications to be of benefit for behavior problems as well as treating seizures (132). Antiseizure medications may be employed in children with autism who do not also have seizures. There is preliminary evidence supporting the hypothesis that there is a subgroup of of autistic children and seizures who preferentially respond to antiseizure medications (133, 134).

Acquired Epileptic Aphasia (Landau-Kleffner Syndrome)

Landau-Kleffner syndrome is typified by the loss of receptive and expressive language in association with paroxysmal EEG changes and, in some cases, seizures (135). Partial seizures in the dominant hemisphere both acutely and postictally may be associated with transient aphasia. However, in this disorder children who have developed normal language then experience a progressive deterioration of language (136). Age of onset ranges from 3 to 8 years, and boys are more frequently affected than girls (137). Diffuse or focal spike-waves with temporal preponderance are present, as are temporal metabolic abnormalities. Magnetoencephalography shows a vertical dipole located in the superior surface of the temporal lobe that is 2–3 cm deep (138). Seizure activity may occur at a much later stage. The aphasia rarely improves with seizure control (139, 140). These children occasionally may have autistic-like features. The first language disturbance is auditory agnosia. Recognition of the progressive nature of the language dysfunction may result in earlier intervention (141). The relationship to young children with a global autistic regression and epileptiform EEG is controversial (142). A consistent cause remains unknown. A relationship between Landau-Kleffner syndrome and continuous spike-wave of slow-wave sleep remains a subject of discussion. Autistic-like features also may be seen in children with epilepsy—generalized tonic-clonic, absence, and partial complex seizures, either primary or secondary (143).

Treatment with standard antiseizure medications may be effective for the seizures but have had little impact on the aphasia. Drugs such as phenytoin, phenobarbital, and carbamazepine may worsen the EEG discharges and neuropsychologic deficit (144). Treatment with high-dose corticosteroids has been the most successful treatment for the aphasia and intellectual disturbance (145, 146). Other treatments have included subpial transection (147, 148), as well as a small series showing possible benefit with the vagus nerve stimulator (149).

Rett Syndrome

Rett syndrome is a unique disorder that affects girls almost exclusively and is due to a mutation at the Xq28 chromosome affecting methyl-CpG-binding protein 2 (MECP2) (150, 151). Rare cases in males have been determined. Three types of MECP2 mutations occur: missense, frameshift, and nonsense. The type of mutation may affect phenotypic expression; for example, awake respiratory dysfunction and lower levels of CSF homovanillic acid (HVA) occurred more often with truncating mutations, whereas scoliosis was more common with missense mutations (150). A large majority (80–85%) of cases of classical, sporadic Rett syndrome test positive for the MECP2 abnormality, whereas under 50% test positive in the variant and familial cases (152, 153).

Abnormalities of CSF biogenic amines have also been demonstrated, suggesting neurotransmitter dysfunction (151, 154). MECP2 appears to target the DLX5 gene on chromosome 7q (155). DLX5 may function to induce expression of glutamic acid decarboxlyase (GAD) and the differentiation of GABA-producing neurons; therefore, alterations in GABAergic neurons may be involved in the pathogenesis of Rett syndrome (156).

In the classical form after an apparently normal early development (112), girls with Rett syndrome lose acquired skills. This deterioration involves loss of acquired purposeful motor and hand skills and loss of communication and cognitive functions between 6 and 30 months. Of particular significance is the loss of acquired speech. Deceleration of head growth, stereotypic hand-wringing movements, and gait apraxia occur between 1 and 5 years (157). Apnea, hyperpnea, and breath-holding spells occur. Seizures usually appear at 3 to 4 years of age. Aberrant behavior, manifesting as irritability, sleeplessness, screaming spells, and self-abusiveness, is common. Subsequently, hypertonicity and spasticity can occur, and progressive scoliosis develops. Atypical or variant forms include girls who have some clinical evidence of Rett syndrome, but not enough to meet all the specific diagnostic criteria.

The progression of the syndrome has been divided into four stages (158, 159). Stage I is the period of apparently normal development lasting 6 to 18 months. Stage II, the regression period with stereotypy and autistic features, lasts 1 to 4 years. Stage III begins at approximately 3 years of age, when seizures and ataxia occur. The deterioration may stop and the patient may appear stationary. Stage IV is associated with severe disability and scoliosis. These stages can overlap. The ultimate prognosis is dependent on the degree of immobility and scoliosis and on the level of subsequent care (160).

Seizures occur in a large majority of Rett syndrome patients. One large series out of Sweden found that 94% of patients with the classic disease had epilepsy (161). These may be generalized tonic, tonic-clonic, atypical absence, complex partial, myoclonic, or atonic seizures (158). Multiple seizure types occur in 30% to 40% of patients and may be intractable (159). The seizures usually appear at the age of 3 or 4 years. After 10 years of age it is uncommon for seizures to begin. Seizure types may appear refractory; however, some patients spontaneously improve on reaching adulthood (158, 160, 162). The incidence of clinical seizures may be overestimated, as demonstrated in one study that looked at video-EEG in Rett syndrome patients and determined that about half of the events identified as typical seizures were nonepileptic (163). EEG may be helpful in the diagnosis of Rett syndrome in stages I and II by ruling out Angelman syndrome, in which seizures occur before 2 years of age (164).

EEG changes similarly stratify into stages but do not correlate with the clinical course. During stage I the EEG may be normal or minimally slow. In stage II a rapid EEG deterioration occurs with slowing, loss of both occipital rhythms, and loss of normal sleep characteristics during quiet (non-rapid-eye-movement, non-REM) sleep. Focal epileptiform activity, first during sleep and then in wakefulness, with subsequent multifocal discharges, then occurs. Stage III is represented by further deterioration with generalized slow spike-wave activity and multifocal discharges during sleep and wakefulness. The EEG remains markedly abnormal during stage IV.

The evolution of EEG changes is distinctive and can aid in the diagnosis of Rett syndrome (165). Multifocal central spikes and spike waves of short duration enhanced by sleep and predating seizure activity is a fairly consistent finding (166–168). These parasagittal spikes are present during the early stages of non-REM sleep and in the early morning hours and can help in differentiating the diagnosis of Rett syndrome from primary autism, in which the EEG usually is normal (169). In some of the episodes, apnea may not be seizure activity (163).

ALPERS DISEASE (POLIODYSTROPHY)

The phrase *progressive infantile poliodystrophy* has been used to designate a pattern of symptoms including seizures and overall deterioration called Alpers disease. The early cases in the literature were heterogeneous, and confusion about diagnosis and nomenclature initially hampered the understanding of this group of diseases (170, 171). Two distinct groups of patients have subsequently emerged. One group has microcephaly with shrunken "walnut" brains, a progressive degeneration (172). The second group indicates a more uniform spectrum of clinical and pathologic phenotypes that are due to several inborn errors that affect energy metabolism, the Krebs cycle, respiratory chain, and mitochondrial function (173–177). Some of these patients have insidious but progressive liver disease (171, 178), while others are without hepatic failure (179). In recent years, when some of these patients have died with liver failure, valproic acid hepatotoxicity has been blamed (171, 180, 181).

Usually thought to be normal at birth, the children develop a progressive illness manifested by developmental delay, failure to thrive, focal myoclonus, seizures with a propensity for status epilepticus, hypotonia, visual disturbances (blindness is common), eventual paralysis, spasticity, and liver failure (177, 182–184). In addition, many of these patients develop multifocal myoclonic twitching or epilepsia partialis continua of the Kojewnikow variety (180, 181, 185). Variable features include deafness, chorea, and ataxia. They often worsen rapidly during an intercurrent illness. Conventional antiseizure agents may be used, though the physician may wish to avoid valproate given the underlying hepatic dysfunction.

At autopsy, there is atrophy of the hemispheres and the cerebellum. The cortex has diffuse foci of degeneration with neuronal necrosis, astrocytosis, and spongiosis with perivascular and pericellular edema. Other affected structures include the basal ganglia, thalamus, brainstem nuclei, dentate nucleus, cerebellar cortex, and lumbar spinal ganglia. The predominant hepatic lesions are microvesicular fatty infiltration and cirrhosis, sometimes with a micronodular pattern (184).

Distinctive EEG features include slow (1 Hz), high-amplitude (200–1,000 μV) background mixed with lower-amplitude polyspikes, often with focal prominence in the occipital area. The polyspikes on the EEG persist despite intravenous doses of barbiturates that suppress clinical seizures. Evoked potentials have been variably abnormal. Flash visual evoked potentials (VEPs) have ranged from normal to absent and often are asymmetric. Brainstem auditory evoked potentials (BAEPs) in some cases have been absent (185).

Several enzyme deficiencies have been reported as a biochemical basis for this disorder. These include abnormalities of the pyruvate dehydrogenase (PDH) complex, pyruvate carboxylase, coenzyme Q, and complexes I and IV, in the second part of the citric acid cycle (after the oxoglutarate dehydrogenase complex) in nicotinamide-adenine dinucleotide (reduced form) (NADH) oxidation, in cytochrome aa3, and in pyruvate carboxylase activity (177). Additional defects in cerebral energy metabolism are likely to be discovered. The types of enzyme defects described thus far have been associated with elevated concentrations of lactic acid in CSF.

COCKAYNE SYNDROME

Cockayne syndrome is characterized by paucity of growth with developmental delay; loss of subcutaneous fat; cold, cyanosed extremities; increased pigmented nevi; and decreased scalp hair. With increasing cachexia the patient's distinctive facies, enophthalmos, and absent fat are prominent features. Mental retardation and microcephaly with ventriculomegaly and questionable normal-pressure hydrocephalus are present. Hypertonicity with various movement disorders and myoclonic jerks is present. Optic atrophy and retinal pigmentary changes occur. The disorder is inherited as an autosomal recessive trait caused by several different mutations on chromosomes 5, 10, 13, and 19. Seizure activity usually has an early onset but can occur initially in adults. Status epilepticus resulting in death has been reported (186, 187).

INFLAMMATORY AND AUTOIMMUNE DISORDERS

Systemic Lupus Erythematosus

Systemic lupus erythematosus (SLE) may manifest primarily or complicate a more systemic presentation.

When neurologic or behavioral symptoms are prominent, the term *neuropsychiatric lupus* [NPSLE] is used. Juvenile-onset lupus carries greater risk of NPSLE and poorer prognosis (188). Eleven percent to 17% of patients with SLE develop seizures unrelated to renal disease, cardiac disease, or drugs. In one large series, 11.6% had seizures, with about a third experiencing seizures at the onset of the disease (189). These generalized or partial seizures usually occur early in the disease. Because a true vasculitis is uncommon, the precise cause is not defined. The pathogenesis of NPSLE is multifactorial and can involve various autoantibodies or immune complexes in mechanisms involving vasculopathic and autoantibody-mediated neuronal injury. Cerebral microinfarcts and subarachnoid hemorrhage have been demonstrated and may be related to antiphospholipid antibodies and lupus anticoagulant that can be present. When seizures are associated with psychiatric symptoms, a generalized vasculitis may be present. However, recently autoantibodies against murine neuronal membrane proteins have been discovered and correlate with psychosis, seizures, or both in lupus patients (190). Infectious causes need to be ruled out in the immunosuppressed patient. Seizures typically appear early in the course and are difficult to control. Phenytoin, ethosuximide, and carbamazepine can cause symptoms similar to those of SLE (191).

Acute Disseminated Encephalomyelitis

The term *acute disseminated encephalomyelitis* (ADEM) describes any immune-mediated encephalomyelitis resulting from infections, allergies, or vaccinations. Typically this is a monophasic illness occurring in pediatric patients, mostly prepubertal, and follows a preceding illness commonly by 1 to 6 weeks. Presenting symptoms include headache, encephalopathy, depressed level of consciousness, paresis, sensory changes, and ataxia. Approximately 25% will present with seizures (192, 193). Laboratory findings may be unremarkable, though about half will have elevated protein on CSF testing, and a mild pleocytosis is not unusual. The most consistent finding is obtained on MRI, with images typically showing fuzzy, poorly defined lesions and a high lesion load in the white matter, associated with thalamus or basal ganglion lesions (194). Good recovery is seen with most patients, but up to half may have some deficit, mild in most cases but potentially severe. Up to 9% may have a residual seizure disorder (106). Corticosteroids are most commonly used to treat this disorder, though intravenous immunoglobulin has been used with good results (195). Seizure treatment is symptomatic, and any of the standard drugs would be appropriate based on the clinical situation.

NEOPLASTIC DISORDERS

Seizures may occur in cancer patients from either direct invasion, secondary electrolyte abnormalities, paraneoplastic syndrome, infection, or drug effect from chemotherapy.

Primary tumors of the central nervous system are a rare cause of seizures. In one series, brain tumors accounted for 2.5% of partial epilepsies and 0.7% of generalized epilepsies (196). Although the majority of seizure-producing tumors are supratentorial, focal motor seizures, with or without secondary generalization, have been seen with cerebellar lesions, particularly gangliogliomas (197, 198). Certain tumors are considered more epileptogenic including ganglioglioma (198), hypothalamic hamartoma (199), dysembryoplastic neuroepithelial [DNET] (200), and some low-grade astrocytomas (201). A large number of seizures prior to lesionectomy and residual hyperintense region in the tumor cavity on postoperative MR imaging are associated with uncontrolled seizures (201).

The incidence of seizures complicating the treatment of systemic cancer in children has been between 4.5% and 14% (202, 203). Seizures have been seen with a variety of neoplasms, with about half as a complication of treatment and the rest by direct tumor invasion (203). Leukemia is the most common neoplasm associated with seizures, accounting for about half overall (204). In patients with leukemia, 47% had a cerebral lesion at the time of first seizure (205). Imaging abnormalities seen in leukemia include sinus and cortical vein thromboses, cerebral hemorrhage, meningeal leukemia, infection, leukemic infiltration, leukoencephalopathy, and radiation necrosis (206). Although seizures may result from metabolic derangements, medications may also be the primary risk; examples of these medications would include cyclosporine, tacrolimus, mehotrexate, busulfan, and thiopeta (204). Paraneoplastic syndromes, such as limbic encephalitis, may lead to seizures. Although these have neurologic problems less frequently in children than in adults, they may still occur and produce seizures (207).

Because of its noninducing properties, lack of protein binding, and lack of drug-drug interaction, gabapentin has been used to treat seizures in children with systemic cancers (204, 208). Many of these same advantages exist with levetiracetam, and the development of a commercial intravenous form may make this the drug of choice in these patients.

CONCLUSIONS

Many disease states may present with generalized, partial, or multifocal seizures in infancy and childhood. In certain instances, seizures are caused by an acute irritation to the nervous system (acute symptomatic seizures); in others, seizures are caused by more chronic neurologic processes (remote symptomatic). Examples of both have been described in this chapter. In either case seizure types are rarely distinctive enough to suggest a specific symptomatic etiology. When seizures are recurrent and due to a remote symptomatic etiology, the EEG features can sometimes be helpful in making a specific diagnosis, such as the "notched delta" pattern in Angelman syndrome or needle-like central spikes in Rett syndrome. More frequently, the epilepsy syndrome and other associated neurologic findings can provide the most useful clues to the presence of remote symptomatic etiology. Epilepsy syndromes that strongly suggest a symptomatic etiology include neonatal seizures, early infantile epileptogenic encephalopathy, West syndrome, and Lennox-Gastaut syndrome. Patients with these epilepsies should have a thorough, but targeted, search for underlying causes. This information can help to guide effective treatment and provides the most useful information for parental counseling.

References

1. Oppenheimer EY, Roosman NP, Dooling EC. The late appearance of hypopigmented maculae in tuberous sclerosis. *Am J Dis Child* 1985; 139:408–409.
2. Gomez MR. Tuberous sclerosis. In: Gomez MR, ed. *Neurocutaneous Diseases*. London: Butterworth, 1987:21–49.
3. Fryer AE, Chalmers AH, Connor JM, et al. Evidence that the gene for tuberous sclerosis is on chromosome 9. *Lancet* 1987; 1:659–661.
4. European Chromosome 16 Tuberous Sclerosis Consortium. Identification and characterization of tuberous sclerosis gene on chromosome 16. *Cell* 1993; 75:1305–1315.
5. Kwiatkowski DJ, Reeve MP, Cheadle JP, et al. Molecular genetics. In: Curatolo P, ed. Tuberoous sclerosis complex: *From Basic Sscience to Clinical Phenotypes*. International Child Neurology Association. London: Mac Keith Press, 2003.
6. Tee AR, Fingar DC, Manning BD, et al. Tuberous sclerosis complex-1 and -2 gene products function together to inhibit mammalian target of rapamycin (mTOR)-mediated downstream signaling. *Proc Natl Acad Sci U S A* 2002; 99(21):13571–13576.
7. Rennebeck G, Kleymenova EV, Anderson R, et al. Loss of function of the tuberous sclerosis 2 tumor suppressor gene results in embryonic lethality characterized by disrupted neuroepithelial growth and development. *Proc Natl Acad Sci U S A* 1998; 95(26):15629–15634.
8. Franz DN. Diagnosis and management of tuberous sclerosis complex. *Semin Pediatr Neurol* 1998; 5:253–268.
9. Riikonen R, Simell O. Tuberous sclerosis and infantile spasms. *Dev Med Child Neurol* 1990; 32:203–209.
10. Ohtsuka Y, Ohmori I, Oka E. Long-term follow-up of childhood epilepsy associated with tuberous sclerosis. *Epilepsia* 1998; 39:1158–1163.
11. Shields WD, Sankar R. Vigabatrin. *Semin Pediatr Neurol* 1997; 4:43–50.
12. Baumgartner JE, Wheless JW, Kulkarni S, et al. On the surgical treatment of refractory epilepsy in tuberous sclerosis complex. *Pediatr Neurosurg* 1997; 27:311–318.
13. Yanai S, Hanai T, Narazaki O. Treatment of infantile spasms with zonisamide. *Brain Dev* 1999; 21(3):157–161.
14. Elterman RD, Shields WD, Mansfield KA, et al. Randomized trial of vigabatrin in patients with infantile spasms. *Neurology* 2001; 23; 57(8):1416–1421.
15. Koh S, Jayakar P, Dunoyer C, et al. Epilepsy surgery in children with tuberous sclerosis complex: presurgical evaluation and outcome. *Epilepsia* 2000; 41(9):1206–1213.
16. Weiner HL, Carlson C, Ridgway EB, et al. Epilepsy surgery in young children with tuberous sclerosis: results of a novel approach. *Pediatrics* 2006; 117(5):1494–1502.
17. Listernick R, Charrow J. Neurofibromatosis type 1 in childhood. *J Pediatr* 1990; 116:845–853.
18. Wertelecki W, Rouleau GA, Superneau DW, et al. Neurofibromatosis 2: clinical and DNA linkage studies of a large kindred. *N Engl J Med* 1988; 319:278–283.
19. Riccardi V. Neurofibromatosis. In: Gomez MR, ed. *Neurocutaneous Diseases*. London: Butterworth, 1987:11–29.
20. Kulkantrakorn K, Geller TJ. Seizures in neurofibromatosis 1. *Pediatr Neurol* 1998; 19:347–350.
21. Boughammoura-Bouatay A, Hizem Y, Chebel S, et al. Type 1 neurofibromatosis and epilepsy. *Tunis Med* 2005; 83(4):243–245.
22. Friedman D, Rothner AD, Estes M, et al. Characterization of seizures in a hospitalized population of persons with neurofibromatosis. *Epilepsia* 1989; 30:670–671.
23. van Emelen C, Goethals M, Dralands L,et al. Treatment of glaucoma in children with Sturge-Weber syndrome. *J Pediatr Ophthalmol Strabismus* 2000; 37(1):2934.
24. Sujansky E; Conradi S. Sturge-Weber syndrome: age of onset of seizures and glaucoma and the prognosis for affected children. *J Child Neurol* 1995; 10(1):49–58.
25. Bebin EM; Gomez MR. Prognosis in Sturge-Weber disease: comparison of unihemispheric and bihemispheric involvement. *J Child Neurol* 1988; 3(3):181–184.
26. Maria BL, Neufeld JA, Rosainz LC, et al. High prevalence of bihemispheric structural and functional defects in Sturge-Weber syndrome. *J Child Neurol* 1998; 13:595–605.
27. Kossoff EH, Buck C, Freeman JM. Outcomes of 32 hemispherectomies for Sturge-Weber syndrome worldwide. *Neurology* 2002; 59(11):1735–1738.
28. Arzimanoglou AA, Andermann F, Aicardi J, et al. Sturge-Weber syndrome: indications and results of surgery in 20 patients. *Neurology* 2000; 55(10):1472–1479.
29. Tuxhorn IE, Pannek HW. Epilepsy surgery in bilateral Sturge-Weber syndrome. *Pediatr Neurol* 2002; 26(5):394–397.
30. Rosenberg S, Artia FN, Campos C, Alonso F. Hypomelanosis of Ito. Case report with involvement of the central nervous system and review of the literature. *Neuropediatrics* 1984; 15:52–55.
31. Hara M, Saito K, Yajima K, Fukuyama Y. Clinico-pathological study on hypomelanosis of Ito: a neurocutaneous syndrome. *Brain Dev* 1987; 9:141.
32. Glover MT, Brett EM, Atherton DJ. Hypomelanosis of Ito: spectrum of the disease. *J Pediatr* 1989; 115:75–80.
33. Pascual-Castroviejo I, Lopez Rodriguez L, de la Cruz Medina M, Salamanca Maesso C, et al. Hypomelanosis of Ito. Neurological complications in 34 cases. *Can J Neurol Sci* 1988; 15:124-129.
34. Placantonakis DG, Ney G, Edgar M, et al. Neurosurgical management of medically intractable epilepsy associated with hypomelanosis of Ito. *Epilesia* 2005; 46(2):329–331.
35. Cohen BA. Incontinentia pigmenti. *Neurol Clin* 1987; 5:361–377.
36. Rossman P. Incontinentia pigmenti. In: Gomez MR, ed. *Neurocutaneous Diseases*. London: Butterworth, 1987:293–300.
37. Happle R. Epidermal nevus syndromes. *Semin Dermatol* 1995:14:111–121.
38. van de Warrenburg BP, van Gulik S, Renier WO, et al. The linear naevus sebaceus syndrome. *Clin Neurol Neurosurg* 1998; 100:126–132.
39. Hager BC, Dyme IZ, Guertin SR, et al. Linear nevus sebaceous syndrome: Megalencephaly and heterotopic gray matter. *Pediatric Neurol* 1991; 7:45–49.
40. Verma NP, Hart ZH, Kooi KA. Electrographic findings in urea-cycle disorders. *Electroencephalogr Clin Neurophysiol* 1984; 57:105–112.
41. Burton BK. Inborn errors of metabolism: a guide to diagnosis. *Pediatrics* 1998; 102:E69.
42. Oechsner M, Steen C, Sturenburg HJ, Kohlschutter A. Hyperammonaemic encephalopathy after initiation of valproate therapy in unrecognized ornithine transcarbamylase deficiency. *J Neurol Neurosurg Psychiatry* 1998; 64:680–682.
43. Engel RC, Buist NRM. The EEGs of infants with citrullinemia. *Dev Med Child Neurol* 1985; 27:199–206.
44. Origuchi Y, Ushijima T, Sakaguchi M, et al. Citrullinemia presenting as uncontrollable epilepsy. *Brain Dev* 1984; 6:328–331.
45. O'Connell P, Leppert M, Hoff M, et al. A linkage map for human chromosome 12. *Am J Hum Genet* 1985; 37:A169 (abstract).
46. Korinthenberg R, Ullrich K, Fullenkemper F. Evoked potentials and electroencephalography in adolescents with phenylketonuria. *Neuropediatrics* 1988; 19:175–178.
47. Pietz J, Benninger CH, Schmidt H, et al. Long-term development of intelligence (IQ) and EEG in 34 children with phenylketonuria treated early. *Eur J Pediatr* 1988; 147:361–367.
48. Menkes JH. Kinky hair disease: twenty-five years later. *Brain Dev* 1988; 10:77–79.
49. Palmer CA, Percy AK. Neuropathology of occipital horn syndrome. *J Child Neurol* 2001; 16(10):764766.
50. Kim BE, Smith K, Petris MJ. A copper treatable Menkes disease mutation associated with defective trafficking of a functional Menkes copper ATPase. *J Med Genet* 2003; 40(4):290–295.
51. Hoover-Fong JE, Shah S, van Hove JL, et al. Natural history of nonketotic hyperglycinemia in 65 patients. *Neurology* 2004; 63:1847–1853.
52. Dalla Bernardina B, Aicardi J, Goutieres F, et al. Glycine encephalopathy. *Neuropädiatrie* 1979; 10:209–225.
53. Jaeken J, Corbeel L, Casaer P, et al. Dipropylacetate (valproate) and glycine metabolism. *Lancet* 1977; 2:617.
54. Lyon G, Adams RD, Kolodny EH. Neurology of hereditary metabolic diseases of children. New York: McGraw-Hill, 1996.
55. Hunt AD Jr, Stokes J Jr, McCrory WW, Stroud HH. Pyridoxine dependency: report of a case of intractable convulsions in an infant controlled by pyridoxine. *Pediatrics* 1954; 13:140–145.
56. Bankier A, Turner M, Hopkins IJ. Pyridoxine dependent seizures—a wider clinical spectrum. *Arch Dis Child* 1983; 58:415–418.
57. Coker S. Postneonatal vitamin B_6-dependent epilepsy. *Pediatrics* 1992; 90:221–223.
58. Bass NE, Wyllie E, Cohen B, Joseph SA. Pyridoxine-dependent epilepsy: the need for repeated pyridoxine trials and the risk of severe electrocerebral suppression with intravenous pyridoxine infusion. *J Child Neurol* 1996; 11:422–424.
59. Cormier-Daire V, Dagoneau N, Nabbout R,et al. A gene for pyridoxine-dependent epilepsy maps to chromosome 5q31. *Am J Hum Genet* 2000; 67(4):991–993.

60. Zadra M, Grandi R, Erli LC, Mirabile D, et al. Treatment of seizures in acute intermittent porphyria: safety and efficacy of gabapentin. *Seizure* 1998; 7:415–416.
61. Salbert BA, Pellock JM, Wolf B. Characterization of seizures associated with biotinidase deficiency. *Neurology* 1993; 43:1351–1355.
62. Wolf B, Heard GS, Weissbecker KA, et al. Biotinidase deficiency: initial clinical features and rapid diagnosis. *Ann Neurol* 1985; 18:614–617.
63. Bale JF, Blackman JA, Sato Y. Outcome in children with symptomatic congenital cytomegalovirus infection. *J Child Neurol* 1990; 5:131–136.
64. Mizrahi EM, Thorp BR. A characteristic EEG pattern in neonatal herpes simplex encephalitis. *Neurology* 1982; 32:1215–1220.
65. Wright R, Johnson D, Neumann M, et al. Congenital lymphocytic choriomeningitis virus syndrome: a disease that mimics congenital toxoplasmosis or cytomegalovirus infection. *Pediatrics* 1997; 100:E9.
66. Brouwers P, Belman AL, Epstein LG. Central nervous system involvement: manifestations, evaluation, and pathogenesis. In: Pizzo PA and Wilfert CM, eds. *Pediatric AIDS*. Baltimore: Williams & Wilkins, 1994:433–455.
67. Belman AL. Acquired immune deficiency in the child's central nervous system. *Pediatr Clin North Am* 1992; 39:691–714.
68. Mintz M, Epstein LG, Koenigsberger MR. Neurologic manifestations of acquired immunodeficiency syndrome (AIDS) in children. *International Pediatrics* 1989; 4:161–171.
69. Narayan P, Samuels OB, Barrow DL. Stroke and pediatric human immunodeficiency virus infection. Case report and review of the literature. *Pediatr Neurosurg* 2002; 37(3):158–163.
70. Visudtibhan A, Visudhiphan P, Chiemchanya S. Stroke and seizures as the presenting signs of pediatric HIV infection. *Pediatr Neurol* 1999; 21(2):53–56.
71. Garg RK. HIV infection and seizures. *Postgrad Med J* 1999; 75:387–390.
72. Wong MC, Suite AND, Labar DR. Seizures in human immunodeficiency virus infection. *Arch Neurol* 1990; 47:640–642.
73. Rish WAS, Haddard FS. The variable natural history of subacute sclerosing panencephalitis: a study of 118 cases from the Middle East. *Arch Neurol* 1979; 36:610–614.
74. Markland CN, Panszi JG. The elective encephalogram in subacute sclerosing panencephalitis. *Arch Neurol* 1975; 32:719–726.
75. Bellini WJ, Rota JS, Lowe LE, et al. Subacute sclerosing panencephalitis: more cases of this fatal disease are prevented by measles immunization than was previously recognized. *J Infect Dis* 2005; 192(10):1686–1693.
76. Labar DR, Harden C. Infection and inflammatory diseases. In:Engel J Jr, Pedley T, eds. *Epilepsy: a Comprehensive Textbook*. Philadelphia: Lippencott-Raven, 1997:2587–2596.
77. Kluczewska E, Jamroz E, Marsza E. Neuroimaging and clinical manifestations of herpes simplex encephalitis in children. *Neurologia i Neurochirurgia Polska* 2003; 37(suppl 2):45–52.
78. Shandera WX, White AC, Chen JC, et al. Neurocysticercosis in Houston, Texas. A report of 112 cases. *Medicine* 1994; 73:37–52.
79. Fourestie V, Douceeron H, Brugieres P, Ancelle T, et al. Neurotrichinosis: a cerebrovascular disease associated with myocardial injury and hypereosinophilia. *Brain* 1993; 116:603–616.
80. Khan WA, Dhar U, Salam MA, et al. Central nervous system manifestations of childhood shigellosis: prevalence, risk factors, and outcome. *Pediatrics* 1999; 103(2):E18.
81. Musumeci SA, Colognola RM, Ferri R, et al. Fragile X syndrome: a particular epileptogenic EEG pattern. *Epilepsia* 1988; 29:41–47.
82. Kluger G, Bohm I, Laub MC, Waldenmaier C. Epilepsy and fragile X mutations. *Pediatr Neurol* 1996; 15:358–360.
83. Stafstrom CE, Patxot OF, Gilmore HE, Wisniewski KE. Seizures in children with Down syndrome: etiology, characteristics and outcome. *Dev Med Child Neurol* 1991; 33:191–220.
84. Chevrie J, Aicardi J. The Aicardi syndrome. In: Pedley T, Meldram J, eds. *Recent Advances in Epilepsy*. 3rd ed. Edinburgh: Churchill-Livingstone, 1986:189–210.
85. Kuriyama M, Shigematsu Y, Konishi K, et al. Septooptic dysplasia with infantile spasms. *Pediatr Neurol* 1988; 4:62–66.
86. Dobyns WB, Truwit CL. Lissencephaly and other malformations of cortical development: 1995 update. *Neuropediatrics* 1995; 26:132–147.
87. Paladin F, Chiron C, Dulac O, et al. Electroencephalographic aspects of hemimegalenocephaly. *Dev Med Child Neurol* 1989; 31:377–383.
88. Gastaut H, Pinsard N, Raybaud C, et al. Lissencephaly (agyria-pachygyria) clinical findings and serial EEG studies. *Dev Med Child Neurol* 1987; 29:167–180.
89. Robb SA, Pohl KR, Baraitser M, Wilson J, et al. The happy "puppet" syndrome of Angelman: review of the clinical features. *Arch Dis Child* 1989; 64:83–86.
90. Laan LA, Renier WO, Arts WF, et al. Evolution of epilepsy and EEG findings in Angelman syndrome. *Epilepsia* 1997; 38:195–199.
91. Geurrini R, DeLorey TM, Bonanni P, et al. Cortical myoclonus in Angelman syndrome. *Ann Neurol* 1996; 40:39–48.
92. Matsumoto A, Kumagai T, Miura K, et al. Epilepsy in Angelman syndrome associated with chromosome 15q deletion. *Epilepsia* 1992; 33:1083–1090.
93. Viani F, Romeo A, Viri M, et al. Seizure and EEG patterns in Angelman's syndrome. *J Child Neurol* 1995; 10:467–471.
94. Ohtsuka Y, Kobayashi K, Yoshinaga H, et al. Relationship between severity of epilepsy and developmental outcome in Angelman syndrome. *Brain Dev* 2005; 27(2):95-100.
95. Rubin DI, Patterson MC, Westmoreland BF, Klass DW. Angelman's syndrome: clinical and electrographic findings. *Electroencephalogr Clin Neurophysiol* 1997; 102:299–302.
96. Valente KD, Andrade JQ, Grossmann RM, et al. Angelman syndrome: difficulties in EEG pattern recognition and possible misinterpretations. *Epilepsia* 2003; 44:1051–1063.
97. Minassian BA, DeLorey TM, Olsen RW, et al. Angelman syndrome: correlations between epilepsy phenotypes and genotypes. *Ann Neurol* 1998; 43:485–493.
98. Williams MS, Rooney BL, Williams J, Josephson K, et al. Investigation of thermoregulatory characteristics in patients with Prader-Willi syndrome. *Am J Med Genet* 1994; 49:302–307.
99. Hall BD, Smith DW. Prader-Willi syndrome. *J Pediatr* 1972; 81:286–293.
100. Wang PJ, Hou JW, Sue WC, et al. Electroclinical characteristics of seizures—comparing Prader-Willi syndrome with Angelman syndrome. *Brain Dev 2005*; 27(2):101–107.
101. Brissenden JE, Levy EP. Prader-Willi syndrome in infant monozygotic twins. *Am J Dis Child* 1973; 126:110–112.
102. Ledbetter DH, Riccardi VM, Airhart SD, et al. Deletions of chromosome 15 as a cause of the Prader-Willi syndrome. *N Engl J Med* 1981; 304:325–329.
103. Knoll JH, Nicholls RD, Magenis RE, et al. Angelman and Prader-Willi syndromes share a common chromosome 15 deletion but differ in parental origin of the deletion. *Am J Med Genet* 1989; 32:285–290.
104. Izmeth MG, Parameshwar E. The Miller-Dieker syndrome: a case report and review of the literature. *J Ment Defic Res* 1989; 33:267–270.
105. Schnizel A. Microdeletion syndromes, balanced translocations, and gene mapping. *J Med Genet* 1988; 25:454–462.
106. Dobyns WB, Reiner O, Carrozzo R, Ledbetter DH. Lissencephaly: a human brain malformation associated with deletion of the LIS1 gene located at chromosome 17p13. *JAMA* 1993; 270:2838–2842.
107. Fogli A, Guerrini R, Moro F, et al. Intracellular levels of LIS1 protein correlate with clinical and neuroradiological findings in patients with classical lissencephaly. *Ann Neurol* 1999; 45:154–161.
108. Caksen H, Tuncer O, Kirimi E, et al. Report of two Turkish infants with Norman-Roberts syndrome. *Genet Couns* 2004; 15(1):9–17.
109. Kamida T, Maruyama T, Fujiki M, Kobayashi H, et al. Total callosotomy for a case of lissencephaly presenting with West syndrome and generalized seizures. *Childs Nerv Syst* 2005; 21:1056–1060.
110. Shoffner JM, Wallace DC. Mitochondrial genetics: principles and practice. *Am J Hum Genet* 1992; 51:1179–1186 (editorial).
111. Garcia-Silva MR, Aicardi J, Goutieres F, Chevrie JJ. The syndrome of myoclonic epilepsy with ragged-red fibres. Report of a case and review of the literature. *Neuropediatrics* 1987; 18:200–204.
112. Naidu S. Rett syndrome: a disorder affecting early brain growth. *Ann Neurol* 1997; 42:3–10.
113. Rosing HS, Hopkins LC, Wallace DC, et al. Maternally inherited mitochondrial myopathy and myoclonic epilepsy. *Ann Neurol* 1985; 17:228–237.
114. Crest C, Dupont S, Leguern E, Adam C, et al. Levetiracetam in progressive myoclonic epilepsy: an exploratory study in 9 patients. *Neurology* 2004; 62(4):640–643.
115. Fabrizi GM, Cardaioli E, Grieco GS, et al. The A to G transition at nt 3243 of the mitochondrial tRNALeu (UUR) may cause an MERRF syndrome. *J Neurol Neurosurg Psychiatry* 1996; 61(1):47–51.
116. Hirano M, Pavlakis SG. Mitochondrial myopathy, encephalopathy, lactic acidosis and stroke-like episodes (MELAS): current concepts. *J Child Neurol* 1994; 9:4–13.
117. Lam CW, Lau CH, Williams JC. Mitochondrial myopathy, encephalopathy, lactic acidosis and stroke-like episodes (MELAS) triggered by valproate therapy. *Eur J Pediatr* 1997; 156(7):562–564.
118. American Psychiatric Association. Diagnostic and statistical manual of mental disorders. 4th ed. Washington, DC: American Psychiatric Association, 1994:70–71.
119. Filipek PA, Accardo PJ, Baranek GT, et al. The screening and diagnosis of autistic spectrum disorders. *J Autism Dev Disord* 1999; 29:437–482.
120. Filipek PA, Accardo PJ, Ashwal S, et al. Practice parameter: screening and diagnosis of autism: report for the Quality Standards Subcommittee of the American Academy of Neurology and the Child Neurology Society. *Neurology* 2000; 55:468–479.
121. Fombonne E. The epidemiology of autism: a review. *Psych Med* 1999:29:769–786.
122. Spratt EG, Macias MM, Lee DO. Autistic spectrum disorders. San Diego, CA: Medlink Neurology, 2004.
123. Courchesne E, Yeung-Courchesne R, Press GA, Hesselink JR, et al. Hypoplasia of cerebellar lobules VI and VII in infantile autism. *N Engl J Med* 1988; 318:1349–1354.
124. Piven J, Saliba K, Bailey J, Arndt S. An MRI study of autism: the cerebellum revisited. *Neurology* 1997; 49(2):547–553.
125. Rapin I. Autism in search of a home in the brain. *Neurology* 1999; 52:902–904.
126. Bachevalier J, Merjanian P. The contribution of medial temporal lobe structures in infantile autism: a neurobehavioral study in primates. In: Bauman M, Kemper T, eds. *The Neurobiology of Autism*. Baltimore: Johns Hopkins University Press, 1994:119–145.
127. DeLong GR. Autism: new data suggest a new hypothesis. *Neurology* 1999; 52:911–916.
128. Bailey A, LeCouteur A, Gottesman I, et al. Autism as a strongly genetic disorder: evidence from a British twin study. *Psychol Med* 1995; 25:63–77.
129. Yaylali I, Tuchmann R, Jaykar P. Comparison of the utility of routine versus prolonged EEG recordings in children with language regression [abstract]. Presented at the American Clinical Neurophysiology Society Annual Meeting, Boston, MA, September, 1996.
130. Gubbay SS, Lobascher M, Kingerlee P. A neurologic appraisal of autistic children: results of a western Australian survey. *Dev Med Child Neurol* 1970; 12:422–429.
131. Gabis L, Pomeroy J, Andriola MR. Autism and epilepsy: cause, consequence, comorbidity, or coincidence? *Epilepsy Behav* 2005; 7(4):652–656.
132. Trevethan E. Seizures and epilepsy among children with language regression and autistic spectrum disorders. *J Child Neurol* 2004; 19(Suppl 1):S49–S57.
133. Tuchman R. AEDs and psychotropic drugs in children with autism and epilepsy. *Ment Retard Dev Disabil Res Rev* 2004; 10(2):135–138.
134. DiMartino A, Tuchman RF. Antiepileptic drugs: affective use in autism spectrum disorders. *Pediatr Neurol* 2001; 25(3):199–207.
135. Landau WM, Kleffner FR. Syndrome of acquired aphasia with convulsive disorder in children. *Neurology* 1957; 7:523–530.
136. Msall M, Shapiro B, Balfour PB, et al. Acquired epileptic aphasia. *Clin Pediatr* 1986; 25:248.

137. Beaumanoir A. The Landau-Kleffner syndrome. In: Roger J, Dravet C, Bureau M, Dreifuss FE, et al, eds. *Epileptic Syndromes in Infancy, Childhood and Adolescence*. London: John Libbey Eurotext, 1985:181–191.
138. Paetau R, Kajola M, Korkman M, et al. Landau-Kleffner syndrome: epileptic activity in the auditory cortex. *Neuroreport* 1991; 2(4): 201–204.
139. Da Silva EA, Chugani DC, Muzik O, Chugani HT. Landau-Kleffner syndrome: metabolic abnormalities in temporal lobe are a common feature. *J Child Neurol* 1997; 12:489–495.
140. Nakano S, Okuno T, Mikawa H. Landau-Kleffner syndrome EEG topographic study. *Brain Dev* 1989; 11:43–50.
141. Nass R, Gross A, Devinsky O. Autism and autistic epileptiform regression with occipital spikes. *Dev Med Child Neurol* 1998; 40:453–458.
142. McVicar KA, Shinnar S. Landau-Kleffner syndrome, electrical status epilepticus in slow wave sleep, and language regression in children. *Ment Retard Dev Disabil Res Rev* 2004; 10(2):144–149.
143. Olsson I, Steffenberg S, Gellberg C. Epilepsy in autism and autistic-like conditions. *Arch Neurol* 1988; 45:666–668.
144. Marescaux C, Hirsch E, Finck S, et al. Landau-Kleffner syndrome: a pharmacologic study of five cases. *Epilepsia* 1990; 31:768–777.
145. Tsuru T, Mori M, Mizuguchi M. Effects of high-dose intravenous corticosteroid therapy in Landau-Kleffner syndrome. *Pediatr Neurol* 2000; 22(2):145–147.
146. Sinclair DB, Snyder TJ. Corticosteroids for the treatment of Landau-Kleffner syndrome and continuous spike-wave discharge during sleep. *Pediatr Neurol* 2005; 32(5):300–306.
147. Morrell F, Whisler WW, Smith MC, et al. Landau-Kleffner syndrome: treatment with subpial intracortical transection. *Brain* 1995; 118:1529–1546.
148. Irwin K, Birch V, Lees J, et al. Multiple subpial transection in Landau-Kleffner syndrome. *Dev Med Child Neurol* 2001; 43(4):248–252.
149. Park YD. The effects of vagus nerve stimulation therapy on patients with intractable seizures and either Landau-Kleffner syndrome or autism. *Epilepsy Behav* 2003; 4(3):286–290.
150. Amir RE,Van den Veyver IB, Wan M, et al. Rett syndrome is caused by mutations in X-linked MECP2, enclosing methyl-CpG-binding protein 2. *Nat Genet* 1999; 23:185–188.
151. Van den Veyver IB, Zoghbi HY. Methyl-CpG-binding protein 2 mutations in Rett syndrome. *Curr Opin Genet Dev* 2000; 10:275–279.
152. Xiang F, Buervenich S, Nicolao P, et al. Mutation screening in Rett syndrome patients. *J Med Genet* 2000; 37(4):250–255.
153. Hoffbuhr K, Devaney JM, LaFleur B, et al. MeCP2 mutations in children with and without the phenotype of Rett syndrome. *Neurology* 2001; 56(11):1486–1495.
154. Zoghbi HY, Milstien S, Beebler IJ, et al.Cerebrospinal fluid biogenic amines and biopterin in Rett syndrome. *Ann Neurol* 1989; 25:56–60.
155. Horike S, Cai S, Miyano M, et al. Loss of silent-chromatin looping and impaired imprinting of DLX5 in Rett syndrome. *Nat Genet* 2005; 37(1):31–40.
156. Stuhmer T, Anderson SA, Ekker M, et al. Ectopic expression of the DLX genes induces glutamic acid decarboxylase and DLX expression. *Development* 2002; 129(1):245–252.
157. The Rett Syndrome Diagnostic Work Group. Diagnostic criteria for Rett syndrome. *Ann Neurol* 1988; 23:425–428.
158. Hagberg BA. Rett syndrome: clinical peculiarities, diagnostic approach, and possible causes. *Pediatr Neurol* 1989; 5:75–83.
159. Trevalhan E, Naidu S. The clinical recognition and differential diagnosis of Rett syndrome. *J Child Neurol* 1988; 3(Suppl):S6–S16.
160. Naidu S, Murphy M, Moser HW, et al. Rett syndrome—natural history in 70 cases. *Am J Med Genet* 1986; 24(Suppl):61–72.
161. Steffenburg U, Hagberg G, Hagberg B. Epilepsy in a representative series of Rett syndrome. *Acta Paediatr* 2001; 90(1):34–39.
162. Coleman M, Brubaker J, Hunter K, Smith G. Rett syndrome: a survey of North American patients. *J Ment Defic Res* 1988; 32:117–124.
163. Glaze DG, Schultz RJ, Frost JD. Rett syndrome: characterization of seizures versus non-seizures. *Electroencephalogr Clin Neurophysiol* 1998; 106(1):79–83.
164. Laan LA, Brouwer OF, Begeer CH, Zwinderman AH, et al. The diagnostic value of EEG in Angelman and Rett syndrome at a young age. *Electroencephalogr Clin Neurophysiol* 1998; 106:404–408.
165. Glaze DG, Frost JD, Zoghbi H, Percy AK. Rett syndrome: correlation of electroencephalographic characteristics with clinical staging. *Arch Neurol* 1987; 44:1053–1056.
166. Garofalo EA, Drury I, Goldstein GW. EEG abnormalities aid diagnosis of Rett syndrome. *Pediatr Neurol* 1988; 4:350–353.
167. Hagne I, Witt-Engerstrom I, Hagberg B. EEG development in Rett syndrome—a study of 30 cases. *Electroencephalogr Clin Neurophysiol* 1989; 72:1–6.
168. Robb SA, Harden A, Boyd SG. Rett syndrome: an EEG study in 52 girls. *Neuropediatrics* 1989; 20:192–195.
169. Aldrich MS, Garofalo EA, Drury I. Epileptiform abnormalities during sleep in Rett syndrome. *Electroencephalogr Clin Neurophysiol* 1990; 75:365–370.
170. Alpers BJ. Progressive cerebral degeneration of infancy. *J Nerv Ment Dis* 1960; 130:442–448.
171. Harding BN. Progressive neuronal degeneration of childhood with liver disease (Alpers-Huttenlocher syndrome): a personal review. *J Child Neurol* 1990; 5:273–287.
172. Laurence KM, Cavanaugh JB. Progressive degeneration of the cerebral cortex in infancy. *Brain* 1968; 91:261–280.
173. Prick MJ, Gabreels FJ, Renier WO, et al. Pyruvate dehydrogenase deficiency restricted to brain. *Neurology* 1981; 31:398–404.
174. Prick MJ, Gabreels FJ, Renier WO, et al. Progressive infantile poliodystrophy. Association with disturbed pyruvate oxidation in muscle and liver. *Arch Neurol* 1981; 38:767–772.
175. Prick MJ, Gabreels FJ, Renier WO, et al. Progressive infantile poliodystrophy (Alpers' disease) with a defect in citric acid cycle activity in liver and fibroblasts. *Neuropediatrics* 1982; 13:108–111.
176. Harding BN, Alsanjari N, Smith SJ. Progressive neuronal degeneration of childhood with liver disease (Alpers' disease) presenting in young adults. *J Neurol Neurosurg Psychiatry* 1995; 58:320–325.
177. Gabreels FJ, Prick MJ, Trijbels JM, et al. Defects in citric acid cycle and the electron transport chain in progressive poliodystrophy. *Acta Neurol Scand* 1984; 70:145–154.
178. Huttenlocher PR, Solitare GB, Adams G. Infantile diffuse cerebral degeneration with hepatic cirrhosis. *Arch Neurol* 1976; 33:186–192.
179. Burgeois M, Goutieres F, Chretien D, et al. Deficiency in complex II of the respiratory chain, presenting as a leukodystrophy in two sisters with Leigh syndrome. *Brain Dev* 1992; 14:404–408.
180. Bickenese A, Dodson WE, May W, Hickey WF. Hepatocerebral degeneration (Alpers' disease) presenting as valproate toxicity. *Ann Neurol* 1990; 28:438–439.
181. Bickenese AR, May W, Hickey WF, Dodson WE. Early childhood hepatocerebral degeneration misdiagnosed as valproate hepatotoxicity. *Ann Neurol* 1992; 32:767–775.
182. Naviaux RK, Nyhan WL, Barshop BA, et al. Mitochondrial DNA polymerase gamma deficiency and mtDNA depletion in a child with Alpers' syndrome. *Ann Neurol* 1999; 45:54–58.
183. Egger J, Harding BN, Boyd SG, Wilson J, et al. Progressive neuronal degeneration of childhood (PNDC) with liver disease. *Clin Pediatr* 1987; 26:167–173.
184. Harding BN, Egger J, Portmann B, Erdohazi M. Progressive neuronal degeneration of childhood with liver disease. A pathological study. *Brain* 1986; 109:181–206.
185. Boyd SG, Harden A, Egger J, Pampiglione G. Progressive neuronal degeneration of childhood with liver disease ("Alpers' disease"): characteristic neurophysiological features. *Neuropediatrics* 1986; 17:75–80.
186. Zimmerman R. Cockayne's syndrome. In: Gomez MR, ed. *Neurocutaneous Diseases*. London: Butterworth, 1987:128–135.
187. Ozdirim E, Topcu M, Ozon A, Cila A. Cockayne syndrome: review of 25 cases. *Pediatr Neurol* 1996; 15:312–316.
188. Carreno L, Lopez-Longo FJ, Monteagudo I, et al. Immunological and clinical differences between juvenile and adult onset of systemic lupus erythematosus. *Lupus* 1999; 8(4):287–292.
189. Appenzeller S, Cendes F, Costallat LT. Epileptic seizures in systemic lupus erythematosus. *Neurology* 2004; 63(10):1808–1812.
190. Tin SK, Xu Q, Thumboo J, et al. Novel brain reactive autoantibodies: prevalence in systemic lupus erythematosus and association with psychoses and seizures. *J Neuroimmunol* 2005; 169(1–2):153–160.
191. Hess E. Drug-related lupus. *N Engl J Med* 1988; 318:1460–1462 (editorial).
192. Murthy SNK, Faden HS, Cohen ME, et al. Acute disseminated encephalomyelitis in children. *Pediatrics* 2002; 110(2):e21.
193. Rust R. Acute disseminated encephalomyelitis. Presented at the American Academy of Neurology Annual Meeting, San Diego, CA, April 2006.
194. Stonehouse M, Gupte G, Wassmer E, Whitehouse WP. Acute disseminated encephalomyelitis: recognition in the hands of general pediatricians. *Arch Dis Child* 2003; 88:122–124.
195. Khurana DS, Melvin JJ, Kothare SV, et al. Acute disseminated encephalomyelitis in children: discordant neurologic and neuroimaging abnormalities and response to plasmapheresis. *Pediatrics* 2005; 116(2):431–436.
196. Fujiwara T, Shigematsu H. Etiologic factors and clinical features of symptomatic epilepsy: focus on pediatric cases. *Psychiatry Clin Neurosci* 2004; 58:S9–S12.
197. Harvey AS, Jayakar P, Duchowny M, Resnick T, et al. Hemifacial seizures and cerebellar ganglioma: an epilepsy syndrome of infancy with seizures of cerebellar origin. *Ann Neurol* 1996; 40(1):91–98.
198. Mesiwala AH, Kuratani JD, Avellino AM, et al. Focal motor seizures with secondary generalization arising in the cerebellum. Case report and review of the literature. *J Neurosurg* 2002; 97(1):190–196.
199. Kuzniecky R, Guthrie B, Mountz J, et al. Intrinsic epileptogenesis of hypothalamic hamartomas in gelastic epilepsy. *Ann Neurol* 1997; 42(1):60–67.
200. Raymond AA, Halpin SF, Alsanjari N, et al. Dysembryoplastic neuroepithelial tumor. Features in 16 patients. *Brain* 1994; 117:461–475.
201. Khan RB, Boop FA, Onar A, et al. Seizures in children with low-grade tumors: outcome after tumor resection and risk factors for uncontrolled seizures. *J Neurosurg* 2006; 104(Suppl 6):377–382.
202. Tasdemiroglu E, Patchell RA, Kryscio R. Neurological complications of childhood malignancies. *Acta Neurochir* 1999; 141(12):1313–1321.
203. Antunes NL, DeAngelis LM. Neurologic consultations in children with systemic cancer. *Pediatr Neurol* 1999; 20(2):121–124.
204. Antunes NL. Seizures in children with systemic cancer. *Pediatr Neurol* 2003; 28(3):190–193.
205. Maytal J, Grossman R, Yusuf FH, et al. Prognosis and treatment of seizures in children with acute lymphoblastic leukemia. *Epilepsia* 1995; 36(8):831–836.
206. Porto L, Kieslich M, Schwabe D, et al. Central nervous system imaging in childhood leukemia. *Eur J Cancer* 2004; 40(14):2082–2090.
207. Pranzatelli M. Paraneoplastic syndromes: an unsolved murder. *Semin Pediatr Neurol* 2000; 7(2):118–130.
208. Khan RB, Hunt DL, Thompson SJ. Gabapentin to control seizures in children undergoing cancer treatment. *J Child Neurol* 2004; 19(2):97–101.

IV

GENERAL PRINCIPLES OF THERAPY

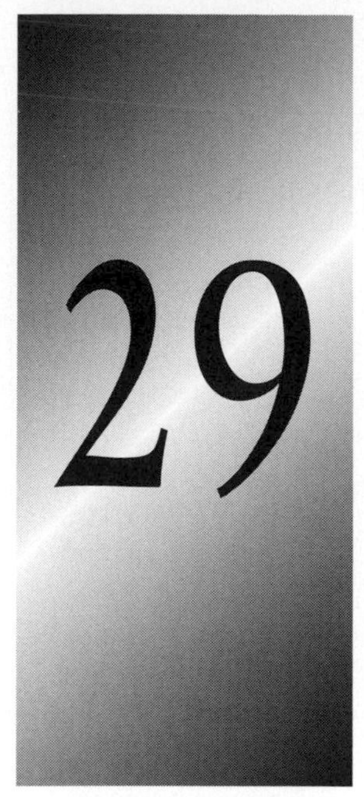

Treatment Decisions in Childhood Seizures

Shlomo Shinnar
Christine O'Dell

In the past, almost all children with a seizure of any type, febrile or afebrile, were placed on long-term therapy with antiepileptic drugs (AEDs). This was based on several assumptions: first, that almost all children with an isolated seizure would go on to have more seizures (1, 2); second, that seizures, even brief ones, could cause brain damage and lead to progressively intractable epilepsy (1–3); third, that AEDs were not only effective but also safe and that treatment was associated with only minimal morbidity; finally, that seizures "beget" seizures, and that early AED therapy not only prevented seizures but also somehow altered the natural history of the disorder and prevented the development of "chronic" epilepsy (3–6). We now know that these assumptions are not true. Research has provided information that has altered the way physicians think about seizures, their consequences, and the drugs used to treat them. The decision whether and for how long to treat a child with AEDs must be weighed against the possible risks of that treatment and must take into account the large body of data that has accumulated: namely, that many children with a single seizure do not go on to experience further seizures (7–20); that many children with epilepsy ultimately go on to become seizure free (21–24); that most seizures are brief, and that even prolonged seizures rarely cause brain damage unless they are associated with an acute neurologic insult (25–28); and that antiepileptic medications can cause untoward effects (18, 29–31).

The decision of whether to initiate treatment in a child with one or more seizures must balance the risks and benefits of treatment in each case (18). Similarly, the patient who is seizure free on medications for some time must weigh the risks of possible seizure recurrence if medications are withdrawn against the risks of continuing long-term AED therapy. This chapter reviews the data relevant to these decisions. The data on the probability of seizure recurrence following a first unprovoked seizure is presented. Next, the issue of withdrawing antiepileptic drugs in children with epilepsy who are seizure free for 2 or more years is considered. This is followed by a review of the risks of not treating (i.e., the risks of subsequent seizures) and of the morbidity of therapy. Finally, recommendations for a therapeutic approach to children with seizures are outlined.

RECURRENCE RISK FOLLOWING A FIRST UNPROVOKED SEIZURE

An understanding of the natural history of children who present with a first unprovoked seizure is necessary in order to develop a rational approach to their management. Over

TABLE 29-1
Risk Factors for Recurrence: Multivariable Analysis using Cox Proportional Hazards Model

Risk Factor	Proportionate Hazards Model	Rate Ratio 95% CI	*P* Value
Overall Group (*N* = 407)			
Abnormal EEG	2.1	1.6, 3.0	<0.001
Remote symptomatic etiology	1.7	1.2, 2.4	0.006
Prior febrile seizures	1.6	1.1, 2.3	0.019
Todd's paresis	1.7	1.0, 2.9	0.038
Seizure while asleep	1.5	1.1, 2.1	0.008
Cryptogenic cases (*N* = 342)			
Abnormal EEG	2.5	1.7, 3.6	<0.0001
Seizure while asleep	1.7	1.2, 2.5	<0.003
Remote Symptomatic Cases (*N* = 65)			
Prior febrile seizures	2.3	1.2, 4.5	<0.02
Age < 3 years	2.4	1.2, 4.9	<0.02

Reprinted with permission from Shinnar et al, 1996 (8).

the past two decades there have been many studies that have attempted to address this issue (7–20). For purposes of this discussion, a first unprovoked seizure is defined as a seizure, or flurry of seizures all occurring within 24 hours, in a patient over one month of age with no prior history of unprovoked seizures (18, 32).

The reported overall recurrence risk following a first unprovoked seizure in children varies from 27% to 71% (7–20). Studies that identified the children at the time of first seizure and carefully excluded those with prior seizures report recurrence risks of 27% to 44% (7–11, 19). Studies that recruited subjects later, either retrospectively or from electroencephalogram (EEG) laboratories, but excluded those with prior seizures, report slightly higher recurrence risks of 48% to 52% (14, 15). Lastly, studies that included children who already had recurrent seizures at the time of identification report the highest recurrence risks, 61% to 71% (12, 13). Once methodological issues and differences in the distribution of risk factors among different studies are taken into account, the results are fairly consistent (9). The majority of recurrences occur early, with approximately 50% of recurrences occurring within 6 months and over 80% within 2 years of the initial seizure (7–20). Late recurrences are unusual.

Similar predictors of recurrent seizures were found in the majority of the studies despite variations in methodology and in subject selection (7–20). Factors that are associated with a differential risk of recurrence include the etiology of the seizure, the electroencephalogram (EEG), whether the first seizure occurred in wakefulness or sleep, and seizure type. Factors not associated with a change in the recurrence risk include age of onset and the duration of the initial seizure. The report of a family history of seizures in a first-degree relative is of unclear significance, with conflicting results in the various studies. Risk factors for seizure recurrence from our large prospective study (8, 20) are shown in Table 29-1.

Selected individual risk factors are discussed in the following subsections.

Etiology

The recent International League Against Epilepsy (ILAE) guidelines for epidemiologic research (32) classify seizures as acute symptomatic, remote symptomatic, cryptogenic, or idiopathic. Acute symptomatic seizures are those associated with an acute insult such as head trauma or meningitis. Remote symptomatic seizures are those without an immediate cause but with an identifiable prior brain injury such as major head trauma (loss of consciousness greater than 30 minutes, depressed skull fracture, or intracranial hemorrhage), meningitis, encephalitis, stroke, or the presence of a static encephalopathy, such as mental retardation or cerebral palsy, which are known to be associated with an increased risk of seizures. Cryptogenic seizures are those occurring in otherwise normal individuals with no clear etiology. Note that factors such as sleep deprivation are considered trigger factors but do not change the classification of the seizure, as they would be associated with seizures only in susceptible individuals. Until recently cryptogenic seizures were also called idiopathic. In the new classification, the term *idiopathic* is reserved for seizures occurring in the context of the presumed genetic epilepsies, such as benign rolandic and childhood absence epilepsy (32–34), but many papers still refer to cryptogenic seizures as idiopathic.

Children with a remote symptomatic first seizure have higher risk of recurrence. In one large prospective study with mean follow-up of over 10 years years, 44 (68%) of 65 children with a remote symptomatic first seizure recurred, compared with 127 (37%) of 347 children with a cryptogenic/idiopathic first seizure ($P < 0.001$) (8, 19). Comparable findings are reported in other studies (9–11, 14, 15).

Electroencephalogram

The EEG is an important predictor of recurrence, particularly in cryptogenic cases (8–11, 14, 17). Epileptiform abnormalities are more important than nonepileptiform ones, but any EEG abnormality increases the recurrence risk in cryptogenic cases (8). In our study, the risk of seizure recurrence by 5 years for children with a cryptogenic first seizure was 27% for those with a normal EEG, 44% for those with nonepileptiform abnormalities, and 62% for those with epileptiform abnormalities (7, 8). In our data (8, 35), any clearly abnormal EEG patterns, including generalized spike-and-wave, focal spikes, and focal or generalized slowing, increased the risk of recurrence, while Camfield et al (14) report that only epileptiform abnormalities substantially increase the risk of recurrence. Hauser et al (10) state that only generalized spike-and-wave patterns are predictive of recurrence, but they studied mostly adolescents and adults and thus would have not included many children with centrotemporal spikes (benign rolandic epilepsy), which is the most common focal spike pattern found in studies focusing on children with a first seizure (8, 31, 14). In children with a cryptogenic first seizure, the EEG appears to be the most important predictor of recurrence (8, 9). Based on these data, a recent practice parameter of the American Academy of Neurology recommended that an EEG be considered a standard as part of the diagnostic evaluation of the child with a first unprovoked seizure (17).

Sleep State at Time of First Seizure

Whether the initial seizure occurs while the child is awake or asleep is associated with a differential recurrence risk, particularly in cryptogenic cases (8). In our series the 5-year recurrence risk was 53% for children whose initial seizure occurred during sleep, compared with 36% for those whose initial seizure occurred while awake ($P < 0.001$) (8). On multivariable analysis, etiology, the EEG and sleep state were the only significant predictors of outcome. The group of children with a cryptogenic first seizure occurring while awake and a normal EEG had a 5-year recurrence risk of only 21%. If seizures did recur, then they usually recurred in the same sleep state as the initial seizure.

Seizure Classification

Some though not all studies indicate that the risk of recurrence following a partial seizure is higher than that following a generalized seizure (9). However, partial seizures are more common in children with a remote symptomatic first seizure and in children with a cryptogenic first seizure who have an abnormal EEG (7). Once the effects of etiology and the EEG are controlled for, partial seizures are not associated with an increased risk of recurrence (7, 8, 10). In the meta-analysis no clear association between seizure type and recurrence risk could be found (9).

Family History

At the present time, there is insufficient data to determine whether a positive family history of epilepsy is a risk factor for recurrence. Although one study, primarily of adults, found a substantially increased risk of recurrence in those with a positive family history of epilepsy (10), others have failed to find a major effect (8, 14). In our study, family history was important only in children with a cryptogenic first seizure who also had an abnormal EEG. This type of patient constitutes a very small fraction of the population (7). These mixed results suggest that the additional risk of a positive family history, if present, will turn out to be small or else limited to specific subgroups.

Duration of First Seizure/Status Epilepticus

The duration of the first seizure does not affect the risk of recurrence (8–10). This is true whether one analyzes it as a continuous variable or separates the children into those who had status epilepticus and those who had a briefer seizure (8). Most cases of status occur as the initial seizure. In our series of 407 children, 48 (12%) had status epilepticus as their seizure, but only 7 (4%) of 171 children with recurrent seizures recurred with status. Although the occurrence of status epilepticus as the first seizure did not alter recurrence risks, a recurrence was more likely to be prolonged. Five (21%) of 24 children with recurrent seizures whose initial seizure was status had an episode of status as their second seizure, compared with 2 (1%) of 147 children with recurrent seizures whose first seizure was brief ($P < 0.001$). None of these experienced any sequela (8). Remission rates were not different in those who presented with an episode of status epilepticus (36).

Age at First Seizure

The majority of studies, in both children and adults, have not found age at first seizure to alter the risk of recurrence

(7–11, 14–16). This was true whether age was analyzed as a continuous variable or broken up into several age ranges. The only exception to this is the National Collaborative Perinatal Project, which found an increased risk of recurrence in children under age 2 with focal motor seizures (13). At the present time, the preponderance of available data is that the age at time of first seizure does not affect the risk of recurrence following a first unprovoked seizure.

Treatment Following a First Seizure

In observational studies such as those just discussed, whether children were treated or not after their first seizure did not alter the recurrence risk (8, 10). However, these were not randomized treatment trials. The physicians presumably treated those children they thought to have a high risk of recurrence. Following an initial seizure, patients are often started on a small dose of medication, and compliance may be lax. Randomized clinical trials comparing AED therapy with placebo following a first unprovoked seizure in children and adults have found that AED therapy can reduce the risk of a second seizure by half (16, 37). However, with longer follow-up, there was no difference between the two groups in terms of the probability of achieving remission (6, 38). Based on a review of the evidence, the American Academy of Neurology practice parameter on the treatment of the child with a first unprovoked seizure concluded that treatment does not prevent the development of chronic epilepsy or alter long-term outcome and should be reserved for those cases where the risks of a second seizure outweigh the morbidity of AED therapy (18).

Conclusions

Knowing these predictors and the recurrence risks, the child with a first unprovoked seizure presents an interesting dilemma. The likelihood that it will be an isolated event that will not repeat itself must be weighed against whether it is the first of many attacks. A thorough evaluation of the patient, including a detailed history and appropriate laboratory studies such as an electroencephalogram (EEG), is indicated regardless of whether AED therapy is started or not (17). Factors such as the seizure type, family history of seizures, and the possible etiology of the seizure must be ascertained. Of particular importance is a careful history of prior events that may be seizures. Many children who first come to medical attention as a result of a convulsive episode are found to have had prior nonconvulsive episodes of absence or complex partial seizures that were not recognized as such by the family (8, 17). These children clearly fall into the category of newly diagnosed epilepsy and not first seizure.

The majority of children with a first unprovoked seizure do not have additional unprovoked seizures. Children with a cryptogenic first seizure and a normal EEG have a particularly favorable prognosis. There are small subgroups of children with multiple risk factors who do have a high risk of recurrence. However, although AED therapy will reduce the likelihood of further seizures, there is no evidence that it alters the long-term prognosis (18). In particular, the data from randomized clinical trials and large epidemiologic studies indicate that delaying therapy will neither alter the response rate to AEDs nor adversely affect the probability of attaining remission (3, 5, 6, 18, 23, 38). Finally, recent data suggest that children who present with a first unprovoked seizure are very unlikely to develop medically refractory epilepsy even if seizures do recur (19, 20). The decision to treat or not after a first seizure must be based on the relative risks and benefits of therapy compared with the risks of further seizures. This risk benefit assessment is discussed at the end of this chapter. The authors rarely treat children with a first unprovoked seizure.

WITHDRAWING AEDS IN CHILDREN WITH EPILEPSY WHO HAVE BEEN SEIZURE FREE FOR 2 OR MORE YEARS

The available data indicate that children who are seizure free on medication for 2 or more years have a very high likelihood of remaining in remission on medication (39). In selected populations, withdrawal may be feasible after an even shorter seizure-free interval (39–42). How long should a child be maintained on medication before the attempt is made to withdraw it? This decision will be influenced by a variety of factors, including the probability of remaining seizure free after withdrawal in a given patient, the potential risk of injury from a seizure recurrence, and the potential adverse effects of continued AED therapy.

The majority of children who are seizure free on medications for at least 2 years will remain seizure free when medications are withdrawn. A large number of well-designed studies involving over 700 children have been done over the past 20 years (39, 43–54). The overall results have been very similar. Between 60% and 75% of children with epilepsy who have been seizure free for more than 2 (39, 43, 44, 49–53) or 4 (44–48) years on medications remain seizure free when antiepileptic medication is withdrawn. Furthermore, the majority of recurrences occur shortly after medication withdrawal, with almost half the relapses occurring within 6 months of medication withdrawal and 60% to 80% within 1 year (39, 53, 54). These studies are supported by a follow-up of patients for 15 to 23 years after medication withdrawal (47, 55). Although late recurrences do occur, they are rare

(47, 53, 55). In a recent randomized study, the increased risk of relapse following AED withdrawal occurred only in the first 2 years after AED withdrawal. The rate of late recurrences was the same in those who remained on AED therapy and those whose AEDs were discontinued (48).

The important question is, Can one identify risk factors such as etiology, age of onset, type of seizure, EEG features, or the specific epilepsy syndrome, that will enable one to identify subgroups of children with an even better prognosis and subgroups with a much less favorable prognosis for maintaining seizure remission off medication? There is much less consensus in this area. A discussion of the potential risk factors that have been looked at and their possible significance is presented next.

Etiology and Neurologic Status

In general, children with epilepsy associated with a prior neurologic insult have a smaller chance of becoming seizure free in the first place than do children with cryptogenic epilepsy (21, 22, 24). In children with remote symptomatic epilepsy who are seizure free on medication, most studies indicate a higher risk of recurrence following discontinuation of medication than in children with cryptogenic epilepsy (44–47, 49, 50, 53). In a recent meta-analysis of this literature, the relative risk of relapse in those with remote symptomatic seizures was 1.55 (95% CI 1.21–1.98) (54). However, almost half of these children will remain seizure free after withdrawal of medication (45, 53, 54). Furthermore, even within this group one can identify subgroups with favorable and unfavorable risk factors (53).

Age of Onset and Age at Withdrawal

Age of onset above 12 years is associated with a higher risk of relapse following discontinuation of medications (39, 42, 45, 49–51, 53, 54). In our data this was the single most important risk factor for recurrence (relative risk 4.24, 95% CI 2.54–7.08). A meta-analysis (54) also found adolescent-onset seizures to be associated with a higher risk of recurrence than childhood-onset (relative risk 1.79, 95% CI 1.46–2.19). There is some controversy as to whether a very young age of onset (under 2 years) may be a poor prognostic factor (45). In our data, a young age of onset was associated with a less favorable prognosis only in those with remote symptomatic seizures and was associated with more severe neurologic abnormalities (53). As most childhood epilepsy is readily controlled with AED therapy, the age at withdrawal of AEDs will be highly correlated with age of onset. However, the age at AED withdrawal does not appear to be important once age of onset is taken into account. In particular, there is no evidence that discontinuation of AEDs during the pubertal period is associated with a higher risk of recurrence (39, 43, 44, 53).

Duration of Epilepsy and Number of Seizures

These two variables are closely interrelated. A long duration of epilepsy may increase the risk of recurrence, though the magnitude of the effect is small (39, 42, 46, 47). One study also reported that having more than 30 generalized tonic-clonic seizures was associated with a high risk of recurrence after discontinuation of therapy (45). In a community-based practice, most children will be easily controlled within a short time after therapy is initiated, so these factors will rarely be important.

Seizure Type

Studies on the effect of seizure type on the risk of recurrence after medication withdrawal in children have produced inconsistent results. Children with multiple seizure types have a poorer prognosis (46, 47). The data regarding partial seizures are conflicting (39, 43–54). At this time it is not clear that any specific seizure type is associated with an increased risk of recurrence following discontinuation of medication.

EEG

In several studies (39, 40, 43–45, 53, 54), the EEG prior to discontinuation of medication was one of the most important predictors of relapse in children with cryptogenic epilepsy. However, the specific EEG abnormalities of significance varied across studies. Two other studies found no correlation between the EEG and outcome (46, 50). A meta-analysis found that an abnormal EEG prior to AED withdrawal was associated with a relative risk of relapse of 1.45 (95% CI 1.18–1.79) (54). The preponderance of evidence indicates that an abnormal EEG is associated with an increased recurrence risk in children with cryptogenic/idiopathic epilepsy.

The EEG obtained at the time of initial diagnostic evaluation may also have predictive value. Certain characteristic EEG patterns associated with specific epileptic syndromes, such as benign rolandic epilepsy or juvenile myoclonic epilepsy, provide additional prognostic information (24, 33, 34, 53). Changes in the EEG over time may also have prognostic value (40, 43).

Epilepsy Syndrome

Epilepsy syndromes are known to be associated with a differential prognosis for remission (24, 33, 34). Regrettably, there is little information on the effect of the specific epilepsy syndrome on the risk of relapse following AED withdrawal. The majority of studies of AED withdrawal

TABLE 29-2
Epileptic Syndromes in Cohort of Children Being Withdrawn from Antiepileptic Drug Therapy After a Seizure-Free Interval: Cryptogenic and Idiopathic Cases

EPILEPTIC SYNDROME		N	RECURRED (%)	P VALUE
Idiopathic epilepsy syndromes		79	22 (28%)	
Primary generalized epilepsy		61	21 (34%)	
	Childhood absence	26	5 (19%)	
	Juvenile absence	9	3 (33%)	
	Juvenile myoclonic epilepsy	4	4 (100%)	0.006
	Other primary generalized	22	9 (41%)	
Idiopathic partial epilepsy		18	1 (4%)	
	Benign rolandic epilepsy	14	0 (0%)	<0.001
	Benign occipital epilepsy	4	1 (25%)	
Cryptogenic epilepsy syndromes		86	26 (30%)	
	Cryptogenic partial epilepsy	50	16 (32%)	
	Temporal lobe epilepsy	7	3 (43%)	
	Other partial epilepsy	43	13 (30%)	
	Unclassified cryptogenic epilepsy	36	10 (28%)	
Total cryptogenic/idiopathic cases		165	48 (29%)	

Adapted from Shinnar et al, 1994 (53).

have not provided information by epilepsy syndrome. The results from our data (53) are shown in Table 29-2. Overall, patients with both idiopathic and cryptogenic epilepsy syndromes have similar prognosis. However, specific syndromes are associated with a differential risk of relapse. Patients with benign rolandic epilepsy have a particularly favorable prognosis, even if their EEGs are still abnormal, whereas all 4 of our patients with juvenile myoclonic epilepsy relapsed. Clearly, future studies will need to focus more on the role of the specific epilepsy syndrome in guiding therapy both in terms of initiating and discontinuing therapy and in the selection of appropriate treatment.

Type of Medication

The majority of studies have not found that the specific AED used affects recurrence rates. One well designed randomized study in adults (52) suggests that the risk of recurrence may be higher in those treated with valproate than in those treated with other medications. The significance of this finding remains unclear. It may be related to the ability of valproate to normalize generalized spike-wave abnormalities, thus making the subject appear to be at lower risk than is actually the case. At the present time, there is insufficient evidence to justify basing the decision to continue or withdraw AEDs on the type of AED the patient is taking.

The serum drug level does not seem to have a great impact on recurrence risk. Children who have not had seizures for several years often have "subtherapeutic" levels, and few have toxic levels. Available studies show little or no correlation between drug level prior to discontinuation and seizure recurrence and outcome (43), or a very modest effect (45).

Duration of Seizure-Free Interval

The chances of remaining seizure free after medication withdrawal is similar whether a 2-year (39, 43, 44, 49–53) or 4-year (39, 44–48) seizure-free interval is used. One study that evaluated seizure-free intervals of one or more years did find that a longer seizure-free period was associated with a slightly lower recurrence risk (44). Note that among children who are 2 years seizure free but remain on medication, approximately 3% to 5% will experience another seizure in the third or fourth year of treatment (21). More recent studies that have utilized a seizure-free interval of 1 year or less have reported higher recurrence risks (39–42). The risk of relapse after a one-year remission compared with a longer seizure–free interval is also higher in patients who continue on AEDs (21).

Remission Following Relapse

The majority of patients who relapse after medication withdrawal will reattain remission after AEDs are restarted though not necessarily immediately (39, 55–57). The prognosis for long-term remission appears to be primarily a function of the underlying epilepsy syndrome. A recent randomized study of medication withdrawal found that the prognosis for seizure control after recurrence in patients with previously well-controlled seizures was no different in those who were withdrawn from AED therapy and relapsed and those who relapsed while remaining on AED therapy (56).

RISKS OF NOT TREATING OR OF DISCONTINUING AEDS

Seizure recurrence is the major risk associated with not treating the child with a single seizure or of discontinuing antiepileptic drug therapy. Although a seizure is a dramatic and frightening event, the main impact of a brief seizure is psychosocial. There is no convincing evidence that a brief seizure causes brain damage (3, 6, 58). Serious injury from a brief seizure is a rare event usually related to loss of consciousness and the resultant fall (57). In general, the physical and emotional consequences of a seizure in a child, who is usually in a supervised environment and is not yet driving, are less serious than in the adult, who faces loss of driving privileges and possible adverse effects on his employment (7, 53, 58–60).

In the past there was concern that delaying treatment would result in a worse long-term prognosis (2, 4). This was based on Gowers's statement that "The tendency of the disease is toward self-perpetuation; each attack facilitates the occurrence of the next by increasing the instability of the nerve elements" (1). Proponents of this view, most notably Reynolds, have argued that treatment after the first seizure is necessary to prevent the development of "chronic" epilepsy (4, 12). Similar concerns have been raised about early discontinuation of AED therapy. Current epidemiologic data and data from controlled clinical trials, some of which have already been discussed in this chapter, indicate that this is not the case (3, 5, 6, 18, 23, 38, 61). Prognosis is primarily a function of the underlying epilepsy syndrome, and although treatment with AEDs does reduce the risk of subsequent seizures, it does not alter the long-term prognosis (18, 38). Several comprehensive reviews of this issue, which is fundamental to one's approach to treating seizures but is outside the scope of this chapter, have been recently published (3, 6, 18).

In children, even status epilepticus, defined as a seizure or a series of seizures lasting more than 30 minutes without the patient's regaining consciousness between seizures (25–28, 32), is rarely associated with brain damage attributable to the status per se (25–28). In mature animals, generalized convulsive status epilepticus produces biochemical and neuropathologic changes (28). However, although immature animals are more susceptible to the development of status with relatively mild insults than are adult ones, they are much less likely to experience brain damage as a result of prolonged seizures (28). Adult rats that had experienced status epilepticus as infants do not show a lower seizure threshold or an increased susceptibility to seizures induced by kindling compared with rats who did not experience seizures as pups (62).

Education is key to empowering the parents and child regardless of which therapeutic option is chosen. Parents need to be reassured that the child will not die during a seizure and that keeping the child safe during the seizure is generally the only action that needs to be taken. Parents will need to be told that most of the child's activities can be continued, although some may need closer supervision by an adult. Specific instructions regarding supervision of activities, such as swimming, should be given to the parents. Counseling of this nature often allays the parents' fear and educates them on safety precautions for the child, thereby reducing the chance for injury from seizures whether or not the child is treated. Educational programs are available for school personnel—teachers, nurses, and students—and information for babysitters is also readily available.

The amount of information and the level of content depends in large part on the medical sophistication of the parents and their ability to attend to the information given them at that particular time. The parents' perception of their child's disorder will be an important factor in their later coping and will ultimately impact on their perception of quality of life. The practitioner's prejudices regarding treatment options will undoubtedly come into play during these discussions, but the different options need to be discussed.

Parents will usually be interested in information that will help them manage the illness or specific problems; lengthy explanations are usually not helpful. It is also important to remember, when giving information to the parents about prognosis, to provide information about how to manage further seizures should they occur. This includes what should be done during a seizure, when it may be necessary to call the physician, and when the child should be taken to the emergency department. Depending on the age of the child, education is needed for the patient. Children may have fear of accidents, fear of the loss of friends, fear of taking "drugs," and other less well-defined fear and apprehension. The practitioner will need to address these issues with the patient and parents for a comprehensive approach to treatment.

RISKS OF INITIATING OR CONTINUING TREATMENT WITH AEDS

Antiepileptic drugs are potent medications whose use is associated with a variety of significant side effects (18, 29–31), which are discussed in detail elsewhere in this volume. The adverse effects of the medications must be

TABLE 29-3
Potential Adverse Consequences of Antiepileptic Drug Therapy and of Seizures

Antiepileptic Drug Therapy	Seizures
Systemic toxicity	Physical injury
Idiosyncratic	Loss of consciousness
Dose Related	Injury from falls
Chronic toxicity	Drowning
Teratogenicity	Status epilepticus
Higher cortical functions	
Cognitive impairment	
Adverse effects on behavior	
Psychosocial	Psychosocial
Need for daily medication	Restrictions on activity
Labeling as chronic illness	Physical
Adverse effect on	Social
psychosocial development	Social stigma of seizure
	Fear of further seizures
Economic/temporal	
Cost of medications	
Cost/time of physician visits	
Cost/time of laboratory tests	

balanced against the risk of further seizures. The potential adverse effects of AED therapy and of having a seizure are summarized in Table 29-3. Physicians are familiar with idiosyncratic drug effects as well as the acute toxicities of the drugs. However, subtle behavioral and cognitive effects are often not recognized in children with epilepsy (30), particularly when they have been on medications since their preschool years. Only when medications are stopped does it become apparent that the child's performance was impaired by the drug. For teenage girls, a discussion of the risks of treatment must include consideration of the potential teratogenicity of these compounds (59, 63, 64). A detailed discussion of this problem will be found elsewhere in this text (Chapter 36). As the major teratogenic effects take place in early gestation, and a large number of pregnancies in this group are unplanned, the physician must always consider this issue in advance. For this reason, the author is particularly aggressive in trying to withdraw medications from adolescent females who have been seizure free for 2 years, even if their other risk factors are not favorable.

A hidden side effect of continued AED treatment is that of being labeled. The person with a single seizure or childhood epilepsy who has not had a seizure in many years and is off medications is considered by himself and society to have outgrown his epilepsy. That individual can lead a normal life with very few restrictions. In contrast, remaining on chronic medication implies ongoing illness to both the patient and those around him. Continued use of medication requires ongoing medical care to prescribe and monitor the medication. It also implies certain restrictions in driving licensure and may have a adverse impact on obtaining employment. In addition to the problems associated with having epilepsy, the perception of any chronic illness will adversely affect the normal psychosocial maturation process, particularly in adolescents (65).

A THERAPEUTIC APPROACH

Given the consequences of long-term drug therapy, it is recommended that an attempt be made to withdraw medications at least once in most children and adolescents with epilepsy who are seizure free regardless of risk factors. In general, avoid starting medications in the children with only one seizure, and aggressively pursue withdrawal of medications in children who are seizure free for 2 or more years. We rarely treat children with a first seizure even if they have risk factors for recurrence. In many cases, treatment may not be necessary even in children with more than one seizure if the seizures are brief and infrequent and the child's underlying syndrome has a favorable prognosis.

Whatever the decision, it should be made jointly by the medical providers and the family after careful discussion, including not only an assessment of the risks and benefits of treatment, but also a review of measures to be taken in the event of a recurrence. Patient and family education is a key factor whether one decides to treat with

AEDs or not, because both seizures and AEDs are associated with some risks. Even children with good prognostic factors may experience another recurrence. Conversely, children with poor risk factors may nevertheless maintain remission off medications. It is far easier to take these risks while the patient is still in the supervised environment of the home and school. Education assists the family in making an informed decision, helps them to participate fully in the plan of care, and prepares them to deal with psychosocial consequences of the diagnosis. Informed decision making by the physician in consultation with the family will maximize the chances of good long-term outcomes in these children.

The approach presented in this chapter emphasizes that both seizures and the therapies available carry some risk and that optimal patient care requires careful balancing of these risks and benefits. Although this approach is presented here in the context of whether or not to treat at all, it is also useful in deciding whether or not to add a second drug or to try experimental drugs in a child whose seizures are not fully controlled on the current therapeutic regimen, whether to consider epilepsy surgery for a child who is medically refractory, or to offer the ketogenic diet as a possible treatment modality. As more information and newer therapies become available, the risk/benefit ratios may well change. In order to provide the best care available, the physician needs both to be aware of the available options and to individualize them to the needs of the specific patient.

ACKNOWLEDGMENTS

Supported in part by grant R01 NS26151 from the National Institute of Neurological Disorders and Stroke, Bethesda, MD, USA.

References

1. Gowers WR. Epilepsy and other chronic convulsive disorders. London: J&A Churchill, 1881.
2. Livingston S. Comprehensive management of epilepsy in infancy, childhood and adolescence. Springfield, Ill: Charles C. Thomas, 1972.
3. Berg AT, Shinnar S. Do seizures beget seizures? An assessment of the clinical evidence in humans. *J Clin Neurophysiol* 1997;14:102–110.
4. Reynolds EH. Do anticonvulsants alter the natural course of epilepsy? Treatment should be started as early as possible. *BrMed J* 1995;310:176–177.
5. Moshe SL, Shinnar S. Early intervention. In: Engel J Jr, ed., *Surgical Treatment of the Epilepsies*. 2nd edition. New York: Raven Press, 1993:123–132.
6. Shinnar S, Berg AT. Does antiepileptic drug therapy prevent the development of "chronic" epilepsy? *Epilepsia* 1996;37:701–708.
7. Shinnar S, Berg AT, Moshe SL, et al. The risk of recurrence following a first unprovoked seizure in childhood: a prospective study. *Pediatrics* 1990;85:1076–1085.
8. Shinnar S, Berg AT, Moshe SL, et al. The risk of seizure recurrence following a first unprovoked afebrile seizure in childhood: an extended follow-up. *Pediatrics* 1996;98: 216–225.
9. Berg A, Shinnar S. The risk of seizure recurrence following a first unprovoked seizure: a quantitative review. *Neurology* 1991;41:965–972.
10. Hauser WA, Anderson VE, Loewenson RB, McRoberts SM. Seizure recurrence after a first unprovoked seizure. *N Engl J Med* 1982;307:522–528.
11. Hauser WA, Rich SS, Annegers JF, Anderson VE. Seizure recurrence after a 1st unprovoked seizure: an extended follow-up. *Neurology* 1990;40:1163–1170.
12. Elwes RDC, Chesterman P, Reynolds EH. Prognosis after a first untreated tonic-clonic seizure. *Lancet* 1985;2:752–753.
13. Hirtz DG, Ellenberg JH, Nelson KB. The risk of recurrence of nonfebrile seizures in children. *Neurology* 1984;34:637–641.
14. Camfield PR, Camfield CS, Dooley JM, Tibbles JAR, et al. Epilepsy after a first unprovoked seizure in childhood. *Neurology* 1985;35:1657–1660.
15. Annegers JF, Shirts SB, Hauser WA, Kurland LT. Risk of recurrence after an initial unprovoked seizure. *Epilepsia* 1986;27:43–50.
16. First Seizure Trial Group. Randomized clinical trial on the efficacy of antiepileptic drugs in reducing the risk of relapse after a first unprovoked tonic-clonic seizure. *Neurology* 1993;43:478–483.
17. Hirtz D, Ashwal S, Berg A, et al. Practice parameter: evaluating a first nonfebrile seizure in children. Report of the Quality Standards Subcommittee of the American Academy of Neurology, the Child Neurology Society and the American Epilepsy Society. *Neurology* 2000;55:616–623.
18. Hirtz D, Berg A, Bettis D, et al. Practice parameter: Treatment of the child with a first unprovoked seizure. Report of the QSS of the AAN and the Practice Committee of the CNS. *Neurology* 2003;60:166–175.
19. Shinnar S, Berg AT, O'Dell C, Newstein D, et al. Predictors of multiple seizures in a cohort of children prospectively followed from the time of their first unprovoked seizure. *Ann Neurol* 2000;48:140–147.
20. Shinnar S, Berg AT, O'Dell C, Sigalova M, et al. Long term outcomes of children with a first unprovoked seizure. *Neurology* 2005;64(suppl 1):A426–A427.
21. Annegers JF, Hauser WA, Elveback LR. Remission of seizures and relapse in patients with epilepsy. *Epilepsia* 1979;20:729–737.
22. Sillanpaa M. Remission of seizures and predictors of intractability in longterm followup. *Epilepsia* 1993;34:930–936.
23. Sander JWAS. Some aspects of prognosis in the epilepsies: a review. *Epilepsia* 1993;34:1007–1016.
24. Berg AT, Hauser WA, Shinnar S. The prognosis of childhood-onset epilepsy. In: Shinnar S, Amir N, Branski D, eds. *Childhood Seizures*. Basel, Switzerland: S. Karger, 1995: 93–99.
25. Maytal J, Shinnar S, Moshe SL, Alvarez LA. The low morbidity and mortality of status epilepticus in children. *Pediatrics* 1989;83:323–331.
26. DeLorenzo RJ, Hauser WA, Towne AR, et al. A prospective population-based epidemiological study of status epilepticus in Richmond, Virginia. *Neurology* 1996;46: 1029–1035.
27. Dodson WE, DeLorenzo RJ, Pedley TA, et al: The treatment of convulsive status epilepticus: Recommendations of the Epilepsy Foundation of America's working group on status epilepticus. *JAMA* 1993;270:854–859.
28. Shinnar S, Babb TL. Long term sequelae of status epilepticus. In: Engel J Jr, Pedley TA, eds. *Epilepsy: A Comprehensive Text*. Philadelphia: Lippincott-Raven Press, 1997:755–763.
29. Reynolds EH. Chronic antiepileptic toxicity: a review. *Epilepsia* 1975;16:319–352.
30. Vining EPG, Mellits ED, Dorsen MM, Cataldo MF, et al. Psychologic and behavioral effects of antiepileptic drugs in children: a double-blind comparison between phenobarbital and valproic acid. *Pediatrics* 1987;80:165–174.
31. Committee on Drugs, American Academy of Pediatrics. Behavioral and cognitive effects of anticonvulsant therapy. *Pediatrics* 1995;96:538–540.
32. Commission on Epidemiology and Prognosis, International League Against Epilepsy. Guidelines for epidemiologic studies on epilepsy. *Epilepsia* 1993;34:592–596.
33. Commission on Classification and Terminology of the International League Against Epilepsy. Proposal for revised classification of epilepsies and epileptic syndromes. *Epilepsia* 1989;30:389–399.
34. Roger J, Dravet C, Bureau M, Dreifuss FE, et al, eds. Epileptic syndromes in infancy, childhood and adolescence. 2nd ed. London: John Libbey–Eurotext, 1992.
35. Shinnar S, Kang H, Berg AT, Goldensohn ES, et al. EEG abnormalities in children with a first unprovoked seizure. *Epilepsia* 1994;35:471–476.
36. Shinnar S, Berg AT, Moshe SL. The effect of status epilepticus on the long term outcome of a cohort of children prospectively followed from the time of their first idiopathic unprovoked seizure. *Dev Med Child Neurol* 1995;37(Suppl 72):116.
37. Camfield P, Camfield C, Dooley J, et al. A randomized study of carbamazepine versus no medication following a first unprovoked seizure in childhood. *Neurology* 1989;39: 851–852.
38. Musicco M, Beghi E, Solari A, Viani F, for the First Seizure Trial Group (FIRST Group). Treatment of first tonic-clonic seizure does not improve the prognosis of epilepsy. *Neurology* 1997;49:991–998.
39. Berg AT, Shinnar S, Chadwick D. Discontinuing antiepileptic drugs. In: Engel J Jr, Pedley TA eds. *Epilepsy: A Comprehensive Textbook*. Philadelphia: Lippincott-Raven, 1997;1275–1284.
40. Braathen G, Melander H. Early discontinuation of treatment in children with uncomplicated epilepsy: a prospective study with a model for prediction of outcome. *Epilepsia* 1997;38:561–569.
41. Arts WFM. The Dutch study of epilepsy in childhood: early discontinuation. *Epilepsia* 1995;36 (Suppl 3):S29.
42. Dooley J, Gordon K, Camfield P, Camfield C, et al. Discontinuation of anticonvulsant therapy in children free of seizures for 1 year: a prospective study. *Neurology* 1996;46:969–974.

43. Shinnar S, Vining EPG, Mellits ED, et al. Discontinuing antiepileptic medication in children with epilepsy after two years without seizures: a prospective study. *N Engl J Med* 1985;313:976–980.
44. Todt H. The late prognosis of epilepsy in childhood: results of a prospective followup study. *Epilepsia* 1984;25:137–144.
45. Emerson R, D'Souza BJ, Vining EP, et al. Stopping medication in children with epilepsy: predictors of outcome. *N Engl J Med* 1981;304:1125–1129.
46. Holowach J, Thurston DL, O'Leary J. Prognosis in childhood epilepsy: Followup study of 148 cases in which therapy had been suspended after prolonged anticonvulsant control. *N Engl J Med* 1972;286:169–174.
47. Holowach-Thurston JH, Thurston DL, Hixon BB, et al. Prognosis in childhood epilepsy: Additional followup of 148 children 15 to 23 years after withdrawal of anticonvulsant therapy. *N Engl J Med* 1982;306:831–836.
48. Medical Research Council Antiepileptic Drug Withdrawal Study Group. Randomised study of antiepileptic drug withdrawal in patients with remission. *Lancet* 1991;337: 1175–1180.
49. Arts WFM, Visser LH, Loonen MCB, et al. Follow-up of 146 children with epilepsy after withdrawal of antiepileptic therapy. *Epilepsia* 1988;29:244–250.
50. Bouma PAD, Peters ACB, Arts RJHM, et al. Discontinuation of antiepileptic therapy: a prospective trial in children. *J Neurol Neurosurg Psychiatry* 1987;50:1579–1583.
51. Juul Jensen P. Frequency of recurrence after discontinuance of anticonvulsant therapy in patients with epileptic seizures: a new followup study after 5 years. *Epilepsia* 1968;9: 11–16.
52. Callaghan N, Garrett A, Goggin T. Withdrawal of anticonvulsant drugs in patients free of seizures for two years. *N Engl J Med* 1988;318:942–946.
53. Shinnar S, Berg AT, Moshe SL, Kang H, et al. Discontinuing antiepileptic drugs in children with epilepsy: a prospective study. *Ann Neurol* 1994;35:534–545.
54. Berg AT, Shinnar S. Relapse following discontinuation of antiepileptic drugs: a meta-analysis. *Neurology* 1994;44:601–608.
55. Shinnar S, O'Dell C, Berg AT. Long term prognosis following discontinuation of antiepileptic drug therapy in childhood onset epilepsy. *Epilepsia* 2004;45(suppl 7): 365–366.
56. Chadwick D, Taylor J, Johnson T. Outcomes after seizure recurrence in people with well-controlled epilepsy and the factors that influence it. The MRC Antiepileptic Drug Withdrawal Group. *Epilepsia* 1996;37:1043–1050.
57. Shinnar S, Berg AT, Moshe SL, et al. What happens to children with epilepsy who experience a seizure recurrence after withdarawal of antiepileptic drugs? *Ann Neurol* 1996;40:301–302.
58. Freeman JM, Tibbles J, Camfield C, Camfield P. Benign epilepsy of childhood: A speculation and its ramifications. *Pediatrics* 1987;79:864–868.
59. Shinnar S. Seizures. In: Friedman SB, Fisher MM, Schonberg SK, Alderman EM, eds. *Comprehensive Adolescent Health Care*. 2nd ed. St. Louis: Quality Medical Publishing, 1997:501–510.
60. Jacoby A, Baker G, Chadwick D, Johnson A. The impact of counseling with a practical statistical model on a patient's decision making about treatment with epilepsy: findings from a pilot study. *Epilepsy Res* 1993;16:207–214.
61. van Donselaar CA, Brouwer OF, Geerts AT, Arts WF, et al. Clinical course of untreated tonic-clonic seizures in childhood: prospective, hospital based study. *Br Med J* 1997;314:401–404.
62. Okada R, Moshe SL, Albala BJ. Infantile status epilepticus and future seizure susceptibility in the rat. *Dev Brain Res* 1984;15:177–183.
63. Yerby MS. Teratogenic effects of antiepileptic drugs: what do we advise patients? *Epilepsia* 1997;38:957–958.
64. Commission on Genetics, Pregnancy and the Child, International League Against Epilepsy. Guidelines for the care of women of childbearing age with epilepsy. *Epilepsia* 1993;34:588–589.
65. Hoare P. Does illness foster dependency: A study of epileptic and diabetic children. *Dev Med Child Neurol* 1984;26:20–24.

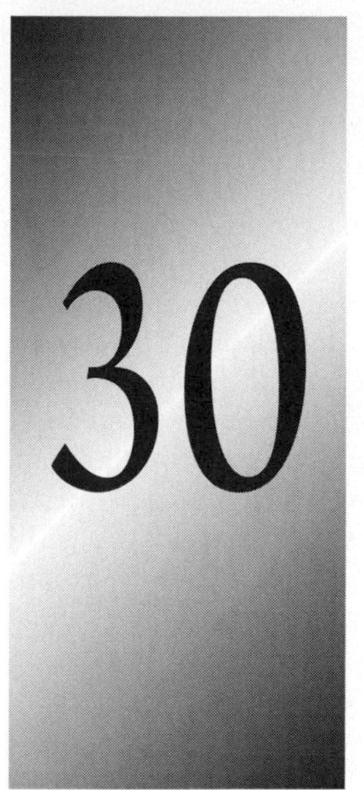

30 Comparative Anticonvulsant Profile and Proposed Mechanisms of Action of Antiepileptic Drugs

H. Steve White
Karen S. Wilcox

For the vast majority of people who develop epilepsy, initial therapy consists of pharmacologic treatment with one or more of the established anticonvulsant drugs. These medications include phenytoin (PHT), carbamazepine (CBZ), valproate (VPA), barbiturates such as phenobarbital (PB), certain benzodiazepines (BZDs), and ethosuximide (ESM). For some patients, complete seizure control with this group of "established" antiepileptic drugs (AEDs) may not ever be achieved at doses that are devoid of various types and severities of AED-related adverse effects.

The 1990s were marked by a number of advances in AED development. Since 1993, several novel AEDs have been commercialized in one or more countries, and several more are in the process of evaluation for worldwide registration. This has been an exciting era for practitioners and their patients who suffer from intractable seizure disorders. For the physician, the new AEDs provide novel therapeutic options for the management of their patients. For the patient with intractable epilepsy, the newer drugs provide renewed hope for complete seizure control and lessening of their AED-associated side-effect profile. This chapter will review the preclinical animal models that led to the initial identification of the "second-generation" AEDs felbamate (FBM), lamotrigine (LTG), gabapentin (GBP), topiramate (TPM), tiagabine (TGB), vigabatrin (VGB), oxcarbazepine (OCBZ), zonisamide (ZNS), levetiracetam (LEV), and pregabalin (PGB), and the proposed molecular mechanisms of action of the new and the established AEDs.

AED DISCOVERY, TESTING, AND PROPOSED MECHANISMS OF ACTION

The process by which new AEDs are discovered has evolved in the seven decades since phenytoin was identified by Putnam and Merritt (1). The strategies employed in the search for new AEDs are varied but, for the most part, have been based largely on three different approaches: (1) random drug screening and efficacy-based AED discovery; (2) rational drug design, wherein structural modifications of an active pharmacophore are synthesized and tested; and (3) mechanistic-based AED development. All three approaches have led to the successful identification of clinically effective drugs. Unfortunately, even with the introduction of 10 new AEDs since 1993, there continues to be a significant need for more efficacious and less toxic AEDs. Regardless of the process by which a chemical entity is brought forth from the medicinal chemistry laboratory, it must first demonstrate some degree of efficacy in an animal model prior to becoming a candidate for clinical trials.

In-Vivo Testing

No single laboratory test will, in itself, establish the presence or absence of anticonvulsant activity or fully predict the clinical utility of an investigational antiepileptic drug. Thus, the true test of a drug's efficacy must always await the results of clinical trials. There are many available animal seizure models that have been described over the years that possess appropriate properties to qualify as predictive seizure models. Historically, the maximal electroshock (MES) test, the subcutaneous pentylenetetrazol (sc PTZ) test, and the electrical kindling model represent the three in-vivo systems that have been most commonly employed in the search for new AEDs (2). Today, newer in-vivo models are being introduced that incorporate known genetic defects that more closely resemble the human condition. In addition, the 6-Hz psychomotor seizure model has recently proven useful in identifying compounds that are effective against partial seizures. In particular, LEV, which is inactive in the MES and sc PTZ models (discussed subsequently), was found to be quite effective against seizures induced following corneal stimulation at 6Hz (3).

To gain a full appreciation for a new AED's overall spectrum of activity (narrow or broad), all investigational AEDs should be screened in a variety of different seizure and epilepsy models.

Correlation of Animal Anticonvulsant Profile and Clinical Utility

The MES test and the kindling model represent two highly predictive models that are useful in the characterization of a drug's potential utility against generalized tonic-clonic and partial seizures, respectively (4–7) (Table 30-1). For some years, positive results obtained in the sc PTZ test were considered suggestive of a drug's potential utility against generalized absence seizures. This interpretation was based largely on the observation that drugs that were active in the clinic (i.e., ETS, trimethadione, VPA, the BZDs) were able to block clonic seizures induced by sc PTZ, whereas drugs such as PHT and CBZ were ineffective against sc PTZ seizures in animals and spike-wave seizures in humans. However, as summarized in Table 30-1, the PTZ test would also suggest that the barbiturates and TGB should also possess efficacy against generalized absence. For the barbiturates (and possibly TGB), this is in direct opposition to what has been reported clinically. For example, phenobarbital worsens human spike-wave discharges (8). On the other hand, PB is useful for the management of myoclonic seizures. In this respect, the sc PTZ test as conducted by most laboratories may have greater utility in the identification of drugs with activity against myoclonic seizures (4).

TABLE 30-1
Correlation Between Clinical Utility and Efficacy in Experimental Animal Models of the Established and Newer AEDs

	Experimental Model			
Seizure Type	MES (Tonic Extension)	sc PTZ (Clonic Seizures)	Spike-Wave Discharges[a]	Electrical Kindling (Focal Seizures)
Tonic and/or clonic generalized seizures	CBZ, PHT, VPA, PB [FBM, GBP, LTG, OCBZ, TPM, ZNS][b]			
Myoclonic/generalized absence seizures		ESM, VPA, PB[c], BZD [FBM, GBP, TGB]		
Generalized absence seizures			ESM, VPA, BZD [LTG, TPM, LEV]	
Partial seizures				CBZ, PHT, VPA, PB, BZD [FBM, GBP, LTG, OCBZ, TPM, TGB, VGB, ZNS, LEV, PGB]

[a]Data summarized from GBL, GAERS, and *lh/lh* spike-wave models (4–7).
[b]Brackets [ ] indicate newer AEDs.
[c]PB blocks clonic seizures induced by sc PTZ but is inactive against generalized absence seizures.

In recent years, three other animal models have emerged that are, to date, perhaps more predictive than the sc PTZ for generalized absence seizures. These include spike-wave seizures induced by the chemoconvulsant gamma-butyrolactone (5), the genetic absence epileptic rat of Strasbourg (GAERS) (6), and the *lethargic* (*lh/lh*) mutant mouse (7, 9). Of these three, the *lh/lh* mouse displays spontaneous spike-wave discharges that are blocked by drugs that have been found clinically effective in reducing spike-wave activity (e.g., the BZDs, ETS, VPA, and LTG). Furthermore, all three models accurately predict the potentiation of spike-wave seizures by drugs that elevate gamma-aminobutyric acid (GABA) concentrations (e.g., VGB and TGB), drugs that directly activate the $GABA_B$ receptor, and the barbiturates. Given this, any drug being evaluated for potential use against absence seizures should be evaluated in one or more of these three models.

The remainder of this chapter will focus primarily on a description of the anticonvulsant profile and comparative mechanisms of action between the established (pre-1993) and second-generation (post-1993) AEDs. Where possible, the reader is referred to more comprehensive reviews and primary citations supporting the proposed mechanisms of action that are addressed.

Mechanism of Action: General Considerations

The mechanisms of action of currently marketed anticonvulsant drugs are not fully understood. Ultimately, there are numerous molecular mechanisms through which drugs can alter neuronal excitability and thereby limit or control seizure activity. However, three primary mechanisms appear to be targeted by most of the established anticonvulsants (10). Thus, as summarized in Table 30-2, drugs that block sustained high-frequency firing through an effect on voltage-sensitive sodium channels can disrupt burst firing; drugs that enhance GABA-mediated neurotransmission can elevate seizure threshold; and drugs that reduce voltage-dependent low-threshold (T-type) calcium currents in thalamocortical neurons can interrupt the thalamic oscillatory firing patterns associated with absence seizures. Likewise, drugs that reduce glutamatergic-mediated excitation can be expected to reduce burst firing elicited

TABLE 30-2
Comparative Mechanistic Profile Between the Established and New AEDs

	Proposed Molecular Mechanism of Action				
AED	Limit SRF[a]/Na^+ Channel Block	Reduce VSCC	Enhance GABA-Mediated Neurotransmission	Reduce Glutamate-Mediated Excitation	Bind to Synaptic Vesicle Protein SV2A
1st Generation					
Phenytoin	+				
CBZ	+				
VPA	+	+(?)	+(?)		
BZDs			+		
PB			+		
ESM		+			
2nd Generation					
FBM	+	+	+	+	
GBP	+[b]	+[c]	+[d]		
LTG	+	+			
OCBZ	+	+			
TPM	+	+	+	+	
ZNS	+	+	+		
VGB			+[e]		
TGB			+[f]		
PGB		+[c]			
LEV					+[g]

[a]Sustained repetitive firing
[b]Mechanism not clearly established; binds to unique site; requires prolonged exposure
[c]Binds to the alpha$_2$delta auxiliary subunit of voltage-sensitive Ca^{2+} channels
[d]Increases brain GABA levels in brains of epileptic patients
[e]Inhibits GABA metabolism via GABA-T
[f]Blocks neuronal and glial uptake of synaptically released GABA
[g]Binds to the SV2A protein on vesicles, mechanism of action not clearly established

TABLE 30-3
Functional Consequences of Proposed Mechanism of Action of Established and Newer AEDs

Molecular Mechanism of Action	AED	Consequences of Action
Na^+ channel blockers	PHT, CBZ, LTG, FBM, OCBZ, TPM, VPA	(1) Block action potential propagation (2) Stabilize neuronal membranes (3) Decrease neurotransmitter release (4) Decrease focal firing (5) Decrease seizure spread
Ca^{2+} channel blockers	ESM, VPA, GBP, LTG, PGB	(1) Decrease neurotransmitter release (N & P types) (2) Decrease slow-depolarization (T-type) (3) Decrease spike-wave discharges
$GABA_A$ receptor allosteric modulators	BZDs, PB, FBM, TPM	(1) Increase membrane hyperpolarization (2) Elevate seizure threshold (3) Attenuate (BZDs) spike-wave discharges (4) Aggravate (barbiturates) spike-wave discharges (5) Decrease focal firing
GABA uptake inhibitors, GABA transaminase inhibitors	TGB, VGB	(1) Increase synaptic GABA levels (2) Increase membrane hyperpolarization (3) Decrease focal firing (4) Aggravate spike-wave discharges
NMDA receptor antagonists	FBM	(1) Decrease slow excitatory neurotransmission (2) Decrease excitatory amino acid neurotoxicity (3) Delay epileptogenesis
AMPA/kainate receptor antagonists	PB, TPM	(1) Decrease fast excitatory neurotransmission (2) Attenuate focal firing
Binds to synaptic vesicle protein, SV2A	LEV	(1) Currently unknown

by synaptic stimulation. Although not a target of standard AEDs, this mechanism does appear to be targeted by some of the new AEDs, including FBM and TPM and the investigational AED remacemide. It should be noted that many of the older established and newer AEDs have been observed to exert a number of different pharmacologic actions that could account for their anticonvulsant action. In those cases where multiple actions have been defined, it is highly likely that the separate mechanisms offer some degree of synergy.

As shown in Table 30-3, inhibition of voltage-sensitive Na^+ and Ca^{2+} channels, augmentation of GABA-mediated inhibition, and inhibition of glutamate-mediated excitatory neurotransmission can produce both synaptic and nonsynaptic effects that, when translated to an in-vivo effect, are likely to contribute to a drug's anticonvulsant action. Unfortunately, the ability of an AED to modulate the function of any one of these neuronal processes can have profound consequences on the abnormal firing of epileptic neurons but also on normal neuronal communication. As a result, the same action(s) that decrease seizure frequency are likely to contribute to a drug's central nervous system (CNS)-related side effect profile. This having been said, some of the drugs display certain properties that lead to a greater separation between therapeutic and toxic effects. For example, it is widely accepted that to be a therapeutically useful Na^+ channel blocker, a drug should possess both voltage- and frequency- dependent actions. These properties confer a certain level of selectivity toward those epileptic neurons that display a paroxysmal depolarization shift and high-frequency sustained repetitive firing (i.e., epileptic neurons within a seizure focus). Thus, at therapeutic concentrations voltage- and use-dependent Na^+ channel blockers would be less likely to affect normal neuronal function than a Na^+ channel blocker that does not display these properties. It is necessary to reconcile this theory with the cognitive impairment that has come to be associated with the voltage- and use-dependent Na^+ channel blockers phenytoin and carbamazepine. This can be done in part by acknowledging the fact that these drugs can, at higher concentrations, attenuate Na^+ currents at resting membrane potentials and thereby modify normal neuronal communication. Furthermore, inhibiting neuronal voltage-sensitive Na^+ channels can produce a subsequent inhibition of depolarization-dependent neurotransmitter release. Given the critical role that the excitatory neurotransmitter glutamate plays in fast excitatory neurotransmission, slight modification of glutamate release in the absence of abnormal neuronal firing may contribute to the cognitive impairment observed in some patients taking these drugs. In this case, drugs that display greater voltage and use dependence would necessarily offer certain potential advantages over less selective Na^+ channel blockers.

Correlation Between Anticonvulsant Profile and Mechanism of Action

A question that is commonly asked is whether a drug's anticonvulsant profile suggests anything about its potential mechanism of action. The short answer to this question is, probably not. However, certain trends have been emerging over the years that are worthy of mention. First of all, activity against MES-induced tonic extension has been suggested to identify drugs that are effective in preventing seizure spread; whereas activity against PTZ-induced clonic seizures is suggestive of a drug's ability to elevate seizure threshold (11). Another common theme among drugs that prevent MES-induced seizures is that a large fraction of the marketed AEDs have been demonstrated to inhibit sustained repetitive firing of neurons through an action at the voltage-sensitive Na^+ channel (12). In addition to the Na^+ channel blockers, two other classes of drugs that are very effective against MES-induced seizures are the N-methyl-D-aspartate (NMDA) and non-NMDA glutamate receptor antagonists. For the NMDA antagonists, this would include both competitive (e.g., CPP, CPPene, and CGS 19755) and noncompetitive (e.g., MK801) antagonists, glycine-site antagonists (e.g., ACEA 1021 and felbamate), and polyamine-site antagonists such as eliprodil and ifenprodil. Drugs active at the non-NMDA receptor and also effective against MES-induced tonic extension include topiramate and the noncompetitive antagonist NBQX.

Interestingly enough, Na^+ channel blockers and nonselective NMDA and non-NMDA antagonists are for the most part inactive against clonic seizures induced by PTZ. Conversely, drugs that enhance GABA-mediated inhibition (e.g., allosteric modulators, uptake inhibitors, and GABA transaminase inhibitors) are active against PTZ-induced clonus and inactive against MES-induced seizures at nontoxic doses. Likewise, drugs that selectively block T-type voltage-sensitive Ca^{2+} channels (e.g., ESM and trimethadione) are active against PTZ-induced clonus but not MES-induced tonic extension.

Whereas the MES and sc PTZ tests may identify a certain mechanistic class of AEDs, the kindled rat model appears to be less discriminating. For example, in the kindled rat, Na^+ channel blockers, $GABA_A$ receptor modulators, Ca^{2+} channel modulators (GBP and PGB), non-NMDA glutamate receptor antagonists (e.g., NBQX), and modulators of synaptic vesicle protein 2A (LEV) display activity, whereas the NMDA receptor antagonists and T-type Ca^{2+} channel antagonists do not. It needs to be noted that the aforementioned correlations between anticonvulsant activity and mechanism of action are based purely on our knowledge regarding the currently available AEDs and experimental compounds that display highly selective mechanisms of action. As new drugs with other well-characterized mechanisms of action become available for testing, it will be interesting to see whether other classes of drugs (e.g., subunit selective NMDA, AMPA, and kainate antagonists; K^+ channel enhancers; other selective Ca^{2+} channel antagonists: N, P, and Q type; and selective adenosine agonists) fall into some rational classification scheme. Last, given that a number of the currently available AEDs are active in a variety of experimental models, one might argue that they are likely to possess multiple mechanisms of action and a broader clinical profile than drugs with a narrow anticonvulsant profile. As discussed subsequently, this certainly appears to be the case for VPA, FBM, and TPM.

The value of such an oversimplified discussion lies not in trying to assess the mechanism of action of a drug based on its anticonvulsant profile, but in providing a logical rationale for assessing efficacy of an investigational AED emerging from a mechanistically driven drug discovery program. Thus, based on the available data with reasonably selective drugs, one would not attempt to demonstrate efficacy with a Na^+ channel blocker or NMDA antagonist using the PTZ test, nor would one initially evaluate a T-type Ca^{2+} channel blocker or GABA uptake blocker against MES seizures. It could be argued that all drugs should be initially screened in the kindled rat, given the broad spectrum of drugs that are active in this model. Since the kindled rat is an extremely labor-intensive model, it would not necessarily be amenable to high-volume screening. One model not discussed thus far that is often employed as a broad-spectrum screen is the audiogenic mouse (e.g. the DBA/2J and the Frings genetically susceptible mouse). Given that the audiogenic mouse model is nondiscriminatory with respect to clinical classes of AEDs, it serves as a useful model for "proof of principle" screening (13). Once an active molecule has been identified, its clinical potential can be further established using more syndrome-specific models.

The remainder of this review will focus on the most widely accepted mechanism(s) that have been observed at therapeutically relevant concentrations of the first- and second-generation AEDs. As previously mentioned, this is not to imply that a minor, less-established action does not contribute to a drug's anticonvulsant profile. The reader is referred to reviews by Rogawski and Porter (14), Macdonald and Meldrum (15), Meldrum (16), and White (12) for a more comprehensive discussion of these effects.

FIRST-GENERATION (PRE-1993) AEDS

Phenytoin (PHT) and Carbamazepine (CBZ)

The anticonvulsant profiles of PHT and CBZ observed in animal seizure models correlate well with their clinical efficacy in generalized tonic-clonic and complex partial seizures (Table 30-1). Thus, both drugs are effective against tonic extension seizures induced by a number of different stimuli, including MES and various chemoconvulsants (17, 18), and both AEDs are effective against fully expressed kindled seizures (14). Unlike ESM, both drugs are ineffective against clonic seizures induced by PTZ. Studies conducted to date provide compelling evidence that therapeutic concentrations of PHT and CBZ prevent sustained repetitive firing resulting from extended depolarization (Table 30-2). In addition, both drugs prevent post-tetanic potentiation (PTP), a process whereby high-frequency stimulation produces a transiently enhanced responsiveness to subsequent stimulation. The ability of PHT and CBZ to block PTP may explain, in part, their ability to limit seizure spread.

The voltage-sensitive Na^+ channel is thought to underlie the ability of neurons to fire repetitively. As such, anticonvulsants that inhibit sustained repetitive firing are likely to exert an effect on voltage-sensitive Na^+ channels. PHT and CBZ have been found to exert an inhibitory effect on voltage-gated Na^+ channels (19–21) that is both use- and voltage-dependent (Table 30-2). These two properties account for the unique ability of PHT, CBZ, and other voltage-dependent Na^+ channel blockers to limit the high-frequency firing that is characteristic of epileptic discharges without significantly altering normal patterns of neuronal firing.

PHT and CBZ have also been demonstrated to produce a shift in the steady-state inactivation curve in mammalian myelinated nerve fibers to more negative voltages (22), thereby effectively reducing the degree of depolarization required to inactivate Na^+ channels. In addition, both drugs delayed the rate of Na^+ channel recovery from inactivation. Whether slight differences between PHT and CBZ in time dependence of the frequency-dependent block account for differences in anticonvulsant efficacy between these drugs has yet to be established. Thus, by stabilizing the Na^+ channel in its inactive form and slowing its rate of recovery from inactivation, both drugs can prevent sustained repetitive firing evoked by prolonged depolarization such as that found in an epileptic focus.

Similarly, voltage-, frequency-, and time-dependent inactivation of Na^+ channels by PHT has also been confirmed in isolated rat hippocampal neurons and *Xenopus* oocytes injected with human brain mRNA (23, 24). All of these studies provide strong experimental evidence supporting an interaction of PHT and CBZ with the voltage-dependent Na^+ channel.

Ethosuximide (ESM)

Unlike PHT and CBZ, ESM is effective against clonic seizures induced by subcutaneously administered PTZ (Table 30-1). It is also active against spike-wave seizures induced by the chemoconvulsant gamma-hydroxybutyrate (6) and against spontaneous spike-wave discharges in the *lh/lh* mouse model of absence (8). ESM is ineffective against tonic extension seizures induced by MES and focal seizures in the kindled rat (25). In this respect, ESM's in-vivo profile is consistent with its clinical efficacy against generalized absence seizures and lack of efficacy in generalized tonic-clonic or partial seizures (Table 30-1).

The mechanism of ESM was not elucidated until 1989, when it was shown to reduce low-threshold T-type Ca^{2+} currents in thalamic neurons isolated from rats and guinea pigs (26). Reduction of the T-type current was voltage-dependent and was observed at clinically relevant ESM concentrations, suggesting that this mechanism may be the basis for efficacy of ESM in controlling absence seizures (Table 30-2). This effect of ESM, which is produced at clinically relevant concentrations, is thought to represent the primary mechanism by which it controls absence epilepsy. Activation of T-channels in thalamic relay neurons generates low-threshold Ca^{2+} spikes that are thought to contribute to the abnormal thalamocortical rhythmicity that underlies the 3-Hz spike-and-wave EEG discharge of absence epilepsy. By preventing Ca^{2+}-dependent depolarization of thalamocortical neurons, ESM as well as dimethadione, the active metabolite of the antiabsence drug trimethadione (27), is thought to block the synchronized firing associated with spike-wave discharges.

Valproic Acid (VPA)

Of the standard AEDs, VPA appears to have the broadest preclinical and clinical profile (Table 30-1). It is active in a variety of animal seizure models including electrical seizures in the MES test, chemically induced clonic seizures in the sc PTZ test, electrically kindled seizures, GBL-induced spike-wave, and spontaneous spike-wave discharges in the *lh/lh* mouse (6, 8, 25). Clinically, VPA is useful in the management of both partial and primary generalized seizures.

Based on VPA's rather broad preclinical and clinical anticonvulsant profile, it might be anticipated that VPA would possess more than one mechanism of action. Indeed, a number of studies suggest that VPA possesses at least three different mechanisms of action. First, in-vitro studies with VPA support an action at the voltage-sensitive Na+ channel (12). For example, VPA has been found to inhibit Na^+ currents in isolated *Xenopus leavis* myelinated nerves (28) and in neocortical neurons in vitro (29). Furthermore, in rat hippocampal neurons VPA decreased peak Na^+ currents in a voltage-dependent manner and produced a 10-mV leftward shift in the Na^+ inactivation curve (30). Such an action may contribute to its ability to prevent MES-induced tonic extension in animals and generalized tonic-clonic and partial seizures in humans. Secondly, VPA, like ESM, has been shown to reduce T-type Ca^{2+} currents in primary afferent neurons (31). This effect, albeit modest and observed at high VPA concentrations, may contribute to VPA's clinical efficacy in absence seizures. Lastly, VPA-mediated elevations of whole-brain GABA levels and potentiation of GABA responses are also found at relatively high drug concentrations (14). This effect, coupled with its effect at the voltage-sensitive Na^+ channel, may also contribute to its efficacy against kindled seizures in rats and against human partial seizures.

Benzodiazepines (BZDs) and Barbiturates

In animal seizure models, the BZDs and barbiturates are effective at low doses against sc PTZ–induced clonic seizures and in the kindled rat model of partial seizures. The barbiturates at low doses and BZDs at higher doses are also active against MES-induced tonic extension. One important distinction between these two classes of compounds lies in their efficacy against spike-wave seizures in the GBL and *lh/lh* models of absence. In both models, the BZDs are effective in reducing spike-wave discharges, whereas the barbiturates actually worsen spike-wave discharges (6, 8).

Once released from GABAergic nerve terminals, the inhibitory neurotransmitter GABA binds to both $GABA_A$ and $GABA_B$ receptors. The $GABA_A$ receptor complex is a multimeric macromolecular protein that forms a chloride-selective ion pore. Thus far, multiple binding sites for GABA, anticonvulsant BZDs, barbiturates, neurosteroids, convulsant beta-carbolines, and the chemoconvulsant picrotoxin have been identified (32). The $GABA_B$ receptor is coupled via a GTP-binding protein to calcium or potassium channels but does not form an ion pore and does not appear to contribute to the anticonvulsant action of either BZDs or barbiturates. The principal anticonvulsant action of the BZDs and barbiturates is thought to be related to their ability to enhance inhibitory neurotransmission by allosterically modulating the $GABA_A$ receptor complex.

GABA receptor current can be enhanced by increasing channel conductance, open and burst frequency, and/or open and burst duration. Studies indicate that the barbiturates act mainly by increasing the mean channel open duration without affecting channel conductances or opening frequency; whereas the binding of a BZD to its allosterically coupled $GABA_A$ binding site increases opening frequency without affecting open or burst duration (33–36). Results from several reconstitution experiments conducted in a variety of laboratories wherein specific GABA receptor subunits were transiently expressed in either *Xenopus* oocytes, Chinese hamster ovary (CHO) cells, or human embryonic kidney cells have suggested a molecular basis for the differential regulation of GABA receptor current by these two classes of drugs. The results from these studies have suggested that the allosteric regulatory site conferring barbiturate sensitivity appears to be contained in the alpha and beta subunits (37, 38). Thus, while GABA receptors formed from alpha1-beta1 subunits are barbiturate-sensitive, they are BZD-insensitive (37, 39). BZD sensitivity is restored when the gamma2 subunit is coexpressed with alpha1 and beta1 subunits (39). Transient coexpression of the gamma2, alpha1, and beta1 subunits in human embryonic kidney cells results in fully functional GABA receptors that are sensitive to the BZDs, barbiturates, beta-carbolines, and picrotoxin. These effects at the $GABA_A$ receptor are likely to account for the efficacy of the BZDs and barbiturates against kindled seizures in rats and partial seizures in humans.

One important difference between these two classes of GABA modulators is that the barbiturates will directly activate a Cl^- current in the absence of GABA; whereas the BZDs will not. This difference, coupled with possible anatomical differences in subunit expression, may explain in part why BZDs attenuate spike-wave seizures in both rodents and humans; whereas the barbiturates actually exacerbate spike-wave discharges (40). For example, clonazepam and diazepam selectively augment $GABA_A$-mediated inhibition in neurons of the nucleus reticularis thalami (NRT), but not other thalamic neurons. Because the inhibitory synapses in the NRT are primarily reciprocal inhibitory circuits, augmentation of inhibition by the BZDs results in decreased output of NRT onto the thalamus. By decreasing the "pacemaker" activity of the thalamic reticular neurons impinging onto the thalamus, the BZDs selectively and effectively prevent spike-wave discharges. In contrast, barbiturates, by increasing the inhibitory drive within the thalamus, enhance the deinactivation of T-currents, which results in a stronger low-threshold burst and increased thalamocortical rhythms. In contrast to the barbiturates, the BZDs do not augment inhibition within the thalamus and thus do not display the same proconvulsant action.

SECOND-GENERATION (POST-1993) AEDs

In some circumstances, the mechanisms of action of those AEDs introduced after 1993 display a marked overlap with those just defined for the pre-1993 AEDs. However, some of these compounds display a unique mechanistic profile relative to the older drugs. Increasingly, AED development has produced novel molecules that enhance inhibitory neurotransmission by acting on GABA receptors, GABA transporters, and GABA metabolism or reduce excitatory neurotransmission mediated by glutamate.

Felbamate (FBM)

Felbamate (2-phenyl-1,3-propanediol dicarbamate) received FDA approval in mid-1993 and was the first new AED approved in the United States since 1978. Results from preclinical studies conducted by the NINDS Anticonvulsant Drug Development Program demonstrated that FBM possessed a broad anticonvulsant profile in animal seizure models (41, 42; Table 30-1). It is effective against tonic extension seizures induced by MES and the glutamate agonists NMDA and quisqualic acid. Like VPA, FBM is also active against clonic seizures induced by a number of chemoconvulsants. In animal models of partial epilepsy, FBM has been found to reduce the seizure severity in corneal kindled rats and PTZ-kindled rats and to raise the seizure threshold in amygdala-kindled rats (43, 44). In addition to its anticonvulsant properties, FBM has also been demonstrated to possess neuroprotectant properties both in vitro and in vivo (45–48). Consistent with FBM's broad preclinical profile is its rather broad clinical spectrum. Upon entry into the U.S. market, FBM was approved for treatment of partial seizures, primary and secondary generalized tonic-clonic seizures, and Lennox-Gastaut syndrome.

FBM also possesses a broad mechanistic profile (12), which provides a basis for understanding its broad preclinical and clinical anticonvulsant profile, as well as its neuroprotectant action. FBM reduces sustained repetitive firing in mouse spinal cord neurons in a concentration-dependent manner. This action suggests an interaction with voltage-dependent Na^+ channels, an effect that was confirmed in rat striatal neurons (49; Table 30-2). FBM, at low concentrations, also appears to inhibit dihydropyridine-sensitive high-threshold voltage-sensitive Ca^{2+} currents (50), an effect that is consistent with decreased excitability. One mechanism that appears to be unique to FBM is related to its ability to modulate glutamate receptor function through an action at the strychnine-insensitive glycine site of the NMDA receptor. FBM has been shown to displace a competitive antagonist at the strychnine-insensitive glycine-binding site of the NMDA receptor in rat brain membranes (51) and postmortem human brains (52). Furthermore, FBM exerts a neuroprotective effect in the rat hippocampal slice that is reversed by glycine (53). Likewise, its anticonvulsant effect is reversed by strychnine-insensitive glycine receptor agonists (54–56). In addition, FBM has been found to inhibit NMDA-evoked currents directly (57). FBM's ability to block NMDA-evoked currents is unique among both the standard and the newer AEDs. Despite its interaction with this receptor complex, FBM does not appear to produce either the behavioral or pathologic impairment of the CNS that has been associated with either competitive or noncompetitive NMDA antagonists (43).

At substantially higher concentrations, FBM has also been reported to enhance GABA-evoked chloride currents (57). The mechanism by which FBM enhances GABA-evoked currents is unknown. For example, FBM in concentrations up to 1 mM does not appear to affect ligand binding to the GABA, BZD, or picrotoxin binding sites on the $GABA_A$ receptor ionophore, nor does it enhance GABA-stimulated $^{36}Cl^{2-}$ flux into cultured mouse spinal cord neurons (58).

FBM remains a mechanistically very interesting AED with an apparently broad anticonvulsant profile. However, its clinical utility has been markedly limited by the serious hematologic and hepatic toxicity reported after its commercialization in the United States (59). A thorough understanding of the mechanisms underlying these idiosyncratic adverse effects and the ability to identify patients at risk will likely lead to an increased use of this highly effective drug in therapy-resistant patients.

Gabapentin (GBP)

The second of the newer generation AEDs to be marketed in the United States is gabapentin (GBP). GBP, 1-(aminomethyl)cyclohexaneacetic acid, was originally designed and synthesized as a drug to enhance GABA-mediated inhibition by mimicking the steric conformation of GABA (60). Thus, GBP is one of the few examples of rational drug design resulting in a potent anticonvulsant.

In animal seizure models, GBP is active in a number of anticonvulsant tests (9, 61–63). It reduces electrically and chemically induced tonic extension seizures, as well as clonic seizures induced by sc PTZ (Table 30-1), and it blocks sound-induced seizures in DBA mice but not absence-like spike-wave seizures. GBP is also effective against fully kindled seizures in the kindled rat. These findings support its clinical efficacy against human partial seizures and secondarily generalized seizures.

Although the chemical structure and steric conformation of GBP were originally designed to enhance GABA-mediated inhibition, GABA mimetic activity was surprisingly absent in early studies. Despite demonstrated efficacy in both animal and human studies and numerous in-vitro studies that have described several potential mechanisms of action, the precise mode of action of GBP remains unknown.

Findings from in-vitro studies suggest that GBP can increase the concentration of GABA in both the glial and neuronal compartments (64). GBP has also been shown to increase in-vivo occipital lobe GABA levels in patients with epilepsy (65, Table 30-2). GBP may increase brain GABA turnover by interacting with a number of different metabolic processes. It has been demonstrated to enhance glutamate dehydrogenase and glutamic acid decarboxylase and inhibit branched-chain amino acid aminotransferase and GABA aminotransferase. Although any one of these effects could singly, or in concert with each other, contribute to the anticonvulsant action of GBP, it is not clear at this point which effects are important (61, 64). After prolonged administration, a voltage- and frequency-dependent limitation of Na^+-dependent sustained action potential firing in mouse cortical neurons was observed at clinically relevant concentrations of GBP (66). GBP's ability to limit sodium-dependent sustained action potential firing in cultured mouse spinal cord neurons was voltage- and frequency-dependent. The precise mechanism of this effect is not known; however, it is unlikely that GBP inhibits sodium currents in a manner similar to that of established sodium channel blockers PHT and CBZ. The delayed effect of GBP against sustained repetitive firing is consistent with the substantial time lag between the appearance of peak plasma and brain concentrations and GBP's time to peak anticonvulsant effect observed following intravenous administration (67). This delay in anticonvulsant effect suggests that prolonged synaptic and/or cytosolic exposure to GBP is important and supports an indirect mechanism of action for GBP.

GBP has also been reported to bind to a novel site in rat brain that is not affected by any of the standard AEDs and is not significantly displaced by NMDA or AMPA (alpha-amino-2,3-dihydro-5-methyl-3-oxo-4-isoxazolepropanoic acid) receptor ligands (61). GBP is displaced stereospecifically by certain L-amino acids, demonstrating a relationship between the GBP binding site and system-L transporter membrane. GBP has also been found to bind to the $alpha_2delta$ regulatory subunit of the voltage-sensitive Ca^{2+} channel (68). The precise function of this auxiliary subunit is not known, but it has been suggested that GBP may modify monamine neurotransmitter release through its interaction with Ca^{2+} channels (64).

In summary, GBP displays a unique anticonvulsant profile in animal studies and has demonstrated efficacy in human trials. Furthermore, results from a number of in-vitro and in-vivo studies would also suggest that the mechanism of action of GBP is unique among the existing AEDs. The two that appear most closely associated with its anticonvulsant action are its ability (1) to enhance GABA turnover and release and (2) to interact with the $alpha_2delta$ regulatory subunit of the voltage-sensitive Ca^{2+} channel.

Lamotrigine (LTG)

Lamotrigine (3,5-diamino-6-{2,3-dichlorophenyl}-1, 2,4-triazine) was the third new generation AED to be marketed in the United States since 1993. LTG was derived from an antifolate drug development program based on the observation that chronic use of phenobarbital, primidone, and phenytoin reduced folate levels (69) and that folates induce seizures in laboratory animals (70). However, despite its structural similarity to other antifolate drugs, LTG displays only weak antifolate activity. Furthermore, results from structure-activity studies suggest that there is little correlation between antifolate activity and anticonvulsant potency (14).

In some respects the preclinical profile of LTG is very similar to that observed with PHT and CBZ (Table 30-1). For example, LTG is active in the kindled rat and against tonic extension seizures in the MES test but is ineffective against sc PTZ–induced clonus (62, 71, 72). However, the preclinical profile of LTG differs significantly from that of PHT and CBZ in one important manner. LTG is effective in the *lh/lh* model of absence (9); whereas PHT and CBZ not only are ineffective but can, upon occasion, actually worsen spike-wave seizures (6, 8, Table 30-1). In this respect, the preclinical profile of LTG supports its clinical utility against partial, generalized tonic-clonic, and generalized absence seizures (73–75).

In in-vitro experiments, LTG selectively blocks veratrine-evoked but not potassium-evoked release of endogenous glutamate (76). These findings suggested that LTG, like PHT, acts at voltage-sensitive Na^+ channels to stabilize neuronal membranes (Table 30-2). Evidence favoring this mechanism includes the documented capacity of LTG to inhibit [^{3}H]batrachotoxin binding and veratrine-stimulated [^{14}C]guanidinium transport into synaptosomes (77, 78), its capacity to inhibit sustained repetitive firing (77), and its demonstrated concentration-dependent inhibition of Na^+ currents in mouse neuroblastoma cells (19). Effects of all three AEDs on Na^+ currents were voltage-dependent, and all three slowed recovery from inactivation.

However, as mentioned above, the clinical profile of LTG appears broader than would be expected based on this single mechanism. Given the lack of efficacy of other Na^+ channel blockers against generalized absence seizures, LTG's efficacy against this seizure type is likely unrelated to this mechanism, unless, as suggested by Coulter (40), LTG exerts an effect on a particular isoform of the brain Na^+ channel that either is anatomically involved in the generation of spike-wave discharges or is expressed in a way that is selectively altered in the thalamocortical circuitry of absence patients. LTG has been found to decrease voltage-gated Ca^{2+} currents (50). This effect may contribute to a decrease in neurotransmitter release and thereby contribute to its anticonvulsant action (Table 30-3). Additional investigations are required to resolve whether this effect contributes to the broader clinical profile of LTG versus that of PHT and CBZ.

Levetiracetam (LEV)

Levetiracetam (LEV; *(S)*-alpha-ethyl-*e*-oxo-pyrrolidine acetamide) is the *(S)*-enantiomer of the ethyl analog of the nootropic drug piracetam. Levetiracetam displays a unique preclinical profile in animal seizure and epilepsy models. For example, it was found to be inactive in the traditional MES and sc PTZ-seizure models but highly active against audiogenic and fully kindled partial seizures (79). Furthermore, LEV has been found to inhibit PTZ-induced spike-wave discharges (80) and spontaneous spike-wave discharges in the genetic absence epilepsy rat from Strasbourg (GAERS) (81). In addition, LEV decreases the afterdischarge duration in the amygdala-kindled rat and inhibits bicuculline-induced increase in hippocampal population spike amplitudes (82–85). Levetiracetam has also been found to be uniquely active in the 6-Hz psychomotor seizure model of pharmacoresistance (3). For example, at a current intensity equivalent to two times the current necessary to evoke a seizure, levetiracetam and valproate were the only two AEDs that retained their ability to block 6-Hz seizures, although there was a marked decrease in the potency of both drugs at two times the critical current needed to induce seizures in 97% of the population (CC_{97}) (3).

In in-vitro studies using rat hippocampal slices, LEV has also been observed to reduce the amplitude and number of repetitive population spikes induced by exposure to high K^+–low Ca^{2+} perfusion medium (86). LEV has also been found to inhibit bicuculline-induced bursts of action potentials and to decrease the frequency of NMDA-evoked bursting in hippocampal pyramidal neurons (87). Despite these observations, a unified molecular mechanism(s) has yet to be clearly defined. This is perhaps not so surprising given LEV's unique anticonvulsant profile. LEV has been demonstrated to bind to a specific, saturable, and stereoselective binding site in rat brain membranes that displays a high density in the hippocampus, cortex, and cerebellum (88). The finding that there is an excellent correlation between LEV binding and anticonvulsant activity in the audiogenic mouse suggests a possible functional role for the LEV binding site. Of the various actions that might be ascribed to LEV, its ability to modulate neuronal high-voltage Ca^{2+} currents (Tables 30-1 and 30-2) appears to be the one most likely to contribute to its ability to dampen neuronal hyperexcitability (89). At higher concentrations, LEV has also been found to prevent the negative modulatory effects of Zn^{2+} and beta-carbolines on GABA- and glycine-gated currents (90). These effects would be expected to prolong the hyperpolarization associated with GABA- and glycine-mediated neurotransmission. More recently, the LEV binding site has been found to be highly homologous with a novel site identified as synaptic vesicle protein 2A (SV2A) (91). The precise mechanism by which modulation of SV2A protein contributes to the anticonvulsant efficacy of LEV is not presently known. SV2A is an abundant protein that is closely associated with synaptic vesicles and is thereby thought to contribute to docking and release of neurotransmitter substances. Thus, it is highly possible that LEV, by binding to SV2A protein, modifies neurotransmitter release.

Oxcarbazepine (OCBZ)

Oxcarbazepine (10,11-dihydro-10-oxo-carbamazepine) is structurally related to CBZ (92). The keto substitution at the 10,11 position of the dibenzazepine nucleus does not affect the therapeutic profile of OCBZ but does contribute to better tolerability in humans (93–96). In vivo, OCBZ is rapidly and completely reduced to its active metabolite (10,11-dihydro-10-hydroxy-carbamazepine, HCBZ), which is thought to be responsible for the anticonvulsant action of OCBZ (97). HCBZ is a racemate that can be separated into two enantiomers, both of which appear to contribute to the anticonvulsant activity of HCBZ (98).

The anticonvulsant profile of OCBZ and HCBZ is virtually identical to that of CBZ (Table 30-1). For example, they are both active against tonic-extension seizures induced by MES and essentially inactive against clonic seizures induced by PTZ, picrotoxin, and strychnine (98, 99). Both compounds were found to possess activity against focal seizures in monkeys with chronic aluminum foci (97). In comparative clinical trials OCBZ was demonstrated to be as efficacious and better tolerated than CBZ (94–96). Clinically, OCBZ seems to represent a less toxic and equally efficacious alternative to CBZ that appears to exert its anticonvulsant effect through a similar mechanism of action. Furthermore, OCBZ appears to be highly efficacious and safe as a first-line treatment in adults with partial and generalized tonic-clonic seizures (100).

OCBZ, HCBZ, and CBZ all appear to share a similar mechanistic profile (Table 30-2). (101). OCBZ and HCBZ, like other drugs that block MES seizures, both block sustained repetitive firing in cultured spinal cord neurons in a voltage- and frequency-dependent manner (102). Additional results from electrophysiologic studies suggest that HCBZ may mediate some of its anticonvulsant effect through an action at high-threshold voltage-gated Ca^{2+} channels (50).

Pregabalin (PGB)

Pregabalin (*S*-(+)-3-isobutyl-gamma-aminobutyric acid) was approved for use as adjunctive therapy for the treatment of partial seizures in 2005. PGB is a structural analog of GABA, but, like the similar compound gabapentin, has no activity at either $GABA_A$ or $GABA_B$ receptors.

The preclinical profile of PGB revealed that it is more potent and bioavailable than gabapentin. In animal models of seizure activity, PGB effectively protects against tonic extension seizures induced by MES, clonic seizures induced by sc PTZ, and audiogenic seizures in the DBA/2 mouse (103). The ability of PGB to block kindled seizures accurately predicted that PGB would be effective against partial seizures. PGB was found to block bicuculline and strychnine-induced seizures only at high concentrations, and it was unable to block absence seizures in the GAERS rat.

Although it is known that PGB binds to the alpha$_2$delta_auxiliary subunit of the voltage-gated calcium channel, it is still not completely clear how it exerts its anticonvulsant activity. Recent work in cultured hippocampal neurons suggests that PGB may reduce spontaneous and evoked neurotransmitter release, most likely by targeting the readily releasable pool of synaptic vesicles (104).

Topiramate (TPM)

Topiramate, 2,3:4,5-bis-O-(1-methylethylidene)-beta-D-fructopyranose sulfamate, is a chemically novel AED. In animal tests, the anticonvulsant profile of TPM most closely approximates those of PHT, CBZ, and LTG. For example, it is active against MES-induced tonic extension seizures. TPM does not prevent seizures induced by sc PTZ; however, it does elevate the seizure threshold for PTZ-induced seizures (105, 106). In the amygdala-kindled rat, TPM reduced both the seizure score and the afterdischarge duration of fully expressed kindled seizures (107) and, with pretreatment, appears to delay the acquisition of kindling (108). This latter effect suggests an antiepileptic vs purely anticonvulsant effect. In the spontaneously epileptic rat, which displays both tonic extension seizures and absence-like spike-wave discharges, TPM was as effective as PHT in reducing tonic extensions and, like ESM, decreased the duration of spike-wave discharges in a dose- and time-dependent fashion (109, Table 30-1). Furthermore, topiramate has been shown to be effective in the GAERS model of absence epilepsy (110). These findings support the apparent broad clinical profile that has emerged for TPM. For example, it appears to be effective against a broad range of seizure types, including partial and generalized tonic-clonic seizures (Table 30-1). In addition, TPM was recently approved for the prophylactic treatment of migraines, further indication of its broad spectrum activity in the CNS. Anecdotal reports have suggested that TPM may be effective against uncomplicated absence seizures, an action supported by findings in the spontaneously epileptic rat (109) but not the *lh/lh* mouse (9).

In studies conducted thus far, TPM has been found to possess multiple potential mechanisms of action ((105, 111, Table 30-2). In cultured hippocampal neurons, therapeutic concentrations (3–30 μM) of TPM inhibit sustained repetitive firing in a use- and concentration-dependent manner (112) and reduce voltage-activated Na^+ currents in cultured neocortical neurons (113).

TPM has also been shown to reduce kainate-evoked inward currents, block kainate-evoked cobalt influx, and block kainic acid receptor-mediated postsynaptic currents in the amygdala, indicating that TPM has antagonistic effects on the kainate/AMPA subtype of glutamate receptor (114–116). The effect of TPM on kainate-evoked currents appears to be unique to TPM among the new AEDs, is consistent with a decrease in neuronal excitability and may, when coupled with its effects against Na^+ currents, contribute to its efficacy against partial and generalized convulsive seizures.

Effects at the Na^+ channel and AMPA/kainate receptor do not necessarily support the ability of TPM to block absence-like spike-wave discharges in the spontaneously epileptic rat and anecdotal reports suggesting efficacy against generalized absence epilepsy. TPM has been reported to enhance GABA-evoked chloride single-channel currents in cultured neocortical neurons (117, 118). Kinetic analysis of single-channel recordings from excised outside-out patches demonstrated that TPM increased the frequency of channel opening and the burst frequency but was without effect on open-channel duration or burst duration. This effect of TPM on $GABA_A$ channel activity was similar to that observed with BZDs; however, the ability of TPM to enhance $GABA_A$-evoked current was not reversed by the BZD antagonist flumazenil. Although consistent with TPM's ability to block spike-wave discharges and its apparent efficacy against absence epilepsy, enhancement of GABA-mediated inhibition would not be predicted from previous in-vitro studies in which TPM did not displace radiolabeled ligand binding to known binding sites on $GABA_A$ receptors (106).

In other preclinical studies, TPM was shown to inhibit certain carbonic anhydrase isoforms, an activity that may, through an alteration of HCO_3 homeostasis, contribute to TPM's mechanism of action (119). Topiramate has also been reported to hyperpolarize hippocampal neurons reversibly in rat hippocampal slices (120) and to inhibit neuronal repetitive firing in rat olfactory cortical neurons by inducing a slow outward membrane current. Both of these effects are thought to be the result of activating an outward current carried by K^+ ions (120, 121). Furthermore, TPM has been observed to decrease high-voltage activated Ca^{2+} currents (HVACC) in CA1 pyramidal (122). This effect at both L- and non L-type Ca^{2+} channels required a short preincubation period.

The results to date suggest that the effects of TPM on Na^+ channels, $GABA_A$ receptors, HVACC, and AMPA/kainate receptors are unique as compared to prototypical modulators of these processes. For example, TPM's effects on all four of these protein complexes can be highly variable. TPM has been observed to produce both immediate and delayed effects; sometimes its effect is reversible and sometimes it is not; in some preparations TPM's action appears to be dependent on the age of neurons in culture. All of these observations, albeit frustrating, are suggestive of a unique interaction with a target protein that may be dependent in part on its molecular structure. Indeed, recent results suggest that the effects of TPM, at least on $GABA_A$ receptor function, depend on the expression of specific subunits (123). Clearly, additional studies are required to elucidate its precise mechanism of action further.

Tiagabine (TGB)

Tiagabine, (R)-N-(4,4-di-(3-methyl-thien-2-yl)but-3-enyl) nipecotic acid hydrochloride, is a selective GABA uptake inhibitor (Table 30-3) that emerged from a mechanistic-based drug discovery program designed to identify lipophilic GABA uptake inhibitors for the treatment of epilepsy (124).

In animals, TGB is effective against several types of chemically induced seizures, including methyl-6, 7-dimethoxy-4-ethyl-beta-carboline-3-carboxylate (DMCM)-induced clonic seizures and sc PTZ-induced tonic (potent inhibitor) and clonic (partial inhibitor) seizures (124, Table 30-1). TGB reduced both seizure severity and afterdischarge duration in the amygdala-kindled rat, was active against audiogenic seizures in DBA/2 mice, and was only partially effective against photically induced myoclonus in the photosensitive baboon. However, it is active in the MES test, but only at doses two- to three-fold higher than that producing motor impairment. TGB, like VGB, also worsens spike-wave discharges in the GAERS, GBL, and *lh/lh* models of absence (9).

In-vitro studies have shown TGB to be a potent inhibitor of neuronal and glial GABA uptake (124, Table 30-2). TGB binds selectively and reversibly to the GAT-1 GABA uptake carrier of both glia and neurons, but it does not stimulate GABA release. It is ineffective at other receptor-binding and uptake sites evaluated to date, including the glutamate receptor, Na^+, and Ca^{2+} channels. Inhibition of GABA uptake by TGB leads to increased synaptic concentrations of GABA and a consequent enhancement and prolongation of GABA-mediated inhibitory neurotransmission, an effect that is assumed to be the basis of TGB's anticonvulsant activity against partial seizures and its ability to aggravate spike-wave seizures in rodents and, potentially, humans. Indeed, TGB treatment has been demonstrated to increase extracellular fluid GABA levels in vivo in both animal (125) and human brains (126). The mechanism of its proconvulsive action is probably much like that of VGB (see following paragraphs) in that elevated synaptic concentrations of GABA at the level of the thalamus are thought to potentiate $GABA_B$ -mediated slow after-hyperpolarization, which leads to enhanced deinactivation of T-currents and increased amplification of thalamocortical rhythms necessary to support spike-wave discharges.

Vigabatrin (VGB)

Vigabatrin (4-amino-5-hexenoic acid or gamma-vinyl GABA), is available in Europe, Mexico, and Canada for the treatment of partial seizures. In experimental seizure models, VGB is active in photosensitive baboons, strychnine- and sound-induced seizures, and amygdala kindling. VGB is essentially inactive in the MES test and in DMCM-induced clonic seizures and worsens spike-wave seizures in the *lh/lh* mouse and GAERS rat (9, 12, 14, 127). Further, direct injection of VGB into the median part of the lateral thalamus of GAERS significantly increased the cumulative duration of spike-and-wave discharges (128, 129). VGB's anticonvulsant activity in the kindled rat and worsening of spike-wave seizures in the *lh/lh* mouse and GAERS correlate well with its clinical utility against partial seizures and its potential exacerbation of spike-wave seizures, respectively.

VGB, a close structural analog of GABA, arose from a synthesis program designed to develop molecules that target GABA alpha-oxoglutarate transaminase (GABA-T; EC 2.6.1.19), the enzyme responsible for GABA metabolism. VGB binds to GABA-T and permanently inactivates the enzyme, thereby increasing brain GABA levels and enhancing GABAergic neurotransmission (Table 30-2). VGB administration to laboratory animals produces a prolonged, dose-related inhibition of GABA-T and corresponding elevation of whole-brain GABA levels (130, 131). An increase in all brain regions examined was observed; however, quantitative differences between brain regions were noted (132). Likewise, in human studies VGB produces a dose-dependent increase in cerebrospinal fluid GABA levels (133–135). In animal studies, there does appear to be a preferential increase in the GABA concentration in the synaptosomal pool over the nonsynaptosomal pool (136). Thus, VGB treatment leads to an increased amount of presynaptic GABA available for release, which indirectly leads to increased GABAergic activity at postsynaptic GABA receptors.

The consequent increased activity of GABA on postsynaptic GABA receptors results in increased inhibition of neurons involved in seizure activity and represents the most likely basis for VGB's clinical activity against partial seizures. The same mechanism that affords efficacy in partial seizures likely contributes to aggravation of generalized absence seizures (9, 40, 123). For example, increased GABA release in the thalamus will lead to a greater activation of $GABA_B$ receptors. Enhanced $GABA_B$ receptor activation leads to a prolonged hyperpolarization and subsequent deinactivation of T-type Ca^{2+} currents, which contribute to the synchronized burst firing of thalamocortical neurons.

Unfortunately, vigabatrin use has been associated with an irreversible visual field defects in both children and adults; see Ben-Menachem 2002 (137) for review and references. Unfortunately the emergence of this idiosyncratic adverse event has had a significant impact on the use of this very effective AED in children with infantile spasms.

Zonisamide (ZNS)

Zonisamide (1,2-benzisoxazole-3-methanesulfonamide) was discovered as a result of routine biological screening of 1,2-benzisoxazole derivatives. ZNS possesses a broad anticonvulsant profile in animal seizure models (14, 138; Table 30-1). It blocks MES seizures in a number of different species and restricts the spread of focal cortical seizures in cats. In addition, ZNS blocked tonic extension seizures in spontaneous epileptic rats and audiogenic seizures in DBA/2 mice (109). In cats and rats, ZNS also suppresses focal seizure activity induced by cortical freezing and tungstic acid gel, respectively. Moreover, in hippocampal-kindled rats, amygdala-kindled rats, and cats ZNS suppresses subcortically evoked seizures. In geniculate-kindled cats, ZNS decreases photically induced myoclonus. In the spontaneous epileptic rat, ZNS did not affect spike-wave discharges (109). Clinically, ZNS appears to possess efficacy against a number of seizure types including partial and secondarily generalized seizures, generalized tonic-clonic, generalized tonic, atypical absence, atonic, and myoclonic seizures (138).

ZNS's broad anticonvulsant profile can likely be accounted for by a similarly broad mechanistic profile (Table 30-2). For example, it blocks sustained repetitive firing in cultured spinal cord neurons (139) through an effect on voltage-sensitive Na^+ channels (140). In voltage-clamped *Myxicola* giant axons, ZNS, like PHT, CBZ, and LTG, appears to retard recovery from fast and slow Na^+ channel inactivation and produces a hyperpolarizing shift in the steady-state inactivation curve. ZNS has also been demonstrated to reduce voltage-dependent T-type calcium currents in cultured neurons (141) and neuroblastoma cells (142). ZNS also appears to modulate GABA-mediated inhibition. For example, ZNS has been reported to decrease (^{3}H)flunitrazepam and (^{3}H)muscimol binding to the BZD and $GABA_A$ receptors, respectively. Similarly, (^{3}H)ZNS binding to rat whole brain membranes is reduced by clonazepam and enhanced by GABA (143). In contrast, ZNS did not affect ion currents evoked by iontophoretically applied GABA (139). Obviously, additional experiments are required to resolve this apparent discrepancy.

Effects on voltage-sensitive Na^+ channels are likely to contribute to ZNS's ability to block MES-induced tonic extension in animals and generalized tonic seizures in humans, whereas effects on low voltage-activated T currents and perhaps GABA receptors are more likely to correlate with its efficacy against generalized absence and myoclonic seizures, respectively.

CONCLUSIONS

In recent years, an improved understanding of the mechanisms associated with epileptiform events and the anticonvulsant activity of AEDs has contributed to the synthesis of new AEDs specifically designed to reduce excitation or to enhance inhibition. This mechanistic approach has been successful in identifying two new drugs that modify GABA-mediated inhibition by either blocking reuptake of synaptically released GABA (i.e., TGB) or inhibiting metabolism of neuronal and glial GABA (i.e., VGB). In addition, knowledge that the binding site for gabapentin (i.e., alpha$_2$delta auxiliary subunit of the voltage-gated calcium channel) correlated with its anticonvulsant profile led to the search for more potent analogs and the subsequent development of pregabalin. These three examples clearly support the validity of the mechanistic approach.

Unfortunately, at the excitatory synapse, the mechanistic approach has been less successful, despite an extensive understanding of the processes underlying excitatory neurotransmission. For example, the drugs developed thus far to target specifically the NMDA-preferring glutamate receptor have not only lacked efficacy in the limited clinical trials conducted to date but have also resulted in intolerable side effects (144). Increased understanding of the molecular biology of not only the NMDA, but also the AMPA and kainate receptors may ultimately lead to the development of selective, less toxic, and clinically efficacious glutamate antagonists. To this point, both felbamate and topiramate demonstrate that a drug that modulates activity at these two molecular targets can be clinically useful for the treatment of patients.

Many of the new AEDs appear to act through a combination of mechanisms that likely extend beyond effects on Na^+ and Ca^{2+} channels and GABA receptors. However, these effects alone are probably not sufficient to account for the apparent efficacy of the newer AEDs in highly refractory seizure patients. Two of the newer drugs (FBM and TPM) appear to possess a unique ability to inhibit glutamate-mediated neurotransmission through an effect on NMDA (FBM) and AMPA/kainate (TPM) receptors. The finding that these drugs limit glutamatergic neurotransmission without producing the typical behavioral disturbances associated with selective glutamate antagonists may suggest that they target a different glutamate receptor subtype. Newly developed molecular biologic techniques will undoubtedly make it possible to address this issue in the future.

Mechanisms of action beyond those discussed are likely to contribute to the underlying efficacy of the new AEDs. The continued search to understand the molecular mode of action of the available drugs thoroughly will indirectly provide important information concerning the underlying causes of seizure disorders. Ultimately the results obtained from these and other studies will continue to assist in the rational design of newer, more effective, and less toxic drugs.

It is worth noting that several investigated AEDs are currently winding their way through the development process and that some of these are likely to come into use in the next few years. Many of these drugs share a similar mechanistic profile with the marketed AEDs. On the other hand, the molecular mechanism of a few of these AEDs has yet to be defined. It is strongly hoped that the "inability" to define a specific mechanism to a given drug would translate into the development of a novel therapy with improved efficacy over the established AEDs.

Perhaps equally important is the finding that several of the drugs in development have been found to prevent neuronal damage secondary to an acute brain insult. It is possible that this action may one day lead to the development of a "disease-modifying" therapy that slows, halts, or prevents the development of epilepsy in the susceptible individual. Such a therapy would be a major leap forward for the patient with newly diagnosed epilepsy, or even the person at risk for developing epilepsy. The challenges associated with the development of a disease-modifying therapeutic are immense, but worthy of pursuit. Last, it is likely that we will eventually identify novel drugs that not only inhibit acute seizures but also interfere with the pathologic processes that underlie the development of drug-resistant epilepsy. Only at that point will we be able to conclude the search for the ideal AED.

References

1. Putnam TJ, Merritt HH. Experimental determination of the anticonvulsant properties of some phenyl derivatives. *Science* 1937; 85:525–526.
2. White HS, Wolf HH, Woodhead JH, Kupferberg HJ, et al. The National Institutes of Health anticonvulsant drug development program: screening for efficacy. In: French J, Leppik I, Dichter MA, eds. *Antiepileptic Drug Development.* Advances in Neurology 76. Philadelphia: Lippincott-Raven Publishers, 1998:29–39.
3. Barton ME, Klein BD, Wolf HH, White HS. Pharmacological characterization of the 6 Hz psychomotor seizure model of partial epilepsy. *Epilepsy Res* 2001; 47(3):217–227.
4. Loscher W, Honack D, Fassbender CP, Nolting B. The role of technical, biological and pharmacological factors in the laboratory evaluation of anticonvulsant drugs. 3. Pentylenetetrazole seizure models. *Epilepsy Res* 1991; 8(3):171–189.
5. Snead OC. Pharmacological models of generalized absence seizures in rodents. *J Neural Transm* 1992; 35:7–19.
6. Marescaux C, Vergnes M. Genetic absence epilepsy in rats from Strasbourg (GAERS). *Ital J Neurol Sci* 1995; 16:113–118.
7. Hosford DA, Clark S, Cao Z, Wilson WA Jr, et al. The role of $GABA_B$ receptor activation in absence seizures of *lethargic (lh/lh)* mice. *Science* 1992; 257:398–401.
8. Mattson RH. General principles: selection of antiepileptic drug therapy. In: Levy RH, Mattson RH, Meldrum BS, eds. *Antiepileptic Drugs.* 4th ed. New York: Raven Press, 1995:123–135.
9. Hosford DA, Wang Y, Utility of the lethargic (lh/lh) mouse model of absence seizures in predicting the effects of lamotrigine, vigabatrin, tiagabine, gabapentin, and topiramate against human absence seizures. *Epilepsia* 1997; 38(4):408–414.
10. Macdonald RL, Kelly KM. *Antiepileptic Drug Mechanisms of Action. Epilepsia* 1995; 36(Suppl 2):S2–S12.
11. Swinyard EA, Woodhead JH, White HS, Franklin MR. General principles: Experimental selection, quantification, and evaluation of anticonvulsants. In: Levy R, Driefuss FE, Mattson R, Meldrum B, et al, eds. *Antiepileptic Drugs.* 3rd ed. New York: Raven Press, 1989:85–102.
12. White HS. Mechanisms of antiepileptic drugs. In Porter R, Chadwick D, eds. *Epilepsies II*, Boston: Butterworth-Heinemann, 1997:1–30.
13. Chapman AA, Croucher MJ, Meldrum BS. Evaluation of anticonvulsant drugs in DBA/2 mice with sound-induced seizures. *Arzneim Forsch/Drug Res* 1984; 34(II, No. 10):1261–1264.
14. Rogawski MA, Porter RJ. Antiepileptic drugs: pharmacological mechanisms and clinical efficacy with consideration of promising developmental stage compounds. *Pharmacol Rev* 1990; 42:223–286.
15. Macdonald RL, Meldrum BS. General principles. Principles of antiepileptic drug action. In: Levy RH, Mattson RH, Meldrum BS, eds. *Antiepileptic Drugs.* 4th ed. New York: Raven Press, 1995:61–77.
16. Meldrum B. Action of established and novel anticonvulsant drugs on the basic mechanisms of epilepsy. *Epilepsy Res* 1996; 11 Suppl.:67–77.
17. Piredda SG, Woodhead JH, Swinyard EA. Effect of stimulus intensity on the profile of anticonvulsant activity of phenytoin, ethosuximide and valproate. *J Pharmacol Exp Ther* 1985; 232(3):741–745.
18. White HS, Johnson M, Wolf HH, Kupferberg HJ. The early identification of anticonvulsant activity: role of the maximal electroshock and subcutaneous pentylenetetrazol seizure models. *Ital J Neurol Sci* 1995; 16:73–77.
19. Lang DG, Wang CM, Cooper BR. Lamotrigine, phenytoin and carbamazepine interactions on the sodium current present in N4TG1 mouse neuroblastoma cells. *J Pharmacol Exp Ther* 1993; 266(2):829–835.
20. Willow M, Catterall WA. Inhibition of binding of [^{2}H]batrachotoxinin A20-a-benzoate to sodium channels by the anticonvulsant drugs diphenylhydantoin and carbamazepine. *Mol Pharmacol* 1982; 22:627–635.
21. Willow M, Kuenzel EA, and Catterall WA. Inhibition of voltage-sensitive sodium channels in neuroblastoma cells and synaptosomes by the anticonvulsant drugs diphenylhydantoin and carbamazepine. *Mol Pharmacol* 1984; 25:228–234.
22. Schwarz JR, and Grigat G. Phenytoin and carbamazepine: potential- and frequency-dependent block of Na currents in mammalian myelinated nerve fibers. *Epilepsia* 1989; 30:286–294.
23. Tomaselli G, Marban E, Yellen G. Sodium channels from human brain RNA expressed in *Xenopus* oocytes: basic electrophysiologic characteristics and their modifications by diphenylhydantoin. *J Clin Invest* 1989; 83:1724–1732.
24. Wakamori M, Kaneda M, Oyama Y, Akaike N. Effects of chlordiazepoxide, chlorpromazine, diazepam, diphenylhydantoin, flunitrazepam and haloperidol on the voltage-dependent sodium current of isolated mammalian brain neurons. *Brain Res* 1989; 494:374–378.
25. White HS, Woodhead JH, Franklin MR, Swinyard EA, et al. General principles: Experimental selection, quantification, and evaluation of antiepileptic drugs. In: Levy RH, Mattson RH, Meldrum BS, eds. *Antiepileptic Drugs.* 4th ed. New York: Raven Press, 1995:99–110.
26. Coulter DA, Hugenard JR, and Prince DA. Characterization of ethosuximide reduction of low threshold calcium current in thalamic neurons. *Ann Neurol* 1989; 25:582–593.
27. Coulter DA, Hugenard JR, Prince DA. Differential effects of petit mal anticonvulsants and convulsants on thalamic neurones: calcium current reduction. *Br J Pharmacol* 1990; 100:800–806.
28. Van Dongen AMJ, Van Erp MG, Voskuyl RA. Valproate reduces excitability by blockage of sodium and potassium conductance. *Epilepsia* 1986; 27(3):177–182.
29. Zona C, Avoli M. Effects induced by the antiepileptic drug valproic acid upon the ionic currents recorded in rat neocortical neurons in cell culture. *Exp Brain Res* 1990; 81:313–317.
30. Van den Berg RJ, Kok P, and Voskuyl RA. Valproate and sodium currents in cultured hippocampal neurons. *Exp Brain Res* 1993; 93:279–287.
31. Kelly KM, Gross RA, Macdonald RL. Valproic acid selectively reduces the low-threshold (T) calcium in rat nodose neurons. *Neurosci Lett* 1990; 116:233–238.
32. Macdonald RL, Olsen RW, $GABA_A$ receptor channels. *Annu Rev Neurosci* 1994; 17:569–602.
33. Rogers CJ, Twyman RE, Macdonald RL. Benzodiazepine and β-carboline regulation of single $GABA_A$ receptor channels of mouse spinal neurones in culture. *J Physiol* 1994; 475:69–82.
34. Study RE, Barker JL. Diazepam and (-)-pentobarbital: fluctuation analysis reveals different mechanisms for potentiation of gamma-aminobutyric acid responses in cultured central neurons. *Proc Natl Acad Sci U S A* 1981; 78:7180–7184.
35. Twyman RE, Rogers CJ, Macdonald RL. Differential regulation of gamma-aminobutyric acid receptor channels by diazepam and phenobarbital. *Ann Neurol* 1989; 25:213–220.
36. Vicini S, Mienville JM, Costa E. Actions of benzodiazepine and β-carboline derivatives on gamma-aminobutyric acid-activated Cl-channels recorded from membrane patches of neonatal rat cortical neurons in culture. *J Pharmacol Exp Ther* 1987; 243:1195–1201.
37. Moss SJ, Smart TA, Porter NM, et al. Cloned GABA receptors are maintained in a stable cell line: allosteric and channel properties. *Eur J Pharmacol* 1990; 189:177–188.
38. Verdoorn TA, Draguhn A, Ymer S, Seeburg PH, et al. Functional properties of recombinant rat $GABA_A$ receptors depend upon subunit composition. *Neuron* 1990; 4(919–928).

39. Pritchett DB, Sontheimer H, Shivers BD, Ymer S, et al. Importance of a novel $GABA_A$ receptor subunit for benzodiazepine pharmacology. *Nature* 1989; 338:582–584.
40. Coulter DA. Antiepileptic drug cellular mechanisms of action: Where does lamotrigine fit in? *J Child Neurol* 1997; 12(Suppl 1):S2–S9.
41. Swinyard EA, Sofia RD, Kupferberg HJ. Comparative anticonvulsant activity and neurotoxicity of felbamate and four prototype antiepileptic drugs in mice and rats. *Epilepsia* 1986; 27:27–34.
42. White HS, Wolf HH, Swinyard EA, Skeen GA, et al. A neuropharmacological evaluation of felbamate as a novel anticonvulsant. *Epilepsia* 1992; 33:564–572.
43. Sofia RD. Felbamate. Mechanisms of action. In: Levy RH, Mattson RH, Meldrum BS, eds. *Antiepileptic Drugs*. 4th ed. New York: Raven Press, 1995:791–797.
44. Wlaz P, Loscher W. Anticonvulsant activity of felbamate in amygdala kindling model of temporal lobe epilepsy in rats. *Epilepsia* 1997; 38(11):1167–1172.
45. Wallis RA, Panizzon KL, Fairchild MD, Wasterlain CG. Protective effects of felbamate against hypoxia in the rat hippocampal slice. *Stroke* 1992; 23:547–551.
46. Wasterlain CG, Adams LM, Hattori H, Schwartz PH. Felbamate reduces hypoxic-ischemic brain damage in vivo. *Eur J Pharmacol* 1992; 212:275–278.
47. Wasterlain CG, Adams LM, Schwartz PH, Hattori H, et al. Post-hypoxic treatment with felbamate is neuroprotective in a rat model of hypoxia-ischemia. *Neurology* 1994; 43:2303–2310.
48. Chronopoulos A, Stafstrom C, Thurber S, Hyde P, et al. Neuroprotective effect of felbamate after kainic acid-induced status epilepticus. *Epilepsia* 1993; 34(2):359–366.
49. Pisani A, Stefani A, Siniscalchi A, Mercuri NB, et al. Electrophysiological actions of felbamate on rat striatal neurones. *Br J Pharmacol* 1995; 116(3):2053–2061.
50. Stefani A, Spadoni F, Bernardi G. Voltage-activated calcium channels: targets of antiepileptic drug therapy? *Epilepsia* 1997; 38(9):959–965.
51. McCabe RT, Wasterlain CG, Kucharczyk N, Sofia RD, et al. Evidence for anticonvulsant and neuroprotectant action of felbamate mediated by strychnine-insensitive glycine receptors. *J Pharmacol Exp Ther* 1993; 264(3):1248–1252.
52. Wamsley JK, Sofia RD, Faull RLM, Narang N, et al. Interaction of felbamate with [^{3}H]DCKA-labeled strychnine-insensitive glycine receptors in human postmortem brain. *Exp Neurol* 1994; 129:244–250.
53. Wallis RA, Panizzon KL Glycine reversal of felbamate hypoxic protection. *Neuroreport* 1993; 4(7):951–954.
54. White HS, Harmsworth WL, Sofia RD, Wolf HH. Felbamate modulates the strychnine-insensitive glycine receptor. *Epilepsy Res* 1995; 20:41–48.
55. Coffin V, Cohen-Williams M, Barnett A, Selective antagonism of the anticonvulsant effects of felbamate by glycine. *Eur J Pharmacol* 1994; 256:R9–R10.
56. De Sarro G, Ongini E, Bertorelli R, Aguglia U, et al. Excitatory amino acid neurotransmission through both NMDA and non-NMDA receptors is involved in the anticonvulsant activity of felbamate in DBA/2 mice. *Eur J Pharmacol* 1994; 262:11–19.
57. Rho JM, Donevan DC, Rogawski MA. Mechanism of action of the anticonvulsant felbamate: Opposing effects on NMDA and $GABA_A$ receptors. *Ann Neurol* 1994; 35:229–234.
58. Ticku MK, Kamatchi GL, Sofia RD. Effect of anticonvulsant felbamate on $GABA_A$ receptor system. *Epilepsia* 1991; 32(3):389–391.
59. Pennell PB, Ogaily MS, Macdonald RL. Aplastic anemia in a patient receiving felbamate for partial seizures. *Neurology* 1995; 45:456–460.
60. Schmidt B. Potential antiepileptic drugs: gabapentin. In: Levy R, Driefuss FE, Mattson R, Meldrum B, et al, eds. *Antiepileptic Drugs*. 3rd ed. New York: Raven Press, 1989: 925–935.
61. Taylor CP. Gabapentin. Mechanisms of action. In: Levy RH, Mattson RH, Meldrum BS, eds. *Antiepileptic Drugs*. 4th ed. New York: Raven Press, 1995:829–841.
62. Dalby NO, Nielsen EB. Comparison of the preclinical anticonvulsant profiles of tiagabine, lamotrigine, gabapentin and vigabatrin. *Epilepsy Res* 1997; 28:63–72.
63. Bartoszyk GD, Meyerson N, Reimann W, Satzinger G, et al. Gabapentin. In Meldrum BS, Porter RJ, eds. *Current Problems in Epilepsy: New Anticonvulsant Drugs*. London: John Libbey, 1986:147:164.
64. Taylor CP, Gee NS, Su T-Z, Kocsis JD, et al. A summary of mechanistic hypotheses of gabapentin pharmacology. *Epilepsy Res* 1998; 29:233–249.
65. Petroff, OAC, Rothman DL, Behar KL, Lamoureux D, et al. Gabapentin increases brain gamma-aminobutyric acid levels in patients with epilepsy. *Ann Neurol* 1995; 38:295–296.
66. Wamil AW, McLean MJ. Limitation by gabapentin of high frequency action potential firing by mouse central neurons in cell culture. *Epilepsy Res* 1994; 17:1–11.
67. Welty DF, Schielke GP, Vartanian MG, Taylor CP. Gabapentin anticonvulsant action in rats: disequilibrium with peak drug concentrations in plasma and brain microdialysate. *Epilepsy Res* 1993; 16:175–181.
68. Gee NS, Brown JP, Dissanayake VUK, Offord J, et al. The novel anticonvulsant drug gabapentin (Neurontin), binds to the $\alpha_2\delta$ subunit of a calcium channel. *J Biol Chem* 1996; 271:5768–5776.
69. Reynolds EH, Milner G, Matthews DM, Chanarin I. Anticonvulsant therapy, megaloblastic haemopoiesis and folic acid metabolism. *Q J Med* 1966; 35:521–537.
70. Hommes OR, Obbens EAMT. The epileptogenic action of sodium folate in the rat. *J Neurol Sci* 1972; 20:269–272.
71. Wheatley P, Miller AA. Effects of lamotrigine on electrically induced after discharge duration in anaesthetised rat, dog and marmoset. *Epilepsia* 1989; 30:34–40.
72. Miller AA, Wheatley P, Sawyer DA, Baxter MG, et al. Pharmacological studies on lamotrigine, a novel potential antiepileptic drug, I: anticonvulsant profile in mice and rats. *Epilepsia* 1986; 27:483–489.
73. Leach JP, Brodie MJ. Lamotrigine. Clinical Use. In: Levy RH, Mattson RH, Meldrum BS, eds. *Antiepileptic Drugs*. 4th ed. New York: Raven Press, 1995:889–895.
74. Yuen AWC. Lamotrigine: a review of antiepileptic efficacy. *Epilepsia* 1994; 35(Suppl 5): S33–S36.
75. Buchanan N. Lamotrigine in the treatment of absence seizures. *Acta Neurol Scand* 1995; 92:348.
76. Leach MJ, Marden CM, and Miller AA. Pharmacological studies on lamotrigine, a novel potential antiepileptic drug, II: neurochemical studies on the mechanism of action. *Epilepsia* 1986; 27:490–497.
77. Cheung H, Kamp D, Harris E. An in vitro investigation of the action of lamotrigine on neuronal voltage-activated sodium channels. *Epilepsy Res* 1992; 13(2):107–112.
78. Riddall DR, Clackers M, and Leach MJ. Correlation of inhibition of veratrine evoked [^{14}C]guanidine uptake with inhibition of veratrine evoked release of glutamate by lamotrigine and its analogues. *Can J Neurol Sci* 1993; 20(Suppl 4):S181.
79. Margineanu DG, Klitgaard H. Levetiracetam: Mechanisms of action. In: Levy RH, Mattson RH, Meldrum BS, Perucca E, eds. *Antiepileptic Drugs*. 5th ed. Philadelphia: Lippincott Williams & Wilkins, 2002:419–427.
80. Gower AJ, Noyer M, Verloes R, Gobert J, et al. ucb L059, a novel anti-convulsant drug: pharmacological profile in animals. *Eur J Pharmacol* 1992; 222(2–3):193–203.
81. Gower AJ, Hirsch E, Boehrer A, Noyer M, et al. Effects of levetiracetam, a novel antiepileptic drug, on convulsant activity in two genetic rat models of epilepsy. *Epilepsy Res* 1995; 22(3):207–213.
82. Loscher W, Honack D, Rundfeldt C. Antiepileptic effects of the novel anticonfulsant levetiracetam (ucb L059) in the kindling model of temporal lobe epilepsy. J Pharmacol *Exp Ther* 1998 Feb;284(2):474–479.
83. Loscher W, Honack D. Profile of ucb L059, a novel anticonvulsant drug, in models of partial and generalized epilepsy in mice and rats. *Eur J Pharmacol* 1993 Mar;232 (2–3):147–258.
84. Margineanu DG, Wülfert E. ucb L059, a novel anticonvulsant, reduces bicuculline-induced hyperexcitability in rat hippocampal CA3 in vivo. *Eur J Pharmacol* 1995; 286:321–325.
85. Margineanu DG, Wülfert E. Inhibition by levetiracetam of a non-GABAA receptor-associated epileptiform effect of biculline in rat hippocampus. *Br J Pharmacol* 1997; 122:1146–1150.
86. Margineanu DG, Klitgaard H. Inhibition of neuronal hypersynchrony in vitro differentiates levetiracetam from classical antiepileptic drugs. *Pharmacol Res* 2000; 42(4): 281–285.
87. Birnstiel S, Wulfert E, Beck SG. Levetiracetam (ucb LO59) affects in vitro models of epilepsy in CA3 pyramidal neurons without altering normal synaptic transmission. *Naunyn Schmiedebergs Arch Pharmacol* 1997; 356(5):611–618.
88. Noyer M, Gillard M, Matagne A, Henichart JP, et al. The novel antiepileptic drug levetiracetam (ucb L059) appears to act via a specific binding site in CNS membranes. *Eur J Pharmacol* 1995; 286(2):137–146.
89. Niespodziany I, Klitgaard H, Margineanu DG. Levetiracetam inhibits the high-voltage-activated Ca(2+) current in pyramidal neurones of rat hippocampal slices. *Neurosci Lett* 2001; 306(1–2):5–8.
90. Rigo JM, Hans G, Nguyen L, Rocher V, et al. The anti-epileptic drug levetiracetam reverses the inhibition by negative allosteric modulators of neuronal GABA- and glycine-gated currents. *Br J Pharmacol* 2002; 136(5):659–672.
91. Lynch BA, Lambeng N, Nocka K, Kensel-Hammes P, et al. The synaptic vesicle protein SV2A is the binding site for the antiepileptic drug levetiracetam. *Proc Natl Acad Sci U S A* 2004; 101(26):9861–9866.
92. Dam M, Ostergaard LH. Other antiepileptic drugs. oxcarbazepine. In: Levy RH, Mattson RH, Meldrum BS, eds. *Antiepileptic Drugs*. 4th ed. New York: Raven Press, 1995:987–995.
93. Gram L, Philbert A. Oxcarbazepine. In: Meldrum BS, Porter RJ, eds. *New Anticonvulsant Drugs*. London: John Libbey & Co., 1986:229–235.
94. Houtkooper MA, Lammertsma A, Meyer JMA. Oxcarbazepine (GP 47.680): a possible alternative to carbamazepine? *Epilepsia* 1987; 28:693–698.
95. Reinikainen KJ, Keranen T, Halonen T, Komulainen H, et al. Comparison of oxcarbazepine and carbamazepine: a double-blind study. *Epilepsy Res* 1987; 1:284–289.
96. Dam M, Ekberg R, Loyning Y, Waltimo O, et al. A double-blind study comparing oxcarbazepine and carbamazepine in patients with newly diagnosed, previously untreated epilepsy. *Epilepsy Res* 1989; 3:70–76.
97. Jensen PK, Gram L, Schmutz M, Oxcarbazepine. *Epilepsy Res* 1991; 3:135–140.
98. Schmutz M, Ferret T, Heckendorn R, Jeker A, et al. GP 47779, the main human metabolite of oxcarbazepine (Trileptal), and both enantiomers have equal anticonvulsant activity. *Epilepsia* 1993; 34(Suppl 2):122.
99. Baltzer V, and Schmutz M. Experimental anticonvulsant properties of GP 47680 and of MHD, its main human metabolite: compounds related to carbamazepine. Meinardi H, Rowan AJ, eds. In: *Advances in Epileptology*. Amsterdam: Swets & Zeitlinger BV, 1978:295–299.
100. Christe W, Kramer G, Vigonius U, Pohlmann H, et al. A double-blind controlled clinical trial: oxcarbazepine versus sodium valproate in adults with newly diagnosed epilepsy. *Epilepsy Res* 1997; 26(3):451–460.
101. McLean MJ, Schmutz M, Wamil AW, Olpe H-R, et al. Oxcarbazepine: mechanisms of action. *Epilepsia* 1994; 35(Suppl 3):S5–S9.
102. Wamil AW, Porter C, Jensen PK, Schmutz M, et al. Oxcarbazepine and its monohydroxy metabolite limit action potential firing by mouse central neurons in cell culture. *Epilepsia* 1991; 32(Suppl 3):65.
103. Vartanian MG, Radulovic LL, Kinsora JJ, Serpa KA, et al. Activity profile of pregabalin in rodent models of epilepsy and ataxia. *Epilepsy Res* 2006; 68(3):189–205.
104. Micheva KD, Taylor CP, Smith SJ. Pregabalin reduces the release of synaptic vesicles from cultured hippocampal neurons. *Mol Pharmacol* 2006; 70(2):444–476.

105. White HS, Brown SD, Woodhead JH, Skeen GA, et al. Topiramate enhances GABA-mediated chloride flux and GABA-evoked chloride currents in murine brain neurons and increases seizure threshold. *Epilepsy Res* 1997; 23:167–179.
106. Shank RP, Gardocki JF, Vaught JL, Davis CB, et al. Topiramate: preclinical evaluation of a structurally novel anticonvulsant. *Epilepsia* 1994; 35(Suppl 2):450–460.
107. Wauquier A, Zhou S. Topiramate: a potent anticonvulsant in the amygdala-kindled rat. *Epilepsy Res* 1996; 24:73–77.
108. Amano K, Hamada K, Yagi K, Seino M. Antiepileptic effects of topiramate on amygdaloid kindling in rats. *Epilepsy Res* 1998; 31(2):123–8.
109. Nakamura J, Tamura S, Kanda T, Ishii A, et al. Inhibition by topiramate of seizures in spontaneously epileptic rats and DBA/2 mice. *Eur J Pharmacol* 1994; 254:83–89.
110. Rigoulot MA, Boehrer A, Nehlig A. Effects of topiramate in two models of genetically determined generalized epilepsy, the GAERS and the Audiogenic Wistar AS. *Epilepsia* 2003; 44(1):14–19.
111. Shank RP, Gardocki JF, Streeter AJ, Maryanoff BE. An overview of the preclinical aspects of topiramate: pharmacology, pharmacokinetics, and mechanism of action. *Epilepsia* 2000; 41 Suppl 1:S3–S9.
112. Coulter DA, Sombati S, DeLorenzo RJ. Selective effects of topiramate on sustained repetitive firing and spontaneous bursting in cultured hippocampal neurons. *Epilepsia* 1993; 34(Suppl 2):123.
113. Zona C, Ciotti MT, Avoli M, Topiramate attenuates voltage-gated sodium currents in rat cerebellar granule cells. *Neurosci Lett* 1997; 231(3):123–126.
114. Severt L, Coulter DA, Sombati S, DeLorenzo RJ. Topiramate selectively blocks kainate currents in cultured hippocampal neurons. *Epilepsia* 1995; 36(Suppl 4):S38.
115. Skradski S, White HS. Topiramate blocks kainate-evoked cobalt influx into cultured neurons. *Epilepsia* 2000; 41 Suppl 1:S45–S47.
116. Gryder DS, Rogawski MA. Selective antagonism of GluR5 kainate-receptor-mediated synaptic currents by topiramate in rat basolateral amygdala neurons. *J Neurosci* 2003; 23(18):7069–7074.
117. Brown SD, Wolf HH, Swinyard EA, Twyman RE, et al. The novel anticonvulsant topiramate enhances GABA-mediated chloride flux. *Epilepsia* 1993; 34(Suppl 2):122–123.
118. White HS, Brown D, Skeen GA, Wolf HH, et al. The anticonvulsant topiramate displays a unique ability to potentiate GABA-evoked chloride currents. *Epilepsia* 1995; 36(Suppl 3): S39–S40.
119. Staley KJ, Soldo BL, Proctor WR. Ionic mechanisms of neuronal excitation by inhibitory $GABA_A$ receptors. *Science* 1995; 269:977–981.
120. Herrero AI, Del Olmo N, Gonzalez-Escalada JR, Solis JM. Two new actions of topiramate: inhibition of depolarizing GABA(A)-mediated responses and activation of a potassium conductance. *Neuropharmacology* 2002; 42(2):210–220.
121. Russo E, Constanti A. Topiramate hyperpolarizes and modulates the slow poststimulus AHP of rat olfactory cortical neurones in vitro. *Br J Pharmacol* 2004; 141(2): 285–301.
122. Zhang X, Velumian AA, Jones OT, Carlen PL. Modulation of high-voltage-activated calcium channels in dentate granule cells by topiramate. *Epilepsia* 2000; 41 Suppl 1: S52–S60.
123. Simeone TA, Wilcox KS, White HS. Subunit selectivity of topiramate modulation of heteromeric GABA(A) receptors. *Neuropharmacology* 2006; 50(7):845–857.
124. Suzdak PD, Jansen JA. A review of the preclinical pharmacology of tiagabine: a potent and selective anticonvulsant GABA uptake inhibitor. *Epilepsia* 1995; 36(6):612–626.
125. Fink-Jensen A, Suzdak PD, Swedberg MBD. The GABA uptake inhibitor tiagabine increases extracellular brian levels of GABA in awake rats. *Eur J Pharmacol* 1992; 220:197–201.
126. During M, Mattson R, Scheyer R, Rask C, et al. The effect of tiagabine HCl on extracellular GABA levels in the human hippocampus. *Epilepsia* 1992; 33(Suppl 3):83.
127. Vergnes M, Marescaux C. Pathophysiological mechanisms underlying genetic absence epilepsy in rats. In: Malafosse A, Genton P, Hirsch E, Marescaux C, et al, eds. *Idiopathic Generalized Epilepsies: Clinical Experimental and Genetic Aspects*. London: John Libbey and Company Ltd., 1994:151–168.
128. Liu Z, Vergnes M, Depaulis A, Marescaux C. Evidence for a critical role of GABAergic transmission within the thalamus in the genesis and control of absence seizures. *Brain Res* 1991; 545:1–7.
129. Marescaux C, Micheletti G, Vergnes M, Rumbach L, et al. Diazepam antagonizes GABAmimetics in rats with spontaneous petit mal-like epilepsy. *Eur J Pharmacol* 1985; 113:19–24.
130. Jung MJ, Lippert B, Metcalf B, Bohlen P, et al. Gamma-vinyl GABA (4-amino-hex-5-enoic acid), a new irreversible inhibitor of GABA-T: effects on brain GABA metabolism in mice. *J Neurochem* 1977; 29:797–802.
131. Schechter PJ, Tranier Y, Jung MJ, Bohlen P. Audiogenic seizure protection by elevated brain GABA concentration in mice: effects of gamma-acetylenic GABA and gamma-vinyl GABA, two irreversible GABA-T inhibitors. *Eur J Pharmacol* 1977; 45:319–328.
132. Chapman AG, Riley K, Evans MC, Meldrum BS. Acute effects of sodium valproate and gamma-vinyl GABA on regional amino acid metabolism in the rat brain: incorporation of 2-[^{14}C]glucose into amino acids. *Neurochem Res* 1982; 7:1089–1105.
133. Ben-Menachem E. Pharmacokinetic effects of vigabatrin on cerebrospinal fluid amino acids in humans. *Epilepsia* 1989; 30(Suppl 3):S12–S14.
134. Grove J, Schechter PJ, Tell G. Increased gamma-aminobutyric acid (GABA), homocarnosine and b-alanine in cerebrospinal fluid of patients treated with gamma-vinyl GABA (4-amino-hex-5-enoic acid). *Life Sci* 1981; 28:2431–2439.
135. Schechter PJ, Hanke NFJ, Grove J, Huebert N, et al. Biochemical and clinical effects of gamma-vinyl GABA in patients with epilepsy. *Neurology* 1984; 34:182–186.
136. Sarhan S, Seiler N. Metabolic inhibitors and subcellular distribution of GABA. *J Neurosci Res* 1979; 4:399–421.
137. Ben-Menachem. Vigabatrin. In Levy RH, Mattson RH, Meldrum BS, Perucca E, et al. Antiepileptic Drugs, 5th ed. Philadelphia: Lippincott Williams & Wilkins, 2002:855–863.
138. Seino M, Naruto S, Ito T, Miyazaki H. Other antiepileptic drugs. Zonisamide. In: Levy RH, Mattson RH, Meldrum BS, eds. *Antiepileptic Drugs*. 4th ed. New York: Raven Press, 1995:1011–1023.
139. Rock DM, Macdonald RL, Taylor CP. Blockade of sustained repetitive action potentials in cultured spinal cord neurons by zonisamide (AD 810, CI 912), a novel anticonvulsant. *Epilepsy Res* 1989; 3:138–143.
140. Schauf CL. Zonisamide enhances slow sodium inactivation in *Myxicola*. *Brain Res* 1987; 413:185–188.
141. Suzuki S, Kawakami K, Nishimura S, Watanabe Y, et al. Zonisamide blocks T-type calcium channel in cultured neurons of rat cerebral cortex. *Epilepsy Res* 1992; 12:21–27.
142. Kito M, Maehara M, and Watanabe K. Mechanisms of T-type calcium channel blockade by zonisamide. *Seizure* 1996; 5(2):115–119.
143. Mimaki T, Suzuki Y, Tagawa T, Tanaka J, et al. [^{3}H]Zonisamide binding in rat brain. *Jpn J Psychiatry Neurol* 1988; 42:640–642.
144. Meldrum BS. Neurotransmission in Epilepsy. *Epilepsia* 1995; 36(Suppl 1):S30–S35.

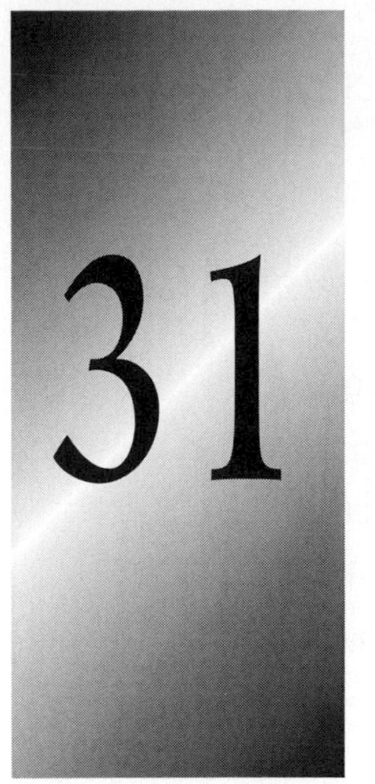

31 Evidence-Based Medicine Issues Related to Drug Selection

Tracy A. Glauser
Diego A. Morita

When selecting an antiepileptic drug (AED) for a patient with epilepsy, a clinician integrates his or herown experience, education, cultural beliefs, and personal values with patient-specific variables and AED-specific variables to select the appropriate AED (Figure 31-1) (1, 2). The overlap between a physician's background and specific AED characteristics can be called the physician's "internal" knowledge base used to make a clinical decision. Similarly, the doctor-patient interaction depends on the physician's background and the patient's characteristics; this "interface" knowledge also plays a role in medication selection.

However, internal and interface knowledge are only two legs of the clinical decision tripod. The third component could be called "external" knowledge—the unbiased third-party evaluation of relevant available scientific evidence about an AED's characteristics or performance within specific patient situations (e.g., partial onset seizures, children, etc.). This last component is represented by various types of rigorous evaluations called systematic reviews, guidelines, or practice parameters. The integration of these three forms of knowledge allows the clinician to make an evidence-based decision and therefore practice evidence-based medicine (EBM).

This chapter will examine a variety of EBM issues related to drug selection for patients with epilepsy. These issues will include a brief review of some historical events leading to the development of the EBM approach; key definitions; description of the evolution, structure, and examples of two types of EBM tools (systematic reviews and practice guidelines); and discussion of the limitations of EBM.

HISTORICAL EVENTS LEADING TO EBM

The development of the controlled clinical trial was essential to the development of modern EBM. From biblical references through bloodletting experiments to James Lind's classic trial of treatments for scurvy, the methodology of the controlled clinical trial slowly developed (3, 4). The subsequent development of EBM in the second half of the twentieth century was a worldwide effort involving numerous people and organizations. Due to space constraints, only three different yet complementary contributions to the development of EBM will be highlighted (3).

The British epidemiologist Professor Archibald Leman Cochrane, CBE, FRCP, FFCM (1909–1988), was a major contributor to the development of EBM. His 1972 book, *Effectiveness and Efficiency: Random Reflections on Health Services*, proposed that, since resources are limited, focus should be on providing health care that

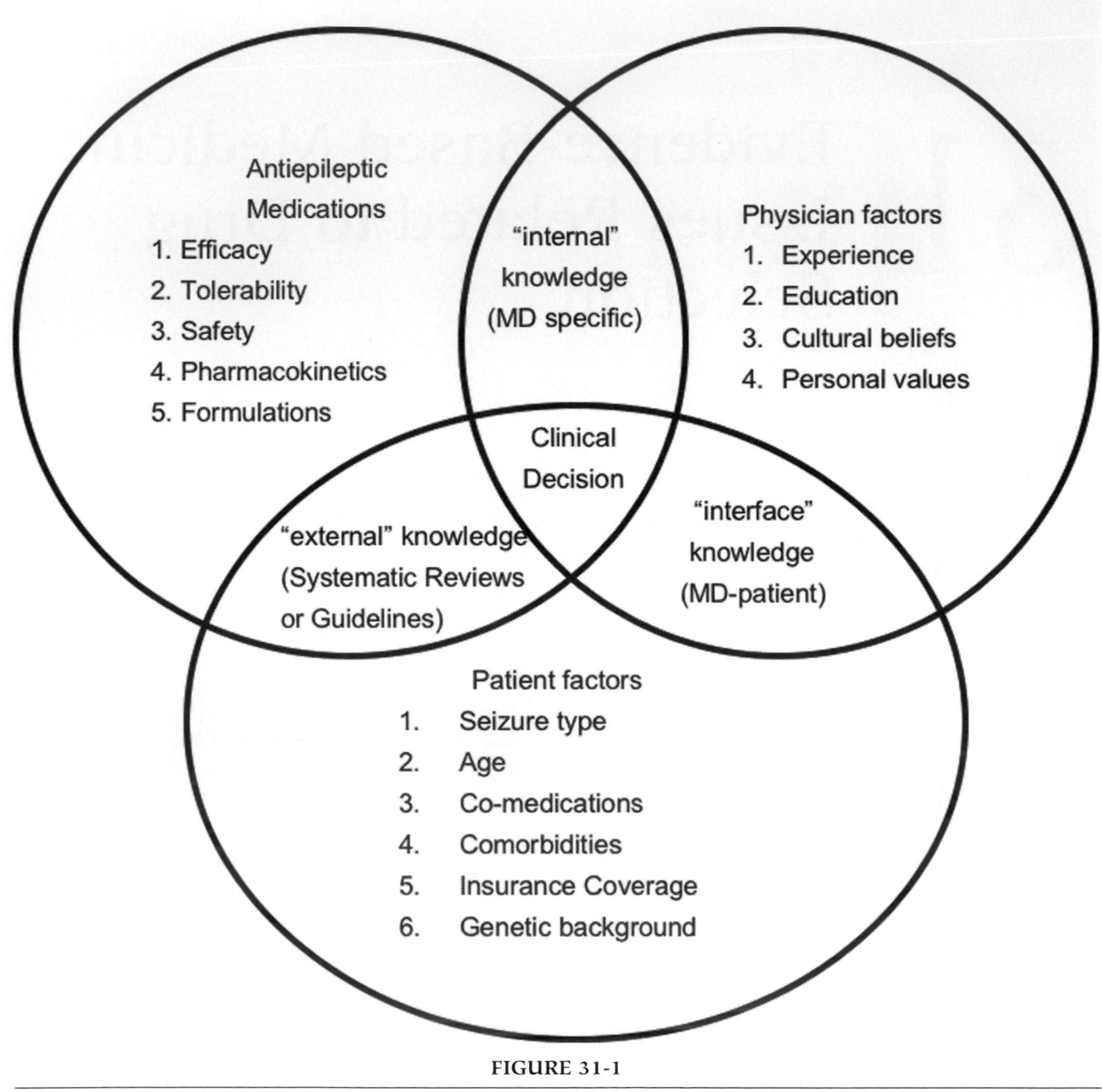

FIGURE 31-1

Factors involved with making drug selection for patients with epilepsy (clinical decision tripod) (adapted from Mulrow CD, Cook DJ, Davidoff F. Systematic reviews: critical links in the great chain of evidence. *Ann Intern Med* 1997; 126[5]:389–391.)

has been shown to be effective (5). Professor Cochrane felt the focus should be on randomized, controlled trials (RCTs) as the most reliable source of information. This approach gained widespread acceptance and led to the development during the 1980s of an international collaboration that developed a database of perinatal trials. After his death in 1988 the movement continued, and in 1992 the first Cochrane center opened in Oxford, UK. The next year, The Cochrane Collaboration was founded. "The Cochrane Collaboration is an international not-for-profit and independent organization, dedicated to making up-to-date, accurate information about the effects of healthcare readily available worldwide. It produces and disseminates systematic reviews of healthcare interventions and promotes the search for evidence in the form of clinical trials and other studies of interventions" (6).

The major output of the Cochrane Collaboration is the Cochrane Database of Systematic Reviews. These reviews are part of the Cochrane Library, which is a collection of databases for clinicians including the Cochrane Database of Systematic Reviews, the Database of Abstracts of Reviews of Effects, the Cochrane Central Register of Controlled Trials (CENTRAL), the Cochrane Methodology Register, the NHS Economic Evaluation Database, Health Technology Assessment Database, and the Cochrane Database of Methodology Reviews (CDMR) (7). The Library is published on CD-ROM and the Internet and updated quarterly (7).

A second major contribution was by the clinical epidemiologist Dr. David Sackett (1934–present). His background was as a physician (MD from the University of Illinois) and epidemiologist (MS in epidemiology from Harvard University). He founded the first department of clinical epidemiology in Canada at McMaster University and played a major role in the development and implementation of problem-based learning for the medical students at McMaster Medical School. He incorporated EBM as an important part of the learning process. In 1994, he left McMaster University for Oxford University in England and the Oxford Centre for Evidence-Based Medicine. His passion for EBM, coupled with his articles (8–16) and books (17, 18) on the need, benefits, and methods of EBM, helped to solidify EBM's place in the medical community (19).

The last major contribution occurred in the United States in the late 1980s. As a result of the skyrocketing cost of health care and the high rate of Americans without health insurance, in 1989 dramatic changes in federally funded health care programs were being proposed, including a cap to total federal health care spending (20). Medical organizations strongly opposed these expenditure targets and argued that a better approach would be to encourage outcome assessment and practice guidelines as cost-effective alternatives (20). In 1989 the final budget reconciliation included legislation that replaced these expenditure targets with Voluntary Performance Standards (20). The goal then was to develop scientifically sound practice parameters that would improve clinical practice and therefore be cost efficient and reduce wasteful spending.

The Agency for Health Care Policy and Research (AHCPR) was established with the goal to develop practice guidelines (20). The Omnibus Budget Reconciliation Act of 1989 also established a National Advisory Council for Health Care Policy Research and Evaluation whose responsibility it was to advise the Administrator of AHCPR and the Secretary of the Department of Health and Human Services on developing, reviewing, and updating guidelines (20). The Institute of Medicine of the National Academy of Sciences was awarded a contract to develop priorities for guidelines along with developing definitions to be used (20). Over the past two decades, multiple professional organizations, nonprofit organizations, and government agencies have developed hundreds of guidelines for a wide variety of diseases (21).

EBM DEFINITIONS

EBM, a term formally introduced in 1992 (22, 23), has been defined as "the conscientious, explicit, and judicious use of current best evidence in making decisions about the care of individualized patients. The practice of evidence-based medicine means integrating individual clinical expertise with the best available external clinical evidence from systematic research" (8).

The two most commonly used EBM tools are the systematic review and the practice guideline.

A systematic review is "A review of a clearly formulated question that uses systematic and explicit methods to identify, select, and critically appraise relevant research, and to collect and analyse data from the studies that are included in the review. Statistical methods (meta-analysis) may or may not be used to analyse and summarise the results of the included studies" (7).

Practice guidelines are "Systematically developed statements to assist practitioner and patient decisions about appropriate health care for specific clinical circumstances" (24).

The American Medical Association (AMA) felt that negative connotations from terminology might limit physicians' acceptance of these policies, standards, and guidelines. As such the AMA preferred to use the term "parameter." The AMA defined "practice parameters" as "strategies for patient management, developed to assist physicians in clinical decision making . . . including standards, guidelines, and other patient management strategies" (20).

EBM TOOLS

Systematic Review

Overview. The most refined example of a systematic review is the Cochrane Review. The development of a Cochrane Review is a multistep collaborative process between the investigators and the Cochrane Review Group's editorial team. After extensive discussions with the editorial team about the topic or title of the review, authors usually attend a protocol workshop to help them understand how to carry out the highly structured review. The next step is to develop and publish a protocol describing how the review will be conducted. All Cochrane Reviews are prepared using a software program called Review Manager (RevMan). The review follows the format described in the *Cochrane Handbook for*

Systematic Reviews of Interventions. As the review is being constructed, additional methodological, statistical, and editorial input is given as needed by the Cochrane Review editorial team. Prior to publication, the review is evaluated by impartial external referees. Once published, authors update the reviews yearly if new relevant information becomes available (25).

Structure. A Cochrane Review is a highly structured document containing well-defined sections. The review begins with a short summary written in plain language for lay people. A structured abstract of the entire review follows. Then relevant background information, objectives of the review, and selection criteria (e.g., types of studies, types of participants, types of interventions, and types of outcome measures) are described, followed by the search strategy for identifying potentially eligible studies. Methods is the next section; the inclusion/exclusion criteria for eligible studies are described, the approach to assessing study quality is presented, how data were extracted and analyzed is depicted, and details about whether any subgroups were studied are presented. The results section describes the type and number of studies identified, along with a detailed assessment of each study's methodologies, and a summary of the data (potentially including a meta-analysis). The interpretation and assessment of the results is contained in the discussion section. Last, the authors provide their own conclusions along with the data's implications for practice for research (25).

Examples. To date, there are 33 epilepsy Cochrane Reviews. Seven systematic reviews have examined AED use in monotherapy (26–32): carbamazepine vs. valproic acid (26), phenytoin vs. valproic acid (28), carbamazepine vs. phenytoin (29), phenytoin vs. phenobarbital (27), carbamazepine vs. phenobarbital (30), oxcarbazepine vs. phenytoin (31), and lamotrigine vs. carbamazepine (32). The outcome focus was on three end points: time to withdrawal, number of patients achieving 12-month seizure freedom, and time to first seizure. Because of the paucity of high-quality studies (class I and class II, as defined in Tables 31-1 and 31-2), the overwhelming majority of data used in these reviews was from class III studies. Many times the reviews found no significant differences for the outcomes examined.

Nine Cochrane Reviews have examined AEDs' use as add-on therapy in drug-resistant partial epilepsy (33–44). These reviews examined topiramate (33), lamotrigine (39), levetiracetam (41), oxcarbazepine (42), zonisamide (34, 37), tiagabine (36), gabapentin (43, 44), calcium antagonists (38), and remacemide (35).

Other Cochrane Reviews have been published for absence seizures (45), infantile spasms (46), Lennox-Gastaut syndrome (47), neonatal seizures (48), corticosteroid use for childhood epilepsy (49), status epilepticus (50, 51), neuropsychological outcomes in children with epilepsy (52), and the ketogenic diet (53).

Non-Cochrane systematic epilepsy reviews have also been published, covering topics such as management of newly diagnosed epilepsy (54–57), tonic-clonic seizures (58), adults with epilepsy and intellectual disability (59), childhood epilepsies (60), AED clinical trials (61), AEDs and cognitive function (62), ketogenic diet (63, 64), quality of life (65), and AED economic issues (66, 67).

Practice Guideline

Overview. The evolution of the systematic review was relatively straightforward compared to the developments leading up to practice guidelines. Guidelines have evolved through multiple stages including individual expert opinion, informal consensus guidelines, formal consensus guidelines, and evidence-based guidelines (68).

Non-evidence-based Guidelines. Over the past hundred years, 36 AEDs have been released worldwide resulting in multiple medical treatment options for people with epilepsy (1). The first wave of AEDs was in the first half of the twentieth century and included phenobarbital, phenytoin, and structurally similar AEDs. In the 1970s a second wave of AEDs included carbamazepine and valproic acid. The latest wave began in the early 1990s and contained 10 new AEDs.

The early growth in AEDs was not accompanied by a concomitant growth in the amount of available scientific evidence regarding each drug's efficacy, safety, and tolerability. Clinicians relied on their own clinical experience coupled with the advice of a few trusted colleagues when selecting a medication for patients with epilepsy. This "individual expert opinion" approach led to diverse (and often strongly held) opinions about the appropriate choice and sequencing of medications for specific groups of patients. During this time, the lack of widely accepted methodology for conducting epilepsy clinical trials and the frequent reporting of treatment outcomes in small groups of patients impaired practitioners from assessing which treatment approaches were superior.

The next evolution was to bring experts together and let them come to a consensus about the appropriate medication or sequencing of medications for particular groups of patients. This approach has been called the "informal consensus development" (68) approach or the "global subjective judgment" approach (69). The methodology involved in developing the conclusions and recommendations for this type of guideline is usually poorly described and poorly implemented. There is frequently little mention of how studies are selected for inclusion, how the recommendations relate to the evidence, or, in general, how the bias of the experts was minimized. Unfortunately this type of guideline remains a commonly used approach because it is easy to construct, fast to develop, and needs little formal statistical analysis (68). Even today, there are multiple examples of this flawed approach in the epilepsy literature; the resulting conclusions must be viewed with a jaundiced eye.

In the late 1970s a new approach was developed called the "formal consensus" (68) or the "expert consensus" approach. This approach is used by the Consensus Development Program sponsored by the National Institutes of Health (NIH) (70–72). Since 1977, these structured two-and-a-half-day conferences have focused on medical technologies and practices in which there is a difference of opinion about best practices (20). These conferences produce evidence-based consensus statements that address controversial issues in medicine that have significant importance to patients, providers, and the general public. From 1977 through 1990, 84 conferences have been held. Only two have focused on seizures or epilepsy: one related to the surgical treatment of epilepsy (73), and one focused on febrile seizures (74, 75). Evidence, including a systematic literature review prepared by the Agency for Healthcare Research and Quality, is presented to an impartial panel. The panel is then sequestered and then renders its recommendations in its statement. Each consensus statement answers approximately four to six questions; the final document is not a policy statement of the NIH or the federal government.

The expert consensus guideline with the largest national impact was the 1993 expert consciences panel sponsored by the Epilepsy Foundation for the management of convulsive seizures and status epilepticus, published in *Journal of the American Medical Association* (76).

Evidence-based Guidelines. Over the last 20 years each medical specialty, nonprofit organization, and government agency that has developed evidence-based guidelines has used the same general approach but slightly different specific methodology. A common backbone for the development of evidence-based guidelines is shown in Figure 31-2. The process starts with selecting a topic and then a panel of experts; these experts develop clinical questions based on the topic. A comprehensive review of the literature is then performed, and identified articles are abstracted according to a stylized format. The abstracted data are placed in evidence tables and the articles are rated. Based upon the identified evidence and a predetermined methodologic approach to interpretation, the panel of experts then develops recommendations and algorithms. The algorithms are distributed for extensive peer review and undergo external validation.

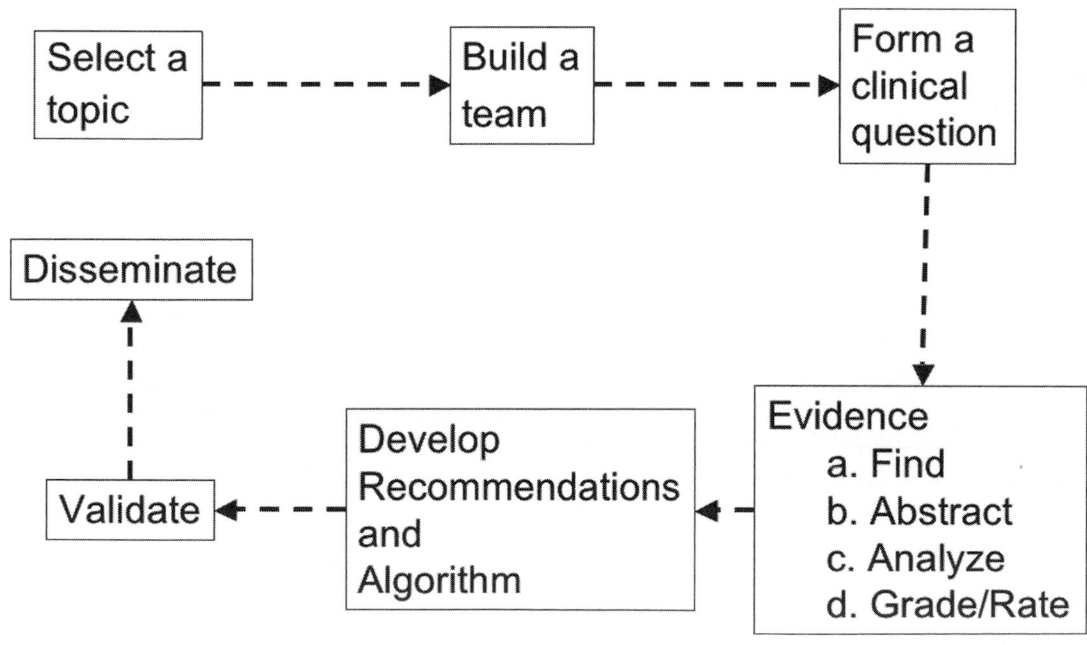

FIGURE 31–2

Sequence of steps involved with developing an evidence-based guideline.

After feedback is received and incorporated, the guidelines are disseminated into the community.

Examples of Evidence-based Guidelines. Since 1996, the American Academy of Neurology (AAN) has produced 14 evidenced-based guidelines focused on some aspect of epilepsy and its evaluation or treatment. There have been treatment guidelines addressing the use of the newer AEDs in new-onset epilepsy (77, 78), the use of the newer AEDs (and felbamate) in refractory epilepsy (79–81), and the treatment of infantile spasms (82). The International League Against Epilepsy (ILAE) published an evidence-based guideline on the treatment of new-onset epilepsy of all seizures types and all ages (1). Other important epilepsy guidelines have been published by the Scottish Intercollegiate Guidelines Network (SIGN; http://www.sign.ac.uk/) (83) and the National Institute for Clinical Excellence (NICE; http://www.nice.org.uk/).

Limitations of Evidence-Based Medicine

Problems with Evidence-based Guidelines. The above approach is a thumbnail sketch of the process. When viewed in detail, many issues arise that impact on the practical application of evidence-based guidelines to clinical care. These issues involve topic selection, conflict of interest, question formation, grading criteria for studies, and criteria for assessing strengths of recommendation.

The process begins with a sponsoring organization picking a topic. The topic must have significance (e.g., there is a gap or controversy between current practice and the existing evidence) and feasibility (there is sufficient medical evidence to try to answer the question). Epilepsy topics often have the former but not the latter. As such, epilepsy guidelines may end up with no clinically relevant conclusion because of lack of evidence. This outcome is frustrating for clinicians seeking guidance for a clinical problem in a specific patient.

The multidisciplinary team of experts can include physicians, nurses, doctors of pharmacy, clinical pharmacologist, statisticians, epidemiologists, health care economists, consumers, and patient representatives. Not every team needs to have all members from each of these constituencies, but the greater the variety of constituencies involved, the more comprehensive and wide ranging the impact of the guideline may be. One problem these teams face are real or perceived conflicts of interest. It is easy to allow bias to subtly affect selection criteria or study interpretation. A guideline's credibility is only as good as the credibility of its authors. Panel members need to declare these real or perceived conflicts of interest in order not to jeopardize the project's credibility. Different guidelines set different time frames. For example, for the AAN, conflicts must be declared for the past 5 years.

Once the topic has been selected and a team assembled, clinical questions must be formed. The clinical question is often formulated as a five-part PECOT-structured question. These letters stand for Patient/Participants/Population, Exposure/Interventions, Comparison, Outcomes, and Time. For example a typical PECOT-structured question would be: "For children with partial onset seizures (P), which antiepileptic drug (E) compared to an adequate comparator (C) provides the highest efficacy (O) over the first year of exposure (T)?" Formulation of this specific clinical question is one of the key aspects of the guideline. Two separate guidelines formulating clinical questions on the same topic can produce different conclusions if their PECOT questions are framed differently. It is critical to understand the question asked by the guideline when assessing the guideline's clinical utility for any particular patient.

Different organizations (and their guidelines) have different strategies on how to score, grade, and rate the evidence found, along with the studies generating it. In general, most scoring systems rank studies according to the number of "major" or "minor" variables present or absent in a study; these variables are factors that impact on the reliability, verifiability, and objectivity of the outcome. For example, major variables include the use of randomization, the use of control groups, the use of masked outcome assessments (blinding), the use of adequate comparators, and adequate enrollment to detect differences (if they exist) between treatment groups. Minor variables include a clearly defined primary outcome variable, clearly stated inclusion and exclusion criteria, addressing of baseline differences between treatment groups, adequate duration of assessment (e.g., in the case of infrequent seizure activity at baseline), and adequate handling of patients who drop out of the study.

In general, studies receiving the top grade are RCTs with the best evidence that meets all major and minor criteria. Studies receiving the next best grade are RCTs that are missing some minor criterion. Trials in the third ranking are those missing some major criterion. The lowest ranked studies are missing most or all major criteria or are only expert opinion. There is significant variability in these grading and rating scales across different guidelines. The AAN and ILAE methods of grading clinical trials are shown in Tables 31-1 and 31-2.

Last, after all the relevant studies have been abstracted, analyzed, and graded, the panel of experts must translate the evidence into recommendations. The strength of these recommendations is determined using a predetermined scoring system, which can vary between organizations (AAN's scoring for strength of recommendations is shown in Table 31-1; ILAE's scoring system is shown in Table 31-3). There are usually four to five levels of recommendations and usually at least one recommendation per question.

TABLE 31-1
Relationship Between Clinical Trial Ratings, Level of Evidence, and Conclusions for AAN Guidelines (77, 78)

Conclusion and Recommendation	Translation of Evidence to Recommendation	Rating of Article
Conclusion: Level A: Established as effective, ineffective or harmful for the given condition in the specified population Recommendation: Should be done or should not be done	Level A rating: Two or more consistent Class I studies	Class I: Prospective, randomized, controlled clinical trial with masked outcome assessment, in a representative population. The following are required: a. Primary outcome(s) is/are clearly defined, b. exclusion/inclusion criteria are clearly defined, c. adequate accounting for drop-outs and crossovers with numbers sufficiently low to have minimal potential for bias d. relevant baseline characteristics are presented and substantially equivalent among treatment groups or there is appropriate statistical adjustment for differences.
Conclusion: Level B: Probably effective, ineffective or harmful for the given condition in the specified population Recommendation: Should be considered or should not be considered	Level B rating: At least one Class I study OR Two consistent Class II studies	Class II: Prospective matched group cohort study in a representative population with masked outcome assessment that meets criteria a–d. above OR an RCT in a representative population that lacks one criteria of a–d.
Conclusion: Level C: Possibly effective, ineffective or harmful for the given condition in the specified population Recommendation: May be considered or may not be considered	Level C rating: At least one Class II study OR Two consistent Class III studies	Class III: All other controlled trials (including well-defined natural history controls or patients serving as own controls) in a representative population, where outcome is independently assessed, or independently derived by objective outcome measurements.
Conclusion: Level U: Data inadequate or conflicting. Given current knowledge, treatment is unproven. Recommendation: None	Level U: Studies not meeting criteria for Class I–Class III	Class IV: Evidence from uncontrolled studies, case series, case reports, or expert opinion.

Although guidelines use a common methodologic backbone, it is hard to compare guidelines from different organizations for the same topic because different PECOT questions are asked, variability in rating and grading scales occurs, and strength of recommendation criteria frequently differ between organizations. Both the ILAE and the AAN/American Epilepsy Society (AES) guidelines use appropriate methodology to provide evidence-based recommendations to specifically address clinically relevant questions. A comparison of the AAN/AES and the ILAE guidelines for the initial monotherapy treatment of epilepsy is shown in Figure 31-3. Although both guidelines dealt with pediatric epilepsy in some form, there were significant differences between the guidelines in terms of drugs examined, scoring system used, and key variables assessed. In addition, cost was never factored into either guideline. This is just one example of how two guidelines addressing the same topic can be dramatically different based on specific aspects of their methodology. These differences in guideline methodology lead to clear differences

TABLE 31-2
Rating Scale of Evidence for Potentially Relevant Studies for ILAE Guideline on Initial Monotherapy for Adults and Children with Epilepsy (1)

Class	Criteria
I	A prospective, randomized, controlled clinical trial (RCT) or meta-analysis of RCTs, in a representative population that meets all 6 criteria: 1. Primary outcome variable: efficacy or effectiveness 2. Treatment duration: ≥48 weeks 3. Study design: Double blind 4. Superiority demonstrated or if no superiority demonstrated the study's actual sample size was sufficient to show non-inferiority of no worse than a 20% relative difference in effectiveness/efficacy (see text for detailed explanation of this detectable noninferiority boundary) 5. Study exit: Not forced by a predetermined number of treatment emergent seizures 6. Appropriate statistical analysis
II	An RCT or meta-analysis meeting all the Class I criteria except that 1. No superiority was demonstrated and the study's actual sample size was sufficient only to show non-inferiority at a 21% to 30% relative difference in effectiveness/efficacy OR 2. Treatment duration: ≥24 weeks but <48 weeks
III	An RCT or meta-nalysis not meeting the criteria for any Class I or Class II category (e.g., an open label study or a double blind study with either a detectable noninferiority boundary of >30% or forced exit criteria)
IV	Evidence from nonrandomized, prospective, controlled or uncontrolled studies, case series, or expert reports.

in guideline conclusions and recommendations. Table 31-4 compares treatment recommendations for pediatric seizure types and epilepsy syndrome for three evidence-based guidelines (ILAE guidelines [1], SIGN [83], and the NICE), two national surveys (Pediatric Expert Consensus survey [84] and a French national survey [85]), and the United States Food and Drug Administration (FDA). Although trends are noted for some AEDs for certain seizure or epilepsy types, there are clear disagreements. It is critical to understand a guideline's questions and methodology before incorporating its recommendations into the evidence-based medicine decision-making process.

Problems with EBM Itself. EBM relies heavily on the power of RCTs. There are many benefits to this: RCTs tend to minimize bias that can affect the trial's outcome, they minimize the impact of variability, and they give better information than anecdotal medicine. In short, RCTs improve the chances of getting the "right answer." However, there are significant limitations with RCTs. The RCT trial may not ask the "right question," may not pick a clinically significant treatment effect, and does not explain the factors underlying intersubject variability in response to therapy. RCTs look for population effects. The study population size in most RCTs is selected to answer only one specific question; any alternative questions and analyses may not show any treatment effect because they are underpowered.

There are critics of the EBM approach in general. Some believe that:

1. Knowledge gained from clinical research and clinical reviews is not directly applicable to the care of individualized patients (23).
2. EBM will be used as an objective (yet incomplete) method by which insurers could approve or deny payment for care (86, 87).
3. EBM is impossible to practice because of the time demands, financial issues, and patient variability seen outside academic centers (8).
4. EBM is "cookbook" medicine (8).
5. EBM is limited because it relies primarily on randomized trials and meta-analyses (8).

Many convincing arguments exist rebutting these concerns. However, EBM is still a young discipline, and much work still must be done before it becomes the standard approach for medical care for patients with epilepsy.

CONCLUSION

Evidence-based medicine is a powerful approach that can help clinicians reach personalized clinical decisions for their patients with epilepsy. Systematic reviews, evidence-based

TABLE 31-3

Relationship Between Clinical Trial Ratings, Level of Evidence and Conclusions for ILAE Guideline on Initial Monotherapy for Adults and Children with Epilepsy (1)

COMBINATION(S) OF CLINICAL TRIAL RATINGS	LEVEL OF EVIDENCE	CONCLUSIONS	RECOMMENDATION (BASED ON EFFICACY AND EFFECTIVENESS DATA ONLY)
≥1 Class I studies or meta-analysis meeting Class I criteria sources OR ≥ 2 Class II studies	A	AED established as efficacious or effective as initial monotherapy	AED should be considered for initial monotherapy—First-line monotherapy candidate
1 Class II study or meta-analysis meeting Class II criteria	B	AED probably efficacious or effective as initial monotherapy	
≥2 Class III double-blind or open label studies	C	AED possibly efficacious or effective as initial monotherapy	AED may be considered for initial monotherapy—Alternative first-line monotherapy candidates
1 Class III double blind or open label study OR ≥1 Class IV clinical studies OR Data from expert committee reports, opinions from experienced clinicians	D	AED potentially efficacious or effective as initial monotherapy	Weak efficacy or effectiveness data available to support the use of the AED for initial monotherapy
Absence of directly applicable clinical evidence upon which to base a recommendation	E	No data available to assess if AED is effective as initial monotherapy	Either no data or inadequate efficacy or effectiveness data available to decide whether AED could be considered for initial monotherapy
Positive evidence of lack of efficacy or effectiveness based on Class I to IV studies OR Significant risk of seizure aggravation based on Class I to IV studies	F	AED established as ineffective or significant risk of seizure aggravation	AED *should not* be used for initial monotherapy

Variable	ILAE	AAN/AES
Team	N = 10, 6 countries	N = 24, 1 country
AEDs examined	31 AEDs	7 newer US AEDs
Study years	1940-present	1987-2003
Scoring system	ILAE system	AAN system
Data reanalysis	Yes, used to rank	No
Key variables	Randomization, blinding, adequate power	Control group
Effective dose	Not discussed	Discussed
Costs	Not considered	Not considered

FIGURE 31-3

Comparison of AAN/AES guideline (77) and ILAE guideline (1) for initial monotherapy in children and adults with new-onset epilepsy.

TABLE 31-4

Comparison of Evidence Based and Consensus Guidelines Recommendations for the Treatment for different pediatric seizure types and epilepsy syndromes. (ref. 84)

Seizure Type or Epilepsy Syndrome	Pediatric Expert Consensus Survey	ILAE	SIGN	NICE	French Study	FDA Approved
Partial-onset	OXC, CBZ	A: OXC; B: *none* C: CBZ, PB, PHT TPM, VPA	PHT, VPA, CBZ LTG, TPM, OXC, VGB, CLB	CBZ, VPA, LTG OXC, TPM,	OXC, CBZ, LTG (adult males)	PB, PHT, CBZ OXC, TPM
BECT	OXC, CBZ	A, B: *none* C: CBZ, VPA	*not specifically mentioned*	CBZ, OXC, LTG, VPA	*not surveyed*	*none*
Childhood absence epilepsy	ESM	A, B: *none*	VPA, ESM, LTG	VPA, ESM, LTG	VPA, LTG	ESM, VPA
Juvenile myoclonic epilepsy	VPA, LTG	A, B, C: *none*	VPA, LTG, TPM	VPA, LTG	VPA, LTG	TPM
Lennox-Gastaut syndrome	VPA, TPM, LTG	*not reviewed*	*not specifically mentioned*	LTG, VPA, TPM	*not surveyed*	FLB, TPM, LTG
Infantile spasms	VGB, ACTH	*not reviewed*	*not specifically mentioned*	VGB, corticosteroids	*not surveyed*	*none*

ACTH, adrenocorticotropin; CBZ, carbamazepine; CLB, clobazam; ESM, ethosuximide; FLB, felbamate; LTG, lamotrigine; OXC, oxcarbazepine; PB, phenobarbital; PHT, phenytoin; TPM, topiramate; VGB, vigabatrin; VPA, valproic acid.

guidelines, and practice parameters are critical tools for practicing evidence-based medicine. However, these "external" knowledge sources should not be used alone; they need to be integrated with a clinician's experience and background, with both AED-specific factors ("internal" knowledge) and patient-specific variables ("interface" knowledge) to select the appropriate antiepileptic medication for a patient.

Clinical decisions should not be driven by only one type of knowledge. For example, ignoring evidence-based guidelines and practice parameters can lead to practicing anecdotal medicine. In contrast, ignoring one's own clinical experience in favor of solely relying on guidelines and practice parameters can lead to a cookbook approach. The physician's background, the patient's characteristics, each AED's characteristics, and evidence-based evaluations are all important components of making the best patient care decisions.

Through better understanding of guidelines and practice parameter methodology, clinicians should feel more comfortable integrating these evidence-based assessments into their clinical decision-making process. Practicing evidence-based medicine should lead to better personalized and comprehensive care of our patients.

References

1. Glauser T, Ben-Menachem E, Bourgeois B, Cnaan A, et al. ILAE treatment guidelines: evidence-based analysis of antiepileptic drug efficacy and effectiveness as initial monotherapy for epileptic seizures and syndromes. *Epilepsia* 2006; 47(7):1094–1120.
2. Mulrow CD, Cook DJ, Davidoff F. Systematic reviews: critical links in the great chain of evidence. *Ann Intern Med* 1997; 126(5):389–391.
3. Claridge JA, Fabian TC. History and development of evidence-based medicine. *World J Surg* 2005; 29(5):547–553.
4. Doherty S. History of evidence-based medicine. Oranges, chloride of lime and leeches: barriers to teaching old dogs new tricks. *Emerg Med Australas* 2005; 17(4): 314–321.
5. Cochrane A. Effectiveness and efficiency. Random reflections on health services. London: Nuffield Provincial Hospitals Trust, 1972.
6. Cochrane Collaboration. What is The Cochrane Collaboration? 2007. Available from: http://www.cochrane.org/docs/descrip.htm.
7. The Cochrane Collaboration. Glossary of terms. In: Higgins J, Green S, eds. *Cochrane Handbook for Systematic Reviews of Interventions 425* (updated May 2005). In: The Cochrane Library, Issue 3. Chichester, UK: John Wiley & Sons, 2005.
8. Sackett DL, Rosenberg WM, Gray JA, Haynes RB, et al. Evidence based medicine: what it is and what it isn't. *BMJ* 1996; 312(7023):71–72.
9. Sackett DL, Straus SE. Finding and applying evidence during clinical rounds: the "evidence cart." *JAMA* 1998; 280(15):1336–1338.
10. Sackett DL. Evidence-based medicine. *Spine* 1998; 23(10):1085–1086.
11. Sackett DL. Evidence-based medicine. *Semin Perinatol* 1997; 21(1):3–5.
12. Sackett DL. Evidence-based medicine and treatment choices. *Lancet* 1997; 349(9051): 572–573.
13. Sackett DL, Rosenberg WM. On the need for evidence-based medicine. *Health Econ* 1995; 4(4):249–254.
14. Sackett DL, Rosenberg WM. On the need for evidence-based medicine. *J Public Health Med* 1995; 17(3):330–334.
15. Sackett DL, Rosenberg WM. The need for evidence-based medicine. *J R Soc Med* 1995; 88(11):620–624.
16. Sackett D. Evidence-based medicine. *Lancet* 1995; 346(8983):1171.
17. Sackett DL, Straus S, Richardson S, Rosenberg W, et al. Evidence-based medicine: how to practice and teach EBM. 2nd ed. London: Churchill Livingstone, 2000.

18. Sackett DL, Richardson SW, Rosenberg W, Haynes RB. *Evidence-Based Medicine*. London: Churchill Livingstone, 1996.
19. Cohen L. McMaster's pioneer in evidence-based medicine now spreading his message in England. *CMAJ* 1996; 154(3):388–390.
20. Rosenberg J, Greenberg MK. Practice parameters: strategies for survival into the nineties. *Neurology* 1992; 42(5):1110–1115.
21. Web site offers database of national guidelines. *Healthcare Benchmarks* 1999; 6(3):30–31.
22. Evidence-based medicine. A new approach to teaching the practice of medicine. Evidence-Based Medicine Working Group. *JAMA* 1992; 268(17):2420–2425.
23. Tonelli MR. The limits of evidence-based medicine. *Respir Care* 2001; 46(12):1435–1440; discussion 1440–1441.
24. Institute of Medicine. Definition of key terms. In: Field MJ, Lohr KN, eds. *Clinical Practice Guidelines: Directions for a New Program*. Washington, DC: National Academy Press, 1990:33–51.
25. Cochrane Collaboration. Cochrane Review structure. 2007. Available from: http://www.cochrane.org/reviews/revstruc.htm.
26. Marson AG, Williamson PR, Clough H, Hutton JL, et al. Carbamazepine versus valproate monotherapy for epilepsy: a meta-analysis. *Epilepsia* 2002; 43(5):505–513.
27. Taylor S, Tudur Smith C, Williamson PR, Marson AG. Phenobarbitone versus phenytoin monotherapy for partial onset seizures and generalized onset tonic-clonic seizures. *Cochrane Database Syst Rev* 2001(4):CD002217.
28. Tudur Smith C, Marson AG, Williamson PR. Phenytoin versus valproate monotherapy for partial onset seizures and generalized onset tonic-clonic seizures. *Cochrane Database Syst Rev* 2001(4):CD001769.
29. Tudur Smith C, Marson AG, Clough HE, Williamson PR. Carbamazepine versus phenytoin monotherapy for epilepsy. *Cochrane Database Syst Rev* 2002(2): CD001911.
30. Tudur Smith C, Marson AG, Williamson PR. Carbamazepine versus phenobarbitone monotherapy for epilepsy. *Cochrane Database Syst Rev* 2003(1):CD001904.
31. Muller M, Marson AG, Williamson PR. Oxcarbazepine versus phenytoin monotherapy for epilepsy. *Cochrane Database Syst Rev* 2006(2):CD003615.
32. Gamble CL, Williamson PR, Marson AG. Lamotrigine versus carbamazepine monotherapy for epilepsy. *Cochrane Database Syst Rev* 2006(1):CD001031.
33. Jette NJ, Marson AG, Hutton JL. Topiramate add-on for drug-resistant partial epilepsy. *Cochrane Database Syst Rev* 2002(3):CD001417.
34. Chadwick DW, Marson AG. Zonisamide add-on for drug-resistant partial epilepsy. *Cochrane Database Syst Rev* 2005(4):CD001416.
35. Leach JP, Marson AG, Hutton JL. Remacemide for drug-resistant localization related epilepsy. *Cochrane Database Syst Rev* 2002(4):CD001900.
36. Pereira J, Marson AG, Hutton JL. Tiagabine add-on for drug-resistant partial epilepsy. *Cochrane Database Syst Rev* 2002(3):CD001908.
37. Chadwick DW, Marson AG. Zonisamide add-on for drug-resistant partial epilepsy. *Cochrane Database Syst Rev* 2002(2):CD001416.
38. Chaisewikul R, Baillie N, Marson AG. Calcium antagonists as an add-on therapy for drug-resistant epilepsy. *Cochrane Database Syst Rev* 2001(4):CD002750.
39. Ramaratnam S, Marson AG, Baker GA. Lamotrigine add-on for drug-resistant partial epilepsy. *Cochrane Database Syst Rev* 2001(3):CD001909.
40. Marson AG, Hutton JL, Leach JP, Castillo S, et al. Levetiracetam, oxcarbazepine, remacemide and zonisamide for drug resistant localization-related epilepsy: a systematic review. *Epilepsy Res* 2001; 46(3):259–270.
41. Chaisewikul R, Privitera MD, Hutton JL, Marson AG. Levetiracetam add-on for drug-resistant localization related (partial) epilepsy. *Cochrane Database Syst Rev* 2001(1):CD001901.
42. Castillo S, Schmidt DB, White S. Oxcarbazepine add-on for drug-resistant partial epilepsy. *Cochrane Database Syst Rev* 2000(3):CD002028.
43. Marson AG, Kadir ZA, Hutton JL, Chadwick DW. Gabapentin add-on for drug-resistant partial epilepsy. *Cochrane Database Syst Rev* 2000(3):CD001415.
44. Marson AG, Kadir ZA, Hutton JL, Chadwick DW. Gabapentin for drug-resistant partial epilepsy. *Cochrane Database Syst Rev* 2000(2):CD001415.
45. Posner EB, Mohamed K, Marson AG. Ethosuximide, sodium valproate or lamotrigine for absence seizures in children and adolescents. *Cochrane Database Syst Rev* 2003(3): CD003032.
46. Hancock E, Osborne J, Milner P. Treatment of infantile spasms. *Cochrane Database Syst Rev* 2003(3):CD001770.
47. Hancock E, Cross H. Treatment of Lennox-Gastaut syndrome. *Cochrane Database Syst Rev* 2003(3):CD003277.
48. Booth D, Evans DJ. Anticonvulsants for neonates with seizures. *Cochrane Database Syst Rev* 2004(4):CD004218.
49. Gayatri N, Ferrie C, Cross H. Corticosteroids including ACTH for childhood epilepsy other than epileptic spasms. *Cochrane Database Syst Rev* 2007(1):CD005222.
50. Prasad K, Al-Roomi K, Krishnan PR, Sequeira R. Anticonvulsant therapy for status epilepticus. *Cochrane Database Syst Rev* 2005(4):CD003723.
51. Appleton R, Martland T, Phillips B. Drug management for acute tonic-clonic convulsions including convulsive status epilepticus in children. *Cochrane Database Syst Rev* 2002(4): CD001905.
52. Cochrane HC, Marson AG, Baker GA, Chadwick DW. Neuropsychological outcomes in randomized controlled trials of antiepileptic drugs: a systematic review of methodology and reporting standards. *Epilepsia* 1998; 39(10):1088–1097.
53. Levy R, Cooper P. Ketogenic diet for epilepsy. *Cochrane Database Syst Rev* 2003(3): CD001903.
54. Ross S, Estok R, Chopra S, French J. *Management of Newly Diagnosed Patients with Epilepsy: a Systematic Review of the Liter ature*. Evidence Report/Technology Assessment No. 39 (Contract 290-97-0016 to MetaWorks, Inc.) AHRQ Publication No. 01-E038. Rockville, MD: Agency for Healthcare Research and Quality, 2001.
55. Consensus statements: medical management of epilepsy. *Neurology* 1998 Nov; 51 5 Suppl 4:S39–S43.
56. Southern Clinical Neurological Society. Management of newly diagnosed patients with epilepsy: a systematic review of the literature. Summary, Evidence Report/Technology Assessment: Number 39. AHRQ Publication Number 01-E037, February 2001. Agency for Healthcare Research and Quality, Rockville, MD. http://www.ahrq.gov/clinic/wpcsums/epilepsum.htm(accessed 9/17/07).
57. Armijo JA, Sanchez B, Gonzalez AB. [Evidence based treatment of epilepsy]. *Rev Neurol* 2002; 35 Suppl 1:S59–S73.
58. Ramsay RE, DeToledo J. Tonic-clonic seizures: a systematic review of antiepilepsy drug efficacy and safety. *Clin Ther* 1997; 19(3):433–446; discussion 367–368.
59. Clinical guidelines for the management of epilepsy in adults with an intellectual disability. *Seizure* 2001; 10(6):401–409.
60. Camfield P, Camfield C. Childhood epilepsy: what is the evidence for what we think and what we do? *J Child Neurol* 2003; 18(4):272–287.
61. Gram L, Bentsen KD, Parnas J, Flachs H. Controlled trials in epilepsy: a review. *Epilepsia* 1982; 23(5):491–519.
62. Brunbech L, Sabers A. Effect of antiepileptic drugs on cognitive function in individuals with epilepsy: a comparative review of newer versus older agents. *Drugs* 2002; 62(4): 593–604.
63. Keene DL. A systematic review of the use of the ketogenic diet in childhood epilepsy. *Pediatr Neurol* 2006; 35(1):1–5.
64. Lefevre F, Aronson N. Ketogenic diet for the treatment of refractory epilepsy in children: a systematic review of efficacy. *Pediatrics* 2000; 105(4):E46.
65. Baker GA, Hesdon B, Marson AG. Quality-of-life and behavioral outcome measures in randomized controlled trials of antiepileptic drugs: a systematic review of methodology and reporting standards [in process citation]. *Epilepsia* 2000; 41(11):1357–1363.
66. Kotsopoulos IA, Evers SM, Ament AJ, de Krom MC. Estimating the costs of epilepsy: an international comparison of epilepsy cost studies. *Epilepsia* 2001; 42(5):634–640.
67. Levy P. Economic evaluation of antiepileptic drug therapy: a methodologic review. *Epilepsia* 2002; 43(5):550–558.
68. Woolf SH. Practice guidelines, a new reality in medicine. II. Methods of developing guidelines. *Arch Intern Med* 1992; 152(5):946–952.
69. Eddy DM. Practice policies: where do they come from? *Jama* 1990; 263(9):1265, 9, 72 passim.
70. Ferguson JH. The NIH Consensus Development Program. The evolution of guidelines. *Int J Technol Assess Health Care* 1996; 12(3):460–474.
71. Ferguson JH. The NIH Consensus Development Program. *Jt Comm J Qual Improv* 1995; 21(7):332–336.
72. Ferguson JH. NIH consensus conferences: dissemination and impact. *Ann N Y Acad Sci* 1993; 703:180–198; discussion 198–199.
73. Surgical treatment of epilepsy. Proceedings of a consensus conference. March 19–21, 1990. *Epilepsy Res Suppl* 1992; 5:1–250.
74. Febrile seizures—long-term management of children with fever-associated seizures. NIH Consensus Development Conference. *Neuropediatrics* 1980; 11(3):192–202.
75. Febrile seizures: long-term management of children with fever-associated seizures. Summary of an NIH Consensus Statement. *Br Med J* 1980; 281(6235):277–279.
76. Epilepsy Foundation of America's Working Group on Status Epilepticus. Treatment of convulsive status epilepticus. *JAMA* 1993; 270(7):854–859.
77. French JA, Kanner AM, Bautista J, Abou-Khalil B, et al. Efficacy and tolerability of the new antiepileptic drugs, I: Treatment of new-onset epilepsy: report of the TTA and QSS Subcommittees of the American Academy of Neurology and the American Epilepsy Society. *Epilepsia* 2004; 45(5):401–409.
78. French JA, Kanner AM, Bautista J, Abou-Khalil B, et al. Efficacy and tolerability of the new antiepileptic drugs I: treatment of new onset epilepsy: report of the Therapeutics and Technology Assessment Subcommittee and Quality Standards Subcommittee of the American Academy of Neurology and the American Epilepsy Society. *Neurology* 2004; 62(8):1252–1260.
79. French JA, Kanner AM, Bautista J, Abou-Khalil B, et al. Efficacy and tolerability of the new antiepileptic drugs, II: Treatment of refractory epilepsy: report of the TTA and QSS Subcommittees of the American Academy of Neurology and the American Epilepsy Society. *Epilepsia* 2004; 45(5):410–423.
80. French JA, Kanner AM, Bautista J, Abou-Khalil B, et al. Efficacy and tolerability of the new antiepileptic drugs II: treatment of refractory epilepsy: report of the Therapeutics and Technology Assessment Subcommittee and Quality Standards Subcommittee of the American Academy of Neurology and the American Epilepsy Society. *Neurology* 2004; 62(8):1261–1273.
81. French J, Smith M, Faught E, Brown L. Practice advisory: the use of felbamate in the treatment of patients with intractable epilepsy: report of the Quality Standards Subcommittee of the American Academy of Neurology and the American Epilepsy Society. *Neurology* 1999; 52(8):1540–1545.
82. Mackay MT, Weiss SK, Adams-Webber T, Ashwal S, et al. Practice parameter: medical treatment of infantile spasms: report of the American Academy of Neurology and the Child Neurology Society. *Neurology* 2004; 62(10):1668–1681.
83. Diagnosis and management of epilepsy in children and young people: A national clinical guidelines. Edinburgh: Scottish Intercollegiate Guidelines Network, March 2005.
84. Wheless JW, Clarke DF, Carpenter D. Treatment of pediatric epilepsy: expert opinion, 2005. *J Child Neurol* 2005; 20 Suppl 1:S1–S56; quiz S9–S60.
85. Semah F, Picot MC, Derambure P, Dupont S, et al. The choice of antiepileptic drugs in newly diagnosed epilepsy: a national French survey. *Epileptic Disord* 2004; 6(4): 255–265.
86. Maynard A. Evidence-based medicine: an incomplete method for informing treatment choices. *Lancet* 1997; 349(9045):126–128.
87. Maynard A. Evidence based medicine. Cost effectiveness and equity are ignored. *BMJ* 1996; 313(7050):170–171.

32 Combination Drug Therapy: Monotherapy Versus Polytherapy

Blaise F. D. Bourgeois

The trends of predominant combination therapy versus predominant monotherapy in the medical treatment of epilepsy can be historically divided into three sequential currents. Following the introduction of phenytoin in 1938, several additional antiepileptic drugs (AEDs) became available, and patients whose seizures were not controlled by one drug were commonly prescribed multiple drugs. It is likely that the rationale for this approach was mostly based on the assumption that AEDs interact synergistically and that multiple drugs can provide more seizure protection together than one drug alone. This reasoning does not take into account the undesirable other side of this equation—namely, that multiple drugs can provide more side effects together than one drug alone. Therefore, the concept of monotherapy and sequential monotherapy gained wide acceptance in the late 1970s and early 1980s, because the frequent negative impact of polytherapy on the number and intensity of side effects was increasingly recognized. Recommendations for monotherapy were based on repeated observations that the severity or number of side effects often diminished following a reduction in the number of AEDs, in most cases without appreciable loss in seizure control (1–6), and that the beneficial effect of adding a second drug after the failure of a first drug was modest (7). Patients who had undergone a temporal lobe resection were randomized to ongoing polytherapy or to reduction to carbamazepine monotherapy (8). The seizure recurrence rate was the same in both groups, but drug-related side effects were less common in the monotherapy group (10%) than in the polytherapy group (30%). The concept of monotherapy was extended to the practice of "high-dose monotherapy" (9). However, two main factors prompted the transition to a third era: (1) the realization that about one-third of patients still remained refractory even to high-dose monotherapy, and (2) the release of several newer AEDs after 1993 with fewer or no pharmacokinetic interactions. In the 1990s, the concept of "rational polytherapy" was promoted, with intense discussion and speculation but few rigorous clinical studies. When single-drug therapy fails to render patients seizure free, the temptation to combine AEDs will endure. Because of this, it will always remain important to evaluate and identify potentially beneficial specific drug combinations and to carefully assess the advantages and disadvantages of AED combinations.

DISADVANTAGES OF COMBINATION DRUG THERAPY

Pharmacokinetic Interactions

Adding or removing a drug from the treatment regimen may alter the established relationship between dose and blood level of drugs already in use, either AEDs or other drugs. In general, pharmacokinetic interactions make more frequent drug level determinations and dosage readjustments necessary, and they also increase the probability of the occurrence of a drug level that is either too low or too high. It is more likely that an interaction will be overlooked when a drug causing an interaction is removed than when it is added. It should also be noted that enzyme-inducing drugs cause interactions that reach their maximum only after days to weeks and are only slowly reversible, whereas enzyme inhibitors cause reactions that reach their full impacts within hours to a few days and are rapidly reversible. Most newer AEDs have a lower potential for interactions, in particular for enzyme induction, and some have practically no interactions. Pharmacokinetic interactions are reviewed in detail in Chapter 39. Pharmacokinetic interactions are only rarely beneficial. For instance, the inhibitory effect of valproate on lamotrigine kinetics can have the theoretical advantages of reducing the fluctuations of the levels of lamotrigine by prolonging its elimination half-life and of reducing the dosage requirements of lamotrigine for a desired blood level. In most instances, however, pharmacokinetic interactions are at best harmless and only if they are anticipated or recognized early. Valproate levels are particularly sensitive to comedication with enzyme-inducing drugs, especially in children. Even at very high doses of more than 100 mg/kg/day, some children cannot achieve therapeutic levels of valproate when in combination therapy with enzyme-inducing drugs (10). The carbamazepine dose-to-level ratio can also be markedly affected by inducing drugs, and the increased dose requirement is associated with an increase in the concentration of the active metabolite carbamazepine-10,11-epoxide. The accelerated biotransformation of such drugs as valproate and carbamazepine usually shortens their half-life and lowers their concentration, causing larger fluctuations in blood levels between doses. Larger fluctuations may increase the risk of seizures just before the dose or increase the risk of toxic side effects at the time of the peak level. Inversely, the inhibition of lamotrigine elimination by valproate increases the level-to-dose ratio of lamotrigine and is likely to be responsible for the observed increase in the incidence of rashes associated with lamotrigine (11), an observation that led to a downward readjustment of the titration rate of lamotrigine dosage in these patients.

Cumulative Toxicity

Experimental data on the pharmacodynamic interactions of AEDs suggest that neurological toxicity is often additive, although it can be at times infra-additive or supra-additive (12) (Table 32-1). This finding implies that two drugs with a concentration in the recommended therapeutic range are more likely to cause side effects than each drug alone at the same concentration. Correspondingly, in several clinical studies in which polypharmacy was reduced, there was an associated decrease in side effects, especially a reduction in sedation (2, 3, 5, 6). This increased alertness was especially apparent after withdrawal of barbiturates or benzodiazepines (4). Controlled monotherapy trials with some of the newer AEDs have demonstrated a lower incidence of side effects than in the corresponding add-on trials with the same drug. The notion of cumulative toxicity becomes particularly important if one considers the fact that toxicity is often subtle and can be associated with chronic impairment of cognitive function (13).

In addition to cumulative toxicity, when two or more drugs are prescribed together, there is a greater likelihood that one of the drug concentrations will eventually be in the toxic range. In a longitudinal study of children with epilepsy, the number of children with one or more drug levels in the toxic range increased with the numbers of drugs prescribed (14). Toxic levels occurred in 14% of those taking one drug, 50% of those taking two drugs, and 100% of those taking three or more drugs. Therefore, polytherapy is likely to increase the frequency of dose-related side effects. It also increases the probability of idiosyncratic adverse effects and organ toxicity. Deckers and coworkers (15) reviewed the literature to reassess the relationship between AED polytherapy and adverse effects. They found some evidence suggesting that the toxicity of polytherapy may be related to total drug load (that is, total dose of all drugs) rather than to the number of drugs. In other words, one drug at a relatively high dose may cause more adverse effects than two drugs at low doses. Combination therapy may result not only in stronger side effects but also in more side effects of different types. For example, a given patient could have thrombocytopenia from valproate, nephrolithiasis from topiramate, and gingival hyperplasia from phenytoin. However, one could also observe cancellation of opposite side effects of different drugs, as for instance a normalization of excessive weight on valproate after the introduction of topiramate, the latter being known to potentially cause excessive weight loss.

Differences in Therapeutic Range

The therapeutic range is a statistical compromise based on studies of groups of patients. It provides loose guidelines

TABLE 32-1
Pharmacodynamic Interactions Between Antiepileptic Drugs in Animal Models

Older Drugs	Interaction Antiepileptic	Neurotoxic	Reference
PHT + PB	Additive	Infra-additive	23
PHT + CBZ	Additive	Additive	24
CBZ + PB	Additive	Additive	25
VPA + PB	Additive	Additive	26
VPA + ESM	Additive	Infra-additive	27
VPA + CBZ	Additive	Infra-additive	26
VPA + PHT	Supra-additive	Additive	28
VPA + CZP	Supra-additive	Supra-additive	29
ESM + CZP	Supra-additive	Supra-additive	29
CBZ + CBZ-E	Additive	Additive	30
PRM + PB	Supra-additive	Infra-additive	31
PB + PEMA	Supra-additive	Supra-additive	31
Newer Drugs	**Interaction Antiepileptic**	**Neurotoxic**	**Reference**
LTG + TPM	Supra-additive	Infra-additive	32
LTG + VPA	Supra-additive	Infra-additive	32
LTG + CBZ	Infra-additive	Additive	32
LTG + PB	Supra-additive	Supra-additive	32
LTG + PHT	Additive	Additive	32
TGB + GBP	Supra-additive	Additive	33
TPM + FBM	Supra-additive	Infra-additive	34
TPM + OXC	Supra-additive	Additive	34
OXC + FBM	Infra-additive	Additive	34
OXC + LTG	Infra-additive	Supra-additive	34
LTG + FBM	Additive	Infra-additive	35
OXC + GBP	Supra-additive	Additive	36
LEV + TPM	Supra-additive	Infra-additive	37
LEV + CBZ	Supra-additive	Infra-additive	37
LEV + OXC	supra-additive	infra-additive	37

Reproduced, with permission from reference Levy and Bourgeois (12).

CBZ, carbamazepine; CBZ-E, carbamazepine epoxide; CZP, clonazepam; ESM, ethosuximide; FBM, felbamate; GBP, gabapentin; LEV, levetiracetam; LTG, lamotrigine; OXC, oxcarbazepine; PB, phenobarbital; PEMA, phenyo-ethyl-malonamide (primidone metabolite); PHT, phenytoin; PRM, primidone; TGB, tiagabine; TPM, topiramate; VPA, valproate.

with regard to the minimal effective concentration and the concentration at which side effects become frequent. Based on the experimental evidence for additive interactions between AEDs, it is unlikely that the therapeutic range of a drug will be the same when it is taken alone as when it is taken in combination with other drugs. Polytherapy is more likely to be associated with toxicity when drug levels are within the therapeutic range. Clinical observations indeed suggest that toxic side effects from carbamazepine or phenytoin (9) and from valproate (16) appear at higher levels when these drugs are taken alone. Therefore, when side effects occur at a certain level of a drug during combination therapy, this finding does not necessarily imply that the side effects will recur at similar levels in monotherapy in the same patient.

Interpretation of Drug Effect

In patients on AED polytherapy, it may be difficult to determine which drug has caused a reduction in seizure frequency and which drug is responsible for side effects, unless the adverse reaction is unique to one of the drugs. Idiosyncratic toxic reactions, such as an allergic rash, do not necessarily appear promptly after the introduction of a new drug; therefore, they may not necessarily be caused by the last drug added to the regimen. This can create a dilemma, especially when two drugs known for their potential for allergic reactions have been introduced within a relatively short time interval. These problems are compounded by frequent dose changes and short periods of observation. A carry-over effect or delayed maximal efficacy of a drug contributes to confusion when several drugs are prescribed simultaneously.

Idiosyncratic Toxic Reactions

Idiosyncratic adverse side effects of drugs are not dose related. Certain idiosyncratic reactions are more likely to occur when two drugs are taken in combination. As mentioned earlier, valproate can increase the incidence of rashes associated with lamotrigine (11). Also, the combination of valproate with other AEDs, more often than valproate monotherapy, can result in a dramatic encephalopathic state that does not result from toxic drug levels or from a pharmacokinetic interaction (16, 17). This is characterized by alteration of consciousness, usually a stuporous state, and by sudden and pronounced slowing of the background activity in the electroencephalogram. It is important to recognize the cause of these stuporous episodes because they are rapidly reversible upon discontinuation of valproate or of the last introduced drug. The mechanism of this encephalopathy has not been elucidated, but it does not appear to be related to hyperammonemia. Finally, one of the disadvantages of taking two or more drugs is the higher cost. For patients who are prescribed multiple drugs for several years, this is a tangible factor and there must be some evidence that the higher cost is associated with an increased benefit.

There can also be an exacerbation of the dose-related side effects of one AED by another. In two reports, an increase in the known tremor associated with valproate therapy was described following the addition of lamotrigine (18, 19). Also, an increase in side effects characteristic of carbamazepine, but not of levetiracetam, was noted in four patients after the addition of levetiracetam to carbamazepine (20), and after the addition of lamotrigine to carbamazepine (21). Finally, three patients experienced chorea while taking phenytoin and lamotrigine in combination only, with resolution when either one of the medications was withdrawn (22).

POTENTIAL ADVANTAGES OF COMBINATION DRUG THERAPY

Compared with single-drug therapy there are two potential advantages of combination drug therapy: better seizure control or a similar degree of seizure control with fewer dose-related side effects. For any combination of AEDs to meet either of these criteria, the particular combination must have either a wider antiepileptic spectrum or a better therapeutic index than either drug alone. For example, a patient with both primarily generalized tonic-clonic seizures and myoclonic seizures who failed to have both seizure types controlled by lamotrigine alone or by clonazepam alone might do well on both drugs. Although lamotrigine may not have controlled the myoclonic seizures and clonazepam may not have controlled the generalized tonic-clonic seizures, together they may complement each other and have a wider antiepileptic spectrum than either one alone. In another hypothetical case, consider a patient whose partial seizures were not controlled by the maximal tolerated doses of either levetiracetam alone or oxcarbazepine alone, leading to both drugs being prescribed together. If the seizures can be controlled by the combination of levetiracetam and oxcarbazepine at doses tolerated by the patient, a superior therapeutic index for the combination of levetiracetam and carbamazepine would have been demonstrated. Unfortunately, there are very few data in the clinical literature demonstrating for any combination of AEDs a better effectiveness than for either drug alone. Furthermore, although a great deal of information is available on the pharmacokinetic interactions between AEDs, less is known about pharmacodynamic interactions—interactions that occur in the central nervous system—because they are more difficult to quantify. However, increasing attention is being paid to the theoretical, experimental, and clinical background for the practice of combining AEDs.

A supra-additive pharmacodynamic interaction (potentiation or synergism) between two drugs with regard to their protective effect against seizures has often been used as supportive evidence that these two drugs represent a superior combination. However, this antiepileptic interaction in itself has little meaning unless the neurotoxic effects are also evaluated. If toxicity is also supra-additive to a same or greater extent as the antiepileptic effect, the therapeutic index of the combination is equal to or inferior to the therapeutic index of each drug alone. In other words, at the same level of neurotoxicity, the drug combination does not provide more seizure protection than either of the two drugs alone. Clinically, it is very difficult to study the individual and combined therapeutic index of AEDs, because both seizure protection and neurotoxic side effects of single drugs and of combinations of drugs must be assessed quantitatively in a homogeneous population of patients with epilepsy. Therefore, most of the available information on the pharmacodynamic effect of combining AEDs has been obtained from animal experiments.

Experimental Studies

Table 32-1 summarizes the results of studies on antiepileptic and neurotoxic interactions between many of the established and newer AEDs, including interactions between drugs and their active metabolites (12, 23–37). All results in these studies are based on the analysis of brain drug concentrations in mice. Seizure protection was assessed by standardized experimental seizure models. Neurotoxicity was assessed by various standardized models of motor incoordination in animals. Although this is a rough assessment of dose-related neurotoxicity, there is no reliable animal model that reflects the scope of dose-related neurotoxicity of AEDs in humans. The methods used for the quantitative assessment of the pharmacodynamic drug interactions were either the isobolographic analysis, the fractional effective concentration index, or both (23, 25, 27).

The majority of the neurotoxic interactions are additive or infra-additive, less commonly supra-additive. Thus, in most instances, neurotoxicity of AEDs is not potentiated when they are combined. Inversely, antiepileptic interactions are mostly additive or supra-additive, less commonly infra-additive. Drug pairs with supra-additive antiepileptic interactions can be advantageous even when the neurotoxic interaction is additive. When the antiepileptic interaction is additive, only combinations with an infra-additive neurotoxic interaction can have a better protective index than the single drug. According to Table 32-1, several pairs of drugs appear to meet these criteria for an advantageous combination in this animal model. When carrying out such studies of pharmacodynamic interactions, drug concentrations and not doses must be used because of the effect of possible pharmacokinetic interactions. For example, earlier studies of the antiepileptic interaction between phenytoin and phenobarbital, based on the analysis of doses administered, suggested a supra-additive interaction. A purely additive interaction was found when brain levels were measured in two independent studies (23, 38). Indeed, an acute elevation of the phenytoin level-to-dose ratio in the presence of phenobarbital could be demonstrated (23).

The combinations of clonazepam with valproate and clonazepam with ethosuximide were also tested in mice (29). Nonprotective and nontoxic doses of clonazepam increased the protective effect and the neurotoxicity of valproate and ethosuximide, indicating supra-additive effects. The two drug combinations had a better protective index than each drug alone despite supra-additive neurotoxicity. Using a similar model, Gordon and coworkers (39) studied pharmacodynamic interactions between felbamate and phenytoin, carbamazepine, valproate, and phenobarbital. They found that nonprotective doses of the latter four drugs decreased the median effective dose (ED_{50}) values of felbamate against maximal electroshock seizures. However, neurotoxicity was not potentiated, and the protective index of felbamate was more than doubled by the addition of any one of the four drugs. Although the analysis was based on doses, the authors did measure plasma drug levels and demonstrated the absence of pharmacokinetic interaction.

Clinical Studies

The results of the above studies in animals cannot be extrapolated to patients. There have been very few clinical studies of AED combinations based on systematic comparisons between the effect of two drugs administered both in monotherapy and their effect in combination. Comparing the effect of adding a second drug with the result of monotherapy with the first drug is not sufficient to demonstrate the superiority of the combination. Success with add-on therapy should be considered as success of alternative therapy until proven otherwise. In 30 adult patients who had failed to respond to the maximal tolerated dose of carbamazepine, phenytoin, phenobarbital, or primidone, a second drug (carbamazepine, phenytoin, phenobarbital, primidone, valproic acid, clonazepam, or clobazam) was added, if necessary up to the maximum tolerated dose (7). A reduction in seizure frequency by 75% or more was observed in 4 patients (13%). However, no patient became seizure free, and 3 patients (10%) experienced an increase in seizure frequency by more than 100%. In a study of 157 patients whose seizures were not controlled on a monotherapy, their treatment was randomized to alternative monotherapy or to adjunctive therapy (40). The outcome in the two groups in terms of seizure control and adverse effects did not differ. Schapel and coworkers (41) evaluated the combination of vigabatrin with lamotrigine in 42 patients with intractable epilepsy. On the combination, the median seizure frequency was reduced by 18% when vigabatrin was added to lamotrigine (n = 27) and by 24% when lamotrigine was added to vigabatrin (n = 15). However, this study does not document superiority of the combination. Because patients did not receive both drugs in monotherapy before the combination, the results may just reflect the effect of the second drug added, not of the combination.

In a sequential study, some patients whose seizures were not controlled by valproate alone and by carbamazepine alone had a response to the combination of these two drugs (42). The combination of carbamazepine and phenytoin was assessed in a well-designed study, which was published only as an abstract (43). Initial treatment in 100 newly diagnosed patients was monotherapy with either carbamazepine or with phenytoin, in a randomized design. Fifty patients were not seizure free after 1 year and were switched to the other drug; 17 (34%) became seizure free. The remaining 33 patients received both medications, and only 5 (15%) were fully controlled. The potential benefit of the combination of carbamazepine with vigabatrin was assessed in newly diagnosed patients whose treatment was randomized to monotherapy with either one of these two drugs (44). Seizure control was not achieved in 25 patients, but 11 of them (44%) became seizure free when switched to the other drug. The remaining still refractory 14 patients were treated with the two drugs in combination, and 5 (36%) achieved full seizure control.

At least two clinical studies provided evidence suggestive of a synergism between valproate and lamotrigine. Brodie and Yuen (45) found evidence suggestive of a synergism between lamotrigine and valproate in a lamotrigine substitution study. In 347 uncontrolled patients on monotherapy with valproate, carbamazepine, phenytoin, or phenobarbital, lamotrigine was added. An attempt was made to withdraw the first drug in patients with a 50% or greater seizure reduction. A synergism between lamotrigine and valproate was suggested on the basis of two observations: (1) a significantly better response after adding lamotrigine to valproate than to carbamazepine or phenytoin ($P < 0.001$), both for partial seizures ($P < 0.02$) and for generalized tonic-clonic seizures (not statistically significant), and (2) a poorer response after valproate was withdrawn. A smaller, but very systematic, study addressed the same combination (18). Valproate was added to a pre-existing drug regimen in 20 patients with refractory complex partial seizures. Only three experienced a >50% reduction in seizure frequency. Valproate was replaced by lamotrigine (added to the same pre-exisitng regimen) in the remaining 17 patients. A >50% seizure reduction was observed in 4 of the 17 patients. When valproate was reintroduced in addition to the lamotrigine in the remaining 13 patients, 8 of the patients had a favorable response, 4 had a >50% seizure reduction, and 4 became seizure free.

Among the drugs used in the treatment of absence seizures, one clinical study suggests that the combination of valproate and ethosuximide is possibly beneficial. Five patients with absence seizures that had remained refractory to ethosuximide or to sodium valproate alone (or to both) became seizure free when the two drugs were combined (46). The experimental evidence discussed earlier also suggests that valproate with ethosuximide is one of the combinations with a favorable protective index.

HOW SHOULD ANTIEPILEPTIC DRUG COMBINATIONS BE SELECTED?

Considering the fact that there are no definitive clinical studies documenting the superiority of any specific drug combination, selecting a combination of two AEDs remains at the present time an educated guess at best. The choice may be based on several considerations that include the mechanisms of action, the clinical spectrum of activity, side effects, and pharmacokinetic interactions.

The mechanism of action of AEDs has been suggested as a consideration for rational combinations (47, 48) based on the concept that drugs to be combined should have different mechanisms of action that could be complementary. This is an elegant hypothesis, which has never been proved experimentally or clinically. For the time being, choosing a drug combination based on the mechanisms of action remains purely hypothetical, and no specific drug pair can be recommended.

When a patient has two or more seizure types that cannot be controlled by one drug alone, two drugs can be selected according to their spectrum of efficacy. For each seizure type, the most effective and best tolerated drug should be selected. An example of epilepsy with multiple seizure types is Lennox-Gastaut syndrome. Valproate has long been a preferred drug in patients with Lennox-Gastaut syndrome, but three drugs have now been shown in double-blind studies to be effective: felbamate (49), lamotrigine (50), and topiramate (51). Combinations between these four drugs might be more effective in reducing drop attacks as well as atypical absences and tonic seizures than only one drug alone. On the other hand, phenytoin and carbamazepine usually are not effective and can even exacerbate certain seizures in these patients (52).

The absence of pharmacokinetic interactions between two drugs certainly makes it easier to use them together. However, pharmacokinetic interactions are known and predictable, and it is the physician's responsibility to make appropriate dosage adjustments, either as a corrective measure or preferably as a preventive measure. Therefore, pharmacokinetic interactions should not be a reason to avoid a drug combination that could be beneficial to the patient. Combinations to be avoided are those between drugs with similar side effects, such as barbiturates and benzodiazepines or barbiturates and topiramate (sedation, cognitive effects), topiramate with zonisamide or acetazolamide (nephrolithiasis, acidosis, weight loss), or carbamazepine with oxcarbazepine (hyponatremia), valproate and gabapentin (weight gain).

As opposed to the classic concept of "high-dose monotherapy" (9), a concept of "low-dose polytherapy" could be advocated. The rationale would be that AEDs share their antiepileptic effect but do not always share their adverse effects. Therefore, if a patient has a good seizure response to two drugs in monotherapy, but with side effects, the two drugs might achieve the same seizure reduction together, at lower doses that could be below the clinical threshold for their side effects. An example would be a child with absence seizures who has thrombocytopenia or tremor at effective doses of valproate and persisting gastrointestinal side effects at effective doses of ethosuximide. The same seizure control without the side effects might be achieved with the two drugs at lower doses. Any two drugs with different side effects, but efficacy against the same seizure type, could be combined according to this concept. This concept is supported by the experimental pharmacodynamic interaction studies described earlier. These studies have demonstrated that the neurotoxic pharmacodynamic interaction often does not parallel the antiepileptic pharmacodynamic interaction (Table 32-1).

In conclusion, in view of the known disadvantages of combination therapy, the benefit of a given drug combination must be well documented in every patient if the combination is to be maintained. To quote Meinardi (53), "at present, however, there are too many gaps in our knowledge to make theoretical planning of [combination] drug therapy more promising than an empirical approach." Drug combinations are best chosen by selecting the best drugs known to be effective against the patient's seizure type or seizure types. Rational polytherapy cannot be predicted and must be documented for every patient according to the following definition: whether the patient does better in terms of seizure control versus side effects while taking drugs A and B together (at any dose) than the patient had done on drug A alone and on drug B alone at their respective optimal doses. However, there may be instances in which it would be appropriate to maintain a drug combination even when the above definition is not met. For instance, a patient may respond partially to a first drug and experience further improvement after addition of the second drug, or the patient may become seizure free after addition of the second drug, despite lack of response to the first drug. In such cases, it is understandable that one may be reluctant to make any change. Finally, in clinical practice, the need to reduce overtreatment of patients with epilepsy may be at least as common as the need to find an appropriate drug combination (54).

References

1. Reynolds EH, Shorvon SD. Single drug or combination therapy for epilepsy? *Drugs* 1981; 21:374–382.
2. Fischbacher E. Effect of reduction of anticonvulsants on well-being. *Br Med J* 1982; 285:423–424.
3. Bennett HS, Dunlop T, Ziring P. Reduction of polypharmacy for epilepsy in an institution for the retarded. *Dev Med Child Neurol* 1983; 25:735–737.
4. Theodore WH, Porter RJ. Removal of sedative-hypnotic antiepileptic drugs from the regimen of patients with intractable epilepsy. *Ann Neurol* 1983; 13:320–324.
5. Albright P, Bruni J. Reduction of polytherapy in epileptic patients. *Arch Neurol* 1985; 42:797–799.
6. Schmidt D. Reduction of two-drug therapy in intractable epilepsy. *Epilepsia* 1983; 24:368–376.
7. Schmidt D. Two antiepileptic drugs for intractable epilepsy with complex-partial seizures. *J Neurol Psychiatry* 1982; 45:1119–1124.
8. Kuzniecky R, Rubin ZK, Faught E, Morawetz R. Anti-epileptic drug treatment after temporal lobe epilepsy surgery: a randomized study comparing carbamazepine and polytherapy. *Epilepsia* 1992; 33:908–912.
9. Lesser RP, Pippinger CE, Lüders H, Dinner DS. High-dose monotherapy in the treatment of intractable seizures. *Neurology* 1984; 34:707–711.
10. Henriksen O, Johannessen SI. Clinical and pharmacokinetic observations on sodium valproate—a 5-year follow-up study in 100 children with epilepsy. *Acta Neurol Scand* 1982; 65:504–523.
11. Besag FMC, Wallace SJ, Dulac O, et al. Lamotrigine for the treatment of epilepsy in childhood. *J Pediatr* 1995; 127:991–997.
12. Levy RH, Bourgeois BFD, Hachad H. Drug-drug interactions (Chapter 111). In: Engel J, Pedley TA, eds. *Epilepsy: A Comprehensive Textbook*. 2nd ed. Philadelphia, PA: Lippincott Williams & Wilkins, 2007.
13. Trimble MR, Thompson PJ. Anticonvulsant drugs, cognitive function, and behaviour. *Epilepsia* 1983; 24 Suppl:S55–S63.
14. Bourgeois BFD. Problems of combination drug therapy in children. *Epilepsia* 1988; 29: S20–S24.
15. Deckers CLP, Hekster YA, Keyser A, Meinardi H, et al. Reappraisal of polytherapy in epilepsy: a critical review of drug load and adverse effects. *Epilepsia* 1997; 38:570–575.
16. Sackellares JC, Lee SI, Dreifuss FE. Stupor following administration of valproic acid to patients receiving other antiepileptic drugs. *Epilepsia* 1979; 20:697–703.
17. Marescaux C, Warter JM, Micheletti G, et al. Stuporous episodes during treatment with sodium valproate: report of seven cases. *Epilepsia* 1982; 23:297–305.
18. Pisani F, Oteri G, Russo MF, Di Perri R, et al. The efficacy of valproate-lamotrigine comedication in refractory complex partial seizures: evidence for a pharmacodynamic interaction. *Epilepsia* 1999; 40:1141–1146.
19. Kanner AM, Frey M. Adding valproate to lamotrigine: a study of their pharmacokinetic interaction. *Neurology* 2000; 55:588–591.
20. Sisodiya SM, Sander JW, Patsalos PN. Carbamazepine toxicity during combination therapy with levetiracetam: a pharmacodynamic interaction. *Epilepsy Res* 2002; 48:217–219.
21. Besag FM, Berry DJ, Pool F, Newbery JE, et al. Carbamazepine toxicity with lamotrigine: pharmacokinetic or pharmacodynamic interaction? *Epilepsia* 1998; 39:183–187.
22. Zaatreh M, Tennison M, D'Cruz O, Beach RL. Anticonvulsants-induced chorea: a role for pharmacodynamic drug interaction? *Seizure* 2001; 10:596–599.
23. Bourgeois BFD. Antiepileptic drug combinations and experimental background: the case of phenobarbital and phenytoin. *Naunyn-Schmiedeberg's Arch Pharmacol* 1986; 333:406–411.
24. Morris JC, Dodson WE, Hatlelid JM, Ferrendelli JA. Phenytoin and carbamazepine alone and in combination: anticonvulsant and neurotoxic effects. *Neurology* 1987; 37:1111–1118.
25. Bourgeois BFD, Wad N. Combined administration of carbamazepine and phenobarbital: effect on anticonvulsant activity and neurotoxicity. *Epilepsia* 1988; 29:482–487.
26. Bourgeois BFD. Anticonvulsant potency and neurotoxicity of valproate alone and in combination with carbamazepine or phenobarbital. *Clin Neuropharmacol* 1988; 11:348–359.
27. Bourgeois BFD. Combination of valproate and ethosuximide: antiepileptic and neurotoxic interaction. *J Pharmacol Exp Ther* 1988; 237:1128–1132.
28. Chez MG, Bourgeois BFD, Pippinger CE, Knowles WD. Pharmacodynamic interactions between phenytoin and valproate: Individual and combined antiepileptic and neurotoxic actions in mice. *Clin Neuropharmacol* 1994; 17:32–37.
29. Bourgeois BFD, VanLente F. Effect of clonazepam on antiepileptic potency, neurotoxicity and therapeutic index of valproate and ethosuximide in mice. *Epilepsia* 1994; 35 Suppl 8:142 (abstract).
30. Bourgeois BFD, Wad N. Individual and combined anti-epileptic and neurotoxic activity of carbamazepine and carbamazepine-10, 11-epoxide in mice. *J Pharmacol Exp Ther* 1984; 231:411–415.
31. Bourgeois BFD, Dodson WE, Ferrendelli JA. Primidone, phenobarbital and PEMA: II. Seizure protection, neurotoxicity and therapeutic index of varying combinations in mice. *Neurology* 1983; 33:291–295.
32. Luszczki JJ, Czuczwar M, Kis J, Krysa J, et al. Interactions of lamotrigine with topiramate and first-generation antiepileptic drugs in the maximal electroshock test in mice: an isobolographic analysis. *Epilepsia* 2003; 44:1003–1013.
33. Luszczki JJ, Swiader M, Parada-Turska J, Czuczwar SJ. Tiagabine synergistically interacts with gabapentin in the electroconvulsive threshold test in mice. *Neuropsychopharmacology* 2003; 28:1817–1830.
34. Luszczki JJ, Czuczwar SJ. Preclinical profile of combinations of some second-generation antiepileptic drugs: an isobolographic analysis. *Epilepsia* 2004; 45:895–907.
35. Luszczki JJ, Czuczwar SJ. Interaction between lamotrigine and felbamate in the maximal electroshock-induced seizures in mice: an isobolographic analysis. *Eur Neuropsychopharmacol* 2005; 15:133–142.
36. Luszczki JJ, Andres MM, Czuczwar SJ. Synergistic interaction of gabapentin and oxcarbazepine in the mouse maximal electroshock seizure model—an isobolographic analysis. *Eur J Pharmacol* 2005; 515:54–61.
37. Luszczki JJ, Andres MM, Czuczwar P, Cioczek-Czuczwar A, et al. Pharmacodynamic and pharmacokinetic characterization of interactions between levetiracetam and numerous antiepileptic drugs in the mouse maximal electroshock seizure model: an isobolographic analysis. *Epilepsia* 2006; 47:10–20.
38. Leppik IE, Sherwin AL. Anticonvulsant activity of phenobarbital and phenytoin in combination. *J Pharmacol Exp Ther* 1977; 200:570–575.
39. Gordon R, Gels M, Wichman J, Diamantis W, Sofia RD. Interaction of felbamate with several other antiepileptic drugs against seizures induced by maximal electroshock in mice. *Epilepsia* 1993; 34:367–371.
40. Beghi E, Gatti G, Tonini C, Ben-Menachem E, et al, BASE Study Group. Adjunctive therapy versus alternative monotherapy in patients with partial epilepsy failing on a single drug: a multicentre, randomized, pragmatic controlled trial. *Epilepsy Res* 2003; 57:1–13.
41. Schapel GJ, Black AB, Lam EL, Robinson M, et al. Combination vigabatrin and lamotrigine therapy for intractable epilepsy. *Seizure* 1996; 5:51–56.
42. Walker JE, Koon R. Carbamazepine versus valproate versus combined therapy for refractory partial complex seizures with secondary generalization. *Epilepsia* 1988; 32:693 (abstract).

43. Hakkarainen H. Carbamazepine vs. diphenylhydatnoin vs. their combination in adult epilepsy. *Neurology* 1980; 30:354.
44. Tanganelli P, Regesta G. Vigabatrin vs. carbamazepine monotherapy in newly diagnosed focal epilepsy: a randomized response conditional cross-over study. *Epilepsy Res* 1996; 25:257–262.
45. Brodie MJ, Yuen AW. Lamotrigine substitution study: evidence for synergism with sodium valproate? 105 Study Group. *Epilepsy Res* 1997; 26:423–432.
46. Rowan AJ, Meijer JW, de Beer-Pawlikowski N, van der Geest P, et al. Valproate-ethosuximide combination therapy for refractory absence seizures. *Arch Neurol* 1983; 40:797–802.
47. Perucca E. Pharmacological principles as a basis for poly-therapy. *Acta Neurol Scand* 1995; 162 Suppl:31–34.
48. Macdonald RL. Is there a mechanistic basis for rational polypharmacy? *Epilepsy Res* 1996; 11:79–93.
49. The Felbamate Study Group in Lennox-Gastaut Syndrome. Efficacy of felbamate in childhood epileptic encephalopathy (Lennox-Gastaut syndrome). *N Engl J Med* 1993; 328:29–33.
50. Motte J, Trevathan E, Arvidsson JF, et al. Lamotrigine for generalized seizures associated with the Lennox-Gastaut syndrome. *N Engl J Med* 1997; 337:1807–1812.
51. Sachdeo RC, Glauser TA, Ritter F, Reife R, et al. A double-blind, randomized trial of topiramate in Lennox-Gastaut syndrome. Topiramate YL Study Group. *Neurology* 1999; 52:1882–1887.
52. Snead OC, Hosey LC. Exacerbation of seizures in children by carbamazepine. *N Engl J Med* 1985; 313:916–921.
53. Meinardi H. Use of combined antiepileptic drug therapy. In: Levy RH, Mattson RH, Meldrum BS, eds. *Antiepileptic Drugs*. 4th ed. New York: Raven Press, 1995:91–97.
54. Bourgeois BFD. Overtreatment in epilepsy–mechanisms and management: reducing overtreatment. *Epilepsy Res* 2002; 52:53–60.

33 Adverse Effects of Antiepileptic Drugs

L. James Willmore
James W. Wheless
John M. Pellock

Children with seizures and epilepsy commonly are treated with an antiepileptic drug. Although efficacy for some specific seizure types sometimes drives drug selection, the side effect profile of drugs and the potential for toxicity are important considerations. Parents and patients must receive adequate data so that they can participate in treatment decisions and provide informed consent. Treatment must balance the goal of complete seizure control with drug toxicity during both acute and chronic treatment (1). Antiepileptic drugs cause nonspecific dose-related responses, unique effects specific to a given drug, or rare but potentially dangerous idiosyncratic reactions. Drug treatment, in the absence of a specific history of allergy, is a task of trial and error. However, specific cellular mechanisms or metabolic abnormalities may account for some adverse drug effects.

Treatment requires accurate diagnosis followed by knowledgeable use of drugs based on pharmacokinetics and pharmacodynamics. Although the commonly used antiepileptic drugs are effective in many patients, efficacy of any selected drug for a specific patient cannot be predicted. Therefore, sequencing of treatment using several drugs often is required. Plasma levels guide treatment in some cases, but titration of dose, using development of dose-related symptoms as an endpoint, should be completed before a drug is declared ineffective.

Common problems can be anticipated, but dangerous, unexpected, and rare individual responses and reactions require physicians to provide detailed information during the process of informed consent. Thus, all persons involved in the care of a patient must be informed in explicit terms about the potential for serious or even fatal reactions to drugs.

Adverse drug reactions (ADRs) are noxious effects occurring at dosages of drugs used appropriately in humans for prophylaxis, diagnosis, or therapy (2). Some of these reactions depend on pharmacokinetic effects, with dose-dependent responses that correlate with plasma blood levels of a drug.

Pharmacodynamic effects occur when target organ responses are altered in a way that is independent of plasma concentration; such effects may be unique to a drug or to an individual patient. Serious non-dose-related ADRs cause drug-induced disease that may be acute or may occur following chronic treatment. Potentially fatal idiosyncratic reactions are listed in Table 33-1 (4).

Neurotoxicity, either dependent on dose or pharmacodynamic in nature, may occur at the time of drug initiation, during dose escalation, or at the time of the peak in plasma levels. These mild and reversible effects include sedation, changes in behavior, tremor, vertigo, diplopia, nystagmus, ataxia, or even dysarthria (1, 5).

Dose-related neurotoxicity becomes a more commonly encountered problem if two or more antiepileptic drugs (AEDs) are used in combination. Monotherapy improves compliance, reduces total cost of medication, and may eliminate interactions that could cause additive adverse effects (6, 7). Monotherapy use of the commonly available AEDs results in seizure control in 50% to 80% of patients with epilepsy (8, 9).

Almost all AEDs have caused idiosyncratic reactions or drug allergy. Such reactions may be severe, unpredictable, and although rare, may be life-threatening (3). Idiosyncratic responses to AEDs in a given patient are associated with cellular, immunologic, or enzymatic characteristics that are unique to that patient. Drug clearance by oxidation requires catalyzed effects of the microsomal membrane-bound mixed function oxidases that contain cytochrome P450 (10). The P450 terminal oxidases receive electrons from reduced nicotinamide adenine dinucleotide phosphate (NADPH) and reduced nicotinamide adenine dinucleotide (NADH). The heterogenicity of the P-450 system causes apparent specificity, with isozyme families produced by the same gene family. Some AEDs are metabolized through such mixed-function oxidases, yielding either stable, unstable, or potentially reactive molecular species. The accumulation of reactive and toxic intermediates as a result of drug treatment is determined by genetically derived enzyme activities. Thus, metabolism of a ring compounds via arene oxidase with impairment of metabolism of the arene oxide product could occur with deficiency of the enzyme epoxide hydrolase. The arene form of phenytoin has been implicated as a cause of hepatotoxicity, teratogenicity, bone marrow toxicity, and allergic skin reactions (11, 12).

AED hypersensitivity syndrome occurs early in the treatment with aromatic antiepileptic compounds. Components include rash, fever, and eosinophilia and may include lymphadenopathy and life-threatening hepatic necrosis (13). Skin rash may or may not be pruritic and is in the form of an exanthema. More severe reactions include exfoliative dermatitis, erythema multiforme, Stevens-Johnson syndrome, or even toxic epidermal necrolysis (14). Adverse reactions of the idiosyncratic type tend to be immune-mediated effects in a susceptible individual (15).

Mechanisms are not completely understood, but most rash and hypersensitivity syndromes probably are related to pharmacogenetic variation in drug biotransformation (16). Immune involvement is suggested by the occurrence of a sensitization interval of 7–10 days after first exposure to a drug (17). In fact, T lymphocytes have been found in the perivascular infiltrate and epidermis (CD8C and CD4C) of patients with carbamazepine-induced toxic epidermal necrolysis (17). Reactive metabolites produced by bioactivation are cytotoxic by binding to microsomal proteins. Such covalent adducts are formed in hepatic cytochrome P-450–medicated reactions (15).

Antibodies to P450 enzymes, with epitopes such as anti-CYP2D6 and anit-CYP3A, have amino acid sequences similar to those of viral or fungal origin that suggest prior host-dependent immune responses to infection that are unique to a person's human lymphocyte antigen (HLA) genotype (15). With exposure to a bioactivated AED, a chemical modification of the P450 enzyme occurs. These effects may be from formation of reactive drug metabolites, free radical species, or impairment of detoxification enzymes. These changes in enzyme function yield altered peptide structures that result in the immune response (15).

TABLE 33-1

REACTION	CBZ	ETH	FBM	GBP	LEV	LTG	OXC	PB	PHT	TPM	TGB	VPA	ZNS
Agranulocytosis	X	X	X					X	X			X	
Blistering skin reactions (Stevens-Johnson Syndrome)	X	X				X		X	X			X	
Aplastic anemia	X	X	X						X			X	
Hepatic failure	X		X					X	X			X	
Allergic dermatitis	X	X	X	X		X	X	X	X	X	X	X	X
Serum sickness	X	X						X	X			X	
Pancreatitis	X												
Nephrolithiasis										X			X
Bone metabolism	X								X				

Abbreviations: CBX, carbamazepine; ETH, ethosuximide; FBM, felbamate; GBP, gabapentin; LEV, levetiracetam; LTG, lamotrigine; OXC, oxcarbazepine; PB, phenobarbital; PHT, phenytoin; TPM, topiramate; TGB, tiagabine; VPA, valproate; ZNS, xonisamide

Impact of enzyme-inducing drugs on bone health must be considered in all patients. Although most institutionalized patients in the modern era are given calcium supplementation and vitamin D, these simple interventions and the need for assessment of bone density in those patients on long-term drug use must be kept in mind (18).

SPECIFIC DRUGS

Phenobarbital

Phenobarbital (see Chapter 48) has been in continual use for at least 95 years. Common side effects in children include behavioral changes with hyperactivity and irritability; adults experience drowsiness. Altered attention, effects on cognition, and even depression may be dose related or occur in specific patients without relationship to plasma level (19–21). Dose-related neurotoxicity includes nystagmus, ataxia, incoordination, dyskinesia, and altered sleep patterns. Idiosyncratic reactions include allergic dermatitis, Stevens-Johnson syndrome, serum sickness, and hepatic failure. Agranulocytosis and aplastic anemia have been reported (3, 4). Folate deficiency in patients treated with AEDs is claimed to be associated with behavioral changes (22). Phenobarbital is known to exacerbate acute intermittent porphyria (23).

Induction of hepatic oxidative metabolism by phenobarbital is a fundamental mechanism for drug interactions. Vitamin D metabolism is induced by phenobarbital; thus, multihandicapped and bedridden children receiving this drug or other AEDs may develop osteoporosis; vitamin D supplementation is important in these children (24). Phenobarbital alters absorption and induces metabolism of vitamin K. Neonates of mothers treated with phenobarbital or other barbiturates need vitamin K supplementation to prevent neonatal hemorrhagic disease. Prophylactic vitamin K must be given during the last month of gestation, at the beginning of labor, and to the infant at birth.

Chronic phenobarbital treatment may cause connective tissue changes, with coarsened facial feature, Dupuytren's contracture, Ledderhose syndrome (plantar fibromas), and frozen shoulder (25). Sedative effects of phenobarbital may cause exacerbation of absence, atonic, and myoclonic seizures, although other mechanisms may be operant (6). Sudden withholding of doses of short-acting barbiturates may precipitate drug withdrawal seizures or even status epilepticus. Given the slow rate of clearance of phenobarbital, such acute withdrawal seizures are less problematic, but it is wise to taper the dose of phenobarbital if the drug is to be discontinued. Some children, and even adults, may experience mild withdrawal symptoms that include tremor, sweating, restlessness, irritability, weight loss, disturbance of sleep, and even psychiatric symptoms. Mothers treated with phenobarbital may deliver infants that have withdrawal, including irritability, hypotonia, and vomiting, for several days after delivery (26).

Phenytoin

Phenytoin is metabolized by hepatic enzymes that are capacity limited (see Chapter 49). This system is commonly saturated at serum concentrations of 8–10 μg/mL. Because of the saturation kinetics of phenytoin, small changes in the maintenance dose will produce large changes in serum concentration (27). Thus the half-life of the drug increases with higher plasma concentrations. Because of saturation kinetics, dose changes must be made with care. One challenge to phenytoin use is alteration of steady state by interaction with other drugs (28).

Dose-related effects of phenytoin include nystagmus, ataxia, altered coordination, cognitive changes, and dyskinesia (3). Infrequently, children may become irritable or hyperactive (29). Children seldom develop nystagmus even when they are overtly ataxic and have elevated serum levels of phenytoin. A constellation of anorexia, weight loss, and vomiting in a child should suggest phenytoin toxicity (29). Although not strictly a pharmacologic problem, phenytoin causes some drug-specific effects that do not appear to be related to dose. Facial features may coarsen, and body hair will change in texture and become dark in color. Acne may worsen, and gingival hypertrophy is common. Other effects of chronic phenytoin use are osteoporosis and lymphadenopathy (30). Folate deficiency may be severe enough to cause megaloblastic anemia; a transient encephalopathy is said to occur by a similar mechanism (22). Prolonged exposure to high plasma levels of phenytoin has been associated with cerebellar atrophy (29, 31). Idiosyncratic reactions that may be fatal include allergic dermatitis, hepatotoxicity (32), serum sickness reaction, and aplastic anemia (3, 30). Drug-induced lupus erythematosus reactions have been observed (33).

Ethosuximide

Ethosuximide (see Chapter 43) has a half-life that would be compatible with single daily dosing, but such large doses of the drug causes nausea, gastric distress, and abdominal pain unless the drug is given with meals and in divided doses. Rash and headaches, and on rare occasion leukopenia, pancytopenia, and aplastic anemia, have occurred (4). Neurologic effects include headache that may be severe, lethargy, agitation, aggressiveness, depression, and memory problems. Psychiatric disorders were attributed to normalization of the electroencephalogram (EEG) by this drug, but such reactions have been described with other drugs as well, making this hypothesis less tenable (34, 35). Drug-induced lupus has been reported to occur in children (36).

Carbamazepine

Carbamazepine (CBZ) (see Chapter 42) is insoluble in aqueous solutions, behaving as a neutral lipophilic substance (37). Carbamazepine is biotransformed, forming CBZ-10,11-epoxide (38). This epoxide is formed at the 10,11-double bond of the azepine ring when CBZ is catalyzed by the hepatic monoxygenases (39). Inhibition of the activity of epoxide hydrolase, as occurs with concomitant administration of valproic acid (VPA), will increase the quantity of the epoxide (40). Carbamazepine causes mild dose-related neurotoxic effects. Most are concentration dependent. Transient effects include nausea, drowsiness, vertigo, ataxia, and speech slurring. Diplopia is a common concentration-dependent effect that is useful for clinical titration (5). Tremor and headache have been reported. Nausea, vomiting, diarrhea, and abdominal pain occur, but infrequently. Hyponatremia is common but rarely of clinical consequence (41). These transient adverse effects may be limited by administering one of the extended release formulations that result in less peak-to-trough variations in blood levels.

Severe reactions to CBZ cause alteration of hematopoietic, skin, hepatic, and cardiovascular systems (5). Rash occurs in 5% to 8% of patients and rarely may progress to exfoliative dermatitis or even a bullous reaction such as Stevens-Johnson syndrome (42). Hematologic changes are common, with leukopenia observed in 10% to 12% of patients treated with CBZ. However, fatal reactions such as aplastic anemia, are rare, with death in 1.1 per 500,000 treated patients per year (43). Patients and parents must be informed about these serious reactions and reassured that frequent monitoring of blood cell counts and liver studies are unnecessary. Communication with the patient and informed consent are the best methods for long-term monitoring (44).

Valproate

Gastrointestinal effects commonly accompanying initiation of VPA (see Chapter 53) treatment include nausea, diarrhea, abdominal pain, and even vomiting (45). Use at meal time, or administration of a slow-release form of the drug, will cause abatement of these symptoms in most patients. Three dose-related effects occur commonly. Tremor with sustention and at rest is age and dose related because this symptom is found less in children (46). Body weight gain is another common side effect, with 20% to 54% of patients reporting this problem (47). Patients report appetite stimulation. Weight change may require discontinuation of this drug. Hair loss is common and transient. Hair appears to be fragile; regrowth of the broken hair results in a curlier shaft (48). Supplementation with multivitamins containing zinc may protect hair.

Thrombocytopenia occurs in a pattern that suggests it is dose related. Platelet counts vary without dose changes necessarily and are commonly asymptomatic. Petechial hemorrhage and ecchymoses do occur, necessitating lowering the dose or even discontinuing the drug (49, 50).

Other less frequently encountered effects include sedation or encephalopathy (51, 52). Acute encephalopathy and even coma may develop on initial exposure to VPA (51). Upon investigation, these patients may be severely acidotic and have elevated urinary organic acid excretion. Because VPA is known to sequester coenzyme A (53), such patients are suspect of having a partially compensated defect in the mitochondrial beta-oxidation enzymes (52, 54). Dermatologic abnormalities are unusual, but may be severe (55).

Acute hemorrhage pacreatitis may develop in younger patients. Fatal outcome has been reported. Abdominal pain reported by patients receiving VPA should lead to measurement of lipase and amylase levels (56).

Age-related changes in pharmacokinetics of VPA should be anticipated because of the high percentage of drug that is protein bound (57). Valproic acid is a branched-chain carboxylic acid that may be metabolized either through mitochondrial mechanisms or via cytoplasmic enzymes. Dehydrogenation of VPA results in the accumulation of 2-en-, 3-en-, and 4-en-VPA compounds. The 4-en metabolites are highest in infants and decline with age. The 2-en compound has anticonvulsant potency (58). Valproic acid binds to albumin at high- and low-affinity sites. This binding is saturable, causing the free fraction to increase with dose.

Assessment of patients developing hepatotoxicity from treatment with VPA suggests that the highest risk is in children younger than 2 years of age being treated with several AEDs. Additional risk characteristics include presumed metabolic disorders or severe epilepsy complicating mental retardation and organic brain disease (59–62). Although this pattern of incidence provides useful clinical guidelines, most clinicians consider them too restrictive or of insufficient detail to allow identification of patients at highest risk (63). Further complicating management strategies, routine laboratory monitoring does not predict the development of fulminant and irreversible hepatic failure (64). Some patients progressing to fatal hepatotoxicity never developed abnormalities of specific hepatic function tests. Conversely, abnormalities of serum ammonia, carnitine, fibrinogen, and hepatic function tests have been reported to occur without the presence of clinically significant hepatotoxicity (65, 66). Reporting clinical symptoms and identification of patients at greatest risk for fatal hepatotoxicity are more reliable means for monitoring. Vomiting was the most frequently reported initial symptom in fatal cases (59, 60). Combined symptoms of nausea, vomiting, and anorexia occurred in 82% of patients with VPA-associated hepatotoxicity, whereas lethargy, drowsiness, and coma were reported in 40% (67, 68). Although some patients may have reversal of hepatotoxicity by early drug discontinuation, fatalities still result following such prompt action (69). No biochemical marker has been identified to differentiate those patients surviving from those with fatal outcome (69). Rescue of patients with hepatic failure by administration of carnitine has been reported (70). Obtain urinary organic acid measurement and metabolic evaluation in high risk patients, as indicated previously, or in any patient without an established reason for mental retardation and seizures (63).

Identifying high risk patients was reported by Dreifuss et al (59, 60). Most fatalities occurred in the first 6 months of treatment, but some patients developed hepatotoxicity up to 2 years after VPA initiation. Children younger than 2 years of age receiving polytherapy had a 1 in 500 to 800 chance of developing fatal VPA hepatotoxicity. Negative predictors were documented. Patients at negligible risk are those older than the age of 10 years treated with VPA alone and free of indication of underlying metabolic or neurologic disorders. Children at intermediate risk were between age 2 and 10 years on monotherapy and all patients requiring polytherapy.

Patients reported with fatal hepatotoxicity, in the majority of cases, had neurologic abnormalities, including mental retardation, encephalopathy, and decline of neurologic function. In those reported patients older than 21 years of age, two of four had degenerative disease of the nervous system. One report stated that 9 of 16 hepatic fatalities were neurologically abnormal (71). In one series, all patients in the 11-to-20 age group were neurologically abnormal. In a recent review, only 7 of 26 adults reported with fatal hepatic failure from valproate were considered to be neurologically normal (72).

Specific biochemical disorders associated with VPA hepatotoxicity include urea cycle defects, organic aciduras, multiple carboxylase deficiency, mitochondrial or respiratory chain dysfunction, cytochrome aa3 deficiency in muscle, pyruvate carboxylase deficiency, and hepatic pyruvate dehydrogenase complex deficiency (brain) (63, 73, 74). Clinical disorders associated with VPA toxicity include GM1 gangliosidosis type 2, spinocerebellar degeneration, Friedreich's ataxia, Lafora body disease, Alpers disease, and MERRF syndrome (myoclonus epilepsy with ragged red fibers) (67). Patients with such disorders must be identified because of higher risk for VPA hepatotoxicity.

Felbamate

Felbamate (FBM) causes headache, insomnia, and weight loss. Drug interactions with FBM are vigorous and may cause clinically significant toxicity or seizure exacerbation. When FBM is added to CBZ, levels of the parent compound decline by 20% to 25%, but the metabolite CBZ-10,11-epoxide increases by as much as 50% (75, 76). These effects suggest induction of cytochrome P450 along with inhibition of some of the action of epoxide hydrolase. This interaction induces CBZ side effects; the combination also causes headache. Following the identification of aplastic anemia and hepatotoxicity and notification of physicians by the Food and Drug Administration (FDA) in August and September 1994, the number of persons being treated with FBM decreased drastically. Kaufman et al (77) reviewed cases of aplastic anemia reported in the United States and suggested an incidence of aplastic anemia of 27–209 per million in those receiving FBM versus 2–2.5 per million persons in the general population. The aplastic anemia risk with FBM treatment is perhaps up to 20 times greater than that for CBZ. Importantly, no case of aplastic anemia has been reported in children younger than 13 years old. The mean time to presentation is 154 days, with very few cases being reported after 6 months of exposure. Similarly, severe hepatotoxicity associated with FBM has been reported, but this risk seems to be similar to that from valproate. Although there is no predilection for age, children have been affected by severe, life-threatening hepatotoxicity associated with FBM.

Recommended guidelines for the use of FBM now stress that this agent should be used for adults and children with severe epilepsy refractory to other therapy, such as patients with Lennox-Gastaut syndrome. Before beginning treatment a careful history concerning past indications of hematologic toxicity, of hepatotoxicity, and of autoimmune diseases should be sought. Women with autoimmune disease account for the largest portion of those who developed aplastic anemia. Baseline routine hematologic and liver function tests should be performed, and patients and their families must be fully informed of the potential risks; in the United States written consent is recommended. Dose escalation should be made slowly, and dosages of adjunctive medication must be corrected for known interactions where possible. Monotherapy with FBM leads to fewer systemic side effects, but it is unknown whether the rare but potentially life-threatening side effects will be decreased by using FBM alone. Clinical monitoring and specific scheduled blood testing should be done frequently, and patients should be educated regarding symptoms that may possibly signify either hematologic toxicity or hepatotoxicity.

Gabapentin

Structurally related to gamma-aminobutyric acid (GABA), gabapentin reaches peak plasma concentrations 2–3 hours after an oral dose. Unique for an AED, gabapentin is not bound to plasma proteins, nor is it metabolized. Its bland pharmacokinetic properties include no hepatic enzyme induction and little effect on plasma levels of other AEDs. Adverse events were detected in treated patients and were typically neurotoxic, but withdrawal from studies was infrequent. Children have similar adverse events profiles as noted in adults. Patients may experience weight gain. Peripheral edema with normal plasma protein and albumin is observed rarely. There is an increase in the incidence of hyperactivity and aggressive behavior, particularly in mentally retarded children (78) (see Chapter 45).

Lamotrigine

CNS-related side effects of lamotrigine include lethargy, fatigue, and mental confusion (79–84). Serious rashes have occurred; the rate of dose ascension appears to be correlated with this type of adverse event (85). Serious rash may be more common in children; current guidelines in the United States require this drug be discontinued if a rash develops (see Chapter 46).

Although erythematous rash with a morbilliform pattern or urticaria or patterns with a maculopapular component are most common (86–91), some patients can develop erythema multiforme and blistering reactions such as the Stevens-Johnson syndrome or toxic epidermal necrolysis. Simple rashes require careful assessment to be sure a hypersensitivity syndrome is not developing. Sensitivity reactions include fever, lymphadenopathy, elevated liver enzymes, and altered numbers of circulating cellular elements of blood (89).

In drug trials in the United States rash was observed in about 10% of patients, with 3.8% having to discontinue and 0.3% being hospitalized (89). Most serious rashes developed within 6 weeks of beginning treatment with lamotrigine. In children treated in drug trials, rash was observed in 12.9% with serious rash in 1.1% with half of those with Stevens-Johnson syndrome (89). Of interest, more than 80% of patients with complete data developing serious rash were being treated with valproate or had been given doses at a rate higher than recommended (89). Rash was suspected to be a drug interaction with valproate, but that drug inhibits metabolism of lamotrigine, causing diminished clearance with resultant high blood levels (90). Apparently when specific treatment guidelines are followed, the incidence of serious rash may possibly be reduced (89, 91, 92). In the United States, if rash develops it is advised that the drug be discontinued. Table 46-1 (in Chapter 46) lists the suggested drug initiation treatment plan for lamotrigine.

Pregabalin

This drug has impact on voltage-gated calcium channels with inhibition of transmembrane calcium flow through binding with the channel's high-affinity alpha$_2$delta subunit (93, 94). Data from postmarketing are not available. Clinical trials revealed most common adverse effects were dizziness, somnolence, and ataxia; weight gain was reported as well (95, 96).

Levetiracetam

Levetiracetam has an effect against partial onset seizures, primary generalized tonic-clonic seizures, juvenile myoclonic epilepsy, and photosensitivity-related epilepsy syndromes. Although a specific mechanism of action has not been reported, the drug does bind to synaptic vesicle protein and has actions on neuronal GABA and glycine-gated currents (97). Side effects reported from the clinical trials include somnolence, headache, anorexia, and nervousness (98). Behavioral changes in children, including psychosis, have been reported; exacerbation of a preexisting tendency has been suggested as a mechanism (99).

Topiramate

Topiramate has a monosaccharide-type structure (see Chapter 52). Treatment emergent adverse effects with add-on studies showed ataxia, impaired concentration, confusion, dizziness, fatigue, paresthesias, somnolence, and abnormal thinking related to topiramate treatment (100). Nephrolithiasis and dose-related weight loss are potential problems that require discussion with patients. Serious rashes have occurred. Reports of development of acute secondary angle closure glaucoma in patients treated with this drug require informing patients and cautioning them to report development of ocular pain or altered visual acuity immediately (101–103). As with other drugs that alter carbonic anhydrase, oligohydrosis with hyperthermia has been reported and children must be monitored for this problem especially in hot weather (104, 105). Many side effects detected in the studies were caused by forced titration to high doses. Adverse cognitive effects occur at higher doses in adults (100). Slowing the pace of dose ascension reduces the impact on cognitive function.

Tiagabine

Most commonly identified side effects in the pivotal trials of tiagabine included dizziness, asthenia, muscle weakness, nervousness, tremor, impaired concentration, lethargy, and depression (106). These occurred during dose titration. Reasons for withdrawal from the trials included occurrence of confusion, somnolence, ataxia, and dizziness (107). Hepatic clearance signals the need to reduce the dose in patients with liver disease (108).

Oxcarbazepine

Oxcarbazepine is a keto analog of CBZ that is rapidly converted to 10,11-dihydro-10-hydroxycarbamazepine, a monohydroxy active metabolite. Dizziness, sedation, and fatigue were side effects that may be dose related. Hyponatremia has occurred with this drug and some vigilance may be required (109). Rash occurs infrequently, and Stevens-Johnson syndrome and toxic epidermal necrolysis are rare (110).

Vigabatrin

Vigabatrin, also known as gamma-vinyl GABA, is an analog of GABA that acts to increase tissue concentration of that inhibitory transmitter by irreversible inhibition of GABA transaminase, the enzyme that degrades GABA. This effect on a specific enzyme makes traditional pharmacokinetics less relevant.

Adverse effects, in general, are those expected with an AED; drowsiness, irritability, ataxia, and headache have been observed. Of concern are severe changes in behavior with agitation, hallucinations, and altered thinking, effects that are thought to be dose related (35). Depression is an important potential problem in treating all patients (111). Loss of peripheral retinal visual function is of concern (112, 113). One report compared 32 adults treated with vigabatrin with 18 patients treated with CBZ. Up to 40% of the vigabatrin-treated patients had concentrically constricted visual fields (113, 114). Because of robust efficacy in children with infantile spasms trials are under way and screening methods for visual change are being developed (115).

Zonisamide

Zonisamide is a sulfonamide drug widely available in Japan and in the United States. Zonisamide is rapidly absorbed by oral intake; protein binding is about 50%, but drug accumulates in erythrocytes. Plasma half-life is prolonged, at around 55 hours, but is reduced to about 30 hours in patients being treated with enzyme-inducing drugs. This drug is extensively metabolized (108).

Adverse effects of drowsiness and altered thinking in clinical trials were associated as well with anorexia, dizziness, ataxia, fatigue, somnolence, confusion, and poor concentration. Zonisamide has been associated with nephrolithiasis (116). Children may develop oligohydrosis and hyperthermia (117). Parents must be taught to be vigilant when a child is exposed to a hot environment and provide skin moisture to aid in convection cooling.

MECHANISMS AND MONITORING

Hypersensitivity reactions may cause cellular changes that resemble the cytotoxic effects of viral hepatitis. This type of hepatic injury is a common component of systemic reactions involving rash, lymphadenopathy, and eosinophilia. Toxic injury at the cellular level may be related to the formation of arene oxide (118).

Even though routine monitoring may detect alterations in liver function, clinical problems are often not apparent (64). Such findings, however, create a dilemma for the physician regarding plans for ongoing assessment and the need for specific action. Biochemical changes observed in patients being treated with valproate seldom herald the development of a fatal reaction. The first detailed report of valproate-induced hepatotoxicity included one patient with symptomatic hepatic dysfunction and three patients with isolated biochemical changes (64). The observation of transient dose-related hepatotoxicity was followed in 1979 by reports of fatalities associated with valproate treatment (119, 120). Unfortunately, although metabolic abnormalities are occasionally uncovered by valproate administration (52, 121, 122), most patients with mild to moderate symptoms caused by a dose-related side effect cannot be differentiated from those with serious idiosyncratic responses in any way other than by outcome. The idiosyncratic effects upon liver function include hyperammonemia (123–125), severe hepatic dysfunction with recovery, and fulminant hepatic failure (60, 122, 126).

Valproic acid occasionally causes stupor or coma (51). Valproate is known to affect mitochondrial function, causing elevations in serum levels of some branched-chain fatty acids (127). Decreased serum carnitine levels observed with valproate administration (53, 127) are accompanied by increased excretion of acetylcarnitine (128). Valproate reduces levels of both free coenzyme A (CoASH) and acetyl-CoA in rat liver (129, 130). This reduction in CoASH is accompanied by an increase in the intrahepatic medium chain acyl-CoA fraction, identified as valproyl-CoA (129). Although valproate increases activity of the medium chain fraction of acyl-CoA hydrolase, valproyl-CoA itself is hydrolyzed poorly (131). Because valproate-induced inhibition of in-vitro fatty acid oxidation is reversed by addition of CoASH and carnitine to the reactants (132), it would appear that VPA causes sequestration of CoASH.

Sequestration of CoASH and formation of valproyl-CoA could impair or block several steps in fatty acid oxidation. Because fatty acid is esterified to acyl-CoA in the cytosol prior to carnitine-mediated transport across the mitochondrial membrane, decreased CoASH would impair formation of acyl-CoA, or conversion of acyl-carnitine to acyl-CoA, favoring omega oxidation with resultant dicarboxylic aciduria. Coenzyme A deficiency also could impair cleavage of 3-ketoacyl-CoA by thiolase activity, causing accumulation of acetoacetyl-CoA, butyryl-CoA, and hexanoyl-CoA, producing ketosis with excretion of ethylmalonic and adipic acids. Because butyryl-CoA and hexanoyl-CoA dehydrogenases are inhibited by an acyl-CoA metabolite of hypoglycin (133), valproyl-CoA may inhibit these dehydrogenases (52, 54, 63).

Drug-induced effects on the hematopoietic system may be caused by hypersensitivity reactions with antibody-mediated peripheral destruction, by secondary effects such as occurs in a lupus-like syndrome, or by toxic marrow inhibition (134–136). Hypersensitivity reactions may be associated with the drug acting as a hapten with a protein. The net result is that IgE is produced. Another possibility is that there may be a direct drug effect by activation of the complement cascade or by a change in the function of lymphocytes. Direct cellular effects may alter lymphocyte populations or reactivity. For example, it has been postulated that phenytoin may alter lymphocytes, because 21% to 25% of patients chronically treated with this drug will have decreased circulating levels of IgA along with depressed lymphocyte phytohemagglutinin transformation (137, 138). Phenytoin hypersensitivity includes characteristic hepatic involvement and lymphadenopathy (139–142). Potential mechanisms include hapten formation, formation of an arene compounds (118), conversion of the aromatic ring by oxidation to phenol metabolites, or chlorination of nitrogen components on the hydantoin ring (136). Indeed, a metabolite of phenytoin from hepatic microsomes appears to be toxic to lymphocytes. A similar mechanism has been proposed for CBZ. Indeed, CBZ is oxidized to several metabolites that may cause toxic effects on granulocytes (143). Lymphocytes from a patient with sequential aplastic anemia had challenge of those cells with metabolites derived from murine hepatocytes; the sensitivity of the lymphocytes suggested an arene oxide metabolite formation as a mechanism (144).

Serious toxic effects that result from the use of AEDs are usually discovered during the course of treatment. Hence, patients must be informed and freely communicate with their physician. It takes a joint effort to use medications to control seizures. Good therapeutic alliances between patient and physician will serve until such time that screening assays are developed to identify patients likely to develop serious adverse drug effects (44).

Clinical Monitoring

Clinical monitoring is adequate especially within the context of incidence of serious adverse reactions. Although routine monitoring of hepatic function revealed elevation of values in 5% to 15% of patients treated with CBZ, fewer than 20 patients with significant hepatic complications were reported in the Unites States from 1978 to 1989 (145). Fewer cases of pancreatitis were reported. Transient leukopenia occurs in up to 12% of adults and children treated with CBZ (5, 143). Aplastic anemia or agranulocytosis, unrelated to benign leukopenia, occurs in 2 per 575,000 with a mortality rate of approximately 1 in 575,000 treated patients per year (145). Only 4 of the 65 cases of agranulocytosis or aplastic anemia occurred in children.

Of patients developing exfoliative dermatitis alone or as part of systemic hypersensitivity, blood test abnormalities were not found until patients developed clinical symptoms. Presymptomatic blood studies fail to predict disease development. Test abnormalities such as benign leukopenia or transient hepatic enzyme elevations do not predict the occurrence of life-threatening reactions. A genetic abnormality in arene oxide metabolism may occur in those patients at higher risk for some types of adverse responses such as hepatitis (118). A screening test for such defects is not available. The data show that routine monitoring, as practiced commonly, does not allow anticipation of life-threatening effects associated with CBZ treatment. Findings for phenytoin and phenobarbital are similar (4).

As new drugs are developed and added to the regimen available for treating children with epilepsy, physicians should review source documents about those medications and devise a strategy for treatment and monitoring. Because data tend to be limited, initiation of treatment with a newly available drug requires special caution. Although the process of informed consent remains informal, patients and parents should be given as much information as possible. Although industry-produced materials may prove useful, in our opinion the physician should provide copies of package inserts coupled with material they prepare describing how the drug is to be used and any monitoring strategy planned. Although the guiding principle about monitoring of patients being treated with established drugs is parsimony in terms of obtaining routine chemical and hematologic studies, based on the knowledge that such monitoring is ineffective in detecting the occurrence of serious adverse events, such is not necessarily the case with a newly introduced drug. As with the established drugs, baseline hematologic and hepatic screening data should be obtained. Communication is still key; the patient must be prepared to contact the physician and the physician must facilitate that communication. Chemical and hematologic monitoring with use of a new drug may be recommended in the materials a company develops in concert with regulatory functions of the FDA. Although recommendations may seem excessively conservative, it may be wise to follow those guidelines until a larger experience is obtained and data become available.

Recommendations for Monitoring

1. Obtain screening laboratory studies before initiation of AED treatment. Data are unavailable regarding the yield of such testing, but baseline studies provide a benchmark and could identify patients with special risk factors that could influence drug selection.
2. Blood and urine monitoring in otherwise healthy and asymptomatic patients treated with AEDs is not necessary.
3. Identify high risk patients before beginning treatment. These patients include those with presumptive biochemical disorders, altered systemic health, neurodegenerative disease, or a history of significant adverse drug reactions. Monitoring must be designed based on the specifics of the clinical situation.
4. Patients without an advocate, or those unable to communicate, require a different strategy. Although data are unavailable, blood monitoring should be obtained for patients with multiple handicaps who are institutionalized. Monitoring should include basic hematology and chemistry with additional studies based upon the patient's clinical situation.
5. For newly introduced drugs, follow recommended guidelines for blood monitoring until the numbers of patients treated in this country increase and data become available.

References

1. Pellock JM. Efficacy and adverse effects of antiepileptic drugs. *Pediatr Clin North Am* 1989:345–348.
2. Karsh FE, Lasagna L. Adverse drug reactions. A critical review. *JAMA* 1975; 234:1236–1241.
3. Plaa GI, Willmore LJ. General principles: toxicology. In: Levy RH, Mattson RH, Meldrum BS, eds. *Antiepileptic Drugs.* New York: Raven Press, 1998:51–60.
4. Schmidt D. Adverse effects of antiepileptic drugs. New York: Raven Press, 1982.
5. Pellock JM. Carbamazepine side effects in children and adults. *Epilepsia* 1987; 28: S64–S70.
6. Lerman P. Seizures induced or aggravated by anticonvulsants. *Epilepsia* 1986; 27: 706–710.
7. Herranz JL, Armijo JA, Artega R. Clinical side effect of phenobarbital, primidone, phenytoin, carbamazepine and valproate during monotherapy in children. *Epilepsia* 1988; 29:794–804.
8. Mattson RH, Cramer JA, Collins JF, et al. Comparison of carbamazepine, phenobarbital, phenytoin, and primidone in partial and secondarily generalized tonic-clonic seizures. *N Engl J Med* 1985; 313:145–151.
9. Elwes RDC, Johnson AL, Shorvon SD, Reynolds EH. The prognosis for seizure control in newly diagnosed epilepsy. *N Engl J Med* 1984; 311:944–947.
10. Galbraith RA, Michnovicz JJ. The effects of cimetidine on the oxidative metabolism of estradiol. *N Engl J Med* 1989; 321:269–274.
11. Gerson WT, Fine DG, Spielberg SP, et al. Anticonvulsant-induced aplastic anemia: increased susceptibility to toxic drug metabolites in vitro. *Blood* 1983; 61:889–893.
12. Strickler SM, Miller MA, Andermann E, Dansky LV, et al. Genetic predisposistion to phenytoin-induced birth defects. *Lancet* 1985; 2:746–749.
13. Schlienger RG, Shear NH. Antiepileptic drug hypersensitivity syndrome. *Epilepsia* 1998; 39 Suppl 7:S3–S7.
14. Licata AL, Louis ED. Anticonvulsant hypersensitivity syndrome. *Comprehens Ther* 1996; 22:152–155.
15. Leeder JS. Mechanisms of idiosyncratic hypersensitivity reacitons to antiepileptic drugs. *Epilepsia* 1998; 39 Suppl 7:S8–S16.
16. Smith TJ, Gill JC, Ambruso DR, Hathaway WE. Hyponatremia and seizures in young children given DDAVP. *Am J Hematol* 1989; 31:199–202.
17. Pirmohamed M, Kitteringham NR, Guenthner TM, et al. An investigation of mechanisms in toxic epidermal necrolysis induced by carbamazepine. *Arch Dermatol* 1992; 130:598–604.
18. Farhat G, Yamout B, Mikati MA, Demirjian S, et al. Effect of antiepileptic drugs on bone density in ambulatory patients. *Neurology* 2002; 58:1348–1353.
19. Meador KJ, Loring DW, Huh K, Gallagher BB, et al. Comparative cognitive effects of anticonvulsants. *Neurology* 1990; 40:391–394.
20. Pellock JM, Culbert JP, Garnett WR, et al. Significant differences of AEDs cognitive and behavioral effects in children. *Ann Neurol* 1988; 24:325 (abstract).
21. Vining EPG, Mellits ED, Dorsen MM, et al. Psychologic and behavioral effects of antiepileptic drugs in children, a double-blind comparison between phenobarbital and valproic acid. *Pediatrics* 1987; 80:165–174.
22. Reynolds EH, Chanarin I, Milner G, Matthews DM. Anticonvulsant therapy, folic acid and vitamin B_{12} metabolism and mental symptoms. *Epilepsia* 1966; 7:261–270.
23. Granick S. Hepatic porphyria and drug-induced or chemical porphyria. *Ann NY Acad Sci* 1965; 123:197.
24. Hunt PA, Wu-Chen ML, Handal JM, et al. Bone disease induced by anticonvulsanat therapy and treatment with calcitrol (1,25-dihydroxyvitamin D3). *Am J Dis Child* 1986; 140:715–718.
25. Mattson RH, Cramer JA, McCutchen CB. Barbiturate related connective tissue disorders. *Arch Intern Med* 1989; 149:911–914.
26. Morselli PL, Franco-Morselli R, Bossi L. Clinical pharmacokinetics in newborns and infants: Age related differences and therapeutic implications. *Clin Pharmacokinetics* 1980; 5:485–527.
27. Bender AD, Post A, Meier JP, Higson JE, et al. Plasma protein binding of drugs as a function of age in adult human subjects. *J Pharmaceut Sci* 1975; 64:1711–1713.
28. Kutt H. Interactions between anticonvulsants and other commonly prescribed drugs. *Epilepsia* 1984; 25 Suppl 2:S118–S131.
29. Pellock JM. Seizures and epilepsy. In: Kelley VC, ed. *Practice in Pediatrics.* Philadelphia, PA: Harper & Row, 1987.
30. Haruda F. Phenytoin hypersensitivity: 38 cases. *Neurology* 1979; 29:1480–1485.
31. Rapport RL, Shaw CM. Phenytoin-related cerebellar degeneration without seizures. *Ann Neurol* 1977; 2:437.
32. Horowitz S, Patwardhan R, Marcus E. Hepatotoxic reactions associated with carbamazepine therapy. *Epilepsia* 1988; 29:149–154.
33. Gleichmann H. Systemic lupus erythematosus triggered by diphenylhydantoin. *Arthritis Rheum* 1982; 25:1387.
34. Wolf P, Inoue Y, Roder-Wanner U, et al. Psychiatric complications of absence therapy and their relation to alteration of sleep. *Epilepsia* 1984; 25:s56–s59.
35. Brodie MJD, McKee PJW. Vigabatrin and psychosis. *Lancet* 1990; 335:1279.
36. Jacobs JC. Systemic lupus erythematosus in childhood. Report of 35 cases, with discussion of seven apparently induced by anticonvulsant medication and the prognosis and treatment. *Pediatrics* 1963; 32:257.
37. Leppik IE. Metabolism of antiepileptic medication: newborn to elderly. *Epilepsia* 1992; 33 Suppl.4:S32–S40.
38. Patsalos PN, Stephenson TJ, Krishna S, elyas AA, et al. Side-effects induced by carbamazepine-10,11-epoxide. *Lancet* 1985; 2:496.
39. Riley RJ, Kitteringham NR, Park BK. Structural requirements for bioactivation of anticonvulsants to cytotoxic metabolites in vitro. *Br J Clin Pharmacol* 1989; 28: 482–487.
40. Pisani F, Caputo M, Fazio A, et al. Interaction of carbamazepine-10,11-epoxide, an active metabolite of carbamazepine, with valproate: a pharmacokinetic study. *Epilepsia* 1990; 31:339–342.
41. Lahr MB. Hyponatremia during carbamazepine therapy. *Clin Pharmacol Ther* 1985; 37:693–696.
42. Coombes BW. Stevens-Johnson syndrome associated with carbamazepine. *Med J Aust* 1965; 1:895–896.
43. Bertolino JG. Carbamazepine. What physicians should know about its hematologic effects. *Postgrad Med* 1990; 88:183–186.
44. Pellock JM, Willmore LJ. A rational guide to routine blood monitoring in patients receiving antiepileptic drugs. *Neurology* 1991; 41:961–964.
45. Dreifuss FE, Langer DH. Side effects of valproate. *Am J Med* 1988; Suppl 1A(84): 34–41.
46. Hyuman NM, Dennis PD, Sinclar KG. Tremor due to sodium valproate. *Neurology* 1979; 29:1177–1180.
47. Dinesen H, Gram L, Andersen T, Dam M. Weight gain during treatment with valproate. *Acta Neurol Scand* 1984; 70:65–69.
48. Jeavons PM, Clark JE, Hirdme GA. Valproate and curly hair. *Lancet* 1977; 1:359.
49. Loiseau P. Sodium valproate, platelet dysfunction and bleeding. *Epilepsia* 1981; 22: 141–146.
50. Sandler RM, Emberson C, Roberts GE, Voak D, et al. IgM platelet autoantibody due to sodium valproate. *Br Med J* 1978; 2:1683–1684.
51. Sackellares JC, Lee SI, Dreifuss FE. Stupor following administration of valproic acid to patients receiving other antiepileptic drugs. *Epilepsia* 1979; 20:697–703.

52. Triggs WJ, Bohan TP, Lin S-N, Willmore LJ. Valproate induced coma with ketosis and carnitine insufficiency. *Arch Neurol* 1990; 47:1131–1133.
53. Millington DS, Bohan TP, Roe CR, Yergey AL, et al. Valproylcarnitine: a novel drug metabolite identified by fast atom bombardment and thermospray liquid chromatography-mass spectrometry. *Clin Chim Acta* 1985; 145:69–76.
54. Triggs WJ, Roe CR, Rhead WJ, Hanson SK, et al. Neuropsychiatric manifestations of defect in mitochondrial beta oxidation response to riboflavin. *J Neurol Neurosurg Psychiatry* 1992; 55:209–211.
55. Roujeau JC, Stern RS. Severe adverse cutaneous reactions to drugs. *N Engl J Med* 1994; 331:1272–1285.
56. Wyllie E, Wyllie R, Cruse RP, Erenberg G, et al. Pancreatitis associated with valproic acid therapy. *Am J Dis Child* 1984; 138:912–914.
57. Perucca E, Grimaldi R, Gatti G, Pirracchio S, et al. Pharmacokinetics of valproic acid in the elderly. *Br J Clin Pharmacol* 1984; 17:665–669.
58. Loscher W, Nau H. Pharmacological evaluation of various metabolites and analogues of valproic acid: anticonvulsant and toxic potencies in mice. *Neuropharmacology* 1985; 24:427–435.
59. Dreifuss FE, Santilli N, Langer DH, Sweeney KP, et al. Valproic acid hepatic fatalities: a retrospective review. *Neurology* 1987; 37:379–385.
60. Dreifuss FE, Langer DH, Moline KA, Maxwell JE. Valproic acid hepatic fatalities. II. US experience since 1984. *Neurology* 1989; 39:201–207.
61. Willmore LJ. Clinical manifestations of valproate hepatotoxicity. In: Levy RH, Penry JK, eds. *Idiosyncratic Reactions to Valporate: Clinical Risk Patterns and Mechanisms of Toxicity.* New York: Raven Press, 1991:3–7.
62. Willmore LJ. Clinical risk patterns: summary and recommendations. In: Levy RH, Penry JK, eds. *Idiosyncratic Reactions to Valproate: Clinical Risk Patterns and Mechanisms of Toxicity.* New York: Raven Press, 1991:163–165.
63. Willmore LJ, Triggs WJ, Pellock JM. Valproate toxicity: risk-screening strategies. *J Child Neurol* 1991; 6:3–6.
64. Willmore LJ, Wilder BJ, Bruni J, Villarreal HJ. Effect of valproic acid on hepatic function. *Neurology* 1978; 28:961–964.
65. Kifune A, Kubota F, Shibata N, Akata T, et al. Valproic acid-induced hyperammonemic encephalopathy with triphasic waves. *Epilepsia* 2000; 41:909–912.
66. Hamer HM, Knake S, Schomburg U, Rosenow F. Valproate-induced hyperammonemic encephalopathy in the presence of topiramate. *Neurology* 2000; 54:230–232.
67. van Egmond H, Degomme P, de Simpel H, Diereck AM, et al. A suspected case of late-onset sodium valproate-induced hepatic failure. *Neuropediatrics* 1987; 18:96–98.
68. Kuhara T, Inoue Y, Matsumoto M, et al. Markedly increased ω-oxidation of valproate in fulminant hepatic failure. *Epilepsia* 1990; 31:214–217.
69. Konig SA, Siemes H, Blaker F, et al. Severe hepatotoxicity during valproate therapy: an update and report of eight new fatalities. *Epilepsia* 1994; 35:1005–1015.
70. Bohan TP, Helton E, McDonald I, Konig S, et al. Effect of L-carnitine treatment for valproate-induced hepatotoxicity. *Neurology* 2001; 56:1405–1409.
71. Scheffner D, Konig St, Rauterberg-Ruland I, Kochen W, et al. Fatal liver failure in 16 children with valproate therapy. *Epilepsia* 1988; 29:530–542.
72. Konig SA, Schenk M, Sick C, et al. Fatal liver failure associate with valproate therapy in a patient with Friedreich's disease: review of valproate hepatotoxicity in adults. *Epilepsia* 1999; 40:1036–1040.
73. Jellinger K, Seitelberger F. Spongy encephalopathies in infancy: spong degeneration of CNS and progressive infantile poliodystrophy. In: Goldensohn ES, Appel SA, eds. *Scientific Approaches to Clinical Neurology.* Philadelphia, PA: Lea & Febiger, 1977:363.
74. Prick M, Gabreels F, Renier W, et al. Pyruvate dehydrogenase deficiency restricted to brain. *Neurology* 1981; 31:398–404.
75. Graves NM, Holmes GB, Fuerst RH, Leppik IE. Effect of felbamate on phenytoin and carbamazepine serum concentrations. *Epilepsia* 1989; 30:225–229.
76. Theodore WH, Raubertas RF, Porter RJ, et al. Felbamate: a clinical trial for complex partial seizures. *Epilepsia* 1991; 32:392–397.
77. Kaufman DW, Kelly JP, Anderson T, et al. Evaluation of case reports of aplastic anemia among patients treated with felbamate. *Epilepsia* 1997; 38:1265–1269.
78. Pellock JM. Utilization of new antiepileptic drugs in children. *Epilepsia* 1996; 37 Suppl 1:S66–S73.
79. Binnie CD, Debets RM, Engelsman M, et al. Double-blind crossover trial of lamotrigine (Lamictal) as add-on therapy in intractable epilepsy. *Epilepsy Res* 1989; 4:222–229.
80. Matsuo F, Bergen D, Faught E, et al. Placebo-controlled study of the efficacy and safety of lamotrigine in patients with partial seizures. *Neurology* 1993; 43:2284–2291.
81. Warner T, Patsalos PN, Prevett M, elyas AA, et al. Lamotrigine-induced carbamazepine toxicity: an interaction with carbamazepine-10,11 epoxide. *Epilepsy Res* 1992; 11:147–150.
82. Jawad S, Richens A, Goodwin G, Yuen WC. Controlled trial of Lamotrigine (Lamictal) for refractory partial seizures. *Epilepsia* 1989; 30:356–363.
83. Schapel GJ, Beran RG, Vajda FJE, et al. Double-blind, placebo-controlled, crossover study of lamotrigine in treatment resistant partial seizures. *J Neurol Neurosurg Psychiatry* 1993; 56:448–453.
84. Messenheimer JA, Ramsay RA, Willmore LJ, et al. Lamotrigine therapy for partial seizures: a multicenter placebo-controlled, double-blind, crossover trial. *Epilepsia* 1994; 35:113–121.
85. Wong ICK, Mawer GE, Sander JWAS. Adverse event monitoring in lamotrigine patients: a pharmcoepidemiologic study in the United Kingdom. *Epilepsia* 2001; 42:237–244.
86. Schlienger RG, Shapiro LE, Shear NH. Lamotrigine-induced severe cutaneous adverse reactions. *Epilepsia* 1998; 39:S22–S26.
87. Pellock JM. Managing pediatric epilepsy syndromes with new antiepileptic drugs. *Pediatrics* 1999; 104:1106–1116.
88. Pellock JM. Overview of lamotrigine and the new antiepileptic drugs: the challenge. *J Child Neurol* 1997; 12:S48–S52.
89. Guberman AH, Besag FMC, Brodie MJ, et al. Lamotrigine-associated rash: risk/benefit consideratins in adults and children. *Epilepsia* 1999; 40:985–991.
90. Willmore LJ, Messenheimer JA. Adult experience with lamotrigine. *J Child Neurol* 1997; 12:s16–s18.
91. Messenheimer JA, Mullens EJ, Giorgi L, Young F. Safety review of adult clinical trial experience with lamotrigine. *Drug Saf* 1998; 18:281–296.
92. Motte J, Trevathan E, Arvidsson JFV, et al. Lamotrigine for generalized seizures associated with the Lennox-Gastaut syndrome. *N Engl J Med* 1994; 337:1807–1812.
93. Gee NS, Brown JP, Dissanayake UV, Offord J, et al. The novel anticonvulsant drug, gabapentin (Neurontin), binds to the alpha2delta subunit of a channel. *J Biol Chem* 1996; 271:5768–5776.
94. Fink K, Dooley DJ, Meder WP, et al. Inhibition of neuronal Ca(2+) influx by gabapentin and pregabalin in the human neocortex. *Neuropharmacology* 2002; 42:229–236.
95. French JA, Kugler AR, Robbins JL, Knapp LE, et al. Dose-response trial of pregabalin adjunctive therapy in patients with partial seizures. *Neurology* 2003; 60: 1631–1637.
96. Beydoun A, Uthman BM, Kugler AR, Greiner MJ, et al, Pregabalin 1008-009 Study Group. Safety and efficacy of two pregabalin regimens for add-on treatment of partial epilepsy. *Neurology* 2005; 64:475–480.
97. Marson AG, Hutton JL, Leach JP, et al. Levetiracetam, oxcarbazepine, remacemide and zonisamide for drug resistant localization-related epilepsy: a systematic review. *Epilepsy Res* 2001; 46:259–270.
98. Harden C. Safety profile of levetiracetam. *Epilepsia* 2001; 42:36–39.
99. Kossoff EHL, Bergey GK, Freeman JM, Vining EP. Levetiracetam psychosis in children with epilepsy. *Epilepsia* 2001; 42(12):1611–1613.
100. Stables JP, Bialer M, Johannessen SI, et al. Progress report on new antiepileptic drugs—a summary of the Second Eilat Conference. *Epilepsy Res* 1995; 22:235–246.
101. Congdon NG, Friedman DS. Angle-closure glaucoma: impact, etiology, diagnosis and treatment. *Curr Opin Ophthalmol* 2003; 14:70–73.
102. Sankar PS, Pasquale LR, Grosskreutz CL. Uveal effusion and secondary angle-closure glaucoma associated with topiramate use. *Arch Ophthalmol* 2001; 119:2110–2111.
103. Thambi L, Kapcala LP, Chambers W, et al. Topiramate-associated secondary angle-closure glaucoma: a case series. *Arch Ophthalmol* 2002; 120:1108.
104. Ben-Zeev B, Watemberg N, Augarten A, et al. Oligohydrosis and hyperthermia: pilot study of a novel topiramate adverse effect. *J Child Neurol* 2003; 18:254–257.
105. Cerminara C, Seri S, Bombardieri R, Pinci M, et al. Hypohidrosis during topiramate threatment: a rare and reversible side effect. *Pediatr Neurol* 2006; 34:392–394.
106. Leppik IE, Gram L, Deaton R, Sommerville KW. Safety of tiagabine: summary of 53 trials. *Epilepsy Res* 1999; 33:235–246.
107. Schachter SC. Tiagabine. *Epilepsia* 1999; 40:S17–S22.
108. Perucca E, Bialer M. The clinical pharmacokinetics of the newer antiepileptic drugs. *Clin Pharmacokinet* 1996; 1:29–46.
109. Dam M. Practical aspects of oxcarbazepine treatment. *Epilepsia* 1994; 35 Suppl 3: S23– S25.
110. Schmidt D, Sachdeo RC. Oxcarbazepine for treatment of partial epilepsy: a review and recommendations for clinical use. *Epilepsy Behav* 2000; 1:396–405.
111. Levinson DF, Devinsky O. Psychiatric adverse events during vigabatrin therapy. *Neurology* 1999; 53:1503–1511.
112. Krauss GL, Johnson MA, Miller NR. Vigabatrin-associated retinal cone system dysfunction. *Neurology* 1998; 50:614–618.
113. Kalviainen R, Nousiainen I, Mantyjarvi M, Nikoskelainen E, et al. Vigabatrin, a gabaergic antiepileptic drug, causes concentric visual field defects. *Neurology* 1999; 53:922–926.
114. Eke T, Talbot J, Lawden MC. Severe persistent visual field constriction associated with vigabatrin. *BMJ* 1997; 314:180–181.
115. Chiron C, Dulac O, Beaumont D, Palacios L, et al. Therapeutic trials of vigabatrin in refractory infantile spasms. *J Child Neurol* 1991; 6 Suppl:2S52–2S59.
116. Kubota M, Nishi-Nagase M, Sakakihara Y, et al. Zonisamide-induced urinary lithiasis in patients with intractable epilepsy. *Brain Dev* 2000; 22:230–233.
117. Knudsen JF, Thambi LR, Kapcala LP, Racoosin JA. Oligohydrosis and fever in pediatric patients treated with zonisamide. *Pediatr Neurol* 2003; 28:184–189.
118. Spielberg SP, Gordon GB, Blake DA, et al. Predisposition to phenytoin hepatotoxicity assessed in vitro. *N Engl J Med* 1981; 305:722–727.
119. Gerber N, Dickinson G, Harland RC, et al. Reye-like syndrome associated with valproic acid therapy. *J Pediatr* 1979; 95:142–144.
120. Suchy FJ, Balistreri WF, Buchino JJ, et al. Acute hepatic failure associated with the use of sodium valproate. *N Engl J Med* 1979; 300:962–966.
121. Hjelm M, de Silva LKV, Seakins JWT, Oberholzer VG, et al. Evidence of inherited urea cycle defect in a case of fatal valproate toxicity. *Br Med J* 1986; 292: 23–24.
122. Kay JDS, Hilton-Jones D, Hyman N. Valproate toxicity and ornithine carbamoyltransferase deficiency. *Lancet* 1986; 2:1283–1284.
123. Stolz A, Kaplowitz N. Biochemical tests for liver disease. In: Zakim D, Boyer TD, eds. *Hepatology.* Philadelphia, PA: WB Saunders, 1990:637–667.

124. Williams C, Tiefenbach S, McReynolds J. Valproic acid-induced hyperammonemia in mentally retarded adults. *Neurology* 1984; 34:550–553.
125. Zaccara G, Paganini M, Campostrini R, Arnetoli G, et al. Hyperammonamia and valproate induced alterations of the state of consciousness: a report of eight cases. *Eur Neurol* 1984; 23:104–112.
126. Zarfani ES, Berthelot P. Sodium valproate in the induction of unusual hepatotoxicity. *Hepatology* 1982; 2:648–649.
127. Murphy JV, Marquardt KM, Shug AL. Valproic acid associated abnormalities of carnitine metabolism [letter]. *Lancet* 1985; 1:820–821.
128. Coude FX, Grimer G, Pelet A, Benoit Y. Action of the antiepileptic drug, valproic acid, on fatty acid oxidation in isolated rat hepatocytes. *Biochem Biophys Res Comm* 1983; 115:730–736.
129. Becker CM, Harris RA. Influence of valproic acid on hepatic carbohydrate and lipid metabolism. *Arch Biochem Biophys* 1983; 223:381–382.
130. Thurston JH, Carroll JE, Hauhart RE, Schiro JA. A single therapeutic dose of valproate affects liver carbohydrate, fat, adenylate, amino acid, coenzyme A, and carnitine metabolism in infant mice: possible clinical significance. *Life Sci* 1985; 36:1643–1651.
131. Moore KH, Decker BP, Schreefel FP. Hepatic hydrolysis of octanoyl-CoA and valproyl-CoA in control and valproate-fed animals. *Int J Biochem* 1988; 20:175–178.
132. Thurston JH, Carroll JE, Norris BJ, et al. Acute in vivo and in vitro inhibition of palmitic acid and pyruvate oxidation by valproate and valproyl-coenzyme A in livers of infant mice. *Ann Neurol* 1983; 14:384–385.
133. Kean EA. Selective inhibition of acyl-CoA dehydrogenases by a metabolite of hypoglycin. *Biochim Biophys Acta* 1976; 422:8–14.
134. Pisciotta AV. Hematological toxicity of carbamazepine. *Adv Neurol* 1975; 11:355–368.
135. Pisciotta AV. Phenytoin: hematological toxicity. In: Woodbury DM, Penry JK, Pippenger CE, eds. *Antiepileptic Drugs*. New York: Raven Press, 1982:257–268.
136. Uetrecht J. Drug metabolism by leukocytes and its role in drug-induced lupus and other idiosyncratic drug reactions. *Crit Rev Toxicol* 1990; 20:213–235.
137. Aarli JA, Tonder O. Effect of antiepileptic drugs on serum and salivary IgA. *Scand J Immunol* 1975; 4:391.
138. Sorrell TC, Forbes IJ. Depression of immune competence by phenytoin and carbamazepine. *Clin Exp Immunol* 1975; 20:273–285.
139. Weisberg LA, Shamsnia M, Elliott D. Seizures caused by nontraumatic parenchymal brain hemorrhages. *Neurology* 1991; 41:1197–1199.
140. Brown M, Schubert T. Phenytoin hypersensitivity hepatitis and mononucleosis syndrome. *J Clin Gastroenterol* 1986; 8:469–477.
141. Kahn HD, Faguet GB, Agee JF, Middleton HM. Drug-induced liver injury: in vitro demonstration of hypersensitivity to both phenytoin and phenobarbital. *Arch Intern Med* 1984; 144:1677.
142. Taylor JW, Stein MN, Murphy MJ, Mitros FA. Cholestatic liver dysfunction after long-term phenytoin therapy. *Arch Neurol* 1984; 41:500.
143. Hart RG, Easton JD. Carbamazepine and hematological monitoring. *Ann Neurol* 1982; 11:309–312.
144. Middleton E Jr, Reed CE, Ellis EF, Adkinson NF, et al. Allergy. principles and practice. 3rd ed. St. Louis, MO: CV Mosby, 1988.
145. Seetharam MN, Pellock JM. Risk-benefit assessment of carbamazepine in children. *Drug Saf* 1991; 6:148–158.

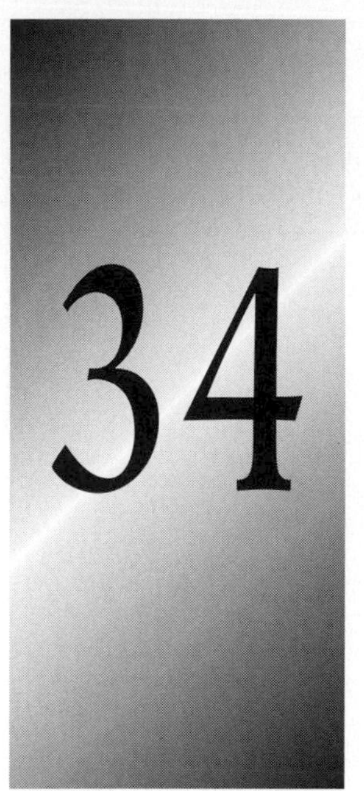

Status Epilepticus and Acute Seizures

David J. Leszczyszyn
John M. Pellock

Status epilepticus (SE) is a true neurologic emergency (1). Both convulsive and nonconvulsive SE affect people of all ages, being more common and carrying greater morbidity and mortality in infants and the elderly (2–5). Recent large population studies have revealed an incidence 2 to 2.5 times greater than previously recognized (6). Large, hospital-based studies have disclosed that SE is underrecognized and is the cause of coma in a significant number of patients who demonstrate no overt seizure activity (7, 8). In addition, the economic burden of SE has recently been estimated at 4 billion dollars. The direct patient care costs are quite high compared with the direct costs of other major health conditions such as acute myocardial infarction and congestive heart failure (9). Prompt recognition and management certainly lead to the best chance for successful outcome. Supported by the refractory nature of seizures lasting longer than 7 minutes and because of the potentially significant morbidity and mortality, there are strong arguments to shorten the functional definition of SE so as to encourage earlier intervention in this important public health issue (10). Several recent advances in treatment have occurred, including improved prehospital care for acute and acute repetitive seizures, new anticonvulsant formulations, use of emergency electroencephalography (EEG), and improved emergency room and intensive care management. These approaches with a particular focus on the treatment of acute seizures as well as a deeper understanding of the pathophysiology and prognosis of SE are discussed.

DEFINITION AND CLASSIFICATION

Although the malady had been recognized for centuries, in 1824 Calmeil first used the term *état de mal* (status epilepticus) to describe the state in which grand mal (generalized tonic-clonic) seizures occurred in rapid succession without recovery between convulsions (11). The International League Against Epilepsy (ILAE) and the World Health Organization currently define SE as a "condition characterized by an epileptic seizure that is so frequently repeated or so prolonged as to create a fixed and lasting condition" (12). The lack of recovery for a fixed period, possible frequent repetition, prolongation, and possible propagation of further seizures are inherent in the definition. Status epilepticus is defined functionally as a seizure lasting more than 30 minutes or recurrent seizures lasting more than 30 minutes from which the patient does not regain consciousness (13). The classification of individual episodes of SE should be based on observation of clinical events combined with electrographic information when possible (Table 34-1). Clinical care requires

TABLE 34-1
Proposed Classification of Status Epilepticus (SE)

Partial	
Convulsive	
• Tonic	Hemiclonic status epilepticus,
• Clonic	hemiconvulsion-hemiplegia-epilepsy, hemi-grand mal status epilepticus, grand mal
Nonconvulsive	
Simple	Focal motor status, focal sensory, epilepsia partialis continuans, adversive status epilepticus
Complex partial	Epileptic fugue state, prolonged epileptic stupor, prolonged epileptic confusional state, temporal lobe status epilepticus, psychomotor status epilepticus, continuous epileptic twilight state
Generalized	
Convulsive	
Tonic-clonic	Grand mal, epilepticus convulsivus
Tonic	
Clonic	
Myoclonic	Myoclonic SE
Nonconvulsive	
Absence	Spike and wave stupor, spike and slow wave or 3-Hz spike-and-wave status epilepticus, petit mal, epileptic fugue, epilepsia minora continua, epileptic twilight state, minor status epilepticus
Undetermined	
Subtle	Epileptic coma
Neonatal	Erratic status epilepticus

TABLE 34-2
Status Epilepticus Precipitating Events

Antiepileptic drug alterations
Withdrawal
Noncompliance
Interactions
Toxicity
Infections
CNS
Systemic
Toxins
Alcohol
Drugs
Poisons
Convulsive agents
Structural
Trauma
Ischemic stroke
Hemorrhagic stroke
Acute hydrocephalus
Hormonal change
Electrolyte imbalance
Diagnostic procedures and medications
Emotional stress
Progressive-degenerative disease
Sleep deprivation
Primary apnea
Cardiac arrhythmias
Fever

Abbreviation: CNS, central nervous system.

intervention for seizures lasting longer than 5 minutes, recognizing that any type of seizure can develop into SE (Table 34-2). The current definition of 30 minutes is not, as described earlier, universally accepted, and several clinical studies have been published using durations of 10 or 20 minutes. Shinnar and colleagues demonstrated that the majority of pediatric seizures lasting 7 minutes or more had not stopped without active treatment by 30 minutes (14). DeLorenzo et al confirmed a nearly 10-fold greater mortality for seizures lasting 30 minutes or greater compared with those lasting 10 to 29 minutes (15). More information is needed to clarify and allow acceptance of a standard operational definition for SE.

This chapter deals primarily with convulsive tonic-clonic SE that is primarily or secondarily generalized using the 30-minute operational definition. This is the most commonly recognized form of SE in children. Partial seizures that evolve to SE most commonly are secondarily generalized convulsive seizures and may occur at any age but probably account for the overwhelming majority of adult cases. Status epilepticus also encompasses several nonconvulsive entities, including complex partial, simple partial, and absence seizures. Complex partial SE usually is characterized by an epileptic twilight state in which there is a cyclical variation between periods of partial responsiveness and episodes of motionless staring and complete unresponsiveness accompanied, at times, by automatic behavior (7, 16, 17). Simple partial SE is characterized by focal seizures that may persist or be repetitive. When this condition lasts for hours or days, it is termed *epilepsia partialis continua*. Absence, or petit mal, status has also been referred to as spike-wave stupor. This type of nonconvulsive SE may be extremely difficult to differentiate from complex partial SE without the aid of an EEG evaluation. Classically, in absence status there is a continuous alteration of consciousness without cyclical variations seen with complex partial SE. The EEG recording exhibits prolonged, sometimes continuous, generalized synchronous 3-Hz spike and wave complexes rather than focal ictal discharges that characterize partial SE (7, 18). The child presenting with a prolonged confused state, fluctuating level of consciousness, or prolonged unconsciousness needs both clinical and EEG evaluations in addition to other studies.

Myoclonic, generalized clonic, and generalized tonic SE are seen primarily in children. Such children usually are those with encephalopathic epilepsies (3, 7, 19), and their consciousness seems to be preserved throughout the attacks. The EEG pattern is bilaterally symmetric with polyspike discharges coinciding with the myoclonic jerks. The term myoclonic SE should not be used when children with severe encephalopathy exhibit repetitive myoclonic jerks not accompanied by ictal discharges on EEG. These patients have subtle, generalized, convulsive SE as defined by Treiman (7). About one-half of the cases of generalized clonic SE occur in normal children and are associated with prolonged febrile seizures; the other half are distributed among those with acute and chronic encephalopathies (20). Generalized tonic SE appears most frequently in children, particularly those with Lennox-Gastaut syndrome. Prolonged generalized tonic convulsions have been precipitated by benzodiazepine administration.

EPIDEMIOLOGY

Status epilepticus is usually a manifestation of symptomatic epilepsy with preexisting neurologic dysfunction or a manifestation of acute disease primarily or secondarily affecting the central nervous system (CNS). In infants and young children, it is uncommon for SE to occur in the unstressed patient with idiopathic epilepsy. A child who has prolonged resistant seizures should receive a full diagnostic evaluation for all etiologies of seizures, along with a search for those precipitating events listed in Table 34-2. Interestingly, there also is evidence for a genetic predisposition for SE (21, 22). The major causes vary with age, such as febrile SE in children 1 to 2 years of age and remote symptomatic etiologies in the 5- to 10-year range (23). Acute symptomatic etiologies most commonly lead to prolonged SE lasting over 1 hour (24, 25). Similarly, recurrent SE is more frequent in children with remote symptomatic etiologies or progressive degenerative disease (23, 26).

A recent prospective population-based study of SE revealed the incidence of SE to be 41 patients per year per 100,000 population, resulting in a total of 50 episodes of SE per year per 100,000. It is projected that between 102,000 and 152,000 events occur in the United States annually, an incidence 2 to 2.5 times greater than that previously proposed by DeLorenzo et al (6) and Hauser et al (27). Approximately one-third of the cases present as the initial seizure of epilepsy, one-third occur in patients with previously established epilepsy, and one-third occur as the result of an acute isolated brain insult. Among those previously diagnosed as having epilepsy, estimates of SE occurrence range from 0.5% to 6.6%. Hauser reported that up to 70% of children who have epilepsy that begins before the age of 1 year experience an episode of SE. Also, within 5 years of the initial diagnosis of epilepsy, 20% of all patients experience an episode of SE. A greater incidence of SE was reported by Shinnar from a cohort of patients with childhood-onset epilepsy. One-third of the patients experienced SE over a 30-year period, 50% presenting as the first seizure and an additional 22% occurring within 12 months of onset of epilepsy. In this group, SE occurred in 44% of those with remote symptomatic epilepsy and 20% of those with idiopathic or cryptogenic epilepsy (28).

Although adults with SE as their first unprovoked seizure are likely to develop subsequent epilepsy (27), a prospective study of children with SE found that only 30% of those initially presenting with SE later developed epilepsy (24). Hesdorffer et al have presented more recent data indicating a greater likelihood of epilepsy following SE in a group of 95 people, one-third of whom were children. Over the ensuing 10-year period following a symptomatic bout of SE, there was a 41% risk of an unprovoked seizure (29).

Among children, SE is most common in infants and young toddlers, with more than 50% of cases of SE occurring in those younger than 3 years of age (30). In the Richmond, Virginia, study, total SE events and incidence per 100,000 individuals per year showed a bimodal distribution with the highest values during the first year of life and after 60 years of age (6, 20, 31). Infants younger than 1 year of age represent a subgroup of children with the highest incidence of SE whether events, total incidents, or recurrence is counted. The recurrence rate of SE in the Richmond study was 10.8% (6), but 38% of patients younger than 4 years old had repeat episodes, findings supported by the Finnish study (28). In another cohort of pediatric epilepsy patients followed by Berg and coworkers for 5 years, only 4.3% had their first episode of SE, whereas 19.6% of those who presented with status had one or more episodes of SE (32). More recently, but again from the prospective pediatric epilepsy cohort in Connecticut, Berg and Shinnar reported on factors influencing SE following a diagnosis of epilepsy. In this study only 10% of the children experienced SE over a median 8-year follow-up period, compared with 20% in the report of Hauser et al and the 22% incidence in the previously described Finnish study. SE occurring prior to the epilepsy diagnosis, younger age, and symptomatic etiology influenced the risk of later SE (33).

Extrapolating these figures worldwide, more than one million cases of SE occur annually. Because SE is a neurologic emergency that requires immediate, effective treatment to prevent residual neurologic complications or death, SE poses a substantial health risk. Mortality rates as high as 30% have been reported in overall studies.

Children have a far lower mortality rate than do adults, with the exception of those in the first year of life (34). Age, etiology, and duration correlate directly with mortality (4, 6, 35). Multiple studies confirm the lower mortality rate in most children following adequate emergency treatment (24, 30, 36–38).

PATHOPHYSIOLOGY

The cellular physiology and neuropathology of SE has been reviewed recently (39, 40) and is discussed in earlier chapters of this book. The mechanisms by which chronic seizures evolve to SE remain unclear (3). There seems to be a loss of inhibitory mechanisms, and neuronal metabolism is not able to keep up with the demand of continuing ictal activity. The pathophysiologic changes that accompany SE can be divided into neuronal (cerebral) and systemic effects. Continuing seizures lead to both biochemical changes within the brain and systemic derangements that further complicate these cerebral changes.

Prolonged convulsive seizures can lead to excitotoxic brain injury. Glutamate, the primary excitatory amino acid neurotransmitter, binds to several neuronal receptors, including the N-methyl-D-aspartate (NMDA) receptor, which is activated by depolarization. The resulting calcium influx causes further depolarization and perpetuates seizures. Glutamate also activates receptors that open channels that conduct sodium and calcium into the cell. Further neuronal damage results through this excessive excitatory neurotransmission. Although gamma-aminobutyric acid (GABA) is the most prevalent inhibitory neurotransmitter in the brain, excessive GABA may in fact increase activity on both $GABA_A$ and $GABA_B$ receptors. Activation of the presynaptic $GABA_B$ receptors can provide feedback inhibition of $GABA_A$ receptors and paradoxically exacerbate seizures. Other neurotransmitters that may be important in the initiation and maintenance of SE include acetylcholine, adenosine, and nitric oxide (39). Neuropeptides such as dynorphin, substance P, and galanin are potent modulators of the process and may affect the maintenance phase of SE (39).

Neuronal injury and cell death from SE are most prominent in areas that are rich in NMDA glutamate receptors, including the limbic region. The increase in intracellular calcium concentration is critical to cell death. Calcium activates proteases and lipases that degrade intracellular elements, leading to mitochondrial dysfunction and cellular necrosis. Laminar necrosis and neuronal damage after prolonged seizures are similar to those following cerebral hypoxia. Although young animals may be less likely to develop brain damage from SE (41, 42), studies using alternative models demonstrate hippocampal cellular injury even in immature rodents (43). It is believed that the glutamate-initiated calcium-dependent cascade is similar to the mechanism of NMDA receptor–mediated cell death during cerebral ischemia. Absence SE associated with excessive inhibitory influences generated by $GABA_B$-mediated hyperpolarization and activation of folinic T-type calcium channels does not cause cerebral injury (44). Furthermore, recent evidence suggests that acute and long-term changes in gene expression may occur following prolonged seizures and may contribute directly to hyperexcitability (45).

Systemic metabolic abnormalities increase the risk of brain damage in convulsive SE. These include alterations of blood pressure, heart rate, acidosis, hypoxia, changes in respiratory function, body temperature, leukocytosis, rhabdomyolysis, and heightened demands on cerebral oxygen and glucose utilization (46). Circulating catecholamine concentrations increase during the initial 30 minutes of SE, resulting in a hypersympathetic state. In some patients there is truly massive catecholamine release, resulting in the formation of cardiac contraction bands, ultimately representing the real cause of death (47). Tachycardia, sometimes associated with severe cardiac dysrhythmias, occurs and (rarely) also may be fatal (48). Furthermore, cardiac output diminishes and total peripheral resistance increases along with mean arterial blood pressure, perhaps because of the sympathetic overload. Hyperpyrexia may become significant during the course of SE, even without prior febrile illness, in both children and adults and may contribute to neuronal injury (49).

Hypoventilation leads to hypoxia and respiratory acidosis. In addition, serum pH and glucose levels are frequently abnormal as lactic acidosis develops following increased anaerobic metabolism. A leukemoid reaction of peripheral blood frequently occurs in the absence of infection. Rhabdomyolysis, which is not uncommonly seen, may compromise renal function. Recovery from this complicated derangement of metabolism is time dependent. More prolonged seizures produce further neuronal injury and death.

PROGNOSIS

The morbidity and mortality of SE are direct consequences of its basic pathophysiology and the efficiency of treatment. Previously, overall mortality figures for SE were quoted as 10% to 30% (35, 50, 51). The mortality rate for the Richmond, Virginia, population was 22% overall. Based on this study, which includes all age groups, there are approximately 126,000 to 195,000 SE events with 22,000 to 42,000 deaths per year in the United States. However, the mortality rate in children was only 3%, and most of the pediatric deaths occurred between the ages of 1 and 4 years (Table 34-3). The pediatric and aged

TABLE 34-3
Childhood Status Epilepticus Prognosis

	Aicardi and Chevrie (50)	Dunn (37)	Maytal et al(24)	DeLorenzo et al(6)
Patients	239	97	193	29
SE Duration	60	30	30	30
Symptomatic (%)	75	72	77	73
Morbidity (%)	>50	23	9.1	11–15
Mortality (%)	11	8	3.6	3

populations had an increased number of recurrences of SE following a single episode. In general, children had chronic neurologic disabilities but rarely went on to die. Among those patients who died, death rarely occurred during the acute episode of SE. Rather, most patients succumbed 15 to 30 days later. Children with chronic epilepsy and low levels of anticonvulsant drugs have the lowest mortality rate overall. This latter finding as well as additional confirmation of a 3% SE-related mortality was reported by Chin et al from the prospective North London Status Epilepticus in Childhood Surveillance Study. This study did not contain morbidity data but did reveal the highest yet reported early SE recurrence—16% within 1 year of the initial episode (52).

The morbidity of SE in children was examined in the same database from Virginia. Before their SE event, 81% of children with no prior history of seizures were neurologically normal, in contrast to only 31% of children with seizure histories. Of the neurologically normal children with no prior seizures, more than 25% deteriorated after their first SE event, in comparison with less than 15% of neurologically normal children with a seizure history. Children who were neurologically abnormal without prior seizure deteriorated further in 6.7%, compared with 11.3% of the abnormal children with a seizure history. Morbidity was determined at the time of hospital discharge, and in some children the abnormalities certainly improve as minor degrees of ataxia, incoordination, or motor deficits can be attributed to the acute therapies or clinical changes after prolonged seizures and may not persist. Determining whether language deficits and school performance difficulties were transient or more permanent was much more difficult. In the prospective study, 11% to 15% had significant morbidity after an episode of SE (Table 34-3). These findings suggest a neurologic morbidity substantially lower than the "greater than 50 percent" rate previously reported in children having SE (50), but the morbidity and mortality of very sick infants is higher than in older children (34).

Hesdorffer and colleagues in Rochester, Minnesota, have recently demonstrated a 41% 10-year risk of having an unprovoked seizure following an acute seizure with SE. This 95-person cohort included 17 individuals younger than 1 year of age and 17 individuals from 1 to 19 years of age. This risk was increased 18.8-fold for SE as a result of anoxic encephalopathy, 7.1-fold for structural causes, and 3.6-fold for metabolic causes over the risk in a population of patients who experienced a less prolonged acute symptomatic seizure (29). Electrographic and biochemical markers for increased morbidity and mortality in SE exist. The duration of the individual seizure, especially if it evolves to nonconvulsive SE (NCSE), has been directly correlated with death or poor outcome as defined by inability to return to prehospital level of function (53). Serum and CSF levels of neuron-specific enolase (NSE) rise above normal after both brief and prolonged seizures. Serum levels following SE are significantly higher and are at their highest in patients following NCSE, where levels higher than 37 ng/mL correlate with poor outcome (54). CSF lactate is certainly elevated following SE, and levels three times greater than the accepted normal have been associated with poor outcome, whereas those elevated 2-fold or less had better outcomes. Elevated CDF proinflammatory cytokines such as tumor necrosis factor-alpha and interleukin-6 have been documented following SE (55). CSF lactate dehydrogenase (LDH) and creatinine kinase do not appear to be valid indicators of prognosis in SE (56). CSF pleocytosis also does not appear to be a valid indicator of prognosis in SE. In all ages it is typically related to the acute illness or injury precipitating the seizure. More than 6 white blood cells (WBCs)/mm^3 or any polymorphonuclear lymphocytes (PMNs) in the adults or more than 8 WBCs/mm^3 (and greater than 4 PMNs/mm^3) in children should prompt a search for an etiology other than the seizure itself (57, 58).

Radiographic findings following SE, typically reversible focal magnetic resonance imaging (MRI) T2-weighted abnormalities, have been recognized for years (59). It had been assumed these findings were benign. The variations in peri- and postictal changes on anatomical and functional imaging examinations have been recently reviewed (60). However, there is a growing collection of case reports suggesting that there is brain injury despite radiographic normalization, as evidenced by persistent EEG abnormalities and proton MR spectroscopy abnormalities (61, 62). One report describing hyperintensities in anterior cerebral white matter suggests that a biphasic clinical course of SE, followed by clinical improvement and then early seizure recurrence, increases the odds for neurologic sequelae (55). Similar changes, particularly evolving mesial temporal sclerosis, are being carefully explored in febrile SE, which represents the single largest etiologic subgroup (63, 64). There is also strong evidence that structural brain injury in the form of ischemic stroke has a synergistic effect with SE, leading to increased mortality (65).

THERAPY

Extrapolating the statistical figures worldwide, more than one million cases of SE occur annually. As a true neurologic emergency, it requires mobilization of significant personal and medical resources and certainly qualifies as a substantial public health concern. With mortality rates as high as 30% reported in all-age-inclusive studies, immediate effective treatment is necessary to prevent residual neurologic complications or death. Age, etiology, and duration correlate directly with mortality (4, 6). The highest mortality is seen in the elderly; fortunately, children have a far lower mortality rate than do adults (4, 24, 27, 35). Some of this improved prognosis is probably a result of fewer coexisting medical conditions. That said, multiple studies confirm a lower mortality rate in children following adequate emergency treatment (24, 30, 36–38).

Acute Seizure Management

SE begins as either a prolonged seizure or continuing acute-repetitive seizures. These usually occur away from a medical center, and our approach for acute seizures is presented. The blurring of the previously clear timeline when long or recurrent seizures become SE has been previously discussed. In an attempt to prevent this progression, medical intervention is suggested when the seizure duration is 5 minutes or more. As such, it is paramount that families become educated on seizure first aid, and they must have an action plan. They or the first responders must note the time of seizure onset as part of their providing support to the child. Many times this support will include at-home benzodiazepine administration, usually in the form of rectal diazepam, but sometimes oral lorazepam or diazepam if consciousness is retained and the patient can safely swallow liquids. Appropriate first-aid recommendations are discussed here for completeness. The Epilepsy Foundation of America (EFA) recommends that the first responders:

- Look for medical identification.
- Protect the person from nearby hazards.
- Loosen ties or shirt collars.
- Protect the head from injury.
- Turn the person on his side to keep the airway clear.
- Reassure when consciousness returns.
- If a single seizure lasts more than 5 minutes, ask whether hospital evaluation is wanted. If multiple seizures, or if one seizure lasts longer than 5 minutes, call an ambulance. If the person is pregnant, injured, or diabetic, call aid at once.

The EFA also recommends that first responders:

- Do not put any hard implement in the mouth.
- Do not try to hold the tongue. It cannot be swallowed.
- Do not try to give liquids during or just after the seizure.
- Do not use artificial respiration unless breathing is absent after muscle jerks subside, or unless water has been inhaled.
- Do not restrain the person.
- The person should be transferred to a medical center as soon as possible if their seizure continues beyond 5 minutes or, if after ceasing, it begins again (66).

The neurologic emergency of SE requires maintenance of respiration, general medical support, and specific treatment of seizures while the etiology is sought (1, 67, 68). One typical and unfortunately frequent mistake made in the treatment of SE is that inadequate doses of drugs are given initially, and physicians wait for more seizures to occur before administering the necessary total dose (67, 69). Additionally, given that febrile seizures are common and such patients regularly present to emergency rooms for evaluation, the progression from prolonged simple febrile seizure to febrile SE is often missed (70). The ideal antiepileptic drug (AED) for the treatment of SE should have the following properties: rapid onset of action, broad spectrum of activity, ease of administration including intravenous (IV) and intramuscular (IM) preparations, minimal redistribution from the CNS, and wide therapeutic safety margin. With confirmed safety and efficacy data (71) and particularly because it is longer acting, lorazepam (LZP) has become more popular in many centers as the initial agent, thus replacing diazepam (DZP). Recent studies in both children and adults also support the use of midazolam (MDZ). Its rapid absorption from varied sites of administration and rapid onset of anticonvulsant activity make MDZ a very attractive agent for use in multiple settings. If, however, SE continues after the initial dosing of a benzodiazepine and persists after a primary AED such as phenytoin (PHT) (as fosphenytoin, FOS) or phenobarbital (PB) is given, a second dose of the same AED should be administered before switching to alternative medications. SE refractory to these established

TABLE 34-4
The Steps of Status Epilepticus Emergency Management

1. Ensure adequate brain oxygenation and cardiorespiratory function
2. Terminate clinical and electrical seizure activity as rapidly as possible
3. Prevent seizure recurrence
4. Identify precipitating factors such as hypoglycemia, electrolyte imbalance, lowered drug levels, infection, and fever
5. Correct metabolic imbalance
6. Prevent systemic complications
7. Further evaluate and treat the etiology of SE

agents carries a graver prognosis (68). Numerous studies suggest that additional bolus administration followed by titrated IV infusions of DZP, MDZ, pentobarbital, or the anesthetic agents lidocaine or propofol, may break these seizures. The use of IV valproic acid (VPA) in the treatment of SE has expanded greatly in the past few years. There are reports, as well, supporting the safety and efficacy of topiramate and levetiracetam in the treatment of refractory SE.

The primary goal of treatment is to stop the convulsive discharges in the brain. Table 34-4 lists the steps of the emergency management of SE (67, 72). The child presenting in SE must have cardiorespiratory function assessed immediately by vital sign determination, auscultation, airway inspection, arterial blood gas determination, and suction if necessary. Although spontaneously breathing on presentation, children may already be hypoxic with respiratory or metabolic acidosis from apnea, aspiration, or central respiratory depression (1). The need for ventilator support depends not only on respiratory status at the time of presentation but also on the conditions before arrival and the ability to maintain adequate oxygenation throughout ongoing seizures and during the IV administration of drugs, all of which cause some amount of respiratory depression. Elective intubation and respiratory support are urged in the neurologically depressed patient. In most patients with placement of an oral airway or nasal canula or both, oxygen is insufficient as respiratory drive is depressed. Significant hypoxia is a principal factor determining morbidity and mortality (6). Rapid assessment of vital signs and general neurologic examination give clues to the etiology of SE. Blood drawn to determine blood gases, glucose, calcium, electrolytes, complete blood count, AED levels, culture, and virologic and toxicologic studies help with the overall determination of etiology. Similarly, urine for drug and metabolic screens should be collected. The roles of CSF NSE, cytokines, and lactate, as well as serum NSE, in the prognostication of outcomes in SE were discussed previously.

Intravenous fluids should be administered judiciously, with appropriate corrections for fever, suction, and chemical abnormality. Fluid restriction is rarely necessary. Immediately following placement of the IV line, 25% glucose (2–4 mL/kg) should be given by bolus. In the case in which IV access cannot be established, the intraosseous route has been shown efficient for both fluid and medication administration (73). Because of the high incidence of febrile SE resulting from CNS infection in infants, a lumbar puncture should be done early in the course of management but not necessarily during the initial phase of stabilization. It is rarely necessary to wait for imaging studies to be performed in this group. If lumbar puncture is deferred for any reason, appropriate antimicrobial coverage for possible meningitis or encephalitis should be considered. Electrocardiographic (ECG) and EEG monitoring is desirable when available (68).

EEG monitoring is extremely useful in both the initial and the subsequent management of SE (72, 74–76). The classification of SE, clues to etiology, and prognosis may be suggested from the EEG and its response to therapy. This includes patients with completely hysterical attacks and those presenting with an overdose of drugs or focal pathology. Definition of seizures as being mainly partial versus primarily or secondarily generalized is easily recognized; in nonconvulsive cases the EEG easily establishes the diagnosis as complex partial or absence. The use of EEG is mandatory in the presence of neuromuscular blockade or whenever recurrence of seizures cannot be documented on a clinical basis (1, 72).

An electroclinical dissociation may exist after large doses of AEDs have been given, so that the clinical manifestations are absent while electrographic seizures continue. The recognition of EEG patterns, such as paroxysmal lateralized epileptiform discharges (PLEDs), periodic epileptiform discharges (PEDs), and evidence of continued post-SE ictal discharges without clinical correlation while the patient remains in a coma, requires ongoing therapy and may be helpful in establishing the etiologic diagnosis and prognosis (8). One recent study of 50 patients with SE reported poor outcomes, including death or persistent vegetative states, in 44% of those whose records demonstrated PEDs, compared with 19% without PEDs (77). ECG alterations seen in adults during and after SE range from ischemic changes to tachyarrythmias. These changes must be promptly and appropriately treated (46, 78). These relatively new findings suggest that EEG be more aggressively used in the evaluation and treatment of SE. Practical limitations must be realized, however, because many treatment sites do not have EEG readily available. Nevertheless, urgent use of this monitoring must be considered when patients do not regain consciousness or when seizures are continuous or recurrent.

DRUG THERAPY OF STATUS EPILEPTICUS

There are multiple regimens for treating SE successfully. Benzodiazepines and FOS (PHT equivalent) as initial therapy are preferred by our group at the Medical College of Virginia of Virginia Commonwealth University (MCV/VCU), but others may wish to continue alternative agents if the patient is known to be on maintenance therapy or has already received smaller doses of PHT or PB (79, 80). LZP, DZP, FOS, and PB are accepted agents for initial and continued therapy of SE. The large SE treatment study done in adults and sponsored by the U.S. Veterans Administration suggests that there is no significant difference between three IV drug regimens: (1) DZP, 0.15 mg/kg, and PHT, 18 mg/kg; (2) LZP, 0.1 mg/kg; or (3) PB, 15 mg/kg, for initial management of generalized convulsive SE when results were measured at 20 minutes (81). Each was superior to PHT, 18 mg/kg, used alone. It is important to note that the rate of PHT administration probably biased the study. The much more rapid speed at which FOS can be administered may significantly change these results. The choice of an initial agent may depend on individual patient characteristics, prior AED therapy, and physician preference. Recommended doses of commonly used drugs for the treatment of convulsive SE are listed in Table 34-5. Protocols presently used by our group at MCV/VCU for the management of SE in children, adolescents, and adults are given in Tables 34-6 and 34-7 (79).

Benzodiazepines

As a group the benzodiazepines are the most potent and efficacious drugs in the treatment of SE (82). Lasting control of SE is achieved in approximately 80% of patients treated with LZP, DZP, or clonazepam (81). Because the IV preparation of clonazepam is not available in the United States, lorazepam and diazepam are most frequently used. A prospective, randomized study determined that IM MDZ is as effective as DZP in stopping seizures and is faster than DZP because it avoids the requirement of starting an IV line (83). Nasal and buccal administration of benzodiazepines have demonstrated efficacy in aborting acute seizures, but no prospective studies support these routes in treating SE (84, 85).

Lorazepam

Lorazepam is a potent benzodiazepine with rapid onset and more prolonged duration of anticonvulsant action than those of DZP. With a half-life of approximately 10 to 15 hours in adults and children, LZP continues to have an effective brain level for 8 to 24 hours. A favorable lipid partition coefficient allows LZP to remain in the brain longer than DZP, which redistributes more rapidly. The recommended IV bolus LZP dose is 0.1 mg/kg up to a total of 5 to 8 mg. Tachyphylaxis develops, making repeated doses less effective (86, 87). LZP is also less useful in patients receiving chronic benzodiazepine therapy.

The efficacy of LZP equals that of DZP in neonates, children, and adults (87–94). Adverse effects include hypoventilation, ataxia, vomiting, amnesia, lethargy, respiratory depression, and hypotension. These symptoms are exacerbated when barbiturates, paraldehyde, or other depressant drugs are administered before LZP. Following rectal administration, LZP has a more delayed onset of action than DZP (93). Sedation that follows IV administration of LZP is longer lasting than that following DZP. Significant sedation is a disadvantage of both drugs when continued observation of level of consciousness is necessary.

Diazepam

Diazepam enters the brain within seconds following IV administration and successfully stops convulsive and

TABLE 34-5
Recommended Initial Intravenous Doses for Status Epilepticus

Patient age	Lorazepam (0.1 mg/kg)	Diazepam (0.3 mg/kg)	Midazolam (0.15–0.3 mg/kg)	Fosphenytoin Phenytoin Equivalents (20 mg/kg)	Phenobarbital (20 mg/kg)	Valproate Sodium (30 mg/kg)
<6 mo	0.3–1.0	1–2	0.5–2	60–200	60–200	90–300*
6–12 mo	0.5–1.2	2–4	1–4	100–250	100–250	150–350*
1–5 yr	0.8–2.5	3–10	1.5–10	160–300	160–300	200–450*
5–12 yr	1.5–6.0	5–15	2.5–15	300–1,200	300–1,200	450–1,500+
13 yr +	3.0–6.0	10–20	5–20	500–1,500+	500–1,500+	500–2,400+

* There is an increased risk of fatal hepatotoxicity in children < 2 years old associated with multiple anticonvulsants use, congenital metabolic disorders, severe seizure disorders with mental retardation, and/or organic brain disease.

TABLE 34-6
Medical College of Virginia Hospitals Status Epilepticus Protocol for Children and Adults

CHILDREN[a]

STEP	TIME FROM START OF INTERVENTION	PROCEDURE
1	0–5 min	Determination of SE. As soon as the diagnosis is made, institute monitoring of temperature, blood pressure, pulse, respirations, ECG, and EEG. Insert oral airway and administer O_2 if necessary. Insert an IV catheter and draw venous blood levels of anticonvulsants, glucose, electrolytes, calcium, BUN, and CBC. Draw arterial blood for antipyretics (acetaminophen). Perform frequent suctioning.
2	6–9 min	Place an IV line with normal saline. Administer a bolus of 2 mL/kg 50% glucose.
3	10–30 min	Initial treatment consists of an infusion by IV lorazepam given at a rate of 1–2 mg/min (0.1 mg/kg) to a maximal dose of 8 mg. This is followed by IV fosphenytoin (FOS) infused at 150 mg/min (or phenytoin [PHT] infused at a rate not to exceed 1 mg/kg/min or 50 mg/min). Monitor ECG and blood pressure. May repeat FOS (PHT) 10 mg/kg before proceeding to next step.
4	31–59 min	If seizures persist, administer a bolus infusion of phenobarbital at a rate not to exceed 50 mg/min until seizures stop or to a loading dose of 20 mg/kg.
5	60 min	If control is not achieved, other options include: • Diazepam (50 mg) is diluted in a solution of 250 mL 0.9% NaCl or D5W and run as a continuous infusion at 1 mL/kg/hr (2 mg/kg/hr) to achieve blood levels of 0.2–8.0 mg/mL. The IV solution is changed every 6 h, as advised by certain authors, and short-length tubing is used. • Pentobarbital with an initial IV loading dose of 5 mg/kg with additional amounts given to produce a "burst suppression" pattern on EEG. Maintenance of pentobarbital anesthesia is continued for approximately 4 h by an infusion of 1–3 mg/kg/hr. The patient is then checked for the reappearance of seizure activity by decreasing the infusion rate. If clinical seizures and/or generalized discharges persist on EEG, the procedure is repeated; if not, the pentobarbital is tapered over 12–24 hours.
6	61–80 min	If seizures are still not controlled, call anesthesia department to begin general anesthesia with halothane and neuromuscular blockade.

Abbreviations: ECG, electrocardiogram; EEG, electroencephalogram; IV, intravenous; BUN, blood urea nitrogen; CBC, complete blood count; D5W, 5% dextrose in water.

[a]Continuous monitoring of EEG is recommended in an obtunded patient to ensure that SE has not recurred. In the management of intractable status, a neurologist who has expertise in SE should be consulted, and advice from a regional epilepsy center should be sought. Lumbar puncture should be performed as soon as possible, especially in a febrile child or infant <1 year old. For infants with a history of neonatal seizures, infantile spasms, or early-onset seizures, pyridoxine 100 mg IV should be administered while EEG monitoring is being performed to diagnose and treat the rare patient with seizures and a vitamin B_6 deficiency.

TABLE 34-6
(Continued)

ADULT[b]

STEP	TIME FROM START OF INTERVENTION	PROCEDURE
1	0–5 min	Determination of SE. As soon as the diagnosis is made, institute monitoring of temperature, blood pressure, pulse, respirations, ECG, and EEG. Insert oral airway and administer O_2 if necessary. Insert an IV catheter and draw venous blood levels of anticonvulsants, glucose, electrolytes, Ca, Mg, BUN, and CBC. Draw arterial blood for ABG analysis. If necessary, nasotracheal suctioning is performed.
2	6–9 min	Place an IV line with normal saline containing vitamin B complex. Administer a bolus of 50 mL 50% glucose.
3	10–30 min	Infuse IV lorazepam given at a rate of 2 mg/min (0.1 mg/kg) to a maximal dose of 8 mg or alternatively administer IV diazepam given at a rate not to exceed 2 mg/min until seizures stop or to a total of 20 mg. This is followed by IV fosphenytoin (FOS) (phenytoin [PHT]), 20 mg/kg, at a rate no faster than 50 mg/min. Monitor ECG and blood pressure.
4	31–59 min	If seizures persist, perform elective endotracheal intubation before starting a bolus infusion of phenobarbital at a rate not to exceed 100 mg/min until seizures stop or to a loading dose of 20 mg/kg.
5	60 min	If control is not achieved, other options include: • Pentobarbital with an initial IV loading dose of 5–10 mg/kg with additional amounts given to produce a "burst suppression" pattern on EEG. Maintenance of pentobarbital anesthesia is continued for approximately 4 hours by an infusion of 1–3 mg/kg/hr. The patient is then checked for the reappearance of seizure activity by decreasing the infusion rate. If clinical seizures and/or generalized discharges persist on EEG, the procedure is repeated; if not, the pentobarbital is tapered over 12–24 hours. • Diazepam (50–100 mg) is diluted in a solution of 500 mL 0.9% NaCl or D5W and run as a continuous infusion to achieve blood levels of 0.2–8.0 mg/mL. The IV solution is changed every 6 h as advised by certain authors and short-length tubing is used.
6	61–80 min	If seizures are still not controlled, call anesthesia department to begin general anesthesia and neuromuscular blockade.

Abbreviations: ECG, electrocardiogram; EEG, electroencephalogram; IV, intravenous; BUN, blood urea nitrogen; CBC, complete blood count; ABG, arterial blood gas; D5W, 5% dextrose in water.

[b,a]Continuous monitoring of EEG is recommended in an obtunded patient to ensure that SE has not recurred. In the management of intractable status, a neurologist who has expertise in SE should be consulted, and advice from a regional epilepsy center should be sought.

nonconvulsive seizures in the majority of adults and children (82). Its primary disadvantages are similar to those of LZP. In addition, because of rapid redistribution, seizures frequently reoccur after 15 to 20 minutes after IV administration, requiring that a second, longer-acting drug be given or a second dose of DZP be administered. Respiratory support should be available when DZP is used to treat SE. Recommended dose estimates by age are given in Table 34-4 based on 10 to 15 mg/m^2, or 0.3 mg/kg. An initial estimate of dose may be made by taking the patient's age and giving 1 mg per year plus 1 mg (1). Diazepam may be given by intraosseous or rectal route or by a continuous IV infusion (95). In addition to respiratory depression, laryngospasm may develop during the administration of diazepam.

As LZP is supplanting DZP in many hospital emergency situations, DZP has taken on another important role—that of prehospital treatment by family or other caregivers for prolonged or acute repetitive seizures. The viscous solution of 5 mg/mL DZP was developed specifically for rectal administration. Its safety and efficacy have been established in two U.S. trials, and considerably

TABLE 34-7 *Medical Complications of Status Epilepticus*
Tachycardia
Bradycardia
Cardiac arrhythmia
Cardiac arrest
Conduction disturbance
Congestive heart failure
Hypertension
Hypotension
Altered respiratory pattern
Pulmonary edema
Pneumonia
Oliguria
Uremia
Renal tubular necrosis
Lower nephron nephrosis
Rhabdomyolysis
Increased creatine phosphokinase
Myoglobinuria
Apnea
Anoxia
Hypoxia
CO_2 narcosis
Intravascular coagulation
Metabolic and respiratory acidosis
Cerebral edema
Excessive perspiration
Dehydration
Endocrine failure
Altered pituitary function
Elevated prolactin
Elevated vasopressin
Hyperglycemia
Hypoglycemia
Increased plasma cortisol
Autonomic dysfunction
Fever

fewer of the DZP gel-treated patients required subsequent emergency medical attention for continued seizures following the treatment of their episode (96, 97). This leads to a reduced cost of care and, in the future, may decrease the prolongation of some seizures to SE (98). Since 2005, and in an effort to improve compliance and enhance safety, the delivery system for branded rectal DZP, Diastat, was changed to the AcuDial system. The dose delivered via the rectal syringe is preset by the pharmacist and can be better tailored to meet the child's need based on age and weight.

Midazolam

Midazolam has been used successfully as a first-line treatment for convulsive SE and for refractory convulsive SE. Clinical evidence supports that IM MDZ is more effective than IM DZP and as effective as IV DZP in abolishing interictal spikes on EEG recordings. At doses from 0.15 to 0.3 mg/kg it effectively terminated convulsive seizure activity (99). More than 100 children with SE are described in the literature as being successfully treated primarily with MDZ, without drug-related cardiac side effects or urgent intubation for ventilatory support (100–102). The dosing of MDZ for SE in children is not established. Suggested values are found in Table 34-5. Although LZP, DZP, and now MDZ are usually considered as the initial drugs of choice, they sometimes are useful as the second or third agent when seizures continue. Respiratory support should be available when any of the benzodiazepines are used because of the cumulative blunting of the respiratory drive centers. Additional intensive monitoring should also be performed to guard against hypotension.

Midazolam undergoes rapid hepatic breakdown, leaving no active metabolites. The elimination half-life of MDZ in children aged 6 months to 10 years ranges from 1.17 to 4 hours, in contrast to longer values in adults (1.8–6.4 hours) and elderly men (5–6 hours) (103). Recall that the active desmethyl metabolite of DZP has a physiologic half-life of 46 to 78 hours. When MDZ is administered as a continuous IV drip, dosing needs to be adjusted upward to achieve continued anticonvulsant or sedative action because of marked tachyphylaxis.

Phenobarbital

Phenobarbital remains the initial drug of choice in some institutions for the treatment of childhood SE (104, 105). Its time to onset of action is longer than that of LZP and DZP, with peak brain levels being reached in 20 to 60 minutes. Slow IV bolus infusion of 20 to 25 mg/kg is suggested initially. Repeated 10 to 20 mg/kg doses may be necessary to be successful (1, 105). Principal side effects are hypotension and respiratory and sensorial depression. PB should be administered by IV infusion no faster than 100 mg/min. In the VA Cooperative Study PB was just as efficacious in treating SE as LZP and LZP plus PHT, and a better first drug (regimen) than PHT alone (81).

Fosphenytoin (Phenytoin Prodrug Equivalent)

Fosphenytoin has replaced injectable PHT at our institution because of its safety advantages. This prodrug is nearly 100% bioavailable and, unlike its product (PHT), is freely soluble in aqueous solutions (106). Given IV, FOS is rapidly converted to PHT by phosphatases in the bloodstream. The PHT then enters the brain, reaching peak brain levels at 15 minutes (107, 108). FOS is an excellent agent for the treatment of convulsive SE, both partial and generalized, but it is ineffective in the treatment of absence status (1). A marked advantage is that it does not depress respiration as other drugs do in this situation (1). The dose is prescribed as milligrams of PHT equivalents (PE). In young children, the initial IV FOS dose should be 15 to 25 mg PE/kg (109). In adolescents and adults, a dose of 18 mg PE/kg provides initial serum PHT levels greater than 25 µg/mL and is effective in maintaining serum levels of 10 µg/mL for 24 hours (110). Cardiac conduction disturbances have not been seen, and hypotension is rare with infusion rates up to 150 mg PE/min (111). According to data from animal and human studies, most systemic adverse effects are due to the derived PHT, so the most common CNS effects include nystagmus, headache, ataxia, and somnolence. Intramuscular administration of FOS at doses from 10 to 20 mg PE/kg may allow for treatment in the field or when no IV access is present, potentially allowing for more rapid seizure control. Therapeutic blood levels can be attained in 20 to 30 minutes following IM injection (112).

Although FOS has many advantages over PHT (IM route, safe when IV site infiltrates, faster rates of administration, and lack of solvent, cardiosuppressive effects), it is not available in all facilities and frequently is not available outside the United States. FOS is significantly more expensive that PHT, but pharmacokinetics studies in patients can demonstrate its overall advantage.

Phenytoin

Phenytoin is an excellent agent for the treatment of convulsive SE, both partial and generalized, but it is not indicated in the treatment of absence status (1). After IV administration PHT reaches peak brain levels at 15 minutes (107, 108). A marked advantage of PHT is that it does not cause significant respiratory depression (1). As demonstrated by the VA study, it is best administered in combination with a benzodiazepine to ensure a rapid anticonvulsant effect, followed by the long-lasting efficacy of PHT (81). The ECG should be monitored during administration because of hypotension and cardiac conduction disturbances, primarily in adults or children with preexisting cardiac disease (1). The rate of infusion should be less than 50 mg/min in adults or 25 mg/min in children. Intravenous injection should be directly into the vein or IV line close to venous access because precipitation is likely to occur in most IV solutions. Intramuscular administration of PHT is discouraged because of crystallization, muscle destruction, and unpredictable absorption (113).

Pentobarbital

Pentobarbital is used at many institutions for refractory SE. Following a loading dose of 20 mg/kg, 1 to 2 mg/kg/hr is given IV to keep the serum level at 20 to 40 µg/mL to produce electrographic suppression or burst-suppression pattern. Pentobarbital's half-life is approximately 20 hours. Most authorities stop pentobarbital coma at 24 to 48 hours to determine whether SE subsides (114). Cardiac output and blood pressure are compromised at levels higher than 40 g/mL. Unfortunately, refractory SE requiring coma with pentobarbital or other anesthetic agents to produce EEG suppression is associated with a higher rate of morbidity and mortality (69).

Other Agents

When SE is resistant to benzodiazepines, PB, and PHT, paraldehyde was previously used (1). Paraldehyde IV solution is no longer commercially available in the United States, but rectal solution is sometimes still used. For rectal administration a 2:1 paraldehyde oil (vegetable or peanut) mixture is administered at 0.3 mL/kg per dose with doses repeated every 2 to 4 hours (115). Intravenous lidocaine may alternatively be used for the treatment of SE. There are no large, double-blind, placebo-controlled studies of the efficacy of lidocaine, but numerous case reports and case series suggest an initial bolus of 1 to 3 mg/kg followed by slow infusion of 4 to 10 mg/kg/hr (107, 116). The principal side effect is cardiovascular dysfunction. Paradoxical convulsions may occur as levels of lidocaine elevate.

In addition to lidocaine, other anesthetic agents have been used for seizure and EEG suppression (1). The foremost of these is propofol, and its use in the treatment of refractory SE has recently been reviewed (117). Based on case reports and two small, open, uncontrolled studies, propofol is no better than other second-line agents for ultimate control of prolonged seizures, but compared with high-dose barbiturate therapy, the time to attain seizure control appears markedly reduced (118). This promising property of propofol is, however, offset in the pediatric population by two drawbacks. The metabolism of this drug is exceedingly rapid, and escalating doses are required to maintain adequate blood levels, without which breakthrough seizures and SE are common. Several cases of severe metabolic acidosis and rhabdomyolysis have also been reported (119). The propofol infusion syndrome in children has been reviewed (120), and there are now clear guidelines for safe use and wide recognition of the need to limit the total dose received.

Intravenous VPA may be given to patients with epilepsy when it is not possible to maintain concentrations by the oral route. Although there still have been no multicenter, controlled trials of IV valproate in SE, the are multiple reports of improvement in patients with refractory SE (121–124). Doses in these studies of seizures and SE were usually an IV bolus of 15 to 30 mg/kg followed by continuous or intermittent infusions at rates of 0.5 to 1.0 mg/kg/hr. We presently recommend administering the available VPA for IV use diluted 1:1 at a rate of 6 mg/kg/min for rapid replacement or when seizures are refractory to other therapies (125). Steady-state concentrations greater than 50 mg/L have been reported after administration of IV VPA 15 mg/kg followed 1 to 3 hours later by either IV VPA or sustained-release oral divalproex sodium 7.0 mg/kg every 8 hours or 4 mg/kg every 6 hours. When VPA concentrations must be maintained above 100 mg/L, the drug may need to be infused every 4 hours (126).

Research efforts concerning the optimal or first-choice drug therapy of SE examine morbidity and mortality, along with the practical issues of drug administration and adverse effects. What Holmes (80) concluded almost 20 years ago is still true today, no one drug of choice may be acceptable to all clinicians. Certainly LZP, DZP, MDZ, PHT, and PB are all useful agents for both the initial and continued therapy of SE (127–129). Thus, one's choice of the initial and subsequent medications for the treatment of SE may depend on the individual patient characteristics, prior AED therapy, and physician preference. Most important, a protocol should be established so that prompt and appropriate emergency treatment can be given in an efficient manner (130). The use of IV VPA in SE is currently being defined. There are also an increasing number of reports supporting agents such as topiramate and levetiracetam in SE (131–133), and ongoing studies are exploring the roles of alternative forms of administering benzodiazepines.

MEDICAL COMPLICATIONS OF STATUS EPILEPTICUS

The treatment of SE requires close monitoring of physiologic variables and excellent nursing to prevent secondary complications (3, 7, 74). Besides the underlying or precipitating disease states associated with SE, subsequent medical complications are quite common. Pulmonary care, proper positioning, and careful observation of seizures, noting the possible changes in seizure pattern, are mandatory. Frequent surveillance and normalization of glucose and electrolytes, particularly in neonates and small infants, is mandatory. Optimal oxygenation and expectant observation and treatment for hyperthermia and other medical complications lead directly to a lessening of morbidity and mortality. Cardiovascular, respiratory, and renal effects may be severe. Medical complications of SE, which may occur in both infants and older children, are listed in Table 34-7.

When hyperthermia is resistant to rectally administered antipyretics and cooling blankets, muscular blockade may be necessary. EEG monitoring is a necessity when this is performed. A rise in blood pressure consistently accompanies seizures but rarely requires antihypertensive medication unless the child is at risk for malignant hypertension. Unfortunately, treatment may result in hypotension and reduce cerebral perfusion pressure. Very infrequently does cerebral edema or increased intracranial pressure become problematic during most cases of SE not associated with an intracranial mass. The use of osmotic diuretics and steroids are therefore rarely indicated in the routine treatment of SE.

NONCONVULSIVE STATUS EPILEPTICUS (NCSE)

Convulsive generalized tonic-clonic SE may evolve into nonconvulsive or subtle SE either without treatment as part of its natural history or because of partially successful drug treatment. The incidence of posttreatment subtle SE has been placed as high as 48% in patients requiring intensive care management (8). NCSE has also been reported as an unrecognized cause of coma in intensive care unit (ICU) patients, with up to 8% of adults and 33% of pediatric patients having EEGs that met criteria for this diagnosis (134, 135). The mortality in such cases has been difficult to isolate from the associated acute medical illnesses, but ranges from 33% to 52%, rising well above that for the SE population as a whole. Multifactorial analysis does suggest, however, that the morbidity and mortality in this group are most closely correlated with the delay in time to diagnosis (duration of seizure) and serum levels of NSE (53, 54). Shnecker and Fountain reviewed the records of 100 consecutive NCSE patients, confirming a similarly high mortality rate of 39% in one subgroup and suggesting that, in addition, severe mental status impairment and acute medical complications influence outcome, but the nature of their EEG discharges do not (136). Treatment of subtle SE is identical to that of refractory SE, and the central theme to improving outcome is early recognition and intensive EEG monitoring.

In addition to postconvulsive subtle seizures, NCSE also presents as prolonged complex partial, absence, myoclonic, or atonic seizures. These confusional or fugue states are a separate entity from the previously described subtle SE. Childhood conditions with periods of frequently occurring seizures that meet the definition of SE include the syndromes of West (infantile spasms/hypsarrhythmia), Lennox-Gastaut, Landau-Kleffner, childhood absence (pyknolepsy), continuous spike-wave during sleep, and continuous occipital spike-wave during sleep (90). Furthermore, neonatal seizures, with their various subtle and sometimes variable symptomatology, may sometimes represent SE. Specific etiologies should always be considered in these cases.

EEG monitoring reveals continuous or noncontinuous generalized, symmetric or diffuse, and irregular 1.5- to 4-Hz multispike-and-wave complexes in absence status, as opposed to the partial discharges seen in SE because of complex partial seizures (60). Clinically, a child in absence status usually demonstrates partial responsiveness with confusion, disorientation, speech arrest, amnesia, and sometimes automatisms (137). Total unresponsiveness with stereotyped automatisms is usually lacking in absence status (137). Complex partial SE is more likely to be fluctuating, sometimes with nearly cyclical impairment of consciousness, including total unresponsiveness and more complex stereotyped automatisms, with wandering eye movements or eye d eviations (138, 139).

The therapy of complex partial SE is similar therapy for convulsive SE. For absence status, IV LZP or DZP is excellent. This medication should then be followed quickly by IV VPA or oral, nasogastric, or rectal doses of ethosuximide or clonazepam. Rarely, combined administration of VPA and clonazepam may produce absence status. Some children with Lennox-Gastaut syndrome have seizures exacerbated by benzodiazepines (127). Case reports demonstrate the response of refractory partial SE to clobazam (140) and refractory absence SE to propofol or IV VPA (141, 142). Respiratory support is less problematic in NCSE than in convulsive forms; however, some patients have difficulty handling secretions in their "twilight state" or spike wave stupor.

CONCLUSIONS

Similar to other seizure types, SE represents a symptom of CNS dysfunction. However, it signifies severe malfunction. The etiology of SE must be sought out, because the highest percentage of SE is symptomatic, particularly in young children. Judicious use of routine laboratory tests coupled with neuroradiologic studies and lumbar puncture should be used in almost every patient. Those patients who remain in prolonged coma may harbor a disease such as intracranial hemorrhage, meningitis, or encephalitis, and in general have a poorer prognosis, as do all patients with prolonged or uncontrollable SE. Recent studies dispute the prior morbidity and mortality figures for SE at approximately two-thirds. A better prognosis seems possible if seizures are controlled more rapidly while optimal support is given. Promptly recognizing medical complications and treating concomitant diseases further improve outcome in all children.

References

1. Pellock JM. Status epilepticus. In: Pellock JM, Myer EC, eds. *Neurologic Emergencies in Infancy and Childhood*. Philadelphia, PA: Harper & Row, 1984.
2. Dodson WE, DeLorenzo RJ, Pedley TA, et al, for the Epilepsy Foundation of America's Working Group on Status Epilepticus. Treatment of convulsive status epilepticus. *JAMA* 1993; 270:854.
3. Pellock JM. Status epilepticus in children: update and review. *J Child Neurol* 1994; 9 Suppl 2:S27–S35.
4. Towne AR, Pellock JM, Ko D, et al. Determinants of mortality in status epilepticus. *Epilepsia* 1994; 35:27.
5. Pellock JM, DeLorenzo RJ. Status epilepticus. In: RJ Porter, D Chadwick, eds. *The Epilepsies 2*. Boston, MA: Butterworth-Heinemann, 1997:267.
6. DeLorenzo RJ, Hauser WA, Towne AR, Boggs JG, et al. A prospective, population-based epidemiologic study of status epilepticus in Richmond, Virginia. *Neurology* 1996; 46:1029–1035.
7. Treiman DM. Status epilepticus. In: Laidlaw J, Richems A, Chadwick D, eds. *A Textbook of Epilepsy*. Edinburgh: Churchhill-Livingstone, 1993:205.
8. DeLorenzo RJ, Waterhouse EJ, Towne AR, et al. Persistent nonconvulsive status epilepticus after the control of convulsive status epilepticus. *Epilepsia* 1998; 39:833–840.
9. Penberthy LT, Towne A, Garnett LK, Perlin JB, et al. Estimating the economic burden of status epilepticus to the health care system. *Seizure* 2005; 14:46–51.
10. Lowenstein DH, Bleck T, Macdonald RL. It's time to revise the definition of status epilepticus. *Epilepsia* 1999; 40:120–122.
11. Calmeil LE. De l'épilepsie, étudiée sous le rapport de son siège et de son influence sur la production de l'aliénation mentale. Master's thesis. Paris: Didot, 1824.
12. Gastaut H. Classification of status epilepticus. In: Delgado-Escueta AV, Porter RJ, Wasterlain CG, eds. *Status Epilepticus: Mechanisms of Brain Damage and Treatment*. New York: Raven Press, 1982.
13. ILAE, 1981.
14. Shinnar S, Berg AT, Moshe SL, Shinnar R. How long do new-onset seizures in children last? *Ann Neurol*. 2001; 49:659–64.
15. DeLorenzo RJ, Garnett L, Towne AR, et al. Comparison of status epilepticus with prolonged seizure episodes lasting from 10 to 29 minutes. *Epilepsia* 1999; 40:164–169.
16. Scher MA, Ask K, Beggarly ME, et al. Electrographic seizures in preterm and full term neonates: clinical correlates, associated brain lesions, and risk for neurologic sequelae. *Pediatrics* 1993; 91:128.
17. Delgado-Escueta AV, Treiman DM. Focal status epilepticus: modern concepts. In: Lüders H, Lesser RP, eds. *Epilepsy Electroclinical Syndromes*. London: Springer, 1987:347.
18. Porter RJ, Penry JK. Petit mal status. In: Delgado-Escueta AV, Wasterlain CG, Treiman DM, et al, eds. *Status Epilepticus*. New York: Raven Press, 1983:61.
19. Lockman LA. Treatment of status epilepticus in children. *Neurology* 1990; 40 Suppl:43–46.
20. DeLorenzo RJ, Towne AR, Pellock JM, et al. Status epilepticus in children, adults, and the elderly. *Epilepsia* 1992; 33 Suppl 4:S15.
21. Corey LA, Pellock JM, Boggs JG, et al. Evidence for a genetic predisposition for status epilepticus. *Neurology* 1998; 50:558–560.
22. Corey LA, Pellock JM, DeLorenzo RJ. Status epilepticus in a population-based Virginia twin sample. *Epilepsia* 2004; 45:159–65.
23. Shinnar S, Pellock JM, Moshe SL, et al. In whom does status epilepticus occur. *Epilepsia* 1997; 38:907–914.
24. Maytal J, Shinnar S, Moshe SL, Alvarez LA. Low-morbidity and mortality of status epilepticus in children. *Pediatrics* 1989; 83:323–331.
25. Driscoll SM, Jack RE, Teasley JE, et al. Mortality in childhood status epilepticus. *Ann Neurol* 1988; 24:318.
26. Driscoll SM, Pellock JM, Towne A, et al. Recurrent status epilepticus in children. *Neurology* 1990; 40:14 Suppl 1:297.
27. Hauser WA, Rich SS, Annegers JF, et al. Seizure recurrence after a first unprovoked seizure: an extended follow-up. *Neurology* 1990; 40:1163.
28. Sillanpaa M, Jalava M, Shinnar S. Status epilepticus in a population-based cohort with childhood-onset epilepsy in Finland. *Epilepsia* 1998; 39 Suppl 6:219–220.
29. Hesdorffer D, Logroscino G, Cascino G, et al. Risk of unprovoked seizure after acute symptomatic seizure: effect of status epilepticus. *Ann Neurol* 1998; 44:908–912.
30. Shinnar S, Pellock JM, Berg AT, et al. An inception cohort of children with febrile status epilepticus: cohort characteristics and early outcomes [abstract]. *Epilepsia* 1995; 36 Suppl 4:31.
31. DeLorenzo RJ, Pellock JM, Towne AR, et al. Pathophysiology of status epilepticus. *J Clin Neurol* 1995; 12:316.
32. Berg AT, Shinnar S, Levy SR, et al. Status epilepticus in children with newly diagnosed epilepsy. *Ann Neurol* 1999; 45:618–623.
33. Berg AT, Shinnar S, Testa FM, Levy SR, et al. Status epilepticus after the initial diagnosis of epilepsy in children. *Neurology* 2004; 63:1027–1034.
34. Morton LD, Watemberg NM, Driscoll-Bannister S, et al. Long-term outcome of status epilepticus in the first year of life. *Epilepsia* 1998; 39 Suppl 6:220 (abstract).
35. Hauser WA. Status epilepticus: epidemiologic considerations. *Neurology* 1990; 40 Suppl:9–13.
36. Pellock JM. Status epilepticus. In: Dodson WE, Pellock JM, eds. *Pediatric Epilepsy: Diagnosis and Therapy*. New York: Demos, 1993:197.

37. Dunn W. Status epilepticus in children: etiology, clinical features, and outcome. *J Child Neurol* 1988; 3:167.
38. Phillips SA, Shanahan RJ. Etiology and mortality of status epilepticus in children. *Arch Neurol* 1989; 46:74–76.
39. Hope O, Blumenfield H. Cellular physiology of status epilepticus. In: Drislane FW, ed. *Status Epilepticus: A Clinical Perspective*. Totowa, NJ: Humana Press, 2005.
40. Fountain NB. Cellular damage and neuropathology of status epilepticus. In: Drislane FW, ed. *Status Epilepticus: A Clinical Perspective*. Totowa, NJ: Humana Press, 2005.
41. Moshe SL. Epileptogenesis and the immature brain. *Epilepsia* 1987; 28 Suppl:53–55.
42. Moshe SL. Brain injury with prolonged seizures in children and adults. *J Child Neurol* 1998; 13 Suppl 1:S3–S6.
43. Thompson K, Wasterlain C. The model of status epilepticus that produces neuronal necrosis in the immature brain. *Neurology* 1994; 44:A272.
44. Fountain N, Lothman EW. Pathophysiology of status epilepticus. *J Clin Neurophysiol* 1995; 12:326–342.
45. Rice AC, DeLorenzo RJ. Kindling induces long-term changes in gene expression. In: Cocoran, Moshe SL, eds. *Kindling 5*. New York: Plenum, 1998:267–284.
46. Simon RP, Pellock JM, DeLorenzo RJ. Acute morbidity and mortality of status epilepticus. In: Engel J, Pedley TA, eds. *Epilepsy: A Comprehensive Textbook*. Philadelphia, PA: Lippencott/Raven. 1997:741–753.
47. Manno EM, Pfeifer EA, Cascino GD, Noe KH, et al. Cardiac pathology in status epilepticus. *Ann Neurol* 2005; 58:954–957.
48. Boggs JG, Painter JA, DeLorenzo RJ. Analysis of electrocardiographic changes in status epilepticus. *Epilepsy Res* 1993; 14:87–94.
49. Liu Z, Gatt A, Mikati M, et al. Effect of temperature on kainic acid-induced seizures. *Brain Res* 1993; 631:51–58.
50. Aicardi JF, Chevrie JJ. Convulsive status epilepticus in infants and children: a study of 239 cases. *Epilepsia* 1987; 11:187.
51. Whitty CWM. Status epilepticus. In: Tryer JH, ed. *The Treatment of Epilepsy*. Philadelphia, PA: JB Lippincott, 1980.
52. Chin RFM, Neville BGR, Peckham C, Bedford H, et al. Incidence, cause, and short-term outcome of convulsive status epilepticus in childhood: prospective popula*Lancet* 2006; 368:222–229.
53. Young GB, Jordan KG, Dolg GS. An assessment of nonconvulsive seizures in the intensive care unit using continuous EEG monitoring: an investigation of variables associated with mortality. *Neurology* 1996; 47:89–89.
54. DeGiorgio CM, Heck CN, Rabinowicz AL, et al. Serum neuron-specific enolase in the major subtypes of status epilepticus. *Neurology* 1999; 52:746–749.
55. Okamoto R, Fujii S, Inoue T, Lei K, et al. Basic clinical course and early white matter abnormalities may be indicators of neurological sequelae after status epilepticus in children. *Neuropediatrics* 2006; 37:32–41.
56. Calabrese VP, Gruemer HD, James K, et al. Cerebrospinal fluid lactate levels and prognosis in status epilepticus. *Epilepsia* 1991; 32:816–821.
57. Barry E, Hauser WA. Pleocytosis after status epilepticus. *Arch Neurol* 1994; 51:190–193.
58. Rider LG, Thapa PB, Del Beccaro MA, et al. Cerebrospinal fluid analysis in children with seizures. *Ped Emerg Care* 1995; 11:226–229.
59. Chan S, Chin SS, Kartha K, et al. Reversible signal abnormalities in the hippocampus and neocortex after prolonged seizures. *Am J Neuroradiol* 1996; 17:1725–1731.
60. Cole AJ. Status epilepticus and periictal imaging. *Epilepsia* 2004; 45 Suppl 4:72–77.
61. Juhasz C, Scheidl E, Szirmai I. Reversible focal MRI abnormalities due to status epilepticus. An EEG, single photon emission computed tomography, transcranial Doppler follow-up study. *Electroencephalogr Clin Neurophysiol* 1998; 107:402–407.
62. Fazekas F, Kapeller P, Schmidt R, et al. Magnetic resonance imaging and spectroscopy findings after focal status epilepticus. *Epilepsia* 1995; 36:946–949.
63. VanLandingham KE, Heinz ER, Cavazos JE, Lewis DV. Magnetic resonance imaging evidence of hippocampal injury after prolonged focal febrile convulsions. *Ann Neurol* 1998; 43:413–26.
64. Lewis DV, Barboriak DP, MacFall JR, Provenzale JM, et al. Do prolonged febrile seizures produce medial temporal sclerosis? Hypotheses, MRI evidence and unanswered questions. *Prog Brain Res* 2002; 135:263–278.
65. Waterhouse EJ, Vaughan JK, Barnes TY, et al. Synergistic effect of status epilepticus and ischemic brain injury on mortality. *Epilepsy Res* 1998; 29:175–183.
66. *Seizure Recognition and First Aid*. Epilepsy Foundation of America, 1989.
67. Pellock JM. Recent advances concerning status epilepticus. *Pediatrics* 1990; 5: 188–195.
68. Van Ness PC. Pentobarbital and EEG burst suppression in treatment of status epilepticus refractory to benzodiazepines and phenytoin. *Epilepsia* 1990; 31:61–67.
69. Delgado-Escueta AV, Porter RJ, Wasterlain CG, eds. Status epilepticus: mechanisms of brain damage and treatment. New York: Raven Press, 1982.
70. O'Dell C, Nordli D, Pellock JM, Lewis DV, et al, and the FEBSTAT Study Team. Recognition of febrile status epilepticus in the emergency department. *Ann Neurol* 2005; 58:S9 (abstract).
71. Alldredge BK, Gelb AM, Isaacs SM, Corry MD, et al. A comparison of lorazepam, diazepam, and placebo for the treatment of out-of-hospital status epilepticus. *N Engl J Med* 2001; 345:631–637.
72. Pellock JM, Myer EC, eds. Neurologic emergencies in infancy and childhood. 2nd ed. New York: Butterworth, 1992.
73. Orlowski JP, Porembha DT, Gallagher BB, et al. Comparison study of intraosseous, central intravenous and peripheral intravenous infusions of emergency drugs. *Am J Dis Child* 1990; 144:112–117.
74. Leppik WA. Status epilepticus: the next decade. *Neurology* 1990; 40 Suppl:4–9.
75. Jaitly R, Sgro JA, Towne AR, et al. Prognostic value of EEG monitoring after status epilepticus: a prospective adult study. *J Clin Neurophysiol* 1997; 14:326–334.
76. Alehan FK, Morton LD, Pellock JM. Electroencephalogram in the pediatric emergency department: is it useful? *Neurology* 1999; 52 Suppl 2:A45.
77. Nei M, Lee JM, Shanker VL, et al. The EEG and prognosis in status epilepticus. *Epilepsia* 1999; 40:157–163.
78. Boggs JG, Marmarou A, Agnew JP, et al. Hemodynamic monitoring prior to and at the time of death in status epilepticus. *Epilepsy Res* 1998; 31:199–209.
79. Pellock JM, DeLorenzo RJ. Status epilepticus. In: Porter RJ, Chadwick D, eds. *The Epilepsies 2*. Boston, MA: Butterworth-Heinemann, 1997:267.
80. Holmes GL. Drug of choice for status epilepticus. I. *Epilepsy* 1990; 3:l.
81. Treiman DM, Meyers PD, Walton NY, Collins JF, et al. A comparison of four treatments for generalized convulsive status epilepticus. Veterans Affairs Status Epilepticus Cooperative Study Group. *N Engl J Med* 1998; 339:792–798.
82. Treiman DM. The role of benzodiazepines in the management of status epilepticus. *Neurology* 1990; 40 Suppl:32–42.
83. Chamberlain J, Alterieri M, Futterman C, et al. A prospective, randomized study comparing intramuscular midazolam with intravenous diazepam for treatment of seizures in children. *Pediatr Emerg Care* 1997; 13:92–94.
84. Wallace S. Nasal benzodiazepines for management of acute childhood seizures? *Lancet* 1997; 25:222.
85. Scott RC, Besag FMC, Neville BGR. Buccal midazolam and rectal diazepam for treatment of prolonged seizures in childhood and adolescence: a randomized trial. *Lancet* 1999; 353:623–626.
86. Homan RW, Unwin DH. Benzodiazepines: lorazepam. In: Levy RH, Dreifuss FE, Mattson RH, et al, eds. *Antiepileptic Drugs*. 3rd ed. New York: Raven Press, 1989:849–854.
87. Crawford TO, Mitchell WG, Snodgrass SR. Lorazepam in childhood status epilepticus and serial seizures: effectiveness and tachyphylaxis. *Neurology* 1987; 37:190–195.
88. Deshnukh A, Wittert W, Schnitzler E, Margutten HH. Lorazepam in the treatment of refractory neonatal seizures. *Am J Dis Child* 1986; 140:1042–1044.
89. Graing DW, McBride MC. Lorazepam versus diazepam for the treatment of status epilepticus. *Pediatr Neurol* 1988; 4:358–361.
90. Lacey DJ, Singer WD, Horwitz SJ, Gilmore H. Lorazepam therapy of status epilepticus in children and adolescents. *J Pediatr* 1986; 198:771–774.
91. Levy RJ, Krall RL. Treatment of status epilepticus with lorazepam. *Arch Neurol* 1984; 41:605–611.
92. Relling MV, Mulhern RK, Dodge RK, et al. Lorazepam pharmacodynamics and pharmacokinetics in children. *J Pediatr* 1989; 114:641–646.
93. Graves NM, Kriel RL. Rectal administration of antiepileptic drugs in children. *Pediatr Neurol* 1987; 3:321–326.
94. Enrile-Bacsal F, Delgado-Escueta AV. IV diazepam drip in tonic-clonic status epilepticus. In: Delgado-Escueta AV, Porter RJ, Wasterlain CG, eds. *Status Epilepticus: Mechanisms of Brain Damage and Treatment*. New York: Raven Press, 1982.
95. Dreifuss F, Rosman N, Cloyd J, et al. A comparison of rectal diazepam gel and placebo for acute repetitive seizures. *N Engl J Med* 1998; 338:1869–1875.
96. Cereghino JJ, Mitchell W, Murphy J, et al. Treating repetitive seizures with a rectal diazepam formulation: a randomized study. The North American Diastat Study Group. *Neurology* 1998; 51:1274–1282.
97. O'Dell C, Shinnar S, Ballaban-Gil KR, Hornick M, et al. Rectal diazepam gel in the home management of seizures in children. *Pediatr Neurol* 2005; 33:166–72
98. Pellock JM. Management of acute seizure episodes. *Epilepsia* 1998; 39(Suppl 1):S28–S35.
99. Egli M, Albani C. Relief of status epilepticus after IM administration of the new short-acting benzodiazepine midazolam (Dormicum). In: *Program and Abstracts of the 12th World Congress of Neurology*. Princeton, NJ: Excerpta Medica, 1981:44 [Abstract 137].
100. Bebin M, Bleck TP. New anticonvulsant drugs. Focus on flunarizine, fosphenytoin, midazolam, and stiripentol. *Drugs* 1994; 48:153–171.
101. Pellock JM. Use of midazolam for refractory status epilepticus in pediatric patients. *J Child Neurol* 1998; 13:581–587.
102. Vilke GM, Sharieff GQ, Marino A, Gerhart AE, et al. Midazolam for the treatment of out-of-hospital pediatric seizures. *Prehosp Emerg Care* 2002; 6:215–217.
103. Greenblatt D, Abernathy D, Locniskar A, et al. Effect of age, gender, and obesity on midazolam kinetics. *Anesthesiology* 1984; 61:27–35.
104. Lombroso CT. The treatment of status epilepticus. *Pediatrics* 1974; 53:536–542.
105. Lockman LA. Treatment of status epilepticus in children. *Neurology* 1990; 40 Suppl:43–46.
106. Quon C, Stampfi H. In-vitro hydrolysis of ACC-9653 (phosphate ester prodrug of phenytoin) by human, dog, rat blood and tissues. *Pharm Res* 1987; 3 Suppl:1349 (abstract).
107. Wilder BJ, Ramsay RE, Hillmore U, et al. Efficacy of intravenous phenytoin in the treatment of status epilepticus: kinetics of central nervous system penetration. *Ann Neurol* 1977; 1:511–518.
108. Ramsey RE, Hammond EJ, Perchalski RJ, et al. Brain uptake of phenytoin, phenobarbital and clonazepam. *Arch Neurol* 1979; 36:535–539.
109. Pellock JM. Seizure disorders. In: Kelley VC, ed. *Practice of Pediatrics*. Hagerstown, MD: Harper & Row, 1987:150.
110. Cranford RE, Leppick IE, Patrick B, et al. Intravenous phenytoin: clinical and pharmacokinetic aspects. *Neurology* 1979; 29:1474–1479.
111. Eldon M, Loewen G, Voightman R, et al. Pharmacokinetics and tolerance of fosphenytoin and phenytoin administration intravenously to healthy subjects. *Can J Neurol Sci* 1993; 20:5180.
112. Knapp LE, Kugler AR. Clinical experience with fosphenytoin in adults: pharmacokinetics, safety, and efficacy. *J Child Neurol* 1998; 13 Suppl 1:S15–S18.
113. Wilensky AJ, Lowden JA. Inadequate serum levels after intramuscular administration of diphenylhydantoin. *Neurology* 1973; 23:318–321.
114. Raskin MC, Younger C, Penowish P. Pentobarbital treatment of refractory status epilepticus. *Neurology* 1987; 37:500–503.

115. Shields WD. Status epilepticus. Pediatr Clin North Am 1989; 36:383–393.
116. Walker I, Slovis C. Lidocaine in the treatment of status epilepticus. *Acad Emerg Med* 1997; 4:918–922.
117. Brown LA, Levin GM. Role of propofol in refractory status epilepticus. *Ann Pharmacother* 1998; 32:1053–1059.
118. Stecker MM, Kramer TH, Raps EC, et al. Treatment of refractory status epilepticus with propofol: clinical and pharmacokinetic findings. *Epilepsia* 1998; 39:18–26.
119. Hanna JP, Ramundo ML. Rhabdomyolysis and hypoxia associated with prolonged propofol infusion in children. *Neurology* 1998; 50:301–303.
120. Wolf AR, Potter F. Propofol infusion in children: when does an anesthetic tool become an intensive care liability. *Pediatr Anesth* 2004; 14:435–38.
121. Price DJ. Intravenous valproate: experience in neurosurgery. *Royal Soc Med Int Cong Symp Ser* 1989; 152:197–203.
122. Marlow N, Cooke RWI. Intravenous sodium valproate in the neonatal intensive care unit. *Royal Soc Med Int Cong Symp Ser* 1989:152:208–210.
123. Peters CN, Pohlmann-Eden B. Intravenous valproate as an innovative therapy in seizure emeregency situations including status epilepticus—experience in 102 adult patients. *Seizure* 2005; 14:164–169.
124. Yu KT, Mills S, Thompson N, Cunana C. Safety and efficacy of intravenous valproate in pediatric status epilepticus and acute repetitive seizures. *Epilepsia* 2003; 44:724–726.
125. Wheless J, Venkataraman V. Safety of high intravenous valproate doses in epilepsy patients. *J Epilepsy* 1999; 11:319–324.
126. Cavanaugh JH, Hussein Z, Lamm J, et al. Effect of multiple oral dose divalproex sodium after intravenous loading dose administration in healthy volunteers. *Drug Invest* 1994; 7:1–7.
127. Shaner DM, McCurdy SA, Herring MO, Gabor AJ. Treatment of status epilepticus: a prospective comparison of diazepam and phenytoin versus phenobarbital and optional phenytoin. *Neurology* 1988; 38:202–207.
128. Gabor AJ. Lorazepam versus phenobarbital: candidates for drug of choice for treatment of status epilepticus. *J Epilepsy* 1990; 3:3–6.
129. Mitchell WG, Crawford TO. Lorazepam is the treatment of choice for status epilepticus. J Epilepsy 1990; 3:7–10.
130. Dodson WE, DeLorenzo RJ Pedley TA, et al, for the Epilepsy Foundation of America's Working Group on Status Epilepticus. Treatment of convulsive status epilepticus. *JAMA* 1993; 270:854.
131. Towne AR, Garnett LK, Waterhouse EJ, Morton LD, et al. The use of topiramate in refractory status epilepticus. *Neurology* 2003; 60:332–334.
132. Perry MS, Holt PJ, Sladky JT. Topiramate loading for refractory status epilepticus in children. *Epilepsia* 47; 1070–1071.
133. Patel N, Landan I, Levin J, Szaflarski J, et al. The use of levetiracetam in refractory status epilepticus. *Seizure* 2006; 15: 137–141.
134. Towne AR, Waterhouse EJ, Boggs JG, Garnett LK, et al. Prevalence of nonconvulsive status epilepticus in comatose patients. *Neurology* 2000; 54:340–345.
135. Hosain SA, Solomon GE, Kobylarz EJ. Electroencephalographic patterns in unresponsive pediatric patients. *Pediatr Neurol* 2005; 32:162–165.
136. Shnecker BF, Fountain NB. Assessment of acute morbidity and mortality in nonconvulsive status epilepticus. *Neurology* 2003; 61:1066–1073.
137. Porter RJ, Penry JK. Petit mal status. In: Delgado-Escueta AV, Wasterlain CG, Treiman DM, et al, eds. *Advances in Neurology, Vol. 34: Status Epilepticus*. New York: Raven Press, 1987:61–67.
138. McBride MC, Dooling EC, Oppenheimer IN. Complex partial status epilepticus in young children. *Ann Neurol* 1981; 9:526–530.
139. Treiman DM, Delgado-Escueta AV. Complex partial status epilepticus. In: Delgado-Escueta AV, Waster-lain CG, Treiman DM, et al, eds. *Advances in Neurology, Vol. 34: Status Epilepticus*. New York: Raven Press, 1987:69–68.
140. Corman C, Guberman A, Benavente O. Clobazam in partial status epilepticus. *Seizure* 1998; 7:243–247.
141. Crouteau D, Shevell M, Rosenblatt B, et al. Treatment of absence status in the Lennox-Gastaut syndrome with propofol. *Neurology* 1998; 51:315–316.
142. Alehan FK, Morton LD, Pellock JM. Treatment of absence status with intravenous valproate. *Neurology* 1999; 52:889–890.

35 The Female Patient and Epilepsy

Mark S. Yerby

Hippocrates noted that while epilepsy at birth tended to be resistant to cure, seizures whose origin was in later childhood tended to cease at puberty. In fact, some early Greek physicians suggested early sexual intercourse for such children in an attempt to provoke a cure. Though many seizure disorders improve during puberty, many worsen. In primarily generalized absence seizure, improvement is common, but a small proportion go on to develop generalized convulsive seizures at puberty (1). Benign focal epilepsy remits during puberty (2). Photic-sensitive epilepsies generally begin during puberty, as do generalized tonic-clonic seizures on awakening (3, 4). Juvenile myoclonic epilepsy also begins at puberty and is more common in girls, and seizures often are more frequent during menses (5). Lennox-Gastaut syndrome often worsens during puberty (6).

PHYSIOLOGY OF SEXUAL MATURATION

At puberty the hypothalamus begins to secrete gonadotropin-releasing hormone (GnRH). This is carried in the portal circulation to the anterior pituitary, which, in turn, releases follicle-stimulating hormone (FSH). Follicle-stimulating hormone promotes the development of ovarian follicles. The ovarian follicles secrete estradiol. Lutenizing hormone (LH) is also secreted by the pituitary, but, unlike FSH, it has a pulsatile secretory pattern. It promotes maturation of the ovarian follicle and ovulation. The remaining follicular cells then become the corpus luteum, which secretes progestins. At the point at which the corpus luteum is developed, the follicular phase ends and the luteal phase of the menstrual cycle begins. Progesterone inhibits secretion of GnRH, FSH, and LH. If there is no fertilization, the corpus luteum regresses, and estrogen and progestin levels decline. With this decline the GnRH secretion resumes and the cycle repeats.

There are direct connections from the temporal lobe to the hypothalamus. Aberrant discharges from the temporal lobe may therefore impact hypothalamic activity and thus pituitary hormone secretion. Direct stimulation of the amygdala's corticomedial zone increases GnRH (7) and stimulation of the basolateral region reduces GnRH (8).

ASSOCIATION OF MENSES WITH EPILEPSY

The term *catamenial epilepsy* (from the Greek *kata*, by; *men*, month) epilepsy refers to seizure exacerbation in relation to the menstrual cycle. Traditionally, the term has been used to refer to seizure exacerbation at the time of menstruation. It has long been a recognized phenomenon. Gowers was the first of the "modern" epileptologists

TABLE 35-1
Rates of Catamenial Epilepsy

Author	Rate in Percent	N
Dickerson, 1941 (13)	10	269
Ansell and Clarke, 1956 (14)	63	42
Laidlaw, 1956 (15)	72	50
Lennox and Lennox, 1960 (16)	48.5	686
Rosciszewska, 1980 (17)	58	69
Marques-Assis, 1981 (18)	27.4	1574
Duncan et al, 1993 (19)	12	40
Panayiotopoulos, 1994 (20)	24	
Towanabut et al, 1998 (21)	9.8	467
Herzog et al, 2004 (22)	39	87
Bazan et al, 2005 (23)	27	39 TLE
	35	14 extra temporal

TABLE 35-2
Patterns of Catamenial Epilepsy

Seizure Frequency During the Menstrual Cycle			
Phase		Ovulation	Anovulation
Menstrual	−3 to +3	0.59*	0.78
Follicular	+4 to +9	0.41	0.49
Ovulation	+10 to −13	0.50*	0.74
Luteal	−12 to −4	0.40	0.74

*$P < 0.001$. Source: Herzog et al, 1997 (25).

to recognize an association of increased seizures with menstruation (9). In 1904 Spratling reported that 25% of women had their seizures during menstruation (10). Turner reported in 1907 "The relationship between fits and menstruation has been well established" (11). Lennox and Cobb (12) wrote that "it is a well known fact that many female patients frequently have seizures near their menstrual period." Subsequent reports were primarily brief case series, and they show significant differences as to whether and to what degree catamenial epilepsy occurred. Although the phenomenon is well described and appreciated, a precise definition of catamenial epilepsy has been elusive. In addition to a lack of precise definition, the length of observation required to make the diagnosis varies widely, and in many studies documentation has been merely the recollection of seizures by patients. Table 35-1 (13–23) gives one an idea of the range of observations.

Using a function definition and a prospective questionnaire, Duncan and colleagues (19) studied forty women of childbearing age with refractory epilepsy. They were asked to record their seizures and the first and last days of their menstrual periods. By defining catamenial epilepsy as the occurrence of at least 75% of seizures each month in the 10-day time frame that included the 4 days preceding menstruation and the 6 days after its onset, only 12.5% were identified who fulfilled the criterion. Nevertheless, after the study was completed, 78% of these patients claimed that most of their seizures occurred near the time of and were exacerbated by menstruation.

Thus, one can see that the notion of what represents an association with menses has a large subjective component. If seizures are random events, then by chance alone many will occur during the menstrual period. That is not to say that the phenomenon does not exist but that its frequency is unclear.

More recent concepts of catamenial epilepsy have been established by prospective observation. Herkes and colleagues (24) followed 12 women for almost four years and found two peaks in seizure occurrence: one just prior to and during menstrual flow, and the other at midcycle. In addition they determined that anovulatory cycles were not associated with an increase in seizures.

Herzog and colleagues (25) have determined that catamenial epilepsies are a heterogenous group. They describe three patterns (Table 35-2). The least frequent are seizures occurring around ovulation. The most common are perimenstrual. There is yet a third group whose cycles tend to be anovulatory, and the exacerbation of seizures occurs throughout the entire luteal phase.

It is interesting to note that the first anticonvulsant drug, potassium bromide, was introduced to treat "hysterical epilepsy" in women. This term was previously used to describe seizures occurring during menstruation. During a presentation by Dr. Sieveking to the Royal Medical and Chirurgical Society of London on May 11, 1857, Sir Charles Locock commented that he had tried bromide for women with (hysterical or catamenial) epilepsy and had successfully prevented seizures in 13 of 14 patents treated (26).

Hormonal Changes in Catamenial Epilepsy

A number of investigators have noted a decrease in progesterone concentrations, particularly during the luteal phase (27–29). It appears as though estrogens potentiate epileptiform discharges on EEG recording (30). Conversely, intravenous progestins reduce epileptiform spikes in women with epilepsy (WWE) (31). A number of investigators have demonstrated a protective effect of progesterone in animal models of epilepsy (32–34). Allopregnanolone, a metabolite of progesterone, has antiseizure activity. It acts as a modulator of $GABA_A$ receptors, thus increasing seizure threshold (35). Cortisol levels are higher and dehydroepiandrosterone sulfate (DHEAS) levels lower in WWE, and these changes are even more pronounced in women whose seizures are poorly controlled (36).

Attempts to use hormonal supplementation for women with catamenial epilepsy has met with mixed results. The use of medroxyprogesterone resulted in seizure reduction in 7 of 14 treated women; however, 11 of them developed amenorrhea (37). A double-blind pacebo-controlled trial of the progestin norethisterone (norethindrone) was not effective (38). The use of intermittent progesterone by Herzog and colleagues (39) resulted in a 68% decline in complex partial seizures. Intravaginal progestone lozenges (200 mg), 3 times daily, were given from days 23 to 25 in women with perimenstrual catamenial epilepsy and from days 15 to 25 for those with exacerbation in the luteal phase. Seventy-two percent of women had a reduction of seizure frequency (40). Unfortunately the lozenges require the patient to remain supine following insertion, and vaginal spotting, breast tenderness, and depression may be seen with progesterone supplementation. It is felt that natural progesterone may be more effective than the synthetic hormone in reducing seizure frequency, and investigations in this area are under way (35).

Management of Catamenial Epilepsy

The effective management of catamenial epilepsy requires a precise diagnosis. Antiepileptic drugs (AEDs) are the first line of defense, and their use should be maximized before alternative therapies are considered. A careful compilation of a woman's seizures and menstrual cycle on a calendar will demonstrate an association if it exists. The present author suggests doing so for at least three cycles in order to confirm the diagnosis.

Once a diagnosis of catamenial epilepsy has been established, one needs to demonstrate a progesterone deficiency prior to supplementing a patient. Differentiating inadequate luteal phase and anovulatory cycles is important in planning further investigations. A progesterone level measured during the midluteal phase (day 20–22 of a 28-day cycle) should be higher than 5.0 ng/mL. Failure to attain this level implies inadequate progesterone production and suggests that supplementation with progesterone may be helpful.

Determining ovulation is a bit more tedious. The failure of the basal body temperature to rise by 0.7°F for at least 10 days during the second half of the cycle implies failure of ovulation. If this occurs, further investigation is required to rule out polycystic ovarian disorder with ultrasound. There are now available a number of "ovulation kits" a woman can purchase over the counter that are quite accurate.

Once the preliminary studies are complete, one can categorize the patient into two groups: one with low progesterone and one with normal progesterone levels. Low-progesterone patients may benefit form progesterone supplementation. A variety of approaches are available. Progesterone creams may be useful, but their concentration and absorption are quite variable, and so is their effectiveness. A natural progesterone creams or lozenge can be prepared by a compounding pharmacist. Herzog (39) recommends 100 to 200 mg three to four times a day. The target progesterone levels are 5–25 ng/mL. Synthetic progestational agents such as medroxyprogesterone may be administered intramuscularly 120–150 mg every 6–12 weeks. Cessation of menses can occur, as can hot flashes, vaginal bleeding, and breast tenderness. Such an approach limits one's ability to adjust the dosage quickly (41, 40). Most authors have not found oral synthetic progesterone effective (42, 43). Many women, unfortunately, suffer from side effects of progesterone, limiting its utility. Sedation, depression, breast tenderness, weight gain, and vaginal spotting have frequently been reported.

For women with normal progesterone levels, one must determine whether they are ovulating or having anovulatory cycles. In ovulatory patients the present author has had some success with the continuous use of oral contraceptives such as Nordette® (levonorgestrel 0.15 mg, ethinyl estradiol 0.03 mg).

In anovulatory patients one must first rule out ovarian dysfunction, particularly polycystic ovaries. If otherwise normal, a short course of clomiphine to restore ovulation may be effective.

Catamenial epilepsy represents a challenge for epileptologists. It is hoped that with more research into the mechanisms by which hormones effect seizures, better therapies may result.

INFERTILITY IN WWE

Infertility and Reproductive Abnormalities

Epidemiologic studies have demonstrated that women with epilepsy have only one-fourth to one-third as many children as women in the general population (44, 45). A variety of hypotheses have been developed to explain this phenomenon. A direct effect of seizures or epileptiform discharges on pituitary and hypothalamus could disrupt ovulation. Electroconvulsive therapy increases prolactin concentrations over 5-fold within 15 to 20 minutes, and in premenopausal women there is an acute increase in LH and FSH. Generalized seizures also increase prolactin serum concentrations within 15 to 20 minutes by a factor 3-fold. This fact has been used to assist physicians in differentiating epileptic from nonepileptic seizures (46).

WWE have higher rates of reproductive and endocrine disorders (RED) than expected. In a large clinical center 50% of WWE were found to have menstrual abnormalities, 20% amenorrheic and 35% anovulatory (47). Herzog and co-workers (48) was among the first to demonstrate RED in women with temporal lobe epilepsy. Women with primary generalized epilepsies also have RED. Five of 20 women studied by Bilo and colleagues (44) had RED: 3 with polycystic ovarian disease and 2 with hypogonadotropic hypogonadism.

AEDs may also interfere with the hypothalamic-pituitary axis. Amenorrhea, oligomenorrhea, and prolonged or irregular cycles have been described in WWE by Isojarvi and colleagues (45). WWE taking valproate were overrepresented; 45% of those on valproate monotherapy and 25% on valproate polytherapy had menstrual disturbances. Polycystic ovaries were found in 4% of valproate-treated women and 80% of women treated with valproate before the age of 29 had polycystic ovaries.

Women with epilepsy have more variation in luteinizing hormone (LH) pulse frequency and lower LH concentrations than controls (46). In addition, women with left-sided ictal epileptiform foci had polycystic ovarian disease, and those with right-sided foci had hypogonadotropic hypogonadism.

Libido is significantly reduced in one-third of men and women with epilepsy (49). Increasing seizure frequency appears to decrease sexual desire, while there is no difference in libido between treated and untreated WWE. Hyposexuality and orgasmic dysfunction has been reported in 8% to 68% of WWE (50). Persons with localization-related epilepsies appear to have higher rates of sexual dysfunction than those with primarily generalized epilepsies. Shukla and colleagues (51) demonstrated 64% of women with partial, compared to 8% of generalized, epilepsies report hyposexuality and sexual dysfunction.

The problem of infertility in WWE is therefore complex. There are multiple factors—seizure type, frequency, and the site of ictal onset, as well as AEDs—that may affect an individual patient. Infertility in a couple deserves a careful evaluation of both partners. For WWE, ultrasonography (to rule out polycystic ovarian disease), serum LH and FSH concentrations, and an evaluation of AED use will help the clinician narrow the focus of treatment. As described previously, there is evidence that valproate may adversely impact the fertility of some women. If the patient's seizures are controlled, discontinuation of valproate is not warranted unless polycystic ovarian disease or hypogondaotropic hypogonadism is found.

ANTIEPILEPTIC DRUGS AND HORMONAL CONTRACEPTIVES

A discussion of pregnancy needs to be preceded by reviewing the problems of contraception. Oral contraceptives have not been associated with exacerbation of epilepsy (43). The effectiveness of hormonal contraceptives can, however, be reduced by enzyme-inducing AEDs (carbamazepine, phenytoin, phenobarbital, felbamate, topiramate). Hormonal contraceptives come in three formulations: oral (estrogen-progesterone combinations, or progesterone only); subcutaneous (levonorgestrel) or intrauterine (Progestasert®) implants; and injectable (Depo-Provera®). All three forms can be adversely impacted by enzyme-inducing AEDs.

AEDs may lower concentrations of estrogens by 40% to 50%. They also increase sex hormone–binding globulin (SHBG), which increases the binding of progesterone and reducing the unbound fraction. The result is that hormonal contraception is less reliable with enzyme-inducing AEDs.

The low- or mini-dose oral contraceptives are therefore to be used with caution. Because it is the progesterone, not the estrogen, that inhibits ovulation, using higher doses of estrogens alone may not be effective. The more rapid clearance of the oral contraceptive, when used in conjunction with an enzyme-inducing AED, will reduce the likelihood of unwanted side effects from higher-dose tablets.

Failures of implantable hormonal contraceptives have also occurred (52). Midcycle spotting or bleeding is a sign that ovulation is not suppressed. If this occurs, alternative or supplementary methods of contraception are required. Contraceptive failure may not always be predictable, even when midcycle spotting does not occur. Failure of basal body temperature to rise at midcycle can be used to document ovulatory suppression.

Medroxyprogesterone injections should be given every 10 instead of 12 weeks to women on enzyme-inducing AEDs. This shorter cycle is less likely to result in unintended pregnancy (53).

For multiparous women with epilepsy, intrauterine devices may be an excellent birth prevention choice. Alternatively, non-enzyme-inducing AEDs may need to be considered (valproate, lamotrigine, gabapentine, or zonisamide). A recent report suggests that topiramate at doses of less than 200 mg/day lacks enough enzyme induction to affect hormonal contraceptives. Higher doses, however, do reduce ethinyl estradiol concentrations by 18% on 200 mg, 21% with 400 mg, and 30% with 800 mg of topiramate a day (54).

The importance of the potential impact of enzyme-inducing AEDs cannot be underestimated. In a survey of 294 general practices in the General Practice Research Database, 16.7% of women with epilepsy aged 15 to 45 were taking an oral contraceptive. Two hundred were on an enzyme-inducing AED, and 56% on low-estrogen (<50 μg) hormonal contraceptives (55).

There has been at least one circumstance in which oral contraceptives affect AED concentration. Sabers and colleagues (56) have demonstrated a marked reduction in lamotrigine concentrations when oral contraceptives are also taken. The average plasma concentration in

22 women on lamotrigine monotherapy and an oral contraceptive was 13 μmol/L. In a similar group of women on lamotrigine monotherapy with no oral contraceptive use the plasma concentrations averaged 28 μmol/L; that is, the contraceptive was correlated with a significant reduction in AED concentration of over 50%. It has been suggested that oral contraceptives may induce the metabolism of glucuronidated drugs such as lamotrigine.

PREGNANCY

The majority of WWE can conceive and bear normal, healthy children. The pregnancies of WWE do present a greater risk for complications of pregnancy; they are more likely to have difficulties during labor, and there is a higher risk of adverse pregnancy outcomes.

Increased Seizure Frequency

One-quarter to one-third of WWE will have an increase in seizure frequency during pregnancy. This increase is unrelated to seizure type, duration of epilepsy, or seizure frequency in a previous pregnancy. Although most studies have demonstrated that the increase trends to occur toward the end of pregnancy, recent reports find that a substantial number (31%) have their increase in the first trimester (57).

Plasma concentrations of anticonvulsant drugs decline as pregnancy progresses, even in the face of constant and, in some instances, increasing doses (58–61). Plasma concentrations tend to rise postpartum (62, 63). Although reduction of plasma drug concentration is not always accompanied by an increase in seizure frequency, virtually all women with increased seizures in pregnancy have subtherapeutic drug levels (64–67). The decline of anticonvulsant levels during pregnancy is largely a consequence of decreased plasma protein binding (59, 68, 69), reduced concentration of albumin, and increased drug clearance (58, 65, 70, 71). The clearance rates are greatest during the third trimester.

Seizures during pregnancy increase the risk of adverse pregnancy outcomes. Generalized, tonic-clonic seizures increase the risk for hypoxia and acidosis (72) as well as injury from blunt trauma. Canadian researchers have found that maternal seizures during gestation increase the risk of developmental delay (73). Although rare, stillbirths have occurred following a single generalized convulsion (74, 75), or series of seizures (76, 77).

Generalized (though not partial) convulsions occurring during labor can have a profound effect on fetal heart rate (78). The increased rate of neonatal hypoxia and low Apgar scores may be related to such events (69). Partial seizures may also have similar effects, if less often (79).

COMPLICATIONS IN THE OFFSPRING

Infants of mothers with epilepsy (IME) are at greater risk for a variety of adverse pregnancy outcomes. These include fetal death, congenital malformations, neonatal hemorrhage, low birth weight, developmental delay, feeding difficulties, and childhood epilepsy.

Infant Mortality

Fetal death (defined as fetal loss after 20 weeks gestation) appears to be as common and perhaps as great a problem as congenital malformations and anomalies. Studies comparing stillbirth rates found higher rates in IME (1.3–14.0%) than in infants of mothers without epilepsy (1.2–7.8%).

Spontaneous abortions, defined as fetal loss prior to 20 weeks of gestation, do appear to occur more commonly in infants of mothers with epilepsy (80). Women with localization-related epilepsies appear to be at greater risk for spontaneous abortions than those with other seizure types (81). Other studies have demonstrated increased rates of neonatal and perinatal death. Perinatal death rates range from 1.3% to 7.8%, compared to 1.0% to 3.9% for controls.

Malformations

Fetal malformations have been associated with in-utero exposure to AED. Congenital malformations are defined as a physical defect requiring medical or surgical intervention and resulting in a major functional disturbance.

IME, exposed to anticonvulsant drugs in utero, are twice as likely to develop birth defects as infants not exposed to these drugs. Malformation rates in the general population range from 2% to 3%. Reports of malformation rates in various populations of exposed infants range from 1.25% to 12.5% (71, 82–92). These combined estimates yield a risk of malformations in a pregnancy of a WWE of 4% to 6%. Cleft lip, cleft palate, or both, and congenital heart disease account for many of the reported cases. Orofacial clefts are responsible for 30% of the increased risk of malformations in these infants (93–95).

A wide variety of congenital malformations have been reported, and every anticonvulsant drug has been implicated as a cause. No anticonvulsant drug can be considered absolutely safe in pregnancy, yet most of these drugs do not produce any specific pattern of major malformations.

An exception to the latter statement is the association of sodium valproate with neural tube defects (NTD). Methodologic problems make frequency estimates imprecise since most published data are case reports, case series, or very small cohorts from registries that were not designed to evaluate pregnancy outcomes. The prevalence of spina bifida (SB) with valproate exposure is approximately 1% to 2% (96), and with carbamazepine 0.5% (97, 98). However, a prospective study in the Netherlands found that IME exposed to valproate had a 5.4% prevalence rate of SB. Average daily valproate doses were higher in the IME with SB (1,640 ± 136 mg/day) than in the unaffected IME (941 ± 48 mg/day) (99). Another group of investigators has found that valproate doses of 1,000 mg/day or less or plasma concentrations of less than 70 μg/mL or less are unlikely to case malformations (87, 90).

WWE, like all women of childbearing age, should take folate supplementation. The dose recommended by the Centers for Disease Control of 400 μg/day may not be high enough for many women who do not metabolize folate effectively. Even with folate supplementation, women taking valproate or carbamazepine should avail themselves of prenatal diagnostic ultrasound to rule out NTD.

Neonatal Hemorrhage

For many years it has been reported that IME are at greater risk for a unique form of neonatal hemorrhage, first described by Van Creveld (100), who suggested that vitamin K deficency might be the cause. It was first delineated as a syndrome by Mountain (101), but there have been numerous reports of in-utero AED exposure associated with neonatal hemorrhage (102–109). It was initially associated with exposure to phenobarbital or primidone but has subsequently also been described in children exposed to phenytoin, carbamazepine, diazepam, mephobarbital, amobarbital, and ethosuximide.

This disorder has been differentiated from other hemorrhagic disorders in infancy in that the bleeding occurs internally, during the first 24 hours after birth. Accurate prevalence figures are lacking.

The hemorrhage appears to be a result of a deficiency of vitamin K-dependent clotting factors II, VII, IX, and X. Maternal coagulation parameters are invariably normal. The fetus, however, will demonstrate diminished clotting factors and prolonged prothrombin and partial thromboplastin times. A prothrombin precursor, protein induced by vitamin K absence (PIVKA), has been discovered in the serum of mothers taking anticonvulsants (110). Assays for PIVKA may permit prenatal identification of infants at risk for hemorrhage (111, 112).

The historical demonstration of an increased risk of neonatal hemorrhage, coupled with a demonstrated deficiency of vitamin K and the PIVKA, led clinicians to believe the relative lack of vitamin K and presence of PIVKA was the cause of this particular neonatal hemorrhage. Three studies demonstrated that oral maternal supplementation increased neonatal vitamin K and reduced hemorrhage (113–115).

The practice of maternal vitamin K supplementation has been challanged. Kaaja and colleagues (2002) found no difference in the rates of neonatal hemorrhage in 667 infants of mothers with epilepsy (0.7%) and 1,334 control infants (0.4%). No mothers in either group were supplimented with vitamin K, but all infants received intramuscular vitamin K at delivery. They felt that on the basis of their experience no evidence of a difference in clinical bleeding could be found; hence, supplementation was not recommended. Hey (117) measured cord blood from 137 infants of mothers with epilepsy taking phenobarbital, phenytoin, or carbamazepine and found that 14 of 105 had prolonged prothrombin times but none had any clinical bleeding. He felt that the lack of clinical bleeding in his series made supplementation with vitamin K inappropriate.

Some background may help clarify the apparent differences in conclusions made by these observers. Vitamin K deficiency is common in a neonates. Maternal vitamin levels are not reflected in cord blood. When Shearer and colleagues (118) measured vitamin K in mothers, they found values ranging from 0.13 to 0.29 ng/mL, but none in the cord blood. Even after IV supplementation raised levels to 45–93 ng/mL, cord values rose only to 0–0.14 ng/mL. This descrepancy between maternal and neonatal vitamin K levels has led researchers to look for PIVKA as a proxy for vitamin K deficency. PIVKA is formed as a result of incomplete carboxylation of protein precursors of vitamin K and so is present when vitamin K is absent or present in very small concentrations.

The problem is in part that there is a confusion between vitamin K deficiency, laboratory evidence of abnormal coagulation parameters, and clinical bleeding. Vitamin K deficiency is common, the presence of PIVKA less so, but clinical bleeding in neonatal life is rare. Shapiro et al (119) demonstrated that PIVKA presence is fairly uncommon in the general population of newborns (2.9%) and more common in premature infants. We have no good data on prevalence of neonatal hemorrhage in infants of mothers with epilepsy, but we do have reasonably accurate case reports.

We also have reasonable causation. Anticonvulsants can act like warfarin and can inhibit vitamin K transport across the placenta. These effects can be overcome by large concentrations of the vitamin. Despite lower coagulation factor levels, the fetus is generally able to obtain enough maternal vitamin K in utero. After birth it must rely on exogenous sources of vitamin K because the newborn gut is sterile. Routine administration of vitamin K at birth is not adequate to prevent hemorrhage if any two of the coagulation factors fall below 5% of normal values (108). Successful treatment requires fresh frozen plasma intravenously.

It is not so much that Kaaja and Hey are incorrect but that it is extremely difficult to measure the effects of infrequent clinical outcomes. Neonatal hemorrhage is also unlikely to be identified unless it is severe and the child clinically ill in those first 24 hours. The marked increase in PIVKA in IME suggests that they are at increased risk for hemorrhage, and the increase in developmental delay and need for additional educational assistance seen so often in this population suggests that small degrees of hemorrhage may effect the development of these infants (73, 120, 121).

To make matters more interesting, Howe and colleagues (122) suggest that vitamin K deficiency in a developing embryo results in a failure of vitamin K–dependent carboxylation processes, resulting in an accumulation of compounds that affect embryonic cartilaginous development. Such children are at risk for midface hypoplasia. They base this hypothesis on the clinical similarities between the midface abnormalities seen in warfarin- and phenytoin-exposed children. Howe suggests that, because maternal supplementation with vitamin K reverses the deficiency, perhaps such supplementation should start prior to conception.

Therefore it is clear that one should offer maternal supplementation to pregnant women with epilepsy. The risk of neonatal hemorrhage, while low, clearly exists, as demonstrated by elevated PIVKA levels, particularly with enzyme-inducing AEDs. There is a lack of an effective intervention once a neonate bleeds. There is the additional possibility of small bleeds that, although not clinically detectable at birth, may have long-term effects. There is a hypothesized possibility of an association of decreased carboxylation secondary to decreased vitamin K and the development of some types of malformations. There is a lack of risk with the recommended vitamin K supplementation (10 mg/day). There is also a clear need for better prevalence data on the true risk of clinical bleeding in infants of mothers with epilepsy.

Low Birth Weight

Low birth weight (less than 2,500 g) and prematurity have been described in infants of mothers with epilepsy. The average rates range from 7% to 10% for low birth weight and 4% to 11% for prematurity (123–127). These studies do not analyze the effect of specific seizure types, frequency, or AED on this aspect of fetal development.

A prospective study that pooled data from three countries (Canada, Japan, and Italy) on 870 infants of mothers with epilepsy found that 7.8% were below the 10th percentile in weight at birth (128). The risk was greater with polytherapy.

Body dimensions of IME have been studied by Wide and colleagues (128). Infants exposed to polytherapy not surprisingly, were shorter and smaller than those exposed to monotherapy. Exposure to monotherapy with carbamazepine revealed a tendency toward small birth weight and head circumference for gestational age, but it was not statistically significant.

Developmental Delay

With epilepsy having a prevalence of 0.6% to 1%, it is estimated that there are 24,000 deliveries to women with epilepsy in the United States each year. If 75% to 95% of these mothers take AEDs, we can expect 18,000 to 22,800 infants exposed to AEDs in utero per year. It is estimated that half of all AED prescriptions are used for conditions other than epilepsy. Though these patient populations may have fewer women of childbearing years, the number of exposed children is substantial.

Most investigators have focused on congenital malformations as the primary adverse outcome for children of mothers with epilepsy. The rates are approximately double those in the general population. We would argue that the magnitude of developmental delay is similar.

Infants of mothers with epilepsy have been reported to have higher rates of mental retardation than controls. This risk is increased 2- to 7-fold according to various authors (130, 131). None of these early studies controlled for parental intelligence; although differences in IQ scores at age 7 between groups of children exposed (FSIQ = 91.7) or not exposed (FSIQ = 96.8) to phenytoin reached statistical significance, the clinical significance of such difference is unclear (132). In comparing 76 IME with 71 unexposed control children, Wide and colleagues (133) found no difference in scores on developmental tests but did find a tendency for phenytoin-exposed children to have a greater reduction in tests of motor coordination.

Leavitt and colleagues found that IME display lower scores in measures of verbal acquisition at both 2 and 3 years of age. Though there was no difference in physical growth parameters between IME and controls, IME scored significantly lower in the Bailey Scale of Infant Development's mental developmental index (MDI) at 2 and 3 years. They also performed significantly less well on the Bates Bretherton early language inventory ($P < 0.02$) and in the Peabody Picture Vocabulary's scales of verbal reasoning ($P < 0.001$) and composite IQ ($P < 0.01$), and they displayed significantly shorter mean lengths of utterance ($P < 0.001$) (134).

Polytherapy-exposed infants performed significantly less well on neuropsychometric testing than those exposed to monotherapy. Socioeconomic status had the strongest association with poor test scores, but maternal seizures during pregnancy were also a significant risk factor (135).

Leonard et al (74) have in part addressed the question of whether maternal seizures or in utero exposure to AEDs are responsible for the developmental delay seen. A group of children of mothers with epilepsy followed to school age were found to have a rate of intellectual deficiency of 8.6%. The Wechsler Intelligence Scale for Children revealed significantly lower scores for children exposed to seizures during gestation (100.3) than for children whose mothers' seizures were controlled (104.1) or controls (112.9). All AEDs are clearly not created equal, and Koch and coworkers (136) have demonstrated that primidone, particularly when used in polytherapy, is associated with lower Wechsler score of intelligence.

Both maternal epilepsy and AED exposure in utero appear to affect development of offspring in a study by Koch et al. (136). Severity of outcomes increased from control, to maternal epilepsy with no AED exposure, to maternal epilepsy AED-exposed children.

An intensive retrospective analysis of 100 consecutive pregnancies seen at a tertiary epilepsy center found that 3.9% of the children were premature, 1.1% had congenital malformations, and 6.2% developmental delay, all despite the fact that 59% of the mothers were seizure free and 98% took folic acid during their pregnancy (137).

Another retrospective study demonstrated that 16% of 594 children of mothers with epilepsy exposed to AED in utero, compared to 11% of 176 children with no AED exposure, required additional educational assistance in school. This was felt to be a reasonable marker for developmental delay. In addition, differences between AEDs were found, with 30% of children exposed to valproate monotherapy, 24% of those exposed to valproate polytherapy, but only 3.2% of children exposed to carbamazepine monotherapy requiring additional educational assistance (120). Monotherapy with other AEDs had rates of 6%, and polytherapy without valproate 16%.

The same cohort of children was studied to determine their IQ scores. Of 251 children tested, the mean IQ for valproate-exposed children was 82, compared to 95 for carbamazepine-exposed and 92 for AED-unexposed children (138).

The authors followed up their initial cohort, eventually studying 249 children of mothers with epilepsy from ages 6 to 16. The numbers in monotherapy were modest: 41 exposed to valproate, 52 to carbamazepine, 21 to phenytoin. Forty-nine were exposed to polytherapy, and there were 80 unexposed children. The investigators used regression analysis to demonstrate that both exposure to valproate and frequent generalized tonic-clonic seizures in pregnancy increased the risk of low verbal IQ scores (139).

Three other studies have found increased rates of developmental delay in children exposed to carbamazepine, ranging from 8% to 20% (140–142). One of these studies used only a single standard deviation from the mean to qualify as developmentally delayed and thus overstates the risk (141).

A retrospective study of mothers with epilepsy delivering in Scotland between 1976 and 2000 used the nonexposed siblings as controls. Developmental delay was demonstrated in 19% of 293 AED-exposed children, compared to just 3% of their nonexposed siblings. The rate of delay in valproate-exposed children was particularly high: 37%. Congenital malformations were found in 14% of exposed and 5% of nonexposed siblings. The investigators also state that facial dysmorphism was present in 52% of exposed and 25% of nonexposed siblings, which makes one wonder about the nature of this population (143).

Reinisch and colleagues conducted double-blind studies examining intelligence in adult men with in-utero exposure to phenobarbital (144). Their mothers by and large had not had epilepsy but took the drug for other indications. Unexposed members of the same birth cohort, matched on a large number of variables, were used as controls. The first study used the Wechsler Adult Intelligence Scale (Danish version); the second, the Danish Military Draft Board Intelligence Test. The authors concluded:

- Men exposed prenatally to phenobarbital had significantly lower verbal intelligence scores (approximately 0.5 SD or 7 IQ points) than predicted.
- Lower socioeconomic status and being the offspring of an "unwanted" pregnancy increased the magnitude of the negative effects to a mean of 20 IQ points less than controls.
- Exposure during the last trimester was the most detrimental.

In one of the best-designed prospective studies of outcomes of mothers with epilepsy, Gaily and colleagues (145) measured the intelligence of 182 children of mothers with epilepsy and 141 controls. The investigators performing the testing were blinded as to the child's exposure. Table 35-3 is from their report.

This study suggests that children exposed to valproate and polytherapy are at higher risk for developmental

TABLE 35-3

IQ Scores of Children of Mothers with Epilepsy and Controls

Group	*N*	Mean VIQ	Mean PIQ	Mean FSIQ
Entire group	182	92.8	100.3	96.0
No AED	45	94.3	98.6	95.6
All mono Rx	107	94.4	101.9	98.0
CBZ mono Rx	86	96.2	103.1	99.7
VPA mono Rx	13	83.5	96.3	89.7
Other mono Rx	8	91.1	96.9	93.6
All poly Rx	30	84.9	97.1	89.5
VPA poly Rx	17	81.5	96.1	86.6
Control	141	94.9	102.4	97.6

Source: Gaily et al, 2004 (145).

delay than children exposed to carbamazepine or unexposed children.

MANAGEMENT OF THE PREGNANT WOMAN WITH EPILEPSY

Those who care for WWE face a dilemma. Seizures need to be prevented; but fetal exposure to anticonvulsant drugs needs to be minimized. Just as important is the fact that maternal seizures increase the risk of injury, miscarriage, epilepsy in the offspring, and developmental delay.

The major organ systems have formed by late in the first trimester. The posterior neuropore closes by day 27, and the palate by the 47th day of gestation. By the time most women realize they are pregnant, malformations already may have developed. WWE of childbearing age need to be informed of the risks of pregnancy associated with anticonvulsant use, prior to conception if at all possible. They also need to know that seizures can be harmful to mother and fetus and that risks can be reduced with proper care.

Many people appear to be unaware that even healthy parents have a 2–3% risk of having a child with a malformation. Given the current state of the art, the best we can do is practice risk reduction. In general, risks can be minimized by the preconceptual use of multivitamins with folate, and using AED in monotherapy with the lowest effective dose and preventing maternal seizures. Monitoring free drug levels, both prior to and during pregnancy, will permit accurate assessment of concentrations in a situation where plasma protein binding is in flux. Dose adjustment, however, should be made on a clinical basis. Plasma anticonvulsant drug concentrations will fall in pregnant women, but only a quarter to one-third will have an increase in seizures. Keep dosage as low as possible during conception and organogenesis. Raising the dosage during the third trimester to reduce the risk of seizures during labor may be advisable.

Supplementation with at least 0.4 mg/day of folate is recommended by the Centers for Disease Control for all women of childbearing age, whether or not they have epilepsy.

Vitamin K_1, 10 mg/day, should be initiated late in the third trimester to prevent neonatal hemorrhage.

Breastfeeding is generally safe in term infants, as they have been exposed to the AED for 9 months and have induced their hepatic microsomal enzyme systems. However, breastfeeding should be done cautiously by women receiving phenobarbital or primidone because of the risk of infant sedation.

Pregnant women taking valproate should avail themselves of prenatal diagnostic techniques: ultrasound and alpha fetoprotein measurement. Ultrasonography has become much more accurate and, in experienced hands, can identify the vast majority of structural defects. Current prenatal testing recommendations are as follows:

1. Anatomic ultrasound at 11–13 weeks (this can identify the most severe defects, such as anencephaly)
2. Maternal serum alpha fetoprotein
3. Repeat anatomic ultrasound at 16 weeks (this can identify abnormalities such as orofacial clefts, heart defects, and caudal neural tube defects)

When a WWE initially presents to her neurologist, pregnant, her gestational age (GA) needs to be established with reasonable accuracy. One cannot rely on last menstrual period (LMP) alone; an early ultrasound should be obtained to date the pregnancy. Once GA is established, a calendar can be planned with dates for monthly AED level checks, prenatal testing, and initiating Vitamin K supplementation determined ahead of time.

CONCLUSION

Young women with epilepsy face multiple issues in addition to the seizures themselves. Epilepsy may affect their libido, ability to reproduce, and effectiveness of hormonal contraceptives. A subset of patients will find that there is a direct effect of their menstrual cycles on their epilepsy. Pregnancy is generally a positive experience, with the vast majority of patients having healthy children. These issues present challenges but can be managed, permitting most young women to enter adulthood with the same expectations as their peers without seizures.

References

1. Juul-Jensen P, Foldspang A. Natural history of epileptic seizures. *Epilepsia* 1983; 24(3):297–312.
2. Blom S, Heijbel J. Benign epilepsy of children with centrotemporal EEG foci: a follow-up study in adulthood of patients initially studied as children. *Epilepsia* 1982; 23:629–632.
3. Jeavons P, Harding GFA. Photosensitive epilepsy: prognosis. *Clin Dev Med* 1975; 56:103–104.
4. Wolf P. Epilepsy and grand mal on awakening. In: Roger J, Dravet C, Bureau M, Dreifuss FE, et al, eds. *Epileptic Syndromes in Infancy, Childhood and Adolescence*. London: John Libbey Eurotext, 1985:242–246.
5. Aicardi J, Chevrie JJ. Myoclonic epilepsies of childhood. *Neuropädiatrie* 1971; 3: 177–190.
6. McKinley I. Epilepsy care: the problem from child to adult. In: Ross E, Chadwick D, Crawford R, eds. *Epilepsy in Young People*. Chichester, UK: John Wiley & Sons Ltd, 1987:3–12.
7. Kaada BR, Feldman RS, Langfeldt T. Failure to modulate autonomic reflex discharge by hippocampal stimulation in rabbits. *Physio Behav* 1971 Aug:7(2):225–231.
8. Friedman MN, Geula C, Holmes GL, Herzog AG. GnRH-immunoreactive fiber changes with unilateral amygdale-kindled seizures. *Epilepsy Res* 2002 Dec; 52(2):73–77.
9. Gowers WR. Epilepsy and other chronic convulsive diseases. Their causes, symptoms and treatment. New York: William Wood, 1885.
10. Spratling 1904.

11. Turner WA. Epilepsy, a study of the idiopathic disease. London: MacMillan, 1907 (reprint New York: Raven Press, 1973):43–46.
12. Lennox WG, Cobb S. Epilepsy. *Medicine* 1928; 7:105–209.
13. Dickerson WW. The effect of menstruation on seizure incidence. *J Nerv Ment Dis* 1941,94:160–169.
14. Ansell B, Clarke E. Epilepsy and menstruation. The role of water retention. *Lancet* 1956; 268(6955):1232–1235.
15. Laidlaw J. Catamenial epilepsy. *Lancet* 1956; 268(6955):1235–1237.
16. Lennox and Lennox 1960.
17. Rosciszewska D. Analysis of seizure dispersion during menstrual cycle in women with epilepsy. *Monogr Neurol Sci* 1980; 5:280–284.
18. Marques-Assis L. Influence of menstruation on epilepsy. *Arq Neuropsiquiatr* 1981; 39:390–395.
19. Duncan S, Read CL, Brodie M. How common is catamenial epilepsy? *Epilepsia* 1993; 34(5):827–831.
20. Panayiotopoulos CP. Juvenile myoclonic epilepsy: a 5-year prospective study. *Epilepsia* 1994; 35:285–296.
21. Towanabut S, Chulavatnatol S, Suthisisang C, Wanakamanee U. The period prevalence of catamenial epilepsy at Prasat Neurological Institute, Bangkok. *J Med Assoc Thai* 1998; 81(12):970–977.
22. Herzog AG, Harden CL, Liporace J, Pennell P, et al. Frequency of catamenial seizure exacerbation in women with localization-related epilepsy. *Ann Neurol* 2004; 56(3):431–434.
23. Bazan AC, Montenegro MA, Cendes F, Min LL, et al. Menstrual cycle worsening of epileptic seizures in women with symptomatic focal epilepsy. *Arq Neuropsiquiatr* 2005; 63(3B):751–756.
24. Herkes GK, Eadie MJ, Sharbrough F, Moyer T. Patterns of seizure occurrence in catamenial epilepsy. *Epilepsy Res* 1993; 15:47–52.
25. Herzog AG, Klein P, Ransil BJ. Three patterns of catamenial epilepsy. *Epilepsia* 1997; 38(10):1082–1088.
26. Temkin O. The falling sickness. Baltimore: Johns Hopkins Press, 1945:286.
27. Murri L, Bonuccelli U, Melis GB. Neuroendocrine evaluation in catamenial epilepsy. *Neurology* 1993; 43:2708–2709.
28. Bonuccelli U. Melis GB, Paoletti AM, Fioretti P, et al. Unbalanced progesterone and estradiol secretion in catamenial epilepsy. *Epilepsy Res* 1989; 3:100–106.
29. Narbone MC, Ruello C, Oliva A, Baviera G, et al. Hormonal disregulation and catamenial epilepsy. *Funct Neurol* 1990; 5:49–53.
30. Logothetis J, Harner R, Morell F, Torres F. The role of estrogens in catamenial exacerbation of epilepsy. *Neurology* 1958; 9:352–360.
31. Backstrom T, Zetterlund B, Blom S, Romano M. Effect of intravenous progesterone infusions on the epileptic discharge frequency in women with partial epilepsy. *Acta Neurol Scand* 1984; 69:240–248.
32. Craig CR. Anticonvulsant activity of steroids: separability of anticonvulsant from hormonal effects. *J Pharmacol Exp Ther* 1966; 153:337–343.
33. Costa PJ, Bonnycastle DD. [The effect of DCA, compound E, testosterone, progesterone and ACTH in modifying "agene-induced" convulsions in dog]. *Arch Int Pharmacodyn Ther* 1952; 91:330–338.
34. Landgren S, Backstrom T, Kalistratov G. The effect of progesterone on the spontaneous interictal spike evoked by the application of penicillin to the cat's cortex. *J Neurol Sci* 1978; 36:119–133.
35. Reddy DS. Pharmacology of catamenial epilepsy. *Methods Find Exp Clin Pharmacol* 2004; 26(7):547–561.
36. Galimberti CA, Magri F, Copello F, Arbasino C, et al. Seizure frequency and cortisol and dehydroepiandrosterone sulfate (DHEAS) levels in women with epilepsy receiving antiepileptic drug treatment. *Epilepsia* 2005; 46(4):517–523.
37. Mattson RH, Cramer JA, Caldwell BV, Siconolfi BC. Treatment of seizures with medroxyprogesterone acetate: preliminary report. *Neurology* 1984; 34:1255–1258.
38. Dana-Haeri J, Richens A. Effect of norethisterone on seizures associated with menstruation. *Epilepsia* 1983; 24:377–381.
39. Herzog 1986.
40. Herzog AG, Progesterone therapy in women with complex partial and secondarily generalized seizures. *Neurology* 1995; 45:1660.
41. Herzog AG. Clomiphene therapy in epileptic women with menstrual disorders. *Neurology* 1988; 38:432–434.
42. Svigos JM. Epilepsy and pregnancy. *Aust NZ J Obstet Gynaecol* 1984; 24:182–185.
43. Mattson RH, Cramer JA, Darney PD, Naftolin F. The use of oral contraceptives by women with epilepsy. *JAMA* 1986; 256(2):238–240.
44. Bilo L, Meo R, Nappi C, Annunziato L, et al. Reproductive endocrine disorders in women with primary generalized epilepsy. *Epilepsia* 1988; 29(5):612–619.
45. Isojarvi JI, Laatikainen TJ, Pakarinen AJ, Juntunen KT, et al. Polycystic ovaries and hyperandrogenism in women taking valproate for epilepsy. *N Engl J Med* 1993; 329(19):1383–1388.
46. Drislane FW, Coleman AE, Schomer DL, Ives J, et al. Altered pulsatile secretion of luteinizing hormone in women with epilepsy. *Neurology* 1994; 44(2):306–310.
47. Herzog AG. Psychoneuroendocrine aspects of temporolimbic epilepsy, Part II: Epilepsy and reproductive steroids. *Psychosomatics* 1999; 40:102–108.
48. Herzog AG, Seibel MM, Schomer DL, Vaitukaitis JL, et al. Reproductive and endocrine disorders in women with partial seizures of temporal lobe origin. *Arch Neurol* 1986; 43:341–346.
49. Morrell MJ. Sexual dysfunction in epilepsy. *Epilepsia* 1991; 32 Suppl 6:S38–S45.
50. Lambert MV. Seizures, hormones and sexuality. *Seizure* 2001; 10(5):319–340.
51. Shukla GD, Srivastava ON, Katiyar BC. Sexual disturbances in temporal lobe epilepsy: a controlled study. *Br J Psychiatry* 1979; 134:288–292.
52. Shane-McWhorter L, Cerveny JD, MacFarlane LL, Osborne C. Enhanced metabolism of levonorgestrel during phenobarbital treatment and resultant pregnancy. *Pharmacotherapy* 1998; 18(6):1360–1364.
53. Crawford P. Epilepsy and pregnancy. *Seizure* 2002; 11(S A):212–219.
54. Doose DR, Jacobs D, Squires L, Wang SS, et al. Oral contraceptive-AED interaction: No effect of topiramate as monotherapy at clinically effective doses of 200 mg or less. *Epilepsia* 2002; 43(S7):205.
55. Shorvon SD, Tallis RC, Wallace HK. Antiepileptic drugs: coprescription of proconvulsant drugs and oral contraceptives: a national study of antiepileptic drug prescribing practice. *J Neurol Neurosurg Psychiatry*. 2002; 72(1):114–115.
56. Sabers A, Ohman I, Christensen J, Tomson T. Oral contraceptives reduce lamotrigine plasma levels. *Neurology* 2003; 61(4):570–571.
57. Cahill WT, Kovilam OP, Pastor D, Khoury JC, et al. Neurologic and fetal outcomes of pregnancies of mothers with epilepsy. *Epilepsia* 2002; 43(Suppl. 7):289.
58. Nau H, Rating D, Koch S, Hauser I, et al. Valproic acid and its metabolites: placental transfer, neonatal pharmacokinetics, transfer via mother's milk and clinical status in neonates of epileptic mothers. *J Pharmacol Exp Ther* 1981; 219(3):768–777.
59. Tomson T, Lindbom U, Ekqvist B, Sundqvist A. Epilepsy and pregnancy: a prospective study of seizure control in relation to free and total plasma concentrations of carbamazepine and phenytoin. *Epilepsia* 1994; 35(1):122–130.
60. Rodriguez-Palomares C, Belmont-Gomez A, Amancio-Chassin O, Estrad-Altamirano A, et al. Phenytoin serum concentration monitoring during pregnancy and puerperium in Mexican epileptic women. *Arch Med Res* 1995; 26(4):371–377.
61. Tomson T, Ohman I, Vitols S. Lamotrigine in pregnancy and lactation: a case report. *Epilepsia* 1997; 38(9):1039–1041.
62. Yerby MS, Friel PN, McCormick K. Antiepileptic drug disposition during pregnancy. *Neurology* 1992:42(Suppl 5):12–16.
63. Ohman I, Vitols S, Tomson T. Lamotrigine in pregnancy: pharmacokinetics during delivery, in the neonate, and during lactation. *Epilepsia* 2000; 41(6):709–713.
64. Dansky LV, Andermann E, Andermann F, Sherwin AL, et al. Maternal epilepsy and congenital malformations: correlation with maternal plasma anticonvulsants levels during pregnancy. In: Janz D, Dam M, Richens A, Bossi L, et al, eds. *Epilepsy, Pregnancy and the Child*. New York: Raven Press, 1982:251–258.
65. Janz D. Antiepileptic drugs and pregnancy: altered utilization patterns and teratogenesis. *Epilepsia* 1982; 23(suppl 1):853–863.
66. Schmidt D, Canger R, Avanzini G, et al. Change of seizure frequency in pregnant epileptic women. *J Neurol Neurosurg Psychiatry* 1983; 46:751–755.
67. Otani K. Risk factors for the increased seizure frequency during pregnancy and the puerpurium. *Fol Psychiatr Neurol Jpn* 1985; 39:33–44.
68. Perruca E, Crema A. Plasma protein binding of drugs in pregnancy. *Clin Pharmacokinet* 1982; 7:336-352.
69. Yerby MS, Koepsell T, Daling J. Pregnancy complications and outcomes in a cohort of women with epilepsy. *Epilepsia* 1985; 26:631–635.
70. Dam M, Christiansen J, Munck O, Mygind KJ. Antiepileptic drugs: metabolism in pregnancy. *Clin Pharmacokinet* 1979; 4:53–62.
71. Philbert A, Dam M. The epileptic mother and her child. *Epilepsia* 1982; 23:85–99.
72. Stumpf DA, Frost M. Seizures, anticonvulsants, and pregnancy. *Am J Dis Child* 1978; 132:746–8.
73. Leonard G, Andermann E, Pitno A, Schopflocher C. Cognitive effects of antiepileptic drug therapy during pregnancy on school age offspring. *Epilepsia* 1997; 38(S3):170.
74. Burnett CWF. A survey of the relation between epilepsy and pregnancy. *J Obstet Gynecol* 1946; 53:539–556.
75. Higgins TA, Comerford JB. Epilepsy in pregnancy. *J Irish Med Assoc* 1974; 67:317–29.
76. Suter C, Klingman WO. Seizure states and pregnancy. *Neurology*.1957; 7:105–118.
77. Klingman, WO, Suter C. Seizure states and pregnancy. *Neurology* 1957 Feb; 7(2):105–118.
78. Teramo K, Hiilesmaa VK, Bardy A, et al. Fetal heart rate during a maternal grand mal epileptic seizure. *J Perinat Med* 1979; 7:3–5.
79. Sahoo S, Klein P. Maternal complex partial seizure associated with fetal distress. *Arch Neurol* 2005; 62(8):1304–1305.
80. Yerby MS, Cawthon ML. Fetal death, malformations and infant mortality in infants of mothers with epilepsy. *Epilepsia* 1996; 37(S5):98.
81. Schumpf N, Ottman R. Risk of epilepsy in offspring of affected women: association with maternal spontaneous abortion. *Neurology* 2001; 57(9):1642–1649.
82. Fedrick J. Epilepsy and pregnancy: A report from the Oxford record linkage study. *Br Med J* 1973; 2:442–448.
83. Kelly TE. Teratogenicity of anticonvulsant drugs I: Review of literature. *Am J Med Genet* 1984; 19:413–434.
84. Nakane Y, Okuma T, Takahashi R, et al. Multi-institutional study on the teratogenicity and fetal toxicity of antiepileptic drugs: Report of a collaborative study group in Japan. *Epilepsia* 1980; 21:663–680.
85. Steegers-Theunissen RP, Reiner WO, Borm GF, Thomas CM, et al. Factors influencing the risk of abnormal pregnancy outcomes in epileptic women: a multicenter prospective study. *Epilepsy Res* 1994; 18(3):261–269.
86. Jick SS, Terris BZ. Anticonvulsants and congenital malformations. *Pharmacotherapy* 1997; 17(3):561–564.
87. Kaneko S, Battino D, Andermann E, Wada K, et al. Congenital malformations due to antiepileptic drugs. *Epilepsy Res* 1999; 33(2–3):145–158.
88. Canger R, Battino D, Canevini MP, Fumarola C, et al. Malformations in offspring of women with epilepsy: A prospective study. *Epilepsia* 1999; 40(9):1231–1236.
89. Thomas SV, Indrani L, Devi GC, Jacob S, et al. Pregnancy in women with epilepsy: preliminary results of Kerala registry of epilepsy and pregnancy. *Neurol India* 2001; 49:60–66.

90. Vajda FJ, O'Brien TJ, Hitchcock A, Graham J, et al. Australian registry of antiepileptic drugs in pregnancy: experience after 30 months. *J Clin Neurosci* 2003; 10(5): 543–549.
91. Wide K, Winbladh B, Kallen B. Major malformations in infants exposed to antiepileptic drugs in utero, with emphasis on carbamazepine and valproic acid: a nation-wide, population-based register study. *Acta Paediatr* 2004 Feb; 93(2):174–176.
92. Morrow J, Russell A, Guthrie E, Parsons L, et al. Malformation risks of antiepileptic drugs in pregnancy: a prospective study from the UK Epilepsy and Pregnancy Register. *J Neurol Neurosurg Psychiatry* 2006; 77(2):193–198.
93. Kelly TE. Teratogenicity of anticonvulsants III: radiographic hand analysis of children exposed in utero to diphenylhydantoin. *Am J Med Genet* 1984b; 19:445–50.
94. Friis ML, Holm NV, Sindrup EH, Fogh-Andersen P, et al. Facial clefts in sibs and children of epileptic patients. *Neurology* 1986; 38:346–50.
95. Abrishamchian AR, Khoury MJ, Calle EE. The contribution of maternal epilepsy and its treatment to the eteiology of oral clefts: a population based case-control study. *Genet Epidemiol* 1994; 11(4):343–351.
96. Lindhout D, Schmidt D. In utero exposure to valproate and neural tube defects. *Lancet* 1986; 327(8494):1392–1393.
97. Rosa FW. Spina bifida in infants of women treated with carbamazepine during pregnancy. *N Engl J Med* 1991; 324:674–677
98. Hiilesmaa VK. Pregnancy and birth in women with epilepsy. *Neurology* 1992; 42 (suppl 5):8–11.
99. Omtzigt JG, Los FJ, Grobbee DE, Pijpers L, et al. The risk of spina bifida aperta after first-trimester exposure to valproate in a prenatal cohort. *Neurology* 1992; 42:119–125.
100. Van Creveld S. Nouveaux aspects de la maladie hémorragique du nouveau né. *Ned Tijdschr Geneeskd* 1957; 101:2109–2112.
101. Mountain KR, Hirsh J, Gallus AS. Maternal coagulation defect due to anticonvulsant treatment in pregnancy. *Lancet* 1970; 1:265–268.
102. Lawerence A. Anti-epileptic drugs and the foetus. *Br Med J* 1963; 1:1267.
103. Douglas H. Haemorrhage in the newborn. *Lancet* 1966; 287(7441):816–817.
104. Kohler HG. Haemorrhage in the newborn of epileptic mothers. *Lancet* 1966; 287(7431):267.
105. Solomon GE, Hilgartner MW, Kutt H. Coagulation defects caused by diphenylhydantoin. *Neurology* 1972; 22:1165–1171.
106. Bleyer WA, Skinner AL. Fatal neonatal hemorrhage after maternal anticonvulsant therapy. *JAMA* 1976; 235:626–627.
107. Griffiths AD. Neonatal hemorrhage associated with maternal anticonvulsant therapy. *Lancet* 1981; 1296–1297.
108. Srinivasan G, Seeler RA, Tiruvury A, et al. Maternal anticonvulsant therapy and hemorrhagic disease of the newborn. *Obstet Gynecol* 1982; 59:250–252.
109. Sutor AH. Vitamin K deficiency-bleeding in infants and children. *Semin Thromb Haemost* 1995; 21:317–329.
110. Davies VA, Argent AC, Staub H. Precursor prothrombin status in patients receiving anticonvulsant drugs. *Lancet* 1985; 325(8421):126–128.
111. Walker NP, Bardlow BA, Atkinson PM. A rapid chromogenic method for the determination of prothrombin precursor in the plasma. *Am J Clin Pathol* 1982; 78:777–780.
112. Argent AC, Rothberg AD, Pienaar N. Precursor prothrombin status in the mother infant pairs following gestational anticonvulsant therapy. *Pediatr Pharmacol* 1984; 4:183–187.
113. Deblay MF, Vert P, Andre M, et al. Transplacental vitamin K prevents hemorrhagic disease of infant of epileptic mother. *Lancet* 1982; 319(8283):1247.
114. Cornelissen M, Steegers-Theunissen R, Kollee L, Eskes T, et al. Supplementation of vitamin K in pregnant women receiving anticonvulsant therapy prevents neonatal vitamin K deciciency. *Am J Obstet Gynecol.* 1993; 168:884–888.
115. Anai T, Hirota Y, Yoshimatsu J, Oga M, et al. Can prenatal vitamin K_1 (phylloquinone) supplementation replace prophylaxis at birth? *Obstet Gynecol* 1993; 81:251–254.
116. Kaaja E, Kaaja R, Matila R, Hiilesmaa V. Enzyme-inducing antiepileptic drugs in pregnancy and the risk of bleeding in the neonate. *Neurology* 2002; 58:549–553.
117. Hey E. Effect of maternal anticonvulsant treatment on neonatal blood coagulation. *Arch Dis Child Fetal Neonatal Ed.* 1999; 81(3):F208–F210.
118. Shearer MJ, Rahim S, Barkhan P, Stimmler L. Plasma vitamin K_1 in mothers and their newborn babies. *Lancet* 1982; 320(8296):460–463.
119. Shapiro AD, Jacobson LJ, Armon ME, Manco-Johnson J, et al. Vitamin K deficiencey in the newborn infant: Prevalence and perinatal risk factors. *Pediatr* 1986; 109:675–680.
120. Adab N, Jacoby A, Smith D, Chadwick D. Additional educational needs in children born to mothers with epilepsy. *J Neurol Neurosurg Psychiatry* 2001; 70:15–21.
121. Meador KJ, Yerby MS. Fetal outcomes following antiepileptic drug use. *The Female Patient* September 2002:S10–S14.
122. Howe AM, Oakes DJ, Woodman PD, Webster WS. Prothrombin and PIVKA-II levels in cord blood from newborn exposed to anticonvulsants during pregnancy. *Epilepsia* 1999; 40(7):980–984.
123. Svigos JM. Epilepsy and pregnancy. *Aust NZ J Obstet Gynaecol* 1984; 24:182–185.
124. Teramo K, Hiilesmaa VK. Pregnancy and fetal complications in epileptic pregnancies: review of the literature. In: Janz D, Dam M, Richens A, Bossi L, et al, eds. *Epilepsy, Pregnancy and the Child.* New York: Raven Press, 1982:53–s59.
125. Nakane Y, Okuma T, Takahashi R, et al. Multi-institutional study on the teratogenicity and fetal toxicity of antiepileptic drugs: Report of a collaborative study group in Japan. *Epilepsia* 1980; 21:663–680.
126. Annegers JF, Elveback LR, Hauser WA, et al. Do anticonvulsants have a teratogenic effect? *Arch Neurol* 1974; 31:364–73.
127. Hvas CL, Henriksen TB, Ostergaard JR, Dam M. Epilepsy and pregnancy: effect of antiepileptic drugs and lifestyle on birthweight. *BJOG* 2000; 107(7):896–902.
128. Battino D, Kaneko S, Andermann E, Avanzini G, et al. Interuterine growth in the offspring of epileptic women: a prospective multicenter study. *Epilepsy Res* 1999; 36(1):53–60.
129. Wide K, Winbladh B, Tomson T, Kallen B. Body dimensions of infants exposed to antiepileptic drugs in utero: observations spanning 25 years. *Epilepsia* 2000; 41(7):854–861.
130. Speidel BD, Meadow SR. Maternal epilepsy and abnormalities of the fetus and newborn. *Lancet* 1972; 300(7782):839–843.
131. Hill RM, Verniaud WM, Horning MG, McCulley LB, Morgan NF. Infants exposed in utero to antiepileptic drugs: A prospective study. *Am J Dis Child* 1974 May; 127(5):645–653.
132. Hill RM, Tennyson L. Premature delivery, gestational age, complications of delivery, vital data at birth on newborn infants of epileptic mothers: review of the literature. In: Janz D, Dam M, Richens A, Bossi L, et al, eds. *Epilepsy, Pregnancy and the Child.* New York: Raven Press, 1982:167–173.
133. Wide K, Henning E, Tomson T, Winbladh B. Psychomotor development in preschool children exposed to antiepileptic drugs in utero. *Acta Paediatr* 2002; 91(4):409–414.
134. Leavitt AM, Yerby MS, Robinson N, Sells CJ, et al. Epilepsy and pregnancy: developmental outcomes at 12 months. *Neurology* 1992; 42(suppl 5):141–143.
135. Losche G, Steinhausen H-C, Koch S, Helge H. The psychological development of children of epileptic parents. II. The differential impact of intrauterine exposure to anticonvulsant drugs and further influential factors. *Acta Paediatr* 1994; 83(9):961–966.
136. Koch S, Tize K, Zimmerman RB, Schroder M, et al. Long-term neuropsychological consequences of maternal epilepsy and anticonvulsant treatment during pregnancy for school age children and adolescents. *Epilepsia* 1999; 40(9):1237–1243.
137. Katz JM, Pacia SV, Devinsky O. Current management of epilepsy and pregnancy: fetal outcome, congenital malformations and developmental delay. *Epilepsy Behav* 2001; 2(2):119–123.
138. Vinten J, Gorry J, Baker GA. The long-term neuropsychological development of children exposed to antiepileptic drugs in utero (the Liverpool and Manchester Neurodevelopmental Study Group). *Epilepsia* 2001; 42(suppl 2):36.
139. Adab N, Kini U, Vinten J, Ayres J, et al. The longer term outcome of children born to mothers with epilepsy. *J. Neurol Neurosurg Psychiatry* 2004; 75(11):1517–1518.
140. Scolnik D, Nulman I, Rovet J. Neurodevelopment of children exposed in utero to phenytoin and carbamazepine monotherapy. *JAMA* 1994; 271:767–770.
141. Jones KL, Lacro RV, Johnson KA, Adams J. Pattern of malformations in the children of women treated with carbamazepine during pregnancy. *New Engl J Med* 1989; 320:1661–1666.
142. Ornoy A, Cohen E. Outcome of children born to epileptic mothers treated with carbamazepine during pregnancy. *Arch Dis Child* 1996; 75:517–520.
143. Dean JC, Hailey H, Moore SJ, Lloyd DJ, et al. Long term health and neurodevelopment in children exposed to antiepileptic drugs before birth. *J Med Genet* 2002; 39(4):251–259.
144. Reinisch JM, Sanders SA, Mortensen EL, Rubin DB. In utero exposure to phenobarbital and intelligence deficits in adult men. *JAMA* 1995; 274(19):1518–1525.
145. Gaily E, Kantola-Sorsa E, Hiilesmaa V, Isoaho M, et al. Normal intelligence in children with prenatal exposure to carbamazepine. *Neurology* 2004; 62(1):28–32.

36 Teratogenic Effects of Antiepileptic Medications

Torbjörn Tomson
Dina Battino

Not so long ago, people with epilepsy were often denied the fundamental right to form a family, prevented by prejudiced legislation and public attitudes. This, fortunately, is no longer the case, thanks to changes in social attitudes as well as improvements in diagnosis and therapy of epilepsy. Today, more and more women with epilepsy become pregnant and have children, and it has been estimated that 0.3–0.4% of all children today are born to mothers with epilepsy (1, 2). The vast majority of these women will have uneventful pregnancies and give birth to perfectly normal children. However, there are specific risks associated pregnancies in women with epilepsy, and the medical management during gestation is a matter of special concern. The maternal and fetal risks associated with uncontrolled seizures generally necessitate continued drug treatment during pregnancy, but these seizure-related risks need to be weighed against the potential adverse outcomes in the offspring due to maternal use of antiepileptic drugs (AEDs). This chapter is dedicated to the latter part in this equation: the teratogenic effects of AEDs. The reader is referred to Chapter 35 for a discussion on how such effects are put into context for a rational management of women with epilepsy of childbearing potential.

The question whether AEDs may be harmful during pregnancy was first raised in a systematic way by Janz and Fuchs in 1964 (3), and the first report of adverse fetal effects of AEDs was published a few years later (4). Since then, all of the major old-generation AEDs, such as phenobarbital, phenytoin, valproate, and carbamazepine, have been shown to be teratogenic. Less is known about the teratogenic potential of the newer-generation AEDs that have been introduced to the market during the last 15 years. Adverse outcomes reported in infants exposed to AEDs in utero include major congenital malformations, minor anomalies and dysmorphism, growth retardation, and impaired cognitive development. Although the pathogenesis is likely to be multifactorial, including genetic predisposition, socio-economic circumstances, seizures, and epilepsy, the available data strongly suggest that AEDs are the major cause for the increased risk of these adverse outcomes.

Other types of adverse pregnancy outcome (e.g., miscarriage, stillbirth, perinatal death, and neonatal haemorrhage) have also been associated with epilepsy. These aspects on pregnancy risks are, however, beyond the scope of this chapter and are dealt with elsewhere.

METHODOLOGICAL ASPECTS

Different methods have been used to assess the fetal risks associated with exposure to AEDs. The most simple is based on spontaneous reporting of pregnancy outcome to manufacturers of AEDs. Such reports may be useful to obtain signals, but they suffer from selective reporting of adverse outcomes and lack of information on the denominator and thus cannot be used for a proper risk assessment. Case-control designs have frequently been used, in which cases with, for example, specific malformations are compared to controls with respect to exposure to AEDs in utero. This design may be useful for uncommon outcomes, but it is associated with the risk of recall bias. Other studies utilize existing registries of, for example, drug prescriptions and cross-link those with registries of birth defects. Such registries can have the advantage of being population-based and sometimes even nationwide. They may thus be representative, but they generally lack information on other factors that could contribute to the outcome. Cohort studies are another common approach. The cohorts are generally identified through the epilepsy diagnosis of the mother. They are often hospital-based and can come from single hospitals, epilepsy centers, or from several collaborating clinics. Such studies can be retrospective or prospective. Retrospective identification of the cohort is associated with the risk of selection bias, whereas prospective studies ideally identify and enroll women with epilepsy before any information on pregnancy outcome is known, thus avoiding the risk of selection bias. A special type of cohort studies, AED and pregnancy registries, has been established lately. These registries are prospective observational studies enrolling women with epilepsy early in pregnancy, collecting information on drug exposure and other potential risk factors before outcome of the pregnancy is known. Women are followed throughout pregnancy, and the outcome, in terms of occurrence of birth defects in the offspring, is recorded. The advantage of such studies is that they may collect a high number of pregnancies, the type of drug exposure is recorded in an unbiased way without prior knowledge of teratogenic outcome, and detailed data on other relevant patient characteristics could be obtained. The internal validity of the risk assessments is therefore likely to be high whereas, the possibility to generalize from the results will depend on how pregnancies were enrolled.

However, even results of properly designed, prospective studies of teratogenic effects of AEDs may be difficult to interpret. The assessment of teratogenic effects is based on observational studies, and the women have not been randomized to different types of treatment. The selection of a particular drug or drug combination, the dosage, and the dosage schedule depend on individual environmental and genetic factors such as type of epilepsy and seizures, seizure frequency, comorbidity, and socioeconomic circumstances. These are factors that could be linked to the risk of malformations. An association between exposure to a certain AED and occurrence of adverse pregnancy outcome is thus not evidence of a causal relationship. The impact of possible confounders, such as type of epilepsy, seizure frequency, family history of birth defects, and exposure to additional risk factors, needs to be assessed, which requires large sample sizes. It is thus important to pay attention to methodological issues such as statistical power, reliability of collected data, and attempts to control for appropriate confounding factors in the analyses, rather than to just compare rates of adverse pregnancy outcome in published studies.

MAJOR CONGENITAL MALFORMATIONS

Epilepsy and Other Potential Confounding Factors

A large number of studies have confirmed an increased frequency of major malformations in offspring of women treated with antiepileptic drugs. The incidence of major congenital malformations has ranged from 4% to 10%, corresponding to a 2- to 4-fold increase from that expected in the general population (Table 36-1) (2, 3, 5–68).

Differences in treatment strategy, study populations, controls, and criteria for malformations can account for the variation in outcome. Whether this increase is caused by the AED treatment or at least to some extent is linked to the underlying epilepsy disorder has been a matter of debate (2). Some studies of malformations in offspring of women with epilepsy have included also those who were untreated during pregnancy. The results of 66 cohort studies that include pregnancies of women with treated as well as untreated epilepsy are summarized in Table 36-1. The table includes retrospective studies that are population-based (5–16) and thus probably representative; retrospective hospital-based (2, 3, 55–68); prospective (22–54) and mixed prospective/retrospective (17–21) cohort studies. Irrespective of study methodology, these studies have consistently reported lower malformation rates among children of untreated mothers with epilepsy (on average 3.0%) than among those who have been exposed to AEDs in utero (6.6%). These observations have been confirmed in a recent meta-analysis of the evidence of epilepsy *per se* as a teratogenic risk (69). For this meta-analysis, ten studies reporting rates of congenital malformations in offspring of untreated women with epilepsy (n = 400) were selected. The malformation rate in this group was not higher than among offspring of nonepileptic healthy controls (n = 2492), odds ratio (OR) 1.92; 95% confidence interval (CI) 0.92–4.00. The OR was 0.99 (CI 0.49–2.01) after removal of some small studies likely to be affected by publication bias. The trend toward an increased risk of malformations among children of untreated women with epilepsy thus disappeared. The authors themselves, however, warned about the potential

TABLE 36-1
Malformation Rates in Offspring of Mothers with Epilepsy With or Without AED Treatment During Pregnancy

	Offspring of Treated Mothers with Epilepsy			Offspring of Untreated Mothers with Epilepsy		
	Total Outcomes	Malformations		Total outcomes	Malformations	
		N	%		*N*	%
Retrospective, population-based[a]	4,323	262	6.1%	1,606	48	3.0%
Mainly prospective cohort[b]	982	95	9.7%	229	4	1.7%
Purely prospective cohorts[c]	8,665	544	6.3%	1,742	46	2.6%
Retrospective cohorts[d]	2,622	188	7.2%	733	33	4.5%
Grand total	16,592	1,089	6.6%	4,310	131	3.0%

The table is based on 66 cohort studies that all include pregnancies of women with treated as well as untreated epilepsy.
[a]Refs. (5–16).
[b](17–21).
[c](22–54).
[d](2, 3, 55–68).

bias derived by incomplete reporting of the exact nature of the epilepsy and lack of information on clinical indications for treatment discontinuation (69). Although, obviously, untreated women with epilepsy are different in many respects from those who are under treatment during pregnancy, the available evidence strongly suggests that treatment is the major cause of increased risk of adverse pregnancy outcomes. Epilepsy-related factors nevertheless cannot be disregarded.

Overall Malformation Rates

Since the 1960s, numerous studies have confirmed malformation rates of 4–10% in offspring of women treated for epilepsy during pregnancy. This is 2–3 times higher than expected in the general population and, as discussed above, also higher than among children of untreated mothers with epilepsy (Table 36-1). With slight variation, this 2–3-fold increase has been a consistent finding despite differences in populations, study design, and outcome criteria. A major limitation in most studies to date is the small sample size. Large cohorts are obviously needed to draw conclusions when the prevalence of birth defects (fortunately) is no more than 4–10%. In fact, surprisingly few studies comprise more than 500 pregnancies, which still, for the purpose of assessing the risk of birth defects, is a fairly small sample. The results of the existing 12 studies, each including at least 500 pregnancies, are summarized in Table 36-2 (7, 9, 16, 20, 31, 34, 42, 70–74). The overall malformation rate was 5.2% among the altogether 12,603 exposed to AEDs in these studies. For comparison, birth defects were reported in 2.7% of 1,820 epilepsy pregnancies without AED exposure from the same studies and 2.7% among offspring of nonepileptic controls (Table 36-2).

Patterns of Malformations

The type of malformations and their frequency in pregnancies of women treated with AEDs, based on studies reporting specific birth defects, is presented in Figure 36-1 (2, 8, 15, 24, 25, 39, 44, 51, 52, 58). The pattern is mostly the same as seen in the general population. Congenital heart defects have been the most common, followed by facial clefts, hypospadia, limb reduction deficits, and neural tube defects. It appears that the pattern of malformations may vary with the type of AED, as indicated in Figure 36-2 (2, 6, 8, 11, 15, 17, 19, 23–25, 27, 28, 31, 32, 39, 40, 45, 51–55, 57, 58, 71–89). Whereas cardiac defects dominate among children exposed to barbiturates and, to a lesser extent, those exposed to phenytoin and carbamazepine, neural tube defects and hypospadia are more common among offspring of mothers who took valproic acid during pregnancy. The risk of neural tube defects in association with valproic acid has been estimated to be 1–2% of exposed infants (13, 90). Valproic acid has also been associated with skeletal abnormalities including radial aplasia (91, 92). An increased risk of neural tube defects of 0.5–1% has also been reported after carbamazepine exposure (93, 94). Changes in prescription patterns and drug selection for women of childbearing age with epilepsy can thus be expected to result in a shift in the pattern of malformations in the offspring of women with epilepsy.

TABLE 36-2

Major Congenital Malformation (MCM) and Minor Anomalies (MA) in Offspring of Mothers with Epilepsy, by Type of Treatment (Polytherapy, Monotherapy, or No AEDs) and of Nonepileptic Controls

Reference	Study Design and Population	Outcome Measure	All Pregnancies of Women with Epilepsy		Pregnancies with AED Exposure		Pregnancies Without AED Exposure		Pregnancies with Monotherapy Exposure		Pregnancies with Polytherapy Exposure		Controls	
			N	%	*N*	%	*N*	%	*N*	%	*N*	%	*N*	%
Weber et al, 1977 (16)	Retrospective population-based	MCM, MA	655	3.8%	569	4.0%	86	2.3%					5,011	2.2%
Nakane et al, 1980 (20)	Mainly prospective	MCM, MA	690	9.1%	478	11.9%	129	2.3%						
Bjerkedal, 1982 (70)	National Registry	MCM, MA	3879	4.6%									3,879	3.8%
Kallen, 1986 (9)	National Registry	MCM, MA	644	6.8%	551	6.9%	93	6.5%	263	4.9%	288	8.7%	903,456	1.9%
Bertollini et al, 1987 (71)	Retrospective	MCM, MA	577	3.5%	577	3.5%			577	3.5%				
Samren et al, 1997 (72)	Pooled prospective	MCM, MA	1,221	8.8%	1,221	8.8%			709	8.0%	512	10%	158	7.6%
Samren et al, 1999 (73)	Retrospective controlled	Severe MCM	1,411	3.7%	1,411	3.7%			899	3.3%	512	4.3%	2,000	1.5%
Kaneko et al, 1999 (34)	Pooled prospective	MCM, MA	983	8.4%	886	9.0%	97	3.1%	495	7.9%	391	10.5%		
Kaaja et al, 2003 (31)	Prospective	Severe MCM	970	3.1%	733	3.8%	237	0.80%	583	3.3%	150	6.0%	9,310	1.5%
Wide et al, 2004 (74)	National Registry	MCM, MA	1,398	6.2%	1,398	6.2%			1,256	5.4%	142	13.4%	582,656	4.0%
Artama et al, 2005 (7)	National Registry	MCM, MA	2,350	3.9%	1,411	4.6%	939	2.8%	1,231	4.2%	180	7.2%		
Morrow et al, 2006 (42)	Prospective pregnancy registry	Severe MCM	3,607	3.9%	3,368	4.0%	239	3.3%	2,598	3.5%	770	5.6%		
Total			18,385	5.0%	12,603	5.2%	1,820	2.7%	8,611	4.5%	2,945	7.6%	1,506,312	2.7%

Studies with >500 cases included.

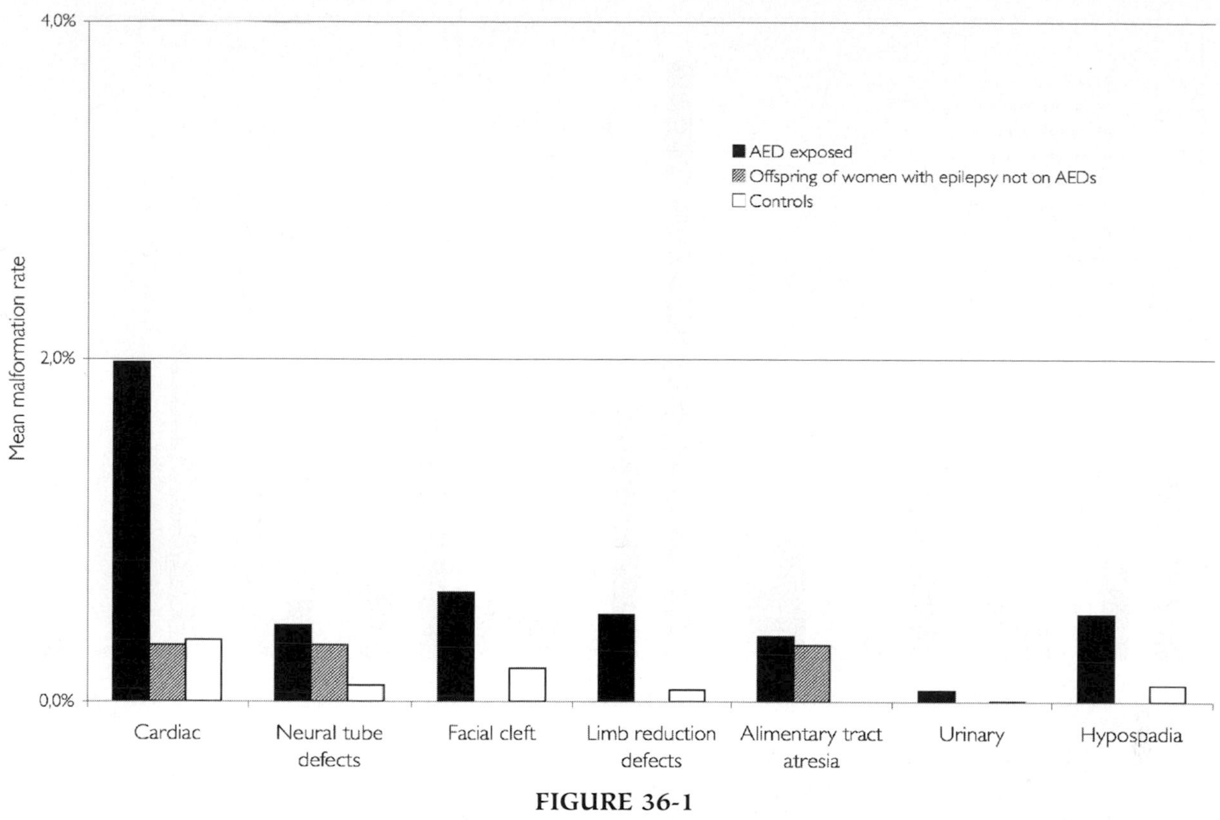

FIGURE 36-1

Rates of different types of malformations in offspring of mothers with epilepsy and under treatment with antiepileptic drugs ("AED exposed"); without treatment during pregnancy ("not on AEDs"); and of nonepileptic control women ("controls"). The figure is based on data from 10 studies, each providing information on specific malformations for these three categories (2, 8, 15, 24, 25, 39, 44, 51, 52, 58).

Risk Factors

Some of the studies summarized in Table 36-2 have applied multivariate analysis in an attempt to elucidate the role of the drug treatment and of other risk factors for the adverse pregnancy outcome. Nakane and coworkers thus identified familial epilepsy, previous miscarriage, partial epilepsy, and exposure to phenobarbital or primidone as risk factors for birth defects (20). Pooling data from five different prospective cohort studies, Samrén and coworkers observed an increased risk with carbamazepine and valproic acid monotherapy compared with unexposed control pregnancies, with phenobarbital in combination with caffeine, as well as with high doses of valproic acid (72). High doses of valproic acid, exposure to monotherapy with valproic acid or primidone, and malformations in siblings were associated with increased risks in the pooled prospective studies from Italy, Japan, and Canada (34). A prospective study from a single center in Finland reported monotherapy with carbamazepine, oxcarbazepine, or valproic acid, low maternal serum folate concentrations and low maternal education as significant risk factors (31). In a population-based nationwide Swedish register study, polytherapy was associated with higher risks than monotherapy, and specifically monotherapy with valproic acid, as compared with carbamazepine (74). A Finnish nationwide study based on drug prescription registries identified polytherapy and monotherapy with valproic acid as associated with an increased risk for birth defects (75).

It is clear from these studies and from Table 36-2 that polytherapy with antiepileptic drugs is associated with a higher malformation rate, 7.6%, than monotherapy, 4.5%. This has been a consistent finding throughout most studies (95). Although, due to confounding factors, alternative interpretations are possible, this observation is supportive evidence for the contribution of the drug treatment to the increased risk of birth defects in children of women with epilepsy. A decreased malformation rate, in parallel with a shift in the therapeutic strategy from polytherapy to monotherapy during pregnancy, is an additional observation supporting a causal relationship between polytherapy and adverse pregnancy outcome (96). Some specific combinations of AEDs have

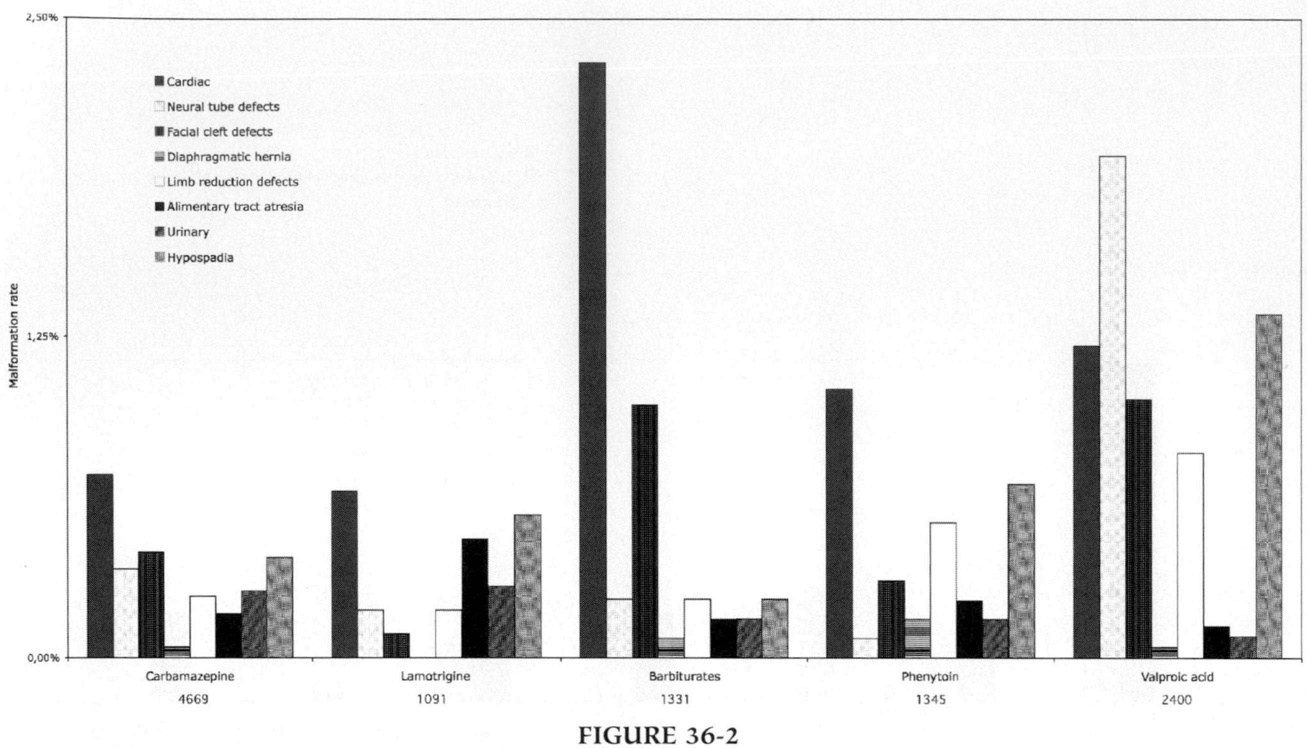

FIGURE 36-2

Rates of different types of malformations in offspring of mothers with epilepsy and under treatment with AEDs, by type of AED used in monotherapy. The graph is based on studies reporting specific malformations by type of monotherapy (2, 6, 8, 11, 15, 17, 19, 23–25, 27, 28, 31, 32, 39, 40, 45, 51–55, 57, 58, 71–89).

been associated with particularly high malformation rates. Among the old-generation anticonvulsants, this has been suggested for the combination of carbamazepine, phenobarbital, and valproic acid (41). More recent studies have also indicated a considerable risk in association with valproic acid in combination with lamotrigine. The International Lamotrigine Pregnancy Registry reported major malformations in 12.5% of children exposed to this specific combination, compared with 2.9% in lamotrigine monotherapy (76). Morrow and collaborators (42) found birth defects among 9.6% of the offspring of mothers treated with valproic acid and lamotrigine combined, versus 3.2% associated with lamotrigine monotherapy and 6.2% in monotherapy with valproic acid. Although interesting, these observations need to be interpreted with great caution, since factors such as differences in drug dosages and severity of the maternal seizure disorder may contribute and were not controlled for.

A dose-effect relationship would be expected with a pharmacologic effect such as the teratogenicity of AEDs. So far this has been shown most convincingly and consistently for valproic acid. Dosages above 800–1,000 mg/day have thus been associated with significantly higher risks for malformations than lower dosages (7, 19, 21, 34, 72, 73, 91, 97). A recent publication from the UK Epilepsy and Pregnancy Register reported a positive dose response for major congenital malformations for lamotrigine as well; doses above 200 mg/day were associated with higher risks (42). This latter observation has, however, not yet been confirmed in other studies.

Genetic factors are obviously also of major importance to explain individual susceptibility to developmental toxicity of AEDs. For example, in some women treated with valproic acid during pregnancy, the history of a pregnancy resulting in a neural tube defect may predict a high risk of further birth defects in subsequent pregnancies (98, 99).

Comparative Teratogenic Potential

Although all major old-generation AEDs have been shown to be teratogenic, the available information on the newer-generation antiepileptics, and, in particular, on potential differences between drugs in teratogenic potential, is more limited and less conclusive. Even in most of the largest cohort studies to date, the numbers on each individual drug as monotherapy have been too small to allow useful comparisons. Unfortunately, pooling of the data is hampered by differences between studies with respect to study populations, methodology, and outcome criteria. An internal comparison between different monotherapies within each of some major, fairly recent studies

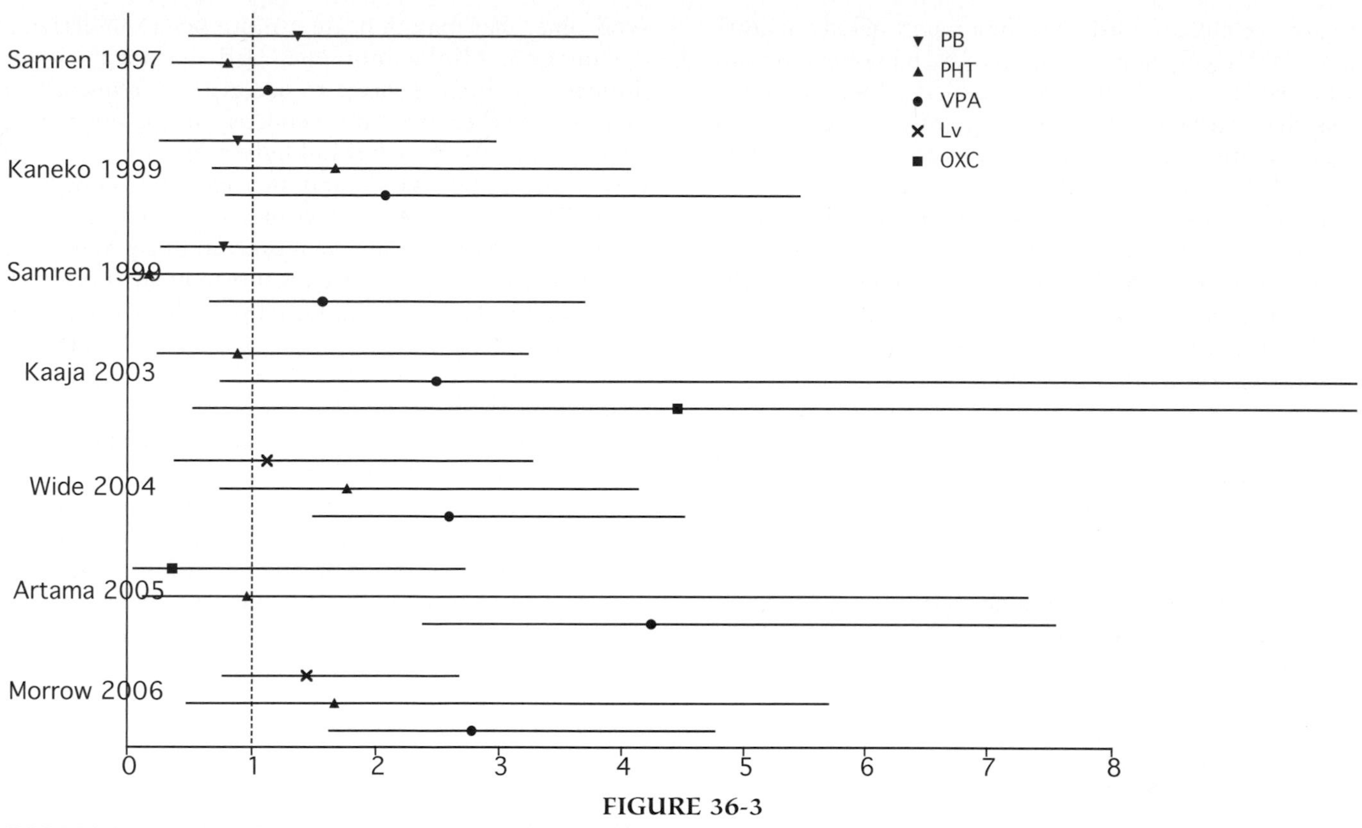

FIGURE 36-3

Odds ratios and 95% confidence intervals for major malformations associated with prenatal exposure to different AEDs in monotherapy relative to the risk associated with exposure to carbamazepine monotherapy (risk = 1) in the same study. The figure presents data from seven recent comparatively large-scale studies.

is presented in Figure 36-3. Although most studies fail to reveal significant differences between drugs, there is a trend for valproic acid to be associated with a higher risk of malformations than carbamazepine. In three of the included studies, this difference is significant (7, 42, 74). In this, as well as many other attempts for comparison between drugs, no distinction is made between different types of major malformations. However, the concept "major malformations" can comprise a wide range of birth defects, some incapacitating, others of very limited consequences. A comparison between AEDs with respect to risks for specific malformations is thus desirable, not least since the types of birth defects are likely to differ (Figure 36-2). It is thus evident that larger studies are needed to obtain more information, in particular, on the new generation AED,s but also to permit multivariate analysis in which potentially contributing factors are included in addition to drug exposure. This will be necessary to advance from observed associations between exposure to a particular drug and pregnancy outcome to an assessment of causal relationships.

For these reasons, prospective AED and pregnancy registries have been set up in the late 1990s. The largest are The North American Antiepileptic Drugs and Pregnancy Registry (NAREP), the United Kingdom Epilepsy and Pregnancy Register, and EURAP, an international registry enrolling pregnancies from 40 countries in Europe, Australia, Asia, Oceania, and South America. Using somewhat different methodologies, each of these registries had enrolled 5,000–8,000 pregnancies by early 2006, and two of them, NAREP and the UK registry, had published the first results on teratogenic outcome. NAREP discloses malformation rates associated with specific treatments as they are found to differ significantly from the background rate. Increased malformation rates in comparison with the general population have so far been identified with phenobarbital (relative risk [RR] 4.2; 95% CI: 1.5–9.4) (100) and valproic acid (RR 7.3; 4.4–12.2) (89). An internal comparison between different specific monotherapies from the same registry has not yet been presented, but the risk with phenobarbital was not significantly increased when compared to three other unspecified monotherapies taken together from the same registry (RR 2.0; 0.9–4.5), whereas the malformation rate with valproic acid was four times higher compared with all other monotherapies taken together (RR 4.0; 2.1–7.4). As yet, NAREP has not revealed any information in relation to the new-generation antiepileptic drugs. The UK register recently published its first report based on 3,607 cases (42). Using multivariate analysis, monotherapy with valproic acid was found to be associated with a higher risk than carbamazepine. The rate of major congenital malformations for pregnancies exposed to valproate monotherapy was 6.2% (95% CI: 4.6–8.2%), compared with 2.2% (1.4–3.4%) for carbamazepine. The malformation rate with lamotrigine monotherapy was 3.2% (2.1–4.9%) based on 647 pregnancies. Interestingly, the malformation rate in offspring of 227 untreated women with epilepsy was 3.5% (1.8–6.8%), very similar to the 3.7% (3.0–4.5%) among the monotherapy exposures in general (n = 2,468). The number of pregnancies with other new-generation antiepileptic drugs was too small for a meaningful assessment of the risks: 31 pregnancies on gabapentin (1 malformation), 28 on topiramate (2 malformations), and 22 on levetiracetam (no malformation).

With the exception of lamotrigine, the information on human teratogenicity of the new generation AEDs is thus particularly scarce and mainly based on case series or uncontrolled studies. In one case series from Argentina, all of 35 pregnancies with oxcarbazepine monotherapy, enrolled at any stage prior to birth, had normal outcome, while one of 20 pregnancies with oxcarbazepine as combination therapy resulted in a cardiac malformation (83). In the drug-prescription registry–based study from Finland, Artama et al (7) reported one urogenital malformation among 99 pregnancies with oxcarbazepine monotherapy. Of 16 retrospectively or prospectively enrolled women taking gabapentin as monotherapy from onset of pregnancy, one resulted in an infant born with one kidney (65). These studies are clearly far too small to allow any firm conclusions as to the teratogenic potential of oxcarbazepine or gabapentin.

Considerably more information is available on lamotrigine through the International Lamotrigine Pregnancy Registry (76), the manufacturer's voluntary reporting system. By March 2004, this registry had included 12 major malformations among 414 prospective lamotrigine monotherapy exposures, 2.9% (1.6–5.1%). Although systematically collected information on the outcome of pregnancies with a specific AED is of importance, the value is limited by possible selection bias and in particular of lack of comparator.

MINOR ANOMALIES AND FETAL ANTIEPILEPTIC DRUG SYNDROMES

Minor anomalies are structural variations that are visible at birth but without medical, surgical or cosmetic importance. Such anomalies frequently occur in normal unexposed infants, but combinations of several anomalies are less common and can form a pattern, or a dysmorphic syndrome, that may indicate a more severe underlying dysfunction. Minor anomalies and dysmorphic syndromes have been reported to occur more frequently in infants of mothers treated for epilepsy during pregnancy. Facial features such as orbital hypertelorism, depressed nasal bridge, low-set ears, and micrognathia, along with distal digital hypoplasia, sometimes in combination with growth retardation and developmental delay, were first reported in association with exposure to phenytoin (101). Subsequently, however, similar patterns have been associated with exposure to carbamazepine (82). Valproate exposure has been claimed to cause a somewhat different dysmorphic syndrome, characterized by thin arched eyebrows with medial deficiency, broad nasal bridge, short anteverted nose, and a smooth long philtrum with thin upper lip (102). Such features have been suggested to be associated with, and indicative of, impaired cognitive development (57, 102). However, there is a considerable overlap in the various dysmorphisms, and their drug specificity has been questioned. A more general term, fetal or prenatal antiepileptic drug syndrome, has therefore been suggested (103). In addition, the pathogenesis is still somewhat controversial, and Gaily et al (104) attributed most of the minor anomalies to genetic factors rather than drug exposure. However, one study examined physical features of infants to women with a history of epilepsy but not taking antiepileptic drugs in pregnancy (105). No infants were found to have features of the fetal antiepileptic drug syndrome, suggesting that such features indeed are related to drug exposure. It should, however, be underlined that minor anomalies are much more difficult to assess objectively than major malformations and that the incidence of minor anomalies in exposed infants varies markedly between studies.

GROWTH RETARDATION

Several studies have reported that exposure to antiepileptic drugs is associated with an impaired intrauterine growth. Reduced birth weight, body length, and head circumference in the offspring of women treated with phenytoin was reported already in the 1970s (106). Reductions in body dimensions, in particular head circumference, have been confirmed in several subsequent studies of larger cohorts (51, 71, 80, 107-111). Most studies report a more pronounced effect in infants exposed to polytherapy (107–111). However, the association with specific antiepileptic drugs in monotherapy varies. Some investigators found an association to phenobarbital and primidone, whereas others report carbamazepine to be most strongly associated to a small head circumference. Wide et al (110) studied body dimensions in infants exposed to antiepileptic drugs in utero in a Swedish population over a period of 25 years, comparing data to the general population.

There was a clear trend toward normalization of the head circumference over the time period, in parallel with a shift from polytherapy toward monotherapy, despite an increasing use of carbamazepine. Other more recent studies also suggest that with present treatment strategies, where monotherapy prevails, microcephaly may no longer be more common among infants of mothers treated for epilepsy during pregnancy (44, 112), although smaller than expected head circumference is reported in some very recent studies (53). The reason for the particular interest in small head circumference, or microcephaly, is that it might signal a functional deficit. However, one study failed to find an association between a small head circumference in children exposed to antiepileptic drugs and cognitive functioning in adulthood (111).

EFFECTS ON POSTNATAL COGNITIVE DEVELOPMENT

A particularly important additional issue is whether exposure to antiepileptic drugs in utero could adversely affect the development of the child after birth. Long-term follow-up studies of large cohorts of exposed individuals are necessary in order to address this issue. Such studies are difficult to perform and also complicated to interpret because of several confounding factors and since environmental factors become more important with increasing age of the child. Only few studies have been published, all with fairly small cohorts, and the results are conflicting. In a prospective population-based study, Gaily et al (113) found no influence on global IQ, and the observed cognitive dysfunction in children exposed to AEDs, mainly phenytoin and carbamazepine, was attributed to maternal seizures and educational level of the parents rather than to the treatment. Wide et al (114), in another population-based prospective study, found no difference in psychomotor development in children exposed to carbamazepine compared with control children of healthy mothers but a trend for phenytoin-exposed children to do slightly worse in some tests of motor coordination. Scolnik et al (115) reported lower global IQ in children exposed to phenytoin but not in those exposed to carbamazepine. Normal intellectual capacity was found in most of 170 individuals exposed to phenobarbital and phenytoin, but 12% of the exposed subjects, in contrast to 1% of unexposed controls, had persistent learning problems (111).

A recent Cochrane Review concluded that the majority of studies on developmental effects of antiepileptic drugs are of limited quality and that there is little evidence about which drugs carry more risks than others to the development of children exposed (116). Some studies in the last years, however, have suggested that exposure to valproic acid might be associated with a particular risk of adverse developmental effects (117, 118). A retrospective survey from the UK found additional educational needs to be considerably more common among children that had been exposed to valproic acid monotherapy than in those exposed to carbamazepine or in unexposed children (117). A more thorough investigation of partly the same cohort of children revealed significantly lower verbal IQ in children exposed to valproic acid monotherapy (mean 83.6, 95% CI 78.2–89.0, $n = 41$) than in unexposed children (90.9, 87.2–94.6, $n = 80$) and children exposed to carbamazepine (94.1, 89.6–98.5, $n = 52$) or phenytoin (98.5, 90.6–106.4, $n = 21$) (118, 120). Multiple regression analysis identified exposure to valproic acid, five or more tonic-clonic seizures in pregnancy, and low maternal IQ to be associated with lower verbal IQ also after adjustment for confounding factors. Valproic acid doses above 800 mg/day were associated with lower verbal IQ than lower doses. Although efforts were made to control for confounding factors, these results should be interpreted with caution given the small numbers, the retrospective nature of the study, and the fact that only 40% of eligible mothers agreed to participate, which might introduce selection bias. The important signals from this report need to be confirmed or refuted in well-designed prospective studies. A recent small population-based prospective study from Finland found a lower verbal IQ in children exposed in utero to valproic acid and to polytherapy in general compared with nonexposed children or children exposed to carbamazepine (120). However, this study could not demonstrate an independent effect of valproic acid because of small numbers (13 children exposed to valproic acid monotherapy) and because the results were confounded by low maternal education and polytherapy. Another small, prospective, population-based Finnish study signals a similar trend for worse outcome in children exposed to valproic acid but also points to the problem of confounding factors, because the mothers using valproic acid in pregnancy scored lower on IQ than other groups (121).

Although conclusive evidence is lacking, the signals concerning potential adverse effects of, particularly, valproic acid on postnatal development need to be considered seriously and be explored in adequately sized prospective studies. However, considering the methodological shortcomings and inconsistencies in the outcome of the available sparse studies of developmental effects of antiepileptic drugs in general, it must be concluded that to date we lack definitive evidence that long-term adverse outcomes in children of epileptic mothers can be ascribed to AEDs.

MECHANISMS OF TERATOGENICITY

A better understanding of the mechanisms behind the developmental toxicity of AEDs is essential for a more rational approach to the treatment of women with epilepsy of childbearing potential. Such advancements might facilitate future development of new, nonteratogenic AEDs, give clues to other protective measures, or help identify individual patients at particular risk. Clinical and experimental data demonstrate an individual variability in the susceptibility to developmental toxicity of AEDs and also in the expression of teratogenic outcome, suggesting a genetic influence (122–128).

All the structural defects, and the retardation of growth and development observed in children exposed to AEDs in utero, have been reproduced after drug exposure to nonepileptic animals of various species (129) confirming the causal role of the antiepileptic drugs in the pathogenesis. As in humans, the pattern of malformations is to some extent different for different AEDs also in animal models, which suggests that multiple mechanisms are involved.

One of the earlier hypotheses suggests that the developmental toxicity of AEDs is related to their interference with folate metabolism. Folates are cofactors involved in the biosynthesis of nucleic acids and in the remethylation of homocysteine to methionine. In experimental studies, a folate-deficient diet has resulted in an increased incidence of malformations in the offspring. Many AEDs, including phenobarbital, phenytoin, primidone, and carbamazepine, are known to reduce folate levels. Some clinical studies (130, 131) have reported an association between low maternal serum folate levels and adverse pregnancy outcome, including malformations. The latter observation, however, is controversial, because other studies have failed to confirm this finding. Pretreatment with folinic acid reduced valproic acid–induced malformations in mouse models (132). In humans, extra periconceptional supplementation with folate has been demonstrated to reduce the risk of neural tube defects (133) and, at higher doses, also the risk of recurrence in high-risk groups (134). These clinical studies, however, did not study prevention of neural tube defects in women with epilepsy or on AEDs.

Although phenytoin and phenobarbital are the antiepileptic drugs that decrease folate levels the most, these drugs have been linked to neural tube defects to a lesser extent than valproic acid and carbamazepine, which have less apparent effects on folate levels. Nevertheless, the available experimental data suggest that interference with embryonic folate metabolism may be involved in some aspects of, in particular, valproic acid teratogenesis, and genetic factors related to folate metabolism may explain differences in susceptibility observed between different strains (132).

The 5,10-methylene tetrahydrofolate reductase (MTHFR) gene has been suggested as one candidate to explain genetic susceptibility to folic acid–sensitive malformations (126). MTHFR is involved in the biotransformation of folate and is highly polymorphic. Some mutations have been associated with increased risks of malformations such as neural tube defects, cleft palate, and congenital heart disease, which are often seen in relation to exposure to AEDs.

A prevailing hypothesis for many years has been that AEDs are metabolized to toxic reactive intermediates, which are responsible for the teratogenic effects (41, 128, 129, 135–143). The toxic intermediate could be an arene oxide produced during oxidation of phenytoin, carbamazepine, or phenobarbital. In general, epoxides are highly reactive and may bind to fetal macromolecules in the embryo and thus cause teratogenic effects. Such epoxides are metabolized by the enzyme epoxide hydrolase and may accumulate and react if the rate of formation of the epoxide exceeds the elimination by epoxide hydrolase. The balance between enzyme activities catalyzing the formation and the elimination of reactive epoxides may be genetically determined and also affected by interactions with AEDs. Interestingly, some specific combinations of AEDs, notably carbamazepine, phenobarbital, and valproic acid, have been associated with a particularly high rate of malformations (41). Hypothetically, carbamazepine's and phenobarbital's inducing effects on the formation of epoxides and valproic acid's inhibitory effect on epoxide hydrolase could explain this particularly high risk. However, some of the most potent teratogenic AEDs, such as trimethadione, lack the premises to form epoxides. Potentiation of phenytoin teratogenesis by drugs inhibiting the cytochrome (CYP) P450-mediated metabolism (144) also argues against a role for the CYP system in teratogenic bioactivation of phenytoin.

Another postulated bioactivating pathway is cooxidation of AEDs to free radical intermediates. After interaction with molecular oxygen, these compounds can liberate reactive oxygen species (ROS), which may cause oxidative stress, thereby initiating teratogenicity. Deficiency of free radical–scavenging enzymes, responsible for eliminating ROS, has been associated with malformations in the offspring of epileptic mothers exposed to anticonvulsants (145–147).

A more recent hypothesis suggests that many AEDs, such as phenytoin, trimethadione, carbamazepine, and phenobarbital, exert their developmental adverse effects by induction of episodes of embryonic cardiac arrhythmia during restricted periods of embryonic development (148). According to this hypothesis, the embryonic hypoxia is followed by reoxygenation and generation of ROS, which will cause tissue damage. Typical developmental toxicity effects, such as orofacial clefts, heart defects, distal digital defects, and growth retardation, can be induced in experimental studies by hypoxia, and AEDs have been shown to affect the embryonic heart in animal models (149, 150). These embryonic cardiac effects have been linked to the drugs' ability to block the rapid component of the delayed rectifying K^+ ion current, I_{Kr} (150). The noninnervated embryonic heart is dependent on I_{Kr} for regulation of the cardiac rhythm during a restricted period and is very susceptible to arrhythmogenic action by I_{Kr} blockers. Drugs, anticonvulsant or otherwise, with such I_{Kr}-blocking properties have been associated with congenital malformations experimentally and in the clinic (150).

Recently, mechanisms involving homeobox (HOX) genes have also been proposed to explain teratogenicity of antiepileptic drugs (132). Retinoic acid signaling regulates the transcription of such genes, essential for early brain development, and may respond to teratogens (151). Such mechanisms include alteration of the expression of retinoic acid receptor (152) and valproic acid inhibition of histone deacetylases (153–157), considered as key elements in the regulation of many genes playing important roles in cell proliferation and differentiation (159–161).

The mechanisms behind developmental toxicity of AEDs are thus presently far from completely understood and are likely to be multiple and also differ between drugs.

CONCLUSIONS

More than 40 years of research on risks associated with the treatment of epilepsy during pregnancy have taught us that use of AEDs is associated with a two- to threefold increase in the risk of major malformations in the offspring. This risk is mainly due to the treatment with AEDs, of which all of the old generation have been shown to be teratogenic. Although the pattern of birth defects apparently varies between drugs, there is limited conclusive evidence on differences in overall teratogenic potential. The available data, however, suggest that the risk of birth defects is higher in association with valproic acid than with carbamazepine. The data in this respect on the new-generation antiepileptic drugs is scarce, with lamotrigine as the only exception. The limited available comparative data indicate that the malformation rates associated with lamotrigine are similar to those seen with carbamazepine. No conclusions can as yet be drawn concerning the teratogenic potential of other new-generation anticonvulsants.

The possibility that exposure to AEDs in utero may adversely affect the intellectual development in the offspring remains a major concern. All available studies have methodological limitations, but there are signals indicating worse outcome, in terms of lower verbal IQ, in children exposed to high doses (> 800 mg/day) of valproic acid. There are no consistent findings indicating similar adverse effects of other old-generation AEDs, whereas we lack data on this issue concerning the new-generation drugs.

Polytherapy with AEDs is associated with higher malformation rates, and probably also increased risks of growth retardation, than is monotherapy. A dose response relationship with respect to birth defects as well as postnatal cognitive development has been demonstrated for valproic acid, and it is reasonable to assume such a relationship also for other drugs. How the teratogenic effects of low dosages of valproic acid (< 800–1,000 mg/day) compare with other antiepileptic drugs remains to be elucidated.

It should be kept in mind that none of these conclusions are based on randomized clinical trials but rather on observational studies. Such studies can demonstrate associations, but because of the existence of confounding factors it is more difficult to provide evidence for a causal relationship. Epilepsy may, in fact, confound the effects of treatment on child well-being because of environmental factors or the effects of its associated genetic background. Even relatively well-established relationships between adverse pregnancy outcomes and drug factors cannot be assumed as if treatment itself were the causal agent, unless they are confirmed by control or matching for confounding variables. Specific clinical indications may confound the assessment of the teratogenicity of individual drugs. Failing to control for appropriate confounders may explain why, apart from the unquestionable teratogenicity of antiepileptic drugs as a group, we lack so much of the needed conclusive data on the developmental toxicity associated with specific AEDs. The ongoing pregnancy registries, which are beginning to accumulate considerable numbers of pregnancies, will allow for more appropriate analyses, including important confounding factors, and thus, in the near future, hopefully provide more conclusive evidence on the differential teratogenic effects of AEDs.

References

1. Gaily E. Development and growth in children of epileptic mothers. A prospective controlled study. *Acta Obstet Gynecol Scand* 1991; 70(7–8):631–632.
2. Holmes LB, Harvey EA, Coull BA, Huntington KB, et al. The teratogenicity of anticonvulsant drugs. *N Engl J Med* 2001; 344(15):1132–1138.
3. Janz D, Fuchs U. Sind antiepileptische Medikamente während der Schwangerschaft schädlich? *Dtsch Med Wochenschr* 1964; 89:241–243.
4. Meadow SR. Anticonvulsant drugs and congenital abnormalities. *Lancet* 1968; 292(7581):1296.
5. Akhtar N, Millac P. Epilepsy and pregnancy: a study of 188 pregnancies in 92 patients. *Br J Clin Pract* 1987; 41(8):862–864.
6. Annegers JF, Hauser I. The frequency of malformations in relative of patients with epilepsy. In: Janz D, Dam M, Bossi L, Helge H, et al, eds. *Epilepsy, Pregnancy, and the Child.* New York: Raven Press, 1982:267–263.
7. Artama M, Auvinen A, Raudaskoski T, Isojarvi I, et al. Antiepileptic drug use of women with epilepsy and congenital malformations in offspring. *Neurology* 2005; 64(11): 1874–1878.
8. Fedrick J. Epilepsy and pregnancy: a report from the Oxford Record Linkage Study. *Br Med J* 1973; 2(5864):442–148.
9. Kallen B. A register study of maternal epilepsy and delivery outcome with special reference to drug use. *Acta Neurol Scand* 1986; 73(3):253–259.

10. Koppe JG, Bosman W, Oppers VM, Spaans F, et al. [Epilepsy and congenital anomalies]. *Ned Tijdschr Geneeskd* 1973; 117(6):220–224.
11. Lowe CR. Congenital malformations among infants born to epileptic women. *Lancet* 1973; 301(7793):9–10.
12. Olafsson E, Hallgrimsson JT, Hauser WA, Ludvigsson P, et al. Pregnancies of women with epilepsy: a population-based study in Iceland. *Epilepsia* 1998; 39(8):887–892.
13. Robert E, Lofkvist E, Mauguiere F, Robert JM. Evaluation of drug therapy and teratogenic risk in a Rhone-Alpes district population of pregnant epileptic women. *Eur Neurol* 1986; 25(6):436–443.
14. Sabers A, Rogvi-Hansen B á, Dam M, Fischer-Rasmussen W, et al. Pregnancy and epilepsy: a retrospective study of 151 pregnancies. *Acta Neurol Scand* 1998; 97(3): 164–170.
15. Speidel BD, Meadow SR. Maternal epilepsy and abnormalities of fetus and newborn. *Lancet* 1972; 300(7782):839–843.
16. Weber M, Schweitzer M, Andre JM, Tridon P, et al. [Epilepsy, anticonvulsants and pregnancy]. *Arch Fr Pediatr* 1977; 34(4):374–383.
17. Al Bunyan M, Abo-Talib Z. Outcome of pregnancies in epileptic women: a study in Saudi Arabia. *Seizure* 1999; 8(1):26–29.
18. Eskazan E, Aslan S. Antiepileptic therapy and teratogenicity in Turkey. *Int J Clin Pharmacol Ther Toxicol* 1992; 30(8):261–264.
19. Mawer G, Clayton-Smith J, Coyle H, Kini U. Outcome of pregnancy in women attending an outpatient epilepsy clinic: adverse features associated with higher doses of sodium valproate. *Seizure* 2002; 11(8):512–518.
20. Nakane Y, Okuma T, Takahashi R, Sato Y, et al. Multi-institutional study on the teratogenicity and fetal toxicity of antiepileptic drugs: a report of a collaborative study group in Japan. *Epilepsia* 1980; 21(6):663–680.
21. Vajda FJ, O'Brien TJ, Hitchcock A, Graham J, et al. The Australian registry of antiepileptic drugs in pregnancy: experience after 30 months. *J Clin Neurosci* 2003; 10(5): 543–549.
22. Dansky L, Anderman E, Anderman F. Major congenital malformation in the offspring of epileptic patients. Genetic and environmental risk factors. In: Janz D, Dam M, Bossi L, Helge H, et al, eds. *Epilepsy, Pregnancy, and the Child*. New York: Raven Press, 1982:223–234.
23. Dansky L. Outcome of pregnancy in epileptic women. Ph.D. Thesis, Mc Gill University, 1989.
24. Dravet C, Julian C, Legras C, Magaudda A, et al. Epilepsy, antiepileptic drugs, and malformations in children of women with epilepsy: a French prospective cohort study. *Neurology* 1992; 42(4 suppl 5):75–82.
25. D'Souza SW, Robertson IG, Donnai D, Mawer G. Fetal phenytoin exposure, hypoplastic nails, and jitteriness. *Arch Dis Child* 1991; 66(3):320–324.
26. Fabris C, Licata D, Stasiowska B, Tanzilli S, et al. [Newborn infants from epileptic mothers: malformation and auxonologic risk]. *Pediatr Med Chir* 1989; 11(1):27–31.
27. Fairgrieve SD, Jackson M, Jonas P, Walshaw D, et al. Population based, prospective study of the care of women with epilepsy in pregnancy. *Br Med J* 2000; 321(7262):674–675.
28. Gramstrom ML. Development of the children of epileptic mothers: preliminary results from the prospective Helsinki study. In: Janz D, Dam M, Bossi L, Helge H, et al, eds. *Epilepsy, Pregnancy, and the Child*. New York: Raven Press, 1982:403–408.
29. Holmes LB, Harvey EA, Brown KS, Hayes AM, et al. Anticonvulsant teratogenesis: I. A study design for newborn infants. *Teratology* 1994; 49(3):202–207.
30. Hvas CL, Henriksen TB, Ostergaard JR, Dam M. Epilepsy and pregnancy: effect of antiepileptic drugs and lifestyle on birthweight. *BJOG* 2000; 107(7):896–902.
31. Kaaja E, Kaaja R, Hiilesmaa V. Major malformations in offspring of women with epilepsy. *Neurology* 2003; 60(4):575–9.
32. Kaneko S, Otani K, Fukushima Y, Ogawa Y, et al. Teratogenicity of antiepileptic drugs: analysis of possible risk factors. *Epilepsia* 1988; 29(4):459–467.
33. Kaneko S, Otani K, Kondo T, Fukushima Y, et al. Malformation in infants of mothers with epilepsy receiving antiepileptic drugs. *Neurology* 1992; 42(4 suppl 5):68–74.
34. Kaneko S, Battino D, Andermann E, Wada K, et al. Congenital malformations due to antiepileptic drugs. *Epilepsy Res* 1999; 33(2–3):145–158.
35. Kelly TE, Edwards P, Rein M, Miller JQ, et al. Teratogenicity of anticonvulsant drugs. II: A prospective study. *Am J Med Genet* 1984; 19(3):435–443.
36. Knight AH, Rhind EG. Epilepsy and pregnancy: a study of 153 pregnancies in 59 patients. *Epilepsia* 1975; 16(1):99–110.
37. Koch S, Hartmann A, Jager E. Major malformation in children of epileptic mothers—due to epilepsy or its therapy? *Epilepsy, Pregnancy and the Child*. New York: Raven Press, 1982:313–315.
38. Koch S, Gopfert-Geyer I, Jager-Roman E, Jakob S, et al. [Anti-epileptic agents during pregnancy. A prospective study on the course of pregnancy, malformations, and child development]. *Dtsch Med Wochenschr* 1983; 108(7):250–257.
39. Koch S, Losche G, Jager-Roman E, Jakob S, et al. Major and minor birth malformations and antiepileptic drugs. *Neurology* 1992; 42(4 suppl 5):83–88.
40. Lander CM, Eadie MJ. Antiepileptic drug intake during pregnancy and malformed offspring. *Epilepsy Res* 1990; 7(1):77–82.
41. Lindhout D, Hoppener RJ, Meinardi H. Teratogenicity of antiepileptic drug combinations with special emphasis on epoxidation (of carbamazepine). *Epilepsia* 1984; 25(1):77–83.
42. Morrow J, Russell A, Guthrie E, Parsons L, et al. Malformation risks of antiepileptic drugs in pregnancy: a prospective study from the UK Epilepsy and Pregnancy Register. *J Neurol Neurosurg Psychiatry* 2006; 77(2):193–198.
43. Nakane Y. Factors influencing the risk of malformations among infants born to epileptic mothers. In: Janz D, Dam M, Bossi L, Helge H, et al, eds. *Epilepsy, Pregnancy, and the Child*. New York: Raven Press, 1982:259–265.
44. Nulman I, Scolnik D, Chitayat D, Farkas LD, et al. Findings in children exposed in utero to phenytoin and carbamazepine monotherapy: independent effects of epilepsy and medications. *Am J Med Genet* 1997; 68(1):18–24.
45. Oguni M, Dansky L, Andermann E, Sherwin A, et al. Improved pregnancy outcome in epileptic women in the last decade: relationship to maternal anticonvulsant therapy. *Brain Dev* 1992; 14(6):371–80.
46. Richmond JR, Krishnamoorthy P, Andermann E, Benjamin A. Epilepsy and pregnancy: an obstetric perspective. *Am J Obstet Gynecol* 2004; 190(2):371–379.
47. Sabers A, Dam M, Rogvi-Hansen B á, Boas J, et al. Epilepsy and pregnancy: lamotrigine as main drug used. *Acta Neurol Scand* 2004; 109(1):9–13.
48. Seino M, Miyakoshi M. Teratogenic risks of antiepileptic drugs in respect to the type of epilepsy. *Folia Psychiatr Neurol Jpn* 1979; 33(3):379–385.
49. Shakir RA, Abdulwahab B. Congenital malformations before and after the onset of maternal epilepsy. *Acta Neurol Scand* 1991; 84(2):153–156.
50. South J. Teratogenic effect of anticonvulsants. *Lancet* 1972; 300(7787):1154.
51. Steegers-Theunissen RP, Renier WO, Borm GF, Thomas CM, et al. Factors influencing the risk of abnormal pregnancy outcome in epileptic women: a multi-centre prospective study. *Epilepsy Res* 1994; 18(3):261–269.
52. Van der Pol MC, Hadders-Algra M, Huisjes HJ, Touwen BC. Antiepileptic medication in pregnancy: late effects on the children's central nervous system development. *Am J Obstet Gynecol* 1991; 164(1 Pt 1):121–128.
53. Viinikainen K, Heinonen S, Eriksson K, Kalviainen R. Community-based, prospective, controlled study of obstetric and neonatal outcome of 179 pregnancies in women with epilepsy. *Epilepsia* 2006; 47(1):186–192.
54. Waters CH, Belai Y, Gott PS, Shen P, et al. Outcomes of pregnancy associated with antiepileptic drugs. *Arch Neurol* 1994; 51(3):250–253.
55. Barry JE, Danks DM. Letter: Anticonvulsants and congenital abnormalities. *Lancet* 1974; 304(7871):48–49.
56. Beck-Mannagetta G, Drees G, Janz D. Malformations and minor anomalies in the offspring of epileptic parents: a retrospective study. In: Janz D, Dam M, Bossi L, Helge H, et al, eds. *Epilepsy, Pregnancy, and the Child*. New York: Raven Press, 1982:317–323.
57. Dean JC, Hailey H, Moore SJ, Lloyd DJ, et al. Long term health and neurodevelopment in children exposed to antiepileptic drugs before birth. *J Med Genet* 2002; 39(4):251–259.
58. Jick SS, Terris BZ. Anticonvulsants and congenital malformations. *Pharmacotherapy* 1997; 17(3):561–564.
59. Katz JM, Pacia SV, Devinsky O. Current management of epilepsy and pregnancy: fetal outcome, congenital malformations, and developmental delay. *Epilepsy Behav* 2001; 2(2):119–123.
60. Laskowska M, Leszczynska-Gorzelak B, Oleszczuk J. Pregnancy in women with epilepsy. *Gynecol Obstet Invest* 2001; 51(2):99–102.
61. Lekwuwa GU, Adewole IF, Thompson MO. Antiepileptic drugs and teratogenicity in Nigerians. *Trans R Soc Trop Med Hyg* 1995; 89(2):227.
62. Majewski F, Steger M, Richter B, Gill J, et al. The teratogenicity of hydantoins and barbiturates in humans, with considerations on the etiology of malformations and cerebral disturbances in the children of epileptic parents. *Int J Biol Res Pregnancy* 1981; 2(1):37–45.
63. Martin PJ, Millac PA. Pregnancy, epilepsy, management and outcome: a 10-year perspective. *Seizure* 1993; 2(4):277–280.
64. Meyer JG. The teratological effects of anticonvulsants and the effects on pregnancy and birth. *Eur Neurol* 1973; 10(3):179–190.
65. Montouris G. Gabapentin exposure in human pregnancy: results from the Gabapentin Pregnancy Registry. *Epilepsy Behav* 2003; 4(3):310–317.
66. Sawhney H, Vasishta K, Suri V, Khunnu B, et al. Pregnancy with epilepsy—a retrospective analysis. *Int J Gynaecol Obstet* 1996; 54(1):17–22.
67. Starreveld-Zimmerman AA, van der Kolk WJ, Meinardi H, Elshove J. Are anticonvulsants teratogenic? *Lancet* 1973; 302(7819):48–49.
68. Watson JD, Spellacy WN. Neonatal effects of maternal treatment with the anticonvulsant drug diphenylhydantoin. *Obstet Gynecol* 1971; 37(6):881–815.
69. Fried S, Kozer E, Nulman I, Einarson TR, et al. Malformation rates in children of women with untreated epilepsy: a meta-analysis. *Drug Saf* 2004; 27(3):197–202.
70. Bjerkedal T. Outcome of pregnancy in women with epilepsy, Norway, 1967 to 1978: congenital malformations. In: Janz D, Dam M, Bossi L, Helge H, et al, eds. *Epilepsy, Pregnancy, and the Child*. New York: Raven Press, 1982:289–296.
71. Bertollini R, Kallen B, Mastroiacovo P, Robert E. Anticonvulsant drugs in monotherapy. Effect on the fetus. *Eur J Epidemiol* 1987; 3(2):164–171.
72. Samren EB, van Duijn CM, Koch S, Hiilesmaa VK, et al. Maternal use of antiepileptic drugs and the risk of major congenital malformations: a joint European prospective study of human teratogenesis associated with maternal epilepsy. *Epilepsia* 1997; 38(9): 981–990.
73. Samren EB, van Duijn CM, Christiaens GC, Hofman A, et al. Antiepileptic drug regimens and major congenital abnormalities in the offspring. *Ann Neurol* 1999; 46(5): 739–746.
74. Wide K, Winbladh B, Kallen B. Major malformations in infants exposed to antiepileptic drugs in utero, with emphasis on carbamazepine and valproic acid: a nation-wide, population-based register study. *Acta Paediatr* 2004; 93(2):174–176.
75. Artama M, Isojarvi JI, Raitanen J, Auvinen A. Birth rate among patients with epilepsy: a nationwide population-based cohort study in Finland. *Am J Epidemiol* 2004; 159(11):1057–1063.
76. Cunnington M, Tennis P. Lamotrigine and the risk of malformations in pregnancy. *Neurology* 2005; 64(6):955–960.
77. Annegers JF, Kurland LT, Elveback LR. Epilepsy, anticonvulsants, and congenital malformations. *Trans Am Neurol Assoc* 1974; 99:184–186.

78. Canger R, Battino D, Canevini MP, Fumarola C, et al. Malformations in offspring of women with epilepsy: a prospective study. *Epilepsia* 1999; 40(9):1231–1236.
79. Diav-Citrin O, Shechtman S, Arnon J, Ornoy A. Is carbamazepine teratogenic? A prospective controlled study of 210 pregnancies. *Neurology* 2001; 57(2):321–324.
80. Fonager K, Larsen H, Pedersen L, Sorensen HT. Birth outcomes in women exposed to anticonvulsant drugs. *Acta Neurol Scand* 2000; 101(5):289–294.
81. Holmes LB, Wyszynski DF. North American antiepileptic drug pregnancy registry. *Epilepsia* 2004; 45(11):1465.
82. Jones KL, Lacro RV, Johnson KA, Adams J. Pattern of malformations in the children of women treated with carbamazepine during pregnancy [see comments]. *N Engl J Med* 1989; 320(25):1661–1666.
83. Meischenguiser R, D'Giano CH, Ferraro SM. Oxcarbazepine in pregnancy: clinical experience in Argentina. *Epilepsy Behav* 2004; 5(2):163–167.
84. Melchior JC, Svensmark O, Trolle D. Placental transfer of phenobarbitone in epileptic women, and elimination in newborns. *Lancet* 1967; 290(7521):860–861.
85. Millar JH, Nevin NC. Congenital malformations and anticonvulsant drugs. *Lancet* 1973; 301(7798):328.
86. Nulman I, Rovet J, Stewart DE, Wolpin J, et al. Neurodevelopment of children exposed in utero to antidepressant drugs. *N Engl J Med* 1997; 336(4):258–262.
87. Omtzigt JG, Los FJ, Grobbee DE, Pijpers L, et al. The risk of spina bifida aperta after first-trimester exposure to valproate in a prenatal cohort. *Neurology* 1992; 42(4 suppl 5): 119–125.
88. Ornoy A, Cohen E. Outcome of children born to epileptic mothers treated with carbamazepine during pregnancy. *Arch Dis Child* 1996; 75(6):517–520.
89. Wyszynski DF, Nambisan M, Surve T, Alsdorf RM, et al. Increased rate of major malformations in offspring exposed to valproate during pregnancy. *Neurology* 2005; 64(6): 961–965.
90. Lindhout D, Schmidt D. In-utero exposure to valproate and neural tube defects. *Lancet* 1986; 327(8494):1392–3.
91. Jager-Roman E, Deichl A, Jakob S, Hartmann AM, et al. Fetal growth, major malformations, and minor anomalies in infants born to women receiving valproic acid. *J Pediatr* 1986; 108(6):997–1004.
92. Verloes A, Frikiche A, Gremillet C, Paquay T, et al. Proximal phocomelia and radial ray aplasia in fetal valproic syndrome. *Eur J Pediatr* 1990; 149(4):266–267.
93. Rosa FW. Spina bifida in infants of women treated with carbamazepine during pregnancy. *N Engl J Med* 1991; 324(10):674–677.
94. Kallen AJ. Maternal carbamazepine and infant spina bifida. *Reprod Toxicol* 1994; 8(3):203–205.
95. Barrett C, Richens A. Epilepsy and pregnancy: Report of an Epilepsy Research Foundation Workshop. *Epilepsy Res* 2003; 52(3):147–187.
96. Lindhout D, Meinardi H, Meijer JW, Nau H. Antiepileptic drugs and teratogenesis in two consecutive cohorts: changes in prescription policy paralleled by changes in pattern of malformations. *Neurology* 1992; 42(4 suppl 5):94–110.
97. Duncan S, Mercho S, Lopes-Cendas I, Seni MH, et al. The effects of valproic acid on the outcome of pregnancy: a prospective study. *Epilepsia* 2003; 44(suppl 8):59 (abstract).
98. Malm H, Kajantie E, Kivirikko S, Kaariainen H, et al. Valproate embryopathy in three sets of siblings: further proof of hereditary susceptibility. *Neurology* 2002; 59(4): 630–633.
99. Duncan S, Mercho S, Lopes-Cendes I, Seni MH, et al. Repeated neural tube defects and valproate monotherapy suggest a pharmacogenetic abnormality. *Epilepsia* 2001; 42(6):750–753.
100. Holmes LB, Wyszynski DF, Lieberman E. The AED (antiepileptic drug) pregnancy registry: a 6-year experience. *Arch Neurol* 2004; 61(5):673–678.
101. Hanson JW, Smith DW. The fetal hydantoin syndrome. *J Pediatr* 1975; 87(2): 285–290.
102. Kini U, Adab N, Vinten J, Fryer A, et al. Dysmorphic features: an important clue to the diagnosis and severity of fetal anticonvulsant syndromes. *Arch Dis Child Fetal Neonatal Ed* 2006; 91(2): F90–F95.
103. Zahn C. Neurologic care of pregnant women with epilepsy. *Epilepsia* 1998; 39 Suppl 8:S26–S31.
104. Gaily E, Granstrom ML, Hiilesmaa V, Bardy A. Minor anomalies in offspring of epileptic mothers. *J Pediatr* 1988; 112(4):520–529.
105. Holmes LB, Rosenberger PB, Harvey EA, Khoshbin S, et al. Intelligence and physical features of children of women with epilepsy. *Teratology* 2000; 61(3):196–202.
106. Hanson JW, Myrianthopoulos NC, Harvey MA, Smith DW. Risks to the offspring of women treated with hydantoin anticonvulsants, with emphasis on the fetal hydantoin syndrome. *J Pediatr* 1976; 89(4):662–668.
107. Hiilesmaa VK, Teramo K, Granstrom ML, Bardy AH. Fetal head growth retardation associated with maternal antiepileptic drugs. *Lancet* 1981; 319(8239):165–167.
108. Battino D, Granata T, Binelli S, Caccamo ML, et al. Intrauterine growth in the offspring of epileptic mothers. *Acta Neurol Scand* 1992; 86(6):555–557.
109. Battino D, Kaneko S, Andermann E, Avanzini G, et al. Intrauterine growth in the offspring of epileptic women: a prospective multicenter study. *Epilepsy Res* 1999; 36(1):53–60.
110. Wide K, Winbladh B, Tomson T, Kallen B. Body dimensions of infants exposed to antiepileptic drugs in utero: observations spanning 25 years. *Epilepsia* 2000; 41(7): 854–861.
111. Dessens AB, Cohen-Kettenis PT, Mellenbergh GJ, Koppe JG, et al. Association of prenatal phenobarbital and phenytoin exposure with genital anomalies and menstrual disorders. *Teratology* 2001; 64(4):181–188.
112. Choulika E, Harvey EA, Holmes LB. Effect of antiepileptic drugs (AED) on fetal growth: assessment at birth. *Teratology* 1999; 59:388.
113. Gaily E, Kantola-Sorsa E, Granstrom ML. Specific cognitive dysfunction in children with epileptic mothers. *Dev Med Child Neurol* 1990; 32(5):403–414.
114. Wide K, Henning E, Tomson T, Winbladh B. Psychomotor development in preschool children exposed to antiepileptic drugs in utero. *Acta Paediatr* 2002; 91(4):409–414.
115. Scolnik D, Nulman I, Rovet J, Gladstone D, et al. Neurodevelopment of children exposed in utero to phenytoin and carbamazepine monotherapy. *JAMA* 1994; 271(10): 767–770.
116. Adab N, Tudur SC, Vinten J, Williamson P, et al. Common antiepileptic drugs in pregnancy in women with epilepsy (Cochrane Review). *The Cochrane Library*. Chichester, UK: John Wiley & Sons, 2004.
117. Adab N, Jacoby A, Smith D, Chadwick D. Additional educational needs in children born to mothers with epilepsy. *J Neurol Neurosurg Psychiatry* 2001; 70(1):15–21.
118. Vinten J, Adab N, Kini U, Gorry J, et al. Neuropsychological effects of exposure to anticonvulsant medication in utero. *Neurology* 2005; 64(6):949–954.
119. Adab N, Kini U, Vinten J, Ayres J, et al. The longer term outcome of children born to mothers with epilepsy. *J Neurol Neurosurg Psychiatry* 2004; 75(11):1575–1583.
120. Gaily E, Kantola-Sorsa E, Hiilesmaa V, Isoaho M, et al. Normal intelligence in children with prenatal exposure to carbamazepine. *Neurology* 2004; 62(1):28–32.
121. Eriksson K, Viinikainen K, Monkkonen A, Aikia M, et al. Children exposed to valproate in utero—population based evaluation of risks and confounding factors for long-term neurocognitive development. *Epilepsy Res* 2005; 65(3):189–200.
122. Finnell RH. Genetic differences in susceptibility to anticonvulsant drug-induced developmental defects. *Pharmacol Toxicol* 1991; 69(4):223–227.
123. Lindhout D, Omtzigt JG. Pregnancy and the risk of teratogenicity. *Epilepsia* 1992; 33(suppl 4):S41–S48.
124. Buehler BA, Delimont D, van Waes M, Finnell RH. Prenatal prediction of risk of the fetal hydantoin syndrome. *N Engl J Med* 1990; 322(22):1567–1572.
125. Raymond GV, Buehler BA, Finnell RH, Holmes LB. Anticonvulsant teratogenesis: 3. Possible metabolic basis. *Teratology* 1995; 51(2):55–56.
126. Dean JC, Moore SJ, Osborne A, Howe J, et al. Fetal anticonvulsant syndrome and mutation in the maternal MTHFR gene. *Clin Genet* 1999; 56(3):216–220.
127. Volcik KA, Shaw GM, Lammer EJ, Zhu H, et al. Evaluation of infant methylenetetrahydrofolate reductase genotype, maternal vitamin use, and risk of high versus low level spina bifida defects. *Birth Defects Res Part A Clin Mol Teratol* 2003; 67(3): 154–157.
128. Strickler SM, Dansky LV, Miller MA, Seni MH, et al. Genetic predisposition to phenytoin-induced birth defects. *Lancet* 1985; 326(8458):746–749.
129. Finnell RH, Dansky LV. Parental epilepsy, anticonvulsant drugs, and reproductive outcome: epidemiologic and experimental findings spanning three decades. 1. Animal studies. *Reprod Toxicol* 1991; 5(4):281–299.
130. Dansky LV, Andermann E, Rosenblatt D, Sherwin AL, et al. Anticonvulsants, folate levels, and pregnancy outcome: a prospective study. *Ann Neurol* 1987; 21(2):176–182.
131. Ogawa Y, Kaneko S, Otani K, Fukushima Y. Serum folic acid levels in epileptic mothers and their relationship to congenital malformations. *Epilepsy Res* 1991; 8(1):75–78.
132. Nau H. Towards the mechanism of valproic acid induced neural tube defects. In: Tomson T, Gram L, Sillanpää M, Johannessen S, eds. *Epilepsy and Pregnancy* Petersfield: Wrightson Biomedical Publishing Ltd, 1997:35–42.
133. Czeizel AE, Bod M, Halasz P. Evaluation of anticonvulsant drugs during pregnancy in a population-based Hungarian study. *Eur J Epidemiol* 1992; 8(1):122–127.
134. Prevention of neural tube defects: results of the Medical Research Council Vitamin Study. MRC Vitamin Study Research Group [see comments]. *Lancet* 1991; 338(8760): 131–137.
135. Martz F, Failinger C 3rd, Blake DA. Phenytoin teratogenesis: correlation between embryopathic effect and covalent binding of putative arene oxide metabolite in gestational tissue. *J Pharmacol Exp Ther* 1977; 203(1):231–239.
136. Rane A, Peng D. Phenytoin enhances epoxide metabolism in human fetal liver cultures. *Drug Metab Dispos* 1985; 13(3):382–385.
137. Pantarotto C, Arboix M, Sezzano P, Abbruzzi R. Studies on 5,5-diphenylhydantoin irreversible binding to rat liver microsomal proteins. *Biochem Pharmacol* 1982; 31(8): 1501–1507.
138. Buehler BA, Rao V, Finnell RH. Biochemical and molecular teratology of fetal hydantoin syndrome. *Neurol Clin* 1994; 12(4):741–748.
139. Lillibridge JH, Amore BM, Slattery JT, Kalhorn TF, et al. Protein-reactive metabolites of carbamazepine in mouse liver microsomes. *Drug Metab Dispos* 1996; 24(5): 509–514.
140. Roy D, Snodgrass WR. Covalent binding of phenytoin to protein and modulation of phenytoin metabolism by thiols in A/J mouse liver microsomes. *J Pharmacol Exp Ther* 1990; 252(3):895–900.
141. Finnell RH, Bennett GD, Slattery JT, Amore BM, et al. Effect of treatment with phenobarbital and stiripentol on carbamazepine-induced teratogenicity and reactive metabolite formation. *Teratology* 1995; 52(6):324–332.
142. Amore BM, Kalhorn TF, Skiles GL, Hunter AP, et al. Characterization of carbamazepine metabolism in a mouse model of carbamazepine teratogenicity. *Drug Metab Dispos* 1997; 25(8):953–962.
143. Bennett GD, Amore BM, Finnell RH, Wlodarczyk B, et al. Teratogenicity of carbamazepine-10,11-epoxide and oxcarbazepine in the SWV mouse. *J Pharmacol Exp Ther* 1996; 279(3):1237–1242.
144. Tiboni GM, Giampietro F, Angelucci S, Moio P, et al. Additional investigation on the potentiation of phenytoin teratogenicity by fluconazole. *Toxicol Lett* 2003; 145(3): 219–229.
145. Wells PG, Winn LM. Biochemical toxicology of chemical teratogenesis. *Crit Rev Biochem Mol Biol* 1996; 31(1):1–40.

146. Wells PG, Kim PM, Laposa RR, Nicol CJ, et al. Oxidative damage in chemical teratogenesis. *Mutat Res* 1997; 396(1–2):65–78.
147. Parman T, Chen G, Wells PG. Free radical intermediates of phenytoin and related teratogens. Prostaglandin H synthase-catalyzed bioactivation, electron paramagnetic resonance spectrometry, and photochemical product analysis. *J Biol Chem* 1998; 273(39):25079–25088.
148. Danielsson B, Skold AC, Azarbayjani F, Ohman I, et al. Pharmacokinetic data support pharmacologically induced embryonic dysrhythmia as explanation to Fetal Hydantoin Syndrome in rats. *Toxicol Appl Pharmacol* 2000; 163(2):164–175.
149. Danielsson BR, Skold AC, Azarbayjani F. Class III antiarrhythmics and phenytoin: teratogenicity due to embryonic cardiac dysrhythmia and reoxygenation damage. *Curr Pharm Des*. 2001; 7(9):787–802.
150. Azarbayjani F, Danielsson BR. Embryonic arrhythmia by inhibition of HERG channels: a common hypoxia-related teratogenic mechanism for antiepileptic drugs? *Epilepsia* 2002; 43(5):457–468.
151. Rodier PM. Environmental causes of central nervous system maldevelopment. *Pediatrics* 2004; 113(4 Suppl):1076–1083.
152. Gelineau-van Waes J, Bennett GD, Finnell RH. Phenytoin-induced alterations in craniofacial gene expression. *Teratology* 1999; 59(1):23–34.
153. Gurvich N, Berman MG, Wittner BS, Gentleman RC, et al. Association of valproate-induced teratogenesis with histone deacetylase inhibition in vivo. *FASEB J* 2005; 19(9):1166–1168.
154. Phiel CJ, Zhang F, Huang EY, Guenther MG, et al. Histone deacetylase is a direct target of valproic acid, a potent anticonvulsant, mood stabilizer, and teratogen. *J Biol Chem* 2001; 276(39):36734–36741.
155. Gottlicher M, Minucci S, Zhu P, Kramer OH, et al. Valproic acid defines a novel class of HDAC inhibitors inducing differentiation of transformed cells. *EMBO J* 2001; 20(24):6969–6978.
156. Eikel D, Hoffmann K, Zoll K, Lampen A, et al. S-2-pentyl-4-pentynoic hydroxamic acid and its metabolite s-2-pentyl-4-pentynoic acid in the NMRI-exencephaly-mouse model: pharmacokinetic profiles, teratogenic effects, and histone deacetylase inhibition abilities of further valproic acid hydroxamates and amides. *Drug Metab Dispos* 2006; 34(4):612–620.
157. Beutler AS, Li S, Nicol R, Walsh MJ. Carbamazepine is an inhibitor of histone deacetylases. *Life Sci* 2005; 76(26):3107–3115.
159. Faiella A, Wernig M, Consalez GG, Hostick U, Hofmann C, Hustert E, et al A mouse model for valproate teratogenicity: parental effects, homeotic transformations, and altered HOX expression. *Hum Mol Genet*. 2000; 9(2):227–36.
160. Massa V, Cabrera RM, Menegola E, Giavini E, Finnell RH. Valproic acid-induced skeletal malformations: associated gene expression cascades. *Pharmacogenet Genomics*. 2005; 15(11):787–800.
161. Kawanishi CY, Hartig P, Bobseine KL, Schmid J, Cardon M, Massenburg G, et al Axial skeletal and Hox expression domain alterations induced by retinoic acid, valproic acid, and bromoxynil during murine development. *J Biochem Mol Toxicol*. 2003; 17(6):346–56.

37 Pharmacokinetic Principles of Antiepileptic Therapy in Children

W. Edwin Dodson

Pharmacokinetics is the study of changes in drug concentrations in the body of a patient over time for the purpose of understanding the time course of drug actions (1–4). The unique pharmacokinetics of each drug result from both drug-related and patient-related factors (Table 37-1). Patient-related factors are responsible for most of the variability in the relationship between drug doses and drug concentrations. However, differences in drug formulation can substantially influence the time course of drug action.

FUNDAMENTAL PHARMACOKINETIC CONCEPTS

Pharmacokinetic principles are based on mathematical models. When a model is selected for a specific pharmacokinetic analysis, assumptions must be made to simplify complex physiologic processes. Models are named according to the number of compartments that are considered and according to the type of kinetics that are applied: linear versus nonlinear. A one-compartment model assumes that the body is a single compartment, whereas a two-compartment model assumes that the body has two compartments: a central (vascular) compartment and a peripheral (tissue) compartment. Although two-compartment models are preferable to one-compartment models, one-compartment models have been used most frequently in pharmacokinetic studies in patients (5).

The physical properties of a drug, such as its size, ionization constant (pK_a), lipid and aqueous solubility, and dissolution rate, determine how the drug interacts with physiologic processes in the body. These interactions result in kinetic patterns of absorption, distribution, metabolism (biotransformation), and excretion that are characteristic for each drug, and they determine the concentration of drug that is available to interact at target sites of drug action in the nervous system (6). Most antiepileptic drugs (AEDs) enter the nervous system by passive processes and interact with brain constituents at relatively low-affinity binding sites. However, recent work on multidrug resistance factors suggests that in some cases these factors may actively promote drug efflux out of epileptogenic tissue. At this point, however, the role of these factors in patients' responses to AEDs has not been delineated (7–9).

Drug elimination comprises all of the mechanisms that act to remove a drug from the body. The elimination of AEDs is largely due to hepatic biotransformation and renal excretion. Although hepatic biotransformation can produce active metabolites, which contribute to drug action, most of the time drug metabolites do not have

TABLE 37-1
Factors That Determine the Pharmacokinetics of a Drug

DRUG-RELATED FACTORS	PATIENT-RELATED FACTORS
Size	Pharmacogenetics
Ionization constant	Age
Lipid solubility	Nutritional state
Aqueous solubility	Disease
Formulation	Comedication
	Route of administration

antiepileptic activity. The total elimination rate is the sum of the elimination rates through all the mechanisms according to the equation

$$k_{el} = k_{renal} + k_{hepatic} + k_{other} \quad (1)$$

Linear Elimination Kinetic

The mechanisms that eliminate most AEDs are capable of removing much more drug than is usually present. In these circumstances, the elimination mechanisms dispose of a constant fractional amount of the drug per unit of time, independent of the drug concentration. These processes have *linear, first-order* kinetics. When the elimination of a drug has linear kinetics, the relationship between the drug dose and the drug concentration in serum is linear and intuitively predictable.

Intravenous Dose and Drug Half-Life

It is easiest to evaluate drug elimination after intravenous (IV) dosing, when drug absorption is not an issue (2, 3). Immediately after an intravenous bolus dose, drug concentrations are very high in serum. At first, the drug level declines very rapidly, but later the rate of decline becomes slower (2, 3, 10) (Figure 37-1). The initial rapid decline (alpha phase) is due to the distribution of drug from the central, vascular compartment into peripheral tissue compartments. Later, the slower decline (beta phase) is determined predominantly by drug elimination. For a two-compartment model, the concentration-time curve after an intravenous dose is described by the equation:

$$C_t = A \cdot e^{-\alpha t} + B \cdot e^{-\beta t} \quad (2)$$

The terminal portion of the concentration-time curve is used to determine the *half-life* ($t_{1/2}$) and the *elimination rate constant* (k_{el}). The half-life is defined as the time that is required for the amount of drug in the body to decline by a factor of one-half. In a single-compartment model,

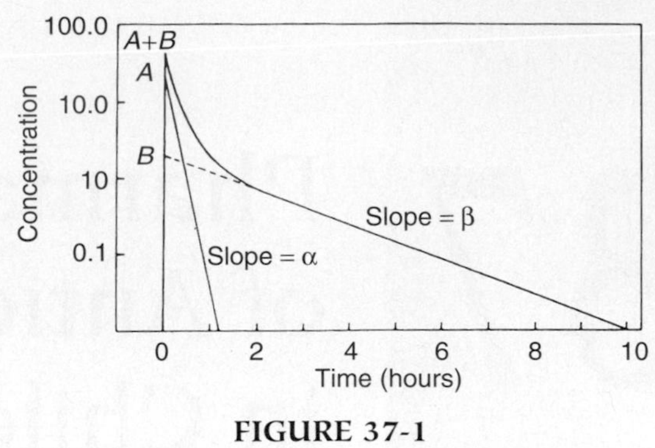

FIGURE 37-1

Semilogarithmic plot of intravenous concentration versus time curve based on a two-compartment model. Curve A is obtained by subtracting the extrapolated terminal portions of curve A + B. For more on exponential curve peeling see Riggs (10) and Greenblatt and Koch-Weser (2, 3).

the elimination rate constant is the slope of the declining curve, but in two-compartment models the elimination rate constant is more complex because of the simultaneous effects of drug distribution into the peripheral compartment. In a two-compartment model, the beta half-life is calculated from the terminal portion of the concentration-time curve. The half-life is related to the elimination rate constant according to the following relationship:

$$k_{el} \cdot t_{1/2} = \ln 2$$

The elimination rate constant has the dimensions of a fraction per unit time; the half-life has the dimension of time.

The half-life is important for several reasons. First, it indicates how much time is required for drug levels to stabilize after the dose is changed (Figure 37-2). Whenever the

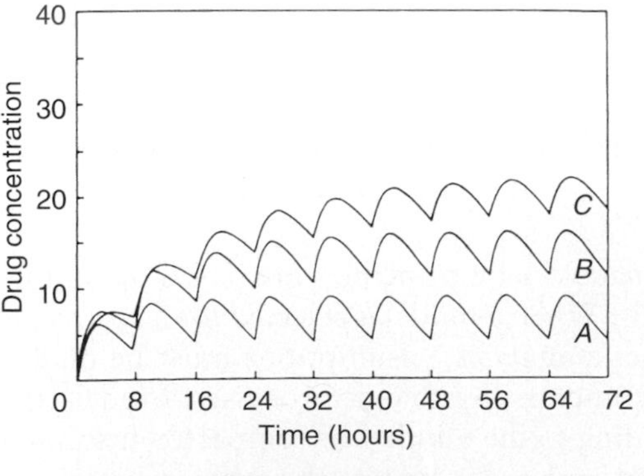

FIGURE 37-2

Effect of varying half-life on time to reach steady state and on the eventual concentration at steady state. The half-lives of curves A, B, and C are 4, 8, and 12 hours, respectively. Increasing the half-life delays steady state and results in higher concentrations.

dose is changed, five half-lives must elapse before a steady state is reached and drug levels stabilize. Second, under steady-state conditions, the drug concentration is directly proportional to the half-life. If the half-life changes, the steady-state concentration changes. Third, the half-life ordinarily dictates how frequently doses should be administered. In most cases doses should be administered at intervals equal to or less than the half-life to limit the fluctuation in drug levels between doses. For drugs that have a short half-life, retarding absorption by the administration of slow-release formulations also limits the fluctuation in drug levels between doses. This is discussed further with other aspects of drug absorption.

Volume of Distribution

The apparent volume of distribution (*Vd*) is the volume that the drug seems to occupy in the body. It is an imaginary volume that does not necessarily conform to anatomical compartments. The volume of distribution is the quotient of the amount of drug in the body divided by the drug concentration. Although the volume of distribution can be calculated several ways, the simplest approach is to extrapolate the terminal phase of the intravenous concentration-time curve back to time zero and use that concentration (the theoretical concentration at time zero) to calculate *Vd* (2, 3). For example, if there is 100 mg of drug in the body and the drug level at time zero is 10 mg/L, the volume of distribution is 10 L. The relative volume of distribution is the *Vd* divided by the patient's weight. If the patient with a *Vd* of 10 L weighed 20 kg, the patient's relative volume of distribution (Vd_{rel}) would be 0.5 L/kg.

The volume of distribution has two important applications. First, it can be used to calculate loading doses. For example, a 100-mg loading dose will result in a level of 20 mg/L in a 10-kg child who has a Vd_{rel} of 0.5 L/kg (dose = $Vd_{rel} \cdot$ concentration · weight). Second, it is an important component of clearance.

Clearance

Clearance (*Cl*) summarizes all of the factors that act to reduce the drug concentration. Clearance is defined as the volume of distribution that is completely rid of drug per unit time; it has the dimensions of volume per time. Operationally, clearance is the product of the volume of distribution times the elimination rate constant: $Cl = Vd \cdot k_{el}$. Clearance is inversely related to half-life; a long half-life causes a low clearance ($Cl = Vd(\ln 2/t_{1/2})$. The relative clearance (Cl_{rel}) is the clearance divided by weight.

The relative clearance is the best parameter for comparing drug dose requirements among different groups of patients. It also provides the most reliable basis for determining initial doses, because clearance accommodates for variations in body water and fat content. However, clearance is rarely used to calculate doses, because the values are harder to remember than doses based on weight.

Steady State

A *steady state* exists when the rate of drug input equals the rate of drug output. When drug administration is initiated at a constant dose, the drug progressively accumulates in the body until the clearance equals the dosing rate. Five half-lives are required to nearly reach a steady state.

Although the administration of large loading doses causes drug levels to increase rapidly, loading doses do not necessarily produce the same concentration that will occur at steady state (Figure 37-3). Steady-state concentrations depend on the maintenance doses, which are administered repeatedly. Thus, a steady state should never be assumed until a constant dose has been administered for a sufficient amount of time.

Under steady-state conditions, the average drug level in serum ($C_m{}^{ss}$) is constant and is equal to the dosing rate divided by the clearance:

$$C_m{}^{ss} = \frac{D}{\tau} \div Cl \qquad (3)$$

After clearance is replaced with its components, *Vd* and $t_{1/2}$, it can be seen that the average drug level at steady state is directly related to the dosing rate and to the half-life and inversely related to the volume of distribution:

$$C_m{}^{ss} = \frac{D}{\tau} \cdot \frac{t_{1/2}}{Vd \cdot \ln 2} \qquad (4)$$

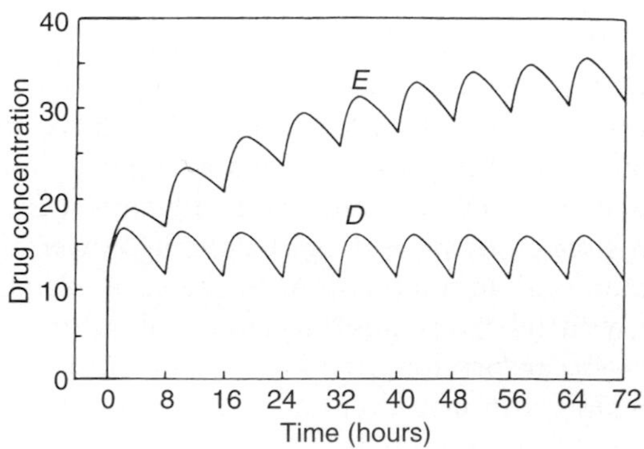

FIGURE 37-3

Effect of varying half-life after loading doses. Note that, independent of the administration of a loading dose, 5 half-lives are required for levels to stabilize. The half-life for curve D is 8 hrs, and that for curve E is 20 hrs.

Drug Absorption

Drug absorption is described both in terms of the *absorption rate* and in terms of the extent of absorption, *bioavailability*. The rate of absorption determines when the peak concentration occurs. Slowing the absorption rate postpones and reduces the peak concentration, attenuating the range of the fluctuations in drug concentrations between doses. Bioavailability (*F*) is a measure of the extent of drug absorption that is independent of time. Bioavailability is the quotient of the areas under the concentration-time curves for a nonintravenous dose divided by that for an IV dose. For example, the area under the curve after an oral dose divided by the area after the same dose IV is the bioavailability of the orally administered formulation. Bioavailability is expressed as either a fraction or a percent.

Several factors reduce the bioavailability of orally administered drugs. Failure to absorb the drug due to gastrointestinal (GI) disease, lack of tablet dissolution, and drug insolubility are obvious reasons. Bioavailability is also reduced when drugs are metabolized in the GI tract or in the liver before they reach the systemic circulation (so-called *first-pass metabolism*).

Bioequivalence is a measure that compares both the extent of absorption and the rate of absorption, but it does not require an IV dose. The bioequivalence of various oral formulations of a drug is determined before generic formulations are authorized for marketing. Operationally, the absorption rate or time to peak concentration and the areas under the concentration-time curves for different formulations are compared. According to the Food and Drug Administration's definition of bioequivalence, different oral formulations of the same drug are bioequivalent if they differ by no more than 20%. However, these tolerance limits may be too broad for some patients with difficult-to-control epilepsy.

The route of drug administration influences the absorption rate and thereby affects the onset of drug action. IV administration increases drug levels fastest, making the drug available for entry into tissues nearly instantaneously. However, drugs that have limited aqueous solubility, such as carbamazepine, cannot be formulated for IV administration. Intramuscular (IM) administration of some drugs results in slower absorption than oral administration. In the case of lipophilic drugs with relatively poor aqueous solubility, such as phenytoin, absorption after IM administration is slow and erratic, although eventually complete. Among the AEDs, phenobarbital is best documented to be rapidly and reliably absorbed after IM administration. Phenobarbital concentrations usually reach peak values in less than 90 minutes in children (11).

Oral administration of AEDs is the cornerstone of the treatment of epilepsy. By and large, drugs with erratic or low bioavailability are not suitable for chronic antiepileptic therapy. Drugs with rapid absorption and short half-lives are manufactured in delayed or slowly absorbed formulations to help sustain drug levels between doses. Examples include valproate (Depakote® Sprinkles) and carbamazepine (Tegretol XR® and Carbatrol). As a general principle, slowly absorbed formulations are preferable for chronic antiepileptic therapy because they attenuate the fluctuations in drug concentrations between doses. The differing absorption rates of different drug formulations have important implications for generic substitution.

Rectal administration of AEDs is important for patients who take drugs that lack parenteral formulations and for emergency situations when drugs cannot be administered either intravenously or orally. Rectal administration is also helpful when epileptic patients undergo surgery and cannot take their medications by mouth (12). Lipophilic antiepileptic drugs such as diazepam are rapidly and well absorbed after rectal administration (13). Typically, drugs in solution are absorbed faster and more reliably than drugs in suppositories. Rectal administration also reduces first-pass hepatic metabolism.

Many AEDs have been given rectally, including diazepam, clonazepam, lorazepam, nitrazepam, ethosuximide, valproic acid, carbamazepine, paraldehyde, and phenytoin (12, 14, 15). Diazepam has an extensive history of rectal administration and has been used to interrupt serial seizures and status epilepticus and to prevent febrile seizures. After rectal administration of diazepam solutions in doses of 0.5 to 1 mg/kg, peak concentrations usually occur in less than 10 minutes (16, 17). The absorption kinetics of carbamazepine in suspension are similar after oral and rectal administration, but rectal administration of carbamazepine suspension produces a strong defecatory urge (18).

Drug Elimination

The route of drug elimination plays an important role in determining a drug's pharmacokinetics as well as its vulnerability to pharmacokinetic interactions. Drugs that are eliminated mainly by hepatic metabolism to inactive metabolites include carbamazepine, ethosuximide, phenytoin, lamotrigine, tiagabine, zonisamide, and various benzodiazepines. Several antiepileptic drugs are eliminated both by hepatic biotransformation and by renal excretion of unmetabolized drug. These include phenobarbital, felbamate, oxcarbazepine, topiramate, and valproate. All of these are subject to substantial hepatic metabolism, and altered hepatic processing affects serum levels substantially. Gabapentin, pregabalin, and vigabatrin are eliminated exclusively by urinary excretion and are impervious to the effects of other drugs on hepatic drug-metabolizing capacity.

TABLE 37-2
Effects of Antiepileptic Drugs on Hepatic Drug-Metabolizing Enzyme Systems

Potent Inducers	Feeble or No Effect	General Inhibitor
Carbamazepine, phenobarbital, phenytoin, primidone	Ethosuximide, gabapentin, lamotrigine, levetiracetam, pregabalin, oxcarbazepine, tiagabine, topiramate, vigabatrin, zonisamide	Felbamate, valproate

The vulnerability of an AED to pharmacokinetic interactions depends how it is eliminated, the extent of induction and/or inhibition of the elimination processes, and the resultant capacity of the drug eliminating mechanisms relative to the amount of drug available for elimination (19). AEDs developed prior to 1990 are more vulnerable to interactions than drugs developed subsequently. Factors that influence the propensity for a drug to participate in pharmacokinetic interactions include which enzymes catalyze its metabolism, which enzymes it induces, and which other drugs are shared as substrates by the enzyme. Drugs that are substrates for the same cytochrome P450 isozyme tend to interact, usually inhibiting each other's elimination. The effects of various antiepileptics on hepatic drug-metabolizing capacity are summarized in Table 37-2.

Drugs that depend on hepatic biotransformation for elimination are prone to pharmacokinetic interactions. Among those drugs that are likely to participate in pharmacokinetic interactions, phenytoin is arguably the most sensitive, because the phenytoin-eliminating enzymes are partially saturated at usual doses and concentrations.

In the past two decades, knowledge about the hepatic cytochrome P450 complex expanded considerably. The components of the P450 system that are most relevant to the metabolism of antiepileptic drugs are CYP2C9, CYP2C19, and CYP3A4. Information about these enzymes and their substrates are summarized in Table 37-3 (20–23). Potent inducers of hepatic drug metabolism increase the activity of these three enzymes plus the activities of epoxide hydrolase and uridine diphosphate glucuronosyl transferase. Uridine diphosphate glucuronosyl transferase catalyzes the formation of glucuronide conjugates and plays a major role in the elimination of lamotrigine, oxcarbazepine, and valproate and a minor role for phenobarbital (19).

Valproic acid has a distinctive pattern of elimination. It is metabolized via beta oxidation like a fatty acid, and it is conjugated with glucuronic acid to facilitate urinary excretion. Underdevelopment of the glucuronidation pathway is the major reason that infants and young children eliminate valproate slowly.

Note that valproate and felbamate are inhibitors of hepatic drug metabolism. This has important implications for pediatric polytherapy of epilepsy. The addition of valproate substantially increases lamotrigine and phenobarbital concentrations. Furthermore, in children valproate approximately doubles the $t_{1/2}$ of tiagabine, with the average $t_{1/2}$ increasing from 3.2 to 5.7 hours (24). Likewise, add-on felbamate increases the concentrations of phenobarbital, phenytoin, and valproate. When either valproate or felbamate is added to phenobarbital, phenytoin, or valproate, the doses of the preexistent drug should be reduced (25).

Nonlinear Kinetics

Although the pharmacokinetics of most AEDs are linear or first order, notable exceptions exist. When the mechanisms that result in drug elimination have linear kinetics, a constant fraction of the drug is absorbed, transported, and eliminated per unit of time. The elimination mechanisms for phenytoin, however, have a low capacity relative to the phenytoin concentrations that are usually present, so these mechanisms are partially *saturated* (26, 27). This partial saturation results in *nonlinear* elimination kinetics and causes the relationship between the phenytoin dose and concentration to be intuitively unpredictable. (Figure 37-4). Other antiepileptic drug pharmacokinetics that are nonlinear include gabapentin absorption and valproate binding. Gabapentin transport into the brain is likely to be saturable as well. Nonlinear kinetic patterns are also designated as saturable, concentration-dependent, or dose-dependent.

When drugs are eliminated by processes with nonlinear kinetics, the fractional rate of drug disposition varies with the dose or drug concentration. As drug concentrations increase, the elimination mechanism becomes progressively saturated. This prolongs the half-life that is measured because a smaller percentage of the drug is eliminated per unit of time as the concentration increases. In this situation, the half-life that is observed should be designated as $t_{50\%}$ to differentiate it from the usual $t_{1/2}$.

When drug elimination has nonlinear kinetics, the apparent half-life ($t_{50\%}$) changes with the dose or concentration. The apparent half-life is directly proportional to the initial concentration that is present when

TABLE 37-3
The Three Major Components of Cytochrome P450 Drug-Metabolizing Enzymes That Participate in the Elimination of AEDs, with Their Substrates

CYP2C9	CYP2C19	CYP3A4
	MAJOR AED SUBSTRATES	
Phenytoin (major)	Phenytoin (minor)	Carbamazepine
Phenobarbital		Benzodiazepines (several)
		Ethosuximide
		Tiagabine
		Zonisamide
	OTHER SUBSTRATES	
Azapropazone	Cimetidine	**Inhibited by**
Cotrimoxazole	Diazepam	Cyclosporine A
Disulfiram	Felbamate	Fluvoxamine
Metronidazole	Fluoxetine	Fluoxetine
Phenylbutazone	Imipramine	Grapefruit juice
Propoxyphene	Omeprazole	Ketoconazole
Stiripental	**Inhibited by**	Macrolide antibiotics (erythromycin and triolean domycin)
Sulfaphenazole	Felbamate	Miconazole
Inhibited by	Fluvoxamine	Nefazadone
Amiodarone	Omeprazole	Sertraline
Fluconazaole	Topiramate	
Fluoxetine		
Fluvoxamine		
Miconazole		
Valproic acid		

These relationships provide the basis for numerous pharmacokinetic interactions (20–23). Shared substrates that produce inhibition of drug metabolism consistently are noted. Other shared substrates that have only mild or inconsistent inhibitory effects are listed as other substrates.

the half-life is measured (28). Thus, increasing doses leads to disproportionate increases in drug concentrations. When drug doses are reduced, the opposite occurs; small reductions in dose can cause precipitous declines in drug concentration. Finally, the amount of drug in the body and the concentration of the drug in blood progressively increase if the dosing rate exceeds the capacity for drug elimination.

$$t_{50\%} = \frac{0.5C_i}{V_{\max}} + \frac{K_M(\ln 2)}{V_{\max}} \qquad (5)$$

The Michaelis-Menten equations that describe the kinetics of enzyme reactions can be applied to describe nonlinear drug elimination (6). The way this is done is to measure drug levels at two or more steady states and then solve for the nonlinear kinetic parameters: the maximal reaction velocity ($V_{\max}$) and the drug concentration (K_M)

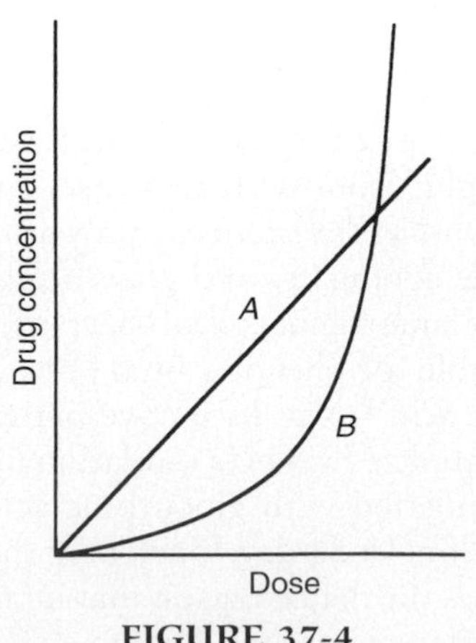

FIGURE 37-4

Dose versus concentration curves for drugs with linear (A) versus nonlinear (B) elimination kinetics.

at which the reaction rate is one-half of the maximal elimination velocity. The critical assumption that underlies these calculations is that at steady state the rate of drug dosing equals the rate of drug elimination. Hence, at steady state the dosing rate equals the reaction velocity. Similarly, the drug concentration is analogous to a substrate concentration. In order to calculate the nonlinear kinetic parameters V_{max} and K_M, it is necessary to know two or more pairs of doses and concentrations. Several methods have been described for calculating V_{max} and K_M (29). These are discussed further in Chapter 49.

$$V = \frac{V_{max} \times C}{K_M + C} \qquad (6)$$

For drugs with nonlinear kinetics, varying the absorption rate changes the apparent bioavailability. Martis and Levy described the effects of bioavailability (F), absorption rate (k_a), K_M, and V_{max} on the rate of phenytoin concentration change (30).

$$\frac{dC}{dt} = K_a F C_0 \exp(-k_a t) - K_1 C - \frac{V_{max} C}{K_M + C} \qquad (7)$$

In this equation k_a is the first-order absorption rate; C_0 is the drug concentration at zero time; C is the concentration at any time t; F is the bioavailability or fraction of the drug that is ultimately absorbed; and K_1 is the overall apparent first-order rate constant.

Equation 7 has been used to evaluate the relationship between absorption rate and apparent bioavailability (31). Based on computer simulations using average values of K_M and V_{max}, the apparent bioavailability declines by 25% as the half time for absorption increases from 0 (intravenous administration) to 1.2 hours.

Drug Protein Binding

Ordinarily, only total (bound plus unbound) AED levels are measured. However, it is the unbound drug concentration in plasma that is in equilibrium with the unbound drug concentration in the brain. The unbound level correlates better with drug action than does the total level (32, 33). Nevertheless, measuring the total drug concentration in plasma usually works well because total concentrations correlate highly with the unbound concentrations in most patients.

Various AEDs differ in the extent to which they are bound to serum constituents (34–37) (Table 37-4). The binding of ethosuximide, phenobarbital, and primidone is so low as to be clinically irrelevant. However, the binding of carbamazepine, phenytoin, and valproate is sufficiently high that significant changes in unbound drug levels occur when binding is altered (34). Conditions that cause hypoalbuminemia, such as renal disease and hepatic disease and certain drug interactions with acidic compounds such as fatty acids, aspirin, and valproate increase the unbound drug concentrations of phenytoin and carbamazepine. Newborns also have reduced drug protein binding because of hypoalbuminemia (35). When drug protein binding is disturbed, therapeutic ranges based on total levels of phenytoin and of carbamazepine no longer apply.

High concentrations of valproate exceed the binding capacity of plasma constituents, resulting in a nonlinear relationship between the total valproate level and the unbound valproate level (38). When total valproate levels are high, the unbound valproate level increases disproportionately.

TABLE 37-4
Binding of Antiepileptic Drugs to Serum Proteins

Drug	Percent Unbound
Carbamazepine	27–40
Clonazepam	15
Diazepam	2
Ethosuximide	90–100
Felbamate	78–64
Gabapentin	100
Lamotrigine	35–45
Levetiracetam	100
Oxcarbazepine	60
Phenobarbital	50–55
Phenytoin	7–15
Pregabalin	100
Primidone	70–100
Tiagabine	4
Topiramate	83–91
Valproic acid (high)	10–30
Valproic acid (low)	8–10
Vigabatrin	100
Zonisamide	50–60

From (27, 36, 37).

MULTIDRUG RESISTANCE

In recent years the possibility has been considered that multidrug resistance factors might play a role in patients' responses to AEDs, especially among patients whose seizures are refractory to AEDs (39, 40). Multidrug resistance factors were first identified in cancer and consist of molecules that transport drugs out of target tissues using energy-dependent processes. By promoting local efflux of drug, they can reduce the drug concentration at target sites of drug action.

Molecules that mediate multidrug resistance include P-glycoprotein (P-gp) and multidrug resistance–associated protein (MDR). Most AEDs are substrates for P-gp (41, 42).

Drug resistance factors have been investigated in several animal models of epilepsy (43–46). Experimentally induced seizures and brain malformations, but not AEDs (47), induce multidrug resistance factors in animals (48, 49). Drug resistance factors have also been identified in human epileptogenic tissue that has been removed surgically, including temporal lobe tissue, cortical dysplasias, and tubers from patients with tuberous sclerosis (9, 50, 51). Multidrug resistance proteins are localized to endothelial cells in brain capillaries and associated astroglia. Whereas in animals multidrug resistance proteins have been shown to reduce the concentrations of AEDs locally, microdialysis of extracellular fluid obtained intraoperatively during epilepsy surgery has shown mixed results (52).

Since multidrug resistance factors are localized to abnormal tissues, they appear to have little or no effect on systemic pharmacokinetics of a drug in the body, such as the volume of distribution, clearance, or half-life. Rather, they may affect the local distribution of the drug within the target epileptogenic areas. If a role in refractory human epilepsy is confirmed for multidrug resistance factors, drugs to inhibit their effects are likely to become topics of great interest.

The expression of multidrug resistance factors is under genetic control. Studies of gene markers linked to polymorphisms of multidrug resistance among patients with refractory epilepsy have generated conflicting results, with some investigators finding genetic markers and others not (8, 53). However, these studies are in the early stages, and they are methodologically complex. Thus, conflicting results at this point do not negate the possibility that genetic influences are important in selected patient populations and might someday help refine treatment (54).

ADJUSTING DOSES AND THE APPLICATION OF DRUG LEVEL MEASUREMENTS

The practical worth of any drug is specified by its *therapeutic index*. The therapeutic index is defined as the dose that produces toxicity divided by the dose that produces the desired therapeutic effect. Most AEDs have a narrow therapeutic index compared to antibiotic drugs such as penicillin. Furthermore, there is great variability in the therapeutic index of AEDs among individual patients because different types of seizures have variable susceptibility to drugs and because patients vary in their sensitivity to dose-related neurotoxicity.

GENERIC AED FORMULATIONS

Generic substitution of AEDs has the potential to reduce the cost of antiepileptic therapy. Generic formulations are produced by several manufacturers and are distributed by more numerous intermediate suppliers. These factors facilitate low cost through open market competition, but they make it difficult to track down the origin of a specific generic formulation.

Despite the need for low-cost antiepileptic therapy, the overriding goal of treating epilepsy with AEDs is to administer enough drug to prevent seizures while maintaining drug levels below those that cause dose-related neurotoxicity in the individual patient. In practical terms, fluctuations in AED levels between doses need to be minimized.

As discussed previously, the magnitude of expected fluctuation in levels between doses depends on two factors: first, the drug's elimination rate or half-life, and second, the absorption rate. Because generic AEDs tend to have faster absorption rates than brand-name products, generic substitution sometimes increases the fluctuations in levels between doses, increasing the risk of both subtherapeutic and toxic levels (Figure 37-5). For certain drugs such as phenobarbital, which has a very long half-life, this is a trivial issue and generic substitution is indicated.

The problems that result from switching among formulations with different absorption rates are most severe for phenytoin, because it has nonlinear kinetics. Different phenytoin formulations with different absorption rates have different apparent bioavailabilities. When a formulation is absorbed rapidly, it produces a higher peak concentration, which in turn causes the apparent half-life to be prolonged. As a result, steady-state concentrations can change significantly when phenytoin formulations are switched. For this reason, generic substitution of phenytoin should be prohibited.

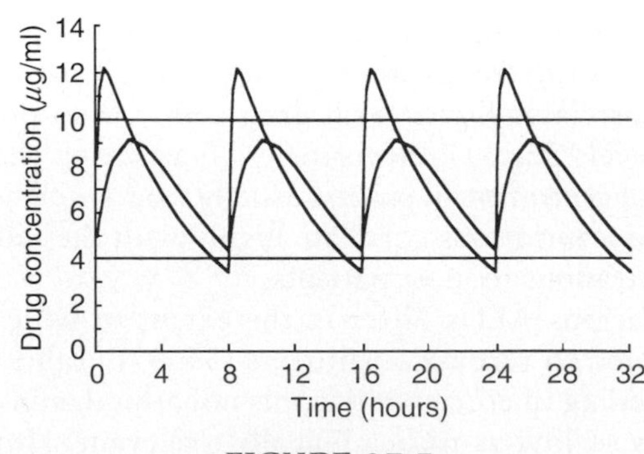

FIGURE 37-5

Effect of rapid versus slow absorption rate on fluctuations in drug levels between doses. Reproduced with permission from (34).

For carbamazepine, which has an intermediate to short half-life (18 hours or less, depending on the patient), the issue of generic substitution is complex. Changing the formulation can modify the extent of fluctuation between doses but does not alter the average concentration at steady state unless there is also a problem with tablet dissolution and bioavailability. For some patients who require only low carbamazepine levels to hold seizures in abeyance, generic substitution works well. For others who have a narrow therapeutic index for carbamazepine, generic substitution is highly problematic. These types of patients are at risk to experience both toxicity and recurrent seizures if they are switched to a formulation that is more rapidly absorbed. Thus the patient and the treating physician should be consulted when generic carbamazepine substitution is contemplated.

EFFECT OF AGE ON AED PHARMACOKINETICS

Age and prior drug exposure affect the child's capacity for drug elimination (55–59). For the purposes of categorizing the affects of age on drug elimination, the following groups have been used: newborns (birth to 6 weeks), infants (6 weeks to 12 months), children (1 year to 11 years), adolescents (11 years to 15 years), adults (> 15 years). These age groupings are somewhat arbitrary, because the pharmacokinetic changes that occur are gradual and because of individual variation in growth and maturation. Adolescence is heralded in individual patients by the transition from Tanner stage 1 to stage 2. For each age group, the children who have prior drug exposure need to be considered separately from those who lack prior drug treatment.

Newborns exposed to drugs in utero usually eliminate antiepileptic drugs at rates that are comparable to those in adults (27). The older AEDs that induce drug-metabolizing pathways in adults also do so prenatally and postnatally. Drugs, such as valproate, that inhibit hepatic drug elimination do so dramatically in newborns and young children. Valproate has extremely long half-lives in newborns and infants who have not been exposed to other inducing agents. Furthermore, most newborns who have seizures do not have prior, intrauterine drug exposure. Consequently, they tend to eliminate AEDs far more slowly than any other age group. Furthermore, the most common cause of neonatal seizures—perinatal asphyxia—may be associated with abnormal hepatic and renal function, which also retard drug elimination. Although the neonatal pharmacokinetic effects of intrauterine exposure to drugs that have become available in the 1990s, such as oxcarbazepine, lamotrigine, gabapentin and topiramate, have not been quantified, they are unlikely to have much impact because they do not induce hepatic drug metabolism.

The postnatal maturation of renal function and hepatic systems for drug conjugation are well recognized. Renal function increases rapidly in the first day after birth and reaches nearly adult capacity by age 3 weeks. Immature hepatic phase II conjugation of nonpolar compounds to water-soluble glucuronides is one reason for slow elimination of antiepileptics, especially valproate, by newborns and infants (60). The maturation of hepatic phase I biotransformation of drugs via the cytochrome P450 system of enzymes varies according to the particular enzymatic pathway.

Different components of the cytochrome P450 system mature at different times during gestation and postnatally (19). The capacity to carry out aromatic oxidations (the principal metabolic pathway for phenytoin and phenobarbital) develops early in gestation. No significant differences have been found between premature and full-term newborns in the development of aromatic oxidations. Postnatally this pathway is induced extensively and has very high capacity by the end of the neonatal period. In fact, infants who have been treated for neonatal seizures have the greatest relative capacity to oxidize these drugs. However, N-dealkylation is more variable (61). Premature newborns have less capacity than full-term newborns to metabolize drugs such as diazepam and methylxanthines via this pathway. Both of these pathways—aromatic oxidations and N-dealkylation—are induced by intrauterine drug exposure to drugs such as phenobarbital and phenytoin but not by exposure to valproate. In the absence of prior drug treatment, the newborn's relative capacity for N-dealkylation is approximately 20% of adult values at birth and gradually increases to adult capacity by age 2 years (62).

The pharmacokinetics of AEDs change during the neonatal period. After loading doses have been given and maintenance drug therapy is under way, several factors act simultaneously to reduce drug concentrations during the neonatal period. These include accelerating drug elimination, changing routes of drug administration, and recovery from hepatic, renal, or gastrointestinal dysfunction caused by systemic disease. Newborns with seizures experience dramatic increases in the clearance of most of the antiepileptic drugs during the neonatal period (27). Increases by factors of 2 to 4 are common for phenobarbital and phenytoin, causing drug levels to decline by 50% to 75% if constant doses are given. The effects of perinatal disease on drug dose requirements are subtle but can be identified in groups of newborns. For example, newborns with perinatal asphyxia have lower relative clearance for phenobarbital than newborns with seizures due to other causes. The relative clearance of phenobarbital of 4.1 mL/kg/h by asphyxiated newborns is approximately 50% lower than the average phenobarbital clearance of 8.7 mL/kg/h by nonasphyxiated newborns (63). This predicts that, at equivalent doses, the levels in asphyxiated newborns will be twice as high.

Switching from intravenous to oral drug administration leads to slower drug absorption, reducing and delaying peak concentrations. In the case of phenytoin, slowed absorption causes a reduction in the apparent bioavailability of 20% to 30% (31).

As drug clearance increases during the neonatal period, it is necessary to increase the dose to sustain uniform drug concentrations. However, most neonatal seizures are symptomatic of disorders that are abating during the neonatal period. Therefore, declining drug levels create fewer problems than might be expected because the intensity of the epileptic process tends to abate concurrently.

After the neonatal period, there are two major differences in the pharmacokinetics of AEDs between children and adults: children have higher relative clearance, and children have greater within-group variability in elimination kinetics (27, 55, 64, 65). The effect of age on relative clearance is similar for most of the AEDs. Infants have the highest relative clearances, which are 3- to 4-fold greater than adult values. With advancing age the relative clearance declines until adult values are reached in late childhood or adolescence (66, 67) (Figure 37-6). Among specific age groups the standard deviation of the average clearance is relatively greater in younger patients. For example, the coefficient of variation (the standard deviation divided by the mean times 100%) for relative clearance of phenytoin is more than 50% for children who are less than 5 years old (66). For this reason the relationships between drug doses and levels are more unpredictable in children than in adults. Often, considerable trial and error are required to adjust children's drug levels.

Drug levels are surprisingly stable during the middle and later years of childhood, because increases in body mass are offset by declining relative drug clearance. This means that children do not outgrow their drug doses frequently. Although the adolescent growth spurt does occasionally necessitate dosage adjustments, dramatic changes in relative drug clearance are scarce during adolescence. Noncompliance is far more common and causes drug levels to vary erratically.

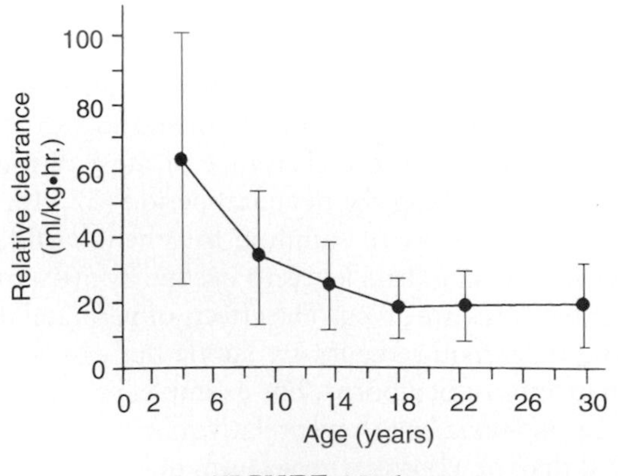

FIGURE 37-6

Effect of age on relative clearance of phenytoin. The vertical bars indicate one standard deviation. Drawn from data reported by Guelen (66). Reproduced with permission from (67).

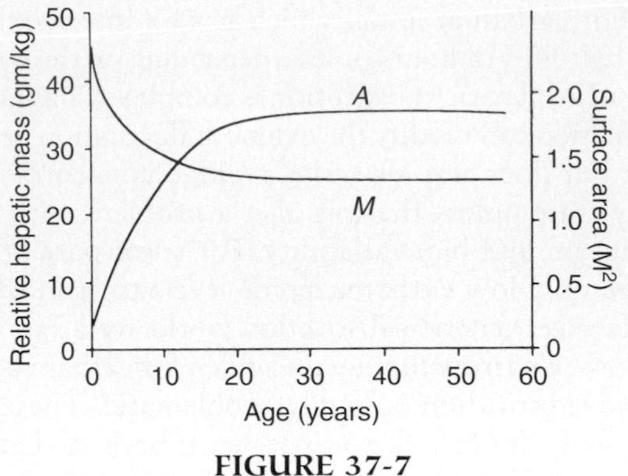

FIGURE 37-7

Relationship between age and body surface area (*A*) and between age and relative hepatic mass (*M*). Data from Korenchevsky (68) were used to create the figure.

The factors that underlie the age-related changes in drug clearance of all of the AEDs correlate with the changes that occur in relative hepatic mass, relative caloric requirements, and surface area relative to body mass during growth to adult size. Children, as compared to adults, have larger surface area relative to body mass, and they are hypermetabolic in order to maintain constant body temperature. With growth and increasing body mass, the surface area relative to body mass decreases, reducing the relative area that is available for radiant heat loss. Concomitantly, the relative hepatic mass and relative production of heat both decline (68) (Figure 37-7). Since most antiepileptic drugs are eliminated by hepatic biotransformation, the declining relative hepatic mass coincides with the decline in drug clearance that occurs with growth. Thus the age-related pattern of declining relative drug clearance seems to be a byproduct of growth in warm-blooded homotherms and results from size-related differences in metabolic rate.

AEDS IN BREAST MILK

Maternal treatment with antiepileptics is not a contraindication to breastfeeding (69–71). However, the issue of maternal drug administration and breastfeeding is somewhat controversial because of conflicting opinions and recommendations in the literature. Data regarding transplacental partition ratios and breast milk to maternal serum concentration have been reviewed at length (71).

TABLE 37-5
Pharmacokinetics of Antiepileptic Drugs Acquired from Maternal Sources

	Half-Life of Transplacental AEDs in Newborn		Percent of Serum Level in Breast Milk	
Drug	Hours	S.D.	Average	S.D.
Carbamazepine	6–44		41	17
Ethosuximide	41		94	6
Gabapentin			70	10
Lamotrigine			40–80	
Phenobarbital	41–628		41	15
Phenylethylmalonamide	35	6	76	15
Phenytoin	7–69		19	16
Primidone	8–83		72	15
Valproic acid	47	15	27	15

From (27, 75).

Newborns who were exposed chronically to inducing drugs in utero are born with induced drug elimination and may also be tolerant to sedative drug actions. If questions arise about the contribution of the antiepileptic drug to a specific symptom in the infant, measuring drug levels in the infant may provide some insight (72).

The amounts of phenytoin, carbamazepine, lamotrigine, vigabatrin, and valproate that are acquired via nursing are generally insignificant (37, 72–78) (Table 37-5). Although isolated case reports describe both neonatal sedation and withdrawal symptoms after prenatal intrauterine and postnatal breast milk–acquired barbiturate exposures, maternal barbiturate therapy is not an absolute contraindication to nursing. Highly lipid-soluble drugs such as diazepam readily penetrate breast milk and theoretically could lead the newborn to accumulate sedating levels, but this rarely occurs. Although the concentration of ethosuximide in breast milk is approximately 90% of the maternal levels, the significance of ingesting this amount is unknown (74, 79).

References

1. Gibaldi M, Perrier D. Pharmacokinetics. New York: Marcel Dekker, 1975.
2. Greenblatt DJ, Koch-Weser J. Clinical pharmacokinetics. *New Eng J Med* 1975; 293: 702–705.
3. Greenblatt DJ, Koch-Weser J. Clinical pharmacokinetics. *New Eng J Med* 1975; 293: 964–970.
4. Greenblatt DJ, Shader RI. Pharmacokinetics in clinical practice. Philadelphia: W.B. Saunders, 1985.
5. Riegelman S, Loo J, Rowland M. Shortcomings in pharmacokinetic analysis by conceiving the body to exhibit properties of a single compartment. *J Pharm Sci* 1968; 57:117–123.
6. Levy RE, Unadkat JD. General principles. Drug absorption, distribution, and elimination. In: Levy R, Mattson R, Meldrum B, Penry JK, et al, eds. *Antiepileptic Drugs*. 3rd ed. New York: Raven Press, 1989:1–22.
7. Brandt C, Bethmann K, Gastens AM, Loscher W. The multidrug transporter hypothesis of drug resistance in epilepsy: Proof-of-principle in a rat model of temporal lobe epilepsy. *Neurobiol Dis* 2006; 24:202–11.
8. Siddiqui A, Kerb R, Weale ME, et al. Association of multidrug resistance in epilepsy with a polymorphism in the drug-transporter gene ABCB1. *N Engl J Med* 2003; 348: 1442–1448.
9. Aronica E, Gorter JA, Jansen GH, et al. Expression and cellular distribution of multidrug transporter proteins in two major causes of medically intractable epilepsy: focal cortical dysplasia and glioneuronal tumors. *Neuroscience* 2003; 118:417–429.
10. Riggs DS. The mathematical approach to physiological problems. Baltimore: Williams and Wilkins, 1972.
11. Brachet-Lierman A, Goutieres F, Aicardi J. Absorption of phenobarbital after intramuscular adminstration of single large doses. *J Pediatr* 1975; 87:624–626.
12. Woody RC, Golladay ES, Fiedorek-SC. Rectal anticonvulsants in seizure patients undergoing gastrointestinal surgery. *J Pediatr Surg* 1989; 24:474–477.
13. de Boer AG, Moolenaar F, de Leede LG, Breimer DD. Rectal drug administration: clinical pharmacokinetic considerations. *Clin Pharmacokinet* 1982; 7:285–311.
14. Graves NM, Kreil RL, Jones-Saete C. Bioavailability of rectally adminsitered lorazepam. *Clin Neuropharmacol* 1987; 10:555.
15. Dulac O, Aicardi J, Rey E, Olive G. Blood levels of diazepam after single rectal administration. *J Pediatr* 1978; 31:1047–1050.
16. Franzoni E, Carboni C, Lambertini A. Rectal diazepam: a clinical and EEG study after a single dose in children. *Epilepsia* 1983; 24:35–41.
17. Graves NM, Kriel RL. Rectal administration of antiepileptic drugs in children. *Pediatr Neurol* 1987; 3:321–326.
18. Graves NM, Kriel RL, Jones-Saete C, Cloyd JC. Relative bioavailability of rectally administered carbamazepine suspension in humans. *Epilepsia* 1985; 26:429–433.
19. Anderson GD. Pharmacogenetics and enzyme induction/inhibition properties of antiepileptic drugs. *Neurology* 2004; 63(Suppl 4):S3–S8.
20. Levy RH. Cytochrome P450 isozymes and antiepileptic drug interactions. *Epilepsia* 1995; 36(Suppl 5):S8–S13.
21. Sproule BA, Naranjo CA, Brenmer KE, Hassan PC. Selective serotonin reuptake inhibitors and CNS drug interactions. A critical review of the evidence. *Clin Pharmacokinet* 1997; 33:454–471.
22. Glue P, Banfield CR, Perhach JL, et al. Pharmacokinetic interactions with felbamate. In vitro–in vivo correlation. *Clin Pharmacokinet* 1997; 33:214–224.
23. Nakasa H, Nakamura H, Ono S, et al. Prediction of drug-drug interactions of zonisamide metabolism in humans from in vitro data. *Eur J Clin Pharmacol* 1998; 54: 177–183.
24. Gustavson LE, Boellner SW, Granneman GR, Qian JX, et al. A single-dose study to define tiagabine pharmacokinetics in pediatric patients with complex partial seizures. *Neurology* 1997; 48:1032–1037.
25. Riva R, Albani F, Contin M, Baruzzi A. Pharmacokinetic interactions between antiepileptic drugs. Clinical considerations. *Clin Pharmacokinet* 1996; 31:470–493.
26. Arnold K, Gerber N. The rate of decline of diphenylhydantoin in human plasma. *Clin Pharmacol Ther* 1970; 11:121–135.

27. Dodson WE. Special pharmacokinetic considerations in children. *Epilepsia* 1987; 8(Suppl 1): S56–S70.
28. Dodson WE. Nonlinear kinetics of phenytoin in children. *Neurology* 1982; 32:42–48.
29. Mullen PW, Foster RW. Comparative evaluation of six techniques for determining Michaelis-Menten parameters relating phenytoin dose and steady-state concentrations. *J Pharm Pharmacol* 1979; 31:100–104.
30. Martis L, Levy RH. Bioavailability calculations for drugs showing simultaneous first-order and capacity-limited elimination kinetics. *J Pharmacokinet Biopharmaceut* 1973; 1:381–383.
31. Dodson WE, Bourgeois BF. Changing kinetic patterns of phenyotin in newborns. In: Wasterlain CG, Vert P, eds. *Neonatal Seizures*. New York: Raven Press, 1990:271–276.
32. Koch-Wesser J, Sellers EM. Binding of drugs of serum albumin (first of two parts). *New Eng J Med* 1976; 294:311–316.
33. Koch-Wesser J, Sellers EM. Binding of drugs of serum albumin (second of two parts). *New Eng J Med* 1976; 294:526–531.
34. Dodson WE. Aspects of antiepileptic drug treatment in children. *Epilepsia* 1988; 29(Suppl 3):S10–S14.
35. Krasner J, Yaffe SJ. Drug-protein binding in the neonate. In: Morselli PL, Garattini S, Sereni F, eds. *Basic and Therapeutic Aspects of Perinatal Pharmacology*. New York: Raven Press, 1975:357–366.
36. Natsch S, Hekster YA, Keyser A, et al. Newer anticonvulsant drugs: role of harmacology, drug interactions and adverse reactions in drug choice. *Drug Saf* 1997; 17:228–240.
37. Rambeck B, Kurlemann G, Stodieck SR, May TW, et al. Concentrations of lamotrigine in a mother on lamotrigine treatment and her newborn child. *Eur J Clin Pharmacol* 1997; 51:481–484.
38. Riva R, Albani F, Franzoni E, Perucca E, et al. Valproic acid free fraction in epileptic children under chronic monotherapy. *Ther Drug Mon* 1983; 5:197–200.
39. Sisodiya SM. Mechanisms of antiepileptic drug resistance. *Curr Opin Neurol* 2003; 16: 197–201.
40. Pedley TA, Hirano M. Is refractory epilepsy due to genetically determined resistance to antiepileptic drugs? *N Engl J Med* 2003; 348:1480–1482.
41. Potschka H, Fedrowitz M, Loscher W. P-glycoprotein-mediated efflux of phenobarbital, lamotrigine, and felbamate at the blood-brain barrier: evidence from microdialysis experiments in rats. *Neurosci Lett* 2002; 327:173–176.
42. Potschka H, Loscher W. In vivo evidence for P-glycoprotein-mediated transport of phenytoin at the blood-brain barrier of rats. *Epilepsia* 2001; 42:1231–1240.
43. Seegers U, Potschka H, Loscher W. Transient increase of P-glycoprotein expression in endothelium and parenchyma of limbic brain regions in the kainate model of temporal lobe epilepsy. *Epilepsy Res* 2002; 51:257–268.
44. Hoffmann K, Gastens AM, Volk HA, Loscher W. Expression of the multidrug transporter MRP2 in the blood-brain barrier after pilocarpine-induced seizures in rats. *Epilepsy Res* 2006; 69:1–14.
45. Volk HA, Loscher W. Multidrug resistance in epilepsy: rats with drug-resistant seizures exhibit enhanced brain expression of P-glycoprotein compared with rats with drug-responsive seizures. *Brain* 2005; 128:1358–1368.
46. Loscher W. Animal models of drug-resistant epilepsy. *Novartis Found Symp* 2002; 243: 149–159.
47. Seegers U, Potschka H, Loscher W. Lack of effects of prolonged treatment with phenobarbital or phenytoin on the expression of P-glycoprotein in various rat brain regions. *Eur J Pharmacol* 2002; 451:149–155.
48. Marchi N, Guiso G, Caccia S, Rizzi M, et al. Determinants of drug brain uptake in a rat model of seizure-associated malformations of cortical development. *Neurobiol Dis* 2006; 24:429–442.
49. Lazarowski A, Lubieniecki F, Camarero S, Pomata H, et al. Multidrug resistance proteins in tuberous sclerosis and refractory epilepsy. *Pediatr Neurol* 2004; 30:102–106.
50. Marroni M, Marchi N, Cucullo L, Abbott NJ, et al. Vascular and parenchymal mechanisms in multiple drug resistance: a lesson from human epilepsy. *Curr Drug Targets* 2003; 4:297–304.
51. Marchi N, Hallene KL, Kight KM, Cucullo L, et al. Significance of MDR1 and multiple drug resistance in refractory human epileptic brain. *BMC Med* 2004; 2:37.
52. Rambeck B, Jurgens UH, May TW, Pannek HW, et al. Comparison of brain extracellular fluid, brain tissue, cerebrospinal fluid, and serum concentrations of antiepileptic drugs measured intraoperatively in patients with intractable epilepsy. *Epilepsia* 2006; 47:681–694.
53. Sills GJ, Mohanraj R, Butler E, McCrindle S, et al. Lack of association between the C3435T polymorphism in the human multidrug resistance (MDR1) gene and response to antiepileptic drug treatment. Epilepsia 2005; 46:643–7.
54. Ott J. Association of genetic loci: Replication or not, that is the question. *Neurology* 2004; 63:955–958.
55. Dodson WE. Antiepileptic drug utilization in children. *Epilepsia* 1984; 25(Suppl 2): S132–S139.
56. Anderson GD. Children versus adults: pharmacokinetic and adverse-effect differences. *Epilepsia* 2002; 43(Suppl 3):53–59.
57. Battino D, Croci D, Granata T, et al. Single-dose pharmacokinetics of lamotrigine in children: influence of age and antiepileptic comedication. *Ther Drug Monit* 2001; 23: 217–222.
58. Eriksson AS, Hoppu K, Nergardh A, Boreus L. Pharmacokinetic interactions between lamotrigine and other antiepileptic drugs in children with intractable epilepsy. *Epilepsia* 1996; 37:769–773.
59. Armijo JA, Bravo J, Cuadrado A, Herranz JL. Lamotrigine serum concentration-to-dose ratio: influence of age and concomitant antiepileptic drugs and dosage implications. *Ther Drug Monit* 1999; 21:182–190.
60. Gal P, Oles KS, Gilman JT, Weaver R. Valproic acid 1. Efficacy, toxicity, and pharmacokinetics in neonates with intractable seizures. *Neurology* 1988; 38:467–471.
61. Aranda JV, MacLeod SM, Renton KW, Eade NR. Hepatic microsomal drug oxidation and electron transport in newborn infants. *J Pediatr* 1974; 85:534–542.
62. Rating D, Jager-Roman E, Nau H, Kuhnz W, et al. Enzyme induction in neonates after fetal exposure to antiepileptic drugs. *Pediatr Pharmacol* 1983; 3:209–218.
63. Gal P, Toback J, Erkan NV, Boer HR. The influence of asphyxia on phenobarbital dosing requirements in neonates. *Dev Pharmacol Ther* 1984; 7:145–152.
64. Mikati MA, Fayad M, Koleilat M, Mounla N, et al. Efficacy, tolerability, and kinetics of lamotrigine in infants. *J Pediatr* 2002; 141:31–35.
65. Miura H. Developmental and therapeutic pharmacology of antiepileptic drugs. *Epilepsia* 2000; 41(Suppl 9):2–6.
66. Guelen PJM. General discussion. In: Schneider J, Janz D, Gardner-Thorpe C, Meinardi H, et al, eds. *Clinical Pharmacology of Anti-Epileptic Drugs*. New York: Springer-Verlag, 1974:2–45.
67. Dodson WE. Kinetics of antiepileptic drugs in children. In: Schoolar JC, Claghorn JL, eds. *The Kinetics of Psychiatric Drugs*. New York: Brunner/Mazel, 1979: 227–242.
68. Korenchevsky V. Physiological and pathological aging. New York: Hafner Publishing Company, 1961:160–162.
69. Roberts RJ. Drug therapy in infants. Philadelphia: WB Saunders, 1984:346–372.
70. Yerby MS. Problems and management of the pregnant woman with epilepsy. *Epilepsia* 1987; 28(Suppl 3):S29–S36.
71. Hagg S, Spigset O. Anticonvulsant use during lactation. *Drug Saf* 2000; 22:425–440.
72. Wong SH. Monitoring of drugs in breast milk. *Ann Clin Lab Sci* 1985; 15:100–105.
73. Nau H, Kuhnz W, Egger HJ, Rating D, et al. Anticonvulsants during pregnancy and lactation. Transplacental, maternal and neonatal pharmacokinetics. *Clin Pharmacokinet* 1982; 7:508–543.
74. Rating D, Nau H, Kuhnz W, Jager-Roman E, et al. Antiepileptika in der Neugeborenenperiode. *Monatsschr Kinderheilkd* 1983; 131:6–12.
75. Tomson T, Ohman I, Vitols S. Lamotrigine in pregnancy and lactation: a case report. *Epilepsia* 1997; 38:1039–1041.
76. Tran A, O'Mahoney T, Rey E, Mai J, et al. Vigabatrin: placental transfer in vivo and excretion into breast milk of the enantiomers. *Br J Clin Pharmacol* 1998; 45: 409–411.
77. Brodie MJ. Management of epilepsy during pregnancy and lactation. *Lancet* 1990; 336:426–427.
78. Johannessen SI. Pharmacokinetics of valproate in pregnancy: mother-foetus-newborn. *Pharm Weekbl Sci* 1992; 14:114–117.
79. Tomson T, Villen T. Ethosuximide enantiomers in pregnancy and lactation. *Ther Drug Monit* 1994; 16:621–623.

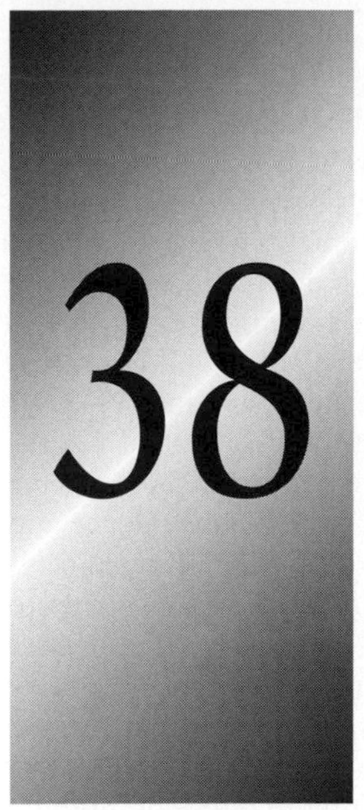

Dosage Form Considerations in the Treatment of Pediatric Epilepsy

William R. Garnett
James C. Cloyd

The successful treatment of pediatric epilepsy requires an accurate diagnosis and seizure classification, individualization of antiepileptic drug (AED) dose, and patient adherence. Because pediatric patients may have difficulty swallowing large, solid dosage forms, the successful treatment of pediatric epilepsy is complicated by the necessity of having a dosage form that can be administered to all pediatric patients, including infants and small children. Because Phase III efficacy trials are usually done in adults, dosage forms convenient for pediatric patients are usually not developed until the compound has been proven efficacious. There has been an increase in the number of AEDs that have dosage forms convenient for use in pediatric patients. Also, because of the nonadherence associated with multiple daily dosing, the pharmaceutical industry has developed extended-release formulations that can be given once or twice a day. This technology has also been applied to AEDs. These dosage forms offer the ability to individualize drug administration; however, ignoring the differences among dosage forms can result in a failure of the patient to receive full therapeutic benefit of the medication.

THEORETICAL ASPECTS IN ANTIEPILEPTIC DOSAGE FORM SELECTION

Intravenous Formulations

When an AED is administered intravenously, high blood drug concentrations may be reached very quickly, allowing the drug to distribute rapidly throughout the body (1, 2). Only drugs that are water soluble or that are soluble in a solvent that has little or no pharmacologic activity can be formulated for an intravenous (IV) dosage form. In some cases (e.g., phenytoin), the solvent may contribute to the toxicity that results from excessively rapid infusion (3). Intravenous dosage forms usually are more expensive than oral formulations. The IV administration of AEDs requires the presence of trained medical personnel and specialized equipment, such as infusion pumps and monitoring equipment, which also add to the cost of therapy. Therefore, IV drug administration is indicated only when rapid attainment of blood levels is needed, as in status epilepticus or when the patient is unable or unwilling to take medications by mouth.

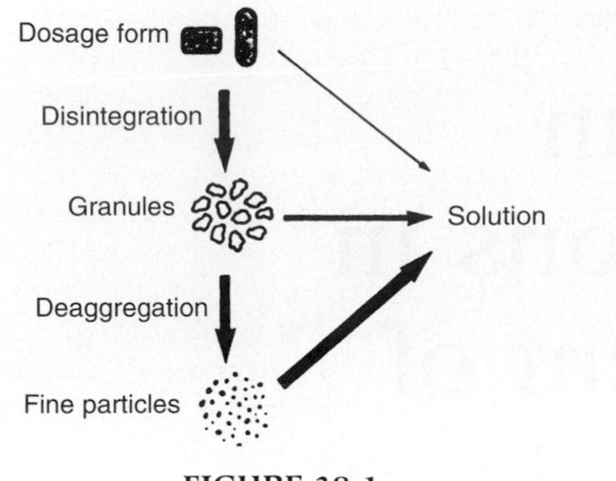

FIGURE 38-1

Drug disintegration and absorption. Reproduced from (1) by permission.

Oral Formulations

Following oral administration, capsules or tablets first must disintegrate, liberating the drug, which then must dissolve in an un-ionized state into intraintestinal fluids before being absorbed (Figure 38-1). While immediate-release drugs are designed to be liberated in the stomach, other drugs, such as Depakote®, are formulated to delay drug liberation until the drug reaches the small intestine. Other medications, such as Tegretol-XR®, Carbatrol®, Depakote-ER, and Phenytek® are liberated throughout the gastrointestinal (GI) tract at controlled rates, providing extended release. The dissolution time (the time to dissolve in GI fluids) may be altered by the surface area of the particles. The smaller the particle size, the faster the rate of dissolution. Liquid dosage forms, such as solution (in which the drug is already dissolved) and suspension (in which the drug is suspended as very small particles), generally display more rapid absorption than solid dosage forms. The rate of absorption for oral formulations usually conforms to the following order: solutions > suspensions > capsules > tablets.

Immediate-release oral solids are designed to disperse all of the medication quickly after ingestion. This usually is followed by rapid absorption. If the drug has a short half-life, multiple daily doses are required to prevent peak concentrations, which may result in side effects, and trough concentrations, which may be associated with seizures. Multiple daily doses may result in poor compliance. There is a trend in pharmaceutical development to develop dosage forms that release drug slowly over time rather than all at once.

Dosage forms that are designed to release their drug content slowly have been referred to as controlled-release, prolonged-release, time-release, slow-release, sustained-release, prolonged-action, or extended-action. Although there is some interchange in these terms, there are technical differences. A controlled-release dosage form is a system in which the rate of release is regulated and is supposed to be constant during GI transit. A sustained-release dosage form releases its contents over an extended period of time. Sustained-release dosage forms provide for the immediate release of an amount of drug that is immediately absorbed and then gradual and continual release of additional drug over the dosing interval. The advantages of controlled-release and sustained-release dosage formulations are (1) reduction in blood drug level fluctuations, (2) enhanced patient convenience and adherence, (3) reduction in adverse side effects, and (4) reduction in health care costs. Potential disadvantages to controlled-release and sustained-release formulations are (1) prolonged effects if the patient develops an adverse drug reaction or is accidentally intoxicated, (2) the possibility of interactions with the contents of the GI tract, and (3) changes in GI motility resulting in "dose dumping," or all of the drug being absorbed at once (4).

Most drugs are weak acids or weak bases and exist in solution as an equilibrium between the ionized and the un-ionized forms. In these cases, it is the un-ionized form in the gut that passively crosses the GI membrane. A continuous flow of blood to the GI tract ensures movement of drug from an area of high concentration in the gut to an area of relatively low concentration in the blood. Once a drug is dissolved, the rate of absorption is determined by the ratio of ionized to un-ionized forms, because it is the un-ionized form that can diffuse across membranes. Weak acids are absorbed more rapidly at pH 1.0 than at pH 8.0, and the converse is true for weak bases, because there is more of the un-ionized form present. The formulation of poorly soluble drugs as salts may enhance solubility and result in better absorption. Physiologically or pharmacologically induced changes in the GI pH may affect the disintegration of tablets or capsules, the dissolution time, and/or the equilibrium between the ionized and un-ionized forms, which alters the rate and/or amount of drug absorption (4).

Some drugs are absorbed by active transport processes. For example, gabapentin is carried across the GI membrane via a transport enzyme (5). Absorption may became saturated with this type of process. When the amount of drug in the GI tract is low relative to the number of transport enzyme-binding sites, the extent of absorption is high and constant. As the amount of drug approaches the capacity limits of the transport enzymes, the fraction of the dose that is absorbed per unit of time decreases. As a result, increases in dose produce less than proportional increases in serum concentration.

Some of the drug may be metabolized as it passes across the gut wall. Further metabolism may take place in the liver before the drug reaches the systemic circulation. This phenomenon is known as first-pass metabolism. Systemic bioavailability depends on the amount of drug absorbed across the gut wall and the degree of first-pass metabolism occurring in the GI tract and the liver before the drug reaches the systemic circulation. If a drug has extensive first-pass metabolism, it may not be suitable for oral administration.

The manufacturing process of the dosage form may affect absorption. There are no legal requirements for the excipients used in solid dosage formulations. Excipients may vary from manufacturer to manufacturer and cause different absorption rates that in-vitro dissolution tests do not detect. A change in the excipients of a phenytoin capsule in Australia resulted in greater bioavailability and an epidemic of phenytoin toxicity (6, 7). Other aspects of manufacturing may differ, such as tablet hardness and friability. The particle size of the active ingredient may also be different. Thus, there may be different rates and amounts of drug absorbed from the same dosage form made by different manufacturers. Sometimes there may be differences in absorption between lots of the same manufacturer.

Oral absorption may be altered by a variety of physiologic and pharmacologic phenomena. For example, food decreases the rate but not the extent of absorption of valproic acid, which results in a delayed time to peak (8). Food enhances the bioavailability of carbamazepine (9). Achlorhydria or the coadministration of drugs that reduce or neutralize gastric acid may alter disintegration and dissolution and affect absorption. Antacids in large doses decrease the absorption of phenytoin (10). For drugs with significant first-pass metabolism, food may alter hepatic blood flow and compete with liver enzymes to increase the systemic bioavailability of drugs. Foods and drugs may affect gastric emptying time and drug absorption.

Absorption usually is greater in the small intestine than in the stomach, because the surface area is larger, the permeability is higher, and the blood flow is greater. Therefore, absorption may be altered by changes in gastric emptying and GI transit times. Diarrhea may decrease the absorption of phenytoin and other slowly absorbed drugs because GI transit rate is increased and reduces drug contact time at intestinal absorption sites (3).

Age per se may alter absorption. In the newborn the intragastric pH and the efficiency of gut enzymes change rapidly (11, 12). Because of relative achlorhydria in the newborn and infant, there should be an increased absorption of acid-labile drugs such as penicillin (13). Age effects on pharmacokinetics are discussed in Chapter 37.

Generic Formulations

When the patent of a drug expires, companies other than the innovator of the drug may manufacture the generic equivalent. The U.S. Food and Drug Administration (FDA) is concerned about generic equivalency, and generic manufacturers must compare their product with that of the innovator. Bioequivalence tests are determined in vivo to prove that there is no difference in the two products. This usually is done by administering a single equal dose of the brand-name formulation and the generic drug to a population of between 24 and 36 normal healthy adults in a randomized, double-blind, crossover design. Multiple blood samples are collected to determine the amount of drug absorbed, as assessed by the total area under the concentration-time curve (AUC) and the rate of drug absorption as determined by the peak concentration (C_{max}), and the time to maximum concentration (T_{max}). The means of these parameters are determined, and a ratio of the log-transformed data is determined. Bioequivalence is accepted when the 90% confidence intervals of the ratios of AUC, C_{max}, and T_{max} fall between 0.8 and 1.25 of those of the branded drug. A popular misconception is that total absorption may vary between 80% and 125%. In fact, a difference in bioavailability between innovator and generic that is greater than 6% would result in confidence intervals that fall below 0.8 or above 1.25. Unfortunately, generics are only compared to the innovator and never to each other for regulatory approval. The lot-to-lot consistency of brand and generic drugs are regulated by in-vitro dissolution rate testing (14).

The FDA Center for Drug Evaluation and Research publishes annually a listing of approved drug products. The official title of this publication is *Approved Drug Products with Therapeutic Equivalence Evaluations*, but it is commonly known as the Orange Book. The FDA has an A rating and B code for generic drugs. An A coded drug is one that is considered to be therapeutically equivalent to other pharmaceutically equivalent products. For example, a drug with an AB rating would be considered to be products meeting bioequivalence reqirements. This applys to all oral generic AEDs. An AA rating applies to conventional dosage forms not presenting bioequivalence problems. This would apply to IV dosage forms such as those for valproic acid. A B code applies to drug products that the FDA does not consider to be therapeutically equivalent to other pharmaceutically equivalent products (15). There are no AEDs with a B code.

Since generic drugs often are less expensive, they may offer an advantage for many patients. The AMA has recognized the equivalency of generic drugs (15). When generic drugs are prescribed, it would be ideal for the patient to remain on the formulation from one supplier. The American Academy of Neurology (AAN) has cautioned against switching suppliers for carbamazepine and phenytoin (16). However, practically this may be difficult to accomplish. Clinicians should know when the source of an AED is being changed. The AAN has recommended that generic switching of AEDs not be done without the consent of the prescriber (17).

Intramuscular Formulations

Absorption of drugs from muscle and subcutaneous tissue is dependent on solubility, ionization, and tissue perfusion. Increases in tissue blood flow increase absorption. Physical activity that changes blood flow rates alters the rate of drug absorption from intramuscular (IM) injections. The location of the injection site also influences the rate of absorption. A standard part of nursing care is to rotate the sites of injection to prevent damage to a particular area. Because different muscle tissues have varying perfusion rates, the rotation of injection sites may result in varying rates of absorption. Injections into muscle tissue have different rates of absorption than injections into fatty tissue. In contrast, the extent of absorption is 100% unless drug is degraded in the tissue. The injection of IM drugs always causes some degree of discomfort, may be irritating to the tissue, and in some cases may result in muscle damage. IM injections require skilled personnel, which limits their use. Therefore, IM injections should be limited to short-term situations.

ALTERNATE ROUTES OF ADMINISTRATION: BUCCAL/SUBLINGUAL, NASAL, AND RECTAL

General Considerations

Occasionally methods of drug administration other than oral and parenteral routes are needed to treat patients. Circumstances such as out-of-hospital therapy of seizure emergencies, or bridge therapy when taking medications by mouth is not possible, require alternate routes of administration. The choice of therapy depends on the drug's physical, chemical, and pharmacokinetic characteristics, the route of administration, and the indication. These characteristics vary substantially among AEDs. For a given drug, factors such as water and lipid solubility, formulation characteristics, the relative size of the absorptive surface area, and retention time at the absorption site will dictate the onset and intensity of effect. Highly lipid-soluble compounds administered as solutions exhibit the most rapid and consistent absorption. Conversely, poorly water-soluble AEDs administered as suspensions or solid dosage forms may exhibit slow absorption that may permit extended dosing intervals if drug can be retained at the site of administration (18).

Buccal/Sublingual Administration

Buccal administration is defined as placement of a drug formulation in the buccal pouch of the oral cavity. The buccal mucosa is rich in blood supply, leading to rapid, systemic drug absorption. The pH of the buccal cavity is approximately 6.5 and the cavity has a surface area of 200 cm^2, which is similar to the areas of the rectal and nasal cavities. Sublingual administration refers to placement of drug, usually as a solid formulation, under the tongue, with absorption occurring at the mucosal epithelium. The absorptive surface area is smaller than that of the buccal cavity, and the drug product can be easily displaced unless disintegration and dissolution are rapid (i.e., within seconds) (18).

Compared with other routes of administration, the practical advantages of buccal administration are obvious: It is much simpler and safer than intravenous or intramuscular injections; it is less embarrassing and inconvenient for patients and caregiviers than intrarectal administration; and it may permit use of larger volumes than would be possible via intranasal administration (18).

Buccal administration, however, has several disadvantages. The maximum rate of absorption is obtained when the solution can be spread uniformly over the buccal pouch and retained in the buccal cavity. This may be difficult to accomplish if the patient's head is moving, as might occur during a seizure, which can result in the pooling or swallowing of the drug solution. Moreover, placement of drug in the buccal pouch during a seizure may be hazardous for both the patient and the caregiver and runs counter to first-aid guidelines for seizures. Regarding sublingual administration, similar problems exist with placement and retention of the formulation under the tongue. When given as solutions, volumes must be small, which often limits the size of the dose. These routes are best suited to treatment of seizure emergencies (18). Research results on this route of administration are discussed in a later section in this chapter.

Intranasal Administration

The advantages of intranasal drug delivery include easy access; lack of need for patient cooperation; and the possibility of rapid and extensive absorption of selected drugs, resulting in a rapid onset of effect. Overall, the needle-free administration of a drug via the intranasal route is simple and convenient. There are several disadvantages: Only small volumes (<200 μL per nostril) can be administered; the absorptive surface area of the nasal cavity (200 cm^2) is limited; and the residence time in the cavity is only about 15 minutes as fluids are drained from the nasal cavity to the throat. The choice of therapeutic agent administered intranasally therefore must be limited to highly potent, lipid-soluble drugs administered as solutions. The limitation in volume and the short residence time make this route best suited for treatment of seizure emergencies (18). Results of research on this route of administration are discussed in a later section in this chapter.

Rectal Formulations

The rectum is a useful route of administration, although there is little intraluminal fluid and the absorptive surface is only 1/10,000 that of the upper GI tract. The disintegration and dissolution problems associated with oral dosage formulations also occur with rectal dosage formulations (19). Solutions and suppositories are the most commonly used rectal dosage forms. Suppositories usually are formulated with a quick-melting base such as cocoa butter. Adequate retention time in the rectum is essential for complete absorption from the rectal dosage forms. Highly lipid-soluble compounds are more rapidly absorbed than less soluble, ionized drugs. The inability to retain the suppository or solution diminishes the usefulness of this route of administration. In contrast to oral administration, first-pass metabolism is significantly reduced with rectal administration—particularly when drug is absorbed from the lower two-thirds of the rectum, where venous drainage bypasses the liver. Rectal administration can be used both for treatment of seizure emergencies and for bridge therapy when a patient is unable to take maintenance AED therapy by mouth. Rectal administration of particular AEDs is discussed in greater detail later in this chapter.

SELECTION OF PARENTERAL AND ORAL ANTIEPILEPTIC DOSAGE FORMS IN PEDIATRIC PATIENTS

The factors that influence the selection of a particular dosage form for a child include the need for rapid attainment of therapeutic blood concentrations, the importance of maintaining therapeutic concentrations throughout a dosing interval, the ability to swallow, the ability to retain a rectal dosage form, the palatability of the oral dosage form, and cost.

Ideally, the drug should be available in a parenteral form for IV and IM administration as well as in oral solid and liquid formulations. The availability of a rectal formulation would allow greater flexibility in dosing. Among the AEDs used for maintenance therapy, only phenytoin, phenobarbital, levetiracetum, and valproic acid are available as parenteral formulations. Diazepam is now available in a gel formulation specifically designed for rectal administration.

For maintenance therapy, oral dosage forms are preferable because they are relatively inexpensive and easy to administer. Therefore, when the patient is able to swallow, the AED should be given orally. If the patient is not able to take a tablet or capsule, consideration should be given to chewable tablets or liquids. Patients with a nasogastric tube may be given liquid AEDs, which negates the need for chronic parenteral therapy. Obviously, liquid medicines should be palatable or capable of being mixed with beverages or enteral feedings without interactions so that the patient is able to ingest the medicine. It is possible to give loading doses of oral medications to attain a therapeutic concentrations more quickly. However, this is often neither rapid enough nor feasible when dealing with an emergency such as status epilepticus.

Phenytoin/Fosphenytoin

Phenytoin is available in parenteral, capsule, chewable tablet, and suspension formulations. Phenytoin is poorly soluble in water; thus, the parenteral formulation contains propylene glycol and ethanol and is buffered to a pH of 12 to keep the drug in solution. The solvents have inherent pharmacologic activity, including cardiac arrhythmias and hypotension. The combination of cosolvent effects and the alkaline pH commonly cause pain and inflammation at the infusion site. Therefore, phenytoin infusions are limited to a rate no faster than 1 to 3 mg/kg/ min in otherwise healthy children (3). Because of the high ionization constant (pK_a) of phenytoin, it is not stable in every IV solution. Phenytoin may be mixed with normal saline in concentration ranges of 2 to 20 mg/mL. Use of an in-line 20-micron filter is recommended to reduce the risk of infusing small particle precipitants. Admixtures should be stored for no longer than 24 hours (20).

Although the parenteral formulation of phenytoin may be given by IM injection, this route is not recommended. The high pK_a of phenytoin results in crystallization in muscle tissue. This results in slow and erratic absorption (21). In addition, IM phenytoin is quite painful and may cause muscle damage (22).

Fosphenytoin is a phenytoin prodrug formed by the addition of a phosphate ester group to the phenytoin molecule. The phosphate ester significantly increases the water solubility of fosphenytoin. The phosphate ester must be cleaved and the compound converted to phenytoin to exert pharmacologic activity. The conversion is done by systemic phosphatases that are found throughout the body. The conversion of fosphenytoin to phenytoin is rapid and complete. The phosphatases are not affected by age, gender, race, hepatic impairment, or renal function (23). An ex-vivo study using blood obtained from premature infants and neonates demonstrated that fosphenytoin is converted to phenytoin in these populations.

Because fosphenytoin is more water soluble than phenytoin, it does not require propylene glycol or ethanol to increase solubility. Fosphenytoin is compatible with all IV fluids, whereas phenytoin should be admixed only with normal saline. Fosphenytoin does not require an inline filter as phenytoin does (24). Fosphenytoin may be given at a much faster IV infusion rate than phenytoin, and the infusion rate does not need to be altered because of age or underlying cardiac disease. The maximum rate of infusion of fosphenytoin is 150 mg/min compared with

50 mg/min for phenytoin. This means that the patient can be loaded in less time. Fosphenytoin is rapidly converted to phenytoin after administration, with a conversion half-life of approximately 15 minutes. Fosphenytoin is highly protein-bound, as is phenytoin. Therefore, fosphenytoin competes with phenytoin for binding sites, which increases the "free" or unbound portion of phenytoin. When both drugs are given at the maximum rate of administration, fosphenytoin achieves bioequivalency with phenytoin in 7 minutes. If the rate of phenytoin is slowed, higher concentrations of phenytoin may be achieved with the administration of fosphenytoin (25). Another advantage of fosphenytoin is that in comparative studies it causes less thrombophlebitis and less burning, pain, or irritation at the injection site. This results in fewer changes in the site of administration (26). The decreased venous irritation is a particular advantage in premature infants, neonates, and children, in whom venous access is a serious problem. The primary side effects of fosphenytoin are pruritus and paresthesias, which are common to phosphate esters and disappear with a reduction in the infusion rate or when the infusion is completed.

Fosphenytoin can safely be given intramuscularly. Peak phenytoin concentrations occur about 3 hours following IM fosphenytoin. However, free phenytoin concentrations in the accepted target range occur in approximately 30 minutes after an IM injection of fosphenytoin (27). There is no pain or necrosis associated with fosphenytoin after IM administration, and the absorption is rapid and complete. Loading doses of 20 mg/kg have been safely given intramuscularly. In adults, volumes exceeding 20 mL have been safely given as a single injection (28). When given as replacement therapy, fosphenytoin is completely converted to phenytoin, whereas oral phenytoin sodium capsules are 92% phenytoin. Therefore, the trough concentrations may increase. If the patient is at the point of enzyme saturation for phenytoin metabolism, there may be a significant increase in blood concentrations (29).

As noted in Chapter 49, the various formulations of phenytoin differ in content of phenytoin (Table 38-1). The capsule and parenteral formulations of phenytoin contain sodium phenytoin and are only 92% phenytoin. The suspension and chewable tablet formulations of phenytoin contain phenytoin acid and are 100% phenytoin. Because of the Michaelis-Menten kinetics of phenytoin, these salt differences should be considered when switching dosage forms. Although it would be anticipated that the rate of absorption of the phenytoin suspension would be faster than the rate of absorption from the capsule, a single-dose study in normal volunteers demonstrated that the time to peak concentration, C_{max}, and AUC time curve for phenytoin extended-release capsules were not different from these parameters for phenytoin suspension when the dose of the suspension was adjusted for the difference in salt concentration (30). It was postulated that the rate of absorption is more dependent on particle size than on formulation. There are also differences in the rate of absorption among the various manufacturers of phenytoin capsules. The innovator's formulation (Dilantin®) provides an extended release. Some of the generic formulations provide faster release. Phenytoin is thus labeled as either prompt-release or extended-release capsules. The FDA recommends that only the extended-release capsules be used for once-a-day dosing (31). The difference in the rate and extent of absorption between the prompt-release and extended-release capsules may affect how rapidly peak concentrations of phenytoin can be obtained. The extended-release capsules display a slower rate and extent of absorption as the dose is increased. This suggests that oral doses need to be larger than IV doses to achieve the same concentration (32). However, if prompt-release capsules are used, phenytoin concentrations are achieved more rapidly, and the prompt-release capsule has been suggested as an alternative in situations where an IV injection is not possible or practical (33). The chewable tablet seems to have a similar absorption profile to phenytoin extended-release capsules when adjusted for salt content.

Although the suspension dosage form has been considered to have rapid settling properties, a recent report measuring settling rates in bottles of phenytoin suspension that were well shaken and then left untouched revealed that no differences in the concentration could be found between the top and bottom of the bottle from time 15 minutes to 4 weeks after resuspension. Only after 5 weeks after resuspension was there a difference between the aliquots taken from the top and the bottom

TABLE 38-1
Phenytoin Content of Various Products

Product Listed	Compound	Phenytoin Strength	Content
Phenytoin capsule	Phenytoin sodium	100 mg	92 mg
Phenytoin capsule	Phenytoin sodium	30 mg	27.5 mg
Fosphenytoin parenteral	Fosphenytoin sodium	50 mg PE/mL	46 mg PE/mL
Phenytoin suspension	Phenytoin	125 mg/5 mL	125 mg/5 mL
Phenytoin chewable tablet	Phenytoin	50 mg	50 mg
Phenytoin parenteral	Phenytoin sodium	50 mg/mL	46 mg

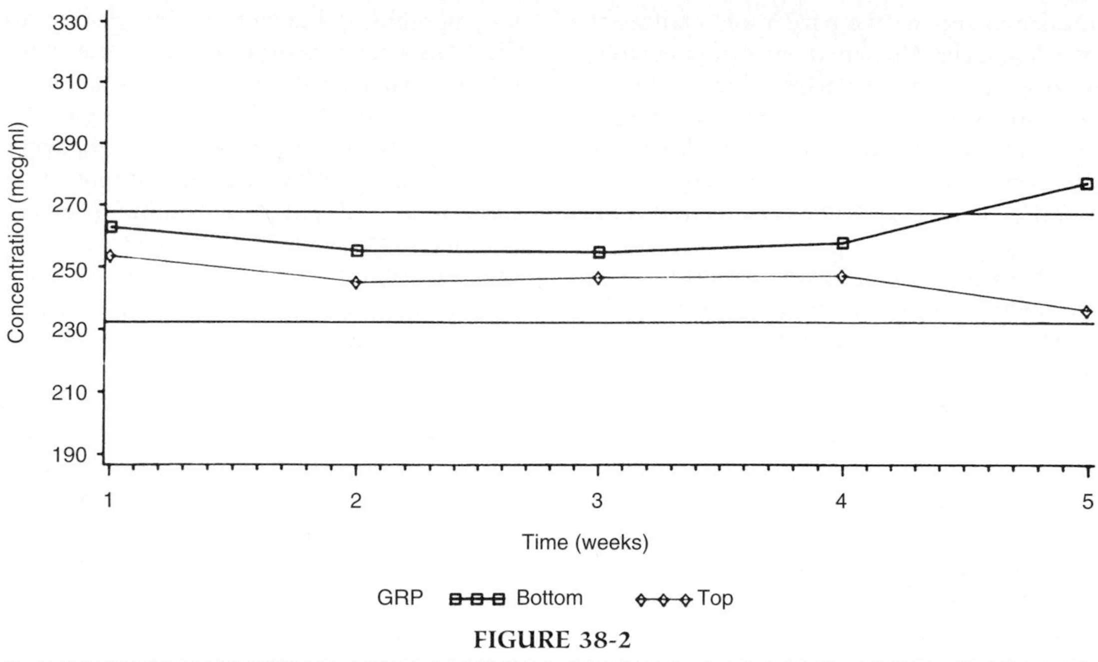

FIGURE 38-2

Long-term concentration vs. time effect of packaged phenytoin suspension. "Bottom" and "Top" indicate that concentrations were measured in suspensions taken from the bottom and top of the bottle, respectively. Reproduced from *Neurology*, February 1989, by permission.

of the bottle (Figure 38-2) (34). In the same study a dose (5.0 mL) was measured every day simulating patient use by a well-shaken technique (vigorous shaking), a poorly shaken technique (inverted once), and an unshaken technique until the bottle was depleted. Only the unshaken technique demonstrated differences in the doses taken (Figure 38-3). It was concluded that phenytoin suspension requires minimal agitation to be uniformly mixed and that it has a slow rate of settling. The problems reported with phenytoin suspension in the past possibly reflect

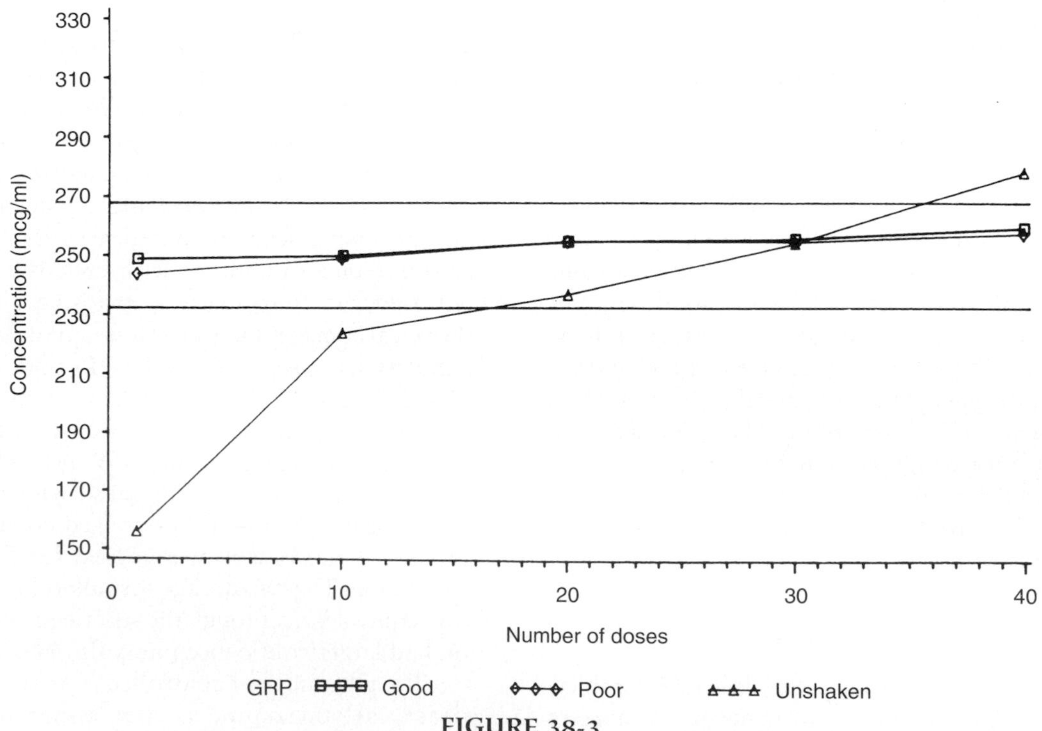

FIGURE 38-3

Effect of shaking techniques on concentration of dose of phenytoin. Reproduced from *Neurology*, February 1989, by permission.

inaccurate measurements by the patient or a failure to understand the Michaelis-Menten kinetics of phenytoin. This dosage form may be very acceptable for young children or for patients with difficulty in swallowing. An accurate measuring device should be used for administration. When changing from oral to nasogastric administration, levels may decrease substantially (see later discussion on nasogastric tubes).

Phenytek™ Capsules contain either 200 mg or 300 mg of the sodium salt of phenytoin. This formulation employs an erodible-matrix delivery system for the extended release of phenytoin. The 200 mg Phenytek™ Capsule has two, and the 300 mg Phenytek™ Capsule has three, erodible-matrix tablets. After ingestion, the capsule shell dissolves to expose the two or three tablets inside. As the outer surfaces of the tablets hydrate, a gel layer containing phenytoin sodium is formed. The initial release of phenytoin sodium from the external layer of the tablets occurs at this stage. Water permeates farther into the erodible matrix, thickening the gel layer and allowing soluble drug to continue diffusing out of the tablets. Once the outer layer of each erodible-matrix tablet is fully hydrated, phenytoin sodium is gradually dissolved in the gastric fluids. Concurrently,water continues to permeate toward the core of the tablet. This multistep process allows solubilized drug to be gradually diffused from the gel layer. In addition, erosion of the tablets over time allows drug to be released by direct exposure to gastric fluids. Phenytoin is released from the tablets in a slow and extended rate with peak concentrations expected in 4 to 12 hours following a single dose. The peak concentrations of prompt-release phenytoin capsules occur within 1.5 to 3 hours. Phenytek™ Capsules are approved for once-a-day dosing. Studies comparing three divided doses of 100 mg of phenytoin to a single daily 300-mg dose of Phenytek™ Capsules indicated that absorption, peak plasma levels, biologic half-life, difference between peak and minimum values, and urinary recovery were equivalent. Two studies comparing the pharmacokinetics of one 300-mg Phenytek™ Capsule to three 100-mg phenytoin (Dilantin®) capsules demonstrated that the two doses were bioequivalent. In the study comparing the effects of food on the bioavailability of phenytoin given as Phenytek™ and Dilantin®, the phenytoin AUC and T_{peak} were slightly lower with Phenytek™. However, the C_{peak} and half-life with Phenytek™ were slightly greater than with Dilantin® Kapseals®, and the products were considered bioequivalent. Phenytek™ Capsules should not be opened and the contents crushed or taken separately (35).

Carbamazepine

Carbamazepine is available as a chewable tablet, tablet, and suspension. A single-dose study in normal volunteers demonstrated that the bioavailability of chewable tablets is comparable to the bioavailability of swallowed tablets (36). The rate of absorption of carbamazepine suspension is faster than that of carbamazepine tablets in single-dose studies in normal volunteers (37). A multidose bioavailability study in epileptic patients comparing equal total daily doses of carbamazepine suspension administered three times a day to tablets administered twice a day also demonstrated that the suspension is absorbed faster than the tablets (Figure 38-4). However, there were no differences in the C_{max}, the AUC time curve, or the peak-to-trough fluctuations for either the parent drug or the 10,11-epoxide metabolite (38) (Table 38-2). If the faster absorption rate is not considered in scheduling dosage administration times, the suspension will produce higher peaks (greater chance of side effects) and lower troughs (greater chance of loss of efficacy) than a comparable dose using carbamazepine tablets.

There are controlled-release and sustained-release dosage forms of carbamazepine. The controlled-release formulation is Tegretol-XR®, which utilizes an osmotic release delivery system. The formulation is provided in a wax matrix with a permeable membrane. This allows water from gastric contents to enter the matrix and increase the osmotic pressure. This forces the drug out at a constant rate. For the 100-mg tablet, 10 mg of drug is released per hour for the first 7 or 8 hours and then the rest of the drug is released. The casing of the tablet is excreted in the feces. Patients should be told that although casings will appear in the stool, the drug is being absorbed. Any disruption to the tablet results in a loss of the controlled-release design. Therefore, this controlled-release formulation must not be crushed, chewed, or opened (39). The sustained-release formulation is Carbatrol®, which uses three different types of beads: immediate-release, extended-release, and enteric-release. This formulation is a capsule, and it may be opened and mixed with food. The ability to use this formulation as a "sprinkle" is an advantage in pediatric patients (40).

Both controlled-release and sustained-release dosage forms have been compared with immediate-release carbamazepine in patients with epilepsy. Patients were converted from four-times-a-day dosing with immediate-release carbamazepine to twice-a-day dosing with both formulations in separate studies. In both studies twice-a-day dosing with controlled-release or sustained-release tablets was bioequivalent to the four-times-a-day dosing with immediate-release tablets (39, 40). The controlled-release formulation was compared with the sustained-release formulation in a randomized crossover study in normal volunteers who were dosed for 5 days on each formulation. The two dosage formulations were found to be bioequivalent, although the sustained-release formulation had larger confidence intervals (41).

The advantage of controlled-release and sustained-release carbamazepine is that either may be given twice a day. This optimizes convenience and promotes

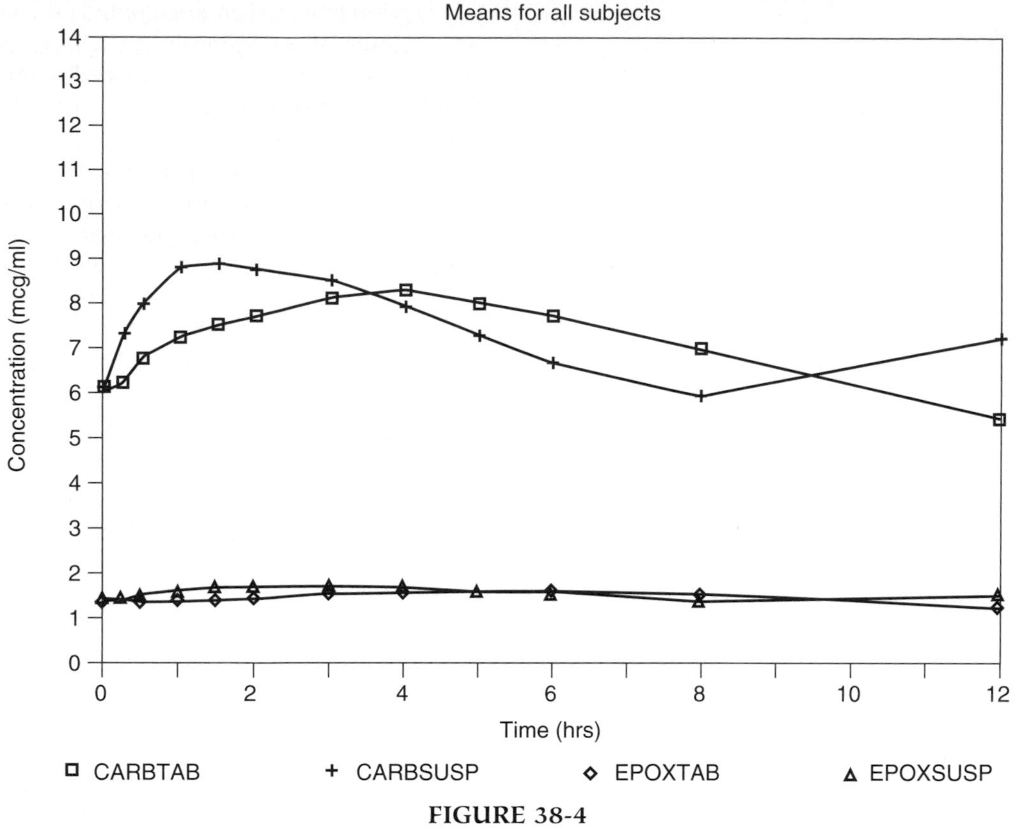

FIGURE 38-4

Twelve-hour concentration vs. time profile of carbamazepine tablets vs. suspension.

adherence. In a pediatric patient who cannot or will not swallow oral solids, the sustained-release formulation can be opened and mixed with food.

Valproic Acid

Valproic acid is available as a soft gelatin capsule containing a liquid, an enteric-coated tablet, a coated particle (sprinkle) capsule, a hydrophylic matrix, controlled release tablet, a syrup, and an IV solution. The bioavailability of the soft gelatin capsule formulation is comparable to that of the solution. The enteric-coated tablet (Depakote) was developed to delay dissolution of the drug until after it leaves the stomach, thereby reducing the incidence of nausea, vomiting, and other types of GI distress. Although the enteric coating does delay and slow absorption, it does not result in true sustained release of valproic acid. For most drugs the minimum (trough) concentration occurs just before the next dose. In contrast, the delayed absorption of enteric-coated valproic

TABLE 38-2
Pharmacokinetic Comparison of Carbamazepine Tablets and Suspension

Statistical Parameter	Tablet	Suspension	Significance	Power	CI (%)
AUC 0–724	192.1	196.9	NS	0.73	12.8
C_{max}					
C_{max}	8.5	9.4	NS	0.97	18.4
T_{max}	3.7	1.5	$P < 0.05$	—	196.0
C_{min}	5.3	5.7	NS	<0.99	14.0
C_{max}					
C_{min}	1.7	1.7	NS	0.92	12.9
$Conc_{ss}$	8.0	8.2	NS	0.73	12.8

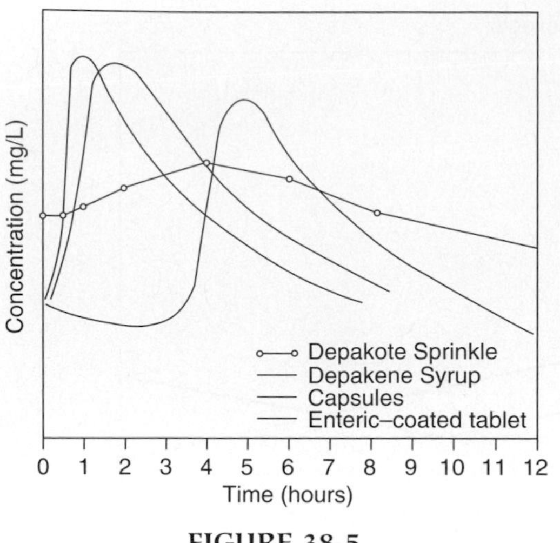

FIGURE 38-5

The effect of formulation on the time course of valproate absorption.

acid produces trough concentrations 2 to 4 hours after the dose when given on an empty stomach (Figure 38-5). Coadministration with food extends the time to the trough concentration from 2 to 8 hours after administration, and peak concentrations may occur just before the next dose (42). These changes in normal absorption profiles must be considered in evaluating blood concentrations, particularly if the timing between drug administration and meals varies. Recently, a diurnal effect on valproic acid absorption from the enteric-coated tablet was also shown (43) (Figure 38-6). Valproic acid is absorbed more slowly, and the amount of drug absorbed is reduced, at night. The enteric-coated dosage form should not be crushed before administering.

A coated particle (sprinkle) formulation of valproic acid is available. The sprinkle formulation is designed to provide slow consistent input, which minimizes peak to trough fluctuations (see Figure 38-5) (44). This dosage form allows the patient or parent to open the capsule and sprinkle the particles over food. It is intended for pediatric use and for patients who have difficulty swallowing solid dosage forms. This dosage form also is particularly useful for patients with large fluctuations between doses who require frequent dosing or who may experience distress with enteric-coated tablets.

Depakote® is an enteric coated dosage form of divalproex sodium. The enteric coating delays the absorption of divalproex sodium until after the drug has left the stomach. This enteric coating is designed to reduce the GI side effects associated with valproic acid. Depakote® is a *delayed-release* formulation; it is not an *extended-release* formulation (45). Depakote-ER® is a hydrophilic-matrix controlled-release tablet system and is an *extended-release* formulation (46). Upon entering the stomach, the film coating dissolves, exposing the hydrophilic polymer matrix tablet. The outer layer of the matrix becomes partially hydrated, forming a gel layer, and drug begins to be released. As fluid enters the tablet, the gel layer increases

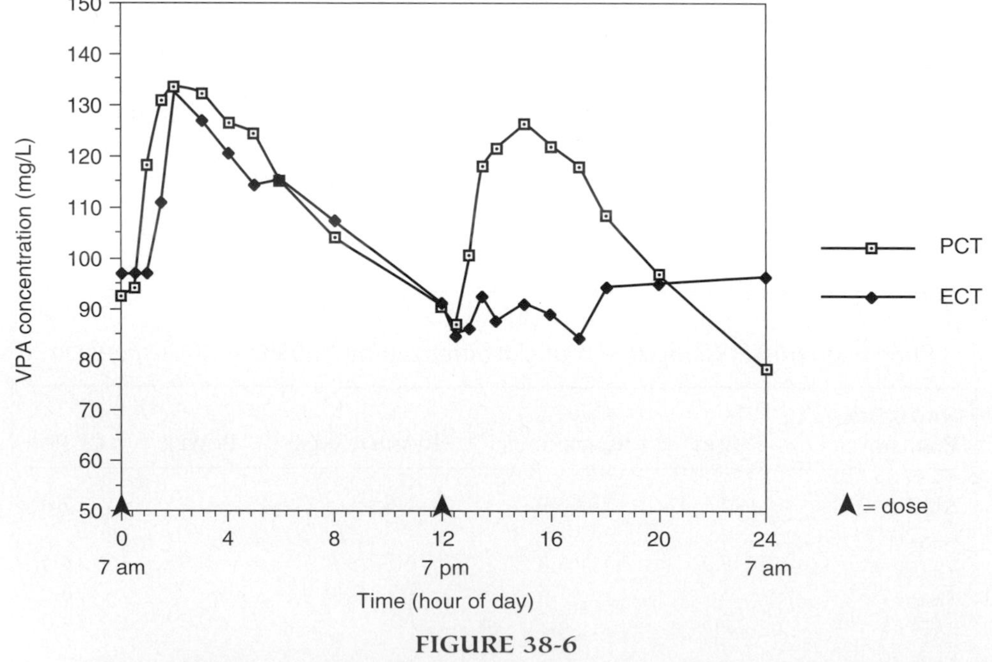

FIGURE 38-6

Twenty-four-hour total valproate concentration-time profile following particle and enteric-coated tablets. Reproduced from (43) by permission.

in thickness, extending the release of the drug. The matrix surface continues to become hydrated, allowing for a continued release of drug. Once the outer layer becomes fully hydrated, it erodes and is released from the tablet. Fluid continues to penetrate toward the tablet core. Thus this system of polymer wetting, polymer hydration, drug diffusion, and polymer erosion results in the release of drug in the stomach, small intestine, and large intestine over an 18- to 24-hour period (47, 48). Depakote-ER® is designed for once a day dosing (46).

The absolute bioavailability of Depakote-ER® administered as a single dose after a meal was approximately 80% to 90% relative to an intravenous infusion. In two multiple-dose studies, when administered either fasting or immediately before smaller meals, Depakote-ER® had an average bioavailability of 81%, compared to 89% for Depakote®. Maximum valproate plasma concentrations (C_{max}) in these studies were achieved on average 7 to 14 hours after the administration of Depakote-ER®. In one of these studies, the average C_{max} and minimum plasma concentration (C_{min}) at steady state of Depakote-ER® given fasting and with smaller meals were 74% and 82%, respectively, relative to Depakote® given twice a day with smaller meals. In the other study, the average C_{max} and C_{min} at steady state of Depakote-ER® were 81% and 85%, respectively, relative to Depakote® given fasting. After multiple dosing, Depakote-ER® given once daily has been shown to produce percent fluctuation (defined as 100% × (C_{max} – C_{min})/average concentration) that is 10% to 20% lower than that of regular Depakote® given twice a day. Depakote-ER® and Depakote® tablets are not bioequivalent (46). It has been recommended that, in converting a patient from Depakote® to Depakote-ER®, the total daily dose of Depakote® be increased by 14% to 20% given as the Depakote-ER® (49, 50).

VALPROATE SODIUM INJECTION (DEPACON®)

Valproate sodium is the sodium salt of valproic acid. It is supplied as a 5-mL single-dose vial containing 100 mg of valproic acid per mL. The initial indication of valproate sodium injection was for patients who were not able to take valproic acid orally. The initial infusion guidelines were to dilute the drug with at least 50 mL of a compatible diluent (dextrose 5% in water, normal saline, or lactated Ringer's solution) and administer as a 60-minute infusion. It was recommended that the drug not be given any faster than 20 mg/min. The initial dose was 10 to 15 mg/kg/day (51). In January 2002, the FDA approved an infusion rate of 1.5 to 3.0 mg/kg/min. Clinical studies have shown that higher loading doses and more rapid rates of infusion are well tolerated in pediatric patients. In a study done at the Virginia Commonwealth University/Medical College of Virginia, 10 patients ranging in age from 2.5 to 16.25 years of age received a total of 38 doses of IV valproate sodium given in doses ranging from 7.5 mg/kg/dose to 42 mg/kg/dose. The mean dose was 23.4 mg/kg/dose. The doses were infused at a rate of 1.5 mg/kg/min to 11 mg/kg/min with a mean rate of infusion of 6 mg/kg/min. No significant side effects were observed. A rapid rate of infusion may be desirable for patients in status epilepticus. Because the protein binding of valproic acid saturates around 50 µg/mL, a rapid rate of infusion would result in higher initial blood concentrations (52, 53). With the saturable binding there would be a higher free fraction. With a higher free fraction, there would be more free drug to diffuse across the blood-brain barrier (53). Rapid intravenous infusions of valproic acid have been used to treat status epilepticus and acute migraine headaches. Parenteral valproic acid should not be given by intramuscular injection.

Phenobarbital and Primidone

Phenobarbital is available in a parenteral form, a tablet, and a solution. The parenteral form can be given by rapid IV infusion or by IM injection. Absorption from the oral formulations seems to be complete and relatively rapid. Primidone is available as a tablet and an oral suspension. Absorption from both formulations appears complete, with peak concentrations occurring 2 to 6 hours after the dose (54).

Ethosuximide

Ethosuximide is available as a capsule and a solution. Absorption appears to be complete from both formulations. Ethosuximide has a long half-life even in children. However, some patients may develop GI side effects with once-a-day dosing and require twice-a-day dosing (54).

NEWER ANTIEPILEPTIC DRUGS

Felbamate

Felbamate (Felbatol®) is indicated for treatment of children with the Lennox-Gastaut syndrome. It is available as a 400-mg tablet, a 600-mg tablets and a 600 mg/5 mL suspension. Absorption is rapid and nearly complete following oral administration. The tablets and the suspension are bioequivalent to the capsules used in clinical trials. The pharmacokinetics of the tablet and the suspension are similar (55).

Gabapentin

Gabapentin (Neurontin®) has been studied in patients with epilepsy 3 years of age and older. In addition to having an indication of the treatment of refractory partial seizures, gabapentin is also indicated for the treatment of postherpetic neuralgia. Gabapentin is supplied as a 100-mg capsule, a 300-mg capsule, a 400-mg capsule, a 600-mg tablet, an 800-mg tablet, and a 250 mg/5 mL oral solution. The bioavailability of gabapentin is not dose proportional; that is, the increase in serum concentration is not proportional to the increase in dose. The administration of two 300-mg capsules and two 400-mg capsules have the same bioavailability as a single 600-mg tablet and a single 800-mg tablet. The manufacturer indicates that gabapentin may be administered by solution, capsule, tablet, or any combination of these formulations (56).

Lamotrigine

Lamotrigine (Lamictal®) is supplied as 25-mg, 100-mg, 150-mg, and 200-mg tablets and as 2-mg, 5-mg, and 25-mg chewable/dispersible tablets. The lamotrigine chewable/dispersible tablets were shown to be equivalent, whether they were administered dispersed in water, chewed and swallowed, or swallowed whole, to the lamotrigine compressed tablets in terms of rate and extent of absorption. The lamotrigine tablets should be swallowed whole because chewing them may leave a bitter taste. The chewable/dispersible tablet may be swallowed whole, chewed, or mixed in water or diluted fruit juice. If the tablets are chewed, consume a small amount of water or diluted fruit juice to aid in swallowing. To disperse the chewable/dispersible tablet, add the tablets to a small amount of liquid—1 teaspoon (5 mL), or enough to cover the medication—in a glass or spoon. Approximately 1 minute later, when the tablets are completely dispersed, mix the solution and take the entire amount immediately (57).

Topiramate

Topiramate (Topamax®) is available as 25-mg, 100-mg, and 200-mg tablets for oral administration and as 15-mg and 25-mg sprinkle capsules. The sprinkle capsule contains coated beads of topiramate in a hard gelatin capsule and may be swallowed whole or opened and sprinkled onto soft food. The sprinkle formulation is bioequivalent to the immediate-release tablet and may be substituted as a therapeutic equivalent. If the sprinkle capsule is to be administered as a sprinkle, the patient should be instructed to hold the capsule upright so that the word TOP can be read. The top should be carefully twisted off. This is best done over the food with which the drug is to be mixed. The entire contents of the capsule should be emptied onto a spoonful of soft food. The patient should swallow the entire contents of the spoonful of food and topiramate mixture. The patient should not chew the food or drug and should follow the ingestion of the food/drug mixture with fluids to ensure that the entire contents are swallowed. The mixture should never be stored for use later (58).

Tiagabine

Tiagabine (Gabatril®) is supplied as 2-mg, 4-mg, 12-mg, 16-mg, and 20-mg tablets. It is sparingly soluble in water. Tiagabine is well absorbed with food, slowing the rate of absorption but not the extent of absorption (59).

Levetiracetam

Levetiracetam (Keppra®) is manufactured as 250-mg, 500-mg, and 750-mg scored tablets. It is very soluble in water, and a solution dosage form is now approved. It may be given with or without food. Levetiracetam recently became available in an intravenous form. The IV dosage form is supplied in vials of 500 mg/5 mL. The drug should be diluted in 100 mL (100 mg/mL) of either sodium chloride 0.9%, lactated Ringer's injection, or Dextrose 5% injection USP. The recommended administration time for IV levetiracetam is 15 minutes (60).

Oxcarbazepine

Oxcarbazepine (Trileptal®) is completely absorbed and rapidly metabolized to its 10-monohydroxy derivative (MHD), which is the pharmacologically active component. Oxcarbazepine is available as 150-mg, 300-mg, and 600-mg tablets and as a 300 mg/5 mL oral suspension. The tablets and the suspension are considered to have the same bioavailability. After a single-dose administration of oxcarbazepine tablets to healthy male volunteers under fasted conditions, the median T_{max} was 4.5 (range 3 to 13) hours. After single-dose administration of oxcarbazepine suspension, the median T_{max} was 6 hours. A 10-mL dosing syringe and press-in bottle adapter are provided with oxcarbazepine suspension. The suspension should be used within 7 weeks of first opening the bottle (61).

Zonisamide

Zonisamide (Zonegran®) is supplied as a 100-mg capsule. Zonisamide may be taken with or without food. Although there is no solution or suspension dosage form of zonisamide commercially available, the capsule may be opened and mixed with apple sauce or juice. The solution is stable for two weeks (62).

Pregabalin

Pregabalin (Lyrica®) is supplied as 25, 50, 75, 100, 150, 200, 225, and 300-mg capsules (63).

RECTAL ADMINISTRATION OF AEDS

The rectal route of administration is a practical alternative when oral or parenteral routes are not available (19) (Table 38-3). Rectal administration is often useful in the treatment of emergent conditions, such as prolonged seizures, clusters of seizures, or status epilepticus, when access to a vein is delayed or when therapy is started at home. Additionally, rectal administration can substitute for oral administration of maintenance AEDs when the latter route is temporarily unavailable because of upper GI illnesses, dental procedures, abdominal surgery, or transient GI intolerance to medication (64). Occasionally, rectal administration is indicated when psychiatric or mentally handicapped patients refuse or are unable to take their medications. A commercial diazepam rectal formulation is available in the United States, and the parenteral solution can also be administered rectally.

Clonazepam

The injectable solution of clonazepam has been administered rectally to volunteers and patients (65, 66). Doses in patients have ranged from 0.05 to 0.1 mg/kg, which produce peak serum concentrations 10 to 120 minutes after administration of the dose. There is no information on the extent of absorption.

Carbamazepine

Carbamazepine has been given rectally as a suspension, a suppository, and a viscous gel solution (37, 67, 68). The commercially available suspension, when diluted and given rectally, is bioequivalent to the tablet given orally, but the peak concentration occurs later than when taken by mouth (37). The suspension is hypertonic, causing a strong urge to defecate. An extemporaneously prepared

TABLE 38-3
Antiepileptic Drugs Available for Rectal Administration

Treatment	Dosage	Drug Usefulness (mg/kg/dose)	Preparation	Pharmacokinetics	Comments
Carbamazepine	Maintenance	Same as oral	Oral suspension (dilute with equal volume of water) Suppository gel (CBZ powder dissolved in 20% alcohol and methyl hydroxy cellulose)	Peak concentration 4–8 h; 80% absorbed	Definite cathartic effect
Clonazepam	?Acute	0.020.1 mg	Parenteral solution	Peak concentration 0.1–2 h	Onset may be too slow for acute use
Diazepam	Acute	0.2–0.5 mg	Parenteral solution	Effect in 2–10 min; peak concentration 2–30 min	Well tolerated; nordiazepam accumulates with repeated doses
Lorazepam	Acute	0.05–0.1 mg	Parenteral solution	Peak concentration 0.5–2 h	Well tolerated
Paraldehyde	Acute	0.3 mL 5 – 25 mg	Oral solution (dilute with equal volume of mineral oil)	Effect in 20 min, peak concentration 2.5 h	Moderate cathartic effect; use glass syringe
Valproic acid	Acute	Same as oral	Oral solution (dilute with equal volume of water)	Peak concentration 1–3 h	Definite cathartic effect
	Maintenance		VPA liquid from capsule mixed into Supocire C lipid base	Peak concentration 2–4 h; 80% absorbed	Well tolerated

suppository has been evaluated in both healthy subjects and patients (67). It was more consistently absorbed than the commercial tablet, with a mean bioavailability of 67 percent and a T_{max} of 12 hours. A viscous gel containing 200 mg of carbamazepine and 250 mg of methylhydroxycellulose dissolved in 5 mL of 20% alcohol was administered in a single patient and produced therapeutic serum concentrations (44). Rectal carbamazepine is absorbed too slowly to be useful in treating status epilepticus, but it may be tried as temporary replacement therapy when the oral route is not available.

Diazepam

Diazepam has been given rectally as a solution or gel and a suppository. Rectal administration of diazepam solutions in children results in rapid and complete absorption, with peak concentrations attained within 5 to 15 minutes after administration (69–71) (Figure 38-7). Given the time needed to establish an IV line, the rectal administration of diazepam solution or gel is a practical alternative to IV diazepam in the acute management of severe seizures (72, 73). A double-blind, placebo-controlled trial demonstrated that a rectal diazepam gel (Diastat®) administered by parents or other caregivers was highly effective in interrupting clusters of seizures and reducing subsequent emergent care (74). Another study has shown that home use of a rectally administered diazepam solution was safe and effective in controlling prolonged seizures and preventing febrile convulsions (75). Rectal diazepam has been shown to reduce health care costs, to reduce caregiver burden, and to reduce parental stress. The most common side effect is somnolence and drowsiness. Suppositories are commercially available in some countries other than the United States, but they are not recommended because absorption is slow and erratic.

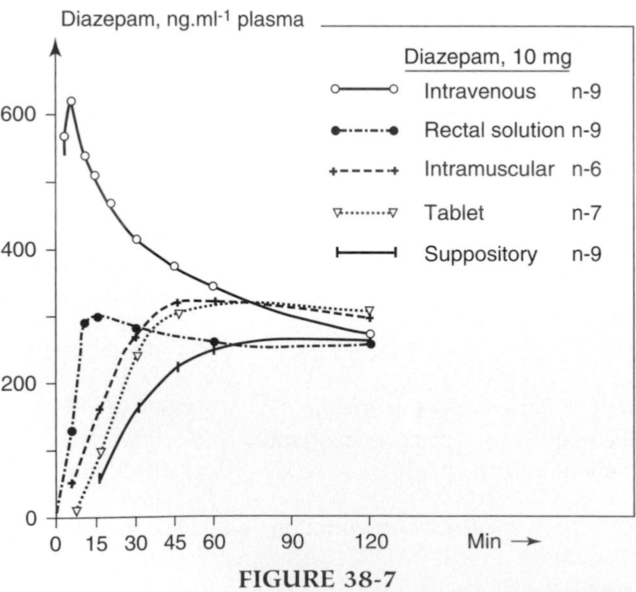

FIGURE 38-7

Plasma concentrations of diazepam following administration in different dosage forms. Reproduced from (30) by permission.

Felbamate

In a single case study, felbamate (FBM) was poorly absorbed rectally. The oral suspension was diluted 1:1 with saline and rectally administered to temporarily replace the oral dosing regimen in a 2-year old child for 4 days (76). FBM concentrations fell throughout rectal administration, indicating little to no absorption. FBM is a lipid-soluble, nonionized medication, making it unclear why it is so poorly absorbed.

Gabapentin

A report involving two children found that the bioavailability of a gabapentin solution given rectally ranged from 17% 29% (77). Therefore, it should not be administered rectally.

Lamotrigine

Two studies have assessed the bioavailability of lamotrigine compressed and chewable/dispersible tablets given rectally (78, 79). The tablets were crushed and suspended in. The bioavailability of these suspensions given rectally was compared to the bioavailability of the corresponding tablets given orally. These studies demonstrated that lamotrigine is absorbed rectally but that the bioavailability is less. The bioavailability of the suspension from the compressed tablet was 0.63 ± 0.33 of that of the same tablet given orally, and the bioavailability was 0.52 ± 0.23 of the oral value for the chewable/dispersible tablet.

Lorazepam

The commercially available parenteral formulation of lorazepam has been given rectally to volunteers and patients (80, 81). Doses of 0.05 mg/kg stopped seizures in eight children. The bioavailability of rectally administered lorazepam was assessed in six volunteers who were given 2 mg of the parenteral solution. The T_{max} was 67 minutes, and the fraction absorbed averaged 86% with a range of 51% to 118%. The slow absorption of the parenteral solution limits the usefulness of rectal lorazepam for treatment of emergent conditions. Diazepam is absorbed more rapidly and is preferred for rectal administration.

Midazolam

Midazolam is absorbed rapidly—T_{max} appears to be 10 to 15 minutes—but its bioavailability is erratic and low,

10% to 20%, which makes it difficult to administer an effective dose (82).

Oxcarbazepine

Clemens et al performed a study in 10 healthy volunteers to characterize the bioavailability of rectally administered oxcarbazepine suspension (300 mg/5 mL) diluted 50% with water. Mean relative bioavailability calculated from plasma AUCs was 8.3% (SD 5.5%) for monohydroxy derivative (MHD) and 10.8% (SD 7.3%) for OXC. The C_{max} and AUC differed significantly between routes for both MHD and OXC ($P < 0.01$). The total amount of MHD excreted in the urine following rectal administration was 10 ± 5% of the amount excreted following oral administration. Oral absorption was consistent with previous studies. The most common side effects were headache and fatigue with no discernable difference between routes. MHD bioavailability following rectal administration of OXC suspension is significantly less than after oral administration, most likely because of OXC's poor water solubility. It is unlikely that adequate MHD concentrations can be reached by rectal administration of diluted OXC suspension (83).

Paraldehyde

Rectally administered paraldehyde has been widely used to control severe seizures, particularly in children (84, 85). However, information on the efficacy, toxicity, and pharmacokinetics is limited. Rectal bioavailability is 75% to 90% versus 90% to 100% for the oral route. Time to peak concentrations after rectal administration is 2.5 hours versus 0.5 hours for oral administration. Paraldehyde should be diluted with an equal volume of olive oil or vegetable oil to reduce mucosal irritation.

Phenobarbital

There is no commercially available rectal dosage form for phenobarbital. Graves and coworkers gave seven volunteers phenobarbital sodium parenteral solution rectally and intramuscularly (86). After rectal administration absorption was 90% complete, with a time to peak concentration of 4.4 hours versus 2.1 hours for the IM injection. Suppositories containing phenobarbital sodium are more rapidly absorbed than phenobarbital acid given either orally or intramuscularly (87, 88).

Phenytoin

Occasionally, there arises a need to administer phenytoin rectally, although no commercial rectal dosage form is available. Several studies of investigational suppository formulations have failed to demonstrate absorption. Rectal administration of phenytoin sodium parenteral solution in dogs produced low but measurable serum concentrations, but absorption was slow (89). Rectal administration of phenytoin is not recommended.

Valproic Acid

Valproic acid absorption has been studied after rectal administration of diluted syrup and suppositories. Rectal absorption of the commercially available syrup is complete, with peak concentrations occurring approximately 2 hours after a dose (90–92). High osmolality necessitates 1:1 dilution of the syrup to minimize catharsis. The syrup has been used to treat status epilepticus when other therapy is ineffective. Various suppository formulations are absorbed well, albeit more slowly than the syrup, with time to peak concentration occurring in 2 to 4 hours (93, 94).

Topiramate

Topiramate is also readily absorbed following rectal administration. In a study of twelve healthy subjects who received either 100 or 200 mg of topiramate orally and a 200 mg dose of topiramate given rectally, the relative bioavailability (F_{rel}), which was determined by calculating the dose-normalized areas under the concentration time curves, was 0.72 ± 0.18 h/L for the rectal dose and 0.76 ± 0.20 h/L for the oral dose.The relative bioavailability for topiramate administered rectally was 0.95 ± 0.17 with a range of 0.68 ± 1.2 (95).

Zonisamide

Nagatomi et al investigated two zonisamide suppositories compared with IV and oral dosing in rats (96). The bioavailability of the hydrophilic base was 96%, and that from the lipophilic base was 108%. The C_{max} following both rectal suppositories was significantly greater than an equal oral dose, and T_{max} occurred faster after the hydrophilic-based suppository (2 hrs) than after either the lipophilic-based or the oral dose (4 hrs).

STUDIES OF OTHER ADMINISTRATION ROUTES

Buccal/Sublingual

Buccal/sublingal administration of diazepam and lorazepam has been recommend by some clinicians as a part of routine clinical practice. However, there are no studies documenting their efficacy. Limited data exist for pharmacokinetic and efficacy for this route of administration.

Buccal administration of midazolam was studied in 10 healthy adults in a study in which 2 mL of the intravenous preparation of midazolam 5 mg/mL flavored with peppermint was held in the mouth for 5 minutes, then spat out. The researchers found that changes on electroencephalography were observed within 5 to 10 minutes of administration of the drug, suggesting rapid absorption and onset of effect (97). In a randomized controlled trial conducted in a hospital emergency department, the safety and efficacy of buccal midazolam were compared with those of rectal diazepam (98). The dose used for each drug was determined by the age of the child, with a target dose of about 0.5 mg/kg (from 2.5 mg for children aged 6 to 12 months; 4 mg for those 1 to 4 years; 7.5 mg for those 5 to 9 years; and 10 mg for those 10 years or older). A total of 219 episodes of acute seizures in 177 children were treated. Therapeutic success was defined as cessation of seizure within 10 minutes of drug administration without respiratory depression and without seizure recurrence within 1 hour. A postivie outcome was achieved in 56% of patients treated with buccal midazolam, compared with 27% of patients treated with rectal diazepam (P <0.001; odds ratio [OR] 4.1, 95% CI 2.2–7.6). Median time to seizure termination was 8 minutes (range: 5–20 minutes) for buccal midazolam and 15 minutes (range: 5–31 minutes) for rectal diazepam (P = 0.01; hazard ratio [HR] 0.7; 95% CI 0.5–0.9).

Greenblatt et al compared the pharmacokinetics of sublingual lorazepam with IV, IM, and oral LZP (99). Ten healthy volunteers randomly received 2 mg of LZP in the following five formulations: IV injection, IM injection, oral tablet, sublingual administration of the oral tablet, and sublingual administration of a specially formulated tablet. Peak plasma concentrations, time to peak concentrations, elimination half life, and relative bioavailability were not significantly different among the formulations. Peak concentrations were highest for the IM route, followed by oral and sublingual; time to peak concentrations was most rapid for the IM route, followed by sublingual and oral. Mean relative bioavailabilities were high for all routes: IM (95.9%), oral (99.8%), sublingual of oral tablet (94.1%) and sublingual of special tablet (98.2%).

It should be noted, however, that the efficacy, safety, duration of effect, and ease of buccal/sublingal administration by nonmedical caregivers have not been evaluated in settings outside of hospitals.

INTRANASAL

Several benzodiazepines possess the physical, chemical, and pharmacokinetic properties required of effective nasal therapies. Among the benzodiazepines considered for intranasal administration, midazolam has been most extensively studied. In one randomized, open-label trial involving 47 children with prolonged (>10 minutes) febrile seizures, the safety and efficacy of intranasal midazolam (0.2 mg/kg) were compared with those of intravenous diazepam (0.3 mg/kg) administered over 5 minutes (100). Intranasal midazolam was as safe and effective as intravenous diazepam and resulted in earlier cessation of seizures as a result of rapid administration.

However, the role of intranasal midazolam in treating seizure emergencies remains to be established. There are no adequately controlled trials demonstrating the safety and efficacy of intranasal midazolam for out-of-hospital treatment. Moreover, the short elimination half-life of midazolam—especially in patients taking enzyme-inducing drugs—raises concern as to whether its duration of effect is satisfactory in out-of-hospital settings.

Intranasal lorazepam has also been studied (101). Intranasal LZP was absorbed with a mean percent bioavailability of 77.7 ± 11.1%. A double-peak concentration-time curve was observed, indicating possible secondary oral absorption. The time to peak concentration was variable, ranging from 0.25–2 hours. Lorazepam's relatively limited lipid solubility as compared with that of midazolam or diazepam results in a slower rate of absorption and onset of action.

Diazepam has a lipid solubility and potency comparable with those of midazolam and a much longer elimination half-life, properties that make it a good candidate for intranasal administration. The bioavailability of a novel intranasal diazepam formulation has been compared with that of intranasal midazolam in healthy volunteers (n = 4) (102). Both midazolam and diazepam were rapidly absorbed, but diazepam's absorption was more extensive and its half-life longer than that of midazolam. Compared with rectally administered diazepam, the nasal diazepam formulation is absorbed to the same extent, but appears to be more rapidly absorbed, resulting in attainment of maximum concentrations as much as 30 minutes earlier (103).

Nasogastric Tubes

A nasogastric (NG) tube offers an alternative route of drug delivery. However, drug may adhere to the tubing, clog the tubing, or not be absorbed. Occlusion of the tube by the drug is also a concern. Tube occlusions may require replacement of the tube, which is both costly and inconvenient for the patient. Recently, it has been demonstrated that sustained-release carbamazepine (Carbatrol®) can be opened, mixed with 0.9% sodium chloride or apple juice as diluents, and reliably delivered through an NG tube or feeding tube 12 French or greater in size (104, 105). Topiramate has also been reported to be effective in patients with status epilepticus when given through an NG tube (106).

However, absorption from nasogastric tubes is not always comparable to orally administered formulations. When patients who are receiving tube feedings are switched from IV phenytoin (fosphenytoin) to oral phenytoin administered via a nasogastric tube, there appears to be decreased absorption of the oral formulation. This seems to occur regardless of whether the suspension or the oral capsule dosage form is used. Although the mechanism has not been clearly documented, it has been postulated that phenytoin may bind to proteins in the enteral feeding. Also, the enteral feeding may increase the GI motility, which may decrease the absorption (107). Sometimes very large oral doses may need to be given to maintain the desired serum concentrations in patients receiving phenytoin and enteral feedings via a nasogastric tube. Some practitioners try to stop the enteral feedings for two hours before and two hours after the dose of phenytoin. IM fosphenytoin would be an alternative (3).

TABLE 38-5
Medication Administration Guidelines for Toddlers

Allow child to choose a position in which to take medications.
Disguise the taste with a small volume of flavored drink or food. Rinse mouth with flavored drink to remove aftertaste.
Use simple commands in the toddler's jargon to obtain cooperation. Allow the toddler to choose which medi cations to take first. Allow toddler to become familiar with the oral dosing device.

SUMMARY

The selection of AED dosage forms is very important in pediatric epilepsy. Patients may be unwilling or unable to take oral solid dosage forms. Therefore, the availability of alternative oral dosage forms such as suspensions, solutions, and sprinkles is important. Patients who experience concentration-dependent side effects or breakthrough seizures may realize improved control by switching to an alternative dosage form. For example, a controlled-release formulation will provide lower peaks and higher troughs, facilitating better seizure control with less toxicity.

Although it has been the practice to crush oral solids and mix the contents with food, this is not always desirable. Some products, such as Phenytek®, Depakote-ER, Depakote®, and Tegretol-XR®, lose the properties they were designed to provide if the structure of the preparation is disrupted. In some cases, the rate or extent of absorption may be altered when the drug is given with food. It also has been a custom to compound pediatric dosage forms extemporaneously. This is an important way to provide drug in a form that young children can take. However, clinicians should be cautious about extemporaneous compounding of pediatric formulations unless they can determine the amount of drug in the formulation, the stability of the product, and the bioavailability. This requires an assay for the compounded product and an assay of the drug in blood. In addition, with compounded drugs, someone should taste the preparation before it is given to the patient. For example, gabapentin has a very bitter taste when it is put into solution. Therefore, when a drug is compounded for pediatric delivery, the new formulation should be tested to ensure that it is being delivered properly. Specialized dosage forms generally are more expensive.

Caregivers should be thoroughly educated in drug administration techniques for children. When carefully instructed, caregivers can properly administer medications (108). Drug administration techniques are summarized in Tables 38-4, 38-5, and 38-6. When doses are given as "teaspoonfuls," caregivers should have a calibrated device for measuring the dose rather than using a common utensil. The volume of "standard" teaspoons varies up to fourfold. Drugs given rectally, such as diazepam, require special caregiver education.

Clinical assessment, selection of a drug, and determination of the dose require special attention in the

TABLE 38-4
Medication Administration Guidelines for Infants

Use a calibrated dropper or oral syringe.

Support the infant's head while holding the infant in lap.

Give small amounts of medication to prevent choking.

If desired, crush non–enteric-coated tablets to a powder and sprinkle on small amounts of food.

Provide physical comforting to calm the infant while administering medications.

TABLE 38-6
Medication Administration Guidelines for Preschool Children

Place tablet or capsule near back of tongue and provide water or a flavored liquid to aid in swallowing.
Do not use chewable tablets if the child's teeth are loose. Use a straw to administer medications that may stain teeth.
Use a rinse with a flavored drink to minimize aftertaste.
Allow child to help make decisions about dosage forms, place of administration, which medication to take first, and the type of flavored drink to use.

pediatric patient, as does the selection of the appropriate formulation and dosage form. This last step in the therapeutic plan plays a pivotal role in the ultimate success of therapy. The objective is to ensure the regular and consistent delivery of drug to the brain. When conventional oral tablets and capsules are inappropriate or impractical, alternate formulations, dosage forms, and routes of administration should be considered. The clinician also must assess the ability of the caregiver to correctly prepare, measure, and administer medications and instruct caregivers about proper drug administration.

References

1. Rowland M, Tozer TN. Clinical pharmacokinetics: concepts and applications. 2nd ed. Philadelphia: Lea & Febiger, 1989.
2. Gibaldi M. Biopharmaceutics and clinical pharmacokinetics. 3rd ed. Philadelphia: Lea & Febiger, 1984.
3. Winter ME, Tozer TN. Phenytoin. In: Burton ME, Shaw LM, Schentag JL, Evans WE, eds. *Applied Pharmacokinetics and Pharmacodynamics: Principles of Therapeutic Drug Monitoring*. 4th ed. Philadelphia: Lippincott.
4. Ansel HC, Popovich NG. Pharmaceutical dosage forms and drug delivery systems. 5th ed. Philadelphia: Lea & Febiger, 1990.
5. Stewart BH, Kugler AR, Thompson PR, Bockbrader HN. A saturable transport mechanism in the intestinal absorption of gabapentin is the underlying cause of lack of proportionality between increasing dose and drug levels in plasma. *Pharm Res* 1993; 10:276–281.
6. Tyrer JH, Eadie MJ, Sutherland JM, Hooper WD. Outbreak of anticonvulsant intoxication in an Australian city. *Br. Med J [Clin Res]* 1970; 4:271–273.
7. Bochner F,Hooper WD,Tyrer JH,Eadie MJ.Factors involved in an outbreak of phenytoin intoxication. *J Neurol Sci* 1972; 16:481–487.
8. Hamilton RA, Garnett WR, Kline BJ, et al. The effect of food on valproic acid absorption. *Am J Hosp Pharm* 1981; 38:1490–1493.
9. Levy R, Pitlick W, Troupin A, et al. Pharmacokinetics of carbamazepine in normal man. *Clin Pharmacol Ther* 1975; 17:657–668.
10. Carter BL, Garnett WR, Pellock JM, et al. Interaction between phenytoin and three commonly used antacids. *Ther Drug Monit* 1981; 3:333–340.
11. Stewart CG, Hampton EM. Effect of maturation on drug disposition in pediatric patients. *Clin Pharm* 1987; 6:548–564.
12. Painter MJ, Pippenger C, MacDonald H, et al. Phenobarbital and diphenylhydantoin levels in neonates with seizures. *J Pediatr* 1978; 92:315–319.
13. Kearns GL, Reed MD. Clinical pharmacokinetics in infants and children: a reappraisal. *Clin Pharmacokinet* 1989; 17(Suppl):29–67.
14. Shargel, L, Wu-Pong W, Yu ABC. Bioavailability and bioequivalence. In: eds. *Applied Biopharmaceutics and Pharmacokinetics,* 5th ed. New York: McGraw-Hill, 2005: 453–499.
15. American Medical Association. Featured report: generic drugs (A-02). http://www.ama.assn.org/ama/pub/category/print/15279.html.
16. American Academy of Neurology. Assessment: generic substitution for antiepileptic medication. *Neurology* 1990; 40:1641–1643.
17. Liow K, Barkley GL, Pollard JR, Harden CL, et al. AAN position statement on AED generics. *Neurology* 2007; 68:1249–1250.
18. Clemens P, Riss JR, Kriel RL, Cloyd JC. Administration of antiepileptic drugs by alternate routes: review. in press.
19. deBoer AG, Moolenaar F, deLeed LGJ, et al. Rectal drug administration: clinical pharmacokinetic considerations. *Clin Pharmacokinet* 1982; 7:285–311.
20. Carmichael RR, Mahoney DC, Jeffrey LP. Solubility and stability of phenytoin sodium when mixed with intravenous solutions. *Am J Hosp Pharm* 1980; 37:95–98.
21. Kostenbauder HD, Rapp RP, McGovern JP, et al. Bioavailability and single-dose pharmacokinetics of intramuscular phenytoin. *Clin Pharmacol Ther* 1975; 18:449–456.
22. Serrano EE, Wilder BJ. Intramuscular administration of diphenylhydantoin. Histologic follow-up. *Arch Neurol* 1974; 31:276–278.
23. Leppik IE, Boucher R, Wilder BJ, Murthy VS, et al. Phenytoin prodrug: preclinical and clinical studies. *Epilepsia* 1989; 30(Suppl):S22–S26.
24. Fisher JH, Cwik MS, Sibley CB, Doyo K. Stability of fosphenytoin sodium with intravenous solutions in glass bottles, polyvinyl chloride, and polypropylene syringes. *Ann Pharmacother* 1997; 31:553–559.
25. Eldon MA, Loewen GR, Viogtman RE, et al. Pharmacokinetics and tolerance of fosphenytoin and phenytoin administered intravenously to healthy subjects. *Can J Neurol Sci* 1993; 20(Suppl 4):S180.
26. Jamerson BD, Dukes GE, Grouwer KLR, et al. Venous irritation related to intravenous administration of phenytoin versus fosphenytoin. *Pharmacotherapy* 1994; 14:47–52.
27. Garnett WR, Kugler AR, O'Hara KA, Driscoll SM, et al. Pharmacokinetics of fosphenytoin following intramuscular administration of fosphenytoin substituted for oral phenytoin in epileptic patients. *Neurology* 1995; 45:A248.
28. Ramsay RE, Wider BJ, Uthman BM, et al. Intramuscular fosphenytoin (Cerebyx) in patients requiring a loading dose of phenytoin. *Epilepsy Res* 1997; 181–187.
29. Wilder BJ, Campbell K, Ramsey RE, et al. Safety and tolerance of multiple doses of intramuscular fosphenytoin substituted for oral phenytoin in epilepsy and neurosurgery. *Arch Neurol* 1996; 53:764–768.
30. Fitzsimmons WE, Garnett WR, Comstock TJ, et al. Comparison of the single dose bioavailability and pharmacokinetics of extended phenytoin sodium capsules and phenytoin oral suspension. *Epilepsia* 1986; 27:464–468.
31. Food and Drug Administration. New prescribing directions for phenytoin. *FDA Drug Bull* 1978; 8:27–28.
32. Jung D, Powell JR, Walson P, Perrier D. Effect of dose on phenytoin absorption. *Clin Pharmacol Ther* 1980; 28:479–485.
33. Goff DA, Spunt KAL, Jung D, Bellur SN, et al. Absorption characteristics of three phenytoin sodium products after administration of oral loading doses. *Clin Pharmacol* 1984; 3:634–638.
34. Sarkar MA, Karnes HT, Garnett WR. Effects of storage and shaking on the settling properties of phenytoin suspension. *Neurology* 1989; 39:202–209.
35. Sherry J. Bioequivalence of Phenytek™ 300 mg capsules. *CNS News* 2002; (Special Report, August):12–16.
36. Maas B, Garnett WR, Comstock TJ, et al. A comparison of the relative bioavailability and pharmacokinetics of carbamazepine tablets and chewable tablet formulations. *Ther Drug Monit* 1987; 9:28–33.
37. Graves NG, Kriel RL, Jones-Saete C, et al. Relative bioavailability of rectally administered carbamazepine suspension in humans. *Epilepsia* 1985; 26:429–433.
38. Garnett WR, Carson, Pellock JM, et al. Comparison of carbamazepine and 10-11-diepoxide carbamazepine plasma levels in children following chronic dosing with Tegretol suspension and Tegretol tablets. *Neurology* 1987; 37(Suppl):93.
39. Thakker KM, Mangat S, Garnett WR, et al. Comparative bioavailability and steady state fluctuations of Tegretol commercial and carbamazepine OROS tablets in adult and pediatric patients. *Biopharm Drug Dispos* 1992; 13:559–569.
40. Garnett WR, Levy B, McLean AM, et al. A pharmacokinetic evaluation of twice-daily extended-release carbamazepine and four-times daily immediate-release carbamazepine in patients with epilepsy. *Epilepsia* 1998; 39:274–279.
41. Stevens RE, Limsakun T, Evans G, Mason DH Jr. Controlled, multidose, pharmacokinetic evaluation of two extended-release carbamazepine formulations (Carbatrol and Tegretol-XR). *J Pharm Sci* 1998 Dec; 87(12):1531–1534.
42. Fischer JH, Barr AN, Palovcek FP, et al. Effect of food on the serum concentration profile of enteric-coated valproic acid. *Neurology* 1988; 38:1319–1320.
43. Cloyd JC. Pharmacokinetic pitfalls of present antiepileptic medications. *Epilepsia* 1991; 32(Suppl 5):S53–S65.
44. Cloyd JC, Kriel RL, Janes-Saete CM, et al. Comparison of sprinkle vs syrup formulations of valproate for bioavailability, tolerance and preference. *J Pediatr* 1992; 120:634–638.
45. Depakote® (divalproex sodium delayed release tablets). In: *Physician's Desk Reference.* 57th ed. Montvale, NJ: Thompson PDR, 2003; 430–437.
46. Depakote-ER® (divalproex sodium extended-release tablets). In: *Physician's Desk Reference.* 57th ed. Montvale, NJ: Thompson PDR, 2003:437–441.
47. Velasco M, Ford JL, Rowe P, Rajabi-Siahboomi AR. Influence of drug: hydroxypropyl methylcellulose ratio, drug and polymer particle size and compression force on the release of diclofenac sodium from HPMC tablets. *J Controlled Release* 1999; 57: 75–85.
48. Ford JL, Rubinstein MH, McCaul F, Hogan JE, et al. Importance of drug type, tablet shape and added diluents on drug release kinetics from hydroxypropylmethylcellulose matrix tablets. *Int J Pharm* 1987; 40:223–234.
49. Dutta S, Zhang Y, Selness DS, et al. Comparison of the bioavailability of unequal doses of divalproex sodium extended-release formulation relative to the delayed release formulation in healthy volunteers. *Epilepsy Res* 2002; 49:1–10.
50. Kernitsky L, O'Hara KA, Jiang P, Pellock JM. Extended-release divalproex in child and adolescent outpatients with epilepsy. *Epilepsia* 2005; 46(3):440–443.
51. Depacon® (valproate sodium injection). In: *Physician's Desk Reference.* 57th ed. Montvale, NJ: Thompson PDR, 2003:416–421.
52. Morton LD, O'Hara KA, Coots PB, Ibrahim M, et al. Intravenous valproate experience in pediatric patients. *Epilepsia* 2002; 43(Suppl 7):62.
53. Cloyd JC, Dutta S, Cao G, et al.Valproate unbound fraction and distribution volume following rapid infusions in patients with epilepsy. *Epilepsy Res* 2003; 53:19–27.
54. Garnett WR. Antiepileptics. In: Schumacher GE, ed. *Therapeutic Drug Monitoring.* Norwalk, CN: Appleton and Lange, 1995:345–395.
55. Felbatol® (felbamate tablets and suspension). In: *Physician's Desk Reference.* 61st ed. Montvale, NJ: Thompson PDR, 2004:1915–1919.
56. Neurontin® (gabapentin capsules, tablets, oral solution). In: *Physician's Desk Reference.* 61st ed. Montvale, NJ: Thompson PDR, 2007:2487–2492.
57. Lamictal® (lamotrigine tablets and chewable/dispersible tablets). In: *Physician's Desk Reference.* 61st ed. Montvale, NJ: Thompson PDR, 2007:1481–1490.
58. Topamax® (topiramate tablets, sprinkle capsules). In: *Physician's Desk Reference*, 61st ed. Montvale, NJ: Thompson PDR, 2007:2404–2413.
59. Gabatril® (tiagabine tablets). In: *Physician's Desk Reference.* 61st ed. Montvale, NJ: Thompson PDR, 2007:984–988.

60. Keppra® (levetiracetam tablets). In: *Physician's Desk Reference*. 61st ed. Montvale, NJ: Thompson PDR, 2007:3314–3323.
61. Trileptal® (oxcarbazepine tablets and oral suspension). In: *Physician's Desk Reference*. 61st ed. Montvale, NJ: Thompson PDR, 2007:2300–2306.
62. Zonegran® (zonisamide capsules). In: *Physician's Desk Reference*. 61st ed. Montvale, NJ: Thompson PDR, 2007:1101–1105.
63. Lyrica (pregabalin capusules. In: *Physician's Desk Reference*. 61st ed. Montvale, NJ: Thompson PDR, 2007:2539–2545.
64. Graves NM, Kriel RL. Rectal administration of antiepileptic drugs in children. *Pediatr Neurol* 1987; 3:321–326.
65. Jensen PK, Abild K, Poulsen MN. Serum concentration of clonazepam after rectal administration. *Acta Neurol Scand* 1983; 68:417–420.
66. Rylance GW, Poulton J, Cherry RC, et al. Plasma concentrations of clonazepam after single rectal administration. *Arch Dis Child* 1986; 61:186–188.
67. Johannessen SI, Henriksen O, Munthe-Kaas AW, et al. Serum concentration profile studies of tablets and suppositories of valproate and carbamazepine in healthy subjects and patients with epilepsy. In: Levy RH, Pitlick WH, Eichelbaum M, Meijer J, eds. *Metabolism of Antiepileptic Drugs*. New York: Raven Press, 1984:61–71.
68. Brouard A, Fonta JE, Masselin S, et al. Rectal administration of carbamazepine gel. *Clin Pharm* 1990; 9:13–14.
69. Moolenaar F, Bakker S, Visser J, et al. Biopharmaceutics of rectal administration of drugs in man. IX. Comparative biopharmaceutics of diazepam after single rectal, oral, intramuscular and intravenous administration in man. *Int J Pharm* 1980; 5:127–137.
70. Lombroso CT. Intermittent home treatment of status and clusters of seizures. *Epilepsia* 1989; 30(Suppl):S11–S14.
71. Dhillon S, Oxley J, Richens A. Bioavailability of diazepam after intravenous, oral and rectal administration in adult epileptic patients. *Br J Clin Pharmacol* 1982; 13:427–432.
72. Hoppu K, Santavuori P. Diazepam rectal solution for home treatment of acute seizures in children. *Acta Paediatr Scand* 1981; 70:369–372.
73. Albano A, Reisdorff J, Wiegenstein JG. Rectal diazepam in pediatric status epilepticus. *Am J Emerg Med* 1989; 70:168–172.
74. Dreifuss FE, Rosman NP, Cloyd JC, Pellock JM, et al. A comparison of rectal diazepam gel and placebo for acute repetitive seizures. *N Engl J Med* 1998; 338(26):1869–1875.
75. Kriel RL, Cloyd JC, Hadsall RS, et al. Home use of rectal diazepam for cluster and prolonged seizures: efficacy adverse reactions, quality of life, and cost analysis. *Pediatr Neurol* 1991; 7:13–17.
76. Grossmann R, Maytal J, Fernando J. Rectal administration of felbamate in a child with Lennox-Gastaut syndrome. *Neurology* 1994; 44(10):1979.
77. Kriel RL, Birnbaum AK, Cloyd JC, et al. Failure of absorption of gabapentin after rectal administration. *Epilepsia* 1997; 38:1242–1244.
78. Birnbaum AK, Kriel RL, Im Y, Remmel RP. Relative bioavailability of lamotrigine chewable dispersible tablets administered rectally. *Pharmacotherapy* 2001; 21:158–162.
79. Birnbaum AK, Kriel RL, Burkhardt RT, Remmel RP. Rectal absorption of lamotrigine compressed tablets. *Epilepsia* 2000; 41:850–853.
80. Dooley JM, Tibbles JAR, Rumney PG, et al. Rectal lorazepam in the treatment of acute seizures in childhood. *Ann Neurol* 1984; 18:312–313.
81. Graves NM, Kriel RL. Bioavailability of rectally administered lorazepam. *Clin Neuropharmacol* 1987; 10:555–559.
82. Malinovsky J-M, Lejus C, Servin F, et al. Plasma concentrations of midazolam after I.V., nasal or rectal administration in children. *Br J Anaesthesia* 1993; 70:617–620.
83. Clemens PL, Cloyd JC, Kriel RL, Remmel RP. Relative bioavailability, metabolism, and tolerability of rectally administered oxcarbazepine suspension. *Clin Drug Investig* 2007; 27:243–250.
84. Anthony RM, Andorn AE, Sunshine I, et al. Paraldehyde pharmacokinetics in ethanol abusers. *Fed Proc* 1977; 36:285.
85. Curless RG, Holzman BH, Ramsay RE. Paraldehyde therapy in childhood status epilepticus. *Arch Neurol* 1983; 40:477–480.
86. Graves NM, Holmes GB, Kriel RL, et al. Relative bioavailability of rectally administered phenobarbital sodium parenteral solution. *Ann Pharmacother* 1989; 23:565–568.
87. Matsukura M, Higashi A, Ikeda T, et al. Bioavailability of phenobarbital by rectal administration. *Pediatr Pharmacol* 1981; 1:259–265.
88. Minkov E, Lambov N, Kirchev D, Bantutova I, et al. Biopharmaceutical investigation of rectal suppositories. Part 2(1): Pharmaceutical and biological availability of phenobarbital and phenobarbital-sodium. *Pharmazie* 1985; 40:257–259.
89. Fuerst RH, Graves NM, Kriel RL, et al. Absorption and safety of rectally administered phenytoin. *Eur J Drug Metab Pharmacokinet* 1988; 13:257–260.
90. Cloyd JC, Kriel RL. Bioavailability of rectally administered valproic acid syrup. *Neurology* 1981; 31:1348–1352.
91. Scanabissi E, DalPozzo D, Franzoni E, et al. Rectal administration of sodium valproate in children. *Ital J Neurol Sci* 1984; 5:189–193.
92. Snead OC, Miles MV. Treatment of status epilepticus in children with rectal sodium valproate. *J Pediatr* 1985; 106:323–325.
93. Moolenaar F, Greving WJ, Huizinga T. Absorption rate and bioavailability of valproic acid and its sodium salt from rectal dosage forms. *Eur J Clin Pharmacol* 1980; 17:309–315.
94. Holmes GB, Rosenfeld WE, Graves NM, et al. Absorption of valproic acid suppositories in human volunteers. *Arch Neurol* 1989; 48:906–909.
95. Conway JM, Birnbaum AK, Kriel R L, Cloyd JC. Relative bioavailability of topiramate administered rectally. *Epilepsy Res* 2003; 54:91–96.
96. Nagatomi A, Mishima M, Tsuzuki O, Ohdo S, et al. Utility of a rectal suppository containing the antiepileptic drug zonisamide. *Biol Pharm Bull* 1997; 20(8):892–896.
97. Scott RC, Besag FMC, Boyd SG, et al. Buccal absorption of midazolam: Pharmacokinetics and EEG pharmacodynamics. *Epilepsia* 1998; 39:290–294.
98. McIntyre J, Robertson S, Norris E, et al. Safety and efficacy of buccal midazolam versus rectal diazepam for emergency treatment of seizures in children: a randomized controlled trial. *Lancet* 2005; 366:205–210.
99. Greenblatt DJ, Divoll M, Harmatz JS, Shader RI. Pharmacokinetic comparison of sublingual lorazepam with intravenous, intramuscular, and oral lorazepam. *J Pharm Sci* 1982; 71(2):248–252.
100. Lahat E, Goldman M, Barr J, et al. Comparison of intranasal midazolam with intravenous diazepam for treating febrile seizures in children: prospective randomized study. *Br Med J* 2000; 321:83–86.
101. Wermeling DP, Miller JL, Archer SM, Manaligod JM, et al. Bioavailability and pharmacokinetics of lorazepam after intranasal, intravenous, and intramuscular administration. *J Clin Pharmacol* 2001; 41:1225–1231.
102. Riss JR, Cloyd JC, Kriel RL. Bioavailability and tolerability of a Novel Intranasal Diazepam Formulation in Healthy Volunteers. American Academy of Neurology, San Diego, CA, April 4, 2006.
103. Cloyd JC, Lalonde RL, Beniak TE, et al. A single-blind, crossover comparison of the pharmacokinetics and cognitive effects of a new diazepam rectal gel with intravenous diazepam. *Epilepsia* 1998; 39:520–526.
104. Garnett WR, Huffman J, Welsh S. Administration of Carbatrol® (carbamazepine extended-release capsules) via feeding tubes. *Epilepsia* 1999; (Suppl):498.
105. Riss JR, Kriel RL, Kammer NM, et al. Administration of Carbatrol® to children with feeding tubes. *Pediatr Neurol* 2002; 27(3):193–195.
106. Towne AR, Garnett LK, Waterhouse EJ, et al. The use of topiramate in refractory status epilepticus. *Neurology* 2003 Jan 28; 60(2):332–334. Review.
107. Au Yeung SC, Ensom MH. Phenytoin and enteral feedings: does evidence support an interaction? *Ann Pharmacother* 2000 Jul-Aug; 34(7–8):896–905. Review.
108. McMahon SR, Rimsza ME, Bay RC. Parents can dose medication accurately. *Pediatrics* 1997; 100:330–333.

39 Principles of Drug Interactions: Implications for Treatment with Antiepileptic Drugs

Barry E. Gidal

Pharmacokinetic interactions, sometimes leading to adverse clinical situations, have long been recognized as an occasionally unavoidable facet of antiepileptic drug (AED) treatment (1, 2). Since the mid-1990s, a number of newer AEDs have entered the marketplace, both in the United States and globally. One general advantage of these newer medications is an improved pharmacokinetic profile, including a reduced potential for participating in drug-drug interactions, as compared to the older medications.

The aim of this chapter is to summarize in-vitro and in-vivo data regarding drug interactions with both the newer as well as the older, traditional AEDs in terms of absorption, distribution, protein binding, and hepatic induction and inhibition. Clinical implications of these interactions will also be discussed.

PATIENTS AT RISK

Patients perhaps at the greatest risk for drug interactions are usually those who are the most severely ill. This includes patients in the intensive care unit, geriatric patients, premature neonates, and young children. Drug interactions may be a significant contributor to both patient morbidity and mortality (3, 4).

Clinicians should recognize that as a group, patients with epilepsy, including both children and adults, tend to receive more medications than does the general population. As the number of concomitant medications increases, so does the likelihood of drug interactions. The patients with the most refractory epilepsy are consequently more likely to encounter problems with drug interactions related to concomitant AED therapy than their controlled counterparts. Although, historically, more attention has been paid to AED-to-AED interactions, there has been increasing attention to the potential for certain AEDs to interact (perhaps adversely) with other concomitant medications that patients may be receiving.

MECHANISMS FOR COMMON DRUG INTERACTIONS

Oral Absorption of Drugs

Most AEDs are well absorbed following oral administration. However, absorption of some compounds can be altered by drug-drug or drug-food interactions. These interactions can affect maximum plasma concentration, time to reach maximum concentration, and even overall extent of absorption. Among the older, traditional AEDs, oral absorption of phenytoin appears to be the most problematic. Of particular concern is the issue of concomitant administration of an AED with an enteral nutrition supplement. Concomitant administration of phenytoin with these nutritional formulations can result in marked reductions in oral bioavailablity (4–6). Because of this interaction, it is commonly suggested that the administration of phenytoin and enteral feedings be separated by at least 2 hours. Unfortunately, this may not be practical, particularly for patients requiring continuous feedings. Alternatively, clinicians can overcome this interaction by simply increasing the phenytoin dosage and using serum drug concentrations as a guide. This approach is also problematic. If for example, enteral feedings are discontinued, or interrupted for a significant period of times, and phenytoin doses are not readjusted downward, there will likely be a marked rise in phenytoin concentrations, potentially leading to drug intoxication. If possible, therefore, this drug-nutrient interaction should be avoided. Concomitant ingestion of food may also delay the rate of absorption of older agents such as valproic acid but is unlikely to impact overall absorption (7).

Generally speaking, oral absorption interactions with the newer-generation AEDs are unlikely to be of clinical significance in most patients. Unlike older, traditional compounds such as phenytoin or carbamazepine, the newer-generation AEDs tend to be quite water soluble and are rapidly and completely absorbed. Indeed, in contrast to the problems described for phenytoin, absorption of newer-generation agents such as gabapentin, lamotrigine, and levetiracetam does not appear to be impaired when coadministered with enteral nutritional supplements (8–9).

When topiramate is administered with food, the rate of absorption is decreased, delaying time to maximum concentration by approximately 2 hours and decreasing mean maximum concentration by approximately 10%, with no significant effect on overall extent of absorption. Conversely, when oxcarbazepine is given with food, the mean maximum serum concentrations of the active monohydroxy metabolite is increased by 23% (10–11). Whether this is clinically meaningful is unclear.

Coadministration of levetiracetam with food delays the time to peak concentration by approximately 1.5 hours and decreases the maximum concentration by 20%; however, the extent of absorption is not affected. Mixing with enteral feeding formulas does not appear to result in significant impairment of absorption, over and beyond that seen with concomitant administration with food (12).

Role of Drug Transporter Proteins

ATP-dependent drug transporters, including members of the multidrug resistance protein (MRP) family and P-glycoprotein (Pgp), have been implicated as a major limiting factor in drug pharmacokinetics (13). Pgp and MRP are located on the apical side of capillary endothelial cells and are thought to extrude drug molecules back into blood (or intestine) from cells. These efflux pumps appear to act in conjunction with drug-metabolizing enzymes such as CYP 3A4 to limit drug access to both the systemic circulation and various cellular compartments (14). This may be clinically important, in that several of the older AEDs, such as carbamazepine, display the ability to induce the activity of CYP 3A4 and Pgp (15). At the intestinal level, induction of both CYP 3A4 and these efflux pumps would serve to significantly reduce the oral bioavailability of a number of medications. While most attention has been focused on the role of these transporters in modulating oral drug absorption, it has also become clear that these transporter proteins are localized in a variety of tissues including the liver, kidney, blood-brain barrier, and placenta. In addition to potentially limiting oral drug absorption or blood-brain barrier penetration, these drug efflux pumps may be important in protecting the fetus from drug/chemical exposure. Several studies have now demonstrated that PgP is expressed in the trophoblast layer of the placenta and may provide an important mechanism of protection to the fetus from maternal drug exposure (16).

IS PROTEIN BINDING RELEVANT?

In most cases, changes in protein binding are not clinically significant, but in some situations these alterations, as a result of either changes in protein concentration (e.g., hypoalbuminemia) or protein binding displacement, may lead to misinterpretation of serum drug concentrations (17).

Protein binding displacement interactions can occur when two highly protein-bound (>90%) agents are administered together and compete for a limited number of binding sites. Typically, the drug with the greater affinity for the binding site displaces the competing agent, increasing the unbound fraction of the displaced drug. It is the unbound drug concentration that is responsible for the drug's pharmacologic activity. Unbound drug concentrations are dependent on the drug dose and drug-metabolizing activity of enzymes (intrinsic clearance). Unbound drug concentrations may rise initially following the concomitant administration of two competing drugs but should return to preinteraction values fairly quickly. In other words, these interactions are transient. Total concentrations of drug, however, will be lower than expected. If serum concentrations are being monitored, this may lead to misinterpretation.

Among the AEDs, the potential for protein-binding interactions is greatest for phenytoin and valproic acid. Both phenytoin and valproic acid are extensively bound to plasma proteins (>90%). Valproic acid is also an inhibitor of cytochrome P450 2C19, one of the enzymes responsible for phenytoin metabolism. When these two agents are coadministered, unbound phenytoin concentrations are higher than typically expected and total (bound + unbound) concentrations are lower (16). When using this combination, it may be prudent to monitor unbound phenytoin concentrations as well as total.

With the exception of tiagabine (96% protein bound), an advantage of the newer-generation AEDs is that they are not extensively protein bound, and therefore these types of pharmacokinetic interactions are not likely.

Metabolism: Implications of Enzyme Induction and Inhibition

Most clinically relevant drug interactions result from alterations in drug metabolism, either in the liver or in the gut. Drug-metabolizing enzyme induction can result in an increased rate of metabolism of the affected drug, leading to both decreased oral bioavailability and increased systemic clearance of extensively metabolized concomitant medications. The clinical result therefore would be potentially subtherapeutic serum concentrations of that drug. Conversely, a number of drugs (including several AEDs) have been shown to be inhibitors of various drug-metabolizing enzymes, and concomitant administration of these agents can slow the rate of metabolism of the affected drug and cause increased serum levels of drug, leading to toxicity.

The metabolic pathways of AEDs can vary; however, most metabolism is achieved via oxidative metabolism and/or glucuronidation (18–20). Oxidative metabolism is accomplished via the cytochrome P450 (CYP) isoenzyme system. This system consists of three main families of enzymes: CYP1, CYP2, and CYP3. There are seven primary isoenzymes that are involved in the metabolism of most drugs: CYP1A2, CYP2A6, CYP2C9, CYP2C19, CYP2D6, CYP2E1, and CYP3A4. Of these, the ones commonly involved with metabolism of AEDs include CYP2C9, CYP2C19, and CYP3A4 (21). Another important metabolic pathway for several AEDs, including valproic acid, lorazepam, and lamotrigine, is conjugation via the enzyme uridine diphosphate glucuronosyltransferase (UGT).

Although they do not necessarily contraindicate AED therapy, these pharmacokinetic interactions can clearly complicate therapy in individuals receiving multiple AEDs. In some cases, it may be difficult to distinguish whether a change in a person's clinical state (change in seizure frequency or appearance of toxicity) is due to an additive pharmacologic effect of the added drug or simply due to a change in serum concentration in the original AED. One approach to rational polytherapy would be to combine agents that do not interact with each other. In this way, the confounders of changes in drug disposition can be excluded from the evaluation of therapeutic response to combined AED treatment. Interactions between AEDs and hepatic enzymes are summarized in Table 39-1 and discussed in the following paragraphs.

Hepatic Enzyme Induction. Compounds that are hepatic inducers increase the synthesis of enzyme protein and thus increase the capacity for drug metabolism. Induction of hepatic enzymes occurs over a gradual period of days to

TABLE 39-1
Effect of Antiepileptic Drugs on CYP Isoenzymes or Other Enzyme Systems

Drug	Effect on Metabolism	Enzymes
Phenobarbital, carbamazepine, phenytoin	Inducers	Broad CYP, UGT inducers
Valproic acid	Inhibitor	CYP 2C19, UGT, Epoxide hydrolase
Gabapentin, pregabalin	No effect	
Lamotrigine	Weak inducer	UGT
Levetiracetam	No effect	
Oxcarbazepine	Inducer (modest)	CYP3A4
Tiagabine	No effect	—
Topiramate	Inhibitor (modest)	CYP2C19
	Inducer (modest)	CYP 3A4
Vigabatrin	None	
Zonisamide	No effect	

weeks and is a reversible process. Addition of an inducer will cause a lowering of serum concentrations of the target drug, conceivably resulting in inadequate therapeutic response. Conversely, removal of an enzyme inducer will cause a rise in the levels of the target drug, potentially causing toxicity.

Among the older-generation AEDs, carbamazepine, phenytoin, and the barbiturates phenobarbital and primidone are inducers of both the cytochrome P450 (CYP) and UGT enzyme systems (18). Combining these agents with other AEDs that are metabolized by either of these enzyme systems can result in markedly enhanced systemic clearance, and reduced serum concentrations of the affected drug, requiring higher doses in order to maintain comparable (as compared to monotherapy) steady-state serum concentrations. An example of this sort of interaction would be the combination of phenytoin and lamotrigine.

Lamotrigine is extensively (>90%) metabolized hepatically by N-glucuronidation via UGT 1A3 and UGT 1A4. Lamotrigine does not appear to significantly alter concentrations of carbamazepine or carbamazepine epoxide (21, 22) nor any of the other AEDs. However, the half-life of lamotrigine is reduced from 24 hours to 15 hours when administered with enzyme-inducing drugs as just described. Following the withdrawal of the enzyme inducers carbamazepine and phenytoin, lamotrigine plasma concentrations have been observed to increase by 50% and 100 %, respectively (23).

Levetiracetam shows limited metabolism in humans, with 66% of the dose renally excreted unchanged. Its major metabolic pathway is via hydrolysis of the acetamide group to yield a carboxylic derivative, which is mainly recovered in the urine. Levetiracetam is not significantly metabolized by CYPs or UGTs and appears to be devoid of pharmacokinetic drug interactions (24, 25). Similarly, the drugs gabapentin and pregabalin appear to be devoid of enzyme-inducing (or inhibition) properties.

Oxcarbazepine is converted to 10-hydroxycarbamazepine (OHCZ), the metabolite primarily responsible for pharmacologic activity. This active metabolite is mostly excreted by direct conjugation to glucuronic acid. Oxcarbazepine does not seem to be a broad-spectrum enzyme inducer, although it does posses modest, specific induction potential toward the CYP3A subfamily, as evidenced by the increased metabolism of estrogens and dihydropyridine calcium channel antagonists (1, 2). Clinicians should be aware that this drug does indeed have modest potential for causing enzyme induction interactions, but that this potential may vary among different patients.

Topiramate is approximately 60% excreted unchanged in the urine. It is also metabolized by hydroxylation and hydrolysis. Two of its metabolites are conjugated as glucuronides. While not considered a potent enzyme inducer, topiramate can increase clearance of valproate by approximately 13% and may lower oral contraceptive serum concentrations (26, 27). Whether these changes in valproic serum concentration are clinically meaningful is unclear. Topiramate metabolic clearance can be increased when it is administered with enzyme-inducing AEDs, thereby reducing half-life and lowering serum concentrations by up to 40%.

Zonisamide is a synthetic 1,2-benzisoaxole derivative that is metabolized in large part by reduction and conjugation reactions. Oxidative reactions involving CYP3A4 and CYP2D6 are also involved. Zonisamide elimination can be altered by other drugs. Specifically, enzyme-inducing drugs such as carbamazepine and phenytoin can significantly increase the clearance of this drug, effectively reducing the half-life of zonisamide by about half.

Hepatic Inhibition. Hepatic enzyme inhibition can occur when two drugs compete for the same enzyme site, reducing the metabolism of the target drug. A resultant increase in the object drug can occur if a substantial portion of the target drug is prevented from occupying the enzyme site. Inhibition is usually a rapid process that is dose/concentration dependent. Addition of an enzyme inhibitor may cause a very rapid rise in serum concentrations of the target drug, potentially leading to acute toxicity (18).

In contrast to enzyme induction, inhibition of selected CYP and/or UGT enzymes can be caused by several AEDs of both the older and newer generations. These combinations may result in unexpectedly high serum concentrations of the affected AED. An example is the interaction of valproic acid and lamotrigine. Lamotrigine's half-life is increased to approximately 59–70 hours when it is coadministered with valproate, resulting from valproate's inhibition of glucuronidation. Inhibition of lamotrigine clearance can occur at valproate doses as low as 125–250 mg/day and becomes maximal at dosages approaching 500 mg/day (28). The clinical implication is that lamotrigine dose and dose escalation will need to be substantially reduced in order to reduce the potential for adverse effects (including perhaps severe rash).

Topiramate may decrease the clearance of phenytoin, suggesting inhibition of CYP2C19. Topiramate has been shown to increase phenytoin serum concentration in some patients. While this interaction is not clinically meaningful in most patients, given the non-linear pharmacokinetics of phenytoin, the potential does exist for this interaction to result in phenytoin intoxication.

A significant advancement of oxcarbazepine over carbamazepine is its lack of *susceptibility* to inhibitory interactions. Consistent with its differing metabolism (as compared to carbamazepine), oxcarbazepine's pharmacokinetics are not altered by erythromycin. Oxcarbazepine

TABLE 39-2
Interactions Between AEDs and Non-AED Medications

Non-AED Medication			
Type	**Drug**	**AED**	**Interaction**
Adrenergic blockers	Alprenolol	PB	PB increases metabolism; dosage of adrenergic blockers may need to be increased.
	Metoprolol Propranolol		
Analgesics	Acetaminophen	CBZ, LTG, PB, PHT	Patients on enzyme inducers such as CBZ, PHT, and PB may be at greater risk of hepatotoxicity following acetaminophen overdose. Acetaminophen appears to slightly increase the elimination of LTG.
	Narcotics	CBZ, PB, PHT	Enzyme inducers (CBZ, PHT, PB) increase the toxicity and decrease the efficacy of meperidine by increasing the conversation to normeperidine.
	Propoxyphene	CBZ	Propoxyphene inhibits CBZ elimination and may lead to CBZ toxicity. Propoxyphene should be avoided if possible.
	Salicylates	PHT, VPA	High-dose salicylates displace PHT and VPA from protein-binding sites and may decrease VPA elimination.
Antiarrythmics	Disopyramide	PB, PHT	PB and PHT may increase hepatic metabolism of disopyramide and require dosage adjustments.
	Mexiletine	CBZ, PB, PHT	Enzyme inducers can substantially decrease mexiletine serum concentrations.
	Quinidine	PB, PHT	Enzyme inducers decrease serum concentrations of quinidine.
Anticoagulants	Warfarin	CBZ, PB, PHT	Inducers increase warfarin metabolism and decrease hypoprothrombinemic effect.
Antidepressants	Tricyclics	CBZ, PB	Induction of tricyclic metabolism. Dosage may require adjustment.
Antidiabetic agents	Tolazamide	CBZ, PB, PHT	Enzyme inducers increase elimination and decrease hypoglycemic effects.
	Tolbutamide Acetohexamide Glibenclamide		
Antimicrobial agents	Ciprofloxacin	PHT	Ciprofloxacin increases serum PHT concentrations, probably by decreasing phenytoin elimination.
	Erythromycin	CBZ, BZD, VPA	Erythromycin decreases biotransformation and can markedly increase serum concentrations.
Antifungal	Fluconazole	PHT	Fluconazole decreases biotransformation of PHT and can result in marked increase in serum concentrations.

TABLE 39-2
(Continued)

Non-AED Medication			
Type	**Drug**	**AED**	**Interaction**
Antineoplastics		PHT	Cytotoxic agents appear to decrease oral absorption of PHT with marked reductions in serum PHT concentrations.
Antituberculous agents	Isoniazid	CBZ, PHT, VPA	Isoniazid decreases CBZ, PHT, and VPA elimination and may lead to toxicity.
	Rifampin	BZD, PHT, VPA	Rifampin increases elimination; dosage adjustments may be necessary.
Carbonic anhydrase inhibitors	Acetazolamide	TPM	Concomitant use may lead to increased risk of nephrolithiasis.
	Dichlorphenamide Methazolamide		
Corticosteroids	Dexamethasone	CBZ, PB, PHT	Enzyme inducers increase metabolism of steroids and decrease efficacy. Decreased PHT absorption and subsequent decrease in serum concentrations.
	Hydrocortisone		
	Methylprednisolone		
	Prednisone		
Miscellaneous	Cimetidine	CBZ, PHT, BZD, ESM	Cimetidine decreases biotransformation of CBZ and PHT and may lead to toxicity.
	Clozapine	CBZ	May result in increased risk of bone marrow suppression.
	Enteral feedings	PHT	Decreased PHT absorption and marked decreased in serum concentration.
	Nafimidone	CBZ, PHT	May result in CBZ toxicity.
	Ritonavir	BDZ, ESM	Ritonavir decreases biotransformation of BDZ and ESM and may lead to toxicity.
Selective serotonin reuptake inhibitors	Fluoxetine	CBZ	Fluoxetine has been reported to result in CBZ toxicity by inhibiting CYP3A3/4.

BDZ = benzodiazepines; CBZ = carbamazepine; LTG = lamotrigine; PB = phenobarbital; PHT = phenytoin; PRM = primidone; VPA = valproic acid; ESM = ethosuximide; TPM = topiramate; MSM = methsuximide.
Source: McInnes and Brodie 1988 (39).

is a weak inhibitor of CYP2C19, however, and, like topiramate, it may increase the plasma concentrations of phenytoin (1).

Because of their primarily renal clearance, and absence of substantial hepatic metabolism, levetiracetam, gabapentin, and pregabalin are not subject to inhibition. In addition, none of these drugs appears to cause inhibition of metabolism of any other medication.

Interactions Between AEDs and Other Medications

Traditionally, most attention regarding AED pharmacokinetic interactions has been directed toward interactions between various combinations of AEDs. It is important for the clinician to recognize the potential impact that AEDs may have on concomitant medications that a patient receive. For example, many psychotropic agents, including tricyclic antidepressants, selective serotonin reuptake inhibitors (SSRIs), and antipsychotic drugs are extensively metabolized by one or more of the CYP isozymes (29). This would imply that higher than expected doses of these drugs may be required in patients receiving enzyme-inducing AEDs such as phenytoin or carbamazepine. Conversely, enzyme-inhibiting drugs such as valproate may inhibit the clearance of certain psychotropic drugs such as amitriptyline, nortriptyline, or paroxetine (1, 2).

For example, AEDs such as carbamazepine and phenytoin have been reported to increase the clearance, and consequently markedly lower the serum concentration, of a number of antipsychotic medications including haloperidol, chlorpromazine, clozapine, risperidone, ziprazidone, and olanzapine (2, 30). Valproate appears to have minimal pharmacokinetic interactions impact on these drugs (31, 32).

Antipsychotic drugs are less likely to *cause* pharmacokinetic interactions with AEDs, although both chlorpromazine and thioridazine have been reported to result in increases in phenytoin serum concentrations. Risperidone has been noted to result in modest decreases in carbamazepine concentrations (33).

Many commonly used antidepressant agents such as tricyclics and SSRIs are also metabolized via the CYP system. Consequently, it would be expected that drugs such as amitriptyline, nortriptyline, imipramine, desipramine, clomipramine, protriptyline, doxepin, sertraline, paroxetine, mianserin, citalopram, and nefazodone may display reduced serum concentrations in patients receiving enzyme-inducing AEDs (1, 2, 34, 35). Conversely, comedication with the enzyme inhibitor valproate may cause substantial (50–60%) increases in serum concentrations of drugs such as amitriptyline and nortriptyline.

AED-antidepressant interactions may be bidirectional, and the clinician should recognize that treatment with certain drugs may result in increased serum concentrations of AEDs, particularly the older, extensively metabolized agents. For example, there are data that suggest that SSRIs such as fluoxetine and sertraline can result in increased phenytoin and carbamazepine serum concentrations.

Examples of other classes of drugs that are extensively metabolized and therefore may be influenced by enzyme-inducing AEDs include stimulants (i.e., methylphenidate), antineoplastics, immunosuppressants, beta receptor antagonists, oral contraceptives, and many antiviral agents such as indinavir, retonavir, and saqquinavir (1, 2, 36–38). Table 39-2 provides a representative list of potential AED–non-AED interactions (39).

SUMMARY

Polypharmacy with multiple concomitant medications is common in patients of all ages who suffer from epilepsy. Clinicians should be aware that many of the older, traditional AEDs such as carbamazepine, phenytoin and the barbiturates have been consistently associated with pharmacokinetic interactions, both with other AEDs, as well as many commonly used medications. In many cases, these interactions may go unrecognized, as routine serum concentration monitoring is not available, or practical in all situations. It would seem prudent therefore for clinicians to monitor clinical response to concomitant medications, and consider potential drug interactions, should sub-optimal patient response (including the appearance of adverse effects) be noted.

Alternatively, clinicians may want to consider using appropriate newer generation AEDs such as that do not seem to interfere, either with drug metabolism, or oral absorption/transport, and thereby avoid these potentially problematic interactions.

References

1. Perucca E. Clinically relevant drug interactions with antiepileptic drugs. *Br J Clin Pharmacol* 2005; 61:246–255.
2. Patsalos P, Perucca E. Clinically important drug interactions in epilepsy: Interactions between antiepileptic drugs and other drugs. *Lancet Neurology* 2003; 2:473–481.
3. Juurlink DN, Mamdani M, Kopp A, Laupacis A, et al. Drug-drug interactions among elderly patients hospitalized for drug toxicity. *JAMA* 2003; 289:1652–1658.
4. Bauer LA. Interference of oral phenytoin absorption by continuous nasogastric feedings. *Neurology* 1982; 32:570–572.
5. Krueger KA, Garnett WR, Comstock TJ, et al. Effect of two administration schedules of an enteral nutrient formula on phenytoin bioavailability. *Epilepsia* 1987; 28:706–712.
6. Nishimura LY, Armstrong EP, Plezia PM, et al. Influence of enteral feedings on phenytoin sodium absorption from capsules. *Drug Intell Clin Pharm* 1988; 22:130–133.
7. Fischer JH, Barr AN, Paloucek FP, Dorociak JV, et al. Effect of food on the serum concentration profile of enteric-coated valproic acid. *Neurology* 1988; 38:1319–1322.
8. Fay MA. Sheth RD. Gidal BE. Oral absorption kinetics of levetiracetam: the effect of mixing with food or enteral nutrition formulas. *Clinical Therapeutics* 2005; 27(5):594–598.
9. Gidal BE, Maly MM, Kowalski J, Rutecki P, et al. Gabapentin absorption: effect of mixing with foods of varying macronutrient content. *Ann Pharmacother* 1998; 32:405–408.
10. Doose DR, Walker SA, Gisclon LG, Nayak RK. Single-dose pharmacokinetics and effect of food on the bioavailability of topiramate, a novel antiepileptic drug. *J Clin Pharmacol* 1996; 36(10):884–891.
11. Degen PH, Flesch G, Cardot JM, Czendlik C, et al. The influence of food on the disposition of the antiepileptic oxcarbazepine and its major metabolite in healthy volunteers. *Biopharm Drug Dispos* 1994; 15(6):519–526.
12. Fay MA. Sheth RD, Gidal BE. Oral absorption kinetics of levetiracetam: the effect of mixing with food or enteral nutrition formulas. *Clinical Therapeutics* 2005; 27(5): 594–598.
13. Lin JH, Yamazaki M. Role of P glycoprotein in pharmacokinetics: clinical implications. *Clinical Pharmacokinet* 2003; 42:59–98.
14. Ceckova-Novotna M, Pavek P, Staud F. P-glycoprotein in the placenta: Expression, localization, regulation and function. *Reprod Toxicol* 2006; 22:400–410.
15. Giessmann T, May K, Modess C, et al. Carbamazepine regulates intestinal P-glycoprotein and multidrug resistance protein MRP2 and influences disposition of talinolol in humans. *Clin Pharmacol Ther* 2004; 76:192–200.
16. Anderson GD. A mechanistic approach to antiepileptic drug interactions. *Ann Pharmacother* 1998; 32:554–563.
17. Benet LZ, Hoener BA. Changes in plasma protein binding have little clinical relevance. *Clin Pharmacol Ther* 2002; 71:115–121.
18. Anderson GD. Pharmacogenetics and enzyme induction/inhibition properties of antiepileptic drugs. *Neurology* 2004; 63:(Suppl 4):S3–S8.
19. Xu C, Li CY, Kong AN. Induction of phase I, II, III drug metabolism/transport by xenobiotics. *Arch Pharm Res* 2005; 28:249–269.

20. Murray M, Petrovich N. Cytochrome P450: decision-making tools for personalized therapeutics. *Curr Opin Mol Ther* 2006; 8:480–486.
21. Pisani F, Xiao B, Faziop A, Spina E, et al. Single-dose pharmacokinetics of CBZ-E in patients on lamotrigine monotherapy. *Epilepsy Res* 1994; 19:245–248.
22. Gidal BE, Rutecki P, Shaw R, Maly MM, et al. Effect of lamotrigine on carbamazepine epoxide/carbamazepine serum concentration ratios in adult patients with epilepsy. *Epilepsy Res* 1997; 28:207–211.
23. Anderson GD, Gidal BE, Gilliam F, Messenheimer J. Time course of lamotrigine de-induction: Impact of step-wise withdrawal of carbamazepine or phenytoin. *Epilepsy Res* 2002; 49:211-217.
24. Gidal BE, Baltes E, Otoul C, Perucca E. Effect of levetiracetam on the pharmacokinetics of adjunctive antiepileptic drugs: a pooled analysis of data from randomized clinical trials. *Epilepsy Res* 2005; 64(1–2):1–11.
25. Perucca E, Gidal BE, et al. Effects of antiepileptic comedication on levetiracetam pharmacokinetics: a pooled analysis of data from randomized adjunctive therapy trials. *Epilepsy Res* 2003; 53:47–56.
26. Rosenfeld WE, Liao S, Anderson G,et al. Comparison of the steady-state pharmacokinetics of topiramate and valproate in patients with epilepsy during monotherapy and concomitant therapy. *Epilepsia* 1997; 38:329–333.
27. Zupanc M. Antiepileptic drugs and hormonal contraceptives in adolescent women with epilepsy. *Neurology* 2006; 66Suppl 3):37–45.
28. Gidal BE, Sheth R, Parnell J, et al. Evaluation of VPA dose and concentration effects on lamotrigine pharmacokinetics: implications for conversion to monotherapy. *Epilepsy Res* 2003; 57:85–93.
29. Spina E, Perucca E. Clinical significance of pharmacokinetic interactions between antiepileptic and psychtropic drugs. *Epilepsia* 2002; 43(Suppl 2):37–44.
30. Jann MW, Ereshefsky L, Saklad SR, et al. Effects of carbamazepine on plasma haloperidol levels. *J Clin Psychopharmacol* 1985; 5:106–109.
31. Spina E, Avenoso A, Facciola G, et al. Plasma concentrations of risperidone and 9-hydroxyrespiridone; effect of comedication with carbamazepine or valproate. *Ther Drug Monit* 2000; 22:481–485.
32. Hesslinger B, Normann C, Langgosch JM, et al. Effects of carbamazepine and valproate on haloperidol levels and on psychopathologic outcome in schizophrenic patients. *J Clin Psychopharmacol* 1999; 19:310–315.
33. Mula M, Monaco F. Carbamazepine-risperidone interactions in patients with epilepsy. *Clin Neuropharmacol* 2002; 25:97–100.
34. Trimble MR, Mula M. Antiepileptic drug interactions in patients requiring psychiatric drug treatment. In: Majkowski J, Bourgeois B, Patsalos P, Mattson R, eds. *Antiepileptic Drugs. Combination Therapy and Interactions*. Cambridge, UK: Cambridge University Press, 2005:350–368.
35. Pihlsgard M, Eliasson E. Significant reduction of sertraline plasma levels by carbamazepine and phenytoin. *Eur J Clin Pharmacol* 2002; 57:915–916.
36. Vecht CJ, Wagner GL, Wilms EB. Treating seizures in patients with brain tumors: drug interactions between antiepileptic drugs and chemotherapeutic agents. *Semin Oncol* 2003; 30(6 Suppl 19):49–52.
37. Flockart DA, Tanus-Santos JE. Implications of cytochrome P450 interactions when prescribing medication for hypertension. *Arch Intern Med* 2002; 162: 405–412.
38. Markowitz JS, Morrison SD, DeVane CL. Drug interactions with psychostimulants. *Int Clin Psychopharmacology* 1999; 14:1–18.
39. McInnes GT, Brodie MJ. Drug interactions that matter—a critical reappraisal. *Drugs* 1988; 36:83–110.

V

ANTIEPILEPTIC DRUGS AND KETOGENIC DIET

40 ACTH and Steroids

Rajesh RamachandranNair
O. Carter Snead, III

The efficacy of adrenocorticotropin (ACTH) therapy in childhood seizures was first observed by Klein and Livingston in 1950 in a series of children with atypical absence seizures (1). In 1958, Sorel and Dusaucy-Bauloye reported that ACTH was effective in children with infantile spasms (IS). These authors not only reported seizure control in children with IS treated with ACTH but also observed improvements in behavior and electroencephalogram (EEG) (2). Subsequently, a number of studies appeared that reported on the efficacy of corticosteroids in IS and confirmed the utility of ACTH in the treatment of this disorder. Both ACTH and corticosteroids have been used in treating a number of epilepsy syndromes, including Ohtahara syndrome, Lennox-Gastaut syndrome and other myoclonic epilepsies, and Landau-Kleffner syndrome (3). The epilepsy syndromes that respond uniquely to ACTH and corticosteroid therapy have an age-related onset during a critical period of brain development, as well as a characteristic regression or plateau of acquired milestones at seizure onset, and long-term cognitive impairment (4). In addition to beneficial effects on the convulsive state, there are some data to suggest that ACTH, corticosteroids, or both also can improve the short-term developmental trajectory and the long-term prognosis for language and cognitive development in at least some of these patients (5–9).

In this review, we will first discuss the evidence in support of the use of steroids in IS. This will be followed by a review of possible mechanisms of the putative anticonvulsant effects of ACTH and corticosteroids. This will be followed by a discussion of the use of these compounds in epilepsy syndromes other than IS. Finally, we will review the therapeutic potential of neuroactive steroids in epilepsy.

INFANTILE SPASMS

In 1841, William West, an English physician, provided the first description of IS in his own 4-month old son (10). Later, the association of IS with the sequelae of severe mental deficiency emerged. In 1952, Gibbs and Gibbs first described the interictal EEG pattern associated with infantile spasms and termed it hypsarrhythmia. This pattern was unique and described as showing high-voltage, chaotic slowing with multifocal spikes, and marked asynchrony (11). Over the years, the triad of infantile spasms, hypsarrhythmia, and mental retardation became known as West syndrome (12).

After 1958, studies began to appear in the literature reporting the effectiveness of corticosteroids in the treatment of this disorder (12). There is a marked variability of response rates to these therapeutic agents that probably is related to the small cohorts reported and the paucity of controlled treatment data. Another confound is that the natural history of IS is poorly understood, particularly the phenomenon of spontaneous remission. Moreover, the literature is replete with marked variations in the dosage of ACTH and/or corticosteroids given, and in treatment duration, of both drugs. In most studies, an objective method of documenting spasm cessation has not been used and response to therapy has been defined in a graded manner, although there is no convincing evidence that spasms respond in a graded fashion to any form of therapy. Usually IS respond in an all-or-none fashion to treatment with ACTH and/or corticosteroids. Finally, most studies have been uncontrolled, unblinded, and retrospective, complicating the establishment of evidence-based recommendations for optimal treatment (12).

The controversies surrounding the treatment of IS outnumber the areas of agreement and encompass the following questions: Which is the most effective therapy: ACTH or corticosteroid? Are other anticonvulsants such as vigabatrin, valproic acid, benzodiazepines, topiramate, zonisamide, or pyridoxine effective against infantile spasms? Is there some other treatment regimen with newer antiepileptic drugs that is effective against infantile spasms? What is the impact of treatment with ACTH compared with corticosteroids on long-term outcome in recurrence of spasms, evolution into other forms of intractable epilepsy, and cognitive or behavioral function? Does treatment change the outcome for a patient with preexisting mental retardation and a structurally abnormal brain? What is the optimal dosage of these drugs, and how long should treatment last? Does the ultimate outcome depend on timing of treatment? Does the efficacy of ACTH depend on the formulation (natural vs. synthetic, sustained vs. short-acting)?

Some of these questions were addressed in a recently published American Academy of Neurology (AAN)/Child Neurology Society (CNS) Practice Parameter on the treatment of infantile spasms (13). In the following few paragraphs we will discuss the key issues addressed by this practice parameter. Important studies published subsequent to the practice parameter also will be discussed in the relevant sections.

Summary of the AAN/CNS Practice Parameter on the Treatment of Infantile Spasms

Three major questions were addressed in the practice parameter.

1. What are the most effective therapies for infantile spasms, as determined by short-term outcome measures, including complete cessation of spasms, resolution of hypsarrhythmia, and likelihood of relapse following initial response?
2. How safe are currently used treatments?
3. Does successful treatment of infantile spasms lead to long-term improvement of neurodevelopmental outcome or a decreased incidence of epilepsy?

Articles included for critical analysis pursuant to answering these questions and formulating treatment recommendations for infantile spasms had the following inclusion criteria (14–27):

1. A clearly stated diagnosis of infantile spasms
2. An EEG demonstrating hypsarrhythmia or modified hypsarrhythmia
3. Age of 1 month to 3 years.

Infantile spasms were classified as either symptomatic or cryptogenic as defined by the International League Against Epilepsy (ILAE).

Outcome measures included short- and long-term measures. Short-term outcome measures were defined as the following:

1. Complete cessation of spasms
2. Resolution of hypsarrhythmia and, where documented, normalization of EEG
3. Relapse rate

In studies with a mean follow-up of >2 years, the following were considered long-term outcome measures:

1. Nonepileptiform EEG
2. Absence of seizures
3. Normal development

A four tiered classification scheme for diagnostic evidence approved by the Quality Standards Subcommittee was utilized as part of the assessment. This schema is outlined in Table 40-1. Depending on the strength of the evidence under this classification system, specific recommendations were made. The strength of these recommendations is shown in Table 40-2.

Based on this critical analysis it was concluded in the practice parameter that ACTH was probably effective in the short-term treatment of IS and in the resolution of hypsarrhythmia (level B). Time to response was usually within 2 weeks, and an "all-or-none" response had been reported in a number of studies. The data were insufficient to recommend optimal dosage and duration of treatment with ACTH for the treatment of IS (level U). As well, data also were insufficient to recommend treatment of IS with oral corticosteroids (level U). ACTH was more effective than oral corticosteroids in causing the cessation of seizures. Side effects reported for ACTH were common and included hypertension, irritability, infection, reversible cerebral shrinkage, and, rarely, death due to sepsis.

TABLE 40-1
American Academy of Neurology Evidence Classification Scheme for a Therapeutic Article

Class I	Evidence provided by a prospective, randomized, controlled clinical trial with masked outcome assessment, in a representative population. The following are required: (a) Primary outcome(s) is/are clearly defined; (b) exclusion/inclusion criteria are clearly defined; (c) dropouts and crossovers are accounted for adequately with numbers sufficiently low to have minimal potential for bias; and (d) relevant baseline characteristics are presented and substantially equivalent among treatment groups, or there is appropriate statistical adjustment for differences.
Class II	Evidence provided by a prospective matched-group cohort study in a representative population with masked outcome assessment that meets (a)–(d) as defined for Class I or a randomized controlled trial in a representative population that lacks one criterion of (a)–(d).
Class III	All other controlled trials (including well-defined natural history controls or patients serving as own controls) in a representative population, where outcome assessment is independent of patients' treatment.
Class IV	Evidence from uncontrolled studies, case series, case reports, or expert opinion.

Although vigabatrin (VGB) is not a steroid, its use in infantile spasms is relevant to this review because steroids and vigabatrin are generally considered to be the only two groups of drugs that work in this disorder—an impression borne out by the Practice Parameter (13). In the analysis that led to the AAN/CNS practice parameter, the evidence for the therapeutic efficacy of vigabatrin in IS was weaker than that for ACTH (level C for vigabatrin vs. level B for ACTH). Hence, vigabatrin was found to be possibly effective for the short-term treatment of IS.

As for the efficacy of ACTH in improving the long-term outcomes in terms of seizure freedom and normal development of children with IS, the data were insufficient (28–31) in that regard (Level U, class III and IV evidence). Similarly, there was insufficient evidence to support the thesis that early initiation of treatment with ACTH improves the long-term outcome of children with IS (Level U, class III and IV evidence).

More recently, the United Kingdom Infantile Spasms Study (32) assessed comparative efficacy of vigabatrin and hormonal treatment of IS in a randomized controlled trial. The primary outcome was cessation of spasms on days 13 and 14. Minimum doses were VGB 100 mg/kg per day, oral prednisolone 40 mg per day, or intramuscular tetracosactide depot 0.5 mg (40 IU) on alternate days. Of 208 infants screened and assessed, 107 were randomly assigned to VGB ($n = 52$) or hormonal treatments (prednisolone $n = 30$, tetracosactide $n = 25$). Patients with no spasms on days 13 and 14 consisted of: 40 (73%) of 55 infants assigned hormonal treatments (prednisolone 21/30 [70%], tetracosactide 19/25 [76%]) and 28 (54%) of 52 infants assigned VGB (difference 19%, CI 1–36%, $P = 0.043$). Adverse events were reported in 30 (55%) of 55 infants on hormonal treatments and 28 (54%) of 52 infants on VGB. This study concluded that cessation

TABLE 40-2
American Academy of Neurology System for Translation of Evidence to Recommendations

Translation of Evidence to Recommendations	Rating of Recommendation
Level A rating requires at least one convincing class I study or at least two consistent, convincing class II studies.	A = established as effective, ineffective, or harmful for the given condition in the specified population.
Level B rating requires at least one convincing class II study or at least three consistent class III studies.	B = probably effective, ineffective, or harmful (or probably useful/predictive or not useful/predictive) for the given condition in the specified population.
Level C rating requires at least two convincing and consistent class III studies.	C = possibly effective, ineffective, or harmful (or possibly useful/predictive or not useful/ predictive) for the given condition in the specified population.
	U = data inadequate or conflicting. Given current knowledge, treatment is unproven.

of spasms was more likely in infants given hormonal treatments than in those given VGB.

Infants enrolled in the United Kingdom Infantile Spasms Study were followed up until clinical assessment at 12–14 months of age (33). Neurodevelopment was assessed with the Vineland Adaptive Behavior Scales (VABS) at 14 months of age. Of 107 infants enrolled, five died, and 101 survivors reached both follow-up assessments. Absence of spasms at final clinical assessment (hormone 41/55 [75%] vs. vigabatrin 39/51 [76%]) was similar in each treatment group. Mean VABS score did not differ significantly (hormone 78.6 vs. vigabatrin 77.5). In infants with no identified underlying etiology, the mean VABS score was higher in those allocated hormone treatment than in those allocated vigabatrin (88.2 vs. 78.9; difference 9.3, 95% CI 1.2–17.3). This study reported that better initial control of spasms by hormone treatment in those with no identified underlying etiology might lead to improved developmental outcome.

Kivity and coworkers assessed the long-term cognitive and seizure outcomes of 37 patients with cryptogenic infantile spasms (onset, age 3 to 9 months) receiving a standardized treatment regimen of high-dose tetracosactide depot, 1 mg intramuscularly (IM) every 48 hours for 2 weeks, with a subsequent 8- to 10-week slow taper and followed by oral prednisone, 10 mg/day for a month, with a subsequent slow taper for 5 months or until the infant reached the age of 1 year, whichever came later (8). Cognitive outcomes were determined after 6 to 21 years and analyzed in relation to treatment lag and pretreatment regression. Normal cognitive outcome was found in all 22 (100%) patients of the early-treatment group (within 1 month), and in 40% of the late-treatment group (1–6.5 months). Normal cognitive outcome was found in all 25 (100%) patients who had no or only mild mental deterioration at presentation, including four in the late-treatment group but in only three of the 12 patients who had had marked or severe deterioration before treatment. This study indicated that early treatment of cryptogenic infantile spasms with a high-dose ACTH protocol was associated with favorable long-term cognitive outcomes. Once major developmental regression lasted for a month or more, the prognosis for normal cognitive outcome was poor.

Practical Considerations Regarding Dosage

Table 40-3 lists the currently available formulations of ACTH. The biologic activity, expressed in international units (IU), permits a comparison of potency in terms of the relative ability of the peptide to stimulate the adrenals, but may not necessarily reflect the ability of the ACTH preparation to affect brain function. The biologic activity of natural ACTH in the brain may differ from that of synthetic ACTH as a result of ACTH fragments and possibly other pituitary hormones with neurobiologic activity in the brain that are present in the pituitary extracts (5). These compounds could enhance the therapeutic efficacy of natural ACTH (34). Any differences in the biologic effects of sustained ACTH levels provided by the depot formulations, as opposed to those of the short-acting preparations, are unknown. Given in high doses, however, long-acting depot preparations are associated with an increased incidence of severe side effects, including death from overwhelming infection.

The most effective dose of ACTH for remission of spasms is controversial. Notably, in comparison to prednisone, no major advantage was demonstrated by

TABLE 40-3
Available Preparations of ACTH

Corticotropin (ACTH 1-39): porcine pituitary extract (short-acting)	
Acthar gel 80 IU/mL	100 IU* = 0.72 mg
Acthar lyophylized powder	100 IU* = 0.72 mg
Cosyntropin/Tetracosactrin (ACTH 1-24): synthetic (short-acting)	
Cortrosyn	100 IU* = 1.0 mg
Cosyntropin/Tetracosactrin (ACTH 1-24): synthetic (long-acting)	
Synacthen depot (CIBA)	100 IU* = 2.5 mg
Cortrosyn-Z (Organon)	100 I U* = 2.5 mg

*Commercial preparations are described in International Units (IU) based on a potency assay in hypophysectomized rats in which depletion of adrenal ascorbic acid is measured after subcutaneous ACTH injection.

low-dose ACTH, whereas high-dose ACTH was reported to be superior (15, 25). High-dose ACTH (60 IU/day or 150 IU/m^2 per day) has been associated with excellent short-term response rates (87–93%) in prospective studies (14, 25). However; in the only randomized, prospective comparison of ACTH, Hrachovy and coworkers found no difference between high dose and low dose (16). A prospective study of synthetic ACTH by Yanagaki and coworkers compared very low-dose ACTH (0.2 IU/kg per day) to low-dose (1 IU/kg per day) and found equivalent efficacy, with response and relapse rates comparable to other studies (18). Heiskala et al. described a protocol that utilized a stepwise increase in dosage, demonstrating that some patients can be controlled on lower doses of carboxymethylcellulose ACTH (3 IU/kg per day) but others required high doses (12 IU/kg per day). Overall, spasms were controlled initially in 65% of patients, but the rate of relapse was high (35).

Some evidence supports a beneficial effect of high-dose ACTH over low-dose ACTH or oral steroids in cognitive outcome. Glaze and coworkers found no difference between low-dose ACTH (20 to 30 IU/day) and prednisone (2 mg/kg per day) with regard to the cognitive outcome (31). However, in a comparison of high-dose ACTH (110 IU/m^2 per day) and steroids, however, Lombroso showed a higher rate of normal cognitive outcome in cryptogenic patients treated with ACTH than in those treated with prednisone alone (55% vs. 17%) (5). Ito and coworkers also showed a positive correlation between dose and developmental outcome comparing different ACTH dosage regimens retrospectively (36).

The optimal ACTH dose may lie between 85 and 250 IU/m^2 per day. Doses of 400 IU/m^2 per day or higher are contraindicated because of a high incidence of life-threatening side effects. The optimal dose of ACTH required to enhance short-term response and long-term cognitive outcome is unknown; however, relatively high doses given early in the disease, accompanied by a second course in the event of relapse, appear warranted. The following high-dose ACTH protocol (21, 25) has been used successfully by us in treating more than 700 children with infantile spasms.

The child is admitted to a day-care unit to initiate ACTH therapy and to teach parents to give the injection, measure urine glucose three times daily with Chemstix, and recognize spasms to keep an accurate seizure calendar. Any diagnostic workup indicated by clinical circumstances is also performed, including screening for occult congenital infections. Before ACTH is started, an endocrine profile, complete blood count, urinalysis, electrolyte panel, baseline renal function, and calcium, phosphorus, and serum glucose levels are obtained. Blood pressure and electrocardiogram are also assessed. The drug is not given if any of these studies show abnormal results. Diagnostic neuroimaging is indicated before initiation of ACTH or steroids because of the association of ACTH treatment with ventriculomegaly. The initial dose of ACTH is 150 IU/m^2/day of ACTH gel, 80 IU/mL, intramuscularly in two divided doses for 1 week. In the second week, 75 IU/m^2 per day is given, followed by 75 IU/m^2 every other day in the third week. Over the next 6 weeks, the dose is gradually tapered. The lot number of the ACTH gel is carefully recorded. Usually, a response is seen within the first 7 days; if no response is noted in 2 weeks, the lot is changed.

Blood pressure must be measured daily at home during the first week and three times weekly thereafter. Control of hypertension is attempted with salt restriction and amlodipine therapy rather than discontinuation of ACTH. The patient is monitored in the outpatient clinic weekly for the first month and then biweekly, with appropriate blood work at each visit. Waking and sleeping EEG patterns are obtained 1, 2, and 4 weeks after the start of ACTH to assess treatment response. As the treatment response is usually all or none, positive results are suggested when properly trained parents report no seizures in a child, whose waking and sleeping EEG patterns are normal. If relapse occurs, the dose may be increased to the previously effective dose for 2 weeks and another tapering begun. If seizures continue, the dose may be increased to 150 IU/m^2 per day and the regimen restarted.

If prednisone is chosen because of its oral formulation and lower incidence of serious side effects, the pretreatment laboratory evaluation described earlier is performed. The initial dose is 3 mg/kg per day in four divided doses for 2 weeks, followed by a 10-week taper (25). A multiple-daily-dose regimen is recommended to produce the sustained elevations of plasma cortisol demonstrated in high-dose ACTH therapy.

Adverse Effects of ACTH and Steroids

ACTH and steroids, particularly at the high doses recommended for infantile spasms, can produce dangerous side effects. These are more frequent and more pronounced with ACTH (37). Cushingoid features and extreme irritability are seen frequently; hypertension is less common but appears to be associated with higher doses. Vigilance is required for signs of sepsis; pneumonia; glucosuria; metabolic abnormalities involving the electrolytes calcium and phosphorus (38–40); and congestive heart failure (41, 42). Cerebral ventriculomegaly, which is not always reversible, can lead to subdural hematoma (43, 44). The cause of the apparent cerebral atrophy is obscure, but its existence emphasizes the importance of diagnostic neuroimaging before initiation of ACTH.

Because hypothalamic-pituitary or adrenocortical dysfunction can result from ACTH therapy, morning levels of cortisol should be monitored during a taper and any medical stress treated with high-dose steroids (45–47).

Treatment with ACTH or steroids also can be immunosuppressant and associated with infectious complications, such as overwhelming sepsis, perhaps as a result of impaired function of polymorphonuclear leukocytes (48). Both agents are therefore contraindicated in the face of serious bacterial or viral infection such as varicella or cytomegalovirus. Because of the potential for fatal *Pneumocystis* pneumonia as an infectious complication of ACTH therapy, prophylaxis with trimethoprim-sulfamethoxazole, accompanied by folate supplementation and frequent blood counts, may be prudent in infants older than 2 months of age. In rare cases, ACTH can exacerbate seizures (49).

Potential Mechanisms of Action of ACTH in Infantile Spasms

ACTH is a 39-amino-acid peptide hormone produced, through post-translational modification of the larger peptide pro-opiomelanocortin (POMC), in the anterior pituitary. POMC expression, processing to ACTH, and ACTH secretion are stimulated by corticotropin-releasing factor (CRF) generated in the hypothalamus, and these processes are under negative feedback control by glucocorticoids (50). ACTH secretion is pulsatile and normally has a pronounced diurnal variation, but secretion also increases substantially in response to a range of stressors. The effects of ACTH are mediated via stimulation of the G-coupled cell surface ACTH receptor, which is expressed primarily on adrenocortical cells. This receptor is a member of the melanocortin family and is alternatively known as the melanocortin-2 (MC-2) receptor. ACTH acutely stimulates the synthesis of cortisol in the adrenal gland. ACTH also increases the long-term capacity of the adrenal gland to generate cortisol by inducing a range of steroidogenic enzymes and hypertrophy of the cortex (51). ACTH additionally has the capacity to cross-react with other melanocortin receptors (52).

The pathogenesis of infantile spasms, and therefore the mechanism of action of ACTH and steroids in this condition, are unknown, principally because there is no available animal model for this disorder. Infantile spasms occur within a narrow developmental window in terms of age of onset and can be found concurrently with a variety of congenital abnormalities of brain, which may be causally linked—so-called symptomatic spasms. However, IS also may occur without apparent cause in children with no pre-existing neurologic abnormality at the onset of spasms (i.e., idiopathic spasms). Those children who are not neurologically normal when the spasms appear, yet have no demonstrable imaging or metabolic abnormality, are said to have cryptogenic spasms.

The effect of ACTH and corticosteroids in infantile spasms is frequently all or none, and the steroid-induced seizure-free state is often sustainable even after drug withdrawal. These observations support the theory that due to various etiologies, a significant stress response is experienced by the developing brain; resulting in this age-dependent epileptic encephalopathy. Within this very narrow developmental window, ACTH and steroids may be able to reset the deranged homeostatic mechanisms of the brain, thereby reducing the convulsive tendency and improving the developmental trajectory.

The Brain-Adrenal Axis There is evidence to suggest that the effects of ACTH in infantile spasms may be independent of steroidogenesis. Efficacy studies have demonstrated superiority of ACTH to corticosteroids in treating infantile spasms and also its efficacy in adrenal-suppressed patients. Substantial physiologic and pharmacologic data indicate that ACTH has direct effects on brain function: increasing dendritic sprouting in immature animals; stimulation of myelination; regulation of the synthesis, release, uptake, and metabolism of dopamine, norepinephrine, acetylcholine, serotonin, and gamma-aminobutyric acid (GABA); regulation of the binding to glutamatergic, serotoninergic, muscarinic type 1, opiate, and dopaminergic receptors; and alteration of neuronal membrane lipid fluidity, permeability, and signal transduction (53–57). Though activation of glucocorticoid receptors has little direct anticonvulsant effect, it modulates the expression and release of a number of neurotransmitters and neuromodulators, including the proconvulsant neuropeptide corticotropin-releasing hormone (CRH). High brain CRH levels would be predicted to reduce the cerebrospinal fluid ACTH and steroids (58). Many authors have reported reduced levels of ACTH in patients with infantile spasms, compared to their age-matched controls (59, 60). In infant animal models CRH causes seizures and death of neurons (61). These effects of CRH are most marked in developing brain (62). Suppression of the after-hyperpolarization and activation of the glutamatergic neurotransmission are the possible mechanisms by which CRH may mediate these effects. In animals, ACTH appears to down-regulate the CRH expression in amygdala. This effect was found to be independent of glucocorticoid receptor activation but required melanocortin receptors (63). ACTH reduces CRH gene expression in specific brain regions. This effect has been demonstrated in the absence of adrenal steroids and resides within the 4-10 fragment of ACTH, a fragment that does not release adrenal steroids. Melanocortin receptor antagonists blocked this effect, suggesting that the melanocortin receptors are the targets of ACTH action (63).

A hypothesis, therefore, can be generated in which a stress response results in enhanced CRH expression, leading to neuronal hyperexcitability and seizures. By suppressing CRH expression, possibly through the action of peptide fragments of ACTH on melanocortin receptors, the CRF-induced hyperexcitability may be reduced, hence ameliorating infantile spasms. Clinical trials of ACTH fragments that have no activity on the adrenal axis have been disappointing (64); however, these clinical trials have utilized the 4-9 peptide fragment rather than the 4-10 peptide fragment studied in animal models. The events that precipitate this proposed endocrine abnormality remain unclear.

THE USE OF ACTH AND CORTICOSTEROIDS IN OTHER SEIZURE DISORDERS

There is limited information concerning treatment of other intractable seizure disorders with ACTH and/or steroids. The Ohtahara and Lennox-Gastaut syndromes are believed to represent earlier and later manifestations, respectively, of a spectrum of infantile epileptic encephalopathies that include infantile spasms. These conditions respond poorly to traditional anticonvulsant drug therapies but are sometimes improved by the antiepileptic drugs used in infantile spasms: ACTH, steroids, benzodiazepines, and valproic acid. ACTH or steroids also may be beneficial in Landau-Kleffner syndrome (65).

Ohtahara Syndrome

The Ohtahara syndrome, also known as early infantile epileptic encephalopathy (EIEE), is characterized by spasms beginning within the first three months of life associated with persistent burst suppression on the EEG in all stages of the sleep-wake cycle. Despite reports of improvement in seizures in Ohtahara syndrome following ACTH, vigabatrin, and/or zonisamide therapy, the long-term prognosis is usually unchanged by any treatment (66). Mortality in this epilepsy syndrome is high, and survivors are usually severely handicapped. If used, ACTH should be administered as described for infantile spasms.

Lennox-Gastaut Syndrome and Other Myoclonic Seizure Disorders

ACTH and steroids have been found to be useful in younger children with various combinations of severe and intractable seizures, particularly atypical absence, myoclonic, tonic, and atonic seizures. This group includes patients with Lennox-Gastaut syndrome, a disorder characterized by mental retardation, generalized slow spike-and-wave discharges, intractable atypical absence, myoclonus, and frequent ictal falls. Snead and coworkers treated 64 children who had myoclonic seizures without EEG evidence of hypsarrhythmia, or other intractable seizures with either prednisone or ACTH. Seventy-three percent of the children treated with ACTH achieved seizure control, as opposed to none of the prednisone-treated children; however, there was a relapse rate of >50% observed on discontinuation of the ACTH (25).

In 45 cases of Lennox-Gastaut syndrome treated with ACTH, the immediate and long-term effects and the various factors affecting them were investigated by a follow-up study (67). Twenty-three (51.1%) of the 45 children became "seizure free" for over 10 days. Ten children relapsed into Lennox syndrome within 6 months, and in the remaining 13 children, seizures were suppressed for over 6 months. Of these 13 patients, seizure relapse was observed in eight from 9 months to 7 years later. The other five children followed a favorable course without relapse. Sinclair treated 10 children with Lennox Gastaut syndrome and intractable seizures with prednisolone at a dose of 1 mg/kg/day for six weeks followed by withdrawal over the next 6 weeks, and achieved seizure freedom in 7 and seizure reduction in 3 children. Long-term outcome was not mentioned (68).

In summary, several uncontrolled, retrospective studies suggest that ACTH is superior to oral steroids in Lennox-Gastaut syndrome. If the decision is made to embark upon such treatment for Lennox-Gastaut syndrome, the regimen described in this chapter for ACTH or prednisone is recommended. Nevertheless, ACTH and steroids should be reserved for the most severe and intractable patients. Usually, the best result is temporary relief, because 70% to 90% of patients with multiple seizure types suffer a relapse during the ACTH taper. As well, older patients with Lennox-Gastaut syndrome do not tolerate high dose ACTH as well as those children under the age of 2 years who are receiving the same regimen for infantile spasms.

Uncontrolled trials of steroids or adrenocorticotropic hormone also have been reported to reduce seizure frequency in severe myoclonic epilepsy of childhood (69), but without a favorable impact on the overall outcome. Myoclonic astatic epilepsy, first described by Doose, is another age-dependent epileptic disorder, characterized by the onset of myoclonic and astatic seizures between 7 months and 6 years of age in a previously normal child, associated with generalized discharges on the EEG. This disorder is resistant to most conventional antiepileptic drugs. Oguni and coworkers retrospectively analyzed 81 patients with myoclonic-astatic epilepsy of early childhood to investigate the most effective treatment. The most effective treatments were ketogenic diet, followed by ACTH and ethosuximide (70).

Landau-Kleffner Syndrome and Related Disorders

Described in 1957, Landau-Kleffner syndrome, also known as acquired epileptic aphasia, is characterized by regression in receptive and expressive language, associated with epileptic seizures (71). The usual presentation occurs between the ages of 2 and 8 years. Behavioral disturbances are frequent, ranging from hyperactivity and aggression to autism and global cognitive deterioration. Some children display sustained agnosia and mutism. Others show a waxing and waning course that parallels the EEG changes. Spontaneous resolution also has been reported. The electroencephalogram typically shows 1- to 3-Hz high-amplitude spikes and slow waves; these may be unilateral, bilateral, unifocal, or multifocal, but often include the temporal region with or without parietal and occipital involvement, and are activated during sleep.

Valproate and benzodiazepines may control the clinical seizures but have only a partial and transient effect on the EEG abnormalities (72). In 1974, McKinney and McGreal described the beneficial effect of ACTH on the characteristic seizures, language regression, and behavioral changes in Landau-Kleffner syndrome (73). Since then, although no controlled prospective trials of ACTH or steroids have been published, case reports and retrospective series have demonstrated improvements in seizure control and language in children treated with varying ACTH or corticosteroid regimens. Marescaux and coworkers reported that corticosteroid treatment resulted in improved speech, suppression of seizures, and normalization of the EEG in three of three children with Landau-Kleffner syndrome (74). Four children with Landau-Kleffner syndrome received early and prolonged ACTH or corticosteroid therapy, with high initial doses (75). In all four cases the EEG promptly became normal, with subsequent long-lasting remission of the aphasia and improvement of seizure control. Three to six years after discontinuation of hormone therapy the children were off medication and free from seizures and language disability. Sinclair and Snyder treated 10 children who had Landau-Kleffner syndrome (8 patients) and continuous spike wave discharge during sleep (2 patients) with steroids. Nine children had significant improvement in language and behavior (76). Use of ACTH or corticosteroids in patients with Landau Kleffner syndrome appears justified; however, further study of dose and duration of therapy is warranted. If ACTH or corticosteroids are chosen to treat LKS, a high-dose regimen, as described in this chapter for infantile spasms, is recommended, with a longer tapering schedule and concomitant use of valproic acid.

Rasmussen Encephalitis

Rasmussen encephalitis is a focal progressive inflammatory condition of the brain, of unclear etiology. Rasmussen encephalitis is characterized by malignant, progressive, and intractable partial seizures with a high incidence of epilepsia partialis continua. Treatments advocated in Rasmussen include anticonvulsants, high-dose steroids, ACTH, intravenous immunoglobulin G (IV IgG), plasmapheresis, antiviral agents, and hemispherectomy (77). Dulac, in 1992 (78), reported the results of high-dose IV methylprednisolone (400 mg/m^2), followed by oral prednisone, in seven patients with epilepsia partialis continua. Six of the seven showed an improvement in seizure control, which was variably sustained over a two-year follow-up period. Hart (79) reported a benefit of steroids, with 10 of 17 patients showing a reduction of 25–75% in seizure frequency. Granata and coworkers reported positive time-limited responses in 11 of 15 patients with Rasmussen encephalitis, using variable combinations of corticosteroids, apheresis, and high-dose IV immunoglobulins (80).

NEUROSTEROIDS

The term *neurosteroid* was coined by Etienne Baulieu (81) and Paul Robel (82) to refer to pregnenolone, 20-alphaOH-pregnenolone, and progesterone synthesized in the brain. A more general definition would include all steroids synthesized in the brain. The phrase "neuroactive steroids" refers to steroids that are active on neural tissue. Therefore, they may be synthesized endogenously in the brain or may be synthesized by classic endocrine tissue but act on neural tissues (83).

Anticonvulsant Properties of Neurosteroids

Grosso and coworkers investigated serum allopregnanolone levels in 52 children with active epilepsy at pubertal Tanner stage I. The interictal serum allopregnanolone levels in the epileptic children were not statistically different from those detected in the control group, whereas postictal levels were significantly higher than the interictal ones. In this subgroup of patients, allopregnanolone levels decreased to the basal values within 12 hours of the seizure. Serum allopregnanolone levels may reflect changes in neuronal excitability, and allopregnanolone appears to be a reliable circulating marker of epileptic seizures. It is possible that increased postictal serum levels of allopregnanolone may play a role in modulating neuronal excitability and represent an endogenous mechanism of seizure control (84).

The brain regulates hormonal secretion and is sensitive to hormonal feedback. This is particularly true of certain highly epileptogenic mesial temporal lobe regions, such as the amygdala and hippocampus (85). The amygdala, in particular, is linked directly to regions of the hypothalamus that are involved in the regulation, production, and secretion of ovarian steroids (86). Neurons containing corticotropin-releasing factor are particularly prominent in the central division of the extended amygdala (87), which shows structural changes in temporal lobe epilepsy (88). Seizures, if occurring in a repetitive manner, are stressful events for the organism, which can cause lack of inhibitory control in the hypothalamus-pituitary axis system (89, 90). Thus, hypothalamus-pituitary axis dysfunction might be induced in epileptic disorders independent of the localization of the focus. Notably, stress and seizures can alter levels of gonadal, adrenal, and neuroactive steroids, which may then influence subsequent seizure activity (91).

Anovulatory cycles are associated with greater seizure frequency (92, 93). This phenomenon may be due to high serum estradiol-to-progesterone ratios that characterize the inadequate luteal phases of anovulatory cycles and to the opposing neuroactive properties of these steroids. Both adult animal models of epilepsy and clinical evidence suggest that estrogen has excitatory and progesterone has inhibitory effects on neuronal excitability and seizures (93). Progesterone protects against seizures in animals and in open-label clinical trials (94, 95). There is also evidence from the work of Lonsdale and Burnham (96) to suggest that an intermediate product of progesterone reduction, 5[alpha]-dihydroprogesterone, exerts potent antiseizure effects in the amygdala kindling model of generalized convulsions in female rats. Androgens also have antiseizure effects. Aromatization of testosterone produces estradiol, which is highly epileptogenic in male rodents (97). Reduction produces androstanediol, which has potent GABAergic properties and inhibits seizures (98).

Putative Mechanism of Action of Neurosteroids

Electrophysiologic and ligand binding experiments showed that the steroids alphaxolone, allopregnanolone, pregnanolone, allotetrahydrodeoxycorticosterone, and tetrahydrodeoxycorticosterone could all interact with the $GABA_A$ receptor. It is now clear that these neurosteroids act as allosteric agonists of the $GABA_A$ receptor and act to enhance GABAergic inhibition in the brain via a single site on the $GABA_A$ receptor. Other neurosteroids (e.g., pregnenolone sulfate and DHEA sulfate, but not nonsulfated steroids), act as noncompetitive antagonists of the $GABA_A$ receptor. Modulation of neurosteroid action can result from regionally specific differences in neurosteoid synthesis, as well as from regionally specific differences in $GABA_A$ receptor subunit composition (99). Further, data suggest that the anticonvulsant effects of progesterone may involve its metabolism to the neuroactive steroid 5-alpha-pregnan-3 alpha-ol-20-one (3 alpha, 5 alpha-THP) and the subsequent actions of this metabolite at $GABA_A$ receptors (91). Although this activity has been attributed to the reduced progesterone metabolite tetrahydroprogesterone (THP), also known as allopregnanolone, a $GABA_A$ receptor-modulating neurosteroid with anticonvulsant properties, a possible role for progesterone receptors also has been raised (100). However, the potent antiseizure properties of progesterone do not require action at the progesterone receptor and can be blocked by preventing reduction of progesterone to its potent GABAergic metabolite tetrahydroprogesterone. Reddy and coworkers used progesterone receptor knockout mice studies to provide strong evidence that the antiseizure effects of progesterone result from its conversion to the neurosteroid THP and not through the actions of progesterone on its receptor (100). The anticonvulsant effects of androgens may be mediated, in part, through actions of the testosterone metabolite and neuroactive steroid 5 alpha-androstane-3 alpha,17 alpha-diol (3 alpha-diol) at $GABA_A$ receptors (91).

Potential for Clinical Use

Since progesterone and 3-reduced pregnane steroids have potent anticonvulsant effects, attempts to develop novel antiepileptic drugs with neurosteroidal properties seem reasonable. In preclinical studies, metabolites of progesterone and deoxycorticosterone, as well as the synthetic neuroactive steroid ganaxolone, exhibit a broad anticonvulsant profile in different animal models (101, 102). Ganaxolone is a member of a novel class of neuroactive steroids, called epalons, which allosterically modulate the $GABA_A$ receptor complex. Ganaxolone is chemically related to progesterone but is devoid of hormonal activity. In animal studies, there appears to be no tolerance to the anticonvulsant activity of ganaxolone when this drug is administered chronically over the course of up to 7 days. In humans, ganaxolone showed a promising pharmacokinetic profile and was well tolerated in a trial with 96 healthy volunteers (103). The steroid proved to be well tolerated, and effective in clinical studies with epilepsy patients (104, 105). Kerrigan and associates (105) found that ganaxolone reduced the frequency of spasms by at least 50% in 33% of 16 children, with medically intractable infantile spasms, who completed the study. Drug-related adverse events (occurring in 10% of the patients) were generally mild and included somnolence, diarrhea, nervousness, and vomiting. The tolerability of ganaxolone at doses up to 36 mg/kg per day was acceptable (106). Ganaxolone monotherapy was evaluated in a randomized, double-blind, presurgical clinical trial. Ganaxolone was administered at a dose of 1,500 mg per day on day 1 and 1,875 mg per day on days 2–8. The tolerability of ganaxolone was similar to that of placebo and the drug showed significant antiepileptic activity, which was measured by the duration of treatment before withdrawal from the study (104). However, like all GABAergic drugs, ganaxolone has the potential to exacerbate absence seizures (107).

References

1. Klein R, Livingston S. The effect of adrenocorticotropic hormone in epilepsy. *J Pediatr* 1950; 37:733–42.
2. Sorel L, Dusaucy-Bauloye A. [Findings in 21 cases of Gibbs' hypsarrhythmia; spectacular effectiveness of ACTH]. *Acta Neurol Psychiatr Belg* 1958; 58:130–141.
3. Hrachovy RA. ACTH and steroids. In: Engel J, Pedley TA, eds. *Epilepsy: a Comprehensive Textbook*. Philadelphia: Lippincott-Raven, 1997:1463–1473.
4. Nabbout R, Dulac O. Epileptic encephalopathies: a brief overview. *J Clin Neurophysiol* 2003; 20:393–397.
5. Lombroso CT. A prospective study of infantile spasms: clinical and therapeutic correlations. *Epilepsia* 1983; 24:135–158.
6. Koo B, Hwang PA, Logan WJ. Infantile spasms: outcome and prognostic factors of cryptogenic and symptomatic groups. *Neurology* 1993; 43:2322–2327.
7. Lux AL, Edwards SW, Hancock E, Johnson AL, et al; United Kingdom Infantile Spasms Study. The United Kingdom Infantile Spasms Study (UKISS) comparing hormone treatment with vigabatrin on developmental and epilepsy outcomes to age 14 months: a multicentre randomized trial. *Lancet Neurol* 2005; 4:712–717.
8. Kivity S, Lerman P, Ariel R, Danziger Y, et al. Long-term cognitive outcomes of a cohort of children with cryptogenic infantile spasms treated with high-dose adrenocorticotropic hormone. *Epilepsia* 2004; 45:255–262.
9. Riikonen R. The latest on infantile spasms. *Curr Opin Neurol* 2005; 18:91–95.
10. West J. On a peculiar form of infantile convulsion. *Lancet* 1841; 1:724–725.
11. Gibbs FA, Gibbs EL. Atlas of electroencephalography, vol 2. Cambridge, MA: Addison-Wesley, 1952.
12. Hrachovy RA, Frost JD Jr. Infantile epileptic encephalopathy with hypsarrhythmia (infantile spasms/West syndrome). *J Clin Neurophysiol* 2003; 20:408–425.
13. Mackay MT, Weiss SK, Adams-Webber T, Ashwal S, et al; American Academy of Neurology; Child Neurology Society. Practice parameter: medical treatment of infantile spasms: report of the American Academy of Neurology and the Child Neurology Society. *Neurology* 2004; 62:1668–1681.
14. Baram TZ, Mitchell WG, Tournay A, et al. High-dose corticotropin (ACTH) versus prednisone for infantile spasms: a prospective, randomized, blinded study. *Pediatrics* 1996; 97:375–379.
15. Hrachovy RA, Frost JD Jr, Kellaway P, Zion TE. Double-blind study of ACTH vs prednisone therapy in infantile spasms. *J Pediatr* 1983; 103:641–645.
16. Hrachovy RA, Frost JD Jr, Glaze DG. High-dose, long-duration versus low-dose, short-duration corticotropin therapy for infantile spasms. *J Pediatr* 1994; 124:803–806.
17. Vigevano F, Cilio MR. Vigabatrin versus ACTH as first-line treatment for infantile spasms: a randomized, prospective study. *Epilepsia* 1997; 38:1270–1274.
18. Yanagaki S, Oguni H, Hayashi K, et al. A comparative study of high-dose and low-dose ACTH therapy for West syndrome. *Brain Dev* 1999; 21:461–467.
19. Hrachovy RA, Frost JD Jr, Kellaway P, et al. A controlled study of ACTH therapy in infantile spasms. *Epilepsia* 1980; 21:631–636.
20. Kusse MC, Van Nieuwenhuizen O, Van Huffelen AC, van der Mey W, et al. The effect of non-depot ACTH(1–24) on infantile spasms. *Dev Med Child Neurol* 1993; 35: 1067–1073.
21. Snead OC III, Benton JW Jr, Hosey LC, et al. Treatment of infantile spasms with high-dose ACTH: efficacy and plasma levels of ACTH and cortisol. *Neurology* 1989; 39:1027–1031.
22. Cossette P, Riviello JJ, Carmant L. ACTH versus vigabatrin therapy in infantile spasms: a retrospective study. *Neurology* 1999; 52:1691–1694.
23. Riikonen R, Simell O. Tuberous sclerosis and infantile spasms. *Dev Med Child Neurol* 1990; 32:203–209.
24. Sher PK, Sheikh MR. Therapeutic efficacy of ACTH in symptomatic infantile spasms with hypsarrhythmia. *Pediatr Neurol* 1993; 9:451–456.
25. Snead OC III, Benton JW, Myers GJ. ACTH and prednisone in childhood seizure disorders. *Neurology* 1983; 33:966–970.
26. Singer WD, Rabe EF, Haller JS. The effect of ACTH therapy upon infantile spasms. *J Pediatr* 1980; 96:485–489.
27. Hrachovy RA, Frost JD Jr, Kellaway P, et al. A controlled study of prednisone therapy in infantile spasms. *Epilepsia* 1979; 20:403–477.
28. Siemes H, Brandl U, Spohr H-L, et al. Long-term follow-up study of vigabatrin in pretreated children with West syndrome. *Seizure* 1998; 7:293–297.
29. Granstrom M-L, Gaily E, Liukkonen E. Treatment of infantile spasms: results of a population-based study with vigabatrin as the first drug for spasms. *Epilepsia* 1999; 40:950–957.
30. Schlumberger E, Dulac O. A simple effective and well-tolerated treatment regime for West syndrome. *Dev Med Child Neurol* 1994; 36:863–872.
31. Glaze DG, Hrachovy RA, Frost JD Jr, et al. Prospective study of outcome of infants with infantile spasms treated during controlled studies of ACTH and prednisone. *J Pediatr* 1988; 112:389–396.
32. Lux AL, Edwards SW, Hancock E, Johnson AL, et al. The United Kingdom Infantile Spasms Study comparing vigabatrin with prednisolone or tetracosactide at 14 days: a multicentre randomized controlled trial. *Lancet* 2004; 364(9447):1773–1778.
33. Lux AL, Edwards SW, Hancock E, Johnson AL, et al; United Kingdom Infantile Spasms Study. The United Kingdom Infantile Spasms Study (UKISS) comparing hormone treatment with vigabatrin on developmental and epilepsy outcomes to age 14 months: a multicentre randomized trial. *Lancet Neurol* 2005; 4:712–717.
34. Snead OC, Chiron C. Medical treatment. In: Dulac O, Chugani HT, Dalla Bernardina B, eds. *Infantile Spasms and West Syndrome*. London: WB Saunders, 1994:244–256.
35. Heiskala H, Riikonen R, Santavuori P, Simell O, et al. West syndrome: individualized ACTH therapy. *Brain Dev* 1996; 18:456–460.
36. Ito M, Okuno T, Fujii T, Mutoh K, et al. ACTH therapy in infantile spasms: relationship between dose of ACTH and initial effect or long-term prognosis. *Pediatr Neurol* 1990; 6(4):240–244.
37. Riikonen R, Donner M. ACTH therapy in infantile spasms: side effects. *Arch Dis Child* 1980; 55:664–672.
38. Riikonen R, Simell O, Jaaskelainen J, Rapola J, et al. Disturbed calcium and phosphate homeostasis during treatment with ACTH of infantile spasms. *Arch Dis Child* 1986; 61:671–676.
39. Rausch HP, Hanefeld F, Kaufmann HJ. Medullary nephrocalcinosis and pancreatic calcifications demonstrated by ultrasound and CT in infants after treatment with ACTH. *Radiology* 1984; 153:105–107.
40. Hanefeld F, Sperner J, Rating D, Rausch H, et al. Renal and pancreatic calcification during treatment of infantile spasms with ACTH. *Lancet* 1984; 1(8382):901.
41. Alpert BS. Steroid-induced hypertrophic cardiomyopathy in an infant. *Pediatr Cardiol* 1984; 5:117–118.
42. Tacke E, Kupferschmid C, Lang D. Hypertrophic cardiomyopathy during ACTH treatment. *Klin Pädiatr* 1983; 195:124–128.
43. Maekawa K, Ohta H, Tamai I. Transient brain shrinkage in infantile spasms after ACTH treatment. Report of two cases. *Neuropädiatrie* 1980; 11:80–84.
44. Glaze DG, Hrachovy RA, Frost JD, Zion TE, et al. Computed tomography in infantile spasms: effects of hormonal therapy. *Pediatr Neurol* 1986; 2:23–27.
45. Rao JK, Willis J. Hypothalamo-pituitary-adrenal function in infantile spasms: effects of ACTH therapy. *J Child Neurol* 1987; 2:220–223.
46. Ross DL. Suppressed pituitary ACTH response after ACTH treatment of infantile spasms. *J Child Neurol* 1986; 1:34–7.
47. Perheentupa J, Riikonen R, Dunkel L, Simell O. Adrenocortical hyporesponsiveness after treatment with ACTH of infantile spasms. *Arch Dis Child* 1986; 61:750–753.
48. Colleselli P, Milani M, Drigo P, Laverda AM, et al. Impairment of polymorphonuclear leucocyte function during therapy with synthetic ACTH in children affected by epileptic encephalopathies. *Acta Paediatr Scand* 1986; 75:159–163.
49. Kanayama M, Ishikawa T, Tauchi A, Kobayashi M, et al. ACTH-induced seizures in an infant with West syndrome. *Brain Dev* 1989; 11:329–331.
50. Raffin-Sanson ML, de Keyzer Y, Bertagna X. Proopiomelanocortin, a polypeptide precursor with multiple functions: from physiology to pathological conditions. *Eur J Endocrinol* 2003; 149:79–90.
51. Lehoux JG, Fleury A, Ducharme L. The acute and chronic effects of adrenocorticotropin on the levels of messenger ribonucleic acid and protein of steroidogenic enzymes in rat adrenal in vivo. *Endocrinology* 1998; 139:3913–3922.
52. Cooper MS, Stewart PM. Diagnosis and treatment of ACTH deficiency. *Rev Endocr Metab Disord* 2005; 6:47–54.
53. Pranzetelli MR. On the molecular mechanism of adrenocorticotrophic hormone in the CNS: neurotransmitters and receptors. *Exp Neurol* 1994; 125:142–161.
54. Palo J, Savolainen H. The effect of high-dose synthetic ACTH on rat brain. *Brain Res* 1974; 70:313–320.
55. Kendall DA, McEwen BS, Enne SJ. The influence of ACTH and corticosterone on [^{3}H] GABA receptor binding in rat brain. *Brain Res* 1982; 236:365–374.
56. Pranzatelli MR. In vivo and in vitro effects of adrenocorticotropic hormone on serotonin receptors in neonatal rat brain. *Dev Pharmacol Ther* 1989; 12:49–56.
57. Riikonen R. Infantile spasms: some new theoretical aspects. *Epilepsia* 1983; 24: 159–168.
58. Hauger RL, Irwin MR, Lorang M, Aguilera G, et al. High intracerebral levels of CRH result in CRH receptor downregulation in the amygdala and neuroimmune desensitization. *Brain Res* 1993; 616:283–292.
59. Baram TZ, Mitchell WG, Snead OC 3rd, Horton EJ, et al. Brain-adrenal axis hormones are altered in the CSF of infants with massive infantile spasms. *Neurology* 1992; 42:1171–1175.
60. Heiskala H. CSF ACTH and beta-endorphin in infants with West syndrome and ACTH therapy. *Brain Dev* 1997; 19:339–342.
61. Baram TZ, Hirsch E, Snead OC 3rd, Schultz L. Corticotropin-releasing hormone-induced seizures in infant rats originate in the amygdala. *Ann Neurol* 1992; 31:488–494.
62. Baram TZ, Hatalski CG. Neuropeptide-mediated excitability: a key triggering mechanism for seizure generation in the developing brain. *Trends Neurosci* 1998; 21:471–476.
63. Brunson KL, Khan N, Eghbal-Ahmadi M, Baram TZ. Corticotropin (ACTH) acts directly on amygdala neurons to down-regulate corticotropin-releasing hormone gene expression. *Ann Neurol* 2001; 49:304–312.
64. Willig RP, Lagenstein I. Use of ACTH fragments of children with infantile spasms. *Neuropediatrics* 1982; 13:55–58.
65. Gupta R, Appleton R. Corticosteroids in the management of the paediatric epilepsies. *Arch Dis Child* 2005; 90(4):379–384.
66. Campistol J, Garcia-Garcia JJ, Lobera E, Sanmarti FX, et al. The Ohtahara syndrome: a special form of age dependent epilepsy. *Rev Neurol* 1997; 25:212–214.
67. Yamatogi Y, Ohtsuka Y, Ishida T, Ichiba N, et al. Treatment of the Lennox syndrome with ACTH: a clinical and electroencephalographic study. *Brain Dev* 1979; 1:267–276.
68. Sinclair DB. Prednisone therapy in pediatric epilepsy. *Pediatr Neurol* 2003; 28: 194–198.
69. Dravet C, Bureau M, Oguni H, Fukuyama Y, et al. Severe myoclonic epilepsy in infancy (Dravet syndrome). In: Roger J, Bureau M, Dravet C, Genton P, et al, eds. *Epileptic*

Syndromes in Infancy, Childhood, and Adolescence. 3rd ed. London/Paris: John Libbey, 2002:81–103.
70. Oguni H, Tanaka T, Hayashi K, Funatsuka M, et al. Treatment and long-term prognosis of myoclonic-astatic epilepsy of early childhood. *Neuropediatrics* 2002; 33:122–132.
71. Landau WM, Kleffner FR. Syndrome of acquired aphasia with convulsive disorder in children. *Neurology* 1957; 7:523–530.
72. Dulac O. Epileptic encephalopathy. *Epilepsia* 2001; 42 Suppl 3:23–26.
73. McKinney W, McGreal DA. An aphasic syndrome in children. *Can Med Assoc J* 1974; 110:637–639.
74. Marescaux C, Hirsch E, Finck S, Maquet P, et al. Landau-Kleffner syndrome: a pharmacologic study of five cases. *Epilepsia* 1990; 31:768–777.
75. Lerman P, Lerman-Sagie T, Kivity S. Effect of early corticosteroid therapy for Landau-Kleffner syndrome. *Dev Med Child Neurol* 1991; 33:257–260.
76. Sinclair DB, Snyder TJ. Corticosteroids for the treatment of Landau-Kleffner syndrome and continuous spike-wave discharge during sleep. *Pediatr Neurol* 2005; 32: 300–306.
77. Dulac O. Rasmussen's syndrome. *Curr Opin Neurol* 1996; 9:75–77.
78. Dulac O, Chinchilla D, Plouin P, Pinel JF, et al. Follow-up of Rasmussen's syndrome treated by high dose steroids. *Epilepsia* 1992; 33:128.
79. Hart YM, Cortez M, Andermann F, Hwang P, et al. Medical treatment of Rasmussen's syndrome (chronic encephalitis and epilepsy); effect of high-dose steroids or immunoglobulins in 19 patients. *Neurology* 1994; 44:1030–1036.
80. Granata T, Fusco L, Gobbi G, Freri E, et al. Experience with immunomodulatory treatments in Rasmussen's encephalitis. *Neurology* 2003; 61:1807–1810.
81. Baulieu EE. Neurosteroids: a function of the brain. In: Costa E, Paul SM, eds. *Neurosteroids and Brain Function.* New York: Thieme Medical Publishers, 1991: 63–73.
82. Paul SM, Purdy RH. Neuroactive steroids. *FASEB J* 1992; 6:2311–2322.
83. Mellon SH. Neurosteroids: biochemistry, modes of action, and clinical relevance. *J Clin Endocrinol Metab* 1994; 78:1003–1008.
84. Grosso S, Luisi S, Mostardini R, Farnetani M, et al. Inter-ictal and post-ictal circulating levels of allopregnanolone, an anticonvulsant metabolite of progesterone, in epileptic children. *Epilepsy Res* 2003; 54:29–34.
85. Herzog AG. A hypothesis to integrate partial seizures of temporal lobe origin and reproductive endocrine disorders. *Epilepsy Res* 1989; 3:151–159.
86. Martin JB, Reichlin S. Clinical neuroendocrinology. 2nd ed. Philadelphia: FA Davis Co. 1987.
87. Heimer L. A new anatomical framework for neuropsychiatric disorders and drug abuse. *Am J Psychiatry* 2003; 160:1726–1739.
88. Aliashkevich AF, Yilmazer-Hanke D, Van Roost D, Mundhenk B, et al. Cellular pathology of amygdala neurons in human temporal lobe epilepsy. *Acta Neuropathol (Berl)* 2003; 106:99–106.
89. Holsboer F. Stress, hypercortisolism and corticosteroid receptors in depression: implications for therapy. *Affect Disord* 2001; 62:77–91.
90. Kudielka BM, Schmidt-Reinwald AK, Hellhammer DH, Kirschbaum C. Psychological and endocrine responses to psychosocial stress and dexamethasone/corticotropin-releasing hormone in healthy postmenopausal women and young controls: the impact of age and a two-week estradiol treatment. *Neuroendocrinology* 1999; 70:422–430.
91. Rhodes ME, Harney JP, Frye CA. Gonadal, adrenal, and neuroactive steroids' role in ictal activity. *Brain Res* 2004; 1000:8–18.
92. Backstrom T. Epileptic seizures in women related to plasma estrogen and progesterone during the menstrual cycle. *Acta Neurol Scand* 1976; 54:321–347.
93. Herzog AG, Klein P, Ransil BJ. Three patterns of catamenial epilepsy. *Epilepsia* 1997; 38:1082–1088.
94. Frye CA. The neurosteroid 3[alpha],5[alpha]-THP has antiseizure and possible neuroprotective effects in an animal model of epilepsy. *Brain Res* 1995; 696:113–120.
95. Herzog AG. Progesterone therapy in women with complex partial and secondary generalized seizures. Neurol 1995; 45:1660–1662.
96. Lonsdale D, Burnham WM. The anticonvulsant effects of progesterone and 5[alpha]-dihydroprogesterone on amygdala-kindled seizures in rats. *Epilepsia* 2003; 44: 1494–1499.
97. Saberi M, Pourgholami MH, Jorjani M. The acute effects of estradiol benzoate on amygdala-kindled seizures in male rats. *Brain Res* 2001; 891:1–6.
98. Rhodes ME, Frye CA. Androgens in the hippocampus can alter and be altered by ictal activity. *Pharmacol Biochem Behav* 2004; 78:483–493.
99. Mellon SH. Neurosteroids: biochemistry, modes of action, and clinical relevance. *J Clin Endocrinol Metab* 1994; 78:1003–1008.
100. Reddy DS, Castaneda DC, O'Malley BW, Rogawski MA. Anticonvulsant activity of progesterone and neurosteroids in progesterone receptor knockout mice. *J Pharmacol Exp Ther* 2004; 310:230–239.
101. Gasior M, Carter RB, Witkin JM. Neuroactive steroids: potential therapeutic use in neurological and psychiatric disorders. *Trends Pharmacol Sci* 1999; 20:107–112.
102. Liptakova S, Velisek L, Veliskova J, Moshe SL. Effect of ganaxolone on flurothyl seizures in developing rats. *Epilepsia* 2000; 41:788–793.
103. Monaghan EP, Navalta LA, Shum L, Ashbrook DW, et al. Initial human experience with ganaxolone, a neuroactive steroid with antiepileptic activity. *Epilepsia* 1997; 38:1026–1031.
104. Laxer K, Blum D, Abou-Khalil BW, Morrell MJ, et al. Assessment of ganaxolone's anticonvulsant activity using a randomized, double-blind, presurgical trial design. Ganaxolone Presurgical Study Group. *Epilepsia* 2000; 41:1187–1194.
105. Kerrigan JF, Shields WD, Nelson TY, Bluestone DL, et al. Ganaxolone for treating intractable infantile spasms: a multicenter, open-label, add-on trial. *Epilepsy Res* 2000; 42:133–139.
106. Rupprecht R, Holsboer F. Neuroactive steroids: mechanisms of action and neuropsychopharmacological perspectives. *Trends Neurosci* 1999; 22:410–416.
107. Snead OC. Ganaxalone, a selective, high-affinity steroid modulator of the gamma-aminobutyric acid-A receptor, exacerbates seizures in animal models of absence. *Ann Neurol* 1998; 44:688–690.

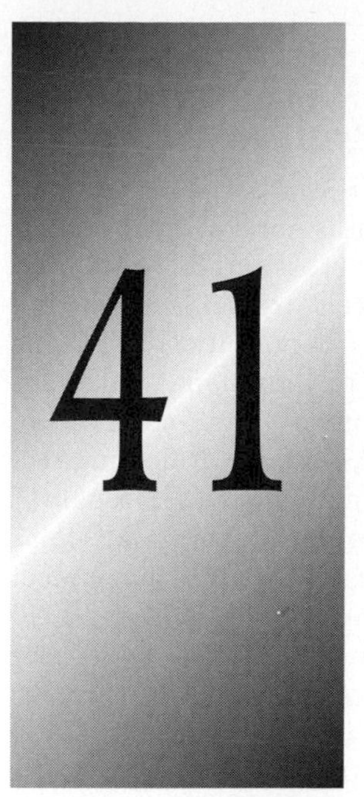

41 Benzodiazepines

Kevin Farrell
Aspasia Michoulas

Benzodiazepines bind to a site on the neuronal $GABA_A$ receptor, a ligand-gated chloride channel, and enhance inhibitory neurotransmission. Their high lipid solubility results in rapid central nervous system (CNS) penetration and they are particularly useful as first-line agents in the management of status epilepticus and seizures occurring repetitively in clusters. Their effectiveness in the chronic treatment of epilepsy is limited by their behavioral effects and their propensity for tolerance in patients with intractable epilepsy.

CHEMISTRY, PHARMACOLOGY, AND MECHANISM OF ACTION

The base compound is a 5-aryl-1,4-benzodiazepine structure composed of three ring systems. Modifications in the structure of ring system have resulted in several compounds with antiepileptic activity but with different efficacy and side effect profiles. Benzodiazepines augment inhibitory neurotransmission by enhancing the activity of GABA at the $GABA_A$ receptor (1). When GABA binds to the $GABA_A$ receptor, it increases the opening of the chloride ion channel, which results in hyperpolarization of the membrane and reduction in neuronal firing (2). Although benzodiazepines bind to the $GABA_A$ receptor, they do not activate it directly but rather modulate GABA binding and enhance its effect by increasing the frequency (not duration) of chloride ion channel opening. This increases the inhibitory tone at GABA synapses, which limits neuronal firing and in turn reduces seizure activity (1). At high concentrations, benzodiazepines also influence sodium channel function in a similar fashion to phenytoin and carbamazepine (3). Thus, benzodiazepines raise the seizure threshold, decrease the duration of epileptiform discharges, and limit their spread (3).

The action of benzodiazepines on the GABA receptor may be influenced both by the maturity of the brain and by disease. GABA synapses are present before glutamate synapses in early fetal development, and it has been suggested that GABA acts as the primary excitatory neurotransmitter in the immature brain (4). The potassium-chloride transport that removes chloride ions is not expressed until later in development, enabling chloride ions to accumulate intracellularly, resulting in GABA synapses that are excitatory (4). The exact timing of the switch from GABA excitatory action to inhibitory action is not known but is believed to occur in utero (4). It has been hypothesized that the excitatory action of GABA in early development modulates neuronal migration and differentiation, and it has been suggested that benzodiazepine use in early pregnancy may have detrimental effects on fetal brain maturation (4).

ADVERSE EFFECTS

Toxicity

Respiratory and cardiovascular depression are the most common adverse effects of benzodiazepines used intravenously. Propylene glycol is a solvent used with intravenous diazepam and lorazepam, but not midazolam, and plays a major role in the respiratory depression associated with the first two drugs (5). Comedication with phenobarbital may exacerbate the cardiovascular and respiratory depression. Intravenous benzodiazepines may precipitate tonic status epilepticus in children with epileptic encephalopathies (6).

Chronic treatment with a benzodiazepine may be associated with sedation, fatigue, ataxia, cognitive dysfunction, drooling, and exacerbation of seizures. Abrupt discontinuation may lead to withdrawal symptoms. Headache and gastrointestinal symptoms can occur but are uncommon. Hematologic abnormalities, hepatic dysfunction, and allergic reactions are uncommon.

Tolerance

Although tolerance probably occurs with all antiepileptic drugs (7), it happens more often with benzodiazepines. The degree of tolerance in animal models is proportional to the agonist efficacy of the benzodiazepine (8). Tolerance to one benzodiazepine does not necessarily result in tolerance to the others (9). The mechanisms underlying tolerance are not clear but may involve down-regulation of $GABA_A$ receptors, altered postsynaptic sensitivity to GABA, or modification in the expression of genes that encode for the various $GABA_A$ receptor subunits (10).

The incidence of tolerance to the antiepileptic effect of benzodiazepines is influenced by the type and severity of the epilepsy. Thus, tolerance to clonazepam is observed much less often in patients with typical absence seizures than in patients with West syndrome or Lennox-Gastaut syndrome (11). Similarly, tolerance to clobazam has been reported in 18% to 65% of patients in open studies (12–14), whereas in children who had been previously untreated or who had received only one drug (15), the incidence of tolerance to clobazam (8%) was similar to tolerance to carbamazepine (4%) and phenytoin (7%).

INDIVIDUAL BENZODIAZEPINES

The use of benzodiazephines in status epilepticus and in the prevention of seizures is outlined in Table 41-1 and Table 41-2 respectively.

Diazepam

Biotransformation, Pharmacokinetics, and Interactions. Rectal diazepam is absorbed via hemorrhoidal veins and then rapidly crosses the blood-brain barrier. Therapeutic blood levels are achieved within 5 minutes and peak levels within 20 minutes (16). Plasma concentrations of 500 ng/mL of diazepam, which are necessary for acute seizure control, were achieved in infants and children within 2–6 minutes following rectal administration of 0.5 to 1 mg/kg (17). Diazepam is absorbed more slowly following oral or intramuscular administration, and these routes are not recommended. Plasma levels decrease by as much as 50% within 20–30 minutes after a single bolus injection (16). This short duration of action following intravenous administration relates to its rapid distribution into fat tissue and to the high protein binding of diazepam.

Diazepam undergoes demethylation to N-desmethyldiazepam, a major metabolite that itself has significant antiepileptic and sedative properties (17). Diazepam and N-desmethyldiazepam are both highly protein bound to albumin (17). The elimination half-life of diazepam is 10 ± 2 hours in infants and 17 ± 3 hours in older children (17). The elimination half-life of N-desmethyldiazepam is longer than that of diazepam, and serum concentrations are two to five times higher in patients receiving long-term treatment (17). The metabolites of diazepam are conjugated with glucuronic acid in the liver and excreted by the kidney.

Diazepam does not significantly influence the pharmacokinetics of other drugs. Valproate comedication decreases protein binding and inhibits the metabolism of diazepam (18), which may result in increased sedation.

Clinical Efficacy. Diazepam is effective in the treatment of both convulsive and nonconvulsive status epilepticus and of acute repetitive seizures. Clinical effect is observed usually within 10 minutes of intravenous administration, which is the optimal route for the treatment of status epilepticus (16, 19). The rapid redistribution following a single dose results in an abrupt decline in brain concentration and reduction in the anticonvulsant effect. Consequently, a long-acting anticonvulsant, for example, phenytoin, should be administered concomitantly in children with status epilepticus. Rectal diazepam is absorbed rapidly, which may be useful in small children in whom intravenous access may be difficult. Limited data suggest continuous diazepam infusion may be effective in the treatment of refractory status epilepticus in children (20–22).

Rectal diazepam gel has been shown to be effective and safe in the management of children with prolonged or acute repetitive seizures (23). Sedation was the most common side effect, but no episodes of serious respiratory

TABLE 41-1
The Use of Benzodiazepines in Status Epilepticus

Drug	Dosage	Comments
Diazepam		
Intravenous	0.2–0.3 mg/kg; max dose 5 mg in infants and 10 mg in older children; can be repeated after 15 minutes	Administer over 2–5 minutes; rapid administration increases risk of apnea
Rectal solution	0.5–1.0 mg/kg; max dose 20 mg	
Rectal gel	2–5 years: 0.5 mg/kg 6–11 years: 0.3 mg/kg >12 years: 0.2 mg/kg	Prefixed unit doses of 5, 10, 15, and 20 mg; prescribed dose should be rounded to nearest available unit dose
Lorazepam		
Intravenous	0.1 mg/kg; max dose 4 mg; can be repeated after 10 minutes	Administer over 2 min
Sublingual	0.05–0.15 mg/kg; max dose 4 mg	Can be used for serial seizures but should not be used for tonic-clonic status epilepticus
Midazolam		
Intravenous bolus	0.15 mg/kg	Administer over 2–5 minutes; if not effective, continuous infusion should be started
Continuous infusion	1–5 μg/kg/min; max dose 18 μg/kg/min	Initiate treatment at 1 μg/kg/min and increase rate by that amount at 15-minute intervals until seizure control
Intramuscular, intranasal, and buccal	0.2 mg/kg	

TABLE 41-2
Benzodiazepine Dosages for Prevention of Seizures

Drug	Initial Dose	Dosage Increase	Maximum Dose
Clobazam	2.5 mg/day < 2 years; 5 mg/day if 2–10 years; 10 mg/day > 10 years	2.5–5 mg/day every 5–7 days; given at night or as b.i.d. dosing	Doses over 30 mg/day rarely improve seizure control
Clonazepam	0.01–0.03 mg/kg/day < 30 kg 0.5 mg/day > 30 kg	0.25–0.5 mg/day every 5–7 days; b.i.d or t.i.d dosing	0.2 mg/kg/day if on enzyme-inducing drugs; 0.1 mg/kg/day in others
Clorazepate	0.3 mg/kg/day	0.3–0.6 mg/kg/day every 5–7 days; b.i.d dosing	3 mg/kg/day (max 60 mg/day)
Nitrazepam	0.1–0.2 mg/kg/day	0.1 mg/kg/day every 5–7 days; b.i.d or t.i.d.	<0.8 mg/kg/day

Abbreviations: b.i.d., twice daily; t.i.d., three times daily.

depression have been reported. Rectal administration can be performed by the parent, which permits treatment at home, decreases emergency room visits, and improves caregivers' global evaluation (24). This is of particular value for children with a history of prolonged seizures (25).

Both oral (26) and rectal diazepam (27) administered intermittently at times of fever have been demonstrated in placebo-controlled studies to be effective in the prevention of recurrent febrile convulsions. Rectal diazepam was as effective as continuous phenobarbital in the prevention of recurrent febrile seizures (28). The potential toxicities associated with antiepileptic drug therapy have generally been considered to outweigh the relatively minor risks associated with simple febrile seizures (29). However, intermittent diazepam may be of value in children who have had a previous prolonged febrile seizure.

Childhood-onset encephalopathies associated with sleep-activated electroencephalographic (EEG) abnormalities may respond to oral diazepam at high doses (30, 31). Oral diazepam (0.5 mg/kg) for 3 to 4 weeks following a rectal diazepam bolus of 1 mg/kg has been reported to be effective in electrical status epilepticus in sleep (ESES) (32). Oral diazepam at a dose of 0.5 mg/kg given 30 minutes before hemodialysis was effective in prevention of hemodialysis-associated seizures in four children who had failed to respond to phenobarbital (33).

Adverse Effects. Sedation and ataxia occur commonly when diazepam is used in the treatment of status epilepticus or in the prevention of recurrent febrile convulsions. Respiratory depression and hypotension may occur following intravenous diazepam, particularly if administered rapidly or used in combination with phenobarbital (17), but are extremely rare following rectal diazepam (34). Mild thrombophlebitis may occur following intravenous administration, particularly if diazepam is mixed with a saline solution or is injected rapidly (17). Diazepam may induce tonic status epilepticus in children with epileptic encephalopathies (35). Intermittent oral diazepam prophylaxis has been associated with ataxia, sedation, lethargy, and irritability (36).

Clinical Use. In the treatment of children with status epilepticus, an initial intravenous dose of 0.2 to 0.3 mg/kg (maximum dose, 5 mg in infants and 15 mg in older children) of diazepam should be given slowly over 2–5 minutes (17). If needed, the dose may be repeated after 15 minutes. When intravenous access in not available, a rectal dose of 0.5 to 0.9 mg/kg has been used to a maximum of 20 mg (37, 38). In refractory status epilepticus, continuous diazepam infusion has been used successfully (20). Treatment was initiated at 0.01 mg/kg/min and increased by 0.005 mg/kg/min every 15 minutes until seizures were controlled or to a maximum dosage of 0.03 mg/kg/min. A subsequent report has described at an infusion rate up to 0.08 mg/kg/min (21). Diazepam may precipitate when the intravenous solution is administered in saline solution, and it may adsorb to polyvinyl tubing. Consequently, fresh solution should be prepared every 6 hours when continuous diazepam infusion is being used (39).

Rectal administration of diazepam should be considered when intravenous access cannot be obtained and when administration by a caregiver may be helpful, for example, when a child with a history of prolonged seizures lives far from medical services. The injectable solution can be administered rectally through a soft plastic intravenous catheter, and doses of 0.5 to 1.0 mg/kg have been reported to be effective in a prehospital setting with a maximum dose of 20 mg (16). Rectal diazepam gel (Diastat®) is available in unit doses of 5, 10, 15, and 20 mg and is easier to handle, faster to administer, and decreases the chance of dosing errors. Rectal doses of 0.5 mg/kg for children 2–5 years of age; 0.3 mg/kg between 6 and 11 years of age, and 0.2 mg/kg above 12 years to a maximum of 20 mg have been used successfully (40). A second dose may be repeated in 4–12 hours, if needed. If administered at home, caregivers should be given instruction as to when they should seek medical attention. The suggested dosage of oral or rectal diazepam used for febrile seizure prophylaxis is 5 mg every 8 hours when the rectal temperature is ≥38.5°C, with a maximum of four consecutive doses to avoid drug accumulation (28).

Lorazepam

Biotransformation, Pharmacokinetics, and Interactions. Lorazepam is a 1,4-benzodiazpine that is metabolized rapidly through hepatic glucuronidation and is excreted by the kidneys (41). It is absorbed more rapidly when administered sublingually than orally or intramuscularly, and peak plasma levels are achieved within 60 minutes (42). The rectal absorption of lorazepam parenteral solution is slow and peak concentrations, which may not be reached for 1–2 hours, are much lower than those achieved following intravenous administration (43). First-pass hepatic transformation decreases the absolute systemic availability of oral lorazepam to 29% of that following intravenous administration (44). Lorazepam is 90% protein bound and rapidly crosses the blood-brain barrier. The maximal EEG effect of intravenous lorazepam is observed approximately 30 minutes after infusion, which is later than with intravenous diazepam, probably as a result of slower entry into the brain (45). Following intravenous administration, there is a rapid fall in blood levels because of the distribution phase. The elimination half-life is 10.5 ± 2.9 hours in children (46) but is longer in neonates (47). Less than 1% is excreted unchanged in the urine.

The clearance of lorazepam is not influenced by acute viral hepatitis (48) or renal disease (49). However, valproate reduces the clearance of lorazepam, possibly as a consequence of inhibition of glucuronidation (50). There are no other significant interactions with antiepileptic drugs (42), and, in contrast to other benzodiazepines, protein binding of lorazepam is not influenced by heparin (51).

Clinical Efficacy. Intravenous lorazepam is more effective than intravenous diazepam in the treatment of status epilepticus; it has fewer side effects and has a longer duration of action (52, 53). Children receiving long-term therapy with another benzodiazepine are less responsive to lorazepam in status epilepticus (54). Sublingual lorazepam has also been shown to be a convenient and effective treatment of serial seizures in children (55). Intravenous or sublingual lorazepam was completely effective in preventing seizures in 29 children receiving high dose busulfan treatment (56). Lorazepam has also been reported to be useful in the treatment of postanoxic myoclonus (57).

Adverse Effects. Sedation is the most common side effect of lorazepam, and ataxia, psychomotor slowing, and agitation may also occur. Respiratory depression may occur but less often than with diazepam (52). The treatment of serial seizures with lorazepam has been associated with drowsiness, ataxia, nausea, and hyperactivity (55). Abrupt discontinuation of lorazepam has been associated with withdrawal seizures, which may occur up to 60 hours following its discontinuation (42). Lorazepam has been reported to cause tonic seizures in patients being treated for atypical absence status epilepticus (58–60).

Clinical Use. The recommended intravenous dose of lorazepam in children is 0.1 mg/kg (maximum dose, 4 mg) (19). The intravenous rate of administration should not exceed 2 mg/min. The dose can be repeated if necessary after 10 minutes. Sublingual doses of 0.05 to 0.15 mg/kg were effective in 8 of 10 children with serial seizures (55).

Midazolam

Biotransformation, Pharmacokinetics, and Interactions. Midazolam is a 1,4-benzodiazepine with a fused imidazole ring. Prior to administration, the benzodiazepine ring of midazolam is open and is water soluble. However, following administration, the benzodiazepine ring closes at physiologic pH and midazolam becomes lipid soluble. These characteristics permit absorption via the intramuscular route (with less pain at the injection site) and rapid transport across the blood-brain barrier. The absorption of intramuscular midazolam is rapid with 80% to 100% bioavailability (61), and peak blood levels are obtained after approximately 25 minutes (61). Pharmacologic effects are observed within 5–15 minutes but may not be maximal for 20 to 60 minutes (62). Intranasal absorption of midazolam also occurs rapidly, with mean time to seizure control of 3.5 minutes (range, 2.5–5.0 minutes) (63). Oral midazolam is absorbed relatively rapidly, with peak blood levels being achieved within 1 hour, but first-pass metabolism in the liver limits the availability to 40% to 50% of the oral dose. It is distributed rapidly and possesses a short elimination half-life (1.5–3 hours) in children. The relatively short half-life makes it less likely to accumulate and therefore more suitable for continuous infusion than diazepam or lorazepam. A longer half-life (6.5 hours) has been observed in critically ill neonates (64).

Midazolam is highly protein bound (96–98%) and is metabolized extensively by the cytochrome P450 3A4 enzyme system. Its metabolism is induced by phenytoin and carbamazepine (65). Medications that inhibit the activity of cytochrome P450 3A4, for example, erythromycin and clarithromycin, may prolong the half-life of midazolam (66). Renal failure does not influence the pharmacokinetics of midazolam (67).

Clinical Efficacy. Intravenous midazolam was effective in the treatment of refractory status epilepticus in 43 of 44 children in two studies (68, 69). The mean infusion rates in these two studies were 2.0 and 2.3 μg/kg/min, with a maximum rate in one study of 18 μg/kg/min. Midazolam appears to be as effective in stopping refractory status epilepticus as pentobarbital or thiopental and is associated with fewer adverse effects (70, 71). Continuous intravenous midazolam infusion was as effective as continuous diazepam infusion in stopping refractory status epilepticus but was associated with a higher incidence of seizure recurrence (21). Continuous midazolam infusion was also effective in stopping refractory nonconvulsive status epilepticus in 82% of episodes but breakthrough seizures, which could only be detected by EEG in most patients, occurred in approximately half of the patients (72). Midazolam administered by continuous intravenous infusion (1.6–6.6 μg/kg/min) was effective in controlling seizures refractory to phenobarbital in four of six neonates and was well tolerated (73).

The high water solubility of midazolam permits administration by a variety of routes. Intramuscular midazolam (15 mg) had a comparable effect to intravenous diazepam (20 mg) in the suppression of interictal spikes in adults within 5 minutes (74). Intramuscular midazolam was effective in stopping 64 of 69 prolonged seizures occurring in 48 children (75). A prospective study reported intramuscular midazolam to be more efficacious than intravenous diazepam in the treatment of acute seizures, with a faster cessation of seizures because of more rapid administration (76). Intranasal administration of midazolam was less effective than intravenous diazepam in one study (77) but stopped prolonged febrile seizures more rapidly in another study (78). In addition, the time to seizure cessation was shorter with intranasal midazolam than with rectal diazepam, and parents felt that the intranasal route was a more favorable means of medication administration (79).

Adverse Effects. Drowsiness and ataxia are the most common side effects. Apnea and hypotension may occur following rapid intravenous administration of a bolus of midazolam, but apnea has been reported in only one patient following intramuscular midazolam (80). Thrombophlebitis occurs less often than with diazepam (80). Paradoxical reactions including agitation, restlessness, and hyperactivity have been reported (81).

Clinical Use. An initial intravenous bolus dose of 0.15 mg/kg (68, 69) may be followed by continuous infusion at an initial rate of 1 μg/kg/min, which may be increased subsequently by 1 μg/kg/min every 15 minutes to achieve seizure control. Seizures are controlled at infusion rates less than 3 μg/kg/minute in most children, but rates up to 18 μg/kg/min have been described (69). Intramuscular administration results in complete and rapid absorption and is particularly usefully if intravenous access is not available or is difficult to obtain quickly. An intramuscular dose of 0.2 mg/kg has been used effectively in children (75). Intranasal and buccal midazolam are safe, effective, and easy to administer, making these routes particularly useful in the home setting. The usual dose is 0.2 mg/kg.

Clonazepam

Biotransformation, Pharmacokinetics, and Interactions. Clonazepam is a 1,4-benzodiazepine, and the bioavailability after oral administration is more than 80% with peak levels occurring between 1 and 4 hours (82). The high lipid solubility results in rapid distribution with easy passage across the blood-brain barrier. The protein binding is 86%. Clonazepam is metabolized initially by reduction to 7-amino-clonazepam and subsequently by acetylation (83). The metabolites, which are pharmacologically inactive, are conjugated to glucuronide and excreted by the kidney. Less than 1% is excreted unchanged in the urine. Clonazepam metabolism involves the hepatic cytochrome P-450 3A4 (84) and comedication with carbamazepine or phenobarbital lowers blood clonazepam levels (82). Acetylation is also a major metabolic pathway and patients who are rapid acetylators are more likely to require higher doses to achieve a response (85). The serum half-life in children is 22–33 hours (86). The plasma half-life following intravenous administration in neonates is 20–43 hours (87).

Clinical Efficacy. Intravenous clonazepam was effective in stopping tonic-clonic status epilepticus in all children in a small open study and was considered to have a longer duration of action than diazepam (88). The initial dose was 0.25 mg, which was repeated up to two times. Intravenous clonazepam was also effective in more than 80% of children and adults with absence status epilepticus (89). Oral clonazepam has been demonstrated in controlled studies to be effective in the treatment of absence (86, 90, 91), myoclonic (90), and atonic seizures (90). Open studies have suggested that clonazepam is also effective in the treatment of photosensitive epilepsy and of primary generalized tonic-clonic seizures, both as monotherapy (92) and in combination with valproic acid (93). In patients with juvenile myoclonic epilepsy, clonazepam is more effective in prevention of myoclonic seizures than of tonic-clonic seizures. This may result in an increased risk of injury to the patient, who is deprived of the warning jerks that presage the onset of the generalized tonic-clonic seizure (94). Clonazepam may also be effective in the treatment of other myoclonic epilepsies, including reflex myoclonic epilepsy, progressive myoclonic epilepsy, posthypoxic intention myoclonus, and epilepsia partialis continua (82). Partial epilepsy may also respond to clonazepam in combination with valproic acid (82). Clonazepam monotherapy is associated with reduction in interictal rolandic discharges in children with benign rolandic epilepsy (95) and is more effective than valproic acid and carbamazepine in that regard (96). The addition of clonazepam was also effective in the treatment of children with partial seizures resistant to carbamazepine (97). Studies have demonstrated mixed results with respect to the efficacy of clonazepam in Lennox-Gastaut syndrome, where it has been considered as a third line choice (98).

Adverse Effects. The most common adverse effects of clonazepam include drowsiness, ataxia, incoordination, and behavioral changes (34, 99). Comedication with phenobarbital usually exacerbates the drowsiness (100). Diplopia, nystagmus, dysarthria, excessive drooling, and hypotonia may also occur. Initiation of therapy at a low dose followed by a slow increase may reduce the neurotoxicity. Increased appetite and weight gain of more than 20% were reported in 9 of 81 children treated with clonazepam (99). Clonazepam may result in increased seizure frequency (101) and has been reported to induce tonic status epilepticus in Lennox-Gastaut syndrome (6).

The development of tolerance to the antiepileptic effect of clonazepam is dependent on the type of epilepsy. Thus, tolerance did not develop in 23 children with partial epilepsy who were treated with clonazepam monotherapy or clonazepam in combination with carbamazepine (97). Similarly, tolerance to clonazepam is observed less often in patients with typical absence seizures than in patients with West syndrome or Lennox-Gastaut syndrome (11). The use of alternate-day clonazepam has been reported to be associated with significantly less tolerance in an animal model (102), an effect also observed in children (103). Discontinuation of clonazepam may be complicated by transient worsening of seizure control, and status epilepticus may occur with abrupt withdrawal (11). Behavioral changes, including restlessness, dysphoria, sleep disturbance, and tachycardia, may also occur during clonazepam withdrawal, which should be done gradually (11).

Clinical Use. To minimize side effects, clonazepam should be started at a dose of 0.01 to 0.03 mg/kg/day in children under 30 kg and given in two or three daily dosages (104). The dose can be increased by 0.25–0.5 mg/day every 5–7 days to a total dose of 0.1 mg/kg/day, or 0.2 mg/kg/day in patients receiving drugs that induce microsomal metabolism. Clonazepam was effective in seven of eight neonates with seizures when administered by slow intravenous infusion in doses of 0.1 mg/kg (87).

Nitrazepam

Biotransformation, Pharmacokinetics, and Interactions. Nitrazepam, a 1,4-benzodiazepine, is rapidly and totally absorbed in the gastrointestinal tract. It is highly protein bound (85–90%) and has an elimination half-life of 24 to 31 hours (105). Nitrazepam is partially metabolized in the liver and then excreted in the urine. There are no clinically significant interactions with other antiepileptic drugs. Oral contraceptives, steroids, and cimetidine reduce nitrazepam clearance, and rifampin increases nitrazepam clearance (105).

Clinical Efficacy. Nitrazepam is generally considered a third line adjunctive medication in the treatment of partial and generalized seizures, including the epileptic encephalopathies of childhood. In a randomized control study in patients with infantile spasms, 75% to 100% reduction in spasm frequency was observed in 52% of patients receiving nitrazepam and 57% of patients receiving adrenocorticotrophin (106), but side effects were less severe in the patients who received nitrazepam. In open studies, nitrazepam has been reported to be effective in the treatment of absence and primary generalized tonic-clonic seizures (107), myoclonic seizures (108)], and partial seizures (107). Nitrazepam has also been reported to be effective in the treatment of Lennox-Gastaut syndrome (105, 109, 110).

Adverse Effects. Drowsiness, ataxia and incoordination, which are common side effects, may be diminished by initiation of treatment at a low dose followed by slow increase. Increased salivation is a well recognized side effect of nitrazepam in children and is related to both hypersecretion of the tracheobronchial tree and abnormal swallowing, due to delay in cricopharyngeal relaxation (111). This may also result in feeding difficulties and aspiration pneumonia, particularly in children (108, 112). Doses of nitrazepam greater than 0.8 mg/kg/day have been found to be associated with an increased risk of death in children (112), and the risk appears highest in children with intractable epilepsy younger than 3.4 years of age (113). Risk factors included feeding difficulties, recurrent respiratory tract infections, and aspiration pneumonia.

Clinical Use. To reduce the risk of side effects, nitrazepam should be started in children at a low dose (0.1–0.2 mg/kg/day) and the dosage increased every 5–7 days to a maximum of 0.8 mg/kg/day (112). Caution should be taken in patients younger than 4 years of age. Discontinuation of nitrazepam should be gradual to minimize the risk of withdrawal seizures.

Clorazepate

Biotransformation, Pharmacokinetics, and Interactions. Clorazepate is a prodrug that is decarboxylated in the stomach to the active medication, N-desmethyldiazepam. Peak concentrations of N-desmethyldiazepam are normally achieved at 0.5 to 2 hours and, with the slow-release preparation, after 12 hours (114, 115). Serum concentrations of N-desmethyldiazepam increase after meals, which may cause somnolence (114). N-Desmethyldiazepam is 97% protein bound, largely to serum albumin (115). Although N-desmethyldiazepam has an elimination half-life of 55–100 hours, administration of clorazepate once daily is associated with unacceptable side effects because of the relatively high peak concentrations that follow its rapid absorption (115). N-Desmethyldiazepam is metabolized extensively by the liver and its elimination half-life is prolonged in patients with liver disease. Drugs that induce hepatic microsomal metabolism enhance the clearance of N-desmethyldiazepam and patients taking these drugs require higher doses of clorazepate.

Clinical Efficacy. Clorazepate was introduced in the 1960s and there have been no controlled studies in children. Improvement in seizure control has been reported in children with partial (116) and generalized seizures (116–118), including children with Lennox-Gastaut syndrome (116).

Adverse Effects. Sedation, ataxia, behavioral changes, and drooling, which are the most common side effects of clorazepate in children, often become less pronounced with time. Comedication with phenobarbital increases the probability of behavioral problems (119) and should be avoided. Idiosyncratic reactions are rare (115).

Tolerance limits the usefulness of clorazepate, but animal studies suggest that tolerance occurs less often with clorazepate than with diazepam or clonazepam (115). Withdrawal seizures and behavioral changes may complicate the discontinuation of therapy, which should occur slowly.

Clinical Use. The initial dose of clorazepate in children is 0.3 mg/kg/day, and the dose is increased gradually to achieve seizure control or until side effects appear, up to a maximum dose of 3 mg/kg/day (115, 117).

Clobazam

Biotransformation, Pharmacokinetics, and Interactions. Clobazam, which differs from the 1,4-benzodiazepines by the presence of a nitrogen atom in the 1 and 5 positions of the diazepine ring, is relatively insoluble and cannot be administered intravenously or intramuscularly. Oral clobazam is absorbed rapidly, and peak concentrations are reached in 1 to 4 hours (120). It is highly lipophilic, distributed rapidly, and approximately 85% protein bound. Factors that influence protein binding, for example, liver disease, may affect the free and total levels of the drug (121). Clobazam is metabolized extensively in the liver to several metabolites including N-desmethylclobazam, which also has antiepileptic activity. The elimination half-life of clobazam is 18 hours, and that of N-desmethylclobazam is 42 hours (121). Thus, blood levels of N-desmethylclobazam are approximately 10 times those of clobazam (122), and N-desmethylclobazam is considered to be responsible for most of the antiepileptic effect in patients receiving clobazam (121).

Comedication with phenytoin, phenobarbital, or carbamazepine increases the N-desmethylclobazam/clobazam ratio (123). Clobazam increases phenytoin concentrations (124) and may result in phenytoin intoxication (125, 126). Clobazam has also been reported to increase valproate levels, which may remain elevated for several weeks after the clobazam has been withdrawn (127), and may result in valproate toxicity (128). Mild increases in phenobarbital, carbamazepine, and carbamazepine epoxide have also been reported (124).

Clinical Efficacy. The use of clobazam in the treatment of epilepsy was pioneered by Gastaut and Low, who reported its effectiveness in patients with partial seizures, idiopathic generalized epilepsy, reflex epilepsy, and Lennox-Gastaut syndrome (129). The antiepileptic effect of clobazam in partial and tonic-clonic seizures has been demonstrated in several placebo-controlled studies (121). In addition, clobazam monotherapy has been demonstrated to be as effective as either carbamazepine or phenytoin in the treatment of children with partial, tonic-clonic seizures, or both, who were previously untreated or who had received only one drug (15). Clobazam appears to have a broad spectrum of antiepileptic activity. In a large retrospective study comprising 1,300 refractory epileptic patients, including 440 children, more than 50% reduction in seizure frequency was observed for each seizure type (except tonic seizures) in 40% to 50% of patients and complete seizure control was obtained in 10% to 30% (128). It has also been reported to be effective in the treatment of reflex epilepsies (130–132), startle epilepsy (133, 134), epilepsy with continuous spike-waves during slow sleep (135), and eyelid myoclonia with absence (136). Complete seizure control was described in 20% of patients with temporal lobe seizures associated with hippocampal sclerosis, and 75% reduction in seizure frequency in a further 25% (137). Clobazam taken intermittently for 10 days each month around the time of menstruation was effective in the treatment of catamenial epilepsy and was not associated with tolerance (138, 139). Administration of intermittent clobazam has also been used successfully by the author in the treatment of seizures that occur periodically in clusters. Prophylactic clobazam has been used prior to bone marrow transplantation in the prevention of seizures induced by high-dose busulfan chemotherapy (140).

Adverse Effects. A major advantage of clobazam over the 1,4-benzodiazepines is the lower incidence of neurotoxicity. In a double-blind comparison of clobazam with phenytoin or carbamazepine in children, the incidence of side effects was similar (15). The side effects of clobazam are generally mild and resolve with dosage reduction. Drowsiness, short attention span, mood change, ataxia, and drooling may occur. These occur less commonly than in patients receiving 1,4-benzodiazepines (13). Marked worsening of behavior has been reported in some patients in open studies but does not appear to occur any more commonly than with carbamazepine or phenytoin (15). Excessive weight gain, which responds to withdrawal of the drug, has been reported (13). Hematologic and hepatic side effects have not been reported, and drug-induced skin rash is extremely rare.

Open studies in children have reported tolerance in 18% to 65% of patients (12–14, 141, 142), but most of these studies comprised patients who had been intractable to several antiepileptic drugs. In a controlled study in children who were previously untreated or who had received only one drug, the incidence of tolerance was similar in patients receiving clobazam (7.5%), carbamazepine (4.2%), and phenytoin (6.7%) (15).

Clinical Use. Clobazam should be started at a dosage of 2.5 mg/day in infants and 5 mg/day in older children. The dose can be increased at 5- to 7-day intervals until the seizures are controlled or side effects occur. Although doses of up to 3.8 mg/kg/day can be administered to children without undue side effects, dosages greater than 1 mg/kg/day are rarely associated with improved seizure control (13). In teenagers and adults, the initial dose is 10 mg/day. The dose can be increased at 5- to 7-day intervals, but those who do not respond to 30 mg/day respond rarely to higher doses (121). Clobazam is usually administered at night or twice a day. To minimize the risk of withdrawal seizures, discontinuation should be done gradually over several weeks. Drug level monitoring is not clinically useful.

References

1. Czapinski P, Blaszczyk B, Czuczwar SJ. Mechanisms of action of antiepileptic drugs. *Curr Top Med Chem* 2005; 5(1):3–14.
2. Wafford KA. GABAA receptor subtypes: any clues to the mechanism of benzodiazepine dependence? *Curr Opin Pharmacol* 2005; 5(1):47–52.
3. MacDonald RL. Benzodiazepines: mechanisms of action. In: Levy RH, Mattson RH, Meldrum BS, eds. Antiepileptic Drugs. 4th ed. New York: Raven Press, 1995: 695–703.
4. Ben-Ari Y, Holmes GL. The multiple facets of gamma-aminobutyric acid dysfunction in epilepsy. *Curr Opin Neurol* 2005; 18(2):141–145.
5. Wilson KC, Reardon C, Theodore AC, Farber HW. Propylene glycol toxicity: a severe iatrogenic illness in ICU patients receiving IV benzodiazepines: a case series and prospective, observational pilot study. *Chest* 2005; 128(3):1674–1681.
6. Bittencourt PR, Richens A. Anticonvulsant-induced status epilepticus in Lennox-Gastaut syndrome. *Epilepsia* 1981; 22(1):129–134.
7. Frey H-H. Experimental evidence for the the development of tolerance to anticonvulsant drug effects. In: Frey H-H, Froscher W, Koella WP, Meinardi H, eds. *Tolerance to the Beneficial and Adverse Effects of Antiepileptic Drugs*. New York: Raven Press, 1986:7–16.
8. Hernandez TD, Heninger C, Wilson MA, Gallager DW. Relationship of agonist efficacy to changes in GABA sensitivity and anticonvulsant tolerance following chronic benzodiazepine ligand exposure. *Eur J Pharmacol* 1989; 170(3):145–155.
9. Ramsey-Williams VA, Wu Y, Rosenberg HC. Comparison of anticonvulsant tolerance, crosstolerance, and benzodiazepine receptor binding following chronic treatment with diazepam or midazolam. *Pharmacol Biochem Behav* 1994; 48(3):765–772.
10. Biggio G, Dazzi L, Biggio F, Mancuso L, et al. Molecular mechanisms of tolerance to and withdrawal of GABA(A) receptor modulators. *Eur Neuropsychopharmacol* 2003; 13(6):411–423.
11. Specht U, Boenigk HE, Wolf P. Discontinuation of clonazepam after long-term treatment. *Epilepsia* 1989; 30:458–463.
12. Keene DL, Whiting S, Humphreys P. Clobazam as an add-on drug in the treatment of refractory epilepsy of childhood. *Can J Neurol Sci* 1990; 17:317–319.
13. Munn R, Farrell K. Open study of clobazam in refractory epilepsy. *Pediatr Neurol* 1993; 9:465–469.
14. Bardy AH, Seppala T, Salokorpi T. Monitoring of concentrations of clobazam and norclobazam in serum and saliva of of children with epilepsy. *Brain Dev* 1991; 13:174–179.
15. Canadian Clobazam Study Group. Clobazam has equivalent efficacy to carbamazepine and phenytoin as monotherapy for childhood epilepsy. *Epilepsia* 1998; 39:952–959.
16. De Negri M, Baglietto MG. Treatment of status epilepticus in children. *Paediatr Drugs* 2001; 3(6):411–420.
17. Schmidt D. Benzodiazepines: diazepam. In: Levy RH, Mattson RH, Meldrum BS, eds. *Antiepileptic Drugs*. 4th ed. New York: Raven Press, 1995:705–724.
18. Dhillon S, Richens A. Valproic acid and diazepam interaction in vivo. *Br J Clin Pharmacol* 1982; 13(4):553–560.
19. Riviello JJ Jr, Holmes GL. The treatment of status epilepticus. *Semin Pediatr Neurol* 2004; 11(2):129–138.
20. Singhi S, Banerjee S, Singhi P. Refractory status epilepticus in children: role of continuous diazepam infusion. *J Child Neurol* 1998; 13(1):23–26.
21. Singhi S, Murthy A, Singhi P, Jayashree M. Continuous midazolam versus diazepam infusion for refractory convulsive status epilepticus. *J Child Neurol* 2002; 17(2):106–110.
22. Bell HE, Bertino JS Jr. Constant diazepam infusion in the treatment of continuous seizure activity. *Drug Intell Clin Pharm* 1984; 18(12):965–970.
23. Dreifuss FE, Rosman NP, Cloyd JC, Pellock JM, et al. A comparison of rectal diazepam gel and placebo for acute repetitive seizures. *N Engl J Med* 1998; 338:1869–1875.
24. Kriel RL, Cloyd JC, Hadsall RS, Carlson AM, et al. Home use of rectal diazepam for cluster and prolonged seizures: efficacy, adverse reactions, quality of life, and cost analysis. *Pediatr Neurol* 1991; 7:13–17.
25. Alldredge BK, Wall DB, Ferriero DM. Effect of prehospital treatment on the outcome of status epilepticus in children. *Pediatr Neurol* 1995; 12:213–216.
26. Rosman NP, Colton T, Labazzo J, Gilbert PL, et al. A controlled trial of diazepam administered during febrile illnesses to prevent recurrence of febrile seizures. *N Engl J Med* 1993; 329(2):79–84.
27. Knudsen FU. Effective short-term diazepam prophylaxis in febrile convulsions. *J Pediatr* 1985; 106(3):487–490.
28. Knudsen F, Vestermark S. Prophylactic diazepam or phenobarbitone in febrile convulsions: a prospective controlled study. *Arch Dis Child* 1978; 53:660–663.
29. Baumann RJ, Duffner PK. Treatment of children with simple febrile seizures: the AAP practice parameter. Pediatr Neurol 2000; 23(1):11–17.
30. De Negri M, Baglietto MG, Battaglia FM, Gaggero R, et al. Treatment of electrical status epilepticus by short diazepam (DZP) cycles after DZP rectal bolus test. *Brain Dev* 1995; 17(5):330–333.
31. Hadjiloizou SM, Bourgeois BFD, Duffy FH, Bergin A, et al. Childhood-onset epileptic encephalopathies with sleep activated EEG and high dose diazepam treatment: review of a 5-year experience at Children's Hospital Boston. *Epilepsia* 2005; 46 Suppl 8:150–151.
32. De Negri M. Electrical status epilepticus during sleep (ESES). Different clinical syndromes: towards a unifying view? *Brain Dev* 1997; 19(7):447–451.
33. Sonmez F, Mir S, Tutuncuoglu S. Potential prophylactic use of benzodiazepines for hemodialysis-associated seizures. *Pediatr Nephrol* 2000; 14(5):367–369.
34. Farrell K. Benzodiazepines in the treatment of children with epilepsy. *Epilepsia* 1986; 27 Suppl 1:S45–S51.
35. Tassinari CA, Daniele O, Michelucci R, Breau M, et al. Benzodiazepines: efficacy in status epilepticus. In: Delgado-Escueta AV, Wasterlain CG, Treiman DM, Porter RJ, eds. *Status Epilepticus: Mechanisms of Brain Damage and Treatment*. New York: Raven Press, 1983:465–475.
36. Verrotti A, Latini G, di Corcia G, Giannuzzi R, et al. Intermittent oral diazepam prophylaxis in febrile convulsions: its effectiveness for febrile seizure recurrence. *Eur J Paediatr Neurol* 2004; 8(3):131–134.
37. Knudsen FU. Rectal administration of diazepam in solution in the acute treatment of convulsions in infants and children. *Arch Dis Child* 1979; 54:855–857.
38. Hoppu K, Santavuori P. Diazepam rectal solution for home treatment of acute seizures in children. *Acta Paediatr Scand* 1981; 70:369–372.
39. MacKichan J, Duffner PK, Cohen ME. Adsorption of diazepam to plastic tubing. *N Engl J Med* 1979; 301(6):332–333.
40. Kriel RL, Cloyd JC, Pellock JM, Mitchell WG, et al. Rectal diazepam gel for treatment of acute repetitive seizures. The North American Diastat Study Group. *Pediatr Neurol* 1999; 20(4):282–288.
41. Herman RJ, Van Pham JD, Szakacs CB. Disposition of lorazepam in human beings: enterohepatic recirculation and first-pass effect. *Clin Pharmacol Ther* 1989; 46:18–25.
42. Homan RW, Treiman DM. Benzodiazepines: lorazepam. In: Levy RH, Mattson RH, Meldrum BS, eds. *Antiepileptic Drugs*. 4th ed. New York: Raven Press, 1995:779–790.
43. Graves NM, Kriel RL, Jones-Saete C. Bioavailability of rectally administered lorazepam. *Clin Neuropharamacol* 1987; 10:555–559.
44. Ochs HR, Greenblatt DJ, Eichelkraut W, DeLuc BW, et al. Contribution of the gastrointestinal tract to lorazepam conjugation and clonazepam nitroreduction. *Pharmacology* 1991; 42:36–48.
45. Greenblatt DJ, Ehrenberg BL, Gunderman J, Scavone JM, et al. Kinetic and dynamic study of intravenous lorazepam: comparison with intravenous diazepam. *J Pharmacol Exp Ther* 1989; 250(1):134–140.
46. Relling MV, Mulhern RK, Dodge RK, Johnson D, et al. Lorazepam pharmacodynamics and pharmacokinetics in children. *J Pediatr* 1989; 114:641–646.
47. McDermott CA, Kowalczyk AL, Schnitzler ER, Mangurten HH, et al. Pharmacokinetics of lorazepam in critically ill neonates with seizures. *J Pediatr* 1992; 120:479–483.
48. Krauss JW, Desmond PV, Marshall JP, Johnson RF, et al. Effects of aging and liver disease on the disposition of lorazepam. *Clin Pharmacol Ther* 1978; 24:411–419.
49. Morrison G, Chiang ST, Koepke HH, Walker BR. Effect of renal impairment and hemodialysis on lorazepam kinetics. *Clin Pharmacol Ther* 1984; 35:646–652.
50. Anderson GD, Gidal BE, Kantor ED, Wilensky AJ. Lorazepam-valproate interaction: studies in normal subjects and isolated perfused rat liver. *Epilepsia* 1994; 35:221–225.
51. Desmond PV, Roberts RK, Wood AJJ, Dunn GD, et al. Effect of heparin administration on plasma binding of benzodiazepines. *Br J Clin Pharmacol* 1980; 9:171–175.
52. Appleton R, Sweeney A, Choonara I, Robson J, et al. Lorazepam versus diazepam in the acute treatment of epileptic seizures and status epilepticus. *Dev Med Child Neurol* 1995; 37(8):682–688.
53. Prasad K, Al-Roomi K, Krishnan PR, Sequeira R. Anticonvulsant therapy for status epilepticus. *Cochrane Database Syst Rev* 2005; (4)(4):CD003723.
54. Crawford TO, Mitchell WG, Snodgrass SR. Lorazepam and childhood status epilepticus and serial seizures: effectiveness and tachyphylaxis. *Neurology* 1987; 37:190–195.
55. Yager JY, Seshia SS. Sublingual lorazepam in childhood serial seizures. *Am J Dis Child* 1988; 142:931–932.
56. Chan KW, Mullen CA, Worth LL, Choroszy M, et al. Lorazepam for seizure prophylaxis during high-dose busulfan administration. *Bone Marrow Transplant* 2002; 29(12):963–965.
57. Vincent FM, Vincent T. Lorazepam in myoclonic seizures after cardiac arrest. *Ann Intern Med* 1986; 104:586 (letter).
58. Amand G, Evrard P. Le lorazepam injectable dans etas de mal epileptiques. *Rev Electroencephalogr Neurophysiol Clin* 1976; 6:532–533.
59. Waltregny A, Dargent J. Preliminary study of parenteral lorazepam in status epilepticus. *Acta Neurol Belg* 1975; 75:219–229.
60. DiMario FJ Jr, Clancy RR. Paradoxical precipitation of tonic seizures by lorazepam in a child with atypical absence seizures. *Pediatr Neurol* 1988; 4(4):249–251.
61. Bell DM, Richards G, Dhillon S, Oxley JR, et al. A comparative pharmacokinetic study of intravenous and intramuscular midazolam in patients with epilepsy. *Epilepsy Res* 1991; 10:183–190.
62. Bebin M, Bleck TP. New anticonvulsant drugs: focus on flunarazine, fosphenytoin, midazolam and stiripentol. *Drugs* 1994; 48:153–171.
63. Lahat E, Goldman M, Barr J, Eshel G, et al. Intranasal midazolam for childhood seizures. *Lancet* 1998; 22; 352:620 (letter).
64. Jacqz-Aigrain E, Wood C, Robieux I. Pharmacokinetics of midazolam in critically ill neonates. *Eur J Clin Pharmacol* 1990; 3:191–192.
65. Backman JT, Olkola KT, Ojala M, Laaksovirta H, et al. Concentrations and effects of oral midazolam are greatly reduced in patients treated with carbamazepine or phenytoin. *Epilepsia* 1996; 37:253–257.
66. Olkkola KT, Aranko K, Luurila H, Hiller A, et al. A potentially hazardous interaction between erythromycin and midazolam. *Clin Pharmacol Ther* 1993; 53(3):298–305.
67. Driessen JJ, Vree TB, Guelen PJ. The effects of acute changes in renal function on the pharmacokinetics of midazolam during long-term infusion in ICU patients. *Acta Anaesthesiol Belg* 1991; 42:149–155.
68. Koul RL, Aithala GR, Chacko A, Joshi R, et al. Continuous midazolam as treatment of status epilepticus. *Arch Dis Child* 1997; 76:445–448.
69. Rivera R, Segnini M, Boltadano A, Perez V. Midazolam in the treatment of status epilepticus in children. *Crit Care Med* 1993; 21:991–994.

70. Holmes GL, Riviello JJ Jr. Midazolam and pentobarbital for refractory status epilepticus. *Pediatr Neurol* 1999; 20(4):259–264.
71. Lohr A Jr, Werneck LC. Comparative non-randomized study with midazolam versus thiopental in children with refractory status epilepticus. *Arq Neuropsiquiatr* 2000; 58(2A):282–287.
72. Claassen J, Hirsch LJ, Emerson RG, Bates JE, et al. Continuous EEG monitoring and midazolam infusion for refractory nonconvulsive status epilepticus. *Neurology* 2001; 57(6):1036–1042.
73. Sheth RD, Buckley DJ, Gutierrez AR, Gingold M, et al. Midazolam in the treatment of refractory neonatal seizures. *Clin Neuropharmacol* 1996; 19(2):165–170.
74. Jawad S, Oxley J, Wilson J, Richens A. A pharmacodynamic evaluation of midazolam as an antiepileptic compound. *J Neurol Neurosurg Psychiatry* 1986; 49:1050–1054.
75. Lahat E, Aladjem M, Eshel G, Bistritzer T, et al. Midazolam in treatment of epileptic seizures. *Pediatr Neurol* 1992; 8:215–216.
76. Chamberlain JM, Altieri MA, Futterman C, Young GM, et al. A prospective, randomized study comparing intramuscular midazolam with intravenous diazepam for the treatment of seizures in children. *Pediatr Emerg Care* 1997; 13(2):92–94.
77. Mahmoudian T, Zadeh MM. Comparison of intranasal midazolam with intravenous diazepam for treating acute seizures in children. *Epilepsy Behav* 2004; 5(2):253–255.
78. Lahat E, Goldman M, Barr J, Bistritzer T, et al. Comparison of intranasal midazolam with intravenous diazepam for treating febrile seizures in children: prospective randomised study. *BMJ* 2000; 321(7253):83–86.
79. O'Regan ME, Brown JK, Clarke M. Nasal rather than rectal benzodiazepines in the management of acute childhood seizures? *Dev Med Child Neurol* 1996; 38(11):1037–1045.
80. Shorvon SD. The use of clobazam, midazolam and nitrazepam in epilepsy. *Epilepsia* 1998; 39 Suppl 1:S15–S23.
81. Roelofse JA, Stegmann DH, Hartshorne J, Joubert JJ. Paradoxical reactions to rectal midazolam as premedication in children. *Int J Oral Maxillofac Surg* 1990; 19(1):2–6.
82. Sato S, Malow BA. Benzodiazepines: clonazepam. In: Levy RH, Mattson RH, Meldrum BS, eds. *Antiepileptic Drugs*. 4th ed. New York: Raven Press, 1995:725–734.
83. Greenblatt DJ, Miller LG, Shader RI. Clonazepam pharmacokinetics, brain uptake, and receptor interactions. *J Clin Psychiatry* 1987; 48 Suppl:4–11.
84. Seree EJ, Pisano PJ, Placidi M, Rahamani R, et al. Identification of human and animal cytochromes P450 involved in clonazepam metabolism. *Fundam Clin Pharmacol* 1993; 7:69–75.
85. DeVane CL, Ware MR, Lydiard RB. Pharmacokinetics, pharmacodynamics, and treatment issues of benzodiazepines: alprazolam, adinazolam, and clonazepam. *Psychopharmacol Bull* 1991; 27:463–473.
86. Dreifuss FE, Penry JK, Rose SW, Kupferberg HJ, et al. Serum clonazepam concentrations in children with absence seizures. *Neurology* 1975; 25:255–258.
87. Andre M, Boutroy MJ, Dubruc C, Thenot JP, et al. Clonazepam pharmacokinetics and therapeutic efficacy in neonatal seizures. *Clin Pharmacol* 1986; 30:585–589.
88. Congdon PJ, Forsythe WI. Intravenous clonazepam in the treatment of status epilepticus in children. *Epilepsia* 1980; 21(1):97–102.
89. Ketz E, Bernoulli C, Siegfried J. Clinical and electroencephalographic trial with clonazepam (Ro 5-4023) with special regard to status epilepticus. *Acta Neurol Scand Suppl* 1973; 53:47–53.
90. Mikkelsen B, Birket-Smith E, Brandt S, Holm P, et al. Clonazepam in the treatment of epilepsy. *Arch Neurol* 1976; 33:322–325.
91. Sato S, Penry JK, Dreifuss FE, et al. Clonazepam in the treatment of absence seizures: a double-blind clinical trial. *Neurology* 1977; 27:371 (abstract).
92. Naito H, Wachi M, Nishida M. Clinical effects and plasma concentrations of long-term clonazepam monotherapy in previously untreated epileptics. *Acta Neurol Scand* 1987; 76:58–63.
93. Mireles R, Leppik IL. Valproate and clonazepam comedication in patients with intractable epilepsy. *Epilepsia* 1985; 26:122–126.
94. Obeid T, Panayiotopoulos CP. Clonazepam in juvenile myoclonic epilepsy. *Epilepsia* 1989; 30:603–606.
95. Takahashi K, Saito M, Kyo K. The effect of clonazepam on Rolandic discharge of benign epilepsy of children with centro-temporal EEG foci. *Jpn J Psychiatry Neurol* 1991; 45:468–470.
96. Mitsudome A, Ohfu M, Yasumoto S, Ogawa A, et al. The effectiveness of clonazepam on the Rolandic discharges. *Brain Dev* 1997; 19(4):274–278.
97. Hosoda N, Miura H, Takanashi S, Shirai H, et al. The long-term effectiveness of clonazepam therapy in the control of partial seizures in children difficult to control with carbamazepine monotherapy. *Jpn J Psychiatry Neurol* 1991; 45:471–473.
98. Schmidt D, Bourgeois B. A risk-benefit assessment of therapies for Lennox-Gastaut syndrome. *Drug Saf* 2000; 22(6):467–477.
99. Hanson RA, Menkes JH. A new anticonvulsant in the management of minor motor seizures. *Dev Med Child Neurol* 1972; 14:3–14.
100. Browne TR. Clonazepam: a review of a new anticonvulsant drug. *Arch Neurol* 1976; 33:326–332.
101. Browne TR. Clonazepam. *N Engl J Med* 1978; 299(15):812–816.
102. Suzuki Y, Edge J, Mimaki T, Walson PD. Intermittent clonazepam treatment prevents anticonvulsant tolerance in mice. *Epilepsy Res* 1993; 15:15–20.
103. Sher PK. Alternate-day clonazepam treatment of intractable seizures. *Arch Neurol* 1985; 42:787–788.
104. Schmidt D. How to use benzodiazepines. In: Morselli PL, Pippenger CE, Penry JK, eds. *Antiepileptic Drug Therapy in Pediatrics*. New York: Raven Press, 1983:271–282.
105. Baruzzi A, Michelucci R, Tassinari CA. Benzodiazepines: nitrazepam. In: Levy RH, Mattson RH, Meldrum BS, eds. *Antiepileptic Drugs*. New York: Raven Press, 1995:735–749.
106. Dreifuss F, Farwell J, Holmes G, et al. Infantile spasms: comparative trial of nitrazepam and corticotrophin. *Arch Neurol* 1986; 43:1107–1110.
107. Vanasse M, Geoffroy G. Treatment of epilepsy with nitrazepam. In: Wada JA, Penry JK, eds. *Advances in Epileptology: The Xth Epilepsy International Symposium*. New York: Raven Press, 1980:503.
108. Millichap JG, Ortiz WR. Nitrazepam in myoclonic epilepsies. *Am J Dis Child* 1966; 112:242–248.
109. Chamberlain MC. Nitrazepam for refractory infantile spasms and the Lennox-Gastaut syndrome. *J Child Neurol* 1996; 11(1):31–34.
110. Hosain SA, Green NS, Solomon GE, Chutorian A. Nitrazepam for the treatment of Lennox-Gastaut syndrome. *Pediatr Neurol* 2003; 28(1):16–19.
111. Wyllie E, Wyllie R, Cruse RP, Rothner AD, et al. The mechanism of nitrazepam-induced drooling and aspiration. *N Engl J Med* 1986; 314:35–38.
112. Murphy JV, Sawasky F, Marquardt KM, Harris DJ. Deaths in young children receiving nitrazepam. *J Pediatr* 1987; 111:145–147.
113. Rintahaka PJ, Nakagawa JA, Shewmon DA, Kyyronen P, et al. Incidence of death in patients with intractable epilepsy during nitrazepam treatment. *Epilepsia* 1999; 40(4):492–496.
114. Wilensky AJ, Ojemann LM, Temkin NR, Troupin AS, et al. Clorazepate kinetics in treated epileptics. *Clin Pharmacol* 1978; 24:22–30.
115. Wilensky AJ. Benzodiazepines: Clorazepate. In: Levy RH, Mattson RH, Meldrum BS, eds. *Antiepileptic Drugs*. 4th ed. New York: Raven Press, 1995:751–762.
116. Guggenheim MA, Donaldson J, Hotvedt C. Clinical evaluation of clorazepate. *Ann Neurol* 1987; 22:412–413.
117. Mimaki T, Tagawa T, Ono J, Tanaka J, et al. Antiepileptic effect and serum levels of clorazepate in children with refractory epilepsy. *Brain Dev* 1984; 6:539–544.
118. Graf WD, Rothman SJ. Clorazepate therapy in children with refractory seizures. *Epilepsia* 1987; 28:606 (letter).
119. Feldman RG. Clorazepate in temporal lobe epilepsy. *JAMA* 1976; 236:2603 (letter).
120. Jawad S, Richens A, Oxley J. Single dose pharmacokinetic study of clobazam in normal volunteers and epileptic patients. *Br J Clin Pharmacol* 1984; 18(6):873–877.
121. Shorvon SD. Benzodiazepines: clobazam. In: Levy RH, Mattson RH, Meldrum BS, eds. *Antiepileptic Drugs*. 4th ed. New York: Raven Press, 1995:763–777.
122. Rupp W, Badian M, Christ O, Hajdu P, et al. Pharmacokinetics of single and multiple doses of clobazam in humans. *Br J Clin Pharmacol* 1979; 7 Suppl 1:51S–57S.
123. Sennoune S, Mesdjian E, Bonneton J, Genton P, et al. Interactions between clobazam and standard antiepileptic drugs in patients with epilepsy. *Ther Drug Monit* 1992; 14:269–274.
124. Goggin T, Callaghan N. Blood levels of clobazam and its metabolites and therapeutic effect. In: Hindmarch I, Stonier PD, Trimble MR, eds. *Clobazam: Human Psychopharmacology and Clinical Applications*. London: Royal Society of Medicine, 1985:149–153.
125. Munn R, Camfield P, Camfield C, Dooley J. Clobazam for refractory childhood seizure disorders—a valuable supplementary drug. *Can J Neurol Sci* 1988; 15:406–408.
126. Zifkin B, Sherwin A, Andermann F. Phenytoin toxicity due to interaction with clobazam. *Neurology* 1991; 41:313–314.
127. Cocks A, Critchley EMR, Hayward HW, Thomas D. The effect of clobazam on blood levels of valproate. In: Hindmarch I, Stonier PD, Trimble MR, eds. *Clobazam: Human Psychopharmacology and Clinical Applications*. London: Royal Society of Medicine, 1985:155–158.
128. Canadian Clobazam Cooperative Group. Clobazam in the treatment of refractory epilepsy: the Canadian experience. A retrospective study. *Epilepsia* 1991; 32:407–416.
129. Gastaut H, Low MD. Antiepileptic properties of clobazam, a 1-5 benzodiazepine, in man. *Epilepsia* 1979; 20:437–446.
130. Senanayake N. "Eating epilepsy"—a reappraisal. *Epilepsy Res* 1990; 5:74–79.
131. Senanayake N. Epilepsia arithmetics revisited. *Epilepsy Res* 1989; 3:167–169.
132. Senanayake N. Epileptic seizures evoked by card games, draughts and similar games. *Epilepsia* 1987; 28:356–361.
133. Tinuper P, Aguglia U, Gastaut H. Use of clobazam in certain forms of status epilepticus and in startle induced epileptic seizures. *Epilepsia* 1986; 27:S18–S26.
134. Aguglia U, Tinuper P, Gastaut H. Startle-induced epileptic seizures. *Epilepsia* 1984; 25:712–720.
135. DeMarco P. Electrical status epilepticus during slow sleep: one case with sensory aphasia. *Clin Electroencephalogr* 1988; 19:111–113.
136. DeMarco P. Eyelid myoclonia with absences in two monovular twins. *Clin Electroencephalogr* 1989; 20:193–195.
137. Montenegro MA, Ferreira CM, Cendes F, Li LM, et al. Clobazam as add-on therapy for temporal lobe epilepsy and hippocampal sclerosis. *Can J Neurol Sci* 2005; 32(1):93–96.
138. Feely M, Gibson J. Intermittent clobazam for catamenial epilepsy: avoid tolerance. *J Neurol Neurosurg Psychiatry* 1984; 47:1279–1282.
139. Feely M, Calvert R, Gibson J. Clobazam in catamenial epilepsy. A model for evaluating anticonvulsants. *Lancet* 1982; 2:71–73.
140. Schwarer A, Sopat S, Watson AL, Cole-Sinclair MF. Clobazam for seizure prophylaxis during busulfan chemotherapy. *Lancet* 1995; 346:1238.
141. Campos P. Uso de clobazam en epilepsias de dificil control en ninos. *Arq Neuropsiqiatr* 1993; 51:66–71 (letter).
142. Shimuzu H, Abe J, Futagi Y, et al. Antiepileptic effects of clobazam in children. *Brain Dev* 1982; 4:57–62.

42 Carbamazepine and Oxcarbazepine

W. Edwin Dodson

CARBAMAZEPINE

Introduced in 1962 for treatment of trigeminal neuralgia, carbamazepine (CBZ) has emerged as a highly effective treatment of epilepsy with partial and secondarily generalized seizures. It has also been reported to benefit neuropathic pain, certain behavior disorders, and affective disorders. At first, CBZ was used to replace sedating antiepileptic drugs, but over time it became the initial therapy for treatment of localization-related epilepsy with partial (focal) seizures and epilepsy with generalized tonic-clonic seizures. Although CBZ produces side effects in many patients, the low incidence of cosmetic, cognitive, and behavioral side effects are advantages. The major disadvantages have been its propensity to interact with other drugs, to cause rashes and to aggravate absence and astatic seizures in patients with generalized epilepsy.

Clinical Efficacy

Carbamazepine is effective in partial (focal seizures), especially complex partial (psychomotor) seizures and generalized tonic-clonic (grand mal) seizures (1, 2). It is ineffective in febrile seizures and absence seizures. Furthermore, children with the Lennox-Gastaut syndrome sometimes have CBZ-induced worsening of several types of seizures, especially atypical absence seizures and astatic seizures, also called drop attacks (3, 4). Nonetheless, numerous studies have shown that CBZ is just as effective as other major anticonvulsants when prescribed for the appropriate type of seizure (5–14). For example, in benign rolandic epilepsy, a pediatric epileptic syndrome characterized by partial seizures, CBZ is effective in 94% of patients, producing complete control in 65%. Given its comparable efficacy to other first-line anticonvulsants, the somewhat unique spectrum of adverse effects associated with CBZ differentiates it from other antiepileptics. Although different rates of response to CBZ have been linked to age and gender, these differences appear to be small.

Carbamazepine has been reported to be more effective in girls than boys, and more effective in older patients than in children (15, 16). The causes for these differences are most likely pharmacokinetic, although they may also relate to distribution of seizure types in various age groups. For example, lower CBZ concentrations have been found among nonresponding children (17). Furthermore, young children have accelerated relative clearance of CBZ as compared to older children. Partial or generalized tonic-clonic seizures are the predominant seizure types in 55% and 90% of children and adults, respectively (18, 19).

The major mechanism of action of CBZ is to limit use-dependent increases in sodium conductance, thereby restricting neuronal high-frequency discharges. This mechanism is shared by phenytoin, oxcarbazepine, lamotrigine, topiramate, and felbamate, but differs from the mechanisms of actions of barbiturates, benzodiazepines, valproate, and succinimides (20). This mechanism at sodium channels correlates with clinical efficacy against partial and generalized tonic-clonic seizures. In experimental animals brain CBZ concentrations of 3.5 to 4.5 μg/g prevent maximal electroshock-induced seizures (21).

Carbamazepine in therapeutic concentrations has few effects on the electroencephalogram (EEG). It does not produce frontal low-voltage fast activity like that caused by barbiturates and benzodiazepines (22). High concentrations of CBZ produce generalized slowing. The effect of CBZ on seizure activity in the EEG varies depending on its efficacy. When CBZ is effective in preventing seizures, focal spikes at first become more brief and sharp and eventually may disappear (23). Discontinuation of CBZ is associated with an increase in the mean dominant rhythm frequency (24). Generalized spike and spike-wave abnormalities either are unaffected by CBZ or worsen (16).

Other uses of CBZ include the treatment of chronic neurogenic pain (25, 26), hemifacial spasm (27), and affective disorders (28–33), although most of the data supporting CBZ use in affective conditions are case reports, retrospective reviews, or open label, uncontrolled trials. Carbamazepine also has been used to treat attention deficit hyperactivity disorder in children and in other psychiatric conditions (34–38). In combination with lithium, CBZ has been used to treat refractory depression, refractory mania, and rapid cycling depression (39–41). Carbamazepine also may be beneficial in the dyscontrol syndrome, a disorder characterized by episodic aggressive outbursts (42, 43). Among impulsive hyperkinetic children with attention deficit disorder, the administration of CBZ is preferred over barbiturates, benzodiazepines and vigabatrin, and other GABA agonists, because the latter cause worsening of behavior in a substantial percentage of patients (18, 44–48).

After patients who have side effects due to other anticonvulsants are switched to CBZ, overall functioning often improves. When this occurs, it has been called a psychotropic action. Subjectively, these changes are described as less dulling of mentation, having a steadier gait, and improved attention and alertness (47). The improvement is most dramatic among patients who are switched from multidrug regimens that include barbiturates to monotherapy with CBZ. On the other hand, CBZ does not enhance cognitive function or behavior in otherwise normal patients unless seizures are occurring frequently enough to impair thinking.

Chemistry

Carbamazepine is a tricyclic compound related to iminostilbene (49). Although the two-dimensional structure of CBZ resembles tricyclic antidepressants, its three-dimensional conformation is more akin to phenytoin. Carbamazepine is a hydroscopic, neutral, lipophilic chemical that is soluble in organic solvents but possesses low water solubility. Due to limited aqueous solubility, CBZ has never been formulated for parenteral administration. Its crystalline structure and the structure-dependent dissolution rate of CBZ are sensitive to its extent of hydration. Exposure to high humidity leads to increasing hydration of CBZ causing the progressive development of a crystalline lattice that resists dissolution and is thereby insoluble. Thus patients who take carbamazepine that has been stored in humid and warm environments are at risk to experience drops in carbamazepine levels.

Biotransformation, Pharmacokinetics, and Interactions in Humans

Carbamazepine is eliminated largely by hepatic metabolism. Unique among unsaturated heterocyclic chemicals, the predominant elimination pathway in humans results in the formation of a stable epoxide that accumulates in serum. This compound, carbamzepine-10-11-epoxide (CBZE), has actions similar to CBZ but it is less potent in experimental models of epilepsy (50). The epoxide is hydrolyzed subsequently to form an inactive 10, 11-dihydroxide, the principal urinary metabolite. Lesser amounts of CBZ are metabolized by aromatic hydroxylation of the lateral rings. Carbamazepine is also a potent broad spectrum inducer of hepatic cytochrome P 450 enzymes, which metabolize other antiepileptic drugs.

Pharmacokinetics

Carbamazepine has linear, predictable elimination kinetics (Table **42-1** and Table **42-2**). In individual patients,

TABLE 42-1
Carbamazepine Reference Information

CARBAMAZEPINE (CBZ)	
Molecular weight	236.26
Conversion factor	CF = 1,000/236.26 = 4.23
Conversion	μg/mL or mg/L × 4.32 = μmol/L
CARBAMAZEPINE-10,11-EPOXIDE (CBZE)	
Molecular weight	252.3
Conversion factor	CF = 1,000/252.3 = 3.96
Conversion:	μg/mL (or mg/L) × 3.96 = μmol/L
RATIO OF CBZE TO CBZ	
Monotherapy	0.10–0.20
Polytherapy	0.15–0.66

From (22, 50).

TABLE 42-2
Carbamazepine Administration and Pharmacokinetics

Type of elimination kinetics	Linear
Special pharmacokinetic features	Autoinduction, dissolution-rate-limited absorption
Maintenance dose	10–20 mg/kg/day
Therapeutic concentration range	4–12 mg/L
Half-life (range)	5–36 hours*
Formulations	
Suspension (Tegretol)	50 mg/mL
Chewable tablet (Tegretol)	100 mg
Tablet (Tegretol, generic)	200 mg
Sustained release granules (Carbatrol)	200, 400
Sustained release (Tegretol XR)	100, 200, 400

From (22).
Half-life varies with duration of therapy (autoinduction), age, pregnancy, and comedication.

but not in groups of patients, the relationship between CBZ dose and concentration are linear and predictable (51–53). However, when standardized doses of CBZ are given to a large group, there is a wide scatter in the concentrations because of individual differences in CBZ elimination. Therefore, little or no correlation is found between CBZ doses and concentrations in groups (54, 55). Because of this, measurement of CBZ concentrations in blood is an important aspect of individualizing CBZ doses.

Elimination. CBZ induces its own metabolism by stimulating the activity of the CYP3A4 isozyme of cytochrome P450, a process called autoinduction (56, 57). Autoinduction causes the elimination rate of CBZ to increase in the days that follow the initiation or modification of doses. Because this process takes several weeks to evolve fully, CBZ pharmacokinetics have also been described as time-dependent kinetics. Among both children and adults who have not previously taken hepatic enzyme-inducing drugs, the half-life of CBZ decreases approximately 50% as autoinduction takes place, with the half-life declining from 36 hours after the first dose to 18 to 20 hours following chronic monotherapy in adults (52, 57). Likewise, studies in children indicate similar magnitudes of change with doubling of CBZ clearance (0.028 L/kg/hr to 0.056 L/kg/hr) after 2 or 3 weeks of therapy (58). Thus in all age groups, autoinduction causes levels to be approximately 50% of what would be predicted from first dose pharmacokinetics. Autoinduction is usually complete 3 to 6 weeks after a change in CBZ dose.

It is important to recognize autoinduction and not to mistake it as noncompliance. If constant doses are given during the first weeks of treatment, the concentration of CBZ increases at first and then declines. When seizures are controlled initially but then recur, autoinduction causing reduced CBZ levels may be the explanation.

The half-life of the epoxide metabolite has been estimated to range from 10 to 20 hours in patients who ceased taking CBZ (57, 59). When CBZE was administered to normal volunteers, a shorter half-life of 6.1 ± 0.9 hours was found (60). Among this same group of subjects the half-life of CBZ was 26 ± 4.6 hours, but autoinduction probably was incomplete.

Carbamazepine elimination is influenced by age, pregnancy, and drug interactions (61). As with other antiepileptic drugs, the relative clearance of CBZ is much higher in young children but declines to adult values in the later years of childhood. Younger patients and pregnant women in their last trimester have higher relative clearance and require higher relative doses than other patients (51). They also have higher ratios of CBZE to CBZ (62).

The ratio of CBZE to CBZ is 10% to 15% in adults. During childhood and pregnancy the ratio is higher, ranging up to 20%. In certain drug interactions involving valproate, the ratio can exceed 50%. Valproate elevates the ratio because it inhibits epoxide hydrolase and increases the epoxide concentration.

Absorption rate varies with formulation. The bioavailability of CBZ has been estimated to be 75% to 85% (52, 63). Food variably increases the rate of absorption (52). Larger doses may be absorbed more slowly than smaller ones. Slow absorption facilitates once daily administration in some patients. However, most authorities recommend more frequent administration to minimize the chance of side effects (64) and to minimize the impact of forgotten doses.

Carbamazepine is absorbed slowly after oral administration of tablets, with peak concentrations occurring 4–8 hours after ingestion (22). This tardy absorption results from slow dissolution of CBZ tablets. For this reason, CBZ absorption has been described as dissolution rate limited (52). Variations in the CBZ formulation significantly affect tablet dissolution rate and thus the absorption rate. Slow-release formulations such as Tegretol XR® and Carbatrol® slow absorption even more than the Tegretol® formulation. Tegretol XR® uses the Oros osmotic mechanism of slow release, whereas Carbatrol® slows dissolution by coating CBZ-containing particles (65). The Oros formulation consists of an osmotic core surrounded by a semipermeable membrane. When water enters the chamber in the center of the tablet, it forces the drug out of the delivery orifice into the gastrointestinal tract.

Carbatrol is a mixture of beads with three different coatings that dissolve at different rates. The so-called immediate coating dissolves quickly and initiates absorption. A slow-release coating of other beads is removed more slowly and releases the CBZ later. Finally, a pH-sensitive coating triggers dissolution in the alkaline pH of the small intestine (66). Crystalline matrix "retard" formulations, marketed as Timonil Retard® or Tegretol Retard® in Europe, also significantly attenuate the fluctuation index between doses (67, 68). In some patients this allows twice daily dosing, which is more convenient, encourages compliance, and reduces the chance of side effects (69).

Suspensions and certain generic formulations are absorbed more rapidly than proprietary Tegretol. For some patients, especially children who have short half-lives for CBZ, rapid absorption confounds their treatment, and switching to slow-release formulations can improve seizure control and reduce side effects.

For most patients slow absorption of CBZ is preferred. Generic formulations tend to be absorbed more rapidly than brand name formulations. For patients who require high, nearly toxic concentrations of CBZ for seizure control, switching to a more rapidly absorbed generic formulation can cause both seizure relapse and side effects due to wider fluctuations in CBZ concentrations between doses. Thus, the decision to substitute generic CBZ must be considered on a case-by-case basis. Generic CBZ is suitable mainly for those patients with mild epilepsy who are treated adequately with low levels.

Rapid elevation of the CBZ concentration is desirable for certain patients such as those who have completed video-EEG recording to determine whether they are candidates for epilepsy surgery or those who need their drugs switched rapidly. The administration of 8 mg/kg of CBZ suspension or tablets produces therapeutic levels in 2 and 5 hours, respectively (69).

Distribution. The volume of distribution for CBZ ranges from 0.93 to 1.28 L/kg (22). The brain-to-plasma ratio of both CBZ and CBZE is approximately 1, with a range of 0.8 to 1.6 (22, 70). Approximately 75% and 50% of CBZ and CBZE are bound to albumin, respectively (22). Concentrations of CBZ and CBZE in cerebrospinal fluid (CSF) are consistent with the protein binding values in serum and CSF concentrations equal the unbound fractions in plasma. The CSF-to-plasma concentration ratios average 0.25 and 0.50 for CBZ and CBZE, respectively. Note that the binding of these compounds is low enough that unless CBZ levels are high, the consequences of altered CBZ binding to constituents of plasma are usually trivial and do justify routine measurement of free CBZ levels (71). Salivary concentrations of CBZ also approximate the unbound concentrations in plasma, although the ratio of CBZ levels in plasma versus saliva varies during the day (72).

Carbamazepine crosses the placenta and penetrates breast milk. Transplacentally acquired CBZ concentrations in newborns at birth correlate highly with those found in maternal plasma (55). Newborns who have been exposed to CBZ in utero experience autoinduction of CBZ metabolism and eliminate CBZ at rates comparable to adults. Among newborns acquiring CBZ transplacentally, the reported half-lives have ranged from 8.2 to 28.1 hours (55). Among mothers taking CBZ, concentrations in their breast milk are so low that nursing infants rarely ingest a substantial dose.

Drug Interactions

Pharmacokinetic drug interactions involve both CBZ metabolism and CBZ binding to serum proteins (73). Numerous drugs including phenytoin, phenobarbital, and primidone induce hepatic enzymes responsible for CBZ biotransformation (74). Phenobarbital has the greatest effect, reducing the average half-life to 10–11 hours in adults. Adult patients taking all three together have an average half-life of 10.6 hours (60). Among patients on polytherapy, CBZ half-lives may be as short as 5 hours, half-lives that are considerably shorter than the average values of 18 to 20 hours reported for adults on CBZ monotherapy (75).

Valproate increases the unbound fraction of both CBZ and CBZE, and it inhibits the hydrolysis of CBZE by epoxide hydrolase, thereby increasing the ratio of CBZE to CBZ (63, 64). Under these circumstances, the valproate concentration correlates with the unbound CBZ fraction (76). Valproate and valpromide reduce the clearance of CBZE by inhibiting hepatic microsomal epoxide hydrolase (77, 78). The highest CBZE concentrations, which sometimes exceed 50% of the CBZ level, occur when CBZ is administered simultaneously with both an inducing agent, such as phenytoin, and with valproate. In these situations CBZE levels may be high enough to contribute to neurotoxicity. Note that routine CBZ levels do not include CBZE.

Patients with "therapeutic" concentrations of both phenytoin and CBZ sometimes develop side effects (57, 65). Evidence has also been found for a pharmacodynamic interaction between CBZ and phenytoin in experimental animals (79). Pharmacodynamic interactions take place in the target organ and are not secondary to changes in drug concentrations. Morris et al found that in mice, the therapeutic index of combined CBZ and phenytoin was no better than either drug given singly (79). Both efficacy in prevention of seizure and neurotoxicity increased when these drugs are given simultaneously. Although comparable data in humans are lacking, it is highly likely that the toxicities of CBZ and phenytoin are additive in humans.

A toxic pharmacodynamic interaction has also been described between CBZ and lamotrigine (80). Patients who had CBZ concentrations greater than 8 μg/mL developed diplopia and dizziness after lamotrigine was added on, even though the CBZ concentration did not change and lamotrigine levels were in the nontoxic range. After the CBZ dose was decreased, the side effects resolved.

CBZ also accelerates the metabolism of folic acid and biotin (81). Folic acid deficiency can cause psychiatric symptoms and should be considered when patients who have been treated chronically with inducing antiepileptic drugs develop psychiatric symptoms (82). Even more critical, folate deficiency during pregnancy has been linked to neural tube defects and folate supplementation has been recommended for all women of childbearing potential (83, 84). Needless to say folate supplementation is doubly important for women with epilepsy.

Several drugs inhibit CBZ elimination and cause CBZ levels to increase (Table 42-3). Isoniazide and CBZ increase the concentration of each other (85). Among the macrolide antibiotics, erythromycin, triacetyloleandomycin, and clarithromycin inhibit the biotransformation of CBZ, causing predictable increases in CBZ levels and neurotoxicity if the CBZ dose is not reduced (86–89). Other macrolide antibiotics have weaker and inconsistent effects on CBZ levels. Several antidepressants and selective serotonin reuptake inhibitors are competitive substrates with CBZ for CYP3A4 (90). Dextropropoxyphene and the antidepressant viloxazine increase CBZ levels after chronic administration (91). Nicotinamide, which is chemically related to isoniazide, also inhibits CBZ elimination, causing CBZ concentrations to increase (92). Carbamazepine does not interact with disulfiram (93) and cimetidine (94), which are metabolized by CYP2C9 and CYP2C19, but not by CYP3A4 (57, 95, 96).

Add-on therapy with CBZ reduces the concentrations of other anticonvulsants that are eliminated by hepatic metabolism, because it is a potent inducer of cytochrome P 450 (97). Carbamazepine causes ethosuximide levels to decline by an average of 17% and lowers valproate levels twice as much, increasing the clearance of valproate by one-third or more (98). The addition of CBZ to phenytoin usually decreases phenytoin concentrations, but the mechanism of the interaction is complex, with CBZ decreasing both the V_{max} and the K_m of phenytoin elimination (99), because it stimulates the activity of cytochromes CYP2C9 and CYP2C19 both of which catalyze phenytoin elimination (98).

TABLE 42-3
Pharmacokinetic Drug Interactions Involving Carbamazepine (CBZ)

DECREASE CBZ
Phenytoin
Phenobarbital
Primidone
INCREASE CBZ
Danazole
Clarithromycin
Diltiazem
Erythromycin
Isoniazide
Nicotinamide
Propoxyphene
Triacetyloleandomycin
Valproic acid
Verapamil
Viloxazine
DRUGS THAT ARE DECREASED BY CBZ
Clonazepam
Doxycycline
Ethosuximide
Haloperidol
Phenytoin*
Steroid contraceptives
Valproic acid
Warfarin

From (213).
*Interaction is variable. Usually CBZ decreases phenytoin levels, but sometimes the opposite is seen (105)

The induction of CBZ elimination by other drugs changes the relationship between CBZ dose and concentration. Among children on monotherapy, each 2 mg/kg/day dosage increases the CBZ concentration by 1 μg/mL. When other antiepileptics are given simultaneously, more than 3 mg/kg/day are required to increase the CBZ concentration by 1 μg/mL (55). Typically, patients receiving polytherapy have lower concentrations despite higher doses (100). Furthermore, patients receiving polytherapy need more frequent doses to avoid intermittent side effects, which occur due to wide fluctuations in serum levels (65).

Changes of drug regimens that involve CBZ. When adding or deleting CBZ, remember that other inducers of hepatic cytochrome P 450 enhance CBZ metabolism and vice versa. Thus, when CBZ is added to an antiepileptic drug regimen, it usually lowers the concentration of other antiepileptic drugs that are subject to hepatic biotransformation. For this reason the dose of the first drug should be held constant as CBZ is added until the concentration of the CBZ exceeds 4 μg/L. Then the original drug can be tapered over a period of three or more weeks, depending on the drug. After this is completed, the CBZ level usually increases if the drug that was replaced was a cytochrome P 450 inducer. This process in which discontinuation of an inducing drug leads to an increase in drug level is called disinduction (70). Note that because discontinuation of benzodiazepines may evoke withdrawal seizures, they should be reduced quite slowly, usually over several months to years. Furthermore, patients with severe epilepsy who are having frequent seizures may need to be hospitalized while their regimens are simplified because of the risk of provoking convulsive status epilepticus by changing the medications.

Adverse effects. Carbamazepine is generally well tolerated (101–103). Although some authorities report side effects in as many as 63% of patients (12, 104), most of the side effects do not warrant discontinuation of therapy. In one pediatric study, 43% had side effects. However, these were usually mild and tolerable such that only 3% discontinued the medication and another 3% required a dosage reduction (103). The most frequent neurologic side effect, drowsiness, occurred in 11%. Gastrointestinal complaints were uncommon. In chronic therapy tolerance develops to the neurologic side effects of CBZ and many of them abate completely (102). As with most other antiepileptic drugs, starting at a low dose and slowly escalating to the desired maintenance doses causes fewer side effects than rapidly raising the dose or starting at full maintenance dose (105).

At concentrations greater than 12 μg/mL side effects are increasingly common. Unbound CBZ levels correlate better with neurotoxicity than total CBZ levels in serum (65). Unbound CBZ concentrations of 1.7 μg/mL or more usually produce side effects. High levels of CBZ cause sedation, vertigo, and ophthalmoplegia resulting in the "3-D" triad of drowsiness, dizziness, and diplopia (6, 8, 23, 106). Brief episodes of toxicity can result from transient elevations of CBZ concentrations due to fluctuations between doses (69, 105–107). In these situations it is necessary to administer smaller, more frequent doses—or better yet, switch to a slow release CBZ formulation. When concentrations are less than 8 μg/mL, dose-related side effects are uncommon unless therapy has been initiated rapidly with high doses or unless the patient is taking other medications that have side effects that are additive to the side effects of CBZ (56, 108). Overdoses have been associated with symptoms resembling the central anticholinergic syndrome similar to that caused by tricyclic antidepressants (109, 110).

Whereas high concentrations are likely to cause neurologic side effects, at usual concentrations CBZ appears to have few if any effects on cognitive function (104, 111, 112).

Hyponatremia caused by CBZ occurs in patients of any age (113) but is more common among the elderly (114, 115). It is usually mild and asymptomatic in children (116). Oxcarbazepine is much more likely to cause hyponatremia than CBZ and can be problematic (116). Interestingly, CBZ-induced hyponatremia is said to be reversed by phenytoin (117).

Chronic side effects of CBZ differ from other anticonvulsants. In contrast to phenobarbital and phenytoin, CBZ monotherapy has not been associated with anticonvulsant-induced osteomalacia (118, 119, 120). Similarly, among the antiepileptic drugs CBZ is one of the least likely to cause cosmetic side effects. Gingival hyperplasia is not a problem with CBZ monotherapy (121).

Carbamazepine variably affects other laboratory tests. It lowers the plasma concentrations of thyroid-binding globulin and both bound and unbound T4 and T3 (122), but clinical hypothyroidism is rare among patients taking CBZ. Among the anticonvulsants used to treat major seizures, CBZ is least likely to elevate the gamma glutamyl transpeptidase (123).

Idiosyncratic neurologic adverse reactions include behavioral reactions, tics, asterixis, dystonia, and worsening of seizures, especially atonic or astatic seizures in children with Lennox-Gastaut syndrome (3, 124–127). Dystonia induced by CBZ at usual doses in brain-damaged children is rare and apparently idiosyncratic (128); it is more common with CBZ poisoning and high levels (129). Patients with cerebellar atrophy develop gaze-evoked nystagmus, dizziness, and ataxia at lower CBZ doses and levels than patients who have normal magnetic resonance imaging (130). Acute idiosyncratic, adverse behavioral reactions have occurred among children with psychiatric disorders. Silverstein et al (131) reported episodic bizarre behavior among seven pediatric patients after CBZ was added. However, five of the seven children tolerated CBZ when it was reintroduced later.

Hematologic side effects. Severe idiosyncratic hematologic toxicity such as aplastic anemia, agranulocytosis, or thrombocytopenia is rare among patients taking CBZ (132–136). The incidence of these complications has been estimated to be less that 1 per 50,000 (137). Thus in spite of previous concerns, experience has shown CBZ to be safe.

On the other hand, CBZ is associated with a dose-dependent reduction in neutrophil counts in 10% to 20% of patients. In adult psychiatric patients leukopenia occurred in 2.1% of patients who took CBZ and was approximately seven times more likely with CBZ than with valproate or with antidepressants (138). For example, in one study of 200 children taking CBZ, leukopenia (white blood count <4,000 per mm^3) occurred in 17% of patients less than 12 years old and 8% of children aged 12 to 17 years (138). These changes sometimes persist but usually do not forebode serious problems (7). Rarely does the neutrophil count decline below 1,200/mm^3 (139). For this reason the justification for costly, routine monitoring of blood counts has been questioned (137).

Although there is agreement about obtaining baseline blood counts, there is no consensus about how often blood counts should be determined during CBZ therapy (137, 138). Some authorities almost never obtain blood counts; others do them weekly at the onset of CBZ therapy and then monthly. Emphasizing that many factors influence the white blood count simultaneously, Silverstein et al recommended doing blood counts monthly during the first six months of therapy and every three months thereafter (138).

When starting CBZ, I check blood counts at baseline and after 6 weeks, 3 months, and 6 months if the counts are adequate. If the leukocyte count is consistently at or greater than 3,500/mm^3 and the granulocytes above 1,200, the frequency of the measurements can be reduced. Because of the possibility of a spurious laboratory result, neutrophil counts lower than 1,200/mm^3 and leukocyte counts of less than 3,500/mm^3 should be repeated to confirm the finding before therapy is modified. If the neutrophil count is confirmed to be less than 1,200/mm^3, the frequency of the observations should be increased. The dose should be reduced or stopped if the neutrophil count is persistently less than 900/mm^3.

If both anemia and neutropenia occur, obtaining a reticulocyte count, serum iron concentration, and iron-binding capacity provides an indirect indication of hematopoietic activity. The combination of a normal or elevated reticulocyte count with a normal or low iron level is reassuring that the bone marrow is active. On the other hand, a low reticulocyte count plus an increased serum iron concentration indicate that hematopoietic activity is reduced. If this occurs, CBZ should be stopped promptly and a hematologist should be consulted regarding a bone marrow evaluation.

Allergic rash is the most common reason that patients are intolerant of CBZ. The incidence of rash has varied from 4% to 10% in various series (12, 18) and may result from the intradermal production of reactive CBZ metabolites (140). Data from Saskatchewan indicate that the risk of serious rash is about the same with CBZ as with phenytoin, approximately 1 to 4 per 10,000 (141). Most CBZ-induced rashes abate after CBZ is discontinued, but severe rashes have been described (142, 143). Approximately 1 in 3,000 patients who are treated for epilepsy develop hypersensitivity to multiple antiepileptic drugs that have aromatic structures, including phenytoin, primidone, and phenobarbital along with CBZ and in some cases sulfonamides (140, 144–146). When multiple drug sensitivities occur, valproate and clobazam have been recommended (147).

Hypersensitivity reactions characterized by fever, renal, and hepatic toxicity are very rare (136, 148–150). Hepatotoxicity due to CBZ like that caused by phenytoin usually has occurred in the setting of a generalized hypersensitivity response (151). Most of the patients who have developed CBZ-induced hepatic dysfunction have taken it for less than 1 month and usually have associated fever or rash (152, 153). The hepatic histopathology usually indicates an inflammatory granulomatous infiltrate, but a different pathologic picture consistent with chemical hepatic insult also occurs (154). Furthermore, some cases have occurred when CBZ was administered with other potentially hepatotoxic agents such as isoniazide (155). In either case, fatalities are uncommon if the drug is stopped promptly (156, 157).

Carbamazepine therapy has been associated with erectile dysfunction possibly due to CBZ-induced hepatic synthesis of sex hormone-binding globulin and that potentially could lead to reduced unbound concentration of testosterone (158).

Other rare idiosyncratic reactions include systemic lupus erythematosus (SLE) and pseudolymphoma (159–162). Most of the cases of pseudolymphoma seem to be manifestations of the CBZ hypersensitivity syndrome.

Monotherapy

Monotherapy with CBZ is often superior to polytherapy. Approximately 80% of patients with only generalized tonic-clonic seizures (grand mal) can be controlled with CBZ alone as can 69% of patients with partial seizures of certain types (16). The most difficult patients are those who have both partial and secondarily generalized seizures in whom single drug therapy succeeds in less than half. Although most authorities agree that these types of patients deserve a trial of therapy with drug combinations, all patients should have a diligent trial of monotherapy before resorting to polytherapy. Among patients with severe epilepsy, combinations of CBZ, phenytoin, and phenobarbital are more efficacious than monotherapy, but severe side effects are prevalent. Cereghino et al (163) found that 68% of adults who took these drugs concurrently had excessive sleepiness, malaise, and impaired abilities to conduct their daily activities.

In the end the impairment due to neurotoxicity must be weighed against the handicap caused by the seizures. The regimen that allows the patient to function optimally is best. Many patients with persistent seizures and side effects taking polytherapy are better off after having their regimens simplified (164, 165). Schmidt was able to switch 83% of patients with intractable complex partial seizures from two medications to CBZ monotherapy with fewer side effects but no increase in seizure frequency; 36% had fewer seizures (166). In another series, 75% of

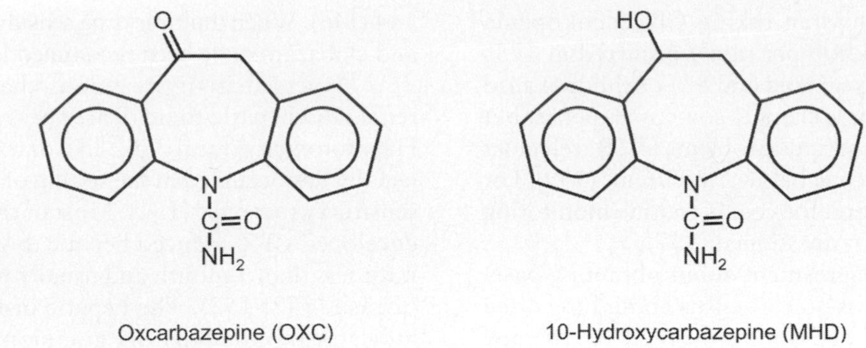

Oxcarbazepine (OXC) 10-Hydroxycarbazepine (MHD)

FIGURE 42-1

Structures of oxcarbazepine and its 10-monohydroxy derivative.

280 patients had adequate seizure control with monotherapy (155). In yet another series involving mentally retarded institutionalized patients, seizure control was no different on monotherapy versus polytherapy (167). Thus many patients who are having both side effects and seizures benefit from simplified regimens.

OXCARBAZEPINE

Oxcarbazepine (OXC; Trileptal) is the 10-keto analog of CBZ. It has gained wide acceptance and use for treatment of epilepsy with partial onset seizures (168–170). The main advantages of OXC over CBZ are its relatively reduced capacity for induction of hepatic cytochrome drug metabolizing enzymes resulting in fewer drug interactions and reduced risk of allergic rash (171, 172). Unlike CBZ, oxcarbazepine does not induce its own metabolism and autoinduction is not an issue. Oxcarbazepine and CBZ appear to share the same mechanisms of action and act to limit high frequency firing by acting on voltage-dependent sodium channels (173). Although case reports and uncontrolled studies have suggested that OXC might be beneficial in childhood bipolar disorder (174), prospective controlled trials are generally lacking or negative. In one report OXC was inferior to valproate and was associated with increased aggression (175, 176). In animal models of combination antiepileptic therapy studied by isobolographic analysis, combinations of OXC with topiramate were favorable whereas OXC with either felbamate or lamotrigine were unfavorable due to additive neurotoxicity that was disproportionately greater than efficacy (177).

Biotransformation, Pharmacokinetics, and Interactions in Humans

Oxcarbazepine is well absorbed after oral administration and then it is rapidly converted by cytosolic arylketone reductase to the active 10-monohydroxy derivative (MHD), which is responsible for most of the antiepileptic effect (178) (Figure 42-1). Concentrations of MHD peak 4 to 12 hours following oral doses of OXC (179). Concentrations of both compounds are linearly related to dose and have been reported to be little affected by interactions with hepatic enzyme-inducing agents (179). Neither compound is highly protein bound, with OXC being 60% bound and MHD 40% bound (180). Whereas the half-life of OXC is 1 to 2.5 hours, the half-life of MHD is 8–10 hours in children (181, 182) with longer values reported in normal volunteers, adults, and elderly patients (179). Moreover, as with other antiepilepsy drugs (AEDs), younger children eliminate OXC and MHD faster than older children and adults, with young children (age 2–5 years) having half-lives for MHD that were 30% shorter than those found in older children (age 6–12 years) (183, 184). Although the conversion of OXC to MDH results in a racemic mixture of enantiomers with the dextrorotary isomer being produced in fivefold greater amounts than the levorotary isomer (185, 186), both stereoisomers are active antiepileptic agents. The MHD is eliminated mainly in urine after conjugation to glucuronic acid. Mild to moderate hepatic dysfunction has no effect on OXC and MHD elimination, but renal impairment can necessitate reducing the dose (179). The therapeutic range of MHD has been proposed to be 50 to 140 μmol/L (187) or 15–35 mg/L (179). Oxcarbazepine and MDH can be monitored in saliva (188, 189). Both OXC and MHD cross the placenta and also enter breast milk in concentrations roughly half of those in plasma (190, 191). Clearance of OXC and MHD increases during pregnancy, causing levels to decrease. The extent of this decrease was greater with OXC monotherapy than with other AEDs and the risk of seizures was higher (192).

Both OXC and its metabolite have a spectrum of activity that is similar to CBZ. Oxcarbazepine is effective as add-on therapy in refractory seizures and as initial monotherapy in new onset seizures (193). Although OXC and CBZ seem to share common mechanisms of action,

TABLE 42-4
Reference Information for Oxcarbazepine

OXCARBAZEPINE (OXC)	
Molecular weight	252.27
Conversion factor	CF = 1,000/252.27 = 3.96
Conversion	μg/mL or mg/L × 3.96 = μmol/L
10-MONOHYDROXY DERIVATIVE METABOLITE (MHD)	
Molecular weight	253.27
Conversion factor	1,000/253.27 = 3.95
Conversion	μg/mL (or mg/L) × 3.95 = μmol/L
C_{max} of MHD	In 3–4 hours
Kinetics	Linear
MHD half-life	8–10 hours (adults)
Time to steady state	2–3 days

From (181).

some patients who are inadequately treated with CBZ improved after they were switched to OXC (194). In a double-blind, randomized study that compared OXC to phenytoin in 193 children aged 5 to 18 years with new onset partial or generalized tonic-clonic seizures, efficacy was equivalent, with approximately 60% of subjects in each group becoming seizure free (195). However, oxcarbazepine was better tolerated as demonstrated by more subjects discontinuing phenytoin due to adverse effects.

Oxcarbazepine Drug Interactions

Oxcarbazepine inhibits CYP2C19 and, although usually clinically irrelevant, it can increase phenytoin concentrations when phenytoin levels are high to begin with. Both OXC and MHD can induce UDP-glucuronyl transferase activity. Oxcarbazepine usually has little or no effect on concentrations of valproate, phenobarbital, CBZ, and low concentrations of phenytoin; however, each of these compounds can decrease the concentration of MHD by 20% to 40% (196). Interactions with lamotrigine have been reported to be negligible among psychiatric patients (197). Oxcarbazepine also induces CYP3A4/5, whereby it can lead to reduced concentrations and effectiveness of low estrogen dose oral contraceptives (179, 198, 199).

Adverse effects. Studies of cognitive adverse effects of CBZ and OXC have found no differences (200). Like CBZ, OXC has been reported to exacerbate seizures in patients with idiopathic epilepsy, including some patients with benign partial epilepsy of childhood (5, 201–203). Oxcarbazepine has a lower incidence of allergic reactions and is less neurotoxic (204–207). However, it causes symptomatic hyponatremia more frequently than CBZ (205–208), with hyponatremia (<125 mEq/L) occurring in 3% of subjects in initial clinical trials (208). Neurologic side effects are most common and include dizziness, headache, diplopia, ataxia, fatigue somnolence, and rash followed by gastrointestinal side effects of nausea and vomiting (174, 177, 209, 210). Rashes reported with OXC include Stevens-Johnson syndrome and toxic epidermal necrolysis in addition to milder maculopapular eruptions (197). Among patients who have had allergic reactions to CBZ, the risk of allergic cross-reactivity with OXC is 25% (197). As with patients taking CBZ monotherapy, those taking OXC monotherapy also are prone to have reduced concentrations of 25-OH vitamin D, which if untreated heightens the risk of osteopenia (211). In contrast to valproate, OXC treatment of girls aged 8 to 18 years was not associated with increased body mass index (212).

References

1. Loiseau P, Duche B. Carbamazepine clinical use. In: Levy RH, Mattson RH, Meldrum BS, eds. *Antiepileptic Drugs*. 4th ed. New York: Raven Press, 1995:555–566.
2. Dodson WE. Carbamazepine efficacy and utilization in children. *Epilepsia* 1987; 28 Suppl 3:S17–S24.
3. Snead OC, Hosey LC. Exacerbation of seizures in children by carbamazepine. *N Engl J Med* 1985; 313:916–921.
4. Sazgar M, Bourgeois BF. Aggravation of epilepsy by antiepileptic drugs. *Pediatr Neurol* 2005; 33:227–234.
5. Livingston S, Villamatar C, Sakata Y, Pauli LL. Use of carbamazepine in epilepsy. *JAMA* 1967; 200:116–119.
6. Livingston S, Pauli LL, Berman W. Carbamazepine (Tegretol) in epilepsy. *Dis Nerv Sys* 1974; 35:103–107.
7. Cereghino JJ, Brock JT, Van Meter JC, Penry JK, et al. Carbamazepine for epilepsy. *Neurology* 1974; 24:401–410.
8. Gram L, Bentsen KD, Parnas J, Flachs H. Controlled trials in epilepsy: a review. *Epilepsia* 1982; 23:491–519.
9. Simonsen N, Zander-Olsen P, Kuhl V, et al. A comparative controlled study between carbamazepine and diphenylhydantion in psychomotor epilepsy. *Epilepsia* 1976; 17:169–176.
10. Kosteljanetz M, Christiansen J, Dam AM, et al. Carbamazepine versus phenytoin. A controlled clinical trial in focal motor and generalized epilepsy. *Arch Neurol* 1979; 36:22–24.
11. Ramsey RE, Wilder BJ, Berger JR, Bruni J. A double-blind study comparing carbamazepine with phenytoin as initial seizure therapy in adults. *Neurology* 1983; 33:904–910.
12. Mitchell WG, Chavez JM. Carbamazepine versus phenobarbital for partial onset seizures in children. *Epilepsia* 1987; 28:56–60.
13. Mattson RH, Cramer JA, Collins JF, et al. Comparison of carbamazepine, phenobarbital, phenytoin, and primidone in partial and secondarily generalized tonic-clonic seizures. *N Engl J Med* 1985; 313:145–151.
14. Verity CM, Hosking G, Easter DJ. A multicentre comparative trial of sodium valproate and carbamazepine in paediatric epilepsy. The Paediatric EPITEG Collaborative Group. *Dev Med Child Neurol* 1995; 37:97–108.
15. Rett A. The so-called psychotropic effect of Tegretol in the treatment of convulsions of cerebral origin in children. In: Birkmayer W, ed. *Epileptic Seizures-Behavior-Pain*. Baltimore, MD: University Park Press, 1976:194–208.
16. Scheffner D, Schiefer I. The treatment of epileptic children with carbamazepine. *Epilepsia* 1972; 13:819–828.
17. Huf R, Schain RJ. Long-term experiences with carbamazepine (Tegretol) in children with seizures. *J Pediatr* 1980; 97:310–312.
18. Gastaut H, Gastaut GE, Silva GEG, Sanchez GFR. Relative frequency of different types of epilepsy: a study employing the classification of the International League Against Epilepsy. *Epilepsia* 1975; 16:457–461.
19. Cavazutti GB. Epidemiology of different types of epilepsy in school age children of Modena, Italy. *Epilepsia* 1980; 21:57–62.

20. Macdonald RL. Carbamazepine mechanisms of action In: Levy RH, Mattson RH, Meldrum BS, eds. *Antiepileptic Drugs*. 4th ed. New York: Raven Press, 1995:491–498.
21. Morselli PL. Carbamazepine absorption, distribution and excretion In: Levy RH, Mattson RH, Meldrum BS, eds. *Antiepileptic Drugs*. 4th ed. New York: Raven Press, 1995:515–528.
22. Rodin EA, Rim CS, Rennick PM. The effects of carbamazepine on patients with psychomotor epilepsy: results of a double-blind study. *Epilepsia* 1974; 15:547–561.
23. Frost JD Jr, Kellaway P, Hrachovy RA, et al. Changes in epileptic spike configuration associated with attainment of seizure control. *Ann Neurol* 1986; 20:723–726.
24. Duncan JS, Smith SJ, Forster A, et al. Effects of the removal of phenytoin, carbamazepine, and valproate on the electroencephalogram. *Epilepsia* 1989; 30:590–596.
25. Swederlow M. Anticonvulsant drugs and chronic pain. *Clin Neuropharmacol* 1984, 7:51–82.
26. Leijon G, Boivie J. Central post-stroke pain—a controlled trial of amitriptyline and carbamazepine. *Pain* 1989, 36:27–36.
27. Shaywitz BA. Hemifacial spasm in childhood treated with carbamazepine. *Arch Neurol* 1974; 31:63–63.
28. Kowatch RA, Suppes T, Carmody TJ, et al. Effect size of lithium, divalproex sodium, and carbamazepine in children and adolescents with bipolar disorder. *J Am Acad Child Adolesc Psychiatry* 2000; 39:713–720.
29. Chang KD, Ketter TA. Special issues in the treatment of paediatric bipolar disorder. *Expert Opin Pharmacother* 2001; 2:613–622.
30. James AC, Javaloyes AM. The treatment of bipolar disorder in children and adolescents. *J Child Psychol Psychiatry* 2001; 42:439–449.
31. Salpekar JA, Conry JA, Doss W, et al. Clinical experience with anticonvulsant medication in pediatric epilepsy and comorbid bipolar spectrum disorder. *Epilepsy Behav* 2006; 9:327–334.
32. Davanzo P, Gunderson B, Belin T, et al. Mood stabilizers in hospitalized children with bipolar disorder: a retrospective review. *Psychiatry Clin Neurosci* 2003; 57:504–510.
33. Post RM, Uhde TW, Rubinow DR, et al. Biochemical effects of carbamazepine: relationship to its mechanisms of action in affective illness. *Prog Neuropsychopharmacol Biol Psychiatry* 1983; 7:263–271.
34. Ballenger JC. The use of anticonvulsants in manic-depressive illness. *J Clin Psychiatry* 1988; 49 Suppl:21–25.
35. Silva RR, Munoz DM, Alpert M. Carbamazepine use in children and adolescents with features of attention-deficit hyperactivity disorder: a meta-analysis. *J Am Acad Child Adolesc Psychiatry* 1996; 35:352–358.
36. Hernandez-Avila CA, Ortega-Soto HA, et al. Treatment of inhalant-induced psychotic disorder with carbamazepine versus haloperidol. *Psychiatr Serv* 1998; 49:812–815.
37. Greil W, Ludwig-Mayerhofer W, Erazo N, et al. Lithium vs carbamazepine in the maintenance treatment of schizoaffective disorder: a randomised study. *Eur Arch Psychiatry Clin Neurosci* 1997; 247:42–50.
38. Greil W, Ludwig-Mayerhofer W, et al. Lithium versus carbamazepine in the maintenance treatment of bipolar disorders—a randomised study. *J Affect Disord* 1997; 43:151–161.
39. Arana GW, Santos AB, Knax EP, Ballenger JC. Refractory rapid cycling unipolar depression responds to lithium and carbamazepine treatment. *J Clin Psychiatry* 1989; 50:356–357.
40. Kramlinger KG, Post RM. The addition of lithium to carbamazepine. Antidepressant efficacy in treatment-resistant depression. *Arch Gen Psychiatry* 1989; 46:794–800.
41. Spurkland I, Vandvik IH. Rapid cycling depression in adolescence. A case treated with family therapy and carbamazepine. *Acta Psychiatr Scand* 1989; 80:60–63.
42. Tunks ER, Dermer SW. Carbamazepine in the dyscontrol syndrome associated with limbic system dysfunction. *J Nerv Ment Dis* 1977; 164:56–63.
43. Foster HG, Hillbrand M, Chi CC. Efficacy of carbamazepine in assaultive patients with frontal lobe dysfunction. *Prog Neuropsychopharmacol Biol Psychiatry* 1989; 13:865–874.
44. Camfield CS, Chaplin S, Doyle A, et al. Side effects of phenobarbital in toddlers: behavioral and cognitive aspects. *J Pediatr* 1979; 95:361–165.
45. Wolf SM, Forsythe A. Behavior disturbance, phenobarbital and febrile seizures. *Pediatrics* 1978; 61:728–731.
46. Troupin AS, Green JR, Levy RH. Carbamazepine as an anticonvulsant: a pilot study. *Neurology* 1974; 24:863–869.
47. Vining EPG, Mellits ED, Cataldo MF, et al. Effects of phenobarbital and sodium valproate on neuropsychological function and behavior. *Ann Neurol* 1983; 14:360.
48. Trimble MR, Cull, C. Children of school age: the influence of antiepileptic drugs on behavior and intellect. *Epilepsia* 1988; 29 Suppl 3:S15–S19.
49. Faigle JW, Feldman KF. Carbamazepine: Chemistry and biotransformation. In Levy RH, Mattson RH, Meldrum BS, eds. *Antiepileptic Drugs*. 4th ed. New York: Raven Press, 1995:499–513.
50. Pynnonen S, Sillanpaa M, Frey H, Iisalo E. Carbamazepine and its 10,11-epoxide in children and adults with epilepsy. *Eur J Clin Pharmacol* 1977; 11:129–133.
51. Levy RH, Pitlick WH, et al. Pharmacokinetics of carbamazepine in normal man. *Clin Pharmacol Ther* 1975; 17:657–668.
52. Perucca E, Bittencourt P, Richens A. Effect of dose increments on serum carbamazepine concentration in epileptic patients. *Clin Pharmacokinet* 1980; 5:576–582.
53. Kerr BM, Levy RH. Carbamazepine: carbamazepine epoxide. In Levy RH, Mattson RH, Meldrum BS, eds. *Antiepileptic Drugs*. 4th ed. New York: Raven Press, 1995:529–541.
54. Rane A, Bengt H, Wilson JT. Kinetics of carbamazepine and its 10,11-epoxide metabolite in children. *Clin Pharmacol Ther* 1976; 19:276–283.
55. Tomson T, Tybring G, Bertilsson L, et al. Carbamazepine therapy in trigeminal neuralgia. *Arch Neurol* 1980; 37:699–703.
56. Levy RH. Cytochrome P450 isozymes and antiepileptic drug interactions. *Epilepsia* 1995; 36 Suppl 5:S8–S13.
57. Eichelbaum M, Ekbom K, Bertilsson L, et al. Plasma kinetics of carbamazepine and its epoxide metabolite in man after single and multiple doses. *Clin Pharmacol* 1975; 8:337–341.
58. Bertilsson L, Bengt H, Gunnel T, et al. Autoinduction of carbamazepine metabolism in children examined by a stable isotope technique. *Clin Pharmacol Ther* 1980; 27: 83–88.
59. Westenberg HGM, van der Kleijn E, Oei TT, de Zoeuw RA. Kinetics of carbamazepine and carbamazepine-epoxide determined by use of plasma and saliva. *Clin Pharmacol Ther* 1978; 23:320–328.
60. Tomson T, Tybring G, Bertilsson E, Bertilsson L. Single-dose kinetics and metabolism of carbamazepine-10,11-epoxide. *Clin Pharmacol Ther* 1983; 33:58–65.
61. Battino D, Bossi L, Croci D, et al. Carbamazepine plasma levels in children and adults: influence of age, dose, and associated therapy. *Ther Drug Monit* 1980; 2:315–322.
62. Brodie MJ, Forrest G, Papeport WG. Carbamazepine 10,11 epoxide concentrations in epileptics on carbamazepine alone and in combination with other anticonvulsants. *Br J Clin Pharmacol* 1983; 16:747–749.
63. Wada JA, Troupin AS, Friel P, Remick R, et al. Pharmacokinetic comparison of tablet and suspension dosage forms of carbamazepine. *Epilepsia* 1978; 19:251–255.
64. Riva R, Albani F, Ambrosetto G, et al. Diurnal fluctuations in free and total steady-state plasma levels of carbamazepine and correlation with intermittent side effects. *Epilepsia* 1984; 25:476–481.
65. Stevens RE, Limsakun T, Evans G, Mason DH Jr. Controlled, multidose, pharmacokinetic evaluation of two extended-release carbamazepine formulations (Carbatrol and Tegretol-XR). *J Pharm Sci* 1998; 87:1531–4.
66. Garnett WR, Levy B, McLean AM, et al. Pharmacokinetic evalution of twice daily extended-release carbamazepine (CBZ) in patients with epilepsy. *Epilepsia* 1998; 39:274–279.
67. Jensen PK, Moller A, Gram L, et al. Pharmacokinetic comparison of two carbamazepine slow-release formulations. *Acta Neurol Scand* 1990; 82:135–7.
68. Canger R, Altamura AC, Belvedere O, et al. Conventional vs controlled-release carabamazepine: a multicentre, double-blind, crossover study. *Acta Neurol Scand* 1990; 82:9–13.
69. Kanner AM, Bourgeois BF, Hasegawa H, Hutson P. Rapid switchover to carbamazepine using pharmacokinetic parameters. *Epilepsia* 1998; 39:194–200.
70. Friis ML, Christiansen J. Carbamazepine, carbamazepine-10,11-epoxide and phenytoin concentrations in brain tissue of epileptic children. *Acta Neurol Scand* 1978; 58: 104–108.
71. Warner A, Privitera M, Bates D. Standards of laboratory practice: antiepileptic drug monitoring. National Academy of Clinical Biochemistry. *Clin Chem* 1998; 44:1085–95.
72. Paxton JW, Aman MG, Werry JS. Fluctuations in salivary carbamazepine and carbamazepine-10,11-epoxide concentrations during the day in epileptic children. *Epilepsia* 1983; 24:716–724.
73. Baciewicz AM. Carbamazepine drug interactions. *Ther Drug Monit* 1986; 8:305–17.
74. Lander CM, Eadie MJ, Tyrer JH. Factors influencing plasma carbamazepine concentrations. *Clin Exp Neurol* 1977; 14:184–193.
75. Eichelbaum M, Kothe KW, Hoffman F, von Unruh GE. Kinetics and metabolism of carbamazepine during combined antiepileptic drug therapy. *Clin Pharmacol Ther* 1979; 26:366–371.
76. Haidukewych D, Zielinski JJ, Rodin EA. Derivation and evaluation of an equation for prediction of free carbamazepine concentrations in patients comedicated with valproic acid. *Ther Drug Monit* 1989; 11:528–32.
77. Kerr BM, Rettie AE, Eddy AC, et al. Inhibition of human liver microsomal epoxide hydrolase by valproate and valpromide: in vitro/in vivo correlation. *Clin Pharmacol Ther* 1989; 46:82–93.
78. Pisani F, Narbone MC, Fazio A, et al. Effect of viloxazine on serum carbazmazepine levels in epileptic patients. *Epilepsia* 1984; 25:482–485.
79. Morris JC, Dodson WE, Hatelid JM, Ferrendelli JA. Phenytoin and carbazazepine, alone and in combination: anticonvulsant and neurotoxic effects. *Neurology* 1987; 37:1111–9.
80. Besag FM, Berry DJ, Pool F, et al. Carbamazepine toxicity with lamotrigine: pharmacokinetic or pharmacodynamic interaction? *Epilepsia* 1998; 39:183–7.
81. Kishi T, Fujita N, Eguchi T, Ueda K. Mechanism for reduction of serum folate by antiepileptic drugs during prolonged therapy. *J Neurol Sci* 1997; 145:109–12.
82. Froscher W, Maier V, Laage M, et al. Folate deficiency, anticonvulsant drugs, and psychiatric morbidity. *Clin Neuropharmacol* 1995; 18:165–82.
83. Lewis DP, Van Dyke DC, Stumbo PJ, Berg MJ. Drug and environmental factors associated with adverse pregnancy outcomes. Part I: Antiepileptic drugs, contraceptives, smoking, and folate. *Ann Pharmacother* 1998; 32:802–17.
84. Chang SI, McAuley JW. Pharmacotherapeutic issues for women of childbearing age with epilepsy. *Ann Pharmacother* 1998; 32:794–801.
85. Wright JM, Stokes EF, Sweeney VP. Isoniazid-induced carbamazepine toxicity and vice versa. *N Engl J Med* 1982; 307:1325–1327.
86. Goulden KJ, Camfield P, Dooley JM, et al. Severe carbamazepine intoxication after adminsitration of erythromycin. *J Pediatr* 1986; 109:135–138.
87. Hedrick R, Williams F, Morin R, et al. Carbamazepine-erythromycin interaction leading to carbamazepine toxicity in four epileptic children. *Ther Drug Monit* 1983; 5:405–407.
88. von Rosensteil NA, Adam D. Macrolide antibacterials. Drug interactions of clinical significance. *Drug Saf* 1995; 13:105–122.
89. Yasui N, Otani K, Kaneko S, et al. Carbamazepine toxicity induced by clarithromycin coadministration in psychiatric patients. *Int Clin Psychopharmacol* 1997; 12: 225–229.

90. Nemeroff CB, DeVane CL, Pollock BG. Newer antidepressants and the cytochrome P450 system. *Am J Psychiatry* 1996; 153:311–320.
91. Hansen BS, Dam M, Brandt J, et al. Influence of dextropropoxyphene on steady state levels and protein binding of three anti-epileptic drugs in man. *Acta Neurol Scand* 1980; 61:357–367.
92. Bourgeois BFD, Dodson WE, Ferrenedelli JA. Interaction between primidone, carbamazepine and nicotinamide. *Neurology* 1982; 32:1122–1126.
93. Krag B, Dam M, Angelo H, Christensen JM. Influence of disulfiram on the serum concentraion of carbamazepine in patients with epilepsy. *Acta Neurol Scand* 1981; 63:395–398.
94. Sonne J, Luhdorf K, Larsen NE, Andreasen PB. Lack of interaction between cimetidene and carbamazepine. *Acta Neurol Scand* 1983, 68:253–256.
95. Nakasa H, Nakamura H, Ono S, et al. Prediction of drug-drug interactions of zonisamide metabolism in humans from in vitro data. *Eur J Clin Pharmacol* 1998; 54:177–183.
96. Bertilsson L, Tybring G, Widen J, et al. Carbamazepine treatment induces the CYP3A4 catalyzed sulphoxidation of omeprazole, but has no or less effect on hydroxylation via CYP2C19. *Br J Clin Pharmacol* 1997; 44:186–189.
97. Warren JW, Benmaman JD, Wannamaker BB, Levy RH. Kinetics of a carbamazepine-ethosuximide interaction. *Clin Pharmacol Ther* 1980; 28:646–651.
98. Bowdle TA, Levy RH, Cutler RE. Effects of carbamazepine on valproic acid kinetics in normal subjects. *Clin Pharmacol Ther* 1979; 26:629–634.
99. Dodson WE. The nonlinear kinetics of phenytoin in children. *Neurology* 1982; 32:42–48.
100. Pippenger CE. Clinically significant carbamazepine drug interactions: an overview. *Epilepsia* 1987; 28 Suppl 3:S71–S76.
101. Collaborative Group for Edidemiology of Epilepsy. Adverse reacion to atniepileptic drugs: a follow-up study of 355 patients with chronic antiepileptic drug treatment. *Epilepsia* 1988; 29:787–793.
102. Herranz JL, Armijo JA, Arteaga R. Clinical side effects of phenobarbital, primidone, phenytoin, carbamazepine, and valproate during monotherapy in children. *Epilepsia* 1988; 29:794–804.
103. Wallace SJ. A comparative review of the adverse effects of anticonvulsants in children with epilepsy. *Drug Saf* 1996; 15:378–393.
104. Andersen EB, Philbert A, Klee JG. Carbamazepine monotherapy in epileptic outpatients. *Acta Neurol Scand Suppl* 1983; 67:29–34.
105. Delcker A, Wilhelm H, Timmann D, Diener HC. Side effects from increased doses of carbamazepine on neuropsychological and posturographic parameters of humans. *Eur Neuropsychopharmacol* 1997; 7:213–218.
106. Keranen T, Silvenius J. Side effects of carbamazepine, valproate and clonazepam during long-term treatment of epilepsy. *Acta Neurol Scand* 1983; 97 Suppl:69–80.
107. Hoppener RJ, Kuyer A, Meijer JW, Hulsman J. Correlation between daily fluctuations of carbamazepine serum levels and intermittent side effects. *Epilepsia* 1980; 21: 341–350.
108. Dulac O, Bouguerra L, Rey E, et al. Monotherapie par la carbamazepine dans les epilepsies de l'enfant. *Arch Fr Pediatr* 1983; 40:415–419.
109. Sullivan JB, Rumack BH, Peterson RG. Acute carbamazepine toxicity resulting from overdose. *Neurology* 1981; 31:621–624.
110. Fisher R-S, Cysyk B. A fatal overdose of carbamazepine: case report and review of literature. *J Toxicol Clin Toxicol* 1988; 26:477–486.
111. Aldenkamp AP, Vermeulen J. Phenytoin and carbamazepine: differential effects on cognitive function. *Seizure* 1995; 4:95–104.
112. Sabers A, Moller A, Dam M, et al. Cognitive function and anticonvulsant therapy: effect of monotherapy in epilepsy. *Acta Neurol Scand* 1995; 92:19–27.
113. Koivikko MJ, Valikangas SL. Hyponatremia during carbamazepine therapy in children. *Neuropediatrics* 1983; 14:93–96.
114. Rado JP, Juhos E, Sawinsky I. Dose-response relations in drug-induced inappropriate secretion of ADH: effects of clofibrate and carbamazepine. *Int J Clin Pharmacol* 1975; 12:315–319.
115. Kalff R, Houtkooper MA, Meyer JW, et al. Carbamazepine and serum sodium levels. *Epilepsia* 1984; 25:390–397.
116. Borusiak P, Korn-Merker E, Holert N, Boenigk HE. Hyponatremia induced by oxcarbazepine in children. *Epilepsy Res* 1998; 30:241–246.
117. Perucca E, Richens A. Water intoxication produced by carbamazepine and its reversal by phenytoin. *Br J Clin Pharmacol* 1980; 9:302–304.
118. Tjellesen L, Gotfredsen A, Christiansen C. Effect of vitamin D2 and D3 on bone-mineral content in carbamazepine-treated epileptic patients. *Acta Neurol Scand* 1983; 68:424–428.
119. Tjellesen L, Nilas L, Christiansen C. Does carbamazepine cause disturbances in calcium metabolism in epileptic patients? *Acta Neurol Scand* 1983; 68:13–19.
120. Wolschendorf K, Vanselow K, Moller WD, Schulz H. A quantitative determination of anticonvulsant-induced bone demineralization by an improved X-ray densitometry technique. *Neuroradiology* 1983; 25:315–318.
121. Lundstrom A, Eeg-Olofsson O, Hamp SE. Effects of antiepileptic drug treatment with carbamazepine or phenytoin on the oral state of children and adolescents. *J Clin Periodontol* 1982; 9:482–488.
122. Bentsen KD, Gram L, Veje A. Serum thyroid hormones and blood folic acid during monotherapy with carbamazepine or valproate. A controlled study. *Acta Neurol Scand* 1983; 67:235–241.
123. Deisenhammer E, Schwarzbach H, Sommer R. Erhohung der gamma-GT bei anticonvulsiver theapie. *Wien Klin Whenschr* 1982; 92:584–585.
124. Silverstein FS, Parrish MA, Johnston MV. Adverse behavioral reactions in children treated with carbamazepine (Tegretol). *J Pediatr* 1982; 101:785–787.
125. Ambrosetti G, Riva R. Hyperammonemia in asterixis induced by carbamazepine: two case reports. *Acta Neurol Scand* 1984; 69:186–189.
126. Bimping-Bita K, Froscher W. Carbamazepine-induced choreoathetoid dyskinesia. *J Neurol Neurosurg Psychiatry* 1982; 45:560.
127. Neglia JP, Glaze DG, Zion TE. Tics and vocalizations in children treated with carbamazepine. *Pediatrics* 1984; 73:841–844.
128. Crosley CJ, Swender PT. Dystonia associated with carbamazepine administration: experience in brain-damaged children. Pediatrics 1979; 63:612–615.
129. Stremski ES, Brady WB, Prasad K, Hennes HA. Pediatric carbamazepine intoxication. *Ann Emerg Med* 1995; 25:624–630.
130. Specht U, May TW, Rohde M, et al. Cerebellar atrophy decreases the threshold of carbamazepine toxicity in patients with chronic focal epilepsy. *Arch Neurol* 1997; 54:427–431.
131. Silverstein FS, Parrish MA, Johnston MV. Adverse reactions to carbamazepine (Tegretol) in children with epilepsy. *Ann Neurol* 1982; 12:198–199.
132. Holmes GL. Carbamazepine: toxicity. In Levy RH, Mattson RH, Meldrum BS, eds. *Antiepileptic Drugs*. 4th ed. New York: Raven Press, 1995:567–579.
133. Mattson RH. Carbamazepine. In: J Engel Jr, Pedley T, eds. *Epilepsy: A Comprehensive Textbook*. Philadelphia, PA: Lippincott-Raven, 1997:1491–1502.
134. Luchins DJ. Fatal agranulocytosis in a chronic schizophrenic patient treated with carbamazepine. *Am J Psychiatry* 1984; 141:687–688.
135. Ponte CD. Carbamazepine-induced thrombocytopenia, rash, and hepatic dysfunction. *Drug Intelligence & Clinical Pharmacy* 1983; 17:642–644.
136. Hart RG, Easton JD. Carbamazepine and hematological monitoring. *Ann Neurol* 1981; 11:309–312.
137. Tohen M, Castillo J, Baldessarini RJ, Zarate C Jr, et al. Blood dyscrasias with carbamazepine and valproate: a pharmacoepidemiological study of 2,228 patients at risk. *Am J Psychiatry* 1995; 152:413–418.
138. Silverstein FS, Boxer L, Johnston MV. Hematological monitoring during therapy with carbamazepine in children. *Ann Neurol* 1983; 13:685–686.
139. Morkunas AR, Miller MB. Anticonvulsant hypersensitivity syndrome. *Crit Care Clin* 1997; 13:727–739.
140. Wolkenstein P, Tan C, Lecoeur S, Wechsler J, et al. Covalent binding of carbamazepine reactive metabolites to P450 isoforms present in the skin. *Chem Biol Interact* 1998; 113:39–50.
141. Tennis P, Stern RS. Risk of serious cutaneous disorders after initiation of use of phenytoin, carbamazepine, or sodium valproate: a record linkage study. *Neurology* 1997; 49:542–546.
142. Roujeau JC, Kelly JP, Naldi L, et al. Medication use and the risk of Stevens-Johnson syndrome or toxic epidermal necrolysis. *N Engl J Med* 1995; 333:1600–1607.
143. Jarrett P, Rademaker M, Havill J, Pullon H. Toxic epidermal necrolysis treated with cyclosporin and granulocyte colony stimulating factor. *Clin Exp Dermatol* 1997; 22:146–147.
144. Mauri-Hellweg D, Bettens F, Mauri D, et al. Activation of drug-specific CD4+ and CD8+ T cells in individuals allergic to sulfonamides, phenytoin, and carbamazepine. *J Immunol* 1995; 155:462–472.
145. Schlienger RG, Shear NH. Antiepileptic drug hypersensitivity syndrome. *Epilepsia* 1998; 39 Suppl 7:S3–S7.
146. De Vriese AS, Philippe J, Van Renterghem DM, et al. Carbamazepine hypersensitivity syndrome: report of 4 cases and review of the literature. *Medicine* 1995; 74:144–151.
147. Hyson C, Sadler M. Cross sensitivity of skin rashes with antiepileptic drugs. *Can J Neurol Sci* 1997; 24:245–249.
148. Hogg RJ, Sawyer M, Hecox K, Eigenbrodt E. Carbamazepine-induced acute tubulointersitial nephritis. *J Pediatr* 1981; 98:830–832.
149. Stewart CR, Vengrow MI, Riley TL. Double quotidian fever caused by carbamazepine. *N Engl J Med* 1980; 302:1262–1264.
150. Eijgenraam JW, Buurke EJ, van der Laan JS. Carbamazepine-associated acute tubulointerstitial nephritis. *Neth J Med* 1997; 50:25–28.
151. Gram L, Bentsen KD. Hepatic toxicity of antiepileptic drugs: a review. *Acta Neurol Scand Suppl* 1982; 97:81–90.
152. Mitchell MC, Boitnott, JK, Arregui A, Maddrey WC. Granulomatous hepatitis assoicated with carbamazepine therapy. *Am J Med* 1981; 71:733–735.
153. Levy M, Goodamn MW, Van Dyne BJ, Sumner HW. Granulomatous hepatitis secondary to carbamazepine. *Ann Inter Med* 1981; 95:64–65.
154. Soffer EE, Taylor RJ, Bertram PD, et al. Carbamazepine-induced liver injury. *South Med J* 1983; 76:681–683.
155. Berkowitz FE, Henderson SL, Fajman N, et al. Acute liver failure caused by isoniazid in a child receiving carbamazepine. *Int J Tuberc Lung Dis* 1998; 2:603–606.
156. Hopen G, Nesthus I, Laerum OD. Fatal carbamazepine-associated hepatitis. Report of two cases. *Acta Med Scand* 1981; 210:333–335.
157. Zucker P, Daum F, Cohen MI. Fatal carbamazepine hepatitis. *J Pediatr* 1977; 91:667.
158. Sachdeo R, Sathyan RR. Amelioration of erectile dysfunction following a switch from carbamazepine to oxcarbazepine: recent clinical experience. *Curr Med Res Opin* 2005; 21:1065–1068.
159. Toepfer M, Sitter T, Lochmuller H, Pongratz D, et al. Drug-induced systemic lupus erythematosus after 8 years of treatment with carbamazepine. *Eur J Clin Pharmacol* 1998; 54:193–194.
160. Nathan DL, Belsito DV. Carbamazepine-induced pseudolymphoma with CD-30 positive cells. *J Am Acad Dermatol* 1998; 38:806–809.
161. Milesi-Lecat AM, Schmidt J, Aumaitre O, et al. Lupus and pulmonary nodules consistent with bronchiolitis obliterans organizing pneumonia induced by carbamazepine. *Mayo Clin Proc* 1997; 72:1145–1147.

162. Yeo W, Chow J, Wong N, et al. Carbamazepine-induced lymphadenopathy mimicking Ki-1 (CD30+) T-cell lymphoma. *Pathology* 1997; 29:64–66.
163. Cereghino JJ, Brock JT, Van Meter JC, et al. The efficacy of carbamazepine combinations in epilepsy. *Clin Pharmacol Ther* 1975; 18:733–741.
164. Lesser RP, Pippenger CE, Luders H, Dinner DS. High dose monotherapy in treatment of intractable seizures. *Neurology* 1984; 34:707–711.
165. Callaghan N, ODwyer R, Keating J. Unnecessary polypharmacy in patients with frequent seizures. *Acta Neurol Scand* 1984, 69:15–19.
166. Schmidt D. Reduction of two drug therapy in intractable epilepsy. *Epilepsia* 1983; 24:368–376.
167. Bennett HS, Dunlop T, Ziring P. Reduction of polypharmacy for epilepsy in an institution for the retarded. *Dev Med Child Neurol* 1983; 25:735–737.
168. Pina-Garza JE, Espinoza R, Nordli D, et al. Oxcarbazepine adjunctive therapy in infants and young children with partial seizures. *Neurology* 2005; 65:1370–1375.
169. Schmidt D, Elger CE. [How is oxcarbazepine different from carbamazpine?]. *Nervenarzt* 2004; 75:153–160.
170. Glauser T, Ben-Menachem E, Bourgeois B, et al. ILAE treatment guidelines: evidence-based analysis of antiepileptic drug efficacy and effectiveness as initial monotherapy for epileptic seizures and syndromes. *Epilepsia* 2006; 47:1094–1120.
171. Sallas WM, Milosavljev S, D'souza J, Hossain M. Pharmacokinetic drug interactions in children taking oxcarbazepine. *Clin Pharmacol Ther* 2003; 74:138–149.
172. McAuley JW, Anderson GD. Treatment of epilepsy in women of reproductive age: pharmacokinetic considerations. *Clin Pharmacokinet* 2002; 41:559–579.
173. Kalis MM, Huff NA. Oxcarbazepine, an antiepileptic agent. Clin Ther 2001; 23: 680–700.
174. Davanzo P, Nikore V, Yehya N, Stevenson L. Oxcarbazepine treatment of juvenile-onset bipolar disorder. *J Child Adolesc Psychopharmacol* 2004; 14:344–345.
175. MacMillan CM, Korndorfer SR, Rao S, et al. A comparison of divalproex and oxcarbazepine in aggressive youth with bipolar disorder. *J Psychiatr Pract* 2006; 12:214–222.
176. Wagner KD, Kowatch RA, Emslie GJ, et al. A double-blind, randomized, placebo-controlled trial of oxcarbazepine in the treatment of bipolar disorder in children and adolescents. *Am J Psychiatry* 2006; 163:1179–1186.
177. Luszczki JJ, Czuczwar SJ. Preclinical profile of combinations of some second-generation antiepileptic drugs: an isobolographic analysis. *Epilepsia* 2004; 45:895–907.
178. May TW, Korn-Merker E, Rambeck B. Clinical pharmacokinetics of oxcarbazepine. *Clin Pharmacokinet* 2003; 42:1023–1042.
179. Northam RS, Hernandez AW. Litzinger MJ, et al. Oxcarbazepine in infants and young children with partial seizures. *Pediatr Neurol* 2005; 33:337–344.
180. Bang LM, Goa KL. Spotlight on oxcarbazepine in epilepsy. *CNS Drugs* 2004; 18: 57–61.
181. Hooper WD, Dickinson RG, Dunstan PR, et al. Oxcarbazepine: preliminary clinical and pharmacokinetic studies on a new anticonvulsant. *Clin Exp Neurol* 1987; 24: 105–112.
182. Dickinson RG, Hooper WD, Dunstan PR, Eadie MJ. First dose and steady-state pharmacokinetics of oxcarbazepine and its 10-hydroxy metabolite. *Eur J Clin Pharmacol* 1989; 37:69–74.
183. Perucca E. Pharmacokinetic variability of new antiepileptic drugs at different ages. *Ther Drug Monit* 2005; 27:714–717.
184. Rey E, Bulteau C, Motte J, et al. Oxcarbazepine pharmacokinetics and tolerability in children with inadequately controlled epilepsy. *J Clin Pharmacol* 2004; 44: 1290–1300.
185. Volosov A, Xiaodong S, Perucca E, et al. Enantioselective pharmacokinetics of 10-hydroxycarbazepine after oral administration of oxcarbazepine to healthy Chinese subjects. *Clin Pharmacol Ther* 1999; 66:547–553.
186. Volosov A, Yagen B, Bialer M. Comparative stereoselective pharmacokinetic analysis of 10-hydroxycarbazepine after oral administration of its individual enantiomers and the racemic mixture to dogs. *Epilepsia* 2000; 41:1107–1111.
187. Johannes Donati F, Gobbi G, Campistol J, et al. Oxcarbazepine Cognitive Study Group. Effects of oxcarbazepine on cognitive function in children and adolescents with partial seizures. *Neurology* 2006; 67:679–682.
188. Kristensen O, Klitgaard NA, Jonsson B, Sindrup S. Pharmacokinetics of 10-OH-carbazepine, the main metabolite of the antiepileptic oxcarbazepine, from serum and saliva concentrations. *Acta Neurol Scand* 1983; 68:145–150.
189. Miles MV, Tang PH, Ryan MA, et al. Feasibility and limitations of oxcarbazepine monitoring using salivary monohydroxycarbamazepine (MHD). *Ther Drug Monit* 2004; 26:300–304.
190. Pennell PB. Antiepileptic drug pharmacokinetics during pregnancy and lactation. *Neurology* 2003; 61 6 Suppl 2:S35–S42.
191. Tomson T. Gender aspects of pharmacokinetics of new and old AEDs: pregnancy and breast-feeding. *Ther Drug Monit* 2005; 27:718–721.
192. EURAP Study Group. Seizure control and treatment in pregnancy: observations from the EURAP epilepsy pregnancy registry. *Neurology* 2006; 66:354–360.
193. Beydoun A. Monotherapy trials of new antiepileptic drugs. *Epilepsia* 1997; 38 Suppl 9: S21–S31.
194. Albani F, Grassi B, Ferrara R, et al. PRIMO Study Group. Immediate (overnight) switching from carbamazepine to oxcarbazepine monotherapy is equivalent to a progressive switch. *Seizure* 2004; 13:254–263.
195. Guerreiro MM, Vigonius U, Pohlmann H, et al. A double-blind controlled clinical trial of oxcarbazepine versus phenytoin in children and adolescents with epilepsy. *Epilepsy Res* 1997; 27:205–213.
196. Novartis. Trileptal Prescribing Information. http://www.pharma.us.novartis.com/product/pi/pdf/trileptal.pdf. (accessed September 2007).
197. Theis JG, Sidhu J, Palmer J, et al. Lack of pharmacokinetic interaction between oxcarbazepine and lamotrigine. *Neuropsychopharmacology* 2005; 30:2269–2274.
198. Fattore C, Cipolla G, Gatti G, Limido GL, et al. Induction of ethinylestradiol and levonorgestrel metabolism by oxcarbazepine in healthy women. *Epilepsia* 1999; 40:783–787.
199. Elwes RD, Binnie CD. Clinical pharmacokinetics of newer antiepileptic drugs. Lamotrigine, vigabatrin, gabapentin and oxcarbazepine. *Clin Pharmacokinet* 1996; 30:403–415.
200. Donati F, Gobbi G, Campistol J, et al. Oxcarbazepine Cognitive Study Group. Effects of oxcarbazepine on cognitive function in children and adolescents with partial seizures. *Neurology* 2006; 67:679–682.
201. Chapman K, Holland K, Erenberg G. Seizure exacerbation associated with oxcarbazepine in idiopathic focal epilepsy of childhood. *Neurology* 2003; 61:1012–1013.
202. Grosso S, Balestri M, Di Bartolo RM, et al. Oxcarbazepine and atypical evolution of benign idiopathic focal epilepsy of childhood. *Eur J Neurol* 2006; 13:1142–1145.
203. Gelisse P, Genton P, Kuate C, et al. Worsening of seizures by oxcarbazepine in juvenile idiopathic generalized epilepsies. *Epilepsia* 2004; 45:1282–1286.
204. Dam M, Ekberg R, Lyning Y, et al. A double-blind study comparing oxcarbazepine and carbamazepine in patients with newly diagnosed, previously untreated epilepsy. *Epilepsy Res* 1989; 3:70–76.
205. Editorial. Oxcarbazepine. *Lancet* 1989; 2:196–198.
206. Nielsen OA, Johannessen AC, Bardrum B. Oxcarbazepine-induced hyponatremia, a cross-sectional study. *Epilepsy Res* 1988; 2:269–271.
207. Pendlebury SC, Moses DK, Eadie MJ. Hyponatraemia during oxcarbazepine therapy. *Hum Toxicol* 1989; 8:337–344.
208. Glauser TA. Oxcarbazepine in the treatment of epilepsy. *Pharmacotherapy* 2001; 21:904–919.
209. Beydoun A, Sachdeo RC, Kutluay E, et al. Sustained efficacy and long-term safety of oxcarbazepine: one-year open-label extension of a study in refractory partial epilepsy. *Epilepsia* 2003; 44:1160–1165.
210. Bourgeois BF, D'Souza J. Long-term safety and tolerability of oxcarbazepine in children: a review of clinical experience. *Epilepsy Behav* 2005; 7:375–382.
211. Mintzer S, Boppana P, Toguri J, DeSantis A. Vitamin D levels and bone turnover in epilepsy patients taking carbamazepine or oxcarbazepine. *Epilepsia* 2006; 47(3):510–515.
212. Rattya J, Vainionpaa L, Knip M, et al. The effects of valproate, carbamazepine, and oxcarbazepine on growth and sexual maturation in girls with epilepsy. *Pediatrics* 1999; 103:588–593.
213. Levy RH, Wurden CJ. Carbamazepine: interactions with other drugs. In: Levy RH, Mattson RH, Meldrum BS, eds. *Antiepileptic Drugs*. 4th ed. New York: Raven Press, 1995:543–551.

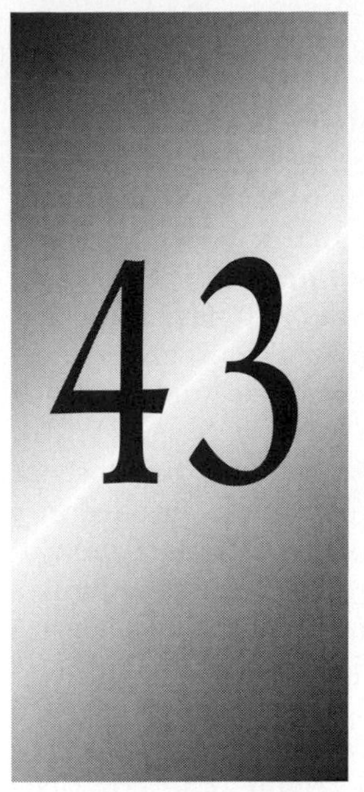

43 Ethosuximide, Methsuximide, and Trimethadione

Blaise F. D. Bourgeois

ETHOSUXIMIDE

Chemistry, Animal Pharmacology, and Mechanism of Action

Ethosuximide (ESM) is 2-ethyl-2-methyl succinimide, a white crystalline powder with a molecular weight of 141.7. The conversion factor from milligrams (mg) to micromoles (μmol) is 7.08 (i.e., 1 mg/L = 7.08 μmol/ L). In animal models, ESM is highly effective against pentylenetetrazol-induced seizures and other models considered to reflect efficacy against absence seizures, including genetically epilepsy-prone rodents, but ESM is ineffective against seizures induced by maximal electroshock, bicuculline, and N-methyl-D-aspartate (1). In view of ESM's narrow clinical spectrum mostly against absence seizures, this selective activity in experimental models has been considered to be a typical example of parallelism between clinical and experimental spectra of activity.

No single unifying mechanism of action of ethosuximide has been identified. The prevailing hypothesis is that thalamic low-threshold T-calcium channels (T for "transient" or "tiny" channels) are involved. It has been demonstrated that ethosuximide, at therapeutic concentrations, can either reduce the number or reduce the conductance of these channels (1–3). However, other studies in thalamocortical neurons of rats revealed an inhibitory effect of ethosuximide on so-called noninactivating sodium currents and on calcium-dependent potassium channels, but not on low-threshold calcium channels (4).

Biotransformation, Pharmacokinetics, and Interactions

Biotransformation. Ethosuximide is mostly metabolized by the liver, with only about 20% being excreted unchanged by the kidneys during chronic intake. The main metabolic pathway consists of hydroxylation and then glucuronidation of the metabolites (5–7). The principal cytochrome P450 oxidase involved is CYP3A. No active metabolites have been identified.

Pharmacokinetics. The bioavailability of ethosuximide is considered to be complete, and was shown to be equivalent for capsules and syrup (6). Peak levels are reached 3–5 hours after intake, slightly faster with the syrup than with the capsules. The apparent volume of distribution of ethosuximide is about 0.7 L/kg throughout age ranges. Because of lack of binding to plasma proteins, concentrations of ethosuximide in the cerebrospinal fluid (CSF), tears, and saliva are similar to the plasma concentration, and those in breast milk are only 10% to 20% lower (6, 8). Serum ethosuximide concentrations in breast-fed infants amount to about 30% to 50% of the levels of their mothers (8).

The elimination half-life of ethosuximide was found to be 40 to 60 hours in adults and 30 to 40 hours in children, with linear kinetics and no evidence of autoinduction (6) (Table 43-1). Accordingly, steady-state levels are reached after 7 to 10 days of daily intake of a stable dose. As with most antiepileptic drugs, the level-to-dose ratio may decrease during pregnancy (8).

Interactions. Enzyme-inducing drugs such as phenytoin, phenobarbital, and carbamazepine can increase the clearance and thus decrease the level-to-dose ratio of ethosuximide (9, 10). Inversely, valproate can inhibit the metabolism of ethosuximide and, at times, significantly raise its plasma level (11). Isoniazid can significantly raise the levels of ethosuximide (12), whereas rifampin may cause a significant decrease in ethosuximide levels (13). Ethosuximide is not known to affect the clearance or levels of any other drug. In particular, there is no known interaction between ethosuximide and oral contraceptives.

Clinical Efficacy

Absence Seizures. Ethosuximide has been used clinically since 1958, mostly as a drug of first choice for typical absence seizures, in particular childhood absence epilepsy (14–16). Other seizure types that may be favorably influenced by ethosuximide include atypical absence and myoclonic seizures, as well as drop attacks.

TABLE 43-1
Clinical Summary of Ethosuximide

Elimination half-life (hours)	
Adults	40–60
Children	30–40
Time to steady-state level (days)	7–10
Suggested therapeutic range (mg/L)	40–100
Initial dose	
Adults (mg/day)	250
Children (mg/kg/day)	5–10
Target dose	
Adults (mg/day)	750–1,000
Children (mg/kg/day)	20–30
Common preparations	250 mg capsules 250 mg/mL syrup
Adverse effects	Gastrointestinal upset, vomiting, hiccups, headache, fatigue, ataxia, depression, psychosis, rare bone marrow depression

In the treatment of typical absence seizures, ethosuximide was shown to achieve a seizure reduction of at least 90% in one-half of the patients, and a reduction of the seizure frequency by at least 50% in 95% of patients (14–16). It appears that response rates improved as more patients achieved levels greater than 40 mg/L. The efficacy of ethosuximide and valproate against absence seizures has been compared in at least two studies, which revealed no difference between the two drugs (17, 18). Sixteen patients not previously treated for absence seizures and 29 refractory patients were enrolled in a double-blind cross-over study of ethosuximide and valproate (18). Frequency and duration of generalized spike-wave bursts on electroencephalographic (EEG) telemetry was used as the measure of efficacy. Ethosuximide and valproate were equally effective in previously untreated patients. No difference in efficacy against absence seizures between valproate, lamotrigine, and ethosuximide could be demonstrated in a recent review of the available evidence (19). This lack of difference could be explained by the methodological quality or statistical power of the studies. Reported evidence suggests that, when ethosuximide and valproate alone are ineffective in fully controlling absence seizures, the combination of the two may be effective (20). This observation is in agreement with experimental evidence from studies in mice that revealed a beneficial pharmacodynamic interaction between ethosuximide and valproate (21). The therapeutic effects of this combination was additive, whereas toxic effects were less than additive, and this resulted in a favorable therapeutic ratio.

Absence status and atypical absence seizures may also respond favorably to high concentrations of ethosuximide, although both are generally less responsive to treatment than typical absence seizures (16).

Other Uses of Ethosuximide in the Treatment of Seizures

Myoclonic seizures associated with various epileptic syndromes, such as Lennox-Gastaut syndrome, severe myoclonic epilepsy of infancy, juvenile myoclonic epilepsy, and myoclonic astatic epilepsy, may also at times respond to ethosuximide (16, 22, 23). A favorable response has been reported with both positive and negative myoclonus (24). Ethosuximide has a role as adjunctive treatment in the management of the Lennox-Gastaut syndrome. In addition to its contribution to a reduction in the atypical absences and the myoclonic seizures, it can be helpful in reducing the frequency of the debilitating drop attacks (25). Two patients with Angelman syndrome and atypical absence seizures that were refractory to valproate had an excellent response to the addition of ethosuximide when levels greater than 100 mg/L were achieved (26).

Adverse Effects

Gastrointestinal Adverse Effects. Benign and fully reversible gastrointestinal side effects are by far the most common adverse reactions to ethosuximide (27). They include mostly abdominal discomfort, vomiting, diarrhea, and hiccups. Some of these effects can improve when the medication is taken at the end of a meal.

Neurologic Adverse Effects. The neurologic side effects of ethosuximide can include headaches, sedation, drowsiness, fatigue, insomnia, and ataxia. Rarely behavioral disturbances may occur, including nervousness, irritability, depression, hallucinations, and even psychosis (12, 28). Psychosis has been found to occur in conjunction with eradication of seizure acitivity, a phenomenon for which the term "forced normalization" has been coined (29). Occasionally, ethosuximide may also cause extrapyramidal reactions, such as dyskinesia (30, 31).

Idiosyncratic Adverse Effects. Ethosuximide has been associated with a dose-related reversible granulocytopenia (26), but very rarely also with more severe bone marrow reactions such as granulocytopenia, thrombocytopenia, or pancytopenia (32). Clinical alertness to possible signs and symptoms is likely to be more effective in recognizing such occurrences than routine monitoring of the blood count (33). Other reported rare idiosyncratic reactions have included systemic lupus erythmatosus (34, 35) and Stevens-Johnson syndrome.

Effect on Offspring. Although malformations have been described in infants whose mothers were treated with ethosuximide, this could not be attributed specifically to ethosuximide alone (8). Ethosuximide crosses the placenta readily. Levels in the milk and in the plasma of breast-fed infants have been discussed in the section on pharmacokinetics.

Clinical Use

The main indication of ethosuximide is in the treatment of childhood absence epilepsy, for which it is a drug of first choice. For this indication, ethosuximide is an effective drug, with mostly benign side effects and only extremely rare severe adverse reactions. However, it should be considered as initial monotherapy only in those children with childhood absence epilepsy who have never experienced a generalized tonic-clonic seizure, against which ethosuximide has no protective effect. Patients with childhood absence epilepsy are at risk for generalized tonic-clonic seizures, especially during the second decade of life. This is also true for patients with juvenile absence epilepsy. Therefore, when treatment of absence seizures is considered or reconsidered in patients older than the age of 10 years, a drug with the appropriate broader spectrum of activity should be used, such as valproate or lamotrigine, or ethosuximide should be combined with another drug that does provide protection against generalized tonic-clonic seizures.

Other clinical uses of ethosuximide have been discussed in the section on efficacy. In these conditions, such as absence status epilepticus, myoclonic seizures in various epilepsy syndromes, atypical absence seizures, and drop attacks in Lennox-Gastaut syndrome, ethosuximide is almost invariably used as adjunctive therapy, because these seizures are generally more refractory to medications and because they tend to occur in conjunction with other seizure types that do not benefit from ethosuximide.

The initial target dose of ethosuximide is about 20–30 mg/kg/day. It is best to initiate treatment at one-third of this dose, preferably after meals, with two subsequent increases by the same amount at intervals of 5–7 days. Available ethosuximide preparations include 250-mg liquid-filled capsules and 250 mg/5 mL syrup. If capsules are preferred, but the patient's weight requires increments of 125 mg, the capsules can be frozen and then easily cut in half. The total daily dose can be divided into two daily doses, or also into three daily doses if this makes it easier for the child to take the medication or if it can be shown to improve gastrointestinal side effects. In absence epilepsy, a response is often noted by parents or teachers within a few days, and provocation of seizures by forced hyperventilation also subsides. In addition, childhood absence epilepsy is one of the rare epilepsies in which a dramatic EEG improvement accompanies clinical improvement. Nevertheless, the EEG response may be incomplete, even if the observable clinical response is complete. Therefore, it is recommended to record an EEG after the patient has achieved full clinical control, and the goal of therapy should be normalization of the EEG, if possible (36). If there is doubt as the whether the patient is free of seizures, a 24-hour ambulatory EEG may be quite helpful.

The suggested therapeutic range of ethosuximide plasma levels is 40–100 mg/L (300–700 μmol/L), but levels below 40 may be fully effective, and levels as high as 150 may be necessary and well tolerated. There are no clear guidelines regarding the need to monitor blood counts for the rare occurrence of bone marrow suppression, and clinical education and observation is likely to provide the best probability of early detection. Once the patient is under good control, there is no need to monitor plasma levels routinely, unless there is a specific question that could be answered by a level. In seizure-free patients with normalized EEG, ethosuximide can be gradually tapered over about 6 weeks after 2 years without seizures, or possibly even after 1 year (37). Because seizure recurrence may be subtle clinically, or significant subclinical spike and wave discharges may require reintroduction of therapy, it is good practice to repeat an EEG 1–3 months after ethosuximide has been discontinued.

METHSUXIMIDE

Chemistry, Animal Pharmacology, and Mechanism of Action

Methsuximide is N,2-dimethyl-2-phenyl-succinimide and has a molecular weight of 203.23. The conversion factor from milligrams (mg) to micromoles (μmol) is 4.92 (i.e., 1 mg/L = 4.92 μmol/L). The efficacy of methsuximide in animal models and mechanisms of action are similar to those of ethosuximide, but the therapeutic index is slightly lower (38).

Biotransformation, Pharmacokinetics, and Interactions

In the liver, methsuximide is rapidly converted to the active metabolite N-desmethylmethsuximide (39), which is then further hydroxylated before renal elimination (40). Less than 1% of the methsuximide dose is excreted unchanged by the kidneys. Peak levels of N-desmethylmethsuximide are reached after 1 to 4 hours (41). The plasma half-life of methsuximide is only 1.0–2.6 hours, with no significant accumulation, whereas the elimination half-life of N-desmethylmethsuximide has been found to be 34–80 hours in adults and 16–45 hours in children (38, 41) (Table 43-2). In human plasma, N-desmethylmethsuximide is 45% to 60% protein bound (42). The suggested therapeutic range of N-desmethylmethsuximide is 10–40 mg/L.

In terms of pharmacokinetic interactions, phenytoin and phenobarbital can raise the levels of N-desmethylmethsuximide, and methsuximide can inversely also raise the levels of phenytoin and phenobarbital, including Phenobarbital-derived from primidone (43, 44). These interactions may be due to competition for enzyme binding. However, methsuximide may also act as an enzymatic inducer, because it can lower levels of carbamazepine (44, 45) and of lamotrigine (46, 47).

Clinical Efficacy

Methsuximide has been used clinically since 1956. In the treatment of absence seizures, published evidence suggests that methsuximide is less effective than ethosuximide, achieving seizure control in one-third or fewer of the patients (38, 48). However, in contrast to ethosuximide, methsuximide has been shown repeatedly to have a role as adjunctive therapy in the treatment of complex partial seizures, with responder rates (≥50% seizure reduction) of at least one-third and up to 80% (44, 48, 49).

TABLE 43-2
Clinical Summary of Methsuximide

Elimination half-life of N-desmethylmethsuximide (hours)	
Adults	34–80
Children	16–45
Time to steady-state level (days)	8–16
Suggested therapeutic range of N-desmethylmethsuximide (mg/L)	10–40
Initial dose	
Adults (mg/day)	300
Children (mg/kg/day)	5–10
Target dose	
Adults (mg/day)	600–1,200
Children (mg/kg/day)	10–30
Common preparations	150- and 300-mg capsules
Adverse effects	Gastrointestinal upset, vomiting, hiccups, drowsiness, depression

Some success with methsuximide has also been reported in children having astatic/myoclonic, tonic, and atypical absence seizures (45), as well as in the treatment of juvenile myoclonic epilepsy (50). Methsuximide has been recommended as a fourth line drug in a review on the treatment of Lennox-Gastaut syndrome (23).

Adverse Effects

Gastrointestinal and neurologic side effects of methsuximide are very similar to those of ethosuximide, but they tend to be more pronounced and less readily reversible without discontinuation of the drug (27). In addition, attacks of hepatic porphyria may be precipitated by methsuximide (51).

Clinical Use

The target dose of methsuximide is 10–30 mg/kg/day. In children, the drug is often introduced as 150 mg once daily after dinner, with weekly dosage increases by 150 mg/day up to the target dose. Because of the long half-life of N-desmethylmethsuximide, the medication can be taken twice daily. The recommended range for plasma levels of N-desmethylmethsuximide is 10–40 mg/L. When methsuximide is taken as adjunctive therapy, attention must be paid to the pharmacokinetic interactions described previously, and the dosages and levels of both methsuximide and the other antiepileptic medications may have to be followed and adjusted as necessary. This may help with the management of side effects, which could be caused also by changes in concentrations of other medications.

TRIMETHADIONE

Oxazolidinediones have a historic role as the first generation antiabsence drugs. They were essentially replaced by the mid-to-late 1960s by the succinimides because of the substantially improved safety and tolerability profile of the latter. The oxazolidinediones are covered here mainly for historic reasons and not for the purpose of recommending trimethadione as an alternative to ethosuximide.

Chemistry, Animal Pharmacology, and Mechanism of Action

Trimethadione is 3,5,5-trimethyl-1,3-oxazolidine-2, 4-dione and has a molecular weight of 143.15. The conversion factor from milligrams (mg) to micromoles (μmol) is 6.99 (i.e., 1 mg/L = 6.99 μmol/L). The main active metabolite, dimethadione (5,5-dimethyloxazolidine-2, 4-dione), has a molecular weight of 129.12. The conversion factor from milligrams (mg) to micromoles (μmol) is 7.75 (i.e., 1 mg/L = 7.75 μmol/L). Like ethosuximide and methsuximide, trimethadione is effective against pentylenetetrazole-induced seizures but not against maximal electroshock-induced seizures (52). In addition, like succinimides, dimethadione was shown to block calcium currents in thalamic neurons (53) and in spinal neurons (54).

Biotransformation, Pharmacokinetics, and Interactions

Trimethadione is almost entirely converted to dimethadione in the liver, and less than 5% of an oral dose of trimethadione is excreted unchanged by the kidneys (55). Dimethadione is excreted mostly unchanged by the kidneys. Protein binding of both trimethadione and dimethadione is low. The plasma half-life of trimethadione in healthy adults was found to be 11–16 hours, and the half-life of dimethadione is much longer, 6–13 days (56) (Table 43-3). Pharmacokinetic interactions with other antiepileptic drugs are not known.

Clinical Efficacy and Use

Trimethadione has been used clinically since 1945 and was the first drug with a specific effect against absence seizures (57). The spectrum of activity of trimethadione and dimethadione is narrow, with no clear evidence of efficacy other than against absence seizures, although their use has been suggested for the other seizure types in patients with Lennox-Gastaut syndrome (58). Best results in the treatment of absence seizures have been observed at levels of dimethadione between 470 and 1,200 mg/L (59–61). The starting dose of trimethadione is about 20 mg/kg/day, and the dose may be increased gradually at intervals of 2 weeks up to 60 mg/kg/day, if tolerated. It is usually given twice daily, although the half-life of dimethadione should allow once-daily intake.

TABLE 43-3
Clinical Summary of Trimethadione and Dimethadione

Elimination half-life of:	
Trimethadione	11–16 hours
Dimethadione	6–13 days
Time to dimethadione steady-state level (days)	20–30
Suggested therapeutic range of dimethadione (mg/L)	500–1,200
Initial dose (mg/kg/day)	20
Target dose (mg/kg/day)	60 (max 2,400)
Adverse effects	Day blindness (hemeralopia), photophobia, dermatitis, Stevens-Johnson syndrome, bone marrow depression, nephrotic syndrome, myasthenic syndrome, pronounced teratogenicity (fetal trimethadione syndrome)

Adverse Effect

Trimethadione has several side effects (56). They include the common side effects of many antiepileptic medications, such as fatigue, sedation, dizziness, ataxia, skin rash, and exfoliative dermatitis. Hemeralopia (day blindness) and photophobia can occur in one-third of patients. Other more specific adverse reactions include a nephrotic syndrome, bone marrow depression, systemic lupus erythematosus, and a myasthenic syndrome. Close monitoring of blood counts and kidney function are necessary. Above all, trimethadione is probably the most teratogenic antiepileptic drug (62, 63). The "fetal trimethadione syndrome" includes, among other features, intrauterine growth retardation, microcephaly, cardiac malformations, malformed ears, and mental retardation.

Less frequent fetal anomalies include genitourinary malformation, epicanthal folds, broad nasal bridge, and cleft palate. Some or all of the features are seen in the offspring of more than two-thirds of pregnant women taking the drug during pregnancy. It is extremely important to discuss this issue before and during treatment with methadiones with any female patient of childbearing potential or with her parents.

References

1. Holland KD, Ferrendelli JA. Succinimides: mechanisms of action. In: Levy RH, Mattson RH, Meldrum BS, Perucca E, eds. *Antiepileptic Drugs*. 5th ed. Philadelphia, PA: Lippincott Williams & Wilkins, 2002:639–645.
2. Coulter DA, Huguenard JR, Prince DA. Characterization of ethosuximide reduction of low-threshold calcium current in thalamic neurons. *Ann Neurol* 1989; 25:582–593.
3. Huguenard JR, Prince DA. Intrathalamic rhythmicity studied *in vitro:* nominal T-current modulation causes robust antioscillatory effects. *J Neurosci* 1994; 14:5485–5502.
4. Leresche N, Parri HR, Erdemli G, Guyon A, et al. On the action of the anti-absence drug ethosuximide in the rat and cat thalamus. *J Neurosci* 1998; 18:4842–4853.
5. Millership JS, Mifsud J, Collier PS. The metabolism of ethosuximide. *Eur J Drug Metab Pharmacokinet* 1993; 18:349–353.
6. Pisani F, Perucca E, Bialer M. Ethosuximide: Chemistry, biotransformation, pharmacokinetics, and drug interactions. In: Levy RH, Mattson RH, Meldrum BS, Perucca E, eds. *Antiepileptic Drugs*. 5th ed. Philadelphia, PA: Lippincott Williams & Wilkins, 2002:646–651.
7. Bachmann K, He Y, Sarver JG, Peng N. Characterization of the cytochrome P450 enzymes involved in the in vitro metabolism of ethosuximide by human hepatic microsomal enzymes. *Xenobiotica* 2003; 33(3):265–276.
8. Kuhnz W, Koch S, Jakob S, Hartmann A, et al. Ethosuximide in epileptic women during pregnancy and lactation. Placental transfer, serum concentrations in nursed infants and clinical status. *Br J Clin Pharmacol* 1984; 18:671–677.
9. Battino D, Costi C, Franceschetti S. Ethosuximide plasma concentrations: influence of age and associated concomitant therapy. *Clin Pharm* 1982; 7:176–180.
10. Giaccone M, Bartoli A, Gatti G, et al. Effect of enzyme inducing anticonvulsants on ethosuximide pharmacokinetics in epileptic patients. *Br J Clin Pharmacol* 1996; 41:575–579.
11. Mattson RH, Cramer SA. Valproic acid and ethosuximide interaction. *Ann Neurol* 1980; 7:583–584.
12. Van Wieringen A, Vrijlandt CM. Ethosuximide intoxication caused by interaction with isoniazid. *Neurology* 1983; 33:1227–1228.
13. Bachmann KA, Jauregui L. Use of single sample clearance estimates of cytochrome P450 substrates to characterize human hepatic CYP status *in vivo*. *Xenobiotica* 1993; 23:307–315.
14. Browne TR, Dreifuss FE, Dyken PR, Goode DJ, et al. Ethosuximide in the treatment of absence (petit mal) seizures. *Neurology* 1975; 25:515–524.
15. Penry JK, Porter RJ, Dreifuss FE. Simultaneous recording of absence seizures with video tape and electroencephalography: a study of 374 seizures in 48 patients. *Brain* 1975; 98:427–440.
16. Sherwin AL. Succinimides: Clinical efficacy and use in epilepsy. In: Levy RH, Mattson RH, Meldrum BS, Perucca E, eds. *Antiepileptic Drugs*. 5th ed. Philadelphia, PA: Lippincott Williams & Wilkins, 2002:652–657.
17. Callaghan N, O'Hare J, O'Driscoll D, O'Neill B, et al. Comparative study of ethosuximide and sodium valproate in the treatment of typical absence seizures (petit mal). *Dev Med Child Neurol* 1982; 24:830–836.
18. Sato S, White BG, Penry JK, et al. Valproic acid versus ethosuximide in the treatment of absence seizures. *Neurology* 1982; 32:157–163.
19. Posner EB, Mohamed K, Marson AG. Ethosuximide, sodium valproate or lamotrigine for absence seizures in children and adolescents. *Cochrane Database Syst Rev* 2005; 19(4): CD003032.
20. Rowan AJ, Meiser JW, De-Beer-Pawlikowski N. Valproate-ethosuximide combination therapy for refractory absence seizures. *Arch Neurol* 1983; 40:797–802.
21. Bourgeois BF. Combination of valproate and ethosuximide: antiepileptic and neurotoxic interactions. *J Pharmacol Exp Ther* 1988; 247:1128–1132.
22. Wallace SJ. Myoclonus and epilepsy in childhood: a review of treatment with valproate, ethosuximide, lamotrigine and zonisamide. *Epilepsy Res* 1998; 29:147–154.
23. Schmidt D, Bourgeois B. A risk-benefit assessment of therapies for Lennox-Gastaut syndrome. *Drug Saf* 2000; 22(6):467–477.
24. Capovilla G, Beccaria F, Veggiotti P, et al. Ethosuximide is effective in the treatment of epileptic negative myoclonus in childhood partial epilepsy. *J Child Neurol* 1999;14:395–400.
25. Snead OC, Horsey L. Treatment of epileptic falling spells with ethosuximide. *Brain Dev* 1987; 9:602–604.
26. Sugiura C, Ogura K, Ueno M, Toyoshima M, et al. High-dose ethosuximide for epilepsy in Angelman syndrome: implication of $GABA_A$ receptor subunit. *Neurology* 2001; 57:1518–1519.
27. Glauser TA. Succinimides: Adverse effects. In: Levy RH, Mattson RH, Meldrum BS, Perucca E, eds. *Antiepileptic Drugs*. 5th ed. Philadelphia, PA: Lippincott Williams & Wilkins, 2002:658–664.
28. Roger J, Grangeon H, Guey J, Lob H. Incidences psychiatriques et psychologiques du traitement par l'éthosuximide chez les épileptiques. *Encéphale* 1968; 5:407–438.
29. Wolf P. Acute behavioral symptomatology at disappearance of epileptiform EEG abnormality: a paradoxical or "forced" normalization. In: Smith DB, Treiman DM, Trimble MR, eds. *Neurobehavioral Problems in Epilepsy.* New York: Raven Press, 1991:127–142.
30. Ehyai A, Kilroy AW, Fenichel GM. Dyskinesia and akathisia induced by ethosuximide. *Am J Dis Child* 1978; 132:527–528.
31. Kirschberg GJ. Dyskinesia—an unusual reaction to ethosuximide. *Arch Neurol* 1975; 32:137–138.
32. Massey GV, Dunn NL, Heckel JL, Myer EC, et al. Aplastic anemia following therapy for absence seizures with ethosuximide. *Pediatr Neurol* 1994; 11:59–61.
33. Pellock JM, Willmore LJ. A rational guide to routine blood monitoring in patients receiving antiepileptic drugs. *Neurology* 1991; 41:961–964.
34. Takeda S, Koizumi F, Takazakura E. Ethosuximide-induced lupus-like syndrome with renal involvement. *Intern Med* 1996; 35:587–591.
35. Ansell BM. Drug-induced lupus erythematosus in a 9-year-old boy. *Lupus* 1993; 2:193–194.
36. Blomquist H, Zeiterund B. Evaluation of treatment in the typical absence seizures. *Acta Paediatr Scand* 1985; 74:409–415.
37. Amit R, Vitale S, Maytal S. How long to treat childhood absence epilepsy. *Clin Electroencephalogr* 1995; 20:163–165.
38. Browne TR. Succinimides: Methsuximide. In: Levy RH, Mattson RH, Meldrum BS, Perucca E, eds. *Antiepileptic Drugs*. 5th ed. Philadelphia, PA: Lippincott Williams & Wilkins, 2002:665–671.
39. Strong JM, Abe T, Gibbs EL, et al. Plasma levels of methsuximide and *N*-desmethylmethsuximide during methsuximide therapy. *Neurology* 1974; 24:250–255.
40. Horning MG. Metabolism of *N*,2-dimethyl-2-phenylsuccinimide (methsuximide) by epoxide-diol pathway in rat, guinea pig, and human. *Res Commun Chem Pathol Pharmacol* 1973; 6:565–578.
41. Miles MV, Tennison MB, Greenwood RS. Pharmacokinetics of *N*-desmethylmethsuximide in pediatric patients. *J Pediatr* 1989; 114:647–650.
42. Wad N, Bourgeois B, Krämer G. Serum protein binding of desmethyl methsuximide. *Clin Neuropharmacol* 1999; 22:239–240.
43. Rambeck B. Pharmacological interactions of methsuximide with phenobarbital and phenytoin in hospitalized epileptic patients. *Epilepsia* 1979; 20:147–156.
44. Browne TR, Feldman RG, Buchanan RA, et al. Methsuximide for complex partial seizures: efficacy, toxicity, clinical pharmacology, and drug interactions. *Neurology* 1983; 33:414–418.
45. Tennison MB, Greenwood RS, Miles MV. Methsuximide for intractable childhood seizures. *Pediatrics* 1991; 87:186–189.
46. May TW, Rambeck B, Jurgens U. Influence of oxcarbazepine and methsuximide on lamotrigine concentrations in epileptic patients with and without valproic acid comedication: results of a retrospective study. *Ther Drug Monit* 1999; 21:175–181.
47. Besag FM, Berry DJ, Pool F. Methsuximide lowers lamotrigine blood levels: a pharmacokinetic antiepileptic drug interaction. *Epilepsia* 2000; 41:624–627.
48. Livingston S, Pauli L. Celontin in the treatment of epilepsy. *Pediatrics* 1957; 19:614–617.
49. Wilder BJ, Buchanan RA. Methsuximide for refractory complex partial seizures. *Neurology* 1981; 31:741–744.
50. Hurst DL. The use of methsuximide for juvenile myoclonic epilepsy. *Ann Neurol* 1995; 38:517 (abstract).
51. Reynolds NC, Miska RM. Safety of anticonvulsants in hepatic porphyries. *Neurology* 1981; 31:480–484.
52. Goodman LS, Toman JEP, Swinyard EA. The anticonvulsant properties of tridione. *Am J Med* 1946; 1:213–228.
53. Coulter DA, Huguenard JR, Prince DA. Specific petit mal anticonvulsants reduce calcium currents in thalamic neurons. *Neurosci Lett* 1989; 98:74–78.
54. Gross RA, Kelly KM, Macdonald RL. Ethosuximide and dimethadione selectively reduce calcium currents in cultured sensory neurons by different mechanisms. *Neurology* 1989; 39:412 (abstract).
55. Butler TC. Quantitative studies of the demethylation of trimethadione (Tridione). *J Pharmacol Exp Ther* 1953; 108:11–17.
56. Pellock JM, Coulter DA. Oxazolidinedione. In: Levy RH, Mattson RH, Meldrum BS, eds. *Antiepileptic Drugs*. 4th ed. New York, Raven Press, 1995:689–694.
57. Lennox MG. The petit mal epilepsies: their treatment with tridione. *JAMA* 1945; 129:1069–1075.
58. Dreifuss FE. Pediatric epileptology: classification and management of seizures in the child. Boston: Wright PSG, 1983.
59. Booker HE. Trimethadione:relation of plasma concentration to seizure control. In: Woodbury DM, Penry JK, Pippenger CE, eds. *Antiepileptic Drugs*. 2nd ed. New York: Raven Press, 1982:697–699.
60. Chamberlin H, Waddell W, Butler T. A study of the product of demethylation of trimethadione in the control of petit mal epilepsy. *Neurology* 1965; 15:499–454.
61. Jensen B. Trimethadione in the serum of patients with petit mal. *Dan Med Bull* 1962; 1:213–228.
62. Nichols MM. Fetal anomalies following maternal trimethadione ingestion. *J Pediatr* 1973; 82:885–886.
63. Rosen RC, Lightner EW. Phenotypic malformations in association with maternal methadione therapy. *J Pediatr* 1978; 92:240–244.

44 Felbamate

Blaise F. D. Bourgeois

At the time of its release in North America in 1993, felbamate was the first new antiepileptic drug (AED) in 15 years. Several relatively unique features characterize the development and release of felbamate. The clinical trials of felbamate were innovative and unconventional. Felbamate was the first AED to undergo a double-blind trial in hospitalized patients withdrawn from AEDs for presurgical long-term monitoring. It was also the first AED submitted to double-blind monotherapy trials. Finally, the efficacy of felbamate was assessed in the first placebo-controlled trial conducted in children with the Lennox-Gastaut syndrome. After 1 year of very successful marketing as a drug with no serious toxicity, felbamate came very close to being completely withdrawn from the market because of several cases of severe bone marrow and liver toxicity, some of which were fatal. The main indication for felbamate at the present time is as a third or fourth drug in children with the Lennox-Gastaut syndrome and similar forms of epilepsy who failed to respond to other AEDs.

CHEMISTRY, ANIMAL PHARMACOLOGY, AND MECHANISM OF ACTION

Felbamate is 2-phenyl-1,3-propanediol dicarbamate. Like the minor tranquilizer meprobamate, felbamate is a dicarbamate. However, felbamate appears to have no sedative or tranquilizing properties at therapeutic levels. Felbamate was found to have a relatively wide spectrum of activity in experimental seizure models. It is effective against seizures produced by systemically administered chemical convulsants, such as pentylenetetrazole and bicuculline, but it is even more potent against seizures elicited by maximal electroshock (1). Felbamate was also shown to possess antiepileptic activity in kindling models (2) and in monkeys with epileptic foci created by injection of aluminum hydroxide (3). The neurotoxicity of felbamate has been found to be exceedingly low in animal models, which resulted in a very high protective index (efficacy-to-toxicity ratio) (1). In various animal species, repeated administration of felbamate suggested an excellent safety profile on various body systems, and no tolerance to the antiepileptic effect could be demonstrated after repeated administration in animals.

Several potential mechanisms of action for the antiepileptic effect of felbamate have been identified. Inhibition of glycine-enhanced N-methyl-D-aspartate (NMDA)-induced intracellular calcium currents was shown in mice (4). Findings regarding the effect of felbamate on the gamma-aminobutyric acid (GABA) receptor have been contradictory; both a lack of effect on ligand binding to the $GABA_A$ receptor (5) and potentiation of GABA responses at high felbamate concentrations (6) have been reported. In addition, inhibition of excitatory NMDA responses was demonstrated at high felbamate levels (6). Use-dependent inhibition of NMDA currents was also demonstrated at therapeutic concentrations of 50–300 μmol/L in rat hippocampal neurons (7). The blockade of the NMDA receptors by felbamate may selectively affect certain subunits (8). The available information suggests that felbamate has a dual action on excitatory and inhibitory brain mechanisms.

BIOTRANSFORMATION, PHARMACOKINETICS, AND INTERACTIONS

After a single dose of felbamate in humans, approximately 50% of the drug is excreted in the urine unmetabolized and unconjugated. Approximately 12% is excreted in the urine as *para*-hydroxyfelbamate and 2-hydroxyfelbamate, and most of the remainder of the dose is recovered in urine as unidentified polar metabolites, some of them being glucuronides or sulfate esters (9). Only 2-hydroxyfelbamate and a monocarbamate metabolite could be quantified in plasma during chronic therapy (10). The concentration of these metabolites is too low (approximately 10% of the felbamate concentration) to contribute to the clinical effect, even if they were pharmacologically active. Because of possible pharmacokinetic interactions, these values for the quantitative aspect of felbamate biotransformation may be different in patients taking enzyme-inducing AEDs concurrently with felbamate. In addition, evidence has been found in humans suggesting the formation of several other metabolites, including atropaldehyde (2-phenylpropenal), which is a potentially cytotoxic metabolite of felbamate (11, 12).

The pharmacokinetics of felbamate have been studied in adults (9,13–17) and in children (16). Based on the administration of ^{14}C-labeled felbamate in adults, an oral bioavailability of at least 90% was estimated (9). Linear absorption at least up to 1,200-mg doses was demonstrated in single-dose pharmacokinetic studies (13, 14). This linearity was also found during chronic administration at doses of 400 to 3,600 mg/day (16). The time to peak concentration is 2 to 6 hours. Felbamate binding to serum proteins is approximately 25% and is independent of the felbamate concentration (18). The elimination half-life of felbamate in adult volunteers not taking other medications ranged from 16 to 22 hours (15). The volume of distribution was calculated to be 0.76 L/kg in adults and 0.91 L/kg in children, and, as for most drugs, the clearance of felbamate was found to be higher in children (19). Brain concentrations of felbamate have been measured in humans and were found to correspond to 60% to 70% of concurrent plasma concentrations (10).

The potential pharmacokinetic interactions between felbamate and other AEDs have been studied quite extensively, and it has been found that felbamate is the cause as well as the object of several pharmacokinetic interactions. When felbamate is added to phenytoin monotherapy, phenytoin levels are raised in a dose-dependent manner (20). Felbamate at a dose of 1,200 mg/day raised phenytoin levels by an average of 24%, and phenytoin levels were raised by an additional 20% at a felbamate dose of 1,800 mg/day. The dose of phenytoin should be reduced by 20% or more when felbamate is added (21). The addition of felbamate also raises valproate levels, probably through an inhibition of the beta-oxidation pathway of valproate metabolism (22). Valproate levels were found to be increased by 28% at a felbamate dose of 1,200 mg/day and by 54% at a felbamate dose of 2,400 mg/day (18). Inversely, felbamate decreases carbamazepine levels by 20% to 25%; however, the level of the active metabolite of carbamazepine (carbamazepine-10,11-epoxide) was found to be raised by 57% after the addition of felbamate (23). A similar interaction was reported with clobazam, with a decrease in clobazam levels and an increase in N-desmethyl-clobazam in the presence of felbamate (24). In a group of healthy volunteers, felbamate increased the area under the phenobarbital plasma concentration-time curve by 22% (25), and an elevation of methsuximide levels by felbamate was also described (26). No conclusive data are available regarding the effect of felbamate on the levels of other AEDs. The clearance of warfarin was shown to be decreased by approximately 50% by the addition of felbamate (27), and felbamate may accelerate the metabolism of oral contraceptive steroids (28, 29).

Other AEDs also affect the elimination of felbamate. The apparent total body clearance of felbamate is doubled by phenytoin, a known potent enzyme inducer (30). This observation suggests that the felbamate dosage requirements are doubled by the concomitant administration of phenytoin, if the same steady-state serum concentration of felbamate is to be maintained. Carbamazepine also seems to increase the clearance of felbamate but only by about 40% (23). No clinically significant effect of valproate on the clearance or elimination half-life of felbamate was demonstrated (15). A recent observation suggests that gabapentin may decrease the clearance of felbamate by approximately one-third, with a corresponding 50% prolongation of the felbamate half-life (31). If confirmed, this would represent the only known pharmacokinetic interaction involving gabapentin. Significant pharmacokinetic interactions between felbamate and drugs other than AEDs have not been reported.

CLINICAL EFFICACY

Four pivotal double-blind controlled trials provided most of the available clinical antiepileptic efficacy data for felbamate: a placebo-controlled trial in patients withdrawn from AEDs for presurgical monitoring, two felbamate monotherapy trials comparing felbamate monotherapy with low dose valproate monotherapy, and a placebo-controlled trial in children with the Lennox-Gastaut syndrome. The so-called presurgical trial was a novel study design. At the end of a period of seizure monitoring with partial or complete withdrawal from their conventional AEDs, 64 adult patients with documented partial onset seizures were randomized to felbamate or placebo (32). In addition to their anticonvulsant regimen at the conclusion of the presurgical evaluation, the patients were either rapidly titrated to felbamate 3,600 mg/day over 3 days or they received placebo. The predetermined efficacy variable of the study was the time to the fourth seizure or completion of a total of 28 days with less than four seizures, with an initial 8-day inpatient period. At the end of the inpatient period, the dose of one AED was adjusted to the premonitoring dose. Thus, patients were discharged neither taking placebo alone nor taking placebo with only a low dose of anticonvulsant. Patients experiencing four seizures within 28 days were restarted on the full dose of the medications they were taking before monitoring. For patients receiving felbamate, the time to the fourth seizure was significantly longer than for those receiving placebo. Four seizures within 28 days occurred in 46% of the patients taking felbamate as opposed to 88% of the patients randomized to placebo. These results clearly established that felbamate has antiepileptic activity in humans with epilepsy, but they did not demonstrate the ability of felbamate to reduce seizure frequency over a longer period in outpatients not withdrawn from AEDs.

The monotherapy studies were designed to compare felbamate with low dose valproate (15 mg/kg/day) against partial seizures (33, 34). The design of these studies was also novel and unique. After felbamate, 3,600 mg/day, or low dose valproate were added in a double-blind parallel manner to the previously administered drug, this drug was withdrawn over 28 days. Because 50% of the patients were to be converted to 15 mg/kg/day of valproate alone, the predetermined endpoint and primary efficacy variable consisted of escape criteria (a predefined degree of seizure exacerbation). The number of patients meeting the escape criteria during the observation period of 112 days was significantly higher in the low dose valproate group than in the felbamate monotherapy group in both studies, showing that felbamate alone has unequivocal efficacy over a period of 112 days against focal onset seizures in adults. However, it is difficult to derive a quantitative assessment of the efficacy. These two studies do not represent a comparison between felbamate and valproate, which was used as a relatively safe placebo. One advantage of such monotherapy studies is that they provide an exclusive assessment of the side effects of the new drug being tested. Adverse experiences were mild to moderate, and their incidence was lower during the monotherapy portion of the trial. However, the monotherapy phase was after day 28. Most drugs cause more side effects during the first month of treatment; therefore, the lower incidence of side effects observed after day 28 may also be attributed to tolerance and not to the fact that the drug regimen had been reduced to monotherapy.

A double-blind, placebo-controlled, add-on study of felbamate was carried out in 73 patients with the Lennox-Gastaut syndrome (mean age, 13 years; range, 4–36 years) (35). An observation period of 56 days was preceded by a 14-day titration period. The previous AED doses remained unchanged, and felbamate was titrated to 45 mg/kg/day or a maximum of 3,600 mg/day. The total number of seizures during a 4-hour period of video-EEG recording, the total number of atonic seizures (drop attacks) as reported by the parents or guardians, and the global evaluations of the patients' quality of life were chosen as the primary efficacy variables. In terms of the total frequency of seizures, felbamate was significantly superior to placebo and was particularly effective in reducing drop attacks, the most debilitating seizure type in these patients. There was an inverse correlation between felbamate plasma levels and the daily number of drop attacks. Additionally, in patients receiving felbamate, the global evaluation scores were significantly higher than in those receiving placebo. When the total number of seizures during a 4-hour period of video-EEG recording was compared, no significant difference between felbamate and placebo was found. The most likely cause of this lack of difference is probably the high spontaneous day-to-day variability in seizure frequency in patients with the Lennox-Gastaut syndrome. This study is of particular interest for two reasons: The Lennox-Gastaut syndrome is notoriously refractory to treatment, and there had been no previous double-blind controlled study of any therapeutic modality in this syndrome. Significant positive behavioral effects in children with Lennox-Gastaut syndrome treated with felbamate have also been reported (36).

A double-blind monotherapy study of felbamate in children with partial seizures was initiated, but it was interrupted when the emergence of serious side effects led to marked restrictions on the use and the promotion of felbamate. The effectiveness of felbamate as an AED that was demonstrated by controlled trials was clearly confirmed by clinical experience during widespread use after its release. Physicians who have used felbamate in many patients with epilepsy comment that felbamate achieved remarkable seizure control, even in some patients who had been previously refractory to AEDs. In addition, uncontrolled reports have suggested that felbamate may be effective in the treatment of absence seizures (37), juvenile myoclonic epilepsy (38), infantile spasms (39–41), and acquired epileptic aphasia (Landau-Kleffner syndrome) (42). In 36 pediatric patients with various forms of epilepsy, the responder rate (≥50% seizure reduction) was 69% at 3 months, 47% at 1 year, and 41% at 3 years

(43). The authors estimated that the best results had been obtained against simple partial seizures with or without secondary generalization, as well as against tonic and atonic seizures.

ADVERSE EFFECTS

Almost exactly a year after felbamate's release, it became evident that the fate of felbamate would be determined much more by its side effects than by its antiepileptic efficacy. Felbamate was initially intensely and broadly marketed as a safe AED that did not display the toxic features of established AEDs and did not require laboratory monitoring. The more common side effects of felbamate in adults and in children, in monotherapy and with concomitant AEDs, are summarized in Table 44-1 (44). The higher incidence of side effects during adjunctive therapy is likely to be due to pharmacokinetic and pharmacodynamic interactions with other AEDs. The gastrointestinal side effects, including anorexia with weight loss, have been by far the most prominent of these side effects. The quoted numbers of 2% to 3% probably underestimate the true incidence of weight loss. The weight loss occurs mostly during the first 3 months of treatment, with subsequent stabilization, and represents approximately 2% to 5% of the body weight. In one series of patients, 34% lost more than 4 kg and 11% lost more than 8 kg (45). Another significant and rather persistent problem in children has been insomnia and irritability. Two children developed involuntary movements, consisting of choreoathetosis in one child and an acute dystonic reaction in the other child (46). A 15-year-old boy taking felbamate was reported to have presented with symptomatic ureteral kidney and bladder stones, which were identified as consisting of felbamate (47). Crystalluria and even renal failure have been observed in cases of felbamate overdoses (48, 49).

TABLE 44-1
Adverse Events Associated with Felbamate Used as Adjunctive Therapy and in Monotherapy in Adults and in Children

	% Patients with Adverse Event	
Adverse Event	Adjunctive Therapy	Monotherapy
Adults		
Nausea	11	4
Anorexia	7	3
Dizziness	6	3
Vomiting	5	2
Weight loss	4	2
Insomnia	4	4
Diplopia	3	0.5
Somnolence	3	1
Headache	3	1
Dyspepsia	2	1
Children		
Anorexia	6	3
Somnolence	6	3
Insomnia	6	1
Vomiting	3	0
Weight loss	2	3
Nausea	2	0
Gait abnormal	2	0

Source: Bourgeois 1997 (44).

The first year of postmarketing use revealed that felbamate was associated with a relatively high incidence of life-threatening side effects. In August of 1994, almost a year after the release of felbamate, the number of cases of aplastic anemia that had accumulated was such that the drug came close to being withdrawn from the market (50, 51). The aplastic anemias were diagnosed between 2.5 and 6 months after the onset of felbamate therapy. A warning was mailed to all physicians in the United States. In addition, several cases of severe and occasionally fatal hepatotoxicity were reported (52). Promotion of felbamate came to a virtual standstill, all ongoing clinical trials were suspended, and a warning was included in the package insert, requiring frequent laboratory monitoring of patients treated with felbamate. Although exact numbers are difficult to determine in such cases, and some degree of underreporting must be assumed, the reported numbers of cases are as follows (51, 53): 34 patients with aplastic anemia were reported and 14 have died; 23 cases were confirmed, of whom 7 have died; among 18 reported patients with hepatotoxicity, felbamate was considered to be the likely cause in 7 (Table 44-2). The estimated denominator is a total of 110,000 patients treated with felbamate in the United States after its release. Using this denominator, the calculated worst-case risk of developing either one of these two complications is approximately 1 in 2,700, with a worst-case risk of death of approximately 1 in 4,800 (Table 44-3). The risk of aplastic anemia could be as much as 10 to 100 times higher than in the general population and 20 times higher than with carbamazepine (53). Although many children have been treated with felbamate, aplastic anemia was not reported in any child younger than the age of 13 years. The only other patient younger than 20 years old was 18 years of age, and this patient was also the youngest patient to die from aplastic anemia. If the risk of aplastic anemia is discounted, the calculated risk of death from a severe felbamate complication in the pediatric age range would be approximately 1 per 20,000. This number is somewhat lower than the rate of valproate

TABLE 44-2
Cases of Aplastic Anemia and Hepatotoxicity Associated with Felbamate Therapy

	Total Number	Number of Deaths
Aplastic anemia		
Reported	34	14 (41%)
Confirmed	23	7 (30%)
FBM only cause	3	
FBM most likely cause	11	
FBM possible cause	9	
Hepatotoxicity		
Reported	18	9 (50%)
FBM likely cause	7	
FBM unlikely cause	9	
Undetermined		2

Sources: Kaufman et al, 1997 (51); Pellock and Brodie 1997 (53); Pellock, 1999 (61). Abbreviation: FBM, felbamate.

hepatic fatalities for monotherapy patients over the age of 2 years and definitely lower than the rate of hepatic fatalities from valproate polytherapy for patients under the age of 10 years (54). This comparison provides a perspective that should help us define the current and future place of felbamate in the treatment of epilepsy. Valproate and carbamazepine have also at some point raised significant concerns of serious idiosyncratic toxicity.

Just as risk factors were identified for valproate, there may also be identifiable risk factors for felbamate toxicity. They may include a history of allergy or cytopenia with previous AEDs, polytherapy, and clinical or serological evidence of a concomitant immune disorder (51). Individuals in whom abnormally high amounts of possibly cytotoxic felbamate metabolites such as atropaldehyde or 2-phenylpropenal accumulate are at higher risk of toxicity (55–59). This and other hypotheses are being explored to identify patients at risk of a severe reaction (60, 61). Fluorofelbamate is a felbamate analog synthesized by substitution of fluorine for hydrogen at position 2 of the propane chain. Fluorofelbamate cannot be metabolized to 2-phenylpropenal and has been investigated as a possibly safer alternative to felbamate (62, 63).

CLINICAL USE

The current clinical experience with felbamate has been reviewed in a recent consensus paper (64). At the present time, the main indication for felbamate is in patients with the Lennox-Gastaut syndrome whose seizures remain uncontrolled despite trials with other AEDs such as valproate, clonazepam, lamotrigine, and topiramate. Felbamate can also be considered as a third-line drug in patients with refractory focal onset seizures (65). If felbamate fails to demonstrate marked seizure reduction after a 2- to 3-month trial, it should be discontinued without delay to reduce or avoid unnecessary exposure of the patient to the risk of a severe reaction. Inversely, in a patient who has been receiving felbamate for 18 months or more, it is probably safe to continue the treatment (65).

To minimize the occurrence of initial adverse reactions, felbamate must be introduced cautiously. Titration of the felbamate dose usually must occur simultaneously with a reduction in the dose of concomitant AEDs because of both pharmacokinetic and probable pharmacodynamic drug interactions. Although precise guidelines have been provided, a slower titration than the one recommended may be at times advisable. A felbamate dose of 1,200 mg/day is recommended during the first week in adults, with a reduction of concomitant AED dose(s) by one-fifth to one-third. During the second week of treatment, the dose is to be increased to 2,400 mg/day. If monotherapy is the goal, the concomitant AED dose should be reduced by another one-third during the second week. During the third week of treatment, if necessary and if tolerated, the

TABLE 44-3
Risk of Aplastic Anemia and Hepatotoxicity Associated with Felbamate Therapy (Denominator is 110,000 Patients)

	Overall Risk	Risk of Death
Aplastic anemia		
Lower limit (n = 3)	1:37,000	
Upper limit (n = 23)	1:4,800	~1:15,800
Most probable (n = 14)	1:7,900	
General population	1:500,000	
Hepatotoxicity	1:15,700–1:6,100	1:31,400–1:12,200
Combined risk (worst case)	1:2,700	1:4,800

felbamate dose is to be increased to 3,600 mg/day. In adult patients, doses of 5,000 to 6,000 mg/day have been commonly used. If felbamate is introduced in a patient who is not taking an enzyme-inducing AED, a slower titration is recommended. After an initial dose of 1,200 mg/day, the dose is increased by increments of 600 mg/day at intervals of 2 weeks. Titration is similar in children, the doses corresponding to 1,200, 2,400, and 3,600 mg/day in adults being 15, 30, and 45 mg/kg/day, respectively. Although it is generally better to keep the titration doses below rather than above these recommended doses, maintenance doses may often safely exceed 45 mg/kg/day in children. Because of felbamate's potential for bone marrow and liver toxicity, complete blood count and transaminases should be ordered before initiation and then at regular intervals. Although no rigid schedule can be established for this monitoring, testing after 1 month and then every 2–3 months would be reasonable, with somewhat longer intervals after the first year.

No definite therapeutic range for plasma felbamate levels has been established. In adults taking 3,600 mg/day of felbamate in monotherapy, plasma levels were 65 to 80 mg/L (33, 32). A tentative target range of 30–60 mg/L (125–250 μmol/L) has been suggested (66). In children, the values for felbamate levels in milligrams per liter (mg/L) were found to be approximately the same as the dose in mg/kg/day (35). Felbamate levels in 41 adult patients were analyzed by Harden and coworkers (67) and divided into low range (9–36 mg/L), mid range (37–54 mg/L), and high range (44–134 mg/L). Anorexia and complaints of severe side effects occurred significantly more often in the high level group, but significantly more patients in this group also reported decreased seizure frequency.

References

1. Swinyard EA, Sofia RD, Kupferberg HJ. Comparative anticonvulsant activity and neurotoxicity of felbamate and four prototype antiepileptic drugs in mice and rats. *Epilepsia* 1986; 27:27–34.
2. White HS, Wolf HH, Swinyard EA, et al. A neuropharmacological evaluation of felbamate as a novel anticonvulsant. *Epilepsia* 1992; 33:564–572.
3. Lockard JS, Levy RH, Moore DF. Drug alteration of seizure cyclicity. In: Wolf P, Dam M, Janz D, Dreifuss FE, eds. *XVIth Epilepsy International Symposium*. Advances in Epileptology. Vol. 16. New York: Raven Press, 1987:725–732.
4. White HS, Harmsworth WL, Sofia RD, et al. Felbamate modulates the strychnine-insensitive glycine receptor. *Epilepsy Res* 1995; 20:41–48.
5. Ticku MK, Kamatchi GL, Sofia RD. Effect of anticonvulsant felbamate on $GABA_A$ receptor system. *Epilepsia* 1991; 32:389–391.
6. Rho JM, Donevan DC, Rogawski MA. Mechanism of action of the anticonvulsant felbamate: opposing effects on NMDA and $GABA_A$ receptors. *Ann Neurol* 1994; 35:229–234.
7. Kuo CC, Lin BJ, Chang HR, Hsieh CP. Use-dependent inhibition of the N-methyl-D-aspartate currents by felbamate: a gating modifier with selective binding to the desensitized channels. *Mol Pharmacol* 2004; 65:370–380.
8. Harty TP, Rogawski MA. Felbamate block of recombinant N-methyl-D-aspartate receptors: selectivity for the NR2B subunit. *Epilepsy Res* 2000; 39:47–55.
9. Shumaker RC, Fantel C, Kelton E, et al. Evaluation of the elimination of [^{14}C]felbamate in healthy men. *Epilepsia* 1990; 31:642.
10. Adusumalli VE, Wichmann JK, Kucharczyk N, et al. Drug concentration in human brain tissue samples from epileptic patients treated with felbamate. *Drug Metab Dispos* 1994; 22:168–170.
11. Thompson CD, Kinter MT, Macdonald TL. Synthesis and in vitro reactivity of 3-carbamoyl-2-phenyl-propionaldehyde and 2-phenylpropenal: putative reactive metabolites of felbamate. *Chem Res Toxicol* 1996; 9:1225–1229.
12. Thompson CD, Gulden PH, Macdonald TL. Identification of modified atropaldehyde mercapturic acids in rat and human urine after felbamate administration. *Chem Res Toxicol* 1997; 10:457–462.
13. Perhach JL, Weliky I, Newton JJ, et al. Felbamate. In: Meldrum BS, Porter RJ, eds. *New Anticonvulsant Drugs*. London, Paris: John Libbey, 1986:117–123.
14. Ward DL, Shumaker RC. Comparative bioavailability of felbamate in healthy men. *Epilepsia* 1990; 31:642.
15. Ward DL, Wagner ML, Perhach JL, et al. Felbamate steady-state pharmacokinetics during co-administration of valproate. *Epilepsia* 1991; 32 Suppl 3:8.
16. Sachdeo RC, Narang-Sachdeo SK, Howard JR, et al. Steady-state pharmacokinetics and dose proportionality of felbamate after oral administration of 1200, 2400, and 3600 mg/day of felbamate. *Epilepsia* 1993; 34:80.
17. Sachdeo R, Narang-Sachdeo SK, Shumaker RC, et al. Tolerability and pharmacokinetics of monotherapy felbamate doses of 1200–6000 mg/day in subjects with epilepsy. *Epilepsia* 1997; 38:887–892.
18. Wagner ML, Graves NM, Leppik IE, et al. The effect of felbamate on valproate disposition. *Epilepsia* 1991; 32:15.
19. Kelley MT, Walson PD, Cox S, Dusci LJ. Population pharmacokinetics of felbamate in children. *Ther Drug Monit* 1997; 19:29–36.
20. Sachdeo R, Wagner M, Sachdeo S, et al. Steady-state pharmacokinetics of phenytoin when co-administered with Felbatol™ (felbamate). *Epilepsia* 1992; 33 Suppl 3:84.
21. Sachdeo R, Wagner ML, Sachdeo S, et al. Coadministration of phenytoin and felbamate: evidence of additional phenytoin dose-reduction requirements based on pharmacokinetics and tolerability with increasing doses of felbamate. *Epilepsia* 1999; 40:1122–1128.
22. Hooper WD, Franklin ME, Glue P, et al. Effect of felbamate on valproic acid disposition in healthy volunteers: inhibition of beta-oxidation. *Epilepsia* 1996; 37:91–97.
23. Howard JR, Dix RK, Shumaker RC, et al. Effect of felbamate on carbamazepine pharmacokinetics. *Epilepsia* 1992; 33 Suppl 3:84–85.
24. Contin M, Riva R, Albani F, Baruzzi AA. Effect of felbamate on clobazam and its metabolite kinetics in patients with epilepsy. *Ther Drug Monit* 1999; 21:604–608.
25. Reidenberg P, Glue P, Banfield CR, et al. Effects of felbamate on the pharmacokinetics of phenobarbital. *Clin Pharmacol Ther* 1995; 58:279–287.
26. Patrias J, Espe-Lillo J, Ritter FJ. Felbamate-methsuximide interaction. *Epilepsia* 1992; 33:84.
27. Tisdel KA, Israel DS, Kolb KW. Warfarin-felbamate interaction: first report [letter]. *Ann Pharmacol* 1994; 28:805.
28. Hachad H, Ragueneau-Majlessi I, Levy RH. New antiepileptic drugs: review on drug interactions. *Ther Drug Monit* 2002; 24:91–103.
29. Perucca E. Clinically relevant drug interactions with antiepileptic drugs. *Br J Clin Pharmacol* 2006; 61:246–255.
30. Wagner ML, Graves NM, Marineau K, et al. Discontinuation of phenytoin and carbamazepine in patients receiving felbamate. *Epilepsia* 1991; 32:398–406.
31. Hussein G, Troupin AS, Montouris G. Gabapentin interaction with felbamate. *Neurology* 1996; 47:1106.
32. Bourgeois B, Leppik IE, Sackellares JC, et al. Felbamate: a double-blind controlled trial in patients undergoing presurgical evaluation of partial seizures. *Neurology* 1993; 43:693–696.
33. Sachdeo R, Kramer LD, Rosenberg A, Sachdeo S. Felbamate monotherapy: controlled trial in patients with partial onset seizures. *Ann Neurol* 1992; 32:386–392.
34. Faught E, Sachdeo RC, Remler MP, et al. Felbamate monotherapy for partial-onset seizures: an active-control trial. *Neurology* 1993; 43:688–692.
35. The Felbamate Study Group in Lennox-Gastaut syndrome. Efficacy of felbamate in childhood epileptic encephalopathy (Lennox-Gastaut syndrome). *N Engl J Med* 1993; 328:29–33.
36. Gay PE, Mecham GF, Coskey JS, Sadler T, Thompson JA. Behavioral effects of felbamate in childhood epileptic encephalopathy (Lennox-Gastaut syndrome). *Psychol Rep* 1995; 77:1208–1210.
37. Devinski O, Kothari M, Rubin R, et al. Felbamate for absence seizures. *Epilepsia* 1992; 33 Suppl 3:84.
38. Sachdeo RC, Murphy JV, Kamin M. Felbamate in juvenile myoclonic epilepsy. *Epilepsia* 1992; 33 Suppl 3:118.
39. Hurst DL, Rolan TD. The use of felbamate to treat infantile spasms. *J Child Neurol* 1995; 10:134–136.
40. Stafstrom CE. The use of felbamate to treat infantile spasms. *J Child Neurol* 1996; 11:170–171.
41. Hosain S, Nagarajan L, Carson D, et al. Felbamate for refractory infantile spasms. *J Child Neurol* 1997; 12:466–468.
42. Glauser TA, Olberding LS, Titanic MK, Piccirillo DM. Felbamate in the treatment of acquired epileptic aphasia. *Epilepsy Res* 1995; 20:85–89.
43. Cilio MR, Kartashov AI, Vigevano F. The long-term use of felbamate in children with severe refractory epilepsy. *Epilepsy Res* 2001; 47:1–7.
44. Bourgeois BFD. Felbamate. *Semin Pediatr Neurol* 1997; 4:3–8.
45. Bergen D, Ristanovic RK, Waikosky K, Kanner A, et al. Weight loss in patients taking felbamate. *Clin Neuropharmacol* 1995; 18:23–27.

46. Kerrick JM, Kelley BJ, Maister BH, Graves NM, et al. Involuntary movement disorders associated with felbamate. *Neurology* 1995; 45:185–187.
47. Sparagana SP, Strand WR, Adams RC. Felbamate urolithiasis. *Epilepsia* 2001; 42:682–685.
48. Rengstorff DS, Milstone AP, Seger DL, Meredith TJ. Felbamate overdose complicated by massive crystalluria and acute renal failure. *J Toxicol Clin Toxicol* 2000; 38:667–669.
49. Meier KH, Olson KR, Olson JL. Acute felbamate overdose with crystalluria. *Clin Toxicol* 2005; 43:189–192.
50. Pennell PB, Ogaily MS, Macdonald RL. Aplastic anemia in a patient receiving felbamate for complex partial seizures. *Neurology* 1995; 45:456–460.
51. Kaufman DW, Kelly JP, Anderson T, Harmon DC, et al. Evaluation of case reports of aplastic anemia among patients treated with felbamate. *Epilepsia* 1997; 38:1265–1269.
52. O'Neil MG, Perdun CS, Wilson MB, McGown ST, et al. Felbamate-associated fatal acute hepatic necrosis. *Neurology* 1996; 46:1457–1459.
53. Pellock JM, Brodie MJ. Felbamate: 1997 update. *Epilepsia* 1997; 38:1261–1264.
54. Bryant AE, Dreifuss FE. Valproic acid hepatic fatalities. III. U.S. experience since 1986. *Neurology* 1996; 46:465–469.
55. Dieckhaus CM, Santos WL, Sofia RD, Macdonald TL. The chemistry, toxicology, and identification in rat and human urine of 4-hydroxy-5-phenyl-1,3-oxazaperhydroin-2-one: a reactive metabolite in felbamate bioactivation. *Chem Res Toxicol* 2001; 14: 958–964.
56. Dieckhaus CM, Thompson CD, Roller SG, Macdonald TL. Mechanisms of idiosyncratic drug reactions: the case of felbamate. *Chem Biol Interact* 2002; 142:99–117.
57. Kapetanovic IM, Torchin CD, Strong JM, et al. Reactivity of atropaldehyde, a felbamate metabolite in human liver tissue in vitro. *Chem Biol Interact* 2002; 142:119–134.
58. Husain Z, Pinto C, Sofia RD, Yunis EJ. Felbamate-induced apoptosis of hematopoietic cells is mediated by redox-sensitive and redox-independent pathways. *Epilepsy Res* 2002; 48:57–69.
59. Popovic M, Nierkens S, Pieters R, Uetrecht J. Investigating the role of 2-phenylpropenal in felbamate-induced idiosyncratic drug reactions. *Chem Res Toxicol* 2004; 17:1568–1576.
60. Pellock JM. Felbamate in epilepsy therapy: evaluating the risks. *Drug Saf* 1999; 21: 225–239.
61. Pellock JM. Felbamate. *Epilepsia* 1999; 40 Suppl 5:S57–S62.
62. Mazarati AM, Sofia RD, Wasterlain CG. Anticonvulsant and antiepileptogenic effects of fluorofelbamate in experimental status epilepticus. *Seizure* 2002; 11:423–430.
63. Parker RJ, Hartman NR, Roecklein BA, et al. Stability and comparative metabolism of selected felbamate metabolites and postulated fluorofelbamate metabolites by postmitochondrial suspensions. *Chem Res Toxicol* 2005; 18:1842–1848.
64. Pellock JM, Faught E, Leppik IE, Shinnar S, et al. Felbamate: Consensus of current clinical experience. *Epilepsy Res* 2006; 71:89–101.
65. French J, Smith M, Faught E, et al. The use of felbamate in the treatment of patients with intractable epilepsy: practice advisory. *Neurology* 1999; 52:1540–1545.
66. Johannessen SI, Battino D, Berry DJ, et al. Therapeutic drug monitoring of the newer antiepileptic drugs. *Ther Drug Monit* 2003; 25:347–363.
67. Harden CL, Trifiletti R, Kutt H. Felbamate levels in patients with epilepsy. *Epilepsia* 1996; 37:280–283.

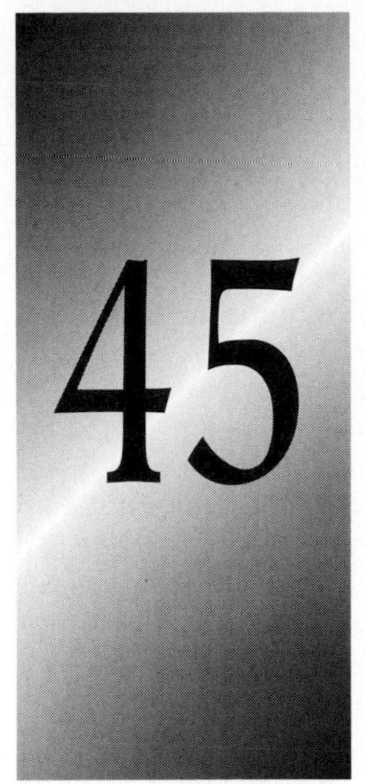

45 Gabapentin and Pregabalin

Gregory L. Holmes
Phillip L. Pearl

Gabapentin (GBP), or 2-[1-aminomethylcyclohexyl]acetic acid, and pregabalin (PGB), or (S)-3-(aminomethyl)-5-methylhexanoic acid, are structural, but not functional analogs of gamma-aminobutyric acid (GABA). GBP (Neurontin®) has U.S. Food and Drug Administration (FDA) approval for adjunctive therapy of partial seizures in children 3 years of age or older, while PGB (Lyrica®) is approved for adjunctive therapy of partial seizures in adults. GBP received FDA approval in 1993 and PGB in 2005.

While the drugs have a number of similarities, there are also some differences in the molecules that are pertinent to children. GBP and PGB will be discussed separately here.

GABAPENTIN

Chemistry, Animal Pharmacology, and Mechanisms of Action

Gabapentin (Figure 45-1) has structural similarities to GABA (Figure 45-2), the major inhibitory neurotransmitter in the human brain. As GABA does not cross the blood-brain barrier, conformational restriction of the GABA molecule, with binding into a cyclohexane system, confers lipid solubility to the molecule and facilitates the penetration of the blood–brain barrier.

Testing in animals has demonstrated that GBP had considerable antiepileptic properties (1, 2). It is effective in the maximal electroshock test in rodents, protects against aspartate- and strychnine-induced and audiogenic tonic-clonic seizures, and prevents seizures in the Mongolian gerbil, a model of reflex epilepsy (1, 2). GBP prolongs time to clonic activity, tonic extension of the extremities, and death in mice after intraperitoneal (ip) injections of N-methyl-D-aspartate (NMDA) but not of kainic acid or quinolinic acid (3). When kainic acid, quinolinic acid, or glutamate was injected into the lateral ventricles of rats, there were no clear effects of GBP on the seizures (4). GBP reduces after-discharge duration in the kindling model (2, 5). GBP has been shown to be effective in preventing seizures following kindling in immature rats (6). These animal studies suggest that GBP should be clinically useful for partial seizures.

While GBP protects mice from clonic convulsions in both the subcutaneous pentylenetetrazol test and the intravenous threshold test (7), in a rat genetic model of absence epilepsy GBP actually increased spike-and-wave bursts (8). In the lethargic (*lh/lh*) mouse model of absence seizures, Hosford and coworkers (9) found that GBP had no effect on absence seizure frequency. Although efficacy against pentylenetetrazol seizures suggests that the drug should be useful in absence seizures, the finding that it is not effective in these animal models of absence seizures raises concerns about the efficacy of the drug in this seizure type. As will be

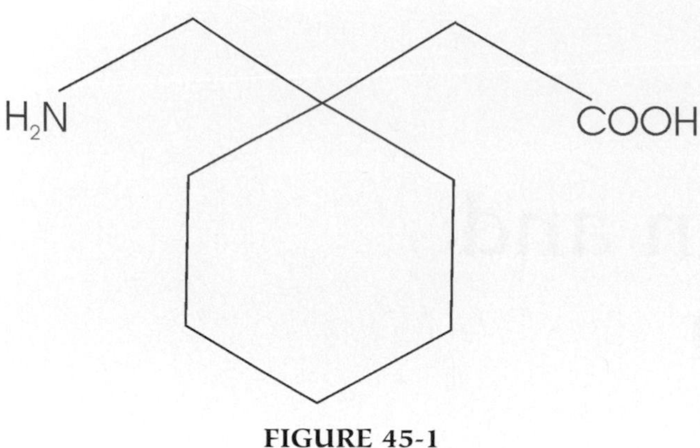

FIGURE 45-1

Molecular structure of gabapentin (GBP).

discussed, GBP has not been demonstrated to be effective in the treatment of childhood absence seizures.

In a developmental study, Mareš and Haugvicová (10) administered GBP before pentylenetetrazol to rats starting at 7 days. GBP suppressed or at least restricted the tonic phase of generalized tonic-clonic seizures at all the developmental stages studied. Cilio et al (11) found that GBP increases latency and decreases intensity of flurothyl induced seizures in immature rats.

GBP exhibits low acute toxicity in mice, rats, and monkeys and no significant systemic toxicity in four species after multidose administration for up to 52 weeks. GBP is not teratogenic and does not affect fertility or general reproductive parameters (5, 12). Pancreatic acinar cell tumors have been found in male Wistar rats receiving very large doses of GBP (2,000 mg/kg). These tumors were not observed in female rats or male or female mice. The tumors were low-grade malignancies, did not metastasize, and did not alter survival. The rat pancreatic tumor is not a generally accepted model of human pancreatic cancer, and human pancreatic tumors have not been reported in patients taking GBP (13).

Despite the similarity of GBP to GABA, binding experiments in rat brain and spinal cord have shown that GBP has no significant affinity for the $GABA_A$ or $GABA_B$ binding sites as measured by [^{3}H]muscimol and [^{3}H]baclofen displacement, respectively (5, 14). GBP does not inhibit binding of [^{3}H]diazepam at the GABA receptor, has only modest inhibitory effects on the GABA-degrading enzyme GABA-aminotransferase, does not elevate GABA content in nerve terminals, and does not affect the GABA uptake inhibitor. However, GBP significantly increases GABA concentrations in human neocortical slices made from tissue resected during epilepsy surgery (15). Petroff and coworkers (16) used magnetic resonance spectroscopy to estimate GABA brain concentrations. GABA was elevated in patients with partial seizures taking GBP compared with patients matched for antiepileptic drug (AED) treatment. There appeared to be a dose-related response; patients taking high-dose GBP had higher levels of GABA than those taking standard doses.

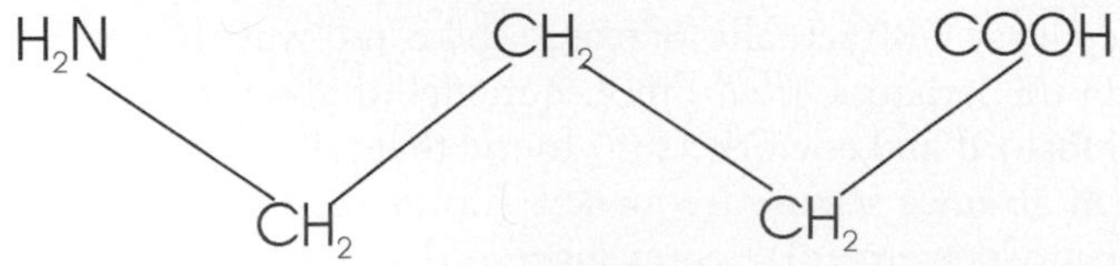

GBP does not have an effect at the NMDA receptors, non-NMDA glutamate receptors, or strychnine-insensitive glycine receptors. Based on the lack of a GBP effect on sustained repetitive firing of action potentials in mouse spinal cord neurons, it does not appear that the drug has an effect on voltage-dependent Na^+ channels (17, 18). While GBP was not found to have any significant effect on any Ca^{2+} channel current subtype (T, N, or L) (18), studies have demonstrated that the drug may act by binding to the alpha$_2$delta1 subunit of the calcium channel (19). Inhibition of Ca^{2+} currents via high-voltage-activated channels containing the alpha$_2$delta1 subunit, leading in turn to reduced neurotransmitter release and attenuation of postsynaptic excitability, is a biologically plausible mechanism and one that is consistently observed at therapeutically relevant concentrations in pre-clinical studies of GBP (Figure 45-3) (20–26).

Because the maximal anticonvulsant effect in the maximal electroshock threshold model is not seen until 2 hours after intravenous (IV) administration, the anticonvulsant effect is probably a result of delayed or indirect pharmacologic action (5, 27). GBP appears to bind to a high-affinity site in membrane fractions of rat brain tissue (28, 29) and is predominantly located on neurons in the brain (28). Binding of GBP is highest in the superficial layers of neocortex and dendritic layers of the hippocampus, with low levels of binding in the white matter and brainstem (28). GBP binding is not affected by valproate, phenytoin, carbamazepine, phenobarbital, diazepam, ethosuximide, or any other neuroactive substance (30). Binding of radiolabeled GBP to this protein is inhibited by leucine, isoleucine, valine, and phenylalanine, which indicates that GBP may bind to a site in the brain that resembles the large neutral amino acid transporter described in other tissues (31). It is possible that this may result in a decrease in the uptake of branched-chain amino acids into neurons; consequently, decreased neuronal glutamate synthesis may occur (32).

H_2N CH_2 COOH CH_2 CH_2

FIGURE 45-2

Molecular structure of gamma-aminobutyric acid (GABA).

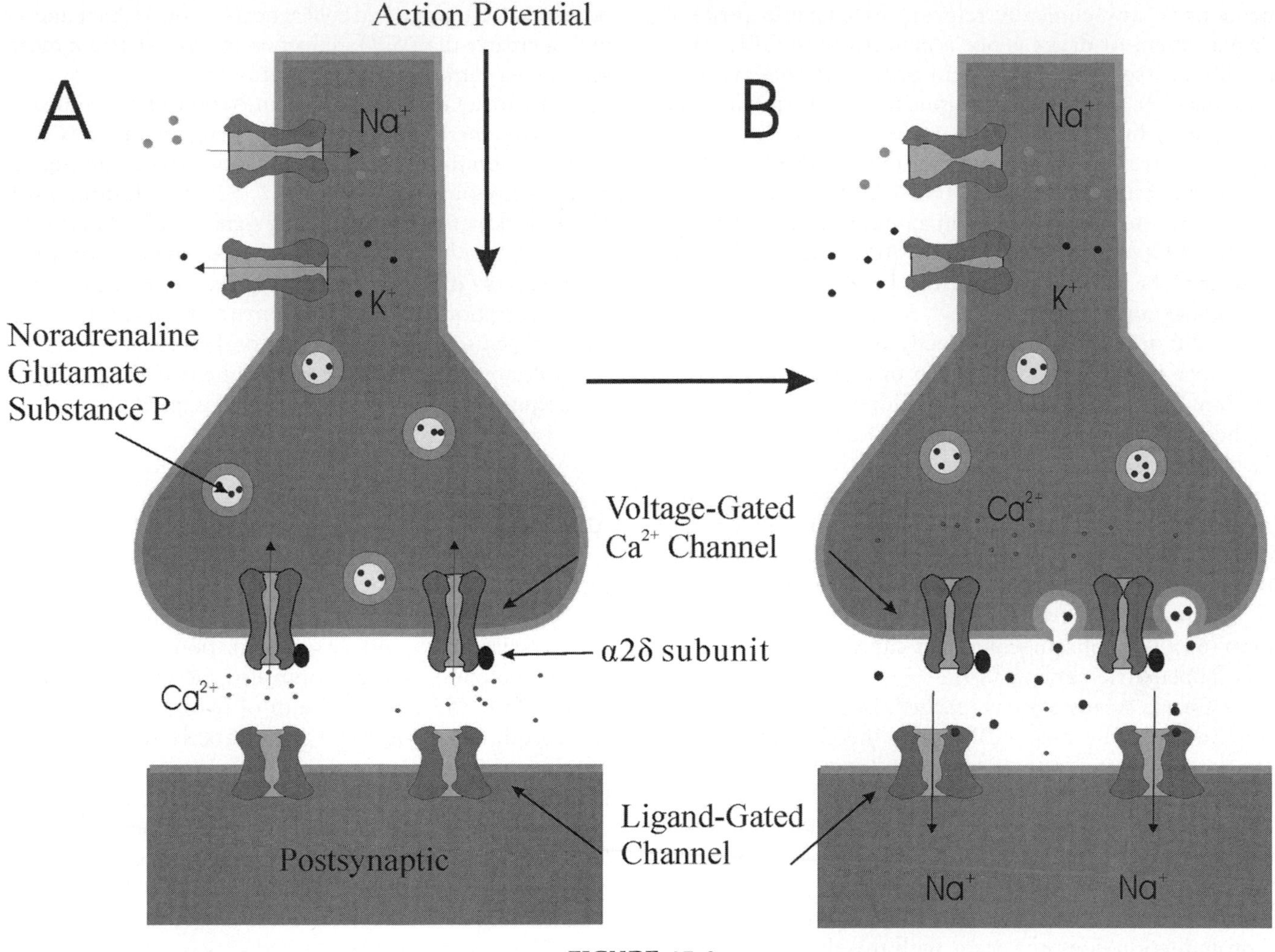

FIGURE 45-3

Mechanism of action for GBP and PGB. (A) The action potential propagates down the axon through activation of voltage-gated Na^+ channels. As the action potential reaches the synapse, voltage-gated Ca^{2+} channels open and allow the influx of Ca^{2+}. (B) Ca^{2+} influx triggers movement of synaptic vesicles to the synapse with release of neurotransmitters into the synaptic cleft. GBP and PGB bind to the alpha$_2$delta subunit of the Ca^{2+} channel and prevents the influx of Ca^{2+}, thus preventing release of the neurotransmitters noradrenaline, glutamate, and substance P.

Biotransformation, Pharmacokinetics, and Interactions in Humans

The absorption of GBP is dose-dependent (33). Sixty percent of a 300-mg dose of GBP is absorbed, compared with 35 percent of a 1,600-mg dose (34, 35). The drug is transported into the blood from the gut by a saturable transport mechanism, the L-system transporter of amino acids (36, 37). Because of this dose-dependent bioavailability, plasma concentrations of the drug are not directly proportional to dose throughout the range of doses studied (37). In adults, mean steady-state maximal and minimal concentrations (C_{max} and C_{min}, respectively) of GBP were proportional with doses up to approximately 1.8 g daily. At higher doses, however, C_{max} and C_{min} continued to increase, but the rate of increase was less than expected (36).

Maximum GBP concentrations occur 2–3 hours after administration of the drug. GBP absorption pharmacokinetics are not altered following multiple-dose administration, and accumulation of the drug following multiple-dose administration is predictable from single-dose data. While food has no effect on absorption (34), aluminum hydroxide–magnesium hydroxide antacid decreases the extent of GBP bioavailability by 20% when administered simultaneously or 2 hours after GBP ingestion (38).

Once absorbed, the drug is widely distributed throughout the body. GBP does not bind to plasma proteins to any clinically relevant extent, and protein displacement of drugs is not a concern with GBP. GBP readily crosses the blood-brain barrier in rodents and humans (39). GBP concentrations in cerebrospinal fluid (CSF) and brain tissue are approximately 20% and 80% of corresponding serum concentrations (35). After 3 months of treatment with 900 or 1,200 mg/day of GBP, brain concentrations of GBP in spinal fluid varied from 6% to 34% of those in plasma (40). There does not appear to be a linear relationship between plasma and CSF concentrations (41).

GBP oral clearance is directly related to creatinine clearance in children (42). When oral clearance is normalized for body weight, young children (<5 years) have higher and more variable values than older children. In 12 children treated with GBP as add-on therapy, Khurana and coworkers (43) found apparent clearance rates to range from 115 mL/kg/hr to 1446 mL/kg/hr with a mean of 372 ± 105 and a median of 292 mL/kg/hr. On a weight basis, 33% larger doses are required for young children (<5 years) to achieve the same exposure as older children (42). GBP pharmacokinetics can vary substantially among pediatric patients (44).

Once a steady state is reached, blood levels should not fluctuate. Because GBP is not metabolized but is excreted unchanged through the kidneys, clearance of the drug is related to creatinine clearance (32, 45). Renal clearance of the drug approximates glomerular filtration rate with an elimination half-life ($t_{1/2}$) in normal healthy adults of 5–9 hours (36). In patients with normal renal function, steady-state can be achieved within 2 days. Autoinduction does not occur with this drug.

Doses of GBP should be decreased in patients with renal impairment in whom the peak plasma concentrations of GBP are increased and occur later than in patients with normal renal function (46, 47). GBP is removed by hemodialysis, and patients undergoing this therapy need to be placed on maintenance doses of the drug. Guidelines are provided in the package insert by the manufacturers.

The usefulness of GBP serum levels has not yet been established (3, 32, 48, 49). The United Kingdom Gabapentin Study Group found that the mean and median plasma GBP concentrations were higher in responders than in nonresponders, but the group did not provide any specific data (50). Sevenius and coworkers (49) found seizure frequency to be decreased in patients with serum GBP concentrations above 2 mg/L. Crawford and coworkers (51) reported a significant therapeutic benefit from 900 mg GBP per day, which resulted in plasma GBP levels of 2–6 µg/mL. Of interest is a patient described by Brodie (48) with renal impairment who reported a 67% reduction in seizure number without side effects while taking 6,000 mg of GBP daily. The patient had a plasma GBP level of 61.2 mg/L. In an open-label study of efficacy of GBP in a pediatric population, Khurana and colleagues (43) found that patients with a greater than 50% reduction in seizures had a mean serum concentration of 3.7 µg/mL.

Because GBP is not protein-bound or metabolized in the liver, there are no significant drug interactions with the other commonly used antiepileptic drugs: carbamazepine, phenytoin, or valproate (7, 52). In addition, GBP pharmacokinetics have not been significantly changed by concomitant administration of other AEDs (45). Studies of the effects of GBP on oral contraceptives report no changes in concentration of the contraceptive components (34, 46). Cimetidine use modestly reduces oral and renal clearance of GBP; however, this is of minimal clinical significance and requires no adjustment in GBP dosages (34).

Clinical Efficacy

Although GBP has been primarily studied in partial seizures in adults, the drug is widely used in children, and there have been a number of studies in children (53, 54).

A total of 792 patients with refractory partial seizures with or without secondary generalization were studied in five double-blind, placebo-controlled, parallel-group studies in adults (55). A minimum of four partial seizures were required per month. Patients received GBP or placebo as add-on therapy for 12 weeks after a 12-week baseline phase, during which concurrent AED therapy was maintained at prestudy levels and baseline seizure frequency was obtained. A total of 307 patients received placebo and 485 received GBP doses of 600, 900, 1,200, or 1,800 mg/day.

The primary efficacy variable was responder rate, which is defined as the percentage of patients experiencing at least a 50% reduction in seizure frequency from baseline to treatment. In this series of placebo-controlled trials, the responder rate in the placebo group was approximately 10%, compared with 20–25% in the patients receiving placebo. The greatest seizure reduction was seen among patients receiving 1,800 mg/day of GBP.

In a study of 129 patients with refractory generalized seizures, Chadwick and colleagues (56) randomized patients to either placebo or 1,200 mg/day of GBP as add-on therapy. While GBP provided greater reduction in the frequency of generalized tonic-clonic seizures than placebo, the results were not statistically significant. GBP was tolerated well in this study.

Appleton et al (57) evaluated GBP as add-on therapy for refractory partial seizures in 247 patients, aged 3–12 years, enrolled from 54 centers in a 12-week double blind, placebo-controlled study and randomized to receive either GBP or placebo. Each patient was receiving one to three AEDs. The response ratio (i.e., reduction of seizure frequency), for all partial seizures was significantly better for GBP-treated patients ($P = 0.04$), and the responder rate, defined as the percentage of patients exhibiting more than

50% reduction in seizure frequency, favored GBP versus placebo, although this did not reach statistical significance. The double-blind trial was subsequently continued into a six month open-label extension study (58). Eighty (34%) of 237 children, aged 3–12 years, who received GPB, showed a >50% reduction in partial seizures.

A large number of patients on GBP have been followed for many years in open-label trials (59–62). Sivenius (60) treated patients with GBP for more than 4 years and found a significant reduction in seizure frequency (>50%) during the follow-up period in five of the seven patients. Likewise, Handforth and Treiman (61) entered 23 patients with intractable epilepsy into an open-label treatment study after a blinded, placebo-controlled, add-on efficacy study. Nine patients had no improvement in seizure control and discontinued the GBP, whereas, the remaining 14 patients continued on the GBP. Seven patients on GBP were followed up for 4 years. Maintenance of the efficacy of GBP was investigated in five long-term, open-label studies in a total of 774 patients (59). A majority of these patients had previously participated in a placebo-controlled study and subsequent short-term, open-label extension, reflecting a retention rate of 66%. The responder rate remained relatively stable over time, and patients who were responders in early phases continued to respond in later phases (12–18 months). The authors also noted that GBP discontinuation did not cause a rebound increase in seizures.

Leiderman and colleagues (63) presented data on 240 patients who entered an open-label trial after completion of a double-blind, placebo-controlled trial of GBP for partial seizures. GBP was continued in 78 (33%) patients for 3 years, 65 (27%) for 4 years, and 40 (17%) for 5 years. The maximum treatment period was 7 years with a mean treatment duration of 843 days. This study demonstrated that GBP can be tolerated for long periods of time.

Patients who have a response to GBP with add-on therapy may be converted to monotherapy. In an ongoing study of an open-label extension of a double-blind, multicenter trial of GBP in partial seizures, 54 of 250 (22%) patients were able to have concurrent antiepileptic drugs discontinued (64). The patients were allowed to take up to 4,800 mg/day.

In a study of the efficacy of GBP in children with refractory partial seizures, Khurana and colleagues (43) reviewed their results in 32 children with refractory partial seizures in which GBP was added to the drug regimen. GBP was given in a dose ranging from 10 to 50 mg/kg/day with a mean dose of 26.7 mg/kg/day for children with partial seizures with or without secondary generalization. Compared to baseline, eleven patients (34.4%) had a greater than 50% reduction in seizure frequency, and four patients (12.5%) had a 25% to 50% decrease.

GBP has been found to be an effective antiepileptic drug in children undergoing cancer therapy (65, 66). In a retrospective analysis, Khan et al (65) reported that seizures were controlled in 74% of 50 children on chemotherapy who developed epilepsy (91% of the leukemia group, 57% of the brain tumor group, and 75% of the other tumor group).

Comparison of GBP with Other AEDs in Partial Seizures. There are few studies comparing GBP with other AEDs in adults, and none that directly compare the antiepileptic efficacy of GBP with those of other AEDs in children. Anhut and coworkers (67) randomized newly diagnosed patients with a minimum of two partial seizures to one of four parallel fixed-dose treatment groups: 136 patients received one of three GBP doses—300, 900, or 1,800 mg/day, and 46 patients received 600 mg/day of carbamazepine (CBZ). The authors found similar efficacy for the two drugs: 42% of the GBP-treated group and 48% of the CBZ-treated group were responders.

Other Seizure Types. GBP has been used in one double-blind study of absence seizures in children (68). Unfortunately, a small dose of GBP (15–20 mg/kg/day) was used in the study. In this study of 33 children, GBP was not effective in reducing seizure frequency. No children had an exacerbation of seizure frequency. There is no information available regarding the usefulness of GBP in neonatal seizures, atonic, or tonic seizures. In rare cases, GBP may exacerbate myoclonic seizures (69, 70).

Adverse Events

In general, GBP is very well tolerated in children. Adverse effects with GBP are uncommon and typically consist of somnolence, dizziness, ataxia, fatigue, nystagmus, headache, tremor, diplopia, and nausea and vomiting (13, 71). In the five placebo-controlled trials in adults, 76% experienced at least one adverse event, compared with 57% of patients treated with placebo. Most of the side effects were mild and transient, and few patients have withdrawn from studies because of adverse side effects (13, 71). In a review of adverse events with GBP, Ramsay (13) noted that in controlled clinical trials, approximately 7% of patients receiving GBP withdrew, compared with 3% of those receiving placebo, with the most common complaints in the GBP-treated patients being somnolence and ataxia. Urinary and fecal incontinence have been reported with GBP (72). Like several other AEDs, GBP can rarely exacerbates seizures (73).

Side effects do not appear to have a strong relationship to dose. In a study of 245 patients randomized to placebo or GBP, Anhut and colleagues (72) found that 69% of patients receiving 900 mg/kg/day and 64% of those receiving 1,200 mg/kg/day had adverse events, compared with 52% in the group that received placebo. Weight gain has been reported in some women but has not been a major issue in children. Severe, life-threatening adverse events have not been reported (13). The most significant serious side effects include rash (0.54%), decreased white blood count (0.19%), increased blood urea nitrogen (0.09%), decreased platelets (0.09%), and angina or electrocardiographic changes (0.04%) (13). Changes in clinical laboratory values during GBP therapy are usually transient, isolated occurrences, most of which have not been considered to be of clinical concern or related to GBP therapy (13, 55). The incidence of rash compares quite favorably with other AEDs.

GBP has been associated with behavioral disturbances in some children (74–78). For the most part, these disturbances appear to be most prominent in children with preexisting behavioral disturbances. Wolf and coworkers (74) described three children with learning disabilities who developed behavioral problems with hyperactive behavior and explosive outbursts consisting of aggressive and oppositional behavior. The behavior improved once GBP was stopped. Lee and colleagues (76) from Children's Hospital in Boston described seven children who received GBP as adjunctive medication and subsequently developed an intensification of baseline behaviors as well as some new behavioral disturbances. These behaviors included tantrums, directed aggression, defiance, and hyperactivity. All of the children had attention deficit hyperactivity disorder and developmental delays before institution of GBP. The exacerbation of GBP-associated behaviors may be dose-related in some patients. since reduction of the dose results in improvement in some children. It is not always necessary to discontinue GBP in children with adverse behavioral changes if it has been useful in reducing seizure frequency (75, 76). The behavioral problems do not appear to be totally confined to children, since hypomania with GBP in an adult patient has been reported (79).

In a 12 week, multi-center, double-blind, placebo-controlled trial of 247 children aged 3–12 years, Appleton et al (58) found that only six (5%) in the GBP group and three (2%) of the placebo group were withdrawn from the study because of adverse events. Compared to the placebo group, children on GBP experienced more somnolence (8.4%) and hostility (7.6%). Behavioral changes (hostility and emotional lability) occurred more in the GBP-treated children than in those receiving placebo. In all patients, the intensity of these behavioral changes was mild to moderate. Findings in the open label extension study were similar (58).

No disturbances of memory or learning have been reported with GBP. In a study of normal subjects, a psychotropic effect characterized by improvement in concentration, numerical memory, complex reactions, and reaction time test was reported with GBP (61). Because of the excellent safety profile and lack of interactions, the drug is increasingly being used in the treatment of epilepsy in children with other medical conditions who are receiving medications.

Clinical Use

The drug comes in 100-, 300-, 400-, 600-, and 800-mg capsules and a solution 250 mg/5 mL. There is no IV form of the drug. Because clearance of GBP is greater in children than in adults, higher doses, on a milligram-per-kilogram basis, are needed in children (43). GBP can be started at 10–15 mg/kg/day and increased every three days, if necessary, until the child is receiving a dose of 30–40 mg/kg/day. The effective dose of GBP in patients 5 years of age and older is 25–35 mg/kg/day. The effective dose in children aged 3–4 years is 40 mg/kg/day. The maximum daily dose has not been established. However, we have had children who tolerated and required over 80 mg/kg/day. Because of the dose-dependent bioavailability and short half-life, most children should take the medication three times a day. While GBP has a saturable, dose-dependent absorption, this becomes a problem with dosing only when high doses of GBP are required. Gidal and coworkers (80) found that there were minimal differences in bioavailability between 3,600 mg/day given three or four times daily. When the dose was increased to 4,800 mg/day, a 22% increase in absorption was found with four-times-a-day dosing compared with dosing given three times a day.

Because there are no drug interactions, doses of other antiepileptic drugs do not need to be adjusted. However, if the patient does well on GBP, it is recommended that other antiepileptic drugs be reduced and eliminated. As mentioned previously, withdrawal of GBP has not been associated with a rebound increase of seizures (61). Nevertheless, it is recommended that GBP be tapered over several months once the decision is made to withdraw the drug.

GBP can be rapidly initiated. In a study of patients 12 years of age or older, GBP was started either gradually (300 mg/day for one day, 600 mg/day for one day, then 900 mg/day), or as an initial dose of 900 mg/day (81). Patients tolerated 900 mg/day as well as the escalation dose. Of the four most common adverse events (somnolence, dizziness, ataxia, fatigue), only one, dizziness, occurred more often in the rapid initiation group.

SUMMARY

GBP was initially released as adjunctive therapy for the treatment of partial seizures in adults. Since the drug has been released, there have been a number of studies demonstrating its efficacy and safety in children. In addition to its antiepileptic properties, the drug has been found to be useful in pain management. GBP has a number of highly desirable properties. There is no protein binding; the drug is not metabolized; and it is excreted unchanged through the urine. There are no significant drug interactions with other antiepileptic drugs, and other antiepileptic drugs do not alter the pharmacokinetics of GBP. The drug appears to have a narrow therapeutic profile. It is effective against partial seizures, although the majority of studies have used the drug as add-on therapy, and it has some efficacy in primarily generalized convulsive seizures. The drug is not effective in the treatment of absence or myoclonic seizures. The side effect profile of the drug is quite attractive. No significant idiosyncratic reactions have been reported. The most common side effects have included dizziness, fatigue, and headache. Rarely, children have adverse behavioral effects such as hyperactivity and agitated behavior. These children usually have preexisting behavioral disturbances.

PREGABALIN

Pregabalin (PGB), like GBP, is a structural, but not functional analog of the inhibitory neurotransmitter GABA Figure 45-4). Pregabalin has been in development for over a decade (82) and is the most recently released antiepileptic drug in the United States at the time of this writing. In addition to its efficacy in partial seizures, the drug is also effective in the treatment of neuropathic pain (83) and anxiety (84).

Chemistry, Animal Pharmacology, and Mechanism of Action

PGB has been tested in a variety of rodent models of seizures (85, 86). PGB inhibits tonic extensor seizures in rats with high-intensity electroshock, low-intensity electroshock seizures in mice, and tonic extensor seizures in the DBA/2 audiogenic mouse model. At high doses, PGB (ED_{50} = 31 mg/kg) prevented clonic seizures from pentylenetetrazole in mice and prevented stage 4–5 behavioral seizures (lowest effective dose = 10 mg/kg) in the kindling model. PGB was not effective in the spontaneous absence-like seizures in the Genetic Absence Epilepsy Rats from Strasbourg (GAERS). In rodents, PGB caused ataxia and decreased spontaneous locomotor activity at dosages 10- to 30-fold higher than those required to stop seizures. PGB has shown efficacy in animal models of anxiety (87).

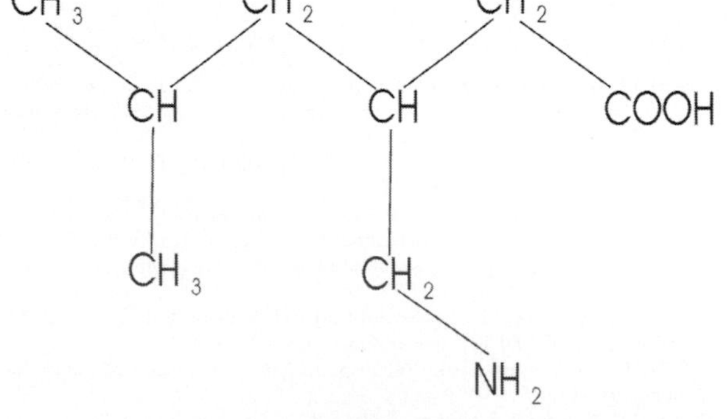

CH_3 CH_2 CH_2
CH CH COOH
CH_3 CH_2
NH_2

FIGURE 45-4

Molecular structure of pregabalin (PGB)

Biotransformation, Pharmacokinetics, and Interactions in Humans

Absorption is extensive, rapid, and proportional to dose (88). PGB absorption from the gastrointestinal tract is proportional to doses up to 150 mg/kg, which contrasts to the partially saturable absorption of GBP in rats (33, 89). The transport of PGB across membranes is largely explained by its substrate action at the L-amino acid transport system (89). However, the lower affinity (K_M) and higher capacity to accumulate PGB appears to facilitate transmembrane absorption in vivo.

Time to maximal plasma concentration is approximately one hour, and steady state is reached within 24–48 hours (88, 90). Absorption with food has no clinically relevant effect on the amount of PGB absorbed.

PGB does not bind to plasma proteins and is excreted virtually unchanged (<2% metabolism) by the kidneys (91). It is not subject to hepatic metabolism and does not induce or inhibit liver enzymes such as the cytochrome P450 system. PGB has a clearance (mL/min) of 45–75 and has a half-life of 5–7 hours (88, 92, 93). PGB demonstrates highly predictable and linear pharmacokinetics in adults.

PGB has no substantial pharmacokinetic drug-drug interactions (82, 90, 94). Brodie et al (94) examined the effect of PGB on steady state concentration of carbamazepine, phenytoin, lamotrigine, and valproate in adult patients with partial seizures. The blood levels were unaffected by PGB. Likewise, PGB steady-state pharmacokinetic parameters were similar among patients on the four drugs. The authors also noted that PGB in combination with carbamazepine, phenytoin, lamotrigine, and valproate was well tolerated.

The drug crosses the blood-brain barrier and binds potently to the alpha$_2$delta subunit of the P/Q voltage-gated calcium channel (Figure 45-3) (95–97). As a result, PGB reduces calcium current at the terminal (95), reducing the release of glutamate (21, 22), noradrenaline (96), and substance P (98). PGB has no effect on $GABA_A$ and $GABA_B$ receptors (82). Likewise, PGB has no discernible effect on GABA uptake or degradation (14, 15, 82).

Clinical Efficacy

Approval for PGB in the United States was based on three multicenter, randomized, double-blind, placebo-controlled trials in which efficacy and tolerability were assessed in patients with refractory epilepsy (99–102). In addition, a large international study evaluated GBP in adult patients with refractory partial seizures (103).

A total of 1,052 patients 12 years or older were entered into the U.S. studies, with 758 receiving PGB and 294 placebo. The patient population had refractory epilepsy and experienced at least six seizures and no 4-week seizure-free period during the 8-week baseline phase. Approximately 75% were on two other AEDs, and about a quarter were on three AEDs. In the first study, patients received PGB 50, 150, 300, or 600 mg/day (99); in the second study, patients received 50 or 600 mg/day (102); in the third study, patients received 600 mg/day (100). Patients receiving doses of 150, 300, or 600 mg/day had statistically fewer seizures than the placebo group, with a clear dose-response relationship. The responder rate, defined in the studies as the percentage of patients with ⩾50% reduction in seizure frequency, approached 50% at 600 mg/day. While direct comparison between PGB and other antiepileptic drugs is difficult, the responder rate with PGB appears to be similar to the response with the other new AEDs (82).

In an international study, 341 patients were randomized to placebo, PGB fixed dose (600 mg/day), or PGB flexible dose 150 mg and 300 mg/day for 2 weeks each and then 450 mg and 600 mg/day for 4 weeks each (103). All patients were refractory patients who were taking one to three AEDs. Both PGB regimens significantly reduced seizure frequency, compared to control, by 35.4% for the flexible dose and 49.3% for the fixed dose, versus 10.6% for placebo. Most adverse events were mild or moderate.

Efficacy of PGB was seen early in the study, with reductions in seizure frequency noted during the first week of therapy. There were no differences in responder rate between twice-daily and three-times-daily dosing.

Adverse Effects

The drug was well tolerated, with most adverse side effects central nervous system based. In adult patients, the adverse effects are dose dependent and occur within the first two weeks of treatment. Up to 33% of patients receiving PGB and 10% of those receiving placebo withdrew from the clinical trials because of adverse events (88). Common side effects associated with PGB, occurring in >10% of patients in epilepsy studies, include dizziness, somnolence, ataxia, asthenia, and weight gain (82, 88). Over 20% of patients report dizziness and somnolence.

Clinical Use

PGB comes in 25-, 50-, 75-, 100-, 150-, 200-, 225-, and 300-mg capsules. In adults, PGB in doses of 150 to 600 mg/day has been shown to be effective as adjunctive therapy in the treatment of partial-onset seizures. There are no guidelines for dosing in children. The authors typically start with a dose of 1–2 mg/kg and slowly titrate upward by 1–2 mg/kg per week until seizure control is achieved or adverse events occur.

PGB is a Schedule V controlled substance. In a study of recreational users (n = 15) of sedative/hypnotic drugs, including alcohol, PGB reported subjective ratings of "good drug effect," "high," and "liking," to a degree that was similar to a single dose of diazepam. In clinical studies with over 5,500 patients, 4% of PGB and 1% of the placebo group reported euphoria as an adverse effect (package insert, Lyrica®). Whether such an adverse side effect occurs in children is not yet known.

ACKNOWLEDGMENT

Supported by the Western Massachusetts Epilepsy Awareness Fund, Friends of Shannon McDermott, the Sara fund, and grants from NINDS (Grants: NS27984 and NS44295).

References

1. Andrews CO, Fischer JH. Gabapentin: a new agent for the management of epilepsy. *Ann Pharmacother* 1994; 28:1188–1196.
2. Goa KL, Sorkin EM. Gabapentin. A review or its pharmacological properties and clinical potential in epilepsy. *Drugs* 1993; 46:409–427.
3. Macdonald RL, Kelly KM. Mechanisms of action of currently prescribed and newly developed antiepileptic drugs. *Epilepsia* 1994; 35:S41–S50.
4. Bartoszyk GD, Meyerson N, Reimann W, Satzinger G, et al. Gabapentin: preclinical profile and first clinical results. In: Meldrum BS, Porter RJ, eds. *Current Problems in Epilepsy*. Vol. 4. *New Anticonvulsant Drugs*. New York: John Libbey, 1986:147.
5. Taylor CP. Gabapentin. Mechanisms of action. In: Levy RH, Mattson RH, Meldrum BS, eds. *Antiepileptic Drugs*. 4th ed. New York: Raven Press, 1995:829.
6. Lado FA, Sperber EF, Moshe SL. Anticonvulsant efficacy of gabapentin on kindling in the immature brain. *Epilepsia* 2001; 42:458–463.
7. McLean MJ. Gabapentin. *Epilepsia* 1995; 36(Suppl 2):S73–S86.
8. Foot M, Wallace J. Gabapentin. In: Pisani F, Perucca E, Avanzini G, Richon A, eds. *New Antiepileptic Drugs*. Amsterdam: Elsevier, 1991:109.
9. Hosford DA, Lin F-H, Kraemer DL, Cao Z, et al. Neuronal network of structures in which $GABA_B$ receptors regulate absence seizures in the lethargic (*lh/lh*) mouse model. *J Neurosci* 1995; 15:7367–7376.
10. Mareš P, Haugvicová R. Anticonvulsant action of gabapentin during postnatal development in rats. *Epilepsia* 1997; 38:893–896.
11. Cilio MR, Bolanos AR, Liu Z, et al. Anticonvulsant action and long-term effects of gabapentin in the immature brain. *Neuropharmacology* 2001; 40:139–147.
12. Taylor CP. Emerging perspectives on the mechanism of action of gabapentin. *Neurology* 1994; 44(Suppl. 5):S10–S16.
13. Ramsay RE. Gabapentin. Toxicity. In: Levy RH, Mattson RH, Meldrum BS, eds. *Antiepileptic Drugs*. 4th ed. New York: Raven Press, 1995:857.
14. Sills GJ. The mechanisms of action of gabapentin and pregabalin. *Curr Opin Pharmacol* 2006; 6:108–113.
15. Errante LD, Williamson A, Spencer DD, Petroff OA. Gabapentin and vigabatrin increase GABA in the human neocortical slice. *Epilepsy Res* 2002; 49:203–210.
16. Petroff OA, Rothman DL, Behar KL, Lamoureux D, et al. The effect of gabapentin on brain gamma-aminobutyric acid in patients with epilepsy. *Ann Neurol* 1996; 39:95–99.

17. Hosford DA, Wang Y. Utility of the lethargic (*lh/lh*) mouse model of absence seizures in predicting the effects of lamotrigine, vigabatrin, tiagabine, gabapentin, and topiramate against human absence seizures. *Epilepsia* 1997; 38:408–414.
18. Rock DM, Kelly KM, Macdonald RL. Gabapentin actions on ligand- and voltage-gated responses in cultured rodent neurons. *Epilepsy Res* 1993; 16:89–98.
19. Gee NS, Brown JP, Dissanayake VUK, Offord J, et al. The novel anticonvulsant drug, gabapentin (Neurontin), binds to the alpha$_2$delta subunit of a calcium channel. *J Biol Chem* 1996; 271:5776.
20. Brown JT, Randall A. Gabapentin fails to alter P/Q-type Ca^{2+} channel-mediated synaptic transmission in the hippocampus in vitro. *Synapse* 2005; 55:262–269.
21. Fink K, Meder W, Dooley DJ, Gothert M. Inhibition of neuronal Ca(2+) influx by gabapentin and subsequent reduction of neurotransmitter release from rat neocortical slices. *Br J Pharmacol* 2000; 130:900–906.
22. Fink K, Dooley DJ, Meder WP, et al. Inhibition of neuronal Ca(2+) influx by gabapentin and pregabalin in the human neocortex. *Neuropharmacology* 2002; 42:229–236.
23. Martin DJ, McClelland D, Herd MB, et al. Gabapentin-mediated inhibition of voltage-activated Ca^{2+} channel currents in cultured sensory neurones is dependent on culture conditions and channel subunit expression. *Neuropharmacology* 2002; 42:353–366.
24. Sutton KG, Martin DJ, Pinnock RD, Lee K, et al. Gabapentin inhibits high-threshold calcium channel currents in cultured rat dorsal root ganglion neurones. *Br J Pharmacol* 2002; 135:257–265.
25. Bayer K, Ahmadi S, Zeilhofer HU. Gabapentin may inhibit synaptic transmission in the mouse spinal cord dorsal horn through a preferential block of P/Q-type Ca^{2+} channels. *Neuropharmacology* 2004; 46:743–749.
26. Oka M, Itoh Y, Wada M, Yamamoto A, et al. Gabapentin blocks L-type and P/Q-type Ca^{2+} channels involved in depolarization-stimulated nitric oxide synthase activity in primary cultures of neurons from mouse cerebral cortex. *Pharm Res* 2003; 20:897–899.
27. Welty DF, Schielke GP, Vartanian MG, Taylor CP. Gabapentin anti-convulsant action in rats: disequilibrium with peak drug concentrations in plasma and brain microdialysate. *Epilepsy Res* 1993; 14:175–181.
28. Hill DR, Suman-Chauhan N, Woodruff GN. Localization of (^{3}H)-gabapentin to a novel site in rat brain: autoradiographic studies. *Eur J Pharmacol* 1993; 244:303–309.
29. Suman-Chauhan N, Webdale L, Hill DR, Woodruff GN. Characterization of [^{3}H]gabapentin in binding to a novel site in rat brain: homogenate binding studies. *Eur J Pharmacol* 1993; 244:293–301.
30. Chadwick D, Browne TR. Gabapentin. In: Engel J, Jr., Pedley TA, eds. *Epilepsy: A Comprehensive Textbook*. Philadephia: Lippincott-Raven Publishers, 1997:1521.
31. Thurlow RJ, Brown JP, Gee NS, Hill DR, et al. [^{3}H]Gabapentin may label a system-L-like neutral amino acid carrier in brain. *Eur J Pharmacol* 1993; 247:341–345.
32. Walker MC, Patsalos PN. Clinical pharmacokinetics of new antiepileptic drugs. *Pharmac Ther* 1995; 67:351–384.
33. Elwes RD, Binnie CD. Clinical pharmacokinetics of newer antiepileptic drugs. Lamotrigine, vigabatrin, gabapentin and oxcarbamazepine. *Clin Pharmacokinet* 1996; 30:403–415.
34. Richens A. Clinical pharmacokinetics of gabapentin. In: Chadwick D, ed. *New Trends in Epilepsy Management: The Role of Gabapentin*. London: Royal Society of Medicine Services, 1993:41.
35. Vollmer KO, Türck D, Bockbrader HN, et al. Summary of Neurontin (gabapentin) clinical pharmacokinetics. *Epilepsia* 1992; 33:77.
36. McLean MJ. Gabapentin. Chemistry, absorption, distribution, and excretion. In: Levy RH, Mattson RH, Meldrum BS, eds. *Antiepileptic Drugs*. 4th ed. New York: Raven Press, 1995:843.
37. Stewart BH, Kugler AR, Thompson PR, Bockbrader HN. A saturable transport mechanism in the intestinal absorption of gabapentin is the underlying cause of the lack of proportionality between increasing dose and drug levels in plasma. *Pharm Res* 1993; 10:276–281.
38. Busch JA, Radulovic LL, Bockbrader HN, Underwood BA, et al. Effect of Maalox TC on single-dose pharmoacokinetics of gabapentin capsules in healthy subjects. *Pharm Res* 1992; 9(suppl.):S135.
39. Ben-Menachem E, Persson LI, Hedner T. Selected CSF biochemistry and gabapentin concentrations in the CSF and plasma in patients with partial seizures after a single oral dose of gabapentin. *Epilepsy Res* 1992; 11:45–49.
40. Ben-Menachem E, Hedner T, Persson LI. Seizure frequency and CSF gabapentin, GABA, and monoamine metabolite concentrations after 3 months treatment with 900 mg or 1200 mg gabapentin daily in patients with intractable complex partial seizures. *Neurology* 1990; 40(Suppl. 1):158.
41. Ben-Menachem E, Soderfelt B, Hamberger A, Hedner T, et al. Seizure frequency and CSF parameters in a double-blind, placebo-controlled trial of gabapentin in patients with intractable complex partial seizures. *Epilepsy Res* 1995; 21:231–236.
42. Ouellet D, Bockbrader HN, Wesche DL, Shapiro DY, et al. Population pharmacokinetics of gabapentin in infants and children. *Epilepsy Res* 2001; 47:229–241.
43. Khurana DS, Riviello J, Helmers S, Holmes G, et al. Efficacy of gabapentin therapy in children with refractory partial seizures. *J Pediatr* 1996; 128:829–833.
44. Tallian KB, Nahata MC, Lo W, Tsao CY. Pharmacokinetics of gabapentin in paediatric patients with uncontrolled seizures. *J Clin Pharm Ther* 2004; 29:511–515.
45. McLean MJ. Gabapentin. *Epilepsia* 1995; 36(Suppl. 2):S73–S86.
46. Comstock TJ, Sica DA, Bockbrader HN, Underwood BA, et al. Gabapentin pharmacokinetics in subjects with various degrees of renal function. *J Clin Pharmacol* 1990; 30:862.
47. Blum RA, Comstock TJ, Sica DA, et al. Pharmacokinetics of gabapentin in subjects with various degrees of renal function. *Clin Pharmacol Ther* 1994; 56:154–159.
48. Brodie MJ. Routine measurement of new antiepileptic drug concentrations: a critique and a prediction. In: French JA, Leppik I, Dichter M, eds. *Antiepileptic Drug Development*. Advances in Neurology 76. Philadelphia: Lippincott-Raven Publishers, 1998:223.
49. Sivenius J, Kälviäinen R, Ylinen A, Riekkinen P. Double-blind study of gabapentin in the treatment of partial seizures. *Epilepsia* 1991; 32:539–542.
50. U.K. Gabapentin Study Group. Gabapentin in partial epilepsy. *Lancet* 1990; 335:1114–1117.
51. Crawford P, Ghadiali E, Lane R, Blumhardt L, et al. Gabapentin as an antiepileptic drug in man. *J Neurol Neurosurg Psychiatr* 1987; 50:682–686.
52. Radulovic LL, Wilder BJ, Leppik IE et al. Lack of interaction of gabapentin with carbamazepine or valproate. *Epilepsia* 1994; 35:155–161.
53. Coppola G. Treatment of partial seizures in childhood: an overview. *CNS Drugs* 2004; 18:133–156.
54. McDonald DG, Najam Y, Keegan MB, Whooley M, et al. The use of lamotrigine, vigabatrin and gabapentin as add-on therapy in intractable epilepsy of childhood. *Seizure* 2005; 14:112–116.
55. Leiderman DB. Gabapentin as add-on therapy for refractory partial epilepsy: results of five placebo-controlled trials. *Epilepsia* 1994; 35:S74–S76.
56. Chadwick D, Leiderman DB, Sauermann W, Alexander J, Garofalo E. Gabapentin in generalized seizures. *Epilepsy Res* 1996; 25:191–197.
57. Appleton R, Fichtner K, LaMoreaux L, et.al. Gabapentin paediatric study group. Gabapentin as add-on therapy in children with refractory partial seizures: a 12-week, multicenter, double-blind, placebo-controlled study. *Epilepsia* 1999; 40:1147–1154.
58. Appleton R, Fichtner K, LaMoreaux L, et al. Gabapentin as add-on therapy in children with refractory partial seizures: a 24-week, multicentre, open-label study. *Dev Med Child Neurol* 2001; 43:269–273.
59. Chadwick D. Gabapentin. Clinical use. In: Levy RH, Mattson RH, Meldrum BS, eds. *Antiepileptic Drugs*. 4th ed. New York: Raven Press, 1995:851.
60. Sivenius J, Ylinen A, Kalviainen R, Riekkinen PJ. Long-term study with gabapentin in patients with drug-resistant epileptic seizures. *Arch Neurol* 1994; 51:1047–1050.
61. Handforth A, Treiman DM. Efficacy and tolerance of long-term, high-dose gabapentin: additional observations. *Epilepsia* 1994; 35:1032–1037.
62. Ojemann LM, Wilensky AJ, Temkin NR, Chmelir T, et al. Long-term treatment with gabapentin for partial epilepsy. *Epilepsy Res* 1992; 13:159–165.
63. Leiderman DB, Koto EM, LaMoreaux LK, McLean MJ, US GBP Study Group. Long-term therapy with gabapentin (GBP. Neurontin): 5-year experience from a US open-label trial. *Epilepsia* 1995; 36:68.
64. Garaofalo E, Hayes A, Greeley C et al. Gabapentin (Neurontin) monotherapy in patients with medically refractory partial seizures: an open-label extension study. *Epilepsia* 1995; 36:S119–S120.
65. Khan RB, Hunt DL, Thompson SJ. Gabapentin to control seizures in children undergoing cancer treatment. *J Child Neurol* 2004; 19:97–101.
66. Khan RB, Hunt DL, Boop FA et al. Seizures in children with primary brain tumors: incidence and long-term outcome. *Epilepsy Res* 2005; 64:85–91.
67. Anhut H, Greiner M, Möckel V, Murray G. Gabapentin (Neurontin) as monotherapy in newly diagnosed patients with partial epilepsy. *Epilepsia* 1995; 36:S119.
68. Trudeau V, Myers S, LaMoreaux L, Anhut H, et al. Gapabentin in naive childhood absence epilepsy: results from two double-blind, placebo-controlled, multicenter studies. *J Child Neurol* 1996; 11:470–475.
69. Asconape J, Diedrich A, DellaBadia J. Myoclonus associated with the use of gabapentin. *Epilepsia* 2000; 41:479–481.
70. Reeves AL, So EL, Sharbrough FW, Krahn LE. Movement disorders associated with the use of gabapentin. *Epilepsia* 1996; 37:988–990.
71. Ramsay RE. Clinical efficacy and safety of gabapentin. *Neurology* 1994; 44(Suppl. 5): S23–S30.
72. Anhut H, Ashman P, Feuerstein TJ, et al. Gabapentin (Neurontin) as add-on therapy in patients with partial seizures: a double-blind, placebo-controlled study. *Epilepsia* 1994; 35:795–801.
73. Mikati M, Khurana D, Riviello J, Holmes G, et al. Efficacy of gabapentin in children with refractory partial seizures. *Neurology* 1995; 45(Suppl. 4):A201–A202.
74. Wolf SM, Shinnar S, Kang H, Gil KB, et al. Gabapentin toxicity in children manifesting as behavioral changes. *Epilepsia* 1995; 36:1203–1205.
75. Tallian KB, Nahata MC, Lo W, Tsao C-Y. Gabapentin associated with aggressive behavior in pediatric patients with seizures. *Epilepsia* 1996; 37:501–502.
76. Lee DO, Steingard RJ, Cesena M, Helmers SL, et al. Behavioral side effects of gabapentin in children. *Epilepsia* 1996; 37:87–90.
77. Glauser TA. Behavioral and psychiatric adverse events associated with antiepileptic drugs commonly used in pediatric patients. *J Child Neurol* 2004; 19 Suppl 1: S25–S38.
78. Glauser TA. Effects of antiepileptic medications on psychiatric and behavioral comorbidities in children and adolescents with epilepsy. *Epilepsy Behav* 2004; 5 Suppl 3: S25–S32.
79. Short C, Cook L. Hypomania induced by gabapentin. *Brit J Psychiatr* 1995; 166:679–680.
80. Gidal BE, DeCerce J, Bockbrader HN, et al. Gabapentin bioavailability: effect of dose and frequence of administration in adult patients with epilepsy. *Epilepsy Res* 1998; 31:91–99.
81. Fisher RS, Sachdeo RC, Pellock J, Penovich PE, et al. Rapid initiation of gabapentin: a randomized, controlled trial. *Neurology* 2001; 56:743–748.
82. Hamandi K, Sander JW. Pregabalin: a new antiepileptic drug for refractory epilepsy. *Seizure* 2006; 15:73–78.
83. Dworkin RH, Corbin AE, Young JP Jr, et al. Pregabalin for the treatment of postherpetic neuralgia: a randomized, placebo-controlled trial. *Neurology* 2003; 60:1274–1283.
84. Pande AC, Crockatt JG, Feltner DE, et al. Pregabalin in generalized anxiety disorder: a placebo-controlled trial. *Am J Psychiatry* 2003; 160:533–540.

85. Vartanian MG, Radulovic LL, Kinsora JJ, et al. Activity profile of pregabalin in rodent models of epilepsy and ataxia. *Epilepsy Res* 2006; 68:189–205.
86. Bryans JS, Wustrow DJ. 3-substituted GABA analogs with central nervous system activity: a review. *Med Res Rev* 1999; 19:149–177.
87. Field MJ, Oles RJ, Singh L. Pregabalin may represent a novel class of anxiolytic agents with a broad spectrum of activity. *Br J Pharmacol* 2001; 132:1–4.
88. Shneker BF, McAuley JW. Pregabalin: a new neuromodulator with broad therapeutic indications. *Ann Pharmacother* 2005; 39:2029–2037.
89. Su TZ, Feng MR, Weber ML. Mediation of highly concentrative uptake of pregabalin by L-type amino acid transport in Chinese hamster ovary and Caco-2 cells. *J Pharmacol Exp Ther* 2005; 313:1406–1415.
90. Ben-Menachem E. Pregabalin pharmacology and its relevance to clinical practice. *Epilepsia* 2004; 45 Suppl 6:13–18.
91. Randinitis EJ, Posvar EL, Alvey CW, Sedman AJ, et al. Pharmacokinetics of pregabalin in subjects with various degrees of renal function. *J Clin Pharmacol* 2003; 43:277–283.
92. Perucca E. Clinical pharmacokinetics of new-generation antiepileptic drugs at the extremes of age. *Clin Pharmacokinet* 2006; 45:351–363.
93. Bialer M, Johannessen SI, Kupferberg HJ, Levy RH, et al. Progress report on new antiepileptic drugs: a summary of the Seventh Eilat Conference (EILAT VII). *Epilepsy Res* 2004; 61:1–48.
94. Brodie MJ, Wilson EA, Wesche DL, et al. Pregabalin drug interaction studies: lack of effect on the pharmacokinetics of carbamazepine, phenytoin, lamotrigine, and valproate in patients with partial epilepsy. *Epilepsia* 2005; 46:1407–1413.
95. Dooley DJ, Donovan CM, Pugsley TA. Stimulus-dependent modulation of [(3)H]norepinephrine release from rat neocortical slices by gabapentin and pregabalin. *J Pharmacol Exp Ther* 2000; 295:1086–1093.
96. Dooley DJ, Donovan CM, Meder WP, Whetzel SZ. Preferential action of gabapentin and pregabalin at P/Q-type voltage-sensitive calcium channels: inhibition of K^+-evoked [^{3}H]-norepinephrine release from rat neocortical slices. *Synapse* 2002; 45:171–190.
97. Bian F, Li Z, Offord J, et al. Calcium channel alpha2-delta type 1 subunit is the major binding protein for pregabalin in neocortex, hippocampus, amygdala, and spinal cord: an ex vivo autoradiographic study in alpha2-delta type 1 genetically modified mice. *Brain Res* 2006; 1075:68–80.
98. Fehrenbacher JC, Taylor CP, Vasko MR. Pregabalin and gabapentin reduce release of substance P and CGRP from rat spinal tissues only after inflammation or activation of protein kinase C. *Pain* 2003; 105:133–141.
99. French JA, Kugler AR, Robbins JL, Knapp LE, et al. Dose-response trial of pregabalin adjunctive therapy in patients with partial seizures. *Neurology* 2003; 60:1631–1637.
100. Beydoun A, Uthman BM, Kugler AR, Greiner MJ, et al. Safety and efficacy of two pregabalin regimens for add-on treatment of partial epilepsy. *Neurology* 2005; 64:475–480.
101. Brodie MJ. Pregabalin as adjunctive therapy for partial seizures. *Epilepsia* 2004; 45 Suppl 6:19–27.
102. Arroyo S, Anhut H, Kugler AR, et al. Pregabalin add-on treatment: a randomized, double-blind, placebo-controlled, dose-response study in adults with partial seizures. *Epilepsia* 2004; 45:20–27.
103. Elger CE, Brodie MJ, Anhut H, Lee CM, et al. Pregabalin add-on treatment in patients with partial seizures: a novel evaluation of flexible-dose and fixed-dose treatment in a double-blind, placebo-controlled study. *Epilepsia* 2005; 46:1926–1936.

46 Lamotrigine

John M. Pellock

Lamotrigine was first approved for marketing in Ireland in 1993 and soon thereafter in most other countries, including the United Kingdom and the United States. It was initially recommended for use as adjunctive therapy in the treatment of partial seizures, but it was soon identified as possessing a much broader scope of antiepileptic action. It is one of the new broad-spectrum antiepileptic drugs (AEDs), resembling valproate in its multiple uses. Lamotrigine is nonsedating and offers several advantages, but it must be used correctly, especially in children (1–3).

CHEMISTRY, ANIMAL PHARMACOLOGY, AND MECHANISM OF ACTION

Lamotrigine (LTG) is the name given to 3,5-diamino-6-(2,3-dichlorophenyl)-1,2,4-triazine. It is a stable white powder with solubility of less than 1 mg/mL in water and 1 mg/mL in ethanol. Lamotrigine was initially developed on the basis of a probably mistaken hypothesis that some AEDs were efficacious because of an antifolate effect. A series of phenyltriazines were investigated by the Wellcome Foundation and led to the development of lamotrigine. Although it has significant antiepileptic action, its action as an antifolate is minimal (4). The identified mechanisms of action of this drug do not explain its broad range of therapeutic efficacy (5). The sole documented cellular mechanism of action is sodium channel block, a mechanism shared by phenytoin and carbamazepine. These drugs are, however, ineffective against absence seizures, and unless the sodium channel block from lamotrigine is quite unique, other mechanisms should explain its broad clinical efficacy (5). This block is both voltage and use dependent. Lamotrigine abolishes hind limb extension in the maximal electroshock model in both mouse and rat, and no tolerance is found after 28 days of dosing. Similar median effective dose (ED_{50}) values are obtained in maximal seizure tests with picrotoxin and bicuculline, but LTG has no effect on pentylenetetrazol (PTZ) threshold or clonus latency after PTZ administration, as is shown with ethosuximide and valproate and would be expected because of LTG's efficacy in absence seizures. Lamotrigine delays the development of electrical kindling in the rat and modifies seizures. A feature that clearly distinguishes it from phenytoin and carbamazepine is its inhibition of visually evoked afterdischarges in the rat, a model in which valproate and ethosuximide are also efficacious. Studies suggest that lamotrigine reduces the effects of glutamate on the rat's spinal cord. The use- and voltage-dependent aspects of lamotrigine interactions at the sodium channel may be hypothesized to be responsible both for LTG's effects in blocking veratridine-induced, but not potassium-induced, glutamate release and in reducing epileptic activity in hippocampal neurons. Coulter suggests that there are as yet undefined mechanisms through which lamotrigine works in addition to the sodium channel effects, which would be primarily responsible for the efficacy observed clinically in partial and generalized tonic-clonic seizures (5).

BIOTRANSFORMATION, PHARMACOKINETICS, AND INTERACTIONS

Lamotrigine is well absorbed, and there is a negligible first-pass metabolic effect, so that its bioavailability is virtually 100 percent. It is uniformly distributed throughout the body with a volume of distribution of 1.1 L/kg in volunteers. It is biotransformed hepatically and excreted in urine primarily as the resultant glucuronide conjugates, with only 8 percent of the compound unchanged in humans. Hepatic dysfunction, and particularly Gilbert's syndrome with its functional impairment of UGT (uridine diphosphate glucuronosyltransferase), result in lower lamotrigine metabolism and subsequent clearance (4). Metabolites are not thought to be active. Lamotrigine is approximately 55% bound to plasma proteins, which is of little clinical significance (4, 6).

The pharmacokinetics of lamotrigine in children are similar to those in adults (6). Lamotrigine exhibits first-order linear pharmacokinetics. Lamotrigine absorption is unaffected by food. In patients, the volume of distribution is between 1.25 and 1.47 L/kg. The serum half-life of lamotrigine is between 24.1 and 35 hours in drug-naïve adults, but it is significantly altered by enzyme-inducing and enzyme-inhibiting drugs, including AEDs in particular. Clinical trials have demonstrated no evidence of autoinduction or saturable metabolism. Young children, less than 5 years, eliminate lamotrigine somewhat faster than older children and adults. A half-life of 7.7 ± 1.8 hours was noted in young children receiving enzyme-inducing AEDs as cotherapy (7).

The most clinically significant pharmacokinetic finding regarding lamotrigine is that metabolism of the agent can be affected by concurrent drugs. The dosing schedule therefore must be altered whenever enzyme-inducing or enzyme-inhibiting agents are being administered before the addition of lamotrigine. Similarly, alterations in dose may be required whenever one of these AEDs is added or removed as lamotrigine is continued. The half-life of 24.1 to 35 hours in healthy adult volunteers is decreased to approximately 14 hours (6.4–32.2 hours) in those receiving enzyme-inducing drugs, such as phenytoin, carbamazepine, phenobarbital, and primidone, and increased to 30.5–88.8 hours in volunteers receiving valproate (6, 8). Whereas valproic acid decreases the clearance of lamotrigine, lamotrigine has been reported to increase the clearance of valproic acid by up to 25 percent in healthy volunteers. Lamotrigine has no significant interaction on carbamazepine or carbamazepine epoxide levels. Lamotrigine has little effect on the plasma levels of oral contraceptives (9), but hormonal therapy (including oral contraceptives) and pregnancy have been noted to interact significantly with lamotrigine, causing a decrease in plasma levels and anticonvulsant effect (10).

CLINICAL EFFICACY

Since the introduction of lamotrigine as a broad-spectrum AED, its use in both partial and generalized seizures has increased in adults and children. Although licensure and specific labeling vary, clinical practice includes use as both adjunctive and monotherapy for the treatment of various types of epilepsy.

The initial trials of lamotrigine were performed in adults with refractory partial onset epilepsy. Using double-blind, add-on, placebo-controlled trials of either crossover or parallel design, data from 457 adult patients with refractory partial epilepsy were used as the basis of the initial efficacy reports (11–19). Five of these six studies with crossover design showed significant reduction in seizure frequency with an overall 50% reduction in 25% of the patients. In these patients, who were formerly primarily on enzyme-inducing concomitant AED therapy, doses of lamotrigine ranged from 200 to 500 mg/day, with a suggestion that doses of 400 to 500 mg were more efficacious than lower doses. In addition to the seizure efficacy, nearly half of the patients reported positive global opinions regarding therapy with lamotrigine versus 22% receiving placebo. Efficacy as monotherapy in adults with partial seizures has also been established in follow-up studies and in two trials comparing monotherapy lamotrigine to that with carbamazepine or phenytoin (20, 21). Forty-three percent of patients treated with lamotrigine and 36% of patients treated with phenytoin were seizure free at the end of 24 weeks, and similar efficacy was noted with carbamazepine, as 39% of patients on lamotrigine and 38% on carbamazepine became seizure free. The rates of withdrawal were greater for those treated with phenytoin and carbamazepine than for patients treated with lamotrigine (19–22). In children, lamotrigine has shown utility in a broad range of pediatric epilepsy syndromes in addition to similar efficacy for partial seizures (23). It has been successfully used to treat primary generalized tonic clonic seizures (24), juvenile myoclonic epilepsy (25, 26), infantile spasms (27), Rett syndrome (28), absence seizures (29, 30), and seizures associated with the Lennox-Gastaut syndrome (31, 32). Myoclonic seizures, however, may not respond as well to lamotrigine therapy (33). In five open-label trials involving 285 pediatric patients, aged 1–13 years, with treatment-resistant epilepsy, 34% of all evaluable patients experienced at least a 50% decrease in seizure frequency at 12 weeks, and 41% experienced the same improvement at 48 weeks (23). Children with absence seizures, both typical and atypical, appeared to have the best response. In addition, the global evaluations reported improvement in 69% of children at 12 weeks and 74% at 48 weeks of follow-up. Rash accounted for a 7.4% discontinuation rate, whereas the overall safety data revealed a 30% discontinuation rate. In a long-term continuation study (34), similar results were noted, with 73% maintaining improvement during the follow-up period of up to 4 years. The improved global functioning, which includes increased attention and alertness, has been reported in both pediatric and adult trials, and this is especially pronounced in children with concomitant developmental and/or attentional problems (23, 31, 35). More recently, positive and negative psychotropic effects have been noted during the treatment of mentally retarded persons with epilepsy (36).

The double-blind, placebo-controlled trial of lamotrigine in the treatment of 169 patients with Lennox-Gastaut syndrome, aged 3–25 years, clearly establishes the drug as being efficacious in this difficult to treat encephalopathic epilepsy of childhood (31). Patients received either lamotrigine 50–400 mg/day (1–15 mg/kg/day), based on weight and the absence or presence of valproate coadministration or placebo as add-on therapy for 16 weeks. At the time of final evaluation, 33 percent of patients taking lamotrigine and 16 percent of patients taking placebo achieved a seizure reduction of at least 50% ($P < 0.01$). Figure 46-1 reveals the median change from baseline and the frequency of all major seizures, drop attacks, and tonic-clonic seizures during this trial. This controlled study clearly demonstrates that lamotrigine may be one of the most effective AEDs in the treatment of patients with Lennox-Gastaut syndrome.

A double-blind, randomized, placebo-controlled trial of lamotrigine add-on therapy for partial seizures in children and adolescents was performed with 201 treatment-resistant patients (37). Lamotrigine significantly reduced the frequency of all partial and secondarily generalized seizures versus placebo (44% vs. 12.8%). Neurotoxicity was only slightly more common in the lamotrigine-treated group. Although the overall rash rate was equal in the placebo group and the actively treated group, two patients receiving lamotrigine developed serious rash that resulted in hospitalization. A similar number of patients from each treatment group withdrew from the study. Thus, lamotrigine was effective for the treatment of partial seizures in children, and the safety profile was similar to that seen in adults. An interim report of an open-label phase of a similar trial performed in infants aged 1–24 months with refractory partial seizures suggests similar success (38).

The efficacy of lamotrigine monotherapy for typical absence seizures in children was studied through a "responder-enriched" study design in children and adolescents with newly diagnosed absence epilepsy. During the initial open-label dose escalation phase of the study, 71.4% of patients in the intent to treat, or 82% as evaluated in the protocol analysis, became seizure free. Individual patients responded at doses ranging from 2 to 15 mg/kg/day. In the placebo-controlled, double-blind phase, more

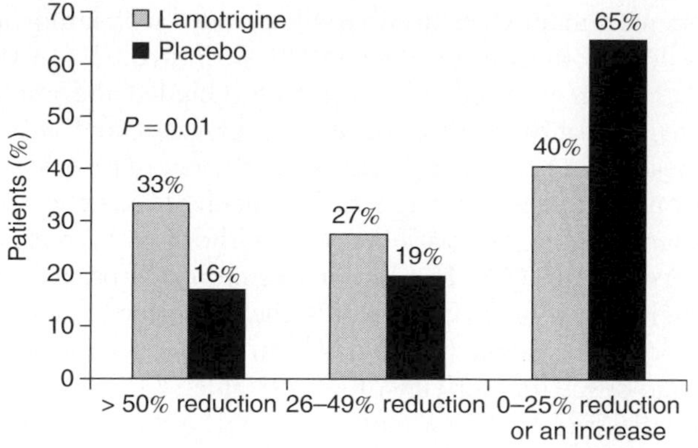

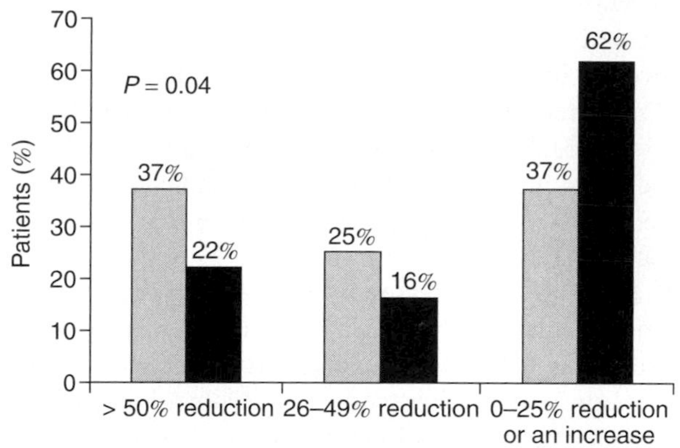

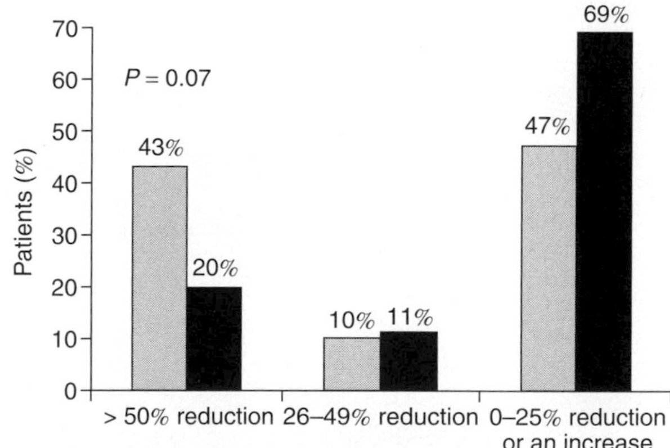

FIGURE 46-1

Median change from base line in the frequency of all types of major seizures, drop attacks, and tonic-clonic seizures during the 16-week treatment period. The values above the bars are the percentages of patients. Because of rounding, not all percentages total 100. From (31).

patients remained seizure-free when treated with lamotrigine (62%) than with placebo (21%; $P = 0.02$). In the 42 children enrolled, adverse effects included abdominal pain, headache, nausea, anorexia, dizziness, and hyperkinesia. Ten patients reported or experienced rashes, but in only one case was the rash considered attributable to lamotrigine. No patients were withdrawn because of adverse events (30). In addition to childhood absence and generalized tonic clonic seizures, the syndrome of juvenile myoclonic epilepsy (JME) has been studied to assess the broad-spectrum activity of lamotrigine. Timmings (25) initially studied 17 patients with JME who had experienced intolerable side effects or were uncontrolled with valproate. No difference in seizure control was observed between the two groups, with patients titrated to maximum daily dose of 500 mg lamotrigine and 2,500 for valproate. In an open-label study, Morris and colleagues (26) reported in patients previously treated with valproate ($n = 63$), 85% became seizure free, and 70% had no myoclonus during 8 weeks of maintenance. In new-onset patients ($n = 29$), 75% became seizure-free and had no myoclonus.

Retrospective reviews (39–42) showed generally positive results for the control of patients with JME and in primary generalized epilepsy. Adverse effects are in the ranges reported in other studies. The control of myoclonic seizures is variable and ranges from excellent to seemingly being exacerbated in individual patients, but some people have the entire spectrum of seizures controlled with lamotrigine (43).

ADVERSE EFFECTS

The toxicity profile of lamotrigine includes common adverse events seen with other AEDs, including dizziness, diplopia, headache, ataxia, blurred vision, nausea, somnolence, and vomiting (1, 2, 4, 19, 35, 37). These classic neurotoxic adverse effects were more commonly seen in trials using adjunctive therapy and less frequently noted when lamotrigine was administered as monotherapy (Table 46-1). During the clinical trials, rash was the most common reason for discontinuation of lamotrigine and subsequently has become the most feared adverse effect, as the potential for developing a life-threatening rash associated with lamotrigine administration has been recognized.

The overall rash rate during the administration of lamotrigine is approximately 10 percent to 12 percent (44, 45). The rash associated with lamotrigine was initially described as maculopapular or erythematous in appearance, displaying characteristics of a delayed hypersensitivity reaction. It was thought to be self-limited, and no alterations in dosing were suggested. Recent work indicates that the immunologic changes associated with lamotrigine-induced rash may be considered an immune-mediated hypersensitivity reaction (44). This rash typically appears within the first 4 weeks of therapy and is rarely seen after 8 weeks. Subsequently, mostly children and fewer adults have developed a more severe erythema multiforme–type eruption, sometimes progressing to desquamation with involvement of mucous membranes resembling Stevens-Johnson or Lyell syndrome. Some patients clearly had

TABLE 46-1
Pooled Tolerability from Controlled Comparative Trials of Lamotrigine Monotherapy

	Incidence, % of Patients		
Adverse Event[a]	Lamotrigine (N = 443)	Carbamazepine (N = 246)	Phenytoin (N = 95)
Headache	20	17	19
Asthenia[b]	16	24	29
Rash	12	14	9
Nausea[c]	10	10	4
Dizziness[b]	8	14	13
Somnolence[b]	8	20	28
Insomnia[c]	6	2	3
Flulike syndrome	5	4	3
Rhinitis	4	4	2
Vomiting	4	4	1

[a]Incidence of the most frequently reported adverse events in patients with newly diagnosed or recurrent epilepsy.
[b]Statistically less common with lamotrigine than with carbamazepine or phenytoin or both.
[c]Statistically more common with lamotrigine than with carbamazepine or phenytoin.
(Glaxo Wellcome Kline, data on file.)

a generalized hypersensitivity reaction, but in others the reaction was limited to the skin. Reviews concerning the incidence of lamotrigine-associated rash confirm that it is slightly higher in children and when lamotrigine is initiated during concomitant therapy with valproate (45). It also has been suggested that rapid increases in rate of titration of lamotrigine will increase the risk of rash (17, 35, 45). Although a potential metabolite has been suggested as responsible for this reaction, none has been proven (46), but the hypersensitivity syndrome has been confirmed by lymphocyte stimulation in vitro (47). At present, it is estimated that approximately one adult in 1,000 and one child in 100–200 treated with lamotrigine may be at risk for this potentially life-threatening dermatologic reaction (45). Prior AED hypersensitivity reactions may be a predisposing condition (48). The incidence of rash in placebo-controlled trials evaluating adjunctive therapy with lamotrigine in pediatric patients (<16 years) was 14% (n = 168) for patients receiving lamotrigine and 12% (n = 171) for patients receiving placebo (49). The overall rate of discontinuation due to any rash in all premarketing clinical trials with lamotrigine as adjunctive therapy was 4.4% (n = 1,081) in children. The prescribing information in the United States for lamotrigine (Lamictal®) contains a boxed warning concerning serious rashes requiring hospitalization and discontinuation of treatment in associated with its use. As stated in the package insert: "Other than age, there are as yet no factors identified that are known to predict the risk of occurrence or the severity of rash associated with lamotrigine. There are suggestions, yet to be proven, that the risk of rash may also be increased by (1) coadministration of lamotrigine with valproate (includes valproic acid and divalproex sodium), (2) exceeding the recommended initial dose of lamotrigine, or (3) exceeding the recommended dose escalation for lamotrigine. However, cases have been reported in the absence of these factors." Postmarketing evaluations continue to show that nearly all cases of life-threatening rashes associated with lamotrigine have occurred within 2 to 8 weeks of treatment, but isolated cases have been reported after prolonged treatment greater than 6 months. The incidence of these serious rashes, including Stevens-Johnson syndrome, is approximately 0.8% (8/1000) in children < 16 years of age and 0.3% (3/1000) in adults. In a prospectively followed cohort of 1,983 pediatric patients taking adjunctive lamotrigine, there was one rash-related death (50). Of particular interest are the data from a registry for all serious cutaneous reactions in western Germany, which has existed since 1990. Since 1996, all of Germany has been included in this registry (51–54). In this academically based registry of an intensive reporting system, it is felt that almost all cases of Stevens-Johnson and toxic epidermal necrolysis are detected prospectively and confirmed by expert review. During the last six months of 1993, when lamotrigine was first marketed in Germany, there were five cases of Stevens-Johnson syndrome or toxic epidermal necrolysis associated with lamotrigine reported in an estimated 4,050 adults patients exposed to lamotrigine. Four patients were also receiving valproate. In the third quarter of 1993, the dosing regimen was amended (starting dose when used with VPA was reduced from 15 mg daily to 25 mg alternative days), and physicians were educated accordingly. Despite the continued increase in use of lamotrigine from 1994 to the present, the incidence of these serious reactions has declined significantly. The German registry data through 2001 estimate Stevens-Johnson occurrence in 0.04% of children and 0.02% of adults (55). These data suggest that careful selection of patients and dose titration may improve the risk/benefit ratio in patients, and especially children, when treated with lamotrigine.

The warning in the prescribing information distributed with lamotrigine that the medication "should ordinarily be discontinued at the first sign of rash" may not be followed outside the United States because of the benign nature of most episodes of rash, even those associated with lamotrigine. When rash is associated with flu-like symptoms and malaise, myalgia, lymphadenopathy, or eosinophilia, this suggests a hypersensitivity reaction. The development of these reactions is more common in those who have experienced prior allergic symptoms to medications, particularly those who have experienced allergic or hypersensitivity reactions to AEDs. It is unclear that the present recommendations suggesting slower dosage titration truly reduce the rate of rash, but recognizing the risk patterns and paying careful attention to titration and dose schedule are mandatory. The clinician's challenge is to work with the family and patient to determine which possible skin changes indicate a serious dermatologic complication. The time course of appearance (within 4–8 weeks), associated symptoms, distribution over the body, and rash characteristics may significantly help in making a decision to discontinue therapy.

Lamotrigine is felt by many to be a nearly ideal AED because of its favorable long-term adverse effect profile, once rash does not occur during the first few months of use. Its relative lack of interactions with other drugs made it a preferred agent in many. In 2006, emerging data from the north American Antiepileptic Drug Pregnancy Registry detected an elevated prevalence of isolated, nonsyndromic cleft palate deformity in infants exposed to lamotrigine monotherapy during the first trimester of pregnancy compared to the reference population (3 in 564; 8.9 per 1000 vs. 0.37 per 1000) (56). This information suggests that lamotrigine should be used in pregnancy when the potential benefits outweigh any possible risk to the developing fetus.

The adverse-effect profile of lamotrigine must be balanced against its broad spectrum efficacy and seemingly positive effects on cognition and behavior (57, 58).

CLINICAL USE

National and international guidelines and expert consensus statements select lamotrigine as a major AED for the treatment of both partial and generalized epilepsy (59–63). Its indication for bipolar mood disorders further enhances lamotrigine's utility in the treatment of children with comorbid behavioral disorders, especially depression (49). Despite the neurobehavioral toxicity noted, it is well tolerated in most adults and children. Direct comparisons reveal positive behavioral and quality of life ratings of patient perceptions. In healthy young adult volunteers, lamotrigine and gabapentin had no performance or other changes, whereas topiramate demonstrated neurocognitive interference after acute and chronic dosing (58). The term *brightening* has been used as patients seem to become less sedated and more alert and attentive.

Because of concomitant AED interactions and the potential to increase life-threatening rash (see the section on adverse effects), the dosing of lamotrigine must be carefully approached. Table 46-2 lists the recommended doses for children and adults (6, 10). Initial dosing, using the 2-mg, 5-mg, or 25-mg tablets, is frequently appropriate in children, especially those receiving valproate. The 2-mg or 5-mg dispersible tablets allows for correct dosing to be accomplished even in most infants. It is recommended that titration of dosage be done every 2 weeks until the desired clinical effect, usual maintenance dose, or clinical toxicity occurs. It is imperative that one prescribe the initial dose in children on enzyme-inducing AEDs at 0.6 mg/kg/day, but this initial dose must be decreased to 0.15 mg/kg/day if valproic acid is being administered (10). Note that the usual maintenance dose while on valproate is approximately one-third that otherwise required if enzyme-inducing AEDs continue to be administered without valproate. Although there is no noted pharmacokinetic interaction with carbamazepine or other AEDs, we have found that as lamotrigine doses are increased in some patients to over 600 mg/day, increased neurotoxicity is observed. This pharmacodynamic interaction can be alleviated by reducing existing higher doses and levels, particularly of carbamazepine, slightly (typically by only 100–200 mg/day) to allow further escalation of lamotrigine.

Initial blood level determination in those experiencing improved seizure control were below 5 μg/mL. Subsequent experience would suggest that levels at least 12–15 μg/mL are well tolerated by some people, especially when lamotrigine is used as monotherapy, with continued seizure improvement as doses are titrated upward. Nevertheless, more neurotoxicity is to be expected at levels in this upper range or above.

FORMULATIONS

The preparations of Lamictal (lamotrigine) available in the United States have increased in number and quality. Tablets are available in doses of 25, 100, 150, and 200 mg and chewable dispersible tablets are available in doses of 2 mg, 5 mg, and 25 mg. It is extremely important for the clinician to be sure to indicate tablet or chewable/dispersible tablet when prescribing medications, depending upon the ability of the child to swallow the dosage form. Generic formulations are now available.

TABLE 46-2
Lamotrigine Dose Recommendations in Children and Adults

Concurrent AED	Weeks 1 and 2	Weeks 3 and 4	Usual Maintenance Dose
Children			
EIAED	0.6 mg/kg/day	1.2 mg/kg/day	5–15 mg/kg/day
Monotherapy	0.3 mg/kg/day	0.6 mg/kg/day	2–8 mg/kg/day
Valproic Acid	0.15 mg/kg/day	0.3 mg/kg/day	1–5 mg/kg/day
Adults			
With EIAEDs but no VPA	50 mg/day (once a day)	100 mg/day (2 divided doses)	300–500 mg/day (2 divided doses). Escalate dose by 100 mg/day every week
With EIAEDs and VPA	25 mg every other day	25 mg/day	100–400 mg/day (2 divided doses). Escalate dose by 25–50 mg/day every 1 or 2 weeks

EIAED: enzyme-inducing antiepileptic drug. Modified from (6, 11).

CONCLUSION

Lamotrigine is a broad-spectrum AED that is effective against both partial and generalized convulsive and nonconvulsive seizures. Its efficacy has been demonstrated in numerous studies in both adult and childhood epilepsy. It joins valproate, felbamate, topiramate, zonisamide, and levetiracetam as broad-spectrum agents. Each agent differs slightly in efficacy profiles and reported adverse effects. Improved behavior and brightening has been commonly reported in those taking lamotrigine, whether adjunctive AEDs have been removed or continued. Careful dose titration should be followed during the initiation of this agent, and removal of concomitant agents will allow optimization of monotherapy and total dosing.

References

1. Pellock JM, ed. Lamotrigine. *J Child Neurol* 1997; 12(Suppl 1):S1–S52.
2. Fitton A, Goa KL. Lamotrigine: an update of its pharmacology and therapeutic use in epilepsy. *Drugs* 1995; 50:691–713.
3. Goa KL, Ross SR, Chrisp P.Lamotrigine. A review of its pharmacological properties and clinical efficacy in epilepsy. *Drugs* 1993; 46:152–176.
4. Binnie CD. Lamotrigine. In: Engel J, Pedley TA, eds. *Epilepsy: A Comprehensive Textbook*. Philadelphia: Lippincott-Raven, 1997:1531–1540.
5. Coulter DA. Antiepileptic drug cellular mechanisms of action: where does lamotrigine fit in? *J Child Neurol* 1997; 12(Suppl 1):S2–S9.
6. Garnett WR. Lamotrigine: pharmacokinetics. *J Child Neurol* 1997; 12(Suppl 1): S10–S15.
7. Vauzelle-Kervdroedan F, Rey E, Cieuta C, et al. Influence of concurrent antiepileptic medication on the pharmacokinetics of lamotrigine as add-on therapy in epileptic children. *Br J Clin Pharmacol* 1996; 41:325–330.
8. Ramsay RE, Pellock JM, Garnett WR, et al. Pharmacokinetics and safety of lamotrigine (Lamictal) in patients with epilepsy. *Epilepsy Res* 1991; 10:191–200.
9. Holdrich T, Whiteman P, Orme M, et al. Effect of lamotrigine on the pharmacology of the combined oral contraceptive pill. *Epilepsia* 1991; 32(Suppl 1):96.
10. Sidhu J. Bulsara S, Job S, et al. A bidirectional pharmacokinetic interaction study of lamotrigine and the combined oral contraceptive pill in healthy subjects. *Epilepsia* 2004; 45(suppl 7):330.
11. Messenheimer JA, Guberman AH. Rash with lamotrigine: dosing guidelines. *Epilepsia* 2000; 41:488.
12. Binnie CD, Debets RM, Engelsman M, et al. Double-blind, crossover trial of lamotrigine (Lamictal) as add-on therapy in intractable epilepsy. *Epilepsy Res* 1989; 4:222–229.
13. Jawad S, Richens A, Goodwin G, Yuen WC. Controlled trial of lamotrigine (Lamictal) for refractory partial seizures. *Epilepsia* 1989; 30:356–363.
14. Loiseau P, Yuen AWC, Duche B, et al. A randomised double-blind placebo-controlled crossover add-on trial of lamotrigine in patients with treatment-resistant partial seizures. *Epilepsy Res* 1990; 7:136–145.
15. Sanders J, Patsalos P, Oxley J, et al. A randomized, double blind, placebo-controlled, add-on trial of lamotrigine in patients with severe epilepsy. *Epilepsy Res* 1990; 6:221–226.
16. Matsuo F, Bergen D, Faught E, et al. Placebo-controlled study of the efficacy and safety of lamotrigine in patients with partial seizures. *Neurology* 1993; 43:2284–2291.
17. Schapel GJ, Beran RG, Vajda FJE, et al. Double-blind, placebo-controlled, crossover study of lamotrigine in treatment resistant partial seizures. *J Neurol Neurosurg Psychiatry* 1993; 56:448–453.
18. Messenheimer JA, Ramsay RA, Willmore LJ, et al. Lamotrigine therapy for partial seizures: a multicenter placebo-controlled, double-blind, crossover trial. *Epilepsia* 1994; 35:113–121.
19. Smith D, Baker G, Davies G, et al. Outcome of add-on treatment with lamotrigine in partial epilepsy. *Epilepsia* 1993; 34:312–322.
20. Willmore LJ, Messenheimer JA. Adult experience with lamotrigine. *J Child Neurol* 1997; 12(Suppl 1):S16–S18.
21. Brodie Mj, Richens A, Yuen AWC. Double-blind comparison of lamotrigine and carbamazepine in newly diagnosed epilepsy. *Lancet* 1995; 345:476–479.
22. Steiner TJ, Silviera C, Yuen AWC. Comparison of lamotrigine (Lamictal) and phenytoin monotherapy in newly diagnosed epilepsy. *Epilepsia* 1994; 35(Suppl 3):S82.
23. Besag FMC, Wallace SJ, Dulac O, et al. Lamotrigine for the treatment of epilepsy in childhood. *J Pediatrics* 1995; 127:991–997.
24. Trevathan E, Keris SP, Hammer AE, Vuong A, et al. Lamotrigine adjunctive therapy among children and adolescents with primary generalized tonic-clonic seizures. *Pediatrics* 2006; 118(2):371–378.
25. Timmings PL, Richens A. Efficacy of lamotrigine as monotherapy for juvenile myoclonic epilepsy: pilot study results. *Epilepsia* 1993; 34(Suppl 2):S160 (abstract).
26. Morris G, Schimschock J, Vuong A, et al. Broad spectrum activity of lamotrigine monotherapy in patients with juvenile myoclonic epilepsy. *Epilepsia* 2000; 41(suppl 7):90.
27. Veggiotti P, Cieuta C, Rey E, et al. Lamotrigine in infantile spasms. *Lancet* 1994; 344:1375–1376.
28. Uldall P, Hansen FJ, Tonnby B. Lamotrigine in Rett syndrome. *Neuropediatrics* 1993; 24:339–340.
29. Ferrie CD, Robinson RO, Knott C, et al. Lamotrigine as an add-on drug in typical absence seizures. *Acta Neurol Scand* 1995; 91:200–202.
30. Frank LM, Enlow T. Holmes GL, et al. Lamictal (lamotrigine) monotherapy for typical absence seizures in children. *Epilepsia* 1999; 40:973–979.
31. Motte J, Trevathan E, Arvidsson JFV, et al. Lamotrigine for generalized seizures associated with the Lennox-Gastaut syndrome. *N Engl J Med* 1997; 337:1807–1812.
32. Ericksson A-S, Nergardh A, Hoppu K. The efficacy of lamotrigine in children and adolescents with refractory generalized epilepsy: a randomized, double-blind, crossover study. *Epilepsia* 1998; 39:495–501.
33. Guerrini R, Dravet C, Genton P, et al. Lamotrigine and seizure aggravation in severe myoclonic epilepsy. *Epilepsia* 1998; 39:508–512.
34. Besag FMC, Dulac O, Alving J, et al. Long-term safety and efficacy of lamotrigine (Lamictal) in pediatric patients with epilepsy. *Seizure* 1997; 6:51–56.
35. Pellock JM: Overview of lamotrigine and the new antiepileptic drugs: the challenge. *J Child Neurol* 1997; 12(Suppl 1):S48–S52.
36. Ettinger AB, Weisbrot DM, Saracco J, et al. Positive and negative psychotropic effects of lamotrigine in patients with epilepsy and mental retardation. *Epilepsia* 1998; 39(8): 874–877.
37. Duchowny M, Pellock JM, Graf WD, et al. A double blind, randomized, placebo-controlled trial of lamotrigine add-on therapy for partial seizures in children and adolescents. *Neurology* 1999; 53:1724–1731.
38. Pina-Garza JE, Womble G, Blum D, et al. Safety and efficacy of lamotrigine in infants age 1–24 months with partial seizures—interim open-label results. Poster presentation at the annual meeting of the American Epilepsy Society, Seattle, WA. December 6–12, 2002.
39. Stein AG, Carrazanna EJ. Exacerbations of juvenile myoclonic epilepsy with lamotrigine. *Neurology* 2001; 56:1424.
40. Prasad A, Knowlton R, Mendez M, et al. A comparison of lamotrigine and topiramate in juvenile myoclonic epilepsy. *Epilepsia* 2002; 43(Suppl 7):198–199 (abstract).
41. Welty TE, Martin JN, Faught E, et al. Comparison of outcomes in patients with juvenile myoclonic epilepsy treated with lamotrigine, topiramate, zonisamide, or levetiracetam. *Epilepsia* 2002; 43 (suppl 7):239 (abstract).
42. Kivity S, Rechtman E. Lamotrigine therapy in patients with juvenile myoclonic epilepsy and valproate related progressive weight gain. *Epilepsia* 2001; 42 (suppl 4):41 (abstract).
43. Dean JC, Muraoka LM, Wiser TH, et al. Outcomes of switch therapy in seizure patients: divalproex sodium to lamotrigine. *Epilepsia* 2001; 42(suppl 7):178 (abstract).
44. Iannetti P, Raucci U, Zuccaro P, Pacifici R. Lamotrigine hypersensitivity in childhood epilepsy. *Epilepsia* 1998; 39:502–507.
45. Guberman AH, Besag F, Brodie MJ, et al. Lamotrigine induced rash: risk/benefit considerations in adults and children. *Epilepsia* 1999; 40:985–991.
46. Anderson GA. Children versus adults: pharmokinetic and adverse effect differences. *Epilepsia* 2002; 43(suppl 3):53–59.
47. Karande S, Gogtay NJ, Kanchan S, Kshirsagar NA. Anticonvulsant hypersensitivity syndrome to lamotrigine confirmed by lymphocyte stimulation in vitro. *Indian J Med Sci* 2006; 60(2):59–63.
48. Hirsch LJ, Weintraub DB, Buchsbaum R, Spencer HT, et al. Predictors of lamotrigine-associated rash. *Epilepsia* 2006; 47(2):318–322.
49. Prescribing information for Lamictal® tablets and Lamictal® chewable dispersible tablets. In: *Physicians' Desk Reference*. Montvale, NJ: Thomson-PDR, 2006 http://us.gsk.com/products/assets/us_lamictal.pdf
50. Messenheimer JA. Rash in adult and pediatric patients treated with lamotrigine. *Can J Neurol Sci* 1998; 25:S14–S18.
51. Mockenhaupt M, Schlingmann J. Schroeder W, et al. Antiepileptic therapy and the risk for severe cutaneous adverse reactions (SCAR). *Neurology* 2000; 54(suppl 3):A84.
52. Rzany B. Mockenhaupt M. Baur S, et al. Epidemiology of erythema exsudativum multiforme majus, Stevens-Johnson syndrome, and toxic epidermal necrolysis in Germany (1990–1992): structure and results of a population-based registry. *J Clin Epidemiol* 1996; 49:769–773.
53. Messenheimer JA. New information confirming the importance of dosing and rash with lamotrigine. Poster presentation at the Lamotrigine Clinical Update session at the American Epilepsy Society Meeting, Los Angeles, CA, December 1–6, 2000.
54. Messenheimer JA. The incidence of AED-related Stevens-Johnson syndrome in the German registry of serious cutaneous reactions: pediatric vs. adult rates. Poster presentation at the Lamotrigine Clinical Update session at the American Epilepsy Society Meeting, Philadelphia, PA, November 30–December 5, 2001.
55. Hoyler S. Kustra RP, Messenheimer JA, et al. Serious cutaneous reactions with antiepileptic drugs: adult and pediatric incidence estimates from registry and prescription data in Germany. Poster presented at the 6th Annual meeting of the College of Neurologic and Psychiatric Pharmacists, Charleston, SC, May 1–3, 2003.

56. Holmes LB, Wyszynski DF, Balwin EJ, Haebecker E, et al. Increased risk for non-syndromic cleft palate among infants exposed to lamotrigine during pregnancy. *Birth Defects Res A Clin Mol Teratol* 2006; 76(5):318 (abstract).
57. Meador KJ, Baker GA. Behavioral and cognitive effects of lamotrigine. *J Child Neurol* 1997; 12(Suppl 1):S44–S47.
58. Mortin R, Kuzniecky R, Ho S, et al. Cognitive effects of topiramate, gabapentin, and lamotrigine in healthy young adults. *Neurology* 1999; 52:321–327.
59. Karceski S, Morrell MJ, Carpenter D. Treatment of epilepsy in adults: expert opinion, 2005. *Epilepsy Behav* 2005; 7 Suppl 1:S1–S64; quiz S65–S67.
60. Glauser T, Ben-Menachem E, Bourgeois B, Cnaan A, et al. ILAE treatment guidelines: evidence-based analysis of antiepileptic drug efficacy and effectiveness as initial monotherapy for epileptic seizures and syndrome. *Epilepsia* 2006; 47(7);1094–1120.
61. Wheless JW, Clarke DF, Carpenter D. Treatment of pediatric epilepsy: expert opinion, 2005. *J Child Neurol* 2005; 20 Suppl 1:S1–S56; quiz S59–S60.
62. French JA, Kanner AM, Bautista J, et al. Efficacy and tolerability of the new antiepileptic drugs, I: treatment of new onset epilepsy: report of the Therapeutics and Technology Assessment Subcommittee and Quality Standards Subcommittee of the American Academy of Neurology and the American Epilepsy Society. *Neurology* 2004; 62:1252–1260.
63. French JA, Kanner, AM, Bautista J, et al. Efficacy and tolerability of the new antiepileptic drugs, I: treatment of new-onset epilepsy: report of the TTA and QSS Subcommittees of the American Academy of Neurology and the American Epilepsy Society. *Epilepsia* 2004; 45:401–409.

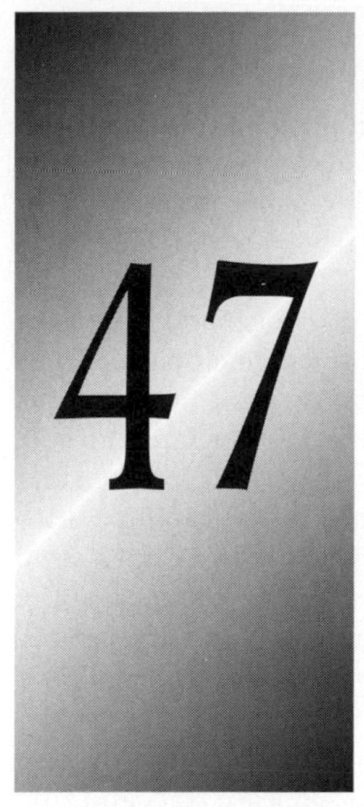

Levetiracetam

Raman Sankar
W. Donald Shields

Levetiracetam (LEV), (−)-(S)-alpha-ethyl-2-oxo-1-pyrrolidine acetamide (Figure 47-1), is an antiepileptic drug (AED) chemically related to the nootropic (cognition-enhancing) agent piracetam (1). Since piracetam was known to suppress myoclonic jerks (2), similar drugs were evaluated for anticonvulsant efficacy, leading to the discovery and development of levetiracetam as an AED.

Levetiracetam (LEV) has been available in the United States since 2000 and is marketed under the trade name Keppra®. It is currently indicated as adjunctive therapy in the treatment of partial-onset seizures in adults and children ≥4 years of age. It was recently approved for treatment of myoclonus as well. However, it is used in patients younger than 4 years, as monotherapy and in other epilepsy types.

CHEMISTRY, ANIMAL PHARMACOLOGY, AND MECHANISM OF ACTION

Preclinical Studies

The pharmacologic activity of levetiracetam has been evaluated in rats and mice. Levetiracetam is not active in the classical acute models of maximal electroshock (MES) and pentylenetetrazole (PTZ) seizures in mice (3). However, LEV does display potent and selective protection against kindling in a broad range of animal models of chronic epilepsy (3–5). This profile distinguishes LEV from most other AEDs, which demonstrate similar activity in both acute and chronic seizure models (3).

The fact that levetiracetam protects animals that have been made epileptic via kindling establishes its anticonvulsant activity (4). However, in addition to its anticonvulsant activity, LEV may also be antiepileptogenic, as suggested by the fact that LEV exposure retards the acquisition of kindling (5). It is important to note that this type of antiepileptogenic activity has been demonstrated by some newer AEDs (6–8), but not by others (9).

Levetiracetam also has a high safety margin, as evidenced by a remarkable separation between the dose that protects against convulsions and the dose that impairs rotarod performance. This observation was borne out of data in corneal electroshock–kindled mice and Genetic Absence Epilepsy Rats from Strasbourg (GAERS), which showed a high therapeutic index for LEV (3). Additionally, LEV demonstrates activity in animal models believed to represent generalized epilepsy. Levetiracetam has been shown to protect against seizures induced by acoustic stimulation in sound-sensitive mice (10) and rats (11) and against spike-and-wave discharges in GAERS rats (11). Levetiracetam was able to terminate self-sustaining status

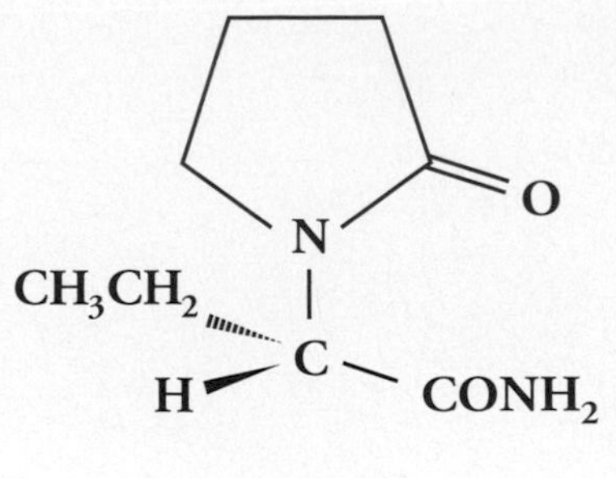

$$CH_3CH_2 \text{ — } C(H)(CONH_2) \text{ — } N \text{ (2-oxopyrrolidine)}$$

FIGURE 47-1

Levetiracetam [(−)-(S)-alpha-ethyl-2-oxo-1-pyrrolidine acetamide].

epilepticus in rats and displayed synergy with diazepam in this model (12). Some limited animal data also indicate neuroprotective effects of LEV in models of status epilepticus (13, 14).

Mechanism of Action

Fortuitously, LEV was discovered to have antiepileptic properties prior to undergoing NIH-standardized animal-model testing, which showed that LEV was not active in the standard models (15). This observation was an indication that LEV has a novel mechanism of action. It also indicates that the NIH-standardized screening may be missing important therapeutic agents and opportunities. Further evidence supporting novel activity lies in the fact that LEV does not produce changes in neuronal excitability by modulation of any of the three main mechanisms underlying classical AED activity (i.e., use-dependent blockade of voltage-gated sodium channels, inhibition of low-threshold [T-type] calcium currents, and augmentation of GABAergic inhibitory responses) (16–18).

In-vitro testing has shown that LEV does not displace ligands specific for 55 different binding sites, including receptor systems, reuptake sites, second messenger systems, and channel proteins (3). The exact mechanism of antiepileptic action of LEV remains to be elucidated; however, the following preclinical studies indicate that certain atypical cellular effects may be involved in reducing neuronal excitability:

- In isolated CA1 hippocampal neurons, LEV inhibits high-voltage–activated calcium currents (19, 20), with selective blockade of N-type calcium channels (20).
- From studies in isolated hippocampal, spinal, and cerebellar neurons, and in sound-susceptible mice, LEV has been shown to suppress negative allosteric modulators (zinc and beta-carbolines) of GABA- and glycine-gated currents (21). Although hyperexcitability may underlie some of the genetic epilepsies that are presently regarded as channelopathies, the acquired epilepsies seem to reveal anatomic and physiologic evidence of seizure-associated circuit rearrangement, which may be, in part, responsible for their intractability. Space in this chapter does not permit extensive discussion of the role of mossy fiber sprouting in the epileptogenic process, but it should be mentioned that mossy fiber sprouting is seen both in experimental models of temporal lobe epilepsy as well as in human hippocampi resected during surgical treatment of mesial temporal lobe epilepsy. Mossy fiber synapses release zinc, and zinc antagonizes GABA-mediated inhibition. The ability of LEV to reverse this interference by zinc of GABAergic inhibition (21) may thus be relevant to its effect on chronic or established epilepsy in animal models.
- One study, in isolated CA1 hippocampal neurons, suggests that LEV may produce a modest reduction in the delayed-rectifier potassium current, thereby lengthening repolarization time (22). A more recent study, however, detected no effect of LEV on the delayed-rectifier potassium current (23).
- Levetiracetam has shown activity in blocking *synchronization* in a slice experiment in which conventional AEDs such as valproic acid, benzodiazepines, and carbamazepine (CBZ) were inactive (24, 25). This is quite interesting because conventional AEDs have been shown to have impact mainly on *hyperexcitability*, even though the two underpinnings of the epileptic state are hypersynchrony and hyperexcitability. How does LEV accomplish this? Could it be antagonizing currents mediated by gap junctions that are responsible for "local" synchrony? We do not know for certain, but the possibility is intriguing.
- Levetiracetam has been shown to bind to a synaptic vesicle–associated protein known as SV2A (26). Mice homozygous for SV2A gene disruption exhibit deficiency in action potential-dependent GABAergic neurotransmission and develop spontaneous seizures (27). It has been proposed that SV2 may enhance neurotransmitter release probability at quiescent synapses by priming vesicles (28). The full details pertaining to the interaction of LEV with vesicle docking and neurotransmitter release remains to be elucidated.

BIOTRANSFORMATION, PHARMACOKINETICS, AND INTERACTIONS IN HUMANS

Over 30 clinical studies have evaluated both the single- and multiple-dose pharmacokinetics of LEV following oral administration. Data from these studies have delineated the pharmacokinetic profile of LEV (29, 30) (Table 47-1).

Absorption and Distribution

Pharmacokinetic data in adults show that LEV is rapidly and almost completely absorbed after oral administration. Absolute oral bioavailability is nearly 100%, and food does not affect the extent of absorption, but does slow the rate of absorption. Peak plasma levels are generally achieved within 1 hour following oral administration in fasted subjects, and steady-state plasma levels are reached after 2 days of twice-daily dosing. Levetiracetam exhibits linear pharmacokinetics at recommended doses (29). Levetiracetam is not extensively bound (10%) to plasma proteins, and its volume of distribution is close to that of intracellular and extracellular body water (29).

Metabolism and Elimination

Levetiracetam is not extensively metabolized in humans (24% of a dose). The main metabolic pathway involves enzymatic hydrolysis of the acetamide group, is independent of the cytochrome P450 system, and results in the formation of the major metabolite of LEV, which is pharmacologically inactive (29,30). Levetiracetam plasma half-life is 7.0 hours and is unaffected by dose or repeated administration. Elimination of both LEV and its major metabolite is via renal excretion, whereby 66% of a dose is excreted as unchanged drug. Total body clearance of LEV is 0.96 mL/min/kg. Renal clearance is 0.6 mL/min/kg and is directly proportional to creatinine clearance (29,30).

In patients with renal impairment, the elimination half-life of LEV is prolonged and total body clearance is decreased 35% to 60%, compared with that in healthy subjects. Thus, daily maintenance doses should be reduced in these patients. Levetiracetam is dialyzable; therefore, supplemental doses should be given to patients following dialysis (29, 30).

Elderly patients experiencing age-related renal function decline may also require dose reduction of LEV based on their estimated creatinine clearance. Patients with hepatic impairment have no changes in LEV pharmacokinetics, and therefore require no dose reduction (29).

TABLE 47-1
Levetiracetam Pharmacokinetic Profile

Parameter	Effect
Absorption	Rapidly and almost-completely (>95%) absorbed No saturable absorption No food interaction
Distribution	
t_{max}	1.3 hr
C_{max}	2.3 μg/mL
AUC	222 μg · hr/mL
Enzyme kinetics	Linear kinetics; C_{max} and AUC are proportional in single doses up to 5000 mg
t_{ss}	After 48 hr
Plasma-protein binding	<10%
Vd	0.5–0.7 L/kg
Metabolism	Minimal; in blood to the inactive deaminated metabolite L057 Not dependent on the hepatic CYP system No auto-induction
Elimination	In urine; 66% as parent drug, 24% as L057
$t_{1/2}$	Adults 6–8 hr, elderly 10–11 hr, children 6 hr

t_{ss}, time to plasma steady-state concentration; $t_{1/2}$, elimination half-life.

Source: From Patsalos PN. Pharmacokinetic profile of levetiracetam: toward ideal characteristics. From (29), with permission.

Pediatric Pharmacokinetics

Pharmacokinetic data in children derive from a multicenter, open-label, single-dose titration study (31). Twenty-four patients (aged 6 to 12 years) received oral LEV as adjunctive therapy at a dose of 20 mg/kg/day. In this pediatric study, LEV clearance was 30 to 40% higher than in adults, resulting in a lower C and area under the curve (AUC) equated for a 1 mg/kg dose. A correspondingly shorter half-life, of 6.01 hours, was observed. Additionally, no significant gender or age differences in pharmacokinetic parameters of LEV were noted. Based on these data, a dose equal to 130% to 140% of the usual daily adult dose in two divided doses, on a weight-normalized level, may be the most appropriate daily maintenance dose in children.

Drug Interactions

Early study of metabolic interactions indicated a low potential for LEV drug interactions (32), and support of this observation has been borne out in additional studies. Pooled data from pivotal Phase III trials confirm that LEV has no known interactions with other AEDs (33). Additionally, LEV does not influence the pharmacokinetics of an oral contraceptive containing ethinyl estradiol and levonorgestrel; on the basis of serum progesterone and luteinizing hormone levels, it does not affect contraceptive efficacy (34). Levetiracetam also does not affect the pharmacokinetics of digoxin (35) and warfarin (36).

CLINICAL EFFICACY

Partial Seizures

The efficacy of LEV in adults has been evaluated extensively. Three randomized, double-blind, placebo-controlled clinical trials conducted in the United States and Europe that enrolled 904 patients were pivotal in supporting LEV efficacy as adjunctive therapy in adults with refractory partial-onset seizures with or without secondary generalization (37–39). All three of these studies evaluated LEV using similar methodology. After an 8-week to 12-week baseline period, patients entered a titration phase where, upon randomization, they had doses titrated upward every 2 weeks over a period of 4 to 6 weeks to a final dose of 1,000, 2,000, or 3,000 mg/day in divided doses, or placebo. Subsequent to titration, a 12-week to 14-week evaluation phase, followed by an optional open-label phase, was completed. A pooled efficacy analysis of these placebo-controlled studies (40) indicates the following. In all three of these studies and in all dose groups, compared with placebo, treatment with LEV resulted in reduced seizure frequency that was statistically significant. Patients receiving LEV achieved a 31% median decrease in seizures from baseline, compared with only a 5.4% median decline in placebo-treated patients ($P < 0.001$). Additionally, 35% of LEV-treated patients achieved 50% seizure reduction, compared with 9.4% of placebo-treated patients ($P < 0.001$). In these studies, increasing response was associated with increasing dose. Whereas the 50% responder rate in placebo-treated patients was 9.4%, 50% responder rates at doses of 1,000, 2,000, and 3,000 mg/day were 28.6%, 35.2%, and 39.5%, respectively. This same trend was seen in patients who were 100% responders (Figure 47-2).

Other blinded, placebo-controlled (41) and open-label trials (42, 43) support efficacy in partial seizures established by the three pivotal trials. In these trials, conducted using doses from 1,000 to 4,000 mg/day, responder rates in patients with partial-onset seizures ranged from around 40% to 60%.

Outside of the traditional clinical trial setting, LEV performance has also been studied in a large, phase IV community-based (KEEPER) trial of 1,030 subjects (44). In this 16-week study involving five office visits, adult outpatients with partial-onset epilepsy received add-on LEV therapy. Overall, 57.9% of patients achieved 50% seizure reduction, and global evaluation scores were improved

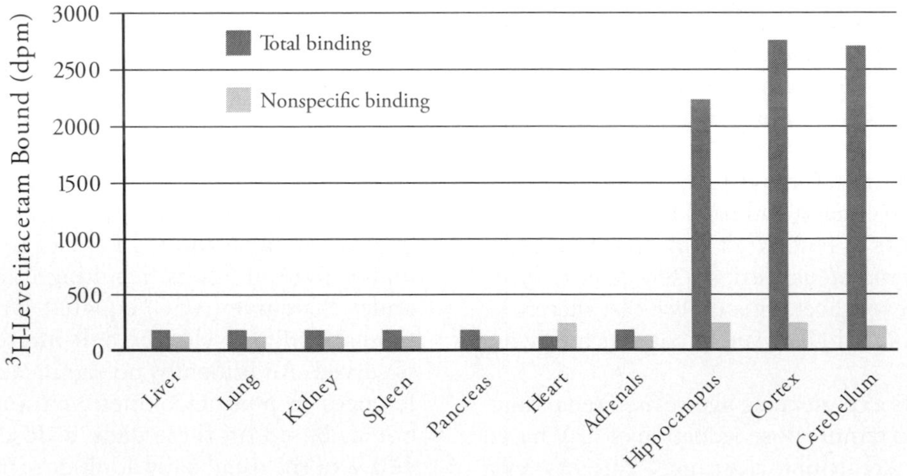

FIGURE 47-2

Pooled response rates by dose from pivotal phase III trials (40).

compared to baseline in nearly 75% of patients. Results of a subset analysis revealed that these findings confirm efficacy results seen in phase III trials. In the SKATE trial, 178 adult patients were treated for 16 weeks with 1,000, 2,000, or 3,000 mg LEV in an open-label, add on study of medically refractory patients. The retention rate at 16 weeks was 84.8%. The 50% responder rate was 46.6% with 16.7% of patients achieving seizure freedom (45).

Monotherapy Studies in Partial Seizures

The data are limited for the use of LEV for monotherapy but there is no reason to assume that it cannot be used as monotherapy in many patients. A responder-selected study of monotherapy was performed in 286 patients. The study began as an add-on study with patients receiving either placebo or 1,500 mg twice daily. Patients who had at least a 50% reduction is seizures entered into a monotherapy phase with a 12-week down-titration of previous medications followed by 12 weeks of monotherapy at 1,500 mg twice daily. In the initial placebo controlled component of the study, 42.1% of the LEV group achieved a 50% reduction compared with 16.7% of controls. In the LEV monotherapy group, the median percent reduction was 73.8%. Nine of the original 181 patients randomized to LEV were seizure free on monotherapy 46). Data from retrospective chart reviews also provide a basis for efficacious monotherapeutic performance. In a review of 45 patients with newly diagnosed partial-onset epilepsy, 5 of 11 patients on LEV therapy for at least 6 months achieved 50% seizure reduction, and 6 became seizure free (47).

A randomized, placebo-controlled trial (48) comparing LEV (n = 288) and controlled-release carbamazepine (CBZ, n = 291) in new-onset epilepsy produced equivalent seizure-freedom rates using conservative doses (LEV, 500 mg twice daily vs. CBZ 200 mg twice daily). One-year remission was achieved by 86% of the patients treated with LEV, while CBZ resulted in remission in 89.3% patients (48).

Generalized Seizures

A number of uncontrolled or retrospective reports suggest that LEV may be of value in patient with generalized seizures. In a small case series of three patients who had failed at least three other AEDs, monotherapy for primary generalized epilepsy (PGE) was assessed (49). All three patients became seizure free for at least 6 months on LEV therapy. Wever reported on ten patients with generalized seizures, including 6 with PGE and 4 with Lennox-Gastaut syndrome. One became seizure free, and 4 more had a > 50% reduction in seizures (50). The add-on monotherapy trials in children by Lagae et al (51) confirmed the efficacy of LEV in both partial and generalized epilepsies. A retrospective study of 59 intractable epilepsy children reported a >50% reduction in 40% of intractable partial seizures, 55% of generalized seizures, and 61% of those with mixed seizures (52).

Two studies that assessed the response of spike-wave density in patients with idiopathic generalized epilepsy with baseline and post-treatment 24-hour EEG have reported impressive results (53, 54). Gallagher et al (53) reported complete cessation of spike-waves in 9 of 10 patients studied in the awake state and significant reduction during sleep. Rocamora et al (54) reported a 72% reduction in median spike-wave duration in their 8 patients. Efficacy of LEV on a variety of epilepsy syndromes involving myoclonus is discussed under a separate heading below. It should be noted, under the present heading, that data submitted to the U.S. Food and Drug Administration (FDA) on the efficacy of LEV on myoclonus associated with juvenile myoclonic epilepsy (JME) has resulted in approval in the United States for that indication. This is consistent with the open-label experience with LEV on JME reported by Specchio et al (55). As of April 1, 2007, LEV has received approval from the FDA for use in primary generalized tonic-clonic seizures in patients 6 years of age or older.

Pediatric Studies

Following the establishment of its efficacy and safety in adults, levetiracetam adjunctive therapy was evaluated in an open-label trial in children. The 24 pediatric patients enrolled in the open-label, single-dose pharmacokinetic study (31) were also evaluated subsequently for levetiracetam efficacy and safety (56). After a 4-week baseline period, these children (mean age 9.4 years) participated in a 6-week titration phase, followed by an 8-week evaluation phase in which doses ranged from 20 to 40 mg/kg/day. Compared with their baseline seizure frequency, 12 of 23 (52%) patients who entered the evaluation phase achieved 50% seizure reduction, and 5 of 23 (21.7%) achieved 75% seizure reduction. Two patients remained seizure free throughout the evaluation period. In another open-label study of 39 pediatric patients (mean age 8.6 years) with refractory epilepsy, adjunctive levetiracetam therapy was evaluated during a 9-month treatment period (57). Results of this study support reduced seizure frequency, improved cognition and behavior, and good tolerability.

A double-blind placebo-controlled trial of LEV as adjunctive therapy was performed in 198 children with medically intractable partial seizures. The reduction of LEV treated patients over placebo treated was significant at 26.8% (P = 0.0002) with a >50% reduction in 44.6% of the LEV group. Significantly, 6.9% of LEV-treated patients became seizure free (58). This study led to FDA approval of LEV as adjunctive therapy for children.

Verrotti et al (59) used LEV in 21 patients with benign rolandic epilepsy (BECTS) and found that all of the patients had at least a 50% reduction in seizures. A longer follow-up study comparing the efficacy of oxcarbazepine (OXC) to LEV in rolandic epilepsy by the same group found 19 of 21 (90.5%) children treated with LEV to be seizure free, compared to 13 of 18 (72.2%) treated with OXC (60).

Case reports suggest that LEV may be helpful in children with seizures due to tuberous sclerosis (61). While one specific case of LEV-responsive Landau Kleffner syndrome has been reported (62), other reports (63, 64) describe the utility of LEV in syndromes of continuous spikes and waves during slow sleep (CSWS). There are no convincing data to advocate the use of LEV in catastrophic childhood epilepsies such as infantile spasms or Lennox-Gastaut syndrome.

Myoclonus

Several open-label studies of LEV in myoclonus due to a variety of underlying disorders have been reported. In a study of juvenile myoclonic epilepsy, 38 patients were enrolled and titrated to a dose of 3,000 mg/day over 2 weeks. Half of the 10 newly diagnosed patients were seizure free, as were 11 of 38 previously refractory patients (55), indicating that LEV may be a reasonable alternative to the more traditional medications such as valproic acid. LEV appears to be effective in many patients with Unverricht-Lundborg disease, with 8 of 13 patients demonstrating a measurable improvement. Most responders were the younger patients in the study (65). The report by Labate et al (66) involved both patients with idiopathic and symptomatic generalized epilepsies and myoclonus. They reported 50% or greater seizure reduction in 82% of the 35 patients studied.

CLINICAL USE IN PEDIATRIC PATIENTS

Levetiracetam is an appropriate medication to use in the pediatric age group. It is approved for add-on therapy for partial seizures in children >4 years and for myoclonus associated with JME. It has also received approval for use in patients 5 years of age or older for primary generalized tonic-clonic seizures. However, it should be noted that special consideration must be given to use of levetiracetam in children. Based on pharmacokinetic data, levetiracetam clearance is enhanced in children as compared to adults. Thus, in patients under the age of 12, 130–140% of the adult daily dose, normalized to body weight, may be appropriate.

The fact that many adult patients will respond to 1,000 mg/day should be taken into account when prescribing for children. It is prudent to start at a low dose, then titrate upward slowly, as this may diminish the propensity for adverse effects. Levetiracetam is currently available as tablets and as a liquid preparation, so it can be readily administered to children of all ages and children with special needs, such as those fed by gastrostomy tube.

Long-Term Studies

Long-term clinical usefulness of LEV has been evaluated. In one study, data from all 1,422 epilepsy patients exposed to LEV during any phase of development were analyzed (67, 68). The median duration of treatment was 399 days (range 1–8 years), and the median reduction from baseline in seizure frequency over the entire treatment period was 39.6%. Furthermore, no decrease in efficacy was observed over time in each cohort exposed to LEV ranging from 6 to 54 months.

Other studies looking at refractory epilepsy patients followed for 1 year support findings of sustained efficacy. In one open-label study of 98 patients, 57 achieved 50% seizure reduction and 14 were seizure free for the first year. This study particularly attempted to investigate types of patients who would not be eligible for clinical trials because of factors such as mental retardation and comorbid neuropsychiatric disorders (69). Another study reported a 26% seizure-free rate at one year, and this benefit correlated with the fact that 77% of patients continued on LEV therapy at 1 year (70).

Quality of Life Studies

The effect of LEV on quality of life has been investigated. Using the 31-item Quality of Life in Epilepsy (QOLIE-31) questionnaire, patients randomized to LEV at 1,000 or 3,000 mg/day or to placebo were studied over an 18-week period. Significant improvements in several areas, including seizure worry, overall quality of life, cognitive functioning, and total score, were seen in patients taking LEV compared with those taking placebo (71). A subsequent evaluation of a subset of these patients who were followed for 4 years indicates that improvements in QOLIE-31 scores remained stable during the 4-year follow-up period (72).

ADVERSE EFFECTS IN ADULTS

The majority of clinical safety data on LEV derive from four large, well-controlled trials (three pivotal phase III and one supportive phase III), which included 769 patients who received levetiracetam and 439 who received placebo (37–39, 41, 73).

A pooled analysis of these four trials found that the most frequently reported treatment-emergent adverse events associated with LEV adjunctive therapy were somnolence, asthenia, infection, and dizzi-

TABLE 47-2
Incidence of Adverse Experiences Reported More by LEV-Treated Patients Than by Placebo-Treated Patients, by Body System

Body System/ Preferred Terms	Levetiracetam (n = 769)		Placebo (n = 439)	
Body as a whole				
Asthenia	113	14.7%	40	9.1%
Headache	105	13.7%	59	13.4%
Infection	103	13.4%	33	7.5%
Pain	52	6.8%	26	5.9%
Nervous system				
Depression	31	4.0%	10	2.3%
Dizziness	68	8.8%	18	4.1%
Somnolence	114	14.8%	37	8.4%
Nausea	34	4.4%	19	4.3%
Insomnia	24	3.1%	11	2.5%
Nervousness	30	3.9%	8	1.8%
Respiratory system				
Pharyngitis	47	6.1%	17	3.9%
Rhinitis	34	4.4%	11	2.5%

Data are for events reported by ≥3% of levetiracetam-treated patients.
Source: (73). Data on file, UCB Pharma

ness (Table 47-2). Overall, a total of 15.0% of patients receiving LEV and 11.6% receiving placebo either discontinued or had a dose reduction as a result of an adverse event (73).

CNS adverse events, often seen in AED-treated patients, occurred in LEV-treated patients. The most common, somnolence and asthenia, were reported by 14.8% and 14.7% of LEV-treated patients, compared with 8.4% and 9.1% of placebo-treated patients, respectively. A total of 3.4% of LEV-treated patients experienced coordination difficulties (reported as ataxia, abnormal gait, or incoordination), compared with 1.6% of placebo-treated patients. Somnolence, asthenia, and coordination difficulties occurred most frequently within the first 4 weeks of treatment. Additionally, 13.3% of LEV-treated patients experienced behavioral symptoms (reported as agitation, hostility, anxiety, apathy, emotional lability, depersonalization, and depression) compared with 6.2% of placebo patients. The majority of these behavioral adverse events were reported early in therapy and occasionally led to withdrawal (73).

Regarding hematologic adverse events, minor but statistically significant decreases compared with placebo in total mean red blood cell (RBC) count, mean hemoglobin, and mean hematocrit were seen in LEV-treated patients. However, all mean values for these parameters remained within normal laboratory ranges. There were small mean decreases in white blood cell (WBC) count from baseline to the final visit in LEV-treated patients. However, no patient required discontinuation due to underlying neutropenia, and the infection adverse events were not related to WBC changes (73).

No significant changes were noted in liver function tests, renal function, or body weight (73).

There are no adequate and well-controlled studies of LEV in pregnant women; thus, it is assigned Pregnancy Category C. Some of the major known mechanisms that mediate AED teratogenicity (74), such as activation of cytochrome P450 systems and inhibition of histone deacetylation, do not apply to LEV. Extensive transfer of LEV from plasma to breast milk (ratio ≈ 1:1) has been described (75, 76), but infants had very low serum concentrations of LEV. Clinical judgment regarding the benefit of LEV therapy should be exercised, and the finding is not generally considered a contraindication to the use of LEV in breastfeeding mothers.

ADVERSE EFFECTS IN PEDIATRIC PATIENTS

Regarding safety, the most common adverse events reported were headache, infection, anorexia, and somnolence. No significant alterations in mean clinical laboratory values or in concomitant AED plasma concentrations were observed. Safety data from various studies (56–58) suggest that, as in adults, LEV is generally well tolerated in children. One area of note, however, is the occurrence of emergent behavioral side effects. Specifically, aggression, emotional lability, oppositional behavior, and psychosis have been described in some children taking levetiracetam (56–58, 77). In the aforementioned study of 24 patients by Glauser et al, the incidence of emotional lability was 12.5% (56). Wheless and Ng studied 39 children and reported that 15 of these patients experienced behavioral side effects. Furthermore, 11 of these 15 patients were developmentally delayed or mentally retarded (57). A small review of four pediatric epilepsy cases by Kossoff et al reports that each of these patients experienced treatment-emergent psychosis that was reversible (77). These studies also indicate that the treatment-emergent behavioral side effects are reversible, have a higher incidence in children with a history of behavioral emotional problems, and may be associated with rapid titration (56–58, 77). A meta-analysis of AED-associated behavioral and psychiatric adverse events suggested that the incidence of such effects with LEV is not substantially different from that associated with most new-generation AEDs (78).

CONCLUSION

Levetiracetam has emerged as an important new anticonvulsant medication for patients with many different types of epilepsy. Initial data led to approval as adjunctive therapy in adults. More recent data have extended this to the pediatric population and to use in myoclonic seizures associated with JME. It has also received approval for use in primary generalized tonic-clonic seizures in patients 6 years of age or older. The recent availability of an intravenous solution with comparable bioavailability to the oral preparations (79, 80) provides flexibility in administration to patients unable to take the oral medications, including patients immediately after surgical procedures. It can be useful in patients with myoclonus or with generalized seizures and is an attractive option in view of the excellent safety and lack of drug interactions associated with its use. These advantages have resulted in extensive use of LEV for the treatment of seizures in patients on complex medical regimens such as cancer chemotherapy or medications to prevent rejection of transplanted organs.

References

1. Genton P, Van Vleymen B. Piracetam and levetiracetam: close structural similarities but different pharmacological and clinical profiles. *Epileptic Disord* 2000; 2:99–105.
2. Brown P, Steiger MJ, Thompson PD, et al. Effectiveness of piracetam in cortical myoclonus. *Mov Disord* 1993; 8:63–68.
3. Klitgaard H, Matagne A, Gobert J, Wülfert E. Evidence for a unique profile of levetiracetam in rodent models of seizures and epilepsy. *Eur J Pharmacol* 1998; 353:191–206.
4. Löscher W, Hönack D. Profile of ucb L059, a novel anticonvulsant drug, in models of partial and generalized epilepsy in mice and rats. *Eur J Pharmacol* 1993; 232:147–158.
5. Löscher W, Hönack D, Rundfeldt C. Antiepileptogenic effects of the novel anticonvulsant levetiracetam (ucb L059) in the kindling model of temporal lobe epilepsy. *J Pharmacol Exp Ther* 1998; 284:474–479.
6. Amano K, Hamada K, Yagi K, Seino M. Antiepileptic effects of topiramate on amygdaloid kindling in rats. *Epilepsy Res* 1998; 31:123–128.
7. Morimoto K, Sato H, Yamamoto Y, Watanabe T, et al. Antiepileptic effects of tiagabine, a selective GABA uptake inhibitor, in the rat kindling model of temporal lobe epilepsy. *Epilepsia* 1997; 38:966–974.
8. Stratton SC, Large CH, Cox B, Davies G, et al. Effects of lamotrigine and levetiracetam on seizure development in a rat amygdala kindling model. *Epilepsy Res* 2003; 53:95–106.
9. Postma T, Krupp E, Li XL, Post RM, et al. Lamotrigine treatment during amygdala-kindled seizure development fails to inhibit seizures and diminishes subsequent anticonvulsant efficacy. *Epilepsia* 2000; 41:1514–1521.
10. Gower AJ, Noyer M, Verloes R, Gobert J, et al. ucb L059, a novel anti-convulsant drug: pharmacological profile in animals. *Eur J Pharmacol* 1992; 222:193–203.
11. Gower AJ, Hirsch E, Boehrer A, Noyer M, et al. Effects of levetiracetam, a novel antiepileptic drug, on convulsant activity in two genetic rat models of epilepsy. *Epilepsy Res* 1995; 22:207–213.
12. Mazarati AM, Baldwin R, Klitgaard H, Matagne A, et al. Anticonvulsant effects of levetiracetam and levetiracetam-diazepam combinations in experimental status epilepticus. *Epilepsy Res* 2004; 58:167–174.
13. Hanon E, Klitgaard H. Neuroprotective properties of the novel antiepileptic drug levetiracetam in the rat middle cerebral artery occlusion model of focal cerebral ischemia. *Seizure* 2000; 10:287–393.
14. Rekling JC. Neuroprotective effects of anticonvulsants in rat hippocampal slice cultures exposed to oxygen/glucose deprivation. *Neurosci Lett* 2003; 335:167–170.
15. Leppik IE. The place of levetiracetam in the treatment of epilepsy. *Epilepsia* 2001; 42(Suppl 4):44–45.
16. Rho JM, Sankar R. The pharmacologic basis of antiepileptic drug action. *Epilepsia* 1999; 40:1471–1483.
17. Zona C, Niespodziany I, Marchetti C, Klitgaard H, et al. Levetiracetam does not modulate neuronal voltage-gated Na^+ and T-type Ca^{2+} currents. *Seizure* 2001; 10:279–286.
18. Poulain P, Margineanu DG. Levetiracetam opposes the action of $GABA_A$ antagonists in hypothalamic neurones. *Neuropharmacology* 2002; 42:346–352.
19. Niespodziany I, Klitgaard H, Margineanu DG. Levetiracetam inhibits the high-voltage-activated Ca^{2+} current in pyramidal neurones of rat hippocampal slices. *Neurosci Lett* 2001; 306:5–8.
20. Lukyanetz EA, Shkryl VM, Kostyuk PG. Selective blockade of N-type calcium channels by levetiracetam. *Epilepsia* 2002; 43:9–18.
21. Rigo J-M, Hans G, Ngiyen L. The anti-epileptic drug levetiracetam reverses the inhibition by negative allosteric modulators of neuronal GABA- and glycine-gated currents. *Br J Pharmacol* 2002; 136:659–672.
22. Madeja M, Margineanu DG, Klitgaard H. Effect of levetiracetam on voltage-gated potassium channels: a novel antiepileptic mechanism of action? *Epilepsia* 2001; 42 (Suppl 2):19.
23. Bischoff U, Schlobohm I. Levetiracetam had no effect on voltage-gated potassium currents in cultured mouse hippocampal neurons. Poster presented at Fifth European Congress on Epileptology, October 7, 2002, Madrid, Spain.
24. Margineanu DG, Klitgaard H. Inhibition of neuronal hyper-synchrony in vitro differentiates levetiracetam from classical antiepileptic drugs. *Phamacol Res* 2000; 42: 281–285.
25. Niespodziany I, Klitgaard H, Margineanu DG. Desynchronizing effect of levetiracetam on epileptiform responses in rat hippocampal slices. *Neuroreport* 2003; 14:1273–1276.
26. Lynch BA, Lambeng N, Nocka K, Kensel-Hammes P, et al. The synaptic vesicle protein SV2A is the binding site for the antiepileptic drug levetiracetam. *Proc Natl Acad Sci USA* 2004; 101:9861–9866.
27. Crowder KM, Gunther JM, Jones TA, Hale BD, et al. Abnormal neurotransmission in mice lacking synaptic vesicle protein 2A (SV2A). *Proc Natl Acad Sci USA* 1999; 96:15268–15273.
28. Custer KL, Austin NS, Sullivan JM, Bajjalieh SM. Synaptic vesicle protein 2 enhances release probability at quiescent synapses. *J Neurosci* 2006; 26:1303–1313.
29. Patsalos PN. Pharmacokinetic profile of levetiracetam: toward ideal characteristics. *Pharmacol Ther* 2000; 85:77–85.
30. Radtke RA. Pharmacokinetics of levetiracetam. *Epilepsia* 2001; 42(Suppl 4):24–27.
31. Pellock JM, Glauser TA, Bebin EM, et al. Pharmacokinetic study of levetiracetam in children. *Epilepsia* 2001; 42:1574–1579.
32. Nicolas J-M, Collart P, Gerin B, et al. In vitro evaluation of potential drug interactions with levetiracetam, a new antiepileptic agent. *Drug Metab Dispos* 1999; 27:250–254.
33. Perucca E, Gidal BE, Baltès E. Effects of antiepileptic comedication on levetiracetam pharmacokinetics: a pooled analysis of data from randomized adjunctive therapy trials. *Epilepsy Res* 2003; 53:47–56.
34. Ragueneau-Majlessi I, Levy RH, Janik F. Levetiracetam does not alter the pharmacokinetics of an oral contraceptive in healthy women. *Epilepsia* 2002; 43:697–702.
35. Levy RH, Ragueneau-Majlessi I, Baltès E. Repeated administration of the novel antiepileptic agent levetiracetam does not alter digoxin pharmacokinetics and pharmacodynamics in healthy volunteers. *Epilepsy Res* 2001; 46:93–99.

36. Ragueneau-Majlessi I, Levy RH, Meyerhoff C. Lack of effect of repeated administration of levetiracetam on the pharmacodynamic and pharmacokinetic profiles of warfarin. *Epilepsy Res* 2001; 47:55–63.
37. Cereghino JJ, Biton V, Abou-Khalil B, Dreifuss F, et al. Levetiracetam for partial seizures: results of a double-blind, randomized clinical trial. *Neurology* 2000; 55:236–242.
38. Shorvon SD, Löwenthal A, Janz D, Bielen E, et al, for the European Levetiracetam Study Group. Multicenter double-blind, randomized, placebo-controlled trial of levetiracetam as add-on therapy in patients with refractory partial seizures. *Epilepsia* 2000; 41:1179–1186.
39. Ben-Menachem E, Falter U, for the European Levetiracetam Study Group. Efficacy and tolerability of levetiracetam 3000 mg/d in patients with refractory partial seizures: a multicenter, double-blind, responder-select-ed study evaluating monotherapy. *Epilepsia* 2000; 41:1276–1283.
40. Privitera M. Efficacy of levetiracetam: a review of three pivotal clinical trials. *Epilepsia* 2001; 42(Suppl 4):31–35.
41. Betts T, Waegemans T, Crawford P. A multicentre, doubleblind randomized, parallel group study to evaluate the tolerability and efficacy of two oral doses of levetiracetam, 2000 mg daily and 4000 mg daily, without titration in patients with refractory epilepsy. *Seizure* 2000; 9:80–87.
42. Grant R, Shorvon SD. Efficacy and tolerability of 1000–4000 mg per day of levetiracetam as add-on therapy in patients with refractory epilepsy. *Epilepsy Res* 2000; 42:89–95.
43. Abou-Khalil B, Hemdal P, Privitera MD. An open-label study of levetiracetam at individualised doses between 1000 and 3000 mg day-1 in adult patients with refractory epilepsy. *Seizure* 2003; 12:141–149.
44. Morrell MJ, Leppik I, French J, Ferrendelli J, et al. The KEEPER trial: levetiracetam adjunctive treatment of partial-onset seizures in an open-label community-based study. *Epilepsy Res* 2003; 54:153–161.
45. Seinhoff BJ, Trinka E, Wieser HG; for the DACH-LEV study group. Levetiracetam in patients with refractory epilepsy: results of the SKATE trial in Austria, Germany and Switzerland. *Seizure* 2005; 14:490–496.
46. Ben-Menachem E, Falter U. Efficacy and tolerability of levetiracetam 3000 mg/d in patients with refractory partial seizures: a multicenter, double-blind, responder-selected study evaluating monotherapy. European Levetiracetam Study Group. *Epilepsia* 2000; 41:1276–1283.
47. Alsaadi TM, Thieman C. Levetiracetam monotherapy for newly diagnosed epilepsy patients. *Seizure* 2003; 12:154–156.
48. Brodie MJ, Perucca E, Ryvlin P, Ben-Menachem E, et al; Levetiracetam Monotherapy Study Group. Comparison of levetiracetam and controlled-release carbamazepine in newly diagnosed epilepsy. *Neurology* 2007; 68:402–408.
49. Cohen J. Levetiracetam monotherapy for primary generalized epilepsy. *Seizure* 2003; 12:150–153.
50. Wever S, Beran RG. A pilot study of compassionate use of levetiracetam in patients with generalized epilepsy. *J Clin Neurosci* 2004; 11:728–731.
51. Lagae L, Buyse G, Cuelemans B. Clinical experience with levetiracetam in childhood epilepsy: an add-on and mono-therapy trial. *Seizure* 2005; 14:66–71.
52. Mandelbaum DE, Bunch M, Kugler SL, Venkatasubramanian A, et al. Efficacy of levetiracetam at 12 months in children classified by seizure type, cognitive status, and previous anticonvulsant drug use. *J Child Neurol* 2005; 20:590–594.
53. Gallagher MJ, Eisenman LN, Brown KM, Erbayat-Altay E, et al. Levetiracetam reduces spike-wave density and duration during continuous EEG monitoring in patients with idiopathic generalized epilepsy. *Epilepsia* 2004; 45:90–91.
54. Rocamora R, Wagner K, Schulze-Bonhage A. Levetiracetam reduces frequency and duration of epileptic activity in patients with refractory primary generalized epilepsy. *Seizure* 2006; 15:428–433.
55. Specchio LM, Gambardella A, Giallonardo AT, Michelucci R, et al. Open label, long-term, pragmatic study on levetiracetam in the treatment of juvenile myoclonic epilepsy. *Epilepsy Res* 2006; 71:32–39.
56. Glauser TA, Pellock JM, Bebin EM. Efficacy and safety of levetiracetam in children with partial seizures: an open label trial. *Epilepsia* 2002; 43:518–524.
57. Wheless JW, Ng Y-T. Levetiracetam in refractory pediatric epilepsy. *J Child Neurol* 2002; 17:413–415.
58. Glauser TA, Ayala R, Elterman RD, Mitchell WG, et al; N159 Study Group. Double-blind placebo-controlled trial of adjunctive levetiracetam in pediatric partial seizures. *Neurology* 2006; 66:1654–1660.
59. Verrotti A, Coppola G, Manco R, Ciambra G, et al. Levetiracetam monotherapy for children and adolescents with benign rolandic seizures. *Seizure* 2007; 16:272–275.
60. Coppola G, Franzoni E, Verrotti A, Garone C, et al. Levetiracetam or oxcarbazepine as monotherapy in newly diagnosed benign epilepsy of childhood with centrotemporal spikes (BECTS): an open-label, parallel group trial. *Brain Dev* 2007; 29:281–284.
61. Collins JJ, Tudor C, Leonard JM, Chuck G, et al. Levetiracetam as adjunctive antiepileptic therapy for patients with tuberous sclerosis complex: a retrospective open-label trial. *J Child Neurol* 2006; 21:53–57.
62. Kossoff EH, Boatman D, Freeman JM. Landau-Kleffner syndrome responsive to levetiracetam. *Epilepsy Behav* 2003; 4:571–575.
63. Capovilla G, Beccaria F, Cagdas S, Montagnini A, et al. Efficacy of levetiracetam in pharmacoresistant continuous spikes and waves during slow sleep. *Acta Neurol Scand* 2004; 110:144–147.
64. Aeby A, Poznanski N, Verheulpen D, Wetzburger C, et al. Levetiracetam efficacy in epileptic syndromes with continuous spikes and waves during slow sleep: experience in 12 cases. *Epilepsia* 2005; 46:1937–1942.
65. Magaudda A, Gelisse P, Genton P. Antimyoclonic effect of levetiracetam in 13 patients with Unverricht-Lundborg disease: clinical observations. *Epilepsia* 2004; 45:687–681.
66. Labate A, Colosimo E, Gambardella A, Leggio U, et al. Levetiracetam in patients with generalised epilepsy and myoclonic seizures: an open label study. *Seizure* 2006; 15:214–218.
67. Ben-Menachem E, Edrich P, Van Vleymen B, Sander JWAS, et al. Evidence for sustained efficacy of levetiracetam as add-on epilepsy therapy. *Epilepsy Res* 2003; 53:57–64.
68. Krakow K, Walker M, Otoul C, Sander JWAS. Long-term continuation of levetiracetam in patients with refractory epilepsy. *Neurology* 2001; 56:1772–1774.
69. Ben-Menachem E, Gilland E. Efficacy and tolerability of levetiracetam during 1-year follow-up in patients with refractory epilepsy. *Seizure* 2003; 12:131–135.
70. Betts T, Yarrow H, Greenhill L, Barrett M. Clinical experience of marketed levetiracetam in an epilepsy clinic—a one year follow up study. *Seizure* 2003; 12:136–140.
71. Cramer JA, Arrigo C, Van Hammee G, Gauer LJ, et al, for the N132 Study Group. Effect of levetiracetam on epilepsy–related quality of life. *Epilepsia* 2000; 41:868–874.
72. Cramer JA, Van Hammee G; N132 Study Group. Maintenance of improvement in health-related quality of life during long-term treatment with levetiracetam. *Epilepsy Behav* 2003; 4:118–123.
73. Harden C. Safety profile of levetiracetam. *Epilepsia* 2001; 42(Suppl 4):36–39.
74. Sankar R. Teratogenicity of antiepileptic drugs: role of drug metabolism and pharmacogenomics. *Acta Neurol Scand* 2007; 116:65–71.
75. Johannessen SI, Helde G, Brodtkorb E. Levetiracetam concentrations in serum and in breast milk at birth and during lactation. *Epilepsia* 2005; 46:775–777.
76. Tomson T, Palm R, Kallen K, Ben-Menachem E, et al. Pharmacokinetics of levetiracetam during pregnancy, delivery, in the neonatal period, and lactation. *Epilepsia* 2007; 48:1111–1116.
77. Kossoff EH, Bergey GK, Freeman JM, Vining EPG. Levetiracetam psychosis in children with epilepsy. *Epilepsia* 2001; 42:1611–1613.
78. Glauser TA. Behavioral and psychiatric adverse events associated with antiepileptic drugs commonly used in pediatric patients. *J Child Neurol* 2004; 19 Suppl 1:S25–S38.
79. Ramael S, Daoust A, Otoul C, Toublanc N, et al. Levetiracetam intravenous infusion: a randomized, placebo-controlled safety and pharmacokinetic study. *Epilepsia* 2006; 47:1128–1135.
80. Baulac M, Brodie MJ, Elger CE, Krakow K, et al. Levetiracetam intravenous infusion as an alternative to oral dosing in patients with partial-onset seizures. *Epilepsia* 2007; 48:589–592.

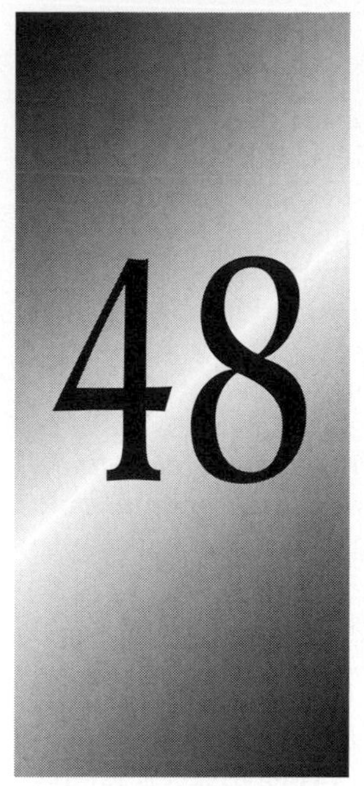

Barbiturates and Primidone

Robert S. Rust

Barbiturates constitute the oldest category of anticonvulsant medications that continue to be widely used in the management of epilepsy and other disorders. Their usefulness derives from a combination of efficacy, safety, and low cost. These virtues account for the fact that barbiturates likely remain among the most widely employed anticonvulsants in the world. Although phenobarbital (PB) is the major focus of this chapter, other drugs are reviewed, particularly mephobarbital, pentobarbital, and primidone. Mephobarbital (MPB) is a useful alternative to PB, more widely employed in some other countries, such as Australia, than in the United States. Like primidone, it undergoes biotransformation to PB. Among the more sedative barbiturates, pentobarbital has been useful in the management of severe and persistent seizures that do not respond to more routine anticonvulsant therapy. Primidone (PRM) is not actually a barbiturate, although it is subject to biotransformation into PB and probably exerts most of its anticonvulsant effects in that form. Because the major antiepileptic effects and side effects can be ascribed to the PB metabolite and because of pharmacokinetic and pharmacodynamic similarities, it is quite appropriate to consider PRM in this chapter.

PHENOBARBITAL

Phenobarbital is 5-ethyl-5-phenyl substituted barbituric acid, with a molecular weight of 232.23. It is a weakly acidic substance with a pK_a that is usually reported as 7.3 (1–4). The free acid has low aqueous and relatively low lipid solubility; however, the sodium salt, which is used for intravenous (IV) and intramuscular (IM) preparations, is freely soluble in slightly alkaline aqueous solutions.

Mechanisms of Action

Phenobarbital exhibits a wide spectrum of anticonvulsant activity, conferring protection to animals subjected either to electroshock or to chemically induced (pentylenetetrazol or bicuculline) experimental seizures (5, 6). This spectrum is shared by most barbiturates and is consistent with their wide spectrum of activity in clinical seizure disorders.

Understanding of the antiepileptic activity of PB has been limited by the incomplete state of our understanding of the mechanisms of epilepsy. Current views suggest that PB modulates the postsynaptic effects of certain neurotransmitters. The modulation is thought to affect both the inhibitory substance gamma-aminobutyric acid (GABA) and such excitatory amino acids as glutamate.

Whether by these or other mechanisms, antiepileptic barbiturates appear to elevate the threshold to chemical or electrical induction of seizures in ways that differ from and are in some respects superior to those of phenytoin (7).

A large body of information has accumulated concerning the ability of barbiturates to depress physiologic excitation in the nervous system and enhance inhibition of synaptic transmission. PB shares with pentobarbital (PnB) the capacity for selective postsynaptic augmentation of GABA-mediated inhibition and depression of glutamate- and quisqualate-mediated excitation in at least some central nervous system (CNS) regions (8–14). Barbiturate augmentation of GABA-stimulated postsynaptic inhibition appears to be due to activation of a subset (alpha-beta) of the $GABA_A$-receptor gated chloride channels (13, 15). These receptors differ from those that are activated by benzodiazepines and are differentially expressed in brain (16). These postsynaptic effects are produced at clinically relevant concentrations (12, 13). Evidence that phenobarbital may elevate concentration of kynurenic acid in relevant brain tissues suggests yet another mechanism whereby this anticonvulsant may control epilepsy. This novel mechanism may be shared by phenytoin, felbamate, and lamotrigine (17).

The reduction of voltage-activated calcium currents may in part account for the sedative and anesthetic effects of barbiturates and may possibly play a role in the efficacy of PnB and very high concentrations of PB in suppressing seizures (13). This is another potential mechanism whereby these agents may work in the setting of intractable status epilepticus with barbiturate coma and may represent one of the mechanisms for production of anesthesia (13).

Pharmacokinetics

Absorption. Phenobarbital is rapidly and nearly completely absorbed after oral or IM administration to infants or children. For most children older than 6 months of age or adults, it is likely that peak serum concentrations of PB are achieved by 2 hours after oral and 2–4 hours after IM bolus administration of the usual age-appropriate maintenance doses. The bioavailability of most oral and parenteral formulations is essentially quantitative (85–100%) through a wide range of doses in otherwise healthy children (>6 months of age) or adults. Rectally administered parenteral solutions of sodium PB are well absorbed at all ages, although the latency to peak concentration may be slightly longer and the bioavailability slightly lower than after IM administration (18).

Distribution. Phenobarbital disseminates into all body tissues. At lower serum pH the ionized fraction of serum PB is smaller, and therefore diffusion into tissues is enhanced, leading to lower serum but higher tissue concentrations. More alkaline serum produces opposite effects (4). Only approximately 50% or less of circulating PB is bound to serum proteins in most patients whose ages are greater than 3 to 6 months. Equilibration of PB across the blood-brain barrier is relatively slow. Twelve to 60 minutes are required for maximal brain-to-plasma PB ratios in adult mammalian brain after IV administration. These data suggest that (1) dosage of PB should be based on lean body mass to avoid overdosing obese individuals (19, 20), and (2) sufficient time for maximal brain penetration should be allowed to occur after bolus administration of PB before administration of additional doses.

Phenobarbital readily crosses the placenta and is secreted in breast milk (21, 22). Breast milk concentrations were 36 ± 20% and 41 ± 16% of maternal serum concentrations in two studies (23, 24). The newborn infants of mothers treated with PB have levels equivalent to those of their mothers immediately after birth (23, 25–28). Estimates of the apparent volume of distribution (*Vd*) of PB vary over nearly a fourfold range but are generally larger in infants and small children than in older individuals (29–31). The *Vd*s for newborns and infants less than 4 months of age treated with IV PB average approximately 0.9 to 1.0 L/kg, independent of body weight, dose, gestational age, or occurrence of asphyxia (29, 32–35). Older children and adults exhibit *Vd*s that range from approximately 0.45 to 0.7 L/kg more or less irrespective of route of administration (36–38).

Metabolism and Elimination. Phenobarbital may be excreted unchanged or may undergo biotransformation before excretion. The most quantitatively important fates for PB metabolism include (1) aromatic hydroxylation to *p*-hydroxyphenobarbital (PBOH) and (2) *N*-glucosidation to 9-D-glucopyranosyl phenobarbital (PNG) (39, 40). On average (with wide interindividual variation), approximately 20% to 30% of a daily dose of PB is converted to the pharmacologically unimportant PBOH, apparently by at least one cytochrome P450 isozyme. In most children and adults, about half of the PBOH is excreted unchanged and about half is excreted as a PBOH-glucuronide conjugate that is formed in liver (41). Although PB is the classic inducer of hepatic microsomal metabolism, it does not appear to induce significant changes in its own metabolic rate or plasma clearance in humans, although slight effects may occasionally be detected (42, 43).

Phenobarbital has the longest half-time of elimination of any of the frequently used anticonvulsants. The two-standard-deviation range for half-time of elimination in children and adults is 24 to 140 hours, resulting in the capacity to eliminate between 11% and 50% of total body PB in 24 hours (42, 44–48). Elimination half-time is longest in premature and full-term newborns, with various studies showing mean values of 100 to 200 hours with standard deviations of 30% to 80% (full range across these studies of 59 to greater than 400 hours) (31, 33, 49–52). Clearance may vary from day to day in individual babies (52); however, the rate of elimination may double by the second week of life and tends to continue to increase for the ensuing few weeks. Infants 6 weeks to 12 months old have the shortest mean half-times of elimination (30–75 hours) of any age group (31, 35, 53, 54). At age 2 months half-time of elimination is usually in the range of 39 to 55 hours. Children 1 to 15 years of age typically have half-time of elimination of 37 to 73 (68 ± 30) hours, while subjects 15 to 40 years of age have 53 to 141 (100 ± 20) hours half-time of elimination (30, 55). Perinatal asphyxia may considerably decrease the clearance by newborns, probably due to the combination of renal and hepatic dysfunction (22, 35, 38, 53, 56–65). Clearance of unmetabolized PB may be higher at higher rates of urine formation (66–68) or in more alkaline urine, as both of these conditions reduce the rate of PB resorption in the distal nephron. Eightfold increase in the rate of urine formation may increase PB clearance by three- to fourfold (69, 70). This effect may be considerably enhanced by the alkalinization of urine with sodium bicarbonate (4).

Interactions with Other Drugs

Although some drugs affect PB kinetics, most of the pharmacokinetically important interactions encountered with the use of PB are those caused by the effects of PB on the kinetics of other drugs. The most common key encountered effect that PB has on the metabolism of other drugs is to increase their biotransformation, thereby increasing their clearance rate. PB is the prototypical inducer of the hepatic mixed-function oxidase system that comprises, among other elements, the numerous isoenzymes of cytochrome P450 and of NADPH-cytochrome c reductase.

A list of drugs for which this effect may be clinically important is provided in Table 48-1 (43, 71–94). In several instances, as indicated in Table 48-1, PB may result in increased concentrations of potentially toxic metabolites. The enhancement of potential valproate toxicity to kidney and liver must be considered in cases in which these drugs are used in combination. Renal tubular injury may be exacerbated by the increased dose of valproate required in some patients taking PB (92, 93), while the chance of hepatic injury may be increased because of PB-induced production of the "4-en" metabolite of valproate, which appears to be toxic to hepatocytes (95–98). Phenobarbital co-administration may increase the risk for valproate-induced hyperammonemic encephalopathy, perhaps by means of unfavorable effects on ammonia clearance (99).

TABLE 48-1
Drugs Subject to Kinetic Alteration When Administered to Patients Receiving Phenobarbital

Shortened Half-Time of Elimination and/or Peak Levels
Acetaminophen (71)*
Amidopyrine (43)
Aniline
Antipyrine (72)*
Bishydroxycoumarin (73)
Carbamazepine, 10,11-carbamazepine epoxide (74–76)
Chloramphenicol (77)
Chlorpromazine (78, 79)
Cimetidine (80)
Cyclosporine (81)
Doxycycline (82)
Ethylmorphine
Flunarizine (83, 84)
Griseofulvin (85)
Haloperidol (86)
Hexobarbital
Meperidine (87)*
Mesoridazine (86)
Methadone (88)*
Methsuximide (89)
Nortriptyline (90)
Theophylline (91)
Valproic acid (92, 93)*
Warfarin (94)

.*May result in increased levels of toxic metabolites.

Although PB induces the metabolism of phenytoin, the degree of that effect is seldom great enough to cause an adjustment of phenytoin dosage (100, 101). Other important potential effects of comedication with PB include inadequate anticoagulation with warfarin (43, 73, 94), reduction of serum levels of exogenously administered prednisone or dexamethasone (102, 103), or failure of oral contraception (104, 105). Coadministration of PB with warfarin or other medications can be managed when the combination is essential. In such cases, care must be taken to adjust anticoagulants with any changes in PB discontinuation (106). The effect of PB on these various drugs may become manifest within days to weeks of initiation of comedication.

Less commonly, other drugs affect PB kinetics. The most important of these in everyday practice is the interaction of PB and valproic acid. Accumulation of PB occurs in most patients who are comedicated with PB and valproate, accompanied by a lower than expected serum level to dosage ratio of valproate. The rate and magnitude of these effects are variable but generally require lowering of PB and increasing of valproate dosages as compared with what might be expected with monotherapy (107). Valproate-related weight gain and thrombocytopenia may also be dose-related. Elevation of PB levels may occur within days of initiation of valproate, but more typically the increase occurs slowly over a number of weeks.

Pharmacodynamic Interactions

Little is known about the pharmacodynamic interactions of PB and other drugs. It was long argued that PB potentiated the antiepileptic effects of phenytoin; therefore, the two drugs were coadministered in many patients for several decades. There is no scientific data upon which such a contention, or the view that PB may potentiate the antiepileptic potency of carbamazepine, can be based (108, 109). Currently, it is more widely held that the combination of these and other antiepileptic drugs more often exacerbates side effects than enhances desirable effects, although there are few objective data to support this clinical impression. The combination of PB with other sedative medications, such as benzodiazepines, may provoke status epilepticus, including tonic motor status in patients with Lennox-Gastaut syndrome (110).

Adverse Effects

Experience has demonstrated that PB generally is a very safe and predictable medication. Nonetheless, it does produce various undesirable effects. The majority of these are reversible effects that can be tolerated but reduce the attractiveness of PB therapy. Serious side effects also occur, but they are rare. The most frequently encountered adverse characteristics of PB are (1) sedation, (2) disturbances of mood and behavior and possibly cognition, and (3) induction of hepatic metabolism, producing various effects on the disposition of a wide variety of other drugs (as discussed in preceding paragraphs). Exacerbation of seizures may possibly occur with weaning and discontinuation of phenobarbital maintenance. Serious allergic reactions may occur.

Sedation and Behavior. Although phenobarbital has the most favorable ratio of antiepileptic potency to sedative properties among the antiepileptic barbiturates, it is certainly more sedating than most other anticonvulsants (111). Drowsiness is most common at the initiation of therapy, afflicting as many as one-third of newly treated patients. Sedation may occur even at very low doses and may persist for several days, occasionally as long as several weeks (45). Sedation may return with dose increases, and there may be a dose-related increment in difficulty awakening in the morning or increase in the frequency with which a nap is required. However, many patients do not experience significant sedation after initially becoming accustomed to the medication, despite many-fold increases in dose (112, 113). Patients receiving chronic PB therapy are least likely to feel drowsy if their serum level falls between 15 and 30 μg/mL, but there is considerable individual variation in tolerance. Some patients complain of little sedation with levels as high as 50 μg/mL, while others find levels of 10 to 15 μg/mL intolerable because of lethargy (114).

Mood Disturbance. Studies have shown that 30% to 42% of children with febrile seizures treated with PB prophylaxis experience deterioration in behavior, the majority having relatively low PB levels (i.e., less than 15 μg/mL). Hyperactivity, irritability, belligerence, intermittent agitation, disruptive and defiant behavior, insomnia, and uncharacteristic episodic sedation are among the most frequent troublesome manifestations—effects that are not related to dose or serum level (115–117). Hyperkinetic characteristics have occurred in as many as 79% of children treated with any drug for epilepsy (118), and disturbances of behavior similar to those noted occur in at least 18% of children who have had at least one febrile seizure without any prophylactic anticonvulsant (119).

Several well-designed studies have failed to find a significant incidence of behavioral deterioration of children treated with PB (120, 121). In a particularly well-designed, double-blind, placebo-controlled study of toddlers, the rate of hyperactivity was no different whether treated with PB or placebo. There were few significant PB-related side effects, and those that did occur (irritability and sleep disturbance) responded to dose reduction (120). The prospective, double-blind, randomized, crossover study of Young and coworkers (122) showed no significant worsening of behavior with either PB or mephobarbital. Drugs that are converted into PB, such as methylphenobarbital and primidone, are regarded by some as less likely to produce behavioral side effects than PB; however, these hypotheses have not been subjected to careful trials in children. One study of the *treatment* of childhood behavioral disturbances with PB or PRM has shown these drugs to be *beneficial* in 33% and 11% of children, respectively (123).

Higher Cortical Function. Very early in what has been nearly nine decades of clinical use of PB, the intellectual function of many epileptic patients improved as their seizures came under better control with PB. With a wider choice of antiepileptic medications and other treatments now available, disturbances of cognition, especially attention and memory, and of skilled motor functions may occur in patients as a consequence of the medication rather than of the epilepsy. In an era of quite limited antiepileptic medication choices, Lennox (124) noted the additional toll that medications might take on epileptic patients with brain injuries, changes readily observed by patients, families, and teachers that were "often subtle and difficult to measure." Nearly 60% of the epileptic patients treated with PB whom Lennox studied did not appear to have such difficulties.

Hillesmaa and coworkers (125) found decreased rate of fetal head growth for human infants of mothers taking PB. Although some early studies documented changes in various measures of intelligence and learning in patients of various ages with some onset of epilepsy, no patterns of deterioration attributable to PB treatment were found. In individual cases IQ measurements increased, while others decreased with PB treatment (126, 127). Dosage in many of these early cases was lower than is now typical, and these studies did not address issues of compliance or attempt to relate intellectual dysfunction to drug levels. A subsequent study suggested, but did not prove, that the everyday intellectual performance of children on PB was deficient as compared with what might be expected given their performance on standardized tests of intellectual function (128). Schain and coworkers (129) found improvement in intelligence subtest scores, attentiveness, and impulse control in children who had their PB replaced with carbamazepine, although these children exhibited the simultaneous and potentially confounding variable of improved seizure control. Subtle but statistically significant lowering of performance- and full-scale IQ, verbal and nonverbal task subtest scores, and deterioration of behavior were found to be a consequence of PB as compared with valproate therapy of epilepsy in a more recent double-blind crossover study (130). Similar results were obtained in another study (131), which also provided evidence on repeat testing for impairment of learning and cognitive development while on PB compared with valproate-treated or untreated control groups.

Several additional studies have aroused concern, especially in the setting of febrile seizure prophylaxis with PB. Hirtz and coworkers (132) and Farwell and colleagues (133) demonstrated that mean IQ scores of large cadres of such children were 5.2 to 8.4 points lower than anticipated, compared with untreated or placebo-treated control groups. A disparity of at least 5 points was shown to persist for as long as 6 months after PB prophylaxis had been discontinued in both studies. Various concerns have been raised about certain aspects of the design of these studies, including low enrollment rates of eligible children, incomplete testing of significant fractions of enrolled children, and particularly the intention-to-treat design. Thus, in the case of one study (133), some children in the placebo group actually received PB, while less than two-thirds of those in the PB-treated group received PB throughout the entire study period (2 years), and one-third of the treatment group had little if any PB exposure or low drug levels during follow-up. An earlier, smaller, but particularly well designed and executed study did not show any such significant effect of PB prophylaxis on infant developmental scales over an 8- to 12-month follow-up interval. However, Stanford-Binet Intelligence scale assessment suggested that in some of these children there were negative effects of PB on performance of certain memory tasks that were drug concentration related, but the effect was not statistically significant (120).

Dependence and Withdrawal. Prolonged administration of PB produces both habituation and dependence; therefore, significant withdrawal signs and symptoms may be provoked by abrupt discontinuation of the drug. Patients may experience anxiety, irritability, insomnia, mood disturbance, emotional lability, hyperexcitability, and tremulousness, various gastrointestinal disturbances, confusion, or delirium. Therefore, chronically administered PB should be withdrawn slowly to prevent these various reactions as well as withdrawal seizures. Seizures that occur during withdrawal of PB (whether the withdrawal is suggested by the physician or undertaken by the noncompliant patient) do not necessarily indicate that the drug remains therapeutically indispensable. In many cases slower rates of withdrawal permit the drug to be withdrawn without seizure recurrence (112, 134, 135). A similar abstinence syndrome may occur in newborn infants of mothers treated with PB, given the ease with which PB crosses the placenta, rendering a level in the neonate that is close to that found in the mother (50). The abstinence syndrome of the newborn may persist for days to weeks and is likely to be better tolerated and of shorter duration in infants whose mothers received the usual antiepileptic doses of PB than in infants of PB-abusing mothers.

Overdosage. Intoxication with PB can occur because of dosing errors, coadministration of valproic acid, accidental ingestion, and suicide attempts. We have observed several instances in which IV PB boluses have been administered in the emergency department to patients on chronic primidone therapy who have presented to the emergency room in status epilepticus, with failure to recognize that primidone is metabolized into PB. Rapid administration of a full loading dose of PB (20 mg/kg) to patients with PB levels of 30 to 40 μg/mL is particularly likely to prompt the development of pulmonary edema and respiratory failure. More frequently encountered are cases in which valproate is added to chronic PB therapy and patients developed progressive lethargy 3 to 5 weeks later with elevated PB levels. Inattention, drowsiness, and dysarthric slurring of speech that may resemble drunkenness are often exhibited by patients acutely intoxicated with PB. Curiously, plasma levels similar to those that produce such effects acutely may be tolerated without evident ill effects after the dose is slowly increased with chronic therapy. Other findings observed in patients that have toxic plasma concentrations (usually >40 μg/mL) include dizziness, constricted pupils, nystagmus, ataxia, or coma (generally with levels above 60 μg/mL).

Phenobarbital levels in excess of 80 μg/mL, although well tolerated in carefully monitored patients with appropriate cardiorespiratory intervention, are potentially lethal if such support is not provided. Such high levels, particularly if acutely achieved, may occasionally produce both cardiac and respiratory dysfunction (136). However, cardiac dysfunction is significantly less likely to occur with PB than with PnB. Indeed, levels in excess of 130 μg/mL appear to be tolerated reasonably well by patients receiving appropriate intensive care support and requiring burst suppression for the management of intractable seizures.

Other Adverse Effects. Phenobarbital therapy has been associated with hypocalcemia more commonly than with vitamin D–deficient osteomalacia (137). This may be the result of mixed-function oxidase induction resulting in enhanced clearance of 25-hydroxy-cholicalciferol (138). The patients who are particularly vulnerable to "phenobarbital rickets" are those who have received many years of PB therapy, are poorly mobile, and have limited exposure to sunlight; diet also may play a role. Symptomatic patients may respond to the administration of 4,000 units of vitamin D each day or 125 μg of vitamin D_3 each week. Prophylactic administration of vitamin D is not recommended (139–142).

Such serious consequences as Stephens-Johnson syndrome, erythema multiforme, or toxic epidermal necrolysis are rare, but they do occur. Malaise, fatigue, fever, and eosinophilia typically accompany allergic rash, which may start centrally and spread to the face and extremities. Variable degrees of hepatic inflammation may accompany the hypersensitivity reaction in children, including fulminant fatal liver necrosis (143–145). Connective tissue disorders including Dupuytren contracture, Ledderhose syndrome (plantar fibromatosis), Peyronie disease, frozen shoulder, and aching joints have been associated with PB.

Clinical Use

Phenobarbital is indicated in the treatment of partial, simple, or complex seizures, as well as primary or secondarily generalized motor seizures (tonic, clonic, tonic-clonic) in all age groups. It is the drug of choice in the treatment of most forms of neonatal seizures and for prophylaxis of febrile seizures, and it is among the most valuable agents for the management of status epilepticus. Well-designed studies of adults have shown that PB, PRM, phenytoin, and carbamazepine are equally effective in the management of generalized motor seizures (146), and although there may be differences in efficacy in treatment of partial seizures, they are slight. The cooperative VA study showed complete control of primary generalized tonic-clonic seizures in 43% of men receiving PB or phenytoin, 45% of those receiving primidone, and 48% of those receiving carbamazepine. Only 16% achieved complete control of partial or secondarily generalized seizures with PB, compared with 43% with carbamazepine (147). Other studies of adults have demonstrated similar results (148, 149). One large noncrossover study of 3-to 14-year-old children with generalized tonic-clonic seizures showed a 22% rate of remission with PB monotherapy, compared with 34% for phenytoin, 40% for carbamazepine, and 16% for valproate. One study showed that localization-related seizures with secondary generalization were completely controlled in only 3% of patients on PB, as compared with 21% with phenytoin, 25% with carbamazepine, and 4% with valproate (150).

Plasma concentrations of PB required for control of generalized tonic-clonic seizures may be bimodally distributed. Schmidt (151) found that the majority of responding patients achieved control at PB levels of 18 ± 10 μg/mL but that a significant minority achieved control at levels of 38 ± 6 μg/mL. One-third of patients considered to have intractable partial complex seizures (e.g., with PB levels less than 20 μg/mL) were found to improve significantly if "adequate" PB or PRM levels were achieved (i.e., levels high enough to achieve control without intolerable side effects). An additional 16% responded if either of these drugs at higher concentrations was combined with phenytoin or carbamazepine (151, 152).

For the management of children under 1 year of age who present with focal or generalized motor seizures excepting infantile spasms, PB represents an attractive "first choice" agent because of its relative ease of administration, reliable kinetics, wide therapeutic window, and safety as compared with phenytoin or valproate. It is less frequently chosen in older children because of sedative qualities and potential effects on behavior. Nonetheless, it remains a valuable reserve agent for older children who cannot be managed effectively with other drugs. There is no clear indication that PB is any less effective than any other major anticonvulsant as alternative therapy for the management of anticonvulsant drug–resistant, localization-related seizures, and it should be among the drugs that are tried in succession in those difficult cases (149, 153). The use of PB as part of polytherapy for such resistant seizures may introduce difficulties because of sedative effects and induction of hepatic enzymes. One study showed that one-third of patients receiving combinations containing PB had improved seizure control when PB was eliminated from the regimen (154).

Initiation of PB Therapy. Phenobarbital loading can be achieved by IV or oral administration. IV loading typically requires administration of 15 to 20 mg/kg for newborns or very young infants and 10 to 20 mg/kg for older infants and children. The drug may be administered as a single dose or in two doses divided by a few hours (34, 155, 156). A number of different approaches to oral loading have been described. Administration of 6 to 8 mg/kg/day for 2 days followed by an age-appropriate daily maintenance dose will quickly render plasma levels of at least 10 μg/mL (148, 157). Bourgeois (158) demonstrated that the PB dose could be increased over 4 days as total daily doses of 3, 3.5, 4, and 5 mg/kg/day on successive days to achieve, in a linear fashion and without significant interim sedation, a serum level of approximately 20 μg/mL at 96 hours. The maintenance dose must be adjusted thereafter to prevent toxic accumulation of PB. Without some form of initial loading, as many as 30 days may be necessary to achieve maximal steady-state PB concentrations (159). Obese adolescent patients may have a volume of distribution of 0.5 L/kg or less, and suitable adjustment in their loading dose must be considered in some cases.

Daily maintenance dose requirements for children are higher, on a weight basis, than those for adults, averaging 2 to 4 mg/kg/day (155, 160). To maintain plasma levels of 10 to 25 μg/mL, Rossi (161) recommended oral maintenance doses of 4.79 ± 1.3 mg/kg in infants aged 2 to 12 months, 3.5 ± 0.99 mg/kg in children aged 1 to 3 years, and 2.31 ± 0.74 mg/kg in those 3 to 6.5 years. The data of others would suggest that for children older than 3 years who weigh less than 40 kg, doses of 1.5 to 3 mg/kg/day are appropriate, whereas doses no greater than 1 to 1.5 mg/kg/day may maintain satisfactory levels for adolescents and adults who weigh more than 40 kg (148, 157). The PB dose may be administered entirely at bedtime or divided throughout the day, depending on degree of sleep disturbance and susceptibility to behavioral abnormalities or sedative effects. Once-daily administration is beneficial to some but not all patients. Multiple daily administration may in some cases improve compliance for forgetful parents.

Neonatal Seizures. Phenobarbital is the most widely employed drug for the management of neonatal seizures. This practice reflects familiarity with the agent and widely shared confidence in the efficacy and safety of PB in neonates rather than any well-established evidence for the superiority of this agent over other anticonvulsants. The choice of PB may be based more on the dosing inconvenience or potential risks associated with other drugs than on any demonstrated superiority of PB (162, 163). Thus, the second most commonly employed agent, phenytoin, carries risks for tissue injury if tissues are infiltrated at the site of IV line placement or for adverse cardiac effects if the rate of administration is excessive, problems that are less frequently encountered with fosphenytoin. However, nonlinear kinetics make oral administration of phenytoin a problem in very small infants.

The initiation of PB therapy for seizures in newborns should start with IV administration of a loading dose of 16 to 20 mg/kg delivered as a single bolus or as two divided boluses. Volume of distribution of an administered bolus of PB to a neonate has been variously estimated at 0.81 to 0.97 L/kg, with 15% to 20% deviation of such mean values, and does not vary as a result of gestational age of the newborn infant (164, 165). From a practical vantage point, a volume of distribution of approximately 1.0 L/kg can safely be presumed in most cases, a loading dose of 20 mg/kg resulting in a peak serum level of 20 μg/mL. Plasma protein binding of phenobarbital averages 22% to 25% in neonates, approximately half the value that is anticipated in older children and adults (166).

Successful control of neonatal seizures is seldom achieved with serum levels less than 16 μg/mL; initial loading should attempt to achieve serum levels ranging from 15 to 25 μg/mL. Electrographic monitoring has shown that many clinically responding newborns show persistence of electrographic seizures after routine loading doses (167). Although the significance of electrographic activity in the newborn without clinical seizures remains uncertain, infants with recalcitrant *clinical* seizures require additional loading boluses delivered as 10 mg/kg at intervals of one to several hours. At plasma concentrations of at least 40 μg/mL as many as 77 percent to 85 percent of neonates respond (168, 169). Serum levels as high as 60 to 80 μg/mL appear to be tolerated by most newborns, although such high levels may necessitate greater degrees of cardiorespiratory support, compromise clinical examination, and interfere with feeding. Svenningson and coworkers (170) found that plasma PB concentrations in excess of 50 μg/mL in newborns were associated with slowing of heart rate to less than 100 beats per minute. This is a potentially serious matter, because the neonate lacks the reflexive capacity to alter stroke volume in compensation for bradycardia.

Newborns respond to an initial loading dosage of 20 mg/kg, a serum level of 20 μg/mL, and oral or IV total daily maintenance dose 2.25 to 4 mg/kg. Although doses of 5 mg/kg/day are widely recommended, the continuation of such a dose through the first few weeks of life generally results in accumulation to serum levels significantly in excess of 20 mg/dL (34, 52, 171). Plasma clearance of PB usually increases after 1 to 2 weeks of life and may require modification of maintenance dosage in some but not all cases.

Status Epilepticus. The ease and relative safety of administration, wide therapeutic window, and long duration of action combine to make PB a particularly attractive choice in the treatment of status epilepticus. Negative aspects of the use of this drug include the relatively low lipid solubility, sedative effects, and the possible provocation of respiratory depression, hypotension, or pulmonary edema. Thus, benzodiazepines and phenytoin are the usual first-line treatments for status epilepticus in children of most ages. On the other hand, PB can be administered more rapidly and in higher concentration than phenytoin, and it can be administered intramuscularly if necessary. IM administration of a full loading dose to a well-perfused location may achieve brain levels adequate for the control of some seizures in less than an hour and is indicated if no better access can be achieved.

The rate of administration of sequential boluses of PB determines the risk for cardiopulmonary complications, which is lower for PB than for PnB or too rapidly administered phenytoin. In general, the rate of IV administration of PB for treatment of status epilepticus should be 2 mg/kg/min for children who weigh less than 40 kg. The rate should be 100 mg/min for children and adults who weigh more than 40 kg. Slower rates may be required in special cases, such as in patients with acute cardiac disease (e.g., tricyclic overdose). In general, respiratory depression is not seen below plasma levels of 60 μg/mL, and hypotension may not arise as a complication of PB until after even higher levels are achieved. Pulmonary edema is an uncommon complication and usually requires very massive PB bolusing over short time intervals to high levels. The most widely accepted practice for PB administration in treatment of status epilepticus in the PB-naïve patient is to administer at total loading dose of 20 mg/kg. This quite reliably produces a plasma level close to 20 μg/mL. It is clear that the administration of only a partial loading dose (e.g., 10 mg/kg) to the anticonvulsant-naïve patient usually is inadequate. Seizures may well diminish or stop, but they often recur as the PB becomes distributed throughout the body. Respiratory support is usually required as the plasma level rises above 50 to 70 μg/mL, and pressor support may be required above levels of 70 to 90 μg/mL, whether as the result of PB, of the causative illness, or both.

Febrile Seizures. Phenobarbital has been the most commonly employed prophylactic agent for prevention of febrile seizures. As febrile seizures are generally without significant immediate or long-term serious medical consequences, there has been significant momentum away from providing prophylactic treatment. Enthusiasm for prophylactic treatment has diminished because (1) approximately two-thirds of children have just one febrile seizure, (2) recurrent febrile seizures have exceedingly low risk for untoward consequences, (3) PB and other agents introduce a risk for various drug-related side effects (115), and (4) it has been difficult to provide convincing proof that prophylaxis is effective. Although there is some evidence supporting the effectiveness of treatment with PB, sodium valproate, or benzodiazepines, it is not conclusive proof. PB is usually judged a safer choice than valproate for administration to very young children, and long-term prophylaxis with benzodiazepines poses unacceptable problems with sedation and tachyphylaxis. However, PB is not without risk, as the death of one child has been ascribed to the use of PB for prophylaxis against febrile seizures (144). The efficacy of PB as prophylactic therapy has recently come into question (172).

There is evidence to suggest that if PB prophylaxis is to be effective, steady-state serum concentrations of 16 to 30 μg/mL are required (173). This study demonstrated a 4% risk for recurrence in children with such levels compared with approximately 20% rates of recurrence for untreated children and for those with PB levels of 8 to 15 μg/mL. Several more recent studies have failed to demonstrate a difference in outcome between groups of children at risk for febrile seizures who received either PB or valproate for prophylaxis compared with children who received no prophylactic anticonvulsant medication (133, 174, 175). However, these studies did not control for the important element of compliance by assessing serum PB levels at time of recurrence. Compliance with PB prophylactic regimens for febrile seizures is notoriously low (176). Herranz (177) found that 20% of children treated with PB prophylaxis for febrile seizures had recurrences at mean levels of 16.4 ± 2.8 μg/mL, compared with 88% of those treated with PRM (mean PB levels 14.1 ± 3.7 μg/mL) and 92% of those treated with valproate (mean levels 35.2 ± 5.9 μg/mL). Side effects were experienced by 7% of those on PB, 53% of those on PRM, and 45% of those on valproate, although most side effects were tolerable.

PB is discontinued gradually in most cases. This is based on evidence that dependence on PB results in provocation of seizures if the rate of decline of PB levels is too rapid. This presumption has been placed in question in one study of patients with partial complex seizures that appeared to demonstrate that the risk for seizures was not dependent on rate of withdrawal but on the achievement of a concentration below 15 to 20 μg/mL (178).

OTHER BARBITURATES

The N-methylbarbiturates (methylphenobarbital and metharbital) and the anesthetic pentobarbital have all been used as anticonvulsants.

Methylphenobarbital

Methylphenobarbital (Mebaral®, MBL), although infrequently used in the United States, is widely employed in some countries, such as Australia. A considerable portion of the administered dose is rapidly cleared as the R-enantiomer; therefore, the dose of racemic MBL should be approximately twice the PB dose required to achieve satisfactory clinical effects (179–181). The single oral dose half-time of elimination for the R-enantiomer has been estimated at 7.5 ± 1.7 hours, compared with 69.8 ± 19.7 hours for the S-enantiomer and 98.0 ± 19.7 hours for the PB metabolite (182).

MBL clearance is almost entirely by biotransformation with urinary excretion of the major metabolites, which are PB and *para*-hydroxymethyl PB (as a phenolic glucuronide conjugate) (180, 183, 184). PB is the only pharmacologically important biotransformation product. The capacity to generate this product may increase with chronic therapy because of increased rate of MBL clearance with faster rates of appearance and higher peak levels of PB. Naïve subjects may excrete less than 11% of their MBL dose as PB, while subjects exposed to MBL or PB may increase that amount to more than 50% (183). Because PB has a smaller volume of distribution and is cleared more slowly than MBL, plasma PB levels may accumulate over time to much higher values than simultaneous serum MBL values. Many or most of the drug interactions experienced with chronic MBL therapy are thought to be due to PB, and any interaction or side effect that has been described for PB can occur with MBL therapy.

The experimental and clinical spectrum of MBL is similar to that of PB (185). It may be administered once or twice daily. Because of the tendency for PB levels to accumulate to higher serum levels than MBL levels over the long term and the greater availability of PB level determinations, most clinicians follow up only the PB level in patients taking MBL. Doses that are calculated to produce therapeutic steady-state PB levels may result in unacceptable drowsiness during the initial phases of therapy, and therefore compliance may be poor. Starting with half the expected dose and accelerating the dose over 1 to 2 weeks avoids this problem but delays the achievement of the desired steady-state peak PB concentrations to as long as 4 to 5 weeks after initiation of therapy. Full initial doses may be started in patients who have recently been treated with PB or other "inducing" anticonvulsants. At steady state, PB concentration is generally 7 to 10 times greater than the total (R + S) MBL concentration in serum.

Pentobarbital

Pentobarbital (PnB) is a 5-ethyl-5 (1-methylbutyl) barbiturate that is clinically employed as a sodium salt (Nembutal®). It is a short-acting barbiturate. The half-time of elimination in adults ranges from 18 to 50 hours and is dose dependent. The partition coefficient for PnB is approximately 11 times greater than that for PB. This reflects much faster lipid solubility, accounting for shorter latency in onset of activity, shorter duration of action, and faster metabolic degradation. The superior lipid solubility may be in part responsible for the fact that PnB is much more potently sedative and hypnotic than PB. Acutely achieved blood concentrations of 0.5 to 3 μg/mL produce approximately the same degree of sedation as PB levels of 5 to 40 μg/mL. PnB levels ≥10 to 18 μg/mL usually induce coma. When PnB is employed as a constant infusion of 0.3 to 4.0 mg/kg/hr after bolus administration of 15 mg/kg over 1 hour, the serum half-time of elimination ranges from approximately 11 to 23 hours in adults (186).

Pentobarbital is indicated for the treatment of status epilepticus that is unresponsive to such first-line therapies as benzodiazepines, phenytoin, or PB. The aim of PnB therapy is to produce coma with suppression-burst pattern on EEG; therefore, the sedative properties of this drug are not deleterious. On the other hand, PnB is more likely than PB to have negative effects on cardiac contractility and to require the addition of cardiotonic medications to support blood pressure and perfusion when employed in the usual doses. Particular caution should be used in the management of patients who have cardiac disease and those whose seizures are the result of hypoxic-ischemic injury or tricyclic overdose, because the negative effects on cardiac function may be particularly deleterious in such settings. Barbiturate anesthesia (with PnB more commonly than thiopental or methohexital) is considered by many neurologists to be the ultimate form of therapy for status epilepticus that has proved intractable to the usual combinations and dosages of short- and long-acting anticonvulsants, including PB (187, 188). Treatment with PnB has not been proven to be superior to the use of very high doses of PB to achieve burst suppression or control of seizures.

Lowenstein and associates (186) reviewed their results with eight retrospectively studied and six prospectively enrolled patients treated with PnB, thiopental, or methohexital anesthesia; only one of these patients was a child. PnB loading with 15 mg/kg over 1 hour to the prospective group resulted in prompt cessation of seizures in patients treated with this protocol. PnB was infused at rates that varied from 0.3 to 4.0 mg/kg/hr, and additional boluses were administered as needed of 5 mg/kg (maximum of 30 mg/kg of bolus drug in the first 12 hours) to achieve and maintain burst suppression. The median peak serum PnB level for patients treated in this fashion was 10.8 μg/mL (range 6.5–21.2 μg/mL). Treatment resulted in a favorable outcome for three of these six adults, whereas one had a poor outcome and two had indeterminate outcomes. Only two of these six required pressors. Significant drop in blood pressure occurred within a few hours of initiation of therapy in 9 of the 14 patients of the entire group reported by these investigators.

Lowenstein and colleagues stopped PnB after approximately 12 hours of treatment, restarting therapy if seizures recurred. Duration of infusion ranged (in the prospective group) from 11 to 77 hours. For those patients who recovered function after cessation of anesthesia, brainstem functions returned in 6 to 24 hours, and various forms of motor activity returned in 1 to 72 hours. Some possible withdrawal phenomena occurred, including repetitive twitching of the extremities, resembling activity observed in some cases of barbiturate overdose and difficult to distinguish on a clinical basis from seizure activity (186, 189, 190). Patients receiving particularly high doses of PnB were found in some instances to have profound weakness and areflexia that persisted for as long as 2 weeks (including as many as 5 days of complete paralysis after cessation of infusion), despite much more rapid recovery of alertness and intellectual interactiveness. This effect may have been the result of PnB-induced dysfunction of peripheral nerve function or release of neurotransmitter in the peripheral synaptic cleft, as has been observed experimentally (191, 192). These transient forms of dysfunction may introduce confusion into attempts to assess patients for "brain death" or to estimate prognosis.

PRIMIDONE

Primidone (PRM), 5-ethyldihydro-5-phenyl-4,6 (1H, 5H) pyrimidine-dione or 2-desoxy-phenobarbital, was synthesized in 1949 and was shown to be effective in the treatment of major motor epilepsy shortly thereafter (193). It is therefore the third oldest anticonvulsant that continues in regular use (194). It has just two carbonyl substituents of the pyrimidine ring rather than the three that are characteristic of barbiturates. Hepatic biotransformation renders two main metabolites of PRM: phenylethylmalonamide (PEMA) and PB. The identification of PB as a metabolite raised questions as to the importance of the other substances in control of seizures, a subject that remains controversial. Although it has remained difficult to clearly demonstrate the contribution that PRM and PEMA make to clinical management of epilepsy independent of the effects of PB, there are both experimental and clinical data that support the view that they are pharmacodynamically important.

Anticonvulsant Activity

The fact that PRM has anticonvulsant properties is suggested by several lines of evidence, including the facts that (1) administration of PRM lowers the plasma level of PB required to protect animals against experimental forms of seizure, and (2) protection against seizures is afforded in the few hours after a single PRM dose is administered before the achievement of significant levels of PEMA or PB (5, 6, 195–197). The potency of PRM is equal to or possibly superior to that of PB in the prevention of electroshock-induced seizures, but it has much less activity against chemically induced (pentylenetetrazol or bicuculline) seizures (6, 194, 195, 197). This is similar to the spectrum of activity exhibited by phenytoin and carbamazepine.

Baumel and coworkers (196) roughly estimated the potency (ED_{50} for prevention of maximal electroshock seizures) of PRM to be 25% more and that of PEMA to be 90% less than that of PB. They also found that PRM had no detectable antichemoconvulsant activity, while PEMA is approximately 0.025 as potent as PB for prevention of that form of experimental seizure. Other researchers in a variety of animal lines have found somewhat different potency ratios of these compounds (5, 197, 198), but PRM and PB generally have had similar antielectroshock potency, while PEMA has been 12- to 18-fold less potent. Experimental evidence (5) suggests that PRM is approximately 2.5 times less neurotoxic than PB and that the two substances are synergistic in seizure control, possibly exerting different mechanisms of action. Bourgeois and coworkers established that a ratio of 1:1 brain concentration of PRM to PB achieved the best therapeutic index (ratio of therapeutic efficacy to toxicity) in control of seizures (5). A therapeutic range for PRM trough concentration of 3 to 12 μg/mL has been suggested (199), but somewhat higher levels may be tolerated. Although PEMA also has anticonvulsant properties, the potency appears to be too low to contribute much to the antiepileptic effects or toxicity of PRM at the usually encountered plasma concentrations of clinical practice (158). Monitoring of serum PEMA levels in patients treated with PRM has no practical value.

Pharmacokinetics

Peak serum PRM levels are achieved in approximately 3 hours in adults and 4 to 6 hours in children after single-dose ingestion of tablets in doses of 12.5 to 20 mg/kg (200). Brand-name tablets probably have nearly complete bioavailability, with 72% to 100% of a single oral dose excreted in urine as PRM or its metabolites (200–202). Absorption of generic preparations may be less reliable (203). Absorption of PRM tablets is reduced by concurrent acetazolamide administration (204). Volume of distribution of PRM and of PEMA after single oral dose has been estimated at 0.86 L/kg and 0.69 L/kg, respectively. There is less than 10% plasma protein binding of either PRM or of PEMA (205, 206).

Biotransformation of PRM is very complicated. PEMA and PB are the two major metabolites with antiepileptic potency. It has been difficult to estimate the relative contribution of PEMA and PB to the pharmacodynamic properties of PRM, including both antiepileptic potency and toxicity, although these properties have been studied carefully in animals (5, 6). Zadavil and Gallagher (207) showed that, on average, approximately 65% of a single IV PRM dose is excreted unchanged in the urine within 5 days of administration to adults, while 7% is excreted as PEMA and 2% is excreted as PB. The rate of conversion of PRM to PB is much slower than that to PEMA. Under steady-state conditions of chronic administration, approximately 25% of monotherapeutically administered PRM can be relied on to be converted to PB (208). The bioconversion of PRM to PB shows age-related variation. In general, the more complete transformation of PRM to PB by children aged 0.5 to 6.5 years often results in disappointingly low PRM to PB serum ratios, although there is considerable individual variability (209, 210).

PRM and its various metabolites are primarily (at least 75–77%) renally excreted (207). The half-time for elimination of orally administered PRM ranges from 10 to 15 hours in adults on monotherapy, but comedication with antiepileptic inducers of hepatic biotransformation enzymes lowers this time to 6.5 to 8.3 hours (201, 204, 207, 211). On average, half-time of elimination for PRM in children ranges from 4. 5 to 11 hours, lower with phenytoin comedication than with PRM monotherapy (200). The hepatic immaturity of newborns accounts for half-times of PRM elimination that vary from 8 to 80 hours.

In one study of steady-state PRM monotherapy, the average trough serum concentration to total daily dose of PRM for PRM, PEMA, and PB were 0.78 ± 0.25, 0.64 ± 0.39, and 1.47 ± 0.53, respectively (212). At steady state, PB levels are almost always higher than PRM levels. Because PB is probably responsible for many of the toxic effects of PRM, especially sedation, attempts have been made to diminish the biotransformation of PRM to PB. As noted previously, a brain ratio of 1:1 for PRM and PB concentrations has been established experimentally as ideal for the achievement of maximal therapeutic efficacy with minimal toxicity (5). Both nicotinamide and isoniazid have been tried for this purpose, but gastrointestinal, hepatic, and other possible toxicities have limited the usefulness of such approaches (213–215). In most clinical situations, PRM levels are of relatively little value as management tools. They may be useful in two situations, however: (1) assigning a cause for possible drug side effects or (2) establishing that the conversion rate of PRM to PB is unfavorably rapid and therefore that the use of the more expensive and inconvenient-to-administer PRM is poorly justified.

Drug Interactions

Coadministration of PRM and some other major antiepileptic drugs to adults decreases excretion of unchanged PRM after a single dose by more than one-third. This is the result of fourfold increase in the conversion rate to PEMA and 50% increase in conversion to PB. Interactions with various anticonvulsants may result in considerable changes in the ratios of PRM, PEMA, and PB. Phenytoin is the most potent accelerator of PRM biotransformation, while carbamazepine has a lesser effect (204, 209, 216, 217). Bourgeois (158) showed that, on average, coadministration of PRM with either phenytoin or carbamazepine, or both, resulted in 50% reduction in the trough PRM level at steady state comparedwith that expected with monotherapy. PEMA levels increased by 17% and PB levels by 60% under those polytherapeutic conditions, and the trough ratio of PB to PRM increased by as much as threefold. Application of the data obtained in Bourgeois's study predicts that with PRM monotherapy a steady-state PB level of 16.5 μg/mL can be expected to be associated with an average PRM level of 10 μg/mL, but that the coadministration of phenytoin or carbamazepine, or both, increases the average PB level to a level of 26.5 μg/mL, while the average PRM level falls to 5 μg/mL. If the total daily dose were increased by approximately 100% to maintain the serum PRM level at 10 μg/mL, the PB level at steady state could be expected to rise to as much as 58.3 μg/mL. Thus, polytherapy with these agents can be expected to lower the therapeutic index of PRM significantly because of the unfavorable ratio of PRM to PB in brain compared with the experimentally ideal 1:1 ratio.

When polytherapy is considered necessary, problems of enzymatic induction are avoided by combining PRM with noninducing agents such as valproate, gabapentin, lamotrigine, topiramate, tiagabine, or benzodiazepines (218). However, combination with valproate produces the unfavorable kinetic problems encountered when PB and valproate are combined (218). Combination with benzodiazepines may produce intolerable sedation. Coadministration of PRM and valproate tends to produce lesser degrees of PB accumulation than are observed with PB and valproate coadministration (as stated previously). This may be because valproate inhibits not only PB clearance but also the conversion of PRM to PB (219). Thus, if it is judged necessary to coadminister valproate with PB, it might be better to administer the latter as PRM. Acetazolamide may diminish the gastrointestinal absorption of PRM, and carbamazepine may in some cases inhibit biotransformation of PRM to PB (215).

Toxicity

Animal studies demonstrate that PRM has less toxicity to the nervous system and other organs than PB (5, 194). Nonetheless, toxic effects, particularly those of the CNS, are common. They are reported at some point in their therapy by one-half to two-thirds of patients who are treated with this drug (147, 220–222). PRM therapy is unsuccessful and is discontinued in 10% to 30% of patients. Discontinuation is much more commonly the result of intolerable side effects than to lack of therapeutic efficacy (147, 221). Side effects of PRM therapy closely resemble those seen with PB. It has been difficult to distinguish the contributions of PRM compared with PB in the elicitation of these problems. Time of onset of side effects and the development of tolerance assist in making this determination.

Sensations variously characterized as sleepiness, light-headedness, dizziness, weakness, or intoxication are very common, if not universal, at the initiation of PRM therapy (211, 223). They develop within a few hours of ingestion of PRM, but there is considerable individual variability in susceptibility to these dose-related effects, which range from mild to severe and incapacitating affectation (224, 225). Cross-tolerance occurs in patients who are in the process of changing from PB to PRM therapy, but those changing from phenytoin or carbamazepine do not experience such cross-tolerance (223). These very early effects are due to PRM, because they occur before any significant accumulation of PB and usually wane within a few days, despite the fact that that is the time at which PB levels begin to rise (226, 227). The severe effects can be avoided by administration of a small "test dose" at the onset of therapy to determine whether the individual patient is highly susceptible. These effects can be minimized in all patients by careful attention to the speed and amplitude of the acceleration of the dosing schedule to achieve full doses (211, 225).

There is a second family of more persistent sedative side effects that develop during the chronic phase of PRM therapy. These chronic side effects are quite similar, if not identical, to those reported by some patients treated with PB. Patients and families report abnormalities of energy level, attentiveness, behavior, and learning. The frequency with which they are reported, and their amelioration in at least some cases when PRM is discontinued, suggest that the medication may be in part or entirely responsible. Rodin and coworkers (228) compared the effects of PRM and carbamazepine as adjuncts to phenytoin therapy and found that PRM produced more significant impairment of performance in a cognitive-perceptual test battery than carbamazepine, especially with regard to concentration and fine motor performance (229). The fact that these types of difficulties are quite similar, if not identical, to the problems reported during PB therapy, and the observation that they are most troublesome during the chronic phase of therapy, when the PB-to-PRM ratio is highest, suggest that PB is the likely culprit. It is unlikely that PEMA, which contributes little to the anticonvulsant potency of PRM, plays any significant role in CNS or other forms of PRM-related toxicity (205).

Virtually all of the other PB-related side effects can occur with PRM therapy, including the various connective tissue problems such as contracture formation, joint problems, and Peyronie's disease. One study has suggested that in children, PRM is less likely to produce any more significant side effects than phenytoin or PB (117). Transient nausea, vomiting, dizziness, and drowsiness may occur with initiation of PRM therapy, a peculiar combination of side effects that are seldom seen in patients who start on PB (147).

Overdosage

Little is known about the relationship between peak PRM concentrations and short-term toxic effects. Acute PRM overdosage (PRM levels exceeding 80–100 μg/mL in tolerant patients) may produce varying degrees of CNS depression ranging from somnolence or lethargy to deep coma, flaccidity, and loss of deep tendon reflexes (227, 230, 231). The degree of these abnormalities tends to correlate with PRM levels rather than PB or PEMA levels in the acute interval, although the ensuing rise in PB levels produces additional CNS depression (227, 232).

Massive overdosage may result in hypotension and acute renal failure in association with crystalluria, especially when serum PRM levels exceed 200 μg/mL (233). Fatal cases of PRM ingestion have been reported. However, with appropriate management (gastric lavage, administration of activated charcoal, forced diuresis, and supportive measures) patients have recovered without permanent sequelae from ingestion of as much as 22 grams of PRM (225). Crystalluria (largely crystallized PEMA) after administration of large amounts of PRM was first observed in rats (194) and is an almost constant feature of serious PRM overdosage in humans (234). It has not been shown to result in chronic renal failure even after massive overdosage with acute renal dysfunction (231). Massive overdosage can be effectively treated with hemoperfusion (233).

Clinical Use

Early uncontrolled, retrospective studies demonstrated that PRM could be used with considerable success as an adjuvant drug in the management of generalized tonic-clonic seizures, localization-related seizures, and myoclonus epilepsies (220, 235–239); however, some more recent controlled studies have shown less favorable results. These data, combined with the availability of a wider range of major anticonvulsants and decreased enthusiasm for polytherapy, have reduced the popularity of this agent. Early comparison studies failed to demonstrate that PRM had some unique value, in the treatment of any particular type of epilepsy or population of patients, compared with PB or phenytoin, drugs that were less expensive and in some ways easier to use (208, 240, 241). Therefore, it appears that the benefits of PRM therapy and the potential toxicity do not support the use of this agent as first-line therapy for any seizure type or syndrome (114).

One possible exception is the treatment of epilepsy occurring in patients with long QT syndrome, because PRM may have some value in the treatment of the cardiac dysrhythmia (242). However, most patients who have seizures in association with the long QT syndrome have them only in association with cardiac decompensation, which may be effectively treated with other medications. On the other hand, PRM continues to be useful as a third-line agent for treatment of occasional patients affected with almost any form of epilepsy for which PB is indicated, including age groups ranging from the neonate (243) to the adult. The exception to this principle is the fact that PRM has little value in the management of status epilepticus, because there is no commercially available parenteral formulation. PRM may be effective in the prophylaxis of febrile seizures (174).

Various direct comparisons of PRM to PB, phenytoin, or carbamazepine treatment in patients of various ages have shown these drugs to have similar efficacy for oral treatment of partial, secondarily generalized, and generalized tonic-clonic seizures (147, 208, 228, 241, 244). However, most of these studies do not control for PB levels. Reinterpretation of one of the best of these studies (208) has suggested that a subgroup of patients may enjoy better control at any given PB level if that level is achieved as the result of PRM rather than PB oral therapy (245). One crossover comparison showed that PRM was superior to orally administered PB in the management of generalized tonic-clonic seizures (246). The VA Epilepsy Cooperative study comparison of PRM to PB, phenytoin, and carbamazepine showed the highest rate of failures in treatment of partial or secondarily generalized seizures occurred with PRM therapy, failure that usually was due to drug discontinuation or poor compliance early in the course of treatment because of intolerable side effects (147). Sapin and coworkers (247) found that PRM exerted antiepileptic effects in neonates that were independent of the effects of PB.

Two potential benefits of the choice of PRM rather than PB are (1) the possibility of achieving seizure control in a given subject at lower serum PB levels than are required with the administration of PB itself, and (2) the possibility that in certain settings PRM is a "better" drug than PB. Others have argued that most or all of the clinically significant antiepileptic effect of PRM is simply due to its conversion into PB (248, 249). This is particularly likely to be true when PRM is administered too infrequently during the day to achieve the most favorable serum ratio of PRM to PB. In most patients this requires administration every 6 hours, which may be inconvenient. Because of unfavorable effects in the PRM-to-PB ratio, there are reasons to believe that there is no advantage to employing PRM in combination with phenytoin, acetazolamide, or carbamazepine. Unfortunately, most patients who now receive PRM are patients with intractable epilepsy on polytherapy with complicated dosing schedules.

When administered to adults as monotherapy, PRM can be administered twice daily because the half-time of elimination for PRM typically is 10 to 15 hours. However, the shorter elimination half-time that is typical of most children and most patients on polytherapy mandates administration of this drug at 6-hour intervals if advantage is to be taken of the presumed antiepileptic potency of PRM. Administration to newborns is little studied, but in the event that administration of PRM were judged important, once-daily dosing is theoretically possible. So great is the variation of elimination half-times observed in the newborn (23) that individualization of dosage for newborns would be prudent, as would careful follow-up to ensure that toxic accumulation of metabolites does not occur.

Treatment Guidelines

If there are no coadministered drugs that interfere with metabolism or distribution, an initial daily PRM dose of approximately 20 mg/kg/day will result, after 2 to 3 weeks, in a steady-state PB level ranging from 10 to 30 μg/mL. Neonates typically require maintenance doses of 15 to 25 mg/kg/day, infants 10–25 mg/kg/day, and children 10–20 mg/kg/day (23). The total daily dose should be divided into three or four times of administration, as noted previously, given the short half-time of elimination of PRM; the peak serum concentration typically is achieved 3 to 5 hours after each dose. Initiation of PRM monotherapy in patients who are not already receiving barbiturates should in many cases start with a low single daily dose at bedtime (e.g., one-fourth of a 250-mg tablet for patients who weigh more than 20 kg) with subsequent upward titration at 3-day intervals (158). Not every patient will require or tolerate steady-state dosage at 20 mg/kg/day. In some cases, relatively large initial doses may be tried to more rapidly achieve serum levels that are effective in controlling seizures. For example, it has been shown that the administration to neonates of 25 mg/kg/day, divided into three doses, produces a serum PRM level of approximately 10 mg/dL by day 3, a level that is sufficient to control the seizures of many neonates independent of the associated PB level (246). Monitoring PRM or PEMA levels confers little therapeutic advantage in most clinical situations.

Changing patients from chronic oral PB therapy to PRM is usually easily accomplished by administering four to five times as much PRM each day as the discontinued total daily PB dose. In patients who are not on PB, rapid initiation of PRM therapy can be achieved by first loading with PB (250). Rapid escalation of oral PB loading can be achieved using PB doses of 3 mg/kg/day on the first day of treatment, 3.5 mg/kg/day on the second day, 4 mg/kg/ day on the third day, and 5 mg/kg/day on the fourth day. This approach results in a linear accumulation of PB in the serum to approximately 20 μg/mL on day 4 without significant sedation. The PB can be discontinued on the following day and replaced with a full maintenance PRM dose of between 12.5 and 20 mg/kg/day (158).

Immediate initiation of PRM at an amount expected to produce serum concentration of 20 to 30 μg/mL can be undertaken by IV loading of 20 mg/kg of PB (producing a serum concentration of 20 μg/mL) and initiation of 20 mg/kg/day of PRM divided into three or four doses. Any patient loaded with enough PB to achieve serum PB concentrations of at least 20 μg/mL within 3 days after initiation will experience significant degrees of sedation (250).

Discontinuation

In general, the considerations that arise with regard to drug discontinuation are similar to those previously noted for PB. One small study suggested that withdrawal-related seizures may be more likely with PRM than with PB (251). Theodore and coworkers (178) found no relationship between the peak dose or rate of withdrawal of PRM or PB and the occurrence of seizures. In their study, seizures were most likely to occur as the PB level fell between 15 and 20 μg/mL.

References

1. Butler TC. Metabolic oxidation of phenobarbital to *p*-hydroxyphenobarbital. *Science* 1954; 120:494.
2. Bush MT. Sedatives and hypnotics: absorption, fate and excretion. In: Rot WS, Hofmann FG, eds. *Physiological Pharmacology*. New York: Academic Press, 1963:185–218.
3. Nishihara K, Katsuyoski U, Saitoh Y, et al. Estimation of plasma unbound phenobarbital concentration by using mixed saliva. *Epilepsia* 1979; 20:37–45.
4. Wade A. Barbiturates. Pharmaceutical handbook. London: The Pharmaceutical Press, 1980.
5. Bourgeois BF, Dodson WE, Ferrendelli JA. Primidone, phenobarbital, and PEMA: I. Seizure protection, neurotoxicity, and therapeutic index of individual compounds in mice. *Neurology* 1983; 33:283–290.
6. Bourgeois BF, Dodson WE, Ferrendelli JA. Primidone, phenobarbital, and PEMA: II. Seizure protection, neurotoxicity, and therapeutic index of varying combinations in mice. *Neurology* 1983; 33:291–295.
7. Morrell F, Bradley W, Ptashne M. Effects of drugs on discharge characteristics of chronic epileptogenic lesions. *Neurology* 1959; 9:492–498.
8. Nicoll RA. Pentobarbital: actions on frog motor neurons. *Brain Res* 1975; 96: 119–123.
9. Macdonald RL, Barker JL. Different actions of anticonvulsant and anesthetic barbiturates resolved by use of cultured mammalian neurons. *Science* 1978; 200:775–777.
10. Ransom BR, Barker JL. Pentobarbital modulates transmitter effects of mouse spinal neurones grown in tissue culture. *Nature* 1975; 254:703–705.
11. Ransom BR, Barker JL. Pentobarbital selectivity enhances GABA-mediated postsynaptic inhibition in tissue cultured mouse spinal neurons. *Brain Res* 1976; 114:530–535.
12. Schulz DW, MacDonald RL. Barbiturate enhancement of GABA-mediated inhibition and activation of chloride ion conductance. *Brain Res* 1981; 209:177–188.
13. French-Mullen JMH, Barker JL, Rogawski MA. Calcium current block by (–)-pentobarbital, phenobarbital, and CHEB but not (+)-pentobarbital in acutely isolated hippocampal CA1 neurons: comparison with effects on GABA-activated Cl^- current. *J Neurosci* 1993; 13:3211–3221.
14. Sawada S, Yamamoto C. Blocking action of pentobarbital on receptors for excitatory amino acids in the guinea pig hippocampus. *Exp Brain Res* 1985; 59:226–231.
15. Newberry NR, Nicoll RA. Comparison of the action of baclofen with gamma-aminobutyric acid on rat hippocampal pyramidal cells. *J Physiol* 1984; 360:161–185.
16. Pritchett DB, Sontheimer H, Shivers BD, et al. Importance of a novel $GABA_A$ receptor subunit for benzodiazepine pharmacology. *Nature* 1989; 338:582–585.
17. Kocki T, Wielosz M, Turski WA, Urbanska EM. Enhancement of brain kynurenic acid production by anticonvulsants—novel mechanism of antiepileptic activity? *Eur J Pharmacol* 2006; 541(3):147–151.
18. Graves NM, Holmes GB, Kriel RL, et al. Relative bioavailability of rectally administered phenobarbital sodium parenteral solution. *DICP* 1989; 23:565–568.
19. Svensmark O, Buchthal F. Accumulation of phenobarbital in man. *Epilepsia* 1963; 4:199–206.
20. Svensmark O, Buchthal F. Dosage of phenytoin and phenobarbital in children. *Dan Med Bull* 1963; 10:234–235.
21. Fouts JR, Hart LG. Hepatic drug metabolism during the perinatal period. *Ann N Y Acad Sci* 1965; 123:245–251.
22. Langset A, Meberg A, Bredesen JE, Lunde PKM. Plasma concentrations of diazepam and *N*-dimethyldiazepam in newborn infants after intravenous, intramuscular, rectal and oral administration. *Acta Paediatr Scand* 1978; 67:699–704.
23. Nau H, Rating D, Hauser I, et al. Placental transfer and pharmacokinetics of primidone and its metabolites phenobarbital, PEMA and hydroxyphenobarbital in neonates and infants of epileptic mothers. *Eur J Clin Pharmacol* 1980; 18:31–42.
24. Kaneko S, Suzuki K, Sato T, Ogawa Y, et al. The problems of antiepileptic medication in the neonatal period: is breastfeeding advisable? In: Janz D, Dam M, Richens A, et al, eds. *Epilepsy, Pregnancy, and the Child.* New York: Raven Press, 1982:343–348.
25. Boreus LO, Jalling B, Kallberg N. Phenobarbital metabolism in adults and in newborn infants. *Acta Paediatr Scand* 1978; 67:193–200.
26. Boreus LO, Jalling B, Wallin A. Plasma concentrations of phenobarbital in mother and child after combined prenatal and postnatal administration of prophylaxis of hyperbilirubinemia. *J Pediatr* 1978; 93:695–698.
27. Bossi L, Battino D, Caccamo ML, et al. Pharmacokinetics and clinical effects of antiepileptic drugs in newborns of chronically treated epileptic mothers. In: Janz D, Dam M, Richens A, et al, eds. *Epilepsy, Pregnancy, and the Child*. New York: Raven Press, 1982:373–381.
28. Rating D, Nau H, Kuhnz W, Jager-Rom E, et al. Antiepileptika in der Neugeborenenperiode. *Monatsschr Kinderheilkd* 1983; 131:6–12.
29. Boreus LO, Jalling B, Kallberg N. Clinical pharmacology of phenobarbital in the neonatal period. In: Morselli PL, Garattini S, Sereni F, eds. *Basic and Therapeutic Aspects of Perinatal Pharmacology*. New York: Raven Press, 1975:331–340.
30. Dodson WE. Antiepileptic drug utilization in pediatric patients. *Epilepsia* 1984; 25: S132–S139.
31. Heinze E, Kampffmeyer HG. Biological half-life of phenobarbital in human babies. *Klin Wochenschr* 1971; 49:1146–1147.
32. Ehrnebo M, Agurell S, Jalling B, Boreus LO. Age differences in drug binding by plasma proteins: studies on human foetuses, neonates and adults. *Eur J Clin Pharmacol* 1971; 3:189.
33. Painter MJ, Pippenger C, MacDonald H, Pitlick W. Phenobarbital and diphenylhydantoin levels in neonates with seizures. *J Pediatr* 1978; 92:315–319.
34. Lockman LA, Kriel R, Zaske D. Phenobarbital dosage for control of neonatal seizures. *Neurology* 1979; 29:1445–1449.
35. Pitlick W, Painter M, Pippenger C. Phenobarbital pharmacokinetics in neonates. *Clin Pharmacol Ther* 1978; 23:346–350.
36. Strandjord RE, Johannessen SI. Serum levels of phenobarbitone in healthy subjects and patients with epilepsy. In: Gardner-Thorpe C, Janz D, Meinardi H, Pippenger CE, eds. *Antiepileptic Drug Monitoring*. Tunbridge Wells (Kent), UK: Pitman Medical, 1977:89–103.
37. Brachet-Lierman A, Gouteres F, Aicardi J. Absorption of phenobarbital after the intramuscular administration of single doses in infants. *J Pediatr* 1975; 87:624–626.
38. Jalling B. Plasma and cerebrospinal fluid concentrations of phenobarbital in infants given single doses. *Dev Med Child Neurol* 1974; 11:781–793.
39. Butler TC, Waddell WJ. Metabolic conversion of primidone (Mysoline) to phenobarbital. *Proc Soc Exp Biol Med* 1956; 93:544–546.
40. Tang BK, Kalow W, Grey AA. Metabolic fate of phenobarbital in man. *N*-glucoside formation. *Drug Metab Dispos* 1979; 7:315–318.
41. Whyte MP, Dekaban AS. Metabolic fate of phenobarbital. A quantitative study of *p*-hydroxyphenobarbital elimination in man. *Drug Metab Dispos* 1977; 5:63–70.
42. Wilensky AJ, Friel PN, Levy RH, Comfort CF, et al. Kinetics of phenobarbital in normal subjects and epileptic patients. *Eur J Clin Pharmacol* 1982; 23:87–92.
43. Conney AH. Pharmacological implications of microsomal enzyme induction. *Pharmacol Rev* 1967; 19:317–366.
44. Butler TC, Mahafee C, Waddell WJ. Phenobarbital: studies of elimination, accumulation, tolerance, and dosage schedules. *J Pharmacol Exp Ther* 1954; 111:425–435.
45. Lous P. Blood serum and cerebrospinal fluid levels and renal clearance of phenemal in treated epileptics. *Acta Pharmacol Toxicol* 1954; 10:166–177.
46. Lous P. Plasma levels and urinary excretion of three barbituric acids after oral administration to man. *Acta Pharmacol Toxicol* 1954; 10:147–165.
47. Morselli PL, Rizzo M, Garrattini S. Interaction between phenobarbital and diphenylhydantoin in animals and in epileptic patients. *Ann N Y Acad Sci* 1971; 179: 88–107.
48. Patel IH, Levy RH, Cutler RE. Phenobarbital-valproic acid interaction. *Clin Pharmacol Ther* 1980; 27:515–521.

49. Domek NS, Barlow CF, Roth LJ. An ontogenetic study of phenobarbital-C 14 in cat brain. *J Pharmacol Exp Ther* 1960; 130:285–293.
50. Melchior JC, Svensmark O, Trolle D. Placental transfer of phenobarbitone in epileptic women, and elimination in newborns. *Lancet* 1967; 11:860–861.
51. Painter MJ, Pippenger CE, MacDonald H, Pitlick WH. Phenobarbital and phenytoin blood levels in neonates. *Pediatrics* 1977; 92:315–319.
52. Painter MJ, Pippenger C, Wasterlain C, Barmada M. Phenobarbital and phenytoin in neonatal seizures: metabolism and tissue distribution. *Neurology* 1981; 31:1107–1112.
53. Heimann G, Gladtke E. Pharmacokinetics of phenobarbital in childhood. *Eur J Clin Pharmacol* 1977; 12:305–310.
54. Jalling B. Plasma concentrations of phenobarbital in the treatment of seizures in the newborn. *Acta Paediatr Scand* 1975; 64:514–524.
55. Dodson WE, Prensky AL, DeVivo D, Goldring S, et al. Management of seizure disorders: selected aspects. Part I. *J Pediatr* 1976; 89:527–540.
56. Baumel I, DeFeo JJ, Lal H. Effects of acute hypoxia on brain-sensitivity and metabolism of barbiturates in mice. *Psychopharmacologia* 1970; 17:1983–1987.
57. Dauber IM, Krauss AN, Symchych PS, Auld PA. Renal failure following perinatal anoxia. *J Pediatr* 1976; 88:851–855.
58. Gal P, Toback J, Erkan NV, Boer HR, et al.The influence of asphyxia on phenobarbital dosing requirements in neonates. *Dev Pharmacol Ther* 1984; 7:145–152.
59. Morselli PL. Antiepileptics. In: Morselli PL, ed. *Drug Disposition During Development*. New York: Spectrum, 1977:311–360.
60. Neuvonen PJ, Elonen E. Effect of activated charcoal on absorption and elimination of phenobarbitone, carbamazepine and phenylbutazone in man. *Eur J Clin Pharmacol* 1980; 17:51–57.
61. Viswanathan CT, Booker HE, Welling PG. Bioavailability of oral and intramuscular phenobarbital. *J Clin Pharmacol* 1978; 18:100–105.
62. Yaffe SJ. Developmental factors influencing interactions of drugs. *Ann N Y Acad Sci* 1976; 281:90–97.
63. Neimann G, Gladtke E. Pharmacokinetics of phenobarbital in childhood. *Eur J Clin Pharmacol* 1977; 12:305.
64. Garrettson LK, Dayton PG. Disappearance of phenobarbital and diphenylhydantoin from serum of children. *Clin Pharmacol Ther* 1970; 11:674–679.
65. Dodson WE. Special pharmacokinetic considerations in children. *Epilepsia* 1987; 28: S56–S70.
66. Waddell WJ, Butler TC. Distribution and excretion of phenobarbital. *J Clin Invest* 1957; 36:1217–1226.
67. Kapetanovic IM, Kupferberg HJ. Inhibition of microsomal phenobarbital metabolism by valproic acid. *Biochem Pharmacol* 1981; 30:1361–1363.
68. Kapetanovic IM, Kupferberg HJ, Porter RJ, et al. Mechanism of valproate-phenobarbital interaction in epileptic patients. *Clin Pharmacol Ther* 1981; 29:480–486.
69. Giotti A, Maynert EW. The renal clearance of barbital and the mechanism of its reabsorption. *J Pharmacol Exp Ther* 1951; 101:296–309.
70. Myschetzky A, Lassen NA. Forced diuresis in treatment of acute barbiturate poisoning. In: Matthew H, ed. *Acute Barbiturate Poisoning*. Amsterdam: Excerpta Medica, 1971:223–232.
71. Davis M, Simmons C, Harrison NG, Williams R. Paracetamol overdose in man: relationship between pattern of urinary metabolites and severity of liver damage. *QJ Med* 1976; 45:181–191.
72. Vesell ES, Page JG. Genetic control of the phenobarbital-induced shortening of plasma antipyrine half-lives in man. *J Clin Invest* 1969; 48:2202–2209.
73. Cucinell SA, Conney AH, Sansur MS, Burns JJ. Drug interactions in man. I. Lowering effect of phenobarbital on plasma levels of bishydroxycoumarin (Dicumarol) and diphenylhydantoin (Dilantin). *Clin Pharmacol Ther* 1965; 6:420–429.
74. Christiansen J, Dam M. Influence of phenobarbital and diphenylhydantoin on plasma carbamazepine levels in patients with epilepsy. *Acta Neurol Scand* 1973; 49:543–546.
75. Lander CM, Eadie MJ, Tyrer JH. Factors influencing plasma carbamazepine concentration. *Clin Exp Neurol* 1977; 14:184–193.
76. Spina E, Martines C, Fazio A, et al. Effect of phenobarbital on pharmacokinetics of carbamazepine-10,11-epoxide, an active metabolite of carbamazepine. *Ther Drug Monit* 1991; 13:109–112.
77. Krasinski K, Kusmiesz H, Nelson JD. Pharmacologic interactions among chloramphenicol, phenytoin and phenobarbital. *Pediatr Infect Dis* 1982; 1:232–235.
78. Lader M. Drug interactions and the major tranquilizers. In: Grahame-Smith DG, ed. *Drug Interactions*. Baltimore: University Park Press, 1977:159–170.
79. Loga S, Curry S, Lader M. Interactions of orphenadrine and phenobarbitone with chlorpromazine: plasma concentrations and effects in man. *Br J Clin Pharmacol* 1975; 2:197–208.
80. Somogyi A, Gugler R. Drug interaction with cimetidine. *Clin Pharmacokinet* 1982; 7:23–41.
81. Carststensen H, Jacobsen N, Dieperink H. Interaction between cyclosporin and phenobarbitone. *Br J Clin Pharmacol* 1986; 21:550–551.
82. Neuvonen PJ, Penttila O, Lehtovaara R, Aho K. Effects of antiepileptic drugs on the elimination of various tetracycline derivatives. *Eur J Clin Pharmacol* 1975; 9:147–154.
83. Fonne R, Meyer UA. Mechanisms of phenobarbital-type induction of cytochrome P-450 isozymes. *Pharmacol Ther* 1987; 33:19–22.
84. Treiman DM, Pledger GW, DeGiorgio C, Tsay J-Y, et al. Increasing plasma concentration tolerability study of flunarizine in comedicated patients. *Epilepsia* 1993; 34:944–953.
85. Beaurey J, Weber M, Vignaud JM. Treatment of tinea capitis: metabolic interference of griseofulvin with phenobarbital. *Ann Dermatol Venereol* 1982; 109:567–570.
86. Linnoila M, Viukari M, Vaisanen K, Auvinen J. Effect of anticonvulsants on plasma haloperidol and thioridazine levels. *Am J Psychiatry* 1980; 137:819–821.
87. Stambaugh JE, Hemphill DM, Wainer IW, Schwartz I. A potentially toxic drug interaction between pethidine (meperidine) and phenobarbital. *Lancet* 1977; 1:398–399.
88. Liu SJ, Wang RIH. Case report of barbiturate-induced enhancement of methadone metabolism and withdrawal syndrome. *Am J Psychiatry* 1984; 141:1287–1288.
89. Rambeck B. Pharmacological interactions of mesuximide with phenobarbital and phenytoin in hospitalized epileptic patients. *Epilepsia* 1979; 20:147–156.
90. Braithwaite RA, Flanagan RA, Richens A. Steady state plasma nortriptyline concentrations in epileptic patients. *Br J Clin Pharmacol* 1975; 2:469–471.
91. Jonkman JHG, Upton RA. Pharmacokinetic drug interactions with theophylline. *Clin Pharmacokinet* 1984; 9:309–334.
92. May T, Rambeck B. Serum concentrations of valproic acid: influence of dose and comedication. *Ther Drug Monit* 1985; 7:387–390.
93. Perruca E, Gatti G, Frigo GM, et al. Disposition of sodium valproate in epileptic patients. *Br J Clin Pharmacol* 1978; 5:495–499.
94. MacDonald MG, Robinson DS. Clinical observations of possible barbiturate interference with anticoagulation. *JAMA* 1968; 204:95–100.
95. Rettie AE, Rettenmeier AW, Howald WN, Baillie TA. Cytochrome P-450-catalyzed formation of delta-four VPA, a toxic metabolite of valproic acid. *Science* 1987; 235: 890–893.
96. Kesterson JW, Granneman GR, Machinist JM. The hepatotoxicity of valproic acid and its metabolites in rats. I. Toxicologic, biochemical and histopathologic studies. *Hepatology* 1984; 4:1143–1152.
97. Kochen W, Schneider A, Ritz A. Abnormal metabolism of valproic acid in fatal hepatic failure. *Eur J Pediatr* 1983; 141:30–35.
98. Prickett KS, Baillie TA. Metabolism of unsaturated derivatives of valproic acid in rat liver microsomes and destruction of cytochrome P-450. *Drug Metab Dispos* 1986; 14:221–229.
99. Segura-Bruna N, Rodruiguez-Campello A, Puente V, Roquer J. Valproate-induced hyperammonemic encephalopathy. *Acta Neurol Scand* 2006; 114(1):1–7.
100. Booker HE, Tormey A, Toussaint J. Concurrent administration of phenobarbital and diphenylhydantoin: lack of interference effect. *Neurology* 1971; 21:383–385.
101. Browne TR, Szabo GK, Evans JE, et al. Phenobarbital does not alter phenytoin steady-state serum concentration or pharmacokinetics. *Neurology* 1988; 38:639–642.
102. Brooks SM, Werk EE, Ackerman SJ, Sullivan I, et al. Adverse effects of phenobarbital on corticosteroid metabolism in patients with bronchial asthma. *N Engl J Med* 1972; 286:1125–1128.
103. Burstein S, Klaiber E. Phenobarbital induced increase in 6β-hydroxycortisol excretion: clue to its significance in human urine. *J Clin Endocrinol Metab* 1965; 25:293–296.
104. Janz D, Schmidt D. Antiepileptic drugs and failure of oral contraceptives. *Lancet* 1974; 1(7866):1113.
105. Levin W, Kuntzman R, Conney AH. Stimulatory effect of phenobarbital on the metabolism of the oral contraceptive 17α-ethynylestradiol-3-methyl ether (Mestranol) by rat liver microsomes. *Pharmacology* 1979; 19:249–255.
106. Kleinman PD, Griner PF. Studies of the epidemiology of anticoagulant drug interactions. *Arch Intern Med* 1970; 126:522–523.
107. Bourgeois BF. Pharmacologic interactions between valproate and other drugs. *Am J Med* 1988; 84:29–33.
108. Leppik IE, Sherwin A. Anticonvulsant activity of phenobarbital and phenytoin in combination. *J Pharmacol Exp Ther* 1977; 200:570–575.
109. Bourgeois BFD, Wad N. Combined administration of carbamazepine and phenobarbital: effect on anticonvulsant activity and neurotoxicity. *Epilepsia* 1988; 29:482–487.
110. Bittencourt PR, Richens A. Anticonvulsant-induced status epilepticus in Lennox-Gastaut syndrome. *Epilepsia* 1981; 22:129–134.
111. Vining EP. Use of barbiturates and benzodiazepines in treatment of epilepsy. *Neurol Clin* 1986; 4:617–632.
112. Buchthal F, Svensmark O, Simonsen H. Relation of EEG and seizures to phenobarbital in serum. *Arch Neurol* 1968; 19:567–572.
113. Hutt SJ, Jackson PM, Belsham A, Higgins G. Perceptual motor behavior in relation to blood phenobarbitone level: a preliminary report. *Dev Med Child Neurol* 1968; 10:626–632.
114. Mattson RH, Cramer JA, Collins JF, VA Epilepsy Cooperative Study #264 Group. Comparison between carbamazepine and valproate for complex partial and secondarily generalized tonic-clonic seizures. *Epilepsia* 1991; 32:S18.
115. Addy DT. Phenobarbitone and febrile convulsions. *Arch Dis Child* 1990; 65:921.
116. Sylvester CE, Marchlewski A, Manaligod JM. Primidone or phenobarbital use complicating disruptive behavior disorders. *Clin Pediatr* 1994; 33:252–253.
117. Herranz JL, Armijo JA, Arteaga R. Clinical side effects of phenobarbital, primidone, phenytoin, carbamazepine, and valproate during monotherapy in children. *Epilepsia* 1988; 29:794–804.
118. Ounsted C. The hyperkinetic syndrome in epileptic children. *Lancet* 1955; 1:303–311.
119. Wolf S, Forsythe A. Behavior disturbance, phenobarbital and febrile seizures. *Pediatrics* 1978; 61:729–731.
120. Camfield CS, Chaplin S, Doyle A. Side effects of phenobarbital in toddlers: behavioral and cognitive aspects. *J Pediatr* 1979; 95:361–365.
121. Mitchell W, Chavez J. Carbamazepine versus phenobarbital for partial onset seizures in children. *Epilepsia* 1987; 28:56–60.
122. Young RSK, Alger PM, Bauer L, Lauderbaugh D. A randomized double-blind crossover study of phenobarbital and methobarbital. *J Child Neurol* 1986; 1:361–363.
123. Hayes SG. Barbiturate anticonvulsants in refractory affective disorders. *Ann Clin Psychiatry* 1993; 5:35–44.
124. Lennox WG. Brain injury, drugs and environment as causes of mental decay in epilepsy. *Am J Psychiatry* 1942; 99:174–180.

125. Hillesmaa VK, Teramo K, Granstrom ML, Bardy AH. Fetal head growth retardation associated with maternal antiepileptic drugs. *Lancet* 1981; 1:165–167.
126. Somerfeld-Ziskind E, Ziskind E. Effect of phenobarbital on the mentality of epileptic patients. *Arch Neurol Psychol* 1940; 43:70–79.
127. Wapner I, Thurston DL, Holowach J. Phenobarbital: its effect on learning in epileptic children. *JAMA* 1962; 182:937.
128. Stores G. Behavioral effects of antiepileptic drugs. *Dev Med Child Neurol* 1975; 17: 647–658.
129. Schain RJ, Ward JW, Guthrie D. Carbamazepine as an anticonvulsant in children. *Neurology* 1977; 27:476–480.
130. Vining EPG, Mellits ED, Dorsen MM, et al. Psychologic and behavioral effects of antiepileptic drugs in children: a double-blind comparison between phenobarbital and valproic acid. *Pediatrics* 1987; 80:165–174.
131. Calandre EP, Dominguez-Granados R, Gomez-Rubio M, Molina-Font JA. Cognitive effects of long-term treatment with phenobarbital and valproic acid in school children. *Acta Neurol Scand* 1990; 81:504–506.
132. Hirtz DG, Sulzbacher SI, Ellenberg JH, Nelson KB. Phenobarbital for febrile seizures—effects on intelligence and on seizure recurrence. *N Engl J Med* 1990; 322:364–369.
133. Farwell J, Young J, Hartz D, et al. Phenobarbital for febrile seizures: effects on intelligence and on seizure recurrence. *N Engl J Med* 1990; 322:364–369.
134. Hollister LE. Nervous system reactions to drugs. *Ann N Y Acad Sci* 1965; 123: 342–353.
135. Isbell H, Fraser HF. Addiction to analgesics and barbiturates. *Pharmacol Rev* 1959; 2:355–397.
136. Berman LB, Jeghers HJ, Schreiner GE, Pallotta AJ. Hemodialysis, an effective therapy for acute barbiturate poisoning. *JAMA* 1956; 161:820–827.
137. Christiansen C, Rodbro P, Lund M. Incidence of anticonvulsant osteomalacia and effect of vitamin D: controlled therapeutic trial. *Br Med J* 1973; 4:695–701.
138. Richens A, Rowe DJF. Disturbance of calcium metabolism by anticonvulsant drugs. *Br Med J* 1970; 4:73–76.
139. Hahn TJ, Birge SJ, Shapp CR, Avioli LV. Phenobarbital-induced alterations in vitamin D metabolism. *J Clin Invest* 1972; 51:741–748.
140. Hunter J. Effects of enzyme induction on vitamin D_3 metabolism in man. In: Richens A, Woodford FP, eds. *Anticonvulsant Drugs and Enzyme Induction*. New York: Elsevier, 1976:77–84.
141. Offermann G, Pinto V, Kruse R. Antiepileptic drugs and vitamin D supplementation. *Epilepsia* 1979; 20:3–15.
142. Perruca E. Clinical implications of hepatic microsomal enzyme induction by antiepileptic drugs. *Pharmacol Ther* 1987; 33:139–144.
143. Welton DG. Exfoliative dermatitis and hepatitis due to phenobarbital. *JAMA* 1950; 143:232–234.
144. Mockli G, Crowley M, Stern R, Warnock ML. Massive hepatic necrosis in a child after administration of phenobarbital. *Am J Gastroenterol* 1989; 84:820–822.
145. Morkunas AR, Miller MB. Anticonvulsant hypersensitivity syndrome. *Crit Care Clin* 1997; 13:727–739.
146. Smith DB, Mattson RH, Cramer JA, et al. Results of a nationwide Veterans Administration Cooperative Study comparing the efficacy and toxicity of carbamazepine, phenobarbital, phenytoin, and primidone. *Epilepsia* 1987; 28 Suppl 3.
147. Mattson RH, Cramer JA, Collins JF, et al. Comparison of carbamazepine, phenobarbital, phenytoin, and primidone in partial and secondarily generalized tonic-clonic seizures. *N Engl J Med* 1985; 313:145–151.
148. Feely M, O'Callagan M, Duggan G, Callagan N. Phenobarbitone in previously untreated epilepsy. *J Neurol Neurosurg Psychiatry* 1980; 43:364–368.
149. Schmidt D, Richter K. Alternative single anticonvulsant drug therapy for refractory epilepsy. *Ann Neurol* 1986; 19:85–87.
150. Forsythe WI. One drug for childhood grand mal: medical audit for three-year remissions. *Dev Med Child Neurol* 1984; 26:742–748.
151. Schmidt D. Two antiepileptic drugs for intractable epilepsy with complex-partial seizures. *J Neurol Neurosurg Psychiatry* 1982; 45:1119–1124.
152. Schmidt D. Single drug therapy for intractable epilepsy. *J Neurol* 1983; 229:221–226.
153. Cornaggia CM, Canevini MP, Giuccioli D, Pruneri C, et al. Carbamazepine, phenytoin and phenobarbital in drug-resistant partial epilepsies. *Ital J Neurol Sci* 1986; 7: 113–117.
154. Callaghan N, O'Dwyer R, Keating J. Unnecessary polypharmacy in patients with frequent seizures. *Acta Neurol Scand* 1984; 69:15–19.
155. Painter MJ. How to use phenobarbital. In: Morselli PL, Pippinger CE, Penry JK, eds. *Antiepileptic Drug Therapy in Pediatrics*. New York: Raven Press, 1983:245–252.
156. Painter MJ. Phenobarbital clinical use. In: Levy RH, Dreifuss FE, Mattson RH, Meldrum BS, Penry JK, eds. *Antiepileptic Drugs*. 3rd ed. New York: Raven Press, 1989: 329–340.
157. Elwes RDS, Johnson AL, Shorvon SC, Reynolds EH. The prognosis for seizure control in newly diagnosed epilepsy. *N Engl J Med* 1984; 311:944–947.
158. Bourgeois BFD. Primidone. In: Wyllie E, ed. *The Treatment of Epilepsy: Principles and Practices*. Philadelphia: Lea & Febiger, 1993:909–913.
159. Tokola RA, Neuvonen PJ. Pharmacokinetics of antiepileptic drugs. *Acta Neurol Scand Suppl* 1983; 97:17–27.
160. Alix D, Berthou F, Riche C, Castel Y. Concentrations plasmatiques de phenobarbital et posologie en fonction de l'age. *Dev Pharmacol Ther* 1984; 7:164–170.
161. Rossi LN. Correlation between age and plasma level dosage for phenobarbital in infants and children. *Acta Paediatr Scand* 1979; 68:431–434.
162. Mizrahi E, Kelloway P. Characterization and classification of neonatal seizures. *Neurology* 1987; 37:1837–1844.
163. Painter MJ, Gaus LM. Neonatal seizures: diagnosis and treatment (review). *J Child Neurol* 1991; 6:101–108.
164. Fischer J, Lockman L, Zoske D, Kriel R. Phenobarbital maintenance dose requirements in treating neonatal seizures. *Neurology* 1982; 31:1042–1044.
165. Donn S, Grasela T, Goldstein G. Safety of a higher loading dose of phenobarbital in the term newborn. *Pediatrics* 1985; 75:1061–1064.
166. Painter MJ, Gaus LM. Phenobarbital. In: Wyllie E, ed. *The Treatment of Epilepsy: Principles and Practices*. Philadelphia: Lea & Febiger, 1993:900–908.
167. Connell J, Oozeer R, DeVries L, Dubowitz L, et al. Clinical and EEG response to anticonvulsants in neonatal seizures. *Arch Dis Child* 1989; 64:459–464.
168. Gal P, Boer HR, Toback J, Erkan NV. Phenobarbital dosing in neonates and asphyxia. *Neurology* 1982; 32:788–789.
169. Gilman J, Gal P, Duchowny M, Weaver R, et al. Rapid sequential phenobarbital treatment of neonatal seizures. *Pediatrics* 1989; 83:674–678.
170. Svenningson NW, Blennow G, Landroth M, Gaddlin P, et al. Brain oriented intensive care treatment in severe neonatal asphyxia. *Arch Dis Child* 1982; 57:176–183.
171. Grasela TH, Donn SM. Neonatal population pharmacokinetics of phenobarbital derived from routine clinical data. *Dev Pharmacol Ther* 1985; 8:374–383.
172. Siemes H. New aspects in prevention of febrile convulsions. *Klin Pädiatr* 1992; 204: 67–71.
173. Faero O, Kastrup KW, Nielsen E, Melchior JC, et al. Successful prophylaxis of febrile convulsions with phenobarbital. *Epilepsia* 1972; 13:279–285.
174. Minagawa K, Miura H. Phenobarbital, primidone and sodium valproate in the prophylaxis of febrile convulsions. *Brain Dev* 1981; 3:385–393.
175. McKinlay I, Newton R. Intention to treat febrile convulsions with rectal diazepam, valproate or phenobarbitone. *Dev Med Child Neurol* 1989; 31:617–625.
176. Schmidt D. Pharmacotherapy of epilepsy—current problems and controversies. *Fortschritte der Neurologie-Psychiatrie* 1983; 51:363–386.
177. Herranz JL, Armijo JA, Arteaga R. Effectiveness and toxicity of phenobarbital, primidone, and sodium valproate in the prevention of febrile convulsions, controlled by plasma levels. *Epilepsia* 1984; 25:89–95.
178. Theodore WH, Porter RJ, Raubertas RF. Seizures during barbiturate withdrawal: relation to blood level. *Ann Neurol* 1987; 22:644–647.
179. Butler TC, Waddell WJ. *N*-methylated derivatives of barbituric acids, hydantoin and oxazolidine used in the treatment of epilepsy. *Neurology* 1958; 8(Suppl 1):106–112.
180. Hooper WD, Kunze HE, Eadie MJ. Pharmacokinetics and bio-availability of methylphenobarbital in man. *Ther Drug Monit* 1981; 3:39–44.
181. Hooper WD, Qing MS. The influence of age and gender on the stereoselective metabolism and pharmacokinetics of methylphenobarbital in humans. *Clin Pharmacol Ther* 1990; 48:633–640.
182. Lim W, Hooper WD. Stereoselective metabolism and pharmacokinetics of methylphenobarbitone in humans. *Drug Metab Dispos* 1989; 17:212–217.
183. Eadie MJ, Bochner F, Hooper WD, Tyrer JH. Preliminary observations on the pharmacokinetics of methyl-phenobarbitone. *Clin Exp Neurol* 1978; 15:131–144.
184. Kunze HE, Hooper WD, Eadie MJ. High performance liquid chromatographic assay of methylphenobarbital and metabolites in urine. *Ther Drug Monit* 1981; 3:45–49.
185. Craig CR, Shideman FE. Metabolism and anticonvulsant properties of mephobarbital and phenobarbital in rats. *J Pharmacol Exp Ther* 1971; 176:35–42.
186. Lowenstein DH, Aminoff MJ, Simon RP. Barbiturate anesthesia in the treatment of status epilepticus: clinical experience with 14 patients. *Neurology* 1988; 38: 395–400.
187. Delgado-Escueta AV, Wasterlain C, Treiman DM, Porter RJ. Current concepts in neurology: management of status epilepticus. *N Engl J Med* 1982; 306:1337–1340.
188. Simon RP. Management of status epilepticus. In: Pedley TA, Meldrum BS, eds. *Recent Advances in Epilepsy*. London: Churchill Livingstone, 1985:.
189. Fraser HF, Wikler A, Essig CF, Isbell H. Degree of physical dependence induced by secobarbital or pentobarbital. *JAMA* 1958; 166:126–129.
190. Essig CF. Clinical and experimental aspects of barbiturate withdrawal convulsions. *Epilepsia* 1967; 8:21–30.
191. Narahashi T, Moore JW, Postron RN. Anesthetic blocking of nerve membrane conductances by internal and external applications. *J Neurobiol* 1969; 1:3–22.
192. Proctor WR, Weakly JN. A comparison of the presynaptic and postsynaptic actions of pentobarbitone and phenobarbitone on the neuromuscular junction of the frog. *J Physiol* 1976; 258:257–268.
193. Handley R, Stewart ASR. Mysoline: a new drug in the treatment of epilepsy. *Lancet* 1952; 1:742–744.
194. Bogue JY, Carrington HC. The evaluation of Mysoline—a new anticonvulsant drug. *Br J Pharmacol* 1953; 8:230–235.
195. Frey HH, Hahn I. Untersuchungen über die Bedeutung des durch Biotransformation gebildeten Phenobarbital für die antikonvulsive Wirkung von Primidon. *Arch Int Pharmacodyn Ther* 1960; 128:281–290.
196. Baumel IP, Gallagher BB, DiMicco D, Goico H. Metabolism and anticonvulsant properties of primidone in the rat. *J Pharmacol Exp Ther* 1973; 186:305–314.
197. Leal KW, Rapport RL, Wilensky AJ, Friel PN. Single dose pharmacokinetics and anticonvulsant efficacy of primidone in mice. *Ann Neurol* 1979; 5:470–474.
198. Frey HH, Loscher W. Is primidone more efficient than phenobarbital? An attempt at a pharmacological evaluation. *Nervenarzt* 1980; 51:359–362.
199. Schottelius DD, Fincham RW. Clinical application of serum primidone levels. In: Pippenger CE, Penry JK, Kutt H, eds. *Antiepileptic Drugs: Quantitative Analysis and Interpretation*. New York: Raven Press, 1978:273–282.
200. Kauffman RE, Habersang R, Lansky J. Kinetics of primidone metabolism and excretion in children. *Clin Pharmacol Ther* 1977; 22:200–205.

201. Gallagher BB, Baumel IP, Mattson RH. Metabolic disposition of primidone and its metabolites in epileptic subjects after single and repeated administration. *Neurology* 1972; 22:1186–1192.
202. Gallagher BB, Baumel IP. Primidone. Absorption, distribution and excretion. In: Woodbury DM, Penry JK, Schmidt RP, eds. *Antiepileptic Drugs*. New York: Raven Press, 1972:357–359.
203. Wyllie E, Pippenger CE, Rothner AD. Increased seizure frequency with generic primidone. *JAMA* 1987; 258:1216–1217.
204. Cloyd JC, Miller KW, Leppik IE. Primidone kinetics: effects of concurrent drugs and duration of therapy. *Clin Pharmacol Ther* 1981; 29:402–407.
205. Baumel IP, Gallagher BB, Mattson RH. Phenylethylmalonamide (PEMA). An important metabolite of primidone. *Arch Neurol* 1972; 27:34–41.
206. Pisani F, Richens A. Pharmacokinetics of phenylethylmalonamide (PEMA) after oral and intravenous administration. *Clin Pharmacol* 1983; 8:272–276.
207. Zavadil P, Gallagher BB. Metabolism and excretion of ^{14}C-primidone in epileptic patients. In: Janz D, ed. *Epileptology*. Stuttgart: Georg Thieme, 1976:129–139.
208. Oleson OV, Dam M. The metabolic conversion of primidone to phenobarbitone in patients under long-term treatment. *Acta Neurol Scand* 1967; 43:348–356.
209. Battino D, Avanzini G, Bossi L, et al. Plasma levels of primidone and its metabolite phenobarbital: Effect of age and associated therapy. *Ther Drug Monit* 1983; 5:73–79.
210. Armijo JA, Herranz JL, Arteaga R, Valiente R. Poor correlation between single-dose data and steady-state kinetics for phenobarbitone, primidone, carbamazepine and sodium valproate in children during monotherapy. Possible reasons for lack of correlation. *Clin Pharmacokinet* 1986; 11:323–335.
211. Booker HE, Hosokowa K, Burdette RD, Darcey B. A clinical study of serum primidone levels. *Epilepsia* 1970; 11:395–402.
212. Bourgeois BFD. Primidone. In: Resor SR, Kutt H, eds. *The Medical Treatment of Epilepsy*. New York: Marcel Dekker, 1992:371–378.
213. Sutton G, Kupferberg HJ. Isoniazid as an inhibitor of primidone metabolism. *Neurology* 1975; 25:1179–1181.
214. Bourgeois BF, Dodson WE, Ferrendelli JA. Isoniazid and other drugs. *Pediatrics* 1982; 70:824–825 (letter).
215. Bourgeois BF, Dodson WE, Ferrendelli JA. Interactions between primidone, carbamazepine, and nicotinamide. *Neurology* 1982; 32:1122–1126.
216. Fincham RW, Schottelius DD, Sahs AL. The influence of diphenylhydantoin on primidone metabolism. *Arch Neurol* 1974; 30:259–262.
217. Reynolds EH, Fenton G, Fenwick P, Johnson AL, et al. Interaction of phenytoin and primidone. *Br Med J* 1975; 2:594–595.
218. Bruni J. Valproic acid and plasma levels of primidone and derived phenobarbital. *Can J Neurol Sci* 1981; 8:91–92.
219. Windorfer JA, Sauer W. Drug interactions during anticonvulsant therapy in childhood: diphenylhydantoin, primidone, phenobarbitone, clonazepam, nitrazepam, carbamazepine and dipropylacetate. *Neuropädiatrie* 1977; 8:29–41.
220. Smith BH, McNaughton FL. Mysoline, a new anticonvulsant drug. Its value in refractory cases of epilepsy. *Can Med Assoc J* 1953; 68:464–467.
221. Sciarra D, Carter S, Vicale CT, Merrit HH. Clinical evaluation of primidone (Mysoline), a new anticonvulsant drug. *JAMA* 1954; 154:827–829.
222. Gallagher BB, Baumel IP, Mattson RH, Woodbury SG. Primidone, diphenylhydantoin and phenobarbital: aspects of acute and chronic toxicity. *Neurology* 1973; 23:145–149.
223. Leppik IE, Cloyd JC, Miller K. Development of tolerance to the side effects of primidone. *Ther Drug Monit* 1984; 6:189–191.
224. Ajax ET. An unusual case of primidone intoxication. *Dis Nerv Syst* 1966; 27: 660–661.
225. Leppik IE, Cloyd JC. Primidone: toxicity. In: Levy RH, Mattson RH, Meldrum BS, eds. *Antiepileptic Drugs*. 4th ed. New York: Raven Press, 1995:487–490.
226. Goldin S. Toxic effects of primidone. *Lancet* 1954; 1:102–103.
227. Brillman J, Gallagher BB, Mattson RH. Acute primidone intoxication. *Arch Neurol* 1974; 30:255–258.
228. Rodin EA, Rim CS, Kitano H, Lewis R, et al. A comparison of the effectiveness of primidone versus carbamazepine in epileptic outpatients. *J Nerv Ment Dis* 1976; 163:41–46.
229. Hartlage LC, Stovall K, Kocack B. Behavioral correlates of anticonvulsant blood levels. *Epilepsia* 1980; 21:185.
230. Dotevall G, Herner B. Treatment of acute primidone poisoning with bemegride and amphenazole. *Br Med J* 1957; 3:451–452.
231. Matzke GR, Cloyd JC, Sawchuk RJ. Acute phenytoin and primidone intoxication: a pharmacokinetic analysis. *J Clin Pharmacol* 1981; 21:92–99.
232. Lin SL, Chung MY. Acute primidone intoxication: report of a case. *J Formosan Med Assoc* 1989; 88:1053–1055.
233. van Heijst AN, de Jong W, Seldenrijk R, van Dijk A. Coma and crystalluria: a massive primidone intoxication treated with haemoperfusion. *J Toxicol Clin Toxicol* 1983; 20:307–318.
234. Lehman DF. Primidone cystalluria following overdose. A report of a case and an analysis of the literature. *Med Toxicol Adverse Drug Exp* 1987; 2:383–387.
235. Butter AJM. Mysoline in treatment of epilepsy. *Lancet* 1953; 1:1024.
236. Calnan WL, Borrell YM. Mysoline in the treatment of epilepsy. *Lancet* 1953; 2: 42–43.
237. Jorgenson G. Mysoline in the treatment of epilepsy. *Lancet* 1953; 2:835.
238. Smith B, Forster FM. Mysoline and Milontin: two new medicines for epilepsy. *Neurology* 1954; 4:137–142.
239. Livingston S, Petersen D. Primidone (Mysoline) in the treatment of epilepsy. *N Engl J Med* 1956; 254:327–329.
240. Millichap JC, Aymat F. Controlled evaluation of primidone and diphenylhydantoin sodium. Comparative anticonvulsant efficacy and toxicity in children. *JAMA* 1968; 204:738–739.
241. White PT, Pott D, Norton J. Relative anticonvulsant potency of primidone. *Arch Neurol* 1966; 14:31–35.
242. DeSilvey DL, Moss AJ. Primidone in the treatment of the long QT syndrome: QT shortening and ventricular arrhythmia suppression. *Ann Intern Med* 1980; 93:53–54.
243. Powell C, Painter MJ, Pippenger CE. Primidone therapy in refractory neonatal seizures. *JPediatr* 1984; 105:651–654.
244. Gruber CM, Brock JT, Dyken M. Comparison of the effectiveness of primidone, mephobarbital, diphenylhydantoin, ethotoin, metharbital, and methylphenylethylhydantoin in motor seizures. *Clin Pharmacol Ther* 1962; 3:23–28.
245. Booker HE. Primidone toxicity. In: Woodbury DM, Penry JK, Schmidt RP, eds. *Antiepileptic Drugs*. 1st ed. New York: Raven Press, 1972:377–383.
246. Oxley J, Hebdige S, Laidlaw J, Wadsworth J, et al. A comparative study of phenobarbitone and primidone in the treatment of epilepsy. In: Johannessen SI, Morselli PL, Pippenger CE, et al, eds. *Advances in Drug Monitoring*. New York: Raven Press, 1980:237–245.
247. Sapin JI, Riviello JJJ, Grover WD. Efficacy of primidone for seizure control in neonates and young infants. *Pediatr Neurol* 1988; 4:292–295.
248. Shorvon S. The treatment of epilepsy by drugs. In: Hopkins A, ed. *Epilepsy*. New York: Demos, 1987:229–282.
249. Eadie MJ. Formation of active metabolites of anticonvulsant drugs. A review of their pharmacokinetic and therapeutic significance. *Clin Pharmacokinet* 1991; 21:27–41.
250. Bourgeois BFD, Lüders H, Morris H, et al. Rapid introduction of primidone using phenobarbital loading: acute primidone toxicity avoided. *Epilepsia* 1989; 30:667.
251. Coulter DL. Withdrawal of barbiturate anticonvulsant drugs: prospective controlled study. *Am J Ment Retard* 1988; 93:320–327.

Phenytoin and Related Drugs

W. Edwin Dodson

Since phenytoin was introduced for the treatment of epilepsy by Merritt and Putnam in 1938, it has become one of the most widely used and extensively investigated antiepileptic drugs. It has been administered to patients of all ages and thus provides a good model for evaluating the effects of age on pharmacokinetics. In addition, phenytoin is unique among the commonly prescribed antiepileptic drugs because of its nonlinear elimination kinetics (Figure 49-1) (1, 2).

CHEMISTRY

Phenytoin is a weak acid, having a pK_a of 8.06 (3) (Table 49-1). Phenytoin sodium is approximately 92% phenytoin, a difference that is sometimes important because of phenytoin's nonlinear elimination kinetics. Phenytoin has limited aqueous solubility, approximately 20 mg/L, unless solubilizing agents are added to the solution. Parenteral formulations of phenytoin are strongly basic and contain the alcohols propylene glycol and ethanol. These formulations are potentially cardiotoxic and thus should be administered slowly intravenously to avoid bradyarrhythmia and hypotension. The phenytoin prodrug fosphenytoin has enhanced solubility and circumvents this hazard; although it is considerably safer for intravenous (IV) administration, it is also considerably more expensive.

CLINICAL EFFICACY

The spectrum of activity of phenytoin includes status epilepticus, partial seizures, partial seizures secondarily generalized, tonic seizures, and generalized tonic-clonic seizures (4, 5). Increasing doses and levels of phenytoin are associated with progressive reduction of seizures in adults (6) and in children (7). When administered following head trauma, phenytoin reduces the risk of seizures within the initial seven days, but it has no effect on the long-term development of epilepsy (8). Long a mainstay in the treatment of status epilepticus, phenytoin has been displaced as the drug to use first by lorazepan (9).

Although the therapeutic range is widely quoted at 10 to 20 mg/L, individual patients may require lower or higher levels for successful treatment. Phenytoin is not effective against generalized absence seizures and may increase their frequency; it is also ineffective in preventing recurrent febrile seizures. Phenytoin has been widely used to treat neonatal seizures, including neonatal status epilepticus (10, 11, 12). After phenobarbital fails to control neonatal seizures, the chance that phenytoin will succeed is approximately 50% (13, 14). However, the

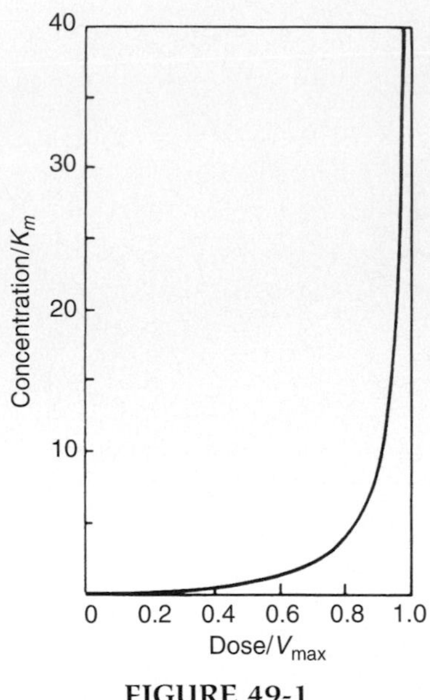

FIGURE 49-1

Dose versus concentration curve for drugs with nonlinear elimination kinetics. Reproduced with permission from (2).

response of neonatal seizures caused by hypoxia, ischemia, or hemorrhage is poor (15). Phenytoin is also used to treat kinesigenic choreoathetosis (16).

PHENYTOIN ADMINISTRATION

Phenytoin is available for parenteral and oral administration (Table 49-1). Although IV phenytoin is effective in stopping status epilepticus and in preventing recurrent seizures, it is slower acting than a benzodiazepine in stopping acute convulsions (17). However, when status has been interrupted by a short-acting drug such as diazepam, phenytoin can be administered next to prevent seizure recurrence. When phenytoin is administered intravenously, it must be given slowly to reduce the risk of cardiovascular toxicity (Table 49-2). For this reason, the safer formulation fosphenytoin is preferred because of the desirability of stopping status epilepticus as rapidly as possible.

Phenytoin has several advantages in the acute treatment of seizures. It is not sedating and thus does not potentiate sedation and respiratory depression as do benzodiazepines and barbiturates. When seizures persist after administration of phenytoin in status, cumulative doses of up to 30 mg/kg can be given initially but should not be exceeded unless it is documented that phenytoin levels are not excessive, because high phenytoin levels can cause seizures. Intramuscular phenytoin is not effective in the acute treatment of seizures.

In chronic oral therapy, phenytoin usually can be administered twice daily. Because of the nonlinear kinetics of phenytoin, it is best to begin with a low average dose and increase the dose stepwise until the desired clinical result is obtained. In young children, initial doses of 8–10 mg/kg/day are reasonable, whereas older children, adolescents, and young adults should begin with 6–8 mg/kg/day (18). As the dose is raised, progressively smaller increases should be made to avoid disproportionate increases in phenytoin level and resultant toxicity. If precise adjustment of phenytoin levels is necessary, the distinction between phenytoin and phenytoin sodium becomes an important consideration when mixing or switching to different products that contain phenytoin. The concentration of phenytoin in contemporary suspensions remains fairly uniform, but, in the past, suspensions were ill advised because of the tendency for phenytoin to settle out. Doses from the top of the bottle were lower than expected, whereas those from the bottom were higher than expected, because the suspended medication settled to the bottom after standing. In all instances when phenytoin dose has been changed, patients should be reexamined to evaluate whether the dose is correct because of the unpredictable relationship between phenytoin dose and concentration.

TABLE 49-1
Phenytoin Reference Information

Molecular weight of sodium phenytoin	274.25
Molecular weight of phenytoin	252.26
pK_a of phenytoin	8.06
Conversion factor	CF = 1000/252.3 = 3.96
Conversion	μg/ml (or mg/L) × 3.96 = μmoles/L
Formulations	
Phenytoin suspension (Dilantin)	50 mg/mL
Phenytoin (Dilantin Infatabs)	50 mg
Phenytoin sodium (Dilantin Capseals)	30, 60, or 100 mg
Type of elimination kinetics	Nonlinear

TABLE 49-2
Aspects of Phenytoin Administration

Intravenous dose	15–20 mg/kg*
Intravenous administration rates	
Rate in adults	< 50 mg/min
Rate in infants and children	< 3 mg/kg/min
Maintenance dose	6–20 mg/kg/day
Therapeutic concentration range	10–20 mg/L

*Administer slowly to avoid cardiovascular toxicity.

TABLE 49-3
Phenytoin Pharmacokinetics

Protein binding	90%
Volume of distribution	
Newborns	0.8–1.2 L/kg
Older children and adults	0.7–0.9 L/kg
Half-life	Concentration-dependent
Nonlinear kinetic parameters	
K_M	5 mg/L
V_{max}	10–20 mg/kg/day

**See text for details.

BIOTRANSFORMATION, PHARMACOKINETICS AND INTERACTIONS IN HUMANS

Phenytoin is largely eliminated by enzymatic biotransformation in the liver to 5-parahydroxyphenyl, 5-phenylhydantoin (HPPH), which is the major metabolite, and to a dihydrodiol that accounts for approximately 10% of phenytoin metabolites in urine. Both of these metabolites are thought to be derived from a highly reactive arene oxide (epoxide) intermediate (19, 15). Negligible amounts of unmetabolized phenytoin are excreted in urine.

Phenytoin is metabolized by the cytochrome P450 enzymes CYP2C9 and CYP2C19 (20, 21). In some families that metabolize phenytoin slowly, mutations have been identified that account for these pharmacokinetic differences (22). Odani et al. identified a mutation of CYP2C9 caused by a substitution of leucine for isoleucine at position 359 that results in a reduction of 33% in maximal capacity to metabolize (V_{max}) phenytoin among Japanese people. Mutations in CYP2C19 reduced V_{max} by as much as 14%.

Phenytoin has nonlinear kinetics in all age groups (1, 23–30). As the dose and concentration of phenytoin increase, the eliminating mechanism becomes progressively saturated, reducing the fraction of phenytoin that is eliminated per unit of time. This leads to a nonlinear relationship between phenytoin dose and concentration (Figure 49-1). Because increasing doses cause disproportional rises in the phenytoin level, smaller increments in dose should be made as the phenytoin level approaches the therapeutic range. Phenytoin kinetics are best characterized by Michaelis-Menten equations. However, the concept of half-life is widely used in clinical pharmacokinetics and therefore merits discussion (Table 49-3).

PHENYTOIN HALF-LIFE

The kinetics of phenytoin elimination are concentration-dependent. Although the half-life of phenytoin is widely quoted and discussed, applying the concept of a half-life to phenytoin kinetics is technically improper, because phenytoin does not have first-order elimination kinetics. The apparent half-life ($t_{50\%}$) of phenytoin changes depending on the concentration range over which it is measured. As a consequence of phenytoin's nonlinear elimination kinetics, increasing concentrations lead to prolongation of the apparent half-life. When phenytoin levels are high, the apparent half-lives can be quite prolonged (25, 30). As the level declines, the rate of phenytoin elimination accelerates and the apparent half-life becomes shorter (Figure 49-2). Thus, at different concentrations, different half-lives can be measured in a single patient. The apparent half-life is sometimes designated by $t_{50\%}$. As was shown in equation 5 in

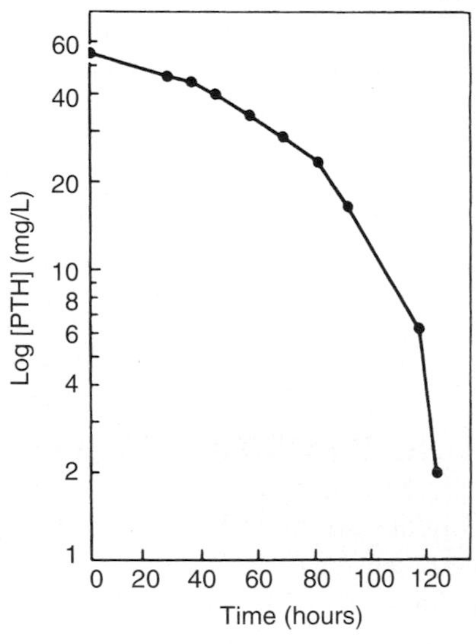

FIGURE 49-2

Log phenytoin concentration versus time curve that was obtained in a 14-month-old who ingested a large dose of phenytoin. Note that the observed half-life becomes progressively shorter as the concentration declines. Reproduced with permission from (18).

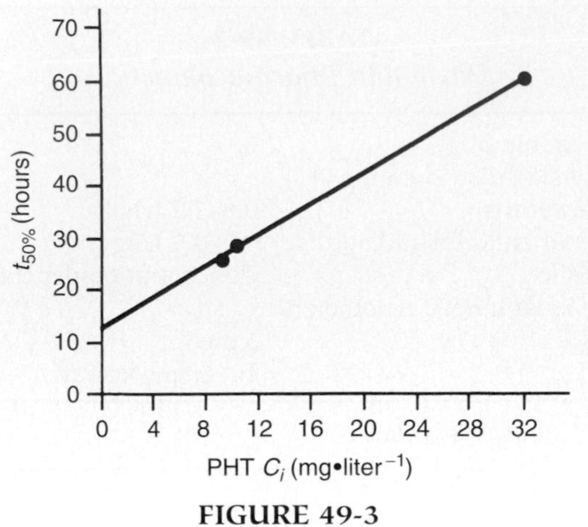

FIGURE 49-3

Relationship of the initial concentration (Ci) to the apparent half-life that was observed in an infant taking phenytoin. As the concentration increased, the apparent half-life (t_{50}%) was prolonged.

Chapter 23, the $t_{50\%}$ is directly related to the concentration at which the $t_{50\%}$ is determined (Figure 49-3).

Because the $t_{50\%}$ of phenytoin varies, it takes longer than expected for patients to reach a steady state. This is particularly a problem when patients take relatively high doses that are close to their maximal phenytoin eliminating capacity (V_{max}). As a rule of thumb, at least two weeks should be allowed before phenytoin levels are considered to be at steady state after the dose is changed. In some patients who have very high levels, even more time may be required.

The changing $t_{50\%}$ of phenytoin is occasionally useful in clinical situations. For example, small increases in the average phenytoin level can be achieved by giving the total daily dose as a single dose (31). This increases the average level slightly because the large single dose produces a higher initial phenytoin concentration, thereby prolonging the $t_{50\%}$. Dividing the daily dose into more frequent daily doses has the opposite effect and slightly lowers the average concentration.

NONLINEAR KINETICS, K_M AND V_{MAX}

Phenytoin kinetics are best characterized by Michaelis-Menten kinetic parameters K_M and V_{max}. Children and adults have similar K_M values of approximately 5 mg/L. However, children have higher capacity to eliminate phenytoin than adults, resulting in higher V_{max} (2, 23, 24, 32). Much of the variation in K_M is caused by drug interactions.

There are several methods for calculating the K_M and V_{max}. The easiest and most reliable method is the direct linear plot (33). This is a graphic solution that can be performed at the bedside. The method depends on knowing the patient's phenytoin level at two or more pairs of doses and steady-state concentrations. The concentrations should be obtained at consistent times after doses. When phenytoin is given twice daily, the best times to measure the level are just prior to a dose and 8 hours after a dose (34). Once K_M and V_{max} are known, it is possible to estimate the relationship between future doses and concentrations.

The direct linear plot technique for calculating K_M and V_{max} is fairly simple and is illustrated in Figure 49-4 (35). The negative value of the phenytoin level is plotted on the horizontal axis and the dose is plotted on the vertical axis. The dose and level pairs are connected by lines that are extended up and to the right, where they intersect. This point of intersection is used as a fulcrum for determining K_M, V_{max}, and other dose-level relationships. A horizontal line drawn from the point of intersection to the vertical axis is V_{max}. A vertical line drawn from the intersection indicates K_M on the horizontal axis. The relationships between other doses and levels are solved by drawing additional lines from the point of intersection as shown in Figure 49-4.

There are many nomograms and related methods for predicting the relationship between phenytoin dose and concentration in various groups of patients (29). Although these provide heuristic exercises in clinical pharmacology, they are untrustworthy guides to phenytoin dosing. In one study, significant errors in predicted levels occurred in 21% to 38% of subjects (36). Large errors are most likely among patients who need high phenytoin levels. For this reason, every patient whose phenytoin dose is changed should be reevaluated after an appropriate interval (29). Although nomograms can reduce trial and error

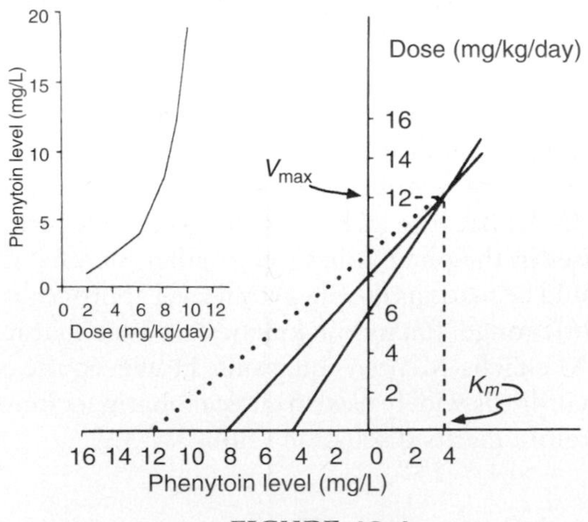

FIGURE 49-4

Direct linear plot (35). In this example K_M = 4 mg/L and V_{max} = 12 mg/kg/day. Predicted values are indicated by the dotted line. Insert indicates the shape of the dose versus concentration curve. See text for details.

in estimating phenytoin doses, they are no substitute for patient follow-up.

PHENYTOIN ABSORPTION

The nonlinear kinetics of phenytoin can affect the apparent extent of phenytoin absorption (bioavailability). Slowing the absorption rate has the practical result of reducing the apparent bioavailabililty (37). Computer simulations indicate that, at average values of K_M and V_{max}, increasing the absorption half-life from 0 to 1.2 hours causes the apparent bioavailability to decrease by approximately 25% (38). If the actual fraction that is absorbed also decreases slightly, the reduction in apparent bioavailability is greater. For example, with 90% absorption and an absorption half-life of 0.9 hours, the apparent bioavailability declines to 69%.

Although phenytoin is well absorbed after oral administration, the rate of absorption depends on the formulation. Changing excipients has been associated with changes in steady-state levels (39). But, even without changes in excipients, other aspects of tablet formulation can affect the absorption rate. Thus switching formulations can change the phenytoin levels significantly. For this reason, generic substitution of phenytoin should be discouraged.

In infants, peak phenytoin concentrations occur 2 to 6 hours after oral dosing (40). In older children, peak concentrations occur 3 to 10 hours following oral doses. The administration of phenytoin with food further delays the time to peak concentrations in patients of all ages (41). However, phenytoin taken postprandially produces 40% higher concentrations than when it is taken before meals (42). Thus the relationship between phenytoin doses and meals should be consistent.

Intramuscular administration of phenytoin is associated with slow and erratic absorption (43). Because of the low solubility of phenytoin, it can crystallize and precipitate at the injection site. Although phenytoin absorption is eventually complete, intramuscular administration of phenytoin is unreliable and should be avoided (44). If intramuscular administration is needed, fosphenytoin should be given.

PHENYTOIN DRUG-PROTEIN BINDING

The unbound drug concentration, not the total drug concentration, determines the drug's action. Phenytoin is normally 90% bound to constituents of serum, mainly to albumin. In diseases with hypoalbuminemia, such as renal disease, hepatic disease, severe malnutrition, burns, and pregnancy (45, 46), unbound phenytoin levels increase such that the total phenytoin levels no longer provide reliable indicators of the unbound levels. In these situations, measuring the unbound phenytoin level is sometimes indicated.

Phenytoin binding is also reduced by bilirubin and acidic compounds such as fatty acids, including valproic acid, and salicylate, which displace phenytoin from protein binding (47). Among developmentally disabled patients, hypoalbuminemia and comedication with valproate have been associated with unbound phenytoin fractions as high as 17% (48). When the unbound phenytoin fraction increases chronically, hepatic metabolism compensates such that the unbound concentration is readjusted to the previous steady-state level. This leads to a decline in the total phenytoin level, but the effect on unbound levels is insignificant. Thus, chronic changes in binding have a negligible effect on unbound phenytoin concentrations unless the dose is changed (49). On the other hand, acute changes in phenytoin binding such as those associated with dialysis may cause transient and symptomatic changes in unbound phenytoin levels. Rapidly fluctuating valproate levels can increase unbound phenytoin levels transiently, resulting in transient phenytoin toxicity (50).

EFFECT OF AGE ON PHENYTOIN PHARMACOKINETICS

The maximal capacity to eliminate phenytoin is affected by genetic factors, age, sex, and drug interactions (51, 52). However, it is important to note that the nonlinear kinetics of phenytoin have confounded most clinical investigations of the effect of age on phenytoin kinetics. When linear kinetic parameters such as half-life or relative clearance are used, the nonlinear kinetics often obscure age-related pharmacokinetic differences (25, 53). In a practical sense, the nonlinear kinetics of phenytoin influence relative dosage requirements more than does age.

Newborns

Newborns who are exposed to phenytoin in utero usually eliminate transplacentally acquired phenytoin at rates that are comparable to those in adults. Studies of urinary metabolites indicate that these newborns rapidly metabolize phenytoin (54). On the other hand, newborns with seizures eliminate phenytoin slowly at first, but later, during the neonatal period, they eliminate it rapidly after their drug-eliminating mechanisms have matured (26).

Among all age groups, premature and full-term newborns who were not exposed in utero to inducing agents have the lowest relative capacity to eliminate phenytoin; thus, they require the lowest doses on average. Phenytoin concentrations and apparent half-lives vary extensively in newborns with seizures, more so than in any other age group. Newborns with seizures have several factors that act simultaneously to produce unstable phenytoin levels. These include nonlinear phenytoin kinetics, postnatal maturation of hepatic function, induction of phenytoin elimination by phenobarbital and other drugs, and slowed phenytoin absorption, which occurs after the newborns have been switched from intravenous to oral dosing. Most newborns who receive phenytoin have been treated previously with phenobarbital. Phenobarbital affects the hepatic biotransformation of phenytoin, increasing both V_{max} and K_M (2, 55). For this reason the changing phenytoin kinetics during the neonatal period preclude the use of steady-state methods for analyzing the nonlinear kinetics of phenytoin. These changes make it necessary to increase the phenytoin dose during the neonatal period if consistently high phenytoin levels are needed.

High phenytoin concentrations occur after intravenous loading doses, often leading to very long apparent half-lives in the first and second week of life. The phenytoin half-lives that have been reported in newborns vary widely, with extremes of 6 hours to more than 200 hours after intravenous therapy (11, 26, 56). Bourgeois and Dodson (2) found that the phenytoin $t_{50\%}$ ranged from 6.9 to 140 hours, with an average value of 57.3 ± 48.2 hours. In newborns aged 3–5 weeks, the $t_{50\%}$ decreased by two-thirds.

After the first week of life, shorter phenytoin half-lives have been reported, but some newborns continue to have prolonged half-lives if phenytoin levels are high (11, 51). Painter et al. (9, 11) reported an average value of 104 ± 17 hours during the second week of life. In a different group of 16 newborns with seizures, half-lives diminished considerably after the first week of life (26). Among children more than 1-week-old, there was good correlation (r = 0.88 to 0.93) between the apparent half-life and the initial phenytoin concentration (26). Correcting for initial concentration revealed that newborns ages 3–5 weeks had the shortest half-life, averaging 19.7 and 12 hours at initial phenytoin concentrations of 18 and 10 mg/L, respectively.

After the first or second week of life, the capacity for phenytoin elimination increases and phenytoin concentrations often decline. Older newborns and young infants require doses as high as 18 to 20 mg/kg/day to achieve therapeutic levels (4). If declining concentrations occur when phenytoin administration is switched from the intravenous to the oral route, the changing dose requirements give the appearance of malabsorption of phenytoin (11, 12).

Newborns absorb phenytoin slowly but completely after oral administration, with less than 3% of administered phenytoin found in feces (57). Studies using stable isotope-labeled phenytoin also indicate complete absorption (58). Similarly, comparisons of levels obtained after intravenous and oral doses indicate complete absorption of orally administered suspensions (59). Thus the decline in phenytoin levels that takes place in the second or third week of life is caused by an increasing capacity for phenytoin biotransformation plus the unique consequences of nonlinear elimination kinetics. Despite numerous statements to the contrary, newborns do not malabsorb phenytoin. Reliable concentrations can be produced by oral administration even in premature newborns (59).

It is technically difficult to actually measure phenytoin bioavailability in newborns because of the changing elimination kinetics during the newborn period. For this reason, computer simulations have been used to provide insight into the problem. These simulations indicate that the changing phenytoin elimination kinetics (V_{max} and K_M)—and the slower absorption rates that occur after phenytoin administration is switched from intravenous to oral routes—both affect the phenytoin level (38). For example, slowing the absorption rate of phenytoin decreases the apparent bioavailabililty by as much as 26%.

The effects of varying the absorption rate and K_M on the apparent extent of phenytoin absorption are modest compared to the large changes that occur when V_{max} increases. Based on computer simulations, increasing V_{max} is expected to produce sizeable reductions in apparent bioavailability even when absorption is complete (38). For example, increasing V_{max} threefold from 5 mg/kg/day to 15 mg/kg/day causes the apparent bioavailability to decrease by 77%. Variations in K_M cause smaller changes in apparent bioavailability; changing K_M from 5 mg/L to 1 mg/L decreases the apparent bioavailability to 67%. Increasing K_M from 5 to 10 mg/L, such as might occur because of an interaction with phenobarbital, has the opposite effect.

Infants and Children

Among all age groups, infants have the highest relative capacity to eliminate phenytoin, causing them to have average dosage requirements that are fourfold greater than adults. V_{max}, but not K_M, changes with increasing age (2, 24) (Figure 49-5). After phenytoin-eliminating capacity peaks during infancy, it declines during childhood to adult values (23). In one study the V_{max} in infants ranged from 11 to 30 mg/kg/day and averaged 17.9 mg/kg/day (2). The average values in older children and adults are approximately 8 to 10 mg/kg/day in various studies. Although most of the variation in K_M is caused by drug interactions, K_M does vary independently as well. In one study 28% of children had a K_M of 2.5 mg/L or less (2). This low value of K_M makes it technically difficult to adjust phenytoin levels when levels are greater than 10 mg/L because the dose versus concentration curve becomes progressively steep and nonlinear (Figure 49-6).

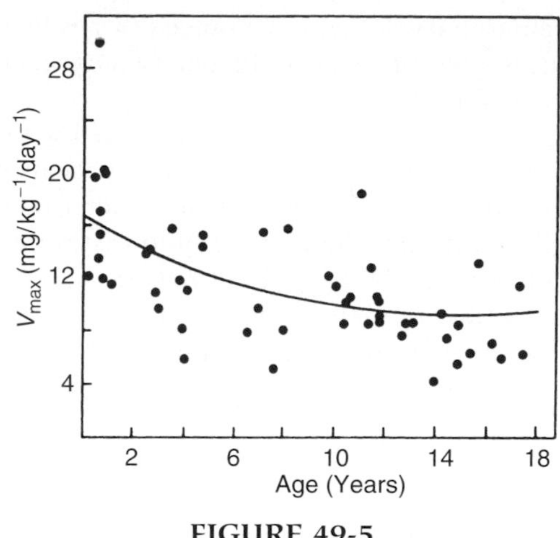

FIGURE 49-5

Relationship between age and V_{max} for phenytoin elimination. Reproduced with permission from (2).

The higher relative clearance for phenytoin in children gradually declines until adult values are reached around ages 10–15. (See Figure 37-6.) During this period, changes in body weight are offset by declining relative drug clearance, such that dosage changes are less frequent than expected. However, within any age group, individual patients deviate significantly from the group average. There are several causes for this variation: foremost among these are drug interactions and intercurrent illness.

Adolescents

No major changes in phenytoin kinetics have been described in adolescence. However, phenytoin concentrations fluctuate during the menstrual cycle. Although these fluctuations are usually modest, concentrations are higher at midcycle, when ovulation occurs, than at the time of menstruation. This suggests that increased concentrations of estrogen and progesterone interfere with phenytoin biotransformation (60). The fluctuations in phenytoin levels are most extensive in patients who have the highest concentrations.

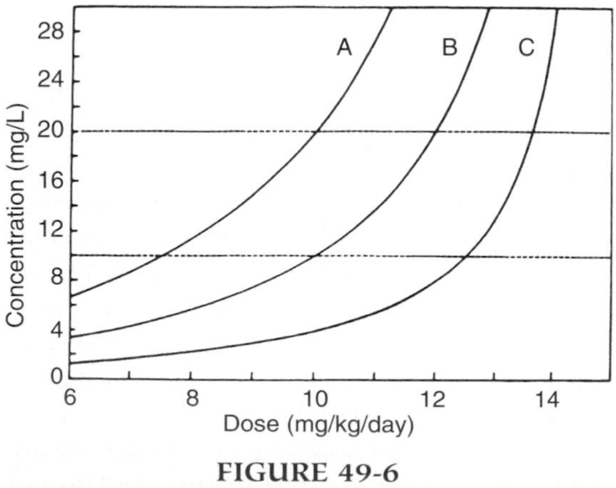

FIGURE 49-6

Dose versus concentration curves for varying values of K_M when V_{max} is held constant at 15 mg/kg/day. Note that, as the values for K_M decline from 10 to 2 mg/L, the curve becomes more nearly vertical through the concentration range of 10 to 20 mg/L. (A) K_M = 10 mg/L; (B) K_M = 5 mg/L; (C) K_M = 2 mg/L.

DRUG INTERACTIONS AND NONLINEAR KINETICS OF PHENYTOIN

Phenytoin is both a cause and a casualty of pharmacokinetic drug interactions. First, it is a potent inducer of many enzymes in the cytochrome P450 drug-metabolizing system (61). By this mechanism, the addition of phenytoin increases the clearance and decreases the concentrations of most other antiepileptics that are eliminated by hepatic metabolism. Examples include carbamazepine, methsuximide, primidone, valproate, and most of the antiepileptic drugs that have been introduced in the 1990s, including felbamate, topiramate, and lamotrigine. Besides enhancing the clearance of these compounds, phenytoin also stimulates the clearance of steroids, including oral contraceptives, and the clearance of vitamins, including vitamin D, folic acid, and vitamin K (61, 62).

Phenytoin elimination is extremely vulnerable to drug interactions by virtue of its dependence on hepatic metabolism for elimination and its nonlinear kinetics (63). Even though general trends can be described, the direction and extent of these interactions are highly unpredictable. For this reason diligent clinical follow-up is required whenever a comedication is added to or deleted from treatment regimens that include phenytoin.

Phenobarbital consistently increases both the V_{max} and K_M of phenytoin elimination (2). Thus phenobarbital has conflicting effects, acting simultaneously as an inducer and as a competitive inhibitor of phenytoin elimination. In groups of patients, the addition of phenobarbital to phenytoin regimens produces no change in the average phenytoin level, but, in individual patients, phenytoin levels can change significantly.

Drug interactions can make the adjustment of phenytoin easier or more difficult, depending on the drug that is involved. The phenobarbital-phenytoin interaction facilitates the titration of phenytoin levels in the upper part of therapeutic range (see Figure 49-5). This pharmacokinetic benefit is due to the increased value of K_M for phenytoin elimination, which leads to a mild degree of flattening of the phenytoin dose versus concentration curve. As a result, the dose to concentration relationship becomes more linear and more predictable. Carbamazepine interacts with phenytoin elimination by inducing cytochrome P450 enzymes CYP2C9 and CYP219 (20, 64, 65). The net effect of this interaction is to reduce both the K_M and V_{max} for phenytoin elimination (2, 66), which is a complex interaction that usually leads to a reduction in phenytoin level. This interaction makes readjustment of phenytoin levels technically difficult because of the reduced K_M value and increased nonlinearity of the dose-to-concentration relationship. Herbal treatment with *Ginkgo biloba* also induces CYP2C9 and has been reported to lower phenytoin levels (67). Valproate interacts with phenytoin by displacing it from binding sites on albumin and increasing the unbound phenytoin fraction. Valproate reduces the K_M of phenytoin elimination but has no effect on V_{max} (2). However, switching from the standard formulation of sodium valproate to a slow-release formulation can cause the phenytoin level to increase. Suzuki et al (68) found that the average phenytoin level went from 14.4 to 18.7 mg/L when the valproate formulation was switched to the slow-release formulation.

Certain drug interactions usually increase the phenytoin level. Chloramphenicol consistently inhibits phenytoin elimination, thus increasing phenytoin levels (69). Conversely, discontinuing chloramphenicol causes phenytoin levels to decline dramatically. Isoniazide also usually increases phenytoin levels. According to the Boston Collaborative Drug Surveillance Program, 27% of the patients who take isoniazide plus phenytoin develop phenytoin toxicity if the phenytoin dose is not adjusted (70).

EFFECT OF ILLNESS ON PHENYTOIN PHARMACOKINETICS

Intercurrent illness can cause changes both in seizure threshold and in drug levels. Among all antiepileptic drugs, phenytoin levels are most liable to change during intercurrent illness. Infectious mononucleosis, influenza immunization, streptococcal pharyngitis, and any illness that causes fever can cause reduced phenytoin levels (71–73). One study indicated that, during febrile illness, phenytoin levels decrease by approximately 50%, declining from 16 to 8 mg/L on the average (73). Changes of this magnitude are expected to contribute to seizure recurrence in some patients.

Chronic renal disease is usually associated with alterations of phenytoin binding. In nephrotic syndrome, phenytoin binding is reduced to 80%, doubling the unbound phenytoin fraction (74). In addition, the half-life of phenytoin is decreased in uremia (75). After successful renal transplantation, phenytoin binding returns to normal (76). Although dialysis removes relatively little phenytoin, dialysis can remove significant amounts of water, thereby altering the patient's serum albumin concentration (77). This can, in turn, reduce the unbound fraction of phenytoin following dialysis even though the total phenytoin level does not change (78). In these situations measuring the unbound phenytoin concentration may be necessary.

Significant hepatic disease is associated with hypoalbuminemia and with increased concentrations of bilirubin and bile acids in serum, which can alter phenytoin binding. In addition, the hepatic biotransformation of phenytoin is variably impaired if hepatic parenchymal function is reduced, such as occurs in hepatitis or passive hepatic congestion due to heart failure. Again, in this case measuring the unbound phenytoin level is sometimes indicated.

ADVERSE EFFECTS

Phenytoin causes some degree of side effects in the majority of patients, but only an estimated 10% to 40% of patients require a change of medication (79). In a study conducted among children in India, the risk of more than one side effect was 32%, 40%, and 19% for children treated with either phenobarbital, phenytoin, or sodium valproate, respectively. However, most of the side effects associated with phenytoin disappeared after phenytoin dosage adjustment (80).

In a British randomized comparison of phenytoin with carbamazepine, phenobarbital, and sodium valproate, all four drugs had equivalent efficacy, but there were substantial differences in side effects. After a high percentage of the children assigned to phenobarbital developed side effects, it was withdrawn from the study. Among the remaining agents, phenytoin was withdrawn in 9% of children compared to 4% withdrawal rates because of unacceptable side effects for carbamazepine and valproate (81).

Overall, the incidence of side effects with phenytoin is similar to that with carbamazepine, but the nature of the side effects differs. In children, the cosmetic side effects of gingival hyperplasia and hirsutism are notably common and aggravating after chronic phenytoin therapy.

Idiosyncratic side effects of phenytoin include blood dyscrasia, allergic reactions, and certain forms of neurotoxicity. Idiosyncratic neurotoxicity is a problem primarily in patients who are abnormal neurologically and who do not manifest the usual signs of phenytoin toxicity. Immune-mediated reactions to phenytoin usually occur within the first two months of therapy. These include rashes, fever, lymphadenopathy, eosinophilia, serum sickness with hepatic and renal dysfunction, and polymyositis (82). Pseudolymphoma consisting of rash, fever, and lymphadenopathy is rare.

Phenytoin is one of many drugs that can cause the antiepileptic drug hypersensitivity syndrome. This syndrome consists of rash, fever, lymphadenopathy, and visceral organ involvement—especially involvement of the liver or the kidneys. The estimated incidence is 1 in 3,000 exposures to phenytoin. Approximately 70% to 80% of patients demonstrate cross-reactivity with phenobarbital, primidone, and carbamazepine (83). The risk of serious skin rashes, defined as rashes extensive enough to require hospitalization, has been estimated at 2.3–4.5 per 10,000 for phenytoin compared to 1–4.1 for carbamazepine (84). Other forms of rash, such as fixed drug eruptions, have been linked to phenytoin as well (85).

Rarely, movement disorders are caused by phenytoin. These usually occur in patients who are neurologically abnormal (86). Both bradykinesia and choreoathetosis have been described. Both can occur on either an idiosyncratic or a dose-related basis, although the latter is more common, with most affected patients having levels greater than 20 mg/L (87, 88, 89). Choreoathetosis has occurred after intravenous therapy and may be long lasting (90, 91). Note that choreoathetosis can also be caused by carbamazepine and by ethosuximide (89, 92, 93).

Dose-related adverse effects of phenytoin may be either acute or delayed, appearing only after chronic treatment. The acute dose-related neurotoxicity of phenytoin was well described by Kutt et al. more than two decades ago (55). Nystagmus occurs at levels of 15–25 mg/L; ataxia occurs at levels greater than 30 mg/L; and mental changes, with lethargy and mental clouding, occur at levels above 40 mg/L. Most patients with levels 20 mg/L have nystagmus. Blood levels above 60 mg/L cause difficulty sitting up. Although rare, ophthalmoplegia is also dose related (94). Paradoxically, seizure frequency increases at phenytoin levels above 30 mg/L in some patients (95, 96). Among patients with severe epilepsy, this becomes a thorny management issue because certain patients require equally high levels for seizure control. The adverse effect of seizure exacerbation has been linked to several other drugs in addition to phenytoin, especially carbamazepine, gabapentin, phenobarbital, vigabatrin, and lamotrigine (97, 98). However, carbamazepine-exacerbated seizures may be controlled by replacing carbamazepine with phenytoin (99).

Phenytoin-induced encephalopathy with dementia is also rare. Usually subacute and insidious, this is more likely to occur in neurologically abnormal patients who do not manifest the usual progression of concentration-related toxic signs. It is usually reversible after phenytoin is discontinued (100–102).

Delayed adverse effects of phenytoin include peripheral neuropathy, reduced vitamin D levels, bone demineralization, and cosmetic changes (103). The cosmetic side effects of hirsutism and gingival hyperplasia are more common with phenytoin than with other antiepileptics. The incidence of gingival hyperplasia is approximately 40%, but percentages as high as 69% have been reported in patients in India with tuberculous meningitis who were treated chronically with phenytoin (104). Although not all studies agree, the risk of gingival hyperplasia appears to be directly related to the phenytoin dose and level and inversely related to age (105, 106). Factors that are unrelated to increased risk of this side effect include sex, age at onset of treatment, and duration of treatment (106). Other factors include genetic predisposition, plaque-induced gingival inflammation, immunological status, and the induction of growth factors. Overall, gingival hyperplasia is more common in children than in adults. Poor oral hygiene further increases the risk; preventive dental hygiene programs reduce the incidence and severity of this problem (107, 108).

The pathogenesis of gingival hyperplasia has not been completely elucidated. Reactive intermediates are thought to play a role. Microsomes from gingival tissue do have the capacity to metabolize phenytoin (109). Phenytoin also increases serum concentrations of basic fibroblast growth factor threefold. Furthermore, basic levels of fibroblast growth factor have correlated better with the extent of gingival overgrowth than age, phenytoin dose, duration of phenytoin administration, and serum phenytoin level (110).

The question of whether chronic phenytoin therapy at ordinary levels causes cerebellar and brain stem atrophy remains unanswered despite years of concern (111–113). The problem is complicated because cerebellar atrophy also occurs in patients with severe epilepsy who have not received phenytoin. In one study of mentally retarded patients, the incidence of cerebellar atrophy (28%) was similar in phenytoin-treated and untreated patients (114). Most cases of persistent ataxia and cerebellar and brain stem atrophy have occurred after chronically high levels of phenytoin and clinical signs of intoxication. However, brief periods of intoxication, and even single episodes of severe phenytoin intoxication, have been followed by cerebellar atrophy with permanent disability (115, 116). The issue is especially complex in mentally handicapped patients, who may not show the usual signs of phenytoin intoxication despite levels that would ordinarily be considered toxic (117). Nonetheless, high phenytoin levels have been temporally linked to the permanent loss of locomotion in mentally handicapped patients who had high levels chronically.

ADVANTAGES AND DISADVANTAGES OF PHENYTOIN

Historically, phenytoin has been one of the most widely used antiepileptic drugs in childhood epilepsy, but, over the past two decades, its use in children has diminished. Phenytoin has several special features that are advantageous compared to other antiepileptic drugs (Table 49-4). These include its availability for parenteral administration

TABLE 49-4
Summary of Special Features Regarding Phenytoin Administration in Childhood Epilepsy

Nonlinear elimination kinetics
Frequent drug interactions
Fosphenytoin preferred for intravenous and intramuscular administration
Need for slow intravenous administration of phenytoin
Unreliable intramuscular absorption of phenytoin
Paradoxical ability to cause seizures at high concentrations
Cosmetic and cognitive side effects
Generic substitution problematic

and its efficacy in status epilepticus. Pediatric physicians have extensive experience with phenytoin, and most are familiar with administering it to children. It is nonsedating. Disadvantages include the cosmetic and cognitive side effects and its complex nonlinear pharmacokinetics. The major adverse cognitive effects include slowing of motor and mental processes and variable impairment of memory.

Fosphenytoin

The intravenous administration of phenytoin has long been hazardous because of the need for alkaline pH and high concentrations of solvents (propylene glycol) in order to keep phenytoin in solution. The invention of fosphenytoin, the disodium phosphate ester of phenytoin, has circumvented both of these problems, resulting in safer phenytoin formulation for parenteral administration (118–120). Despite substantially increased cost compared to phenytoin, fosphenytoin has gained wide acceptance because of safety considerations (121,122).

Fosphenytoin can be administered intravenously and intramuscularly and can be used to administer phenytoin parenterally for extended periods if necessary (123–125). The phosphate ester is hydrolyzed rapidly by nonspecific hepatic phosphatases, releasing phenytoin. Although the half-life of the hydrolysis is approximately 8–15 minutes (126), the concentration of unbound phenytoin increases more rapidly because fosphenytoin displaces phenytoin from binding sites in blood (127, 128). As a result, the newly liberated phenytoin is largely unbound until the fosphenytoin concentration declines.

The fosphenytoin dose is prescribed and administered as equimolar amounts of phenytoin, called "phenytoin equivalents." Thus the loading and maintenance doses of fosphenytoin in phenytoin equivalents are identical to phenytoin doses (129). Fosphenytoin infusion causes fewer adverse effects than intravenous phenytoin (125). Unique side effects compared to phenytoin are pruritus and perineal paresthesias (130). Hypotension occurs less often following fosphenytoin intravenous infusion than with phenytoin but may occur later, after the infusion (131, 132). Compared to intravenous phenytoin, fosphenytoin infusion is less likely to be painful or to cause erythema, irritation at the infusion site, or venous cording (132, 133). It has not been reported to cause purple glove syndrome as intravenous phenytoin can. Occurring mainly in elderly patients, purple glove syndrome consists of progressive edema, pain, and discoloration of the limb following intravenous phenytoin infusion. (134).

Other Antiepileptic Compounds Related to Phenytoin

The other hydantoins with antiepileptic potential use include mephenytoin (Mesantoin), a N-methylated compound, and ethotoin (Peganone), which is N-ethylated (135). Information about the use of these drugs in children is scant. Whereas phenytoin has two phenyl groups in the 5 position of the hydantoin ring, mephenytoin has both a phenyl and an ethyl group, like phenobarbital; ethotoin has a single phenyl group in the same position. Like other N-alkylated compounds, both ethotoin and mephenytoin are dealkylated in the body. The spectrum of activity of these compounds is similar to that of phenytoin, but their side effects differ; both compounds have a lower incidence of gingival hyperplasia and hirsutism. The genetic basis for variability in mephenytoin metabolism has been described (135).

Mephenytoin use was discouraged by potentially fatal blood dyscrasias that occurred in an estimated 1% of patients; it is no longer marketed in the United States. The N-demethylated metabolite nirvanol is a racemic mixture of dextro- and levorotary isomers and accumulates in serum. Nirvanol, possibly the dextrorotary isomer, is responsible for most of the anticonvulsant activity of mephenytoin. Nirvanol has a long half-life in adults, ranging from 77 to 176 hours (135–137). Among adults nirvanol levels of 25–40 mg/L have been associated with improved seizure control (138). Both of these compounds have largely become pharmacogenetic probes for characterizing cytochrome P450 isozymes (139).

Since 1949 only 33 references regarding ethotoin have been listed in *Index Medicus* and there are no references on its use since 1993. Nonetheless, ethotoin remains useful for patients with intractable epilepsy, where its role is bottom tier (140). It has nonlinear kinetics; one study reported V_{max} to range from 50 to 95 mg/kg/day and K_M to range from 9 to 43 mg/L in children (141). Among patients switched from phenytoin to ethotoin, gingival hyperplasia recedes. The incidence of hirsutism and ataxia is also said to be lower with ethotoin. Doses have ranged from approximately 20 to 50 mg/kg/day. The best contemporary source of information about how to use ethotoin is online at Wikipedia (http://en.wikipedia.org/wiki/Ethotoin) and at the pharmaceutical website where prescribing information is posted (http://www.ovationpharma.com/images/products/pdf/peganone_pi.pdf).

References

1. Arnold K, Gerber N. The rate of decline of diphenylhydantoin in human plasma. *Clin Pharmacol Ther* 1970; 11:121–135.
2. Dodson WE. The nonlinear kinetics of phenytoin in children. *Neurology* 1982; 32:42–48.
3. Glazko AJ. Phenytoin: chemistry and methods of determination. In: Levy RH, Mattson RH, Meldrum BS, Penry JK, eds. *Antiepileptic Drugs*, 3rd ed. New York: Raven Press, 1989; 159–176.
4. Cranford RE, Leppik IE, Patrick B, Anderson CB, et al. Intravenous phenytoin in acute treatment of seizures. *Neurology* 1979; 29:1474–1479.
5. Cloyd JC, Gumnit RJ, McLain W. Status epilepticus. The role of intravenous phenytoin. *JAMA* 1980; 244:1479–1481.
6. Lund L. Anticonvulsant effect of diphenylhydantoin relative to plasma levels. *Arch Neurol* 1974; 31:289–294.
7. Borofsky LG, Louis S, Kutt H. Diphenylhydantoin in children. *Neurology* 1973; 23: 967–972.
8. Chang BS, Lowenstein DH. Quality Standards Subcommittee of the American Academy of Neurology. Practice parameter: antiepileptic drug prophylaxis in severe traumatic brain injury: report of the Quality Standards Subcommittee of the American Academy of Neurology. *Neurology* 2003; 60:10–16.
9. Prasad K, Al-Roomi K, Krishnan PR, Sequeira R. Anticonvulsant therapy for status epilepticus. *Cochrane Database Syst Rev* 2005; (4):CD003723.
10. Koren G, Brand N, Halkin H, Dany S, et al. Kinetics of intravenous phenytoin in children. *Ped Pharmacol* 1984; 4:31–38.
11. Painter MJ, Pippenger C, MacDonald H, Pitlick W. Phenobarbital and diphenylhydantoin levels in neonates with seizures. *J Pediatr* 1978; 92:315–319.
12. Painter MJ, Pippenger C, Wasterlain C, et al. Phenobarbital and phenytoin in neonatal seizures: metabolism and tissue distribution. *Neurology* 1981; 31:1107–1112.
13. Gilman JT, Gal P, Duchowny MS, Weaver RL, et al. Rapid sequential phenobarbital treatment of neonatal seizures. *Pediatrics* 1989; 83:674–678.
14. Camfield PR, Camfield CS, Gordon K, Dooley JM. If a first antiepileptic drug fails to control a child's epilepsy, what are the chances of success with the next drug? *J Pediatr* 1997; 131:821–824.
15. Connell J, Oozeer R, de Vries L, Dubowitz L-M, et al. Clinical and EEG response to anticonvulsants in neonatal seizures. *Arch Dis Child* 1989; 64:459–464.
16. Homan RW, Vasko MR, Blaw M. Phenytoin plasma concentration in paroxysmal kinesigenic choreoathetosis. *Neurology* 1980; 30:673–676.
17. Treiman DM, Meyers PD, Walton NY, Collins JF, et al. A comparison of four treatments for generalized convulsive status epilepticus. Veterans Affairs Status Epilepticus Cooperative Study Group. *N Engl J Med* 1998; 339:792–798.
18. O'Mara NB, Jones PR, Anglin DL, Cox S, et al. Pharmacokinetics of phenytoin in children with acute neurotrauma. *Crit Care Med* 1995; 23:1418–1424.
19. Browne TR, LeDuc B. Phenytoin: chemistry and biotransformation. In: Levy RH, Mattson RH, Meldrum BS, eds. *Antiepileptic Drugs*, 4th ed. New York: Raven Press, 1995: 283–300.
20. Levy RH. Cytochrome P450 isozymes and antiepileptic drug interactions. *Epilepsia* 1995; 36(Suppl 5):S8–S13.
21. Nakasa H, Nakamura H, Ono S, Tsutsui M, et al. Prediction of drug-drug interactions of zonisamide metabolism in humans from in vitro data. *Eur J Clin Pharmacol* 1998; 54:177–1783.
22. Odani A, Hashimoto Y, Otsuki Y, Uwai Y, et al. Genetic polymorphism of the CYP2C subfamily and its effect on the pharmacokinetics of phenytoin in Japanese patients with epilepsy. *Clin Pharmacol Ther* 1997; 62:287–292.
23. Chiba K, Ishiizaki T, Muri H, Minagawa K. Michaelis-Menten pharmacokinetics of diphenylhydantoin and application in the pediatric age patient. *J Pediatr* 1980; 96: 479–484.
24. Chiba K, Ishiizaki T, Muri H, Minagawa K. Apparent Michaelis-Menten kinetic parameters of phenytoin in pediatric patients. *Ped Pharmacol* 1980; 1:171–180.
25. Dodson, WE. Phenytoin elimination in childhood: effect of concentration dependent kinetics. *Neurology* 1980; 30:196–199.
26. Bourgeois BFD, Dodson WE. Phenytoin elimination in newborns. *Neurology* 1983; 33:173–178.
27. Bauer LA, Blouin RA. Phenytoin Michaelis-Menten pharmacokinetics in Caucasian paediatric patients. *Clin Pharmacokinet* 1983; 8:545–549.
28. Yukawa E. Higuchi S. Aoyama T. Population pharmacokinetics of phenytoin from routine clinical data in Japan. *J Clin Pharm Ther* 1989; 14:71–77.
29. Yuen GJ, Latimer PT, Littlefield LC, Mackey RW. Phenytoin dosage predictions in paediatric patients. *Clin Pharmacokinet* 1989; 16:254–260.
30. Jacobsen D. Alvik A. Bredesen JE. Brown RD. Pharmacokinetics of phenytoin in acute adult and child intoxication. *J Toxicol Clin Toxicol* 1986–1987; 24:519–531.
31. Zaccara G, Galli A. Effectiveness of simplified dosage schedules on management of ambulant epileptic patients. *Eur Neurol* 1979; 18:341–344.
32. Eadie MJ, Tyrer JH, Bochner F, Hooper WD. The elimination of phenytoin in man. *Clin Exp Pharmacol Ther* 1976; 3:217–224.
33. Mullen PW, Foster RW. Comparative evaluation of six techniques for determining Michaelis-Menten parameters relating phenytoin dose and steady-state concentrations. *J Pharm Pharmacol* 1979; 31:100–104.
34. Dodson WE. Phenytoin kinetics in children. *Clin Pharmacol Ther* 1980; 27:704–707
35. Mullen PW. Optimal phenytoin therapy: a new technique for individualizing dosage. *Clin Pharmacol Ther* 1978; 23:228–232.
36. Chan E. Single-point phenytoin dosage predictions in Singapore Chinese. *J Clin Pharm Ther* 1997; 22:47–52.
37. Martis L, Levy RH. Bioavailability calculations for drugs showing simultaneous first-order and capacity-limited elimination kinetics. *J Pharmacokinet Biopharmaceut* 1973; 1:381–383.
38. Dodson WE, Bourgeois BF. Changing kinetic patterns of phenytoin in newborns. In: Waterlain CG, Vert P, eds. *Neonatal Seizures*. New York: Raven Press, 1990:271–276.
39. Tryer JH, Eadie MJ, Sutherland JM, et al. Outbreak of anticonvulsant intoxication in an Australian city. *Br Med J* 1970; 4:271–273.
40. Albani M. Phenytoin in infancy and childhood. In: Delgado-Escuata AV, Wasterlain CG, Treiman DM, Porter RJ, eds. *Advances in Neurology, Vol. 34: Status Epilepticus*. New York: Raven Press, 1983:457–464.
41. Albani M, Wernicke I. Oral phenytoin in infancy: dose requirement, absorption, and elimination. *Pediatr Pharmacol* 1983; 3:229–236.
42. Melander A, Brante G, Johansson O, Lindberg T, et al. Influence of food on the absorption of phenytoin in man. *Eur J Clin Pharmacol* 1979; 15:269–274.
43. Serrano EE, Roye DB, Hammer RH, Wilder BJ. Plasma diphenylhydantoin values after oral and intramuscular administration of diphenylhydantoin. *Neurology* 1973; 23:311–317.
44. Kostenbauder HB, Rapp RP, McGovren JP, Foster TS, et al. Bioavailability and single-dose pharmacokinetics of intramuscular phenytoin. *Clin Pharmacol Ther* 1975; 18:449–456.
45. Koch-Weser J, Sellers EM. Binding of drugs to serum albumin (second of two parts). *New Engl J Med* 1976; 294:526–531.
46. Reidenberg MM, Odar-Cederlof I, von Bahr C, Borga O, et al. Protein binding of diphenylhydantoin and desmethylimiporamine in plasma from patients with poor renal function. *New Engl J Med* 1971; 285:264–267.
47. Fredholm BB, Rane A, Persson B. Diphenylhydantoin binding to proteins in plasma and its dependence on free fatty acid and bilirubin concentration in dogs and newborn infants. *Pediatr Res* 1075; 9:26–30.
48. Mamiya K, Yukawa E, Matsumoto T, et al. Synergistic effect of valproate coadministration and hypoalbuminemia on the serum-free phenytoin concentration in patients with severe motor and intellectual disabilities. *Clin Neuropharmacol* 2002; 25:230–233.
49. Olanow CW, Finn AL, Prussak C. The effects of salicylate on the pharmacokinetics of phenytoin. *Neurology* 1981; 31:341–342.
50. Rodin EA, DeSousa G, Haidkewych D, Lodhi R, et al. Dissociation between free and bound phenytoin levels in presence of valproate sodium. *Arch Neurol* 1981; 38:240–242.
51. Anderson GD. Children versus adults: pharmacokinetic and adverse-effect differences. *Epilepsia* 2002; 43(Suppl 3):53–59.
52. Anderson GD. Sex differences in drug metabolism: cytochrome P-450 and uridine diphosphate glucuronosyltransferase. *J Gend Specif Med* 2002; 5:25–33.
53. Houghton GW, Richens A, Leighton M. Effect of age, height, weight, and sex on serum phenytoin concentration in epileptic patients. *Br J Clin Pharmacol* 1975; 2:25125–6.
54. Rane A. Urinary excretion of diphenylhydantoin metabolites in newborn infants. *J Pediatr* 1974; 85:534–545.
55. Kutt H, Winters W, Kokenge R, McDowell F. Diphenylhydantoin metabolism a, blood levels, and toxicity. *Arch Neurol* 1964; 11:642–648.
56. Loughnan PM, Greenwald A, Purton WW, Aranda JV, et al. Pharmacokinetic observations of phenytoin disposition in the newborn and young infant. *Arch Dis Child* 1977; 52:302–309.
57. Leff RD, Fischer LJ, Roberts RJ. Phenytoin metabolism in infants following intravenous and oral administration. *Dev Pharmacol Ther* 1986; 9:217–223.
58. Painter MJ. Personal communication.
59. Frey OR, von Brenndorff AI, Probst W. Comparison of phenytoin serum concentrations in premature neonates following intravenous and oral administration. *Ann Pharmacother* 1998; 32:300–303.
60. Shavit G, Korczyn AD, Kivity S, Bechar M, et al. Phenytoin pharmacokinetics in catamennial epilepsy. *Neurology* 1984; 34:959–961.
61. Kutt H. Phenytoin: interactions with other drugs: clinical aspects. In: Levy RH, Mattson RH, Meldrum BS, eds. *Antiepileptic Drugs*, 4th ed. New York: Raven Press, 1995:315–328.

62. Howe AM, Lipson AH, Sheffield LJ, Haan EA, et al. Prenatal exposure to phenytoin, facial development, and a possible role for vitamin K. *Am J Med Genet* 1995; 58: 238–244.
63. Kutt H. Interactions between anticonvulsants and other commonly prescribed drugs. *Epilepsia* 1984; 25(Suppl 2):S118–S131.
64. Sproule BA, Naranjo CA, Brenmer KE, Hassan PC. Selective serotonin reuptake inhibitors and CNS drug interactions. A critical review of the evidence. *Clin Pharmacokinet* 1997; 33:454–471.
65. Nakasa H, Nakamura H, Ono S, Tsutsui M, et al. Prediction of drug-drug interactions of zonisamide metabolism in humans from in vitro data. *Eur J Clin Pharmacol* 1998; 54:177–183.
66. Leppik IE, Pepin SM, Jacobi J, Miller KW. Effect of carbamazepine on the Michaelis-Menten parameters of phenytoin. In: Levy RH, Mattson RH, Meldrum BS, eds. *Metabolism of Antiepileptic Drugs*. New York: Raven Press, 1984:217–222.
67. Kupiec T, Raj V. Fatal seizures due to potential herb-drug interactions with *Ginkgo biloba*. *J Anal Toxicol* 2005; 29:755–758.
68. Suzuki Y, Nagai T, Mano T, Arai H, et al. Interaction between valproate formulation and phenytoin concentrations. *Eur J Clin Pharmacol* 1995; 48:61–63.
69. Rose JQ, Choi HK, Schentag JJ, Kinkel WR, et al. Intoxication caused by interaction of chloramphenicol and phenytoin. *JAMA* 1977; 237:2630–2631.
70. Miller RR, Porter J, Greenblatt DJ. Clinical importance of the interaction of phenytoin and isoniazid. *Chest* 1979; 75:356–358.
71. Braun CW, Goldstone JM. Increased clearance of phenytoin as the presenting feature of infectious mononucleosis. *Ther Drug Mon* 1980; 2:355–357.
72. Leppik IE, Ramani V, Sawchuk RJ, Gumnit RJ. Increased clearance of phenytoin during infectious mononucleosis. *New Engl J Med* 1979; 300:481–482.
73. Leppik IE, Fisher J, Kreil R, Sawchuck RJ. Altered phenytoin clearance with febrile illness. *Neurology* 1986; 36:1367–1370.
74. Gugler R, Azarnoff DL, Shoeman DW. Diphenylhydantoin: correlation between protein binding and albumin concentration. *Klin Wshcr* 1975; 53:445–446.
75. Letteri JM, Mellik H, Louis S, Kutt H, et al. Diphenylhydantoin metabolism in uremia. *New Engl J Med* 1971; 285:648–652.
76. Kang H, Leppik IL. Phenytoin binding and renal transplantation. *Neurology* 1984; 34:83–86.
77. Martin E, Gambertoglio JG, Adler DS, Tazer TN, et al. Removal of phenytoin by hemodialysis in uremic patients. *JAMA* 1977; 238:1750–1753.
78. Dodson WE, Loney LC. Hemodialysis reduces the unbound phenytoin in plasma. *J Pediatr* 1982; 101:465–468.
79. Herranz JL, Armijo JA, Arteaga R. Clinical side effects of phenobarbital, primidone, phenytoin, carbamazepine, and valproate during monotherapy in children. *Epilepsia* 1988; 29:794–804.
80. Thilothammal N, Banu K, Ratnam RS. Comparison of phenobarbitone, phenytoin with sodium valproate: randomized, double-blind study. *Indian Pediatr* 1996; 33: 549–555.
81. de Silva M, MacArdle B, McGowan M, Hughes E, et al. Randomised comparative monotherapy trial of phenobarbitone, phenytoin, carbamazepine, or sodium valproate for newly diagnosed childhood epilepsy. *Lancet* 1996; 347:709–713.
82. Haruda F. Phenytoin hypersensitivity: 38 cases. *Neurology* 1979; 29:1480–1485.
83. Schlienger RG, Shear NH. Antiepileptic drug hypersensitivity syndrome. *Epilepsia* 1998; 39(Suppl 7):S3–S7
84. Tennis P, Stern RS. Risk of serious cutaneous disorders after initiation of use of phenytoin, carbamazepine, or sodium valproate: a record linkage study. *Neurology* 1997; 49:542–546.
85. Sharma VK, Dhar S, Gill AN. Drug-related involvement of specific sites in fixed eruptions: a statistical evaluation. *J Dermatol* 1996; 23:53053–4
86. Luhdorf K, Lund M. Phenytoin-induced hyperkinesia. *Epilepsia* 1977; 18:409–415.
87. Prensky AL, DeVivo DC, Palkes H. Severe bradykinesia as a manifestation of toxicity to antiepileptic medications. *J Pediatr* 1971; 78:700–704
88. Challub EG, DeVivo DC, Volpe JJ. Phenytoin-induced dystonia and choreoathetosis in two retarded epileptic children. *Neurology* 1976; 26:494–498.
89. Krishnamoorthy KS, Zaleraitis EL, Young RSK, Bermad PG. Phenytoin-induced choreoathetosis in infancy: case reports and a review. *Pediatrics* 1983; 72:831–834.
90. Kurata K, Kido H, Kobayashi K, Yamaguchi N. Long-lasting movement disorder induced by intravenous phenytoin administration for status epilepticus. A case report. *Clin Neuropharmacol* 1988; 11:467–471.
91. Howrie DL, Crumrine PK. Phenytoin-induced movement disorder associated with intravenous administration for status epilepticus. *Clin Pediatr* 1985; 24:467–469.
92. Chaudhary N, Ravat SH, Shah PU. Phenytoin-induced dyskinesia. *Indian Pediatr* 1998; 35:274–276.
93. Koukkari MW, Vanefsky MA, Steinberg GK, Hahn JS. Phenytoin-related chorea in children with deep hemispheric vascular malformations. *J Child Neurol* 1996; 11: 490–491.
94. Spector RH, Davidoff RA, Schwartzman RJ. Phenytoin-induced ophthalmoplegia. *Neurology* 1976; 26:1031–1034.
95. Levy LL, Fenichel GM. Diphenylhydantoin-activated seizures. *Neurology* 1965; 15: 716–722.
96. Stilman N, Masdeu JC. Incidence of seizures with phenytoin toxicity. *Neurology* 1985; 35:1769–1772.
97. Wallace SJ. A comparative review of the adverse effects of anticonvulsants in children with epilepsy. *Drug Saf* 1996; 15:378–393.
98. . Perucca E, Gram L, Avanzini G, Dulac O. Antiepileptic drugs as a cause of worsening seizures. *Epilepsia* 1998; 39:5–17.
99. Miyamoto A, Takahashi S, Oki J, Itoh J, et al. Exacerbation of seizures by carbamazepine in four children with symptomatic localization related epilepsy. *No To Hattatsu* 1995; 27;23–28.
100. Logan WJ, Freeman JM. Pseudodegenerative disease due to diphenylhydantoin intoxication. *Arch Neurol* 1969; 21:631–637.
101. Vallarta JM, Bell DB, Reichert A. Progressive encephalopathy due to chronic hydantoin intoxication. *Am J Dis Child* 1974; 128:27–34.
102. Tindall RSA, Willerson J. Subacute phenytoin intoxication syndrome. *Arch Intern Med* 1978; 138:1168–1169.
103. Pack AM, Morrell MJ, Marcus R, et al. Bone mass and turnover in women with epilepsy on antiepileptic drug monotherapy. *Ann Neurol* 2005; 57:252–257.
104. Patwari AK, Aneja S, Chandra D, Singhal PK. Long-term anticonvulsant therapy in tuberculous meningitis—a four-year follow-up. *J Trop Pediatr* 1996; 42:98–103.
105. Seymour RA, Thomason JM, Ellis JS. The pathogenesis of drug-induced gingival overgrowth. *J Periodontol* 1996; 23:165–175.
106. Casetta I, Granieri E, Desidera M, Monetti VC, et al. Phenytoin-induced gingival overgrowth: a community-based cross-sectional study in Ferrara, Italy. *Neuroepidemiology* 1997; 16:296–303.
107. Addy V, McElnay JC, Eyre DG, Campbell N, et al. Risk factors in phenytoin-induced gingival hyperplasia. *J Periodontol* 1983; 54:373–377.
108. Stinnett E, Rodu B, Grizzle WE. New developments in understanding phenytoin-induced gingival hyperplasia. *J Am Dent Assoc* 1987; 114:814–816.
109. Zhou LX, Pihlstrom B, Hardwick JP, Park SS, et al. Metabolism of phenytoin by the gingiva of normal humans: the possible role of reactive metabolites of phenytoin in the initiation of gingival hyperplasia. *Clin Pharmacol Ther* 1996; 60:191–198.
110. Sasaki T, Maita E. Increased bFGF level in the serum of patients with phenytoin-induced gingival overgrowth. *J Clin Periodontol* 1998; 25:42–47.
111. Crooks R, Mitchell T, Thom M. Patterns of cerebellar atrophy in patients with chronic epilepsy: a quantitative neuropathological study. *Epilepsy Res* 2000; 41:63–73.
112. Lee SK, Mori S, Kim DJ, et al. Diffusion tensor MRI and fiber tractography of cerebellar atrophy in phenytoin users. *Epilepsia* 2003; 44:1536–1540.
113. De Marcos FA, Ghizoni E, Kobayashi E, Li LM, et al. Cerebellar volume and long-term use of phenytoin. *Seizure* 2003; 12:312–315.
114. Botez MI, Attig E, Vezina JL. Cerebellar atrophy in epileptic patients. *Can J Neurol Sci* 1988; 15:299–303.
115. Masur H, Elger CE, Ludolph A C, Galanski M. Cerebellar atrophy following acute intoxication with phenytoin. *Neurology* 1989; 39:432–433.
116. Lindvall O, Nilsson B. Cerebellar atrophy following phenytoin intoxication. *Ann Neurol* 1984; 16:258–260.
117. Iivanainen M, Viukari M, Helle EP. Cerebellar atrophy in phenytoin-treated mentally retarded epileptics. *Epilepsia* 1977; 18:375–386.
118. Ramsay RE, DeToledo J. Intravenous administration of fosphenytoin: options for the management of seizures. *Neurology* 1996; 46(Suppl 1):S17–S9.
119. Kriel RL, Cifuentes RF. Fosphenytoin in infants of extremely low birth weight. *Pediatr Neurol* 2001; 24(3):219–221.
120. Marchetti A, Magar R, Fischer J, Sloan E, et al. A pharmacoeconomic evaluation of intravenous fosphenytoin (Cerebyx) versus intravenous phenytoin (Dilantin) in hospital emergency departments. *Clin Ther* 1996; 18:953–966.
121. Miller MH. Fosphenytoin: worth the cost? *Ann Emerg Med* 1997; 29:823.
122. Kriel RL, Cifuentes RF. Fosphenytoin in infants of extremely low birth weight. *Pediatr Neurol* 2001; 24(3):219–221.
123. Wilder BJ, Campbell K, Ramsay RE, Garnett WR, et al. Safety and tolerance of multiple doses of intramuscular fosphenytoin substituted for oral phenytoin in epilepsy or neurosurgery. *Arch Neurol* 1996; 53:764–768.).
124. Pellock JM. Fosphenytoin use in children. *Neurology* 1996; 46(Suppl 1):S14–S6.
125. Boucher BA, Feler CA, Dean JC, Michie DD, et al. The safety, tolerability, and pharmacokinetics of fosphenytoin after intramuscular and intravenous administration in neurosurgery patients. *Pharmacotherapy* 1996; 16:638–645.
126. Browne TR, Kugler AR, Eldon MA. Pharmacology and pharmacokinetics of fosphenytoin. *Neurology* 1996; 46(Suppl 1):S3–S7.
127. Lai CM, Moore P, Quon CY. Binding of fosphenytoin, phosphate ester prodrug of phenytoin, to human serum proteins and competitive binding with carbamazepine, diazepam, phenobarbital, phenylbutazone, phenytoin, valproic acid or warfarin. *Res Commun Mol Pathol Pharmacol* 1995; 88:51–62.
128. Fischer JH, Patel TV, Fischer PA. Fosphenytoin: clinical pharmacokinetics and comparative advantages in the acute treatment of seizures. *Clin Pharmacokinet* 2003; 42:33–58.
129. Fierro LS, Savulich DH, Benezra DA. Safety of fosphenytoin sodium. *Am J Health Syst Pharm* 1996; 53:2707–2712.
130. Ramsay RE, DeToledo J. Intravenous administration of fosphenytoin: options for the management of seizures. *Neurology* 1996; 46(Suppl 1):S17–S9.
131. Browne TR. Fosphenytoin (Cerebyx). *Clin Neuropharmacol* 1997; 20:1–12.
132. Luer MS. Fosphenytoin. *Neurol Res* 1998; 20:178–182.
133. Jamerson BD, Dukes GE, Brouwer KL, Donn KH, et al. Venous irritation related to intravenous administration of phenytoin versus fosphenytoin. *Pharmacotherapy* 1994; 14:47–52.
134. O'Brien TJ, Cascino GD, So EL, Hanna DR. Incidence and clinical consequence of the purple glove syndrome in patients receiving intravenous phenytoin. *Neurology* 1998; 51:1034–1039.
135. Kupferberg HJ. Other hydantoins: mephenytoin and ethotoin. In: Levy RH, Mattson RH, Meldrum BS, eds. *Antiepileptic Drugs*, 4th ed. New York: Raven Press, 1995: 351–357.

136. Bourgeois BF, Kupfer A, Wad N, Egli M. Pharmacokinetics of R-enantiomeric normephenytoin during chronic administration in epileptic patients. *Epilepsia* 1986; 27:412–418.
137. Bourgeois BF, Kupfer A, Wad N, Egli M. Pharmacokinetics of R-enantiomeric normephenytoin during chronic administration in epileptic patients. *Epilepsia* 1986; 27:412–418.
138. Troupin AS, Ojemann LM, Dodrill CB. Mephenytoin: a reappraisal. *Epilepsia* 1976; 17:403–414.
139. Suzuki H, Kneller MB, Rock DA, et al. Active-site characteristics of CYP2C19 and CYP2C9 probed with hydantoin and barbiturate inhibitors. *Arch Biochem Biophys* 2004; 429:1–15.
140. Biton V, Gates JR, Ritter FJ, Loewenson RB. Adjunctive therapy for intractable epilepsy with ethotoin. *Epilepsia* 1990; 31:433–437.
141. Carter CA, Helms RA, Boehm R. Ethotoin in seizures of childhood and adolescence. *Neurology* 1984; 34:791–795.

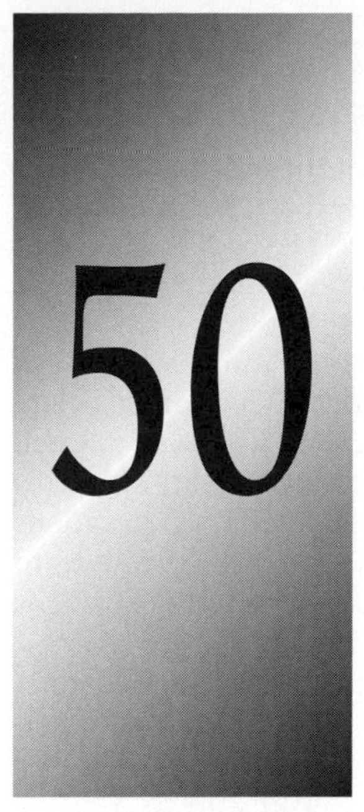

Sulthiame

Dietz Rating
Nicole Wolf
Thomas Bast

CHEMISTRY, ANIMAL PHARMACOLOGY, AND MECHANISM OF ACTION

Sulthiame (STM) is a sulfonamide derivate, N-(4-sulfamoylphenyl)-1,4-butansultam (Figure 50-1), a crystalline powder, with a molecular weight of 290 g/mol (1).

STM has no antibacterial properties, and although it is a weak carbonic anhydrase inhibitor it has no diuretic activity at therapeutic doses.

^{35}S-STM is well absorbed from the gastrointestinal tract in rats; 80% of the dose of STM is excreted unchanged in the urine during the next 48 hours and only a small amount is found as an inactive hydroxylated derivative in urine (2). STM readily penetrates into tissues and brain and reaches concentrations similar to those found in plasma. STM half-lives in animal studies are variable and range from ~4 hours in rabbits to 4.5–7.3 hours in dogs and ~15–30 hours in rats (2).

Long-term observations in rats and dogs did not show toxic effects on organs such as liver, kidney, or bone marrow. The acute toxicity after oral intake calculated as LD_{50} is >5,000 mg/kg in rats and mice and in rabbits ~1,000 mg/kg (3).

Tests investigating adverse effects on reproduction were performed by feeding rats with STM at doses ranging from 30 to 300 mg/kg. With higher doses, animals became lethargic, appetite decreased, and pregnant animals gained less weight. A significant and dose-dependent decrease in fetal weight with doses higher than 100 mg/kg was observed, and even fetuses exposed to a dose of 30 mg/kg STM were, albeit not significantly, smaller than controls (D. Lorke, personal communication 1985).

In a model designed to investigate the influence of antiepileptic drugs (AEDs) on the developing brain, neuronal apoptosis increased in the brain of newborn rats exposed to standard anticonvulsants such as phenytoin (PHT), phenobarbital (PB), carbamazepine (CBZ), vigabatrin, or valproate (VPA). With STM, neuronal death was comparable with exposure to VPA or vigabatrin, however not as prominent as with PHT or PB (4, 5).

STM was proven to be effective against maximal electroshock (MES) (ED_{50} = 35 mg/kg) and penthylentetrazol-induced seizures (ED_{50} = 260 mg/kg) in mice, however it was ineffective against strychnine-induced seizures (3). The therapeutic index (LD_{50}/ED_{50}) of STM in MES was 10 times higher than that of PB and 4 to 5 times higher than that of PHT. In a primate model—photosensitive baboons (20–125 mg/kg i.v.)—STM did not show anticonvulsant properties (6). In amygdaloid-kindled seizures in rats, Albertson and coworkers reported no efficacy (7); whereas another group found some effects, which were, however, much weaker and not comparable to those of CBZ, PHT, PB, or zonisamide demonstrated by the same group (8).

FIGURE 50-1

Structural formula of sulthiame.

Like acetazolamide—although 10–20 times weaker (3)—STM has carbonic anhydrase–inhibiting properties (9, 10). A familiar and still accepted explanation for the anticonvulsant effect of STM is the inhibition of carbonic anhydrase activity, mainly in glial cells. Subsequently, carbon dioxide concentrations increase, leading to acidification of both intracellular and extracellular space. By acting via N- methyl-D-aspartate (NMDA) receptors and calcium currents, this acidification reduces the excitability of neurons. In addition, there seems to be an independent effect of STM on the function of neuronal ion channels. In isolated neurons from guinea pig hippocampus, STM reduced inactivating sodium currents without changing potassium currents. Therapeutic concentrations of 1 to 10 µg/mL decreased sodium currents to about 20% and led to impairment of repetitive generation of action potentials and a reduction of the maximum discharge frequency by 20% to 40% (11).

BIOTRANSFORMATION, PHARMACOKINETICS, AND INTERACTIONS IN HUMANS

A total of 80% to 90% of oral STM is excreted mostly unchanged in urine, and 10% to 20% is lost with feces after biliary secretion (2). In humans, 32% of a single dose of STM is excreted by the urine within the first 24 hours. The protein binding of STM amounts to 29%.

STM serum peak levels were reached after 4 hours (range, 2–8 hours) after a first single oral dose of 5 mg/kg in children with epilepsy taking other AEDs (12). May et al calculated the STM interquartile range (25th to 75th percentile) of serum concentrations as being between 2.3 and 5.8 (mean, 4.7) µg/mL in 86 patients (2–89 years) on chronic 9.1 ± 4.67 mg/kg STM therapy in combination with other AEDs, mainly CBZ, VPA, or PB (13). In various studies, a linear correlation between STM serum concentrations and the dose/body weight in children and adults could be demonstrated with an STM dose of 4 to 16.7 mg/kg (9, 13, 14). Children need higher doses per kilogram of body weight than adults to reach comparable serum levels (13). After a single first STM load, serum half-life was calculated to be 3.7 hours (range, 2–7 hours) (12). May et al found somewhat longer STM half lifes (8.65 ± 3.0 hours) at steady-state in children and adults on stable comedication with CBZ, VPA, or PB. Half-lives are shorter in children than in adults (7 ± 2 hours vs. 12 ± 2 hours) (13).

The decline of plasma concentrations followed in most cases a first-order kinetic; only a few patients' data were in favor of saturated kinetics. Steady state is reached 3 to 4 days after beginning treatment with STM. This short half-life explains the considerable daily fluctuations in STM concentrations, which explains the failure to establish a correlation between STM drug concentrations and anticonvulsive effect (13, 15).

Sulthiame is known for its interaction with phenytoin (16–18). In one study, adult patients with epilepsy on a stable dose of 300 mg PHT daily were started on a concomitant administration of 200 to 800 mg of STM. This caused a rise in serum PHT after one week and prolonged PHT half-life substantially (17). In some patients with already critical PHT serum concentrations, adding STM can provoke PHT intoxication (19). Olesen and Jensen already speculated that this increase of PHT levels is due to a direct inhibition by STM of the *para*-hydroxylation of PHT (18), which was later proven (20). CBZ decreases STM concentrations, probably secondary to enzyme induction (13). STM increased CBZ-epoxide by >30% in 6 of 39 patients, whereas CBZ levels remained unchanged, and PHT levels increased by >30% in 3 of 5 patients (21). No interactions with VPA were observed (13).

CLINICAL EFFICACY AND SPECTRUM OF ACTIVITY

Sulthiame is one of the older AEDs, developed in the 1950s and introduced into the market in the 1960s. Therefore, much of our knowledge today comes from case studies and open trials of that period. Only two prospective studies evaluating the efficacy of STM in benign epilepsy of childhood with centrotemporal spikes (BECTS) (22) and West syndrome (23, 24) were performed according to recent recommendations of the International League Against Epilepsy (ILAE).

History

Results of the first open trials, mainly in adult patients with temporal lobe seizures according to the classification then in force, were published in 1960 (24–26); 23 of 81 patients treated with STM (200–1,200 mg/day) became seizure free (28%), 9 of the 23 taking STM monotherapy; the mean length of follow-up was 6 months (25). Of these 9 patients, 3 stopped STM medication. Seizures relapsed but could be controlled again after reintroduction of STM. Such a high success rate of 28% could not be reproduced in other trials (26, 27).

In 1960, Doose et al were the first to demonstrate the efficacy of STM in children with epilepsy (28, 29); 129 children with focal, mainly "psychomotor" seizures, secondarily generalized tonic-clonic seizures, as well as generalized grand mal seizures and petit mal with or without grand mal, were treated and observed for over 6 months. Doose et al made the surprising observation that the best effects of STM were seen in children with psychomotor seizures, being regarded as especially difficult to treat at that time. With STM monotherapy, 13 of 24 children with psychomotor seizures and a further 24 of 41 children with focal seizures (simple and complex partial seizures with or without grand mal) became seizure free; in 7 children a reduction in seizure frequency of >50% was seen. In reading this old study with our present knowledge, we understand how close Doose et al were to discover independently the concept of benign epilepsy with centrotemporal spikes (BECTS), which was proposed first in 1958 by Nayrac et al and 2 years later by Nayrac and Beaussart (30) and Gibbs and Gibbs (31). It is of historical interest that the focal discharges in the first electroencephalogram (EEG) of a 10-year-old patient later shown to normalize under treatment with 400 mg/day STM would be classified today as rolandic spikes (Figure 50-2) (26).

In 1974, Green et al published a double-blind, crossover study comparing the efficacy of STM with that of PHT, which was defined as the "standard of comparison for anticonvulsant testing" (16). The design of this study is quite unusual, and lack of detailed data makes it impossible to draw one's own conclusions.

In this study, 67 patients with partial seizures with or without secondary generalization were included. In an open phase, all patients were first placed on a monotherapy with PHT for 2 months before the blinded phase started, during which patients were randomized to either PHT or STM. Whereas PHT was titrated to an individual dose during the open phase, in the blinded phase a ratio of 4:1 STM to PHT was calculated, meaning either that patients remained taking the same dose of PHT, or that a fourfold dose of STM was added, resulting in STM doses of 3.7 to 64.0 mg/kg. In most cases, this dose was 17 to 50 mg/kg (mean, 31.2 mg/kg), being well above recommended doses even at that time. A total of 10 of 67 patients were already lost during the first open phase on PHT monotherapy, and 36 more during the blinded part of the study—11 taking PHT and 25 taking STM. Only 21 of 67 patients completed the study, 11 taking PHT, 10 taking STM. Of these 21 patients, 10 had fewer seizures with PHT, 9 with STM. Nevertheless, the authors stated that "sulthiame has very little value as a primary anticonvulsant agent" and concluded that "it seems logical . . .to ascribe the benefit of sulthiame in the control of seizures to the fact that it raises serum PHT levels. . . . it is easier, more precise and less expensive to increase PHT serum level by administrating more PHT than by giving sulthiame."

Callaghan et al (14) came to similar conclusions when analyzing 10 adult patients (14–75 years of age; mean, 32.7 years) allocated to 3 to 10 mg/kg/day STM. They concluded that "STM did not appear to be of benefit to patients with severe and frequent seizures. The improvement (seen) was related to an increase in serum phenytoin levels" (14).

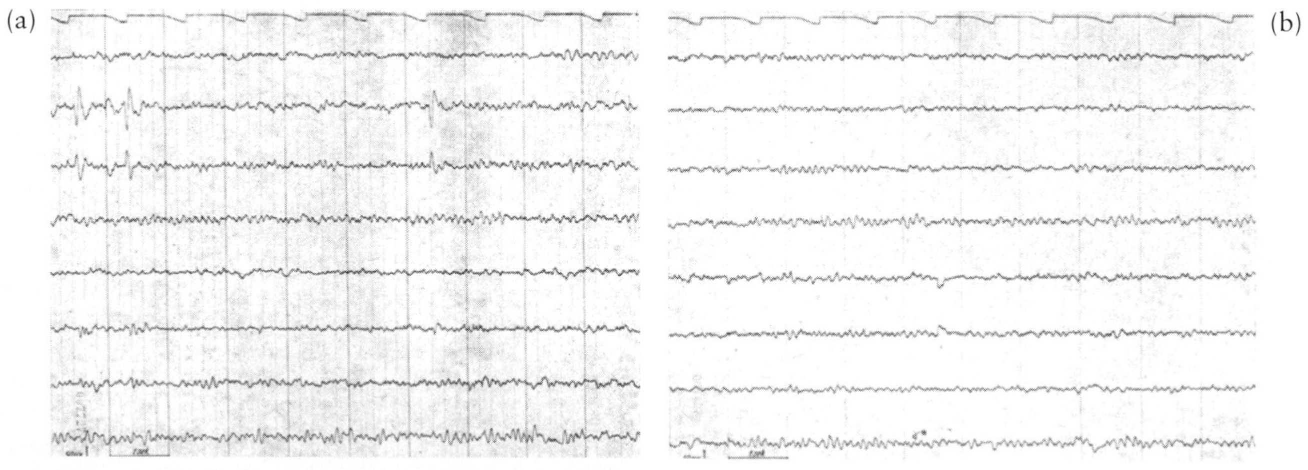

FIGURE 50-2

Electroencephalogram in a 10-year-old boy (a) before and (b) after a 30-day treatment with 400 mg of sulthiame.

These interpretations stopped further clinical trials with STM for a long time in most parts of Europe and North America.

Spectrum of Efficacy

STM is proven to have specific action in BECTS. After BECTS was recognized as a distinct epileptic syndrome in children (30–32), the efficacy of STM was reevaluated by Doose et al (33). In a retrospective open study with a follow up from 7 months to 7 years they reported that 48 of 56 children (85%) with typical benign partial epilepsy became permanently seizure-free with 4 to 6 mg/kg/day STM.

A 6-month prospective, randomized, double-blind, placebo-controlled multicenter study of STM in BECTS, following the recommendation of the ILAE, was published in 2000 (22); 194 patients were screened, and 66 children (40 males, 26 females; age 8.3; range, 3.1–10.7 years) with the diagnosis of BECTS and two or more seizures during the past 6 months were randomized to either STM or placebo for 6 months of treatment. The primary effectiveness was the rate of treatment failure events per group, which were defined as the first seizures after a 7-day run-in period, intolerable adverse effects, development of another epileptic syndrome, or termination of the study by the parents or the investigator. The trial was stopped when the first interim analysis showed a significant superiority of STM treatment; 25 of 31 patients in the STM group (80.6%) but only 10 of the 35 placebo-treated group (28.6%) completed the trial ($P < 0.0001$). In only 4 children taking STM but in 21 taking placebo, the failure event was a seizure. Two parents of the placebo group withdrew. All other failure events were due to termination of the trial by the investigators after the interim analysis.

The efficacy of STM in typical and atypical benign idiopathic partial epilepsies was shown by case reports from single centers and in some prospective as well as retrospective open studies (34–36).

In an open prospective trial between 1988 and 2001 and a follow-up of more than 12 months, 21 children with BECTS, atypical rolandic epilepsy, Landau-Kleffner syndrome, or continuous spike waves during slow sleep (CSWS) were treated with STM. In 15 children STM was the first and only treatment, whereas 10 children had had another treatment before STM. Of 21 children with seizures, 13 became seizure free, including 10 of 16 patients with BECTS. In 6 of 10 STM was the first drug (36).

A total of 125 children with various epileptic syndromes treated with STM as monotherapy or add-on between 1989 to 1998 were analyzed retrospectively in a multicenter study; 24 of 26 patients with benign rolandic epilepsy of childhood (including 3 atypical cases) and all 13 children with benign occipital epilepsy of childhood were treated with STM only. A total of 29 of these 39 children became seizure free, and a further 6 of 39 showed a reduction of seizures of >50% (37).

In a retrospective analysis, 111 consecutive patients with BECTS seen at five pediatric neurology outpatient clinics and one private clinic were collected. All patients were treated with either STM or CBZ according to the institutional policy. Efficacy was defined by seizure freedom for more than 2 years. In 67% of patients treated with STM "seizures disappeared," whereas in 74% treated with CBZ "seizures abated." Authors stated no significant difference regarding efficacy between the two drugs. It is noteworthy that 5 of 8 patients who were switched to STM after failing CBZ became seizure free, whereas none of the 3 patients having failed STM became seizure free after treatment had been changed to CBZ (38).

In another single center study, 35 patients with typical rolandic epilepsy treated either by STM ($n = 17$) or CBZ ($n = 16$) or other AED ($n = 2$; primidone, PHT) were analyzed. A total of 15 of 17 patients in the STM group, but only 9 of 16 in the CBZ group became seizure free. The author speculated that in 3 of the 15 STM children, and in 6 of the 9 CBZ children, this outcome could have been due to the natural outcome of BECTS (34).

Of 8 children with atypical benign partial epilepsy, 5 became seizure free with STM, 1 with CBZ and 1 with ACTH. In 2 children, it was believed that the epilepsy was worsened by CBZ. Both became seizure free when switched to STM (34).

Gross-Selbeck reported further data on Landau-Kleffner syndrome (LKS) and CSWS treated with various AEDs, including STM. Two of four children with LKS showed a normalization of EEG under STM alone or in combination with clobazam; in the two others the EEG markedly improved. One of three children with CSWS on STM ± clobazam became seizure free and showed a substantial amelioration of the EEG abnormalities (34). Wakai et al report on a 5-year-old, previously normal boy who developed a loss of acquired language, auditory agnosia, and atypical absences and complex partial seizures as well as CSWS. When he received 80 mg/day of STM, there was an excellent outcome regarding all clinical symptoms, accompanied by an improvement of EEG changes and disappearance of CSWS (39).

The second prospective, randomized, double-blind, placebo-controlled, multicenter study on STM, following the guidelines of the ILAE, was done in patients with West syndrome (23); 33 infants with newly diagnosed typical West syndrome (clinically infantile spasms and hypsarrhythmia in the EEG) were included in the study. To exclude pyridoxine-dependent seizures, all received for the first 3 days of the baseline phase 150 to 300 mg/kg pyridoxine. On day 4 they were randomized to either STM or placebo. STM was started with 5 mg/kg/day and increased to 10 mg/kg/day when after 3 days no response was recorded. At the end of day 9, an EEG was recorded and study medication revealed. In the 16 patients in the placebo group, neither spasms nor hypsarrhythmia disappeared. In the STM group 6 of 17 infants showed a complete clinical and EEG response. In the follow-up period none of these six children on STM monotherapy relapsed ($P < 0.022$). Three patients of the STM group who failed during the trial period became free of seizures after the STM dose was increased to 15–16.4 mg/kg/day. All but one patient of the placebo group received STM in the open follow-up. Four of these 15 patients also became seizure free.

Lerman and Nussbaum (35) reported on the use of STM in patients with epilepsies with myoclonic seizures comprising cases of Lennox-Gastaut syndrome, myoclonic petit mal, myoclonic seizures in Unverricht-Lundborg disease, and juvenile myoclonic epilepsy (JME). In the retrospective analysis of 12 adolescents and young adults with juvenile myoclonic epilepsy, 8 were controlled completely on STM alone (doses, 400–800 mg/day). In 4 of these 8 patients STM was the first drug; in the remaining 4 STM replaced previous drugs, even combinations of several AEDs (35). Ten patients with JME were treated by STM only; 7 of 10 became seizure-free, and another 3 of 10 had a reduction of seizures by >50% (37). Kurlemann et al, investigating STM efficacy in newly diagnosed epilepsies, reported on one child with a childhood absence epilepsy who became seizure free by STM monotherapy as the first drug (40).

STM was shown in old (15, 24–26, 41–45) and new open, prospective and retrospective studies to have effects as add-on treatment in cryptogenic or symptomatic localization-related epilepsy in adults as well as in children (21, 37, 40, 46). A total of 17 of 42 children aged 3 to 18 years with a symptomatic localization-related epilepsy treated by STM became seizure free, and another 12 of 42 had a reduction in seizures of >50% (37). Kurlemann et al reported on 48 consecutive children seen at one institution and suffering from simple or complex partial seizures; 28 of 48 (65.1%) treated by STM, which was the first AED in most patients, became seizure free (40). In an institutional analysis of 49 children with a pharmacoresistant focal epilepsy, 8 became seizure free after add-on STM and 6 more patients had a reduction of seizures by >50% (follow-up in most cases >21 months) (46).

Recently, in a prospective open-label study with 48 adult patients with refractory epilepsy classified either as cryptogenic or symptomatic localization-related epileptic syndromes, STM was given as add-on at a dose of 200 to 600 mg/day. STM and concomitant AEDs were adjusted at the discretion of the investigator as indicated by patient tolerability. A total of 36 of 48 patients completed the titration and continuation phase and could be analyzed. Overall seizure frequency against baseline level was significantly reduced by 36%, with a significant reduction in complex partial and generalized seizures, in the number of clusters and number of days affected by seizures ($P < 0.01$ to 0.001). Twenty-two patients experienced at least a >50% reduction in seizure frequency; three became completely seizure free. After more than 2 years, 17 patients having a >50% reduction of seizure frequency still received STM (21).

Effect of STM on Epileptiform EEG Activity

At least in Europe, the impact of focal discharges in BECTS on cognitive function, language performance, and overall intellectual development is a highly discussed issue. Transition of rolandic spikes to CSWS is possible (34, 47, 48). Normal neuropsychological and motor functions before and declining with the onset of CSWS have been described (49). There are reports that CBZ—although effective to treat seizures in BECTS—does not substantially alter the EEG pattern and may even lead to deterioration, including transition to CSWS. Therefore, the influence of STM on the EEG abnormalities in BECTS as well as in CSWS is of special interest.

In a prospective double-blind trial on STM versus placebo in BECTS, 179 sleep EEGs were recorded at screening and after 4 weeks, 3 months, and 6 months of therapy. All EEGs were analyzed by a blinded reviewer using a standard protocol and building a score by collecting data on epileptiform activity (number of foci, proportion, propagation). At screening, no difference was found between the two groups. A total of 80 foci were identified in 59 patients with sufficient EEG data. Most of them had only one focus, 15 had two, and 3 had three independent foci. The number of patients with EEG normalization was significantly higher in the STM group than in the placebo group. EEG normalization was transient in 12 of 31 in the STM and 4 of 35 in the placebo group and persistent in 9 in the STM and 1 in the placebo group. Using a complex score for intraindividual comparisons during follow-up, the STM group displayed a significant improvement of this EEG score at 4 weeks and at 3 and at 6 months (50).

In another study, the EEG in 21 of 25 children with BECTS and related disorders was controlled 3 to 6 months after the introduction of STM. In 4 of 21 a total disappearance; in a further 9 of 21 a marked decrease of discharges in the EEG was seen. Of these 13 children with EEG improvement, a second control EEG remained normal, respectively further improved, in 9 cases. In the EEG of the 4 remaining children epileptiform discharges increased again compared to the first control (36). In another group of patients with benign partial epilepsies of childhood, EEG data before and during STM treatment were available in 20 of 39 patients. Complete EEG normalization was obtained in 13 patients 1 to 3 months after initiation of treatment. This EEG normalization was transient in all patients, although seizure control was maintained (37). Similar data were reported in an open trial in 27 children with BECTS; in 70.4% the EEG was normalized.(40) In his retrospective study, Gross-Selbeck emphasized the EEG features and treatment-induced EEG changes in BECTS. Of 33 patients suffering from typical and atypical rolandic epilepsy, 16 were treated with CBZ. In this group, the EEG showed no clear improvement, the patients suffered even temporary EEG deterioration, whereas in 14 of 17 patients treated with STM the EEG showed clear improvement and normalized in 7 children (34). In a study comparing CBZ and STM, EEG normalization was defined only for patients who became seizure free and in whom an EEG was done during the first year after the last seizure. EEG data were available in 19 patients who became seizure free with CBZ; in 8 of those 19 the EEG was normalized. In the STM group EEG data were available for 7, who responded to STM; 5 of 7 had a normalized EEG (38).

Since the first description of subclinical electrical status epilepticus during sleep (ESES) in children by Patry et al (51), later called CSWS, there is an ongoing debate on the relationship between BECTS and related syndromes such as atypical rolandic epilepsy, CSWS, or Landau-Kleffner syndrome. CSWS has been observed to develop in children with prior idiopathic partial epilepsies—either BECTS (34, 47) or idiopathic childhood occipital epilepsy (48). It was suggested to try STM in these conditions. In a study on STM in typical and atypical rolandic epilepsy and related epilepsy syndromes ($n = 21$), 4 children with cognitive disturbances associated with "focal sharp waves" but without recognized clinical seizures were included and treated with STM. A total of 19 of 21 of all children were investigated by formal neuropsychological testing before and under STM therapy. Neither stagnation nor decline of individual performance was observed. In the four cases without seizures, an improvement of test performance could be documented; but the authors stated that it was not possible to conclude with certainty whether this was the natural evolution or the result of decreased epileptiform discharges (36). Gross-Selbeck reported improvement of language and overall intellectual development in children with atypical benign partial epilepsy and Landau-Kleffner syndrome after STM, which was accompanied by an EEG improvement not obtained with various other AEDs tried previously (34).

Besides its effect on idiopathic rolandic spikes, STM also seems to be effective against focal discharges in symptomatic epilepsy. In adult patients with temporal lobe epilepsy (TLE) (age, 16–43 years) the EEG showed "considerable improvement" in 20 of 35 "marked responders" (>75% reduction of seizure frequency), follow-up being at least 6 months (52). But there is also contradicting evidence. In a prospective blinded study the number of epileptiform discharges during the first 20 minutes of each waking tracing or the first 20 minutes of sustained sleep EEG was counted. More patients treated with STM showed an increase in epileptiform patterns than those taking PHT (53). Whereas 8 of 13 patients completing the trial had fewer epileptiform patterns compared to baseline at the end of the PHT phase, in 11 of 16 patients the number of epileptiform patterns increased when taking STM. Recently, Kurlemann et al reported on 48 children suffering from symptomatic epilepsies with simple or complex partial seizures and found—besides the clinical improvement—an EEG normalization in 65% of the patients receiving STM (40).

ADVERSE EFFECTS

Data coming from prospective studies are insufficient to draw final conclusions on adverse effects in STM, because the number of patients is limited and the observation time short. There are no severe, life-theatening adverse effects described. In prospective and retrospective studies, most often hyperventilation or dyspnea are reported. Somnolence or drowsiness or apathy and paresthesias in the fingers and periorally are other frequently encountered side effects. Hyperventilation and apathy are certainly dose related. This does not seem to be true for paresthesias. Still, all three symptoms may disappear even if the STM dose remains unchanged. Fenton et al reported on one adult with a pronounced hyperventilation and an increased ventilation at rest. The ventilatory capacity was normal and pCO_2 was substantially reduced but returned to normal after cessation of STM (43). Tröger et al found a decrease in serum bicarbonate and pH and elevated base excess, that is, signs of a mild compensated metabolic acidosis (54). This adverse effect can easily be explained by the inhibition of carbonic anhydrase activity by STM.

Already in the older literature of the 1960s and 1970s psychiatric problems were reported with the higher doses of STM used at that time. In a retrospective multicenter study on 125 patients with different epilepsies and epileptic syndromes, adverse effects associated with STM were regarded "as minimal" (37); main adverse effects were hyperventilation (19), paresthesias (8), and drowsiness (5). However, psychiatric syndromes (3), anorexia (2), sensation of fear (2), and forced normalization (1) were reported. STM discontinuation was necessary in 4 because of psychiatric problems (3), hyperventilation (1), and paresthesias (1). Tröger et al reported a 4.5-year-old boy receiving 15 mg/kg/day of STM developing hallucinatory symptoms after 3 weeks. The authors claimed that drug-associated metabolic acidosis caused this symptom; it disappeared within 1 day after discontinuation of STM (54). Poor concentration, depressed mood, fatigue, and lack of drive were observed in a 9-year-old boy with BECTS treated with STM in a dose of 5 mg/kg/day. The Developmental Test of Visual Perception (Frostig) revealed a significant drop in performance (55). In rare cases children taking STM became unable to conduct even simple mathematical tasks that they had been able to perform without any difficulty before (own observation, unpublished). Already in 1964, Fenton et al reported the "inability to think clearly" in three adults under STM (43). All these disturbances resolved within a few days, or even within hours after discontinuation of STM (23). Comparing CBZ and STM in an open, multicenter trial on 111 patients, 11 of 73 taking CBZ discontinued the treatment because of adverse reactions and 4 of 27 taking STM discontinued treatment because of paresthesias (n = 3) or severe behavioral problems (n = 1) (38).

It had been speculated that STM, as a weak carbonic anhydrase inhibitor, like acetazolamide or zonisamide, may change the urinary pH, thus increasing the risk of urolithiasis. Nevertheless it was shown that urinary pH remains in the normal range with STM treatment (56). In concordance with these findings crystalluria is less often observed in children taking STM than in those taking acetazolamide or zonisamide, indicating an elevated risk of developing urolithiasis (57).

There is one report on a reversible adverse effect on liver function. A 10-year-old child receiving 4.3 mg/kg/day STM developed a progressive elevation of liver enzymes alanine aminotransferase (ALT), aspartate aminotransferase (AST), and gamma-glutamyl transpeptidase (GGT) to a maximum of 946 U/L, 416 U/L, and 68 U/L, respectively, without any other clinical signs of hepatic disturbance except for a mild increase in bilirubin to 1.2 mg/dL. All laboratory findings normalized within 6 weeks after discontinuation of STM (58). There are no other reports on adverse effects influencing hepatic function, blood count, or renal function.

CLINICAL USE (INCLUDING PREPARATIONS, DOSAGE, TITRATION, AND PRECAUTIONS) AND LABORATORY MONITORING

For the treatment of BECTS and related epileptic syndromes a dose of 4 to 8 mg/kg/day of STM is recommended. In West syndrome, the STM dose should be increased from 5 to10 mg/kg/day up to 20 (to 25) mg/kg/day. Whether in older children the intake of more than 10 mg/kg/day is of any benefit is still under discussion. Though half-lives are short and require, in theory, three daily doses, we believe from our clinical experience that two doses per day are sufficient in most cases.

Alhough no specific adverse effects are described, blood count and renal and hepatic functions should be checked every 6 to 12 months, as in any long-term treatment. In the special case of severe hyperventilation it is worthwhile to check base excess, bicarbonate level, and pCO_2; in some children the addition of bicarbonate may be useful to help continuing treatment with STM.

Serum levels need not be controlled in patients treated with STM. The dose should be titrated according to efficacy and side effects.

STM is available at least in Argentinia, Australia, Austria, Czech Republic, Germany, Hungary, Israel, Slovakia, and Switzerland.

No allergic reactions were reported in cases with known sulfonamide intolerance. STM should be used with caution in acute porphyria, hyperthyroidism, hypertension, and decreased renal function (46). There are no data regarding teratogenicity of STM in humans. In rats STM significantly reduced placental and fetal weight secondary to reduced food intake by pregnant animals treated with 100 to 300 mg/kg/day. A slight, however significant, reduction in the birth weight of rat pups is found even after 30 mg/kg/day STM during pregnancy. No malformations have been reported so far.

References

1. Wirth W, Hoffmeister F, Friebel H, Sommer S. Zur Pharmakologie des N-(4'-sulfamoylphenyl)-butansultam-1,2-thiazinene-dioxide). *Dtsch Med Wochenschr* 1960; 85:2195–2199.
2. Duhm B, Maul W, Medenwald H, Patzschke K, et al. Tierexperimentelle Untersuchungen mit ^{35}Smarkiertem N-(4'- sulfamylphenyl)butansultam-1,4). *Z Naturforsch B* 1965; 20:434–445.
3. Wirth W, Hoffmeister F, Sommer S. The pharmacology of Ospolot. *Deutsche Medizinische Monatsschrift* 1961; 6:309–312.
4. Bittigau P, Sifringer M, Genz K, Reith E, et al. Antiepileptic drugs and apoptotic neurodegeneration in the developing brain. *Proc Natl Acad Sci U S A* 2002; 99:15089–15094.
5. Bittigau P, Sifringer M, Ikonomidou C. Antiepileptic drugs and apoptosis in the developing brain. *Ann N Y Acad Sci* 2003; 993:103–114.
6. Meldrum BS, BChir MB, Horton RW, Toseland PA. A primate model for testing anticonvulsant drugs. *Arch Neurol* 1975; 32:289–294.
7. Albertson TE, Peterson SL, Stark LG. Anticonvulsant drugs and their antagonism of kindled amygdaloid seizures in rats. *Neuropharmacology* 1980; 19:643–652.
8. Song HK, Hamada K, Yagi K, Seino M. Effects of single and repeated administration of sulthiame on amygdaloid kindled seizures in rats. *Epilepsy Res* 1997; 27:81–87.
9. Egli M, Hess R, Wad N. Therapeutische Serumkonzentration von Sulthiam. *Nervenarzt* 1978; 49:402–404.
10. Tanimukai H, Inui M, Hariguchi S, Kaneko Z. Antiepileptic property of inhibitors of carbonic anhydrase. *Biochem Pharmacol* 1965; 14:961–970.
11. Madeja M, Wolf C, Speckmann EJ. Reduction of voltage-operated sodium currents by the anticonvulsant drug sulthiame. *Brain Res* 2001; 900:88–94.
12. Baier WK, Doose H. Sulthiame. In: Resor SR, Kutt H, eds. *The Medical Treatment of Epilepsy*. New York: Marcel Dekker, 1992:419–422.
13. May TW, Korn-Merker E, Rambeck B, Boenigk HE. Pharmacokinetics of sulthiame in epileptic patients. *Ther Drug Monit* 1994; 16:251–257.
14. Callaghan N, Feely MP, O'Callaghan M, Duggan B. A prospective longitudinal study of serum levels of sulthiame and phenytoin, together with an evaluation seizure control. In: Penry JK, ed. *Epilepsy. The Eighth International Symposium*. New York: Raven Press, 1977:119–123.
15. Feely MP, O'Callaghan M, O'Driscoll D, Callaghan N. Sulthiame in previously untreated epilepsy. *Ir J Med Sci* 1982; 151:175–179.
16. Green JR, Troupin AS, Halperm LM, Friel P, et al. Sulthiame: evaluation as an anticon vulsant. *Epilepsia* 1974; 15:329–349.
17. Hansen JM, Kristensen M, Skovsted L. Sulthiame (Ospolot) as inhibitor of diphenylhydatoin metabolism. *Epilepsia* 1968; 9:17–22.
18. Olesen OV, Jensen ON. Drug interaction between sulthiame (Ospolot (R)) and phenytoin in the treatment of epilepsy. *Dan Med Bull* 1969; 16:154–158.

19. Houghton GW, Richens A. Proceedings: inhibition of phenytoin metabolism by sulthiame. *Br J Pharmacol* 1973; 49:157–158.
20. Houghton GW, Richens A. Phenytoin intoxication induced by sulthiame in epileptic patients. *J Neurol Neurosurg Psychiatry* 1974; 37:275–281.
21. Koepp MJ, Patsalos PN, Sander JW. Sulthiame in adults with refractory epilepsy and learning disability: an open trial. *Epilepsy Res* 2002; 50:277–282.
22. Rating D, Wolf C, Bast T. Sulthiame as monotherapy in children with benign childhood epilepsy with centrotemporal spikes: a 6-month randomized, double-blind, placebo-controlled study. Sulthiame Study Group. *Epilepsia* 2000; 41:1284–1288.
23. Debus OM, Kurlemann G. Sulthiame in the primary therapy of West syndrome: a randomized double-blind placebo-controlled add-on trial on baseline pyridoxine medication. *Epilepsia* 2004; 45:103–108.
24. Engelmeier MP. Über die klinische Erprobung antiepileptischer Medikamente unter besonderer Berücksichtigung des Ospolot. *Dtsch Med Wochenschr* 1960; 85:2207–2211.
25. Raffauf HJ. Die Behandlung zerebraler Anfallsleiden mit Ospolot. *Dtsch Med Wochenschr* 1960; 85:2203–2207.
26. Fluegel F, Bente D, Itil T. Zur Stellung des Butansultamderivates Ospolot in der Behandlung zerebraler Anfallsleiden. *Dtsch Med Wochenschr* 1960; 85:2199–2203.
27. Rabe F, Penin H, Matthes A. Erfahrung mit Ospolot in der Epilepsiebehandlung. *Dtsch Med Wochenschr* 1987; 18:953–959.
28. Doose H, Ehmsen U. Bericht über die Erfahrungen mit Ospolot bei der Behandlung kindlicher Epilepsien an der Universitätskinderklinik Kiel. *Symposien aktueller therapeutischer Probleme* 1963; 4:189–203.
29. Doose H, Kluge D, Ehmsen U. Erfahrungen mit Ospolot bei der Behandlung kindlicher Epilepsien. *Med Klin* 1964; 59:271–274.
30. Nayrac P, Beaussart M. Les pointes-ondes prérolandiques: expression EEG très particulière. *Rev Neurol (Paris)* 1958; 99:201–206.
31. Gibbs EL, Gibbs FA. Good prognosis of mid-temporal epilepsy. *Epilepsia* 1960; 1:448–453.
32. Dalla Bernardina B, Sgro V, Fejerman N. Epilepsy with centro-temporal spikes and related syndromes. In: Roger J, Bureau M, Dravet Ch, Genton P, et al, eds. *Epileptic Syndromes in Infancy, Childhood and Adolescence*. 3rd ed. London: John Libbey, 2002:181–202.
33. Doose H, Baier WK, Ernst JP, Tuxhorn I, et al. Benign partial epilepsy—treatment with sulthiame. *Dev Med Child Neurol* 1988; 30:683–684.
34. Gross-Selbeck G. Treatment of "benign" partial epilepsies of childhood, including atypical forms. *Neuropediatrics* 1995; 26:45–50.
35. Lerman P, Nussbaum E. The use of sulthiame- in myoclonic epilepsy of childhood and adolescence. *Acta Neurol Scand Suppl* 1975; 60:7–12.
36. Engler F, Maeder-Ingvar M, Roulet E, Deonna T. Treatment with sulthiame (Ospolot) in benign partial epilepsy of childhood and related syndromes: an open clinical and EEG study. *Neuropediatrics* 2003; 34:105–109.
37. Ben Zeev B, Watemberg N, Lerman P, Barash I, et al. Sulthiame in childhood epilepsy. *Pediatr Int* 2004; 46:521–524.
38. Kramer U, Shahar E, Zelnik N, Lerman-Sagie T, et al. Carbamazepine versus sulthiame in treating benign childhood epilepsy with centrotemporal spikes. *J Child Neurol* 2002; 17:914–916.
39. Wakai S, Ito N, Ueda D, Chiba S. Landau-Kleffner syndrome and sulthiame. *Neuropediatrics* 1997; 28:135–136.
40. Kurlemann G, Fiedler B, Debus O. Sultiam in der Therapie epileptischer Anfälle im Kindesalter. *Zeitschrift für Epileptologie* 2005; 18:122 (abstract).
41. Bray CA, Bower BD. Ospolot in epilepsy. *Dev Med Child Neurol* 1963; 18:409-411.
42. Ingram TT, Ratcliffe SG. Clinical trial of Ospolot in epilepsy. *Dev Med Child Neurol* 1963; 5:313–315.
43. Fenton G, Serafetinides EA, Pond DA. The effect of sulthiame, a new anticonvulsant drug in the treatment of temporal lobe epilepsy. *Epilepsia* 1964; 23:59–67.
44. Gordon N. The use of Ospolot in the treatment of epilepsy. *Epilepsia* 1964; 23:68–73.
45. Garland H, Sumner D. Sulthiame in treatment of epilepsy. *Br Med J* 1964; 5381:474–476.
46. Korn-Merker E, Boenigk HE. Sultiam—auch zur Behandlung nicht benigner fokaler Epilepsien. *Pädiatrische Praxis* 1994; 47:433–438.
47. Dalla Bernardina B, Fontana E, Michelizza B, Colamaria V, et al. Partial epilepsies of childhood, bilateral synchronization, continuous spike-waves during slow sleep. In: Manelis, Bental E, Loeber JN, Dreifuss FE, eds *Advances in Epileptology*. New York: Raven Press, 1989:295–302.
48. Panayiotopoulos CP. Severe syndromes of mainly linguistic and neuropsychological deficits, seizures or both and marked EEG abnormalities from the Rolandic and neighbouring regions. In: Panayiotopoulos CP, ed. *Benign Childhood Partial Seizures and Related Epileptic Syndromes*. London: John Libbey, 1999:337–360.
49. Tassinari CA, Rubboli G, Volpi L, Billard C, Bureau M. Electrical status epilepticus during slow sleep (ESES or CSWS) including acquired epileptic aphasia (Landau-Kleffner syndrome). In: Roger J, Bureau M, Dravet Ch, Genton P, et al, eds. *Epileptic Syndromes in Infancy, Childhood and Adolescence*. 3rd ed. London: John Libbey, 2002:265–284.
50. Bast T, Volp A, Wolf C, Rating D. The influence of sulthiame on EEG in children with benign childhood epilepsy with centrotemporal spikes (BECTS). *Epilepsia* 2003; 44:215–220.
51. Patry G, Lyagoubi S, Tassinari CA. Subclinical "electrical status epilepticus" induced by sleep in children. A clinical and electroencephalographic study of six cases. *Arch Neurol* 1971; 24:242–252.
52. Smyth VO. The use of Ospolot in temporal lobe epilepsy. A preliminary communication. *Epilepsia* 1964; 90:293–295.
53. Wilkus RJ, Green JR. Electroencephalographic investigations during evaluation of the antiepileptic agent sulthiame. *Epilepsia* 1974; 15:13–25.
54. Tröger U, Fritzsch C, Darius J, Gedschold J, et al. Sulthiame-associated mild compensated metabolic acidosis. *Int J Clin Pharmacol Ther* 1996; 34:542–545.
55. Weglage J, Pietsch M, Sprinz A, Feldmann R, et al. A previously unpublished side effect of sulthiame in a patient with Rolandic epilepsy [letter]. *Neuropediatrics* 1999; 30:50 (letter).
56. Go T. Effect of antiepileptic drug monotherapy on urinary pH in children and young adults. *Childs Nerv Syst* 2006; 22:56–59.
57. Go T. Effect of antiepileptic drug polytherapy on crystalluria. *Pediatr Neurol* 2005; 32:113–115.
58. Brockmann K, Hanefeld F. Progressive elevation of liver enzymes in a child treated with sulthiame. *Neuropediatrics* 2001; 32:165–166.

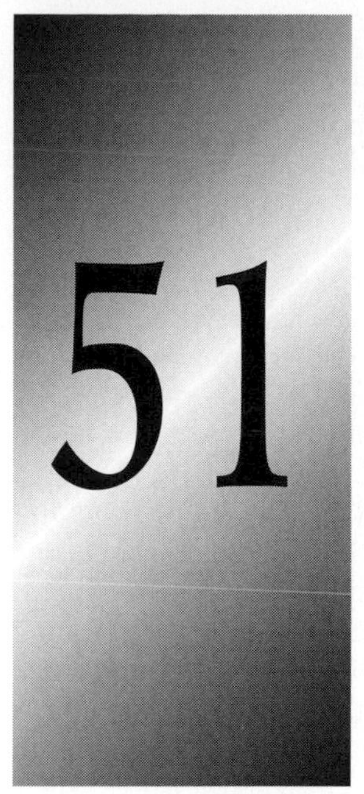

Tiagabine

Shlomo Shinnar
Richard Civil
Kenneth W. Sommerville

In the last few years, a new generation of antiepileptic drugs (AEDs) has been developed (1, 2), with much interest in drugs that work on the gamma-aminobutyric acid (GABA) system. GABA is the primary inhibitory neurotransmitter in the mammalian nervous system (3, 4). Increasing the effects of the GABA system is theorized to prevent seizures. This type of prevention has already been noted with the barbiturates and benzodiazepines, which act on the GABA receptor. Valproate, a GABA analog, is an effective AED against a variety of seizure disorders, although its precise mechanism of action remains unclear (5, 6). Recent attempts to utilize the GABA system have focused on GABA metabolism and have resulted in the development of two new drugs. One drug, vigabatrin (Chapter 54), available in much of the world but still experimental in the United States because of concerns about retinal toxicity, is an irreversible inhibitor of GABA transaminase (1, 5, 7). By blocking degradation vigabatrin raises the levels of GABA. The second drug, tiagabine (Gabitril), was approved by the FDA for the adjunctive treatment of partial seizures in adults and adolescents in 1997.

Tiagabine was developed as a designer drug to block GABA uptake by presynaptic neurons and glial cells (1, 3, 8–13). This blocking should increase GABA concentration in the synapse, resulting in longer duration of action in the synaptic cleft without substantially altering total brain GABA levels. Tiagabine has undergone extensive clinical trials in adults with intractable partial seizure disorders (14–19). Less information is available on the use of tiagabine in children, although some clinical trials were done (20–23). In this manuscript, we review the available data on tiagabine with an emphasis on its use in the pediatric age group. Because tiagabine is a relatively new drug and its use in epilepsy has decreased over time, the pediatric data are relatively sparse. This chapter reviews the available data, including the recent safety data, with an emphasis on the pediatric aspects.

PHYSICOCHEMICAL CHARACTERISTICS

Tiagabine hydrochloride is a whitish, odorless crystalline powder with the chemical name (-)-(R)-1-[4,4-Bis (3-methyl-2-thienyl)-3-butenyl] nipecotic acid hydrochloride. The chemical formula is $C_{20}H_{25}NO_2S_2 \cdot HCl$, and the structure is shown in Figure 51-1. It is 3% soluble in water and is insoluble in hexane. The nipecotic acid moiety of the molecule has an asymmetric carbon, and the R (−) enantiomer is four times more potent that the S (+) enantiomer. The name *tiagabine* refers to the R (−) enantiomer, which consists of nipecotic acid joined to a lipophilic anchor.

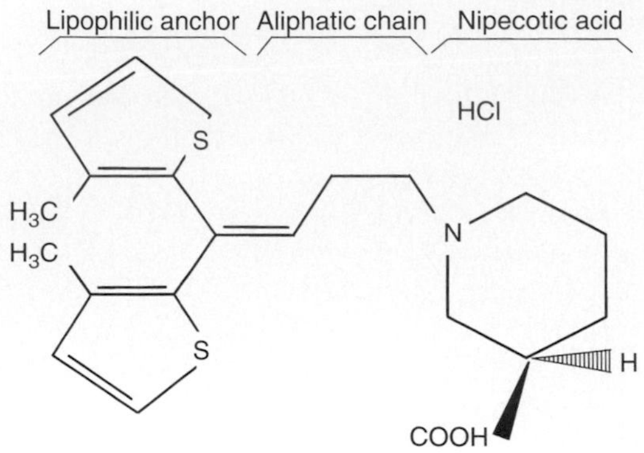

FIGURE 51-1

Chemical structure of tiagabine HCl.

Animal experiments demonstrated that nipecotic acid was anticonvulsant and could preferentially block glial and neural GABA uptake in mice (24). However, nipecotic acid had to be injected intracerebrally in animals because it did not cross the blood-brain barrier. The addition of a lipophilic anchor to nipecotic acid allowed passage across the brain barrier and maintained the desired property of blocking GABA uptake. The resulting compound is tiagabine hydrochloride and is referred to as tiagabine.

MECHANISM OF ACTION

Tiagabine increases the amount of GABA available in the extracellular space by preventing GABA uptake into presynaptic neurons, as schematically shown in Figure 51-2. The increased GABA enhances inhibitory effects on receptors of postsynaptic cells. This effect was confirmed in hippocampal rat slices, in which tiagabine prolonged GABA-mediated inhibitory postsynaptic potentials (25).

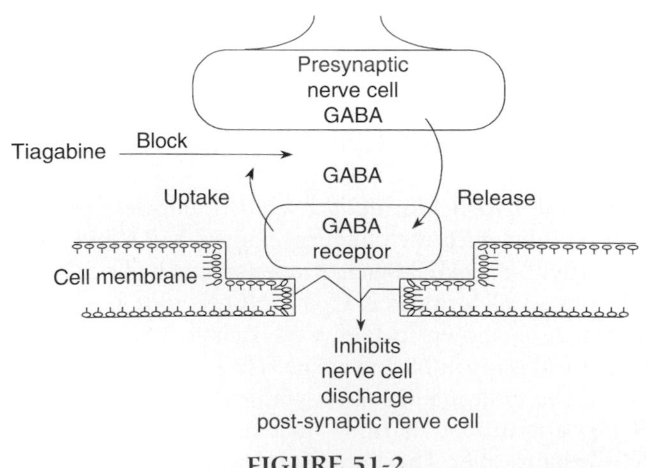

FIGURE 51-2

Tiagabine inhibits the uptake of gamma-aminobutyric acid (GABA) in the synaptic cleft.

In-vitro work in adult rats has shown that tiagabine blocks GABA uptake by binding in a stereospecific and saturable fashion to the GABA recognition sites in neurons and glial cells (26). Tiagabine binds to a class of high-affinity binding sites that most likely represent the GABA transporter GAT-1 (27).

The action of tiagabine is confined to blocking GABA uptake. Tiagabine is not itself taken into neurons or glia. Tiagabine is highly selective for the GABA system and does not affect other neurotransmitters. Tiagabine binds weakly to the benzodiazepine and H_1 receptors, but only at concentrations 20 to 400 times those required to inhibit GABA uptake (26). This binding is unlikely to be clinically relevant.

Tiagabine is an anticonvulsant in a variety of animal models of epilepsy, including pentylenetetrazol (PTZ)-induced seizures (11), DMCM-induced seizures (8), and, at high doses, seizures induced by maximal electroshock (11) (DMCM, methyl 6,7-dimethoxy-4-ethyl-beta-carboline-3-carboxylate, is a proconvulsant that is an inverse agonist of the benzodiazepine receptor).

Tiagabine has shown other anticonvulsant activity in animal models. Tiagabine suppresses amygdala-kindled seizures in rats (8) and is effective in treating convulsive status epilepticus in cobalt-lesioned rats (28). Tiagabine also has moderate efficacy in the genetically determined generalized epilepsy in photosensitive baboons. Tiagabine may have a proconvulsant effect that has been noted with other AEDs. Spike-and-wave discharges were noted after control of motor status at doses of more than 5 mg/kg in both lesioned and normal rats (28). In a strain of rats (WAG/Rij) that are genetically prone to epilepsy—a strain that is considered an animal model of generalized nonconvulsive absence epilepsy—type II spike wave discharges were increased at dose of 3 mg/kg and 10 mg/kg, but not at doses of 1 mg/kg, which is closer to the therapeutic range (29). In these epilepsy-prone rats, the increase in spike-wave discharges was not correlated with behavioral abnormalities in the animals. These data suggest that tiagabine may exacerbate absence seizures. However, tiagabine is effective in blocking PTZ-induced seizures, which often predicts efficacy against generalized seizures.

The adult animal data suggest that tiagabine may have efficacy in treating some types of both partial and generalized seizure disorders. Data are lacking on the effects of tiagabine on experimental seizure models in the developing brain of animals. This lack is unfortunate, because some AEDs have age-dependent effects on seizures (30–32), but it is a common problem with all AEDs in early clinical usage.

METABOLISM AND PHARMACOKINETICS

Animal studies have shown that tiagabine is rapidly absorbed and has a short half-life, 1 to 3 hours in rats and 1 to 2 hours in dogs. Bioavailability is 25% in dogs and 50–75% in rats (9). Tiagabine, like many other AEDs, is metabolized by the hepatic cytochrome P450 system (33). Metabolites include 5-oxotiagabine, which is excreted in the urine. Tiagabine is also conjugated with glucuronic acid, and metabolites are excreted via urine and via feces through the biliary system (9).

Studies in adult volunteers have shown that tiagabine is rapidly absorbed from the gastrointestinal tract and peak plasma concentrations (C_{max}) are achieved within 2 hours. Absorption is linear and independent of the dose (34). The rate—but not the extent of absorption—is reduced by food. The time to peak plasma concentration (T_{max}) after a meal is more than twice that in the fasting state. However, although the C_{max} is lower, the area under the curve (AUC) is similar (35). Clinical trials were therefore performed with patients taking tiagabine after a meal in order to reduce the possible peak-related toxicities without altering the total amount of drug absorbed.

In normal volunteers, the mean half-life of tiagabine is 4 to 9 hours and is independent of the dose. Because tiagabine is metabolized by the hepatic cytochrome P450 system, it has a shorter half-life in patients taking drugs that induce that system, such as barbiturates, carbamazepine, and phenytoin (36). When given in single or multiple doses, tiagabine does not appear to induce or inhibit hepatic microsomal enzyme systems (34, 37).

Tiagabine is extensively metabolized by the hepatic microsomal system because less than 2% is excreted unchanged in the urine (34, 38, 39). Radiolabeled [^{14}C]tiagabine studies in human volunteers showed that 25% was excreted in the urine and 63% in the feces (40). Tiagabine has no identified active metabolites (40). Tiagabine does not appear to accumulate appreciably in plasma with multiple dosing. In Phase I studies of healthy volunteers given daily doses over a 5-day period, both the peak levels and the AUC increased proportionally with the dose, as would be expected in a drug with linear pharmacokinetics (34). The therapeutic half-life, as distinct from the serum half-life, is unclear. Microdialysis studies in patients given oral tiagabine demonstrated extracellular GABA levels in the brain that rise within about 1 hour after oral dosing (41) but are not sustained more than a few hours and do not completely correlate with the serum concentrations (40). The duration of the antiepileptic activity, which is presumably mediated by these changes in GABA, remains unclear and has not been precisely studied.

Tiagabine is heavily protein bound, although it does not appear either to displace or to be displaced by most of the commonly used drugs (42, 43). In-vitro studies showed that tiagabine is over 95% protein bound, primarily to albumin and a glycoprotein.

Tiagabine pharmacokinetics were studied in patients with epilepsy who were taking tiagabine as add-on therapy. Steady state tiagabine doses ranged from 24 to 80 mg/day in four divided doses (44). All patients were taking enzyme-inducing concomitant AEDs. Results showed that tiagabine had linear kinetics in this population also, with a linear dose-response curve for peak concentrations (C_{max}) as well as for the AUC. Although the kinetics remained linear, the half-life of tiagabine was shorter in patients taking AEDs that induce the cytochrome P450 system than for those on monotherapy or taking noninducing AEDs (36). This difference is expected and explains why the dosages used in this study were considerably higher than those tolerated by healthy volunteers who were not taking enzyme-inducing AEDs. The dosage ranges in this study exceeded the upper doses of 56 mg/day used in the randomized clinical trials in the descriptions that follow.

The most important drug interaction of tiagabine to date is the effect of enzyme-inducing AEDs. The half-life of tiagabine was shorter and the AUC smaller for the same dose in patients receiving enzyme-inducing AEDs (carbamazepine, phenytoin, phenobarbital, primidone) than in those on tiagabine monotherapy (9, 36, 45). The pharmacokinetics of tiagabine in patients taking an AED that was not enzyme inducing, such as valproate, were similar to those in healthy volunteers. Dosages of tiagabine need to be substantially higher in patients taking concurrent enzyme-inducing AEDs than with monotherapy or noninducing AEDs. Similar guidelines have been suggested for the recently approved AED lamotrigine (46, 47). Although the half-life of tiagabine is shortened by the concurrent use of enzyme-inducing AEDs, it is not prolonged by the concurrent use of valproate, as is the case with lamotrigine and phenobarbital (46–49).

Tiagabine has little effect on other AEDs. Tiagabine does not appear to affect the kinetics of carbamazepine or phenytoin (42). However, tiagabine did reduce the peak concentration and the AUC of valproate by approximately 10% (49). The reason for this reduction is expected to be of little or no clinical importance. Because tiagabine is metabolized by the 3A isoform subfamily of the hepatic cytochrome P450 system (33), there is potential for interaction with other drugs with similar metabolism, including other AEDs, cimetidine, theophylline, warfarin, and digoxin. However, no clinically significant interactions have been found between tiagabine and these drugs (43). Surprisingly, a recent study showed no interaction with erythromycin (50).

Oral contraceptives are also metabolized by the cytochrome P450 system. In one study, tiagabine, given at a dose of 8 mg/day as monotherapy to healthy young women, did not affect the metabolism of oral contraceptives (37, 43). Higher doses of tiagabine would not be expected to have an interaction because tiagabine is neither an inducer nor an inhibitor of the cytochrome P450 system, but data are lacking to confirm this impression.

Tiagabine pharmacokinetics behave predictably in hepatic and renal disease (51, 52). There is no effect from renal impairment, and there is reduced clearance and a longer half-life with hepatic impairment. Patients with hepatic disease require lower doses to attain similar concentrations than healthy subjects.

Single-dose tiagabine pharmacokinetics have been studied in children (20). In this study, 25 children ages 3–10 with complex partial seizures who were taking one AED were given a single dose of 0.1 mg/kg of tiagabine, and plasma concentrations were checked over the next 24 hours. The mean half-life of tiagabine was 3.2 hours in the 17 children on enzyme-inducing concomitant AEDs (carbamazepine or phenytoin) and 5.7 hours for the 8 children on valproate (noninducing AED). This result is comparable to the adult data. Clearance rates, peak plasma concentrations, and AUC of tiagabine were affected by the concurrent AEDs in a manner similar to adults. The clearance of tiagabine was two times higher in children than in noninduced adults with epilepsy when the rate was adjusted for body weight. However, when adjusted according to body surface area, clearance rates of tiagabine in children were 1.5 times higher than in noninduced adults with epilepsy. The results indicate that tiagabine pharmacokinetics in children ages 2 and older are similar to those in adults, including the effects of concurrent AEDs. Infants have not been studied.

The initial studies of tiagabine were done in patients who were also on other AEDs, primarily enzyme-inducing ones such as carbamazepine. Subsequently, it has been used in conjunction with AEDs that are not enzyme inducing, as well as in monotherapy. The effect of enzyme-inducing AEDs is clearly much stronger than had been appreciated. It appears that the dose of tiagabine for someone who is not on enzyme-inducing AEDs is less than half that for someone who is. Failure to appreciate this difference when tiagabine is used in conjunction with the newer AEDs that are not enzyme inducers can result in significant toxicity.

DATA ON HUMAN ADULT EFFICACY

Add-On Therapy in Adults with Partial Seizures

The clinical data regarding the efficacy of tiagabine as add-on therapy come from five placebo-controlled clinical trials in patients with intractable partial seizures. In all five trials, tiagabine was statistically significantly more effective than placebo in the treatment of one or more partial seizure types (53). Two of the studies were crossover and three were parallel group. Most of the patients were adults ages 18–75; however, adolescents starting at age 12 were also included. Thus, efficacy data are available in this age group, although in a relatively small number of patients. Pediatric trials in younger children are in progress, and the available data are discussed separately.

The first Phase II multicenter study was a crossover design performed in Europe with 94 patients ages 18–65 with refractory complex partial seizures (14). The study had an "enrichment" design. Patients started with a dose of 8 mg/day of tiagabine and titrated the dose to either reduce seizures sufficiently or produce unacceptable adverse events with a maximum dose of 52 mg/day. Patients who improved in this phase were then enrolled in a double-blind trial. Of the 94 patients enrolled, 20 discontinued participation during the open-label phase, and another 28 failed to qualify for the double-blind phase for lack of sufficient reduction in seizures. The average total daily dose of tiagabine in the 42 patients in the double-blind phase was 33 mg/day, and most were taking a concomitant enzyme-inducing AED. Even with this relatively small sample size, the frequency of complex partial seizures only and partial seizures with secondary generalization was significantly reduced when the tiagabine and placebo phases were compared. Details of the second crossover trial have not yet been published, but the results were similar to the first study (53).

The three randomized Phase III multicenter, placebo-controlled, double-blind, parallel-group studies in adults included two studies in the United States and one in Europe. All of these studies showed that tiagabine was significantly superior to placebo as adjunctive treatment of partial seizures.

The first U.S. study (15) was a dose-response study, with patients receiving placebo, or 16, 32 or 56 mg/day of tiagabine in addition to their regular stable AED regimen. Tiagabine was significantly better than placebo at both 32 and 56 mg for median change from baseline and proportion of patients achieving at least 50% reduction in complex partial seizures (in both, $P < 0.03$). Tiagabine was effective for both median change from baseline and proportion with >50% reduction in the groups receiving 16, 32, and 56 mg for simple partial seizures.

Partial seizures with secondary generalization were reduced compared to placebo, but this reduction did not reach significance, possibly because of fewer patients and numbers of seizures. A clear dose response was present in this study. The minimum effective dose of tiagabine necessary to achieve a reduction of 50% in complex partial seizure frequency was 32 mg/day, with the group at 56 mg/day showing a better response. Doses greater than 56 mg were not studied in this trial. Note that the patients in this study and in the other two randomized studies were all taking one to three concurrent AEDs, at least one of which was required to be an inducer of the cytochrome P450 enzyme system. Thus, as discussed in the metabolism section, the doses required in monotherapy, or with a single concomitant noninducer such as valproate, are substantially smaller than when used together with an enzyme-inducing AED such as carbamazepine. The patients in this study were, by and large, a very refractory group with a median duration of epilepsy of 20 years, who had failed to respond to a median of seven AEDs prior to study entry.

The second U.S. multicenter, randomized, double-blind, placebo-controlled parallel-group trial compared placebo to 32 mg/day of tiagabine as add-on therapy in 318 patients (16). In this dose-frequency trial, the tiagabine patients received a total of 32 mg/day as 16 mg twice a day or as 8 mg four times a day. Both groups were superior to placebo ($P < 0.001$) in the number of patients achieving a reduction greater than 50% in complex partial seizures. Both groups were also superior to placebo for simple partial seizures, for either reduction from baseline or proportion, with a reduction in seizures of at least 50%. Taken together with the prior study, the data suggested that the add-on dose of 32 mg/day was likely to be in the low therapeutic range for enzyme-induced patients.

The multicenter European double-blind, parallel-group study was the only adjunctive trial to evaluate tiagabine given three times daily (TID) (54). Tiagabine was given as 10 mg TID or 8 mg TID if a dose of 30 mg/day was not tolerated. There were 154 patients randomized to tiagabine ($n = 77$) or placebo ($n = 77$). The tiagabine-treated group had a significant reduction in both the number of complex and simple partial seizures.

Tiagabine consistently demonstrated efficacy against partial seizures in these trials, but the dose ranges chosen were probably too low in enzyme-induced patients to establish its upper therapeutic range and maximum efficacy. These trials included 67 adolescents ages 12–18 and therefore can be regarded as demonstrating efficacy and safety for this age group as well.

These placebo-controlled trials showed that tiagabine is superior to placebo. The challenge for the practicing clinician is to determine the role of a new AED in the treatment of patients for whom there are a number of other AEDs to consider. Tiagabine has been compared to add-on carbamazepine or phenytoin in a double-blind multicenter study. Placebo and active drug were given in a double-dummy design of patients on baseline carbamazepine receiving add-on tiagabine or phenytoin, or patients on baseline phenytoin receiving add-on tiagabine or carbamazepine. Patients were allowed to titrate to their best-tolerated dose within a wide range to mimic clinical practice.

Preliminary results of the patients taking baseline carbamazepine were recently reported (55). There was no difference in efficacy between the tiagabine group ($n = 106$) and the phenytoin group ($n = 100$) for any partial seizure type in the intent-to-treat analysis. However, phenytoin patients had greater discontinuations for adverse events (17%) than those on tiagabine (10%). Overall discontinuation rates also favored tiagabine (31% vs. 22%). However, further studies are needed before the precise role of tiagabine in treating refractory partial seizures can be determined.

Monotherapy Trials

There have been three studies of tiagabine monotherapy in adults with partial seizures (56, 57). The first was a double-blind randomized pilot study of 11 patients who had their AEDs discontinued while they were in the hospital undergoing monitoring for presurgical evaluation (57). Patients receiving tiagabine had fewer seizures than those receiving placebo during the treatment period. In the second study (56), which was an open-label, dose-ranging study, 19 of 31 patients (61%) successfully converted to tiagabine monotherapy. In the third study, which included 198 randomized patients with partial seizures, patients were randomized to daily doses of tiagabine as either 6 or 36 mg/day. Baseline AEDs were discontinued after tiagabine was added on. Seizure frequency was reduced in both the low- and high-dose groups, with the high-dose group having a significantly higher proportion of patients who experienced a reduction in seizure frequency that was greater than 50% (56). The following open-label pediatric data have also been promising (22).

Human Pediatric Efficacy Data

In a open-label pilot study (22), 25 children with refractory complex partial seizures from a single-dose pharmacokinetics study (20) were enrolled in an open-label, long-term study. Children were initially taking a dose of 0.1 mg/kg/day of tiagabine. They were also continuing a baseline concomitant AED. The dosage was increased every two weeks by 0.1 mg/kg/day until clinical efficacy or toxicity was reached. The results of this study have been encouraging for the use of tiagabine in children. As of January 1996, 23 of 25 children were still taking tiagabine. Of 21 patients treated for greater than 6 months, 19 (90%) had a reduction in the frequency of complex partial seizures that was greater than 50% compared with historical seizure rates. These children had previously uncontrolled partial seizures. For these children, the median 4-week historical baseline rate for complex partial seizures was 5 (range 1–90) and mean 21.1. Conversion to tiagabine monotherapy had been possible for 16 of the children, and they had been seizure-free at least two months on a mean dose of 0.31 mg/kg/day.

The other pediatric study was a dose-ranging, multicenter, add-on study, conducted at three European sites, of 52 children ages 2–15 with epilepsy with a variety of seizure types and epilepsy syndromes refractory to other AEDs (21). The results are unfortunately difficult to interpret because of the heterogeneous nature of the epilepsy disorders in the study. Twenty-two of the children had generalized epilepsies, including Lennox-Gastaut syndrome; others had myoclonic seizure disorders, infantile spasms, or childhood absence. Before entry into the trial, the children had been unsuccessfully tried on 3–16 other AEDs, including carbamazepine, valproate, and vigabatrin for more than 80% of them.

This study differed from the U.S. open-label study. After a placebo lead-in period of three weeks, tiagabine was given at more rapid escalating doses than in the U.S. study of 0.25 mg/kg/day up to 1.5 mg/kg/day. Dose escalation in the U.S. study was by 0.1 mg/kg/day at no faster than weekly intervals. Patients who completed this phase either entered a long-term extension study or were withdrawn from tiagabine. Of the 53 patients enrolled, 47 entered the tiagabine-dosing phase. Of these, 20 completed the trial and 20 withdrew for lack of efficacy ($n = 16$), adverse events ($n = 3$), or other reasons ($n = 1$). Seven patients were still in the dosing phase when the preliminary report was published (21). Seventeen of 20 patients completing the study entered the long-term extension.

The drug was generally well tolerated (see the following discussion of safety). The study showed no improvement for children with generalized epilepsy, but those with partial seizures improved at doses ranging from 0.37 to 1.25 mg/kg/day. However, the results of this small-scale trial in a very refractory population did not demonstrate a statistically significant effect. These results suggest even more strongly that a controlled trial is needed to determine the place of tiagabine in treating children with partial seizures. The results from the open-label U.S. experience are encouraging, but they need further confirmation.

SAFETY

Animal Safety Data

In the preclinical animal studies of tiagabine, there was a large therapeutic window because doses producing sedation were 2.5- to 30-folder greater than the doses treating seizures (58). Other studies in animals have shown no evidence of abnormalities relevant to humans or of carcinogenicity, mutagenicity, or teratogenicity (9).

Adult Data

Phase I studies in healthy volunteers showed that multiple doses of tiagabine were well tolerated up to 10 mg/day (39) and that side effects greater than those with placebo were noted when the initial dose reached 12 mg/day (59). The side effects included difficulty concentrating, lightheadedness, impaired visual perception, and confusion. The side effects increased at higher initial doses. These doses may be lower than what might be tolerated by patients taking enzyme-inducing concomitant AEDs, in whom the clearance of tiagabine is greater.

Clinical trials of tiagabine therapy in patients with epilepsy have shown an adverse-events profile that was favorable and comparable to many of the current AEDs. The most common adverse events involved the central nervous system and were usually mild to moderate and transient. In the U.S. multicenter dose-response trial, adverse events sufficient to require discontinuation of the drug occurred twice as often in the groups receiving 32 mg/day (15%) and 56 mg/day (16%) of tiagabine as in the groups receiving placebo (8%) or 16 mg (7%) of tiagabine (15). The side effects with significantly higher incidence in tiagabine-treated patients were dizziness, tremor, and difficulty concentrating or mental lethargy. Adverse events in the second U.S. study, which used a dosage regimen of 32 mg/day (either twice or four times per day), were similar to those in the first study but milder (16). Again, the percentage of patients withdrawn from the study as a result of adverse events was higher in the combined tiagabine groups (10%) than in the placebo group (7%). Nervousness, difficulty with immediate recall (amnesia), and emotional lability were other events of the central nervous system (CNS) that were significantly greater with tiagabine. Abdominal pain, vomiting, and other pain were also significantly increased, but they were usually not attributed to tiagabine. Myalgia was increased with placebo compared to tiagabine given four times per day.

Three monotherapy studies again showed that CNS-related adverse events were the most common (56). These studies may have used higher doses of tiagabine than necessary for clinical practice. One study was a small, inpatient presurgical population; one was an open-label pilot study titrating to the maximally tolerated dose; the third was a controlled high- vs. low-dose conversion-to-monotherapy study. The conversion study enabled an evaluation of dose-related side effects, in which dizziness, trouble concentrating, nervousness, and paresthesia were significantly increased in the high-dose group (36 mg/day). A key finding for safety in the open-label pilot study was that patients converting to monotherapy from enzyme-inducing AEDs demonstrated deinduction of tiagabine clearance. The dose of tiagabine may need to be reduced when monotherapy is reached because tiagabine concentrations rise without an increase in dose when the inducing AED is discontinued. This does not occur if the concomitant AED is a single noninducer such as valproate.

Neuropsychologic testing has been performed in add-on studies and in the controlled conversion-to-monotherapy study (18, 19, 60). Compared with placebo, tiagabine had no adverse effects on neuropsychologic test scores in both an add-on Finnish study using 30 mg/day (18) and in the multicenter U.S. dose-response study using 16, 32, and 56 mg/day (19). The multicenter U.S. high- vs. low-dose conversion to monotherapy study showed results related to both dose and whether monotherapy was attained (60). Patients achieving monotherapy improved in mood in the low-dose group, whereas abilities improved in the high-dose group. There was worse performance for mood in the high-dose group if monotherapy was not reached. The reasons for improvement did not correlate with control of seizures and may have been from benefits of withdrawing the baseline concomitant AED, better tolerance of tiagabine, or both.

Long-term safety data from the open-label studies have also been reassuring. There have been no clinically relevant changes in laboratory values for hematological or hepatic function. The most commonly reported adverse events were dizziness, somnolence, accidental injury, asthenia (lack of energy), and headache, which are similar to those in the randomized studies (17). Accidental injury and headache are common in populations with severe epilepsy. These adverse events were usually mild and transient and did not require discontinuation of tiagabine therapy. In the long-term open-label clinical trials of tiagabine in the United States, 220 of 1437 patients (15%) have discontinued therapy for adverse events (61).

Recently, loss in the peripheral visual field has been reported in patients treated with vigabatrin (62). Theoretically, this is a concern for all GABAergic drugs, including tiagabine. However, the mechanism of action of tiagabine is different than that of vigabatrin. Tiagabine does not cause total GABA levels in the brain to rise and is only associated with a transient rise in extracellular GABA concentrations (41). Review of the database on tiagabine safety and a study of visual fields by Novo Nordisk have found no comparable visual abnormalities that are attributable to tiagabine therapy to date (K Sommerville, MD, personal communication).

Safety data have also been published on tiagabine overdose (63, 64). There were 22 overdoses in clinical trials as of the end of 1996, with the highest single dose of 800 mg. The most common symptoms were ataxia, confusion, somnolence, agitation, hostility, speech difficulty, weakness, impaired consciousness, and myoclonus. All patients completely recovered. One adolescent had generalized tonic-clonic status epilepticus from a 400-mg overdose but recovered after treatment with phenobarbital. Only supportive care is generally recommended. These findings suggest that the margin of safety with tiagabine is large.

The experience in pregnancy is limited to 21 cases from clinical trials as of October 1996 (65): 9 fetuses were carried to term; 8 were healthy, and 1 had a hip displacement attributed to a breech presentation. There were 5 elective abortions, 4 women had miscarriages, 1 had a blighted ovum, and another had a salpingectomy for an ectopic pregnancy. The remaining patient drowned in a bathtub during a seizure after discontinuing tiagabine three months earlier. Postmortem examination showed a healthy fetus of 5 months.

DATA ON PEDIATRIC SAFETY

The safety data in children have also been reassuring. Children in the U.S. open-label pharmacokinetics trial tolerated the drug well in single doses of 0.1 mg/kg (20). Nine of 25 (36%) children reported adverse events, with somnolence being the most common ($n = 7$). One other patient reported a headache, and another had pain at the site of the heparin lock used for sampling blood. All adverse events were mild in severity and resolved without treatment. These children have also tolerated tiagabine very well in a subsequent open-label, long-term study (22). As of January 1996, 23 children were taking tiagabine on an ongoing basis, without discontinuation for adverse events.

The data from the European pediatric study that used higher doses and a more rapid titration were also comparable to adult data (20). Three of 47 children were withdrawn from tiagabine for adverse events, including ataxia ($n = 2$), somnolence ($n = 1$), and depression ($n = 1$). Two additional children had been hospitalized, but both had complete recoveries and were discharged on the same dose of tiagabine. The common adverse events were CNS related and were similar to those in adults. Most were mild to moderate in severity and resolved without requiring discontinuation of the drug.

TIAGABINE AND STATUS EPILEPTICUS

Soon after the introduction of tiagabine into clinical use, there were reports of possible nonconvulsive status epilepticus associated with tiagabine therapy (66, 67). One report described two patients with confusion and reduced consciousness and simultaneous generalized spike wave discharges on electroencephalogram (EEG) (67). The authors suggested that this reaction may be from $GABA_B$ receptor agonism and that frontal lobe foci (present in both patients) may be a risk factor. The reports, however, did not confirm that the patients had nonconvulsive status epilepticus or that tiagabine was the cause. The first patient improved slightly after intravenous diazepam and then spontaneously improved 3 hours later. The second patient deteriorated 5 days after a reduction in tiagabine dose of 25%, suggesting that the possible nonconvulsive status was precipitated by a dose reduction.

An additional 13 cases of possible spike-wave discharges and impaired mental status associated with tiagabine therapy have been intensively reviewed (68). The medical histories and pretreatment EEGs were located and reviewed by an advisory panel. Eight of the cases were thought to have preexisting generalized spike-wave abnormalities that worsened with poorly tolerated increases in tiagabine dose. These patients improved with dose reductions and usually continued on tiagabine at lower doses. Three patients had nonconvulsive status epilepticus that could be attributed to their underlying condition. The remaining two patients either improved with a higher tiagabine dose or did not have spike-wave discharges. The panel concluded that the evidence so far is that, in the majority of reported cases, tiagabine did not cause the spike-wave discharges, but rather exacerbated preexisting spike-wave patterns in association with poorly tolerated doses. At high doses, a confusional state occurs. However, a few of the cases clearly were nonconvulsive status.

With the wider use of tiagabine, as well as its off-label use in psychiatric conditions in patients with no prior history of seizure, additional safety data have accumulated (61, 69). Koepp et al. (69) retrospectively reviewed the records of patients with intractable seizures treated with tiagabine and compared them to those not treated with tiagabine. They found that 7 of 90 subjects (8%) treated with tiagabine had electroclinically confirmed nonconvulsive status epilepticus compared with 32 of 1165 patients (3%) who were not treated with tiagabine. Although this review was retrospective and may have included ascertainment bias, the results are of concern. More recently, there have been reports of frank convulsions in both children and adults who were being prescribed tiagabine off label for psychiatric conditions not associated with seizures, such as anxiety. Although most cases were in the context of a high dosage or a very rapid titration and other signs of toxicity, a few cases occurred in a low dose in patients without clear risk factors for epilepsy. This has led to a change in the label to reflect that convulsions can be a rare but serious side effect of tiagabine (61).

CONCLUSIONS

Results in multiple controlled trials have consistently shown tiagabine to be an effective AED for patients with partial seizures. The profile of side effects appears to be favorable. Pediatric data remain limited. The data suggest that tiagabine is effective in partial seizure disorders in adults and children. At this point ,it is fairly clear that tiagabine should not be used in generalized seizure disorders because of its potential to exacerbate generalized spike-wave discharges in both primary and secondarily generalized epilepsies. Tiagabine has great theoretical appeal as a "designer drug" that enhances the availability of GABA at the postsynaptic membrane without interfering with overall GABA metabolism and without altering GABA levels in the brain. However, as with other GABA agents, the results to date have been mixed. Tiagabine has a number of favorable characteristics, including a spectrum of efficacy in animal models and a relative lack of sedation or changes in neuropsychologic testing, which make it an exciting new drug. However, this is offset by a tendency at higher doses to exacerbate seizures sometimes and by the potential to actually trigger seizures in select patients. Unlike many other AEDs whose typical clinical usage is to push to efficacy or clinical toxicity, tiagabine is a drug that, with rare exceptions, should not be used at doses exceeding those recommended. Although it is too early to know the precise role of tiagabine, physicians caring for patients with seizures can add tiagabine as one of the therapeutic options in selected patients with partial seizures. The availability of multiple new agents improves our ability to care for children and adults with seizures.

References

1. Dichter MA, Brodie MJ. New antiepileptic drugs. *N Engl J Med* 1996; 334:1583–1590.
2. Wyllie E, ed. New developments in antiepileptic drug therapy. *Epilepsia* 1995; 36 (Suppl 2):S1–S118.
3. Suzdak PD, Jansen JA. A review of the preclinical pharmacology of tiagabine: a potent and selective anticonvulsant GABA uptake inhibitor. *Epilepsia* 1995; 36:612–626.
4. Meldrum B. Pharmacology of GABA. *Clin Neuropharmacol* 1982; 5:293–316.
5. MacDonald RL, Kelly KM. Antiepileptic drug mechanisms of action. *Epilepsia* 1995; 36(Suppl 2):S2–S12.
6. Farriello RG, Varasi M, Smith MC. Valproic Acid: mechanisms of action. In: Levy RH, Mattson RH, Meldrum BS, eds. *Antiepileptic Drugs*, 4th ed. New York: Raven Press, Ltd., 1995:581–588.
7. Ben-Menachem E. Vigabatrin. *Epilepsia* 1995; 36(Suppl 2):S95–S104.
8. Giardina WJ. Anticonvulsant action of tiagabine, a new GABA-uptake inhibitor. *J Epilepsy* 1994; 7:161–166.
9. Ostergaard LH, Gram L, Dam M. Potential antiepileptic drugs: tiagabine. In: Levy RH, Mattson RH, Meldrum BS, eds. *Antiepileptic Drugs*, 4th ed. New York: Raven Press, Ltd., 1995:1057–1061.
10. Mengel HB. Tiagabine. *Epilepsia* 1994; 35(Suppl 5):S81–S84.
11. Neilsen EB, Suzdac PD, Andersen KE, Knutsen LJ, et al. Characterization of tiagabine (NO-328), a new potent and selective GABA uptake inhibitor. *Eur J Pharmacol* 1991; 196:257–266.
12. Andersen KE, Braestrop C, Gronwald FC, et al. The synthesis of novel GABA uptake inhibitors. 1. Elucidation of the structure-activity studies leading to the choice of (R)-1-[4,4-bis(3-methyl-2-thienyl)-3-butenyl]-3-piperidinecarboxylic acid (tiagabine) as an anticonvulsant drug candidate. *J Med Chem* 1993; 36:1716–1725.
13. Thompson SM, Gähwiler BH. Effects of the GABA uptake inhibitor tiagabine on inhibitory synaptic potentials in rat hippocampal slice cultures. *J Neurophysiol* 1992; 67:1698–1701.
14. Richens A, Chadwick D, Duncan J, et al. Adjunctive treatment of partial seizures with tiagabine: a placebo-controlled trial. *Epilepsy Res* 1995; 21:37–42.
15. Uthman BM, Rowan AJ, Ahmann PA, Leppik IE, et al. Tiagabine for complex partial seizures: a randomized, add-on, dose-response trial. *Arch Neurol* 1998; 55:56–62.
16. Sachdeo R, Leroy R, Krauss G., et al. Tiagabine therapy for complex partial seizures: a dose-frequency study. *Arch Neurol* 1997; 54:595–601.
17. Leppik IE. Tiagabine: the safety landscape. *Epilepsia* 1995; 36(Suppl 6):S10–S13.
18. Kalviainen R, Salmenpera T, Aikia M, et al. Tiagabine monotherapy in newly diagnosed partial epilepsy: follow-up with cognitive tests, EEG, quantitative MRI, and CSF amino acids. *Epilepsia* 1994; 35(Suppl 7):74.
19. Dodrill CB, Arnett JL, Sommerville KW, et al. Cognitive and quality of life effects of differing doses of tiagabine in epilepsy. *Neurology* 1997; 48:1025–1031.

20. Gustavson LE, Boellner SW, Granneman GR, et al. A single-dose study to define the tiagabine pharmacokinetics in pediatric patients with complex partial seizures. *Neurology* 1997; 48:1–6.
21. Uldall P, Bulteau C, Pederson SA, Dulac O, et al. Single-blind study of safety, tolerability, and preliminary efficacy of tiagabine as adjunctive treatment of children with epilepsy. *Epilepsia* 1995; 36(Suppl 3):S147.
22. Boellner S, McCarty J, Mercante D, et al. Pilot study of tiagabine in children with partial seizures. *Epilepsia* 1996; 37(Suppl 4):92.
23. Biton V, Alto G, Pixton G, Sommerville K. Tiagabine monotherapy in adults and children in a long-term study. *Epilepsia* 1996; 37(Suppl 5):1–7.
24. Croucher MJ, Meldrum BS, Krogsgaard-Larsen P. Anticonvulsant activity of GABA uptake inhibitors and their prodrugs following central or systemic administration. *Euro J Pharmacol* 1983; 89:217–228.
25. Rekling JC, Jahnsen H, Laursen AM. The effect of two lipophilic gamma-aminobutyric acid uptake blockers in CA1 of the rat hippocampal slice. *Br J Pharmacol* 1990; 99:103–106.
26. Braestrup C, Nielsen EB, Sonnewald U, Knutsen LJS, et al. (R)-N-[4,4-bis(3-methyl-2-thienyl)but-3-en-1-yl ninecotic acid binds with high affinity to the brain gamma-aminobutyric acid uptake carrier. *J Neurochem* 1990; 54:639–647.
27. Borden LA, Murali Dhar TG, Smith KE, Weinshank RL, et al. Tiagabine, SKF 89976-A, CI-966 and NNC-711 are selective for the cloned GABA transporter GAT-1. *Eur J Pharmacol* 1994; 269:2219–224.
28. Walton NY, Gunawan S, Treiman DM. Treatment of experimental status epilepticus with the GABA uptake inhibitor, tiagabine. *Epilepsy Res* 1994; 19:237–244.
29. Coenen AM, Blezer EH, van Luijtelaar EL. Effects of the GABA uptake inhibitor tiagabine on eletroencephalogram, spike-wave discharges and behaviour of rats. *Epilepsy Res* 1995; 21:89–94.
30. Velisek L, Veliskova J, Ptachewich Y, Shinnar S, et al. Effects of MK-801 and phenytoin on flurothyl-induced seizures during development. *Epilepsia* 1995; 36:179–185.
31. Velisek L, Veliskova J, Ptachewich Y, Ortiz J, et al. Age-dependent effects of gamma-aminobutyric acid agents on flurothyl seizures. *Epilepsia* 1995; 36:636–643.
32. Sheridan PH, Jacobs MP. Conference Review. The development of antiepileptic drugs for children: Report from the NIH workshop, Bethesda, Maryland, February 17–18, 1994. *Epilepsy Res* 1996; 23:87–92.
33. Bopp BA, Nequist GE, Rodrigues AD. Role of the cytochrome P450 3A subfamily in the metabolism of [^{14}C] tiagabine in human hepatic microsomes. *Epilepsia* 1995; 36(Suppl 3):S159.
34. Gustavson LE, Mengel HB. Pharmacokinetics of tiagabine, a gamma-aminobutyric acid-uptake inhibitor, in healthy subjects after single and multiple doses. *Epilepsia* 1995; 36:605–611.
35. Mengel HB, Gustavson LE, Soerensen HJ, McKelvy JF, et al. Effect of food on the bioavailability of tiagabine HC1. *Epilepsia* 1991; 32(Suppl 3):6.
36. Richens A, Gustavson LE, McKelvy JF, Mengel H, et al. Pharmacokinetics and safety of single-dose tiagabine HC1 in epileptic patients chronically treated with four other antiepileptic drug regimens. *Epilepsia* 1991; 32(Suppl 3):12.
37. Mengel HB, Houston A, Back DJ. An evaluation of the interaction between tiagabine and oral contraceptives in female volunteers. *J Pharm Med* 1994; 4:141–150.
38. Gustavson LE, Mengel HB, Pierce MW, Chu S-Y. Tiagabine, a new gamma-aminobutyric acid uptake inhibitor antiepileptic drug: pharmacokinetics after single oral doses in man. *Epilepsia* 1990; 31:642.
39. Mengel HB, Pierce M, Mant T, Gustavson L. Tiagabine, a GABA-uptake inhibitor: safety and tolerance of multiple dosing in normal subjects. *Acta Neurol Scand* 1990; 82 (Suppl 133):35.
40. Bopp BA, Gustavson LE, Johnson MK, et al. Disposition and metabolism of orally administered ^{14}C-tiagabine in humans. *Epilepsia* 1992; 33(Suppl 3):83.
41. During M, Mattson R, Scheyer R, Rask C, et al. The effect of tiagabine HC1 on extracellular GABA levels in the human hippocampus. *Epilepsia* 1992; 33(Suppl 3):83.
42. Gustavson LE, Cato A, Boellner SW, et al. Lack of pharmacokinetics drug interactions between tiagabine and carbamazepine or phenytoin. *American Journal of Therapeutics* 1998; 5:9–16.
43. Mengel HB, Jansen JA, Sommerville K, Jonkman JHG, et al. Tiagabine: evaluation of the risk of interaction with theophylline, warfarin digoxin, cimetidine, oral contraceptives, triazolam, or ethanol. *Epilepsia* 1995; 36(Suppl 3):S160.
44. So EL, Wolff D, Graves NM, Leppik IE, et al. Pharmacokinetics of tiagabine as add-on therapy in patients taking enzyme-inducing drugs. *Epilepsy Res* 1995; 22: 221–226.
45. Brodie MJ. Tiagabine pharmacology in profile. *Epilepsia* 1995; 36(Suppl 6):S7–S9.
46. Messenheimer JA. Lamotrigine. *Epilepsia* 1995; 36(Suppl 2):S87–S94.
47. Yuen AWC. Lamotrigine: interaction with other drugs. In: Levy RH, Mattson RH, Meldrum BS, eds. *Antiepileptic Drugs*, 4th ed. New York: Raven Press, Ltd., 1995: 883–888.
48. Dodson WE. Principles of antiepileptic drug therapy. In: Shinnar S, Amir N, Branski D, eds. *Childhood Seizures*. Basel, Switzerland: S Karger, 1995:78–92.
49. Gustavson LE, Sommerville KW, Cato A, Boellner SW, et al. Lack of a clinically significant pharmacokinetics drug interaction between tiagabine and valproate. *Online J Curr Clin Trials* February 18, 1997; document 203.
50. Thompson MS, Groes L, Schwietert HR, Jonkman JHG, et al. An open label sequence listed two period crossover pharmacokinetics trial evaluating the possible interaction between tiagabine and erythromycin during multiple administration to healthy volunteers. *Epilepsia* 1997; 38(Suppl 3):64.
51. Cato A, Gustavson LE, Qian J, et al. Effect of renal impairment on the pharmacokinetics and tolerability of tiagabine. *Epilepsia* 1998; 39(Suppl 1):43–47.
52. Lau AH, Gustavson LE, Sperelakis R, Lam NP, et al. Pharmacokinetics and safety of tiagabine in subjects with various degrees of hepatic function. *Epilepsia* 1997; 38:445–451.
53. Ben-Menachem. International experience with tiagabine add-on therapy. *Epilepsia* 1995; 36(Suppl 6):S14–S21.
54. Schachter SC, Sommerville KW. Tiagabine. A potent new drug for partial seizures. Presented at Third Eilat conference on new antiepileptic drugs, May 28–29, 1996, Eilat, Israel.
55. Vasquez B, Sachdeo RC, Chang, et al. Tiagabine or phenytoin as first add-on therapy for complex partial seizures. *Neurology* 1998; 50(Suppl 4):A199.
56. Schachter SC. Tiagabine monotherapy in the treatment of partial epilepsy. *Epilepsia* 1995; 36(Suppl 6):S2–S6.
57. Alarcon G, Binnie CD, Elwes RDC, Polkey CE. Monotherapy antiepileptic drug trials in patients undergoing presurgical assessment: methodological problems and possibilities. *Seizure* 1995; 4:293–301.
58. Pierce MW, Suzdak PD, Andersen KE, et al. Tiagabine. In: Pisani F, Perucca E, Avansini A, eds. *New Antiepileptic Drugs*, Amsterdam: Elsevier, 1991:157–160.
59. Mengel HB, Mant TGK, McKelvy JM, Pierce MW. Tiagabine: Phase I study of safety and tolerance following single oral doses. *Epilepsia* 1990; 31:642–643.
60. Dodrill CE, Arnett JL, Shu V, et al. Effects of tiagabine monotherapy on abilities, adjustment, and mood. *Epilepsia* 1998; 39:33–42.
61. Gabitril™ prescribing information, Cephalon, 2005.
62. Eke T, Talbot JF, Lawden MC. Severe persistent visual field constriction associated with vigabatrin. *BMJ* 1997; 314:180–181.
63. Parks BR, Flowers WG, Dostrow VG, et al. Experience with clinical overdoses of tiagabine. Antiepileptic drug treatment: state of the art and further perspectives. Bredlefeld, Germany, April 24–27, 1997.
64. Leach JP, Stolarek I, Brodie MJ. Deliberate overdose with the novel anticonvulsant tiagabine. *Seizure* 1995 Jun; 4(2):155–157.
65. Collins SD, Sommerville KW, Donnelly J, et al. Pregnancy and tiagabine exposure. *Neurology* 1997; 48(Suppl 2):A38.
66. Schapel G, Chadwick D. Tiagabine and non-convulsive status epilepticus. *Seizure* 1996; 5:153–156.
67. Eckardt KM, Steinhoff BJ. Non-convulsive status epilepticus in two patients receiving tiagabine treatment. *Epilepsia* 1998; 39:671–674.
68. Shinnar S, Berg AT, Treiman DM, et al. Status epilepticus and tiagabine therapy: review of safety data and epidemiologic comparisons. *Epilepsia* 2001; 42:372–379.
69. Koepp MJ, Edwards M, Collins J, Farrel F, et al. Status epilepticus and tiagabine therapy revisited. *Epilepsia* 2005; 46:1625–1632.

52 Topiramate

Tracy A. Glauser

Topiramate (TPM) is one of the second-generation antiepileptic medications approved in many countries during the 1990s. It has efficacy against a broad spectrum of seizure types, is effective as monotherapy or adjunctive therapy, and is used extensively in both adults and children. Other favorable characteristics include linear pharmacokinetics, few drug-drug interactions, and a well-described adverse-events profile, with recognizable and reversible adverse events. Overall, TPM has emerged as a valuable antiepileptic drug (AED) for a variety of pediatric and adult epilepsies.

CHEMISTRY, ANIMAL PHARMACOLOGY, AND MECHANISM OF ACTION

Chemistry

Topiramate, 2,3:4,5-bis-O-(1-methylethylidene)-beta-D-fructopyranose sulfamate, a sulfamate-substituted monosaccharide derived from the D-enantiomer of fructose, is structurally distinct from other anticonvulsant drugs (Figure 52-1) (1, 2). TPM is a white crystalline powder with a molecular weight of 339.37; it is soluble in water and organic solvents at physiologic pH (3); and it has a pK_a of 8.7 at 25°C (4).

Animal Pharmacology

Efficacy

TPM was initially tested in two traditional animal models of epilepsy, the maximal electroshock test (MES) and the pentylenetetrazol (PTZ) seizure test. The MES test has been hypothesized to identify agents effective against partial-onset and generalized tonic-clonic (GTC) seizures and those that have the capacity to prevent the spread of seizures (5, 6). In rats and mice, TPM blocked MES seizures with a potency similar to that of phenytoin (PHT), carbamazepine (CBZ), phenobarbital (PB), and acetazolamide (1). In the subcutaneous PTZ test, a chemically induced seizure model hypothesized to identify agents that raise the seizure threshold, TPM, like PHT, was either ineffective or only weakly effective (1). This activity profile suggests that TPM exerts its anticonvulsant effects by blocking the spread of seizures rather than by raising the seizure threshold. However, TPM did increase seizure threshold in response to an intravenous infusion of PTZ in mice (7), suggesting that TPM possessed an even broader spectrum of action than was originally thought.

TPM was effective in blocking seizures in four other rodent models of epilepsy. In rats, TPM inhibited amygdala-kindled seizures, indicating a potential for activity against complex partial seizures (5, 8). In the

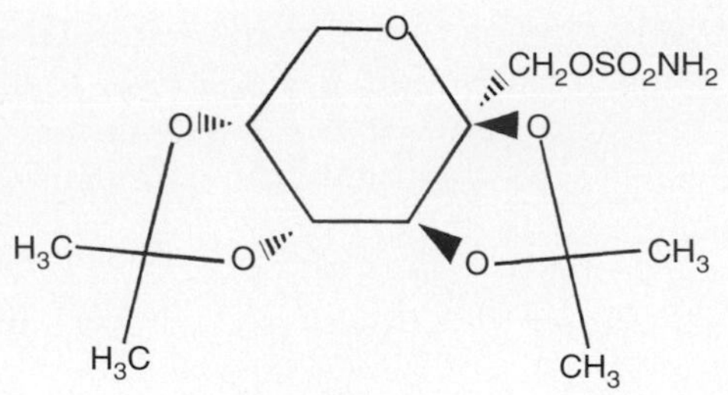

FIGURE 52-1

Topiramate; 2,3:4,5-bis-O-(1-methylethylidene)-beta-fructopyranose sulfamate.

DBA/2 mouse, a strain genetically prone to seizures, TPM blocked sound-induced clonic seizures when administered before the auditory stimulus (9). In the spontaneously epileptic rat (SER), a hereditary model of epilepsy, TPM inhibited tonic and absence-like seizures (9). TPM was also effective in a rat model of post-traumatic epilepsy (10).

TPM's profile of activity in experimental models of epilepsy suggests a multifactorial mechanism of action. The MES test in rats was used to study the development of tolerance to the anticonvulsant effects of TPM. No tolerance was noted after 14 days of TPM, administered at nearly twice the effective dose (ED_{50}) (1, 11).

Toxicity

Acute studies. TPM was well tolerated following acute administration in mice, rats, and dogs (4, 12). The estimated LD_{50} after oral TPM administration in mice and rats ranged from 2338 to 3745 mg/kg. Dogs were more sensitive than mice or rats to the acute toxic effects of TPM, which were primarily central nervous system (CNS) related.

Multiple-dose studies. Multiple-dose (3- and 12-month) toxicity studies were performed in rats and dogs. In these studies, reversible gastric mucosal hyperplasia changes were seen that were similar to those reported with carbonic anhydrase inhibitors (13–15). No evidence of dysplasia, aplasia, or any change suggesting tumor formation was apparent. In studies of rats and mice, formation of urinary microcalculi, associated with TPM use, was also consistent with carbonic anhydrase inhibition (16).

Reproductive studies. Fertility was not affected by TPM in male or female rats (R. Reife, personal communication), and TPM did not affect pup survival at doses up to 100 mg/kg/day (4).

Teratology studies. In teratology studies, TPM caused right-sided ectrodactyly (congenital absence of all or part of a digit) in rats and rib and vertebral malformations in rabbits (R. Reife, personal communication). These effects of TPM are similar to those reported with acetazolamide and other carbonic anhydrase inhibitors (17–19).

Protective index. TPM was selected for development as an AED, based on its high protective index (PI) and its potency and duration of action in tests in rodents (1, 2). The PI can be determined from the ratio of the median toxic dose (TD_{50}) from a neurotoxicity test, such as the rotarod test or the loss of righting reflex test, to the MES ED_{50}. A higher, more advantageous ratio was obtained in rats and mice with TPM than with PHT, CBZ, or PB. For example, with oral doses, the PI for TPM in rats was greater than 116, whereas the values for PB, CBZ, and PHT were 3.5, 20.8, and greater than 60.8, respectively (1).

Mechanisms of Action

In vitro, TPM demonstrates an ability to modulate ionic channels, enhance inhibitory neurotransmission, and reduce excitatory transmission processes involved in the generation of seizures. Preclinical studies indicate that TPM has at least six mechanisms of action that may contribute to its anticonvulsant activity.

1. *Modulation of voltage-dependent sodium channels*: In cultured rat hippocampal neurons displaying spontaneous activity, micromolar concentrations of TPM reduced the duration and frequency of action potentials associated with sustained repetitive firing (20). TPM also blocked action potentials induced by depolarizing electric currents. (20).
2. *Modulation of glutamate-mediation neurotransmission*: TPM produced concentration-dependent decreases in kainate-evoked inward currents (excitatory currents) in cultured hippocampal neurons without affecting the activity of glutamate receptors of the *N*-methyl-D-aspartate (NMDA) subtype (those modulated by benzodiazepines) (20, 21). In cultured rat amygdalar neurons, TPM postsynaptically antagonizes the action of kainate receptors of the GluR5 subtype (22). TPM protects against seizures in mice induced by the convulsant substance ATPA, a GluR5 kainate receptor agonist (23). TPM has no effect on the NMDA-mediated glutamate receptor type (20).
3. *Promotion of gamma-aminobutyric acid (GABA) activity:* In cultured murine cerebellar granule cells, micromolar concentrations of TPM, in combination with GABA, augmented GABA-stimulated chloride flux into chloride-depleted neurons (i.e., enhanced inhibitory neurotransmission) compared with

GABA alone (7, 24). The effect of TPM on $GABA_A$ receptors was not blocked by the benzodiazepine antagonist flumazenil, suggesting that a novel or nonbenzodiazepine modulatory site may be involved (7, 25). As measured by magnetic resonance spectroscopy in vivo, TPM increases GABA content in the human brain (26, 27).

4. *Enhancement of potassium channel conduction:* In rat neurons, TPM increases potassium channel conductance (28).
5. *Modulation of voltage-dependent calcium channels:* In rat neurons, TPM inhibits L-type high voltage-activated calcium channels, possibly through a second messenger. (29)
6. *Carbonic anhydrase inhibition:* The sulfamate moiety of TPM is structurally similar to that of the carbonic anhydrase inhibitor acetazolamide. However, the potency of TPM as an inhibitor of erythrocyte carbonic anhydrase is much lower than that of acetazolamide (1). In vitro, TPM does not appear to exert an anticonvulsant effect through inhibition of carbonic anhydrase (1).

This broad activity profile in vitro suggests that TPM may be effective against a number of seizure types.

BIOTRANSFORMATION, PHARMACOKINETICS, AND INTERACTIONS IN HUMANS

Absorption and Distribution

In adults and children, TPM has linear pharmacokinetics with low intersubject variability. In adult studies, TPM is rapidly absorbed from the gastrointestinal tract after administration of single oral doses ranging from 100 to 1,200 mg (30). Its estimated bioavailability is approximately 80% (31, 32); its absorption is not significantly affected by food (30).

The volume of distribution of TPM ranges from 0.6 to 0.8 L/kg, which is consistent with a distribution in total body water (33). For most patients, 90% of the maximal plasma concentration (C_{max}) is achieved within 2 hours after oral administration (30), although this can range from 1.4 to 4.3 hours (30), depending on the dose. Mean values for C_{max} and area under the concentration-time curve (AUC), which are reflections of drug absorption and clearance, increase linearly with respect to dose in adults (34). TPM is not highly bound to plasma proteins (9%–17%) (35).

Metabolism and Elimination

In monotherapy, TPM is not extensively metabolized (34). Six trace metabolites of TPM were identified that represented less than 5% of the sample radioactivity (36). The metabolites, formed by hydroxylation, hydrolysis, and glucuronidation, do not display significant antiepileptic activity (34, 36). In adults, the elimination half-life ($t_{1/2}$) values for TPM when used as monotherapy range from 19 to 25 hours (37).

Renal excretion is a major route of TPM elimination (36). In adults, within a dose range of 200 to 1,200 mg, at least 51% of the dose is estimated to be excreted by the kidneys (30). Because TPM's renal clearance is much lower than its glomerular filtration rate (30), it has been proposed that TPM may undergo tubular reabsorption. In adults, the $t_{1/2}$ values for TPM, calculated from plasma (mean, 21.5 hours) and urine (mean, 18.5 hours) data, appear to be independent of dose (30). In patients with renal failure (creatinine clearance <30 mL/min/1.73 m^2), an approximately twofold increase in AUC and $t_{1/2}$ occurs (38). Therefore, adults with renal impairment may require reduced TPM dosages. During hemodialysis, TPM is cleared from plasma roughly nine times faster than in patients with normal renal function, implying that patients may need additional doses after hemodialysis (39).

Information on TPM pharmacokinetics in children and adolescents was determined from a single-center, open-label outpatient trial of 18 patients with epilepsy (12, 40). Patients ages 4–17 years received an oral TPM dose of up to 9 mg/kg/day in addition to their standard regimen of AEDs. As in adults, pharmacokinetics were linear in children, and plasma clearance was not affected by TPM dose. Compared with adults, clearance values were 54% greater in children when TPM was administered in the presence of enzyme-inducing drugs and 44% greater in the absence of enzyme-inducing drugs (40). Because overall TPM clearance was approximately 50% greater in children than in adults, for any given dose based on weight (mg/kg), steady state TPM plasma concentrations would be predicted to be approximately 33% lower in children than in adults.

Two studies have examined TPM pharmacokinetics in young children. TPM's mean plasma clearance, in a study of five children ages 2–2.5 years, was slightly higher than that reported for children and adolescents; the plasma clearance was higher in infants on concomitant enzyme-inducing AEDs than in those on nonenzyme-inducing concomitant AEDs (41). In another study of 22 children (ages 6 months to 4 years), TPM's oral clearance was significantly higher in infants and young children on concomitant enzyme-inducing AEDs (85.4 ± 34.0 mL/h/kg) compared with those taking valproic acid (VPA) (49.6 ± 13.6 mL/h/kg) or nonenzyme-inducing AEDs (46.5 ± 12.8 mL/h/kg) (42).

Drug Interactions

TPM and AEDs

In general, administration of TPM does not have major effects on the plasma concentrations of other

AEDs. TPM has no effect on most cytochrome P450 isozymes in in-vitro studies (43, 44). There were no TPM effects detected on concomitant drug levels in add-on clinical trials (45, 46). In one study, PHT levels rose 30% to 50% in three patients when TPM was added at a dose of 400–800 mg/day; these patients had baseline PHT levels of 15 μg/mL or higher, and it is proposed that TPM probably inhibited CYP2C19, the secondary enzyme for PHT metabolism (37).

Effects on other antiepilepsy drugs are negligible (43, 44, 47). When TPM was administered concomitantly with CBZ, there were no significant changes in total or unbound CBZ plasma concentrations (47). Similar results were found for lamotrigine (48). Although TPM has little net influence on VPA clearance, it can shift the proportions of several VPA metabolic pathways, but the clinical significance of this is uncertain. An increase in a potentially toxic metabolite, 4-ene-valproate, has been proposed as a factor in the rare cases of hyperammonemic encephalopathy observed with combination TPM-VPA therapy (49). TPM had no effect on plasma PB concentrations (50). No studies are available on the effects of TPM on felbamate, gabapentin, or tiagabine.

In contrast, studies have shown that administration of concomitant AEDs may affect plasma concentrations of TPM. Conversion of patients to TPM monotherapy from concomitant therapy with TPM and PHT (an enzyme-inducing AED) resulted in appreciably higher mean steady state values for TPM C_{max} and AUC (51). Similarly, withdrawal of CBZ from patients receiving concomitant TPM and CBZ resulted in an approximately twofold increase in TPM plasma levels (47). Therefore, there is a potential need for TPM dosage adjustment when enzyme-inducing AEDs are either added or discontinued. Barbiturates may have a similar effect but have not been studied. Conversely, simultaneous administration of TPM and VPA (an inhibitor of hepatic enzymes) resulted in slightly (17%) higher values for TPM C_{max} and AUC (52).

TPM and Non-AEDs

TPM at doses of 200 mg/day or more reduced serum levels of ethinyl estradiol derived from an oral contraceptive by 30% (53), but, in another series of women, TPM doses of 50, 100, and 200 mg/day had no significant effect (54). This TPM effect on oral contraceptives is less than that of the effect of either CBZ, PHT, or PB; unlike these other antiepileptic medications, TPM does not lower progestin levels (54).

Coadministration of TPM and digoxin in healthy adults results in a small reduction in digoxin C_{max} (16%) and AUC (12%) (55). The apparent oral clearance of digoxin increased by 13% without a corresponding change in the renal clearance, suggesting that TPM may affect the systemic availability of digoxin.

The clearances for lithium, amitriptyline, and risperidone increase and the levels decrease slightly when they are given with TPM (43). Metformin AUC increased by 25% in healthy volunteers given TPM (44). TPM has no pharmacokinetic effects on concomitant propranolol, sumatriptan, or dihydroergotamine (43).

CLINICAL EFFICACY

A summary of the randomized controlled trials involving TPM across a broad spectrum of seizure types, usages (monotherapy, adjunctive therapy), and ages (adults and children) is shown in Table 52-1.

Monotherapy in Adults and Children with Partial-Onset and Generalized-Onset Seizures

The efficacy of TPM monotherapy has been assessed in four randomized controlled monotherapy trials (56–61). The first trial was a single-center study in which adult outpatients with refractory partial-onset seizures were randomized to either TPM 100 mg/day (low dose) or TPM 1000 mg/day (high dose), converted over 5 weeks from one or two standard AEDs to TPM monotherary, and then followed for 11 more weeks (56). The study's primary outcomes of time until study exit and successful completion of 112 study days were significantly better for the high-dose TPM group compared with the low-dose TPM group. During the study, 13% of the high-dose TPM patients, but no low-dose TPM patients, became seizure free (56).

Subsequently, two multicenter randomized, controlled trials of TPM monotherapy in children and adults with recently diagnosed epilepsy employed a similar high-dose versus low-dose design, but both studies used lower TPM dosages (57, 58). The study population included both adults and children with partial-onset seizures and generalized-onset tonic-clonic seizures. The first trial randomized 252 patients (age 3 years and older), with epilepsy for less than three years, to either a low dose (25 mg/day if weight was less than 50 kg; 50 mg/day if weight was greater than 50 kg) or a high dose (200 mg/day if weight was less than 50 kg; 500 mg/day if weight was greater than 50 kg) (58). At baseline, patients were either on no medication (56%) or on one drug that was withdrawn within six weeks. The primary endpoint, a comparison of time to second seizure between these doses, was not statistically significant; however, when the time to first seizure was added as a covariate for the data analysis, the high dose proved superior in efficacy (P = 0.01). A secondary outcome variable, the percentage of patients who were seizure free during the six-month trial, favored the high-dose group (54% vs. 39%, P = 0.02).

The second randomized controlled trial enrolled 470 patients (age 6 years and older), with untreated epilepsy (two or more lifetime unprovoked seizures, with one or two partial-onset seizures or generalized-onset tonic-clonic seizures in a three-month retrospective baseline), to either TPM 50 mg/day or TPM 400 mg/day (57). The primary endpoint, time to first seizure, was better in the high-dose group ($P = 0.0002$). The treatment arms demonstrated a significant difference ($P = 0.046$) in favor of the high-dose arm by study day 14, when patients were receiving 100 mg/day (high dose) and 25 mg/day (low dose). The seizure-free rates for the high and low doses at 12 months were 76% and 59%, respectively ($P = 0.001$) (57). The trial included a large cohort ($n = 151$, 32%) of children and adolescents 6–15 years of age. The primary efficacy endpoint of time to first seizure favored the higher TPM dose in the cohort of children and adolescents ($P = 0.002$). The probability that children and adolescents were seizure-free at six months was 78% in the group given the 50-mg target dose and 90% in the group with the higher dose ($P = 0.04$). At 12 months, the probability of being seizure free was higher in the high-dose group compared to the low-dose group (85% vs. 62%, respectively, $P = 0.002$) (60).

A fourth TPM monotherapy trial used a different design (59). Patients were eligible if their epilepsy was diagnosed within the previous three months. Study investigators identified whether CBZ (600 mg/day) or VPA (1250 mg/day) would have been their preferred therapy based on the patient's clinical presentation. A total of 613 study patients were randomized to double-blind treatment with either the investigator's preferred therapy (CBZ or VPA) as the active control drug, TPM 100 mg/day, or TPM 200 mg/day. Designed to detect inferiority, the study found no evidence of it between either TPM dose or the active control (CBZ or VPA) for any of the efficacy measures examined: time to exit, time to first seizure, and the proportion of patients who were seizure free during the last six months of treatment. Because 100 mg/day of TPM proved just as effective as 200 mg/day, the authors suggested 100 mg/day as an initial target dose for patients with new-onset seizures. In the subset of pediatric partial-onset seizure patients, the time to first seizure was similar for patients in the TPM, CBZ, or VPA arms, as were the proportions of seizure-free patients during the last six months of treatment (61).

Adjunctive Therapy in Adults and Children with Partial-Onset Seizures

TPM has been extensively studied as adjunctive therapy in adults with refractory partial-onset seizures with or with-

TABLE 52-1

Summary of Randomized Controlled Trials Involving Topiramate in Patients with Epilepsy

Type of TPM use	Seizure type	Age group	Number of studies	Design*	Result	Ref
Monotherapy	Partial onset—treatment resistant	Adult	1	High dose vs. low dose	High dose > low dose	56
Monotherapy	Partial onset—recently diagnosed	Adults and children	2	High dose vs. low dose	High dose > low dose	57, 58, 60
Monotherapy	Partial onset—recently diagnosed	Adults and children	1	TPM vs CBZ OR TPM vs VPA	TPM not inferior to CBZ or VPA	59, 61
Adjunctive	Partial onset	Adult	8	Placebo controlled	TPM > placebo	45, 46, 62–67
Adjunctive	Partial onset	Child	1	Placebo controlled	TPM > placebo	70
Adjunctive	Generalized tonic clonic seizures of non-focal origin	Adults and children	1	Placebo controlled	TPM > placebo	72
Adjunctive	Seizure types associated with Lennox–Gastaut syndrome	Adults and children	1	Placebo controlled	TPM > placebo	75

TPM = topiramate, CBZ = carbamazepine, VPA = valproic acid, * = see text for details

out secondary generalization. Eight multicenter, randomized, placebo-controlled trials of adjunctive TPM therapy for adults with treatment-resistant, partial-onset seizures have documented TPM's efficacy compared to placebo at dosages of 200 mg/day or greater (45, 46, 62–67). Initial clinical trials examined the effects of doses ranging from 200 mg/day to 1600 mg/day. The minimum effective daily dose was 200 mg/day (45); intent-to-treat analyses identified 400 mg/day as the most effective dose (45, 67); and doses from 600 mg/day to 1,000 mg/day provided no additional benefit, but they increased the rate of adverse effects (45, 46, 67). It is possible, however, that individual patients may benefit from higher dosages. An initial target dose of 200 mg/day to 400 mg/day is recommended for adults. Pooled analyses of placebo-controlled studies in adults indicate that TPM is effective regardless of race, gender, baseline seizure rate, or concomitant AEDs (68). Subsequent trials examined slower titration rates (64, 66) or lower target dose (65, 66).

Long-term data are available from some of these controlled trials. In one report, 64% of the 214 adults with refractory partial-onset seizures who decided to take TPM after completion of blinded, controlled trials continued on it for another 30 months. Among the approximately one-third of these patients who converted to TPM monotherapy, 28 (13% of the 214) were seizure free for at least the last three months (69).

The efficacy of adjunctive TPM in children, aged 1–16 years with treatment-resistant, partial-onset seizures with or without secondary generalization, was examined in a multicenter, double-blind, randomized, placebo-controlled trial (70). An 8-week baseline was followed by a 16-week double-blind treatment phase (an 8-week titration period followed by an 8-week stabilization period) with a weight-based target dose of 6 mg/kg/day. Forty-one TPM-treated and 45 placebo-treated children ages 2–16 years completed treatment. The median percentage of reduction from the baseline in the average monthly partial-onset rate in the TPM-treated group was 33%, compared to 11% in the placebo group ($P = 0.034$) (70). For the 83 children with partial-onset seizures, with or without secondary generalization, who continued long-term open-label TPM therapy after the double-blind trial phase, the mean TPM dosage was 9 mg/kg/day. Seizure frequency over the last three months of therapy was reduced by 50% or more in 57% of the children; 14% of children were seizure free for six months or more at the last visit (71).

Adjunctive Therapy in Adults and Children with Generalized-Onset Tonic-Clonic Seizures of Nonfocal Origin

A double-blind, placebo-controlled, multicenter study demonstrated TPM's efficacy against treatment-resistant, uncontrolled, GTC seizures of nonfocal origin in 80 children and adults (72). Inclusion and exclusion criteria were that patients were ages 4 years or older, had experienced three or more GTC seizures during an 8-week baseline phase, had electroencephalogram (EEG) findings consistent with generalized epilepsy, and were taking no more than two standard AEDs at study entry. Patients meeting these criteria were randomized to either TPM or placebo adjunctive treatment, titrated to target dosages of 6 mg/kg/day over 8 weeks, and maintained at that dose for 12 weeks.

A total of 80 patients (ages 3–59 years) were randomized; the median baseline average monthly rate of GTC seizures was 5.0 in the TPM group and 4.5 in the placebo group. The mean TPM dosage during the stabilization period was 5.0 mg/kg/day. The median percentage of reduction from baseline in average monthly GTC seizure rate at the end of the 20-week double-blind phase was higher for the TPM group compared with the placebo group (57% vs. 9%, $P = 0.019$). More TPM-treated patients experienced a reduction of 50% or greater in GTC seizures compared to the placebo-treated controls (56% vs. 20%, $P = 0.001$). A similarly designed study was published only in abstract form (73).

In an analysis of long-term follow-up of 131 adults and children from the previously described studies, 63% had a decrease of 50% in seizure frequency during a mean follow-up period of 387 days (range, 14–909 days) and 16% were seizure free for the past six months (74). The cohort's mean TPM dose was 7 mg/kg/day (range, 1–16 mg/kg/day). At the last visit, 82% of the patients ($n = 107$) were still taking TPM (74).

Adjunctive Therapy in Patients with Lennox-Gastaut Syndrome

TPM's efficacy as adjunctive therapy in patients with Lennox-Gastaut syndrome was established in a multicenter, double-blind placebo-controlled trial (75). Study patients had to have active drop attacks (either tonic or atonic seizures), a history of or active atypical absence seizures, and a prior EEG showing a slow spike wave pattern and be taking one or two concomitant AEDs at the time of study entry. Following a 4-week baseline, eligible patients were randomized to either TPM or placebo adjunctive therapy. Study dosages were increased at weekly intervals over 3 weeks to 6 mg/kg/day and then maintained at that dose for 8 weeks.

A total of 98 patients, ages 2–42 years (an average of 11 years) were randomized. The two groups were evenly matched in the median monthly frequency of drop attacks (90 for the TPM group, 98 in the placebo group) and median monthly frequency of all seizure types (267 for the TPM group and 244 in the placebo group). The median average TPM dosage during the stabilization period was 5.8 mg/kg/day (75).

During blinded treatment, patients in the TPM group had a greater median percentage of reduction from baseline in drop attacks (15%) compared to the placebo group (–5%; $P = 0.041$). TPM-treated patients experienced a larger improvement in seizure severity compared with controls (52% vs. 28%; $P = 0.040$) based on parental global evaluations (75).

In the open-label extension phase of this trial, the mean TPM dose for the 97 patients was 11 mg/kg/day, with a mean duration of 539 days (range, 44–1,225 days). At the last clinic visit, drop attacks were reduced by 50% or greater in 55% of patients; 15% of patients had no drop attacks for six months or more (76).

Monotherapy and Adjunctive Therapy in Patients with Infantile Spasms (West Syndrome)

TPM's efficacy against infantile spasms has been reported in at least 10 open-label trials (77–86). In the first reported study, 11 patients with treatment-resistant infantile spasms documented by 24-hour video EEG, utilized an initial dose of 25 mg TPM, followed by a "rapid-dose" titration schedule of 25-mg increments every 2–3 days over a 4-week period until either a maximal tolerated dose was reached, spasms were controlled, or a maximal dose of 24 mg/kg/day was achieved. A total of five patients (45%) became spasm free, with repeat 24-hour video EEG demonstrating absence of infantile spasms and hypsarrhythmia (77). A majority of the patients (64%, 7 of 11) were able to achieve TPM monotherapy; the others were able to reduce their intake of concomitant AEDs (77).

Four of seven infants with West syndrome became seizure free with TPM therapy, as reported in a retrospective study of TPM in patients with intractable epilepsy (78). A third study reported the efficacy of TPM in 13 infants with West syndrome as part of a multicenter study of 224 unselected patients with a variety of epilepsy types. Two (15%) West syndrome infants became seizure free; seven (54%, 7 of 13) had a reduction greater than 50% in their seizures. TPM was used as initial monotherapy in nine patients, with doses as much as 16 mg/kg/day (79). An open-label, multicenter retrospective study of 28 infants treated with TPM included 8 infants with West syndrome; 88% (7 of 8) improved with TPM therapy, and 3 patients received TPM monotherapy (80). One study of 18 patients with spasms (14 infantile, 4 late-onset) found 6 responders, but none were seizure free (82). In contrast, 19 patients with West syndrome were included in an open, prospective, pragmatic study of TPM in 59 infants with epilepsy. Four of the six patients with cryptogenic West syndrome became seizure free (14-month median follow-up). Among the remaining 13 patients with symptomatic West syndrome, 4 patients were responders, but only one (8%) became seizure free (81). Two of nine patients with infantile spasms became seizure free, and another two patients experienced a reduction of greater than 50% in seizure frequency in a prospective open-label trial of TPM in 47 children (ages 6–60 months) with refractory epilepsy (83). Following initiation of TPM therapy in 4 infants with infantile spasms (in a retrospective review of TPM use in 13 children ages less than 2 years), 2 infants became spasm free, 1 infant had a reduction greater than 75% in spasms, and the other infant had no response to TPM (84). Twenty patients with infantile spasms were treated with TPM monotherapy, with an initial dose of 1 mg/kg/day up to a maximal dose of 12 mg/kg/day (85). Six patients (30%) became spasm free and hypsarrhythmia free on video EEG; the patients with idiopathic spasms did better (4 of 8, 50% spasm free) compared to those with only symptomatic spasms (2 of 12, 17% spasm free) (85).

The largest study of TPM in children with infantile spasms was a 2006 prospective open-label study using TPM as initial therapy in 54 patients with newly diagnosed infantile spasms (86). Overall, 57% (31 of 54) of patients were seizure free for more than 24 months. Among these patients, 9 were on TPM monotherapy and 22 patients received TPM with nitrazepam, valproic acid, or both. The average dosage applied was 5.2 mg/kg per day (range 1.6–26 mg/kg/day). The authors concluded that TPM was an "effective and safe first-choice drug not only as adjunctive but also as monotherapy of infantile spasms in children younger than 2 years" (86).

Adjunctive Therapy in Patients with Severe Myoclonic Epilepsy of Infancy (Dravet Syndrome)

Four studies have examined TPM's efficacy for children with severe myoclonic epilepsy in infancy (SMEI) (81, 82, 87, 88). A trial examined TPM's effectiveness in 18 patients with SMEI, with a starting dose of 1 mg/kg/day, which was increased every 1–2 weeks, with a maximum dose of 6–8 mg/kg/day. The study showed that 17% (3 of 18) of the patients became seizure free, and 56% (10 of 18) had a reduction greater than 50% in seizure frequency (mean 10.5 months, with a range of 6–18 months) (87). A prospective multicenter, open-label adjunctive therapy study of 18 patients (ages 2–21 years, mean 9 years), with SMEI initiated TPM at 0.5–1 mg/kg/day, used 2-week increments of 1–3 mg/kg/day and a maximum dose of 12 mg/kg/day. Similar to the previous study, 3 patients (3 of 18, 17%) became seizure free, and 10 patients (10 of 18, 56%) had a reduction greater than 50% in seizures (mean 11.9 months, with a range of 2–24 months). No patient experienced worsening of seizures with TPM therapy (88). In a subset of a study with 207 children with refractory epilepsy, 3 of 5 SMEI patients responded to TPM therapy (82). Six patients with SMEI were included in an open, prospective, pragmatic study of TPM in 59 infants with epilepsy; only 2 of the 6 SMEI patients responded, and none became seizure-free (81).

Adjunctive Therapy in Patients with Juvenile Myoclonic Epilepsy

A posthoc analysis of two multicenter, double-blind, randomized, placebo-controlled, trials of TPM for GTC seizures of nonfocal origin revealed that 22 patients with juvenile myoclonic epilepsy had been randomized to either TPM ($n = 11$, target dose, 400 mg/day in adults) or placebo ($n = 11$). A significantly higher number of patients in the TPM-treated arm experienced a reduction of 50% or greater in GTC seizures compared to the placebo arm (8 of 11, 73% vs. 2 of 11, 18%; $P = 0.03$). Although reductions were noted in the number of myoclonic and absence seizures and total number of generalized seizures in the TPM arm, the difference did not reach statistical significance (89).

A second study examined TPM's efficacy in 22 patients with juvenile myoclonic epilepsy (ages 13–53 years). The target TPM dosage was as much as 200 mg/day. Among the 16 patients who completed one year of follow-up, 10 patients (62.5%) were free of GTC seizures, and myoclonia was controlled in 11 patients (90).

Adjunctive Therapy in Patients with Other Epilepsy Syndromes

There are small studies suggesting that TPM is effective for absence epilepsy (91), Doose syndrome (82), and progressive myoclonic epilepsies (92).

Adjunctive Long-Term Open-Label Treatment

Prospective open-label series may be more predictive of results in clinical practice because long-term extension studies include only patients who have successfully completed randomized trials (a subset that is probably not reflective of the general population). Among 292 adults with refractory seizures treated with adjunctive, open-label TPM, in dosages of 100–1,600 mg/day, and followed for a mean of 2.2 years (84–804 days), mean reductions greater than 50% in both partial- and generalized-onset seizures were observed, and 10% were seizure free for at least six months (93). Discontinuations were more often due to adverse effects (32%) than to lack of efficacy (19%), a pattern typical for TPM treatment (93–96).

A 6-month Canadian multicenter open-label study of 209 adults given TPM as adjunctive therapy reported that patients had a reduction of 41% in median seizure frequency during the final 8 weeks, with 10% becoming seizure free and with improvements in quality of life measurements (97).

A multicenter, retrospective review of open-label TPM adjunctive therapy in 277 children (average age, 8.4 years; range, 1–16 years) with treatment-resistant epilepsy evaluated TPM's long-term efficacy. Overall, after 27.5 months of treatment (range, 24–61 months), 4% (11 of 277) of children were seizure free and 20% (56 of 277) had a reduction of greater than 50% in seizure frequency. TPM's long-term efficacy was greater in patients with partial-onset epilepsy than in those with generalized-onset epilepsy (98).

ADVERSE EFFECTS

TPM's profile for adverse events is similar for adults and children. TPM-related adverse events in 199 children participating in double-blind, placebo-controlled trials (the events occurred with a greater frequency of more than 5% in the TPM treatment group than in the placebo group) were somnolence, anorexia, fatigue, nervousness, concentration or attention difficulties, aggression, difficulty with memory, and weight loss (99). The mean TPM dose was 6.2 mg/kg/day for a mean of 107 days (99).

In general, TPM is associated with a lower incidence of adverse events (i.e., better tolerated) when it is used as monotherapy than in adjunctive therapy. A slower titration is better tolerated than a rapid titration. The slower rate of TPM titration (i.e., increases at 2-week intervals) that is used in some of these pediatric studies resulted in a lower frequency of adverse events compared to the higher frequency observed with a more rapid rate of titration that is used in many of the adult studies and the trial in patients with Lennox-Gastaut syndrome (100). During the double-blind portion of the placebo-controlled studies involving children, the use of TPM did not result in any discontinuations due to an adverse event (100).

One framework to examine these adverse events is to group them by system: the most common adverse events involve the CNS (cognitive effects, somnolence, fatigue, effects on mood, psychosis, and, rarely, hyperammonemic encephalopathy and acute bilateral secondary angle-closure glaucoma), gastrointestinal system (anorexia, weight loss), and systemic (paresthesias, metabolic acidosis, renal stones). Some of the adverse events are definitely dose related (e.g., cognitive problems, paresthesias, anorexia, and decreases in serum bicarbonate), some are proposed to be dose related (e.g., gastrointestinal symptoms, renal stones, and psychiatric effects), and others are seen mostly during dose initiation and are thus unrelated to final dose (e.g., dizziness, somnolence, fatigue, and ataxia) (101, 102). Serious adverse effects are rare.

CNS Adverse Events

In clinical trials, the most commonly reported treatment-emergent adverse events were CNS-related, and most were rated as mild or moderate in severity. In clinical practice, cognitive adverse events are those most likely to limit TPM therapy (95, 96). Cognitive events are less common with a slow titration and when TPM is used as monotherapy (56–58). In the comparative trial of patients with new-onset seizures treated with either monotherapy CBZ 600 mg/day, monotherapy valproate 1250 mg/day, monotherapy TPM 100, or monotherapy TPM 200 mg/day, no cognitive side effect exceeded 8% in any group, although valproate was slightly better tolerated (59). In an adjunctive TPM therapy trial with a slow upward titration of 25–50 mg/week to a target dose of 200 mg, only 5% of patients experienced "concentration or attention difficulty" (66). In contrast, TPM's cognitive effects were clearly seen during the early, high-dose, rapid-titration, adjunctive therapy clinical trials; "thinking abnormal" occurred in 13% to 33% of patients, while 15% to 25% had "concentration impaired" (68, 101).

A common misperception is that cognitive effects are universally present; in fact, many patients are completely unaffected, even at higher dosages, and group differences are strongly influenced by a subset of patients who are severely affected (103). Patients with intellectual disabilities do not appear to be at greater risk than other patients for the cognitive effects of TPM (104, 105). In addition to slowing the titration rate and using TPM as monotherapy, another effective strategy is to reduce concomitant medications if adverse cognitive events appear (106).

The specific types of cognitive adverse events associated with TPM appear qualitatively different from those with other AEDs. Examples of TPM-related cognitive adverse events include impaired expressive language function, impaired verbal memory, a general slowing of cognitive processing (without apparent sedation or mood change), mild dysnomia, hesitation in verbal replies, and declines in word fluency (68, 107–111). Nineteen patients withdrawn from polytherapy TPM experienced improvements in verbal fluency, working memory, and other functions associated with the frontal lobe (112). Patients with dominant-hemisphere seizure foci or pathology may be more likely to experience word-finding difficulty (110).

Other TPM-related CNS adverse events included sleepiness and fatigue. Between 15% and 35% of subjects experienced transient, nontherapy-limiting sleepiness during short-term clinical trials (45, 46, 63, 64, 95). Fatigue was reported in approximately 16% of study patients during TPM monotherapy trials using 25–500 mg/day, but there was no relationship to TPM dose (31). In adult adjunctive TPM clinical trials, fatigue was seen in 13% of patients taking placebo, 15% of patients receiving TPM 200–400 mg/day, and 30% of patients taking TPM 600–1000 mg/day (44). In children, fatigue was seen in 16% of patients taking adjunctive TPM and 5% taking placebo (44).

In the first five controlled trials using adjunctive TPM therapy, depression was reported in 15% of participants; this was similar to that in the placebo group (101). In an open-label series, 11.9% of patients were described as having depression, hyperirritability, or aggressiveness (96). In another report, 5% had depression and 5.7% displayed irritability or aggressive behavior (113). In this latter report, patients with psychiatric histories were more likely to experience these adverse events (113).

The incidence of psychosis in TPM clinical trials was 0.8%, which is not significantly different from the psychosis rate in the placebo group or the reported rates of psychosis in patients with treatment-resistant epilepsy (114). However, another study reported the rate of psychotic symptoms in 94 patients treated with TPM as 12% (115). Psychiatric adverse events (such as depression and psychosis) are related to a high starting dose and rapid titration (116).

Hyperammonemic encephalopathy has been reported in a few patients taking concurrent TPM and VPA. These patients developed stupor, worsening of seizures, and focal neurologic signs and had slowing of their EEG background rhythm. Recovery was rapid after either TPM or VPA was removed. (49, 117–119).

TPM-related acute bilateral secondary angle-closure glaucoma has been seen in all ages, from children to elderly (120, 121). Symptoms usually start a week after (mean, 7 days; range, 1–49 days) from initiation of therapy and include blurred vision, eye pain, headache, nausea, vomiting, pupillary changes, and hyperemia (121). Early recognition and immediate cessation of TPM are key to successful management (121).

Gastrointestinal Adverse Events

Many patients taking TPM lose weight, a result that is probably related to anorexia. The extent and duration of this weight loss is variable. In adults, the average decrease in body weight is 4.6%; this loss usually reaches a plateau by 18 months of therapy (68, 122). Obese adults tend to lose more weight on TPM than nonobese adults (123). Weight loss is not always beneficial and can be therapy limiting. Underweight adults and children who cannot voluntarily increase caloric intake may not tolerate this adverse event. In placebo-controlled TPM trials involving children, weight loss occurred in 9% of the TPM group versus 1% of the placebo group (99).

Systemic Adverse Effects

TPM's most common systemic adverse events include paresthesias, metabolic acidosis, hypohydrosis, and renal stones. These effects are associated with TPM's inhibition of carbonic anhydrase isozymes II and IV (124).

Paresthesias more commonly occur with monotherapy use compared to adjunctive therapy use. It is speculated that this is because of higher serum levels of TPM in the monotherapy trials (56, 58). In contrast to epilepsy studies, in clinical trials for migraine, 35% of subjects had paresthesias at 50 mg/day and 49% at 200 mg/day (44). Tingling or numbness involved hands and feet or sometimes the whole body.

TPM can lower serum bicarbonate levels in a dose-dependent effect. The package insert reports that 32% of adults taking 400 mg/day have serum bicarbonate levels less than 20 mEq/L and that the effect is more prevalent in children (44). Another study reports an average decrease of 5.1 mEq/L (26.8 to 21.7) (125). Most patients are asymptomatic because serum pH can ordinarily compensate. In some circumstances, a patient could experience a clinically significant nonanion-gap hyperchloremic acidosis that would manifest with ketosis, renal or respiratory insufficiency, or status epilepticus (126).

Hypohidrosis and oligohidrosis with TPM therapy can be asymptomatic or appear as heat intolerance (127). One study found that 5% (5 of 102) children taking TPM experienced symptomatic hypohidrosis with hyperthermia (128). The adverse event is reversible with TPM withdrawal (129.) The mechanism is not definite, but it is proposed to relate to carbonic anhydrase inhibition at the level of the sweat gland (129).

An incidence of nephrolithiasis of 1.5% during TPM treatment is similar to that during treatment with another carbonic anhydrase inhibitor, acetazolamide (12, 130). Most cases of nephrolithiasis are resolved by the spontaneous passage of renal stones, and 83% of the 18 patients with stones elected to continue TPM treatment (101). Like acetazolamide, TPM has a sulfamate moiety; however, carbonic anhydrase inhibition by TPM is relatively weak.

One study examined 14 children treated simultaneously with TPM and the ketogenic diet (known to predispose patients to metabolic acidosis) for periods of 33–544 days (131). Nine children experienced a decrease of less than 20% in serum bicarbonate levels, (mean, 7.6 meq/L; range, 5.3–12.3 meq/L). Two children required bicarbonate supplements, but no patient had nephrolithiasis (131).

Teratogenicity

TPM is rated as Pregnancy Category C by the U.S. Food and Drug Administration (FDA) (44). The Category C label means that animal reproduction studies have shown an adverse effect on the fetus, there are no adequate and well-controlled studies in humans, and the benefits from the use of the drug in pregnant women may be acceptable despite its potential risks (132).

CLINICAL USE

FDA Indications

TPM is indicated as initial monotherapy in patients ages 10 years and older, with partial-onset or primary GTC seizures, as adjunctive therapy for adults; for pediatric patients ages 2–16 years with partial-onset seizures or primary GTC seizures; and for patients ages 2 years and older with seizures associated with Lennox-Gastaut syndrome. It is also indicated in adults for the prophylaxis of migraine headache (44).

Formulations

TPM is available in oral preparations, either as a tablet (25 mg, 50 mg, 100 mg, and 200 mg strengths) or as a sprinkle capsule (15 mg and 25 mg) (44). There is no intravenous preparation commercially available.

Dosing

Attention to the initial dose of TPM, subsequent titration rates, and the maintenance target dose are important to maximize tolerability and, subsequently, to maximize effectiveness. TPM should be titrated until there is a clear clinical response consisting of either seizure control without intolerable adverse events or persisting seizures with intolerable side effects. In patients showing some seizure reduction without intolerable adverse events, the dose of TPM can be further increased. If adverse experiences do occur, titration can be slowed; on the other hand, titration can be more rapid if the suppression of seizures is urgently needed. A small subset of patients (1% to 3%) appears unable to tolerate even the lowest doses of TPM.

For children with epilepsy, commonly used initial TPM doses range from 0.5 to 1 mg/kg/day. Subsequent weekly increases in dosage are in increments of 0.5–1 mg/kg/day. As monotherapy, typical TPM target doses are in the range of 3 mg/kg/day, whereas in adjunctive therapy TPM target doses range from 6 to 9 mg/kg/day. With these slow rates of titration, it may take 6 to 8 weeks to begin to see efficacy, and it is important to explain this time frame to the parents of the patient to avoid undue anxiety and frustration.

An open-label, naturalistic TPM monotherapy clinical trial involving 114 children (ages less than 12 years) at 127 centers throughout Europe and the Middle East found 3.3 mg/kg/day (range, 1.3–13.0 mg/kg/day) as the median final dose of TPM (133). However, infants and some children may require significantly higher initial and target doses. Some infants and children benefit from TPM doses up to 50 mg/kg/day—particularly in the presence of a concomitant enzyme-inducing AED such as CBZ.

For adults with epilepsy, commonly used initial TPM doses range from 25 to 50 mg/day. Subsequent increments of 25–50 mg/day are done every 1–2 weeks. For initial monotherapy, TPM target doses as low as 100 mg/day may be effective, whereas, in adjunctive therapy, TPM target doses range from 400–600 mg/day. In an open-label, naturalistic TPM monotherapy clinical trial involving 441 adults at 127 centers throughout Europe and the Middle East, the median final TPM dose was 125 mg/day (range, 25–700 mg/day) (133).

Precautions

Measurement of baseline and periodic bicarbonate levels is recommended (44). Periodic measurements could occur when the initial target dose is reached, after large dose increases, and in circumstances predisposing the patient to metabolic acidosis. Minor decreases in bicarbonate usually do not require any action; in general, clinical judgment should guide whether dose reduction or alkali treatment is needed. No other routine laboratory testing is recommended.

Women taking more than 200 mg/day of TPM along with oral contraceptives should take precautions. The absence of breakthrough bleeding is not a reliable sign of secure birth control, but its occurrence may suggest a need for a higher estrogen dose or a second method.

Contraindications

The only absolute contraindication is hypersensitivity to components of the compound (44).

Plasma Concentrations

Most large clinical laboratories (in hospitals or independent laboratories) offer TPM plasma concentrations. Optimal treatment response is most likely to occur at TPM plasma concentrations ranging from 3.2 to 28.8 µg/mL for children ages 5 and younger (134), 1.5–20.4 µg/mL for older children (ages 6–12 years) on TPM monotherapy (134), and 2–10.5 µg/mL (6–31 µmol/L) for adults with treatment-resistant partial epilepsy (135).

CONCLUSION

TPM is an antiepileptic medication with efficacy in multiple animal models; it possesses multiple mechanisms of action, demonstrates a favorable pharmacokinetic profile in humans, exhibits efficacy against a variety of seizure types in children and adults in both clinical trials and clinical practice, and has a well-defined profile for adverse events.

TPM has efficacy in the MES and the PTZ seizure tests along with multiple other rodent models of epilepsy. Its multiple mechanisms of action include, but are not limited to, state-dependent blockade of Na^+ channels, potentiation of GABA-mediated (inhibitory) neurotransmission, and antagonism of glutamate (excitatory) receptors of the kainate (non-NMDA) subtype. It exhibits a favorable pharmacokinetic profile, including rapid absorption, long duration of action, and minimal interaction with other AEDs. In clinical trials involving adults and children with epilepsy, TPM exhibited efficacy against partial-onset and generalized-onset seizures. It has demonstrated efficacy in patients with epilepsy, ranging from those with newly diagnosed, untreated epilepsy to patients with long-standing, treatment-resistant epilepsy. TPM has demonstrated efficacy as monotherapy and in adjunctive therapy. TPM has a well-characterized adverse event profile with recognizable and reversible adverse events. Overall, TPM has emerged as a valuable AED for children and adults with epilepsy.

References

1. Shank RP, Gardocki JF, Vaught JL, Davis CB, et al. Topiramate: preclinical evaluation of structurally novel anticonvulsant. *Epilepsia* 1994; 35(2):450–460.
2. Maryanoff BE, Nortey SO, Gardocki JF, Shank RP, et al. Anticonvulsant O-alkyl sulfamates. 2,3:4,5-Bis-O-(1- methylethylidene)-beta-D-fructopyranose sulfamate and related compounds. *J Med Chem* 1987; 30(5):880–887.
3. Kramer LD, Reife R. Topiramate. In: Engel JPT, ed. *Epilepsy: A Comprehensive Textbook*. Philadelphia: Lippincott-Raven, 1997:1593–1598.
4. Reife R. Topiramate, a novel antiepileptic agent. In: Shorvon S, Dreifuss, F, Fish, D, Thomas, D, eds. *Treatment of Epilepsy*. Oxford, UK: Blackwell Science, 1996.
5. White HS. Clinical significance of animal seizure models and mechanism of action studies of potential antiepileptic drugs. *Epilepsia* 1997; 38(Suppl 1):S9–S17.
6. Rogawski M, Porter R. Antiepileptic drugs: pharmacological mechanisms and clinical efficacy with consideration of promising developmental state compounds. *Pharmacol Rev* 1990; 42:223–286.
7. White HS, Brown SD, Woodhead JH, Skeen GA, et al. Topiramate enhances GABA-mediated chloride flux and GABA-evoked chloride currents in murine brain neurons and increases seizure threshold. *Epilepsy Res* 1997; 28:167–179.
8. Wauquier A, Zhou S. Topiramate: a potent anticonvulsant in the amygdala-kindled rat. *Epilepsy Res* 1996; 24(2):73–77.
9. Nakamura J, Tamura S, Kanda T, Ishii A, et al. Inhibition by topiramate of seizures in spontaneously epileptic rats and DBA/2 mice. *Eur J Pharmacol* 1994; 254(1–2): 83–89.
10. Edmonds H, Jiang D, Zhang YP, Vaught JL. Topiramate in rat model of post traumatic epilepsy. *Epilepsia* 1991; 32(Suppl 3):15.
11. Kimishima K, Wang Y, Tanabe K. Anticonvulsant activities and properties of topiramate. *Japan J Pharmacol* 1992; 58(Suppl 1):211.
12. Glauser TA. Topiramate. *Semin Pediatr Neurol* 1997; 4(1):34–42.
13. Hersey SJ, High WL. On the mechanism of acid secretory inhibition by acetazolamide. *Biochim Biophys Acta* 1971; 233:604–609.
14. Cho CH, Chen SM, Chen SW. Pathogenesis of gastric ulceration produced by acetazolamide in rats. *Digestion* 1984; 29:5–11.
15. Ryberg B, Bishop AE, Bloom SR. Omeprazole and ranitidine, antisecretagogues with different modes of action, are equally effective in causing hyperplasia of enterochromaffin-like cells in rat stomach. *Regul Peptides* 1989; 2:235–2246.
16. Molon-Noblot S, Boussiquet-Leroux C, Owen RA. Rat urinary bladder hyperplasia induced by oral administration of carbonic anhydrase inhibitors. *Toxicol Pathol* 1992; 20:93.
17. Hirsch KS, Scott WJ, Hurley LS. The presence of carbonic anhydrase during the sensitive stage of rat development. *Teratology* 1973; 17:38A.

18. Scott WJ, Hirsch KS, DeSesso JM, Wilson JG. Comparative studies on acetazolamide teratogenesis in pregnant rats, rabbits, and rhesus monkeys. *Teratology* 1981; 24:37–42.
19. Nakatsuka T, Komatsu T, Fujii T. Axial skeletal malformations induced by acetazolamide in rabbits. *Teratology* 1992; 45:629–636.
20. Coulter DA, Sombati S, DeLorenzo RJ. Selective effects of topiramate on sustained repetitive firing and spontaneous bursting in cultured hippocampal neurons. *Epilepsia* 1993; 34(Suppl 2):123.
21. Severt L, Coulter DA, Sombati S, DeLorenzo RJ. Topiramate selectively blocks kainate currents in cultured hippocampal neurons. *Epilepsia* 1995; 36(Suppl 4):38.
22. Gryder DS, Rogawski MA. Selective antagonism of GluR5 kainate-receptor-mediated synaptic currents by topiramate in rat basolateral amygdala neurons. *J Neurosci* 2003; 23(18):7069–7074.
23. Kaminski RM, Banerjee M, Rogawski MA. Topiramate selectively protects against seizures induced by ATPA, a GluR5 kainate receptor agonist. *Neuropharmacology* 2004; 46(8):1097–1104.
24. Brown SD, Wolf HH, Swinyard EA, Twyman RE, et al. The novel anticonvulsant topiramate enhances GABA-mediated chloride flux. *Epilepsia* 1993; 34(Suppl 2):122–123.
25. White HS, Brown SD, Skeen GA, Twyman RA. The investigational anticonvulsant topiramate potentiates GABA-evoked currents in mouse cortical neurons. *Epilepsia* 1995; 36(Suppl 4):34.
26. Kuzniecky R, Hetherington H, Ho S, Pan J, et al. Topiramate increases cerebral GABA in healthy humans. *Neurology* 1998; 51(2):627–629.
27. Petroff OA, Hyder F, Mattson RH, Rothman DL. Topiramate increases brain GABA, homocarnosine, and pyrrolidinone in patients with epilepsy [see comments]. *Neurology* 1999; 52(3):473–478.
28. Herrero AI, Del Olmo N, Gonzalez-Escalada JR, Solis JM. Two new actions of topiramate: inhibition of depolarizing GABA(A)-mediated responses and activation of a potassium conductance. *Neuropharmacology* 2002; 42(2):210–220.
29. Zhang X, Velumian AA, Jones OT, Carlen PL. Modulation of high-voltage-activated calcium channels in dentate granule cells by topiramate. *Epilepsia* 2000; 41:(Suppl 1): S52–S60.
30. Doose DR, Walker SA, Gisclon LG, Nayak RK. Single-dose pharmacokinetics and effect of food on the bioavailability of topiramate, a novel antiepileptic drug. *J Clin Pharmacol* 1996; 36(10):884–891.
31. Waugh J, Goa KL. Topiramate: as monotherapy in newly diagnosed epilepsy. *CNS Drugs* 2003; 17(13):985–992.
32. Nayak RK, Gisclon LG, Curtin CA, Benez LZ. Estimation of the absolute bioavailability of topiramate in humans without intravenous data. *J Clin Pharmacol* 1994; 34:1029.
33. Easterling DE, Zakszewski T, Moyer MD, Margul BL, et al. Plasma pharmacokinetics of topiramate, a new anticonvulsant in humans. *Epilepsia* 1988; 29:662.
34. Johannessen SI. Pharmacokinetics and interaction profile of topiramate: review and comparison with other newer antiepileptic drugs. *Epilepsia* 1997; 38(Suppl 1):S18–S23.
35. Perucca E. Pharmacokinetic profile of topiramate in comparison with other new antiepileptic drugs. *Epilepsia* 1996; 37(Suppl 2):S8–S13.
36. Wu WN, Heebner JB, Streeter AJ. Evaluation of the absorption, excretion, pharmacokinetics and metabolism of the anticonvulsant topiramate in healthy men. *Pharmaceut Res* 1994; 11 (Suppl 10):S336.
37. Sachdeo RC, Sachdeo SK, Levy RH, Streeter AJ, et al. Topiramate and phenytoin pharmacokinetics during repetitive monotherapy and combination therapy to epileptic patients. *Epilepsia* 2002; 43(7):691–696.
38. Gisclon LG, Riffitts JM, Sica DA, Gehr T, et al. The pharmacokinetics (PK) of topiramate (T) in subjects with renal impairment (RI) as compared to matched subjects with normal renal function (NRF). *Pharm Res* 1993; 10 (Suppl 10):S397.
39. Gisclon LG, Curtin CR. The pharmacokinetics (PK) of topiramate (T) in subjects with end stage renal disease undergoing hemodialysis. *Clin Pharmacol Ther* 1994; 55 (2):196.
40. Rosenfeld WE, Doose DR, Walker SA, Baldassarre JS, et al. A study of topiramate pharmacokinetics and tolerability in children with epilepsy. *Pediatr Neurol* 1999; 20(5):339–344.
41. Glauser TA, Miles MV, Tang P, Clark P, et al. Topiramate pharmacokinetics in infants. *Epilepsia* 1999; 40(6):788–791.
42. Mikaeloff Y, Rey E, Soufflet C, d'Athis P, et al. Topiramate pharmacokinetics in children with epilepsy aged from 6 months to 4 years. *Epilepsia* 2004; 45(11):1448–1452.
43. Bialer M, Doose DR, Murthy B, Curtin C, et al. Pharmacokinetic interactions of topiramate. *Clin Pharmacokinet* 2004; 43(12):763–780.
44. Ortho-McNeil Neurologics. TOPAMAX prescribing information. 2006. June 20, 2006 cited; Available from: http://www.topamax-epilepsy.com/utilities/images/tpamax.pdf#zoom=100
45. Faught E, Wilder BJ, Ramsay RE, Reife RA, et al. Topiramate placebo-controlled dose-ranging trial in refractory partial epilepsy using 200-, 400-, and 600-mg daily dosages. Topiramate YD Study Group. *Neurology* 1996; 46(6):1684–1690.
46. Privitera M, Fincham R, Penry J, Reife R, et al. Topiramate placebo-controlled dose-ranging trial in refractory partial epilepsy using 600-, 800-, and 1,000-mg daily dosages. Topiramate YE Study Group. *Neurology* 1996; 46(6):1678–1683.
47. Sachdeo RC, Sachdeo SK, Walker SA, Kramer LD, et al. Steady-state pharmacokinetics of topiramate and carbamazepine in patients with epilepsy during monotherapy and concomitant therapy. *Epilepsia* 1996; 37(8):774–780.
48. Doose DR, Brodie MJ, Wilson EA, Chadwick D, et al. Topiramate and lamotrigine pharmacokinetics during repetitive monotherapy and combination therapy in epilepsy patients. *Epilepsia* 2003; 44(7):917–922.
49. Hamer HM, Knake S, Schomburg U, Rosenow F. Valproate-induced hyperammonemic encephalopathy in the presence of topiramate. *Neurology* 2000; 54(1):230–232.
50. Doose DR, Walker SA, Pledger G, Lim P, et al. Evaluation of phenobarbitol and primidone/phenobarbitol (primidone's active metabolite) plasma concentrations during administration of add-on topiramate therapy in five multicenter, double-blind, placebo-controlled trials in outpatients with partial seizures. *Epilepsia* 1995; 36(Suppl 3): S158.
51. Gisclon LG, Curtin CR, Kramer LD. The steady-state (SS) pharmacokinetics (PK) of phenytoin (Dilantin) and topiramate in comparison with other new antiepileptic drugs. *Epilepsia* 1994; 35(Suppl 8):54.
52. Rosenfeld WE, Liao S, Kramer LD, Anderson G, et al. Comparison of the steady-state pharmacokinetics of topiramate and valproate in patients with epilepsy during monotherapy and concomitant therapy. *Epilepsia* 1997; 38(3):324–333.
53. Rosenfeld WE, Doose DR, Walker SA, Nayak RK. Effect of topiramate on the pharmacokinetics of an oral contraceptive containing norethindrone and ethinyl estradiol in patients with epilepsy. *Epilepsia* 1997; 38(3):317–323.
54. Doose DR, Wang SS, Padmanabhan M, Schwabe S, et al. Effect of topiramate or carbamazepine on the pharmacokinetics of an oral contraceptive containing norethindrone and ethinyl estradiol in healthy obese and nonobese female subjects. *Epilepsia* 2003; 44(4):540–549.
55. Liao S, Palmer M. Digoxin and topiramate drug interaction study in male volunteers. *Pharm Res* 1993; 10(Suppl 10):S405.
56. Sachdeo RC, Reife RA, Lim P, Pledger G. Topiramate monotherapy for partial onset seizures. *Epilepsia* 1997; 38(3):294–300.
57. Arroyo S, Dodson WE, Privitera MD, Glauser TA, et al. Randomized dose-controlled study of topiramate as first-line therapy in epilepsy. *Acta Neurol Scand* 2005; 112(4):214–222.
58. Gilliam FG, Veloso F, Bomhof MA, Gazda SK, et al. A dose-comparison trial of topiramate as monotherapy in recently diagnosed partial epilepsy. *Neurology* 2003; Jan 28; 60(2):196–202.
59. Privitera MD, Brodie MJ, Mattson RH, Chadwick DW, et al. Topiramate, carbamazepine and valproate monotherapy: double-blind comparison in newly diagnosed epilepsy. *Acta Neurol Scand* 2003; 107(3):165–175.
60. Glauser TA, Dlugos DJ, Dodson WE, Grinspan A, et al. Topiramate monotherapy in newly diagnosed epilepsy in children and adolescent. *J Child Neurol* 2007 Jun; 22(6): 693–699.
61. Wheless JW, Neto W, Wang S. Topiramate, carbamazepine, and valproate monotherapy: double-blind comparison in children with newly diagnosed epilepsy. *J Child Neurol* 2004; 19(2):135–141.
62. Sharief M, Viteri C, Ben-Menachem E, Weber M, et al. Double-blind, placebo-controlled study of topiramate in patients with refractory partial epilepsy. *Epilepsy Res* 1996; 25(3):217–224.
63. Tassinari CA, Michelucci R, Chauvel P, Chodkiewicz J, et al. Double-blind, placebo-controlled trial of topiramate (600 mg daily) for the treatment of refractory partial epilepsy. *Epilepsia* 1996; 37(8):763–768.
64. Korean Topiramate Study Group. Topiramate in medically intractable partial epilepsies: double-blind placebo-controlled randomized parallel group trial. Korean Topiramate Study Group. *Epilepsia* 1999; 40(12):1767–1774.
65. Yen DJ, Yu HY, Guo YC, Chen C, et al. A double-blind, placebo-controlled study of topiramate in adult patients with refractory partial epilepsy. *Epilepsia* 2000; 41(9): 1162–1166.
66. Guberman A, Neto W, Gassmann-Mayer C. Low-dose topiramate in adults with treatment-resistant partial-onset seizures. *Acta Neurol Scand* 2002; 106(4):183–189.
67. Ben-Menachem E, Henriksen O, Dam M, Mikkelsen M, et al. Double-blind, placebo-controlled trial of topiramate as add-on therapy in patients with refractory partial seizures. *Epilepsia* 1996; 37(6):539–543.
68. Reife R, Pledger G, Wu SC. Topiramate as add-on therapy: pooled analysis of randomized controlled trials in adults. *Epilepsia* 2000; 41(Suppl 1):S66–S71.
69. Rosenfeld WE, Sachdeo RC, Faught RE, Privitera M. Long-term experience with topiramate as adjunctive therapy and as monotherapy in patients with partial onset seizures: retrospective survey of open-label treatment. *Epilepsia* 1997; 38 (Suppl 1):S34–S6.
70. Elterman RD, Glauser TA, Wyllie E, Reife R, et al. A double-blind, randomized trial of topiramate as adjunctive therapy for partial-onset seizures in children. *Neurology* 1999; 52(7):1338–1344.
71. Ritter F, Glauser TA, Elterman RD, Wyllie E. Effectiveness, tolerability, and safety of topiramate in children with partial-onset seizures. *Epilepsia* 2000; 41(Suppl 1):S82–S85.
72. Biton V, Montouris GD, Ritter F, Riviello JJ, et al. A randomized, placebo-controlled study of topiramate in primary generalized tonic-clonic seizures. Topiramate YTC Study Group. *Neurology* 1999; 52(7):1330–1337.
73. Ben-Menachem E, Group TTY-ES. A double-blind trial of topiramate in patients with generalised tonic-clonic seizures of non-focal origin. *Epilepsia* 1997; 38 (Suppl 3):60.
74. Montouris GD, Biton V, Rosenfeld WE. Nonfocal generalized tonic-clonic seizures: response during long-term topiramate treatment. Topiramate YTC/YTCE Study Group. *Epilepsia* 2000; 41(Suppl 1):S77–S81.
75. Sachdeo RC, Glauser TA, Ritter F, Reife R, et al. A double-blind, randomized trial of topiramate in Lennox-Gastaut syndrome. *Neurology* 1999; 52(9):1882–1887.
76. Glauser TA, Levisohn PM, Ritter F, Sachdeo RC. Topiramate in Lennox-Gastaut syndrome: open-label treatment of patients completing a randomized controlled trial. Topiramate YL Study Group. *Epilepsia* 2000; 41(Suppl 1):S86–S90.
77. Glauser TA, Clark PO, Strawsburg R. A pilot study of topiramate in the treatment of infantile spasms. *Epilepsia* 1998; 39(12):1324–1328.
78. Thijs J, Verhelst H, Van Coster R. Retrospective study of topiramate in a paediatric population with intractable epilepsy showing promising effects in the West syndrome patients. *Acta Neurol Belg* 2001; 101(3):171–176.

79. Herranz JL. Topiramate: a broad spectrum antiepileptic administered to 224 patients with refractory epilepsies. *Rev Neurol* 2000; 31(9):822–828.
80. Watemberg N, Goldberg-Stern H, Ben-Zeev B, Berger I, et al. Clinical experience with open-label topiramate use in infants younger than 2 years of age. *J Child Neurol* 2003; 18(4):258–262.
81. Grosso S, Galimberti D, Farnetani MA, Cioni M, et al. Efficacy and safety of topiramate in infants according to epilepsy syndromes. *Seizure* 2005; 14(3):183–189.
82. Mikaeloff Y, de Saint-Martin A, Mancini J, Peudenier S, et al. Topiramate: efficacy and tolerability in children according to epilepsy syndromes. *Epilepsy Res* 2003; 53(3): 225–232.
83. Al Ajlouni S, Shorman A, Daoud AS. The efficacy and side effects of topiramate on refractory epilepsy in infants and young children: a multi-center clinical trial. *Seizure* 2005; 14(7):459–463.
84. Valencia I, Fons C, Kothare SV, Khurana DS, et al. Efficacy and tolerability of topiramate in children younger than 2 years old. *J Child Neurol* 2005; 20(8):667–669.
85. Kwon YS, Jun YH, Hong YJ, Son BK. Topiramate monotherapy in infantile spasm. *Yonsei Med J* 2006; 47(4):498–504.
86. Zou LP, Ding CH, Fang F, Sin NC, et al. Prospective study of first-choice topiramate therapy in newly diagnosed infantile spasms. *Clin Neuropharmacol* 2006; 29(6): 343–349.
87. Nieto-Barrera M, Candau R, Nieto-Jimenez M, Correa A, et al. Topiramate in the treatment of severe myoclonic epilepsy in infancy. *Seizure* 2000; 9(8):590–594.
88. Coppola G, Capovilla G, Montagnini A, Romeo A, et al. Topiramate as add-on drug in severe myoclonic epilepsy in infancy: an Italian multicenter open trial. *Epilepsy Res* 2002; 49(1):45–48.
89. Biton V, Bourgeois BF. Topiramate in patients with juvenile myoclonic epilepsy. *Arch Neurol* 2005; 62(11):1705–1708.
90. Sousa Pda S, Araujo Filho GM, Garzon E, Sakamoto AC, et al. Topiramate for the treatment of juvenile myoclonic epilepsy. *Arq Neuropsiquiatr* 2005; 63(3B): 733–737.
91. Cross JH. Topiramate monotherapy for childhood absence seizures: an open-label pilot study. *Seizure* 2002; 11(6):406–410.
92. Aykutlu E, Baykan B, Gurses C, Bebek N, et al. Add-on therapy with topiramate in progressive myoclonic epilepsy. *Epilepsy Behav* 2005; 6(2):260–263.
93. Abou-Khalil B, Group TYS. Topiramate in the long-term management of refractory epilepsy. *Epilepsia* 2000; 41(Suppl 1):S72–S76.
94. Lhatoo SD, Wong IC, Polizzi G, Sander JW. Long-term retention rates of lamotrigine, gabapentin, and topiramate in chronic epilepsy. *Epilepsia* 2000; 41(12):1592–1596.
95. Tatum WO, 4th, French JA, Faught E, Morris GL, 3rd, et al. Postmarketing experience with topiramate and cognition. *Epilepsia* 2001; 42(9):1134–1140.
96. Bootsma HP, Coolen F, Aldenkamp AP, Arends J, et al. Topiramate in clinical practice: long-term experience in patients with refractory epilepsy referred to a tertiary epilepsy center. *Epilepsy Behav* 2004; 5(3):380–387.
97. Baker GA, Currie NG, Light MJ, Schneiderman JH. The effects of adjunctive topiramate therapy on seizure severity and health-related quality of life in patients with refractory epilepsy—a Canadian study. *Seizure* 2002; 11(1):6–15.
98. Grosso S, Franzoni E, Iannetti P, Incorpora G, et al. Efficacy and safety of topiramate in refractory epilepsy of childhood: long-term follow-up study. *J Child Neurol* 2005; 20(11):893–897.
99. Ormrod D, McClellan K. Topiramate: a review of its use in childhood epilepsy. *Paediatr Drugs* 2001; 3(4):293–319.
100. Glauser TA. Topiramate. *Epilepsia* 1999; 40(Suppl 5):S71–S80.
101. Shorvon SD. Safety of topiramate: adverse events and relationships to dosing. *Epilepsia* 1996; 37(Suppl 2):S18–S22.
102. Majkowski J, Neto W, Wapenaar R, Van Oene J. Time course of adverse events in patients with localization-related epilepsy receiving topiramate added to carbamazepine. *Epilepsia* 2005; 46(5):648–653.
103. Meador KJ, Loring DW, Hulihan JF, Kamin M, et al. Differential cognitive and behavioral effects of topiramate and valproate. *Neurology* 2003; 60(9):1483–1488.
104. Singh BK, White-Scott S. Role of topiramate in adults with intractable epilepsy, mental retardation, and developmental disabilities. *Seizure* 2002; 11(1):47–50.
105. Kerr MP, Baker GA, Brodie MJ. A randomized, double-blind, placebo-controlled trial of topiramate in adults with epilepsy and intellectual disability: impact on seizures, severity, and quality of life. *Epilepsy Behav* 2005; 7(3):472–480.
106. Naritoku DK, Hulihan JF, Schwarzman LK, Kamin M, et al. Effect of cotherapy reduction on tolerability of epilepsy add-on therapy: a randomized controlled trial. *Ann Pharmacother* 2005; 39(3):418–423.
107. Martin R, Kuzniecky R, Ho S, Hetherington H, et al. Cognitive effects of topiramate, gabapentin, and lamotrigine in healthy young adults. *Neurology* 1999; 52(2):321–327.
108. Thompson PJ, Baxendale SA, Duncan JS, Sander JW. Effects of topiramate on cognitive function. *J Neurol Neurosurg Psychiatry* 2000; 69(5):636–641.
109. Meador KJ. Effects of topiramate on cognition. *J Neurol Neurosurg Psychiatry* 2001; 71(1):134–135.
110. Mula M, Trimble MR, Thompson P, Sander JW. Topiramate and word-finding difficulties in patients with epilepsy. *Neurology* 2003; 60(7):1104–1107.
111. Meador KJ, Loring DW, Vahle VJ, Ray PG, et al. Cognitive and behavioral effects of lamotrigine and topiramate in healthy volunteers. *Neurology* 2005; 64(12):2108–2114.
112. Kockelmann E, Elger CE, Helmstaedter C. Significant improvement in frontal lobe associated neuropsychological functions after withdrawal of topiramate in epilepsy patients. *Epilepsy Res* 2003; 54(2–3):171–178.
113. Kanner AM, Wuu J, Faught E, Tatum WO, 4th, et al. A past psychiatric history may be a risk factor for topiramate-related psychiatric and cognitive adverse events. *Epilepsy Behav* 2003; 4(5):548–552.
114. Khan A, Faught E, Gilliam F, Kuzniecky R. Acute psychotic symptoms induced by topiramate. *Seizure* 1999; 8(4):235–237.
115. Crawford P. An audit of topiramate use in a general neurology clinic. *Seizure* 1998; 7(3):207–211.
116. Mula M, Trimble MR, Lhatoo SD, Sander JW. Topiramate and psychiatric adverse events in patients with epilepsy. *Epilepsia* 2003; 44(5):659–663.
117. Latour P, Biraben A, Polard E, Bentue-Ferrer D, et al. Drug-induced encephalopathy in six epileptic patients: topiramate? valproate? or both? *Hum Psychopharmacol* 2004; 19(3):193–203.
118. Cheung E, Wong V, Fung CW. Topiramate-valproate-induced hyperammonemic encephalopathy syndrome: case report. *J Child Neurol* 2005; 20(2):157–160.
119. Longin E, Teich M, Koelfen W, Konig S. Topiramate enhances the risk of valproate-associated side effects in three children. *Epilepsia* 2002; 43(4):451–454.
120. Fraunfelder FW, Fraunfelder FT, Keates EU. Topiramate-associated acute, bilateral, secondary angle-closure glaucoma. *Ophthalmology* 2004; 111(1):109–111.
121. Alore PL, Jay WM, Macken MP. Topiramate, pseudotumor cerebri, weight-loss and glaucoma: an ophthalmologic perspective. *Semin Ophthalmol* 2006; 21(1):15–17.
122. Rosenfeld W, Slater J. Characterization of topiramate-associated weight changes in adults with epilepsy. *Epilepsia* 2002; 43 (Suppl 7):220–221.
123. Ben-Menachem E, Axelsen M, Johanson EH, Stagge A, et al. Predictors of weight loss in adults with topiramate-treated epilepsy. *Obes Res* 2003; 11(4):556–662.
124. Dodgson SJ, Shank RP, Maryanoff BE. Topiramate as an inhibitor of carbonic anhydrase isoenzymes. *Epilepsia* 2000; 41(Suppl 1):S35–S39.
125. Garris SS, Oles KS. Impact of topiramate on serum bicarbonate concentrations in adults. *Ann Pharmacother* 2005; 39(3):424–426.
126. Groeper K, McCann ME. Topiramate and metabolic acidosis: a case series and review of the literature. *Paediatr Anaesth* 2005; 15(2):167–170.
127. Ben-Zeev B, Watemberg N, Augarten A, Brand N, et al. Oligohydrosis and hyperthermia: pilot study of a novel topiramate adverse effect. *J Child Neurol* 2003; 18(4):254–257.
128. Yilmaz K, Tatli B, Yaramis A, Aydinli N, et al. Symptomatic and asymptomatic hypohidrosis in children under topiramate treatment. *Turk J Pediatr* 2005; 47(4):359–363.
129. de Carolis P, Magnifico F, Pierangeli G, Rinaldi R, et al. Transient hypohidrosis induced by topiramate. *Epilepsia* 2003; 44(7):974–976.
130. Wasserstein AG, Rak I, Reife RA. Nephrolithiasis: during treatment with topiramate. *Epilepsia* 1995; 36(Suppl 3):S153.
131. Takeoka M, Riviello JJ, Jr., Pfeifer H, Thiele EA. Concomitant treatment with topiramate and ketogenic diet in pediatric epilepsy. *Epilepsia* 2002; 43(9):1072–1075.
132. U.S. Food and Drug Administration. Pregnancy "Category C" Labeling. Washington, D.C.; 2006.
133. Guerrini R, Carpay J, Groselj J, van Oene J, et al. Topiramate monotherapy as broad-spectrum antiepileptic drug in a naturalistic clinical setting. *Seizure* 2005; 14(6): 371–380.
134. Schwabe MJ, Wheless JW. Clinical experience with topiramate dosing and serum levels in children 12 years or under with epilepsy. *J Child Neurol* 2001; 16(11):806–808.
135. Christensen J, Andreasen F, Poulsen JH, Dam M. Randomized, concentration-controlled trial of topiramate in refractory focal epilepsy. *Neurology* 2003; 61(9):1210–1218.

53 Valproate

Blaise F. D. Bourgeois

Valproic acid, or valproate (VPA), has been used in the treatment of epilepsy for more than 40 years (1). During this time, it undoubtedly has established itself as one of the major antiepileptic drugs (AEDs), mainly because it was the first (and until the 1990s the only) drug with a broad spectrum of activity against different seizure types, and because of its relatively low sedative effect. In addition to being the first drug to be highly effective against several primarily generalized seizure types, such as absences, myoclonic seizures, and generalized tonic-clonic seizures, VPA also was found to have some effectiveness in the treatment of partial seizures, Lennox-Gastaut syndrome, infantile spasms, neonatal seizures, and febrile seizures. Thus, VPA became particularly popular among pediatric neurologists. In addition to its place in the treatment of epilepsy, VPA has gained acceptance in the treatment of affective disorders in psychiatry and in the prophylaxis of migraine headaches. Effectiveness in the treatment of Sydenham's chorea has also been suggested (2), indications that will not be included in this chapter.

CHEMISTRY, ANIMAL PHARMACOLOGY, AND MECHANISM OF ACTION

Valproic acid (Figure 53-1) is a colorless liquid of molecular weight (MW) 144.21 with low solubility in water. Sodium valproate (MW 166.19) is a highly water-soluble and highly hygroscopic, white, crystalline material. Sodium hydrogen divalproate (divalproex sodium) is a mixture of equal parts of valproic acid and sodium valproate. Being a short-chain branched fatty acid, VPA differs chemically from all other known AEDs. The anticonvulsant effect of VPA was discovered serendipitously when it was used as a solvent for compounds being tested in an animal model of seizures (3). The antiepileptic activity of VPA has been well demonstrated in several animal models (4–6). The effects of VPA include protection against maximal electroshock (MES)-induced seizures; seizures induced chemically by pentylenetetrazol (PTZ), bicuculline, glutamic acid, kainic acid, strychnine, ouabain, nicotine, and intramuscular penicillin; and seizures induced by kindling (7). This broad spectrum of efficacy of VPA in animal models suggests that it is effective in

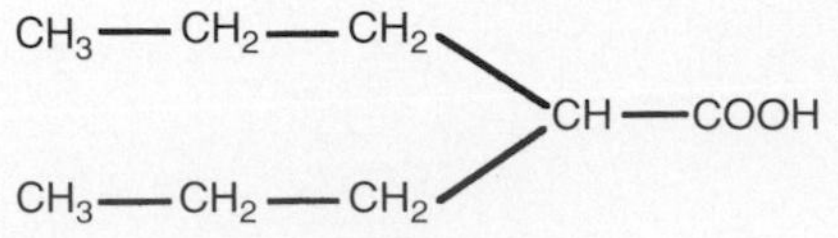

$$CH_3-CH_2-CH_2 \searrow CH-COOH \swarrow CH_3-CH_2-CH_2$$

FIGURE 53-1

Structural formula of valproic acid (N-dipropylacetic acid).

both preventing the spread and lowering the threshold of seizures, and this is consistent with the broad spectrum of antiepileptic activity of VPA in humans.

Extensive studies have been carried out to elucidate the mechanism of action of VPA. Several effects of VPA have been demonstrated at the cellular level, but the precise mechanism underlying the antiepileptic effect of VPA has not been identified, more than one mechanism may be involved, and none of the identified actions has been widely accepted as the predominant relevant mechanism (8). VPA raises brain levels of the inhibitory neurotransmitter gamma-aminobutyric acid (GABA) (5, 9). This increase may be due to the inhibition of GABA-transaminase, the first step in GABA deactivation (10); inhibition of succinic semialdehyde dehydrogenase, the second step in GABA deactivation (11); or an increase in activity of glutamic acid decarboxylase, an enzyme involved in the synthesis of GABA (9). However, because it occurs at much higher than usual therapeutic doses and because its time course lags behind the anticonvulsant effect (12), elevation of GABA is unlikely to be the predominant mechanism of the antiepileptic effect of VPA. In addition to its effect on GABA levels, VPA reduces sustained repetitive high-frequency firing by blocking voltage-sensitive sodium channels (13) or by activating calcium-dependent potassium conductance (14). It was also demonstrated in mice that VPA can decrease brain levels of the excitatory amino acid aspartate (15), as well as decreased expression of the glutamate transporter-1 in rat hippocampus (16). It is not known to what extent these actions contribute to the clinical effect of VPA.

BIOTRANSFORMATION, PHARMACOKINETICS, AND INTERACTIONS

Biotransformation

The main pathways of VPA biotransformation in humans include glucuronidation of VPA itself, beta-oxidation, hydroxylation, ketone formation, and desaturation (Figure 53-2). Both beta-oxidation and desaturation can result in the formation of double bonds. By far the most abundant metabolites are VPA glucuronide and 3-oxo-VPA, which represent about 40% and 33%, respectively, of the urinary excretion of a VPA dose (17). Two desaturated metabolites of VPA, 2-ene-VPA and 4-ene-VPA, have anticonvulsant activity that is similar in potency to that of VPA itself (18). Because there is delayed but significant accumulation of 2-ene-VPA in the brain and it is cleared more slowly than VPA itself (19), the formation of 2-ene-VPA may provide a possible explanation for the discrepancy between the time courses of VPA concentrations and the antiepileptic activity of VPA (20). It appears that 2-ene-VPA does not possess the pronounced embryotoxicity (21) and hepatotoxicity (22) of 4-ene-VPA, and it may thus represent a better AED than VPA itself. The strongly hepatotoxic 4-ene-VPA is produced under the action of cytochrome P450 enzymes. These enzymes are induced by other AEDs such as phenobarbital, phenytoin, and carbamazepine (17, 23), and this may explain the increased risk of hepatotoxicity in patients receiving these drugs together with VPA (24). However, elevation of 4-ene-VPA levels has not yet been documented in patients with VPA hepatotoxicity or in conjunction with short-term adverse effects or hyperammonemia (25).

Pharmacokinetics

The main pharmacokinetic parameters of VPA are summarized in Table 53-1.

The bioavailability of oral preparations of VPA is virtually complete when compared with the intravenous route (26). The purpose of the enteric coating of tablets is to prevent the gastric irritation associated with release of valproic acid in the stomach. When VPA syrup was administered rectally, it was found to have the same bioavailability as the oral preparation (27, 28). Compared with oral syrup, the bioavailability of VPA suppositories was found to be 80% in volunteers (29). The time to peak level was longer for the suppositories than for the syrup (3.1 hours vs. 1.0 hour). In a study in patients treated chronically with VPA, administration of VPA suppositories was well tolerated for several days, and the bioavailability was the same as for the oral preparations (30). The available evidence suggests that there is no need for a dosage change or a change in regimen when oral VPA administration is transiently replaced by rectal administration. The bioavailability of the divalproex extended-release preparation is 8% to 20% lower than that of other divalproex preparations (31, 32).

The rate of absorption of VPA after oral administration is quite variable depending on the formulation. Administration of syrup and uncoated regular tablets or capsules is followed by rapid absorption, and peak levels are achieved within 2 hours. Absorption from enteric-coated tablets is delayed, but once absorption begins, it is rapid. The onset of absorption varies as a function of the state of gastric emptying at the time of ingestion, and

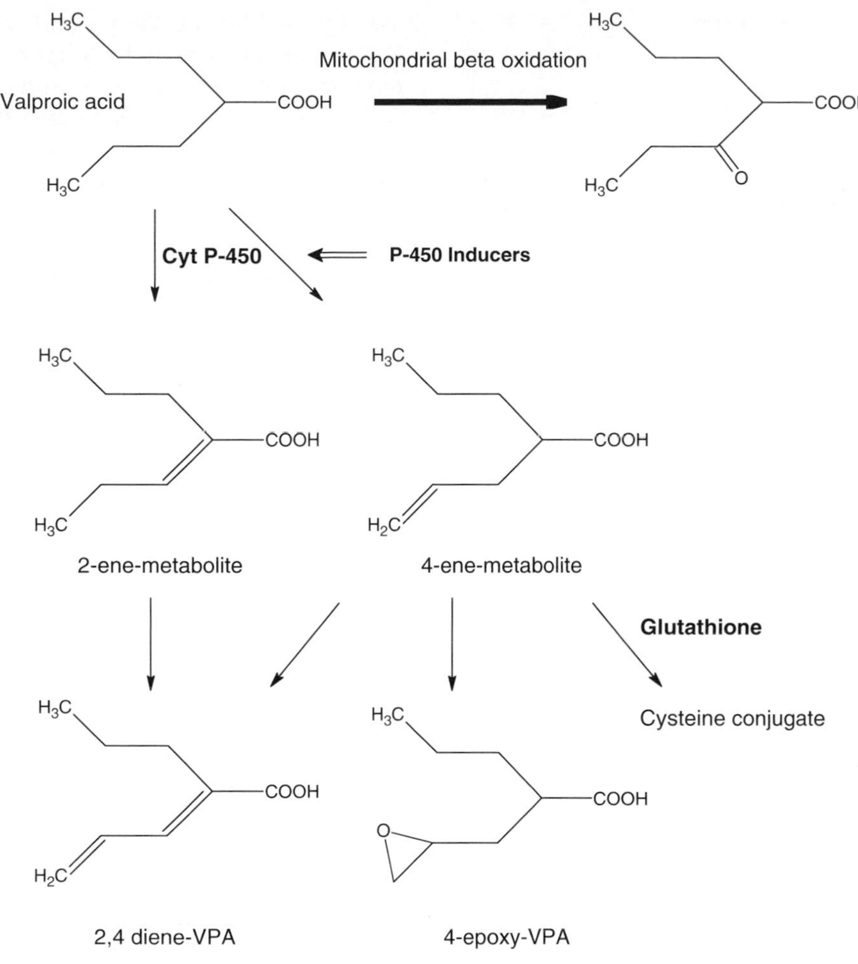

FIGURE 53-2

Main biotransformation pathways of valproate. (Courtesy of Dr. Raman Sankar)

TABLE 53-1
Pharmacokinetic Parameters of Valproate

Bioavailability	>90%
Time to peak level[a]	1–8 hours
Volume of distribution	0.16 L/kg
Serum protein binding[b]	70–93%
Elimination half-life[c]	5–15 hours
Therapeutic range	50–100 (−150) mg/L 350–700 (−1,000) μmol/L

[a]The longer values are for enteric-coated and slow-release preparations.
[b]Concentration dependent; lower at higher total concentrations.
[c]Shorter values are for comedication with inducing drugs.

peak levels may be reached only 3 to 8 hours after oral ingestion of enteric-coated tablets (33–35). Figure 53-3 shows the serum levels of a patient who received a first oral dose of 500 mg of enteric-coated divalproex sodium. No VPA was detectable in serum until 8 hours after the oral intake, and this was followed by a rapid rise of serum levels (36).

Because of this delayed absorption, serum levels of VPA in patients taking VPA chronically (twice or three times daily) continue to decrease for 2 or more hours after drug ingestion. Therefore, the lowest VPA levels of a 24-hour cycle are not the assumed "trough levels" before the morning dose, but actually occur in the late morning or early afternoon (30). The absorption of enteric-coated sprinkles was compared with the absorption of VPA syrup in 12 children, and no difference in overall bioavailability was found between the two formulations. However,

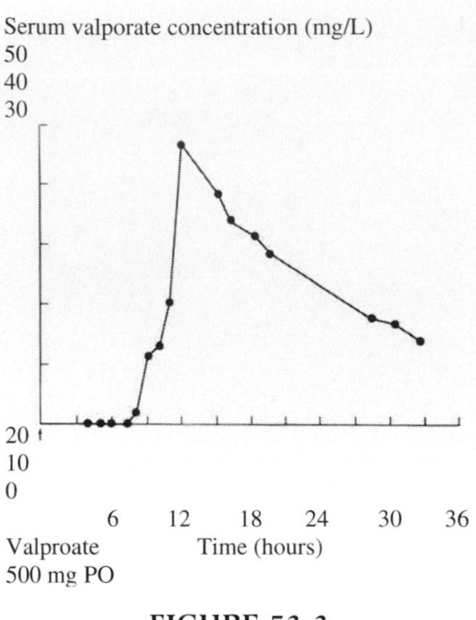

FIGURE 53-3

Valproate serum concentrations after a 500-mg single first oral dose of enteric-coated divalproex sodium in a 60.4-kg woman. Reproduced with permission from (36).

the absorption of VPA was slower from the sprinkles, with an average time to maximal VPA concentrations of 4.2 hours after ingestion of sprinkles, as compared with 0.9 hours after ingestion of syrup (37).

The volume of distribution of VPA is relatively small (0.13–0.19 L/kg in adults and 0.20–0.30 L/kg in children). This suggests that VPA has a relatively lower affinity for binding outside the blood compartment than for binding to serum proteins. Indeed, VPA is highly bound to serum proteins. This binding appears to be saturable at therapeutic concentrations, and the free fraction of VPA increases as the total concentration increases. For instance, Cramer et al (38) found that the average free serum fraction of VPA in adults was only 7% at 50 mg/L and 9% at 75 mg/L, increasing to 15% at 100 mg/L, 22% at 125 mg/L, and 30% at 150 mg/L. Based on these values, with a threefold increase in the total concentration of VPA from 50 to 150 mg/L, the free level of VPA would increase more than 10 times from 3.5 mg/L to 45 mg/L. Because the clearance of VPA is related to the free concentration, there is a linear relationship between the daily maintenance dose of VPA and steady-state free levels. But, as expected on the basis of saturable binding, a curvilinear relationship between VPA maintenance dose and total steady-state concentrations was found by Gram and coworkers (39), with relatively smaller increases in concentrations at higher doses.

The elimination half-life of VPA varies as a function of comedication. In the absence of inducing drugs, the half-life in adults is 13 to 16 hours (34, 40), whereas the half-life in adults receiving polytherapy with inducing drugs averaged 9 hours (26); half-lives in children are slightly shorter. Cloyd and coworkers (41) found an average half-life of 11.6 hours in children receiving monotherapy and 7.0 hours with polytherapy. Hall and coworkers (42) determined that VPA half-lives were significantly related to age, but volume of distribution and clearance were not. Newborns eliminate VPA slowly, with half-lives that are longer than 20 hours (43).

Interactions. Pharmacokinetic interactions involving VPA fall into three categories, based on the fact that (1) the metabolism of VPA is sensitive to enzymatic induction, (2) VPA itself can inhibit the metabolism of other drugs, and (3) VPA has a high affinity for serum proteins and can displace other drugs. Pharmacokinetic interactions with VPA have been reviewed previously (44). Concomitant administration of enzyme-inducing AEDs such as carbamazepine, phenytoin, phenobarbital, and primidone has been repeatedly shown to result in lower VPA levels in relation to the maintenance dose (45). The addition of both carbamazepine (46, 47) and phenytoin (47) significantly lowers VPA levels, usually by at least one-third to one-half. These interactions are particularly pronounced in children, resulting in VPA level reductions of 50% or more (48, 49). When children receiving polytherapy had other drugs discontinued, VPA levels rose 122% after withdrawal of phenytoin, 67% after withdrawal of phenobarbital, and 50% after withdrawal of carbamazepine (50). The antibiotic meropenem can decrease VPA levels to a clinically relevant degree (51). In general, when an inducing drug is added or withdrawn in a patient taking VPA, the dose of VPA must be increased or decreased, respectively, by a factor of about 2, if the same level is to be maintained. Inversely, levels of VPA are raised by felbamate (52, 53). The increase in VPA levels was found to be 28% at a felbamate dose of 1,200 mg/day and 54% at a dose of 2,400 mg/day. In addition to felbamate, clobazam has also been found to reduce the clearance and elevate the levels of VPA (54).

When VPA affects the kinetics of other drugs, the interaction is either an enzymatic inhibition or a displacement from serum proteins. Levels of phenobarbital have been found to increase by 57% (55) to 81% (56) after the addition of VPA. Levels of ethosuximide can also be raised by the addition of VPA, mostly in the presence of additional AEDs (57). Although VPA does not raise levels of carbamazepine itself, levels of the active metabolite, carbamazepine-10,11-epoxide may double (58, 59). The elimination of lamotrigine is markedly inhibited by VPA, with a twofold to threefold prolongation of the lamotrigine half-life (60). This interaction is competitive and rapidly reversible, but it seems to persist at low VPA concentrations (61, 62). Lamotrigine must be introduced at lower doses in patients taking VPA.

A pharmacokinetic interaction occurs between VPA and phenytoin because both drugs have a high affinity for serum proteins. VPA increases the free fraction of phenytoin (63, 64). Because the free serum level of phenytoin determines the brain concentration, total phenytoin concentrations in the usual therapeutic range may, in the presence of VPA, be associated with clinical toxicity. In contrast to inducing AEDs, VPA is not associated with failure of oral contraceptives (65). Acetylsalicylic acid can both displace VPA from serum proteins and alter its metabolism (66). It appears that this interaction can be sufficient to cause clinical VPA toxicity (67).

CLINICAL EFFICACY

Absence Seizures

Valproate is a prime example of a broad-spectrum antiepileptic drug, with at least some degree of efficacy against most seizure types (68). During the first years of routine clinical use of VPA, it soon became apparent that it is a highly effective drug in the treatment of primarily generalized idiopathic seizures such as absence seizures, generalized tonic-clonic seizures, and myoclonic seizures (69). The primary indication of VPA when it was first released in North America in 1978 was the treatment of absence seizures. When VPA was administered to patients with typical and atypical absence seizures, a reduction of spike-and-wave discharges was repeatedly demonstrated (70–75). Comparison of the efficacy of VPA and ethosuximide in the treatment of absence seizures revealed equal efficacy in at least two studies (76, 77). Sixteen patients not previously treated for absence seizures and 29 refractory patients were enrolled in a double-blind crossover study of VPA and ethosuximide, in which the measure of efficacy was the frequency and duration of generalized spike wave bursts on electroencephalogram (EEG) telemetry (77). Ethosuximide and VPA were equally effective in previously untreated patients. An open randomized comparison of VPA and lamotrigine revealed that VPA achieved seizure control much faster than lamotrigine, but the overall seizure freedom at 1 year did not differ (78). According to other reports, simple absence seizures could be completely controlled by VPA monotherapy in 11 of 12 patients (79), in 10 of 12 patients (50), in 14 of 17 patients (80), and in 20 of 21 patients (81). Overall review of the available evidence cannot demonstrate a difference in efficacy between VPA, lamotrigine, and ethosuximide against absence seizures, possibly because of the methodological quality or statistical power of the studies (82). It appears that absence seizures are more likely to be fully controlled if they occur alone than if they are mixed with another seizure type (50, 81). Overall, treatment with VPA appears to be less effective against atypical or "complex" absences than against simple absences (79, 83). VPA can also be used effectively in patients with recurrent absence status (84).

Generalized Tonic-Clonic Seizures

In addition to establishing itself as a first-line drug in the treatment of absence seizures, VPA was found to be highly effective in the treatment of certain generalized convulsive seizures (85–88). In 36 patients with primarily generalized tonic-clonic seizures, of whom 24 had been treated previously with other AEDs, VPA was used in monotherapy (79). In 33 of these patients, seizures were fully controlled. Among 42 patients with intractable seizures, the generalized tonic-clonic seizures were fully controlled by add-on VPA in 14 patients (07). VPA was compared with phenytoin in 61 previously untreated patients with generalized tonic-clonic, clonic, or tonic seizures (89). The seizures came under control during the time of observation in 73% of patients receiving VPA and in 47% of patients treated with phenytoin. Discounting seizures that occurred before therapeutic plasma drug levels had been reached, this response increased to 82% for VPA and 76% for phenytoin. In another randomized study comparing valproate and phenytoin in patients with previously untreated tonic-clonic seizures, a 2-year remission was achieved in 27 of 37 patients with VPA and in 22 of 39 patients with phenytoin (86). Monotherapy with VPA was assessed in two studies of patients with primary (or idiopathic) generalized epilepsies (81, 82). Among patients who had only generalized tonic-clonic seizures, complete seizure control was achieved in 51 of 70 patients (82) and in 39 of 44 patients (81), respectively. Monotherapy with VPA in children with generalized tonic-clonic seizures was also found to be highly effective (90).

Myoclonic Seizures

VPA is currently a drug of first choice for most myoclonic seizures, particularly those occurring in patients with primary or idiopathic generalized epilepsies (79–81). In a group of 23 patients with myoclonic epilepsy of adolescence, 16 came under full control with VPA monotherapy (79). In the same study, 22 patients with myoclonic epilepsy of adolescence and abnormality on intermittent photic stimulation, of whom 17 had failed to respond to previous medications, full seizure control was achieved in 17 patients. Photosensitivity on the EEG is easily suppressed by VPA, regardless of the associated clinical seizure type (91). Among a group of patients with primary generalized epilepsies treated with VPA monotherapy, 22 patients had myoclonic seizures and 20 of those had at least one other seizure type, either absence or tonic-clonic seizures. The myoclonic seizures were controlled by VPA monotherapy in 18 of these 22 patients (81). Patients with juvenile myoclonic epilepsy have an excellent response to VPA (92), which still remains a drug of first choice for this condition in most patients, at least in terms of efficacy. Benign myoclonic epilepsy of infancy, which belongs to the group of primary or idiopathic generalized epilepsies, also responds well to treatment with VPA (90). Postanoxic intention myoclonus is usually refractory to treatment, but some success has been achieved with VPA (93–95). A combination of VPA and clonazepam was advocated in the treatment of the myoclonic and tonic-clonic seizures in patients with severe progressive myoclonus epilepsy (96).

Infantile Spasms and Lennox-Gastaut Syndrome

The available information on the use of VPA in the treatment of generalized encephalopathic epilepsies of infancy and childhood, such as West syndrome and Lennox-Gastaut syndrome, is much less extensive than for the more benign idiopathic primary generalized epilepsies. Like all other antiepileptic medications, VPA is less effective in the treatment of these severe forms of generalized epilepsy. In a larger series of patients treated with VPA, 38 had myoclonic astatic epilepsy, a term used by the authors synonymously with Lennox-Gastaut syndrome (79). Of these patients, seven became and remained seizure free with VPA. In addition, a 50% to 80% improvement was achieved after the addition of VPA in one-third of these patients, and other AEDs were withdrawn or reduced. In the same series, seizures were fully controlled in three of six patients with myoclonic absence epilepsy, all of them on combination therapy. In another series involving 100 children treated with VPA (50), seizure control was achieved in 12 of 27 children with "absences and other seizures" and in 9 of 39 children with atonic seizures.

The majority of reports on the use of VPA for the treatment of infantile spasms include small numbers of patients (97–99), or they include patients receiving corticotropin and VPA simultaneously (100, 101). VPA was used without corticotropin in one series of 19 infants with infantile spasms (102). With VPA as their first drug, 8 of these 19 infants experienced good seizure control and did not require corticotropin. These patients received VPA doses ranging from 20 to 60 mg/kg/day. The patients who experienced an initial failure with either VPA or corticotropin were subsequently switched to the other drug. Comparison of the two groups revealed a tendency toward a better response to corticotropin, but the incidence and severity of side effects was lower with VPA. A low dose of 20 mg/kg/day of VPA was used in a series of 18 infants with infantile spasms not previously treated with corticotropin (103). In 12 of these patients, the short-term results were described as good to excellent. On follow-up, 7 patients had residual seizure activity, and moderate to severe mental retardation was diagnosed in 16. The authors concluded that the efficacy of VPA was similar to the efficacy of corticotropin and that VPA was associated with fewer side effects.

Partial Seizures

Systematic assessment of the efficacy of VPA against partial seizures began only after its role in the treatment of generalized seizures had been established. Preliminary information had been provided by subgroups of patients in studies not dealing primarily with partial seizures, all of which suggested some benefit (50, 79, 104). The first direct comparison of VPA with carbamazepine in the treatment of partial seizures was an open study in 31 previously untreated adults (105). Eleven patients receiving VPA and 8 patients receiving carbamazepine were controlled, but follow-up was less than 1 year in 12 of the 31 patients. Comparison between carbamazepine, phenytoin, and VPA in monotherapy in a prospective study of 79 patients with previously untreated simple partial or complex partial seizures revealed no difference in efficacy among the three drugs (106). A group of 140 adults with previously untreated seizures were randomized to monotherapy with phenytoin or VPA (107). The seizures were tonic-clonic in 76 patients and predominantly complex partial in 64. Determination of 2-year remission rate or time to first seizure revealed no difference between the two drugs in either subgroup. A retrospective study of VPA monotherapy in 30 patients with simple partial and complex partial seizures in whom previous drugs had failed revealed a remarkable response (108). Seizure control was achieved in 12 patients, a more than 50% seizure reduction occurred in 10 patients, and only 9 patients were not improved.

Mattson and coworkers (109) carried out the most comprehensive controlled comparison of VPA and carbamazepine monotherapy in the treatment of partial and secondarily generalized seizures. This multicenter, double-blind, randomized trial included 480 adult patients in whom several seizure indicators, as well as neurotoxicity and systemic toxicity, were assessed quantitatively. Four of five efficacy indicators were significantly in favor of carbamazepine against complex partial seizures, and a combined composite score for efficacy and toxicity was higher for carbamazepine than for VPA at 12 months, but not at 24 months. Outcomes for secondarily generalized seizures did not differ between the two drugs. Two comparative studies of VPA were carried out specifically in children (110, 111). A total of 260 children with newly diagnosed primary generalized or partial epilepsy were randomized to VPA or carbamazepine and followed for 3 years (110). The doses were titrated as needed and as tolerated according to clinical response. Equal efficacy was found for the two drugs against generalized and partial seizures, and adverse events were mostly mild for both drugs. The four drugs, phenobarbital, phenytoin, carbamazepine, and VPA, were compared in 167 children with untreated tonic-clonic or partial seizures entered into a randomized, unblinded study (111). Based on time to first seizure and to 1-year remission, there was no difference in efficacy at 1, 2, or 3 years. Unacceptable side effects necessitating withdrawal occurred in 6 of 10 patients on phenobarbital, which was prematurely eliminated from the study, in 9% of children taking phenytoin, and in 4% each of children taking carbamazepine or VPA. When trials comparing VPA and carbamazepine were subjected to a meta-analysis, carbamazepine was more effective than VPA for time to first seizure and for time to 12 months of remission (112). Valproate therapy was evaluated in 143 adult patients with poorly controlled partial epilepsy randomized to monotherapy with VPA at low levels (25–50 mg/L) or high levels (80–150 mg/L) (113). The reduction in the frequency of both complex partial and secondarily generalized tonic-clonic seizures was significantly higher among patients in the high-level group.

Other Uses of Valproate in the Treatment of Seizures

Several studies have assessed the efficacy of VPA in the prevention of febrile seizures (114–120). In some studies VPA was found to be as effective as phenobarbital, and in other studies it was more effective than phenobarbital, placebo, or no treatment in reducing seizure recurrence. Nevertheless, based on risk-versus-benefit ratio considerations, VPA cannot be recommended for the prophylaxis of febrile seizures. Treatment with intermittent diazepam during febrile episodes was as effective as prophylactic VPA in children with a high risk of recurrence of febrile seizures (121). A small group of newborns with seizures have also been treated with VPA either rectally (122) or orally (43). Overall results were favorable. A loading dose of 20 to 25 mg/kg was followed by a maintenance dose of 5 to 10 mg/kg every 12 hours (43). Newborns treated with VPA were found to have a longer elimination half-life (26.4 hours) and higher levels of ammonia.

ADVERSE EFFECTS

Although adverse effects of AEDs are commonly divided into those that are dose related and those that are idiosyncratic, the distinction is not always easy, particularly with VPA. Some reactions, such as tremor, are indeed fairly predictable and dose related. However, certain adverse events that only occur in a small fraction of patients, and therefore appear to be idiosyncratic, may be more likely to occur at high doses or levels of VPA, such as thrombocytopenia, certain cases of confusion or stupor, and neural tube defects. Finally, certain side effects that are too common to be considered idiosyncratic could never be clearly shown to be dose related, such as hair changes and weight gain. The main adverse effects of VPA are summarized in Table 53-2.

TABLE 53-2
Adverse Effects of Valproate

Adverse Effects
Neurologic
Tremor, drowsiness, lethargy, confusion, reversible dementia, brain atrophy, encephalopathy
Gastrointestinal
Nausea, vomiting, anorexia
Gastrointestinal distress
Hepatic failure
Pancreatitis
Hematologic
Thrombocytopenia
Decreased platelet aggregation
Fibrinogen depletion
Metabolic/Endocrinologic
Hyperammonemia
Hypocarnitinemia
Hyperinsulinism
Menstrual irregularities
Polycystic ovaries
Teratogenicity
Major malformations, including neural tube defect and possible developmental delay in offspring
Miscellaneous
Hair loss
Edema
Nocturnal enuresis
Decreased bone mineral density

Neurologic Adverse Effects

A tremor with the characteristics of essential tremor is relatively common with VPA (123, 124). It is dose-related and occurs in about 10% of patients. If it does not improve sufficiently with dose reduction, propranolol may be effective (124). Asterixis (125) and reversible parkinsonism (126–128) have also been described. Drowsiness, lethargy, and confusional states are uncommon with VPA, but may occur in some patients, usually at levels greater than 100 mg/L. There have also been well-documented cases of reversible dementia (126, 129, 130) and pseudoatrophy of the brain (130–132). Treatment with VPA has been associated with a rather specific and unique adverse effect characterized by an acute mental change that can progress to stupor or coma (133, 134). It is usually associated with generalized delta slowing of the EEG tracing. The mechanism is not known with certainty, and hyperammonemia or carnitine deficiency can be associated (135). This encephalopathic picture is more likely to occur when VPA is added to another AED, and it is usually reversible within 2 to 3 days upon discontinuation of VPA or of the other AED. Overall, VPA does not appear to be associated with a high incidence of dose-related effects on cognition or behavior (136–140). A possible psychotropic effect of VPA (141) was not confirmed in a controlled study (142).

Gastrointestinal Adverse Effects

The most frequent gastrointestinal adverse effects of VPA are nausea, vomiting, gastrointestinal distress, and anorexia. They may be due in part to direct gastric irritation by VPA, and the incidence is lower with enteric-coated tablets. Excessive weight gain is another common problem (143–146). It is not due entirely to increased appetite, and decreased beta-oxidation of fatty acids has been postulated as a mechanism (147). More recently, obese VPA-treated men were found to have higher serum insulin levels than obese control subjects (148, 149). The mechanism for this may be interference with hepatic insulin metabolism rather than increased insulin secretion or insulin resistance (150). In addition, patients who developed obesity while taking VPA had higher leptin levels and lower ghrelin and adiponectin levels (149). Despite recommendations for diet and exercise, weight gain tends to be a bothersome side effect, especially in young women. Excessive weight gain seems to be less of a problem in children, and one study suggests that VPA does not cause more weight gain than carbamazepine in children (151).

Fatal hepatotoxicity remains the most feared adverse effect of VPA (24, 152, 153). The two main risk factors are young age and polytherapy. The risk of fatal hepatotoxicity while receiving polytherapy with VPA was found to be approximately 1 in 600 younger than the age of 3 years, 1 in 8,000 from 3 to 10 years, 1 in 10,000 from 11 to 20 years, 1 in 31,000 between 21 and 40 years, and 1 in 107,000 older than the age of 41 years (24). The risk is much lower for monotherapy and varies between 1 in 16,000 (3–10 years old) and 1 in 230,000 (21–40 years old). No fatalities have been reported for certain age groups. Because a benign elevation of liver enzymes is common with VPA, and the severe hepatotoxicity is usually not preceded by a progressive elevation of liver enzymes, laboratory monitoring is of little value, although it is commonly done routinely. The diagnosis of hepatic failure due to VPA depends mostly on recognition of the clinical features, which include nausea, vomiting, anorexia, lethargy, jaundice, edema, and at times loss of seizure control. Although increased production of toxic metabolites has been considered as a cause of VPA hepatotoxicity, this has not yet been documented (154, 155). There has also been evidence of a protective effect of carnitine administration (especially intravenously) in cases of severe VPA hepatotoxicity (156). A panel of pediatric neurologists concluded that daily L-carnitine supplementation is strongly suggested in several situations, including certain secondary carnitine deficiency syndromes, symptomatic VPA-associated hyperammonemia, multiple risk factors for VPA hepatotoxicity, or renal-associated syndromes, infants and young children taking VPA, patients with epilepsy using the ketogenic diet who have hypocarnitinemia, patients receiving dialysis, and premature infants who are receiving total parenteral nutrition (157).

Another serious complication of VPA treatment is the development of acute hemorrhagic pancreatitis (158–163). Suspicion should be raised by the occurrence of vomiting and abdominal pain. Serum amylase and lipase are the most helpful diagnostic tests, and abdominal ultrasound may be considered. However, amylase may be elevated in 20% of asymptomatic patients taking VPA (164), and pancreatitis has been described in a patient with normal amylase but elevated lipase (165).

Hematologic Adverse Effects

Hematologic alterations are relatively common with VPA therapy, but they seldom lead to discontinuation of the drug (166–168). By far the most frequently diagnosed hematologic adverse event is thrombocytopenia (169, 170), which tends to improve with dosage reductions. The thrombocytopenia, in conjunction with other VPA-mediated disturbances of hemostasis, such as impaired platelet function, fibrinogen depletion, and coagulation factor deficiencies (171–174), may cause excessive bleeding. The common practice of discontinuing VPA about 1 month before elective surgery is therefore recommended, especially surgeries considered to be associated with higher blood losses, although several reports have found no objective evidence of excessive operative bleeding during neurosurgical procedures in patients maintained on VPA (175–177). In addition to the described hematologic changes, VPA can also occasionally cause neutropenia (178), bone marrow suppression (179), and systemic lupus erythematosus (180).

Metabolic and Endocrinologic Changes, Effect on Offspring

Hyperammonemia is a very common finding in asymptomatic patients receiving chronic VPA therapy, and routine monitoring of ammonia is not warranted. Because ammonia levels were initially measured in symptomatic patients, their elevation was thought to be the cause of the symptoms (181–183). It was later found that hyperammonemia is very common in asymptomatic patients, particularly in those taking VPA together with an enzyme-inducing AED (184, 185). The origin of the excessive ammonium may be renal (186). Although hyperammonemia can be reduced by L-carnitine supplementation (187), there is no documentation that this is necessary or clinically beneficial (188). Chronic treatment with VPA, especially in polytherapy, also tends to lower carnitine levels (189, 190). A role for carnitine deficiency in the development of severe adverse effects of VPA has never been established. One patient who developed an acute encephalopathy and cerebral edema after acute administration of VPA was found to have low carnitine levels (191). A beneficial role of L-carnitine supplementation in acute VPA overdoses has been suggested (192, 193).

VPA can cause menstrual irregularities (194), hormonal changes such as hyperandrogenism and hyperinsulinism (195–199), and pubertal arrest in women (200). Another concern has been the association between VPA therapy and polycystic ovaries (195–197, 201). To what extent these observations are significant and reproducible is an open and debated issue (202–207).

When taken during pregnancy, VPA is associated with an increased of major malformations and of developmental delay in the offspring (208–211). Treatment with VPA during the first trimester of pregnancy is associated with an estimated 1% to 2% risk of neural tube defect in the newborn (212–215). This risk appears to be greater at higher doses of VPA (216) and may also result from a pharmacogenetic susceptibility (217). Folate supplementation seems to reduce the risk (218), and a daily dose of at least 1 mg should be considered in all female patients of childbearing age who are taking VPA (see Chapters 35 and 36). Finally, a more recent concern has been that developmental delay may result from exposure to VPA in utero (219, 220).

Miscellaneous Adverse Effects

Excessive hair loss may be seen early during treatment with VPA, and, although the hair tends to grow back, it may become different in texture (221) or color (222). Facial or limb edema can occur in the absence of VPA-induced hepatic injury (223). Children may develop secondary nocturnal enuresis during VPA therapy (118, 143, 224–226). Hyponatremia (227) has also been reported in one patient. The occurrence of rashes with VPA is extremely rare (228). Bone mineral density can also be decreased by VPA, with increased risk for fractures (229–233). The precise mechanism has not been elucidated, and VPA, unlike enzyme-inducing drugs, does not cause bone loss through hypovitaminosis D.

CLINICAL USE

Many different preparations of VPA are available, although not all preparations are available in all countries. Preparations of VPA include valproic acid capsules, tablets, and syrup (immediate release), enteric-coated tablets of sodium valproate or sodium hydrogen divalproate (divalproex sodium) (delayed release), divalproex sodium enteric-coated sprinkles, extended-release oral preparations, magnesium valproate and valpromide (the amide of VPA) for oral administration, valproate suppositories, and a parenteral formulation of sodium valproate for intravenous use. The sprinkles consist of capsules containing enteric-coated particles of divalproex sodium. These capsules can be swallowed as such, or they can be opened and the contents can be sprinkled on food. This is a convenient formulation for younger children.

An initial VPA dose of approximately 15 mg/kg/day is recommended, with subsequent dose increases, as necessary and as tolerated, by 5 to 10 mg/kg/day at weekly intervals. The optimal VPA dose or concentration may vary according to the patient's seizure type (234). Daily doses between 10 and 20 mg/kg are often sufficient for VPA monotherapy in primary generalized epilepsies (50, 80, 81, 89). Children may require higher doses in milligrams per kilogram of body weight per day (56, 79). Doses of 30 to 60 mg/kg/day (in children even more than 100 mg/kg/day) may be necessary to achieve adequate VPA levels in patients who are also taking enzyme-inducing AEDs. If therapeutic levels of VPA are to be achieved rapidly or in patients who are unable to take oral medications, VPA can be administered intravenously (235, 236). This route has also been suggested for the treatment of status epilepticus (237–242), with an initial dose of 15 mg/kg followed by 1 mg/kg/hr (243), but more rapid administration, up to 6 mg/kg/min, has been successfully given (244). In those receiving intravenous replacement therapy or bolus dosing, subsequent administration should be given within 6 hours because of the precipitous fall in levels and return of clinical symptoms. Because of the relatively short elimination half-life of VPA, it is common practice to divide the daily dose into two or three single doses. However, the pharmacodynamic profile of VPA may explain why equally good results were achieved with a single daily dose of VPA (79, 245, 246).

The value of serum levels of VPA is relatively limited. First, there is a considerable fluctuation in VPA levels because of the short half-life, and the reproducibility in a given patient is not good. Second, there seems to be a poor correlation between VPA serum levels and clinical effect at a given time, because the pharmacodynamic effect of VPA may lag significantly behind its blood concentrations (81, 100, 247, 248). Although the recommended therapeutic range for VPA serum levels is usually 50 to 100 mg/L (350–700 μmol/L), levels up to 150 mg/L are often both necessary and well tolerated.

In selected cases, and particularly during combination therapy with enzyme-inducing drugs, serum VPA levels can be valuable, but the result of a single measurement has limited value and must be interpreted cautiously (249). In patients receiving chronic VPA therapy, it is common practice to monitor routinely liver enzymes and complete blood count with platelets, at least 1 to 3 months after initiation, and then about every 6 months if results are normal. Severe hepatotoxicity is unlikely to be detected by routine monitoring of liver enzymes, and hematologic abnormalities are more likely to be discovered.

References

1. Carraz G, Gau R, Chateau R, Bonnin J. Communication a propos des premiers essais cliniques sur l'activité antiépileptique de l'acide *n*-dipropylacétique (sel de Na+). *Ann Med Psychol* 1964; 122:577–585.
2. Daoud AS, Zaki M, Shakir R, Al-Saleh Q. Effectiveness of sodium valproate in the treatment of Sydenham's chorea. *Neurology* 1990; 40:1140–1141.
3. Meunier H, Carraz G, Meunier V, Eymard M. Propriétés pharmacodynamiques de l'acide *n*-propylacétique. *Thérapie* 1963; 18:435–438.
4. Pellegrini A, Gloor P, Sherwin AL. Effect of valproate sodium on generalized penicillin epilepsy in the cat. *Epilepsia* 1978; 19:351–360.
5. Chapman A, Keane PE, Meldrum BS, Simiand J, et al. Mechanism of anticonvulsant action of valproate. *Prog Neurobiol* 1982; 19:315–399.
6. Frey HH, Löscher W, Reiche R, Schultz D. Antiepileptic potency of common antiepileptic drugs in the gerbil. *Pharmacology* 1983; 27:330–335.
7. Leveil V, Naquet R. A study of the action of valproic acid on the kindling effect. *Epilepsia* 1977; 18:229–234.
8. Löscher W. Valproic acid: mechanisms of action. In: Levy RH, Mattson RH, Meldrum BS, Perucca E, eds. *Antiepileptic Drugs*. 5th ed. Philadelphia: Lippincott Williams & Wilkins, 2002:767–779.
9. Löscher W. Correlation between alterations in brain GABA metabolism and seizure excitability following administration of GABA aminotransferase inhibitors and valproic acid—a reevaluation. *Neurochem Int* 1981; 3:397–404.
10. Fowler LJ, Beckford J, John RA. An analysis of the kinetics of the inhibition of rabbit brain GABA-transaminase by sodium N-dipropylacetate and some other simple carboxylic acids. *Biochem Pharmacol* 1975; 24:1267–1270.
11. Harvey PKB, Bradford HF, Davisson AN. The inhibitory effect of sodium n-dipropylacetate on the degradative enzymes of the GABA shunt. *FEBS Lett* 1975; 52F: 251–254.
12. Kerwin RW, Olpe HR, Schmutz M. The effect of sodium-n-dipropylacetate on GABA dependent inhibition of rat cortex *in vivo*. *Br J Pharmacol* 1980; 71:545–551.
13. McLean MJ, MacDonald RL. Sodium valproate, but not ethosuximide, produces use and voltage-dependent limitation of high frequency repetitive firing of action potentials of mouse central neurons in cell culture. *J Pharmacol Exp Ther* 1986; 237:1001–1011.
14. Franceschetti S, Hamon B, Heinemann U. The action of valproate on spontaneous epileptiform activity in the absence of synaptic transmission and on evoked changes on [Ca^{++}] and [K^+] in the hippocampal slice. *Brain Res* 1986; 386:1–11.
15. Schechter PJ, Trainer Y, Grove J. Effect of N-dipropyl-acetate on amino acid concentration in mouse brain: correlations with anticonvulsant activity. *J Neurochem* 1978; 3:1325–1327.
16. Ueda Y, Willmore LJ. Molecular regulation of glutamate and GABA transporter proteins by valproic acid in rat hippocampus during epileptogenesis. *Exp Brain Res* 2000; 133:334–339.
17. Levy RH, Rettenmeier AW, Anderson GD. Effects of polytherapy with phenytoin, carbamazepine, and stiripentol on formation of 4-ene-valproate, a hepatotoxic metabolite of valproic acid. *Clin Pharmacol Ther* 1990; 48:225–235.
18. Löscher W, Nau H. Pharmacological evaluation of various metabolites and analogues of valproic acid. *Neuropharmacology* 1985; 24:427–435.
19. Pollack GM, McHugh WB, Gengo FM, Ermer JC, et al. Accumulation and washout kinetics of valproic acid and its active metabolites. *J Clin Pharmacol* 1986; 26:668–676.
20. Nau H, Löscher W. Valproic acid: brain and plasma levels of the drug and its metabolites, anticonvulsant effects and γ-aminobutyric acid (GABA) metabolism in the mouse. *J Pharmacol Exp Ther* 1982; 220:654–659.
21. Nau H, Hauck RS, Ehlers K. Valproic acid-induced neural tube defects in mouse and human: aspects of chirality, alternative drug development, pharmacokinetics, and possible mechanisms. *Pharmacol Toxicol* 1991; 69:310–321.
22. Kesterson JW, Granneman GR, Machinist JM. The hepatotoxicity of valproic acid and its metabolites in rats. I. Toxicologic, biochemical and histopathologic studies. *Hepatology* 1984; 4:1143–1152.
23. Rettie AE, Rettenmeier AW, Howald WN, Baillie TA. Cytochrome P450-catalyzed formation of D^4-VPA, a toxic metabolite of valproic acid. *Science* 1987; 235: 890–893.
24. Bryant AE, Dreifuss FE. Valproic acid hepatic fatalities. III. U.S. experience since 1986. *Neurology* 1996; 46:465–469.
25. Paganini M, Zaccara G, Moroni F, et al. Lack of relationship between sodium valproate-induced adverse effects and the plasma concentration of its metabolite 2-propylpenten-4-oic acid. *Eur J Clin Pharmacol* 1987; 32:219–222.
26. Perucca E, Gatti G, Frigo GM, et al. Disposition of sodium valproate in epileptic patients. *Br J Clin Pharmacol* 1978; 5:495–499.
27. Cloyd JC, Kriel RL. Bioavailability of rectally administered valproic acid syrup. *Neurology* 1981; 31:1348–1352.
28. Thorpy MJ. Rectal valproate syrup and status epilepticus. *Neurology* 1980; 30: 1113–1114.
29. Holmes GB, Rosenfeld WE, Graves NM, et al. Absorption of valproic acid suppositories in human volunteers. *Arch Neurol* 1989; 46:906–909.
30. Issakainen J, Bourgeois BFD. Bioavailability of sodium valproate suppositories during repeated administration at steady-state in epileptic children. *Eur J Pediatr* 1987; 146:404–407.
31. Dutta S, Zhang Y, Selness D, et al. Comparison of the bioavailability of unequal doses of divalproex sodium extended release formulation relative to the delayed-release formulation in healthy volunteers. *Epilepsy Res* 2002; 49:1–10.
32. Sommerville KS, Dutta S, Biton V, Zhang Y, et al. Bioavailability of a divalproex extended-release formulation versus the conventional divalproex formulation in adult patients receiving enzyme-inducing antiepileptic drugs. *Clin Drug Invest* 2003; 23:661–670.
33. Klotz U, Antonin KH. Pharmacokinetics and bioavailability of sodium valproate. *Clin Pharmacol Ther* 1977; 21:736–743.
34. Gugler R, Schell A, Eichelbaum M, Froscher W, et al. Disposition of valproic acid in man. *Eur J Clin Pharmacol* 1977; 12:125–132.
35. Levy RH, Conraud B, Loiseau P, et al. Meal-dependent absorption of enteric-coated sodium valproate. *Epilepsia* 1980; 21:273–280.
36. Bourgeois BFD. Pharmacokinetics and pharmacodynamics of antiepileptic drugs. In: Wyllie E, ed. *The Treatment of Epilepsy: Principles and Practice*. 4th ed. Philadelphia: Lippincott Williams & Wilkins, 2006:655–664.
37. Cloyd J, Kriel R, Jones-Saete C, et al. Comparison of sprinkle versus syrup formulations of valproate for bioavailability, tolerance, and preference. *J Pediatr* 1992; 120:634–638.
38. Cramer JA, Mattson RH, Bennett DM, Swick CT. Variable free and total valproic acid concentrations in sole- and multidrug therapy. *Ther Drug Monit* 1986; 8:411–415.
39. Gram L, Flachs H, Würtz-Jorgensen A, Parnas J, Andersen B. Sodium valproate, serum level and clinical effect in epilepsy: a controlled study. *Epilepsia* 1979; 20:303–312.
40. Perucca E, Grimaldi R, Gatti G, et al. Pharmacokinetics of valproic acid in the elderly. *Br J Clin Pharmacol* 1984; 17:665–669.
41. Cloyd JC, Fischer JH, Kriel RL, Kraus DM.Valproicacid pharmacokinetics in children. IV. Effects of age and antiepileptic drugs on protein binding and intrinsic clearance. *Clin Pharmacol Ther* 1993; 53:22–29.
42. Hall K, Otten N, Johnston B, et al. A multivariable analysis of factors governing the steady-state pharmacokinetics of valproic acid in 52 young epileptics. *J Clin Pharmacol* 1985; 2:261–268.
43. Gal P, Oles KS, Gilman JT, Weaver R. Valproic acid efficacy, toxicity and pharmacokinetics in neonates with intractable seizures. *Neurology* 1988; 38:467–471.
44. Bourgeois BFD. Pharmacologic interactions between valproate and other drugs. *Am J Med* 1988; 84 Suppl 1A:29–33.
45. May T, Rambeck B. Serum concentrations of valproic acid: influence of dose and comedication. *Ther Drug Monit* 1985; 7:387–390.
46. Bowdle TA, Levy RH, Cutler RE. Effect of carbamazepine on valproic acid kinetics in normal subjects. *Clin Pharmacol Ther* 1979; 26:629–634.
47. Reunanen MI, Luoma P, Myllyla V, Hokkanen E. Low serum valproic acid concentrations in epileptic patients on combination therapy. *Curr Ther Res* 1980; 28:456–462.
48. De Wolff FA, Peters ACB, van Kempen GMJ. Serum concentrations and enzyme induction in epileptic children treated with phenytoin and valproate. *Neuropediatrics* 1982; 13:10–13.
49. Cloyd JC, Kriel RL, Fischer JH. Valproic acid pharmacokinetics in children. II. Discontinuation of concomitant antiepileptic drug therapy. *Neurology* 1985; 35:1623–1627.
50. Henriksen O, Johannessen SI. Clinical and pharmacokinetic observations on sodium valproate—a 5-year follow-up study in 100 children with epilepsy. *Acta Neurol Scand* 1982; 65:504–523.
51. Coves-Orts FJ, Borras-Blasco J, Navarro-Ruiz A, Murcia-Lopez A, et al. Acute seizures due to a probable interaction between valproic acid and meropenem. *Ann Pharmacother* 2005; 39:533–537.
52. Wagner ML, Graves NM, Leppik IE, et al. The effect of felbamate on valproate disposition. *Epilepsia* 1991; 32:15.
53. Hooper WD, Franklin ME, Glue P, et al. Effect of felbamate on valproic acid disposition in healthy volunteers: inhibition of β-oxidation. *Epilepsia* 1996; 37:91–97.
54. Theis JGW, Koren G, Daneman R, Sherwin AL, et al. Interactions of clobazam with conventional antiepileptics in children. *J Child Neurol* 1997; 12:208–213.
55. Suganuma T, Ishizaki T, Chiba K, Hori M. The effect of concurrent administration of valproate sodium on phenobarbital plasma concentration/dosage ratio in pediatric patients. *J Pediatr* 1981; 99:314–317.

56. Redenbaugh JE, Sato S, Penry JK, Dreifuss FE, et al. Sodium valproate: pharmacokinetics and effectiveness in treating intractable seizures. *Neurology* 1980; 30:1–6.
57. Mattson RH, Cramer JA. Valproic acid and ethosuximide interaction. *Ann Neurol* 1980; 7:583–584.
58. Levy RH, Moreland TA, Morselli PL, et al. Carbamazepine/valproic acid interaction in man and rhesus monkey. *Epilepsia* 1984; 25:338–345.
59. Pisani F, Fazio A, Oteri G, et al. Sodium valproate and valpromide: differential interactions with carbamazepine in epileptic patients. *Epilepsia* 1986; 27:548–552.
60. Yuen AWC, Land G, Weatherley BC, Peck AW. Sodium valproate acutely inhibits lamotrigine metabolism. *Br J Clin Pharmacol* 1992; 33:511–513.
61. Gidal BE, Anderson GD, Rutecki PR, et al. Lack of an effect of valproate concentration on lamotrigine pharmacokinetics in developmentally disabled patients with epilepsy. *Epilepsy Res* 2000; 42:23–31.
62. Kanner AM, Frey M. Adding valproate to lamotrigine: a study of their pharmacokinetic interaction. *Neurology* 2000; 55:588–591.
63. Rodin EA, De Sousa G, Haidukewych D, et al. Dissociation between free and bound phenytoin levels in presence of valproate sodium. *Arch Neurol* 1981; 38:240–242.
64. Pisani FD, Di Perri RG. Intravenous valproate: effects on plasma and saliva phenytoin levels. *Neurology* 1981; 31:467–470.
65. Mattson RH, Cramer JA, Darney PD, Naftolin F. Use of oral contraceptives by women with epilepsy. *JAMA* 1986; 256:238–240.
66. Abbott FS, Kassam J, Orr JM, Farrell K. The effect of aspirin on valproic acid metabolism. *Clin Pharmacol Ther* 1986; 40:94–100.
67. Goulden KJ, Dooley JM, Camfield PR, Fraser AD. Clinical valproate toxicity induced by acetylsalicylic acid. *Neurology* 1987; 37:1392–1394.
68. Bourgeois BFD. Valproic acid: clinical efficacy and use in epilepsy. In: Levy RH, Mattson RH, Meldrum BS, Perucca E, eds. *Antiepileptic Drugs*. 5th ed. Philadelphia: Lippincott Williams & Wilkins, 2002:808–817.
69. Jeavons PM, Clark JE, Maheshwari MC. Treatment of generalized epilepsies of childhood and adolescence with sodium valproate (Epilim). *Dev Med Child Neurol* 1977; 19:9–25.
70. Adams DJ, Lüders H, Pippenger CE. Sodium valproate in the treatment of intractable seizure disorders: a clinical and electroencephalographic study. *Neurology* 1978; 28:152–157.
71. Henrick CE, Maheshwari MC. Sodium valproate (Epilim) and photosensitivity. A preliminary report. *Electroencephalogr Clin Neurophysiol* 1975; 39:429.
72. Braathen G, Theorell K, Persson A, Rane A. Valproate in the treatment of absence epilepsy in children. *Epilepsia* 1988; 29:548–552.
73. Maheshwari MC, Jeavons PM. The effect of sodium valproate (Epilim) on the EEG. *Electroencephalogr Clin Neurophysiol* 1975; 39:429.
74. Mattson RH, Cramer JA, Williamson PD, Novelly R. Valproic acid in epilepsy: clinical and pharmacological effects. *Ann Neurol* 1978; 3:20–25.
75. Villareal HJ, Wilder BJ, Willmore LJ, et al. Effect of valproic acid on spike and wave discharges in patients with absence seizures. *Neurology* 1978; 28:886–891.
76. Callaghan N, O'Hare J, O'Driscoll D, O'Neill B, et al. Comparative study of ethosuximide and sodium valproate in the treatment of typical absence seizures (petit mal). *Dev Med Child Neurol* 1982; 24:830–836.
77. Sato S, White BG, Penry JK, et al. Valproic acid versus ethosuximide in the treatment of absence seizures. *Neurology* 1982; 32:157–163.
78. Coppola G, Auricchio G, Federico R, Carotenuto M, et al. Lamotrigine versus valproic acid as first-line monotherapy in newly diagnosed typical absence seizures: an open-label, randomized, parallel-group study. *Epilepsia* 2004; 45:1049–1053.
79. Covanis A, Gupta AK, Jeavons PM. Sodium valproate: monotherapy and polytherapy. *Epilepsia* 1982; 23:693–720.
80. Feuerstein J. A long-term study of monotherapy with sodium valproate in primary generalized epilepsy. *Br J Clin Pract* 1983; 27 Suppl 1:17–23.
81. Bourgeois B, Beaumanoir A, Blajev B, et al. Monotherapy with valproate in primary generalized epilepsies. *Epilepsia* 1987; 28 Suppl 2:S8–S11.
82. Posner EB, Mohamed K, Marson AG. Ethosuximide, sodium valproate or lamotrigine for absence seizures in children and adolescents. *Cochrane Database Syst Rev* 2005; (4):CD003032.
83. Erenberg G, Rothner AD, Henry CE, Cruse RP. Valproic acid in the treatment of intractable absence seizures in children. A single-blind clinical and quantitative EEG study. *Am J Dis Child* 1982; 136:526–529.
84. Berkovic SF, Andermann F, Guberman A, Hipola D, et al. Valproate prevents the recurrence of absence status. *Neurology* 1989; 39:1294–1297.
85. Dulac O, Steru D, Rey E, Perret A, et al. Monothérapie par le valproate de sodium dans les épilepsies de l'enfant. *Arch Fr Pediatr* 1982; 39:347–352.
86. Turnbull DM, Howel D, Rawlins MD, Chadwick DW. Which drug for the adult epileptic patient: phenytoin or valproate? *Br Med J* 1985; 290:816–819.
87. Spitz MC, Deasy DN. Conversion to valproate monotherapy in nonretarded adults with primary generalized tonic-clonic seizures. *J Epilepsy* 1991; 4:33–38.
88. Ramsey RE, Wilder BJ, Murphy JV, Holmes GL, et al. Efficacy and safety of valproic acid versus phenytoin as sole therapy for newly diagnosed primary generalized tonic-clonic seizures. *J Epilepsy* 1992; 5:55–60.
89. Wilder BJ, Ramsey RE, Murphy JV, et al. Comparison of valproic acid and phenytoin in newly-diagnosed tonic-clonic seizures. *Neurology* 1983; 33:1474–1476.
90. Dulac O, Steru D, Rey E, Arthius M. Sodium valproate monotherapy in childhood epilepsy. *Brain Dev* 1986; 8:47–52.
91. Jeavons PM, Bishop A, Harding GFA. The prognosis of photosensitivity. *Epilepsia* 1986; 27:569–575.
92. Delgado-Escueta AV, Enrile-Bacsal F. Juvenile myoclonic epilepsy of Janz. *Neurology* 1984; 34:285–294.
93. Fahn S. Post-anoxic action myoclonus: improvement with valproic acid. *N Engl J Med* 1978; 299:313–314.
94. Bruni J, Willmore LJ, Wilder BJ. Treatment of postanoxic intention myoclonus with valproic acid. *Can J Neurol Sci* 1979; 6:39–42.
95. Rollinson RD, Gilligam BS. Post-anoxic action myoclonus (Lance-Adams syndrome) responding to valproate. *Arch Neurol* 1979; 36:44–45.
96. Iivanainen M, Himberg JJ. Valproate and clonazepam in the treatment of severe progressive myoclonus epilepsy. *Arch Neurol* 1982; 39:236–238.
97. Barnes SE, Bower BD. Sodium valproate in the treatment of intractable childhood epilepsy. *Dev Med Child Neurol* 1975; 17:175–181.
98. Olive D, Tridon P, Weber M. Action du dipropylacétate de sodium sur certaines variétés d'encéphalopathies épileptogènes du nourrisson. *Schweiz Med Wochenschr* 1969; 99:87–92.
99. Rohmann E, Arndi R. The efficacy of Ergenyl (dipropyl acetate) in clonic, jackknife, and salaam spasms. *Kinderaerztl Prax* 1976; 44:109–113.
100. Brachet-Liermain A, Demarquez JL. Pharmacokinetics of dipropylacetate in infants and young children. *Pharm Weekbl* 1977; 112:293–297.
101. Yokoyama S, Kodama S, Ogini H. Study of the treatment of infantile spasms. *Brain Dev* 1976; 8:447–453.
102. Bachman DS. Use of valproic acid in treatment of infantile spasms. *Arch Neurol* 1982; 39:49–52.
103. Pavone L, Incorpora G, LaRosa M, LiVolti S, et al. Treatment of infantile spasms with sodium dipropylacetic acid. *Dev Med Child Neurol* 1981; 23:454–461.
104. Bruni J, Albright P. Valproic acid therapy for complex partial seizures: its efficacy and toxic effects. *Arch Neurol* 1983; 40:135–137.
105. Loiseau P, Cohadon S, Jogeix M, Legroux M, et al. Efficacité du valproate de sodium dans les épilepsies partielles. *Rev Neurol (Paris)* 1984; 140:434–437.
106. Callaghan N, Kenny RA, O'Neill B, Crowley M, et al. A prospective study between carbamazepine, phenytoin and sodium valproate as monotherapy in previously untreated and recently diagnosed patients with epilepsy. *J Neurol Neurosurg Psychiatry* 1985; 48:639–644.
107. Turnbull DM, Rawlins MD, Weightman D, Chadwick DW. A comparison of phenytoin and valproate in previously untreated adult epileptic patients. *J Neurol Neurosurg Psychiatry* 1982; 45:55–59.
108. Dean JC, Penry JK. Valproate monotherapy in 30 patients with partial seizures. *Epilepsia* 1988; 29:140–144.
109. Mattson RH, Cramer JA, Collins JF; Dept. of VA Epilepsy Cooperative Study No. 264 Group. A comparison of valproate with carbamazepine for the treatment of complex partial seizures and secondarily generalized tonic-clonic seizures in adults. *N Engl J Med* 1992; 327:765–771.
110. Verity CM, Hosking G, Easter DJ. A multicentre comparative trial of sodium valproate and carbamazepine in pediatric epilepsy. The Paediatric EPITEG Collaborative Group. *Dev Med Child Neurol* 1995; 37(2):97–108.
111. deSilva M, MacArdle B, McGowan M, et al. Randomised comparative monotherapy trial of phenobarbitone, phenytoin, carbamazepine, or sodium valproate for newly diagnosed childhood epilepsy. *Lancet* 1996; 347:709–713.
112. Marson AG, Williamson PR, Clough H, Hutton JL, et al; Epilepsy Monotherapy Trial Group. Carbamazepine versus valproate monotherapy for epilepsy: a meta-analysis. *Epilepsia* 2002; 43:505–513.
113. Beydoun A, Sackellares JC, Shu V. Safety and efficacy of divalproex sodium monotherapy in partial epilepsy: a double-blind, concentration-response design clinical trial. Depakote monotherapy for partial seizures study group. *Neurology* 1997; 48:182–188.
114. Cavazzutti GB. Prevention of febrile convulsions with dipropylacetate (Depakine). *Epilepsia* 1975; 16:645–648.
115. Ngwane E, Bower B. Continuous sodium valproate or phenobarbital in the prevention of "simple" febrile convulsions. *Arch Dis Child* 1980; 55:171–174.
116. Minagawa K, Miura H. Phenobarbital, primidone and sodium valproate in the prophylaxis of febrile convulsions. *Brain Dev* 1981; 3:385–393.
117. Lee K, Melchoir JC. Sodium valproate versus phenobarbital in the prophylactic treatment of febrile convulsions in childhood. *Eur J Pediatr* 1981; 137:151–153.
118. Herranz JL, Armijo JA, Arteaga R. Effectiveness and toxicity of phenobarbital, primidone and sodium valproate in the prevention of febrile convulsions, controlled by plasma levels. *Epilepsia* 1984; 25:89–95.
119. Mamelle N, Mamelle JC, Plasse JC, Revol M, et al. Prevention of recurrent febrile convulsions—a randomized therapeutic assay: sodium valproate, phenobarbital and placebo. *Neuropediatrics* 1984; 15:37–42.
120. Rantala H, Tarkka R, Uhari M. A meta-analytic review of the preventive treatment of recurrences of febrile seizures. *J Pediatr* 1997; 131(6):922–925.
121. Lee K, Taudorf K, Hvorslev V. Prophylactic treatment with valproic acid or diazepam in children with febrile convulsions. *Acta Paediatr Scand* 1986; 75:593–597.
122. Steinberg A, Shaley RS, Amir N. Valproic acid in neonatal status convulsion. *Brain Dev* 1986; 8:278–279.
123. Hyuman NM, Dennis PD, Sinclar KG. Tremor due to sodium valproate. *Neurology* 1979; 29:1177–1180.
124. Karas BJ, Wilder BJ, Hammond EJ, Bauman AW. Treatment of valproate tremors. *Neurology* 1983; 33:1380–1382.
125. Bodensteiner JB, Morris HH, Golden GS. Asterixis associated with sodium valproate. *Neurology* 1981; 31:186–190.
126. Armon C, Miller P, Carwile S, et al. Valproate-induced dementia and parkinsonism: prevalence in actively ascertained epilepsy clinic population. *Neurology* 1991; 41:22.
127. Sasso E, Delsoldato S, Negrotti A, Mancia D. Reversible valproate-induced extrapyramidal disorder. *Epilepsia* 1994; 35:391–393.

128. Easterford K, Clough P, Kellett M, Fallon K, et al.. Reversible parkinsonism with normal β-CIT-SPECT in patients exposed to sodium valproate. *Neurology* 2004; 62:1435–1437.
129. Zaret BS, Cohen RA. Reversible valproic acid-induced dementia: a case report. *Epilepsia* 1986; 27 Suppl 3:234–240.
130. Shin C, Gray L, Armond C. Reversible cerebral atrophy: radiologic correlate of valproate-induced parkinson-dementia syndrome. *Neurology* 1992; 42 Suppl 3:277 (abstract).
131. McLachlan RS. Pseudoatrophy of the brain with valproic acid monotherapy. *Can J Neurol Sci* 1987; 14:294–296.
132. Papazian O, Canizales E, Alfonso I, et al. Reversible dementia and apparent brain atrophy during valproate therapy. *Ann Neurol* 1995; 38:687–691.
133. Sackellares JC, Lee SI, Dreifuss FE. Stupor following administration of valproic acid to patients receiving other antiepileptic drugs. *Epilepsia* 1979; 20:697–703.
134. Marescaux C, Warter JM, Micheletti G, et al. Stuporous episodes during treatment with sodium valproate: report of seven cases. *Epilepsia* 1982; 23:297–305.
135. Verrotti A, Trotta D, Morgese G, Chiarelli F. Valproate-induced hyperammonemic encephalopathy. *Metab Brain Dis* 2002; 17:367–373.
136. Sonnen AEH, Zelvelder WH, Bruens JH. A double blind study of the influence of dipropylacetate on behaviour. *Acta Neurol Scand* 1975; 60 Suppl:43–47.
137. Aman M, Werry J, Paxton J, Turbott S. Effect of sodium valproate on psychomotor performance in children as a function of dose, fluctuations in concentration and diagnosis. *Epilepsia* 1987; 28:115–125.
138. Vining EPG, Mellits ED, Dorsen MM, et al. Psychologic and behavioral effects of antiepileptic drugs in children: a double-blind comparison between phenobarbital and valproic acid. *Pediatrics* 1987; 80:165–174.
139. Gallassi R, Morreale A, Lorusso S, et al. Cognitive effects of valproate. *Epilepsy Res* 1990; 5:160–164.
140. Stores G, Williams PL, Styles E, Zaiwalla Z. Psychological effects of sodium valproate and carbamazepine in epilepsy. *Arch Dis Child* 1992; 67:1330–1337.
141. Betts TA, Crowe A, Alford C. Psychotropic effect of sodium valproate. *Br J Clin Pract* 1982; 18:145–146.
142. Sommerbeck KW, Theilgaard A, Rasmussen KE, et al. Valproate sodium: evaluation of so-called psychotropic effect. A controlled study. *Epilepsia* 1977; 18:159–167.
143. Dinesen H, Gram L, Anderson T, Dam M. Weight gain during treatment with valproate. *Acta Neurol Scand* 1984; 70:65–69.
144. Dean JC, Penry JK. Weight gain patterns in patients with epilepsy: comparison of antiepileptic drugs. *Epilepsia* 1995; 36 Suppl 4:72 (abstract).
145. Novak GP, Maytal J, Alshansky A, Eviatar L, et al. Risk of excessive weight gain in epileptic children treated with valproate. *J Child Neurol* 1999; 14:490–495.
146. Biton V, Mirza W, Montouris G, et al. Weight change associated with valproate and lamotrigine monotherapy in patients with epilepsy. *Neurology* 2001; 56:172–177.
147. Breum L, Astrup A, Gram L, et al. Metabolic changes during treatment with valproate in humans: implications for weight gain. *Metabolism* 1992; 41:666–670.
148. Pylvänen V, Knip M, Pakarinen AJ, et al. Fasting serum insulin and lipid levels in men with epilepsy. *Neurology* 2003; 60:571–574.
149. Greco R, Latini G, Chiarelli F, Iannetti P, et al. Leptin, ghrelin, and adiponectin in epileptic patients treated with valproic acid. *Neurology* 2005; 65:1808–1809.
150. Pylvänen V, Pakarinen AJ, Knip M, Isojärvi J. Characterization of insulin secretion in valproate-treated patients with epilepsy. *Epilepsia* 2006; 47:1460–1464.
151. Easter D, O'Bryan-Tear CG, Verity C. Weight gain with valproate or carbamazepine—a reappraisal. *Seizure* 1997; 6(2):121–125.
152. Scheffner D, König S, Rauterberg-Ruland I, et al. Fatal liver failure in 16 children with valproate therapy. *Epilepsia* 1988; 29 Suppl 5:530–542.
153. König SA, Siemes H, Bläker F, et al. Severe hepatotoxicity during valproate therapy: an update and report of eight new fatalities. *Epilepsia* 1994; 35:1005–1015.
154. Sugimoto T, Muro H, Woo M, Nishida N, et al. Valproate metabolites in high-dose valproate plus phenytoin therapy. *Epilepsia* 1996; 37:1200–1203.
155. Sugimoto T, Muro H, Woo M, Nishida N, et al. Metabolite profiles in patients on high-dose valproate monotherapy. *Epilepsy Res* 1996; 25:107–112.
156. Bohan TP, Helton E, Mcdonald I, et al. Effect of L-carnitine treatment for valproate-induced hepatotoxicity. *Neurology* 2001; 56:1405–1409.
157. DeVivo D, Bohan T, Coulter D, et al. L-Carnitine supplementation in childhood epilepsy: current perspectives. *Epilepsia* 1998; 39:1216–1225.
158. Camfield PR. Pancreatitis due to valproic acid. *Lancet* 1979; 1:1198–1199.
159. Coulter DL, Allen RJ. Pancreatitis associated with valproic acid therapy for epilepsy. *Ann Neurol* 1980; 7:693–720.
160. Williams LHP, Reynolds RP, Emery JL. Pancreatitis during sodium valproate treatment. *Arch Dis Child* 1983; 58:543–544.
161. Wyllie E, Wyllie R, Cruse R, Erenberg G, Rothner AD. Pancreatitis associated with valproic acid therapy. *American Journal of Diseases of Children* 1984; 138:912–914.
162. Asconapé JJ, Penry JK, Dreifuss FE, Riela A, et al. Valproate-associated pancreatitis. *Epilepsia* 1993; 34:177–183.
163. Grauso-Eby NL, Goldfarb O, Feldman-Winter LB, McAbee GN. Acute pancreatitis in children from valproic acid: case series and review. *Pediatr Neurol* 2003; 28:145–148.
164. Bale JF, Gay PE, Madsen JA. Monitoring of serum amylase levels during valproic acid therapy. *Ann Neurol* 1982; 11:217–218.
165. Otusbo S, Huruzono T, Kobae H, Yoshimi S, et al. Pancreatitis with normal serum amylase associated with sodium valproate case report. *Brain Dev* 1995; 17(3):219–221.
166. May RB, Sunder TR. Hematologic manifestations of long-term valproate therapy. *Epilepsia* 1993; 34:1098–1101.
167. Hauser E, Seidl R, Freilinger M, Male C, et al. Hematologic manifestations and impaired liver synthetic function during valproate monotherapy. *Brain Dev* 1996; 18(2):105–109.
168. Acharya S, Bussel JB. Hematologic toxicity of sodium valproate. *J Pediatr Hematol Oncol* 2000; 22:62–65.
169. Neophytides AN, Nutt JG, Lodish JR. Thrombocytopenia associated with sodium valproate treatment. *Ann Neurol* 1978; 5:389–390.
170. Barr RD, Copeland SA, Stockwell ML, Morris N, Kelton JC. Valproic acid and immune thrombocytopenia. *Arch Dis Child* 1982; 57:681–684.
171. Gidal B, Spencer N, Maly M, et al. Valproate-mediated disturbances of hemostasis: relationship to dose and plasma concentration. *Neurology* 1994; 44:1418–1422.
172. Kreuz W, Linde M, Funk R, et al. Valproate therapy induces von Willebrand disease type I. *Epilepsia* 1991; 33:178–184.
173. Pohlmann-Eden B, Peters CN, Wennberg R, Dempfle CE. Valproate induces reversible factor XIII deficiency with risk of perioperative bleeding. *Acta Neurol Scand* 2003; 108:142–145.
174. Teich M, Longin E, Dempfle CE, Konig S. Factor XIII deficiency associated with valproate treatment. *Epilepsia* 2004; 45:187–189.
175. Winter SL, Kriel RL, Novachec TF, et al. Perioperative blood loss: the effect of valproate. *Ped Neurol* 1996; 15:19–22.
176. Ward MM, Barbaro NM, Laxer KD, Rampil IJ. Preoperative valproate administration does not increase blood loss during temporal lobectomy. *Epilepsia* 1996; 37:98–101.
177. Anderson GD, Lin YX, Berge C, Ojemann G. Absence of bleeding complications in patients undergoing cortical surgery while receiving valproate treatment. *J Neurosurg* 1997; 87(2):252–256.
178. Jaeken J, van Goethem C, Casaer P, Devlieger H, et al. Neutropenia during sodium valproate treatment. *Arch Dis Child* 1979; 54:985–986.
179. Smith FR, Boots M. Sodium valproate and bone marrow suppression. *Ann Neurol* 1980; 8:197–199.
180. Asconapé JJ, Manning KR, Lancman ME. Systemic lupus erythematosus associated with use of valproate. *Epilepsia* 1994; 35:162–163.
181. Coulter DL, Allen RJ. Hyperammonemia with valproic acid therapy. *J Pediatr* 1981; 99:317–319.
182. Batshaw ML, Brusilow SW. Valproate-induced hyperammonemia. *Ann Neurol* 1982; 11:319–321.
183. Zaret BS, Beckner RR, Marini AM, Wagle W, et al. Sodium valproate-induced hyperammonemia without clinical hepatic dysfunction. *Neurology* 1982; 32:206–208.
184. Haidukewych D, John G, Zielinski JJ, Rodin EA. Chronic valproic acid therapy and incidence of increases in venous plasma ammonia. *Ther Drug Monit* 1985; 7:290–294.
185. Zaccara G, Paganini M, Campostrini R, et al. Effect of associated antiepileptic treatment on valproate-induced hyperammonemia. *Ther Drug Monit* 1985; 7:185–190.
186. Warter JM, Brandt C, Marescaux C, et al. The renal origin of sodium valproate-induced hyperammonemia in fasting humans. *Neurology* 1983; 33:1136–1140.
187. Gidal BE, Inglese CM, Meyer JF, et al. Diet- and valproate-induced transient hyperammonemia: effect of L-carnitine. *Pediatr Neurol* 1997; 16(4):301–305.
188. Bohles H, Sewell AC, Wenzel D. The effect of carnitine supplementation in valproate-induced hyperammonaemia. *Acta Paediatr* 1996; 85(4):446–449.
189. Laub MC, Paetake-Brunner I, Jaeger G. Serum carnitine during valproate acid therapy. *Epilepsia* 1986; 27 Suppl 5:559–562.
190. Coulter DL. Carnitine deficiency in epilepsy: risk factors and treatment. *J Child Neurol* 1995; 10 Suppl 2:S32–S39.
191. Triggs WJ, Gilmore RL, Millington DS, et al. Valproate associated carnitine deficiency and malignant cerebral edema in the absence of hepatic failure. *Int J Clin Pharmacol Ther* 1997; 35(9):353–356.
192. Ishikura H, Matsuo N, Matsubara M, et al. Valproic acid overdose and L-carnitine therapy. *J Anal Toxicol* 1996; 20(1):55–58.
193. Murakami K, Sugimoto T, Woo M, Nishida N, et al. Effect of L-carnitine supplementation on acute valproate intoxication. *Epilepsia* 1996; 37(7):687–689.
194. Margraf JW, Dreifuss FE. Amenorrhea following initiation of therapy with valproic acid. *Neurology* 1981; 31:159 (abstract).
195. Isojarvi JI, Laatikainen TJ, Pakarinen AJ, Juntunen KT, et al. Polycystic ovaries and hyperandrogenism in women taking valproate for epilepsy. *N Engl J Med* 1993; 19:1383–1388.
196. Isojarvi JI, Laatikainen TJ, Knip M, Pakarinen AJ, et al. Obesity and endocrine disorders in women taking valproate for epilepsy. *Ann Neurol* 1996; 39:579–584.
197. Isojarvi JI, Rattya J, Myllyla VV, et al. Valproate, lamotrigine, and insulin-mediated risks in women with epilepsy. *Ann Neurol* 1998; 43:446–451.
198. Isojärvi JI, Tauboll E, Pakarinen AJ, et al. Altered ovarian function and cardiovascular risk factors in valproate-treated women. Am J Med 2001; 111:290–296.
199. Luef G, Abraham I, Trinka E, et al. Hyperandrogenism, postprandial hyperinsulinism and the risk of PCOS in a cross sectional study of women with epilepsy treated with valproate. *Epilepsy Res* 2002; 48:91–102.
200. Cook JS, Bale JF, Hoffman RP. Pubertal arrest associated with valproic acid therapy. *Pediatr Neurol* 1992; 8:229–231.
201. Sharma S, Jacobs HS. Polycystic ovary syndrome associated with treatment with the anticonvulsant sodium valproate. *Curr Opin Obstet Gynecol* 1997; 9(6):391–392.
202. Bauer J, Jarre A, Klingmuller D, Elger CE. Polycystic ovary syndrome in patients with focal epilepsy: a study in 93 women. *Epilepsy Res* 2000; 41:163–167.
203. Genton P, Bauer J, Duncan S, et al. On the association of valproate and polycystic ovaries. *Epilepsia* 2001; 42:295–304.
204. Isojärvi JI, Tauboll E, Tapanainen JS, et al. On the association between valproate and polycystic ovary syndrome: a response and an alternative view. *Epilepsia* 2001; 42:305–310.
205. Morrell MJ, Giudice L, Flynn KL, et al. Predictors of ovarian failure in women with epilepsy. *Ann Neurol* 2002; 52:704–711.
206. Luef G, Abraham I, Haslinger M, et al. Polycystic ovaries, obesity and insulin resistance in women with epilepsy. A comparative study of carbamazepine and valproic acid in 105 women. *J Neurol* 2002; 249:835–841.

207. Meo R, Bilo L. Polycystic ovary syndrome and epilepsy: a review of the evidence. *Drugs* 2003; 63:1185–1227.
208. Vajda FJ, O'Brien TJ, Hitchcock A, Graham J, et al. Critical relationship between sodium valproate dose and human teratogenicity: results of the Australian register of anti-epileptic drugs in pregnancy. *J Clin Neurosci* 2004; 11:854–858.
209. Wyszynski DF, Nambisan M, Surve T, Alsdorf RM, et al. Antiepileptic drug pregnancy registry. Increased rate of major malformations in offspring exposed to valproate during pregnancy. *Neurology* 2005; 64:961–965.
210. McMahon CL, Braddock SR. Septo-optic dysplasia as a manifestation of valproic acid embryopathy. *Teratology* 2001; 64:83–86.
211. Mawer G, Clayton-Smith J, Coyle H, et al. Outcome of pregnancy in women attending an outpatient epilepsy clinic: adverse features associated with higher doses of sodium valproate. *Seizure* 2002; 11:1059–1031.
212. Bjerkedal T, Czeizel A, Goujard J, et al. Valproic acid and spina bifida. *Lancet* 1982; 2:1096 (letter).
213. Lindhout D, Meinardi H. Spina bifida and in utero exposure to valproate. *Lancet* 1984; 2:396 (letter).
214. Omtzigt JGC, Los FJ, Grobbee DE, et al. The risk of spina bifida aperta after first-trimester exposure to valproate in a prenatal cohort. *Neurology* 1992; 42 Suppl 5:119–125.
215. Yerby MS. Management issues for women with epilepsy: neural tube defects and folic acid supplementation. *Neurology* 2003; 61 Suppl 2:S23–S26.
216. Samren EB, van Duijn CM, Hiilesmaa VK, et al. Maternal use of antiepileptic drugs and the risk of major congenital malformations. *Epilepsia* 1997; 38:981–990.
217. Duncan S, Mercho S, Lopes-Cendes I, et al. Repeated neural tube defects and valproate monotherapy suggest a pharmacogenetic abnormality. *Epilepsia* 2001; 42:750–753.
218. Wegner C, Nau H. Alteration of embryonic folate metabolism by valproic acid during organogenesis. *Neurology* 1992; 42 Suppl 5:17–24.
219. Adab N, Jacoby A, Smith D, Chadwick D. Additional educational needs in children born to mothers with epilepsy. *J Neurol Neurosurg Psychiatry* 2001; 70:15–21.
220. Adab N, Kini U, Vinten J, et al. The longer term outcome of children born to mothers with epilepsy. *J Neurol Neurosurg Psychiatry* 2004; 75:1575–1583.
221. Jeavons PM, Clark JE, Harding GFA. Valproate and curly hair. *Lancet* 1977; 1:359.
222. Herranz JL, Arteaga R, Armijo JA. Change in hair colour induced by valproic acid. *Dev Med Child Neurol* 1987; 23:386–387.
223. Ettinger A, Moshe S, Shinnar S. Edema associated with long-term valproate therapy. *Epilepsia* 1990; 31:211–213.
224. Herranz JL, Arteaga R, Armijo JA. Side effects of sodium valproate in monotherapy controlled by plasma levels: a study in 88 pediatric patients. *Epilepsia* 1982; 23: 203–214.
225. Panayiotopoulos CP. Nocturnal enuresis associated with sodium valproate. *Lancet* 1985; 1:980–981.
226. Choonra IA. Sodium valproate and enuresis. *Lancet* 1985; 1:1276.
227. Branten AJ, Wetzels JF, Weber AM, Koene RA. Hyponatremia due to sodium valproate. *Ann Neurol* 1998; 43(2):265–267 (letter).
228. Hyson C, Sadler M. Cross sensitivity of skin rashes with antiepileptic drugs. *Can J Neurol* 1997; 24(3):245–249.
229. Sato Y, Kondo I, Ishida S, Motooka H, et al. Decreased bone mass and increased bone turnover with valproate therapy in adults with epilepsy. *Neurology* 2001; 57:445–449.
230. Boluk A, Guzelipek M, Savli H, et al. The effect of valproate on bone mineral density in adult epileptic patients. *Pharmacol Res* 2004; 50:93–97.
231. Oner N, Kaya M, Karasalihoglu S, Karaca H, et al. Bone mineral metabolism changes in epileptic children receiving valproic acid. *J Paediatr Child Health* 2004; 40:470–473.
232. Kumandas S, Koklu E, Gumus H, Koklu S, et al. Effect of carbamezapine and valproic acid on bone mineral density, IGF-I and IGFBP-3. *J Pediatr Endocrinol Metab* 2006; 19:529–534.
233. Vestergaard P, Rejnmark L, Mosekilde L. Epilepsia. Fracture risk associated with use of antiepileptic drugs. *Epilepsia* 2004; 45:1330–1337.
234. Lundberg B, Nergardh A, Boreus LO. Plasma concentrations of valproate during maintenance therapy in epileptic children. *J Neurol* 1982; 228:133–141.
235. Devinsky O, Leppik I, Willmore LJ, et al. Safety of intravenous valproate. *Ann Neurol* 1995; 38(4):670–674.
236. Boggs JG, Preis K. Successful initiation of combined therapy with valproate sodium injection and divalproex sodium extended-release tablets in the epilepsy monitoring unit. *Epilepsia* 2005; 46:949–951.
237. Hovinga CA, Chicella MF, Rose DF, Eades SK, et al. Use of intravenous valproate in three pediatric patients with nonconvulsive or convulsive status epilepticus. *Ann Pharmacother* 1999; 33:579–584.
238. Chez MG, Hammer MS, Loeffel M, Nowinski C, et al. Clinical experience of three pediatric and one adult case of spike-and-wave status epilepticus treated with injectable valproic acid. *J Child Neurol* 1999; 14:239–242.
239. Sheth RD, Gidal BE. Intravenous valproic acid for myoclonic status epilepticus. *Neurology* 2000; 54:1201–1202.
240. Sinha S, Naritoku DK. Intravenous valproate is well tolerated in unstable patients with status epilepticus. *Neurology* 2000; 55:722–724.
241. Überall MA, Trollmann R, Wunsiedler U, Wenzel D. Intravenous valproate in pediatric epilepsy patients with refractory status epilepticus. *Neurology* 2000; 54:2188–2189.
242. Limdi NA, Shimpi AV, Faught E, Gomez CR, et al. Efficacy of rapid IV administration of valproic acid for status epilepticus. *Neurology* 2005; 64:353–355.
243. Giroud M, Gras D, Escousse A, Dumas R, et al. Use of injectable valproic acid in status epilepticus: a pilot study. *Drug Invest* 1993; 5:154–159.
244. Wheless JW, Vazquez BR, Kanner AM, Ramsay RE, et al. Rapid infusion with valproate sodium is well tolerated in patients with epilepsy. *Neurology* 2004; 63:1507–1508.
245. Gjerloff I, Arentsen J, Alving J, Secher BG. Monodose versus 3 daily doses of sodium valproate: a controlled trial. *Acta Neurol Scand* 1984; 69:120–124.
246. Stefan H, Burr W, Fichsel H, Fröscher W, et al. Intensive follow-up monitoring in patients with once daily evening administration of sodium valproate. *Epilepsia* 1974; 25:152–160.
247. Rowan AJ, Binnie CD, Warfield CA, Meinardi H, et al. The delayed effect of sodium valproate on the photoconvulsive response in man. *Epilepsia* 1979; 20:61–68.
248. Burr W, Fröscher W, Hoffmann F, Stefan H. Lack of significant correlation between circadian profiles of valproic acid serum levels and epileptiform electroencephalographic activity. *Ther Drug Monit* 1984; 6:179–181.
249. Chadwick DW. Concentration-effect relationships of valproic acid. *Clin Pharmacokinet* 1985; 10:155–163.

54 Vigabatrin

Günter Krämer
Gabriele Wohlrab

Gamma-aminobutyric acid (GABA) is the major inhibitory neurotransmitter in the mammalian brain. Vigabatrin (gamma-vinyl-GABA, 4-amino-5-hexenoic acid; VGB) was synthesized in 1974 as a structural GABA analog with a vinyl appendage. The aim was to achieve an enzyme-activated inhibition of GABA catabolism (1). It has been regarded as a prime example of a drug developed on a rational scientific basis for treatment of a disease (2). VGB was first marketed as an antiepileptic drug (AED) for adults in the United Kingdom in 1989 and thereafter in most European countries (3). The application was extended in 1990 to the use of VGB in children suffering from refractory epilepsy, and later to its use as monotherapy for infantile spasms. Although VGB has been approved in over 65 countries worldwide, its usage has declined after the detection of persistent peripheral visual field defects (VFD) in up to more than 50% of the patients, with restrictions in its approval.

CHEMISTRY

VGB is a white to off-white crystalline amino acid that is highly water soluble and only slightly soluble in ethanol and methanol. The molecular weight is 129.16, and the conversion factor is 7.75 (mg/L $\times$ 7.75 = μmol/L). VGB exists as a racemic mixture of S(+)- and R(–)-enantiomers in equal proportions. The S(+)-enantiomer is responsible for the pharmacologic action, whereas the R(–)-enantiomer is inactive (4, 5). The only available forms of VGB are oral formulations (tablets and sachets, containing 500 mg).

ANIMAL PHARMACOLOGY

The anticonvulsant effect of VGB has been demonstrated in numerous animal models. Whereas it is inactive in models such as maximal electroshock or pentylenetetrazol, it protects against bicuculline-induced myoclonic activity, strychnine-induced tonic seizures, isoniazid-induced generalized seizures, audiogenic seizures in mice, light-induced seizures in the baboon, and amygdala-kindled seizures in the rat (6).

The usual animal preclinical safety studies carried out in rats, mice, dogs, and monkeys demonstrated no significant adverse effects on the liver, kidney, lung, heart, or gastrointestinal tract. Studies revealed no evidence of mutagenic or carcinogenic effects. However, in the brain, microvacuolation has been observed in white matter tracts of rats, mice, and dogs at doses of 30–50 mg/kg/day. In the monkey, these lesions were minimal or equivocal.

This effect is caused by a separation of the outer lamellar sheath of myelinated fibers, a change characteristic of intramyelinic edema. In both rats and dogs the intramyelinic edema was reversible upon discontinuation of VGB, and even with continued treatment histologic regression was observed. In rodents, minor residual changes consisting of swollen axons and mineralized microbodies have been observed (7, 8).

VGB-associated retinotoxicity has been observed in albino rats, but not in pigmented rats, dogs, or monkeys. The retinal changes in albino rats were characterized as focal or multifocal disorganization of the outer nuclear layer with displacement of nuclei into the rod and cone area. The other layers of the retina were not affected. Although the histologic appearance of these lesions was similar to that found in albino rats following excessive exposure to light, the retinal changes may also represent a direct drug-induced effect (7).

Although there is no evidence of intramyelinic edema in humans, the U.S. Food and Drug Administration (FDA) halted clinical studies with VGB in the United States because of these findings for 5 years between 1983 and 1988. Tests done to confirm lack of significant adverse effect on neurologic function include evoked potentials, computed tomography (CT) and magnetic resonance imaging (MRI) scans, cerebrospinal fluid (CSF) analyses, and, in a small number of cases, neuropathologic examinations of brain specimens (8, 9).

Further animal experiments have shown that VGB has no negative influence on fertility or pup development. No teratogenicity was seen in rats at doses up to 150 mg/kg (three times the human dose) or in rabbits in doses up to 100 mg/kg. However, in rabbits, a slight increase in the incidence of cleft palate at doses of 150–200 mg/kg was seen. Therefore, the usage of VGB is not recommended for women with childbearing potential (10).

In neonatal rat brains, the application of VGB (50, 100, or 200 mg/kg twice daily on three consecutive days) elicited apoptotic neurodegeneration in a dose-dependent manner at a threshold dose of 100 mg/kg of body weight. However, the same apoptotic processes have also been shown for other AEDs such as valproate (VPA), phenytoin (PHT), and phenobarbital, which are commonly used AEDs in pediatric epilepsies (11, 12).

MECHANISM OF ACTION

VGB acts by replacing GABA as a substrate of GABA-transaminase (GABA-T) (13). However, because VGB possesses an inert appendage at the gamma-position, it prevents the transamination of GABA to form succinic acid semialdehyde by irreversible and covalent binding to GABA-T, causing its permanent inactivation (14, 15). This results in prolonged elevation of brain GABA levels without any major influence on other enzymes involved in GABA synthesis and metabolism. The effect is maximal 3 to 4 hours after administration and maintained for at least 24 hours. Thus, the major pharmacologic effects of VGB are determined not by the half-life of the drug itself but by that of GABA-T. Restoration of normal enzyme activity by resynthesis after withdrawal of VGB takes several days (16). In addition, VGB significantly reduces the activity of the plasma alanine aminotransferase (ALAT) between 20% and 100% (17, 18).

In patients with epilepsy, a dose-related (up to 3 g/day) elevation of free GABA, total GABA, and homocarnosine (a dipeptide of GABA) CSF levels could be demonstrated (19). ^{1}H-MR spectroscopy has shown that the brain GABA content in the occipital region of patients with epilepsy increased two- to threefold (20–22). Increasing VGB dosage from 3 to 6 g/day did not result in a further increase in brain GABA concentrations, most probably because of a feedback inhibition of glutamic acid decarboxylase (GAD), the GABA-synthesizing enzyme, at high GABA concentrations.

In young children no studies of GABA levels in CSF during VGB treatment have been performed, and GABA levels in brain have not been measured by MR spectroscopy. In a study using ^{11}C-flumazenil (FMZ)-positron emission tomography (PET) imaging, 15 children (age 1–8 years) with drug-resistant epilepsy were studied to determine whether prolonged treatment with VGB interferes with age-related changes of in-vivo $GABA_A$-receptor bindings (23). Seven of these children were treated with VGB (1,000–2,500 mg/day) for at least 3 months, used as add-on therapy with one other AED. Eight age-matched children, treated with one to three other AEDs, were used as a control group. The VGB-treated children were observed to have significantly lower hemispheric FMZ volume of distribution (*Vd*) in all cortical regions and the cerebellum. This led to the conclusion that VGB induces a decrease in $GABA_A$-receptor binding in the cortex and cerebellum of the developing epileptic brain. Further studies of this age-specific drug effect concerning the reversibility and functional consequences are urgently needed because of the important role of the GABAergic system in developmental nervous system plasticity.

BIOTRANSFORMATION, PHARMACOKINETICS, AND DRUG INTERACTIONS IN HUMANS

Pharmacokinetics

Infants and Children. VGB is rapidly and almost completely absorbed from the gastrointestinal tract. Absorption is faster and more complete in older than in younger children, and therefore, the bioavailability of the drug is higher. Accordingly, the area under the curve (AUC) values for both isomers are significantly lower in infants than in children, which in turn are lower than in adults. A pharmacokinetic study after a single racemic 50 mg/kg VGB dose in six infants (5–24 months) and six children (4–14 years) with intractable epilepsy showed results comparable to those in adults for the children, mainly with regard to the elimination of the active S(+)-enantiomer, which seems to be age independent (24). In contrast to adults, in whom t_{max} of the inactive R(–)-enantiomer is about twice that of the active S(+)-enantiomer, no differences were found for t_{max} of the two allosteric forms in children. However, the mean AUC of the R(–)-enantiomer was also significantly greater. Larger apparent volumes of distribution (V/F values) were found for the active S(+)-enantiomer only in younger children. No differences were observed between infants and children aged 4 to 14 years. Smaller V/F values have been measured in adults.

Although the drug-metabolizing capacity is reduced in newborns—particularly in those born prematurely—and increases rapidly during the first weeks of life, the mean values of C_{max} and AUC were significantly lower for the active S(+)-enantiomer following single oral doses of 125 mg of VGB racemate in six neonates. No difference was found for the time to reach peak plasma concentrations (t_{max}). Repeated administration of 125 mg twice daily over 4 days showed no evidence of accumulation of either enantiomer (25).

In children, the renal excretion of unchanged drug is the main route of elimination; no metabolites of VGB have been identified. The mean $t_{1/2}$ of the S(+)-enantiomer is significantly longer than that of the inactive R(–)-enantiomer, but only in younger children (26). The $t_{1/2}$ and clearance (CL/F) values are shorter and higher in young children.

In conclusion, despite lower AUC values in children, pharmacokinetics of VGB appeared to be little influenced by age, and VGB accumulation during multiple dose administration (5 days) did not occur (24). These findings support the use of similar doses per kilogram according to age between 1 month and 15 years of age.

Adults. Food does not influence absorption (27), and peak plasma concentrations (C_{max}) are reached within 0.5 to 2 hours after single doses (28). Areas under the plasma concentration time curve (AUC) as well as C_{max} indicate linear pharmacokinetics over the dose range of 0.5 to 4 g. VGB is widely distributed in the body with a volume of distribution of 0.8 L/kg; levels in the cerebrospinal fluid (CSF) are approximately 10% of those in the blood (29).

VGB is neither bound to proteins nor does it influence the protein binding of other drugs or cytochrome P450-dependent enzymes. Elimination is primarily renal with a renal clearance of unchanged drug accounting for 60% to 70% of the total clearance, which indicates an oral bioavailability of at least that magnitude. The elimination half-life ($t_{1/2}$) is between 5 and 7 hours, but in patients taking hepatic enzyme-inducing drugs, slightly shorter half-life values of 4–6 hours have been observed (29, 30).

Because about 60% of the drug is removed from the blood during hemodialysis, VGB should be administered thereafter (31). The passage of both enantiomers of VGB across the human placenta is slow, and the concentration ratio in breast milk compared to plasma for the active S(+)-enantiomer is below 0.5 (32).

Drug Interactions

VGB has no effect on the plasma concentrations of VPA (33) and felbamate (FBM) (34). Usually there is also no effect on carbamazepine (CBZ) levels, but an increase of up to 27% has been described by two authors (35, 36), who studied pediatric and adult patients. A decrease of up to 50% was observed by other investigators (37, 38). After a latency of some weeks VGB reduces PHT levels about 25% without altered absorption (39) or plasma protein binding (40). In children with epilepsy, the drop of PHT levels can be even more pronounced (41). Serum levels of phenobarbital and primidone can also be slightly reduced by VGB (30). VPA has no effect on VGB plasma levels (33), and this has also been described for the other established AEDs (42), although a shorter half-life of VGB in patients on enzyme-inducing drugs has been observed (29, 30). FBM leads to a slight increase of the active S(+)-enantiomer (34). Regarding other drugs than AEDs, VGB has no effect on oral steroid contraceptives (43), and there is no information on effects of other drugs on VGB (44).

Drug Monitoring

VGB can be determined in biologic fluids by high-performance liquid chromatography (HPLC) and gas chromatography–mass spectroscopy (45). A sensitive HPLC method for the simultaneous determination of VGB and gabapentin (GBP) in serum and urine has been described (46). The value of plasma level determinations for therapeutic drug monitoring of VGB is mainly limited because of its mechanism of action, with irreversible enzyme inhibition resulting in a biologic half-life of several days. Consequently, in a study of 16 children with refractory epilepsy there was no strong correlation between VGB dosages, plasma concentrations, and clinical efficacy. Those patients who responded to VGB showed a good correlation between seizure reduction and VGB dosage, but there was no positive correlation between seizure reduction and either inhibition of platelet

GABA-T activity or plasma concentration (47). This was confirmed by another study in 36 patients with VGB dosages between 1,000 and 4,000 mg/day (48). Correspondingly, a proposed tentative target range for the serum concentration of VGB of between 6 and 278 µmol/L is very broad (49).

CLINICAL EFFICACY

Infants and Children

Partial and Generalized Epilepsies. Following the "usual clinical procedure" to test new AEDs, VGB has been used in refractory epilepsies as an add-on medication to approved AEDs. In most countries, no randomized, placebo-controlled, double-blind trials (evidence class I) in infants and children were published before approval, which was granted on the basis of compassionate experience and open-label studies. Small open trials (41, 50–59) resulted in a response with >50% reduction in seizure frequency in 23% to 89% of patients. The efficacy was generally similar to that reported in adults. One prospective study (58), encompassing 175 children (neonates, children, and adolescents from age 1 week to 19 years) with partial seizures, led to about 30% of patients becoming seizure free and 70% achieving a >50% reduction in seizure frequency. The highest percentage of responders was found in patients with tuberous sclerosis complex (85%), and the lowest in patients with tumors (45%). VGB was effective against both simple and complex partial seizures and secondary generalization.

A randomized withdrawal study of placebo (VGB blindly stopped) versus VGB (continued) in children who had responded earlier to VGB was published by Chiron et al. (60). The seizure frequency was compared to the prerandomization period. A more than 50% increase in seizure frequency induced drop out. The patients remaining in the study were more numerous (93%) than on placebo (46%)($P < 0.01$) and seizure frequency was lower on VGB than placebo ($P < 0.05$).

Two dose-response studies performed in a total of 81 children with refractory epilepsy (61, 62) demonstrated an optimal efficacy with a dose between 40 and 80 mg/kg/day (mean, 60 mg/kg/day), which is slightly higher than in adults (35–65 mg/kg/day). Further increase of the dose in nonresponders, although well tolerated, did not result in a higher number of patients being controlled. On the basis of pharmacokinetic and dose-response studies, the following dosage regimen for children was recommended and approved: starting dose: 40 mg/kg/day, increasing to 80 to 100 mg/kg/day, depending on response.

The satisfying results obtained with VGB in children with drug-resistant epilepsy have prompted some investigators to use it as first-line treatment in partial epilepsy. Three open, prospective and randomized studies with a follow-up of 6 months, and 2 years, respectively (63–65; evidence class III), compared the efficacy of VGB (n = 104) and CBZ (n = 100) in monotherapy in newly diagnosed children with partial epilepsy. Both therapeutic groups included patients with idiopathic, cryptogenic, and symptomatic partial epilepsy at comparable levels. In these trials the evaluation of the efficacy of VGB and CBZ did not reveal any significant differences. Interictal electroencephalographic (EEG) abnormalities decreased in VGB patients more than in CBZ patients. In conclusion, VGB seemed to be an effective AED as primary monotherapy in partial childhood epilepsy.

Long-term efficacy data of VGB treatment in children up to 10 years of age have also been published. One of these studies investigated a cohort of 196 children with drug-resistant epilepsy and VGB as add-on therapy over a period of 1.5 to 5.5 years (66). The evaluation of the long-term prognosis was focused on the incidence of increased seizure frequency, loss of efficacy, and appearance of new seizure types. Increase of seizure frequency occurred in only 10% of patients, with half occurring during the first month of treatment. Patients with atypical absences had the highest incidence of increase in seizure frequency (38%) compared with less than 8% of those with partial seizures. Nonprogressive myoclonic epilepsy and Lennox-Gastaut syndrome (LGS) showed the greatest increase in seizure frequency, 38% and 29%, respectively. Loss of efficacy was reported in 12% of children who were taking VGB (25–50% of responders, some of whom had been seizure free). Three-quarters of these patients had never had their seizures controlled prior to the introduction of VGB. Loss of efficacy was not connected to any specific seizure type except atypical absences and clonic seizures. The average time reported for loss of efficacy was 7 months. In 38%, the loss of efficacy was simultaneous to an attempt to decrease concomitant antiepileptic medication. Eleven percent of the children developed new seizure types, mainly myoclonic and new partial seizures, after a very variable time lag. Partial seizures were better tolerated than the initial seizure type and had little impact on the patient's overall clinical development.

Based on the long-term study of patients with intractable epilepsies of childhood, a sustained beneficial effect of VGB on seizure frequency can be expected in children with partial rather than with generalized seizures. A comparison of lamotrigine (LTG; n = 132), VGB (n = 80), and GBP (n = 39) as add-on therapy in children with intractable epilepsy was performed in a 10-year follow-up study (67). Thirty-tree percent of the children taking LTG were seizure free or had a sustained reduction of seizure frequency of >50%. In contrast, only 19% of the VGB and 15% of the GBP-group still responded to the additional drug. The main difference was found in patients with generalized epilepsy, respectively, in patients classified as having LGS, myoclonic-astatic epilepsy, or unclassified epilepsies. On the other hand, no significant difference in efficacy was found in children with partial seizures.

The long-term retention rate seems to be lower for VGB than for LTG in children with difficult-to-treat epilepsies (68). Comparing efficacy and retention at 5 years in an open label study, the initial efficacy showed no difference (VGB n = 56, responder 32%; LTG n = 39, responder 28%) after 6 weeks, and 4 months, respectively. In contrast, the retention at 5 years was still 25.6% in the LTG group, but was reduced to 8.9% in the VGB group. A loss of efficacy occurred in 10 of the initial 18 responders, usually within the first 9 months after initial response.

Several anecdotal case reports have described favorable effects in neonatal seizures due to Ohtahara syndrome (69), partial seizures in Sturge-Weber syndrome (70), Landau-Kleffner syndrome (71), and infantile spasms in Down syndrome (72) as well as an improved outcome in Aicardi syndrome (73). However, the numbers of patients in these reports are too small for a meaningful analysis.

In conclusion, VGB has proved to be a useful AED for add-on treatment of partial seizures with and without secondary generalization, refractory to first-line AEDs. Loss of efficacy, increase of seizures in specific seizure types, and side effects (see following) must be kept in mind. The following studies allow for a better definition of the profile of activity of VGB in different types of drug-resistant epilepsies, including the epileptic syndromes specific to childhood and for the assessment of the tolerability of VGB in children.

Infantile Spasms (West Syndrome). One single randomized placebo-controlled study provided class I evidence for the efficacy of VGB in infantile spasms (IS) (74). This trial, which included children with newly diagnosed IS (n = 20 in each group) showed that at the end of the 5-day double-blind phase, seven (35%) patients treated with VGB were spasm free and five (25%) had resolution of hypsarrhythmia compared with two (10%) and one (5%), respectively, in the placebo-group (P = 0.063). Relapse was seen in four (20%) of the VGB-treated patients. At the end of the study 42% of the 36 patients who entered the open phase were spasm free with VGB monotherapy. No patient withdrew from the study because of side effects.

In addition, three randomized controlled studies provide class III evidence. The first class III study (75) compared VGB (100–150 mg/kg/day) with adrenocorticotropic hormone (ACTH or tetracosactide; 10 IU/day) as first-line therapy in 42 infants with IS. The alternative drug was administered in nonresponders (within 20 days) or in case of intolerance to the initial therapy. Cessation of IS was observed in 48% (11 of 23) of the VGB-treated patients and 74% (14 of 19) of those treated with ACTH. The response to VGB was seen within 14 days. Follow-up data for up to 44 months showed only one relapse. In the ACTH group six patients showed a relapse 40–45 days after cessation of ACTH and replacement by a benzodiazepine.

In a multicenter study (76) including 142 patients, spasms ceased completely within 2 weeks in 23% of the patients, and this effect increased to 65% by the end of a 3-month open label period. Infants were randomly assigned to receive low-dose (18–36 mg/kg/day) or high-dose (100–148 mg/kg/day) treatment. A marked difference in response in dependency to the VGB dosage was observed. Within the first 2 weeks, 8 of 75 patients (10.6%) of the low-dose and 24 of 67 (35.8%) of the high-dose group responded. The response increased considerably during the follow-up period (42% at 4 weeks, 55% at 2 months, and 65% at 3 months), in the course of which the infants allocated to the high-dose treatment showed an earlier cessation of spasms.

The third class III study was a multicenter, randomized controlled trial comparing VGB with prednisolone or tetracosactide in a 14-day trial and a 14-month follow-up (77, 78). Of 52 patients randomized to the VGB group, 28 (54%) were spasm free within 2 weeks. The efficacy of VGB was lower than for the hormone-treated patients, with 21 of 30 (70%) of the patients receiving prednisolone and 19 of 25 (76%) assigned tetracosactide becoming spasm free. Adverse events were reported in 28 of 52 (54%) infants taking VGB, mainly drowsiness and gastrointestinal complaints. Thirty of 55 (55%) children taking hormonal treatment suffered from side effects, mainly irritability and gastrointestinal problems as well. Of the 55 infants allocated to hormonal treatment, 27 received VGB after day 14 because of failure to achieve cessation of spasms (12 of 27), seizure relapse (14 of 27), and one for treatment of focal seizures, respectively. Of the 52 primarily given VGB, 22 received a hormone therapy, 3 due to a relapse. The response rate was 9 of 12 (75%) for VGB and 14 of 19 for hormone treatment, respectively. There were five deaths during the follow-up period. One child died of *Staphylococcus aureus* septicemia on day 15 of treatment with prednisolone. The deaths of the other four children were related to their underlying disease.

Except for the low dose option performed by the U.S. Infantile Spasms Vigabatrin Study Group (76), all prospective studies used cessation of IS by caregiver observation as the primary efficacy endpoint. Initial doses of VGB varied between 50 and 150 mg/kg/day, but in all studies dose was titrated up to 150 mg/kg/day. The relapse rate in these four randomized controlled studies ranged from 8% to 20%.

In addition to these controlled studies, there have been many reports on VGB treatment in newly diagnosed or refractory IS. They included different patient groups regarding symptomatic or cryptogenic etiology. In six open label uncontrolled prospective (class IV) observations (79–84) with between 23 and 116 enrolled patients, the overall response rate varied between 26% and 66.7%. For cryptogenic cases the response ranged from 50% to 100%, and for infants with symptomatic West syndrome from 19% to 57%. The relapse rate was low, ranging from a single case to 14%. The percentage of complete cessation of IS without relapse was comparable for newly diagnosed patients, 43% (81) and 45% (80), and refractory patients, 43% (85) and 48% (79).

In a retrospective survey of the safety and efficacy data from IS patients treated initially with VGB monotherapy at 59 European centers (86), the dosage varied from 20 to 400 mg/kg/day (mean dose, 99 mg/kg/day) and the duration of therapy ranged from 0.2 to 28.6 months. Complete disappearance of IS was reported in 131 of 192 (68%) of the patients. Treatment with VGB did not result in any improvement in 24 (12.5%) of the patients and 1 patient deteriorated. Of the subgroups of IS types, patients with tuberous sclerosis had the highest response rate (27 of 28 = 97%), followed by patients with cryptogenic IS (69.4%) and symptomatic IS of other causes (59.7%). Infants younger than 3 months at the onset responded better (18 of 20 infants, 90%) than those with a later seizure onset (65%). Of the 131 patients with complete initial response to VGB, 28 (21.3%) relapsed at a mean period of 4 months. There were few adverse events reported, and they were generally mild (somnolence, insomnia, hypotonia, hyperkinesia). Therefore drug withdrawal was necessary only in a few patients (~1%).

In all studies the time from initiation of therapy to cessation of spasms ranged from 2 to a maximum of 35 days, and sometimes was observed after only 1 or 2 doses. The placebo-controlled studies performed by Vigevano and Eltermann (75, 76) as well as several different open-label studies (81, 82) proposed a 2-week cutoff for qualifying responders. The time to EEG response was 7 to 35 days and 11% to 83% of the children had resolution of hypsarrhythmia.

The prospective studies cited used VGB in dosages between 18 and 200 mg/kg/day. Mitchell and Shah (87) presumed a dose-independent response to VGB in infantile spasms. They reported a complete cessation of infantile spasms and resolution of hypsarrhythmia at doses ranging from 25 to 135 mg/kg/day in 12 of 20 patients. In contrast an Asian study (88) mentioned a relapse rate of 56% within 6 months, in all patients who received a reduced dosage (average, 59 mg/kg/day) in comparison to the initial dose. It was concluded that at least 70 mg/kg/day will be necessary to achieve adequate seizure control.

Tuberous Sclerosis Complex. VGB has been found most effective in the treatment of IS due to tuberous sclerosis complex (TSC). This has been shown in a multicenter retrospective survey (86), which showed a response rate of 96% (27 of 28 children obtained a complete cessation of spasms). These results were confirmed by a prospective randomized trial comparing VGB and hydrocortisone (89). The monotherapy study in 22 newly diagnosed patients with IS and confirmed diagnosis of tuberous sclerosis was performed with an optional crossover for nonresponders. It showed a highly significant difference between oral hydrocortisone (15 mg/kg/day) and VGB (150 mg/kg/day) both before and after crossover. In patients taking VGB the efficacy was 100% (11 of 11), whereas it was less than half (5 of 11) for patients taking hydrocortisone. All 7 patients who crossed from hydrocortisone to VGB (6 for inefficacy, 1 for adverse events) also became completely seizure free. In addition, there was a statistically significant difference for the mean time to disappearance of IS favoring VGB (3.5 days vs. 13 days), and side effects were less common.

Hancock and Osborne (90) reviewed 16 studies with 77 patients with TCS investigating the use of VGB in IS. Of the 313 patients without TCS, 170 (54%) had complete cessation of their IS; of the 77 patients with TCS, 73 (95%) had complete cessation. They concluded that VGB should be considered as first-line monotherapy for the treatment of IS in infants with either a confirmed diagnosis of TCS or those at high risk, that is, those with a first-degree relative with TCS. In a later review the same authors (91) concluded that they found no single treatment to be proven to be more efficacious in treating IS than any of the others, with the exception of VGB in the treatment of IS in TCS in one underpowered study. Other researchers found that the VGB-induced cessation of the spasms was associated with a marked improvement of behavior and mental development (92). They hypothesized that the complete cessation of the generalized epileptic phenomena of IS seems to be a key factor for the mental outcome, even when partial seizures persist.

The particular efficacy of VGB in TSC suggests that the epileptogenesis in TSC may be related to the impairment of GABAergic transmission. However, the mechanisms underlying this etiology-related efficacy are still unknown (93). In TSC, seizures have a focal or a multifocal origin. IS might represent the secondary generalization of partial seizures and VGB may be especially able to control this secondary generalization (85). Summarizing the relevant data, Riikonen (94), who prefers steroid therapy in IS of other etiology, suggests VGB as the treatment of choice in IS caused by TSC. This opinion is shared by some other authors (95) but not by all. Recent U.S. practice parameters for the medical treatment of IS include the following two recommendations (96): (1) Vigabatrin is possibly effective for the short-term treatment of infantile spasms (level C, class III and IV evidence); (2) vigabatrin is also possibly effective for the short-term treatment of infantile spasms in the majority of children with tuberous sclerosis (level C, class III and IV evidence).

Lennox-Gastaut Syndrome. In the treatment of children with Lennox-Gastaut syndrome (LGS), study results have been controversial and the interpretation of the results has been difficult. LGS is characterized by multiple seizure types that are frequently not analyzed individually in terms of VGB response. In the first European open, add-on, noncontrolled clinical study, 26 children with LGS were included. Good seizure response was observed in less than 30% (6 of 26), and 13 of 26 were unchanged or even worse (50). Only a small number of children with LGS has been included in other studies, and most of them have not been regarded as treatment successes: In a single-blind, placebo-controlled trial (62), 2 of 7 showed a greater than 50% seizure reduction, but 2 showed increases in seizure frequency. Other small studies reported a good response in 3 of 6 (51), or none of 6 patients (97).

A good response rate to VGB in LGS was observed in only one open add-on study (98). Twenty children aged 2 to 20 years with refractory LGS were first treated with high-level VPA monotherapy, and afterwards for 12 months with add-on VGB. Eighty-five percent experienced a more than 50% reduction in seizures and 40% became seizure free under VGB. A decrease of at least 50% was observed in all seizure types (tonic, atonic, atypical absences, tonic-clonic, and complex partial seizures), except myoclonic seizures, which increased by 5%. VGB may therefore have a limited role as add-on treatment in the management of LGS but not in case of myoclonic seizures as the main seizure type.

Adults

Clinical studies with VGB have included more than 2,000 adult patients. After initial open and single-blind dose-finding studies, several randomized, double-blind, placebo-controlled crossover studies in adult patients with refractory partial epilepsies and add-on therapy with VGB were conducted.

An early Australian study in 97 patients with uncontrolled partial seizures comparing 2 and 3 g/day showed a similar efficacy, with 42% of the patients experiencing a 50% or greater reduction of their seizure frequency in comparison to placebo (=responders). In addition, the number of seizure-free days and longest seizure-free period were significantly longer during VGB and more patients had less severe and shorter seizures (99).

In addition to crossover studies, several double-blind, placebo-controlled parallel group studies were carried out. The therapeutic efficacy of VGB add-on in treatment-resistant epilepsy, as assessed as the percentage of patients having at least a 50% reduction in seizure frequency, was quite similar across the studies, with about 40% of patients being responders (for review of the earlier studies see references 100–102). In the first of more recent studies from the United States, 92 patients received VGB 3 g/day add-on and were compared to 90 patients in the placebo group (103). Significantly more patients receiving VGB were responders with 50% to 99% reduction of seizure frequency (37% vs. 18%) or seizure freedom (6% vs. 1%). The second study examined three different VGB daily doses (1, 3, or 6 g) in a total of 174 patients (104). Whereas only 7% in the placebo group were responders, the corresponding figures for the VGB groups were 24%, 51%, and 54%.

A double-blind, double-dummy substitution trial comparing add-on VGB (2–4 g daily) and VPA (1–2 g daily) in CBZ-resistant partial epilepsy allowing withdrawal of CBZ in responders showed similar percentages of responders (53% vs. 51%) and maintenance of alternative monotherapy (27% vs. 31%) (105).

Two open, single-center randomized monotherapy studies using CBZ as comparator included 100 (106) and 51 patients (107), respectively. Both studies failed to show differences in efficacy but demonstrated a more favorable side-effect profile of VGB (prior to the knowledge of VFD related to VGB). In addition, several open, long-term studies on the add-on use of VGB in adult patients with treatment-resistant partial epilepsy have been reported. The length of the follow-up varied between 9 and 78 weeks. Most of the patients included had a favorable initial response to VGB, which was maintained in 22% to 75% of the patients.

More recently, two larger randomized, double-blind, parallel-group studies have been carried out to compare the efficacy of VGB as monotherapy with CBZ and VPA in newly diagnosed epilepsy. In the VGB/CBZ study, 53% of the 229 patients receiving 2 g of VGB daily and 57% of the 230 patients receiving 600 mg of CBZ daily achieved a 6-month period of remission. However, significantly more patients receiving VGB withdrew due to lack of efficacy than with CBZ, and time to first seizure after the first 6 weeks from randomization also showed CBZ to be more effective. It was concluded that VGB cannot be recommended as a first-line drug for monotherapy of newly diagnosed partial epilepsies (108).

In the VGB/VPA study in a total of 215 patients (age range, 12–76 years), an initial open monotherapy with CBZ was followed by a blinded add-on of VGB (1–4 g/day) or VPA (0.5–2 g/day), and polytherapy in those patients resistant to optimal CBZ monotherapy before CBZ was withdrawn and monotherapy with VGB or VPA was maintained in the final study phase. The therapeutic efficacy was similar for the two study drugs (109).

In most double-blind trials in adults, the daily dose of VGB was 2 to 3 g. Initial studies suggested that 1 g might also have some therapeutic efficacy, and there are patients who benefit from doses of 4 g or more. In the U.S. study comparing daily doses of 1, 3, and 6 g, no improvement in efficacy was observed in patients given 6 g versus 3 g, but side effects increased substantially (104). Although VGB is usually administered twice daily, a double-blind pilot study in 50 patients comparing once-daily versus twice-daily add-on administration demonstrated no statistical difference (110).

During long-term treatment with VGB, development of tolerance after an initially beneficial effect is observed in about one-third (111) of the patients.

ADVERSE EFFECTS

In humans, based on histopathologic findings from autopsies and surgical brain samples of patients with an estimated 350,000 patient-years of VBG exposure, no definite case of VGB-induced intramyelinic edema corresponding to the animal data (presented in the section on animal pharmacology) has been identified (112). A single observation reported about normal ophthalmologic and neurologic findings in two children, investigated at the age of 6.10 and 7.9 years, who were exposed to VGB prenatally (113).

Most side effects during VGB treatment are usually mild and well tolerated even with high doses. In adults and older children, fatigue, drowsiness, dizziness, nystagmus, agitation, amnesia, abnormal vision, ataxia, weight increase, confusion, depression, and diarrhea were most often reported (104). In children and infants receiving VGB, drowsiness, somnolence, insomnia, hyperexcitability and agitation, weight gain, and hypertonia or hypotonia were the most frequently reported adverse events (9, 51, 114). A VGB-induced encephalopathy with stupor, confusion, and EEG slowing has been described in single cases (115–117), one of them suffering from an underlying leukodystrophy (Morbus Alexander).

An adverse event possibly related to the GABAergic mechanism of action is an increased incidence of psychosis (118), sometimes as forced normalization. A retrospective survey of behavior disorders in 81 patients described 50 cases meeting the criteria for either psychosis ($n = 28$) or depression ($n = 22$). A comparison with psychotic events in epilepsy patients never treated with VGB described an increased risk for more severe epilepsies, right-sided EEG focus, and suppression of seizures (119). A formal testing of mood disturbances in 73 adult patients with refractory epilepsy before and under treatment with VGB revealed that mood problems were the main reason for discontinuation (120). Repeated testing with a series of eight cognitive measures in a double-blind, placebo-controlled, parallel group dose-response study in patients with difficult to control focal seizures detected a decreased performance in only one cognitive test (Digit Cancellation Test) (121).

A review of U.S. and non-U.S. double-blind, placebo-controlled trials of VGB as add-on therapy for refractory partial epilepsy in a total of 717 patients revealed a significantly higher incidence of depression and psychosis without differences between treatment groups for aggressive reactions, manic symptoms, agitation, emotional lability, anxiety, or suicide attempt (122). Depression and psychosis were usually observed during the first 3 months. Depression was usually mild, and psychosis was reported to respond to reduction or discontinuation of VGB or to treatment with neuroleptics.

As a secondary effect of treatment with VGB a significant increase of alpha-aminoadipic acid in plasma and urine occurs that may mimic alpha-aminoadipic aciduria, a known rare metabolic disease. Therefore, when a genetic metabolic disease is suspected, amino acid chromatography should be performed before initiation of VGB treatment (123). In addition, VGB can interfere with urinary amino acid analysis through inhibition of catabolism of beta-alanine (124).

In 1997, three patients with severe, symptomatic, persistent visual field constriction (VFC) associated with the use of VGB were described (125). In the meantime it has been demonstrated that VFC is a very common side effect of VGB, at least in adults, and is associated with retinal cone system dysfunction (126). The most important data for adult patients are from a randomized monotherapy trial in newly diagnosed patients comparing VGB and CBZ (127). Of 32 patients receiving long-term VGB monotherapy, 13 (40%) had concentric VFC. The main reason it took almost a decade to detect this severe neurotoxicity has been that the vast majority of even severe defects were asymptomatic. However, in the meantime, it could be demonstrated that in the absence of spontaneous complaints about VFC, symptoms can be elicited by structured questioning, at least in adult patients (128).

Because VGB is often administered during different developmental stages at even higher doses (related to the body weight) and formal visual field testing is often difficult or even impossible, the risk of VGB-induced VFC is a major challenge for pediatric patients with epilepsy. Several case reports have confirmed the possibility of their occurrence in childhood. Based on an observation of 2 patients (129), Vanhatalo et al (130) performed Goldman kinetic perimetry tests on 91 visually asymptomatic Finnish children (age 5.6 to 17.9 years) with a history of VGB treatment at any level. Visual field constriction

(VFC), defined as visual field extent <70 degrees in the temporal median, was considered abnormal. This finding was observed in repeated test sessions in 17 of 91 children (18.7%). A significant inverse correlation was emphasized between the temporal extent of the visual fields and the total dose and the duration of VGB treatment. The shortest duration of VGB treatment associated with VCF was 15 months, the lowest total dosage 914 g. There was no correlation found with age at treatment onset or with total duration of the treatment.

Comparable results were reported in case reports using the same investigation procedure but encompassing smaller patient numbers. Ianetti et al (131) reported 4 of 21 children with VFC, prevailing in the nasal hemifield. One child showed a greater improvement after drug discontinuation. In further reports the range of abnormal findings was 5 of 12 children (41.6%) (132) and 10 of 14 children (71.4%) (133). In 4 of these cases, there was a preexisting visual pathway damage, and in 2 of these, optic disc pallor increased in association with constricted visual fields (133). A prospective long-term follow-up study investigated 29 children before VGB treatment and at 6-month periods up to 6.5 years and reported a variation of ocular pathology (retinal pigmentation, hypopigmented retinal spots, vascular sheathing, and optic atrophy) in 4 of 29 patients (19%) during the follow-up period. Perimetry was not performed (134). In addition to retinotoxic effects of VGB, a reduced ocular blood flow has been described (135).

In an interventional case series report, 138 patients, mainly infants, were evaluated regularly for evidence of possible VGB toxicity (136). Sequential clinical and electroretinographic (ERG) evaluations were performed every 6 months. Three children showed definite clinical findings of peripheral retinal nerve fiber layer atrophy, with relative sparing of the central or macular portion of the retina and relative nasal optic nerve atrophic changes. Some macular wrinkling was evident in one case. Progressive ERG changes showing decreased responses, especially the 30-Hz flicker response, supported the presence of decreased retinal function. The authors concluded that a recognizable and characteristic form of peripheral retinal atrophy and nasal or "inverse" optic disc atrophy can occur in a small number of children being treated with VGB. Because these changes are accompanied by electrophysiologic evidence of retinal dysfunction, discontinuation of VGB should be strongly considered.

Reversibility of VFC has been described in a few pediatric and adult patients, verified by repeated examinations (137–140). Versino and Veggiotti described a 10-year-old girl, developing clinical symptoms ("bumping into objects") 2 years after starting VGB treatment. Symptoms ceased 5 months after VGB discontinuation and perimetry significantly improved. On the other hand, due to the difficulties in testing children, improvement in perimetry examinations might be an artifact of a learning effect. Nevertheless, from a cognitive age of 9 years on, perimetry seems to be the most sensitive modality for identifying VGB toxicity (141). Abnormal ERG (142) and field-specific visual-evoked potentials (VEP), as described by Spencer and Harding (143), may be useful in monitoring children who are too young to cooperate for perimetry or who are handicapped.

Currently the minimum duration and doses of VGB treatment that can produce side effects are unknown. Short-course therapy, for instance of 6 months in children with IS (72), might reduce the risk of developing visual field constriction. However, today there are no clear data about the incidence of VFC in children treated with VGB for IS during infancy and early childhood. If VGB treatment is continued in spite of the establishment of VFC, there seems to be no progression in the majority of patients, which led to the hypothesis that VGB-associated VFC may be an idiosyncratic rather than dose-dependent toxic side effect (144). Recent U.S. practice parameters for the medical treatment of IS recommend serial ophthalmologic screening. However, data are insufficient to make recommendations regarding the frequency or type of screening that would be of value in reducing the prevalence of this complication in children (level U, class IV studies) (96).

In addition to the persistent VFC, discrete nonhemorrhagic focal lesions in the splenium of the corpus callosum have been described in six patients with epilepsy and treatment with VGB or PHTor both. In two of the patients, the lesions disappeared on follow-up MRI after withdrawal of VGB, PHT, or both (145).

The precipitation or exacerbation of myoclonic seizures, absence seizures, and nonconvulsive status have been reported (146, 147). Therefore, the prescription of VGB in idiopathic generalized epilepsies is not recommended and has been mentioned as a contraindication in some countries. The main mechanism of aggravation of epilepsy is the occurrence of an inverse pharmacodynamic effect. Children treated for epilepsy are particularly likely to suffer from paradoxical aggravation as a result of medical intervention (148). Comparable to CBZ, VGB therapy in patients with idiopathic generalized epilepsies (IGE), for instance in typical or atypical absence seizures, can result in an increase in absence seizure frequency and in absence status (66, 149). Myoclonic seizures are generally aggravated by the same drugs that aggravate IGEs. Induction and increase of myoclonic seizures, myoclonic-astatic seizures, and absence seizures are described particularly in children with Angelman syndrome (150).

CONCLUSION

VGB shows good pharmacokinetic properties with rapid onset of action and mostly tolerable side effects, especially in infancy. VGB is a very efficient AED in infants with IS, especially caused by TSC. In infants with IS, who responded to VGB, the drug could be withdrawn without a relapse after a spasm-free period of 6 months (limited data). In addition, VGB has proved to be an efficacious AED for partial seizures with and without secondary generalization, previously drug resistant to first-line AEDs. VGB is still a therapeutic option when other AEDs have failed or were poorly tolerated. However, the concern of severe of concentric VFC requires a careful risk-benefit analysis and some recent authors have omitted VGB as a treatment option in children with partial epilepsies (151).

Guidelines for prescribing VGB in children (152) may help in deciding whether to prescribe the drug. They, along with others, recommend performing visual field examination with a Goldman perimeter or a Humphrey field analyzer in children with a cognitive age of >9 years before prescribing VGB and, ideally, every 6 months while they continue to take the drug.

A clear statement concerning the indication for VGB in children is made by Wallace (153). She declared that "in clinical use, VGB should be prescribed only in very strictly defined circumstances: partial seizures refractory to other medications, and infantile spasms. Particular caution is necessary, when VGB is being considered in a young child who either is known to have, or is at risk of having, a visual defect due to other causes. Though, obviously, those who already have no vision would not be excluded from treatment with VGB."

References

1. Bey P. Mechanism-based enzyme inhibitors as an approach to drug design. In: Palfreyman MG, McCann PP, Lovenberg W, Temple JR Jr, et al, eds. *Enzymes as Targets for Drug Design*. San Diego: Academic Press, 1989:59–83.
2. Cereghino JJ. New antiepileptic drugs. In: Dodson WE, Pellock, JM, eds. *Pediatric Epilepsy; Diagnosis and Therapy*. New York: Demos, 1993:343–355.
3. Krämer G, Schmidt D, eds. Vigabatrin, Pharmakologie–Wirksamkeit–Verträglichkeit. Berlin: Springer, 1994.
4. Ben-Menachem E. Vigabatrin. In: Levy RH, Mattson RH, Meldrum BS, Perucca E, eds. *Antiepileptic Drugs*. 5th ed. Philadelphia: Lippincott Williams & Wilkins, 2002: 855–863.
5. Richens A. Pharmacology and clinical pharmacology of vigabatrin. *J Child Neurol* 1991; 6 Suppl 2:2S7–2S10.
6. Ben-Menachem E, French J. Vigabatrin. In: Engel J Jr, Pedley TA, eds. *Epilepsy. A Comprehensive Textbook*. Philadelphia: Lippincott-Raven, 1997:1609–1618.
7. Butler WH. The neuropathology of vigabatrin. *Epilepsia* 1989; 30 Suppl 3:S15–S17.
8. Cannon DJ, Buttler WH, Mumford JP, Lewis PJ. Neuropathologic findings in patients receiving long-term vigabatrin therapy for chronic intractable epilepsy. *J Child Neurol* 1991; 6 Suppl 2:2S17–2S24.
9. Fisher RS, Kerrigan JF III. Vigabatrin. Toxicity. In: Levy RH, Mattson RH, Meldrum BS, eds. *Antiepileptic Drugs*. 4th ed. New York: Raven Press, 1995:931–939.
10. Morrell MJ. The new antiepileptic drugs and women: efficacy, reproductive health, pregnancy, and fetal outcome. *Epilepsia* 1996; 37 Suppl 6:S34–S44.
11. Bittigau P, Sifringer M, Genz K, Reith E, et al. Antiepileptic drugs and apoptotic neurodegeneration in the developing brain. *Proc Natl Acad Sci U S A* 2002; 99: 15089–15094.
12. Bittigau P, Sifringer M, Ikonomidou C. Antiepileptic drugs and apoptosis in the developing brain. *Ann N Y Acad Sci* 2003; 993:103–114.
13. Lewis P. Introduction. Vigabatrin: a new antiepileptic drug. *Br J Clin Neuroparmacol* 1989; 27 Suppl 1:1S.
14. Lippert B, Metcalf BW, Jung MJ, Casar P. 4-amino-hex-5-enoic acid, a selective catalytic inhibitor of 4-aminobutyric-acid aminotransferase in mammalian brain. *Eur J Biochem* 1977; 74:441–445.
15. Patsalos PN, Duncan JS. The pharmacology and pharmacokinetics of vigabatrin. *Rev Contemp Pharmacother* 1995; 6:447–456.
16. Jung MJ, Palfreyman MG. Vigabatrin. Mechanisms of action. In Levy RH, Mattson RH, Meldrum BS, eds. *Antiepileptic Drugs*. 4th ed. New York: Raven Press, 1995: 903–913.
17. Foletti GB, Delisle M-C, Bachmann C. Reduction of plasma alanine aminotransferase during vigabatrin treatment. *Epilepsia* 1995; 36:804–809.
18. Richens A, McEwan JR, Deybach JC, Mumford JP. Evidence for both in vivo and in vitro interaction between vigabatrin and alanine transaminase. *Br J Clin Pharmacol* 1997; 43:163–168.
19. Schechter PJ, Hanke, NFJ, Grove J, Huebert N, et al. Biochemical and clinical effects of γ-vinyl GABA in patients with epilepsy. *Neurology* 1984; 34:182–186.
20. Mattson RH, Petroff O, Rothman D, Behar K. Vigabatrin: effects on human brain GABA levels by nuclear magnetic resonance spectroscopy. *Epilepsia* 1994; 35 Suppl 5: S29–S31.
21. Petroff OAC, Rothman DL, Behar RL, Mattson RH. Human brain GABA levels rise after initiation of vigabatrin therapy but fail to rise further with increasing dose. *Neurology* 1996; 46:1459–1463.
22. Petroff OAC, Hyder F, Collins T, Mattson RH, et al. Acute effects of vigabatrin on brain GABA and homocarnosine in patients with complex partial seizures. *Epilepsia* 1999; 40:958–964.
23. Juhasz C, Muzik O, Chugani D, Shen C, et al. Prolonged vigabatrin treatment modifies developmental changes of GABA A-receptor binding in young children with epilepsy. *Epilepsia* 2001; 42:1320–1326.
24. Rey E, Pons G, Richard MO, Vauzelle F, et al. Pharmacokinetics of the individual enantiomers of vigabatrin (gamma-vinyl-GABA) in epileptic children. *Br J Clin Pharmacol* 1990; 30:253–257.
25. Vauzelle-Kervroëdan F, Rey E, Pons G, d'Athis P, et al. Pharmacokinetics of the individual enantiomers of vigabatrin in neonates with unconztrolled seizures. *Br J Clin Pharmacol* 1996; 42:779–781.
26. Battino D, Estienne M, Avanzini G. Clinical pharmacokinetics of antiepileptic drugs in pediatric patients. *Clin Pharmacokinet* 1995; 29:341–369.
27. Frisk-Holmberg M, Kerth P, Meyer P. Effect of food on the absorption of vigabatrin. *Br J Clin Pharmacol* 1889; 27 Suppl:23S–25S.
28. Haegele KD, Schechter PJ. Kinetics of the enantiomers of vigabatrin after an oral dose of the racemate or the inactive S-enantiomer. *Clin Pharmacol Ther* 1986; 40:581–586.
29. Ben-Menachem E, Persson LI, Schechter PJ, Haegele KD, et al. Effects of single doses of vigabatrin on CSF concentrations of GABA, homocarnosine, homovanillic acid and 5-hydroxyindoleacetic acid in patients with complex partial epilepsy. *Epilepsy Res* 1988; 2:96–101.
30. Browne TR, Mattson TH, Penry JK, Smith DB, et al. Vigabatrin for refractory complex partial seizures: multicenter single-blind study with long-term follow-up. *Neurology* 1987; 37:184–189.
31. Bachmann D, Ritz R, Wad N, Haefeli E. Vigabatrin dosing during haemodialysis. *Seizure* 1996; 5:239–242.
32. Tran A, O'Mahoney T, Rey E, Mai J, et al. Vigabatrin: placental transfer in vivo and excretion into breast milk of the enantiomers. *Br J Clin Pharmacol* 1998; 45: 409–411.
33. Armijo JA, Arteaga R, Valdizán EM, Herranz JL. Coadministration of vigabatrin and valproate in children with refractory epilepsy. *Clin Neuropharmacol* 1992; 15:459–469.
34. Reidenberg P, Glue P, Banfield CR, Colucci R, et al. Pharmacokinetic interaction studies between felbamate and vigabatrin. *Br J Clin Pharmacol* 1995; 40:157–160.
35. Majkowski J. Interactions between new and old generations of antiepileptic drugs. *Epileptologia* 1994; 2 Suppl 1:33–42.
36. Steinborn B. Pharmacokinetic interactions of carbamazepine with some antiepileptic drugs during epilepsy treatment in children and adolescents. *Rocz Akad Med Bialymst* 2005; 50 Suppl 1:9–15.
37. Sánchez-Alcarez A, Quintana B, Rodriguez I, López E. Plasma concentrations of vigabatrin in epileptic patients. *J Clin Pharm Ther* 1996; 21:393–398.
38. Sánchez-Alcarez A, Quintana B, López E, Rodriguez I, et al. Effect of vigabatrin on the pharmacokinetics of carbamazepine. *J Clin Pharm Ther* 2002; 27:427–430.
39. Gatti G, Bartoli A, Marchiselli R. Vigabatrin-induced decrease in phenytoin concentration does not involve a change in phenytoin bioavailability. *Br J Clin Pharmacol* 1993; 36:603–606.
40. Rimmer EM, Richens A. Interaction between vigabatrin and phenytoin. *Br J Clin Pharmacol* 1989; 27:27S–33S.
41. Dalla Bernardina B, Fontana E, Vigevano F, Fusco L, et al. Efficacy and tolerability of vigabatrin in children with refractory partial seizures: a single-blind dose-increasing study. *Epilepsia* 1995; 36:687–691.
42. Szylleyko OJ, Hoke JF, Eller MG, Weir Sj, et al. A definitive study evaluating the pharmacokinetic of vigabatrin in patients with epilepsy. *Epilepsia* 1993; 34 Suppl 6:41–42.
43. Bartoli A, Gatti G, Cipolla G, et al A double-blind, placebo-controlled study on the effect of vigabatrin on in vivo parameters of hepatic microsomal enzyme induction and on the kinetics of steroid oral contraceptives in healthy female volunteers. *Epilepsia* 1997; 38:702–707.
44. Krämer G. Pharmacokinetic interactions of new antiepileptic drugs. In: Stefan H, Krämer G, Mamoli B, eds. *Challenge Epilepsy—New Antiepileptic Drugs*. Berlin: Blackwell Science, 1998:87–103.
45. Rey E, Pons G, Olive G. Vigabatrin. Clinical pharmacokinetics. *Clin Pharmacokinet* 1992; 23:267–278.

46. Wad N, Krämer G. Sensitive high-performance liquid chromatographic method with fluorometric detection for the simultaneous determination of gabapentin and vigabatrin in serum and urine. *J Chromatogr B Analyt Technol Biomed Life Sci* 1998; 705: 154–158.
47. Arteaga R, Herranz JL, Valdizan EM, Armijo JA. Gamma-vinyl-GABA (vigabatrin): relationship between dosage, plasma concentrations, platelet GABA-transaminase inhibition, and seizure reduction in children. *Epilepsia* 1992; 33:923–931.
48. Lindberger M, Luhr O, Johannessen SI, Larsson S, et al. Serum concentrations and effects of gabapentin and vigabatrin: observations from a dose titration study. *Ther Drug Monit* 2003; 25:457–462.
49. Johannessen SI, Battino D, Berry DJ, Bialer M, et al. Therapeutic drug monitoring of the newer antiepileptic drugs. *Ther Drug Monit* 2003; 25:347–363.
50. Livingston JH, Beaumont D, Arzimanoglou A, Aicardi J. Vigabatrin in the treatment of epilepsy in children. *Br J Clin Pharmacol* 1989; 27 Suppl 1:109–112.
51. Dulac O, Chiron C, Luna D, Cusmai R, et al. Vigabatrin in childhood epilepsy. *J Child Neurol* 1991; 6 Suppl 2:530–537.
52. Uldall P, Alving J, Gram L, Beck S. Vigabatrin in pediatric epilepsy—an open study. *J Child Neurol* 1991; 6 Suppl 2:538–544.
53. Uldall P, Alving J, Gram L, Høgenhaven H. Vigabatrin in childhood epilepsy: a 5-year follow-up study. *Neuropediatrics* 1995; 26:253–256.
54. Fois A, Buoni S, Di Bartolo RM, Di Marco V, et al. Vigabatrin treatment in children. *Child Nerv Syst* 1994; 10:244–248.
55. Wong V. Open label trial with vigabatrin in children with intractable epilepsy. *Brain Dev* 1995; 17:249–252.
56. Arteaga R, Herranz JL, Armijo JA. Add-on vigabatrin in children with refractory epilepsy; a 4-year follow-up study. *Clin Drug Invest* 1996; 12:287–297.
57. Sheth RD, Buckley D, Penney S, Hobbs GR. Vigabatrin in childhood epilepsy: comparable efficacy for generalized and partial seizures. *Clin Neuropharmacol* 1996; 19:297–304.
58. Nabbout RC, Chiron C, Mumford J, Dumas C, et al. Vigabatrin in partial seizures in children. *J Child Neurol* 1997; 12:172–177.
59. Dimova PS, Korinthenberg R. Efficacy of lamotrigine and vigabatrin in drug-resistant epilepsies of childhood. *Pediatr Neurol* 1999; 21:802–807.
60. Chiron C, Dulac O, Gram L. Vigabatrin withdrawal randomized study in children. *Epilepsy Res* 1996; 25:209–215.
61. Herranz JL, Arteaga R, Farr IN, Valdizan E, et al. Dose-response study of vigabatrin in children with refractory epilepsy. *J Child Neurol* 1991; 6 Suppl 2:545–551.
62. Luna D, Dulac O, Pajot N, Beaumont D. Vigabatrin in the treatment of childhood epilepsies: a single-blind placebo-controlled study. *Epilepsia* 1989; 30:430–437.
63. Zamponi N, Cardinali C. Open comparative long-term study of vigabatrin vs carbamazepine in newly diagnosed partial seizures in children. *Arch Neurol* 1999; 56:605–607.
64. Gobbi G, Pini A, Bertani G, Menegati E, et al. Prospective study of first-line vigabatrin monotherapy in childhood partial epilepsies. *Epilepsy Res* 1999; 35:29–37.
65. Sobaniec W, Kulak W, Strzelecka J, Śmigielska-Kuzia J, et al. A comparative study of vigabatrin vs. carbamazepine in monotherapy of newly diagnosed partial seizures in children. *Pharmacol Rep* 2005; 57:646–653.
66. Lortie A, Chiron C, Dumas C, Mumford JP, et al. Optimizing the indication of vigabatrin in children with refractory epilepsy. *J Child Neurol* 1997; 12:253–259.
67. McDonald DG, Najam Y, Keegan MB, Whooley M, et al. The use of lamotrigine, vigabatrin and gabapentin as add-on therapy in intractable epilepsy of childhood. *Seizure* 2005; 14:112–116.
68. Kluger G, Berz K, Holthausen H. The long-term use of vigabatrin and lamotrigine in patients with severe childhood onset epilepsy. *Eur J Paed Neurol* 2001; 5:37–40.
69. Baxter PS, Gardner-Medwin D, Barwick DD, Ince P, et al. Vigabatrin monotherapy in resistant neonatal seizures. *Seizure* 1995; 4:57–59.
70. Buchanan N, Kearney B. Vigabatrin in Sturge-Weber syndrome. *Med J Aust* 1993; 158:652.
71. Appleton R, Hughes A, Beirne M, Acomb B. Vigabatrin in the Landau-Kleffner syndrome (letter). *Dev Med Child Neurol* 1993; 35:457–459.
72. Nabbout RC, Melki I, Gerbaka B, Dulac O, et al. Infantile spasms in Down syndrome: good response to a short course of vigabatrin. *Epilepsia* 2001; 42:1580–1583.
73. Chau V, Karvelas G, Jacob P, Carmant L. Early treatment of Aicardi syndrome with vigabatrin can improve outcome. *Neurology* 2004; 63:1756–1757.
74. Appleton RE, Peters ACB, Mumford JP, Shaw DE. Randomised, placebo-controlled study of vigabatrin as first-line treatment of infantile spasms. *Epilepsia* 1999; 40: 1627–1633.
75. Vigevano F, Cilio MR. Vigabatrin versus ACTH as first-line treatment for infantile spasms: a randomized, prospective study. *Epilepsia* 1997; 38:1270–1274.
76. Elterman RD, Shields WD, Mansfield KA, Nakagawa J; US Infantile Spasms Vigabatrin Study Group. Randomized trial of vigabatrin in patients with infantile spasms. *Neurology* 2001; 57:1416–1421.
77. Lux AL, Edwards SW, Hancock E, Johnson A, et al. The United Kingdom infantile spasm study comparing vigabatrin with prednisolone or tetracosactide at 14 days: a multicenter, randomised controlled trail. *Lancet* 2004; 364:1773–1778.
78. Lux AL, Edwards SW, Hancock E, Johnson A, et al. The United Kingdom infantile spasm study (UKISS) comparing hormone treatment with vigabatrin on developmental and epilepsy outcomes to age 14 months: a multicenter randomized trial. *Lancet* 2005; 4:712–717.
79. Siemes H, Brandl U, Spohr HL, Völger S, et al. Long-term follow-up study of vigabatrin in pretreated children with West syndrome. *Seizure* 1998; 7:293–297.
80. Covanis A, Theodorou V, Lada C, Skiadas K, et al. The first-line use of vigabatrin to achieve complete control of seizures. *J Epilepsy* 1998; 11:265–269.
81. Wohlrab G, Boltshauser E, Schmitt B. Vigabatrin as a first-line drug in West syndrome: clinical and electroencephalographic outcome. *Neuropediatrics* 1998; 29:133–136.
82. Granström ML, Gaily E, Liukkonen E. Treatment of infantile spasms: results of a population-based study with vigabatrin as the first drug for spasms. *Epilepsia* 1999; 40:950–957.
83. Fejerman N, Cersosimo R, Caraballo R, Grippo J, et al. Vigabatrin as a first-choice drug in the treatment of West syndrome. *J Child Neurol* 2000; 15:161–165.
84. Kankirawatana P, Raksadawan N, Balangkura K. Vigabatrin therapy in infantile spasms. *J Med Assoc Thai* 2002; 85 Suppl 2:S778–S783.
85. Chiron C, Dulac O, Beaumont D, Palacios L, et al. Therapeutic trial of vigabatrin in refractory infantile spasms. *J Child Neurol* 1991; 6 Suppl 2:552–557.
86. Aicardi J, Sabril IS Investigator and Peer Review Groups, Mumford J, Dumas C, Wood S. Vigabatrin as initial therapy for infantile spasms: a European retrospective survey. *Epilepsia* 1996; 37:638–642.
87. Mitchell WG, Shah NS. Vigabatrin (VGB) for infantile spasms: non-dose dependent response. *Epilepsia* 2000; 41:187.
88. Tay SKH, Ong HT, Low PS. The use of vigabatrin in infantile spasms in Asian children. *Ann Acad Med Singapore* 2001; 30:26–31.
89. Chiron C, Dumas C, Jambaqué I, Mumford J, et al. Randomized trial comparing vigabatrin and hydrocortisone in infantile spasms due to tuberous sclerosis. *Epilepsy Res* 1997; 26:389–395.
90. Hancock E, Osborne JP: Vigabatrin in the treatment of infantile spasms in tuberous sclerosis: literature review. *J Child Neurol* 1999; 14:71–74.
91. Hancock E, Osborne JP: Treatment of infantile spasms. *Cochrane Database Syst Rev* 2002; 2:CD001770. DOI: 10.1002/14651858, CD001770.
92. Jambaqué I, Chiron C, Dumas C, Mumford J, et al. Mental and behavioural outcome of infantile epilepsy treated by vigabatrin in tuberous sclerosis patients. *Epilepsy Res* 2000; 38:151–160.
93. Curatolo P, Verdecchia M, Bomberdieri R. Vigabatrin for tuberous sclerosis complex. *Brain Dev* 2001; 23:649–653.
94. Riikonen R. The latest on infantile spasms. *Curr Opin Neurol* 2005; 18:91–95.
95. Curatolo P, Bomberdieri R, Cerminara C. Current management for epilepsy in tuberous sclerosis complex. *Curr Opin Neurol* 2006; 19:119–123.
96. Mackay MT, Weiss SK, Adams-Webber T, Ashwal S, et al. Practice parameter: medical treatment of infantile spasms. Report of the American Academy of Neurology and the Child Neurology Society. *Neurology* 2004; 62:1668–1681.
97. Gibbs JM, Appleton RE, Rosenbloom L. Vigabatrin in intractable childhood epilepsy: a retrospective study. *Pediatrc Neurol* 1992; 8:338–340.
98. Feucht M, Brantner-Inthaler S. γ-Vinyl-GABA (vigabatrin) in the therapy of Lennox-Gastaut syndrome: an open study. *Epilepsia* 1994; 35:993–998.
99. Beran RG, Berkovic SF, Buchanan N, Danta G, et al. A double-blind, placebo-controlled crossover study of vigabatrin 2g/day and 3 g/day in uncontrolled partial seizures. *Seizure* 1996; 5:259–265.
100. Grant SM, Heel RC. Vigabatrin. A review of its pharmacodynamic and pharmacokientic properties, and therapeutic potential in epilepsy. *Drugs* 1991; 41:889–926.
101. Ferrie CD, Panayiotopoulos CP. The clinical efficacy of vigabatrin in adults. *Rev Contemp Pharmacother* 1995; 6:457–468.
102. Ferrie CD, Robinson CD. The clinical efficacy of vigabtrin in children. *Rev Contemp Pharmacother* 1995; 6:469–476.
103. French JA, Mosier M, Walker S, Sommerville K, et al; and the Vigabatrin Protocol 024 Investigative Cohort. A double-blind, placebo-controlled study of vigabatrin three g/day in patients with uncontrolled complex partial seizures. *Neurology* 1996; 46:54–61.
104. Dean C, Mosier M, Penry K. Dose-response study of vigabatrin as add-on therapy in patients with uncontrolled complex partial seizures. *Epilepsia* 1999; 40:74–82.
105. Brodie MJ, Mumford JP; 012 Study Group. Double-blind substitution of vigabatrin and valproate in carbamazepine-resistant partial epilepsy. *Epilepsy Res* 1999; 34:199–205.
106. Kälviäinen R, Äikiä M, Saukkonen AM, Mervaala E, et al. Vigabatrin vs carbamazepine monotherapy in patients with newly diagnosed epilepsy. A randomized, controlled study. *Arch Neurol* 1995; 52:989–996.
107. Tanganelli P, Regesta G. Vigabatrin vs. carbamazepine monotherapy in newly diagnosed focal epilepsy: a randomized response conditional cross-over study. *Epilepsy Res* 1996; 25:257–262.
108. Chadwick D, for the Vigabatrin European Monotherapy Study Group. Safety and efficacy of vigabatrin and carbamazepine in newly diagnosed epilepsy: a multicentre randomised double-blind study. *Lancet* 1999; 354:13–19.
109. Aventis (formerly Hoechst Marion Roussel, now sanofi-Aventis). Data on file, 1999.
110. Zahner B, Stefan H, Blankenhorn V, Krämer G, et al. Once-daily versus twice-daily vigabatrin: Is there a difference? The results of a double-blind pilot study. *Epilepsia* 1999; 40:311–315.
111. Michelucci R, Veri L, Passarelli D, Zamagni M, et al. Long-term follow-up study of vigabatrin in the treatment of refractory epilepsy. *J Epilepsy* 1994; 7:88–93.
112. Cohen JA, Fisher RS, Brigell MG, Peyster RG, et al. The potential for vigabatrin-induced intramyelinic edema in humans. *Epilepsia* 2000; 41:148–157.
113. Sorri I, Herrgård E, Viinikainen K, Pääkkönen A, et al. Ophthalmologic and neurologic findings in two children exposed to vigabatrin in utero. *Epilepsy Res* 2005; 65: 117–120.
114. Gherpelli JLD, Guerreiro MM, da Costa JC, Rotta NT, et al. Vigabatrin in refractory childhood epilepsy. The Brazilian multicenter study. *Epilepsy Res* 1997; 29:1–6.
115. Sälke-Kellermann A, Baier H, Rambeck B, Boenigk HE, et al. Acute encephalopathy with vigabatrin. *Lancet* 1993; 342:185.
116. Sharif MK, Sander JWA, Shorvon SD. Acute encephalopathy with vigabatrin. *Lancet* 1993; 342:619.

117. Haas-Lude K, Wolff M, Riethmüller J. Niemann G, et al. Acute encephalopathy associated with vigabatrin in a six-month-old girl. *Epilepsia* 2000; 41:628–630.
118. Sander JWAS, Hart YM, Trimble MR, Shorvon SD. Vigabatrin and psychosis. *J Neurol Neurosurg Psychiatry* 1991; 54:435–439.
119. Thomas L, Trimble M, Schmitz B, Ring H. Vigabatrin and behaviour disorders: a retrospective survey. *Epilepsy Res* 1996; 25:21–27.
120. Aldenkamp AP, Vermeulen J, Mulder OG, Overweg J, et al. γ-Vinyl GABA (vigabatrin) and mood disturbances. *Epilepsia* 1994; 35:999–1004.
121. Dodrill CB, Arnett JL, Sommerville KW, Sussman NM. Effects of differing dosages of vigabatrin (Sabril) on cognitive abilities and quality of life in epilepsy. *Epilepsia* 1995; 36:164–173.
122. Levinson DF, Devinsky O. Psychiatric adverse events during vigabatrin therapy. *Neurology* 1999; 53:1503–1511.
123. Vallat C, Rivier F, Bellet H, Magnan de Bornier B, et al. Treatment with vigabatrin may mimic α-aminoadipic aciduria. *Epilepsia* 1996; 37:803–805.
124. Preece MA, Sewell IJ, Taylor JA, Green A. Vigabatrin—interference with urinary amino acid analysis. *Clin Chim Acta* 1993; 218:113–116.
125. Eke T, Talbot JF, Lawdon MC. Severe persistent visual field constriction associated with vigabatrin. *BMJ* 1997; 314:180–181.
126. Krauss GL, Johnson MA, Miller NR. Vigabatrin-associated retinal cone system dysfunction. Electroretinogram and ophthalmologic findings. *Neurology* 1998; 50:614–618.
127. Kalviäinen R, Nousiainen I, Mäntyjärvi M, Nikoskelainen E, et al. Vigabatrin, a gabaergic antiepileptic drug, causes concentric visual field defects. *Neurology* 1999; 53:922–926.
128. Schmidt T, Rüther K, Schmitz B. Are vigabatrin-associated visual field constrictions symptomatic? *J Neurol* 2004; 251:887–888.
129. Vanhatalo S, Pääkkönen L. Visual field constriction in children treated with vigabatrin. *Neurology* 1999; 52:1713–1714.
130. Vanhatalo S, Nousiainen I, Eriksson K, Rantala H, et al. Visual field constriction in 91 Finnish children treated with vigabatrin. *Epilepsia* 2002; 43:748–756.
131. Iannetti P, Spalice A, Perla FM, Conicella E, et al. Visual field constriction in children with epilepsy on vigabatrin treatment. *Pediatrics* 2000; 106: 838–842.
132. Wohlrab G, Boltshauser E, Schmitt B., Schriever S, et al. Visual field constriction is not limited to children treated with vigabatrin. *Neuropediatrics* 1999; 30:130–132.
133. Russel-Eggit IM, Mackay DA, Taylor DS, Timms C, et al. Vigabatrin-associated visual field defects in children. *Eye* 2000; 14:334–339.
134. Koul R, Chacko A, Ganesh A, Bulusu S, et al. Vigabatrin associated retinal dysfunction in children with epilepsy. *Arch Dis Child* 2001; 85:469–473.
135. Hosking SL, Roff Hilton EJ, Embleton SJ, Gupta AK. Epilepsy patients treated with vigabatrin exhibit reduced ocular blood flow. *Br J Ophthalmol* 2003; 87:96–100.
136. Buncic JR, Westall CA, Panton CM, Munn JR, et al. Characteristic retinal atrophy with secondary "inverse" optic atrophy identifies vigabatrin toxicity in children. *Ophthalmology* 2004; 111:1935–1942.
137. Versino M, Veggiotti P. Reversibility of vigabratin-induced visual-field defect. *Lancet* 1999; 354:486.
138. Giordano L, Valseriati D, Vignoli A, Morescalchi F, et al. Another case of reversibility of visual-field defect induced by vigabatrin monotherapy: is young age a favorable factor? *Neurol Sci* 2000; 21:185–186.
139. Vanhatalo S, Alen R, Riikonen R, Rantala H, et al. Reversed visual field constrictions in children after vigabatrin withdrawal—true retinal recovery or improved test performance only? *Seizure* 2001; 10:508–511.
140. Fledelius HC. Vigabatrin-associated visual field constriction in a longitudinal series. Reversibility suggested after drug withdrawal. *Acta Ophthalmol Scand* 2003; 81:41–46.
141. Gross-Tsur V, Banin E, Shahar E, Shalev RS, et al. Visual impairment in children with epilepsy treated with vigabatrin. *Ann Neurol* 2000; 48:60–64.
142. Westall CA, Nobile R, Morong S, Buncic RJ, et al. Changes in the electroretinogram resulting from discontinuation of vigabatrin in children. *Doc Ophthalmol* 2003; 107:299–309.
143. Spencer EL, Harding GF. Examining visual field defects in the pediatric population exposed to vigabatrin. *Doc Ophthalmol* 2003; 107:281–287.
144. Best JL, Achseon JF. The natural history of vigabatrin associated visual field defects in patients electing to continue their medication. *Eye* 2005; 19:41–44.
145. Kim SS, Chang K-H, Kim ST, Suh DC, et al. Focal lesion of the splenium of the corpus callosum in epileptic patients: antiepileptic drug toxicity? *Am J Neuroradiol* 1999; 20:125–129.
146. Appleton RE. Vigabatrin in the management of generalized seizures in children. *Seizure* 1995; 4:45–48.
147. Vogt H, Krämer G. Vigabatrin und Lamotrigin. Erfahrungen mit zwei neuen Antiepileptika an der Schweizerischen Epilepsie-Klinik. *Schweiz Med Wochenschr* 1995; 125:125–132.
148. Genton P. When antiepileptic drugs aggravate epilepsy. *Brain Dev* 2000; 22:75–80.
149. Panayiotopoulos CP, Agathonikou A, Sharoqi IA, Parker AP. Vigabatrin aggravates absences and absence status. *Neurology* 1997; 49:1467.
150. Künzle C, Steinlin M, Wohlrab G, Boltshauser E, et al. Adverse effects of vigabatrin in Angelman syndrome. *Epilepsia* 1998; 39:1213–1215.
151. Guerrini R. Epilepsy in children. *Lancet* 2006; 367:499–524.
152. Vigabatrin Paediatric Advisory Group. Guideline for prescribing vigabatrin in children has been revised. *BMJ* 2000; 320:1404–1405.
153. Wallace SJ. Newer antiepileptic drugs: advantages and disadvantages. *Brain Dev* 2001; 23:277–283.

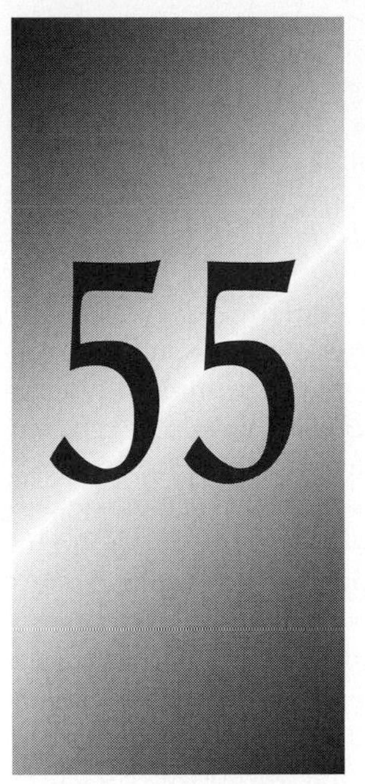

55 Vitamins, Herbs, and Other Alternative Therapies

Orrin Devinsky
Daniel Miles
Josiane LaJoie

Complementary and alternative medicine (CAM) is increasing in popularity. In 1997, CAM costs in the United States were close to $50 billion (1). In a 2002 survey of more than 30,000 U.S. adults, 62% reported using CAM therapy in the past year (2). The most common were prayer, natural products, deep breathing exercises, meditation, chiropractic care, yoga, massage, and diet-based therapies. CAM is used by 20% to 25% of parents for their children (3–5), with common forms being vitamin supplements, other nutritional supplements or elimination diets, herbs, homeopathy, prayer, massage, and aromatherapy (3, 5–7).

In a Canadian pediatric neurology clinic, CAM was used by 44% of the children (8). The most common CAM therapies were chiropractic manipulations (15%), dietary therapy (12%), herbal remedies (8%), homeopathy (8%), and prayer or faith healing (8%). Caregivers' sociodemographic variables or pediatric health-related quality of life was not significantly associated with CAM use. Parents reported benefits in 59% of CAM-treated children. Side effects were reported in 1 of 46 patients. Its use in children with certain chronic illnesses is 50% to 70% (9). A survey of parents of children with cerebral palsy showed that 56% used one or more CAMs (10). Notably, an increased severity of cerebral palsy correlated with the increased use of CAM. CAM is used in an estimated 14% to 32% of children with epilepsy (11). As with other pediatric groups, we have observed higher rates of CAM use in children with refractory epilepsy.

As CAM use rises in both pediatric and adult patients, a large communication gap exists between lay persons and traditional health care providers. Although pediatricians and pediatric subspecialists recognize that many patients use or are interested in CAM therapies, many do not feel comfortable discussing or recommending them (12, 13). Fewer than 40% of parents report CAM use to pediatricians (4). The exact frequency of alternative medicine use among children is difficult to ascertain largely because the majority of parents do not disclose their use of these substances to their children's medical providers. Individuals may feel that their complaints will not be taken seriously or that they will be made to feel that their actions are irrational in regard to alternative medicine. Parents are also concerned that others may think they are harming their children. The decision to use alternative medicine also depends on the cultural or religious beliefs of the families.

In this chapter we review some of the many complementary and alternative therapies used for epilepsy (Table 55-1). A recent, multiauthored volume on CAM in epilepsy summarizes many of the relevant findings (6). Many studies focus on adult patients, making extrapolation to pediatric populations problematic. In any case,

TABLE 55-1
Common Forms of Complementary and Alternative Medicine Therapies

Acupuncture*
Aromatherapy
Ayurveda*
Biofeedback*
Chelation therapy*
Chiropractic care*
Craniosacral care*
Deep breathing exercises
Diet-based therapies
  Atkins diet
  Ketogenic diet
  Low glycemic diet
Energy healing therapy*
Folk medicine*
Guided imagery
Herbs
Homeopathic treatment
Hypnosis*
Massage*
Meditation
Megavitamin therapy
Minerals
Naturopathy*
Neurofeedback*
Prayer
Progressive relaxation
Qi gong
Reiki*
Self-healing ritual
Tai chi
Vitamins
Yoga

*These therapies require the involvement of a practitioner.

reliable information on specific CAMs in epilepsy is lacking, making refutations difficult or clear recommendations impossible. Claims for efficacy often outstrip the available data.

STRESS

Stress is associated with a diverse set of conditions that can cause or aggravate many disorders. Stress is reported as a provocative factor for seizures by both patients and physicians (14). In self-report studies, stress is a leading seizure precipitant (15, 16). Both emotional and physical stressors may be involved. However, the scientific study of stress and seizures is difficult because stress is subjective and difficult to quantify, can indirectly affect seizure activity (e.g., hyperventilation, sleep deprivation, and medication noncompliance), and can be induced by seizures and the social-emotional consequences of epilepsy. Further, electroencephalograms (EEGs) recorded while the patient is under stress do not show increased epileptic activity (17).

Stress affects individuals to different degrees, ranging from clinically significant anxiety disorders to problems of everyday life that seem overwhelming. Epilepsy patients with clinical anxiety disorders should be referred for psychologic or psychiatric care. A psychologist, social worker, or other mental health professional can use behavioral strategies to reduce stress and improve emotional well-being and adjustment (6 pp. 25–32). Anxiolytic or antidepressant agents are underused in epilepsy patients owing to underdiagnosis and inflated fear of seizure exacerbation with selective serotonin reuptake inhibitors or other agents (e.g., buspirone) (18). Benzodiazepines can be valuable short-term agents, but withdrawal seizures are a concern in patients with epilepsy. For all epilepsy patients with anxiety symptoms, however, nonpharmacologic approaches are worth pursuing.

Many CAM therapies for epilepsy focus on stress reduction. Reducing stress and its physiologic effects can be achieved through a variety of techniques, such as exercise (19), yoga (6, 20), and specific relaxation techniques, such as progressive muscle relaxation (21). Few controlled studies exist to demonstrate the efficacy of these therapies. In small, uncontrolled studies, exercise either reduced seizure frequency (19, 22, 23) or had no significant effect on it (24, 25). However, exercise may also induce seizures (26–28). A nonblinded study showed that epilepsy patients who performed Sahaja yoga reduced their seizure frequency by 86% and showed fewer signs of stress, whereas those who did simulated yoga or had no intervention had no significant reductions (29). This study has not been replicated. Given the high frequency with which patients report stress as a provocative factor for seizures, stress reduction is a reasonable goal for patients.

PSYCHOTHERAPY

Psychotherapy can help manage specific psychologic problems as well as reveal how social interactions and self-perception contribute to stress. Group psychoeducational therapy (30–32), interpersonal psychotherapy (6, 33), and cognitive behavioral therapy (34–36) are used in adult and pediatric patients with epilepsy. Small studies with limited data support their effectiveness in reducing seizure frequency (37). In one uncontrolled study (38), 16 patients with refractory epilepsy learned behavioral techniques to interrupt the beginning of a seizure and to "neutralize provoking factors." Self-reported seizure reductions of at least 60% were reported by 80% of the participants. Psychotherapy is also used to treat psychogenic, nonepileptic seizures (39, 40). Cognitive-behavioral interventions may help epileptic patients with anxiety and depression (35).

FEEDBACK THERAPY

Andrews-Reiter Method

The Andrews-Reiter method, developed by Donna Andrews and Joel Reiter, was a new comprehensive neurobehavioral approach for using biofeedback to treat epilepsy. Their initial positive results from six patients with refractory complex partial seizures (41) were replicated at the Victoria Epilepsy Center (MacKinnon J, personal communication, 2002) and others (42, 43). The Andrews-Reiter method was developed to treat patients with refractory epilepsy and antiepileptic drug (AED) side effects who declined surgery or were not good candidates for it. This approach targets the onset of seizures in developing preventive techniques (44).

An essential part of the Andrews-Reiter treatment is to change the patient's response to preseizure warnings and auras by recognizing them and instituting a new, seizure-preventing response (6). Triggers may be physical (e.g., chemical imbalance, disturbed sleep, and missed medication), external (people, places, or situations that cause pressure or stress), or internal (emotional reactions and stressful states). The Andrews-Reiter treatment program includes cognitive and behavioral counseling to reduce seizure activity through enhanced awareness of premonitory or aura symptoms, identifying emotional, behavioral, physiologic, or environmental mechanisms that trigger seizure activity, progressive relaxation and reinforcement, deep diaphragmatic breathing, and EEG and electromyographic (EMG) biofeedback (44).

Neurofeedback Therapy

Operant conditioning of the EEG (i.e., neurofeedback or neurotherapy) is a noninvasive treatment for patients with refractory epilepsy. Neurofeedback may increase the seizure threshold through producing EEG changes. Initially, a quantitative EEG assessment is obtained to identify abnormal regions that can be targeted during treatment. Neurofeedback is a learning procedure with the goal of altering recorded EEG patterns. It is based on the law of effect, that is, provide positive reinforcement of EEG patterns that approach a normal configuration, and negative reinforcement of abnormal (epileptic) EEG patterns. In practice, a computer processes the EEG signals, identifies the critical components, and then modifies a display on a screen in front of the patient, which provides an integrated response dependent upon the EEG pattern. This process can be reduced to a simple game involving the completion of a task followed by the scoring of points. For children, these points can lead to meaningful rewards, such as privileges or money. The ultimate reward is learning to change the underlying circuitry of the brain to raise the seizure threshold. Although a natural consequence of neurofeedback is relaxation, it is not a relaxation technique; on the contrary, neurofeedback is more akin to a "cerebral workout" (6).

In animal studies, increasing the sensorimotor rhythm through operant conditioning eliminated or significantly reduced seizures induced by convulsant chemical compounds (45). In other animal experiments, sensorimotor rhythm training increased sleep spindles and improved sleep organization (46). These findings led to a pilot study of neurofeedback for a boy with refractory tonic-clonic seizures; he became seizure free after 3 months (47).

The clinical data on neurofeedback is based on uncontrolled, nonblinded studies in which operant conditioning reduced seizure frequency by over 50% and also reduced seizure severity (6). There is no relation between AED levels and the outcome of the conditioning (6). Studies using sham feedback, relaxation training, or alternate EEG criteria for reward showed no benefits.

Neurofeedback is an expensive and time-consuming process. It can be administered in 1-hour sessions, one to three times per week for periods ranging from 3 months to more than 1 year. It is usually about $100 per session and is often covered by health insurance under the "outpatient mental health" benefit (6).

Craniosacral Therapy

Craniosacral therapy was created by Dr. William Sutherland in the early 1900s to examine, assess, and correct cranial bone movements (6). Current practice focuses on the cranial and sacral bones and the membrane structures that connect them. This system is hypothesized to have a craniosacral rhythm, created by the flow of cerebrospinal fluid through the membrane complex.

A practitioner of craniosacral therapy assesses this rhythm and seeks to treat subtle imbalances in the nervous and skeletomuscular systems to restore health. A minimal amount of force (approximately the weight of a nickel) over a long period of time (30 seconds to several minutes) is used during craniosacral therapy. Widespread regions of the body, including many soft tissue structures, are often treated (6).

Although craniosacral therapy is used to treat epilepsy, there have been no controlled trials. The technique can probably reduce stress and muscular tension, but evidence to support the specific craniosacral rhythm mechanism of action is lacking. The reliability of palpating a craniosacral rhythm is poor between practitioners (48, 49). This fundamental skill is the basis of therapy. In one study (49), two registered osteopaths with postgraduate training in craniosacral techniques simultaneously palpated the head and sacrum of 11 normal subjects. Intrarater reliability at either the head or the sacrum was fair to good (correlation coefficients, 0.52−0.73). Interexaminer reliability was poor to nonexistent (correlation coefficients, −0.09−0.31).

VITAMINS

The use of vitamins, minerals, and other dietary supplements in the care of children with epilepsy takes multiple forms, including treatment of seizures in the case of vitamin-deficient or vitamin-dependent seizure disorders involving, for example, pyridoxine, biotin, and folinic acid, the replacement or supplementation of vitamin stores, such as folate and carnitine, depleted by the adverse effects of AEDs, and the use of multivitamins for general health maintenance.

Biotin

Biotin, a water-soluble B vitamin, was discovered to be an essential nutrient in the 1930s, when animal studies of diets containing large quantities of raw egg whites resulted in toxicity manifested by severe dermatitis, hair loss, and poor motor coordination. Biotin administration reversed the symptoms. Subsequently, avidin, a glycoprotein in egg whites, was found to irreversibly bind biotin, preventing its absorption. Cooking eggs destroys the ability of avidin to bind biotin.

Biotin deficiency, which is rare, can result from eating raw eggs, total parenteral nutrition without biotin supplementation, AED use, and prolonged antibiotic use. Antiepileptic medications associated with biotin deficiency include phenytoin, primidone, and carbamazepine; these agents can inhibit transport across the intestinal mucosa and accelerate the metabolism of biotin. Alteration of intestinal flora results in biotin deficiency with antibiotic use. Human biotin deficiency is manifested by seborrheic dermatitis, fungal infections, a perioral, erythematous, macular rash, fine brittle hair, hair loss, depression, mental status changes, myalgias, and paresthesias.

In addition to biotin therapy to counteract the adverse effects of AEDs, biotin is used to treat seizures secondary to biotinidase deficiency. Biocytin, the product of proteolysis of biotin-containing proteins and peptides, is cleaved by biotinidase into lysine and biotin, which is then free to be absorbed across the intestinal mucosa and used in multiple carboxylation reactions. Mutation of the gene that encodes for biotinidase is localized to chromosome 3p25 and results in seizures, ataxia, neuropathy, auditory dysfunction, breathing irregularities, and optic atrophy, as well as skin rashes, hair loss, and chronic candidiasis. Seizures are the presenting symptom in 38% of patients with biotinidase deficiency and are found in up to 55% of patients at some time before treatment (50). Generalized seizures (tonic-clonic, clonic, and myoclonic) and infantile spasms can occur (51, 52). Biotinidase deficiency is readily screened for by enzyme assay, and is part of newborn screening in many states and countries around the world. Recommended daily treatment is 5 to10 mg of biotin.

Pyridoxine

Pyridoxine, or vitamin B_6, is a cofactor involved in the metabolism of amino acids and multiple neurotransmitters, including gamma-aminobutyric acid (GABA). Glutamate decarboxylase, the enzyme responsible for the conversion of glutamate to GABA, requires pyridoxine. Insufficient concentrations of pyridoxine or glutamate decarboxylase dysfunction result in diminished production of GABA and increased concentrations of the excitatory neurotransmitter glutamate, producing circumstances favoring seizure activity. Seizures associated with pyridoxine are classified as pyridoxine deficient, pyridoxine dependent, or pyridoxine responsive.

Pyridoxine-deficient seizures were first reported in 1950 when children given a diet lacking in pyridoxine experienced seizures that resolved rapidly with intravenous doses of 50 mg pyridoxine (53). Later case reports were associated with baby formulas containing insufficient levels of pyridoxine. Vitamin B_6-deficient seizures typically begin in the first 4 months of life. The seizures are refractory to AEDs, and a family history of seizures is unlikely. These seizures typically respond to a single dose of pyridoxine (1–5 mg) and do not recur if dietary intake is adequate.

Neonatal seizures refractory to standard AEDs are the characteristic manifestation of pyridoxine-dependent epilepsy, a rare genetic disorder that can present as late as the second year of life. These neonatal seizures may take the form of partial, atonic, or generalized myoclonic episodes, as well as infantile spasms (54). Status epilepticus or seizures may occur in utero. EEG findings include focal, multifocal, and generalized epileptiform discharges. If seizures in early life are resistant to standard treatment, consider pyridoxine-dependent seizures and give an intravenous dose of 50 to 100 mg of pyridoxine. The response to pyridoxine may be dramatic and rapid; EEG monitoring during administration may reveal an abrupt cessation of seizure activity. Children responding to the intravenous dose of vitamin B_6 should then be maintained on daily supplementation to ensure seizure control and promote normal development. Confirmation of the diagnosis requires cessation of treatment with recurrence of seizure activity, then restarting vitamin B_6 and regaining a seizure-free state. An atypical form of pyridoxine-dependent seizures characterized by later onset may be manifested by seizures with febrile illness and episodes of status epilepticus. Intravenous pyridoxal phosphate, the active form of vitamin B_6, may be more effective than the oral form of pyridoxine in treating pyridoxine-dependent seizures (55).

Pyridoxine-responsive seizures were first described in 1968 (56). Pyridoxine is used to treat infantile spasms associated with diminished GABA concentrations in children and evidence of pyridoxine deficiency. There are no randomized, controlled trials of this use, but two prospective, open-label studies of pyridoxine treatment for infantile spasms revealed response rates of 13% to 29% (57, 58), raising the question of whether response to pyridoxine therapy exceeds the spontaneous remission rate. Data are insufficient to determine whether vitamin B_6 is effective in treating infantile spasms (59).

Folate

Folate is another vitamin that plays an important role in the health care of individuals with epilepsy, primarily in relation to AED side effects and the care of women of childbearing age, but also in the treatment of seizures in rare metabolic disorders. Folate is essential for DNA synthesis, and inadequate concentrations are associated with an increased risk of fetal neural tube defects. Certain AEDs (phenytoin, carbamazepine, and barbiturates) can decrease folate absorption. The American College of Obstetricians and Gynecologists in 1996 and the American Academy of Neurology in 1998 published statements recommending folate supplementation in women with a history of a previous pregnancy affected by a neural tube defect and girls and women of childbearing age with epilepsy. Dosage recommendations range from 0.4 to 4 mg daily. Folate deficiency is also associated with elevated homocysteine levels, which increase the risk of cardiovascular disease in both men and women.

Seizures are associated with two disorders of folate activity, cerebral folate deficiency, and folinic acid-responsive seizures. Folinic acid-responsive seizures are most often noted in the neonatal period. The medically refractory seizures are at times mistakenly thought to be related to perinatal hypoxic-ischemic injury because of the presence of atrophy and abnormalities of the white matter seen on magnetic resonance imaging (MRI) of the brain. Analysis of cerebrospinal fluid with high-performance liquid chromatography revealed an as yet unidentified compound (60). Seizures responded to treatment within 24 hours of folinic acid administration.

AMINO ACIDS AND SUPPLEMENTS

Gamma-Aminobutyric Acid

The fact that GABA is an inhibitory neurotransmitter has led to both the development of aids that enhance the effect of GABA and attempts to increase its cerebral concentrations via oral supplementation. GABA is not well absorbed across the blood-brain barrier, even when nitric oxide and other free radicals thought to increase the permeability of the blood-brain barrier are used simultaneously, and increased brain GABA levels are not known to affect seizure activity (61, 62).

Carnosine

Research into the use of carnosine in the treatment of epilepsy has led to conflicting results. In one study (63), higher levels of homocarnosine were found in children with refractory epilepsy than in those with medically controlled epilepsy. In other studies (64, 65), greater concentrations of homocarnosine were associated with better seizure control. The usefulness of carnosine in the treatment of epilepsy remains uncertain.

Taurine

Taurine is an amino acid that acts as an inhibitory neurotransmitter in multiple metabolic pathways, including cell membrane stabilization, regulation of cellular calcium levels, and detoxification. Genetic variations of taurine metabolism occur in some epilepsies (66). Although taurine in higher concentrations is associated with lower seizure susceptibility, and in lower concentrations with increased seizure activity, there is no conclusive evidence that taurine supplementation improves seizure control (67). One unblinded study of 25 children with intractable epilepsy treated with taurine reported complete seizure control in only 1 patient, a greater than 50% decrease of seizure frequency in another, and a less than 50% decrease of seizures in 4 patients, but no effect in 18 patients (68). No more than transient effects were noted in another unblinded study of 9 patients with intractable seizures. Five patients were seizure free for about 2 weeks, seizure frequency was temporarily reduced by 25% in 1 patient, and no effect was noted in the remaining 3 patients (69).

Carnitine

Treatment of mice with carnitine before exposure to a proconvulsant agent had a protective effect on the brain, with reduced seizure frequency noted, but no human research has shown similar results (70). Carnitine-deficient states can be associated with the use of valproate. Clinically significant carnitine deficiency is not common, but may be associated with fatigue, weakness, cardiomyopathy, hypotonia, poor growth, and hyperammonemia. Carnitine supplementation is recommended for patients with deficiency syndromes, but the use of carnitine prophylactically is not advised (71).

Glycine

Glycine, another inhibitory neurotransmitter, may reduce seizure frequency at a dose of 200 mg a day (72), and one study showed a reduction of seizures provoked by strychnine in animals (73). However, most reports show no significant anticonvulsant effect of glycine (74, 75).

HERBS

The use of herbal therapy has dramatically increased during the last decade. Despite their common use, little is known about the efficacy or side effects of these compounds. This is due not only to the paucity of controlled trials and rigorous research, but also to the lack of an oversight agency. Moreover, side effects tend to go unreported, or their incidence can be increased by the lack of knowledge on proper dosing and administration, misidentification of a particular herb, or poor manufacturing and quality control. New studies are in progress, but long-term effects will not be known for many years. The lack of information on these supplements makes it even more difficult for the practitioner to advise patients appropriately. Nevertheless, from increasing experience, knowledge about these substances continues to expand. Most of the available information must be adapted from the adult population, keeping in mind the unique differences in the physiology and underlying conditions of the pediatric population. Extreme caution must be taken when these substances are a component of treatment, because they can have profound side effects, negatively affect other conventional medications, or worsen preexisting conditions. All herbs have potential risks and side effects during pregnancy and, in particular, can negatively affect the unborn fetus; therefore their use during pregnancy and lactation is contraindicated (76).

Many popular herbs have been used in patients with epilepsy, but the mechanisms of their antiseizure activity are often unknown. Some herbs in toxic doses may actually provoke seizures. Comorbid conditions should be taken into account, because many of these supplements may interact with other medications or may be contraindicated in certain individuals. Of note, blue cohosh (*Caulophyllum thalictroides*) is an herb that has some properties similar to those of nicotine and is primarily used to induce labor. Its seeds are bright blue and eye-catching to children, who are at particular risk for poisoning if they ingest larger than recommended quantities (76). It is beyond the scope of this chapter to describe each individual herb in detail. Table 55-2 provides information about some of the more popular herbs.

Kava (*Piper methysticum*) is used for the alleviation of anxiety. It can also be used as an antiepileptic supplement. It potentially exhibits various mechanisms of action, including the inhibition of L-type calcium channels and sodium channels, increase of K^+ outward current, and enhancement of GABAergic inhibitory neurotransmission in animal studies (77). Although many studies have evaluated its efficacy in anxiety, there are few large studies involving patients with epilepsy. Kava's toxicity is increased when it is combined with alcohol, benzodiazepines, and barbiturates (78). Cases of hepatotoxicity have been reported. Its use is contraindicated in children less than 12 years of age.

Gotu kola (*Centella asiatica*) has a variety of uses. Animal studies suggest that it is protective against seizures via action at D2 receptors and possible cholinergic mechanisms, and it delays penetylenetetrazol-induced seizures. Some reports suggest that this herb may also improve children's cognitive status, but the sample sizes were small (76).

More than 30 herbs have been found to block seizures in animal experiments (79). Mistletoe (*Viscum*), for example, is protective against pentylenetetrazol- and bicuculline-induced seizures in animal models (80), but has no significant effect in the *N*-methyl-D-aspartic acid (NMDA) tonic seizure model. Data from human studies, however, are insufficient to recommend its use. It is an extremely toxic substance that may cause cardiac, neurologic, and gastrointestinal side effects.

Some herbs should not be used despite their popularity. Ginkgo biloba has been grown in China for more than 200 years. Typically, it is used in the treatment of cognitive deficits such as in Alzheimer's and multi-infarct dementia. It is believed to act as a free-radical scavenger. It reportedly can reduce the seizure threshold, induce seizures, or both (81). Ginkgo biloba should be avoided in patients with epilepsy because it can decrease the effectiveness of certain AEDs, including carbamazepine, phenytoin, and phenobarbital (81). The herb should not be used in individuals taking tricyclic antidepressants, which can also lower the seizure threshold (81). Ginkgo biloba must be used with caution in patients taking anticoagulants because of possible bleeding (82, 83).

Valerian (*Valeriana officinalis*) is commonly used as an anxiolytic and sleep aid. It is thought to inhibit the degradation and reuptake of GABA. Studies on its efficacy, safety, and potential drug interactions are sparse. Because valerian binds to the same receptors as benzodiazepines and may cause sedation, it should not be combined with benzodiazepines or sedatives such as barbiturates. Tremor, headache, cardiac disturbances, and gastrointestinal upset have been reported in patients using valerian in high doses or for a prolonged period of time (84).

Primrose oil and borage, both used for various conditions, are known to lower the seizure threshold (81). Another widely used herb, St. John's wort, which is used to treat depression, is believed to inhibit GABA and other neurotransmitters. Theoretically, this mechanism

TABLE 55-2
Common Herbs Used as Adjunctive Treatment in Epilepsy

Herb	Latin Name	Common Uses	Place of Origin	Chemistry	Systemic Effects	CNS Effects	Pregnancy Issues
American hellebore	*Veratum viride*	Antiemetic, neuralgia, pneumonia	United States	Similar to steroids	Blood pressure alteration, gastrointestinal and respiratory problems, salivation; high risk of side effects, narrow therapeutic index	Paresthesias, weakness, paralysis, seizure	Teratogenic
Behen	*Moringa oleifera*	Antimicrobial, gastrointestinal ailments	India	Contains glucosinolates, fatty acids	Gastrointestinal problems	Dizziness	Possible abortive effect
Betony	*Stachys officinalis*	Respiratory and gastrointestinal ailments,	Europe, North Africa, Siberia	Part of mint family, related to tannins	Hypotension, gastrointestinal problems, hepatic dysfunction	—	Uterine contractions
Black cohosh	*Cimicifuga racemosa*	Menstrual pain	North America	Estrogen effect	Hypotension, gastrointestinal problems; not for long-term use	Sedation, headache	Increased risk of spontaneous abortion
Blue cohosh	*Caulophyllum thalictroides*	Induce labor	Midwest and Eastern United States, Canada	Similar to nicotine	Hypertension, gastrointestinal problems, increases glucose; poisonous to children, cardiotoxic to neonates	Seizures	Uterine contractions, teratogenic
Calotropis	*Calotropis procera*	Antineoplastic	Asia, India, Africa, Pakistan, Sunda Islands	Related to steroids	Gastrointestinal steroids bradycardia; highly toxic	Seizures	—
European peony	*Paeonia officinalis*	Pain, headache	Southern Europe, Asia	Contains tannins, flavonoids	Hypotension	No anticonvulsant effect in studies	Uterine contractions
Ginkgo	*Ginkgo biloba*	Cognitive impairment	China	Platelet-activating factor antagonist	Bleeding	Seizures	—

TABLE 55-2
(Continued)

Herb	Latin Name	Common Uses	Place of Origin	Chemistry	Systemic Effects	CNS Effects	Pregnancy Issues
Goto kola	*Centella asiatica*	Antimicrobial, antineoplastic, CNS depressant, wound healing	South East Asia, India, Sri Lanka, China, Madagascar, South Africa, Southeastern United States, Mexico, parts of South America	Consists of triterpene acids and sugar residues, affects D2 receptors and cholinergic system	Contact dermatitis, infertility, hyperglycemia, hyperlipidemia	—	Should not be used in pregnancy
Groundsel	*Senecio vulgaris*	Worm infestation	Europe, Asia, Africa, Australia, Americas	Contains alkaloids, flavonoids	Hepatic dysfunction, carcinogenic; should not be taken internally	—	—
Kava	*Piper methysticum*	Anxiety	South Pacific	Inhibits L-type Ca^{2+} and Na^+ channels, increases K^+ outward current, enhances GABA transmission; member of black pepper family	Hypertension, gastrointestinal and respiratory problems, hepatic dysfunction, leucopenia, thrombocytopenia, dermatitis; should not be used in children <12 years	Acute dystonic reaction	Loss of uterine tone
Lily of the valley	*Convallaria majalis*	Arrhythmia, cardiac insufficiency	—	Related to steroids	Gastrointestinal problems, cardiac arrhythmia; many drug interactions, highly toxic, not recommended for use	Headache, stupor, changes in color perception	—
Melatonin*	—	Sleep disorders, jet lag	—	Derivative of serotonin	—	Drowsiness	Should not be used in pregnancy

Mistletoe	*Viscum album*	Cancer, seizures, heart disease, headache	England, Europe, Asia	Contains choline, histamine, tyramine	Blood pressure alteration, gastrointestinal problems, bradycardia, cardiac arrest; highly toxic	Coma, seizures, sedation, psychosis	Uterine contractions
Mugwort	*Artemisia vulgaris*	Change of fetal position in utero (breech), menstrual problems, depression	Northern Europe, Asia, North America	Part of daisy family	Dermatitis, allergy; not recommended for use	—	Uterine contractions, increased risk of abortion
Pipsissewa	*Chimaphilia umbellale*	Seizures, antispasmodic, diuretic	Europe, Asia, North America	—	Gastrointestinal problems, rash; problems, rash; not recommended for use	—	Should not be used in pregnancy
Skullcap	*Scutellaria laterifolia*	Cancer, sedative	North America	Contains flavonoids	Hepatic dysfunction, cardiac arrhythmia	Confusion, seizures	Should not be used in pregnancy
Valerian	*Valeriana officinalis*	Anxiety, sleep	Europe, Mexico, India, Japan	Inhibits degradation and reuptake of GABA	Gastrointestinal problems, hepatic dysfunction; many drug interactions	Sedation, tremor, headache; should not be used in children <14 years	Uterine contractions
Yew	*Taxus baccata*	Antimicrobial	Europe	Contains taxines, flavonoids	Cardiotoxic, arrhythmia, severely toxic	—	Causes spontaneous abortion

CNS, Central nervous system; GABA, gamma-aminobutyric acid.
*not an herb

TABLE 55-3
Herbs That May Cause Seizures

Bearberry (*Arcostaphylos uva-ursi*)
Borage (*Borago officinalis*)
Ephedra (*Ephedra sinica*)
Gingko (*Gingko biloba*)
Ginseng (*Panax ginseng*)
Ma Huang (*Herba ephedra*)
Monkshood (*Aconitum* sp.)
Primrose (*Oenothera biennis*)
Yohimbe (*Pausinystalia yohimbe*)

can make seizures worse (84). Herbs containing thujone, such as wormwood and sage, which are used to treat gastrointestinal disorders, may have proconvulsant effects. Table 55-3 lists some herbs that may cause seizures.

Some herbs can interfere with the hepatic P450 system (Table 55-4) and, when used together with antiepileptic medications, produce toxic side effects or decrease their effectiveness. Other herbs can lower anticonvulsant levels or otherwise interact with AEDs (Table 55-5).

MELATONIN

Melatonin is an indolamine that is synthesized from tryptophan in the pineal gland. It is released in a circadian pattern, with peak levels in the early morning hours (85). Its apparent main function is to signal the brain to induce sleep. Melatonin is used for a variety of conditions, including sleep disorders, jet lag, and autism. By regulating sleep patterns it appears to be helpful in attaining better seizure control, and from animal models, melatonin is helpful in preventing seizure-related brain damage. A variety of proposed mechanisms are thought to account for melatonin's antiepileptic effect. It appears to increase GABA's concentration in the brain and protects against seizure-induced brain damage by inhibiting calcium influx into neurons and by free-radical scavenging properties (86–89). When given orally, its blood concentration peaks within 1 hour, and usually returns to baseline within 4 to 8 hours (90).

TABLE 55-4
Herbs That Inhibit the P450 System

American hellebore
Chamomile
Echinacea
Garlic
Licorice
Milk thistle
Mugwort
Pipsissewa
Pycnogel
St. John's wort*
Trifolium pratense (red clover)

*Effect on the P450 system is controversial.

TABLE 55-5
Herbs and Their Effects on Antiepileptic Drugs

Herb	Drug	Effect
Septilin	Carbamazepine	Decreases drug level
Sho-seiryu-to	Carbamazepine	Delays drug absorption
Paeoniae radix	Phenytoin	Delays drug absorption
Thujone (wormwood, sage)	Phenobarbital	Reduces drug efficacy
Ginkgo	Phenytoin, phenobarbital, carbamazepine	Reduces drug efficacy

Melatonin's effectiveness has been shown in animal models. It inhibits kainic acid-induced seizures in rats. It also inhibits lipid peroxidation, is a potent free-radical scavenger, and reduces seizure-induced brain damage (91). Melatonin also blocks potassium cyanide-induced seizures in mice (92). Melatonin stimulates brain glutathione peroxidase activity, which is an antioxidative enzyme that metabolizes the precursor of the hydroxyl and peroxyl radicals to water. It also raises the electroconvulsive threshold in animal models and potentiates the anticonvulsive activity of carbamazepine and phenobarbital (93). In addition, melatonin significantly reduces neurobehavioral changes in mice, as well as morphologic changes in association with seizures, mostly in the CA3 region of the rat hippocampus (94).

Most clinical studies have looked at the use of melatonin in a limited number of subjects. Its effectiveness and safety profile in epilepsy patients was supported by several open-label trials. Peled et al (95) found that five of six children with intractable epilepsy had significant improvement not only in seizure control but also in their cognitive function. Bazil et al (96) showed that patients with epilepsy had a peak level of melatonin that was 50% of controls' peak level and that the peak occurred 3 hours before that of controls. Some studies have shown a lack of melatonin's efficacy, which may be related to inadequate dosing or other factors (97, 98).

TABLE 55-6
Some Homeopathic Remedies Used for Seizues

Febrile Seizures	Nonfebrile Seizures
Aconitum napellus	*Atropa belladonna*
Aethusa cynapium	*Chamomilla vulgaris*
	Cuprum metallica
	Glonoinum
	Ignatia amara
	Zincum metallicum

PHYTOTHERAPY

Practitioners of phytotherapy believe that there is an imbalance in the body and that specific herbs may restore this balance. Many plants are known for their anticonvulsant properties. Approximately 150 preparations of plants have been investigated. Individual plants are usually used but can be combined if necessary. In most cases, the active compound has not yet been identified. Studies have shown that some natural plant coumarins and triterpenoids exhibit anticonvulsant properties (99, 100). Several show promise against seizures (see Table 55-6), but further study is needed before their routine use.

Albizia lebbek increases levels of GABA in the brain. *Piper nigrum* may have antagonistic actions at NMDA receptors. The efficacy of *Casimiroa edulis* has been shown in animal studies to be similar to that of phenytoin and phenobarbital. *Ipomoea stans* is similar in effectiveness to valproic acid. The action of *Piper guineese* and *Psidium guyanensis* is similar to that of phenobarbital (101). The toxicity or side effects of these plants are largely unknown. Some plants may interact with antiepileptic medications; *Ruta chalepensis,* for example, may increase the hypnotic effects of phenobarbital. More work on the use of phytotherapy in epilepsy is needed.

ASIAN MEDICINE

Traditional Chinese medicine has been used for thousands of years and has been gaining interest in the Western world for quite some time. It is partly based on the view that the body is closely related to its surrounding outside world. The organs inside of the body are themselves considered to be interconnected via an interlacing network of channels and collaterals (102). Most therapies are composed of several herbs. The use of combination therapy is thought to improve the effectiveness and lessen any possible side effects. From the Chinese perspective, certain types of seizures are considered to be due to an exogenous or endogenous "wind." In children, the pathogenesis is attributed to the insufficiency of the spleen, stagnation of phlegm, and reversed flow of *qi* (known as the vital forces of the body), and stirring up of the endogenous wind (103). Some open-label studies of traditional Chinese herbal mixtures have shown a reduction in seizures and fewer side effects compared with standard AEDs, but well-controlled double-blind studies are lacking. Numerous combinations of Chinese herbs are used to combat seizures; only a few will be discussed.

Tianma gouteng yin is composed of amino acids, alkaloids, and fatty acids in addition to other compounds. Interestingly, it has been found to act as an NMDA-receptor antagonist. Not only does it have direct influences at the receptor, but it also helps to prevent neuronal injury and death (102). When quingyangsen (root) was given as an adjunct to standard AED treatment, almost 30% of patients had seizure control ranging from 2 to 9 months after initiating therapy (104). This compound has also been shown to block seizures in animal models (105). Zhenxianling contains different flowers, animal parts, and human placenta in addition to other substances. A study using Zhenxianling in 239 patients with refractory epilepsy, of whom 147 were aged 1.5 to 20 years, showed that 66% had a greater than 75% seizure reduction and an additional 30% had a greater than 50% reduction of their seizures (106). These effects were seen 1 to 5 days after treatment. In 15 patients with absence seizures, 11 had their seizure frequency reduced by 50% to 75%. A few studies have been performed using longdanxiegan tang, or a modified version, in absence epilepsy. Approximately 90% of patients taking this herb showed significant clinical or EEG improvement (107, 108).

In a study using capsules composed of a variety of Chinese supplements, a significant improvement was found among children with different types of epilepsy (103). More than 900 children were treated with these capsules, and their response was compared with that of only 160 patients treated with phenobarbital. In children taking the capsules, 57% had their seizures reduced by more than 75%. An additional 26% had a seizure reduction of 50% to 75%. The duration of individual seizures was also significantly diminished. In the control group, 40% of patients achieved a 75% seizure decrease and 12% had a 50% reduction in seizures. Approximately 1% had worsening seizure control. Fifty percent of children with absence and benign rolandic seizures had a 75% decrease in seizures. Two cases of infantile spasms were included in this study. One patient had a 75% reduction of seizures and the other a 50% to 75% decrease. Of those in the treatment group who previously had abnormal EEGs, 54% had normal EEGs at the end of the study period.

In Japan, kampo medicines are herbal remedies used to combat various medical conditions, including epilepsy. Most of these therapies are mixtures of different herbs, some of which are similar to those used in traditional Chinese medicine. Sho-saiko-to is an herbal formula commonly used to treat liver disorders; it also is recommended as a possible treatment for intractable epilepsy. Another formula similar to this compound, the Chinese bupleurum–cinnamon combination (chai-hu-keui-chi-tang), has shown some preliminary benefit in epilepsy. These formulas contain the same nine herbs with minor variations in their relative amounts. They appear to have equivalent effects (109). Sho-saiko-to has been administered to adults and children. The pediatric dose depends on the child's weight (110). There are no well-designed clinical studies on the benefit of this formula in epilepsy. In one study (111), it was given to 24 patients who were taking multiple drugs for uncontrolled epilepsy. Six of the 24 patients had no seizures within 10 months of the herbal therapy. An additional 13 patients were improved, three had no change, and two did not complete the study. Improvements were seen as soon as 1 month. Tonic-clonic seizures seemed to have the best response rate. Another study (112) revealed possible cognitive improvements with the use of this supplement, but the study was flawed and not optimally designed. Animal studies (113) have shown that it can inhibit pentylenetetrazol-induced seizures as well as cobalt-induced seizures and neuronal damage. Other studies (114, 115) revealed that there were no changes in barbiturate potentiation.

Adverse effects have rarely been reported. The formula has caused pneumonitis or hepatitis, or both, in a number of patients with liver disease, and has caused fatalities. Patients using this supplement must be advised to report coughs and fevers to their health care providers; prompt and careful follow-up is necessary (116, 117). Occasionally, gastrointestinal upset or mild transient symptoms are present. In addition to side effects, some of these supplements have been known to contain toxic ingredients that are not named on the label. These herbal remedies have been found to contain such elements as lead, arsenic, and mercury, which, if consumed in greater than safe amounts, can lead to serious consequences (118, 119). Although some report significant success with the use of these products, extreme caution should be maintained.

ACUPUNCTURE

Acupuncture has been practiced in Asia for more than two thousand years. In the United States, where it has increased in popularity over the past 30 to 40 years, it is used by approximately one million individuals. This ancient therapy is used mostly for pain management, but also for a number of different conditions, including epilepsy. Up to 70% of people who undergo acupuncture treatments do not inform their health care providers (120). Acupuncture involves the use of fine needles (now made of stainless steel) that are inserted into the skin at defined points of the body. For epilepsy, points along the scalp are key, as acupuncturists consider the scalp a direct projection of the cerebral cortex. Different points are selected depending on the different types and symptoms of seizures (121).

Acupuncture is presumed to restore balance to the disruption of the natural flow of energy that the body requires to function normally. Acupuncture releases endorphins, adrenocorticotropic hormone (ACTH), and other neurochemicals, such as GABA (122). Some studies show that afterward there is an increase of the serotonin level, which may lead to improved cognitive function (123). Specific sites are used to combat different conditions. The point naokong (GB19) is located near the occipital protuberance. It is selected for acupuncture in a variety of medical conditions in addition to epilepsy, and has been used in children. It is said to have tranquilizing effects, regulate blood flow, and calm "endopathic wind."

In terms of efficacy, there is a paucity of well-performed and well-controlled clinical trials for evaluating the usefulness of acupuncture in epilepsy, as well as other medical conditions. This is due in part to the individualization of therapy. Acupuncture differs between individuals, making standardization difficult. Even sham acupuncture is difficult to assess, because nonspecific needling can lead to the stimulation of neurohormonal responses (124).

Kloster et al (125) compared the effects of sham acupuncture and actual acupuncture in patients with intractable epilepsy. There was a small but statistically nonsignificant reduction in seizure frequency in both groups, perhaps due to the small sample size. No significant EEG changes were appreciated. Stavem et al (126) also failed to show that acupuncture significantly reduced seizures or had any effect on the patients' quality of life. Adverse effects are rare, the most common being infection and trauma. Other rare complications such as pneumothorax, cardiac tamponade, hepatitis, and spinal cord injuries have also been reported. The transmission of human immunodeficiency virus (HIV) has rarely been reported. The importance of sterilization and universal precautions cannot be emphasized enough (120).

In a child who had almost continuous simple partial seizures, acupuncture improved the seizures after seven sessions, and almost completely eliminated them by 30 sessions (127). Six months later, the patient was reported to be seizure free. In another study (121) involving almost 100 children and adults, 66% had a greater than 75% reduction in seizures, and an additional 24% had a 50% to 75% reduction. Yang (128) reported the use of acupuncture in eight children with status epilepticus. Different acupoints were used depending on the case. Seizures ceased within 10 minutes in all cases. No recurrences were reported in three patients for up to 2 years and in one patient for 8 years. Acupuncture may be a useful adjunctive therapy in epilepsy, but better designed studies are needed to fully evaluate its effectiveness.

HOMEOPATHY

There is little scientific evidence for the efficacy of homeopathy in epilepsy, and even less information is available on its use in children. It has been used for more than 200 years, and more than 500 homeopathic remedies have been used to treat seizures. Homeopathy is based on the principle that substances causing medical conditions can also be used to combat them. Symptoms are believed to represent the body's attempt to restore itself to health, and homeopathy aims to treat the patient's symptoms. It relies on the body's own powers for self-healing; therefore an individual's mental and physical state is important and taken into account prior to the administration of remedies. The identification of imbalances within the person in conjunction with his or her symptoms aids the homeopathist in choosing supplements that will restore the body's ability to heal itself. When dealing with children, choosing the correct treatment is further complicated by the fact that the homeopathist must rely on parental observations instead of directly obtaining information from the child.

The remedies used are derived mainly from plants, minerals, and animals. Remedies derived from toxins that are believed to cause illness are diluted before administration (129). Formulas containing *Aconitum napellus* and *Aethusa cynapium* are thought to be helpful in febrile seizures and other seizures associated with illnesses (Table 55-6). There are supplements that may be helpful in febrile and nonfebrile seizures (130). Reliable information on the risks associated with homeopathic remedies is lacking.

NATUROPATHY

Naturopathic medicine was established more than a hundred years ago and uses forms of Western medicine in addition to natural therapies. It uses noninvasive techniques and is based on the principle that natural substances can help the body's intrinsic ability to heal itself. Naturopath practitioners place a large emphasis on attempting to remove the underlying cause of the disease. Consuming the proper foods for sufficient nutrition of the body is one way of using natural substances. Nutritional supplements in the form of vitamins and minerals are often used (6). Certain herbs are prescribed to support the liver and kidneys, through which many AEDs are metabolized. In addition, some vitamins can interfere with certain AEDs. Information on the efficacy of naturopathic medicine in epilepsy is limited.

CONCLUSION

Alternative medicine is a growing field that comprises several different approaches. Most facets have not been well studied, making recommendations for their use in patients with epilepsy difficult. Side effects and complications are mostly underreported. Open communication between patients and health care professionals is vital in ensuring the well-being of patients. Patients should be encouraged to make their physicians aware of any other treatments they are receiving. They should also be advised not to discontinue their conventional medications without discussing their plans with their primary caregivers. Further research is required to better evaluate the role of alternative medicine in the treatment of epilepsy.

References

1. Eisenberg DM, Davis RB, Ettner SL, Yager A, et al. Trends in alternative medicine use in the United States, 1990-7: results of a follow-up national survey. *JAMA* 1998; 280:1569–1575.
2. Barnes PM, Powell-Griner E. Complementary and alternative medicine use among adults: United States, 2002. Advance data from vital and health statistics. US Department of Health and Human Services: Centers for Disease Control and Prevention, National Center for Health Statistics. No. 343, Hyattsville, MD. May 27, 2004.
3. Ottolini MC, Hamburger EK, Loprieato JO, et al. Complementary and alternative medicine use among children in the Washington, DC area. *Ambul Pediatr* 2001; 1:122–125.
4. Sibinga EM, Ottolini MC, Duggan AK, Wilson MH. Parent–pediatrician communication about complementary and alternative medicine use for children. *Clin Pediatr* 2004; 4:367–373.
5. Lim A, Cranswick N, Skull S, South M. Survey of complementary and alternative medicine use at a tertiary children's hospital. *J Pediatr Child Health* 2005; 41:424–427.
6. Devinsky O, Schachter S. Pacia S, eds. Complementary and alternative therapies for epilepsy. New York: Demos, 2005:33–42, 53–6, 65–80, 81–94, 113–9, 165–76, 285–90.
7. Losier A, Taylor B, Fernandez CV. Use of alternative therapies by patients presenting to a pediatric emergency department. *J Emerg Med* 2005; 28:267–271.
8. Soo I, Mah JK, Barlow K, Hamiwka L, et al. Use of complementary and alternative medical therapies in a pediatric neurology clinic. *Can J Neurol Sci* 2005; 32:524–528.
9. Spigelblatt L, Laine-Ammara G, Ples IB, Guyer A. The use of alternative medicine by children. *Pediatrics* 1994; 94:811–814.
10. Hurvitz EA, Leonard C, Ayyangar R, Nelson VS. Complementary and alternative medicine use in families of children with cerebral palsy. *Dev Med Child Neurol* 2003; 45:364–370.
11. Waaler PE, Blom BH, Skeidsvoll H, Mykletun A. Prevalence, classification and severity of epilepsy in children in western Norway. *Epilepsia* 2000; 41:802–810.
12. Fearon J. Complementary therapies: knowledge and attitudes of health professionals. *Pediatr Nurs* 2003; 15:24–27.
13. Kemper KJ, O'Connor KG. Pediatricians' recommendations for complementary and alternative medical (CAM) therapies. *Ambul Pediatr* 2004; 4:482–487.
14. Haut SR, Vouyiouklis M, Shinnar S. Stress and epilepsy: a patient perception survey. *Epilepsy Behav* 2003; 4:511–514.
15. Spatt J, Langbauer G, Mamoli B. Subjective perception of seizure precipitants: results of a questionnaire study. *Seizure* 1998; 7:391–395.
16. Spector S, Cull C, Goldstein LH. Seizure precipitants and perceived self-control of seizures in adults with poorly-controlled epilepsy. *Epilepsy Res* 2000; 38:207–216.
17. Lai C-W, Trimble MR. Stress and epilepsy. *J Epilepsy* 1997; 10:177–186.
18. Jones JE, Hermann BP, Barry JJ, Gilliam F, et al. Clinical assessment of Axis I psychiatric morbidity in chronic epilepsy: a multicenter investigation. *J Neuropsychiatry Clin Neurosci* 2005; 17:172–179.

19. Nakken KO, Loyning A, Loyning T, Gloerson G, et al. Does physical exercise influence the occurrence of epileptiform EEG discharges in children? *Epilepsia* 1997; 38:279–284.
20. Panjwani U, Gupta HL, Singh SH, Selvamurthy W, et al. Effect of Sahaja yoga practice on stress management in patients of epilepsy. *Indian J Physiol Pharmacol* 1995; 39:111–116.
21. Lehrer PM, Carr R, Sargunaraj D, Woolfolk RL. Stress management techniques: are they all equivalent, or do they have specific effects? *Biofeedback Self Regul* 1994; 19:353–401.
22. Denio LS, Drake ME Jr, Pakalnis A. The effect of exercise on seizure frequency. *J Med* 1989; 20:171–6.
23. Eriksen HR, Ellertsen B, Gronningsaeter H, Nakken KO, et al. Physical exercise in women with intractable epilepsy. *Epilepsia* 1994; 35:1256–1264.
24. Nakken KO, Bjorholt PG, Johannessen SI, Loyning T, et al. Effects of physical training on aerobic capacity, seizure occurrence, and serum level of antiepileptic drugs in adults with epilepsy. *Epilepsia* 1990; 31:88–94.
25. Esquivel E, Chaussain M, Plouin P, Ponsot G, et al. Physical exercise and voluntary hyperventilation in childhood absence epilepsy. *Electroencephalogr Clin Neurophysiol* 1991; 79:127–132.
26. Ogunyemi AO, Gomez MR, Klass DW. Seizures induced by exercise. *Neurology* 1988; 38:633–634.
27. Schmitt B, Thun-Hohenstein L, Vontobel H, Boltshauser E. Seizures induced by physical exercise: report of two cases. *Neuropediatrics* 1994; 25:51–53.
28. Sturm JW, Fedi M, Berkovic SF, Reutens DC. Exercise-induced temporal lobe epilepsy. *Neurology* 2002; 59:1246–1248.
29. Panjwani U, Selvamurthy W, Singh SH, Gupta HL, et al. Effect of Sahaja yoga practice on seizure control & EEG changes in patients of epilepsy. *Indian J Med Res* 1996; 103:165–172.
30. Ogata A, Amano K. A psychosocial approach to epileptic patients. *Epilepsia* 2000; 41 Suppl 9:36–38.
31. Olley BO, Osinowo HO, Brieger WR. Psycho-educational therapy among Nigerian adult patients with epilepsy: a controlled outcome study. *Patient Educ Couns* 2001; 42:25–33.
32. Snead K, Ackerson J, Bailey K, Schmitt MM, et al. Taking charge of epilepsy: the development of a structured psychoeducational group intervention for adolescents with epilepsy and their parents. *Epilepsy Behav* 2004; 5:547–556.
33. Chmelarova D. [Use of psychotherapy in patients with combined epileptic and nonepileptic seizures]. *Cas Lek Cesk* 2005; 144:557–559; discussion 559.
34. Martinovic Z. Adjunctive behavioural treatment in adolescents and young adults with juvenile myoclonic epilepsy. *Seizure* 2001; 10:42–47.
35. Au A, Chan F, Li K, Leung P, et al. Cognitive-behavioral group treatment program for adults with epilepsy in Hong Kong. *Epilepsy Behav* 2003; 4:441–446.
36. Goldstein LH, McAlpine M, Deale A, Toone BK, et al. Cognitive behaviour therapy with adults with intractable epilepsy and psychiatric co-morbidity: preliminary observations on changes in psychological state and seizure frequency. *Behav Res Ther* 2003; 41:447–460.
37. Ramaratnam S, Baker GA, Goldstein L. Psychological treatments for epilepsy. *Cochrane Database Syst Rev* 2003; (4):CD002029.
38. Schmid-Schonbein C. Improvement of seizure control by psychological methods in patients with intractable epilepsies. *Seizure* 1998; 7:261–270.
39. Goldstein LH, Deale AC, Mitchell-O'Malley SJ, Toone BK, et al. An evaluation of cognitive behavioral therapy as a treatment for dissociative seizures: a pilot study. *Cogn Behav Neurol* 2004; 17:41–49.
40. Zaroff CM, Myers L, Barr WB, Luciano D, et al. Group psychoeducation as treatment for psychological nonepileptic seizures. *Epilepsy Behav* 2004; 5:587–592.
41. Reiter JM, Lambert RD, Andrews DJ, et al. Complex-partial epilepsy: a therapeutic model of behavioral management and EEG biofeedback. *Self-Control Epilepsy* 1990; 1:27–38.
42. Andrews DJ, Schonfeld WH. Predictive factors for controlling seizures using a behavioral approach. *Seizure* 1992; 1:111–116.
43. Meencke HJ, Schmid-Schonbein C, Heinen G. Methods and results of a treatment program on self-control of epileptic seizures. Presented at the 54th Annual Meeting of the American Epilepsy Society, Los Angeles, CA, December 2000.
44. Reiter JM, Andrews DJ, Janis C. Taking control of your epilepsy: a workbook for patients and professionals. Available from Andrews/Reiter Epilepsy Research Program, 1103 Sonoma Avenue, Santa Rosa, CA 95405; 1987.
45. Sterman MB. Studies of EEG biofeedback training in man and cats. In: *Highlights of the 17th Annual Conference*. VA Cooperative Studies in Mental Health and Behavioral Sciences. Washington D.C.: U.S. Government, 1972:50–60.
46. Sterman MB, Howe RD, Macdonald LR. Facilitation of spindle-burst sleep by conditioning of electroencephalographic activity while awake. *Science* 1970; 167:1146–1148.
47. Sterman MB, Friar L. Suppression of seizures in an epileptic following sensorimotor EEG feedback training. *Electroencephalogr Clin Neurophysiol* 1972; 33:89–95.
48. Hanten WP, Dawson DD, Iwata M, Seiden W, et al. Craniosacral rhythm: reliability and relationships with cardiac and respiratory rates. *J Orthop Sports Phys Ther* 1998; 27:213–218.
49. Moran RW, Gibbons P. Intraexaminer and interexaminer reliability for palpation of the cranial rhythmic impulse at the head and sacrum. *J Manipulative Physiol Ther* 2001; 24:183–190.
50. Salbert B, Pellock J, Wolf B. Characterization of seizures associated with biotinidase deficiency. *Neurology* 1993; 43:1351–1354.
51. Kalayci O, Coskun T, Tokatli A, Demir E, et al. Infantile spasms as the initial symptom of biotinidase deficiency. *J Pediatr* 1994; 124:103–104.
52. Wolf B, Heard G, Wissbecker K, McVoy JR, et al. Biotinidase deficiency: initial clinical features and rapid diagnosis. *Ann Neurol* 1985; 18:614–617.
53. Snyderman SE, Carretero R, Holt LE. Pyridoxine deficiency in the human being. *Fed Proc* 1950; 9:372–373.
54. Hunt AD, Stockes J, McCrory WW. Pyridoxine dependency: report of a case of intractable convulsions in an infant controlled by pyridoxine. *Pediatrics* 1954; 13:140–145.
55. Wang HS, Kuo MF, Chou ML, Hung PC, et al. Pyridoxal phosphate is better than pyridoxine for controlling idiopathic intractable epilepsy. *Arch Dis Child* 2005; 90:512–515.
56. Hansson O, Hagberg B. Effect of pyridoxine treatment in children with epilepsy. *Acta Soc Med Uppsala* 1968; 73:35–43.
57. Ohtsuka Y, Matsuda M, Ogino T, Kobayashi K, et al. Treatment of the West syndrome with high-dosage pyridoxal phosphate. *Brain Dev* 1987; 9:418–421.
58. Pietz J, Benninger C, Schafer H, Sontheimer D, et al. Treatment of infantile spasms with high-dosage vitamin B_6. *Epilepsia* 1993; 34:757–763.
59. Mackay MT, Weiss SK, Adams-Webber T, Ashwal S, et al; American Academy of Neurology; Child Neurology Society. Practice parameter: medical treatment of infantile spasms. Report of the American Academy of Neurology and the Child Neurology Society. *Neurology* 2004; 62:1668–1681.
60. Torres OA, Miller VS, Buist NM, Hyland K. Folinic acid-responsive neonatal seizures. *J Child Neurol* 1999; 14:529–532.
61. Shyamaladevi N, Jayakumar AR, Sujatha R, Paul V, et al. Evidence that nitric oxide production increases gamma-amino butyric acid permeability of blood-brain barrier. *Brain Res Bull* 2002; 57:231–236.
62. Oztas B, Kilic S, Dural E, Ispir T. Influence of antioxidants on the blood-brain barrier permeability during epileptic seizures. *J Neurosci Res* 2001; 66:674–678.
63. Takahashi H. Studies on homocarnosine in cerebrospinal fluid in infancy and childhood. Part II. Homocarnosine levels in cerebrospinal fluid from children with epilepsy, febrile convulsions or meningitis. *Brain Dev* 1981; 3:263–270.
64. Petroff OA, Hyder F, Collins T, Mattson RH, et al. Acute effects of vigabatrin on brain GABA and homocarnosine in patients with complex partial seizures. *Epilepsia* 1999; 40:958–964.
65. Petroff OAC, Hyder F, Rothman DL, Mattson RH. Brain homocarnosine and seizure control of patients taking gabapentin or topiramate. *Epilepsia* 2006; 47:495–498.
66. Collins BW, Goodman HO, Swanton CH, Remy CN. Plasma and urinary taurine in epilepsy. *Clin Chem* 1988; 34:671–675.
67. Durelli L, Mutani R. The current status of taurine in epilepsy. *Clin Neuropharmacol* 1983; 6:37–48.
68. Fukuyama Y, Ochiai Y. Therapeutic trial by taurine for intractable childhood epilepsies. *Brain Dev* 1982; 4:63–69.
69. Konig P, Kriechbaum G, Presslich O, et al. Orally-administered taurine in therapy-resistant epilepsy. *Wien Klin Wochenschr* 1977; 89:111–113.
70. Igisu H, Matsuoka M, Iryo Y. Protection of the brain by carnitine. *Sangyo Eiseigaku Zasshi* 1995; 37:75–82.
71. De Vivo DC, Bohan TP, Coulter DL, Dreifuss FE, et al. L-Carnitine supplementation in childhood epilepsy: current perspectives. *Epilepsia* 1998; 39:1216–1225.
72. Department of Neurology, Massachusetts General Hospital. Epilepsy and nutritional supplementation [pamphlet]. 1994.
73. Gascon G, Patterson B, Yearwood K, Slotnick H. N,N Dimethylglycine and epilepsy. *Epilepsia* 1989; 30:90–93 (letter).
74. Haidukewych D, Rodin EA. N,N-Dimethylglycine shows no anticonvulsant potential. *Ann Neurol* 1984; 15:405 (letter).
75. Roach ES, Gibson P. Failure of N,N-dimethylglycine in epilepsy. *Ann Neurol* 1983; 14:347 (letter).
76. Groenwald J, ed. PDR for herbal medicines. 3rd ed. Montvale, NJ: Thomson PDR. 2004.
77. Grunze H, Langosch J, Schirrmacher K, Bingmann D, et al. Kava pyrones exert effects on neuronal transmission and transmembranous cation currents similar to established mood stabilizers: a review. *Prog Neuropsychopharmacol Biol Psychiatry* 2001; 25:1555–1570.
78. Almeida JC, Grimsley EW. Coma from the health food store: interaction between kava and alprazolam. *Ann Intern Med* 1996; 125:940–941.
79. Tyagi A, Delanty N. Herbal remedies, dietary supplements, and seizures. *Epilepsia* 2003; 44:228–235.
80. Amabeoku GJ, Leng MJ, Syce JA. Antimicrobial and anticonvulsant activities of *Viscum capense*. *J Ethnopharmacol* 1998; 61:237–241.
81. Miller LG. Herbal medicinals: selected clinical considerations focusing on known or potential drug-herb interactions. *Arch Intern Med* 1998; 158:2200–2211.
82. Rosenblatt M, Mindel J. Spontaneous hyphema associated with ingestion of *Ginkgo biloba* extract. *N Engl J Med* 1997; 336:1108 (letter).
83. Vale S. Subarachnoid hemorrhage associated with *Ginkgo biloba*. *Lancet* 1998; 352:36 (letter).
84. Mar C. Clinical evidence: an evidence based review of the ten most commonly used herbs. *West J Med* 1999; 171:168–171.
85. Brzezinski A. Melatonin in humans. *N Engl J Med* 1997; 336:186–195.
86. Kabuto H, Yokoi I, Ogawa N. Melatonin inhibits iron-induced epileptic discharges in rats by suppressing peroxidation. *Epilepsia* 1998; 39:237–243.
87. Niles LP, Pickering DS, Arciszewski MA. Effect of chronic melatonin administration of GABA and diazepam binding in rat brain. *J Neurol Transm* 1987; 70:117–124.
88. Castroviejo DA, Rosenstein RE, Romeo HE, Cardinali DP. Changes in gaba-amino-butyric acid high affinity binding to cerebral cortex membranes after pinealectomy or melatonin administration to rats. *Neuroendocrinology* 1986:43:24–31.
89. Ross C, Davies P, Whitehouse W. Melatonin's role as an anticonvulsant and neuronal protector: experimental and clinical evidence. *Neurology* 1998:13:501–519.
90. Ross C, Whitehouse W. Melatonin treatment for sleep disorders in children with neurodevelopmental disorders: an observational study. *Dev Med Child Neurol* 2002; 44:339–344.

91. Mohanan PV, Yamamoto HA. Preventative effect of melatonin against brain mitochondria DNA damage, lipid peroxidation and seizures induced by kainic acid. *Toxicol Lett* 2002; 129:99–105.
92. Yamamoto H, Tang H. Antagonistic effect of melatonin against cyanide induced seizures and acute lethality in mice. *Toxicol Lett* 1996; 87:19–24.
93. Borowicz KK, Kaminski R, Gasior M, Kleinrok Z, et al. Influence of melatonin upon the protective action of conventional anti-epileptic drugs against maximal electroshock in mice. *Eur Neuropsychopharmacol* 1999; 9:185–190.
94. Tan DX, Manchester LC, Reiter RJ, Qi W, et al. Melatonin protects hippocampal neurons in vivo against kainic acid-induced damage in mice. *J Neurosci Res* 1998; 54:382–389.
95. Peled N, Shorer Z, Peled E, Pillar G. Melatonin effect on seizures in children with severe neurologic deficit disorders. *Epilepsia* 2001; 42:1208–1210.
96. Bazil CW, Short D, Crispin D, Zheng N. Patients with intractable epilepsy have low melatonin, which increases following seizures. *Neurology* 2000; 55:1746–1748.
97. Sheldon SH. Pro-convulsant effects of oral melatonin in neurologically disabled children. *Lancet* 1998; 351:1254 (letter).
98. Camfield P, Gordon K, Dooley J, Camfield C. Melatonin appears ineffective in children with intellectual deficits and fragmented sleep: six "N of 1" trials. *J Child Neurol* 1996:11:341–343.
99. Chaturvedi AK, Parmar SS, Bhatnagar SC, Misra G, et al. Anticonvulsant and antiinflammatory activity of natural plant coumarins and triterpenoids. *Res Commun Chem Pathol Pharmacol* 1974; 9:11–22.
100. Chaturvedi AK, Parmar SS, Nigam SK, Bhatnagar SC, et al. Anti-inflammatory and anti-convulsant properties of some natural plant triterpenoids. *Pharmacol Res Commun* 1976; 8:199–210.
101. Nsour WM. Review on phytotherapy in epilepsy. *Seizure* 2000; 9:96–107.
102. Sucher NK. Insights from molecular investigations of traditional Chinese herbal stroke medicines: implications for neuroprotective epilepsy therapy. *Epilepsy Behav* 2006; 8:350–362.
103. Ma R, Li S, Li X, Hu S, et al. Clinical observation on 930 child epilepsy cases treated with anti-epilepsy capsules. *J Tradit Chin Med* 2003; 23:109–112.
104. Ding Y, Xiaoxian H. Traditional Chinese herbs in treatment of neurological and neurosurgical disorders. *Can J Neurol Sci* 1986; 13:210–213.
105. Guo Q, Kuang P. Studies of Qingyangshen (II): modulatory effect of co-treatment with qingyangshen and diphenylhydantoin sodium on rat hippocampal *c-fos* expression during seizures. *J Tradit Chin Med* 1996; 16:48–50.
106. Tiancai W. Effects of Chinese medicine Zhenxianling in 239 cases of epilepsy. *J Tradit Chin Med* 1996; 16:94–97.
107. Li X. The herbal treatment of petit mal epilepsy based on traditional Chinese medicine liver and spleen therapies. *Liaoning J Tradit Chinese Med* 1998; 25:310.
108. Deng S. Clinical observation on 36 petit mal cases treated by tonifying method. *J Tradit Chin Med* 1997; 7:418.
109. Sugaya E. Introduction. In: Hosoya E, Yamamura Y, eds. *Recent Advances in the Pharmacology of Kampo (Japanese Herbal) Medicine: Proceedings of Satellite Meeting on Kampo Medicine of the 10th International Congress of Pharmacology* (August 19–21, 1988). Auckland and Amsterdam: Excerpta Medica, 1988:54.
110. Tajiri H, Kozaiwa K, Ozaki Y, Miki K, et al. Effect of Sho-saiko-to (xiao-chai-hu-tang) on HBeAg clearance in children with chronic hepatitis B virus infection and with sustained liver disease. *Am J Chin Med* 1991; 19:121–129.
111. Narita Y, Satowa H, Kokubu T, Sugaya E. Treatment of epileptic patients with the Chinese herbal medicine "saiko-keshi-to." *IRCS Med Sci* 1982; 10:88–89.
112. Nagakubo S, Niwa S, Kumagai N, Fukuda M, et al. Effects of TJ-960 on Sternberg's paradigm results in epileptic patients. *Jpn J Psychiatry Neurol* 1993; 47:609–619.
113. Sugimoto A, Ishige A, Sudo K, et al. Protective effect of "Sho-siko-to-go-keishi-ka-shaduyaku-to" (TJ-960) against cerebral ischemia. In: Hosoya E, Yamamura Y, eds. *Recent Advances in the Pharmacology of Kampo (Japanese Herbal) Medicine: Proceedings of Satellite Meeting on Kampo Medicine of the 10th International Congress of Pharmacology* (August 19–21, 1988). Aukland and Amsterdam: Excerpt Medica, 1988:112–119.
114. Takato M, Takamura K, Sugaya A, Tsuda T, et al. Sugaya E. Effect of the Chinese medicine "saiko-keishi-to" on audiogenic seizure mice, kindling animals, and conventional pharmacological screening procedures. *IRCS Med Sci* 1982; 10:85–87.
115. Sugaya E, Ishige A, Sekiguchi K, Iizuka S, et al. Inhibitory effect of a mixture of herbal drugs (TJ-960, SK) on pentyenetetrazole-induced convulsions in E1 mice. *Epilepsy Res* 1988; 2:337–339.
116. Yarnell E, Abascal K. An herbal formula for treating intractable epilepsy. *Alternative & Complementary Therapies* 2000; 6:203–206.
117. Kamiyama T, Nouchi T, Kojima S, Murata N, et al. Autoimmune hepatitis triggered by administration of an herbal medicine. *Am J Gastroenterol* 1997; 92:703–704.
118. Haung WF, Wen KC, Hsiao ML. Adulteration by synthetic therapeutic substances of tradition Chinese medicines in Taiwan. *J Clin Pharmcol* 1997; 37:344–350.
119. Espinoza EO, Mann MJ, Bleasdell B. Arsenic and mercury in traditional Chinese herbal balls. *N Engl J Med* 1995; 333:803–804.
120. Pearl D, Schillinger E. Acupuncture: its use in medicine. *West J Med* 1999; 171:176–180.
121. Shi ZY, Gong BT, Jia YW, Huo ZX.. The efficacy of electroacupuncture on 98 cases of epilepsy. *J Tradit Chin Med* 1987; 7:21–22.
122. Wu D. Mechanism of acupuncture in suppressing epileptic seizures. *J Tradit Chin Med* 1992; 12:187–192.
123. Dos Santos J Jr, Tabosa A, do Monte FH, Blanco MM, et al. Electoacupuncture prevents cognitive deficits in pilocarpine-epileptic rats. *Neurosci Lett* 2005; 384:234–238.
124. Le Bars D, Dickenson AH, Besson JM. Diffuse noxious inhibitory controls (DNIC). I. Effects on dorsal horn convergent neurons in the rat. *Pain* 1979; 6:283–304.
125. Kloster R, Larsson PG, Lossius R, Nakken KO, et al. The effect of acupuncture in chronic intractable epilepsy. *Seizure* 1999; 8:170–174.
126. Stavem K, Kloster R, Rossberg E, Larsson PG, et al. Acupuncture in intractable epilepsy: lack of effect on health-related quality of life. *Seizure* 2000; 9:422–426.
127. Lu F. Experience in the clinical application of Naokong (GB19). *J Tradit Chin Med* 2005; 25:10–12.
128. Yang J. Treatment of status epilepticus with acupuncture. *J Tradit Chin Med* 1990; 10:101–102.
129. Koehler G. The handbook of homeopathy. London: Thursons, 1983.
130. Lockie A. Family guide of homeopathy: symptoms and natural solutions. New York: Fireside/Simon Schuster, 1998.

56 Zonisamide

John F. Kerrigan
John M. Pellock

Zonisamide (ZNS) was first synthesized by Dainippon Pharmaceutical Company in Osaka, Japan, in 1974 (1). ZNS was originally developed in an effort to discover medications for psychiatric illness (2–4). However, screening for anticonvulsant effectiveness in the maximal electroshock seizures (MES) model showed positive results, and ZNS subsequently entered human epilepsy trials, with Phase I studies in Japan in 1979 and Phase II trials in 1985. ZNS was approved for marketing in Japan in 1989. Enthusiasm for ZNS in the United States was dampened by the occurrence of renal calculi in early trials, which was attributed to the mechanism of carbonic anhydrase (CA) inhibition. However, subsequent pivotal trials led to approval for marketing by the U.S. Food and Drug Administration (FDA) in March 2000, with an indication for adjunctive therapy for adults with partial epilepsy. As of 2006, the estimated worldwide exposure to ZNS exceeds 2 million patient-years (5).

Very few controlled trials examining the efficacy of ZNS in children have been performed. However, published open-label reports describing ZNS effectiveness with various seizure types and epilepsy syndromes that occur in the pediatric age range have demonstrated that ZNS should be included among the broad-spectrum group of antiepileptic drugs (AEDs).

CHEMISTRY, ANIMAL PHARMACOLOGY, AND MECHANISMS OF ACTION

Chemistry

ZNS (1,2-benzisoxazole-3-methanesulfonamide) is a synthetic amine sulfonamide compound (Figure 56-1(A)) (2). ZNS is the only compound in this chemical class among AEDs. Several features of the chemical structure of ZNS deserve comment. All sulfonamide antibiotic compounds include an arylamine domain at the N4-position, which contributes to allergic reactions in susceptible individuals (Figure 56-1(B)) (6). However, ZNS is a nonarylamine sulfonamide and therefore lacks the chemical domain with the greatest potential to produce hypersensitivity reactions. ZNS shares structural similarity with acetazolamide (Figure 56-1(C)) and likewise shares an ability to inhibit the function of CA. Although the role of CA inhibition has been questioned as a mechanism of anticonvulsant action, there appears to be little debate that it contributes significantly to the side effect profile of ZNS. Lastly, ZNS bears structural similarity to other

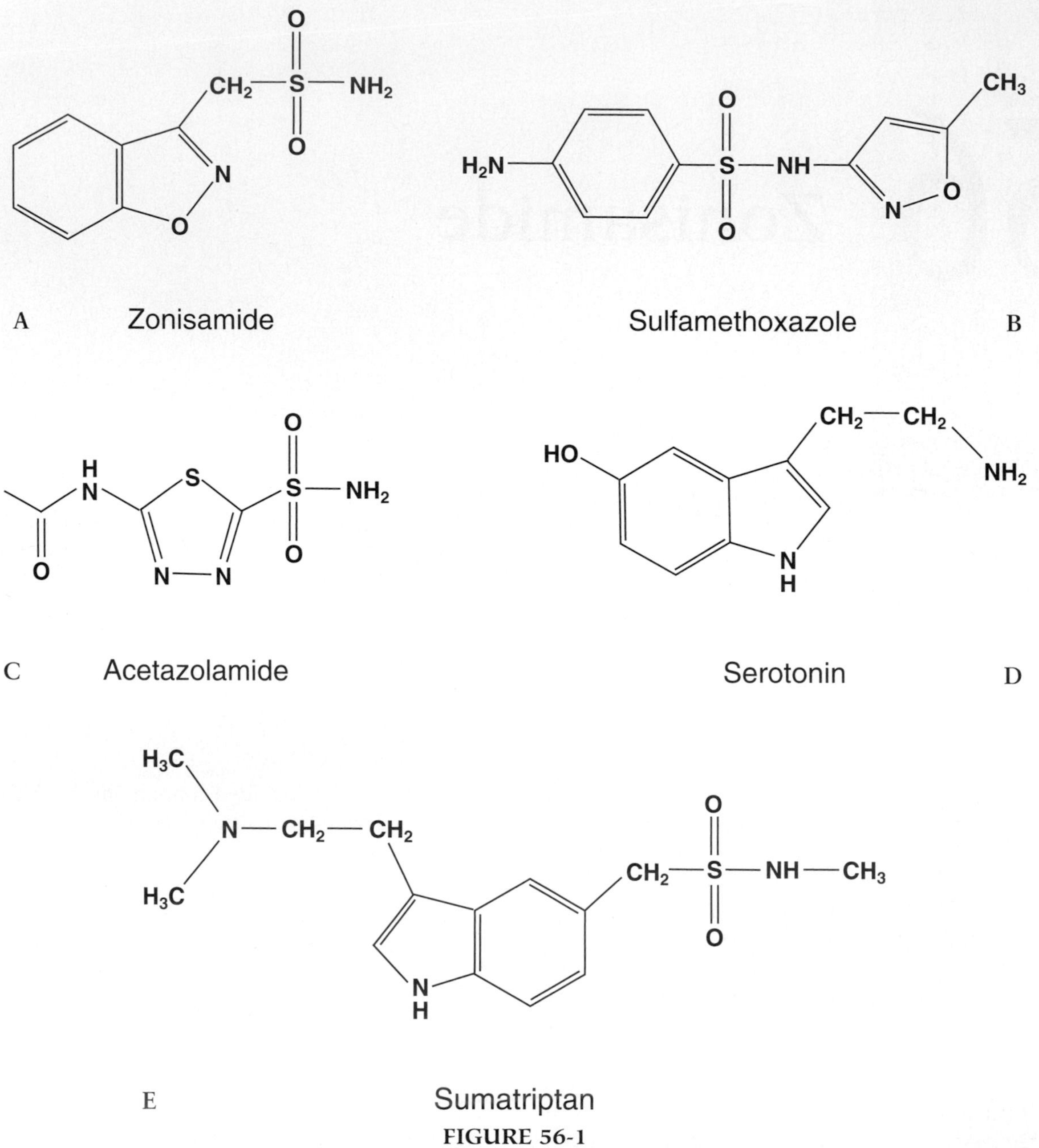

A Zonisamide

Sulfamethoxazole B

C Acetazolamide

Serotonin D

E Sumatriptan

FIGURE 56-1

Chemical structures of (A) the AED zonisamide; (B) the antimicrobial sulfamethoxazole; (C) the CA inhibitor acetazolamide; (D) the neurotransmitter serotonin; (E) the migraine medication sumatriptan.

compounds of neurologic interest, including serotonin (Figure 56-1(D)) and sumatriptan (Figure 56-1(E)).

Mechanisms of Action: Seizure Protection

Like many of the new AEDs, a number of different mechanisms of action have been proposed for ZNS. The mechanism or mechanisms that are of greatest importance in inhibiting seizure activity in humans remain unknown.

ZNS inhibits repetitive neuronal firing in spinal cord neurons that are depolarized during microelectrode recordings (7). This effect occurred at concentrations (3 μg/mL) that are less than the blood levels typically achieved in human subjects taking ZNS. The mechanism of this effect may be partial blockade of activity-dependent sodium channels, which has been shown in the giant axon of *Myxicola infundibulum* (8). (It is of interest that this critical observation was made in an invertebrate fanworm inhabiting the intertidal zone; it does not appear to have been reported in any other experimental system.)

ZNS also reduces voltage-dependent calcium currents by blocking the T-type calcium channel in a concentration-dependent fashion (9, 10). A methylated analog of ZNS, shown to be ineffective in blocking MES seizures, was likewise ineffective in blocking calcium currents (9). The relevance of T-type calcium channels as potential therapeutic targets of ZNS is suggested by studies in an animal model that examined the consequences of a single episode of status epilepticus, in which hippocampal CA1 pyramidal cells are converted into an abnormal burst-firing mode by up-regulation of T-type calcium channels (11). In addition, the study of dentate granule cells derived from temporal lobe tissue from patients undergoing surgery for refractory epilepsy has shown the presence of calcium currents mediated by T-type calcium channels (12).

In-vitro and animal studies also suggest that ZNS may modulate synaptic transmission as well. ZNS inhibited potassium-mediated glutamate release in the hippocampus in a microdialysis model in rats (13). Also in microdialysis experiments, ZNS functions to increase extracellular levels of dopamine and serotonin (possibly by enhancing synaptic release) in rat hippocampus and striatum (14–18).

ZNS may affect synaptic transmission by altering gene expression of neurotransmitter transporter proteins. In a rat model of hippocampal seizures elicited by injection of $FeCl_3$ into the amygdala, ZNS caused (1) up-regulation of excitatory amino-acid carrier-1 (EAAC-1), which has the potential effect of enhancing the removal of excitatory amino acids such as glutamate from the synaptic cleft, and (2) down-regulation of the expression of gamma-aminobutyric acid (GABA) transporter-1 (GAT-1), which could enhance inhibitory neurotransmission by increasing synaptic levels of GABA (19). This change in EAAC-1 and GAT-1 expression was present in both epileptic and control animals.

Although chemically related to acetazolamide, it appears that the mechanism for treating seizures may not be by CA inhibition, because drug concentrations for ZNS needed to be 100- to 1,000-fold higher than that of acetazolamide to reach an equivalent inhibitory effect on CA (20, 21). On the other hand, the profile of side effects of ZNS includes signs and symptoms attributable to CA inhibition.

ZNS has also been studied in seizure and epilepsy models in intact animals (22). ZNS can prevent the tonic extensor components of MES in several different species (3). ZNS inhibited the focal cortical discharge provoked by acute electrical stimulation of the visual cortex in cats (23), as well as seizures provoked by electrical stimulation in cats that have undergone kindling of the visual cortex (24). ZNS also prevents spread from the ictal focus in cats that have undergone focal freezing lesions of the cortex (23).

In addition to antiseizure effects, ZNS may have effectiveness as an antiepileptogenic compound as well (see also the discussion in the following section on possible neuroprotective effects). ZNS suppressed the kindling process, as well as inhibiting seizures resulting from kindling, in adult rats (25). ZNS also inhibited the development of elevated levels of chemical markers for oxidative damage in iron-induced focal epileptogenic foci in rat brain (26). This finding requires further study, but it raises the possibility that ZNS may help prevent the emergence of seizure foci following traumatic brain injury or intracranial hemorrhage.

Mechanisms of Action: Neuroprotection

ZNS has also been a subject of investigation for possible neuroprotective effects. In an in vitro model, ZNS demonstrates dose-dependent reductions in hydroxyl and nitric oxide free radicals (27). The same group has also shown that ZNS has reduced nitric oxide synthase activity in the hippocampus of rats exposed to N-methyl-D-aspartate (NMDA) (28). Recent studies have shown that pretreatment with ZNS reduces the half-life of free radicals in the hippocampus of rats. This finding was present in normal animals and in those undergoing an acute episode of status epilepticus induced by kainic acid (29, 30). These results suggest that ZNS has the capacity to protect the brain from free-radical-mediated injury.

ZNS reduces hypoxic-ischemic brain injury in neonatal rats (31). In this model, the carotid artery was ligated on one side, and the animal was then exposed to prolonged hypoxia (8% O_2 for 2.5 hours). ZNS was administered by intraperitoneal injection (75 mg/kg) prior to hypoxemia. Cortical infarction size, as a percentage of volume, was 6% in the ZNS-treated animals compared to 68% in control animals. Neuronal loss in the hippocampus was also reduced in ZNS-treated animals. Seizure recordings showed no significant difference between the two groups, suggesting that the neuroprotective effect was independent of any impact of the drug on seizure activity.

ZNS reduced cerebral infarction in a transient middle cerebral artery occlusion model in adult rats (32). Pretreatment with ZNS has shown neuroprotective effects following transient cerebral ischemia in the adult gerbil, as determined by memory performance with water maze and subsequent histologic study. These findings correlated with reduced extracellular glutamate in the hippocampus of the ZNS-treated animals (33).

BIOTRANSFORMATION, PHARMACOKINETICS, AND INTERACTIONS

ZNS has several properties that are desirable for an AED. These include a long half-life (making once daily dosing a feasible option), limited plasma-protein binding (minimizing displacement of other AEDs because of competition for protein binding sites), and an absence of autoinduction of the hepatic enzymes responsible for its metabolism (34).

Absorption

Absorption of ZNS following oral administration appears to be highly efficient, probably approaching 100%, based on recovery of radiolabeled drug in urine (35, 36). Absorption is rapid, with peak blood levels occurring 2–6 hours following dosage administration (37). When taken with food, peak levels are delayed slightly (4–6 hours), but the bioavailability is no different (37).

Distribution

The volume of distribution following oral administration is 1.0 to 1.9 L/kg in healthy adult volunteers. ZNS is only approximately 50% noncovalently bound to plasma proteins, which limits competition for binding sites with highly protein-bound medications such as phenytoin and valproic acid (37). Accordingly, drug-drug interaction resulting from alterations of free drug levels because of competition for binding sites is minimized.

On the other hand, ZNS has a particularly high binding affinity to the intracellular compartment of erythrocytes. The tendency of ZNS to sequester in erythrocytes has potential practical clinical importance, with a risk of false elevations of reported ZNS serum levels in hemolyzed specimens (38).

Distribution in the brain has been studied in rats with autoradiography following injection of ^{14}C-ZNS), showing preferential uptake in cerebral cortex relative to subcortical structures, including striatum, thalamus, hypothalamus, and cerebellum (39). However, further specificity with respect to binding sites is not yet available.

Metabolism and Drug-Drug Interactions

Among the drugs used to treat epilepsy, ZNS has a relatively long elimination half-life, with a mean of approximately 60 hours in healthy adult volunteers (range 52 to 69 hours) (40, 41). This favorable serum half-life enables twice-daily or even once-daily dosing schedules, but it also implies a prolonged time to steady state, as much as 10–14 days (22).

Zonisamide is partially metabolized by either acetylation, to produce N-acetyl ZNS, or by reduction to 2-sulfamoylacetylphenol (SMAP), then followed by glucuronidation and urinary excretion (40, 42–45) (see Figure 56-2). Study of the disposition of radio-labeled ZNS in human adult volunteers has shown that 62% of ZNS was recovered in the urine, of which 35% was unmetabolized ZNS, 15% N-acetyl ZNS, and 50% as the glucuronide derivative of SMAP (46).

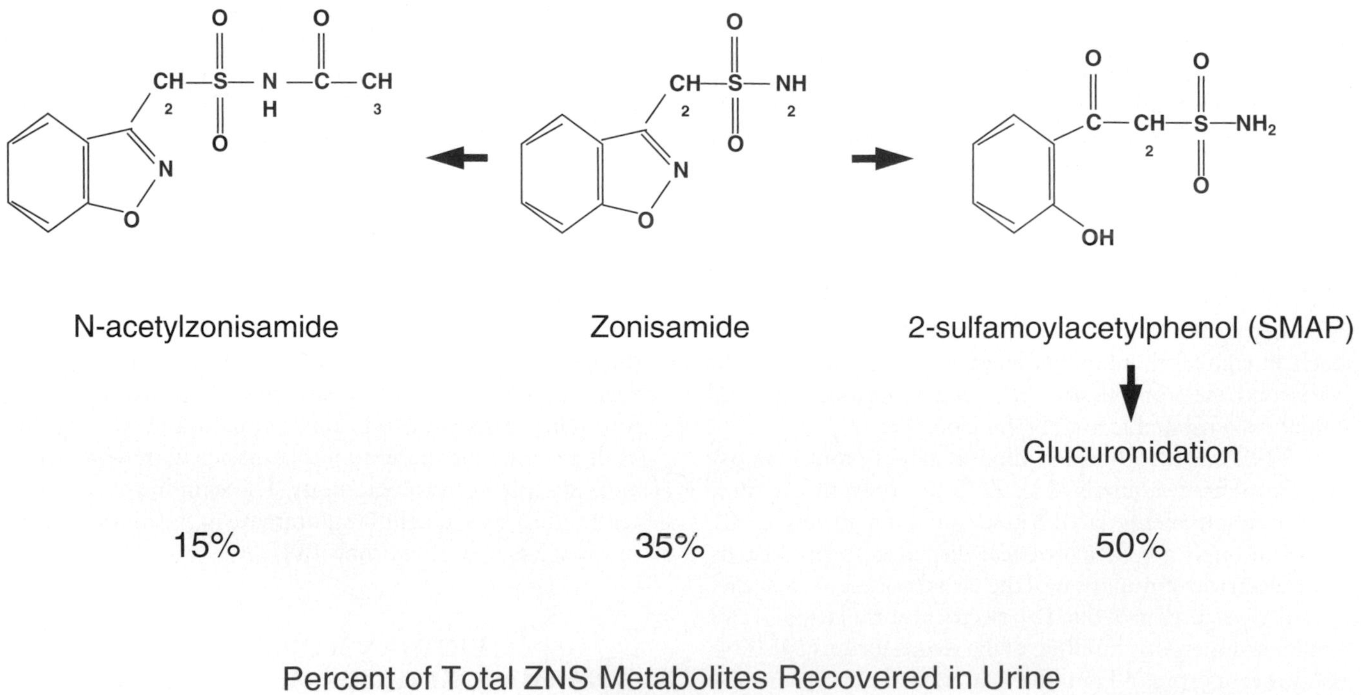

FIGURE 56-2

Metabolic pathways for zonisamide.

ZNS is metabolized by the hepatic cytochrome P450 system, specifically by the 3A subfamily, and predominately by the 3A4 isoenzyme (45, 47). However, ZNS does not induce its own metabolism, nor does it induce or inhibit other elements of the cytochrome P450 system (46). Because of the relatively low plasma-protein binding of ZNS, as well as its lack of hepatic enzyme induction, ZNS has little or no effect on the blood levels of other AEDs (48).

Other AEDs, however, can affect ZNS blood levels by virtue of their cytochrome P450-inducing or -inhibiting features. The elimination half-life of ZNS is decreased to 27 hours in adult patients fully induced by coadministration of phenytoin, to 38 hours in patients taking carbamazepine or phenobarbital, and to 46 hours in patients taking sodium valproate (46, 48–50). Non-AED compounds such as cimetidine can inhibit hepatic metabolism of ZNS (51). Other non-AED compounds, such as erythromycin, midazolam, and nifedipine, are also preferentially metabolized by the 3A4 isoenzyme and can therefore compete with ZNS for metabolism, resulting in increased ZNS blood levels (52). Certain dietary items, such as grapefruit juice, may have this same effect. Dexamethasone can act to induce the P450 reduction pathway for ZNS (47).

Detailed pharmacokinetic studies of ZNS within the pediatric age range have not been performed. However, as the metabolizing capacity of young children generally exceeds that of adults on a per-kilogram basis, higher doses may be required to reach the same target drug level (53). ZNS is likely to have a shorter serum half-life in children compared to adults.

Serum Levels

The significance of ZNS serum levels with respect to efficacy appear limited (37, 54). However, levels greater than 40 μg/mL were more likely to be associated with dose-related side effects, specifically drowsiness (54). This study also showed relatively small changes between blood levels at the peak (4 hours after once-daily morning dose) and the trough (prior to once-daily morning dose). The ratio of the peak to the trough levels showed a mean of 1.28 ± 0.15 in this sample of 72 children on initial ZNS monotherapy, which is consistent with the relatively long half-life of this AED.

A therapeutic ZNS level of 15 to 40 μg/mL has been suggested (50, 55).

CLINICAL EFFICACY

Pivotal Adult Trials

Not unexpectedly, Class I studies demonstrating the efficacy of ZNS for treating epilepsy enrolled predominantly adult subjects with partial seizures. In 2005 Brodie reported the results of a multicenter, randomized, double-blind, placebo-controlled trial in patients with refractory partial seizures (56). The group consisted of patients aged 12 to 77 years, who were taking one to three preexisting AEDs at the time of enrollment. Subjects were randomized to placebo or ZNS at one of three doses (100 mg/day, 300 mg/day, or 500 mg/day).

Efficacy varied directly with ZNS dose. The median reduction in seizure frequency for complex partial seizures was 51.2% for the study group taking 500 mg/day and 16.3% for the placebo group ($P < 0.0001$). The responder rate (the percentage of patients having at least a 50% improvement in seizure frequency) for complex partial seizures was 52.3% for ZNS at 500 mg/day and 21.3% for the placebo group ($P < 0.001$). The most frequent treatment-emergent adverse events during titration to 500 mg/day were somnolence (14.4%), headache (6.8%), dizziness (11.9%), and nausea (7.6%). The frequency of adverse events was generally lower at lower ZNS doses (and with placebo) and during the fixed-dose phase of the trial.

Additional pivotal studies with ZNS utilizing a randomized, placebo-controlled, add-on design have been performed in adult patients with refractory, partial-onset epilepsy (57–59). Representative results of these four studies are shown in Table 56-1.

Continued observation of these refractory partial-epilepsy patients with open-label extensions of the pivotal trials has provided further evidence that ZNS is effective and well tolerated with long-term follow-up (5, 60, 61).

Early Pediatric Trials in Japan

The initial observations concerning the use of ZNS in children with epilepsy arises from open-label clinical trials and practice experience in Japan, subsequently published in either Japanese or English, and reviewed by Glauser and Pellock (53). In this detailed meta-analysis examining efficacy and safety of ZNS in children in the Japanese publications, the available studies were broken down into those employing ZNS monotherapy (either newly diagnosed or previously treated cases) (62–67), adjunctive therapy with ZNS for treatment-resistant cases (68–72), or studies with a mixed group of patients receiving either ZNS monotherapy or ZNS adjunctive therapy (73–75). Results were then further analyzed by seizure type (partial-onset or generalized-onset seizures), and the percentage of responders (those with an improvement of at least 50% in seizure frequency) was reported. These results are shown in Table 56-2.

A component of one study included a group of 32 children that was randomized to monotherapy treatment with either ZNS (n = 16) or valproate (n = 16) (53, 73). These patients had generalized seizures and had previously failed seizure control with one to three AEDs. No significant difference in efficacy was observed. The

TABLE 56-1
Seizure Efficacy for ZNS in Randomized, Placebo-Controlled, Add-On Trials in Adults with Refractory Partial Epilepsy

Study (First Author)	Number of Subjects	Age Range (Years)	Maximum ZNS Dose	Median Reduction in Total Seizure Frequency (% Change from Baseline)	Median Reduction in Total Seizure Frequency (% Change from Baseline)	P Value
				ZNS Group	Placebo Group	
Schmidt 1993 (57)	139	18–59	20 mg/kg/day	22.5%	−3.0%	<0.05
Faught 2001 (58)	203	13–68	400 mg/day	40.5%	9.0%	= 0.009
Sackellares 2004 (59)	152	17–67	600 mg/day	25.5%	−6.6%	= 0.0005
Brodie 2005 (60)	351	12–77	500 mg/day	51.3%	18.1%	<0.0001

responder rate was 50% for ZNS treatment (at a mean dose of 7.3 mg/kg/day) and 44% for valproate (at a mean dose of 27.6 mg/kg/day).

Recent Studies on ZNS Efficacy in Children

Initial Monotherapy. In an uncontrolled trial of initial monotherapy in 72 children (mean age, 8.3 years; range, 3 months to 15 years) with newly diagnosed cryptogenic partial epilepsy, Miura treated patients with ZNS at an initial dose of 2 mg/kg/day, escalating at weekly intervals to a maintenance dose of 8 mg/kg/day (54). Dosing was provided once daily. At this initial target dose, 49 of 72 cases (68%) were completely controlled. After further dosage adjustment, 57 of 72 cases (79%) were completely controlled. The mean duration of ZNS treatment was 27 months (range, 6 to 43 months). Although a clear relationship between ZNS blood levels and clinical effectiveness was not seen, patients who were symptomatic with dose-related side effects (predominantly drowsiness) had blood levels greater than 40 μg/mL.

Seki and colleagues studied 77 children (ages 8 months to 15 years) with various seizure types, 68 of whom were included for analysis of ZNS efficacy (76). Fifty had

TABLE 56-2
Anti-Epilepsy Treatment with Zonisamide in Children

Inclusion Criteria for Open-Label Study	Partial-Onset Seizures RR	Partial-Onset Seizures *n*	Generalized-Onset Seizures RR	Generalized-Onset Seizures *n*
Patients on ZNS Monotherapy Only	78%	209	71%	49
Patients on ZNS as Adjunctive Therapy Only	34%	137	15%	54
Patients on Either Monotherapy or Adjunctive Therapy	60%	718	42%	291

Summary results of open-label trials in Japan as reviewed by Glauser and Pellock 2002 (53), noting the responder rate for children with either partial-onset or generalized-onset seizures according to the inclusion criteria for the study (ZNS monotherapy only, ZNS adjunctive therapy only, or combined ZNS monotherapy and adjunctive therapy).
n = Number of patients in each summary category. RR = Responder rate.

previously not taken any AEDs. All patients were on ZNS monotherapy. Doses were initiated at 2 mg/kg/day (divided twice daily), and increased by 1–2 mg/kg/day at 1–2 week intervals, up to a dose of 12 mg/kg/day. Forty-eight patients (of 68 patients, 62%) had localization-related epilepsy, and 20 (38%) had generalized epilepsies. Of the patients with localization-related epilepsy, 40 of 48 (83%) showed an "excellent" response (at least 3 months seizure-free); for patients with generalized epilepsy, 18 of 20 (90%) were seizure-free for at least 3 months.

Follow-up Monotherapy. Wilfong has described an uncontrolled case series of 131 children and adolescents treated with open-label ZNS monotherapy (77). Patients with both partial and generalized seizure types were included, although limited detail regarding seizure type and epilepsy syndrome was provided. Eighty-nine patients (68%) had previously been treated with at least one AED. When all patients are grouped together, 30% were completely seizure free, and an additional 47% had an improvement of at least 50% in seizure frequency. Forty-three patients (33%) reported at least one adverse effect while on ZNS, but only 3 (2.3%) had to discontinue ZNS therapy (sleeplessness and increased seizures, failure to gain weight, and behavioral changes in one patient each).

Add-on Polytherapy. Kim and colleagues have reported an uncontrolled, retrospective study of ZNS use in 68 children and adolescents treated for epilepsy (median age, 6.9; range, 1.9 to 18.1 years) (78). ZNS was used initially as monotherapy in 11.8% and as adjunctive polytherapy in 88.2%. The median ZNS dose was 8.0 mg/kg/day (range, 1.5 to 23.2 mg/kg/day). Of the 68 patients, 69.1% had exclusively generalized seizures, 10.3% exclusively partial seizures, 14.7% both generalized and partial, and 5.9% had seizures of undetermined type. Data to determine efficacy were available in 62 patients: 25.8% were completely seizure free, 21.0% had a reduction of at least 50% in overall seizure frequency, 16.1% were improved in seizure frequency by less than 50%, 22.6% showed no change, and 14.5% were reported as having increased seizure frequency. There were no clear trends with regard to efficacy and seizure type or etiology. Adverse events were reported by 61.8% of patients, predominantly during dose escalation. These were generally central nervous system (CNS) related, with behavioral or psychiatric symptoms (such as aggression, agitation, and decreased attention) reported in 23.5%, cognitive dysfunction in 12.0%, and sedation in 10.3%.

A retrospective study by Santos and Brotherton included 50 patients (range, 9 months to 20 years; mean age, 9.1 years) (79). With one exception, all had previously failed at least one other AED, and 47 subjects (94%) were taking at least one other AED with ZNS. The study group experienced a wide diversity of seizure types. For the entire population, 16% became seizure free, and an additional 22% had an improvement of at least 50% in seizure frequency. Efficacy was not broken down by seizure type. Adverse events were experienced by 62% of patients, including loss of appetite in 14 (28% of total study population), weight loss in 5 (10%), and kidney stones in 2 (4%). Fourteen patients (28% of total study population) discontinued ZNS because of adverse effects. Mean dosage for ZNS was 15.9 mg/kg/day (range, 3.3 to 35 mg/kg/day).

In another retrospective chart review of ZNS add-on therapy in 35 children with refractory epilepsy, Mandelbaum and colleagues determined that 11% of the study population was completely seizure-free, and 31% had an improvement in seizure frequency of at least 50% (80). When efficacy was analyzed by seizure type (generalized, partial, or mixed), there were no clear trends. The authors conclude that ZNS is a broad-spectrum AED.

Efficacy in Specific Seizure Types or Epilepsy Syndromes in Children

Partial Seizures. Miura has reported an uncontrolled series of 72 children (mean age, 8.3 years; range, 0.3–15 years) treated with initial ZNS monotherapy for cryptogenic localization-related epilepsy (54). The initial maintenance dose of ZNS was increased incrementally to 8 mg/kg/day and could be increased thereafter for patients not responding with complete seizure control. At 8 mg/kg/day of ZNS, 49 patients (68.1%) were completely controlled. Of the remaining patients, an additional 8 achieved complete seizure control with an increased dose of ZNS (79.2% of study group completely controlled on ZNS monotherapy). CNS-related side effects (drowsiness) tended to occur with blood levels greater than 40 μg/mL. A therapeutic range of 15–40 μg/mL was suggested.

Absence. T-type calcium channels have been implicated as an important mechanistic component of absence seizures (81). The ability of ZNS to functionally block these channels makes ZNS a potentially attractive AED for treating this seizure type (9, 10). Wilfong and Schultz have retrospectively reviewed the charts of 45 patients under 18 years of age treated with ZNS for absence seizures (82). Study subjects included both typical and atypical absence seizures and were not further analyzed according to epilepsy syndrome. However, 88.9% of patients had failed prior AED therapy. The mean ZNS dose was 9.0 mg/kg/day (range, 2–24 mg/kg/day). Twenty-three of 45 patients (51.1%) were 100% seizure-free for absence seizures, and 14 (31.1%) had a reduction in absence seizures of at least 50%. The efficacy with regard to treating other seizure types in this series of patients was not provided.

Juvenile Myoclonic Epilepsy(JME). Kothare examined the use of ZNS for seizure control in 15 patients with JME, utilizing a retrospective chart review method (83). There was no control group. ZNS was used as monotherapy in 13 patients (87%) and as add-on therapy in 2 patients. Dosing for ZNS ranged from 200 to 500 mg/day (2.0 to 8.5 mg/kg/day). For patients taking ZNS monotherapy, 80% had a decrease of at least 50% in total seizure frequency. When broken down by the individual seizure types commonly seen with JME, 69% of patients were seizure free for generalized tonic-clonic seizures, 62% were seizure-free for myoclonic seizures, and 38% were seizure free for absence seizures. One patient on monotherapy discontinued ZNS because of lack of efficacy, and 3 patients reported adverse events (weight loss, headache, dizziness), which resolved with continuing therapy.

West Syndrome or Infantile Spasms (IS). Several uncontrolled, open-label studies have reported the use of ZNS in patients with IS (West syndrome) (77, 80, 84–90).

Suzuki published a prospective, multicenter, open-label, uncontrolled trial with treatment of 13 infants with newly diagnosed IS (84). By protocol, all patients were initially treated with high-dose pyridoxine. Two responded, and the remaining 11 patients were then treated with ZNS, with a dose escalation program to reach seizure control or a maximum of 10 mg/kg/day. Eight of 11 patients (73%) had symptomatic IS. A positive response was defined as complete cessation of seizures and disappearance of hypsarrhythmia on electroencephalogram (EEG).

Four of 11 patients (36%) were initial responders. Interestingly, all had resolution of spasms within days of taking the initial dose at 3–5 mg/kg/day. However, 2 of these patients later relapsed. There were no adverse events reported during ZNS treatment. Of the 7 nonresponders, 5 of 7 later responded to an intramuscular adrenocorticotropic hormone (ACTH) treatment protocol.

Yanagaki treated 23 infants with West syndrome, ages 4–11 months, as either initial or adjunctive therapy, with a dose-ranging protocol to study an increased titration rate. Initial doses varied from 3 mg/kg/day to 10 mg/kg/day, to achieve a final target dose of 9–11 mg/kg/day for the entire group (90). A positive response (defined as a complete cessation of spasms and disappearance of hypsarrhythmia for at least 3 months) was observed in 7 patients (30%). Of these, 4 were cryptogenic and 3 were symptomatic cases. A mild degree of hyperthermia (temperature above 37.5°C), but without obvious signs of infection, was observed in 3 of the 10 patients in the highest initial dose treatment group, but the medication was continued in all, with simple environmental cooling.

Based on this collective open-label experience, it has been noted that the likelihood of success with ZNS for IS is higher in patients with cryptogenic IS in comparison to those with symptomatic IS. Notably, those who responded often did so quickly and at relatively low doses of 4–8 mg/kg/day (87).

Lennox-Gastaut Syndrome (LGS). In comparison to IS, there is relatively little published information directly addressing the use of ZNS for treating patients with LGS. Some of the retrospective, tertiary clinic-based surveys previously noted contain large numbers of patients with cryptogenic or symptomatic generalized epilepsy, but LGS is not broken out as an identified subgroup (78, 80).

Yamauchi has recently described a large cadre of patients followed prospectively as part of an uncontrolled, multicenter, postmarketing surveillance study consisting of 1,631 patients, including enrollment of 774 children (ages 15 years or less) (91). Within the entire study population, 79 patients are described as having LGS. Details regarding ZNS dosing, including whether ZNS was used as monotherapy or polytherapy, are not broken out for the LGS subgroup. However, in response to ZNS treatment, 27.9% of LGS patients experienced an improvement in total seizure frequency of at least 50%, whereas 51.9% are described as unchanged.

Myoclonic Seizures and Progressive Myoclonus Epilepsy. Yamauchi (see preceding discussion) also describes open-label efficacy of ZNS broken down by seizure type in a large postmarketing surveillance study (91). Fifty-six subjects experienced myoclonic seizures. Of these, 19.6% are described as completely free of myoclonic seizures, and an additional 32.2% showed an improvement of at least 50% in myoclonic seizure frequency. Details regarding ZNS dosing are not provided for this subgroup.

Generally favorable results have been described in several small, uncontrolled, open-label reports of ZNS treatment of the refractory seizures associated with progressive myoclonus epilepsies, including Unverricht-Lundborg disease (92, 93) and Lafora disease (93, 94).

Importantly, ZNS is not one of the AEDs that may exacerbate myoclonic seizures, which is a list that includes lamotrigine, carbamazepine, phenytoin, gabapentin, pregabalin, and vigabatrin (95).

ADVERSE EFFECTS

Dose-Related Effects

Premarketing Phase II and Phase III trials in Japan in 1,008 patients (of whom, 403 patients [40%], were ages 15 years or less) demonstrated that the most frequent treatment-emergent adverse events were drowsiness (24%), ataxia (13%), decreased appetite (11%), gastrointestinal symptoms (7%), decrease in spontaneity (6%), and slowing of mental activity (5%) (96).

Ohtahara has described the side effect profile of ZNS in 928 children participating in an open-label postmarketing surveillance study (97). The children had a statistically significant lower likelihood of all adverse events (24.3% of pediatric population) in comparison to adult patients in the study (40.1%; $P < 0.001$).

Not surprisingly, the likelihood of adverse events increased with polypharmacy. In one large multicenter trial of ZNS in Japanese children (72), the incidence of adverse events of any kind was 14% in those taking ZNS monotherapy, 37% in those taking one other AED in addition to ZNS, and 53% in those taking two additional AEDs [reviewed in (53)]. The likelihood of adverse effects appeared to correlate with serum level of ZNS; mean levels of ZNS for symptomatic patients were generally greater than 20 μg/mL. Target doses of 8 mg/kg/day and lower were well tolerated.

Idiosyncratic Effects

Hyperthermia and Oligohydrosis. Decreased sweating and increased core temperature, a potential consequence of CA inhibition, is a recognized adverse event with ZNS therapy. This side effect appears to be more common in children and more likely to occur in hot weather (98). Postmarketing assessment of the likelihood of oligohidrosis, hyperthermia, or both in the United States suggested an incidence of 1 case per 4,590 patient-years (0.02% per patient-year) (98). Surveillance of the Japanese market for 11 years after ZNS approval suggested an incidence of 1 case per 10,000 pediatric-years (0.01% per pediatric-year) (98). Knudsen analyzed the Adverse Events Reporting System of the FDA for cases with oligohidrosis, fever, or both (99). Six cases were identified, all in children or adolescents. The reporting rate was calculated to be 1 case per 769 pediatric-years (0.13% per pediatric-year). Ascertainment of the cases in these reports depends on physician report and is biased in favor of medically serious episodes. Conversely, one Japanese report identified decreased sweating in 12 of 70 patients (17%) taking ZNS, based on historical reports by the patients' parents (100). In summary, the preponderance of data suggests that the incidence of serious episodes of oligohidrosis and hyperthermia is low, but milder instances are encountered during routine clinical practice.

Renal Calculi. Renal stones occurred in 1.9% of 700 adult patients treated with ZNS in U.S. and European studies (101). A more recent study, also in adult patients, identified stones in 4% of 750 patients (1.2% symptomatic and 2.8% asymptomatic) (102). The incidence of renal calculi in children taking ZNS is unknown. An increased risk of renal stones is most likely attributable to the effect of ZNS as a CA inhibitor, resulting in alkalinization of the urine and an increased risk of calcium phosphate stones. An increased risk for kidney stones is likely in those with a prior history of stones or in those with a family history of renal calculi.

Rash. Although ZNS is a sulfonamide, it does not include the arylamine group that increases risk for hypersensitivity skin reactions (6). Accordingly, the risk of allergic drug rash appears to be substantially lower with the use of ZNS in comparison to the sulfonamide antibiotics, for which hypersensitivity can occur in as much as 6% of the population (6). Postmarketing surveillance reports show an incidence of serious rash associated with ZNS treatment of approximately 0.25% (5). Even so, caution and careful observation with use of ZNS in a patient with a recognized history of hypersensitivity to sulfonamide drugs are warranted.

Cognitive and Behavioral Side Effects. There is a lack of research into the potential impact of ZNS on cognition, particularly in children. A pilot study in nine adult patients with refractory partial-onset epilepsy, undergoing psychometric testing prior to and 12 weeks following the addition of ZNS, showed impairments in verbal learning without overt signs of overmedication (103). The degree of impairment correlated directly with ZNS plasma levels, particularly with blood levels greater than 30 μg/mL. However, retesting at 24 weeks failed to show significant changes in cognition function relative to baseline, suggesting a drug tolerance effect.

Adverse effects of ZNS on behavior and psychiatric functioning have been reported. In a retrospective report based on open-label use of ZNS for epilepsy in 68 pediatric patients, Kim and colleagues determined behavioral or psychiatric side effects in 23.5% of patients (78). Difficulties described included aggression, agitation, irritability, poor attention, hallucinations, hyperactivity, dysphoria, paranoia, and psychosis. All of these behavioral side effects resolved with lowering the dose or discontinuing ZNS. Only 5 patients in the entire study population (7.4%) discontinued because of side effects, suggesting that behavioral problems were handled successfully by a reduction in dose in most instances.

A postmarketing surveillance study in Japan of 1,512 patients (including 928 children ages more than 16 years) revealed irritable or excitable behavioral episodes in 45 patients (3.0%), depression in 8 (0.5%), and anxiety or hypochondria in 14 (0.9%) (97).

Teratogenicity. There is insufficient data regarding ZNS and any associated risk of fetal malformations (104). A small prospective registry study of pregnant epileptic women taking ZNS examined 26 offspring (105). The 4 children born to mothers taking ZNS monotherapy were normal. The remaining 22 offspring were exposed to AED polytherapy, including ZNS: 2 had significant malformations, 1 with anencephaly, and 1 with an atrial septal defect. Both of these mothers had low ZNS serum concentrations (6.1 μg/mL and 6.3 μg/mL, respectively) during the first trimester.

CLINICAL USE

A recent survey of recommendations for AED management by selected pediatric epilepsy specialists in the United States shows that ZNS is favorably regarded as a first-line option for initial monotherapy in children with myoclonic and generalized tonic-clonic seizures and as a second-line option for initial treatment of patients with IS, LGS, symptomatic generalized tonic-clonic seizures, and for children with partial seizures who have failed prior AED treatment (106).

Formulations for ZNS currently available in the United States include 25-mg, 50-mg, and 100-mg capsules. Liquid suspensions can be specially formulated, but there are no data regarding stability and shelf-life.

Initial dosing is usually at 1–2 mg/kg/day, and the conventional recommendation is to increase the dose by 1–2 mg/kg/day every 2 weeks. ZNS is correctly regarded as an AED for which it is suggested to "start low and go slow." Clinical experience has shown that tolerance is improved and the likelihood of dose-related side effects is lower with incremental dosing. The maximum dose is determined by patient tolerance and seizure control; however, a total daily dose of 10 mg/kg/day is a reasonable initial target, and doses up to 20 mg/kg/day are commonly used. In light of the long serum half-life, ZNS can be administered once or twice daily.

Anticipatory guidance should include a recommendation about the need for the child to stay well hydrated, in an effort to reduce the likelihood of renal calculi, and the need to be aware of the importance of environmental heat as a possible risk factor for oligohidrosis and hyperthermia.

SUMMARY

ZNS is properly regarded as a broad-spectrum AED. Although not often chosen as the drug of first choice for the newly diagnosed patient, ZNS is an important option for treating children with epilepsy who have failed initial therapy. It may be a particularly good choice for patients with myoclonic seizures as a component of their epilepsy. Although evidence from open-label trials and practice experience is compelling, controlled studies examining the efficacy of ZNS in children and its impact on cognition and behavior would be most welcome.

References

1. Seino M. Review of zonisamide development in Japan. *Seizure* 2004; 13 (Suppl 1): S2–S4.
2. Uno H, Kurokowa M, Masuda Y, Nishimura H. Studies on 3-substituted 1,2-benzisoxazole derivatives. VI. Synthesis and their anticonvulsant properties. *J Med Chem* 1979; 22:180–183.
3. Masuda Y, Karasawa T, Shiraishi Y, Hori M, et al. 3-Sulfamoylmethyl-1,2-benzisoxazole, a new type of anticonvulsant drug: pharmacological profile. *Arzneimittel-Forschung* 1980; 30:477–483.
4. Masuda Y, Ishizaki I, Shimizu M. Zonisamide: pharmacology and clinical efficacy in epilepsy. *CNS Drugs Rev* 1998; 4:341–360.
5. Leppik IE. Practical prescribing and long-term efficacy and safety of zonisamide. *Epilepsy Res* 2006; 68(Suppl 2); S17–S24.
6. Brackett CC, Singh H, Block JH. Likelihood and mechanisms of cross-allergenicity between sulfonamide antibiotics and other drugs containing a sulfonamide functional group. *Pharmacotherapy* 2004; 24:856–870.
7. Rock DM, Macdonald RL, Taylor CP. Blockade of sustained repetitive action potentials in cultured spinal cord neurons by zonisamide (AD 810, CI 912), a novel anticonvulsant. *Epilepsy Res* 1989; 3:138–143.
8. Schauf CL. Zonisamide enhances slow sodium inactivation in *Myxicola*. *Brain Res* 1987; 413:185–188.
9. Suzuki S, Kawakami K, Nishimura S, Watanabe Y, et al. Zonisamide blocks T-type calcium channels in cultured neurons of rat cerebral cortex. *Epilepsy Res* 1992; 12:21–27.
10. Kito M, Maehara M, Watanabe K. Mechanisms of T-type calcium channel blockade by zonisamide. *Seizure* 1996; 5:115–119.
11. Su H, Sochivko D, Becker A, Chen J, et al. Upregulation of a T-type Ca^{2+} channel causes a long-lasting modification of neuronal firing mode after status epilepticus. *J Neurosci* 2002; 22:3645–3655.
12. Beck H, Steffens R, Heinemann U, Elger CE. Properties of voltage-activated Ca^{2+} currents in acutely isolated human hippocampal granule cells. *J Neurophysiol* 1997; 77:1526–1537.
13. Okada M, Kawata Y, Mizuno K, Wada K, et al. Interaction between Ca^{2+}, K^+, carbamazepine and zonisamide on hippocampal extracellular glutamate monitored with a microdialysis electrode. *Br J Pharmacol* 1998; 124:1277–1285.
14. Okada M, Kaneko S, Hirano T, Ishida M, et al. Effects of zonisamide on extracellular levels of monoamine and its metabolite, and on Ca^{2+} dependent dopamine release. *Epilepsy Res* 1992; 13:113–119.
15. Okada M, Kaneko S, Hirano T, Mizuno K, et al. Effects of zonisamide on dopaminergic system. *Epilepsy Res* 1995; 22:193–205.
16. Kawata Y, Okada M, Murakami T, Mizuno K, et al. Effects of zonisamide on K^+ and Ca^{2+} evoked release of monoamine as well as K^+ evoked intracellular Ca^{2+} mobilization in rat hippocampus. *Epilepsy Res* 1999; 35:173–182.
17. Okada M, Hirano T, Kawata Y, Murakami T, et al. Biphasic effects of zonisamide on serotonergic system in rat hippocampus. *Epilepsy Res* 1999; 34:187–197.
18. Gluck MR, Santana LA, Granson H, Yahr MD. Novel dopamine releasing response of an anti-convulsant agent with possible anti-Parkinson's activity. *J Neural Transm* 2004; 111:713–724.
19. Ueda Y, Doi T, Tokumaru J, Willmore LJ. Effect of zonisamide on molecular regulation of glutamate and GABA transporter proteins during epileptogenesis in rats with hippocampal seizures. *Brain Res Mol Brain Res* 2003; 116:1–6.
20. Masuda Y, Karasawa T. Inhibitory effect of zonisamide on human carbonic anhydrase in vitro. *Arzneimittel-Forschung* 1993; 43:416–418.
21. Masuda Y, Noguchi H, Karasawa T. Evidence against a significant implication of carbonic anhydrase inhibitory activity of zonisamide in its anticonvulsant effect. *Arzneimittel-Forschung* 1994; 44:267–269.
22. Leppik IE. Zonisamide: chemistry, mechanism of action, and pharmacokinetics. *Seizure* 2004; 13(Suppl 1):S5–S9.
23. Ito T, Hori M, Masuda Y, Yoshida K, et al. Sulfamoylmethyl-1,2-benzisoxazole, a new type of anticonvulsant drug: electroencephalographic profile. *Arzneimittel-Forschung* 1980; 30:603–609.
24. Wada Y, Hasegawa H, Okuda H, Yamaguchi N. Anticonvulsant effects of zonisamide and phenytoin on seizure activity of the feline visual cortex. *Brain Dev* 1990; 12: 206–210.
25. Hamada K, Song HK, Ishida S, Yagi K, et al. Contrasting effects of zonisamide and acetazolamide on amygdaloid kindling in rats. *Epilepsia* 2001; 42:1379–1386.
26. Komatsu M, Hiramatsu M, Willmore LJ. Zonisamide reduces the increase in 8-hydroxy-2'-deoxyguanosine levels formed during iron-induced epileptogenesis in the brains of rats. *Epilepsia* 2000; 41:1091–1094.
27. Mori A, Noda Y, Packer L. The anticonvulsant zonisamide scavenges free radicals. *Epilepsy Res* 1998; 30:153–158.
28. Noda Y, Mori A, Packer L. Zonisamide inhibits nitric oxide synthase activity induced by N-methyl-D-aspartate and buthionine sulfoximine in the rat hippocampus. *Res Commun Mol Pathol Pharmacol* 1999; 105:23–33.

29. Tokumaru J, Ueda Y, Yokoyama H, Nakajima A, et al. In vivo evaluation of hippocampal anti-oxidant ability of zonisamide in rats. *Neurochem Res* 2000; 25:1107–1111.
30. Ueda Y, Doi T, Tokumaru J, Nakajima A, et al. In vivo evaluation of the effect of zonisamide on the hippocampal redox state during kainic acid-induced seizure status in rats. *Neurochem Res* 2005; 30:1117–1121.
31. Hayakawa T, Higuchi H, Nigami H, Hattori H. Zonisamide reduces hypoxic-ischemic brain damage in neonatal rats irrespective of its anticonvulsive effect. *Eur J Pharmacol* 1994; 257:131–136.
32. Minato H, Kikuta C, Fujitani B, Masuda Y. Protective effect of zonisamide, an antiepileptic drug, against transient focal cerebral ischemia with middle cerebral artery occlusion-reperfusion in rats. *Epilepsia* 1997; 38:975–980.
33. Owen AJ, Ijaz S, Miyashita H, Wishart T, et al. Zonisamide as a neuroprotective agent in an adult gerbil model of global forebrain ischemia: a histological, in vivo microdialysis and behavioral study. *Brain Res* 1997; 770:115–122.
34. Biton V. Zonisamide: newer antiepileptic agent with multiple mechanisms of action. *Expert Rev Neurotherapeutics* 2004; 4:935–943.
35. Perucca E, Bialer M. The clinical pharmacokinetics of the newer antiepileptic drugs. Focus on topiramate, zonisamide and tiagabine. *Clin Pharmacokinet* 1996; 31:29–46.
36. Perucca E. Pharmacokinetic variability of new antiepileptic drugs at different ages. *Ther Drug Monit* 2005; 27:714–717.
37. Mimaki T. Clinical pharmacology and therapeutic drug monitoring of zonisamide. *Ther Drug Monitor* 1998; 29:593–597.
38. Willmore LJ. Commentary on Leppik. *Seizure* 2004; 13(Suppl 1):S10.
39. Mimaki T, Tanoue H, Matsunaga Y, Miyazaki H, et al. Regional distribution of 14C-zonisamide in rat brain. *Epilepsy Res* 1994; 17:233–236.
40. Ito T, Yamaguchi T, Miyazaki H, Sekine Y, et al. Pharmacokinetic studies of AD-810, a new antiepileptic compound: phase I trials. *Arzneimittel-Forschung* 1982; 32:1581–1586.
41. Kochak GM, Page JG, Buchanan RA, Peters R, et al. Steady-state pharmacokinetics of zonisamide, an antiepileptic agent for treatment of refractory complex partial seizures. *J Clin Pharmacol* 1998; 38:166–171.
42. Stiff DD, Zemaitis MA. Metabolism of the anticonvulsant agent zonisamide in the rat. *Drug Metab Dispos* 1990; 18:888–894.
43. Stiff DD, Robicheau JT, Zemaitis MA. Reductive metabolism of the anticonvulsant agent zonisamide, a 1,2-benzisoxazole derivative. *Xenobiotica* 1992; 22:1–11.
44. Nakasa H, Komiya M, Ohmori S, Rikihisa T, et al. Characterization of human liver microsomal cytochrome P450 involved in the reductive metabolism of zonisamide. *Mol Pharmacol* 1993; 44:216–221.
45. Nakasa H, Ohmori S, Kitada M. Formation of 2-sulphamoylacetylphenol from zonisamide under aerobic conditions in rat liver microsomes. *Xenobiotica* 1996; 26:495–501.
46. Eisai Inc., Zonegran (zonisamide) FDA Approved Labeling Text, March 27, 2000.
47. Nakasa H, Komiya M, Ohmori S, Rikihisa T, et al. Rat liver microsomal cytochrome P-450 responsible for reductive metabolism of zonisamide. *Drug Metab Dispos* 1993; 21:777–781.
48. Ojemann LM, Shastri RA, Wilensky AJ, Friel PN, et al. Comparative pharmacokinetics of zonisamide (CI-912) in epileptic patients on carbamazepine or phenytoin monotherapy. *Ther Drug Monit* 1986; 8:293–296.
49. Wagner JG, Sackellares JC, Donofrio PD, Berent S, et al. Nonlinear pharmacokinetics of CI-912 in adult epileptic patients. *Ther Drug Monit* 1984; 6:277–283.
50. Sackellares JC, Donofrio PD, Wagner JG, Abou-Khalil B, et al. Pilot study of zonisamide (1,2-benzisoxazole-3-methanesulfonamide) in patients with refractory partial seizures. *Epilepsia* 1985; 26:206–211.
51. Nakasa H, Komiya M, Ohmori S, Kitada M, et al. Formation of reductive metabolite, 2-sulfamoylacetylphenol, from zonisamide in rat liver microsomes. *Res Commun Chem Pathol Pharmacol* 1992; 77:31–41.
52. Eisai Inc., data on file.
53. Glauser TA, Pellock JM. Zonisamide in pediatric epilepsy: review of the Japanese literature. *J Child Neurol* 2002; 17:87–96.
54. Miura H. Zonisamide monotherapy with once-daily dosing in children with cryptogenic localization-related epilepsies: clinical effects and pharmacokinetic studies. *Seizure* 2004; 13(Suppl 1):S17–S23.
55. Wilensky AJ, Friel PN, Ojemann LM, Dodrill CB, et al. Zonisamide in epilepsy: a pilot study. *Epilepsia* 1985; 26:212–220.
56. Brodie MJ, Duncan R, Vespignani H, Solyom A, et al. Dose-dependent safety and efficacy of zonisamide: a randomized, double-blind, placebo-controlled study in patients with refractory partial seizures. *Epilepsia* 2005; 46:31–41.
57. Schmidt D, Jacob R, Loiseau P, Deisenhammer E, et al. Zonisamide for add-on treatment of refractory partial epilepsy: a European double-blind trial. *Epilepsy Res* 1993; 15:67–73.
58. Faught E, Ayala R, Montouris GG, Leppik IE. Randomized controlled trial of zonisamide for the treatment of refractory partial-onset seizures. *Neurology* 2001; 57:1774–1779.
59. Sackellares JC, Ramsay RE, Wilder BJ, Browne TR III, et al. Randomized, controlled clinical trial of zonisamide as adjunctive treatment for refractory partial seizures. *Epilepsia* 2004; 45:610–617.
60. Brodie MJ. Zonisamide clinical trials: European experience. *Seizure* 2004; 13(Suppl 1): S66–S70.
61. Faught E. Review of United States and European clinical trials of zonisamide in the treatment of refractory partial-onset seizures. *Seizure* 2004; 13(Suppl 1):S59–S65.
62. Shuto H, Sugimoto T, Yasuhara A, et al. Efficacy of zonisamide in children with refractory partial seizures. *Curr Therapeut Res* 1989; 45:1031–1036. [As cited in reference (53)]
63. Hosoda N, Miura H, Takanashi S, et al. Clinical efficacy and blood concentration with once-daily zonisamide monotherapy in pediatric patients with partial seizures [in Japanese]. *TDM Kenkyu* 1993; X:240–241. [As cited in reference (53)]
64. Hosoda N, Miura H, Takanashi S, et al. Clinical effects and blood concentration of zonisamide in epileptic children with partial seizures treated with a once-daily dose of zonisamide monotherapy. *Jpn J Ther Drug Monit* 1994; O-18:68. [As cited in reference (53)]
65. Hosoda N, Miura H, Takanashi S, et al. Once-daily dose of zonisamide monotherapy in the control of partial seizures in children with cryptogenic localization-related epilepsies: clinical effects and their pharmacokinetic basis. *Jpn J Psychiatry Neurol* 1994; 48:335–337. [As cited in reference (53)]
66. Kumagai N, Seki T, Yamawaki H, Suzuki N, et al. Monotherapy for childhood epilepsies with zonisamide. *Jpn J Psychiatry Neurol* 1991; 45:357–359.
67. Hayakawa T, Nejihashi Y, Kishi T, et al. Serum zonisamide concentration in fresh cases of childhood epilepsy following zonisamide monotherapy [in Japanese]. *J Jpn Epilepsy Soc* 1994; 12:249–254. [As cited in reference (53)]
68. Fukushima K, Yagi K, Seino M, et al. Phase II clinical trial of a new antiepileptic drug, zonisamide (ZNA) in pediatric epilepsy patients [in Japanese]. *Jpn J Pediatr* 1987; 40:3389–3397. [As cited in reference (53)]
69. Kanazawa K, Segoku A, Kawai I. A clinical trial of zonisamide, a new antiepileptic drug, on adults and children with refractory epilepsy [in Japanese]. *J Clin Therapeut Med* 1987; 3:1181–1186. [As cited in reference (53)]
70. Takahashi I, Yamamoto N, Furune S, et al. Efficacy of zonisamide for intractable epilepsy in childhood [in Japanese]. *J Jpn Epilepsy Soc* 1987; 5:100–105. [As cited in reference (53)]
71. Tagawa T, Mimaki T, Yabuuchi H, et al. Treatment of childhood epilepsies with zonisamide (AD-810) [in Japanese]. *J Pediatr Pract* 1988; 51:539–543. [As cited in reference (53)]
72. Oguni H, Hayakawa T, Fukuyama Y. Clinical trial of zonisamide, a new antiepileptic drug, in cases of refectory childhood epilepsy [in Japanese]. *J Jpn Epilepsy Soc* 1989; 7:43–50. [As cited in reference (53)]
73. Oguni H, Hayashi K, Fukuyama Y, et al. Phase III clinical study of the new antiepileptic drug AD-810 (zonisamide) in patients with childhood epilepsy [in Japanese]. *Jpn J Pediatr* 1988; 41:439–450. [As cited in reference (53)]
74 Suzuki N, Seki T, Yamawaki H, et al. Therapy of partial epilepsy with AD-810 (zonisamide). *Jpn J Pediatr* 1987; 40:3147–3152. [As cited in reference (53)]
75. Sakamoto K, Kurokawa T, Tomita S, et al. Effects of zonisamide on children with epilepsy. *Curr Therapeut Res* 1988; 13:378–383. [As cited in reference (53)]
76. Seki T, Kumagai N, Maezawa M. Effects of zonisamide monotherapy in children with epilepsy. *Seizure* 2004; 13(Suppl 1):S26–S32.
77. Wilfong AA. Zonisamide monotherapy for epilepsy in children and young adults. *Pediatr Neurol* 2005; 32:77–80.
78. Kim HL, Aldridge J, Rho JM. Clinical experience with zonisamide monotherapy and adjunctive therapy in children with epilepsy at a tertiary care referral center. *J Child Neurol* 2005; 20:212–219.
79. Santos CC, Brotherton T. Use of zonisamide in pediatric patients. *Pediatr Neurol* 2005; 33:12–14.
80. Mandelbaum DE, Bunch M, Kugler SL, Venkatasubramanian A, et al. Broad-spectrum efficacy of zonisamide at 12 months in children with intractable epilepsy. *J Child Neurol* 2005; 20:594–597.
81. Kim D, Song I, Keum S, Lee T, et al. Lack of the burst firing of thalamocortical relay neurons and resistance to absence seizures in mice lacking alpha (1G) T-type Ca(2+) channels. *Neuron* 2001; 31:35–45.
82. Wilfong A, Schultz R. Zonisamide for absence seizures. *Epilepsy Res* 2005; 64: 31–34.
83. Kothare SV, Valencia I, Khurana DS, Hardison H, et al. Efficacy and tolerability of zonisamide in juvenile myoclonic epilepsy. *Epileptic Disord* 2004; 6:267–270.
84. Suzuki Y, Nagai T, Ono J, Imai K, et al. Zonisamide monotherapy in newly diagnosed infantile spasms. *Epilepsia* 1997; 38:1035–1038.
85. Yanai S, Hanai T, Narazaki O. Treatment of infantile spasms with zonisamide. *Brain Dev* 1999; 21:157–161.
86. Kishi T, Nejihashi Y, Kajiyama M, Ueda K. Successful zonisamide treatment for infants with hypsarrhythmia. *Pediatr Neurol* 2000; 23:274–277.
87. Suzuki Y. Zonisamide in West syndrome. *Brain Dev* 2001; 23:658–661.
88. Suzuki Y, Imai K, Toribe Y, Ueda H, et al. Long-term response to zonisamide in patients with West syndrome. *Neurology* 2002; 58:1556–1559.
89. Lotze TE, Wilfong AA. Zonisamide treatment for symptomatic infantile spasms. *Neurology* 2004; 62:296–298.
90. Yanagaki S, Oguni H, Yoshii K, Hayashi K, et al. Zonisamide for West syndrome: a comparison of clinical responses among different titration rate. *Brain Dev* 2005; 27:286–290.
91. Yamauchi T, Aikawa H. Efficacy of zonisamide: our experience. *Seizure* 2004; 13(Suppl 1): S41–S48.
92. Henry TR, Leppik IE, Gumnit RJ, Jacobs M. Progressive myoclonus epilepsy treated with zonisamide. *Neurology* 1988; 38:928–931.
93. Kyllerman M, Ben-Menachem E. Zonisamide for progressive myoclonus epilepsy: long-term observations in seven patients. *Epilepsy Res* 1998; 29:109–114.
94. Yoshimura I, Kaneko S, Yoshimura N, Murakami T. Long-term observations of two siblings with Lafora disease treated with zonisamide. *Epilepsy Res* 2001; 46: 283–287.
95. Wheless JW, Sankar R. Treatment strategies for myoclonic seizures and epilepsy syndromes associated with myoclonic seizures. *Epilepsia* 2003; 44(Suppl 11):27–37.
96. Yagi K. Overview of Japanese experience—controlled and uncontrolled trials. *Seizure* 2004; 13(Suppl 1):S11–S15.
97. Ohtahara S, Yamatogi Y. Safety of zonisamide therapy: prospective follow-up survey. *Seizure* 2004; 13(Suppl 1):S50–S55.

98. Low PA, James S, Peschel T, Leong R, et al. Zonisamide and associated oligohydrosis and hyperthermia. *Epilepsy Res* 2004; 62:27–34.
99. Knudsen JF, Thambi LR, Kapcala LP, Racoosin JA. Oligohydrosis and fever in pediatric patients treated with zonisamide. *Pediatr Neurol* 2003; 28: 184–189.
100. Okumura A, Hayakawa F, Kuno K, Watanabe K. Oligohydrosis caused by zonisamide [in Japanese]. *No To Hattatsu* 1996; 28:44–47.
101. Peters DH, Sorkin EM. Zonisamide: a review of its pharmacodynamic and pharmacokinetic properties and therapeutic potential in epilepsy. *Drugs* 1993; 45: 760–787.
102. Bennett WM. Risk of kidney stones in patients treated with zonisamide. *Neurology* 2002; 58(Suppl 3):S298–S299 [Abstract].
103. Berent S, Sackellares JC, Giordani B, Wagner JG, et al. Zonisamide (CI-912) and cognition: results from preliminary study. *Epilepsia* 1987; 28:61–67.
104. Perucca E. Birth defects after prenatal exposure to antiepileptic drugs. *Lancet Neurol* 2005; 4:781–786.
105. Kondo T, Kaneko S, Amano Y, Egawa I. Preliminary report on teratogenic effects of zonisamide in the offspring of treated women with epilepsy. *Epilepsia* 1996; 37:1242–1244.
106. Wheless JW, Clarke DF, Carpenter D. Treatment of pediatric epilepsy: expert opinion, 2005. *J Child Neurol* 2005; 20(1):S1–S56.

57 The Ketogenic Diet

Douglas R. Nordli, Jr.
Darryl C. De Vivo

The ketogenic diet (KD) is a high-fat, low-carbohydrate regimen with adequate protein. It has been used for more than 70 years on thousands of patients. It is effective and safe, but, like any medical treatment for epilepsy, it must be judiciously applied and carefully monitored.

There are biblical passages that some regard as referring to the salutary effects of starvation on seizure control, but the earliest scientific reports emerged in the 1920s. Geyelin at the Presbyterian Hospital carefully studied the beneficial effects of starvation on seizures (1). Shortly thereafter, Wilder proposed a high-fat diet to mimic the effects of starvation (2). At the time, it was known that ketone bodies could be found in the urine of patients with diabetes and that they were produced when fatty acids were oxidized. This led to the notion that ketone bodies were metabolic waste products of fatty acid degradation. Because this high-fat diet increased the production of ketone bodies, the regimen became known as a ketogenic diet or "keto." Its anticonvulsant effect was attributed to a sedative effect of the ketone bodies on the nervous system; this notion is easy to understand because the available anticonvulsants of that era—bromides and phenobarbital—were both sedatives.

In the 1950s, however, it was discovered that a separate pathway synthesized the ketone bodies, acetoacetate (AcAc) and 3-hydroxybutyrate; in 1961 Krebs suggested that ketone bodies were fuels for respiration. In 1967 Owen and colleagues proved that ketone bodies were the major fuel for brain metabolism during starvation (3). Appleton and De Vivo later showed in experimental animals that the utilization of ketone bodies during starvation altered brain metabolites and increased cerebral energy reserves (4). Huttenlocher showed that the level of ketosis correlated with efficacy (5).

There are several different variations of the KD, but the mostly widely used regimen uses long-chain triglycerides (LCT) in the form of heavy cream, butter, and meat fat. We review the scientific basis, effectiveness, and safety of the LCT diet.

SCIENTIFIC BASIS OF THE DIET

Improved Cerebral Energy Reserves and Increased Gamma-Aminobutyric Acid (GABA) Synthesis

Ketone bodies derive from the metabolism of nonesterified fatty acids. During the fasting state, the fall in blood glucose reduces plasma insulin production, stimulates lipolysis in fatty tissues, and increases the flux of nonesterified fatty acids to the liver. Nonesterified fatty acids can be esterified or metabolized to ketone bodies.

The fate of fatty acids in the liver is determined, at least in part, by the carbohydrate status of the host (6). A critical component of this regulation is malonyl-CoA, an intermediate in the pathway of lipogenesis. (7, 8). Malonyl-CoA inhibits carnitine acyltransferase I, which is needed to shuttle long-chain fatty acyl-CoA into the mitochondria for oxidation. The production of glucose from glycogen provides the carbon source for lipogenesis and, in particular, malonyl-CoA. If glucose is reduced, so is malonyl-CoA. The reduction in malonyl-CoA decreases the inhibition on (or increases the net activity of) carnitine acyltransferase. This allows more movement of fatty acids into the mitochondria, where fatty acyl-CoA is converted to acetyl-CoA, and later acetoacetate. Acetoacetate is in equilibrium with beta-hydroxybutyrate, the major ketone body utilized by the brain.

Passage of ketone bodies into the brain may be the critical factor limiting the rate of brain utilization of ketone bodies. Movement of ketone bodies into the brain relies on the monocarboxylic transport system (MCT-1). This is up-regulated during fasting in adults and during milk feeding in neonates (9, 10). Fasting studies in humans demonstrated that the brain's ability to extract ketone bodies is inversely related to the age of the subject (3). In contrast to glucose, ketone bodies can pass directly into mitochondria without being processed in the cytosol. Also, in contrast to glucose, ketone bodies may be used directly by neurons for metabolism (11).

Once inside the mitochondria, beta-hydroxybutyrate is converted to AcAc, and then to AcAc-CoA. The enzyme that facilitates this is 3-oxoacid-CoA transferase or succinyl-CoA-acetoacetate-CoA transferase. As the name implies, this conversion requires commensurate conversion of succinyl-CoA to succinate. It is possible that reduced blood glucose and increased blood ketone may be needed to induce the activity of this enzyme (12).

Scientific studies of the KD have revealed important biochemical and metabolic observations. Appleton and De Vivo (4) developed an animal model to permit study of the effect of the KD on cerebral metabolism (Figure 57-1). Adult male albino rats were placed on either a high-fat diet containing (by weight) 38% corn oil, 38% lard, 11% vitamin-free casein, 6.8% glucose, 4% U.S. P. salt mixture, and 2.2% vitamin diet fortification mixture, or on a high-carbohydrate diet containing (by weight) 50% glucose, 28.8% vitamin-free casein, 7.5% corn oil, 7.5% lard, 4% U.S. P. salt mixture, and 2.2% vitamin diet fortification mixture. Parallel studies were conducted to evaluate electroconvulsive shock responses and biochemical alterations. These studies revealed that the mean voltage necessary to produce a minimal convulsion remained constant for 12 days before the high-fat diet was started and for about 10 days after beginning the feedings (69.75 ± 1.88 volts). After the animal was on the high-fat diet for 10–12 days, the intensity of the convulsive response to the established

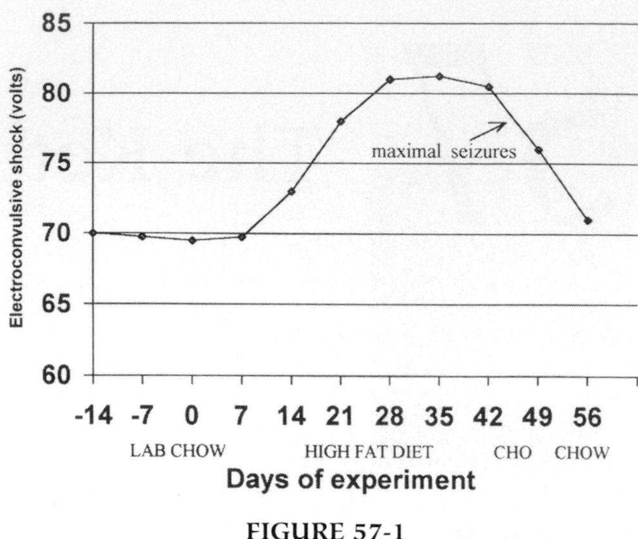

FIGURE 57-1

The effect in adult rats of dietary manipulation on the electroconvulsive threshold. Abstracted from the original, Appleton DB, De Vivo DC, *Epilepsia* 15:211–227, 1974 (4), with permission.

voltage decreased, necessitating an increase in voltage to reestablish a minimal convulsive response. Approximately 20 days after the animal began the high-fat diet, a new convulsive threshold was achieved (81.25 ± 2.39 volts) ($P < 0.01$). When the high-fat diet was replaced by the high-carbohydrate diet, a rapid change in response to the voltage was observed. Within 48 hours the animal exhibited a maximal convulsion to the electrical stimulus, which had previously produced only a minimal convulsion, and the mean voltage to produce a minimal convulsion returned to the prestudy value (70.75 ± 1.37 volts).

Blood concentrations of beta-hydroxybutyrate, acetoacetate, chloride, esterified fatty acids, triglycerides, cholesterol, and total lipids increased in the rats fed on the high-fat diet. Brain levels of beta-hydroxybutyrate and sodium were also significantly increased in the fat-fed rats.

De Vivo et al reported the change in cerebral metabolites in chronically ketotic rats and found no changes in brain water content, electrolytes, or pH (13). As expected, fat-fed rats had significantly lower blood glucose concentrations and higher blood beta-hydroxybutyrate and acetoacetate concentrations. More importantly, brain concentrations of adenosine triphosphate (ATP), glycogen, glucose-6-phosphate, pyruvate, lactate, beta-hydroxybutyrate, citrate, alpha-ketoglutarate, and alanine were higher and the brain concentrations of fructose 1, 6-diphosphate, aspartate, adenosine diphosphate (ADP), creatine, cyclic nucleotides, acid-insoluble CoA, and total CoA were lower in the fat-fed group.

The biochemical implications of these results can be grouped into three major categories:

1. Glycolysis and glucose flux are reduced during ketosis. As Wilder originally postulated, the effects of eating a high-fat, low-carbohydrate diet are similar to the biochemical consequences of starvation (2). In this regard, the reduction in glycolysis makes physiologic sense, because the starving organism wants to make every attempt to preserve the rather meager stores of glycogen and to provide the brain with an alternate, more substantial fuel for metabolism (ketone bodies from fats). Measurements of glucose flux in children and adults during ketosis have confirmed the reduced utilization of glucose. Haymond et al. performed sequential glucose flux studies in 11 children (5 control, 6 with epilepsy) and 10 adult volunteers using tagged glucose (14). All subjects were studied after a fast while consuming either a normal diet or the KD. The authors found that glucose flux and ketonemia were inversely related, particularly when corrected for estimated brain mass. This was consistent with the replacement of glucose by ketone bodies for cerebral metabolism.
2. Tricarboxylic acid (TCA) cycle flux is increased by chronic ketosis. The enzyme alpha-ketoglutarate dehydrogenase is the rate-limiting enzyme in TCA cycle function. The major inhibitor of this enzyme is the concentration of the product of the reaction, succinyl-CoA. This product is relatively reduced in the fat-fed group (down 26%), implying that alpha-ketoglutarate dehydrogenase should be functioning at maximal capacity. Yet concentrations of alpha-ketoglutarate, the substrate for this enzyme, was found to be elevated 11% in the fat-fed group. The most plausible explanation is that the TCA cycle is driven to its maximal capacity and is overwhelming the ability of this rate-limiting enzyme to deal with substrate.
3. Cerebral energy reserves are increased by chronic ketosis.

Cerebral energy reserves were calculated from these measurements using the following equation (15):

$$\text{Energy reserve} = (\text{PCr} + \text{ADP}) + 2(\text{ATP} + \text{glucose}) + 2.9(\text{glycogen}) \quad (1).$$

Applying the values determined for phosphocreatine (PCr), ADP, ATP, glucose, and glycogen enabled the calculation of the reserves. Energy reserves were significantly higher in the fat-fed rats (26.4 ± 0.6) compared to those in the controls (23.6 ± 0.2) ($P < 0.005$).

Ketone bodies are thermodynamically more efficient fuels than glucose because they avoid the less efficient glycolytic pathway (Figure 57-2) (16). Animals fed an equivalent amount of calories in the form of high-fat diets are therefore expected to have more efficient energy production. Assuming that energy demands do not substantially change during fasting, the increased efficiency of ketone body utilization most likely contributes to higher energy reserves.

Pan et al used ^{31}P spectroscopic imaging at 4.1T to demonstrate an elevated ratio of phosphocreatine or inorganic phosphorus in patients on the KD and concluded that there was improvement of energy metabolism with use of the diet (17). Seven patients with intractable

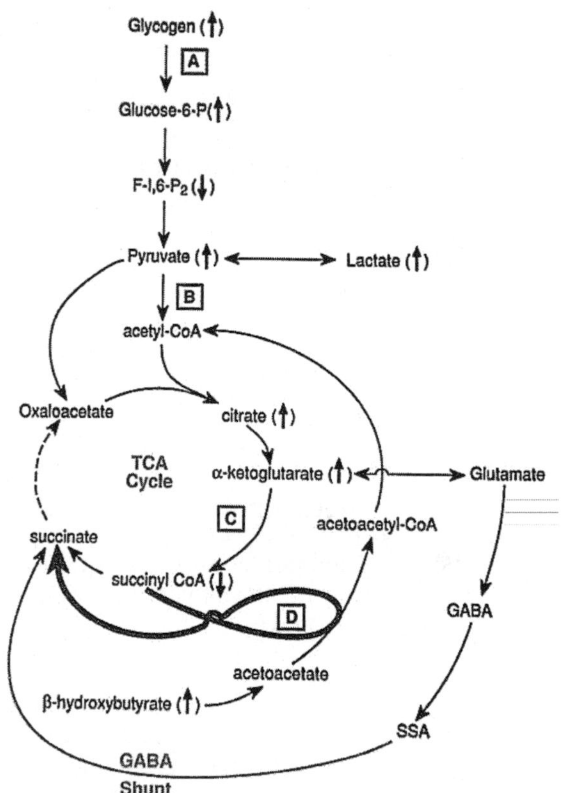

FIGURE 57-2

Summary of the relevant metabolic pathways affected by the ketogenic diet. The arrows ↑ and ↓ indicate significant differences of brain metabolites between ketotic animals and nonketotic animals. (A) phophofructokinase; (B) pyruvate dehydrogenase; (C) alpha-ketoglutarate dehydrogenase; (D) 3-oxoacid-CoA transferase; TCA, tricarboxylic acid; SSA, succinic semialdehyde. The biochemical observations imply that cerebral energetics is improved by chronic ketosis. These findings also suggest that flux rates through the tricarboxylic acid cycle and the gamma-aminobutyrate (GABA) shunt may be maximized and that GABA effects may be augmented. Used with permission from Nordli and De Vivo, 1997 (16).

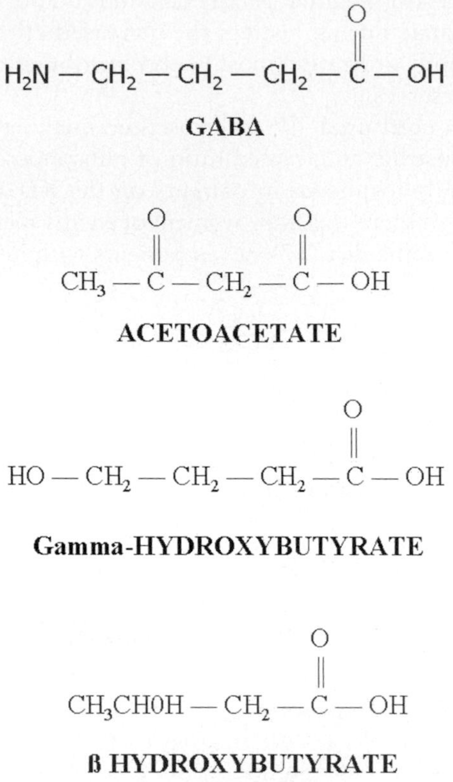

$$H_2N - CH_2 - CH_2 - CH_2 - \overset{O}{\overset{\|}{C}} - OH$$

GABA

$$CH_3 - \overset{O}{\overset{\|}{C}} - CH_2 - \overset{O}{\overset{\|}{C}} - OH$$

ACETOACETATE

$$HO - CH_2 - CH_2 - CH_2 - \overset{O}{\overset{\|}{C}} - OH$$

Gamma-HYDROXYBUTYRATE

$$CH_3CHOH - CH_2 - \overset{O}{\overset{\|}{C}} - OH$$

ß HYDROXYBUTYRATE

FIGURE 57-3

Chemical structural similarities of GABA, acetoacetate, gamma-hydroxybutyrate, and beta-hydroxybutyrate.

epilepsy (four with Lennox-Gastaut syndrome, one with absence seizures, one with primary generalized tonic-clonic seizures, and one with partial complex seizures) were studied before and after institution of the KD. Coronal ^1H anatomic imaging was performed to provide a correlate to the ^{31}P data. Ratios of PCr:ATP were measured at baseline and compared with those obtained after the KD. These showed a small but significant increase from 0.61 ± 0.08 to 0.69 ± 0.08 ($P < 0.05$). The ratio of PCr to inorganic phosphorus also changed from 2.45 ± 0.27 at baseline to 2.99 ± 0.44 during the diet ($P < 0.05$). The authors calculated an increase in the ΔG of ATP hydrolysis from 12.5 kcal/mol to 12.85 kcal/mol, or 2.5%.

In summary, the available biochemical data suggest that the KD favorably influences cerebral energetics by increasing cerebral energy reserves. This may be an important mechanism behind the increased resistance to seizures in ketotic brain tissue and the favorable cognitive effect sometimes seen with the KD.

Direct Anticonvulsant Effects of Ketone Bodies

There are direct anticonvulsant effects of the ketone bodies that perhaps relate to the chemical structural similarities of GABA, beta-hydroxybutyrate, and acetoacetate (Figure 57-3). Rats given intraperitoneal acetone showed reduction in seizures in the maximal electroshock, pentylenetetrazole, generalized-kindled seizures, focal-kindled seizures and AY-9944 models (18). Acetoacetate and acetone also suppressed seizures in Frings audiogenic, seizure-susceptible mice (19).

Possible Neuroprotective Effects Mediated by Mitochondrial Uncoupling Protein

In a model thought to mimic human idiopathic epilepsy, EL mice were shown to have a delayed development of seizures, implying an antiepileptogenic effect of the KD (20). This and the results of other studies also suggested a possible neuroprotective effect of the KD, perhaps involving inhibition of caspase-3-mediated apoptosis (21, 22). Others have examined the effect of the KD on mitochondrial uncoupling protein in the hippocampi of juvenile mice. Mitochondrial respiration rates were found to be substantially higher, and Western blots showed significant increases in uncoupling protein levels, particularly in the dentate gyrus of KD-fed mice. This, combined with the results of reactive oxygen species studies, suggested that the KD might be neuroprotective by diminishing reactive oxygen species production through activation of mitochondrial uncoupling proteins (23).

INITIATION OF THERAPY

Prior to the initiation of the KD, a nutrition support team or registered dietitian performs a comprehensive assessment. The nutritionist or dietitian asks whether there have been any gastrointestinal problems, food allergies, or feeding difficulties, such as problems with sucking, swallowing, or chewing. They also note the patient's weight, height, usual weight, weight pattern since birth, and head circumference. Next, weight-for-age and height-for-age are plotted and ideal body weight-for-height is determined. Laboratory data are used other tools for nutritional assessment of the patient, and we routinely obtain serum protein, lipid profile, electrolytes, free and total carnitine, hemoglobin, hematocrit, and red blood indices.

The nutritionist or dietitian reviews the method of delivery of the KD, taking into consideration factors such as the patient's age, stage of development, and expected tolerance of the regimen. In the usual case, the KD is offered in a normal, by-mouth fashion, with the expectation being that the patient will eat and drink as is appropriate for his or her developmental stage. The consistency of the KD can be altered to adjust for feeding difficulties. In very rare circumstances, the nutritional support team may recommend the use of a feeding tube. If patients are to be fasted, they should be hospitalized for the initiation of the KD. Close observation is important because a child with an occult underlying inborn error of metabolism, particularly one that interferes with utilization of ketone bodies, could quickly decompensate (24). The hospitalization also provides the opportunity for family members to be instructed on the maintenance of the diet.

Although this is the traditional method of starting the KD for many, others argue that a fast is not necessary and that equivalent or superior results can be obtained without fasting (25). In one study, Bergqvist and colleagues randomized children who were starting the KD into two groups: one group began with a 24- to 48-hour fast, and the other had a gradual initiation of the KD without a fast (26), They found no difference in efficacy between the two groups, but those who had a gradual initiation of the KD without fasting had less weight reduction, fewer episodes of hypoglycemia, less treatments for acidosis, and a reduced need for intravenous (IV) fluid treatment for dehydration.

The LCT diet consists of three or four parts fat to one part nonfat (carbohydrate and protein) calculated on the basis of weight. It is computed to provide 75 to 100 kcal/kg per body weight and 1–2 g dietary protein/kg of body weight per day. Caloric requirements are adjusted to minimize weight gain and to maximize ketonemia. If a 3:1 (fat-to-nonfat) ratio is insufficient to produce the required ketosis, a ratio of 4:1 is used.

THE CONVENTIONAL KD OR LCT DIET

Prior to initiating the conventional KD or LCT diet, a dietary prescription is made. Calculation of this prescription is straightforward. For example, if a 10-kg 2-year-old child is to be started on a 3:1 diet, one begins by estimating the calorie requirements of the child:

$$10 \text{ kg} \times 100 \text{ kcal/kg/day} = 1000 \text{ kcal/day} \quad (2)$$

Alternatively, consulting a table of recommended daily allowances (RDA) may derive this figure. In either case, it may require adjustment based on the child's individual metabolic needs. In general, starting prescriptions should begin with 75–80% of RDA needs, but these figures may need to be modified depending on the child's level of activity.

The 3:1 ratio of the diet stipulates that 4 grams of food must contain 3 grams of fat and 1 gram of nonfat. The nonfat consists of both carbohydrate and protein. One gram of fat has the caloric equivalent of nine calories, whereas 1 gram of protein or carbohydrate has the calorie equivalent of approximately four calories. Four grams of food (arbitrarily referred to as one unit here) on a 3:1 diet is equal to 31 calories:

$$1\text{g fat} = 9 \text{ calories} \times 3 = 27 \text{ calories}$$

$$1\text{g protein and carbohydrate} = 4 \text{ calories} \times 1 = 4 \text{ calories}$$

$$\text{Total calories} = 27 + 4 = 31 \text{ calories per unit} \quad (3)$$

To calculate the daily fat intake, one first divides the daily requirements of calories by this number of 31 calories per unit, which generates the number of units required for the day:

$$1000 \text{ calories/day}/31 \text{ calories/unit} = 32.25 \text{ units/day} \quad (4)$$

Next, multiplying by 27 calories of fat per unit provides the daily fat requirement:

$$32.26 \text{ units/day} \times 27 \text{ calories of fat per unit} = 871 \text{ calories of fat per day} \quad (5)$$

which is equivalent to 96 grams.

The protein requirement depends on the age of the child: children ages 1–3 years require 1.2 g protein/kg/day, children ages 4–6 years require 1.1 g protein/kg/day, and children ages 7 and up require 1 g protein/kg/day. For this child, the requirement would be 10 kg × 1.2 g/kg or 12 g/day (48 calories). Alternatively, one may consult the RDA table to determine the protein requirement.

So far, the combination of 871 calories of fat and 48 calories of protein leaves only 81 calories (i.e., 1,000 – 919) that are not accounted for in the daily allowance. The carbohydrate intake is calculated to supply the necessary remaining calories (81 calories), which is approximately 20 g.

The diet prescription for this 10-kg patient on a 3:1 LCT diet is the following:

Fat: 96 grams per day or 32 grams per meal

Protein: 12 grams per day or 4 grams per meal

Carbohydrate: 20 grams per day or 7 grams per meal

Meal Preparation

Meal preparation is key to the success of the diet for patients who are fed by mouth. The meals can be generated using calculations either by a trained dietitian or utilizing a computerized program. The advantage of involving a dietitian for the KD is that meals are calculated under strict guidelines to ensure that they meet the prescription of the diet and also the child's complete dietary needs. The dietitian may also provide valuable insights into the timing of meals and snacks to help maximize consistent control of ketosis and seizures. If parents utilize a home computer program, a dietitian should oversee these recipes to ensure that the nutritional elements are complete and within the doctor's prescription.

When the diet is begun, the number of meal options should be limited to help eliminate errors. Over time, meal options can be increased to provide variety. Variety is important because it increases satisfaction and thereby helps encourage continuation on the diet. Some institutions use a fruit and vegetable exchange system, which allows these foods to be organized by categories and substituted without the need for arduous recalculations. While on the KD, children need daily supplements of calcium and a multivitamin. Care must be taken so that these supplements (and all medications) are appropriately low in carbohydrates. The diet ratio, total calories, or both may need to be altered with the help of the physician to maximize seizure control. Dietary protein may also need adjustment to ensure proper growth. (27)

Liquid KD

For infants who are bottle-fed or older children who are tube-fed, the KD can be adapted to a liquid form. The ingredients are available through a pharmacy, and the preparation is simple for parents to learn. There are two regimens that can be prescribed for the liquid KD: KetoCal® and the modular formula with a product manufactured by Ross Laboratories, Columbus, Ohio: Ross Carbohydrate Free (RCF®). KetoCal®, manufactured by Nutricia North America (Rockville, Maryland), is a nutritionally complete formula powder that provides a 4:1 ketogenic ratio. It contains 30 g of protein/L, 144 g of fat/L, and 6 g of carbohydrate/L. This diet regimen has a makeup of 90% fats (all of which are LCT), 1.6% carbohydrates, and 8.4% protein. In addition, each liter provides 1,600 mg of calcium, 600 mg of sodium, 2,160 mg of potassium, and 22 mg of iron. This supplies 100% of the recommended vitamins and minerals, even at 75% of the RDA. No additional vitamin or mineral supplementation is necessary.

As an alternative, Ross Carbohydrate Free (RCF®) is a soy-based formula with iron that provides essential proteins and nutrients for the diet. It contains 40 g of protein/L, 72 g of fat/L, and 0.08 g of carbohydrate/L. In addition, each liter supplies 1,400 mg of calcium, 591 mg of sodium, 1,460 mg of potassium, and 24.3 mg of iron. RCF is used in conjunction with Ross Polycose® Glucose Polymers for carbohydrate and Microlipid® from Sherwood Services AG (St. Louis, MO) to provide the fat portion of the liquid KD. This is an emulsion of 50% fat that contains safflower oil and provides 1 gram of fat per 2 mL. The formula made from the mixture of RCF®, Polycose®, and Microlipid® can be given at scheduled bolus feedings or as a continuous enteral tube feeding. This formula method is utilized less often than the KetoCal® formula solely because of the ease of use of the latter. The RCF® regimen is lactose- and gluten-free and therefore is useful in patients with known sensitivities to these substances. When using KetoCal® or RCF® in combination with food, the formulas should contribute approximately 50% of the patient's total energy needs; the remaining half should come from food sources. The need for supplementation should be considered when a combination of food and liquid forms of the diet is prescribed.

Maintenance of Therapy

After discharge from the hospital, the child and family are closely monitored. Typically, a dietitian contacts the family, often by telephone, within one week from discharge to assess the patient's tolerance of the diet and the caregiver's comfort level. The call is also used to assess for unforeseen needs related to the KD or new questions that may have arisen in the interim. The first scheduled outpatient visit is typically one month from the initiation of the diet, with return visits every three months thereafter. At each visit, note is made of tolerance, apparent palatability, bowel habits, seizure control, and urinary ketone measures. The patient's height, weight, and head circumference are measured and plotted at each visit.

Modified Atkins Diet for Seizures

The Atkins diet can be modified for use in patients with intractable epilepsy. It is similar to the KD in that there is a higher proportion of fat and a lower proportion of carbohydrates compared with that in regular diets. Prior to starting on the Atkins Diet, the patient and caregivers read the book, *New Diet Revolution,* by Robert Atkins, MD. The dietitian evaluates a 3- to 7-day log of the patient's habitual diet, paying attention to the amount of carbohydrates. The amount of carbohydrates is halved for 1 week following this assessment. Seizure control is evaluated, and, if appropriate, carbohydrates are again cut by a quarter to a half to improve seizure control. Once the diet is initiated, ketones are checked periodically using a urine dipstick.

The scope of use for the Atkins diet is not well known. In a study of 20 patients with intractable epilepsy, the Atkins diet was effective and well tolerated. On the Atkins diet, all 20 children had at least moderate ketones within 4 days. In the 16 patients who completed the 6-month study, 13 (65%) had a seizure reduction of greater than 59% and 7 (35%) had a seizure reduction of greater than 90%; 4 patients (25%) were seizure-free (28).

RESULTS

Livingston reported extensive (41-year) experience with the diet in the treatment of myoclonic seizures of childhood (29). He stated that it completely controlled seizures in 54% of his patients and markedly improved control in another 26%. Therefore, only 20% of patients did not respond. In Livingston's experience, the diet was ineffective in controlling either true "petit mal" or temporal lobe epilepsy, although others have found the diet helpful in a wide variety of seizure types (30).

Other investigators using both the "classic" diet and its variants have reported results similar to Livingston's. In 63 studies of 55 patients conducted by Schwartz et al., a total of 51 studies (81%) showed a reduction greater than 50% in seizure frequency regardless of the type of diet used (31). Others, however, have found that the MCT diet is slightly less efficacious, with 44% of patients achieving a reduction greater than 50% in the number of seizures (32). A corn oil KD was found to be equally beneficial compared with the MCT diet (33). Seizure control appears to be inconsistently accompanied by electroencephalographic improvement (34).

In a prospective study of the diet, 150 children with intractable seizures were treated. Seizure frequency, adverse effects, and reasons for diet discontinuation were noted. Three months after initiation, 83% of children remained on the diet and 34% had a reduction greater than 90% in seizures. After 1 year, 55% remained on the diet and 27% had a reduction greater than 90% in seizures (35).

Clinical experience suggests that, in addition to improved seizure control, the diet may have a calming effect on behavior and may stabilize mood. Although one study with rodents failed to duplicate this effect, another showed reduction in the Porsolt test scores, interpreted as a reduction in "behavioral despair" (36, 37).

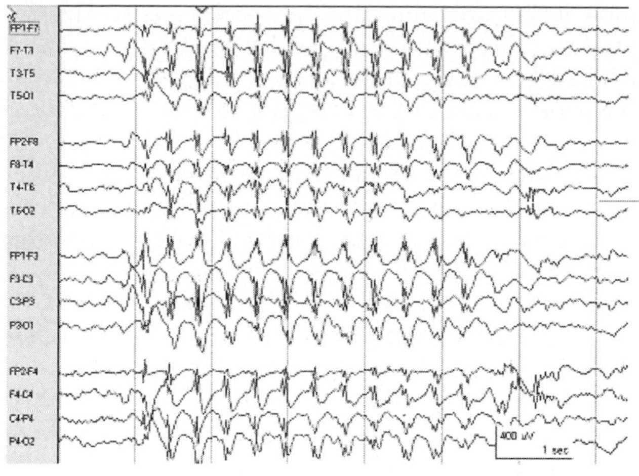

FIGURE 57-4

The EEG of a 5-year-old with glucose transporter protein deficiency. There are bursts of generalized spike-wave activity with a regular repetition rate. These bursts correlated with clinical absence attacks. After several days of the ketogenic diet there was a marked dimunition in the frequency of the seizures and epileptiform activity.

INDICATIONS FOR USE

Primary Therapy

The KD is first-line therapy for the treatment of seizures in association with glucose transporter protein deficiency and pyruvate dehydrogenase deficiency. (38–40) (Figure 57-4). In both cases, the diet effectively treats seizures while providing essential fuel for brain metabolic activity. In this manner, the diet is not only an anticonvulsant treatment, but also treats the other nonepileptic manifestations of these diseases.

Secondary Treatment

The KD may be considered as an alternate treatment, usually after the failure of valproate (VPA), for generalized epilepsies, particularly those with myoclonic seizures, including severe myoclonic epilepsy of infancy and myoclonic absence epilepsy (41, 42). Given the effectiveness of the diet in the treatment of myoclonic epilepsies, it could be considered as first-line treatment for patients with these conditions, but no comparative studies exist. The KD can be beneficial in infants with West syndrome who are refractory to corticosteroids and other medications (43–45). Based on Keith's data and our own experience, the KD may also be useful in the treatment of children with refractory absence epilepsy without myoclonus (46). Additionally, in one study in which a modified Atkins diet was used to treat children with intractable epilepsy, four out of five children with absence had a reduction greater than 50% and three went at least one month without seizures (28).

Further Possible Indications

Partial Seizures. It is very difficult to determine the efficacy of the diet in the treatment of partial seizure disorders. Livingston stated that the diet was not effective in treating patients with partial seizures. Keith did not classify his patients in a manner that allows one to determine the effectiveness in partial seizures. In current use, the diet is usually prescribed for children with other forms of refractory epilepsy. In kindled animals, a model of focal epilepsy, the diet was shown to have at least transient anticonvulsant properties (47). This bolsters the consideration of its use in children with refractory partial epilepsy. Nevertheless, although the diet may be considered in this group, there is no compelling clinical data to favor its use. Therefore, children with refractory partial seizures should be evaluated to determine if they are candidates for focal resective surgery. If they are, surgery need not be delayed to institute a trial of the KD. On the other hand, if drugs have failed and the patient is deemed to be a poor surgical candidate, the diet should be considered. It would seem inappropriate to treat children with otherwise benign seizure disorders, such as febrile seizures, benign rolandic epilepsy, benign occipital epilepsy, and benign familial neonatal convulsions with the KD.

Other Possible Indications. Preliminary experience showing some beneficial effects of the KD have been reported in the following disorders: Lafora body disease (48), partial seizures in children with tuberous sclerosis (49, 50), Rett syndrome (51), glycogenosis type V (52), and subacute sclerosing panencephalitis (53).

ADVERSE EFFECTS OF THE KD

The diet has several adverse effects that are important to note. In general the KD can cause nausea and vomiting, fatigue, loss of appetite, and hypoglycemia. These tend to be short-term effects that are seen most frequently during the initiation of the diet and usually resolve within the first few weeks of treatment.

A variety of long-term side effects can occur, some of which can be identified by screening, but others only by clinical symptoms. Renal calculi may develop and may be exacerbated by concurrent treatment with carbonic anhydrase inhibitors. Although these medications may be cautiously continued in patients, their use will effectively double the incidence of kidney stone formation, when examined as a function of patient-years exposure(54). Discontinuation or reductions of these medications should be considered, particularly if the patient has a family history of urolithiasis, hematuria, or elevated urine calcium-to-creatinine ratio. Bicarbonate levels have been monitored in patients on the KD concurrently treated with topiramate (55). These were found to decrease markedly at the time of diet initiation. The authors recommended monitoring of bicarbonate levels in these children and supplementation for symptomatic patients. Metabolic acidosis may occur in general in patients on the KD, but the lower limit of safe levels of acidosis is not clearly established. We check for acidosis if there are clinical symptoms (lethargy or fatigue), and, if they are confirmed, we recalculate the dietary prescription. If the patient is on concurrent carbonic anhydrase inhibitors, these are further reduced. It may also be necessary to increase total calories or reduce the ratio of the diet. Elevated blood lipids can occur, and one study found increases at 6 months of treatment with the KD in low-density lipoprotein (LDL), very low-density lipoproteins (VLDL), non-high-density lipoprotein cholesterol, triglycerides, and total apolipoprotein B. At the same time, mean HDL cholesterol decreased while apoA-I increased. These changes were still significant, but were less pronounced, at 12 months and 2 years (56). The clinical significance of this for atherosclerosis is not yet known.

Osteopenia and slowed growth rates are other possible consequences of the diet (57). Patients on the KD exhibit a significantly reduced quantity of bone mass, which improves in response to vitamin D supplementation. Growth rate is carefully tracked, and calories and protein are altered to ensure proper growth (58). Vitamin deficiency should be evaluated, and supplementation should be consistent throughout treatment on the diet. A low-carbohydrate multivitamin and a calcium supplement are recommended for patients on the diet. Selenium deficiency was reported in nine children on the KD, and cardiomyopathy was attributed to this deficiency in one patient (59). Lipemia retinalis developed in two of Livingston's patients (60). Bilateral optic neuropathy has been reported in two children who were treated with a 4:2 classic KD. These patients were not originally given vitamin B supplements. Vision was restored in both after administration of supplements. Thinning of hair and alopecia may occur.

Constipation occurs in some patients because of the decrease in carbohydrates and bulk. To treat constipation, increase fluids, utilize Group A vegetables. These have fewer carbohydrates and therefore allow for a larger portion size. If constipation continues, suppositories or daily oral stool softeners may be useful.

Severe adverse effects of the KD are pancreatitis, death, and coma. A lethal case of pancreatitis was reported in a patient with gemfibrozil-controlled hypertriglyceridemia that developed after initiation of the diet (61). Kang et al. reported deaths in 3.1% of their patients, caused by sepsis, cardiomyopathy, and lipoid pneumonia (62).

Precautions

The KD may be lethal in circumstances in which cerebral energy metabolism is deranged. An example of this is pyruvate carboxylase deficiency, a condition in which patients may present early in life with refractory myoclonic seizures (24). Mitochondrial disorders or diseases that involve the respiratory chain, such as myoclonic epilepsy with ragged red fibers (MERRF); syndrome of mitochondrial encephalomyopathy, lactic acidosis, and strokelike episodes (MELAS); and cytochrome oxidase deficiency, would also probably be contraindications for use of the KD, because of the increased stress on respiratory chain and TCA cycle function. Patients who have problems with fatty acid oxidation would also be adversely affected by the KD, but such patients do not, as a rule, present with seizures.

Stopping the KD

The KD should be stopped gradually. A sudden stop of the diet or sudden administration of glucose may aggravate seizures and precipitate status epilepticus. Livingston advocates maintaining the diet at a ratio of 4:1 for 2 years and, if successful, weaning down to a 3:1 diet for 6 months, followed by 6 months of a 2:1 diet. At this point, a regular diet is given. We have not utilized such a rigorous protocol.

Potential Adverse Drug Interactions

Carbonic anhydrase inhibitors such as acetazolamide, zonisamide, and topiramate should be avoided, particularly in the early stages of treatment with the KD. VPA is an inhibitor of fatty acid oxidation and mitigates hepatic ketone body production. When possible, therefore, we avoid use of this agent, but one retrospective study found no difference in relatively small numbers of patients (total of 71) who were taking (24) or not taking (47) VPA (63). Adrenocorticotropic hormone (ACTH) is not used while patients are on the KD.

Carnitine supplementation is complex. It is often used to supplement the diet of patients with various metabolic derangements whose defects allow a buildup of undesirable intermediates (64). One study summarized the findings of serial measurements of serum carnitine in patients on the KD. Multiple anticonvulsant medications were found to lower the total serum carnitine level, but actual deficiency was uncommon. Most patients had a gradual improvement in levels with long-term treatment and did not appear to require supplementation with carnitine (65). These factors must be weighed in each patient, and the decision to use the supplementation should be individualized. A measure of the serum carnitine concentration may be helpful in making this decision.

ILLNESS PROTOCOL

While on the KD, children may have periodic normal childhood illness or periodic interruptions of the feedings for other reasons, such dental procedures. All medications should be evaluated for carbohydrate content, and elixirs should be avoided because they usually contain high levels of sugars.

Children may require an increased amount of liquid during an illness because of increased insensible losses and fluid intake should be adjusted accordingly. Table 57-1 outlines common problems and associated suggestions:

DURATION OF TREATMENT AND STOPPING THE KD

The KD occasionally shows results immediately, but for many patients it may take several months to achieve optimal effect. While on the diet, patients need adjustments to account for increase caloric needs or ratio. We usually encourage parents to give the KD a trial for at least 3–6 months. If the diet is not sufficiently effective, we wean the diet by decrements of 0.5 over several months. The diet is abruptly stopped only in urgent circumstances.

TABLE 57-1
Common Ketogenic Diet Issues

Problem	Suggestions
Vomiting	Stop ketogenic meals; offer fluids to avoid dehydration, including fluids without glucose; refer to pediatrician for evaluation if vomiting is protracted. If vomiting continues for more than 24 hours and no serious medical illness is found, offer unflavored Pedialyte until patient can tolerate ketogenic foods, starting with lower fat ratio, and increase as child recovers.
Diarrhea	Increase binding foods if possible (bananas, rice, applesauce, toast). Dietitian may be able to add these temporarily. If needed, use a lower ratio until child recovers.
Fever or pain	Acetaminophen suppositories have no carbohydrate; all medications should be checked for carbohydrate content.
Hospitalization	If intravenous fluids are necessary, make sure to use glucose-free solutions. If clinical signs of hypoglycemia are present and stat measurement confirms this, give single bolus of glucose (1 g/kg of body weight). 75 mL of D5 = 3.75 grams of carbohydrate = 20 mL of orange juice.
General anesthesia	Give carbohydrate-free intravenous solutions, monitor serum pH and bicarbonate levels (66).

If there is a complete response and patients are seizure free on the diet, the diet is often continued for 2 years and then weaned over several months, again usually by decrements of 0.5 ratio.

CONCLUSIONS

It is remarkable that 70 years and scores of drugs later, the KD still retains a role in the modern treatment of children with refractory epilepsy. However, even with our new pharmacologic armamentarium, there remain patients whose epilepsy is resistant to the effects of antiepileptic medications. Indeed, once several antiepileptic drugs (AEDs) with multiple mechanisms of action have failed, it is unlikely that another will demonstrate good efficacy. In a sense, these patients may be declaring that they are not candidates for drugs and that they require alternate forms of treatment, such as the KD or surgery. Yet, it is still difficult to determine who these patients are at the onset, and the only reliable way to determine the refractory nature of their epilepsy is by trying treatment with various AEDs. Improvements in the classification of epilepsy, animal models, clinical studies, and deeper insights into the basic pathogenesis of refractory epilepsy will most likely provide useful information in this regard. In the meantime, physicians caring for children with epilepsy must still carefully weigh the known risks and benefits of all forms of treatment and use their best clinical judgment in order to arrive at the optimal regimen for their patients.

ACKNOWLEDGMENTS

The authors would like to thank Sarah Mass Ahlm and Robyn Blackford for a thorough review of the chapter, many useful suggestions, and help with background research. Robyn Blackford is a registered dietitian who works with the KD and had many helpful and practical comments regarding the daily use of the diet. Sarah Ahlm is a registered social worker who has been very involved in the clinical management and counseling of patients on the diet.

References

1. Geyelin HR. Fasting as a method for treating epilepsy. *Medical Record* 1921; 99:1037–1039.
2. Wilder RM. Effects of ketonuria on the course of epilepsy. *Mayo Clin Bull* 1921; 2:307–314.
3. Owen OE, Morgan AP, Kemp HG, Sullivan JM, et al. Brain metabolism during fasting. *J Clin Invest* 1967; 46:1589–1595.
4. Appleton DB, DeVivo DC. An animal model for the ketogenic diet. *Epilepsia* 1974; 15(2):211–227.
5. Huttenlocher PR. Ketonemia and seizures: metabolic and anticonvulsant effects of two ketogenic diets in childhood epilepsy. *Pediatr Res* 1976; 10(5):536–540.
6. Robinson AM, Williamson DH. Physiological roles of ketone bodies as substrates and signals in mammalian tissues. *Physiol Rev* 1980; 60(1):143–187.
7. McGarry JD, Mannaerts GP, Foster DW. A possible role for malonyl-CoA in the regulation of hepatic fatty acid oxidation and ketogenesis. *J Clin Invest* 1977; 60(1):265–270.
8. McGarry JD, Takabayashi Y, Foster DW. The role of malonyl-coa in the coordination of fatty acid synthesis and oxidation in isolated rat hepatocytes. *J Biol Chem* 1978; 253(22):8294–8300.
9. Pan JW, Telang FW, Lee JH, de Graaf RA, et al. Measurement of beta-hydroxybutyrate in acute hyperketonemia in human brain. *J Neurochem* 2001; 79(3):539–444.
10. Cremer JE, Braun LD, Oldendorf WH. Changes during development in transport processes of the blood-brain barrier. *Biochim Biophys Acta* 1976; 448(4):633–637.
11. Pan JW, de Graaf RA, Petersen KF, Shulman GI, et al. 2, 4-13 C2-beta-Hydroxybutyrate metabolism in human brain. *J Cereb Blood Flow Metab* 2002; 22(7):890–898.
12. Fredericks M, Ramsey RB. 3-Oxo acid coenzyme A transferase activity in brain and tumors of the nervous system. *J Neurochem* 1978; 31(6):1529–1531.
13. DeVivo DC, Leckie MP, Ferrendelli JS, McDougal DB, Jr. Chronic ketosis and cerebral metabolism. *Ann Neurol* 1978; 3(4):331–337.
14. Haymond MW, Howard C, Ben-Galim E, DeVivo DC. Effects of ketosis on glucose flux in children and adults. *Am J Physiol* 1983; 245(4):E373–E378.
15. Lowry OH, Passonneau JV, Hasselberger FX, Schulz DW. Effect of ischemia on known substrates and cofactors of the glycolytic pathway in brain. *J Biol Chem* 1964; 239:18–30.
16. Nordli DR, De Vivo DC. The ketogenic diet revisited: back to the future. *Epilepsia* 1997; 38:743–749.
17. Pan JW, Bebin EM, Chu WJ, Hetherington HP. Ketosis and epilepsy: ^{31}P spectroscopic imaging at 4.1 T. *Epilepsia* 1999; 40(6):703–707.
18. Likhodii SS, Serbanescu I, Cortez MA, Murphy P, et al. Anticonvulsant properties of acetone, a brain ketone elevated by the ketogenic diet. *Ann Neurol* 2003; 54(2):219–226.
19. Rho JM, Anderson GD, Donevan SD, White HS. Acetoacetate, acetone, and dibenzylamine (a contaminant in 1-(+)-beta-hydroxybutyrate) exhibit direct anticonvulsant actions in vivo. *Epilepsia* 2002; 43(4):358–361.
20. Todorova MT, Tandon P, Madore RA, Stafstrom CE, et al. The ketogenic diet inhibits epileptogenesis in EL mice: a genetic model for idiopathic epilepsy. *Epilepsia* 2000; 41(8):933–940.
21. Noh HS, Kim YS, Lee HP, Chung KM, et al. The protective effect of a ketogenic diet on kainic acid-induced hippocampal cell death in the male ICR mice. *Epilepsy Res* 2003; 53(1–2):119–128.
22. Gasior M, Rogawski MA, Hartman AL. Neuroprotective and disease-modifying effects of the ketogenic diet. *Behav Pharmacol* 2006; 17(5-6):431–439.
23. Sullivan PG, Rippy NA, Dorenbos K, Concepcion RC, et al. The ketogenic diet increases mitochondrial uncoupling protein levels and activity. *Ann Neurol* 2004; 55(4):576–580.
24. DeVivo DC, Haymond MW, Leckie MP, Bussman YL, et al. The clinical and biochemical implications of pyruvate carboxylase deficiency. *J Clin Endocrinol Metab* 1977; 45(6):1281–1296.
25. Vaisleib, II, Buchhalter JR, Zupanc ML. Ketogenic diet: outpatient initiation, without fluid, or caloric restrictions. *Pediatr Neurol* 2004; 31(3):198–202.
26. Bergqvist AG, Schall JI, Gallagher PR, Cnaan A, et al. Fasting versus gradual initiation of the ketogenic diet: a prospective, randomized clinical trial of efficacy. *Epilepsia* 2005; 46(11):1810–1819.
27. Carroll J, Koenigsberger D. The ketogenic diet: a practical guide for caregivers. *J Am Diet Assoc* 1998; 98(3):316–321.
28. Kossoff EH, McGrogan JR, Bluml RM, Pillas DJ, et al. A modified Atkins diet is effective for the treatment of intractable pediatric epilepsy. *Epilepsia* 2006; 47(2):421–424.
29. Livingston S, Pauli LL, Pruce I. Ketogenic diet in the treatment of childhood epilepsy. *Dev Med Child Neurol* 1977; 19:833–834.
30. Schwartz RH, Eaton J, Bower BD, Aynsley-Green A. Ketogenic diets in the treatment of epilepsy: short-term clinical effects. *Dev Med Child Neurol* 1989; 31(2):145–151.
31. Schwartz RM, Boyes S, Aynsley-Green A. Metabolic effects of three ketogenic diets in the treatment of severe epilepsy. *Dev Med Child Neurol* 1989; 31(2):152–160.
32. Sills MA, Forsythe WI, Haidukewych D, MacDonald A, et al. The medium chain triglyceride diet and intractable epilepsy. *Arch Dis Child* 1986; 61:1168–1172.
33. Woody RC, Brodie M, Hampton DK, Fiser RH, Jr. Corn oil ketogenic diet for children with intractable seizures. *J Child Neurol* 1988; 3(1):21–24.
34. Janaki S, Rashid MK, Gulati MS, Jayaram SR, et al. A clinical electroencephalographic correlation of seizures on a ketogenic diet. *Indian J Med Res* 1976; 64(7):1057–1063.
35. Freeman JM, Vining EP, Pillas DJ, Pyzik PL, et al. The efficacy of the ketogenic diet-1998: a prospective evaluation of intervention in 150 children. *Pediatrics* 1998; 102(6):1358–1363.
36. Zhao Q, Stafstrom CE, Fu DD, Hu Y, et al. Detrimental effects of the ketogenic diet on cognitive function in rats. *Pediatr Res* 2004; 55(3):498–506.
37. Murphy P, Likhodii S, Nylen K, Burnham WM. The antidepressant properties of the ketogenic diet. *Biol Psychiatry* 2004; 56(12):981–983.
38. DeVivo DC, Trifiletti RR, Jacobson RI, Ronen GM, et al. Defective glucose transport across the blood-brain barrier as a cause of persistent hypoglycorrhachia, seizures, and developmental delay. *New Engl J Med* 1991; 325:713–721.
39. Wexler ID, Hemalatha SG, McConnell J, Buist NR, et al. Outcome of pyruvate dehydrogenase deficiency treated with ketogenic diets. Studies in patients with identical mutations. *Neurology* 1997; 49(6):1655–1661.

40. Klepper J, Diefenbach S, Kohlschutter A, Voit T. Effects of the ketogenic diet in the glucose transporter 1 deficiency syndrome. Prostaglandins, leukotrienes, and Essential Fatty acids. *Prostaglandins Leukot Essent Fatty Acids* 2004; 70(3):321–327.
41. Caraballo RH, Cersosimo RO, Sakr D, Cresta A, et al. Ketogenic diet in patients with Dravet syndrome. *Epilepsia* 2005; 46(9):1539–1544.
42. Oguni H, Tanaka T, Hayashi K, Funatsuka M, et al. Treatment and long-term prognosis of myoclonic-astatic epilepsy of early childhood. *Neuropediatrics* 2002; 33(3): 122–132.
43. Nordli DR, Jr., Kuroda MM, Carroll J, Koenigsberger DY, et al. Experience with the ketogenic diet in infants. *Pediatrics* 2001; 108(1):129–133.
44. Kossoff EH, Pyzik PL, McGrogan JR, Vining EP, et al. Efficacy of the ketogenic diet for infantile spasms. *Pediatrics* 2002; 109(5):780–783.
45. Eun SH, Kang HC, Kim DW, Kim HD. Ketogenic diet for treatment of infantile spasms. *Brain Dev* 2006; 28(9):566–571.
46. Keith HM. Convulsive disorders in children: with reference to treatment with ketogenic diet. Boston: Little, Brown, 1963.
47. Hori A, Tandon P, Holmes GL, Stafstrom CE. Ketogenic diet: effects on expression of kindled seizures and behavior in adult rats. *Epilepsia* 1997; 38(7):750–758.
48. Cardinali S, Canafoglia L, Bertoli S, Franceschetti S, et al. A pilot study of a ketogenic diet in patients with Lafora body disease. *Epilepsy Res* 2006; 69(2):129–134.
49. Coppola G, Klepper J, Ammendola E, Fiorillo M, et al. The effects of the ketogenic diet in refractory partial seizures with reference to tuberous sclerosis. *Eur J Paediatr Neurol* 2006; 10(3):148–151.
50. Kossoff EH, Thiele EA, Pfeifer HH, McGrogan JR, et al. Tuberous sclerosis complex and the ketogenic diet. *Epilepsia* 2005; 46(10):1684–1686.
51. Giampietro PF, Schowalter DB, Merchant S, Campbell LR, et al. Widened clinical spectrum of the Q128P MECP2 mutation in Rett syndrome. *Childs Nerv Syst* 2006; 22(3):320–324.
52. Busch V, Gempel K, Hack A, Muller K, et al. Treatment of glycogenosis type V with ketogenic diet. *Ann Neurol* 2005; 58(2):341.
53. Bautista RE. The use of the ketogenic diet in a patient with subacute sclerosing panencephalitis. *Seizure* 2003; 12(3):175–177.
54. Kossoff EH, Pyzik PL, Furth SL, Hladky HD, et al. Kidney stones, carbonic anhydrase inhibitors, and the ketogenic diet. *Epilepsia* 2002; 43(10):1168–1171.
55. Takeoka M, Riviello JJ, Jr., Pfeifer H, Thiele EA. Concomitant treatment with topiramate and ketogenic diet in pediatric epilepsy. *Epilepsia* 2002; 43(9):1072–1075.
56. Kwiterovich PO, Jr., Vining EP, Pyzik P, Skolasky R, Jr., et al. Effect of a high-fat ketogenic diet on plasma levels of lipids, lipoproteins, and apolipoproteins in children. *JAMA* 2003 20; 290(7):912–920.
57. Peterson SJ, Tangney CC, Pimentel-Zablah EM, Hjelmgren B, et al. Changes in growth and seizure reduction in children on the ketogenic diet as a treatment for intractable epilepsy. *J Am Diet Assoc* 2005; 105(5):718–725.
58. Liu YM, Williams S, Basualdo-Hammond C, Stephens D, et al. A prospective study: growth and nutritional status of children treated with the ketogenic diet. *J Am Diet Assoc* 2003; 103(6):707–712.
59. Bergqvist AG, Chee CM, Lutchka L, Rychik J, et al. Selenium deficiency associated with cardiomyopathy: a complication of the ketogenic diet. *Epilepsia* 2003; 44(4):618–620.
60. Livingston S. Comprehensive management of epilepsy in infancy, childhood and adolescence. Springfield, IL: Charles C. Thomas, 1972.
61. Buse GJ, Riley KD, Dress CM, Neumaster TD. Patient with gemfibrozil-controlled hypertriglyceridemia that developed acute pancreatitis after starting ketogenic diet. *Curr Probl Surg* 2004; 61(2):224–226.
62. Kang HC, Chung DE, Kim DW, Kim HD. Early- and late-onset complications of the ketogenic diet for intractable epilepsy. *Epilepsia* 2004; 45(9):1116–1123.
63. Lyczkowski DA, Pfeifer HH, Ghosh S, Thiele EA. Safety and tolerability of the ketogenic diet in pediatric epilepsy: effects of valproate combination therapy. *Epilepsia* 2005; 46(9):1533–1538.
64. De Vivo DC, Bohan TP, Coulter DL, Dreifuss FE, et al. L-carnitine supplementation in childhood epilepsy: current perspectives. *Epilepsia* 1998; 39(11):1216–1225.
65. Berry-Kravis E, Booth G, Sanchez AC, Woodbury-Kolb J. Carnitine levels and the ketogenic diet. *Epilepsia* 2001; 42(11):1445–1451.
66. Valencia I, Pfeifer H, Thiele EA. General anesthesia and the ketogenic diet: clinical experience in nine patients. *Epilepsia* 2002; 43(5):525–529.

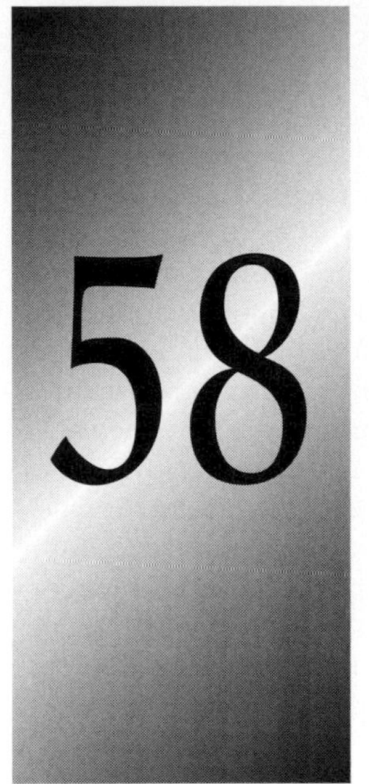

58 Inflammation, Epilepsy, and Anti-Inflammatory Therapies

Stéphane Auvin
Raman Sankar

An understanding of the etiologic role played by the immune system in the genesis or modification of the human epilepsies is complicated by the paucity of high-quality data based on clinical research. It is reasonable to propose a major role for inflammation in the intractable epilepsy associated with Rasmussen encephalitis, and yet present treatment remains surgical. On the other hand, immunomodulatory therapy involving adrenocorticotropic hormone (ACTH) or corticosteroids is more convincingly established for the treatment of infantile spasms, a syndrome that is not generally attributed to an inflammatory etiology. The clinical literature abounds with scattered and anecdotal reports on the efficacy of ACTH, corticosteroids, or intravenous immunoglobulin (IVIG) in a variety of difficult-to-treat epilepsy syndromes, but almost always as a treatment of last resort; no randomized, placebo-controlled, and blinded studies are available. The foregoing statements are obvious to most clinicians but are recounted here to describe the challenge facing the writers on this important and rapidly evolving topic. It is clear that the topic requires a review of what has been established by basic scientific inquiry before a description of the clinical data and speculation on future developments.

BASIC SCIENCE

Inflammation and Epilepsy

There is a reciprocal relationship between seizures and inflammatory cytokines (1). In many experimental systems, proinflammatory stimuli exhibit proconvulsant properties. On the other hand, seizure or status epilepticus (SE) that is induced by chemical or electrical stimulation has been demonstrated to enhance the expression of proinflammatory cytokines such as interleukin-1beta (IL-1beta), interleukin-6 (IL-6), and tumor necrosis factor-alpha (TNF-alpha) (1).

The proconvulsant effects of inflammation have been studied in animals using the bacterial endotoxin lipopolysaccharide (LPS), which induces a broad inflammatory response, or by employing specific cytokines. The latter have also been used to study effects on excitability in in-vitro preparations. LPS is a component of the outer membrane of gram-negative bacteria and is recognized by cells of the immune system. The effects of LPS in the central nervous system (CNS) are conceivably related to stimulating production of several microglial cytokines (2, 3), although a direct effect through Toll-like receptor (TLR) is also possible (4). IL-1beta has been the most studied cytokine. IL-1beta is a proinflammatory cytokine involved in immune defense against infection.

Inflammatory Enhancement of Seizure Susceptibility. Seizure susceptibility to pentylenetetrazol (PTZ) is enhanced in mice by preadministration of LPS, and this phenomenon is blocked by anti-inflammatory drugs (5, 6). Using LPS from *Shigella*, Yuhas et al first showed that LPS enhanced the sensitivity of mice to PTZ-induced seizures via mechanisms involving TNF-alph, IL-1beta, and nitric oxide (5). LPS produced a decrease in seizure threshold in a dose- and time-dependent manner. The role of nitric oxide (NO), prostaglandins (PGs), and the endogenous opioid systems in mediating the effect of LPS was suggested by the ability of specific antagonists of those systems to mitigate the effect of LPS (6). Heida et al. (7) showed that the combination of LPS and subconvulsant doses of kainic acid (KA) resulted in convulsions in approximately 50% of animals, with very low mortality in P14 rat pups. In the genetically epileptic Wistar Albino Glaxo/Rijswijk rat strain (WAG/Rij, a rat model for absence epilepsy), the high voltage spike-wave discharges increased in number and duration proportionate to dose of LPS (10–350 μg/kg) administered (8). In the same model, repetitive administration of LPS daily for 5 days initially increased the number of spike-wave discharges, but a tolerance was observed on the fifth day. The LPS-induced increase in spike-wave discharges was not directly correlated with the elevation of the core body temperature (8).

Cytokines and Seizure Activity. Vezzani et al. (9) demonstrated the reciprocal relationship between IL-1beta and seizure activity. Induction of seizures by KA or bicuculline injection resulted in expression of IL-1beta and microglial activation. Injection of human recombinant IL-1beta into the hippocampus 10 minutes preceding the application of KA prolonged the seizures induced by KA, whereas coinjection of an IL-1beta receptor antagonist (IL-1RA) or an N-methyl-D-aspartate (NMDA) antagonist prevented this effect. The IL-1RA demonstrated powerful anticonvulsant effect (10). IL-1beta also lowered the threshold for hyperthermic seizures and even produced seizures by itself (11). IL-1beta receptor–deficient mice were resistant to experimental hyperthermic seizure model. This resistance appeared to be independent of genetic background and was attributed to lack of IL-1beta signaling, because exogenous cytokine reduced seizure threshold in wild-type, but not receptor-deficient, mice independent of strain. In addition, high IL-1beta doses induced seizures only in IL-1beta receptor–expressing mice (11).

Transgenic mice with glial fibrillary acidic protein (GFAP) promoter–driven astrocyte production of the cytokines IL-6 and TNF-alpha were studied in terms of their susceptibility to experimentally induced seizures (12). GFAP-IL6, but not GFAP-TNF, mice showed markedly enhanced sensitivity to glutamatergic- but not cholinergic-induced seizures. Consistently, intrahippocampal injection of TNF-alpha in mice inhibits seizure (13).

A recent study of surgically resected tissue involving focal cortical dysplasia found a significant number of cells of macrophage and microglia line that were immunocytochemically recognizable as CD68- and human leukocyte antigen (HLA)-DR-positive (14). Another study of brain tissue removed surgically for the treatment of intractable epilepsy found immunocytochemical evidence for IL-1beta signaling in a substantial population of neurons and glia surrounding focal cortical dysplasia or glioneuronal tumors (15). Such was not the case in histologically normal perilesional tissue or normal control cortex, suggesting that this signaling probably does not represent seizure-induced activation of cytokines and may, in fact, have a causative role in the epileptogenicity of the dysplastic lesion.

Potential Mechanisms Underlying Altered Excitability

Several studies have observed a relationship between cytokines and neurotransmitter systems that modulate neuronal excitability. Evidence has been found to support the interaction of cytokines, especially IL-1beta, with glutamatergic and gamma-aminobutyric acid (GABA)ergic systems, both directly (at the level of receptors and ion channels) and indirectly (via neuromodulatory systems). Direct mechanisms include effects on glutamate and GABA receptor trafficking that amplify excitatory response and limit inhibitory response.

Direct interaction with the glutamatergic systems can take place by at least two routes: (1) enhancement of extracellular glutamate concentrations and (2) increased function of the NMDA and/or -amino-5-methyl-3-hydroxy-4-isoxazolepropionic acid (AMPA) receptors. IL-1beta has been shown to inhibit glutamate reuptake in cultures of rat and human astrocytes (16, 17). IL-1beta activates inducible NO synthase, leading to production of NO and subsequent increase in glutamate release (18, 19). In addition, cytokines can enhance substance P release (20), and substance P, in turn, can augment cytokine expression (21). Substance P can also enhance glutamate release and contribute to maintenance of seizure activity in hippocampal networks (22).

The proconvulsant activity of IL-1beta via NMDA receptors was first suggested in animal models when IL-1beta activity was found to be blocked by a selective competitive antagonist of NMDA receptors (9). The interaction between IL-1beta and NMDA receptors was described in further detail in a latter report (23). IL-1beta increased NMDA receptor function through activation of tyrosine kinases and subsequent NR2A/B subunit phosphorylation, resulting in an increase of NMDA-induced calcium influx. Furukawa and Mattson (24) used whole-cell perforated patch-clamp recording of cultured hippocampal neurons to show that treatment with TNF-alpha caused an increase in calcium current by approximately 30%. Beattie et al. (25) showed that glial interaction of TNF-alpha causes an increase in surface expression of neuronal AMPA receptors responsible for an increase of synaptic efficacy. The newly expressed AMPA receptors were shown to have lower stoichiometric amounts of GluR2, making the receptors permeable to calcium ions. More recently, TNF-alpha was considered to regulate neuronal homeostasis. In fact, TNF-alpha increases excitatory pathway by stoichiometric modification of synaptic AMPA receptor even as it causes $GABA_A$ receptor endocytosis (26).

Effect of IL-1beta and TNF-alpha in mediating AMPA-induced excitotoxicity has been demonstrated in an organotypic hippocampal slice culture (27). Either potentiation of excitotoxicity or neuroprotection was observed, depending on the concentration of the cytokines and the timing of exposure. Preincubation with low concentrations of IL-1beta (1 ng/mL) followed by coexposure with AMPA enhanced the effect of AMPA, whereas a higher concentration (10 ng/mL) afforded neuroprotection. Although IL-1beta per se did not produce these effects, the effects caused by IL-1beta in combination with AMPA could be blocked by IL-1beta antagonism. By using TNF-alpha receptor knockout mice, it was shown that the potentiation of AMPA-induced toxicity by TNF-alpha involves TNF receptor-1, whereas the neuroprotective effect is mediated by TNF receptor-2.

Effects on the GABAergic System. In an in vitro study, IL-1beta produced a decrease in synaptic inhibition by about 30% in CA3 pyramidal cells and dentate granule cells (28). Such an effect was confirmed by Wang et al in a subsequent study (29). Such diminution of GABA-mediated currents by TNF-alpha may be explained by its enhancement of GABA receptor endocytosis (25, 26).

Inflammation, Neuronal Injury, and Epileptogenesis

The reciprocal relationship between seizures and inflammation was alluded to earlier. Although inflammation may exacerbate seizure activity and possibly excitotoxicity, it can also be induced by many experimental seizure models. A question of considerable translational importance is whether the inflammatory process set in motion by an initial bout of SE (or other epileptogenic insults, such as traumatic brain injury) contributes to the process of epileptogenesis. If this question can be answered affirmatively, novel targets for antiepileptogenic therapy may be identified.

Experimentally induced seizures in rodents trigger a prominent inflammatory response in brain areas recruited in the onset and propagation of epileptic activity involving microglia, astrocytes, and, in some instances, neurons (1). Seizures induced either chemically (systemic and focal kainate injection, lithium-pilocarpine) or electrically increase cytokines in rodent brain. Proinflammatory cytokines are induced in brain also by audiogenic and kindled seizures (30, 31) and remain up-regulated in the brain for several days. In the lithium-pilocarpine model, the expression of IL-1beta, NF-kappaB, and COX-2 started by 12 hours postinjection, persisted for 24 hours (SE period), and returned to basal levels by 3 and 6 days (during the latent period) (32). The regional distribution of the inflammatory markers occurred mainly in structures prone to develop neuronal damage. The authors suggested that seizure-related IL-1beta, NF-kappaB, and COX-2 expression may contribute to the pathophysiology of epilepsy by inducing neuronal death and astrocytic activation (32). Neuronal COX-2 gene induction has been proposed as a key signaling event during epileptogenesis in the kindling model (33).

The effect of cytokines in modulating glutamatergic excitotoxicity via NMDA (23) and AMPA (27) mechanisms has been alluded to earlier. Work in the author's laboratory has shown that an inflammatory stimulus by systemic LPS preceding SE induced by lithium-pilocarpine resulted in enhancement of neuronal injury without being accompanied by an elevation in temperature or prolongation of the status (34). We have also found an increase in the incidence of spontaneous recurrent seizures in rat pups that received LPS prior to lithium-pilocarpine SE and have also observed that administration of LPS accelerated kindling acquisition and intensified kindled seizures in a rapid kindling protocol (unpublished results). On the other hand, Sayyah et al have reported that both LPS (35) and IL-1beta (36) displayed anticonvulsant and antiepileptogenic properties when administered intracerebroventricularly (ICV). The same authors have also documented the ability of systemically administered LPS to enhance seizure susceptibility (6). Thus, with the exception of those studies that involved ICV administration of provocateurs, the likelihood is that inflammatory response contributes to epileptogenesis, and interventions that antagonize different aspects of downstream signaling (COX-2, NOS) tend to be antiepileptogenic.

The role of inflammation as a causative factor in human epileptogenesis is beginning to be explored. An association of prolonged febrile convulsions and temporal lobe epilepsy with hippocampal sclerosis with a polymorphism in the promoter of IL-1beta gene (IL-1beta-511T) was first reported from a study in Japan by Kanemoto and colleagues (37). Such an association could not be confirmed in populations of European ancestry (38–40). However, an important difference accounting for the discrepancy could be the difference in the prevalence of prolonged febrile convulsions in these populations (41).

CLINICAL PRACTICE

Anti-Inflammatory Therapies in Clinical Epilepsy

The treatment of epilepsy with immunomodulatory agents has mainly involved ACTH, glucocorticoids, and IVIG. Use of IVIG has all but replaced plasmapheresis. Indeed, this approach has generally been resorted to for syndromes that are known to respond poorly to antiepileptic drugs (AEDs), such as infantile spasms or epilepsy with electrical SE during slow-wave sleep (ESES), or in individuals with any type of seizure syndrome that has failed to respond adequately to AEDs. Klein and Livingston first reported the use of ACTH in children with intractable seizures (42). The pharmacology of all these agents (ACTH, glucocorticoids, and IVIG) is so complex and diverse that we cannot be certain that the basis of their efficacy is their immunomodulatory ability. In fact, the response of Rasmussen encephalitis to immunomodulatory approaches has been less than satisfactory and enduring, even though a strong role for inflammation is suspected in this syndrome. We shall present a brief summary of our present state of knowledge regarding the use of immunotherapy in specific epilepsy syndromes. If there is a "bottom line" conclusion, it will be stated early in the discussion so that the reader has the option not to traverse a confusing, contradictory, and occasionally contentious body of literature to arrive at that conclusion. Where possible, we shall bring to the reader's attention potential mechanisms of action that may or may not rely on immune mechanisms.

Infantile Spasms

The strongest tradition to date for the use of immunomodulatory therapy exists for the use of ACTH in this catastrophic epilepsy syndrome of infancy. Even here, the strongest statement made by an august group of clinicians who adopted the methods of evidence-based medicine to evaluate the clinical literature was that ACTH is *probably effective* for the *short-term treatment* (italics ours) of infantile spasms, but there is insufficient evidence to recommend the optimal dosage and duration of treatment. There is insufficient evidence to determine whether oral corticosteroids are effective (43). The conclusions reflect the difficulty in undertaking the study of a relatively rare and age-specific, but not etiology-specific, disorder of considerable variability in the premorbid state.

Previous studies have attempted to clarify whether ACTH treatment is superior to treatment with corticosteroids, whether a higher dose of ACTH (150 IU/m^2) is superior to a lower dose (40 IU/m^2), and whether an optimal duration of therapy can be determined. The practice parameters from the American Academy of Neurology (AAN) and the Child Neurology Society do not endorse corticosteroids as effective, based on the weight of available evidence. It should be stressed that lack of evidence in support of steroids is not proof of lack of efficacy. However, it may be suggestive of a mode of action for ACTH that is not entirely dependent on its ability to induce steroidogenesis. Many of the available studies are covered in some detail in Chapter 16 and need not be duplicated under this heading.

How does ACTH mitigate infantile spasms? The mechanism(s) remain(s) elusive. A major hypothesis has centered around the ability of ACTH to reduce the endogenous synthesis of corticotropin-releasing hormone, which, when injected, produces severe seizures in immature rats (44, 45). This theory does account for the time course of action of ACTH and for the all-or-none response to treatment, and it is also supported by the findings of reduced ACTH and cortisol levels in the spinal fluids of patients with infantile spasms (46, 47). Could ACTH be functioning, at least in part, by its effect on melanocortin receptors, independent of steroid release? There are peptides that are ACTH fragments and can function as agonists at those receptors without mediating steroidogenesis, but no clinical trials with such compounds have been undertaken yet.

Another attractive idea proposes that ACTH stimulates the synthesis of deoxycorticosterone, which is bioconverted to the tetrahydroxy derivative, a potent agonist at the $GABA_A$ receptor site (48, 49). This theory is consistent with the known ameliorative action of infantile spasms by vigabatrin and supports the present interest in ganaxalone, a neurosteroid derivative that is a highly selective agonist for the delta subunit containing $GABA_A$ receptors, which are extrasynaptic and mediate tonic inhibition.

None of the previously discussed mechanisms exclude the possibility that the administration of ACTH mitigates infantile spasms by modifying a wide range of cytokines (immunomodulation), which in turn may also influence brain excitability by interactions with glutamatergic and GABAergic mechanisms as described earlier. Thus, both aspects related to immune function and other aspects of the pharmacology of ACTH (and steroids) may be important in why this approach to the treatment of infantile spasms has endured.

Scattered reports describe the use of IVIG in the treatment of infantile spasms, but the data do not permit conclusions in support of this treatment modality (50, 51). One study reported benefit from a single treatment with IVIG in children with refractory juvenile spasms (52). The practice parameters from the AAN and the Child Neurology Society did not recognize IVIG as a valid therapy for infantile spasms.

Lennox-Gastaut Syndrome

The reports describing the use of ACTH (53) and IVIG (51) in the treatment of Lennox-Gastaut syndrome (LGS) are extremely limited. It is likely that most specialists will consider using the ketogenic diet or vagus nerve stimulation in medically refractory patients with LGS. One report described a favorable response in 7 of 10 patients treated with prednisone (54). It is not clear that the benefit was lasting. The use of corticosteroids in managing medically intractable LGS was likely more common before the availability of new-generation AEDs with demonstrated benefit in this syndrome. Anecdotal series describing the use of IVIG in LGS (55, 56) have reported favorable effects, and the therapy is generally better tolerated than either ACTH or corticosteroids. More details on the treatment options for LGS are available in Chapter 21.

Syndromes with Electrical SE During Slow-Wave Sleep: Landau-Kleffner Syndrome, Tassinari Syndrome of Continuous Spike Waves During Slow-Wave Sleep

A spectrum of clinical disorders have been associated with the electoencephalogram (EEG) signature of electrical SE during slow-wave sleep (ESES): the clinical syndromes include the distinctive Landau-Kleffner syndrome (LKS) and the syndrome of continuous spike waves during slow-wave sleep (CSWS) (57, 58), the latter sometimes also referred to as the Tassinari syndrome (59). LKS exhibits many clinical features that are typically associated with idiopathic epilepsy syndromes, whereas CSWS generally presents in a manner that suggests a symptomatic epilepsy syndrome (60). These syndromes are covered in detail in Chapter 24.

Clinical practice tends to approach the pharmacologic aspects of management of these syndromes in a more or less similar fashion, concentrating on the EEG trait of ESES. In the published literature, the immunologic approach seems to work better in LKS (60). The treatment of LKS with corticosteroids in high doses for a protracted period was advocated by Marescaux and colleagues (61). Sinclair and Snyder (62) reported a favorable outcome in 9 of 10 patients with LKS who were treated with prednisone, which compares favorably to the surgical approach of multiple subpial transections (63, 64). Such a robust response has never been achieved in CSWS. One study (65) reported two patients whose language functions recovered rapidly with the initiation of intravenous corticosteroid therapy, followed by conversion to oral therapy. It is uncertain whether intravenous therapy adds much benefit to the more common oral treatment (61, 62, 66).

Successful therapy of LKS with IVIG (67–69) was reported in isolated cases. In a subsequent review, Mikati, one of the authors who had reported two of the three published cases (67, 69), stated that only 2 of 11 patients with LKS had responded adequately to treatment with IVIG (70).

There is no literature to substantiate the specific use of ACTH, corticosteroids, or IVIG in ESES that presents as CSWS. The initial report by De Negri and colleagues (71) advocating nightly diazepam treatment has been adopted by many clinicians, and abstracts have been published in support of this approach. There has not been a peer-reviewed publication yet that describes this therapy and its outcome in a manner that moves it toward wider acceptance.

Rasmussen Encephalitis

Rasmussen syndrome probably represents the best example of an epilepsy syndrome with a major component of the histopathology of resected tissue representing an inflammatory encephalopathy. The report suggesting a role for auto antibodies to the GluR3 subunit of the glutamate receptor (72) initially resulted in much anticipation for the development of successful immunomodulating therapy. This initial enthusiasm has diminished considerably since then, with lack of consistent identification of such antibodies in many patients (73) and the less than gratifying sustained clinical response to steroids, plasmapheresis, or IVIG (74). Surgery remains the most effective treatment (see also Chapter 27).

CONCLUSIONS

There is a lack of convergence between our scientific advances thus far in linking inflammatory processes with epilepsy and our ability to translate those findings to clinical practice. There is a paucity of scientific evidence to support the development of sound clinical guidelines for implementing immunomodulatory therapy, whereas the toxicities associated with extended treatment with ACTH or corticosteroids are considerable. Although IVIG is generally better tolerated, there is insufficient evidence to support its logical placement in a therapeutic algorithm for any epilepsy syndrome. Where the weight of evidence in support of efficacy for a treatment is somewhat stronger (e.g., ACTH in infantile spasms), it is still not clear whether it is the immunomodulating effect that is critical or some other aspect of the pharmacology of the treatment that is responsible for the observed benefits. In most cases, we do not know the status of markers of inflammation before and after therapy. It is still not entirely clear which markers of inflammation are especially relevant to our pursuit of ameliorating epilepsy by immunomodulation. Indeed, this is also true to a large extent in terms of our ability to explain what aspect of the effect of a particular AED on a neurotransmitter system or a channel is responsible for its efficacy in a particular epilepsy syndrome. Ultimately, clinical decisions are based on the empiric findings of efficacy and the demonstration of safety (or acceptable risk that is not out of proportion to the benefit). That is the equation that has relegated immune therapy as a late option in most epilepsy syndromes.

What may the future hold? Future research should be directed toward identifying inflammation-related biomarkers that correlate with the epileptic process in humans. In animal models, some immunomodulatory drugs tantalize us with the holy grail of antiepileptogenic therapy (75). In clinical practice, many of these agents (cyclosporine, tacrolimus) are associated with the potential for encephalopathy, seizures, or both, as well as other risks to the patient in terms of infection and organ toxicity. Improvement in the toxicity profile of this class of agents can do much to stimulate well-designed clinical trials.

References

1. Vezzani A, Granata T. Brain inflammation in epilepsy: experimental and clinical evidence. *Epilepsia* 2005; 46:1724–1743.
2. Lee, SC, Liu W, Dickson DW, Brosnan CF, et al. Cytokine production by human fetal microglia and astrocytes. Differential induction by lipopolysaccharide and IL-1 beta. *J Immunol* 1993; 150:2659–2667.
3. Turrin, NP, Gayle D, Ilyin SE, Flynn MC, et al. Pro-inflammatory and anti-inflammatory cytokine mRNA induction in the periphery and brain following intraperitoneal administration of bacterial lipopolysaccharide. *Brain Res Bull* 2001; 54:443–453.
4. Lehnardt S, Massillon L, Follett P, Jensen FE, et al. Activation of innate immunity in the CNS triggers neurodegeneration through a Toll-like receptor 4-dependent pathway. *Proc Natl Acad Sci U S A* 2003; 100:8514–8519.
5. Yuhas Y, Nofech-Mozes Y, Weizman A, Ashkenazi S. Enhancement of pentylenetetrazole-induced seizures by *Shigella dysenteriae* in LPS-resistant C3H/HeJ mice: role of the host response. *Med Microbiol Immunol (Berl)* 2002; 190:173–178.
6. Sayyah M, Javad-Pour M, Ghazi-Khansari M. The bacterial endotoxin lipopolysaccharide enhances seizure susceptibility in mice: involvement of proinflammatory factors: nitric oxide and prostaglandins. *Neuroscience* 2003; 122:1073–1080.
7. Heida JG, Boisse L, Pittman QJ. Lipopolysaccharide-induced febrile convulsions in the rat: short-term sequelae. *Epilepsia* 2004; 45:1317–1329.
8. Kovacs Z, Kekesi KA, Szilagyi N, Abraham I, et al. Facilitation of spike-wave discharge activity by lipopolysaccharides in Wistar Albino Glaxo/Rijswijk rats. *Neuroscience* 2006; 140:731–742.
9. Vezzani A, Conti M, De Luigi A, Ravizza,T, et al. Interleukin-1beta immunoreactivity and microglia are enhanced in the rat hippocampus by focal kainate application: functional evidence for enhancement of electrographic seizures. *J Neurosci* 1999; 19:5054–5065.
10. Vezzani A, Moneta D, Richichi C, Aliprandi M, et al. Functional role of inflammatory cytokines and antiinflammatory molecules in seizures and epileptogenesis. *Epilepsia* 2002; 43(Suppl 5):30–35.
11. Dubé C, Vezzani A, Behrens M, Bartfai T, et al. Interleukin-1beta contributes to the generation of experimental febrile seizures. *Ann Neurol* 2005; 57:152–155.
12. Samland H, Huitron-Resendiz S, Masliah E, Criado J, et al. Profound increase in sensitivity to glutamatergic- but not cholinergic agonist-induced seizures in transgenic mice with astrocyte production of IL-6. *J Neurosci Res* 2003; 73:176–187.
13. Balosso S, Ravizza T, Perego C, Peschon J, et al. Tumor necrosis factor-alpha inhibits seizures in mice via p75 receptors. *Ann Neurol* 2005; 57:804–812.
14. Boer K, Spliet WG, van Rijen PC, Redeker S, et al. Evidence of activated microglia in focal cortical dysplasia. *J Neuroimmunol* 2006; 173:188–195.
15. Ravizza T, Boer K, Redeker S, Spliet WG, et al. The IL-1beta system in epilepsy-associated malformations of cortical development. *Neurobiol Dis* 2006; 24:128–143.
16. Ye ZC, Sontheimer H. Cytokine modulation of glial glutamate uptake: a possible involvement of nitric oxide. *Neuroreport* 1996; 7:2181–2185.
17. Hu S, Sheng WS, Ehrlich LC, Peterson PK, et al. Cytokine effects on glutamate uptake by human astrocytes. *Neuroimmunomodulation* 2000; 7:153–159.
18. Casamenti F, Prosperi C, Scali C, Giovannelli L, et al. Interleukin-1beta activates forebrain glial cells and increases nitric oxide production and cortical glutamate and GABA release in vivo: implications for Alzheimer's disease. *Neuroscience* 1999; 91:831–842.
19. Hewett SJ, Csernansky CA, Choi DW. Selective potentiation of NMDA-induced neuronal injury following induction of astrocytic iNOS. *Neuron* 1994; 13:487–494.
20. Cioni C, Renzi D, Calabro A, Annunziata P. Enhanced secretion of substance P by cytokine-stimulated rat brain endothelium cultures. *J Neuroimmunol* 1998; 84:76–85.
21. Martin FC, Charles AC, Sanderson MJ, Merrill JE. Substance P stimulates IL-1 production by astrocytes via intracellular calcium. *Brain Res* 1992; 599:13–18.
22. Liu H, Mazarati AM, Katsumori H, Sankar R, et al. Substance P is expressed in hippocampal principal neurons during status epilepticus and plays a critical role in the maintenance of status epilepticus. *Proc Natl Acad Sci U S A* 1999; 96:5286–5291.
23. Viviani B, Bartesaghi S, Gardoni F, Vezzani A, et al. Interleukin-1beta enhances NMDA receptor-mediated intracellular calcium increase through activation of the Src family of kinases. *J Neurosci* 2003; 23:8692–8700.
24. Furukawa K, Mattson MP. The transcription factor NF-kappaB mediates increases in calcium currents and decreases in NMDA- and AMPA/kainate-induced currents induced by tumor necrosis factor-alpha in hippocampal neurons. *J Neurochem* 1998; 70: 1876–1886.
25. Beattie EC, Stellwagen D, Morishita W, Bresnahan JC, et al. Control of synaptic strength by glial TNFalpha. *Science* 2002; 295:2282–2285.
26. Stellwagen D, Beattie EC, Seo JY, Malenka RC. Differential regulation of AMPA receptor and GABA receptor trafficking by tumor necrosis factor-alpha. *J Neurosci* 2005; 25: 3219–3228.
27. Bernardino L, Xapelli S, Silva AP, Jakobsen B, et al. Modulator effects of interleukin-1beta and tumor necrosis factor-alpha on AMPA-induced excitotoxicity in mouse organotypic hippocampal slice cultures. *J Neurosci* 2005; 25:6734–6744.
28. Zeise ML, Espinoza J, Morales P, Nalli A. Interleukin-1beta does not increase synaptic inhibition in hippocampal CA3 pyramidal and dentate gyrus granule cells of the rat in vitro. *Brain Res* 1997; 768:341–344.
29. Wang S, Cheng Q, Malik S, Yang J. Interleukin-1beta inhibits gamma-aminobutyric acid type A (GABA(A)) receptor current in cultured hippocampal neurons. *J Pharmacol Exp Ther* 2000; 292:497–504.
30. Gahring LC, White HS, Skradski SL, Carlson NG, et al. Interleukin-1alpha in the brain is induced by audiogenic seizure. *Neurobiol Dis* 1997; 3:263–269.
31. Plata-Salaman CR, Ilyin SE, Turrin NP, Gayle D, et al. Kindling modulates the IL-1beta system, TNF-alpha, TGF-beta1, and neuropeptide mRNAs in specific brain regions. *Mol Brain Res* 2000; 75:248–258.
32. Voutsinos-Porche B, Koning E, Kaplan H, Ferrandon A, et al. Temporal patterns of the cerebral inflammatory response in the rat lithium-pilocarpine model of temporal lobe epilepsy. *Neurobiol Dis* 2004; 17:385–402.
33. Tu B, Bazan NG. Hippocampal kindling epileptogenesis upregulates neuronal cyclooxygenase-2 expression in neocortex. *Exp Neurol* 2003; 179:167–175.
34. Sankar R, Auvin S, Mazarati A, Shin D. Inflammation contributes to seizure-induced hippocampal injury in the neonatal rat brain. *Acta Neurol Scand* 2007; 115:16–20.
35. Sayyah M, Najafabadi IT, Beheshti S, Majzoob S. Lipopolysaccharide retards development of amygdala kindling but does not affect fully-kindled seizures in rats. *Epilepsy Res* 2003; 57:175–180.
36. Sayyah M, Beheshti S, Shokrgozar MA, Eslami-far A, et al. Antiepileptogenic and anticonvulsant activity of interleukin-1 beta in amygdala-kindled rats. *Exp Neurol* 2005; 191:145–153.
37. Kanemoto K, Kawasaki J, Miyamoto T, Obayashi H, et al. Interleukin (IL)1beta, IL-1alpha, and IL-1 receptor antagonist gene polymorphisms in patients with temporal lobe epilepsy. *Ann Neurol* 2000; 47:571–574.
38. Heils A, Haug K, Kunz WS, Fernandez G, et al. Interleukin-1beta gene polymorphism and susceptibility to temporal lobe epilepsy with hippocampal sclerosis. *Ann Neurol* 2000; 48:948–950.
39. Buono RJ, Ferraro TN, O'Connor MJ, Sperling MR, et al. Lack of association between an interleukin 1 beta (IL-1beta) gene variation and refractory temporal lobe epilepsy. *Epilepsia* 2001; 42:782–784.
40. Tilgen N, Pfeiffer H, Cobilanschi J, Rau B, et al. Association analysis between the human interleukin 1beta (-511) gene polymorphism and susceptibility to febrile convulsions. *Neurosci Lett* 2002; 334:68–70.
41. Kanemoto K, Kawasaki J, Yuasa S, Kumaki T, et al. Increased frequency of interleukin-1beta-511T allele in patients with temporal lobe epilepsy, hippocampal sclerosis, and prolonged febrile convulsion. *Epilepsia* 2003; 44:796–799.
42. Klein R, Livingston S. The effect of adrenocorticotropic hormone in epilepsy. *J Pediatr* 1950; 37:733–742.
43. Mackay MT, Weiss SK, Adams-Webber T, Ashwal S, et al; American Academy of Neurology; Child Neurology Society. Practice parameter: medical treatment of infantile spasms: report of the American Academy of Neurology and the Child Neurology Society. *Neurology* 2004; 62:1668–1681.
44. Brunson KL, Khan N, Eghbal-Ahmadi M, Baram TZ. Corticotropin (ACTH) acts directly on amygdala neurons to down-regulate corticotropin-releasing hormone gene expression. *Ann Neurol* 2001; 49:304–312.
45. Brunson KL, Eghbal-Ahmadi M, Baram TZ. How do the many etiologies of West syndrome lead to excitability and seizures? The corticotropin releasing hormone excess hypothesis. *Brain Dev* 2001; 23:533–538.
46. Baram TZ, Mitchell WG, Snead OC, 3rd, Horton EJ, et al. Brain-adrenal axis hormones are altered in the CSF of infants with massive infantile spasms. *Neurology* 1992; 42: 1171–1175.
47. Baram TZ, Mitchell WG, Hanson RA, Snead, OC 3rd, et al. Cerebrospinal fluid corticotropin and cortisol are reduced in infantile spasms. *Pediatr Neurol* 1995; 13: 108–110.
48. Reddy DS, Rogawski MA. Stress-induced deoxycorticosterone-derived neurosteroids modulate GABA(A) receptor function and seizure susceptibility. *J Neurosci* 2002; 22: 3795–3805.
49. Rogawski MA, Reddy DS. Neurosteroids and infantile spasms: the deoxycorticosterone hypothesis. *Int Rev Neurobiol* 2002; 49:199–219.
50. Ariizumi M, Baba K, Hibio S, Shiihara H, et al. Immunoglobulin therapy in the West syndrome. *Brain Dev* 1987; 9:422–425.

51. van Engelen BG, Renier WO, Weemaes CM, Strengers PF, et al. High-dose intravenous immunoglobulin treatment in cryptogenic West and Lennox-Gastaut syndrome; an add-on study. *Eur J Pediatr* 1994; 153:762–769.
52. Bingel U, Pinter JD, Sotero de Menezes M, Rho JM. Intravenous immunoglobulin as adjunctive therapy for juvenile spasms. *J Child Neurol* 2003; 18:379–382.
53. Yamatogi Y, Ohtsuka Y, Ishida T, Ichiba N, et al. Treatment of the Lennox syndrome with ACTH: a clinical and electroencephalographic study. *Brain Dev* 1979; 1: 267–276.
54. Sinclair DB. Prednisone therapy in pediatric epilepsy. *Pediatr Neurol* 2003; 28: 194–198.
55. van Rijckevorsel-Harmant K, Delire M, Rucquoy-Ponsar M. Treatment of idiopathic West and Lennox-Gastaut syndromes by intravenous administration of human polyvalent immunoglobulins. *Eur Arch Psychiatry Neurol Sci* 1986; 236:119–122.
56. Gross-Tsur V, Shalev RS, Kazir E, Engelhard D, et al. Intravenous high-dose gammaglobulins for intractable childhood epilepsy. *Acta Neurol Scand* 1993; 88:204–209.
57. Galanopoulou AS, Bojko A, Lado F, Moshé SL. The spectrum of neuropsychiatric abnormalities associated with electrical status epilepticus in sleep. *Brain Dev* 2000; 22: 279–295.
58. McVicar KA, Shinnar S. Landau-Kleffner syndrome, electrical status epilepticus in slow wave sleep, and language regression in children. *Ment Retard Dev Disabil Res Rev* 2004; 10:144–149.
59. Tassinari CA, Bureau M, Dravet C, Dalla Bernardina B, et al. Epilepsy with continuous spikes and waves during slow sleep—otherwise described as ESES (epilepsy with electrical status epilepticus during slow sleep). In: Roger J, Bureau M, Dravet C, Dreifuss FE, Perret A, Wolf P, eds. *Epileptic Syndromes In Infancy, Childhood And Adolescence*. London: John Libbey; 1992:245–256.
60. Van Hirtum-Das M, Licht EA, Koh S, Wu JY, et al. Children with ESES: variability in the syndrome. *Epilepsy Res* 2006; 70(Suppl 1):S248–S258.
61. Marescaux C, Hirsch E, Finck S, Maquet P, et al. Landau-Kleffner syndrome: a pharmacologic study of five cases. *Epilepsia* 1990; 31:768–777.
62. Sinclair DB, Snyder TJ. Corticosteroids for the treatment of Landau-Kleffner syndrome and continuous spike-wave discharge during sleep. *Pediatr Neurol* 2005; 32:300–306.
63. Morrell F, Whisler WW, Smith MC, Hoeppner TJ, et al. Landau-Kleffner syndrome. Treatment with subpial intracortical transection. *Brain* 1995; 118(Pt 6):1529–1546.
64. Grote CL, Van Slyke P, Hoeppner JA. Language outcome following multiple subpial transection for Landau-Kleffner syndrome. *Brain* 1999; 122(Pt 3):561–566.
65. Tsuru T, Mori M, Mizuguchi M, Momoi MY. Effects of high-dose intravenous corticosteroid therapy in Landau-Kleffner syndrome. *Pediatr Neurol* 2000; 22:145–147.
66. Lerman P, Lerman-Sagie T, Kivity S. Effect of early corticosteroid therapy for Landau-Kleffner syndrome. *Dev Med Child Neurol* 1991; 33:257–260.
67. Fayad MN, Choueiri R, Mikati M. Landau-Kleffner syndrome: consistent response to repeated intravenous gamma-globulin doses: a case report. *Epilepsia* 1997; 38:489–494.
68. Lagae LG, Silberstein J, Gillis PL, Casaer PJ. Successful use of intravenous immunoglobulins in Landau-Kleffner syndrome. *Pediatr Neurol* 1998; 18:165–168.
69. Mikati MA, Saab R. Successful use of intravenous immunoglobulin as initial monotherapy in Landau-Kleffner syndrome. *Epilepsia* 2000; 41:880–886.
70. Mikati MA, Shamseddine AN. Management of Landau-Kleffner syndrome. *Paediatr Drugs* 2005; 7:377–389.
71. De Negri M, Baglietto MG, Battaglia FM, Gaggero R, et al. Treatment of electrical status epilepticus by short diazepam (DZP) cycles after DZP rectal bolus test. *Brain Dev* 1995; 17:330–333.
72. Rogers SW, Andrews PI, Gahring LC, Whisenand T, et al. Autoantibodies to glutamate receptor GluR3 in Rasmussen's encephalitis. *Science* 1994; 265:648–651.
73. Watson R, Jiang Y, Bermudez I, Houlihan L, et al. Absence of antibodies to glutamate receptor type 3 (GluR3) in Rasmussen encephalitis. *Neurology* 2004; 63:43–50.
74. Granata T, Fusco L, Gobbi G, Freri E, et al. Experience with immunomodulatory treatments in Rasmussen's encephalitis. *Neurology* 2003; 61:1807–1810.
75. Moia LJ, Matsui H, de Barros GA, Tomizawa K, et al. Immunosuppressants and calcineurin inhibitors, cyclosporin A and FK506, reversibly inhibit epileptogenesis in amygdaloid kindled rat. *Brain Res* 1994; 648:337–341.

59 Antiepileptic Drugs in Development

John R. Pollard
Jacqueline A. French

In the last decade and a half, nine antiepileptic drugs (AEDs) have been approved for use, more than doubling the available agents for patients with epilepsy (1). There is no doubt that this has enhanced the options for physicians as they attempt to optimize therapy. New drugs tend to be safer, better tolerated, broader in spectrum, and less likely to cause drug-drug interactions than older drugs. Yet, in many people's estimation, the number of children with uncontrolled seizures has not changed. Clearly, there is still a need for newer and better drugs. Fortunately, the pipeline of drugs in development is rich in new compounds. These compounds have come from many sources. One source that has been providing new compounds throughout the history of antiepileptic drug development is the discovery of analogs of existing compounds (2). Examples include brivaracetam and seletracetam (analogs of levetiracetam), eslicarbazepine acetate (an analog of oxcarbazepine), as well as several analogs of valproic acid (VPA). Some compounds have been discovered through focus on novel mechanisms. An example is talampanel, the first antiepileptic drug that works through alpha-amino-5-methyl-3-hydroxy-4-isoxazolepropionic acid (AMPA) antagonism. Other compounds are found through high-throughput screening programs. For these drugs, the mechanism of action may be less clear. This chapter briefly describes the AEDs currently in development, including information about mechanism of action, if known, as well as early trial data and pharmacokinetics.

BRIVARACETAM

Chemistry, Animal Pharmacology, and Mechanism of Action

Brivaracetam, ((2S)-2-[(4R)-2-oxo-4-propylpyrrolidinyl] butanamide), is a pyrrolidone derivative in the same class as levetiracetam (LEV) and piracetam (3). Brivaracetam has a higher affinity (pK_i = 7.1) than LEV (pK_i = 6.1) for the synaptic vesicle protein 2A (SV2A). SV2A is a membrane glycoprotein found in synaptic and endocrine vesicles. The cellular physiology that leads to subsequent anticonvulsant effect is under active investigation (4). In addition to binding SV2A, the drug has been shown to inhibit voltage-dependent sodium currents (5).

Presuming that the SV2A binding site is important for antiepileptic efficacy, brivaracetam should be more potent than LEV in suppressing seizures. Indeed, several animal models seem to confirm this. Brivaracetam is more potent in the corneal-kindled mouse model (reduced afterdischarge and seizure severity after suprathreshold stimulation compared to LEV), in the audiogenic seizure model, and also in a rat model that is thought to mimic absence seizures in humans: Genetic Absence Epilepsy Rats of Strasbourg (GAERS) (6, 7). In this model, almost complete suppression of spike wave discharges is seen at high doses. Unlike LEV, there is some effect in the maximal electroshock (MES) model. Like LEV, brivaracetam potently suppresses the development of kindling. Animal data also indicate that the drug should be well tolerated. Although effective doses in seizure models were in the range of 1.2–2.4 mg/kg when the drug was administered intraperitoneally, doses of as much as 212 mg/kg have been administered safely. The drug is also active in animal models of neuropathic pain and essential tremor (3).

Biotransformation, Pharmacokinetics, and Interactions in Humans

Brivarecetam is well tolerated in humans in Phase I. Doses ranging from 10 to 600 mg demonstrate linear pharmacokinetics. The volume of distribution is close to that of body water. Plasma protein binding is low, and the half-life is approximately 8–10 hours. The extent of absorption is not affected by a high-fat meal, but the rate of absorption is slowed. The drug is extensively metabolized in the liver via hydrolysis and hydroxylation—the latter via cytochrome P450 (CYP) isoenzymes 2C8, 3A4, and 2C19—and the metabolites are predominantly cleared renally.

In vitro, brivaracetam inhibits epoxide hydrolase and CYP 2C19 and is also a weak inducer of CYP3A4. Drug-drug interactions studies were performed at relatively high doses of brivaracetam. When administered to patients on steady doses of carbamazepine (CBZ), the CBZ-epoxide levels increased in a dose-dependent fashion, whereas the CBZ levels were slightly reduced. In healthy male volunteers, the interaction between phenytoin and brivaracetam resulted in a slightly lower phenytoin serum concentration. In addition, serum concentration of brivaracetam was reduced slightly in the presence of CBZ. When tested with concomitant oral contraceptive use, there was a moderate reduction of estrogen and progestin components, but no change in the suppression of ovulation. In hepatically impaired patients, the half-life of the drug is prolonged. Renally impaired and elderly subjects do not need dose adjustment, although one metabolite increased in serum concentration.

Clinical Efficacy

The drug was tested in patients with a photoparoxysmal response. Each patient received a single dose of study medication. Even at the lowest administered dose of 10 mg, there was substantial suppression of the photoparoxysmal response. At doses of 10–80 mg, there was only one nonresponder, with all other patients (3 or 4 per group) having partial or complete suppression of the photosensitive response (and the nonresponder did not have an adequate predose expression of photosensitivity). The pharmacodynamic half-life against photosensitivity increased with dose. At 10 mg, the first effect was seen at 30 minutes, and the effect lasted for 30 hours, whereas the duration of effect was 60 hours at the highest dose tested (8). A Phase II multicenter, double-blind, randomized, placebo-controlled, dose-ranging trial is in progress at the time of writing, in which brivaracetam is being tested at doses of 150 and 50 mg/day in one study and 5, 20, and 50 mg/day in the other, in both studies against placebo, as twice daily (BID) administration. The U.S. Food and Drug Administration (FDA) approved orphan drug testing status for brivaracetam for the treatment of symptomatic myoclonus. The drug is also in Phase II clinical trials of patients with postherpetic neuralgia. It is being tested at doses of 200 and 400 mg/day in BID administration.

Adverse Effects

To date, adverse events have been central nervous system (CNS)-related, consisting of dizziness, somnolence, and fatigue, and increase with escalating dose.

ESLICARBAZEPINE ACETATE

Chemistry, Animal Pharmacology, and Mechanism of Action

Eslicarbazepine acetate (S-(-)-10-acetoxy-10,11-dihydro-5H-dibenzo(*b,f*)azepine-5-carboxamide) is structurally related to carbamazepine (CBZ) and oxcarbazepine (OXC) (2). This drug is a prodrug of S-10-monohydroxy derivative (S-MHD), with a "simpler" metabolism than CBZ and OXC. The first studies in humans were in 2000, with the first Phase II studies in 2002. Phase III is underway. Eslicarbazepine acetate shares the dibenzazepine nucleus with OXC and CBZ. It is metabolized exclusively via hydrolysis to S-licarbazepine, with minor traces of the R enantiomer. It is therefore not subject to autoinduction. It is active in MES and amygdala kindling, equipotent to CBZ, and more potent than OXC. Like CBZ, it acts as stabilizer of the inactive conformation of voltage-gated sodium channels through interaction with site 2 of the channel. The result is preferential impairment of rapidly firing neurons (9–11).

Biotransformation, Pharmacokinetics, and Interactions in Humans

In humans, the drug is rapidly converted to the active metabolite eslicarbazepine. To a much lesser extent, it is also converted to its R enantiomer as well as OXC. Plasma levels of the parent compound are typically undetectable. Time to maximum concentration (T_{max}) is

2–3 hours after dosing. Terminal half-life is 9–17 hours. Steady state is reached in 4–5 days, longer than expected from the half-life because of the biotransformation. The PK is not affected by age, gender, or food. Protein binding is low. In-vitro studies showed no inhibitory effect on cytochrome P450, but there was mild induction of UGT1A1, which may indicate a potential for interaction with the oral contraceptive pill. Studies suggest that there is no clinically significant interaction with warfarin and digoxin (12–14).

Clinical Efficacy

To date, 1,200 subjects or patients have been exposed to the drug. A Phase II add-on study in adults and another in children have been completed. In the adult studies, doses from 400 to 1,200 mg were given in once-daily (QD) and BID regimens. Of note, patients on CBZ and OXC were not excluded from the trial. Side effects included headache, somnolence, dizziness, and perioral paresthesia. A double-blind study was performed in 143 patients with more than four seizures per month, with doses up to 1,200 mg BID or QD. Significant seizure reduction was demonstrated. There was a low discontinuation rate because of adverse events (15). Three Phase III studies are comparing 400, 800, and 1,200 mg QD. A Phase II study for acute mania and recurrence prevention in bipolar disorder is also underway.

Clinical Use and Laboratory Monitoring

Important for children, an oral suspension (50mg/ml) has been developed that is bioequivalent to the 200- and 800-mg tablets.

FLUOROFELBAMATE

Chemistry, Animal Pharmacology, and Mechanism of Action

Fluorofelbamate (2-phenyl-2-fluoro-1,3 propanediol dicarbamate) is a felbamate analog that was designed to avoid the toxicities of its parent compound (7). Fluorine is substituted for hydrogen in the 2-position of the propanediol moiety of felbamate in an attempt to block production of at least one toxic metabolite, atropaldehyde. Some preclinical data suggest that this was successful.

This drug has a broad spectrum of activity against all models of electrically induced seizures and has activity against picrotoxin-induced seizures in mice and sound-induced seizures in the audiogenic seizure–prone Frings mouse. The ED_{50} is between 1 and 8 times that of felbamate in the various models. In a sustained status epilepticus animal model, it was effective even at a late stage that is usually refractory to anticonvulsants (16). In animals, weight loss was seen, similar to that seen with felbamate.

There is some evidence in cell culture, slice model, and hypoxic rat pups that this drug has some neuroprotective capacity (17).

The mechanism of action is unknown but may be due to interactions at the glutamate receptor sites or sodium channels. Both of these hypotheses are supported by electrophysiological data.

Biotransformation, Pharmacokinetics, and Interactions in Humans

A Phase I study has been performed in 54 patients. The drug was well tolerated, and the exposure was dose-proportional. T_{max} was 1 hour, and elimination half-life ($T_{1/2}$) was 17 hours. Kinetics were linear.

GANAXALONE

Chemistry, Animal Pharmacology, and Mechanism of Action

Ganaxalone (3alpha-hydroxy-3beta-methyl-5alpha-pregnan-20-one) is a synthetic analogue of allopregnanolone, a metabolite of progesterone that has no progesterone activity. It is an allosteric modulator of the $GABA_A$ receptor complex (18). The exact binding site is unknown, but binding to the benzodiazepine site has been ruled out. It has activity in both the 6-Hz and pentylenetetrazol (PTZ) models (19, 20).

Biotransformation, Pharmacokinetics, and Interactions in Humans

Metabolism is via CYP 3A4. Drug interactions have not been seen, but specific interaction studies have not been performed. There are no major metabolites. There is no evidence of induction in human trials, and the half-life is 10–20 hours. BID dosing is expected (21).

Clinical Efficacy

There have been 14 Phase I studies in 210 healthy volunteers. However, after these studies were completed, there was a change in formulation. Bioavailability with the initial formulation was low, with a significant food effect. There have been 500 patients (79 children) exposed in 11 Phase II studies, including exposures for as long as 4 years. In a 3-month pediatric refractory seizure add-on study, 20 subjects aged 6 months to 7 years were titrated up to 12 mg/kg. Sixteen patients completed the study; 25% showed a $>$ 50% reduction in seizures, and one patient was seizure free. An additional 25% showed a 25–50% reduction (22). Two other open-label pediatric studies were conducted in 60 patients aged 2–13 years, with about half having a history of infantile spasms. The most common background drugs were valproic acid, CBZ, and clonazepam. A 50% seizure reduction was seen in one-third of the patients; 17 patients were on the drug for more than 1 year, and the most common adverse events were somnolence and agitation. Eight subjects reported increased seizure frequency. One subject had agitation, hostility, and hallucinations. A presurgical trial in adults was performed. There were 24 patients on ganaxalone vs. 28 on placebo. Outcome was completion of the trial without meeting exit criteria. Although there was a trend in favor of ganaxalone, this did not reach statistical significance. One patient discontinued because of agitation (23). Additional studies in infantile spasms and adult partial seizures are planned.

ISOVALERAMIDE

Chemistry, Animal Pharmacology, and Mechanism of Action

Isovaleramide (3-methylbutanamide) is a branched-chain aliphatic amide that is structurally similar to valproic acid. This is one of a series of valproate-like compounds that has the potential to be broad spectrum but may avoid some of the issues related to valproate administration, including weight gain, hepatic toxicity, difficult pharmacokinetics, and teratogenicity. As with valproic acid, the mechanism of action is unknown. Studies of neurotransmitter binding and uptake have been negative, so a direct receptor-mediated effect is unlikely.

It is effective in oral doses in multiple models, including MES, PTZ in rodents, bicuculline- and picrotoxin-induced seizures in mice, generalized seizure in corneal-kindled rats, seizure score and afterdischarge duration in amygdala-kindled rats, spontaneous EEG spike wave of absence seizures in rats, and sound-induced audiogenic seizures in Frings mice. It also delays kindling in amygdala-kindled rats. Bialer et al. characterize the spectrum of anticonvulsant activity as comparable to that of valproic acid. There was also activity in models of spasticity, pain, and anxiety.

Adverse effects seen in animal species at high doses include transient ataxia and hypoactivity. Doses that caused these effects were significantly higher than that expected to be used in humans. Notably, reproductive toxicity was lower for isovaleramide than for valproic acid. In addition, unlike valproic acid, isovaleramide did not inhibit mitochondrial beta-oxidation and respiration at concentrations up to 1mM (2, 7).

Biotransformation, Pharmacokinetics, and Interactions in Humans

In Phase I studies the bioavailability of single doses ranging from 100–1,600 mg was almost 100%. The half-life of the drug is about 30 minutes −2.4 hours, with a T_{max} of 40 minutes, but sustained-release formulations are possible. There is no protein binding. Only 2–4% of the drug was excreted unchanged in the urine at 24 hours, so, as with valproic acid, hepatic metabolism predominates. In marked contrast to valproic acid, isovaleramide does not inhibit any of the major human P450 isoforms.

Clinical Efficacy

In Phase I studies there were no serious adverse events and no changes in any assessed clinical value. A Phase II trial for treatment of migraine in about 300 patients was completed in 2004 and showed no statistically significant activity, but the drug was well tolerated.

LACOSAMIDE

Chemistry, Animal Pharmacology, and Mechanism of Action

Lacosamide (formerly harkoseride, 2-acetamido-N-benzyl-3-methoxypropionamide) is a trifunctional amino acid derivative that has activity in epilepsy, neuropathic pain, and stroke. It shows affinity for the glycine strychnine-insensitive receptor site of the NMDA receptor complex, but this is not yet confirmed as the molecular anticonvulsant site of action (4, 24).

This drug is active in the MES model, the 6-Hz refractory seizure model, hippocampal kindling, sound-induced seizures in Frings mice, and self-sustaining status epilepticus. Developmental toxicity occurred in rats only at a maternally toxic dose. No teratogenicity or adverse effects on male or female reproductive function was identified preclinically (7).

Biotransformation, Pharmacokinetics, and Interactions in Humans

Absorption is rapid and complete and occurs in the gastrointestinal tract. Bioavailability is good and similar in the fed and fasted states. 30–40% of the drug is excreted unchanged by the kidneys, 30% is excreted as an inactive metabolite, and less than 0.5% is recovered in the feces. Peak concentrations are attained at about 1–5 hours after an oral dose. Lacosamide is protein bound by less than 15%, and the half-life is approximately 13 hours. The drug is being developed as an intravenous formulation as well. When an infusion is administered over a 1-hour period, the kinetics are similar to oral dosing. Formal interaction studies performed in volunteers have shown no drug-drug interactions in either direction with CBZ, valproic acid, levonorgestrel, or ethinylestradiol (7).

Clinical Efficacy

Three Phase II trials have been completed in epilepsy. Efficacy against partial seizures was demonstrated at doses between 100 and 600 mg/day divided BID (25). Several studies have also been carried out for painful diabetic neuropathy and showed significant reduction in pain scores at 400 and 600 mg/day, compared to placebo.

Adverse Effects

The most common adverse effects from the trials were seen with increasing frequency at higher doses and led to a moderate dropout incidence at the 600-mg dose. These included dizziness, somnolence, diplopia, fatigue, and headache. The intravenous formulation caused paresthesias as well as the symptoms listed for the oral dosing.

Clinical Use and Laboratory Monitoring

As previously noted, the drug is being developed in an intravenous formulation as well as an oral formulation. This adds potential for treatment of patients who cannot take medication orally.

RETIGABINE

Chemistry, Animal Pharmacology, and Mechanism of Action

Retigabine, N-[2-amino-4-(4-fluorobenzylamino)-phenyl]carbamic acid ethyl ester, is a structurally novel anticonvulsant related to flupirtine (an analgesic and antispastic drug available only in Europe). Although it was discovered by screening in animal models of acute seizures, it was subsequently discovered to have a unique mechanism of action, which has galvanized interest in the compound. It has activity at the KCNQ2/3 and KCNQ3/5 potassium channels and is thought to stabilize hyperexcitable cells by altering steady-state activation of the M-current (26). In addition, it has an ancillary mechanism, potentiating GABA-evoked currents, which may not be relevant in human doses (27, 28). The mechanism may be of particular interest to pediatric neurologists, given the recent discovery that benign familial neonatal convulsions may be associated with mutations in genes encoding these channels.

Retigabine is effective in all three classes of models: electrical induction, chemical induction, and genetic epilepsy. It is also effective against kindling. It is most effective in the amygdala-kindling model in rats (29, 30).

Potentially this drug also has neuroprotective effect, as it produces protection against electroshock amnesia and learning in a cerebral ischemia model. It is also effective against neuropathic pain in two animal models (31, 32). In animal studies CNS side effects were sedation, accompanied by hyperexcitability, and decreased body temperature.

Biotransformation, Pharmacokinetics, and Interactions in Humans

Phase I studies to assess pharmacokinetic properties indicated bioavailability of 60% (not affected by food), a T_{max} of 1.5 hours, and a half-life of 8–9 hours. Clearance is reduced in black subjects by about 25%. The drug has demonstrated linear pharmacokinetics in healthy subjects and patients. The drug is hepatically metabolized via N-glucuronidation and N-acetylation, and metabolites are excreted in the urine. The N-acetyl metabolite is active and shows anticonvulsant effect in animals.

There are several potential minor drug-drug interactions. Concurrent administration with phenobarbital caused an increase of 10% in the area under the curve for a single dose (33). Lamotrigine (LTG) half-life was slightly reduced after several days of retigabine (34). Neither of these interactions were significant enough to alter Phase II studies. A Phase II study of 60 patients to evaluate drug interactions revealed that retigabine clearance was increased by 30% in the setting of coadministration of phenytoin or CBZ. Higher doses of retigabine would likely be necessary in the setting of enzyme-inducing medications.

Clinical Efficacy

In five Phase II studies and one Phase IIb study, 600 patients have been studied. In a randomized, double-blind, placebo-controlled, parallel group adjunctive therapy trial in partial epilepsy, doses of 600, 900, and 1,200 mg/day in three daily doses produced a median reduction in seizures of 23%, 29%, and 35% compared to 13% in the placebo group. The responder rate (reduction greater than 50% in seizures) was 23%, 32%, and 33% for these doses, respectively, compared to 16% for placebo. Studies have not been performed in syndromes other than partial, so spectrum of activity is not known.

Adverse Effects

CNS-related adverse effects were asthenia, dizziness, somnolence, tremor, speech disorder, amnesia, vertigo, and abnormal thinking. Dropout rate was slightly greater than 40% in the highest dosage group (7, 35). At the time of writing of this chapter, trials in children had not been initiated.

Clinical Use and Laboratory Monitoring

To date there is only a single preparation, which is tablets.

RUFINAMIDE

Chemistry, Animal Pharmacology, and Mechanism of Action

Rufinamide, 1-[(2,6-difluorophenyl)methyl]triazole-4-carboxamide, is a structurally novel agent for which the mechanism of action is unknown. Studies suggest it interacts with the inactivated state of the voltage-gated sodium channel, limiting high-frequency firing of action potentials in neurons (4).

It is active in models such as MES, PTZ, picrotoxin, and bicuculline, with an oral ED_{50} of 5–17 mg/kg. It is also effective in delaying kindling. It is not mutagenic or teratogenic in animal models.

Biotransformation, Pharmacokinetics, and Interactions in Humans

The drug has undergone extensive investigation: 1,965 epilepsy patients have been exposed to rufinamide in clinical studies. Population pharmacokinetic (PK) analysis has been performed on 1,072 patients. There is a moderate increase in exposure when the drug is administered with food (36). However, at steady state, food does not seem to influence bioavailability. Absorption is reduced slightly as doses increase. Intrasubject variability is low.

The bioavailability of tablets is approximately 85%, and T_{max} is reached at 3–4 hours after ingestion. It is bound to plasma proteins by about 34% and has a half-life of 6–10 hours. It is almost completely metabolized, and very little is excreted unchanged. The metabolism is via hydrolysis via a non-P450-mediated interaction. The breakdown products are nonactive and mostly excreted in the urine. Children and elderly patients do not have different pharmacokinetic parameters. Renal function has no impact on clearance.

There is no autoinduction. In population PK analysis, valproic acid decreased apparent oral clearance of rufinamide by 22%, possibly by a greater percentage in children. Any combination of phenytoin, phenobarbital, and primidone increased clearance of rufinamide by 25%, again possibly more so in children. Rufinamide can cause the clearance of phenytoin to decrease slightly, but this may be significant only at higher starting serum concentrations of phenytoin. Rufinamide is a slight inducer of CYP 3A4, leading to slightly increased clearance of ethinyl estradiol and norethindrone.

Clinical Efficacy

There have been two Phase II trials in refractory partial epilepsy. Both were in adults, but patients above age 15 years in one trial and 16 in the other were included. In one study, 3,200 mg/day led to a median reduction of 20.4% in seizures vs. a median increase of 1.6% for placebo. The dose ranges in these studies was 400–3,200 mg/day (37, 38). A study in refractory primary generalized tonic-clonic convulsions did not show a difference from placebo.

Rufinamide was shown to have clinical benefit in the treatment of seizures associated with the Lennox-Gastaut syndrome in a randomized, double-blind, placebo-controlled trial that enrolled 139 patients aged 4–30 years, who were taking up to three background AEDs. A dose of 45 mg/kg/day was used. Inclusion criteria included presence of drop attacks (tonic or atonic) , more than 90 seizures per month, and an EEG demonstrating slow spike-wave activity. Reduction from baseline monthly tonic-atonic seizure frequency was 42.5% in the rufinamide group compared to 1.4% increase in the placebo group ($P < 0.0001$). There was a dropout rate of 14% in the rufinamide-treated patients vs. 8% for placebo, with the most common treatment-related adverse events leading to discontinuation being vomiting, somnolence, and rash (39). There did not appear to be an impact of rufinamide on weight.

Adverse Effects

In trials, headache, dizziness, fatigue, somnolence, and nausea were the most common side effects. In the Lennox-Gastaut patients, rash was a rare side effect.

Clinical Use and Laboratory Monitoring

There is a liquid formulation as well as a tablet formulation of the drug.

At the time of writing of this chapter, Eisai had received an "approvable" letter from the FDA both for adjunctive treatment of partial-onset seizures with and without secondary generalization in adults and adolescents aged 12 years and older and for adjunctive treatment of seizures associated with Lennox-Gastaut syndrome in children aged 4 years and older and in adults.

RWJ-333369 (CARISBAMATE)

Chemistry, Animal Pharmacology, and Mechanism of Action

Carisbamate, or RWJ 333369, is a carbamate with the chemical formula (S)-2-O-carbamoyl-1-o-chlorophenyl-ethanol. The drug is highly potent in MES and various chemical models, including bicuculline and PTZ, and is active in genetic epilepsy models (4, 40).

Biotransformation, Pharmacokinetics, and Interactions in Humans

Phase I explored doses from 200 to 1,500 mg/day. Pharmacokinetics are linear with a 12-hour half-life. There is a mild food effect. After food, C_{max} was reduced by about 11%. The drug is metabolized by a non-CYP-dependent route (UGT). There are virtually no circulating metabolites. CBZ induces the compound by about 40%, but carisbamate does not impact CBZ. There is an increase of 20% in LTG and VPA metabolism, but neither of these impacts the metabolism of carisbamate.

Clinical Efficacy

A Phase II add-on study in refractory patients is complete, at doses up to 1,600 mg/day: 537 subjects were randomized; up to three background AEDs were permitted. This study showed a statistically significant reduction in seizures. Dropout rate from adverse events was dose dependent and up to 20% at the highest dose. The most common adverse events were primarily CNS related events, including dizziness, somnolence, nausea, vertigo, and diplopia. Headache increased at the highest dose only.

SELETRACETAM

Chemistry, Animal Pharmacology, and Mechanism of Action

Seletracetam is one of two SV2A ligands currently in development at the pharmaceutical firm UCB. Seletracetam has a 10-fold higher affinity to the SV2A binding site than LEV and a 50-fold greater potency in inhibiting high-voltage-activated calcium channels (6, 41). There is minor inhibition of the plateau phase of NMDA currents (42). Indirect suppression of glycine inhibition is also seen and is significantly greater than that observed with LEV. Seletracetam has no effect on sodium channels (43).

Seletracetam is more potent than LEV in corneal-kindling, hippocampal-kindling, and audiogenic seizures. There is no effect in the acute screening tests, MES and PTZ. There is also efficacy in the GAERS model at relevant human concentrations. Interestingly, the protective index is substantially higher than that seen for LEV, using the corneal-kindling and the GAERS model (44).

Biotransformation, Pharmacokinetics, and Interactions in Humans

The pharmacokinetic parameters are favorable, and like those of LEV, they are linear and dose-proportional. Absorption is rapid and nearly complete, and there is a slight decrease in rate but not extent of absorption with food. The volume of distribution is close to that of body water.

Seletracetam undergoes hydrolysis and is eliminated in the urine, 60% as metabolite and 40% as parent compound. There is no hepatic metabolism, and drug interactions are not expected. The half-life is 8 hours, and there is less than 10% protein binding.

In Phase I, seletracetam was well tolerated. Treatment-emergent adverse events were CNS related, not dose related. The maximum tolerated dose was not reached in a single, rising-dose study, so the maximum tolerated dose is estimated to be greater than 600 mg.

Clinical Efficacy

A Phase IIa study was done in patients with photoparoxysmal response. There were 4–8 patients per dosing group, although some were tested at two doses. Doses of 0.5– 20 mg were explored, and all doses produced some suppression. Modeling of the dose effect showed an increasing effect as doses increased, with a plateau effect reached at 10–20 mg. Subsequently. two exploratory, open-label, dose-exploration studies were performed. One study enrolled 30 patients who could be taking as many as three background AEDs, not including LEV. The second study enrolled 60 patients, all of whom were receiving LEV in addition to up to two additional AEDs. Doses up to 160 mg were tested, and assessments of efficacy, safety, and tolerability were made. Unfortunately, results were not available at the time of writing of this chapter.

In addition to the oral formulation, both intravenous and intramuscular dosing are currently under discussion.

STIRIPENTOL

Stiripentol, 4,4-dimethyl-1-[(3,4 methylenedioxy)phenyl]-1-penten-3-ol, is an antiepileptic compound that has been used in France and Canada for more than 10 years in catastrophic pediatric epilepsy syndromes. Meanwhile, broader development and availability have been hampered by the fact that the drug causes significant inhibition of the metabolism of several commonly prescribed AEDs. This has caused two problems. The first is potential toxicity related to elevated serum concentrations of the inhibited drugs. The second is difficulty in discriminating direct antiepileptic effects of stiripentol vs. seizure reduction because drug-drug interactions lead to higher serum concentrations of other concomitantly prescribed medications. Nonetheless, several investigators believe that stiripentol may have an important place in management of these patients, who are very difficult to treat.

Chemistry, Animal Pharmacology, and Mechanism of Action

There are multiple proposed mechanisms of action for stiripentol (7, 45). It inhibits synaptosomal uptake of

GABA and glycine and inhibits GABA transaminase (46). It also enhances beta-hydroxybutyrate dehydrogenase activity. It is said to increase duration of GABAergic currents in a dose-related fashion, with the duration of channel opening increased, similar to the mechanism of action of barbiturates (47).

The drug is active in PTZ and MES models in mice and in the alumina gel Rhesus monkey (48, 49).

Biotransformation, Pharmacokinetics, and Interactions in Humans

The drug reaches T_{max} within 2 hours. It is 99% protein bound and, as the dose increases in patients on other AEDs, the serum concentration increases in an exponential fashion (50–52).

As previously noted, development has been complicated by multiple drug interactions. Stiripentol inhibits cytochrome P450 isoenzymes 3A4, 1A2, and 2C19. This results in the plasma concentrations of many concurrent AEDs being potentiated, but with better tolerability than would be expected by giving the parent compound. For example, CBZ is better tolerated, because the ratio of CBZ epoxide to CBZ is reduced in a dose-dependent fashion (53–55). For clobazam, addition of stiripentol leads to significantly higher concentration of the metabolite norclobazam, which is also better tolerated, and a lower concentration of hydroxyl norclobazam, a less well-tolerated metabolite. This is because there is more inhibition of 2C19, which is involved in the nor-to-hydroxy reaction (56). Clearance of stiripentol is increased in the presence of enzyme-inducing medications.

Clinical Efficacy

There have been 1,000 patients treated over 11 years. Clinical studies were discontinued in adults but continued in children, and stiripentol is used currently in Canada and France.

In an open-label trial of 212 children, there were 49% responders, with long-term data up to 2.5 years. The better responders were those with partial epilepsy who were also receiving CBZ, and children with severe myoclonic epilepsy of infancy (SMEI) who were also receiving VPA and CBZ. Subsequently, a randomized, controlled trial was performed, but, as previously noted, it was difficult to separate the effect of stiripentol directly from the effect of potentiation of concomitant AEDs.

The double-blind study started with open add-on treatment of 67 patients with stiripentol. The responders were then randomized to withdrawal to placebo or continuation of stiripentol. The primary endpoint, the number of discontinuations, was not significantly different, but there was a reduction in seizure frequency. The CBZ dose was increased in the placebo arm in order to mimic the effects of stiripentol, but this was not well tolerated.

Another study in SMEI randomized 41 patients to placebo or stiripentol, in patients on valproic acid and clobazam. Nine patients on stiripentol became seizure free, vs. none of the placebo patients (57). A long-term study followed. The best effect was not on frequency, but on duration of seizures. Efficacy was best for patients under 2 years old. Currently, 200 patients with SMEI receive stiripentol as compassionate use in France. and the drug has been designated as an orphan drug by the European Agency for the Evaluation of Medicinal Products (EMEA). A subsequent trial is under way as a European Integrated project.

TALAMPANEL

Chemistry, Animal Pharmacology, and Mechanism of Action

Talampanel, R(-)-enantiomer of 7-acetyl-5-(4-aminophenyl)-8,9-dihydro-8 methyl-7H-1,3-dioxolo(4,5H)-2, 3-benzodiazepine (58), is a novel AED whose mechanism of action involves noncompetitive AMPA antagonism (59, 60). This and similar compounds, unlike other benzodiazepines, are highly selective for the AMPA receptor and have no activity at the $GABA_A$ receptor. There is also no evidence of activity at other common AED targets. Talampanel is effective in a broad range of animal models such as MES and PTZ and against seizures induced by excitatory amino acids that are agonists at the kainate and AMPA sites of the NMDA receptor (61). It also is protective against fully kindled seizures but does not retard the development of kindling (62). There is no evidence of effect in the WAG/Rij spike wave rat model. In animal models, the therapeutic window is small.

Biotransformation, Pharmacokinetics, and Interactions in Humans

After an oral dose, peak plasma concentration is achieved in 2.5 hours. Protein binding ranges from 67% to 88%. At dosages that cause the plasma concentration to exceed 200 ng/ml, the half-life is approximately 7–8 hours. Elimination is by biotransformation, including acetylation (63). An N-acetyl metabolite is produced, which is active, and may contribute both to efficacy and side effects. Patients may have different genotypes in respect to acetylation. Those who are slow acetylators may have reduced clearance of talampanel; conversely, fast acetylators may need a higher dose.

This drug may have a slight effect on metabolism of CBZ. Conversely, inducing medications reduce the serum concentration of talampanel.

Clinical Efficacy

Two clinical trials have investigated the efficacy of talampanel in epilepsy. The first study was a crossover design, which randomized 49 patients. Talampanel serum concentrations were very variable and depended on concomitant AEDs. The mean seizure reduction was 21% over the placebo period. CBZ levels rose slightly during talampanel treatment (64). The second study investigated doses up to 50 mg three times per day (TID), as add-on therapy in patients experiencing at least three seizures per month. Patients were stratified according to their AED (inducers vs. noninducers), and doses were escalated to either 35 mg TID or a maximum of 50 mg TID or placebo. Results are not published.

The drug was relatively well tolerated, but dizziness and ataxia were seen.

VALROCEMIDE

Chemistry, Animal Pharmacology, and Mechanism of Action

Valrocemide (valproyl glycinamide) is a VPA analog that combines valproic acid and glycine derivatives (65). The mechanism of action has not been established. The molecule was synthesized to improve brain penetration and eliminate the inhibition of beta-oxidative metabolism seen with valproic acid.

Valrocemide is effective in a wide variety of animal models of epilepsy, with a good protective index and low neurotoxicity in the rotarod test. It is effective in MES, PTZ, corneal kindling, and the 6-Hz model. It is either equipotent to or more potent than VPA in all of these models (59, 66–69). Studies in mice strains susceptible to VPA teratogenicity imply a lower potential for teratogenicity. The typical teratogenicity studies in rats and rabbits were also negative (2). Importantly, it is also effective in animal models of neuropathic pain and bipolar disorders. In addition, the brain:plasma ratio is about four times higher than that for VPA, indicating better penetration.

Biotransformation, Pharmacokinetics, and Interactions in Humans

Phase I doses of as much as 4 g were explored. It was safe and well tolerated. Pharmacokinetics are linear. About 10–20% of valrocemide oral dose is excreted unchanged in the urine; 40% is excreted as valproyl glycine. It is also metabolized in small amounts to valproic acid (about 5%). The half-life is 7 hours. When a dose of 3 g/day is given, VPA levels of 15 mg/L may result. T_{max} is about 1.2 hours. Metabolism appears to be induced by enzyme-inducing AEDs. In-vitro studies using probes for effect on hepatic isozymes did not predict any effect on CYP 1A2, 2C9, 2C19, or 2D6. However, 3A4 was mildly induced. Unlike valproic acid, valrocemide does not inhibit epoxide hydrolase.

Clinical Efficacy

In a Phase IIa trial, 22 patients were exposed to the drug in doses up to 2,000 mg BID. Clearance was higher in epilepsy patients, most likely because the drug is inducible. Adverse events were mild to moderate and impacted the CNS and the gastrointestinal system.

A new, controlled-release formulation has been developed.

CONCLUSION

There are as many new AEDs in the pipeline at this time as at any time in the past. These should serve to improve the management of children with epilepsy into the next decade and beyond. The diverse mechanisms and profiles of the drugs discussed in this chapter represent enormous promise for expanded efficacy, safety, and tolerability. In addition, it is to be hoped that one or several will turn out to be magic bullets for specific difficult epilepsy syndromes encountered in children.

References

1. French JA, Kanner AM, Bautista J, et al. Efficacy and tolerability of the new antiepileptic drugs II: treatment of refractory epilepsy: report of the Therapeutics and Technology Assessment Subcommittee and Quality Standards Subcommittee of the American Academy of Neurology and the American Epilepsy Society. *Neurology* 2004; 62(8):1261–1273.
2. Bialer M. New antiepileptic drugs that are second generation to existing antiepileptic drugs. *Expert Opin Investig Drugs* 2006; 15(6):637–647.
3. Malawska B, Kulig K. Brivaracetam UCB. *Curr Opin Investig Drugs* 2005; 6(7):740–746.
4. Rogawski MA. Diverse mechanisms of antiepileptic drugs in the development pipeline. *Epilepsy Res* 2006; 69:273–294.
5. Zona C, Pieri M, Klitgaard H, Margineanu D. UCB 34714, a new pyrrolidone derivative, inhibits Na^+-currents in rat cortical neurons in culture. *Epilepsia* 2004 45 (Suppl 7):146.
6. Kenda BM, Matagne AC, Talaga PE, et al. Discovery of 4-substituted pyrrolidone butanamides as new agents with significant antiepileptic activity. *J Med Chem* 2004; 47(3):530–549.
7. Bialer M, Johannessen SI, Kupferberg HJ, Levy RH, et al. Progress report on new antiepileptic drugs: a summary of the Seventh Eilat Conference (EILAT VII). *Epilepsy Res* 2004; 61(1–3):1–48.
8. Kasteleijn-Nolst Trenite DGPD, Masnou P, Genton P, Steinhoff BJ, et al. Proof of principle in the new AED UCB 34714: use of the photosensitivity model. *Epilepsia* 2004; 45(Suppl 7): 309 (Abstract 2.349).
9. Bonifacio MJ, Sheridan RD, Parada A, Cunha RA, et al. Interaction of the novel anticonvulsant, BIA 2-093, with voltage-gated sodium channels: comparison with carbamazepine. *Epilepsia* 2001; 42(5):600–608.

10. Ambrosio AF, Silva AP, Malva JO, Soares-da-Silva P, et al. Inhibition of glutamate release by BIA 2-093 and BIA 2-024, two novel derivatives of carbamazepine, due to blockade of sodium but not calcium channels. *Biochem Pharmacol* 2001; 61(10):1271–1275.
11. Parada A, Soares-da-Silva P. The novel anticonvulsant BIA 2-093 inhibits transmitter release during opening of voltage-gated sodium channels: a comparison with carbamazepine and oxcarbazepine. *Neurochem Int* 2002; 40(5):435–440.
12. Almeida L, Falcao A, Maia J, Mazur D, et al. Single-dose and steady-state pharmacokinetics of eslicarbazepine acetate (BIA 2-093) in healthy elderly and young subjects. *J Clin Pharmacol* 2005; 45(9):1062–1066.
13. Almeida L, Soares-da-Silva P. Safety, tolerability and pharmacokinetic profile of BIA 2-093, a novel putative antiepileptic agent, during first administration to humans. *Drugs R D* 2003; 4(5):269–284.
14. Almeida L, Soares-da-Silva P. Safety, tolerability, and pharmacokinetic profile of BIA 2-093, a novel putative antiepileptic, in a rising multiple-dose study in young healthy humans. *J Clin Pharmacol* 2004; 44(8):906–918.
15. Almeida L, Maia J, Soares-da-Silva P. A double-blind, add-on, placebo-controlled, exploratory trial of eslicarbazepine acetate in patients with partial-onset seizures. *Epilepsia* 2005; 46(Suppl 8):167–168.
16. Mazarati AM, Sofia RD, Wasterlain CG. Anticonvulsant and antiepileptogenic effects of fluorofelbamate in experimental status epilepticus. *Seizure* 2002; 11(7):423–430.
17. Wallis R, Panizzon K, Niquet J, Masaratis L, et al. Neuroprotective effects of the anticonvulsant, fluorofelbamate. *Epilepsia* 2000; 41(Suppl. 7):16.
18. Carter RB, Wood PL, Wieland S, et al. Characterization of the anticonvulsant properties of ganaxolone (CCD 1042; 3alpha-hydroxy-3beta-methyl-5alpha-pregnan-20-one), a selective, high-affinity, steroid modulator of the gamma-aminobutyric acid(A) receptor. *J Pharmacol Exp Ther* 1997; 280(3):1284–1295.
19. Gasior M, Ungard JT, Beekman M, Carter RB, et al. Acute and chronic effects of the synthetic neuroactive steroid, ganaxolone, against the convulsive and lethal effects of pentylenetetrazol in seizure-kindled mice: comparison with diazepam and valproate. *Neuropharmacology* 2000; 39(7):1184–1196.
20. Kaminski RM, Livingood MR, Rogawski MA. Allopregnanolone analogs that positively modulate GABA receptors protect against partial seizures induced by 6-Hz electrical stimulation in mice. *Epilepsia* 2004; 45(7):864–867.
21. Monaghan EP, Navalta LA, Shum L, Ashbrook DW, et al. Initial human experience with ganaxolone, a neuroactive steroid with antiepileptic activity. *Epilepsia* 1997; 38(9):1026–1031.
22. Kerrigan JF, Shields WD, Nelson TY, et al. Ganaxolone for treating intractable infantile spasms: a multicenter, open-label, add-on trial. *Epilepsy Res* 2000; 42(2–3):133–139.
23. Laxer K, Blum D, Abou-Khalil BW, et al. Assessment of ganaxolone's anticonvulsant activity using a randomized, double-blind, presurgical trial design. Ganaxolone Presurgical Study Group. *Epilepsia* 2000; 41(9):1187–1194.
24. Lees G, Stohr T, Errington AC. Stereoselective effects of the novel anticonvulsant lacosamide against 4-AP induced epileptiform activity in rat visual cortex in vitro. *Neuropharmacology* 2006; 50(1):98–110.
25. Ben-Menachem EBV, Jatuzis D, Abou-Khalil B, Doty P, et al. SP667 Study Group. Efficacy and safety of adjunctive oral lacosamide for the treatment of partial-onset seizures in patients with epilepsy. *Neurology* 2005; 64(6)(Suppl 1):A187.
26. Tatulian L, Delmas P, Abogadie FC, Brown DA. Activation of expressed KCNQ potassium currents and native neuronal M-type potassium currents by the anti-convulsant drug retigabine. *J Neurosci* 2001; 21(15):5535–5545.
27. Rundfeldt C. The new anticonvulsant retigabine (D-23129) acts as an opener of K+ channels in neuronal cells. *Eur J Pharmacol* 1997; 336(2–3):243–249.
28. Rundfeldt C. Characterization of the K^+ channel opening effect of the anticonvulsant retigabine in PC12 cells. *Epilepsy Res* 1999; 35(2):99–107.
29. Rostock A, Tober C, Rundfeldt C, et al. D-23129: a new anticonvulsant with a broad spectrum activity in animal models of epileptic seizures. *Epilepsy Res* 1996; 23(3):211–223.
30. Tober C, Rostock A, Rundfeldt C, Bartsch R. D-23129: a potent anticonvulsant in the amygdala kindling model of complex partial seizures. *Eur J Pharmacol* 1996; 303(3):163–169.
31. Blackburn-Munro G, Jensen BS. The anticonvulsant retigabine attenuates nociceptive behaviours in rat models of persistent and neuropathic pain. *Eur J Pharmacol* 2003; 460(2–3):109–116.
32. Rivera-Arconada I, Martinez-Gomez J, Lopez-Garcia JA. M-current modulators alter rat spinal nociceptive transmission: an electrophysiological study in vitro. *Neuropharmacology* 2004; 46(4):598–606.
33. Ferron GM, Patat A, Parks V, Rolan P, et al. Lack of pharmacokinetic interaction between retigabine and phenobarbitone at steady-state in healthy subjects. *Br J Clin Pharmacol* 2003; 56(1):39–45.
34. Hermann R, Knebel NG, Niebch G, Richards L, et al. Pharmacokinetic interaction between retigabine and lamotrigine in healthy subjects. *Eur J Clin Pharmacol* 2003; 58(12):795–802.
35. Plosker GL, Scott LJ. Retigabine: in partial seizures. *CNS Drugs* 2006; 20(7):601–608; discussion 609–610.
36. Cardot JM, Lecaillon JB, Czendlik C, Godbillon J. The influence of food on the disposition of the antiepileptic rufinamide in healthy volunteers. *Biopharm Drug Dispos* 1998; 19(4):259–262.
37. Rufinamide: CGP 33101, E 2080, RUF 331, Xilep. *Drugs R D* 2005; 6(4):249–252.
38. Vazquez B, Sachdeo R, Maxoutova A. Efficacy and safety of rufinamide as adjunctive therapy in adult patients with therapy-resistant partial-onset seizures. *Epilepsia* 2000; 37(Suppl 7):255.
39. Glauser T, Kluger G, Sachedo R, Krauss G, et al. Efficacy and Safety of rufinamide adjunctive therapy in patients with Lennox-Gastaut syndrome (LGS): a multicenter, randomized, double-blind, placebo-controlled, parallel trial: LBS.001. *Neurology;* 2005; 64:1826.
40. Nehlig A, Rigoulot M-A, Boehrer A. A new drug, RWJ 333369, displays potent antiepileptic properties in genetic models of absence and audiogenic epilepsy. *Epilepsia* 2005; 46 (Suppl 8):215.
41. Pisani A, Bonsi P, Martella G. Selectracetam (ucb44212), a new pyrrolidone derivative, inhibits high-voltage-activated Ca^{2+} currents and intracellular $[Ca^{2+}]$ increase in rat cortical neurons *in vitro*. *Epilepsia* 2005; 46(Suppl 8):119–120.
42. Rigo J, Nguyen L, Hans G. Selectracetam (ucb44212): effect on inhibitory and excitatory neurotransmission. *Epilepsia* 2005; 46(Suppl 8):110–111.
43. Zona C, Niespodzianky I, Pieri M. Selectracetam (ucb44212), a new pyrrolidone derivative, lacks effect on Na+ currents in rat brain neurons *in vitro*. *Epilepsia* 2005; 46(Suppl 8):116.
44. Matange A, Michel P, Kenda BM, Klitgaard H. Ucb44212, a new pyrrolidone derivative, suppresses seizures in animal models for chronic epilepsy *in vivo*. *Epilepsia* 2003; 46(Suppl 6):121.
45. Trojnar MK, Wojtal K, Trojnar MP, Czuczwar SJ. Stiripentol. A novel antiepileptic drug. *Pharmacol Rep* 2005; 57(2):154–160.
46. Poisson M, Huguet F, Savattier A, Bakri-Logeais F, et al. A new type of anticonvulsant, stiripentol. Pharmacological profile and neurochemical study. *Arzneimittelforschung* 1984; 34(2):199–204.
47. Quilichini PP, Chiron C, Ben-Ari Y, Gozlan H. Stiripentol, a putative antiepileptic drug, enhances the duration of opening of GABA-A receptor channels. *Epilepsia* 2006; 47(4):704–716.
48. Lockard JS, Levy RH, Rhodes PH, Moore DF. Stiripentol in acute/chronic efficacy tests in monkey model. *Epilepsia* 1985; 26(6):704–712.
49. Shen DD, Levy RH, Moor MJ, Savitch JL. Efficacy of stiripentol in the intravenous pentylenetetrazol infusion seizure model in the rat. *Epilepsy Res* 1990; 7(1):40–48.
50. Levy RH, Lin HS, Blehaut HM, Tor JA. Pharmacokinetics of stiripentol in normal man: evidence of nonlinearity. *J Clin Pharmacol* 1983; 23(11–12):523–533.
51. Levy RH, Loiseau P, Guyot M, Blehaut HM, et al. Stiripentol kinetics in epilepsy: nonlinearity and interactions. *Clin Pharmacol Ther* 1984; 36(5):661–669.
52. Levy RH, Loiseau P, Guyot M, Blehaut HM, et al. Michaelis-Menten kinetics of stiripentol in normal humans. *Epilepsia* 1984; 25(4):486–491.
53. Kerr BM, Martinez-Lage JM, Viteri C, Tor J, et al. Carbamazepine dose requirements during stiripentol therapy: influence of cytochrome P-450 inhibition by stiripentol. *Epilepsia* 1991; 32(2):267–274.
54. Tran A, Vauzelle-Kervroedan F, Rey E, et al. Effect of stiripentol on carbamazepine plasma concentration and metabolism in epileptic children. *Eur J Clin Pharmacol* 1996; 50(6):497–500.
55. Cazali N, Tran A, Treluyer JM, et al. Inhibitory effect of stiripentol on carbamazepine and saquinavir metabolism in human. *Br J Clin Pharmacol* 2003; 56(5):526–536.
56. Giraud C, Treluyer JM, Rey E, et al. In vitro and in vivo inhibitory effect of stiripentol on clobazam metabolism. *Drug Metab Dispos* 2006; 34(4):608–611.
57. Chiron C, Marchand MC, Tran A, et al. Stiripentol in severe myoclonic epilepsy in infancy: a randomised placebo-controlled syndrome-dedicated trial. STICLO study group. *Lancet* 2000; 356(9242):1638–1642.
58. De Sarro G, Gitto R, Russo E, Ibbadu GF, et al. AMPA receptor antagonists as potential anticonvulsant drugs. *Curr Top Med Chem* 2005; 5:31–42. http://www.bentham.org/ctmc/sample/ctmc5-1/0004R.pdf (accessed August 13, 2007).
59. Levy RH, Mattson RH, Meldrum BS, et al., eds. *Antiepileptic Drugs.* 5th ed. Philadelphia, PA: Lippincott Williams & Wilkins, 2002: 922–924.
60. Bleakman D, Ballyk BA, Schoepp DD, et al. Activity of 2,3-benzodiazepines at native rat and recombinant human glutamate receptors in vitro: stereospecificity and selectivity profiles. *Neuropharmacology* 1996; 35(12):1689–1702.
61. Czuczwar SJ, Swiader M, Kuzniar H, Gasior M, et al. LY 300164, a novel antagonist of AMPA/kainate receptors, potentiates the anticonvulsive activity of antiepileptic drugs. *Eur J Pharmacol* 1998; 359(2–3):103–109.
62. Borowicz KK, Luszczki J, Szadkowski M, Kleinrok Z, et al. Influence of LY 300164, an antagonist of AMPA/kainate receptors, on the anticonvulsant activity of clonazepam. *Eur J Pharmacol* 1999; 380(2–3):67–72.
63. Langan YM, Lucas R, Jewell H, et al. Talampanel, a new antiepileptic drug: single- and multiple-dose pharmacokinetics and initial 1-week experience in patients with chronic intractable epilepsy. *Epilepsia* 2003; 44(1):46–53.
64. Chappell AS, Sander JW, Brodie MJ, et al. A crossover, add-on trial of talampanel in patients with refractory partial seizures. *Neurology* 2002; 58(11):1680–1682.
65. Blotnik S, Bergman F, Bialer M. The disposition of valproyl glycinamide and valproyl glycine in rats. *Pharm Res* 1997; 14(7):873–878.
66. Isoherranen N, Woodhead JH, White HS, Bialer M. Anticonvulsant profile of valrocemide (TV1901): a new antiepileptic drug. *Epilepsia* 2001; 42(7):831–836.
67. Bialer M, Johannessen SI, Kupferberg HJ, Levy RH, et al. Progress report on new antiepileptic drugs: a summary of the Third Eilat Conference. *Epilepsy Res* 1996; 25(3):299–319.
68. Bialer M, Johannessen SI, Kupferberg HJ, Levy RH, et al. Progress report on new antiepileptic drugs: a summary of the Fifth Eilat Conference (EILAT V). *Epilepsy Res* 2001; 43(1):11–58.
69. Hadad S, Bialer M. Pharmacokinetic analysis and antiepileptic activity of two new isomers of N-valproyl glycinamide. *Biopharm Drug Dispos* 1997; 18(7):557–566.

VI

EPILEPSY SURGERY AND VAGUS NERVE STIMULATION

60 Surgical Evaluation

Michael Duchowny

Epilepsy surgery is an important treatment for children with medically resistant seizures. Successful surgical therapy offers hope for reversing long-standing medical and psychosocial disability and for achieving a more productive and independent life (1).

Identifying appropriate pediatric surgical candidates and evaluating their seizure patterns are rarely straightforward exercises, because children manifest a wide range of seizure types with polymorphous clinical presentations. When electroencephalogram (EEG) findings are nonlocalizing or nonspecific, a comprehensive battery of investigations is often needed to assist in seizure localization. This chapter reviews the indications and special features of epilepsy surgery in the pediatric population, emphasizing currently available procedures for determining surgical candidacy.

CANDIDATE IDENTIFICATION AND SELECTION

Refractory Seizures

Partial seizures are a common form of epilepsy. Their incidence in the Danish registry is 135 cases per 100,000 unselected patients (2), accounting for 60% of the cumulative lifetime prevalence of all epileptic seizures (3, 4). Fortunately, most patients are controlled medically, but there remains a large pool of children with recurrent seizures who are at risk for personal injury, diminished quality of life, and, occasionally, death. For the 5% to 10% of chronic epilepsy patients who are disabled by their disorder, surgery is a justifiable option (5).

To establish intractability, it is first necessary to show that appropriate antiepileptic drugs (AEDs) are ineffective. Serum concentrations should optimally be administered to achieve high therapeutic levels, and polytherapy must be chosen judiciously. Although there are many new and investigational AEDs for partial seizure disorders, children who do not respond to traditional agents are unlikely to go into remission.

Special factors in children may compromise the goal of complete remission. Medication noncompliance in the adolescent population and parental anxiety are two common concerns. At the same time, physician factors, such as medication omissions and dosing errors, can undermine otherwise successful treatment efforts and allow seizures to persist indefinitely (6).

Nonepileptic disorders and psychogenic seizures affect approximately 10% of adolescent and adult epilepsy patients and are a common cause of "pseudointractability" (7). Mimickers of epilepsy are particularly common in children and show a diverse clinical spectrum (8). Two common pitfalls are mistaking complex partial seizures for primary absence epilepsy and failing to identify precipitating factors such as sleep deprivation. More rarely, supplementary motor area seizures may be mistaken for psychogenic nonepileptic seizures because their clinical semiology consists of bilateral motor convulsive movement with preserved awareness. Supplementary motor area seizures are simple partial seizures arising from a discrete and operable focus in the interhemispheric fissure (9). Neurodegenerative disorders, inborn errors of metabolism, and indolent gliomas are occasionally associated with refractory seizures.

Surgical referral is indicated for all children with partial seizures that do not respond to conventional AEDs and the ketogenic diet and that interfere with daily functioning. Family dynamics and perceptions of well-being often influence referral patterns. It has recently been confirmed that children rendered seizure free by excisional procedures achieve enhanced quality of life in multiple functional domains (10).

Gilman and coworkers (6) reexamined the diagnosis of medical intractability in 21 children referred for epilepsy surgery who had significant treatment omissions, such as nonutilization of a first-or second-line AED or lack of therapeutic drug level. Correcting these omissions did not benefit 19 children (90%), whereas 2 children improved on high-dose AED monotherapy. This experience suggests that, although the occasional medically refractory child responds to additional therapeutic intervention, definitive remission is rare.

Pediatric Risk Factors

Several seizure-related factors are associated with medical intractability (11). Frequent seizures (daily or weekly), clustering (12), and early seizure onset (particularly in infancy) favor seizure persistence (13). Infantile hemiconvulsive status epilepticus is linked to later temporal lobe epilepsy in some individuals (14–16). Motor convulsions in nonconvulsive disorders worsen prognosis in direct proportion to the overall number of convulsive episodes (17). Children with brain damage are particularly prone to persistent seizures (12, 18), with the greatest risk in more severely damaged patients (19).

The negative consequences of medically uncontrolled childhood epilepsy were starkly revealed in early prospective cohort studies begun shortly after World War II of 100 children with temporal lobe epilepsy (20). When seizures persisted into adolescence, patients regressed behaviorally and cognitively, and few symptomatic individuals ever led functionally independent lives. Psychosocial disturbance was most troublesome, and less than 5% of the children with significant psychopathology ever functioned normally if their schooling was interrupted (20).

Deleterious Effects of Repeated Seizure Activity

Although psychosocial and intellectual deterioration are not uniformly associated with chronic epilepsy, seizures are deleterious to the developing nervous system. Recurrent seizures induce both transient and long-lasting disruptions of neural circuitry and permanent memory dysfunction (21). Kainic acid exposure increases binding sites in fascia dentata and the CA3 regions of the hippocampus (22), while even brief seizures are capable of inducing mossy fiber sprouting, synaptic reorganization, long-lasting alterations in gene expression, and potentiated neural excitability (23, 24). Similar findings are noted in anterior temporal lobectomy specimens (25, 26), emphasizing that regulatory disturbance of neural excitation and abnormal cellular architecture accompany human epilepsy as well. Hippocampal damage identical to that in chronic temporal lobe epilepsy is also seen in patients with dementia (27).

Other factors predispose children to limbic dysfunction and cellular change. Prolonged early febrile seizures are a recognized antecedent of hippocampal sclerosis (HS) and temporal lobe epilepsy (28). Developmental staging is critical because older individuals are less likely to be damaged (29). Bacterial meningitis and viral encephalitis predispose children to HS after infections only prior to age 4 years (30, 31).

HS, the predominant histopathologic feature of adults with temporal lobe epilepsy, is also prevalent in childhood. In a study of 53 children with chronic temporal lobe seizures who underwent detailed magnetic resonance imaging (MRI) evaluations, 30 children demonstrated either HS or abnormal hippocampal signal without evidence of a mass lesion (16). HS was subsequently confirmed pathologically in 11 of 13 patients treated surgically.

SYNDROMES ASSOCIATED WITH MEDICALLY INTRACTABLE EPILEPSY

Epilepsy syndromes were included in the 1989 International League Against Epilepsy classification (32), and that classification is presently in widespread use to categorize epileptic seizures (33). Identification of specific epilepsy syndromes helps define long-term prognosis, assist genetic analysis, and facilitate surgical referral.

Sturge-Weber Syndrome

Sturge-Weber syndrome is a neurocutaneous disorder manifested by venous angiomas of the leptomeninges and ipsilateral facial angiomatosis (portwine stain, nevus flammeus), which are associated with varying degrees of mental deficiency; ocular defects, including glaucoma and buphthalmos; and epilepsy (34). Partial seizures are particularly common (35), and patients often have uncontrolled seizures and deteriorate clinically. Depressed glucose metabolism on positron emission tomography (PET) (36) and decreased regional blood flow on ^{133}Xe single-photon emission computed tomography (SPECT) (37) confirm severe functional derangement of cerebral cortex underlying the angioma.

Tuberous Sclerosis Complex

Tuberous sclerosis complex (TSC) is a phakomatous disorder causing multiorgan dysfunction, severe psychomotor delay, hypopigmentary skin lesions, adenoma sebaceum, and shagreen patches. Eighty-five percent of patients have infantile spasms and partial epilepsy (38), a high proportion of which are drug-resistant. Excisional procedures designed to remove cortical tissue in proximity to the epileptogenic tuber successfully induce seizure remission (39). Multiple tubers are not a surgical contraindication, because sustained seizure relief is still possible (40).

Although intractable focal epilepsy is often viewed as being either lesional or nonlesional, TSC patients are more precisely characterized as "multilesional" in that they harbor several potential epileptogenic lesions. However, removal of a single tuber often successfully improves or alleviates seizures. The preoperative evaluation is therefore oriented toward identifying the epileptogenic surgical tuber while simultaneously assessing the epileptogenic potential of other lesions.

The identification and removal of an epileptogenic tuber utilizes standard preoperative investigational and planning protocols. Video-EEG characterizes primary seizure origin and functional spread patterns. Ictal recording is particularly valuable for localizing seizure onset in rapid secondarily generalized tonic spasms (41) and lateralizing apparent bilaterally synchronous discharges (42).

Hyperperfused cortical regions on ictal SPECT are used to corroborate electrographic seizure origin and are highly localizing when the EEG demonstrates sustained rhythmic focal fast discharges or spiking (43, 44). A significant proportion of surgical candidates experience a good outcome if the MRI, EEG, and SPECT findings are convergent, whereas the risk of developing a new focus postoperatively is acceptably small (45–47). Early seizure control reverses profound mental retardation and severe autism (48).

The long-term prognosis for seizure recurrence in TSC patients rendered seizure free by surgery is unknown. Although any of the remaining tubers could activate in later life, similar risks exist for all surgery in patients with malformations of cortical development. Alternatively, it is also possible that removal of the primary epileptogenic region could modify potential secondary epileptogenic areas, as may occur in other brain lesions (49). Persistent multifocal abnormalities underscore the need for caution and long-term seizure surveillance.

Cortical Dysplastic Lesions (CDLs)

Dysplasias of the cerebral cortex represent abnormal patterns of neuronal migration and cellular morphogenesis and are an important cause of intractable childhood epilepsy. High-field-strength magnetic resonance (MR) and functional imaging can detect subtle abnormalities in cryptogenic disorders (Figure 60-1). Although the generalized dysplasias, such as lissencephaly and band heterotopia, are rarely amenable to excisional procedures, focal lesions often merit surgical consideration (50, 51).

Very young patients with intractable partial seizures have a high proportion of CDLs and are prone to severe developmental deterioration. Dysplastic changes in infants with catastrophic seizures are often multilobar and show a predilection for the posterior hemispheres (52, 53). Treatment with multilobar excision or hemispherectomy is often required for full seizure control.

Syndrome of Gelastic Epilepsy and Hypothalamic Hamartoma

The syndrome of gelastic seizures and hypothalamic hamartoma is characterized by laughing seizures in early life in association with a hamartoma of the posterior hypothalamus. The lesion consists of heterotopic and hyperplastic tissues arising in the interpeduncular cistern or within the hypothalamus near the tuber cinereum and mammillary bodies (54). Patients manifest complex partial seizures or tonic, atonic, and clonic motor convulsions (55). Few are controlled by medication. Precocious puberty in some patients indicates a neurosecretory potential for the lesion. Progressive mental decline during the second decade of life is the rule.

Despite the uniform occurrence of the hypothalamic lesion in affected patients, it has been difficult to prove unequivocally that the hamartoma is intrinsically epileptogenic. Supportive evidence has come from several sources. Ictal SPECT during gelastic seizures reveals hyperperfusion within the hamartoma, hypothalamus, and thalamus, but not the cortex (56, 57). Direct EEG recording from the hamartoma reveals focal spiking (57, 58), whereas electrical stimulation of the hamartoma reproduces gelastic seizures (57).

Both surgical excision (59, 60) and radiofrequency lesioning (57) successfully alleviate seizures. Seizure freedom facilitates progressive improvement in the EEG and eventual disappearance of the paroxysmal activity (59). Improved cognitive ability and behavior have also been reported (59).

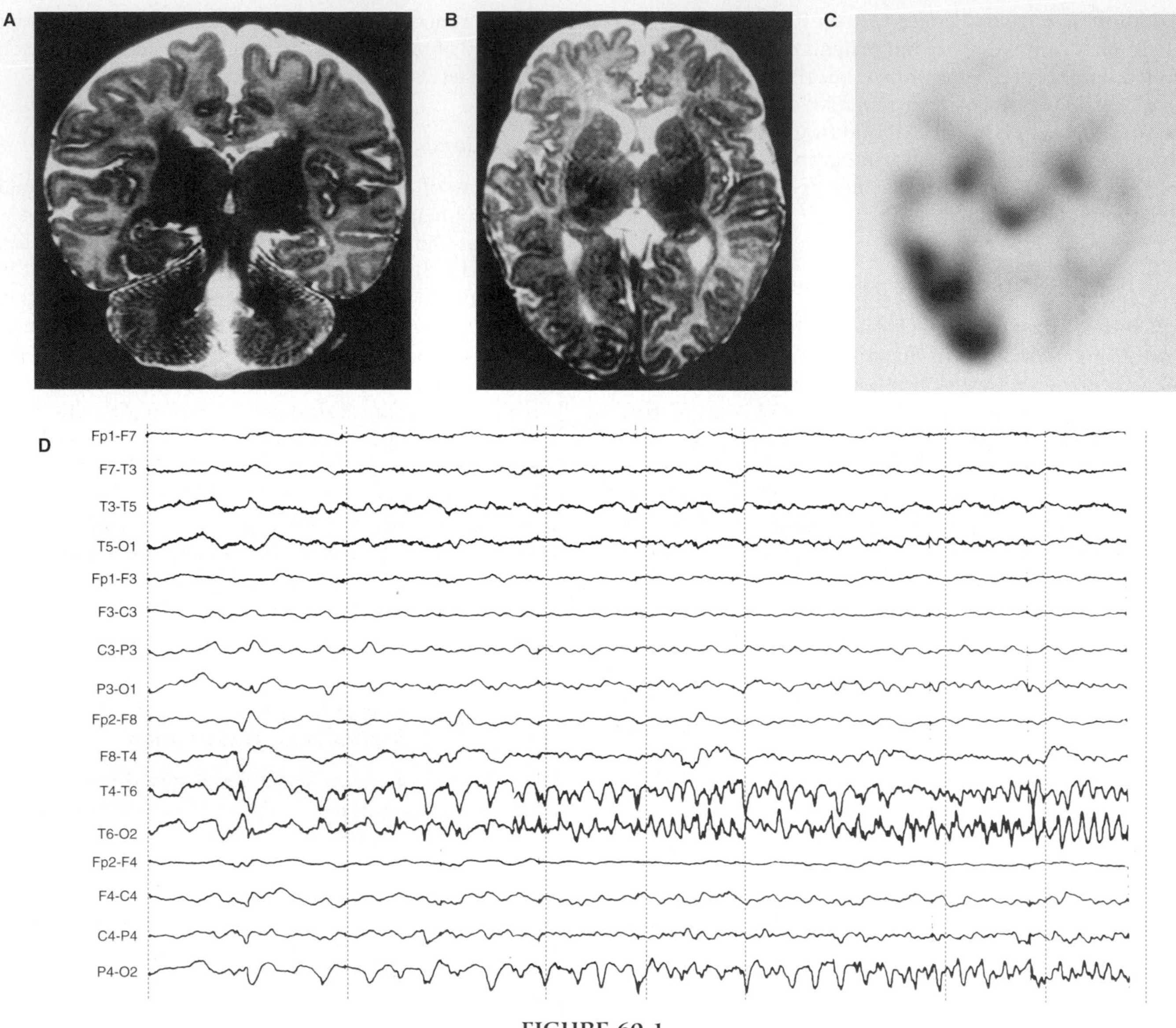

FIGURE 60-1

A 3-month-old male candidate for epilepsy surgery because of neurologic deterioration associated with medically resistant partial seizures and infantile spasms. (A) T2-weighted coronal MR image. There is asymmetric thickening of the cortex in the right parahippocampal and occipitotemporal gyri consistent with cortical dysplasia. (B) T2-weighted axial MR image. There is asymmetric increased myelin deposition in the right occipital and posterior temporal lobes as indicated by the hypointense white matter signal (in comparison to the normal hyperintensity of cerebral white matter in a 3-month-old patient). Areas of hypermyelination are known to occur in conjunction with cortical dysplasia. (C) Axial ^{99m}Tc HMPAO ictal SPECT. There is increased activity in the right occipital and posterior temporal lobes, corresponding to the regions of abnormality on MR images. (D) Ictal EEG recorded during injection for SPECT study, demonstrating repetitive rhythmic sharp waves in the right temporo-occipital region. The electrographic discharge was accompanied by contraversive eye deviation and facial grimacing.

In contrast, focal resection of epileptogenic cortical regions is rarely beneficial (61). A rationale for corticectomy is rooted in abnormal cortical epileptogenic activity and a belief that ictal laughter and confusion are cortically organized complex partial seizure manifestations. Patients with hypothalamic hamartomas also manifest extralesional abnormalities of gray and white matter throughout the hemispheres (62), but, although these regions form aberrant intraneuronal networks, their elimination is alone insufficient for seizure freedom.

It should be emphasized that, despite the remarkable advances in surgical technique, removing hypothalamic hamartomas is not without risk. Hypothalamic disturbance and Korsakoff's dementia are potential consequences of damage to the mammillary bodies, and sessile hamartomas are technically difficult. The Gamma Knife offers a noninvasive alternative for ablating small, deep-seated lesions (63).

Hemimegalencephaly

Hemimegalencephaly is a rare disorder of brain growth in which one cerebral hemisphere undergoes striking enlargement in conjunction with gyral thickening and accelerated myelination. Histologic analysis reveals bizarre giant neurons and heterotopias similar to those of TSC and high-grade cortical dysplasia (64). Fulminant hemiconvulsive seizures and mental deterioration lead to early death in some affected individuals (65), whereas others experience a more benign course (66).

Chronic Focal (Rasmussen) Encephalitis

First described by Rasmussen in 1958 (67, 68), chronic focal encephalitis is a rare but striking cause of epilepsia partialis continua and progressive hemiplegia and characteristically is drug-resistant. Serial neuroimaging reveals progressive atrophy associated with nonspecific focal inflammatory changes in brain tissue and cerebral vasculature (69, 70). A viral etiology has not been established despite repeated attempts to culture an agent (67). Acquired autoimmune dysfunction is suggested by the partial resolution of symptoms after immunotherapy and the recent identification of antibodies to the GluR3 receptor in some patients. Hemispherectomy prevents progression in patients with unilateral hemispheric involvement (70).

West Syndrome

West syndrome, a disorder of brief clonic or tonic spasms, developmental delay, and EEG hypsarrhythmia, is a catastrophic early-onset epilepsy that is often drug resistant. Treatment with corticosteroids and vigabatrin induces remission in approximately half of affected individuals, leaving a sizable proportion with continuing seizures.

The occurrence of spasms in patients with confirmed structural lesions or evidence of localized functional derangement often leads to consideration of excisional surgery (53, 71). The ability to induce surgical remission in an apparently generalized disorder implies that the spasms are a form of secondarily generalized epilepsy. PET abnormalities in dysplastic cortical regions (36) and the cessation of generalized and partial epileptic seizures support this hypothesis (72).

Malformations of cortical developmental and acquired tumors are identified in a high proportion of patients. The restricted region of cortical dysfunction is not inextricably linked to gross structural pathology; many patients with EEG hypsarrhythmia show only microscopic changes and a normal MRI. The potential preoperative pool thus includes all patients with focal cortical dysfunction, with or without a discrete anatomic abnormality.

The utilization of excisional procedures to treat infants with West syndrome has been facilitated by high-resolution MR imaging of cortical dysplasia and other subtle malformations of cortical development. In nonlesional cases, PET studies may identify focal hypometabolic regions that are subsequently proven to be foci of cortical dysplasia. The ability to identify abnormal metabolic cortex is especially critical in the absence of gross structural lesions (73). Localized cerebral hypoperfusion can also be demonstrated by SPECT (74). For unknown reasons, dysplastic lesions producing infantile spasms show a predilection for the posterior cerebral hemispheres.

Successful excisional surgery to treat patients with West syndrome was first performed in infants with documented spasms and localized hypometabolism on PET. Resections were carried out on patients lacking focal anatomic lesions if there was evidence of localized metabolic abnormality. Resected tissue demonstrated histopathologic findings consistent with cortical dysplasia (73).

More recently, Shewmon et al (75) confirmed the efficacy of surgery in 28 infants who were experiencing active spasms at time of operation. Twenty-six (93%) obtained immediate postoperative seizure relief, and only three relapsed. At long-term follow-up, 11 patients were seizure free, with 5 still taking medication.

There are no universally accepted selection criteria for patients with infantile spasms. Perfectly symmetric spasms are rare, and it is important to document any clinical or electrographic feature suggesting a lateralized process. Apart from clinical signs such as hemiparesis, successful candidates should manifest partial seizures or asymmetric spasms, with or without asymmetry of the hypsarrhythmic EEG (76). Asymmetric spasms and partial seizures can coexist as the principal seizure pattern or occur concurrently (77). Partial seizures trigger spasms in some patients (78).

SURGERY IN INFANCY

Despite compelling evidence that very young patients can deteriorate rapidly, surgery is often postponed until later childhood or adolescence (79, 80). Rapid deterioration is especially common in infants with exceptionally frequent seizures. Hemispherectomy is indicated when there is hemispheric damage and widespread unilateral epileptic involvement (81). Approximately 85% of hemispherectomy patients achieve seizure freedom. Smaller resections are restricted to patients with localized ictal patterns and convergent neuroimaging findings (82, 83). In an early report, three of five infants with partial epilepsy undergoing resections became seizure free, two improved significantly, and none deteriorated (84). The favorable experience has been confirmed in larger series of infants undergoing excisional procedures (85, 86).

SURGICAL CONTRAINDICATIONS

Degenerative and Metabolic Disorders

Metabolic and degenerative disorders are important surgical contraindications. Most of these disorders present in the first decade of life and are occasionally associated with partial seizures.

Benign Focal Epilepsies

Syndromes of benign partial epilepsy resolve by the end of the second decade. Benign rolandic epilepsy and benign focal epilepsy of childhood with occipital spikes are relatively common and easily diagnosed by their distinctive clinical and EEG features (87, 88).

Medication Noncompliance

Noncompliance is usually established by the referring physician and rarely surfaces as an issue during the preoperative evaluation. Noncompliant patients are unsuitable surgical candidates.

Psychosis

The occurrence of psychotic symptoms in children with partial seizures is controversial and rarely reported. Chronic thought disorders in the adult are rarely improved after surgery, and peri-ictal disturbances generally remit with seizure control (89). It is not known whether psychotic symptoms can be prevented by early surgical intervention.

Mental Retardation

Patients with chronic epilepsy manifest variable cognitive impairment, but surgery is rarely withheld if patients can comply with the preoperative evaluation. Retarded individuals clearly benefit from seizure freedom.

Dysfunctional Families

Cooperation with epilepsy surgery team members is fundamental to the success of elective surgery. Psychodynamically dysfunctional families are rarely comfortable during intensive or prolonged hospitalizations and may not be able to evaluate the risks and benefits of surgery objectively. Dysfunctional families require psychologic and social intervention and support before surgical workup.

PREOPERATIVE EVALUATION

Neuropathologic Considerations

Disorders of cortical development underlie the majority of intractable seizures in childhood, whereas acquired lesions (i.e., atrophic, sclerotic, or both) are less common. Extensive resections (hemispherectomy or multilobar excision) prove necessary because developmental lesions are associated with widespread anatomic and functional derangement. Although temporal lobectomy is frequently used to treat adults, pediatric patients are more prone to extratemporal seizures and catastrophic presentations (1, 90). Direct comparisons of children and adults with cortical dysplasia and epilepsy reveal that onset of seizure at a younger age is associated with a higher incidence of developmental delay, larger structural lesions, and higher seizure frequency (91).

Not unexpectedly, seizures from a developmentally abnormal cortex are more difficult to characterize by scalp EEG; high-field-strength MR imaging can assist localization by detecting subtle dysplastic lesions. Even so, many low-grade dysplastic lesions and neuronal heterotopias remain undetected (92). Functional localization using PET and SPECT can identify epileptogenic regions through abnormal metabolism or ictal blood flow (93–96).

CLINICAL SEIZURE SEMIOLOGY

Frontal Lobe Epilepsy (FLE)

The clinical and electrographic manifestations of FLE are extremely heterogeneous. Frontal lobe seizures are typically brief (<5 minutes) and stereotyped. Clustering and sleep onset are common; prolonged seizure episodes and auras are unusual. Patients may experience brief nonspecific fears or sensations immediately before seizure onset.

Motor seizures of frontal lobe origin may be tonic or clonic, reflecting involvement of Brodmann areas 6 or 4. Seizures arising in motor strip produce contralateral clonic activity, with or without Jacksonian spread to adjacent cortical areas. Very young children are more prone to secondary generalization. Tonic contraversive arm, head, or eye movements suggest involvement of dorsolateral frontal cortex anterior to motor strip. Tonic version is commonly the result of secondary spread of epileptic activity to the frontal cortex.

Ictal head version is a common manifestation of frontal lobe seizure and occurs when the sternocleidomastoid muscle is activated. This muscle has two heads (sternal and clavicular) that rotate the head and neck in opposite trajectories (contralateral turning vs. ipsilateral tilting) (97). Either or both heads may become active, resulting in complex ictal patterns.

Stereotyped psychomotor patterns are more typical of seizures arising in the premotor cortex. Symptoms include bicycling movements, repetitive arm postures and gestures, and disturbances of phonation, including speech arrest and vocalization (98, 99). Activation of anterior and orbitofrontal cortexes are associated with prominent automatisms and complex behavioral sequences. Truncal postural change is not unusual, and patients often appear frightened or agitated. Seizures are typically nocturnal, with frequent arousals that, together with the lack of epileptiform discharges, have suggested paroxysmal nocturnal dystonia.

Supplementary motor area (SMA) seizures often begin in childhood (9); they cause bilateral proximal tonic limb posturing with fully preserved consciousness. The routine EEG may be normal or nondiagnostic, yielding a false impression of psychogenic seizures. Intracortical propagation of SMA discharges may falsely localize seizure onset to the dorsolateral convexity.

Temporal Lobe Epilepsy (TLE)

Seizures of temporal lobe origin are common in childhood. Although they are well characterized in adolescents and adults, the manifestations of TLE are less well documented in infants and children. Many features are seen in adults, but diagnostic pitfalls abound.

Complex partial seizures of temporal lobe origin impair or distort consciousness. Auras are common, although rarely described by the preverbal or nonverbal patient. Automatisms typically consist of gestural or oroalimentary movements in infancy, whereas verbal and complex behavioral automatisms are characteristic of older patients (100).

Secondary motor seizures occur frequently in infants and may be the only seizure manifestation. Their incidence declines with advancing age, while behavioral arrest and stereotyped automatisms increasingly predominate. Video-EEG is often required to diagnose secondary motor phenomena (100, 101).

Parietal Lobe Epilepsy (PLE)

Seizures of parietal lobe origin are relatively uncommon, and their true incidence is probably underestimated because symptoms arise only after extraparietal spread. Two clinically distinct propagation patterns are recognized: motor convulsions with spread to the frontal lobes and complex partial seizures with temporal lobe involvement (102–104). Both patterns may occur in the same patient (104). Panic attacks may be the sole manifestation of right parietal lobe seizures (105).

The EEG is often silent or subtly abnormal. Ictal SPECT may confirm anterior parietal seizure origin in patients with sensorimotor symptoms; psychoparetic symptoms arise posteriorly (104).

Occipital Lobe Epilepsy (OLE)

Occipital seizures produce visual symptomatology, including hallucinations, amaurosis, visual field deficits, and forced eye and eyelid movement (102). Seizure activity may spread frontally or, more rarely, to the temporal lobe and produce regional symptoms. Many children with OLE have benign syndromes that are easily controlled and that remit during adolescence (106, 107).

SCALP EEG

The EEG evaluation remains the single most useful tool for evaluating pediatric epilepsy surgery patients. Experienced pediatric EEG personnel should evaluate the EEG, because the interpretation of pediatric seizure patterns is complex (108). Although patients referred for surgery usually have had extensive EEG evaluations, electroclinical diagnoses should always be reconfirmed by careful review of prior EEG recordings. Video-EEG is essential for documenting seizure manifestations. The appearance of electrographic discharges before clinical seizure onset suggests remote seizure onset (108).

Ictal patterns in the childhood epilepsies are more often regional than localized, and children display a wide variety of artifacts that obscure EEG interpretation. There is a close relationship between ictal and interictal electrographic findings, but less than half of all interictal spikes are detected at the scalp (108). Pediatric surgical candidates often manifest bilaterally synchronous or multifocal discharges. Regionalization serves as a basis for planning further invasive studies. MR and functional imaging often help confirm equivocal electrophysiologic data.

STRUCTURAL IMAGING

Magnetic resonance imaging is the modality of choice for evaluating pediatric epilepsy surgery candidates. Its high specificity and sensitivity provide clues to the pathologic basis of many developmental disorders, including CDLs, migrational disturbances, and developmental tumors (e.g., dysembryoplastic neuroepithelial tumors or gangliogliomas).

MRI presently detects pathologic substrates in more than 80% of children with intractable partial epilepsy (92). Thirty of 98 children and adolescents with partial epilepsy undergoing both computed tomography (CT) and MRI investigations had lesions responsible for their epilepsy that were detected by MRI, but not by CT (109).

MRI studies also reveal a high incidence of HS in childhood. In a study of 53 children with TLE undergoing detailed MRI investigations, 30 children showed either HS or regions of abnormal signal in the absence of a mass lesion (110). Hippocampal volume loss can also be documented (111). One developmentally delayed infant with a normal MRI reportedly developed a unilaterally increased signal in the hippocampus within 24 hours of an episode of status epilepticus (112). Cortical dysgenesis was identified in the temporal lobe specimen.

Neuroimaging of pediatric epilepsy surgery candidates should employ techniques to maximize yield. T1-weighted data are optimally acquired in an oblique coronal orientation, orthogonal to the long axis of the hippocampi (113). Sequencing should include thin (1- to 1.5-mm) images without gaps, especially through the hippocampal regions. Further sequences, such as fluid attenuated inversion recovery (FLAIR), help detect subtle abnormalities. We routinely perform MRI after video-EEG monitoring to facilitate more detailed examination of the candidate seizure region.

FUNCTIONAL IMAGING

Functional imaging of the epileptogenic region may help define the seizure focus, especially when other modalities yield equivocal or divergent findings. Several techniques are presently available.

PET

PET utilizes radioactive tracers with short half-lives linked to cerebral blood flow. ^{18}Fluorodeoxyglucose (FDG) is a marker of the interictal focus, correlating with the epileptogenic region (usually the temporal lobe) in approximately 80% of adult cases (114). Ictal capture is unlikely and should not be induced by convulsant agents because of technical limitations of the scanning process.

The requirement for sedation and the higher proportion of extratemporal seizures limit the clinical utility of PET in children. Newer isotopes that bind to receptor-specific compounds such as ^{11}C-flumazenil, which is linked to the benzodiazepine receptor, hold promise for enhanced localization (115).

Although less widely employed in the pediatric setting, PET studies have also been employed successfully to localize seizure origin in cases of West syndrome (73) and other epileptic encephalopathies (116), Sturge-Weber syndrome (117), TSC (118), frontal lobe epilepsy (119), and generalized tonic-clonic seizures (120). PET studies are particularly useful in children with extratemporal epilepsy and childhood syndromes with apparently generalized epileptic discharges.

PET has also been utilized successfully for presurgical localization of eloquent cortex in children with seizures. PET mapping of eloquent language, motor, and visual areas was accomplished in 15 children by coregistering PET images of task-activated cerebral blood flow onto MR images (121). All patients had lesional epilepsy. PET mapping was well tolerated in all cases.

The absolute reliability of PET as a stand-alone localizing tool in the pediatric epilepsy surgical evaluation has been questioned (122). Whereas FDG-PET studies in older children and adolescents have produced results similar to those in adults (123), with one exception (116), there are no longitudinal studies of PET in younger children. It has also been shown that [^{11}C]flumazenil PET is significantly more sensitive than 2-deoxy-2-[^{18}F] fluoro-D-glucose for detecting cortical regions of seizure onset and frequent spiking in children with extratemporal epilepsy, and that both radioisotopes have low sensitivity when there is rapid seizure spread (124).

Single-Photon Emission Computerized Tomography

Imaging with SPECT utilizes isotopes such as hexylmethylpropylene amine oxime (HMPAO) for qualitative measures of regional cerebral perfusion (rCP). Early studies were performed in the interictal state, but ictal injections are acknowledged to yield more accurate localization of the epileptogenic region (125). The high yield of ictal SPECT has supplanted PET in the functional evaluation of pediatric epilepsy surgery candidates (126).

The widespread availability of SPECT cameras in nuclear medicine facilities, the low cost of gamma-emitting isotopes, and the introduction of more stable radiopharmaceuticals have facilitated SPECT studies at many pediatric epilepsy centers. SPECT has been employed successfully to evaluate a wide spectrum of pediatric epilepsy surgical syndromes including Sturge-Weber syndrome (127), tuberous sclerosis complex (44), Rasmussen syndrome (128), hemimegalencephaly (129) and focal cortical dysplasia (130).

Ictal SPECT studies remain the procedure of choice to localize a high proportion of children with partial epilepsy (131). Ictal SPECT studies revealed hyperperfusion in 14 of 15 children with temporal lobe epilepsy undergoing preoperative evaluation (132). In 4 children, ictal SPECT provided additional localizing information that was absent from ictal EEG recordings. Similarly, Cross et al (133) reported abnormalities on ictal SPECT in 13 of 14 children with both temporal and extra-temporal seizures. The timing of injection was a critical variable, with injections more than 30 seconds postictally being less likely to yield reliable measurements of regional cerebral blood flow. Pediatric ictal SPECT studies have also been shown to reliably colocalize the epileptogenic zone demonstrated by intracranial EEG recording and to correlate with higher rates of surgical success (134).

In contrast, interictal SPECT injections are a significantly less reliable localizing tool in pediatric patients (135). Normal studies or uncertainty regarding regions of hypoperfusion may potentially be misleading and are rarely relied upon for surgical decision making. Ictal SPECT studies may be used to confirm localizing data from EEG and MRI investigations or to define the epileptogenic region in children with normal or discordant EEG and imaging data. SPECT may also play a role in clarifying the extent of the epileptogenic region and assist in placement of intracranial electrodes.

Proton Magnetic Resonance Spectroscopy (MRS)

MRS studies in epilepsy use N-acetyl aspartate (NAA), creatine, and phosphocreatine-containing compounds, as several lines of evidence indicate that NAA is primarily intraneuronal and an indicator of neuronal well-being (136). ^{1}H-MRS can be added to routine imaging and provides important lateralizing information, especially in temporal lobe epilepsy (137). Recent MRS studies document neuronal dysfunction in neocortical dysplastic lesions, and correction of metabolic derangement at mirror temporal foci improves after successful surgery (138).

Functional MR Imaging (fMRI)

fMRI is based on noninvasive detection of small regions of increased cerebral blood flow through decreases in deoxyhemoglobin concentration. Three applications are especially promising for patients with epilepsy: delineation of ictal events, localization of the primary epileptogenic region, and identification of a functionally critical cortex (139).

At present, pediatric applications of fMRI are limited. Subjects must be awake, fully cooperative, and not easily distracted. In many candidates, who are developmentally delayed or suffer from behavioral and/or motor disabilities, fMRI data are not easily acquired. fMRI is, however, increasingly being incorporated into the preoperative evaluation of children. fMRI has reliably been used to localize language, sensory, motor, and visual functions in children and can influence surgical planning (140).

Language mapping utilizing developmentally appropriate paradigms generates localizing data in children that is similar to adults. Cooperative children as young as age 5 years have been studied successfully (141). It has been shown that networks for auditory processing are regionally localized and lateralized by age 5 years (142). Receptive language sites are located primarily along the superior temporal sulcus, similar to those of the adult, suggesting that language localization and network formation is established in early life. False lateralization of language cortex to the homologous nondominant hemisphere may occur in children undergoing fMRI in the postictal state (143).

Sensorimotor cortex can be positively identified utilizing paradigms in which the child taps a finger or toe, wiggles the tongue, or has an extremity brushed. All of these paradigms are simple to apply and achieve reliable results, even in very young children. The location of sensorimotor function by fMRI agrees with localization data obtained by direct cortical stimulation.

NEUROBEHAVIORAL AND PSYCHOSOCIAL ASSESSMENT

Candidate Selection

Neurobehavioral and psychosocial disabilities are common in pediatric epilepsy surgical candidates. A high proportion display mental handicap, short attention span, or high activity level (80, 144). There is a clear link between brain damage and the presence of these features, with the most damaged patients showing earlier seizure onset and a higher frequency of recurrence (12). Older children and adolescents with TLE may develop psychotic thought disorders, especially with left-sided seizure origin (89); adults may experience hyposexuality and personality disturbances (145).

The high incidence of psychosocial and behavioral problems makes baseline assessment of these areas of functioning critical to the preoperative evaluation. However, level of cooperation is often poor, and cognitive deficits may not permit standardized testing.

There is also greater difficulty lateralizing and localizing function in the immature nervous system. Whereas neuropsychologic assessment in adults can lateralize dysfunction, similar procedures are rarely successful in children. The frontal lobes are not fully mature until the second decade, and temporal lobe findings are often nonspecific. Developmental lesions may produce widespread functional disturbance.

The contribution of psychosocial assessment to pediatric epilepsy surgery is more realistically directed in two ways. First, preoperative baseline level of function can be documented for future comparisons. Second, psychosocial assessment provides a descriptor of overall maturational brain status.

Testing Protocol

There is no single neurobehavioral protocol for children being worked up for epilepsy surgery. At the Palm Desert II Epilepsy Surgery Conference, 82 centers completed detailed questionnaires about neuropsychologic testing (146). Forty-two (52.4%) included information about pediatrics, although children were often a small minority. Most centers employed adult test batteries with pediatric norms rather than devising their own batteries. There was uniformity of testing for intelligence and certain measures of cognition but a striking diversity in tests of certain verbal skills and nondominant-hemisphere function. The Wisconsin Card Sorting Test and the Controlled Oral Word Association Test (FAS Fluency) were most commonly used. A more complete listing of tests is found elsewhere (147).

INVASIVE EEG STUDIES

Intracranial EEG Recording

In children, as anomalous development occurs throughout the neocortex (148) and is frequently in proximity to eloquent cortex, even seizures of temporal lobe origin are rarely evaluated properly by adult evaluation paradigms (149, 150).

Several additional factors in children explain the higher incidence of more complex workups and higher rates of electrode implantation. Electrocorticographic (ECoG) monitoring, the only tool for physiologically assessing seizure foci intraoperatively, is performed under general anesthesia and frequently is nondiagnostic (108). Electrographically active regions may extend beyond known anatomic boundaries (151), are particularly extensive in infants and very young children (148, 152, 153), and are more likely to involve eloquent cortical regions (154, 155). Dysplastic tissue is rarely visible in the operating room, making visually guided surgery problematic.

Depth electrodes, which are used primarily to sample temporolimbic structures, have limited utility for neocortical foci. Subdural electrodes provide more comprehensive coverage and are well tolerated, even in very young children and infants (155, 156).

Indications for Implanting Electrodes

There are no universal criteria for invasive EEG monitoring in pediatric patients. Invasive monitoring is often indicated for nonlesional cases (157), whereas scalp EEG, in conjunction with imaging and ECoG, is usually sufficient to evaluate seizures associated with gross structural lesions. Excisional procedures have been performed in patients undergoing only intraoperative ECoG monitoring and PET (53).

Possible indications for invasive EEG recording include the following:

1. *Partial seizures with normal or nonlocalizing imaging data.* Nonlesional epilepsy patients become seizure free only if the ictal onset zone and interictal abnormalities are completely resected. Subdural recording helps define the limits of the epileptogenic region, because depth electodes cannot sample wide regions of epileptogenic cortex.
2. *Epileptogenic zone larger than the structural lesion.* The true physiologic limits of the epileptic focus in patients with developmental lesions require careful documentation (158). Invasive recording assists surgical planning (159). In 42 children with lesional epilepsy, 90 percent were seizure free after complete excision of the lesion and entire epileptogenic region, whereas half were seizure free with lesion removal and incomplete resection of electrophysiologically abnormal tissue (160).
3. *Noncongruence of data.* Defining the epileptogenic zone with noncongruent seizure semiology, interictal-ictal EEG, and imaging data may not be possible. Invasive EEG recording can help resolve incongruities.
4. *Multiple lesions and/or multifocal interictal epileptiform activity.* Children with multiple structural lesions and/or multifocal interictal spike discharges are surgical candidates when seizures arise from a single operable epileptogenic zone (40, 161, 162). Multiple epileptogenic regions can exert complex ictal interactions, rendering localization difficult from scalp EEG data alone.
5. *Involvement of regions subserving eloquent cortical function.* Regions of eloquent cortex that are contiguous to the epileptic focus require mapping with subdural electrodes. Sensory cortex may be identified intraoperatively by median nerve stimulation. In children, language function is optimally defined extraoperatively.

Functional Cortical Stimulation

The high incidence of extratemporal and multilobar epilepsy in children requires definition of cortical function in many surgical candidates. The standard adult paradigm, whereby baseline stimulation is increased in 0.5- to 1.0-mA steps until an afterdischarge, functional response, or 15-mA ceiling is obtained, is rarely successful in younger patients (163, 164). Electrical responsiveness increases in direct proportion to age, while threshold for functional responsiveness decreases until adolescence (164).

Cortical responses are more reliably elicited in children by increasing both stimulus intensity and duration in a stepwise fashion (164). Increasing both domains rather than intensity alone causes the stimulus to converge toward the chronaxie on the strength-duration curve. Responses obtained at the chronaxie are elicited at the lowest possible expenditure of energy, a clear advantage when working in immature cortex. In comparison to the adult paradigm, only dual stimulation successfully evokes both afterdischarges and functional responses in patients 4 years of age and younger (164).

Sensorimotor Mapping

Dual-stimulation mapping of sensorimotor responses in pediatric epilepsy surgery candidates reveals anatomic representation of cortical function similar to that in the adult. Despite the similarities, however, there are several important maturational features (165). Children under the age of 4 years have predominantly tonic rather than clonic movements, and movement of the tongue is unusual. Below the age of 6 years, hand movement but not individual finger movement is observed. As a rule, tonic finger movements appear earlier than clonic movements, a developmental sequence that mirrors the ontogenetic expression of motor seizure patterns in childhood (100, 166).

Below the age of 2 years, facial motor responses may be bilateral (165), resembling a grimace that lasts several seconds. Bilateral facial movement is absent in older children, suggesting that bilateral facial innervation is a postnatal pattern that predates axonal and/or synaptic elimination (167, 168). Ipsilateral lower facial innervation is gradually lost with maturation. Bilateral facial movement is supported by the observation of facial sparing in congenital but not acquired hemiplegia (169).

Patients with aberrant cortical development exhibit unexpected anomalies of the motor homunculus (165). A hand region superior to primary shoulder region and double shoulder region above and below hand and finger cortex have been described. Aberrant cortical motor organization is more common in patients with other anomalies of cortical development (170). Experimental studies in the primate brain indicate that prenatal lesions are capable of inducing anomalous cortical sulci and functional reorganization at remote cortical sites in both cerebral hemispheres (171, 172).

Language Mapping

Much of our knowledge of the organization of primary language cortex in the child comes from studies of recovery from childhood aphasia (173). Complete or near-complete recovery is possible based on age at which the lesion occuerred and size and location of the damage (174). Recovery involves interhemispheric reorganization and a switch to right-hemisphere dominance. Language recovers well after early postnatal lesions, but deficits in nonlinguistic skills suggest that recovery is rarely complete or predictable (175).

Although postnatal lesions of the dominant hemisphere in early childhood lead to significant reorganization of language cortex, there is little information about language representation in children with partial seizures and anomalous cortical development. Clarification has obvious implications when seizures originate within or adjacent to language cortex (176).

A recent investigation of electrical stimulation of language cortex in 34 predominantly pediatric patients with implanted subdural grid electrodes, identified 28 with MRI and/or histologic evidence of developmental pathology (155). Patients with developmental lesions had language cortex in frontal and temporal sites anatomically similar to those in the adult. The "adult" representation has been documented in an epilepsy patient as young as 4 years old and a 2-year-old being mapped for tumoral surgery. The actual amount of surface area of cortex devoted to language (based on the number of subdural electrodes showing language representation) is also similar to that of the adult (154, 177), which suggests that language sites are designated in early life and conserved anatomically over the lifespan. The increasing language competence of the child is therefore not attributable to increased cortical surface area.

The relatively fixed position of language cortex in children with anomalous disorders of cortical development contrasts sharply with the relocation of language following early peri- or postnatally acquired lesions (178). Relocation of language sites occurs if language cortex is destroyed before the age of 6 years. By contrast, developmental lesions do not ablate language cortex and therefore do not lead to relocation. Epileptic bombardment also does not displace language cortex from predetermined sites.

PREOPERATIVE PREDICTORS OF SEIZURE OUTCOME

Clinical, EEG, imaging, and neuropsychologic features have been used to predict outcome of adults selected for temporal lobectomy (1), and multivariate algorithms for predicting success have been described (179). Children exhibit more diverse causes for intractable seizures, making extrapolation from the adult experience difficult. Pediatric candidates with a well-circumscribed interictal EEG focus, localized seizure pattern on monitoring, and tumoral epilepsy have a greater likelihood of seizure freedom (180). Although younger age at surgery is not associated with reduced chances of success, younger patients more often manifest poorly localized EEG patterns (180), and completeness of resection of the epileptogenic area (1) may not be possible.

Studies of preoperative factors for pediatric temporal lobectomy have not identified specific predictors of seizure outcome (181). The absence of statistically significant adult variables such as duration of epilepsy, daily seizures, motor convulsions, and mental retardation suggests caution before excluding potential candidates. The lower predictive power of preoperative variables in pediatric epilepsy surgical candidates, in direct contrast with the adult experience, suggests that all children with surgically amenable intractable seizures are potential surgical candidates.

References

1. Engel JJ. Epilepsy surgery. *Curr Opin Neurol* 1994; 7:140–147.
2. Juul Jensen P, Foldspang A. Natural history of epileptic seizures. *Epilepsia* 1983; 24:297–312.
3. Hauser WA, Annegers JF, Kurland LT. Prevalence of epilepsy in Rochester, Minnesota: 1940–1980. *Epilepsia* 1991; 32:429–445.
4. Hauser WA. Recent developments in the epidemiology of epilepsy. *Acta Neurol Scand* 1995; 162(Suppl):17–21.
5. National Institutes of Health Consensus Conference. Surgery for epilepsy. *JAMA* 1990; 264:729–733.
6. Gilman JT, Duchowny M, Jayakar P, Resnick TJ. Medical intractability in children evaluated for epilepsy surgery. *Neurology* 1994; 44:1341–1343.
7. Desai BT, Porter RJ, Penry JK. Psychogenic seizures. A study of 42 attacks in six patients, with intensive monitoring. *Arch Neurol* 1982; 39:202–209.
8. Sassower K, Duchowny M. Psychogenic seizures and nonepileptic phenomena in childhood. In: Devinsky O, Theodore W, eds. *Epilepsy and Behavior*. New York: Wiley-Liss, 1991:223–235.
9. Bass N, Wyllie E, Comair Y, et al. Supplementary sensorimotor area seizures in children and adolescents. *J Pediatr* 1995; 126:537–544.
10. Sabaz M, Lawson JA, Cairns DR, Duchowny MS, et al. The impact of epilepsy surgery on quality of life in children. *Neurology* 2006; 66(4):557–561.
11. Chevrie JJ, Aicardi J. Convulsive disorders in the first year of life: persistence of epileptic seizures. *Epilepsia* 1979; 20: 643–649.
12. Aicardi J. Epilepsy in brain-injured children. *Dev Med Child Neurol* 1990; 32:191–202.
13. Lindsay J, Ounsted C, Richards P. Long-term outcome in children with temporal lobe seizures. IV: Genetic factors, febrile convulsions and the remission of seizures. *Dev Med Child Neurol* 1980; 22:429–439.
14. Gastaut H, Poirier F, Payan H, et al. HHE syndrome, hemiconvulsions, hemiplegia, epilepsy. *Epilepsia* 1959; 1:418–447.
15. Cendes F, Andermann F, Dubeau F, et al. Early childhood prolonged febrile convulsions, atrophy and sclerosis of mesial structures, and temporal lobe epilepsy: an MRI volumetric study. *Neurology* 1993; 43:1083–1087.
16. Harvey AS, Grattan Smith JD, Desmond PM, Chow CW, et al. Febrile seizures and hippocampal sclerosis: frequent and related findings in intractable temporal lobe epilepsy of childhood. *Pediatr Neurol* 1995; 12:201–206.
17. Emerson R, D'Souza BJ, Vining EP, et al. Stopping medication in children with epilepsy. Predictors of outcome. *N Engl J Med* 1981; 304:1125–1129.
18. Huttenlocher PR, Hapke RJ. A follow-up study of intractable seizures in childhood [see comments]. *Ann Neurol* 1990; 28:699–705.
19. Hadjipanayis A, Hadjichristodoulou C, Youroukos S. Epilepsy in patients with cerebral palsy. *Dev Med Child Neurol* 1997; 39:659–663.
20. Ounsted C, Lindsay J, Norman R. Biological factors in temporal lobe epilepsy. Clinics in Developmental Medicine 22. Philadelphia: Lippincott, 1966; London: SIMP with Heinemann Medical.
21. Ben Ari Y. Activity-dependent forms of plasticity. *J Neurobiol* 1995; 26:295–298.
22. Represa A, Niquet J, Pollard H, Ben Ari Y. Cell death, gliosis, and synaptic remodeling in the hippocampus of epileptic rats. *J Neurobiol* 1995; 26:413–425.
23. Represa A, Ben Ari Y. Molecular and cellular cascades in seizure-induced neosynapse formation. *Adv Neurol* 1997; 72:25–34.
24. Sloviter RS. Hippocampal pathology and pathophysiology in temporal lobe epilepsy. *Neurologia* 1996; 4:29–32.
25. Sutula T, Cascino G, Cavazos J, et al. Mossy fiber synaptic reorganization in the epileptic human temporal lobe. *Ann Neurol* 1989; 26:321–330.
26. Houser CR. Granule cell dispersion in the dentate gyrus of humans with temporal lobe epilepsy. *Brain Res* 1990; 535:195–204.
27. Bloom JC, Sabbagh MN, Bondi MW, Hansen L, et al. 1997. Hippocampal sclerosis contributes to dementia in the elderly. *Neurology* 1997; 48:154–160.
28. Verity CM, Ross EM, Golding J. Outcome of childhood status epilepticus and lengthy febrile convulsions: findings of national cohort study. *Br Med J* 1993:225–228.
29. Sagar HJ, Oxbury JM. Hippocampal neuron loss in temporal lobe epilepsy: correlation with early childhood convulsions. *Ann Neurol* 1987; 22:334–340.
30. Ounsted C, Glaser GH, Lindsay J, Richards P. Focal epilepsy with mesial temporal sclerosis after acute meningitis. *Arch Neurol* 1985; 42:1058–1060.
31. Marks DA, Kim J, Spencer DD, Spencer SS. Characteristics of intractable seizures following meningitis and encephalitis. *Neurology* 1992; 42:1513–1518.
32. Commission on Classification and Terminology of the International League Against Epilepsy. Proposal for classification of epilepsies and epileptic syndromes. *Epilepsia* 1985; 26:268–278.
33. Duchowny M, Harvey AS. Pediatric epilepsy syndromes: an update and critical review. *Epilepsia* 1996; 37:S26–S40.
34. Alexander GL, Norman R. The Sturge-Weber syndrome. Bristol: Wright and Son, 1960.
35. Peterman AF, Hayles AB, Dockrty MD, Love JG. 1958. Encephalotrigeminal angiomatosis (Sturge-Weber disease): clinical study of thirty-five cases. *JAMA* 1958; 67: 2169–2176.
36. Chugani HT, Mazziotta JC, Phelps ME. Sturge-Weber syndrome: a study of cerebral glucose utilization with positron emission tomography. *J Pediatr* 1989; 114:244–253.
37. Vaernet K. Temporal lobotomy in children and young adults. In: Parsonage M, ed. *XIVth Epilepsy International Symposium*. New York: Raven Press, 1983:255–61.
38. Monaghan HP, Krafchik B, Mac Gregor D, Fitz C. Tuberous sclerosis complex in children. *Am J Dis Child* 1981; 135:912–917.
39. Perot P, Weir B, Rasmussen T. Tuberous sclerosis. Surgical therapy for seizures. *Arch Neurol* 1966; 15:498–506.
40. Erba G, Duchowny MS. 1990. Partial epilepsy and tuberous sclerosis: indications for surgery in disseminated disease. In: Duchowny MS, Resnick TJ, Alvarez LA, eds. *Pediatric Epilepsy Surgery*. New York: Demos, 1990:315–322.
41. Ohmori I, Ohtsuka Y, Ohno S, Oka E. Analysis of ictal EEGs of epilepsy associated with tuberous sclerosis. *Epilepsia* 1998; 39:1277–1283.
42. Seri S, Cerquiglini A, Pisani F, Michel CM, et al. Frontal lobe epilepsy associated with tuberous sclerosis. *J Child Neurol* 1998; 13:33–38.
43. Koh S, Jayakar P, Resnick T, Alvarez L, et al. The localizing value of ictal SPECT in children with tuberous sclerosis complex and refractory partial epilepsy. *Epileptic Disord* 1999; 1:41–46.
44. Koh S, Jayakar P, Dunoyer C, Whiting S, et al. Epilepsy surgery with tuberous sclerosis complex: presurgical evaluation and outcome. *Epilepsia* 2000; 41:1206–1213.
45. Erba G, Duchowny MS. Partial epilepsy and tuberous sclerosis: Indications for surgery in disseminated disease. In: Duchowny MS, Resnick TJ, Alvarez LA, eds. *Pediatric Epilepsy Surgery*. New York: Demos, 1990:315–322.
46. Bye AM, Matheson JM, Tobias VH, Mackenzie RA. Selective epilepsy surgery in tuberous sclerosis. *Aust Paediatr J* 1989; 25:243–245.
47. Bebin EM, Kelly PJ, Gomez MR. Surgical treatment for epilepsy in cerebral tuberous sclerosis. *Epilepsia* 1993; 34:651–657.
48. Gillberg C, Uvebrant P, Carlsson G, Hedstrom A, et al. Autism and epilepsy (and tuberous sclerosis?) in two pre-adolescent boys: neuropsychiatric aspects before and after epilepsy surgery. *J Intellect Disabil Res* 1996; 40:75–81.
49. Morrell F. Varieties of human secondary epileptogenesis. *J Clin Neurophysiol* 1989; 6:227–275.
50. Guerrini R, Canapicchi R, Zifkin BG, et al. Dysplasias of cerebral cortex and epilepsy. Philadelphia: Lippincott-Raven, 1996.
51. Duchowny M. Epilepsy surgery in children. *Curr Opin Neurol* 1995; 8:112–116.
52. Guerrini R, Dubeau F, Dulac O, et al. Bilateral para-sagittal parietooccipital polymicrogyria and epilepsy. *Ann Neurol* 1997; 41:65–73.
53. Chugani HT, Shields WD, Shewmon DA, et al. Infantile spasms: I. PET identifies focal cortical dysgenesis in cryptogenic cases for surgical treatment [see comments]. *Ann Neurol* 1990; 27:406–413.
54. Breningstall GN. Gelastic seizures, precocious puberty, and hypothalamic hamartoma. *Neurology* 1985; 35:1180–1183.
55. Berkovic SF, Andermann F, Melanson D, Ethier RE, et al. Hypothalamic hamartomas and ictal laughter: evolution of a characteristic epileptic syndrome and diagnostic value of magnetic resonance imaging. *Ann Neurol* 1988; 23:429–439.
56. Arroyo S, Santamaria J, Sanmarti F, Lomena F, et al. Ictal laughter associated with paroxysmal hypothalamopituitary dysfunction. *Epilepsia* 1997; 38:114–117.
57. Kuzniecky R, Guthrie B, Mountz J, Bebin M, et al. Intrinsic epileptogenesis of hypothalamic hamartomas in gelastic epilepsy. *Ann Neurol* 1997; 42:60–67.
58. Munari C, Kahane P, Francione S, Hoffmann D, et al. Role of the hypothalamic hamartoma in the genesis of gelastic fits (a video-stereo-EEG study). *Electroencephalogr Clin Neurophysiol* 1995; 95:154–160.
59. Nishio S, Morioka T, Fukui M, Goto Y. Surgical treatment of intractable seizures due to hypothalamic hamartoma. *Epilepsia* 1994; 35:514–519.
60. Valdueza JM, Cristante L, Dammann O, Bentele K, et al. Hypothalamic hamartomas: with special reference to gelastic epilepsy and surgery. *Neurosurgery* 1994; 34:949–958.
61. Cascino GD, Andermann F, Berkovic SF, Kuzniecky RI, et al. Gelastic seizures and hypothalamic hamartomas: evaluation of patients undergoing chronic intracranial EEG monitoring and outcome of surgical treatment. *Neurology* 1993; 43:747–750.
62. Sisodiya SM, Free SL, Stevens JM, Fish DR, et al. Widespread cerebral structural changes in two patients with gelastic seizures and hypothalamic hamartoma. *Epilepsia* 1997; 38:1008–1010.
63. Whang CJ, Kim CJ. Short-term follow-up of stereotactic Gamma Knife radiosurgery in epilepsy. *Stereotact Funct Neurosurg* 1995; 1:202–208.

64. Robain O, Chiron C, Dulac O. Electron microscopic and Golgi study in a case of hemimegalencephaly. *Acta Neuropathol Berl* 1989; 77:664–666.
65. King M, Stephenson JB, Ziervogel M, Doyle D, et al. Hemimegalencephaly—a case for hemispherectomy? *Neuropediatrics* 1985; 16:46–55.
66. Vigevano F, Fusco L, Holthausen H, Lahl R. The morphological spectrum and variable clinical picture in children with hemimegalencephaly. In: Tuxhorn I, Holthausen H, Boenigk H. eds. *Pediatric Epilepsy Syndromes and Their Surgical Treatment*. London: John Libbey, 1997:377–391.
67. Rasmussen T, Olszewski J, Lloyd-Smith D. Focal seizures due to chronic localized encephalitis. *Neurology* 1958; 8:435–445.
68. Rasmussen T, McCann W. Clinical studies of patients with focal epilepsy due to "chronic encephalitis." *Trans Am Neurol Assoc* 1968; 93:89–94.
69. Andermann F. Clinical indications for hemispherectomy and callosotomy. *Epilepsy Res* 1992; Suppl 5:189–199.
70. Rasmussen T, Andermann F. Update on the syndrome of "chronic encephalitis" and epilepsy. *Cleve Clin J Med* 1989; 56:S181–S184.
71. Chugani HT. Infantile spasms. *Curr Opin Neurol* 1995; 8:139–144.
72. Shields WD, Shewmon DA, Chugani HT, Peacock WJ. The role of surgery in the treatment of infantile spasms. *J Epilepsy* 1990; 3:S321–S324.
73. Chugani HT, Shields WD, Shewmon DA, Olson DM, et al. Infantile spasms: I. PET identifies focal cortical dysgenesis in cryptogenic cases for surgical treatment [see comments]. *Ann Neurol* 1990; 27(3):406–413.
74. Cascino GD, Buchhalter JR, Sirven JI, So EL, et al. Peri-ictal SPECT and surgical treatment for intractable epilepsy related to schizencephaly. *Neurology* 2004; 63(12):2426–2428.
75. Shewmon DA, Shields WD, Sankar R, Yudovin SL, et al. Follow-up on infants with surgery for catastrophic epilepsy. In: Tuxhorn I, Holthausen H, Boenigk H, eds. *Pediatric Epilepsy Syndromes and Their Surgical Treatment*. London: John Libbey, 1997: 513–525.
76. Kramer U, Sue WC, Mikati MA. Focal features in West syndrome indicating candidacy for surgery. *Pediatr Neurol* 1997; 16:213–217.
77. Donat JF, Wright FS. Simultaneous infantile spasms and partial seizures. *J Child Neurol* 1991; 6:246–250.
78. Carrazana EJ, Lombroso CT, Mikati M, Helmers S, et al. Facilitation of infantile spasms by partial seizures. *Epilepsia* 1993; 34:97–109.
79. Duchowny MS. Surgery for intractable epilepsy: issues and outcome. *Pediatrics* 1989; 84:886–894.
80. Shields WD, Peacock WJ, Roper SN. Surgery for epilepsy. Special pediatric considerations. *Neurosurg Clin N Am* 1993; 4:301–310.
81. Peacock WJ. Hemispherectomy for the treatment of intractable seizures in childhood. *Neurosurg Clin N Am* 1995; 6:549–563.
82. Wyllie E, Comair YG, Kotagal P, Raja S, et al. Epilepsy surgery in infants. *Epilepsia* 1996; 37:625–637.
83. Duchowny M, Jayakar P, Resnick T, et al. Epilepsy surgery in patients under age 3 years. *Ann Neurol* 1996; 40:286.
84. Duchowny MS, Resnick TJ, Alvarez LA, Morrison G. Focal resection for malignant partial seizures in infancy. *Neurology* 1990; 40:980–984.
85. Wyllie E. Surgery for catastrophic localization-related epilepsy in infants. *Epilepsia* 1998; 39:737–743.
86. Duchowny M, Jayakar P, Resnick T, et al. Epilepsy surgery in the first three years of life. *Epilepsia* 1998; 39:737–743.
87. Heijbel J, Blom S, Bergfors PG. Benign epilepsy of children with centrotemporal EEG foci. A study of incidence rate in outpatient care. *Epilepsia* 1975; 16:657–664.
88. Gastaut H. A new type of epilepsy: benign partial epilepsy of childhood with occipital spike-waves. *Clin Electroencephalogr* 1982; 13:13–22.
89. Trimble M. Behavioural complications of limbic epilepsy: implications for an understanding of the emotional motor system in man. *Prog Brain Res* 1996; 107:605–616.
90. Duchowny M, Harvey AS, Jayakar P, et al. The preoperative evaluation of pediatric temporal lobe epilepsy. In:Tuxhorn I, Holthausen H, and Boenigk H, eds. *Pediatric Epilepsy Syndromes and Their Surgical Treatment*. London: John Libbey, 1997:261–273.
91. Wyllie E. Children with seizures: when can treatment be deferred? *J Child Neurol* 1994; 2:8–13.
92. Kuzniecky R, Murro A, King D, et al. Magnetic resonance imaging in childhood intractable partial epilepsies: pathologic correlations. *Neurology* 1993; 43:681–687.
93. Harvey AS, Berkovic SF. Functional neuroimaging with SPECT in children with partial epilepsy. *J Child Neurol* 1994; 9:S71–S81.
94. Chugani HT. The use of positron emission tomography in the clinical assessment of epilepsy. *Semin Nucl Med* 1992; 22:247–253.
95. Cross JH, Gordon I, Jackson GD, et al. Children with intractable focal epilepsy: ictal and interictal ^{99}TcM HMPAO single photon emission computed tomography. *Dev Med Child Neurol* 1995; 37:673–681.
96. Cross JH, Gordon I, Connelly A, et al. Interictal ^{99}Tc(m) HMPAO SPECT and ^{1}H MRS in children with temporal lobe epilepsy. *Epilepsia* 1997; 38:338–345.
97. Jayakar P, Duchowny M, Resnick T, Alvarez L. Ictal head deviation: lateralizing significance of the pattern of head movement. *Neurology* 1992; 42:1989–1992.
98. Salanova V, Morris HH, Van Ness P, Kotagal P, et al. Frontal lobe seizures: electroclinical syndromes. *Epilepsia* 1995; 36:16–24.
99. Riggio S, Harner RN. Repetitive motor activity in frontal lobe epilepsy. *Adv Neurol* 1995; 66:153–164.
100. Jayakar P, Duchowny MS. Complex partial seizures of temporal lobe origin in early childhood. In: Duchowny MS, Resnick TJ, Alvarez LA, eds. *Pediatric Epilepsy Surgery*. New York: Demos, 1990:41–46.
101. Duchowny MS. Complex partial seizures of infancy. *Arch Neurol* 1987; 44:911–914.
102. Williamson PD, Boon PA, Thadani VM, et al. Parietal lobe epilepsy: diagnostic considerations and results of surgery. *Ann Neurol* 1992; 31:193–201.
103. So NK. Atonic phenomena and partial seizures. A reappraisal. *Adv Neurol* 1995; 67:29–39.
104. Ho SS, Berkovic SF, Newton MR, et al. Parietal lobe epilepsy: clinical features and seizure localization by ictal SPECT. *Neurology* 1994; 44:2277–2284.
105. Alemayehu S, Bergey GK, Barry E, et al. Panic attacks as ictal manifestations of parietal lobe seizures. *Epilepsia* 1995; 36:824–830.
106. Fois A, Tomaccini D, Balestri P, et al. Intractable epilepsy: etiology, risk factors and treatment. *Clin Electroencephalogr* 1988; 19:68–73.
107. Panayiotopoulos CP. Benign childhood epilepsy with occipital paroxysms: a 15-year prospective study. *Ann Neurol* 1989; 26:51–56.
108. Jayakar P, Duchowny M, Resnick TJ, Alvarez LA. Localization of seizure foci: pitfalls and caveats. *J Clin Neurophysiol* 1991; 8:414–431.
109. Resta M, Dicuonzo PF, Spagnolo P, et al. Imaging studies in partial epilepsy in children and adolescents. *Epilepsia* 1994; 35:1187–1193.
110. Grattan Smith JD, Harvey AS, Desmond PM, Chow CW. Hippocampal sclerosis in children with intractable temporal lobe epilepsy: detection with MR imaging. *AJR Am J Roentgenol* 1993; 161:1045–1048.
111. Kuks JB, Cook MJ, Fish DR, Stevens JM, et al. Hippocampal sclerosis in epilepsy and childhood febrile seizures [see comments]. *Lancet* 1993; 342:1391–1394.
112. Nohria V, Lee N, Tien RD, et al. Magnetic resonance imaging evidence of hippocampal sclerosis in progression: a case report. *Epilepsia* 1994; 35:1332–1336.
113. Duncan JS. Imaging and epilepsy. *Brain* 1997; 120:339–377.
114. Engel JJ. PET scanning in partial epilepsy. *Can J Neurol Sci* 1991; 18:588–592.
115. Savic I, Thorell JO, Roland P. [^{11}C]flumazenil positron emission tomography visualizes frontal epileptogenic regions. *Epilepsia* 1995; 36:1225–1232.
116. Parker AP, Ferrie CD, Keevil S, Newbold M, et al. Neuroimaging and spectroscopy in children with epileptic encephalopathies. *Arch Dis Child* 1998; 79:39-43.
117. Chugani HT, Mazziotta JC, Phelps ME. Sturge-Weber syndrome: a study of cerebral glucose utilization with positron emission tomography. *J Pediatr* 1989; 114:244–253.
118. Juhasz C, Chugani DC, Padhye UN, Muzik O, et al. Evaluation with alpha-[^{11}C]methyl-L-tryptophan positron emission tomography for reoperation after failed epilepsy surgery. *Epilepsia* 2004; 45(2):124–130.
119. da Silva EA, Chugani DC, Muzik O, Chugani HT. Identification of frontal lobe epileptic foci in children using positron emission tomography. *Epilepsia* 1997; 38:1198–1208.
120. Korinthenberg R, Bauer-Schied C, Burkart P, Martens-Le Bouar H, et al. ^{18}FDG-PET in epilepsies of infantile onset with pharmacoresistant generalized tonic-clonic seizures. *Epilepsy Res* 2004; 60:53–61.
121. Duncan JD, Moss SD, Bandy DJ, Manwaring K, et al. Use of positron emission tomography for presurgical localization of eloquent brain areas in children with seizures. *Pediatr Neurosurg* 1997; 26:144–156.
122. Snead OC 3rd, Chen LS, Mitchell WG, Kongelbeck SR, et al. Usefulness of [^{18}F] fluorodeoxyglucose positron emission tomography in pediatric epilepsy surgery. *Pediatr Neurol* 1996; 14:98–107.
123. Gaillard WD, White S, Malow B, et al. FDG-PET in children and adolescents with partial seizures: role in epilepsy surgery evaluation. *Epilepsy Res* 1995; 20:77–84.
124. Muzik O, da Silva EA, Juhasz C, Chugani DC, et al. Intracranial EEG versus flumazenil and glucose PET in children with extratemporal lobe epilepsy. *Neurology* 2000; 54:171–179.
125. Duncan R, Patterson J, Roberts R, Hadley DM, et al. Ictal/postictal SPECT in the presurgical localisation of complex partial seizures. *J Neurol Neurosurg Psychiatry* 1993; 56:141–148.
126. Harvey AS, Bowe JM, Hopkins IJ, Shield LK, et al. Ictal ^{99m}Tc-HMPAO single photon emission computed tomography in children with temporal lobe epilepsy. *Epilepsia* 1993; 34:869–877.
127. Chiron C, Raynaud C, Tzourio N, Diebler C, et al. Regional cerebral blood flow by SPECT imaging in Sturge-Weber disease: an aid for diagnosis. *J Neurol Neurosurg Psychiatr* 1989; 52:1402–1409.
128. English R, Soper N, Shepstone BJ, Hockaday JM, et al. Five patients with Rasmussens's syndrome investigated by single-photon-emission computed tomography. *Nucl Med Commun* 1989; 10:5–14.
129. Vies JSH, Demandt E, Ceulemans B, de Roo M, et al. Single photon emission computed tomography (SPECT) in seizure disorders in childhood. *Brain Dev* 1990; 12: 385–389.
130. Gupta A, Raja S, Kotagal P, Lachwani D, et al. Ictal SPECT in children with partial epilepsy due to focal cortical dysplasia. *Pediatr Neurol* 2004; 31:89–95.
131. Hertz-Pannier L, Chiron C, Vera P, Van de Morteele PF, et al. Functional imaging in the work-up of childhood epilepsy. *Childs Nerv Syst* 2001; 17:223–228.
132. Harvey AS, Bowe JM, Hopkins IJ, Shield LK, et al. Ictal ^{99m}Tc-HMPAO single photon emission computed tomography in children with temporal lobe epilepsy. *Epilepsia* 1993; 34:869–877.
133. Cross JH, Gordon I, Jackson GD, Boyd SG, et al. Children with intractable focal epilepsy: ictal and interictal ^{99}Tc^{M} HMPAO single photon emission computed tomography. *Dev Med Child Neurol* 1995; 37:673–681.
134. Kaminska A, Chiron C, Ville D, Dellatolas G, et al. Ictal SPECT in children with epilepsy: comparison with intracranial EEG and relation to postsurgical outcome. *Brain* 2003; 126:248–260.
135. Harvey AS, Berkovic SF. SPECT imaging of regional cerebral blood flow in children with partial epilepsy. *Acta Neuropediatrica* 1994; 1:9–27.
136. Connelly A, Jackson GD, Duncan JS, King MD, Gadian DG. Magnetic resonance spectroscopy in temporal lobe epilepsy. *Neurology* 1994; 44:1411–1417.

137. Gadian DG, Connelly A, Duncan JS, et al. ¹H magnetic resonance spectroscopy in the investigation of intractable epilepsy. *Acta Neurol Scand* 1994; 152 (Suppl):116–121.
138. Cendes F, Andermann F, Dubeau F, Matthews PM, et al. Normalization of neuronal metabolic dysfunction after surgery for temporal lobe epilepsy, evidence from proton MR spectroscopic imaging. *Neurology* 1997; 49:1525–1533.
139. Connelly A. Ictal imaging using functional magnetic resonance. *Magn Reson Imaging* 1995; 13:1233–1237.
140. Bernal B, Altman NR. Speech delay in children: a functional MR imaging study. *Radiology*. 2003 Dec; 229(3):651–658
141. Gaillard WD, Balsamo LM, Ibrahim Z, Sachs BC, et al. fMRI identifies regional specialization of neural networks for reading in young children. *Neurology* 2003; 60: 94–100.
142. Ahmad Z, Balsamo LM, Sachs BC, Xu B, Galliard WD. Auditory comprehension of language in young children: neural networks identified with fMRI. *Neurology* 2003 May 27; 60(10):1598–1605.
143. Jayakar P, Bernal B, Santiago Medina L, Altman N. False lateralization of language cortex on functional MRI after a cluster of focal seizures. *Neurology* 2002; 58(3):490–492.
144. Holmes GL, King DW. Epilepsy surgery in children. *Wien Klin Wochenschr* 1990; 102:189–97.
145. Lindsay J, Ounsted C, Richards P. Long-term outcome in children with temporal lobe seizures. III: Psychiatric aspects in childhood and adult life. *Dev Med Child Neurol* 1979; 21: 630–636.
146. Jones-Gotman M, Smith ML, Zatorre RJ. Neuropsychological testing for localizing and lateralizing the epileptogenic region. In: Engel J, ed. *Surgical Treatment of the Epilepsies*. New York: Raven Press, 1993:245–62.
147. Levin B, Feldman E, Duchowny M, Brown M. Neuropsychological assessment of children with epilepsy. *Int Pediatr* 1991; 6:214–219.
148. Wyllie E. Developmental aspects of seizure semiology: problems in identifying localized-onset seizures in infants and children [editorial]. *Epilepsia* 1995; 36:1170–1172.
149. Duchowny M, Levin B, Jayakar P, et al. Temporal lobectomy in early childhood. *Epilepsia* 1992; 33:298–303.
150. Duchowny M, Jayakar P, Resnick T, Levin B, et al. Posterior temporal epilepsy: electroclinical features. *Ann Neurol* 1994; 35:427–431.
151. Farrell MA, DeRosa MJ, Curran JG, et al. Neuropathologic findings in cortical resections (including hemispherectomies) performed for the treatment of intractable childhood epilepsy. *Acta Neuropathol Berl* 1992; 83:246–259.
152. Mischel PS, Nguyen LP, Vinters HV. Cerebral cortical dysplasia associated with pediatric epilepsy. Review of neuropathologic features and proposal for a grading system. *J Neuropathol Exp Neurol* 1995; 54:137–153.
153. Adelson PD, Peacock WJ, Chugani HT, et al. Temporal and extended temporal resections for the treatment of intractable seizures in early childhood. *Pediatr Neurosurg* 1992; 18:169–178.
154. DeVos KJ, Wyllie E, Geckler C, Kotagal P, et al. Language dominance in patients with early childhood tumors near left hemisphere language areas. *Neurology* 1995; 45:349–356.
155. Duchowny M, Jayakar P, Harvey AS, et al. Language cortex representation: effects of developmental versus acquired pathology. *Ann Neurol* 1996; 40:31–38.
156. Kramer U, Riviello JJ, Carmant L, et al. Morbidity of depth and subdural electrodes: children and adolescents versus young adults. *J Epilepsy* 1994; 7:7–10.
157. Wyllie E, Luders H, Morris HH, et al. Subdural electrodes in the evaluation for epilepsy surgery in children and adults. *Neuropediatrics* 1988; 19:80–86.
158. Palmini A, Andermann F, Olivier A, Tampieri D, et al. Focal neuronal migration disorders and intractable partial epilepsy: results of surgical treatment. *Ann Neurol* 1991; 30:750–757.
159. Jayakar P, Duchowny M, Resnick TJ. Subdural monitoring in the evaluation of children for epilepsy surgery. *J Child Neurol* 1994; 2:61–66.
160. Jayakar P, Duchowny M, Alvarez L, Resnick T. Intraictal activation in the neocortex: a marker of the epileptogenic region. *Epilepsia* 1994; 35:489–494.
161. Bebin EM, Kelly PJ, Gomez MR. Surgical treatment for epilepsy in cerebral tuberous sclerosis. *Epilepsia* 1993; 34:651–657.
162. Bye AM, Matheson JM, Tobias VH, Mackenzie RA. Selective epilepsy surgery in tuberous sclerosis. *Aust Paediatr J* 1989; 25:243–245.
163. Alvarez LA, Jayakar P. 1990. Cortical stimulation with subdural electrodes: special considerations in infancy and childhood. *J Epilepsy* 1990; 3(Suppl):125–130.
164. Jayakar P, Alvarez LA, Duchowny MS, Resnick TJ. A safe and effective paradigm to functionally map the cortex in childhood. *J Clin Neurophysiol* 1992; 9:288–293.
165. Duchowny M, Jayakar P. Functional cortical mapping in children. *Adv Neurol* 1993; 63:149–154.
166. Brockhaus A, Elger CE. Complex partial seizures of temporal lobe origin in children of different age groups. *Epilepsia* 1995; 36:1173–1181.
167. Innocenti GM, Caminitti R. Postnatal shaping of callosal connections from sensory areas. *Brain Res* 1980; 38:381–394.
168. Rakic P, Bourgeois JP, Eckenhoff MF, Zecevic N, et al. Concurrent overproduction of synapses in diverse regions of the primate cerebral cortex. *Science* 1986; 232:231–232.
169. Lenn NJ, Freinkel AJ. Facial sparing as a feature of prenatal-onset hemiparesis. *Pediatr Neurol* 1989; 5:291–295.
170. Maegaki Y, Yamamoto T, Takeshita K. Plasticity of central motor and sensory pathways in a case of unilateral extensive cortical dysplasia: investigation of magnetic resonance imaging, transcranial magnetic stimulation, and short-latency somatosensory evoked potentials. *Neurology* 1995; 45:2255–2261.
171. Goldman PS. Neuronal plasticity in primate telencephalon: anomalous projections induced by prenatal removal of frontal cortex. *Science* 1978; 202:767–768.
172. Goldman PS, Galkin TW. Prenatal removal of frontal association cortex in the fetal rhesus monkey: anatomical and functional consequences in postnatal life. *Brain Res* 1978; 152:451–485.
173. Rapin I. Acquired aphasia in children. *J Child Neurol* 1995; 10:267–270.
174. Woods BT, Carey S. Language deficits after apparent clinical recovery from childhood aphasia. *Ann Neurol* 1979; 6:405–409.
175. Alajouanine TH, Lhermitte F. Acquired aphasia in children. *Brain* 1965; 88:653–662.
176. Berger MS, Kincaid J, Ojemann GA, Lettich E. Brain mapping techniques to maximize resection, safety, and seizure control in children with brain tumors. *Neurosurgery* 1989; 25:786–792.
177. Lesser RP, Luders H, Dinner DS. The location of speech and writing functions in the frontal language area: results of extraoperative cortical stimulation. *Brain* 1985; 107:275–291.
178. Basser LS. Hemiplegia of early onset and the faculty of speech with special reference to the effects of hemispherectomy. *Brain* 1962; 85:427–460.
179. Dodrill C, Wilkus R, Ojemann G. Multidisciplinary prediction of seizure relief from cortical resection surgery. *Ann Neurol* 1986; 20:2–12.
180. Vossler DG, Wilkus RJ, Ojemann GA. Preoperative EEG correlates of seizure outcome from epilepsy surgery in children. *J Epilepsy* 1995; 8:236–245.
181. Goldstein R, Harvey AS, Duchowny M, et al. Preoperative clinical, EEG, and imaging findings do not predict seizure outcome following temporal lobectomy in childhood. *J Child Neurol* 1996; 11:445–450.

61 Advanced Neuroimaging: PET-MRI Fusion and Diffusion Tensor Imaging

Noriko Salamon

Neuroimaging for presurgical evaluation of pediatric epilepsy has changed in the last 20 years with the development of modern imaging techniques. Magnetic resonance imaging (MRI) is now the recommended study of choice for patients with epilepsy (1–3). More than 70% of epileptogenic lesions are identified by MRI, including mesial temporal sclerosis, severe cortical dysplasia, vascular malformation, and tumors (4). However, subtler types of cortical dysplasia or cortical dysplasia associated with tumors and mesial temporal sclerosis can be overlooked (5). Advanced imaging techniques including positron emission tomography (PET)-MRI fusion and diffusion tensor imaging (DTI) provide additional findings. In this chapter, the examples of PET-MRI fusion and DTI in mesial temporal sclerosis, tumors, various types of cortical dysplasia, and tuberous sclerosis complex (TSC) are discussed.

PET-MRI FUSION

PET is a well-established tool for presurgical evaluation of epilepsy (6–9). The most commonly used tracers for epilepsy are 2-deoxy-2[^{18}F] fluoro-D-glucose (FDG) and [^{11}C] flumazenil (FMZ) (6–10). Other agents, such as [^{11}C]methyl-L-tryptophan, can be used to define the epileptogenic focus in TSC patients (11). One of the weaknesses of PET imaging is the poor delineation of the anatomical structures. Using the fusion technique, the functional information can be superimposed onto the precise anatomical landmark on MRI. This combined modality technique is useful and increases the sensitivity of neuroimaging in patients with epilepsy.

At some institutions, PET-MRI fusion is performed for all patients undergoing evaluation for epilepsy surgery (12). At the University of California at Los Angeles (UCLA), axial DICOM images of the PET and MRI coronal MPRAGE are transferred into a postprocessing program (Vitrea Vital Image). The images are automatically coregistered (Fusion-7-Mirada), and color coding is applied. Red indicates higher and blue indicates lower FDG metabolic regions.

DTI

DTI is an emerging MRI method that is potentially useful for uncovering subtle changes in the brain, but few studies have linked DTI changes with histopathology in patients with epilepsy (13). Diffusion-weighted images can provide information on the molecular movements in the microstructure, which is not visible by conventional T1- or T2-weighted MRI. There are two factors that characterize the DTI phenomenon: diffusivity and anisotropy. The mean diffusivity is often referred to as the apparent diffusion coefficient (ADC). Anisotropy decreases in random microstructures, such as the white matter of cortical dysplasia, and under TSC tubers. Eriksson et al (14) found decreased regional anisotropy in 9 of 11 patients with cortical dysplasia. In addition, decreased anisotropy was also found in the areas beyond the signal abnormality or in areas where conventional MRI T1 or T2 signal were normal. In animal studies, changes in DTI measurements have been associated with changes in myelin (15) and during cortical development high anisotropy in neonates followed by rapid decreases have been attributed to dendrite growth (16).

MESIAL TEMPORAL SCLEROSIS

Hippocampal sclerosis is the most common type of mesial temporal lobe epilepsy amenable to surgery. In the recent literature (17), about 50% of patients with hippocampal sclerosis have dual pathology, with evidence of neocortical microscopic cortical dysplasia in the postsurgical specimen. In MRI, these cases are shown as temporal lobe atrophy or subtle T2-weighted signal abnormality in the temporal lobe. Mitchell et al (18) found temporal pole T2-weighted high signal abnormality in 57% (31 of 57 cases) of pediatric patients with hippocampal sclerosis. This suggests that the developmental cytoarchitecture is disorganized in many children with hippocampal sclerosis. These findings are easily picked up by FDG-PET study as an area of hypometabolism. (Figure 61-1).

Adachi et al. showed anterior temporal lobe hyperintense T2-weighted signal in 54 of 112 patients with temporal lobe epilepsy. Two cases had focal lesion in the contralateral side, but the electroencephalographic (EEG) seizure foci were seen in the same side as temporal pole signal abnormality (18).

DTI adds further structural imaging information in the otherwise normal-appearing gray or white matter regions. Extrahippocampal white matter abnormality was found in the genu of the corpus callosum and external capsule as decreased fractional anisotropy (FA) values in adults with mesial temporal sclerosis (19).

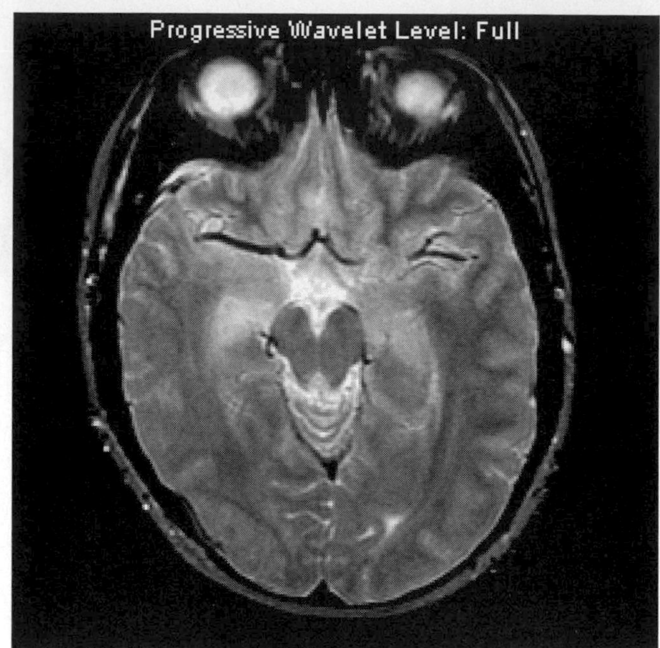

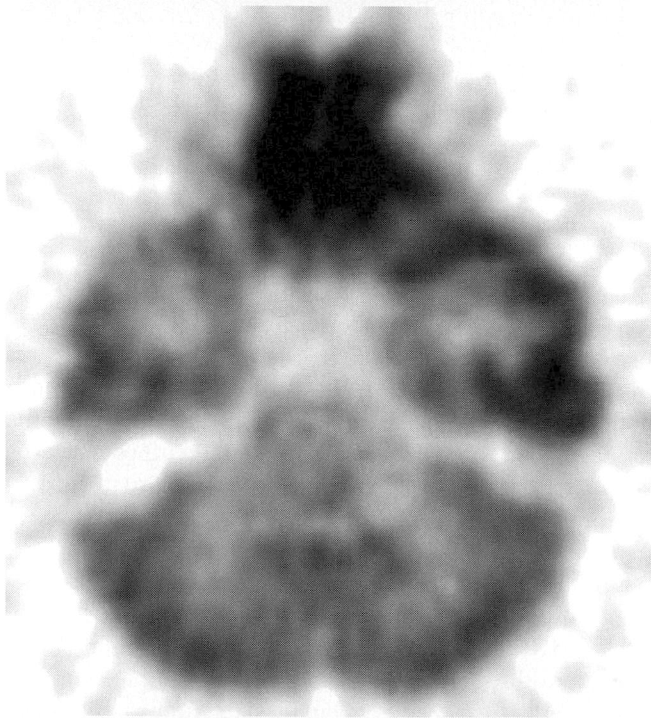

FIGURE 61-1

Right mesial temporal sclerosis: the patient is a 16-year-old male; complex partial seizure started at age 9. (A) T2-weighted hyperintense signal in the right hippocampus; the right temporal lobe is smaller than the left. (B) Larger area of hypometabolism in PET.

TUMORS

Approximately 80% of the tumors seen in patients with intractable epilepsy are in the temporal lobe (20). The common tumors include gangliogliomas, dysembryoplastic neuroepithelial tumors (DNT), pilocytic astrocytomas, oligodendrogliomas, and pleomorphic xanthoastrocytomas. These lesions can be associated with cortical dysplasia (21). One series showed that DNT was associated with focal cortical dysplasia (FCD) in 83% (22). The identification of associated cortical dysplasia is important for preoperative evaluation, because this tissue may need to be included in the surgical margin for good results.

In our series, FDG-PET-MRI fusion showed a larger area of hypometabolism in 50% of the patients with ganglioglioma compared with conventional imaging. These lesions are associated with type I cortical dysplasia, and the MRI showed very subtle T2W hyperintense signal in the neighboring tissues.

CORTICAL DYSPLASIA

Cortical dysplasia is a developmental anomaly characterized by architectural and cellular abnormalities of the cortex. This anomaly is a significant cause of medically intractable pediatric epilepsy. Histopathologically, cortical dysplasia is a spectrum of abnormalities that can be classified into (1) architectural dysplasia, containing cortical dyslamination and heterotopic neurons in the white matter; (2) cytoarchitectural dysplasia, with features of architectural dysplasia in addition to giant neurons or cytomegalic neurons; (3) Taylor's focal cortical dysplasia, with dysmorphic neurons without or with balloon cells, in addition to features of cytoarchitectural dysplasia (23–24). The Taylor-type focal cortical dysplasia is considered the most severe end of the spectrum of histopathologic abnormalities, and the presence of dysmorphic neurons is related to higher epileptogenicity (23). Palmini et al proposed a classification of cortical dysplasia (25). These different histological types of cortical dysplasia are associated with varied surgical success (25, 27). In addition, conventional MRI is not sensitive enough to detect all types of cortical dysplasia (Table 61-1).

TABLE 61-1
Various Types of Cortical Dysplasia

A. Mild MCD (formerly described as microdysgenesis and not detectable by current MRI techniques)

- Type I: ectopic neurons in or adjacent to layer I
- Type II: microscopic neuronal heterotopias outside layer I

B. FCD

FCD type I (non-Taylor) no dysmorphic neuron or balloon cell and mostly temporal

- Type IA isolated architectural abnormalities (dyslamination plus mild MCD)
- Type IB isolated architectural abnormalities plus giant or immature, but not dysmorphic neurons (cytoarchitectural dysplasia)

FCD type II (Taylor) mostly extratemporal

- Type IIA: architectural abnormalities with dysmorphic neurons without balloon cells
- Type IIB: architectural abnormalities with dysmorphic neurons with balloon cells

The degree of hypometabolism can correlate with the degree of dysplasia (28). PET-MRI fusion has been helpful to define the extent of the abnormality and correlates well with the preoperative electrocorticography. Because PET is very sensitive for the subtle type of cortical dysplasia, PET-MRI fusion is even more helpful (Figure 61-2).

TSC

Approximately 80% of patients with TSC have epilepsy (29). To achieve the best developmental outcome, early seizure control is critical (30). The subset of TSC children with normal development before the onset of seizures, with a single seizure type, and with late-onset partial seizures or transient infantile spasms, fared the best of all children with TSC, both in terms of seizure control and functional outcome (31).

For those children with TSC and drug-resistant epilepsy, surgical resection of the epileptogenic tuber in a timely manner should be considered. Surgical resection is now considered a viable option at leading epilepsy centers, but the process of selecting the epileptogenic tuber among the many others is daunting. The multicentric nature of epilepsy in TSC has mostly prevented surgical consideration until recent times. The earliest known case report of epilepsy surgery in TSC was reported in 1989 (32), with the first epilepsy surgery series in 1993 (33). Subsequent studies have suggested that early intervention and single-tuber seizure focus lead to better seizure and functional outcome postsurgically (34).

Recent developments in multistaged, often bilateral, invasive monitoring have yielded promising results for some patients with TSC (35). However, by the nature of the invasive, multistaged, and bilateral monitoring, it is clear that these patients have already progressed to multifocal seizures from multiple different tubers. Thus, the ideal situation remains early surgery when medications fail, with noninvasive presurgical studies, and single-stage resection before secondary epileptogenesis occurs, for the best seizure and developmental outcome for children with TSC and epilepsy.

An ideal diagnostic method will not only identify but also localize the epileptogenic tuber for epilepsy surgery noninvasively, to allow for repeat studies to assess any change over time in the dynamic epileptogenic process. PET scan utilizing alpha-[^{11}C]methyl-l-tryptophan is reported to define the epileptogenic focus, but it is unfortunately more specific rather than sensitive in selecting the

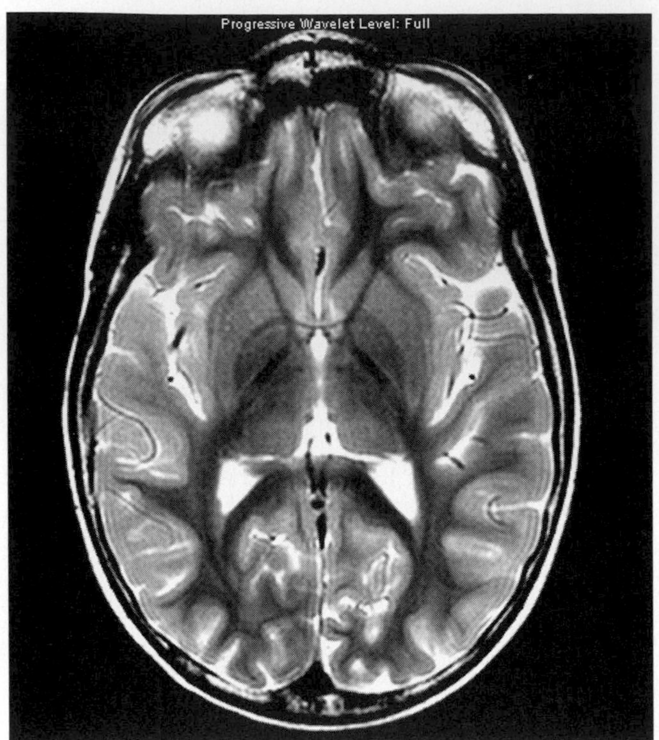

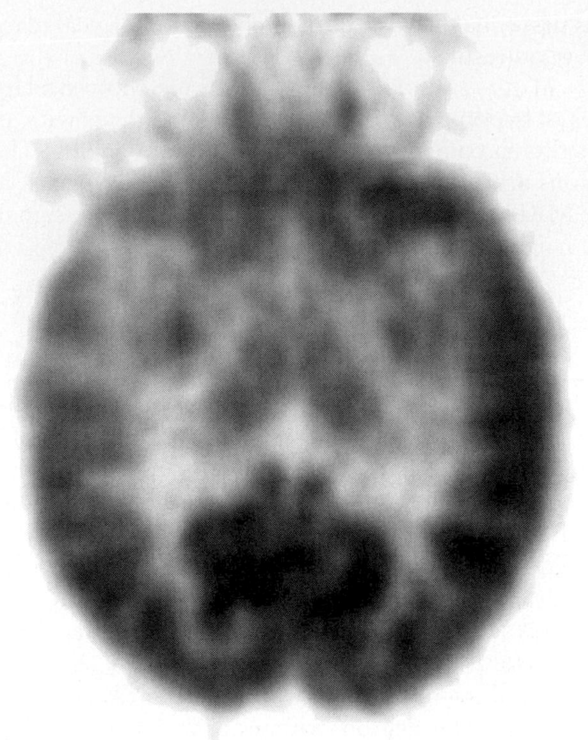

FIGURE 61-2

Subtle cortical dysplasia. An 8-year-old male with intractable epilepsy. (A) Very subtle white matter hyperintensity in the right temporal lobe. (B) FDG-PET shows clear hypometabolism in the area of suspicion.

epileptogenic tuber (11) and is not available at most centers. Ictal single-photon emission computed tomography (SPECT) can, in theory, identify the ictal zone, but it poses logistic challenges and offers limited spatial resolution. Lastly, because of the quick propagation potential of neocortical epilepsy, seizures often appear nonlateralized on video-EEG.

The UCLA experience using FDG-PET and MRI fusion is shown in Figure 61-3. The epileptogenic tuber has a larger area of hypometabolism than the nonepileptogenic tuber. DTI is another noninvasive tool that increases MRI sensitivity for subtle structural abnormalities in the brain such as epileptogenic TSC tubers. Jansen et al. (36) used DWI methods and successfully localized the epileptogenic tuber in four children, identified as an increase in ADC values. The ability of DWI to provide data on increased ADC, as well as to estimate reductions in anisotropy the two parameters that are felt to be independent (37), may theoretically improve the sensitivity and specificity of this neuroimaging technique.

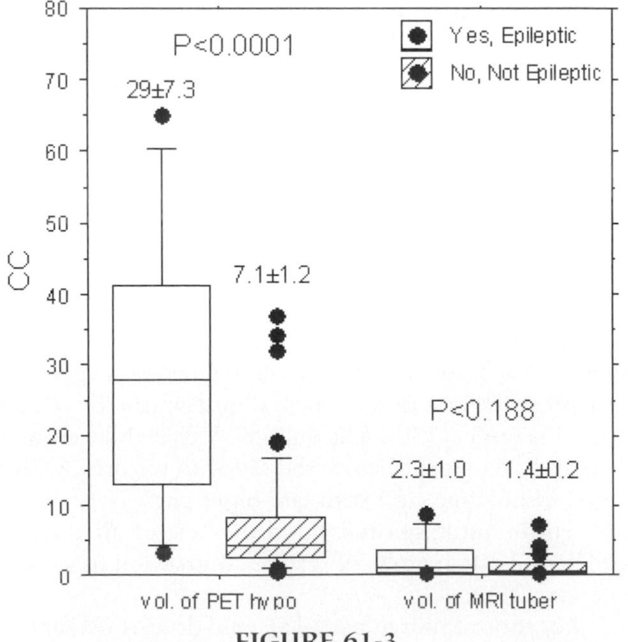

FIGURE 61-3

Volume of PET hypometabolism and MR tubers between epileptogenic vs. nonepiletogenic tubers.

CONCLUSION

Neuroimaging will continue to develop, with faster scan time and higher resolution, but these advances alone may not considerably increase the detection of otherwise cryptic epileptogenic lesions such as subtle cortical dysplasia. Instead, combining various modalities, such as PET-MRI fusion, and utilizing new techniques, such as DTI, will help identify epileptogenic structural lesions. Whatever modality is used, all imaging findings should be verified with pathology and electrophysiology to understand better the pathophysiology of epileptogenic lesions.

References

1. Kuzniecky RI. Neuroimaging in pediatric epilepsy *Epilepsia* 1996; 37(Suppl 1):S10–S21.
2. Raybaud C, Guye M, Mancini J, et al. Neuroimaging in epilepsy in children. *Magne Reson Imaging Clin N Am* 2001; 9:121–147.
3. Grant PE. Imaging of the developing epileptic brain. *Epilepsia* 2005; 46(Suppl 7):S7–S14.
4. Li LM, Fish DR, Sisodiya SM, et al. High resolution magnetic resonance imaging in adults with partial or secondary generalized epilepsy attending a tertiary referral unit. *J Neurol Neurosurg Psychiatry* 1995; 59(4):384–387.
5. Colombo N, Tassi L, Galli C, et al. Focal cortical dysplasias: MR imaging, histopathologic, and clinical correlations in surgically treated patients with epilepsy. *Am J Neuroradiol* 2003; 24:724–744.
6. Chugani HT, Shields WD, Shewmon DA, et al. Infantile spasms: 1. PET identifies focal cortical dysgenesis in cryptogenic cases for surgical treatment. *Ann Neurol* 1990; 27:406–413.
7. Chugani HT, Shewmon DA, Shields WD, et al. Surgery for intractable infantile spasms: neuroimaging perspectives. *Epilepsia* 1993; 34:764–771.
8. Chugani HT, Shewmon D, Khanna S, et al. Interictal and postictal focal hypometabolism on positron emission tomography. *Pediatr Neurol* 1993; 9:10–15.
9. Chugani HT, Da Silva E, Chugani DC. Infantile spasms: III. Prognostic implications of bitemporal hypometabolism on positron emission tomography. *Ann Neurol* 1996; 39:643–649.
10. Juhasz C, Nagy F, Muzik O, et al. 11C-Flumazenil PET in patients with epilepsy with dual pathology. *Epilepsia* 1999; 40:566–574.
11. Chugani DC, Chugani HT, Muzik O, et al. Imaging epileptogenic tubers in children with tuberous sclerosis complex using alpha [11C] methyl-L tryptophan positron emission tomography. *Ann Neurol* 1998; 44:858–866.
12. Chandra PS, Salamon N, Huang J, et al. FDG-PET/MRI coregistration and diffusion tensor imaging distinguish epileptogenic tubers and cortex in patients with tuberous sclerosis complex: a preliminary report. *Epilepsia* 2006; 47(9):1543–1549.
13. Pierpaoli C, Basser PJ. Toward a quantitative assessment of diffusion anisotropy. *Magn Reson Med* 1996; 36(6):893–906.
14. Eriksson SH, Rugg-Gunn FJ, Symms MR, et al. Diffusion tensor imaging in patients with epilepsy and malformations of cortical development. *Brain* 2001; 124(Part 3):617–626.
15. Sun SW, Liang HF, Trinkaus K, et al. Non invasive detection of cuprizone-induced axonal damage and demyelination in the mouse corpus callosum. *Magn Reson Med* 2006; 55(2):302–308.
16. Mukherjee P, Miller JH, Shimony JS, et al. Diffusion tensor MR imaging of gray and white matter development during normal human brain maturation. *Am J Neuroradiol* 2002; 23(9):1445–1456.
17. Diehl B, LaPresto E, Najm I, et al. Neocortical temporal FDG-PET hypometabolism correlates with temporal lobe atrophy in hippocampal sclerosis associated with microscopic cortical dysplasia. *Epilepsia* 2003; 44(4):559–564.
18. Adachi Y, Yagishita A, Arai N. White matter abnormalities in the anterior temporal lobe suggests the side of the seizure foci in temporal lobe epilepsy. *Neuroradiology* 2006; 48(7):460–464.
19. Gross DW, Concha L, Beaulieu C. Extrahippocampal white matter abnormalities in mesial temporal lobe epilepsy demonstrated with diffusion tensor imaging. *Epilepsia* 2006; 47(8):1360–1363.
20. Luyken C, Blumcke I, Fimmers R, et al. The spectrum of long term epilepsy associated tumors: long term seizures and tumor outcome and neurosurgical aspects. *Epilepsia* 2003; 44:822–830.
21. Blumcke I, Lobach M, Wolf HK, et al. Evidence for developmental precursor lesion in epilepsy associated ganglioneuronal tumors. *Microsc Res Tech* 1999; 46:53–58.
22. Takahashi A, Hong SC, Seo DW, et al. Frequent association of cortical dysplasia in dysembryoplastic neuroepithelial tumor treated by epilepsy surgery. *Surg Neurol* 2005; 64(5):419–427.
23. Taylor DC, Falconer MA, Brutin CJ, et al. Focal cortical dysplasia of the cerebral cortex in epilepsy. *J Neurol Neursurg Psychiatry* 1971; 34:369–387.
24. Barkovich AJ, Kusniecky RI, Jackson GD, et al. Classification system for malformation of cortical development. Update 2001. *Neurology* 2001; 57:2168–2178.
25. Palmini A, Najm I, Avanzini G, et al. Terminology and classification of the cortical dysplasias. *Neurology* 2004; 62(Suppl 3):S2–S8.
26. Fauser S, Schulze-Bonhage A, Honegger J, et al. Focal cortical dysplasias: surgical outcome in 67 patients in relation to histological subtypes and dual pathology. *Brain* 2004; 127:2406–2418.
27. Palmini A, Gambaradella A, Andermann F, et al. Operative strategies for patients with cortical dysplasia lesions and intractable epilepsy. *Epilepsia* 1994; 35(Suppl 6): S57–S71.
28. Cepeda C, Andre VM, Flores-Hernandez J, et al. Pediatric cortical dysplasia: correlations between neuroimaging, electrophysiology and location of cytomegalic neurons and balloon cells and glutamate/GABA synaptic circuits. *Dev Neurosci* 2005; 27(1): 59–76.
29. Curatolo P, Cusmai R, Cortesi F, et al. Neuropsychiatric aspects of tuberous sclerosis. *Ann NY Acad Sci* 1991; 615:8–16.
30. Jambague I, Chiron C, Dumas C, et al. Mental and behavioral outcome of infantile epilepsy treated by vigabatrin in tuberous sclerosis patients. *Epilepsy Res* 2000; 38: 51–60.
31. Curatolo PM, Verdecchia M. Neurological manifestations In: Curatolo P, ed. *Tuberous Sclerosis Complex: From Basic Science To Clinical Phenotypes*. Cambridge University Press, 2003; 26–45.
32. Bye Am, Matheson JM, Tobias VH, et al. Selective epilepsy surgery in tuberous sclerosis. *Aust Paediatr J* 1989; 25:243–245.
33. Bebin EM, Kelly PJ, Gomez MR. Surgical treatment for epilepsy in cerebral tuberous sclerosis. *Epilepsia* 1993; 34:651–657.
34. Romanelli P, Verdecchia M, Rodas R, et al. Epilepsy surgery for tuberous sclerosis. *Pediatr Neurol* 2004; 31(4):239–247.
35. Romanelli P, Najjar S, Weiner HL, et al. Epilepsy surgery in tuberous sclerosis: multistage procedures with bilateral or multilobar foci. *J Child Neurol* 2002; 17:689–692.
36. Jansen FE, Braun KP, van Nieusenhuizen O, et al. Diffusion weighted magnetic resonance imaging and identification of the epileptogenic tuber in patient with tuberous sclerosis. *Arch Neurol* 2003; 60(11):1580–1584.
37. Wieshmann UC, Clark CA, Symms MR, et al. Reduced anisotropy of water diffusion in structural cerebral abnormalities demonstrated with diffusion tensor imaging. *Magn Res Imaging* 1999; 17:1269–1274.

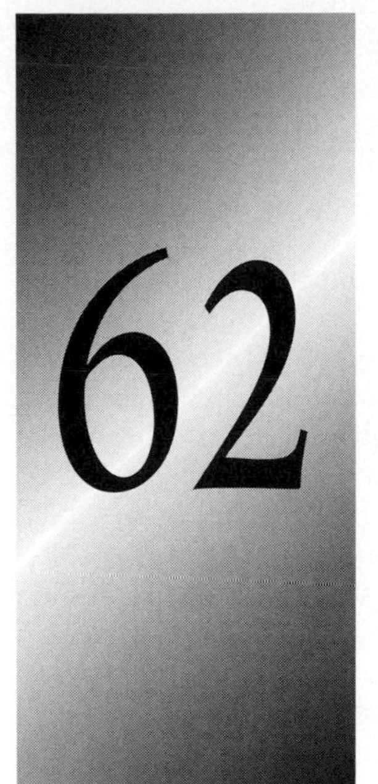

Surgical Treatment of Therapy-Resistant Epilepsy in Children

Gary W. Mathern
Olivier Delalande

As advocated by physicians and patient activist groups, the treatment goal for patients with epilepsy is to eliminate both seizures and adverse side effects of treatment (1). For young children, an additional aim is to eliminate seizures quickly, at the youngest possible age, in order to optimize cognitive development and improve long-term behavior and quality of life (2). Although physicians concede that complete seizure control is not always possible for every child, it has become increasingly recognized that the difference in quality of life is so significantly better without seizures that this therapeutic objective should be as close to the standard of care as possible.

Epilepsy neurosurgery is an important clinical tool used in the treatment of patients whose epilepsy is resistant to antiepileptic drugs (AEDs). Of historical note, epilepsy neurosurgery predates the discovery of electroencephalography (EEG) as well as most of the AEDs used today. For example, Victor Horsley, working with John Hughlings Jackson and David Ferrier, performed resective brain surgery in London in the 1880s (3). Wilder Penfield carried out his first temporal lobectomy around 1928 (4, 5). By comparison, Hans Berger's initial EEG studies were published in 1929 (6), Foerster and Altenburger reported the first electrocorticogram (ECoG) in 1934 (7), and Merritt and Putnam discovered phenytoin in 1938 (8). Thus, epilepsy neurosurgery is not a new treatment. What is relatively new to clinical neurology is the application of epilepsy neurosurgery for infants and children. With the introduction of continuous EEG video-telemetry and modern neuroimaging techniques, such as magnetic resonance imaging (MRI), [^{18}F]2-fluoro-2-deoxyglucose (FDG) positron emission tomography (PET), and ictal single-photon emission computed tomography (SPECT), the late 1980s and early 1990s saw the development of multidisciplinary specialty groups involving pediatric neurologists, neurosurgeons, psychologists, and psychiatrists focused on the diagnosis and operative and nonoperative management of children with therapy-resistant epilepsy (9–12). While the initial clinical protocols mirrored those used by adult epilepsy surgery programs, what has evolved over the past 15 years is a unique conceptual approach to the surgical treatment of children with medically refractory epilepsy (13).

The purpose of this chapter is to highlight what constitutes the distinctive elements of epilepsy neurosurgery in children. Covered topics will include the goals of surgery for the developing brain, clinical characteristics of children undergoing surgery, special challenges related to operating on young children, outcomes and complications, and when the pediatrician and neurologist should consider referral of therapy-resistant patients to a pediatric specialty epilepsy center.

THERAPY-RESISTANT EPILEPSY: INCIDENCE AND NATURAL HISTORY

Population based epidemiology studies classify children with epilepsy into three general etiologic categories that are relevant in understanding which patients are likely to become therapy resistant (14–18). These categories include patients whose epilepsy is from suspected or confirmed genetic etiologies (termed *idiopathic*; e.g., absence seizures, rolandic epilepsy), and these account for about 30% of new-onset cases. Seizures due to structural brain lesions (termed *symptomatic*; e.g., stroke, cortical dysplasia) occur in around 20% of children, and seizures that have unknown or as yet unidentified etiologies (termed *cryptogenic*) constitute nearly 50% of new-onset pediatric epilepsy cases. Seizure control with AEDs differs depending on the epilepsy etiology category. In the first two years of AED treatment, idiopathic pediatric epilepsy patients can expect a 95% chance of near seizure control (less than 1 seizure per month), and the rate for cryptogenic cases is 90%. By comparison, children with symptomatic epilepsy, who are the most common surgical candidates, can expect near seizure control with 50% probability. The type of symptomatic substrate, as identified by neuroimaging, can also provide a guide to the probability of AEDs controlling seizures. Higher rates of seizure control were achieved with AED therapy in patients with epilepsy related to strokes and vascular malformations than in patients with low-grade tumors, cortical dysplasia, or hippocampal atrophy (19–21). In fact, a recent study found that all children with temporal lobe epilepsy and positive MRI scans showing lesions eventually become medically refractory over a follow-up of more than 10 years (22, 23). Hence, it is estimated that in a general pediatric neurology practice the number of new-onset epilepsy patients whose seizures will not be controlled with medications should be about 16% (expected etiologies times AED failure rate). Of those with therapy-resistant epilepsy, the ones that might be potential surgical candidates (i.e., symptomatic epilepsy) should be 9% to 10% of all new-onset epilepsy cases, or just over half of those with refractory epilepsy. Thus, most patients with new-onset epilepsy will be controlled by AEDs, but a small percentage will not. Population studies with follow-up intervals of nearly 40 years indicate that children less than age 16 years with symptomatic epilepsy are the least likely to become seizure free as adults, generally do not complete higher education, and are unemployed (24, 25). In fact, the development of new AEDs has not substantially affected the rate of medical intractability (26). Hence, young children with symptomatic epilepsy are at greatest risk for not being controlled with currently available drugs and are the group that should be strongly considered for possible epilepsy neurosurgery.

Based on the clinical response to AED treatment, physicians can predict with relative confidence when a child is deemed "therapy-resistant." Once a child has failed to reach seizure remission after 2 to 3 medications in mono- or polytherapy, the probability that other drugs will stop seizures is less than 5%, and even less if that child has symptomatic epilepsy (26–28). In addition, 5% to 10% of cases with seizure control on AEDs have sufficiently severe adverse side effects that parents discontinue or change to less effective medical therapy (29). Hence, therapy resistance does not mean failure of all AEDs, as that would take many years with all the available drugs. Instead, therapy resistance can be determined by response to a few medications and knowledge of the underlying substrate as determined by neuroimaging (20, 21, 23).

It is important to note that deciding who might be a surgical candidate is not always straightforward in children with severe epilepsy. For example, children, especially infants, with unilateral hemispheric symptomatic substrates may present with what appear to be generalized clinical seizures, including infantile spasms and bihemispheric EEG abnormalities (30, 31). This may confuse practicing physicians into thinking they are dealing with a nonoperative process when in fact the child is an excellent surgical candidate with a high chance of seizure control (Figure 62-1). Likewise, children may begin with focal epilepsy from a cortical abnormality that rapidly (sometimes within days) progresses to status epilepticus with minimal focal features (32). Analysis of video-EEGs in children indicates that ictal behavior is often less lateralizing in young children than in adults (33, 34). Similarly, children may present with focal EEG patterns and an apparent negative MRI (initially diagnosed as cryptogenic), when in fact they harbor focal cortical pathologies, converting them into symptomatic epilepsy that is surgically treatable. This is especially true for cortical dysplasia, which can be very difficult to identify in the young, rapidly growing brain because of cerebral cortical development and white matter myelination (Figure 62-2). Another clinical presentation, often unique to children, consists of those who have multiple lesions of which only one or two may be epileptogenic, as is often the case in children with multiple tubers from tuberous sclerosis complex (35–37). Hence, pediatric patients with surgically treatable conditions can present with generalized seizures with focal pathologies, with focal pathologies and EEG with an apparent negative initial MRI, and with multiple lesions the removal of one or two of which could result in excellent seizure control. Such unique presentations should be considered in considering when to refer a child with therapy-resistant epilepsy to a specialty center.

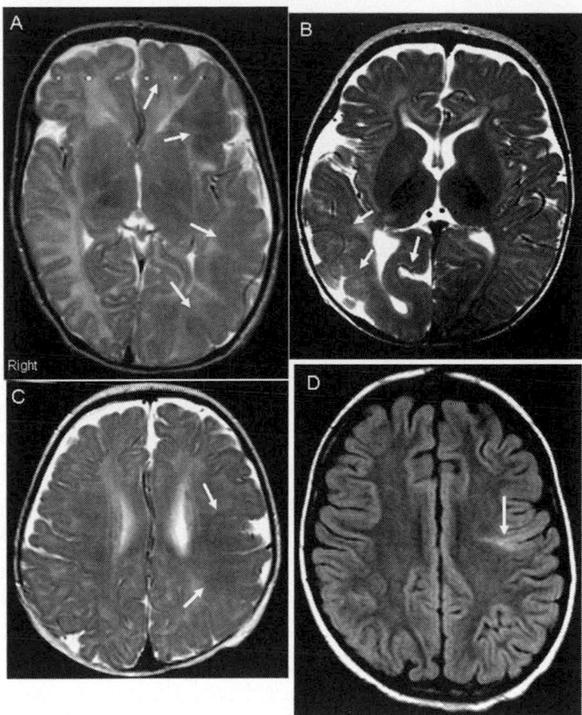

FIGURE 62-1

MRI scans of pediatric patients with different types of cortical dysplasia. Right side of patient for all figures is shown in panel A. (A) This 2.5-month-old began to have seizures shortly after birth, consisting of body twitches and eye deviation. Scalp EEG disclosed interictal abnormalities and ictal onsets over the left hemisphere corresponding to a region of hemimegalencephaly. Notice the enlarged left cerebral hemisphere with multiple areas of thickened cortex (arrows). Histopathology confirmed severe cortical dysplasia with cytomegalic neurons. (B) This 1-year-old began to have seizures within 2 weeks of birth that eventually progressed to infantile spasms, and EEG abnormalities were localized over the right cerebral hemisphere. MRI disclosed cortical abnormalities involving the right posterior temporal and occipital lobes (arrows) representing multilobar disease. Histopathology after surgical resection confirmed severe cortical dysplasia without balloon cells. (C) This 6-month-old began to have seizures shortly after birth, there was motor asymmetry on examination with mild weakness of the right arm and hand, and seizures consisted of right greater than left tonic motor events. MRI revealed a focal region of cortical and subcortical abnormality involving the left frontal and parietal cortex (arrows). Histopathology confirmed severe cortical dysplasia with cytomegalic neurons and balloon cells. (D) This 7.5-year-old began to have seizures at age 4.8 years that involved focal motor onsets of the right body. MRI revealed a focal region of abnormality in the left frontal lobe with a "tail" extending from the cortex into the white matter (arrow). Histopathology confirmed severe cortical dysplasia with balloon cells.

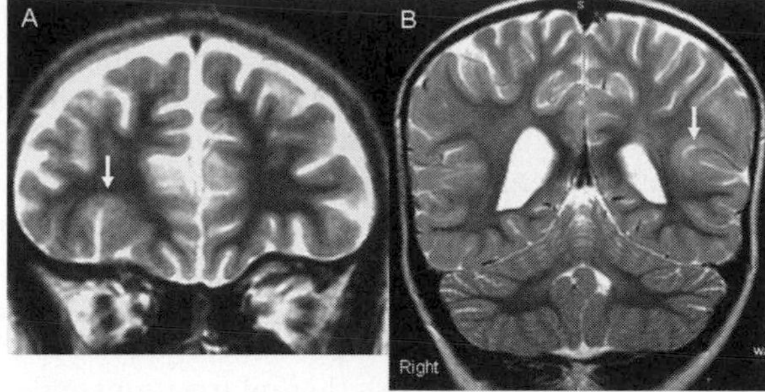

FIGURE 62-2

MRI scans of pediatric patients with difficult-to-diagnose regions of cortical dysplasia. Right side of both patients is shown in panel B. (A) This 8-year-old had a long history of refractory complex partial epilepsy and significant behavioral problems. He had previously attacked his family with a knife and tried to set the house on fire, and outside MRI scans had been read as "normal." Scalp EEG showed bihemispheric abnormalities with more findings referrable to the right frontal and temporal regions. Notice the region of thickened cortex in the right orbital frontal region (arrow). Histopathology showed severe cortical dysplasia with balloon cells. There was a 90+% decrease in seizures with surgery; however, he still has persistent, although less severe, behavioral problems at home and school. (B) This 3.5-year-old presented with new-onset seizures that rapidly progressed over a few weeks into status epilepticus. She was hospitalized at an outside facility receiving pharmacologic therapy with two MRI scans read as "normal." After transfer, EEG abnormalities were found mostly in the left central-parietal region. Re-review of the MRI scans disclosed an area of thickened cortex at the posterior margin of the Sylvian fissure. Histopathology confirmed mild cortical dysplasia, and the child has been seizure free since surgery.

RISKS OF THERAPY-RESISTANT EPILEPSY IN CHILDREN

Severe developmental delay or regression and increased seizure-related mortality are the major recognized risks of therapy-resistant epilepsy in children (38, 39). Clinical studies indicate that there are at least five independent factors that are associated with developmental delay and lower IQ scores in children with early-onset epilepsy. These are (1) seizure type; (2) age at seizure onset; (3) seizure frequency; (4) seizure duration; and (5) number of AEDs. Children with generalized symptomatic epilepsy (e.g., infantile spasms) and partial seizures originating from one or two lobes of the brain are more likely to have significantly lower IQ scores (>2 standard deviations of the mean) than those with idiopathic epilepsy (e.g., absence, rolandic). Likewise, children whose epilepsy begins before age 1 year, have daily or greater seizure frequency, have uncontrolled seizures for more than

2 years, and use more than three AEDs are at increased risk for developing epilepsy-induced encephalopathy (39, 40). Epilepsy-induced encephalopathy is irreversible, and there is consensus among specialists that early therapeutic intervention, such as resective neurosurgery, is especially critical in infants and young children to prevent catastrophic developmental regression (2, 41). There is emerging clinical data in surgical cohorts that early surgery is associated with better cognitive outcomes (38, 42–46). Even adolescents with therapy-resistant epilepsy are less likely to finish high school, find employment, get married, and be productive citizens than are seizure-free patients (24).

Another important consideration in deciding the timing for epilepsy surgery in children is developmental cerebral cortical plasticity. The developing human brain is capable of significant reorganization of neurologic function, including language and motor skills, after insult and surgery (47–50). In most children, developmental cerebral cortical plasticity may reduce the anticipated neurologic deficits following resective surgery, but it should be noted that the amount of plasticity cannot be predicted before surgery (51).

Therapy-resistant epilepsy in children is also associated with significant seizure-related mortality. There is a higher than expected death rate in children with therapy-resistant epilepsy, with a risk of dying that is more than five times greater than that of the general population in the first 15 to 20 years after diagnosis (52, 53). Clinical trials in therapy-resistant cases indicate that the rate of death from seizures is conservatively 0.5% per patient year (1 in 200), and this risk accumulates over time (54). The causes of death related to seizures include status epilepticus, aspiration pneumonia, drowning, falls, or sudden unexplained deaths due to epilepsy (SUDEP). It is the poor natural history of therapy-resistant epilepsy in children, with increased cognitive morbidity and mortality, that prompts physicians and parents to consider alternate therapies, including epilepsy neurosurgery. In addition, the risks of surgery should be weighed against the risk of cognitive problems and seizure-related mortality in deciding surgical candidacy.

WHEN TO REFER CHILDREN FOR AN EPILEPSY SURGERY EVALUATION

Expert consensus recommends that children with therapy-resistant seizures or disabling medication side effects should be referred to a pediatric epilepsy center that includes surgery as one of the therapeutic options (2). The purpose of the referral is to evaluate children to be sure they have a correct epilepsy diagnosis, and consider optional therapies in an attempt to stop refractory epilepsy. Thus, not all children referred to a pediatric epilepsy center end up with surgery. Changes in medical management, after a through diagnostic evaluation, can often control seizures, and children are returned to their community physicians (37). Likewise, alternate nonsurgical options can be considered, such as the ketogenic diet (55).

The timing of the referral to a pediatric center is important for children, especially infants who are at greatest risk of epilepsy-induced encephalopathy. It is recommended that children with uncontrolled seizures or infantile spasms under age 2 years should be promptly referred to a specialty center regardless of MRI findings (2). An MRI showing a lesion in any child, regardless of seizure control with AEDs, should also be referred to a pediatric epilepsy center, as these substrates often become therapy-resistant, or the lesion itself should be closely followed for signs of progression (56). Also, focal epilepsy in childhood can be from low-incidence etiologies that should be referred to a specialty center with experience in these pathologies. These etiologies may include children with hemimegalencephaly (57), Rasmussen syndrome (58), Sturge-Weber syndrome (59), tuberous sclerosis complex (35, 36), Landau-Kleffner syndrome, hypothalamic hamartomas (60), and polymicrogyria (57, 59–62).

The evaluation of prospective pediatric epilepsy surgery candidates involves EEG, structural and functional imaging, and appropriate psychologic and psychiatric evaluations (63, 64). EEG studies include interictal and ictal scalp and video recordings to capture seizures and their behaviors. MRI with specific epilepsy protocols is recommended as the primary imaging modality to identify subtle cortical abnormalities not appreciated on routine MRI scans (see Figure 62-2). The MRI sequences may include diffusion tensor imaging (DTI) and thin slices using spoiled gradient recalled (SPGR) sequences or surface coils to capture small cortical defects (56). Other MRI sequences may be required in the first two years of life because of immature myelination, and serial scans may be necessary to identify abnormalities during early postnatal brain development when the clinical team suspects a localized pathologic substrate on the basis of seizure semiology and EEG characteristics. Functional imaging studies may include ictal and interictal SPECT, FDG-PET, and magnetoencephalography (MEG) (37, 65–68). Age-appropriate neuropsychologic/developmental assessments are another important aspect of the pre- and post-surgery evaluation (38, 69). In approximately 25% to 30% of children the seizures cannot be adequately localized with noninvasive studies, and they undergo intracranial electrode placement (grid or depth studies) for ictal seizure localization prior to resection (70).

Not all procedures are necessary for all children, and the decision on the elements of the presurgery evaluation will vary by patient based on age and clinical syndrome. The main criteria for assessing the child with therapy-resistant epilepsy will be a risk/benefit analysis in which the risks of progressive cognitive delay and death from the seizures is weighed against the probability of seizure control with resection of brain tissue (benefit) and any probable neurologic deficits resulting from surgery (risk). Those judgments involve input from all members of the specialty epilepsy clinical team (surgeons and nonsurgeons) in carefully detailed discussions with the child and family. Thus, there are no set paradigms in deciding who is an epilepsy surgery candidate, and the risk-benefit ratio will vary from one family to another. Also, the presurgery evaluation is expected to change as new technologies and methods are introduced and validated in pediatric patients (1, 67). Postsurgery evaluations should include structural MRI scans and neuropsychologic, psychiatric, and behavioral assessments, along with physical, occupational, and speech therapy. It is recommended that children continue to be followed at the pediatric epilepsy center for as long as necessary to assess and treat these children with chronic conditions even if their seizures are controlled (2).

TABLE 62-1
Incidence of Symptomatic Substrates in Pediatric Epilepsy Surgery

Etiology	Percent of Cases
Cortical dysplasia	42%
Tumor	19%
Infection/stroke/trauma	10%
Hippocampal sclerosis	6%
Tuberous sclerosis complex	5%
Hypothalamic hamartoma	4%
Sturge-Weber syndrome	3%
Rasmussen syndrome	3%
Vascular lesions	1%
Other (gliosis, rarer pathology, normal)	7%

ILAE Pediatric Sub-Commission survey of 20 centers in Europe, Australia, and North America for 2004, patients aged less than 18 years (n = 543 patients). From Harvey et al, 2005 (70).

CLINICAL CHARACTERISTICS OF PEDIATRIC EPILEPSY NEUROSURGERY PATIENTS

To repeat, the goals of surgical treatment are the same as those of medical therapy. They are to stop seizures with minimal or no additional serious neurologic side effects so that the developing brain can reach its greatest cognitive potential (2). This is especially relevant for pediatric epilepsy surgery in that 45% to 50% of children undergoing surgery have their first seizure before age 1 year (70) and thus are at significant risk of epileptic encephalopathy (71). The best chance for stopping symptomatic therapy-resistant epilepsy is with resective neurosurgery. The optimal surgical candidates are those individuals in whom the seizures arise from portions of the brain that are already severely damaged or nonfunctional such that the resulting neurologic outcome is likely to be no worse than their currently existing medical condition. However, in some children the epilepsy can be so early in life and unrelenting that large resections, such as hemispherectomy, with accompanying physical neurologic deficits may be necessary in order to prevent severe cognitive developmental delay. This is especially true for children with hemispheric cortical dysplasia and hemimegalencephaly with infantile spasms, and slightly older children with Rasmussen syndrome.

The clinical characteristics of the symptomatic etiologies in pediatric patients are different from those in adults (Table 62-1). In a recent International League Against Epilepsy (ILAE)-sponsored survey of 20 pediatric epilepsy surgery centers from Europe, North America, and Australia (70), the most common pathologic finding in over 40% of pediatric surgical patients was cortical dysplasia. This pathology consists, at a minimum, of cortical dyslamination and columnar disorganization that is nearly always coupled with excessive, heterotopic neurons in the subcortical white matter (72, 73). Cortical dysplasia can be mild or severe; in the latter case the tissue contains abnormal, cytomegalic neurons and balloon cells. As shown by MRI, cortical dysplasia can be hemispheric, multilobar, or lobar/focal (see Figures 62-1 and 62-2), with lobar/focal dysplasia in the frontal and temporal lobes the most common (74). Larger areas of cortical dysplasia are associated with younger ages at seizure onset and surgery (75).

The next most frequent etiologies in pediatric epilepsy surgery patients are low-grade tumors (76), and these typically consist of gangliogliomas and dysembryoplastic neuroepithelial tumors (DNETs) in over half the cases (Figure 62-3). Other relatively common etiologies in pediatric epilepsy surgery patients include atrophic pathologies from stroke, infections, and cerebral trauma, hippocampal sclerosis, and patients with tuberous sclerosis complex (Figures 62-3 through 62-5). Hypothalamic hamartomas, Sturge-Weber, Rasmussen syndrome, and vascular lesions are less frequently found pathologies in pediatric epilepsy surgery patients.

In hypothalamic hamartomas, surgical treatment with or without endoscopy leads to favorable results when performed as soon as possible after the diagnosis of therapy-resistant epilepsy has been established (77). Such a precocious approach is recommended in order to avoid the devastating influence that continuous

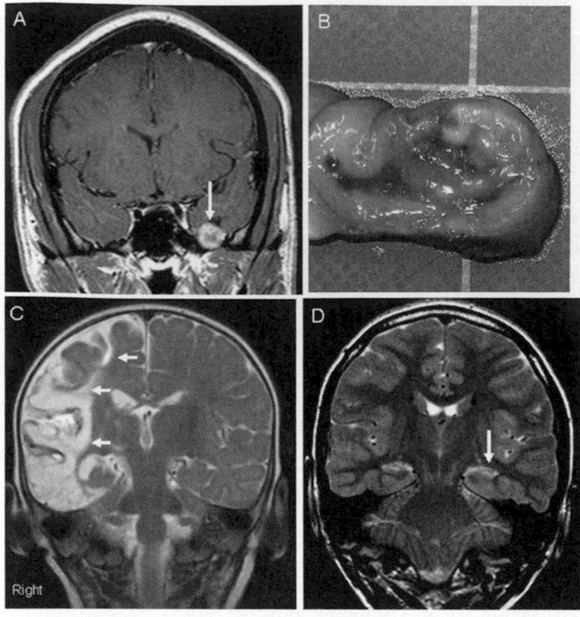

FIGURE 62-3

MRI examples of other frequently found symptomatic substrates associated with surgically treated pediatric epilepsy cases. (A, B) This 15-year-old began to have complex partial seizures at age 10 years. MRI disclosed a contrast-enhancing mass lesion in the inferior left temporal pole (A, arrow). Examination of the fresh surgical specimen (B) showed a cystic hard mass that was shown by histopathology to be a ganglioglioma. (C) This 2-year-old presented with new-onset seizures from herpes encephalitis at age 9 months that destroyed most of the right cerebral hemisphere (arrows). Seizures were daily before hemispherectomy, which stopped all events. (D) This 12-year-old had a prolonged complex febrile convulsion at 9 months of age. She remained seizure free until age 6 years, when she developed complex partial epilepsy consisting of staring and lip smacking. MRI revealed signal change in the left hippocampus, and hippocampal sclerosis was established at histopathology.

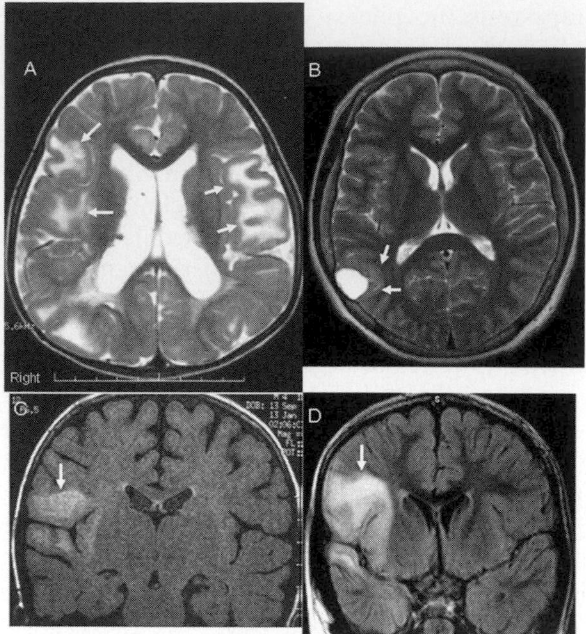

FIGURE 62-4

MRI examples of other less frequent symptomatic substrates associated with surgically treated pediatric epilepsy cases. (A) This 2.5-year-old presented at 7 months of age with infantile spasms from multiple tubers associated with tuberous sclerosis complex (arrows). Removal of the left frontal tuber has controlled all seizures for over 3 years. (B) This 14.5-year-old began to have seizures at age 3 years. Despite failing many different AEDs, he never had an MRI scan until age 14 years, when a cystic mass was found in the right posterior temporal region that included cortical changes into the white matter (arrows). The lesion did not enhance with contrast. Histopathology showed signs of old hemorrhage without evidence of tumor or arteriovenous malformation (AVM), most suggestive of an atypical cavernous angioma. (C, D) This 5-year-old began to have seizures 9 months earlier that within weeks evolved to constant motor clonus of the left face and hand. MRI within two weeks of seizure onset showed fluid-attenuated inversion recovery (FLAIR) changes in the right perisylvian region (arrow in C), and this region enlarged two months later (arrow in D). Clinical presentation and histopathology were most consistent with Rasmussen syndrome (58). This child is seizure free 2 years after cerebral hemispherectomy.

epileptic activity exerts on the developing nervous system. Nonsurgical techniques (such as Gamma Knife, radiofrequency thermocoagulation, or interstitial radiosurgery), have also been proposed in order to avoid surgery-related complications such as hemiplegia, third cranial nerve palsy, visual field deficit, and central insipid diabetes (62, 78, 79).

Types of epilepsy neurosurgical procedures also are quite varied in pediatric patients (Table 62-2). In the 2004 ILAE survey, 81% of operative cases were resective surgeries involving removing portions of the brain for seizure control, compared with 19% for palliative operations (vagal nerve stimulators and corpus callosotomy) (80–83). Of the resective cases, lobar and focal resections were the most common (48%), and the regions most fequently involved with pathology were the temporal (23%) and frontal (17%) lobes. In other words, in children undergoing epilepsy neurosurgery, 70% of cases involve extratemporal resection, which is a much higher proportion than typically observed in adult epilepsy surgery cohorts (84). Hemispherectomy was the second most common resective

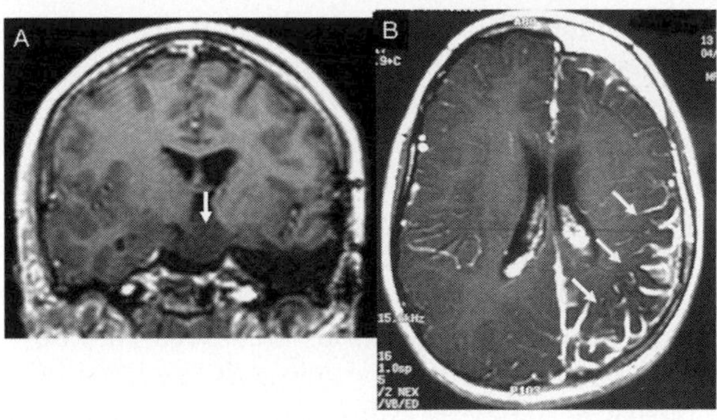

FIGURE 62-5

Examples of less frequently encountered pathologies in children. (A) This child had refractory epilepsy with developmental delay. Evaluation at an outside hospital found EEG evidence of ictal onsets in the left temporal region, and a left temporal lobectomy was performed. Seizure persisted from the hypothalamic hamartoma (arrow) successfully treated with an endoscopic approach. (B) This child presented with a portwine stain over the forehead. MRI with contrast discloses the typical enhancement pattern seen with Sturge-Weber, which was treated by hemispherectomy.

surgical procedure, followed by multilobar resections (85). In order to decrease complication rates, newer surgical procedures are designed to reduce the volume of brain removal and increase the ratio of disconnection to resection. Such techniques reduce the size of the skin incision and bone flap, which offers the advantages of preventing excessive blood loss and avoiding the exposure of large venous sinuses. This concept, for example, has replaced the term *hemispherectomy* with *hemispherotomy*.

The age at surgery was associated with differences in type of etiology and surgical procedures. Children under age 4 years at the time of surgery are more likely to have hemispherectomy or multilobar cortical resections (50% of all procedures) for cortical dysplasia (60% of all etiologies), and children had daily or greater seizure frequency. From ages 4 to 12 years the more likely operative procedure would be a focal resection (50%) for cortical dysplasia and tumors (60%), and children would have daily or slightly less frequent seizures. From ages 12 to 18 years the operative procedure will most likely be a focal resection (60%) for cortical dysplasia, tumors, or hippocampal sclerosis (67%), and seizure frequency will be several per week. Palliative procedures, such as vagal nerve stimulators and corpus callosotomy, are evenly distributed by age at surgery.

TABLE 62-2
Types of Surgery in Pediatric Epilepsy

TYPE OF SURGERY	PERCENT
Lobar/focal resections	48%
Hemispherectomy	16%
Multilobar resections	13%
Vagal nerve stimulator implants	16%
Corpus callosotomy	3%
Other: multiple subpial transections (MST), grids no resection, etc.	4%

ILAE Pediatric Sub-Commission survey of 20 centers in Europe, Australia, and North America for 2004, patients aged less than 18 years (n = 543 patients). From Harvey et al, 2005 (70).

SPECIAL OPERATIVE CONSIDERATIONS IN CHILDREN

Neurosurgical procedures can pose special challenges for smaller children, and this is especially true for epilepsy surgery, where younger cases undergo larger cortical resections, which are associated with significant perioperative blood loss relative to total vascular volume (85–89). In children, brain weight is proportionally larger compared to body volume than in adults (90, 91). At age 2 years, for example, the brain is approximately 70% of its adult size, whereas body weight is about 12%. At 10 years of age brain weight is 95% of adult value, but body weight is 50%. Infants weigh 6 to 10 kg at 6 months and 8 to 12 kg by 1 year. Estimated total blood volume (at 75 mL/kg) is 450 to 750 mL at 6 months and 600 to 900 mL at 1 year. By comparison, 10-year-olds weigh 23 to 51 kg, and estimated blood volumes range from 1,700 to 3,800 mL. Expected blood loss varies by operation and generally ranges from 200 to 500 mL for a focal or lobar resection, and 1,500 mL or more for anatomic hemispherectomy. Thus, in a 6-month-old, even relatively small epilepsy surgery procedures can result in blood loss equal to half or more of total blood volume, and larger operations, such as anatomic hemispherectomy, will involve more than a total body transfusion of red cells. Moreover, blood loss and other complications appear to be more common in cases of hemimegalencephaly, where the cortex is very vascular and dysmature (44, 92, 93). Anticipating these operative and postsurgery problems requires a dedicated surgical team that includes neuroanesthesiologists and pediatric intensive care physicians who proactively treat problems before they occur, have adequate vascular access, monitor for ongoing blood loss during surgery, and have a surgical approach that minimizes operative blood loss (85).

Waiting for the child to grow larger before performing epilepsy neurosurgery does not reduce operative risks over the first 3 years of life, and significantly increases the probability for poorer cognitive outcomes. Two-year-olds weigh 10 to 15 kg, whereas 3-year-olds from 11.5 to 17.8 kg with calculated vascular volumes of 750 to 1,100 mL for 2-year-olds and 860 to 1,300 mL for 3-year-olds. Thus, hemispherectomy and other larger neurosurgical operations, where blood loss is expected to range from 500 to 1,000 mL with newer disconnection procedures, is still associated with possible operative blood transfusion in young children, especially in those with large cortical dysplasia and hemimegalencephaly. In other words, the risk of surgery is not significantly reduced in a 2- or 3-year-old compared with an infant. Hence, although operating in young children is riskier than in adolescents and adults, the increased operative risks are justified in order to prevent permanent epilepsy-related cognitive and developmental deficits.

OUTCOME

Depending on the type of surgery and etiology, resective neurosurgery is expected to achieve seizure remission (no seizures) in 60% to 80% of pediatric cases in the first two years after surgery (94–96). This exceeds the 5% or less chance of seizure remission with AED therapies (26, 84, 97, 98). Postsurgery seizure remission is higher in those children with localized lesions and pathologies requiring focal or lobar resections than those with multilobar resections and more diffuse pathologies such as hemimegencephaly (9, 45). Analysis of the pediatric epilepsy surgery data base from the University of California, Los Angeles (UCLA), for example, found that 73% of children were seizure free after hemispherectomy compared with 65% after multilobar resections (99). So far, there is currently no evidence that seizure control is influenced by duration of seizures before surgery. However, developmental outcomes do appear to be influenced by duration of epilepsy prior to surgery (100). Children that achieve seizures control through surgery with less than 2 years of seizure duration have higher developmental quotients than those with seizure durations over 2 years (44, 45). What is unclear is the impact of epilepsy surgery on quality of life and altering abnormal behaviors, which will require further study in pediatric epilepsy surgery patients (101, 102).

OPERATIVE COMPLICATIONS

Resective neurosurgery is not without possible complications, but the risk from operative therapy is generally less than from long-term uncontrolled epilepsy. Reported operative mortality varies from 0.24% for temporal lobe surgery to 2.5% for hemispherectomy performed using older techniques (96). The operative mortality with newer hemispherectomy techniques is under 1%. The reported risk of permanent surgical morbidity varies by type of surgery from 1.1% for temporal lobe surgery to about 5% for frontal lobe resections (26). For temporal lobe epilepsy surgery, the major serious complication is infarct and possible hemiparesis. For frontal lobe resections, corpus callosotomy, and multiple subpial resections, the major serious complications are increased motor or language deficits. Of interest, patients rendered seizure free postsurgery have a risk of epilepsy-related mortality comparable to that of patients who are seizure free with AEDs alone (103, 104). Thus, in correctly identified pediatric patients, the operative morbidity and mortality is less than the risks associated with the natural history of therapy-resistant epilepsy.

CONCLUSIONS

Epilepsy neurosurgery has a very important role in the treatment of therapy-resistant epilepsy, especially for the young developing brain at risk for seizure induced encephalopathy. The goal of surgical treatment for pediatric patients is to stop seizures as quickly as possible with minimal or acceptable side effects and to optimize cognitive development leading to improved behavior and quality of life. Rational decisions regarding epilepsy surgery in children involve a benefit-and-risk assessment of all treatment alternatives with parents so that they can reach an informed decision. That discussion and decision are best performed at a specialty pediatric epilepsy surgery center with the input of a team of pediatric neurologists and surgeon. Surgery is medically justified because children with refractory seizures have an increased risk of serious neurologic morbidity and mortality related to their epilepsy. Generally, the most refractory cases are those patients with symptomatic substrates, and they are often excellent surgical candidates. Seizure control can be expected in 60% to 70% of patients postsurgery and varies by operative technique and whether the goal of surgery was palliative or curative. Operative morbidity and mortality are generally under 5%, which is less than the mortality expected from 10 years of therapy-resistant epilepsy. There are no age restrictions for epilepsy surgery, nor is epilepsy surgery restricted to a single epilepsy syndrome or type of operation (105, 106).

ACKNOWLEDGMENTS

GWM was supported by National Institutes of Health grants RO1 NS38992, R21 HD050707, and P01 NS02808.

References

1. Jacobs MP, Fischbach GD, Davis MR, Dichter MA, et al. Future directions for epilepsy research. *Neurology* 2001; 57(9):1536–1542.
2. Cross JH, Jayakar P, Nordli D, et al. Proposed criteria for referral and evaluation of children for epilepsy surgery: recommendations of the Subcommission for Pediatric Epilepsy Surgery. *Epilepsia* 2006; 47(6):952–959.
3. Horsley V. Brain surgery. *BMJ* 1886; 2:670–675.
4. Penfield W, Baldwin M. Temporal lobe seizures and the technique of subtotal temporal lobectomy. *Ann Surg* 1952; 136:625–634.
5. Temkin O. The falling sickness: a history of epilepsy from the Greeks to the beginnings of modern neurology. Baltimore: The Johns Hopkins Press. 1945:380.
6. Karbowski K. Sixty years of clinical electroencephalography. *Eur Neurol* 1990; 30(3): 170–175.
7. Foerster O, Altenburger H. Elektrobiologische Vorgange an der menschlichen Hirnrinde. *Dtsch Z Nervenheilkd* 1934:277–288.
8. French JA. Antiepileptic drug development. In: Wyllie E, ed. *The Treatment of Epilepsy.* Philadelphia: Lippincott Williams & Wilkins, 2001:719.
9. Mathern GW, Giza CC, Yudovin S, et al. Postoperative seizure control and antiepileptic drug use in pediatric epilepsy surgery patients: the UCLA experience, 1986–1997. *Epilepsia* 1999; 40(12):1740–1749.
10. Wyllie E, Luders H, Morris HH 3rd, et al. Clinical outcome after complete or partial cortical resection for intractable epilepsy. *Neurology* 1987; 37(10):1634–1641.
11. Morrison G, Duchowny M, Resnick T, et al. Epilepsy surgery in childhood. A report of 79 patients. *Pediatr Neurosurg* 1992; 18(5–6):291–297.
12. Goldring S. A method for surgical management of focal epilepsy, especially as it relates to children. *J Neurosurg* 1978; 49(3):344–356.
13. Engel J Jr. Surgery for seizures. *N Engl J Med* 1996; 334(10):647–652.
14. Arts WF, Brouwer OF, Peters AC, et al. Course and prognosis of childhood epilepsy: 5-year follow-up of the Dutch study of epilepsy in childhood. *Brain* 2004; 127(Pt 8):1774–1784.
15. Berg AT, Testa FM, Levy SR, et al. Neuroimaging in children with newly diagnosed epilepsy: a community-based study. *Pediatrics* 2000; 106(3):527–532.
16. Berg AT, Shinnar S, Levy SR, et al. Two-year remission and subsequent relapse in children with newly diagnosed epilepsy. *Epilepsia* 2001; 42(12):1553–1562.
17. Berg AT, Shinnar S, Levy SR, et al. Defining early seizure outcomes in pediatric epilepsy: the good, the bad and the in-between. *Epilepsy Res* 2001; 43(1):75–84.
18. Berg AT, Shinnar S, Levy SR, et al. Early development of intractable epilepsy in children: a prospective study. *Neurology* 2001; 56(11):1445–1452.
19. Cardoso TA, Coan AC, Kobayashi E, et al. Hippocampal abnormalities and seizure recurrence after antiepileptic drug withdrawal. *Neurology* 2006; 67(1):134–136.
20. Stephen LJ, Kwan P, and Brodie MJ. Does the cause of localisation-related epilepsy influence the response to antiepileptic drug treatment? *Epilepsia* 2001; 42(3):357–362.
21. Semah F, Picot MC, Adam C, et al. Is the underlying cause of epilepsy a major prognostic factor for recurrence? *Neurology* 1998; 51(5):1256–1262.
22. Szabo CA, Rothner AD, Kotagal P, et al. Symptomatic or cryptogenic partial epilepsy of childhood onset: fourteen-year follow-up. *Pediatr Neurol* 2001; 24(4):264–269.
23. Spooner CG, Berkovic SF, Mitchell LA, et al. New-onset temporal lobe epilepsy in children: lesion on MRI predicts poor seizure outcome. *Neurology* 2006; 21:2147–2153.
24. Sillanpaa M, Jalava M, Kaleva O, et al. Long-term prognosis of seizures with onset in childhood. *N Engl J Med* 1998; 338(24):1715–1722.
25. Sillanpaa M, Schmidt D. Natural history of treated childhood-onset epilepsy: prospective, long-term population-based study. *Brain* 2006; 129:617–624.
26. Chapell R, Reston J, Snyder D. Management of treatment-resistant epilepsy. Evidence Report/Technology Assesment No 77. AHRQ Publication No. 03-0028. Vol. 1. Rockville, MD: Agency for Healthcare Research and Quality, 2003:323.
27. Kwan P, Brodie MJ. Early identification of refractory epilepsy. *N Engl J Med* 2000; 342(5):314–319.
28. Kwan P, Brodie MJ. Refractory epilepsy: a progressive, intractable but preventable condition? *Seizure* 2002; 11(2):77–84.
29. Singhvi JP, Sawhney IM, Lal V, et al. Profile of intractable epilepsy in a tertiary referral center. *Neurol India* 2000; 48(4):351–6.
30. Chugani HT, Shewmon DA, Peacock WJ, et al. Surgical treatment of intractable neonatal-onset seizures: the role of positron emission tomography. *Neurology* 1988; 38(8): 1178–1188.
31. Chugani HT, Shields WD, Shewmon DA, et al. Infantile spasms: I. PET identifies focal cortical dysgenesis in cryptogenic cases for surgical treatment. *Ann Neurol* 1990; 27(4):406–413.
32. Koh S, Mathern GW, Glasser G, et al. Status epilepticus and frequent seizures: incidence and clinical characteristics in pediatric epilepsy surgery patients. *Epilepsia* 2005; 46(12):1950–1954.
33. Nordli DR Jr, Bazil CW, Scheuer ML, et al. Recognition and classification of seizures in infants. *Epilepsia* 1997; 38(5):553–560.
34. Fogarasi A, Janszky J, Tuxhorn I. Peri-ictal lateralizing signs in children: blinded multiobserver study of 100 children < or =12 years. *Neurology* 2006; 66(2):271–274.
35. Chandra PS, Salamon N, Huang J, et al. FDG-PET/MRI coregistration and diffusion-tensor imaging distinguish epileptogenic tubers and cortex in patients with tuberous sclerosis complex. *Epilepsia* 2006; 47:1543–1549.
36. Weiner HL, Carlson C, Ridgway EB, et al. Epilepsy surgery in young children with tuberous sclerosis: results of a novel approach. *Pediatrics* 2006; 117(5):1494–1502.
37. Wu JY, Sutherling WW, Koh S, et al. Magnetic source imaging localizes epileptogenic zone in children with tuberous sclerosis complex. *Neurology* 2006; 66:1270–1272.
38. Battaglia D, Chieffo D, Lettori D, et al. Cognitive assessment in epilepsy surgery of children. *Childs Nerv Syst* 2006; 22(8):744–759.
39. Nolan MA, Redoblado MA, Lah S, et al. Intelligence in childhood epilepsy syndromes. *Epilepsy Res* 2003; 53(1–2):139–150.
40. Vasconcellos E, Wyllie E, Sullivan S, et al. Mental retardation in pediatric candidates for epilepsy surgery: the role of early seizure onset. *Epilepsia* 2001; 42(2):268–274.
41. Hrachovy RA, Frost JD Jr. Infantile epileptic encephalopathy with hypsarrhythmia (infantile spasms/West syndrome). *J Clin Neurophysiol* 2003; 20(6):408–425.
42. Devlin AM, Cross JH, Harkness W, et al. Clinical outcomes of hemispherectomy for epilepsy in childhood and adolescence. *Brain* 2003; 126(Pt 3):556–566.
43. Gleissner U, Sassen R, Schramm J, et al. Greater functional recovery after temporal lobe epilepsy surgery in children. *Brain* 2005; 128(Pt 12):2822–2829.
44. Jonas R, Nguyen S, Hu B, et al. Cerebral hemispherectomy: hospital course, seizure, developmental, language, and motor outcomes. *Neurology* 2004; 62(10):1712–1721.
45. Jonas R, Asarnow RF, LoPresti C, et al. Surgery for symptomatic infant-onset epileptic encephalopathy with and without infantile spasms. *Neurology* 2005; 64(4):746–750.
46. Korkman M, Granstrom ML, Kantola-Sorsa E, et al. Two-year follow-up of intelligence after pediatric epilepsy surgery. *Pediatr Neurol* 2005; 33(3):173–178.
47. Curtiss S, de Bode S, Mathern GW. Spoken language outcomes after hemispherectomy: factoring in etiology. *Brain Lang* 2001; 79(3):379–396.
48. de Bode S, Firestine A, Mathern GW, et al. Residual motor control and cortical representations of function following hemispherectomy: effects of etiology. *J Child Neurol* 2005; 20(1):64–75.
49. van Empelen R, Jennekens-Schinkel A, Gorter JW, et al. Epilepsy surgery does not harm motor performance of children and adolescents. *Brain* 2005; 128(Pt 7):1536–1545.
50. Soufflet C, Bulteau C, Delalande O, et al. The nonmalformed hemisphere is secondarily impaired in young children with hemimegalencephaly: a pre- and postsurgery study with SPECT and EEG. *Epilepsia* 2004; 45(11):1375–1382.
51. de Bode S, Mathern GW, Bookheimer S, et al. Locomotor training remodels fMRI sensorimotor cortical activations in children after cerebral hemispherectomy. *Neurorehab Neural Repair* 2007 Mar 16; Epub.
52. Patwardhan RV, Mathern GW. Surgical treatment of therapy-resistant epilepsy. *American Academy of Neurology Continuum: Livelong Learning in Neurology* 2004; 10(4):100–118.
53. Tellez-Zenteno JF, Ronquillo LH, Wiebe S. Sudden unexpected death in epilepsy: evidence-based analysis of incidence and risk factors. *Epilepsy Res* 2005; 65(1–2): 101–115.
54. Racoosin JA, Feeney J, Burkhart G, et al. Mortality in antiepileptic drug development programs. *Neurology* 2001; 56(4):514–519.
55. Marsh EB, Freeman JM, Kossoff EH, et al. The outcome of children with intractable seizures: a 3- to 6-year follow-up of 67 children who remained on the ketogenic diet less than one year. *Epilepsia* 2006; 47(2):425–430.
56. Raybaud C, Shroff M, Rutka JT, et al. Imaging surgical epilepsy in children. *Childs Nerv Syst* 2006; 22(8):786–809.
57. Salamon N, Andres M, Chute DJ, et al. Contralateral hemimicrencephaly and clinical-pathological correlations in children with hemimegalencephaly. *Brain* 2006; 129: 352–365.
58. Bien CG, Granata T, Antozzi C, et al. Pathogenesis, diagnosis and treatment of Rasmussen encephalitis: a European consensus statement. *Brain* 2005; 128(Pt 3):454–471.
59. Di Rocco C, Tamburrini G. Sturge-Weber syndrome. *Childs Nerv Syst* 2006; 22(8): 909–921.
60. Fohlen M, Lellouch A, Delalande O. Hypothalamic hamartoma with refractory epilepsy: surgical procedures and results in 18 patients. *Epileptic Disord* 2003; 5(4):267–273.
61. Harvey AS, Freeman JL, Berkovic SF, et al. Transcallosal resection of hypothalamic hamartomas in patients with intractable epilepsy. *Epileptic Disord* 2003; 5(4):257–265.
62. Rekate HL, Feiz-Erfan I, Ng YT, et al. Endoscopic surgery for hypothalamic hamartomas causing medically refractory gelastic epilepsy. *Childs Nerv Syst* 2006; 22(8):874–880.
63. Guerrini R. Epilepsy in children. *Lancet* 2006; 367(9509):499–524.
64. Sheth RD. Epilepsy surgery. Presurgical evaluation. *Neurol Clin* 2002; 20(4): 1195–1215.
65. Cascino GD, Buchhalter JR, Mullan BP, et al. Ictal SPECT in nonlesional extratemporal epilepsy. *Epilepsia* 2004; 45 Suppl 4:32–34.
66. Sood S, Chugani HT. Functional neuroimaging in the preoperative evaluation of children with drug-resistant epilepsy. *Childs Nerv Syst* 2006; 22(8):810–820.
67. Knowlton RC, Elgavish R, Howell J, et al. Magnetic source imaging versus intracranial electroencephalogram in epilepsy surgery: a prospective study. *Ann Neurol* 2006, 59(5):835–842.
68. Grondin R, Chuang S, Otsubo H, et al. The role of magnetoencephalography in pediatric epilepsy surgery. *Childs Nerv Syst* 2006; 22(8):779–785.
69. McLellan A, Davies S, Heyman I, et al. Psychopathology in children with epilepsy before and after temporal lobe resection. *Dev Med Child Neurol* 2005; 47(10):666–672.
70. Harvey AS, Mathern GW, Nordli D, et al. Epilepsy surgery in children: results from an international survey. *Epilepsia* 2005; 46(Suppl. 6):82.
71. Stafstrom CE, Lynch M, Sutula TP. Consequences of epilepsy in the developing brain: implications for surgical management. *Semin Pediatr Neurol* 2000; 7(3):147–157.
72. Palmini A, Najm I, Avanzini G, et al. Terminology and classification of the cortical dysplasias. *Neurology* 2004; 62(6 Suppl 3):S2–S8.
73. Mischel PS, Nguyen LP, and Vinters HV. Cerebral cortical dysplasia associated with pediatric epilepsy. Review of neuropathologic features and proposal for a grading system. *J Neuropathol Exp Neurol* 1995; 54(2):137–153.

74. Tassi L, Colombo N, Garbelli R, et al. Focal cortical dysplasia: neuropathological subtypes, EEG, neuroimaging and surgical outcome. *Brain* 2002; 125(Pt 8):1719–1732.
75. Cepeda C, Andre VM, Levine MS, et al. Epileptogenesis in pediatric cortical dysplasia: the dysmature cerebral developmental hypothesis. *Epilepsy Behav* 2006; 9(2):219–235.
76. Khan RB, Boop FA, Onar A, et al. Seizures in children with low-grade tumors: outcome after tumor resection and risk factors for uncontrolled seizures. *J Neurosurg* 2006; 104(6 Suppl):377–382.
77. Procaccini E, Dorfmuller G, Fohlen M, et al. Surgical management of hypothalamic hamartomas with epilepsy: the stereoendoscopic approach. *Neurosurgery* 2006; 59(4 Suppl 2):ONS336–ONS346.
78. Maixner W. Hypothalamic hamartomas—clinical, neuropathological and surgical aspects. *Childs Nerv Syst* 2006; 22(8):867–873.
79. Regis J, Scavarda D, Tamura M, et al. Epilepsy related to hypothalamic hamartomas: surgical management with special reference to Gamma Knife surgery. *Childs Nerv Syst* 2006; 22(8):881–895.
80. Benifla M, Rutka JT, Logan W, et al. Vagal nerve stimulation for refractory epilepsy in children: indications and experience at The Hospital for Sick Children. *Childs Nerv Syst* 2006; 22(8):1018–1026.
81. Patwardhan RV, Stong B, Bebin EM, et al. Efficacy of vagal nerve stimulation in children with medically refractory epilepsy. *Neurosurgery* 2000; 47(6):1353–1357; discussion 1357–1358.
82. Wong TT, Kwan SY, Chang KP, et al. Corpus callosotomy in children. *Childs Nerv Syst* 2006; 22(8):999–1011.
83. Feichtinger M, Schrottner O, Eder H, et al. Efficacy and safety of radiosurgical callosotomy: a retrospective analysis. *Epilepsia* 2006; 47(7):1184–1191.
84. Wiebe S, Blume WT, Girvin JP, et al. A randomized, controlled trial of surgery for temporal-lobe epilepsy. *N Engl J Med* 2001; 345(5):311–318.
85. Cook SW, Nguyen ST, Hu B, et al. Cerebral hemispherectomy for pediatric epilepsy patients: a comparison of three techniques by pathologic substrate in 115 patients. *J Neurosurg* 2004; 100(2 Suppl Pediatrics):125–141.
86. Brian JE Jr, Deshpande JK, McPherson RW. Management of cerebral hemispherectomy in children. *J Clin Anesth* 1990; 2(2):91–95.
87. Gonzalez-Martinez JA, Gupta A, Kotagal P, et al. Hemispherectomy for catastrophic epilepsy in infants. *Epilepsia* 2005; 46(9):1518–1525.
88. Kossoff EH, Vining EP, Pyzik PL, et al. The postoperative course and management of 106 hemidecortications. *Pediatr Neurosurg* 2002; 37(6):298–303.
89. Kossoff EH, Vining EP, Pillas DJ, et al. Hemispherectomy for intractable unihemispheric epilepsy etiology vs outcome. *Neurology* 2003; 61(7):887–890.
90. Piastra M, Pietrini D, Caresta E, et al. Hemispherectomy procedures in children: haematological issues. *Childs Nerv Syst* 2004; 20(7):453–458.
91. Pietrini D, Zanghi F, Pusateri A, et al. Anesthesiological and intensive care considerations in children undergoing extensive cerebral excision procedure for congenital epileptogenic lesions. *Childs Nerv Syst* 2006; 22(8):844–851.
92. Battaglia D, Di Rocco C, Iuvone L, et al. Neuro-cognitive development and epilepsy outcome in children with surgically treated hemimegalencephaly. *Neuropediatrics* 1999; 30(6):307–313.
93. Di Rocco C, Iannelli A. Hemimegalencephaly and intractable epilepsy: complications of hemispherectomy and their correlations with the surgical technique. A report on 15 cases. *Pediatr Neurosurg* 2000; 33(4):198–207.
94. Caplan R, Siddarth P, Mathern G, et al. Developmental outcome with and without successful intervention. *Int Rev Neurobiol* 2002; 49:269–284.
95. Tellez-Zenteno JF, Dhar R, Wiebe S. Long-term seizure outcomes following epilepsy surgery: a systematic review and meta-analysis. *Brain* 2005; 128(Pt 5):1188–1198.
96. Tonini C, Beghi E, Berg AT, et al. Predictors of epilepsy surgery outcome: a meta-analysis. *Epilepsy Res* 2004; 62(1):75–87.
97. Bien CG, Kurthen M, Baron K, et al. Long-term seizure outcome and antiepileptic drug treatment in surgically treated temporal lobe epilepsy patients: a controlled study. *Epilepsia* 2001; 42(11):1416–1421.
98. Tuxhorn I, Holthausen H, Boenigk H, eds. Paediatric epilepsy syndromes and their surgical treatment. London: John Libbey, 1997.
99. Leiphart JW, Peacock WJ, Mathern GW. Lobar and multilobar resections for medically intractable pediatric epilepsy. *Pediatr Neurosurg* 2001; 34(6):311–318.
100. Chapman K, Wyllie E, Najm I, et al. Seizure outcome after epilepsy surgery in patients with normal preoperative MRI. *J Neurol Neurosurg Psychiatry* 2005; 76(5):710–713.
101. Caplan R, Siddarth P, Bailey CE, et al. Thought disorder: a developmental disability in pediatric epilepsy. *Epilepsy Behav* 2006; 8(4):726–735.
102. Ott D, Siddarth P, Gurbani S, et al. Behavioral disorders in pediatric epilepsy: unmet psychiatric need. *Epilepsia* 2003; 44(4):591–597.
103. Sperling MR, Harris A, Nei M, et al. Mortality after epilepsy surgery. *Epilepsia* 2005; 46 Suppl 11:49–53.
104. Sperling MR, O'Connor MJ, Saykin AJ, et al. Temporal lobectomy for refractory epilepsy. *JAMA* 1996; 276(6):470–475.
105. Duchowny M, Jayakar P, Resnick T, et al. Epilepsy surgery in the first three years of life. *Epilepsia* 1998; 39(7):737–743.
106. Wyllie E, Comair YG, Kotagal P, et al. Epilepsy surgery in infants. *Epilepsia* 1996; 37(7):625–637.

63 Outcome of Epilepsy Surgery in Childhood

Shekhar Patil
J. Helen Cross
William Harkness

The primary aim of epilepsy surgery is relief from seizures, and there are various parameters that may predict the likelihood of seizure freedom. In addition, there are various secondary aims that need to be considered in order to outline realistic expectations to the family. This is particularly relevant in children, where the range of abilities and behavioral phenotypes of those coming to surgery is wide. In the past, predictions of outcome were based on adult series, but there is now a growing literature of outcome in children that can be referred to. As longitudinal data become available, outcome can be measured in both the short and the long term.

COMPLICATIONS OF SURGERY

As a result of advances in neuroimaging, neurosurgical techniques, and neuroanaesthesia, surgical morbidity has been reduced. Nonetheless, no surgical procedure can be carried out without risk, and this truth needs to be clearly communicated to patients and or their families as part of the consent process. Complications (1–5) may occur in the perioperative period (within 30 days of the procedure) or may be delayed. Intraoperative problems (2–5) may include excessive blood loss, derangement of clotting, fluid and electrolyte imbalance, and resultant neurologic deficits. Postoperatively there may be CSF leakage, subdural or intracerebral hemorrhage, hydrocephalus, wound and bone infection, and meningitis (chemical or bacterial). Hydrocephalus may occur as either an early or a late complication of hemispherectomy. In our experience, however, this has been seen in only 9% of our own series of 91 children (unpublished data) 6 weeks to 6 months following surgery.

Risk of infection, hematoma formation, or cerebral edema may increase with the insertion of subdural grids (6, 7) or depth electrodes for seizure localization. The rate of infection ranges between 10% and 12%, depending on the series, and the rate of hemorrhage between 3% and 10%. In the series by Onal (6) et al, 8 out of 35 children implanted developed a hemorrhage, either a subdural or an intracerebral hemorrhage, removed where necessary at the time of explantation of the grid. Five of the hematomas were evacuated, and the rest managed conservatively. They highlight the fact that occurrence of hematomas is directly proportional to the size of the grid and the extent of the bone flap and the importance in avoiding venous compression by the edges of the grid. Also of note is the delayed occurrence of subdural hematomas.

SEIZURE OUTCOME

The primary aim of resective surgery for intractable epilepsy is to achieve seizure freedom. Seizure outcome is related to a number of factors including pathologic substrate, the extent of that substrate and the completeness of its resection, and the type of procedure performed. Factors that have usually been attributed to a poor outcome are a longer duration of epilepsy, normal pathology on histologic evaluation, male sex, an extra temporal focus, and incomplete resection. It is likely, however, that it is the completeness of resection (8–10), whether structurally or electrically defined, that is the most important factor for determining whether a child will become seizure free.

In 2001 the first randomized controlled trial in adults (11) conclusively proved the benefit of epilepsy surgery in temporal lobe epilepsy compared to antiepileptic therapy. Adult studies have demonstrated the greater likelihood of seizure freedom following temporal as opposed to extratemporal resection. Similar results have been demonstrated in pediatric series, although, as yet, no randomized study has taken place (12–14). The seizure-free outcome for temporal lobectomy varies from 60% to 78% depending on the series and the spectrum of operated population (15–32). Foreign tissue lesions may be more common in series with predominantly young patients nearing 5 years of age, whereas hippocampal sclerosis is more common in older populations. Overall, the presence of unilateral EEG abnormalities, extent of resection, and presence of imaging abnormalities predict a good outcome, whereas bilateral or multifocal epileptiform discharges, incomplete resection, and possibly selective resection of mesial temporal structures predict a poor outcome.

A series of children undergoing temporal lobe resection for hippocampal sclerosis revealed similar outcome in those under 12 years of age as in adults, although adult criteria were used for surgical selection (33). A wider series of children with higher degrees of comorbidities appeared to have a lesser chance of seizure freedom (34). Such has previously been attributable to dual pathology, with similar predictors of outcome as seen in adults (antecedent prolonged febrile convulsion, normal IQ), In a more recent series, however, reviewing the outcome in children undergoing temporal lobectomy for a primary diagnosis of hippocampal sclerosis showing a seizure-free rate of 58%, good seizure outcome was unrelated to the preoperative IQ, but predicted by history of febrile status and absence of additional MRI with or without histopathologic abnormalities (32). Low IQ should therefore not be an exclusion criterion for epilepsy surgery (35–37). Other series of a wider range of procedures have agreed with this.

Another group that is being increasingly seen in epilepsy centers consists of children with dual pathology; for instance, mesial temporal sclerosis in addition to cortical dysplasia or other developmental pathologies within the temporal lobe. From 5% to 30% of patients with temporal lobe epilepsy are reported as having dual pathology (38–41), tending to be more frequent in children (33, 41). Surgery in this population has similar results as in individuals with typical temporal lobe epilepsy, provided that there is complete resection of the hippocampus and the second pathology.

Extratemporal resections account for a greater proportion of resectional surgeries performed in children than in adults. As the outcome of such resections is considered to be poorer, it could be assumed that the global outcome in children would be less favorable than in adults. This is well depicted by the study of Fish et al (42), with good outcome in 29% of children and adolescents following frontal lobe resection, compared to 59% with temporal lobe resection. Pediatric series have reported outcome from frontal lobe resections comparable to the adult series. The difference in outcomes between frontal lobe and temporal lobe resections tends to be multifactorial and is probably reflected by poorly defined localization of the epileptogenic zone, the possibility of incomplete or limited resection because of the proximity the eloquent cortices, and involvement of insular cortex less amenable to resective surgery. With the increasing use of intracranial grids as a part of presurgical evaluation, the rates for seizure freedom are showing an improving trend but, as yet, remain lower than the outcomes in temporal lobe surgery. Even with similar pathology, patients with frontal lobe resections for cortical dysplasia (43–47) tend to have a poor outcome in comparison to other resections. There is also variability according to the grade of cortical dysplasia. Some studies report that children with Taylor-type dysplasia have better outcomes (48), approaching 75% seizure freedom at one-year follow up, as opposed to 45–50% for other types of dysplasia, and even within this group of Taylor-type dysplasia those with balloon cells tend to do better than the nonballoon type of dysplasia (49). Others report a better outcome for mild or type I cortical dysplasia (50). However, although the short term outcome (51–54) is reasonably good, the longer-term (53) view may be quite different.

Apparent seizure outcome may relate to the time elapsed following surgery prior to evaluation. The occurrence of seizures in the acute postoperative period in children undergoing extra temporal resections and hemispherectomy is considered to be a poor prognostic sign, with eventual poor seizure outcome at 24 months (55–57). However, most studies report a very good short-term outcome in the first year. This initial advantage gradually fades with time, with cumulative relapses of around 25% (28). In fact, in the latter study (28), the only predictor of a poor outcome was the latency to remission after surgery. A further study (58) puts the outcome at the first follow-up at the end of one year following surgery as a reliable indicator of a long-term outcome, meaning that a good outcome at the first follow-up usually translates to eventual better outcome in the longer term with very few relapses, but of note was the group of 93% undergoing temporal resections versus 7% with extratemporal resections in their cohort of 399 patients. A study (59) by Mathern et al compared a group of 64 children with cortical dysplasia and 71 children with other etiologies such as infection and ischemic etiology to a group of 34 children with temporal lobe resections. At early follow-up, the seizure control in all the groups was equal, but in the long term, at 5 years the children with cortical dysplasia had deteriorated. In another long term review (53), at 10 years seizure freedom was seen in 72% children with developmental tumors and 32% of children with cortical dysplasia, although outcome at two years was indicative of outcome at 10 years.

Parietal and occipital lobe resections have not been reported in large numbers, in contrast to temporal and frontal lobe (60–65). The seizure outcome in occipital epilepsy is related to the pathology, with poor outcome in the developmental malformation group. Identification of a clear demarcation of the epileptogenic zone, presence of a localized lesion on MRI, an acquired pathology, and concordance of investigations carried as part of the presurgical evaluation are positive predictors of a good surgical outcome in occipital lobe epilepsy. Most of the series have studied small populations, but in a large series (65) of 81 patients concentrating on posterior epilepsies, the only predictors of good outcome were shorter duration of epilepsy and a normal neurologic examination prior to surgery. All the studies document an overall benefit of surgery over antiepileptic drug (AED) therapy. Comparative data of series (66) with a long-term follow-up show excellent outcome for temporal lobe resections, followed by posterior epilepsies, whereas median long-term seizure freedom in frontal lobe epilepsies was only 27%.

An important consideration is for children with possible multifocal disease such as tuberous sclerosis. These children tend to have a good outcome if the preoperative evaluation localizes a single tuber or area to be epileptogenic; resection may then alleviate the epilepsy, sometimes with seizure freedom (67, 68). Similar good results have been seen of late with multistage procedures and nonlocalizing scalp EEG; however, the long-term outcome of such procedures has not been evaluated (69). In the only study (70) of long-term follow-up in 22 postsurgical patients of TS followed for 1–14 years, the predictors of favorable outcome were localized and unifocal ictal onset with normal development.

In children undergoing hemispherectomy (71–78), the outcome is related to the completeness of disconnection and the pathology of the substrate. Children with developmental malformations such as hemimegalencephaly and extensive or hemicortical dysplasia have lower rates of seizure freedom, varying between 37% and 58%, as compared to children with acquired pathologies such as Rasmussen encephalitis and vascular pathologies, who tend to have a good outcome, with seizure-free rates between 67% and 88%. Series with older children have reported a greater proportion of those with acquired pathologies and show a good overall outcome, whereas series with young children, especially infants with early-onset epilepsy, appear to have more developmental malformations and less seizure freedom.

A question often asked by parents preoperatively is the likelihood of surgery allowing the drugs to be either reduced or stopped. There is little data on this aspect of care; however, from adult studies, a seizure recurrence is quoted in nearly a third of patients at the end of five years following complete withdrawal of AEDs (79, 80). The risk of relapse in the study by Schiller et al (79) was higher in face of a normal imaging. In another mixed adult and pediatric cohort of 396 postsurgical patients (81), the risk for seizure recurrence in patients who discontinue AED was not different from the risk in those who continue to take the drugs. Data in children are sparse (82, 83), but suggest that although there are predictive factors with regard to seizure freedom, reduction or withdrawal of anticonvulsants cannot be guaranteed, and such information should be included in the counseling of families preoperatively. Hamiwka et al (53), reporting 10-year outcome for children undergoing surgery for cerebral malformations, reported 71% still to be taking anticonvulsant medication at that time, whereas the group of Mathern et al (59) reported 75% to be on anticonvulsants after 5 years. Another group, however, showed that in 20 of 33 patients the drugs could be either reduced or stopped (84), and thus for each individual patient the decision to reduce or discontinue anticonvulsants should be based on the pathophysiologic substrate identified prior to surgical treatment, the completeness of excision of that substrate, any peri- or postoperative complications, and the seizure outcome. Naturally, the views of the family and child are pivotal to this decision and are likely to depend on psychosocial as well as clinical issues.

A number of children are not suitable candidates for primary resective surgery—for example, children with Lennox-Gastaut syndrome who are incapacitated with drop attacks, children with bihemispheric malformations, and children with Landau-Kleffner syndrome. These children may benefit from palliative surgeries such as corpus callosotomy and multiple subpial transections (MST). Outcome for callosotomy is more favorable in children with atonic and tonic attacks, with approximately 60–80% benefiting from the procedure with more than 50% drop in the seizure frequency (85–87). Studies have shown a seizure freedom rate with callosotomy and on concomitant AED between 10% and 20%. The main role of multiple transections is in patients with epileptogenic zone within the eloquent cortex. This procedure can be combined with cortical resection. Seizure freedom with isolated MST (88, 89) is highly improbable, but with additional procedure of resection, seizure-free outcome may be seen in 40–50% of patients.

The final group to consider is those patients in whom surgery is either turned down or not deemed to be an option. Natural history data in individuals with medically refractory localization-related epilepsy who do not undergo surgery paint a uniformly dismal picture, quoting the seizure freedom rate of approx 8–11% at one-year follow-up (11, 90), whereas in longer-term follow-up, the study by Selwa et al (91) in predominantly an adult population showed a seizure free outcome ranging from 15% to 21% in their cohort of 34 cases. This was again confirmed in a further study, with seizure freedom that varied between 14% and 21% in unoperated localization-related epilepsy (92). Thus, the true benefit of surgery over best medical therapy may yet be unknown. Another consideration is whether surgery affects the long-term risk of mortality. After epilepsy surgery, patients who have recurrent seizures had a standard mortality ratio of 5.75 as compared to the patients with seizure freedom. This benefit of seizure freedom following surgery tends to counter the negative effect of intractable epilepsy on survival (93). As most of the data from adult studies are used to predict the outcomes in pediatric population, this benefit in survival may be seen in children with intractable epilepsy rendered seizure free following surgery.

NEURODEVELOPMENTAL OUTCOME

Neuropsychologic evaluation is an important aspect of presurgical evaluation. The neuropsychologic profile can sometimes aid the laterality and localization of seizures, and knowledge of the degree of cognitive impairment serves as a baseline for postoperative assessment and outcome. This is important from the point of postoperative functioning, as the evaluations of mental reserve capacity allows for a predictive postoperative profile that can be used for counseling and advising on the risks of surgery. This can be used as a tool to evaluate the surgical outcome and quality of life–related issues.

It is of prime importance to consider the potential effects of epilepsy surgery on the development and cognition of any child. There is growing evidence that early-onset, poorly controlled epilepsy has an adverse impact on cognition, hampering normal development (94, 95). Vargha-Khadem (96, 97) showed that patients with early cerebral damage show a greater deficit if associated with onset of epilepsy under the age of 5 years, implying a negative effect of epilepsy on the brain development. It could therefore be presumed that early treatment with epilepsy surgery could give a window of opportunity to allow for more optimal development of the brain, but this has been difficult to quantify. Duchowny et al (98) concluded that cortical resection in very young children with catastrophic epilepsy does not guarantee an optimal or improved neurologic development, and perceptions of accelerated development in patients rendered seizure free was not confirmed on formal developmental assessment. This is not surprising when one considers that IQ is a measure of development relative to peers of normal development, and therefore a maintained, though not increased, IQ indicates maintained progress relative to peers, preferable to the deterioration that could possibly be expected with continuing seizures. Freitag et al (99) proposed early intervention to at least stabilize the developmental velocity. A recent study by Battaglia et al (100) found that the cognitive level is generally unchanged in a majority of cases postsurgery, with very few patients showing either a sustained improvement or impairment. Their study showed a stable cognitive outcome in 71.5% of children, with improvement seen in 13.3%. There is also no consensus as to whether there is an optimal time for intervention. It does seem from studies (99, 101), however, that early intervention does not really impact on the eventual cognitive outcome, although in children with infantile spasms a shorter duration of epilepsy leads to better neurodevelopmental outcome (102).

Focal Resections

Data to date suggest that temporal lobe resection in carefully selected candidates is unlikely to have a cognitive impact in children. In one of the largest reported multicenter series on outcome of temporal lobectomy (103), approximately 82% of children did not experience any significant change in their presurgical scores for verbal or performance IQ regardless of the side of surgery, but the individual analysis does show an increase in the performance IQ regardless of the laterality of surgery. A significant decline in global IQ following temporal lobectomy is unlikely to occur (104), but in those with a decline in cognition the investigators propose the influence of the underlying pathology on the eventual outcome. There was no correlation between the seizure laterality and verbal or nonverbal cognitive functioning, and temporal lobe seizures had an equal effect on the verbal reasoning and nonverbal problem-solving capacity irrespective of their side of onset. Earlier studies (105–107) had suggested postoperative decline in verbal memory in the short term, but in the long term and, in particular, in the pediatric population, two studies (107, 108), failed to show any change in the memory at 12 and 24 months after surgery from the preoperative scores. That this deficit is clearly reversible has been well demonstrated more recently by a prospective study (109) that showed a greater recovery of memory deficits in children than in adults undergoing temporal lobectomy. Their data suggest an increased neuronal plasticity in childhood, with a proposal of a strong argument in favor of early surgery.

Literature review shows a dearth of information on other lobar resections. There are very few studies on postsurgical series in children with frontal lobe and posterior epilepsies (100). Preoperative groups with frontal lobe epilepsy have deficits in the domain of executive functioning and motor coordination. Lendt et al (111, 112) compared the one-year postsurgical cognitive profiles in groups of 12 children, one group with temporal and the other with frontal lobe epilepsy. Both groups showed important gains in attention, processing speed, memory, and bimanual coordination. Surgery did not lead to any additional impairment. The neuropsychologic profile in frontal lobe epilepsy (113) is akin to that of adults with frontal lobe lesions. Surgical outcome has no bearing on the postoperative neuropsychologic profile in children with frontal lobe epilepsy in both good- and poor-seizure-outcome groups. Some gains, albeit insignificant, are made in the domain of motor coordination. Data from other studies lend weight to offering surgery to suitable candidates, as the benefits from epilepsy surgery far outweigh the risks of inflicting minor deficits in the form of working memory and visual constructional skills (114, 115).

The posterior epilepsies are relatively rare in children. In terms of cognition, the posterior cortex plays an important role in attention and visuoconstructional abilities (116, 117). In general the group of patients with posterior epilepsies (100) has a low IQ compared to groups of temporal or frontal lobe epilepsy. The deficit is especially in the domain of visuoconstruction performance; also of note is the fact that the effects are even more disabling in children with early-onset damage to the posterior cortex. Sinclair et al (77) studied a group of children undergoing extratemporal resections, and within this group the children with frontal lobe epilepsy were relatively better preserved, with a mean full-scale IQ nine points higher than in the children with posterior epilepsies, and the postsurgical outcome mirrored the preoperative assessment. Postoperatively, except for an improvement in the sphere of verbal learning, there was no change in the intellectual functioning and memory. Similar results of a stable postoperative cognitive profile were seen in a group of 26 children (118). Even though the group is quite small, the data show no impairment or adverse effects of surgery on the intelligence or memory. Mabbott and Smith (119) assessed memory in a series of 44 children and adolescents undergoing temporal or extratemporal resection and found no significant decline in memory in either group of children. Children have variable performance on the tasks used for assessment. Within the surgical groups, some children perform poorly within tasks, while others perform well on the same tasks. The observed variability may be dependent on several factors, probably including age, duration of epilepsy, nature of material used to test memory, and number of medications. Also of note is the effect of age at onset; children with older age of seizure onset performed better on tasks of verbal memory and face recognition.

Hemispherectomy

Many children coming to this procedure have developmental malformations as their underlying responsible pathology, such as hemimegalencephaly (120) or widespread hemispheric cortical dysplasia. The remaining patients have other etiologies such as Rasmussen encephalitis or vascular pathology. Both the groups tend to have a low IQ/DQ preoperatively; but the deficit is most marked in the group with developmental malformations (121–23). This is particularly relevant, considering the data suggest that age of onset of epilepsy is likely to have a major impact on ultimate developmental outcome, and the onset tends to be earlier in the group with developmental malformations (124, 125). Most studies do not show any significant longitudinal change with regards to developmental and cognitive outcome following hemispherectomy. There are a few studies that do report some gain (98, 120–122), whereas others have reported loss of skills postoperatively, predominantly in those with acquired pathology (124). In a group of 71 children (124), 11 children showed a decline of more than 15 points in the IQ at follow-up, but eight of the 11 children had Rasmussen syndrome, and the decline may have been a result of the progressive nature of the disease. Even in this study almost 80% of the children had a postoperative neuropsychologic profile similar to or slightly better than the preoperative score.

The majority of children who come to hemispherectomy are developmentally delayed, as verified by data from the literature. This has not been a criterion to exclude them from a surgical program. Evidence to date suggests that, although we aim to optimize neurodevelopment, we are more likely to prevent possible further cognitive damage from ongoing epilepsy. Data to date suggest the final outcome to be usually comparable to the preoperative level of functioning, suggesting a maintenance of the developmental trajectory. Children who are well maintained preoperatively tend to do better than those with poor developmental skills (126). A recent meta-analysis (127) showed a better outcome in children than in adults, and the short-term cognitive outcomes were maintained in the longer term. Overall, children undergoing left hemispherectomy (128) with early-onset epilepsy and developmental malformations have a poor cognitive profile as compared to children with right hemispheric lesions, and this translates to a similar postoperative profile.

FUNCTIONAL OUTCOME

When deciding on whether resective surgery should be offered, the likelihood of inflicting a possible neurologic deficit should be carefully considered. The presurgical evaluation is undertaken with meticulous care to reduce the chance of causing this deficit, by outlining the eloquent cortices and, if necessary, using invasive monitoring with subdural grids and functional stimulation. Recently, with the advent of functional imaging to complement the presurgical evaluation and mapping of the motor and language cortex, the need for invasive monitoring for delineation of eloquent cortex has been reduced. In each individual case the risk-benefit ratio needs to be carefully considered.

Reorganization (129–132) of the eloquent cortices has a bearing on the eventual area of resection. Early-onset epilepsy may be presumed to lead to a greater chance of relocalization of function, but studies have shown that language and motor function (129–132) may be localized within dysplastic cortex. In such cases the risk of postoperative functional deficit is very high. The majority of children with congenital hemiplegia (associated with a structural brain pathology) and early-onset epilepsy can expect little change between pre- and postoperative functional status, although a visual field defect is inevitable if not present preoperatively. Surgery for right-sided lesions (128) in the acquired pathology group tends to have a better outcome; overall, however, the outcome is poor in the developmental pathologies as compared to the acquired pathologies. Curtiss et al (133) showed a better outcome for right-sided hemispherectomies with underlying acquired pathologies, but even the left hemispherectomies may have better postoperative performance on the subdomains of language function, suggesting that the right hemisphere can support language reorganization, with better receptive language than expressive (134). Also in the study by Curtiss et al (133), postoperative seizure outcome had a positive impact on language development in children with developmental pathologies.

Frank aphasia and major language dysfunction are usually not seen after standard temporal lobe resection. The only deficit seen in patients with dominant temporal lobe resection is in naming and, probably, verbal learning (135). This too usually resolves within 6–12 months of surgery. Verbal fluency is unaffected in both dominant and nondominant resection.

Hemiparesis is an expected effect of hemispherectomy, but focal motor deficits may be seen in focal, lobar, or multilobar resections encroaching upon eloquent cortex. The degree of motor deficit will vary with time, and many deficits improve, suggesting that the cause is reversible, such as edema or ischemia, or that in the longer term some reorganization can take place. In a group (136) of 15 children posthemispherectomy, etiology-specific differences in reorganization of the remaining cortex were shown. Ambulation is important for independence, and in those undergoing hemispherectomy (137), children who are ambulant prior to surgery continue to remain so after surgery irrespective of developmental and acquired pathologies. In terms of other musculature, they do show slight deterioration in their function within the first few months after surgery, but they usually recover to near the presurgical level of functioning except for finger dexterity and power in the distal upper limb musculature.

Formal discussion with the parents and the child regarding the expected motor, visual, or language deficit will eventually decide the optimum time for surgery. The risk-benefit assessment should be discussed at length before offering surgery. This is particularly true for children with progressive conditions such as Rasmussen encephalitis and Sturge-Weber syndrome.

BEHAVIORAL AND PSYCHIATRIC OUTCOME

The prevalence of behavioral problems in intractable childhood epilepsy is high (138), and a proportion of these children will enter a surgical program for evaluation. Psychiatric disorder (34) is reported in 29% of children with idiopathic generalized seizures and in 58% of children with seizures and structural brain abnormality. Davies et al (139) showed that the presence of psychiatric disorder and behavioral problems adds to the already significant disability in these children. At times, behavior can be the most challenging aspect of epilepsy management.

Surgery for epilepsy has a variable impact on the psychiatric and behavioral outcome postoperatively. Few of the patients improve, few worsen, and few remain the same, while (140) a further proportion develop new symptoms following surgery for epilepsy (34, 141). Although new symptoms may evolve in previously normal children, it is generally seen that absence of psychiatric disorder preoperatively predicts a good postoperative psychiatric outcome. Thus, epilepsy surgery has a predominantly positive effect on the behavioral outcome in children with intractable epilepsy beginning early in life. Psychiatric and behavioral outcomes in slightly older children are unclear, with variable results, as mentioned previously. Following surgery there appears to be a risk of precipitating new psychiatric disorders with a *Diagnostic and Statistical Manual* (DSM) *IV* diagnosis in a proportion of these children.

When hemispherectomy was first described by MacKenzie in 1938 and subsequently by Krynau in the 1950s, it was noted that significant improvement in behavior could be achieved. In one study (142) 36 of 50 children had severe behavioral problems that resolved in 54% of the children postsurgery and improved in a further 40%. White (143), looking at 144 surgeries for infantile hemiplegia and epilepsy, saw behavior improve in 80% of the 108 patients with behavioral dysfunction. Later studies show behavioral difficulty in 33% of children preoperatively, with improvement in all but one child and new symptoms emerging in five children. In the study by Pulsifer et al (124), there was no difference in the pre- and postoperative scores as measured by the Child Behavior Check List (CBCL).

The rate of behavioral disorders in children coming to temporal lobe resection is high (34), with 83% demonstrating a DSM IV diagnosis at any point pre- and postoperatively. Though poor postoperative seizure control heralds a poor outcome in psychiatric symptoms in adults, studies in children fail to confirm this observation, although in the group of McLellan et al (34), 24% of seizure-free children lost the DSM IV diagnosis, whereas only 4% from the poor-seizure-outcome group lost their diagnosis. Szabo et al (141), in their small series of five patients, did not find any significant change between the pre- and postoperative behavior in children with pervasive developmental disorder undergoing temporal lobectomy for the treatment of epilepsy. Whether the natural history of the disorder may be influenced by early surgery and seizure control remains under debate (144). Lendt et al (145) looked at a cohort of 56 children, with a study group and a control group of 28 children each. The 28 children underwent surgery, and the control group was managed medically. On review of the CBCL scores, there was normalization of behavior in the study group; at the same time, the control group had new emergent behavioral issues. This study highlights the likelihood of impact of surgery on behavioral outcome as opposed to the natural history of the condition.

CONCLUSIONS

Surgery for epilepsy in childhood can confer considerable benefits, not only with regard to seizure control but also with regard to neurodevelopmental and behavioral outcome. The degree to which the latter can be achieved, however, is difficult to assess in each individual case. Such needs to be considered carefully, and the likely outcome, however uncertain, in all domains should be outlined to the family prior to any final decision. Further prospective data collection is required to enable more accurate preoperative counseling.

References

1. Salanova V, Markand O, Worth R. Temporal lobe epilepsy surgery: outcome, complications, and late mortality rate in 215 patients. *Epilepsia* 2002; 43(2):170–174.
2. Kelley RE, DellaBadia J, Minagar A, Kelley BJ, et al. Neuroimaging of the complications of epilepsy surgery. *J Neuroimaging* 2004; 14(1):33–41.
3. Rydenhag B, Silander HC. Complications of epilepsy surgery after 654 procedures in Sweden, September 1990–1995: a multicenter study based on the Swedish National Epilepsy Surgery Register. *Neurosurgery* 2001; 49(1):51–57.
4. Behrens E, Schramm J, Zentner J, Konig R. Surgical and neurological complications in a series of 708 epilepsy surgery procedures. *Neurosurgery* 1997; 41(1):1–9; discussion 9–10.
5. Benbadis S, Chelune GJ, Stanford LD, Comair YG. Outcome and complications of epilepsy surgery. In: Wyllie E, ed. *The Treatment of Epilepsy: Principles and Practice*. 2nd ed. Philadelphia. Wiliams & Wilkins; 1997:1103–1120.
6. Onal C, Otsubo H, Araki T, et al. Complications of invasive subdural grid monitoring in children with epilepsy. *J Neurosurg* 2003; 98(5):1017–1026.
7. Hamser HM. Complications of invasive video-EEG monitoring with subdural grid electrodes. *Neurology* 2002; 58(1):97–103.
8. Hader WJ, Mackay M, Otsubo H, et al. Cortical dysplastic lesions in children with intractable epilepsy: role of complete resection. *J Neurosurg* 2004; 100(2 Suppl Pediatrics):110–117.
9. Paolicchi JM, Jayakar P, Dean P, et al. Predictors of outcome in pediatric epilepsy surgery. *Neurology* 2000; 54(3):642–647.
10. Wyllie E, Luders H, Morris HH 3rd, et al. Clinical outcome after complete or partial cortical resection for intractable epilepsy. *Neurology* 1987; 37(10):1634–1641.
11. Wiebe S, Blume WT, Girvin JP, Eliasziw M. A randomized, controlled trial: surgery for temporal-lobe epilepsy. *N Engl J Med* 2001; 345(5):311–318.
12. Davidson S, Falconer MA. Outcome of surgery in 40 children with temporal lobe epilepsy. *Lancet* 1975; 1(7919):1260–1263.
13. Terra-Bustamante VC, Inuzuca LM, Fernandes RM, et al. Temporal lobe epilepsy surgery in children and adolescents: clinical characteristics and post-surgical outcome. *Seizure* 2005; 14(4):274–281.
14. Blume WT. Temporal lobe epilepsy surgery in childhood: rationale for greater use. *Can J Neurol Sci* 1997; 24(2):95–98.
15. Mittal S, Montes JL, Farmer JP, et al. Long-term outcome after surgical treatment of temporal lobe epilepsy in children. *J Neurosurg* 2005; 103(5 Suppl):401–412.
16. Sotero de Menezes MA, Connolly M, Bolanos A, et al. Temporal lobectomy in early childhood: the need for long-term follow-up. *J Child Neurol* 2001; 16(8):585–590.
17. Duchowny M, Levin B, Jayakar P, et al. Temporal lobectomy in early childhood. *Epilepsia* 1992; 33(2):298–303.
18. Jarrar RG, Buchhalter JR, Meyer FB, Sharbrough FW, et al. Long-term follow-up of temporal lobectomy in children. *Neurology* 2002; 59(10):1635–1637.
19. Cross JH. Epilepsy surgery in childhood. *Epilepsia* 2002; 43 Suppl 3:65–70.
20. Harkness W. Temporal lobe resections. *Childs Nerv Syst* 2006; 22(8):936–944.
21. Sinclair DB, Aronyk K, Snyder T, et al. Pediatric temporal lobectomy for epilepsy. *Pediatr Neurosurg* 2003; 38(4):195–205.
22. Hennessy MJ, Elwes RD, Rabe-Hesketh S, et al. Prognostic factors in the surgical treatment of medically intractable epilepsy associated with mesial temporal sclerosis. *Acta Neurol Scand* 2001; 103:344–350.
23. Cataltepe O, Turanli G, Yalgnizoglu D, Topcu M, et al. Surgical management of temporal tumor-related epilepsy in children. *J Neurosurg* 2005; 102(3 Suppl):280–287.
24. Kuzniecky R, Ho SS, Martin R, et al. Temporal lobe developmental malformations and hippocampal sclerosis: epilepsy surgical outcome. *Neurology* 1999; 52:479–484.
25. Clusmann H, Kral T, Gleissner U, et al. Analysis of different types of resections for pediatric patients with temporal lobe epilepsy. *Neurosurgery* 2004; 54(4):847–860.
26. Salanova V, Markand O, Worth R. Temporal lobe epilepsy: analysis of failures and the role of reoperation. *Acta Neurol Scand* 2005; 111(2):126–133.
27. Sinclair DB, Aronyk K, Snyder T, et al. Pediatric temporal lobectomy for epilepsy. *Pediatr Neurosurg* 2003; 38(4):195–205.
28. Spencer SS, Berg AT, Vickrey BG, Sperling MR, et al. Predicting long-term seizure outcome after resective epilepsy surgery. The Multicenter Study. *Neurology* 2005; 65:912–918.
29. Terra-Bustamante VC, Fernandes RM, Inuzuca LM, et al. Surgically amenable epilepsies in children and adolescents: clinical, imaging, electrophysiological, and post-surgical outcome data. *Childs Nerv Syst* 2005; 21(7):546–551.
30. Wyllie E, Chee M, Granstrom ML, et al. Temporal lobe epilepsy in early childhood. *Epilepsia* 1993; 34(5):859–868.
31. Zaatreh MM, Firlik KS, Spencer DD, Spencer SS. Temporal lobe tumoral epilepsy: characteristics and predictors of surgical outcome. *Neurology* 2003; 61(5):636–641.
32. Fung CW, Scott RC, Harding B, et al. Clinical spectrum of paediatric patients with mesial temporal lobe epilepsy: hippocampal sclerosis and post surgical outcome. *Epilepsia* 2005; 46(Suppl 6):51 (abstract).
33. Mohamed A, Wyllie E, Ruggieri P, Kotagal P, et al. Temporal lobe epilepsy due to hippocampal sclerosis in pediatric candidates for epilepsy surgery. *Neurology* 2001; 56(12):1643–1649.
34. McLellan A, Davies S, Heyman I, et al. Psychopathology in children with epilepsy before and after temporal lobe resection. *Dev Med Child Neurol* 2005; 47(10):666–672.
35. Levisohn PM. Epilepsy surgery in children with developmental disabilities. *Semin Pediatr Neurol* 2000; 7(3):194–203.
36. Gleissner U, Johanson K, Helmstaedter C, Elger CE. Surgical outcome in a group of low-IQ patients with focal epilepsy. *Epilepsia* 1999; 40(5):553–559.
37. Gleissner U, Clusmann H, Sassen R, Elger CE, et al. Postsurgical outcome in pediatric patients with epilepsy: a comparison of patients with intellectual disabilities, subaverage intelligence, and average-range intelligence. *Epilepsia* 2006; 47(2):406–414.

38. Cendes F, Cook MJ, Watson C, et al. Frequency and characteristics of dual pathology in patients with lesional epilepsy. *Neurology* 1995; 45(11):2058–2064.
39. Li LM, Cendes F, Watson C, et al. Surgical treatment of patients with single and dual pathology: relevance of lesion and of hippocampal atrophy to seizure outcome. *Neurology*. 1997; 48(2):437–444.
40. Li LM, Cendes F, Andermann F, et al. Surgical outcome in patients with epilepsy and dual pathology. *Brain* 1999; 122(Pt 5):799–805.
41. Salanova V, Markand O, Worth R. Temporal lobe epilepsy: analysis of patients with dual pathology. *Acta Neurol Scand* 2004; 109(2):126–131.
42. Fish DR, Smith SJ, Quesney LF, Andermann F, et al. Surgical treatment of children with medically intractable frontal or temporal lobe epilepsy: results and highlights of 40 years' experience. *Epilepsia* 1993; 34(2):244–247.
43 Leiphart JW, Peacock WJ, Mathern GW. Lobar and multilobar resections for medically intractable pediatric epilepsy. *Pediatr Neurosurg* 2001; 34(6):311–318.
44. Kral T, Kuczaty S, Blumcke I, et al. Postsurgical outcome of children and adolescents with medically refractory frontal lobe epilepsies. *Childs Nerv Syst* 2001; 17(10):595–601.
45. Bast T, Ramantani G, Seitz A, Rating D. Focal cortical dysplasia: prevalence, clinical presentation and epilepsy in children and adults. *Acta Neurol Scand* 2006; 113(2): 72–81.
46. Kral T, Clusmann H, Blumcke I et al. Outcome of epilepsy surgery in focal cortical dysplasia. *J Neurol Neurosurg Psychiatry* 2003; 74(2):183–188.
47. Kloss S, Pieper T, Pannek H, Holthausen H, et al. Epilepsy surgery in children with focal cortical dysplasia (FCD): results of long-term seizure outcome. *Neuropediatrics* 2002; 33(1):21–26.
48. Tassi L, Colombo N, Garbelli R, et al. Focal cortical dysplasia: neuropathological subtypes, EEG, neuroimaging and surgical outcome. *Brain* 2002; 125(Pt 8):1719–1732.
49. Lawson JA, Birchansky S, Pacheco E. Distinct clinicopathologic subtypes of cortical dysplasia of Taylor. *Neurology* 2005; 64(1):55–61.
50. Fauser S, Schulze-Bonhage A, Honegger J, et al. Focal cortical dysplasias: surgical outcome in 67 patients in relation to histological subtypes and dual pathology. *Brain* 2004; 127(Pt 11):2406–2418.
51. Sisodiya SM. Surgery for malformations of cortical development causing epilepsy. *Brain* 2000; 123(Pt 6):1075–1091.
52. Luders H, Schuele SU. Epilepsy surgery in patients with malformations of cortical development. *Curr Opin Neurol* 2006; 19(2):169–174.
53. Hamiwka L, Jayakar P, Resnick T et al. Surgery for epilepsy due to cortical malformations: ten-year follow-up. Epilepsia. 2005 Apr; 46(4):556-60.
54. Park CK, Kim SK, Wang KC, et al. Surgical outcome and prognostic factors of pediatric epilepsy caused by cortical dysplasia. *Childs Nerv Syst* 2006; 22(6):586–592.
55. Mani J, Gupta A, Mascha E, Lachhwani D, et al. Postoperative seizures after extratemporal resections and hemispherectomy in pediatric epilepsy. *Neurology* 2006; 66(7):1038–1043.
56. Park K, Buchhalter J, McClelland R, Raffel C. Frequency and significance of acute postoperative seizures following epilepsy surgery in children and adolescents. *Epilepsia* 2002; 43(8):874–881.
57. Koh S, Nguyen S, Asarnow RF, et al. Five or more acute postoperative seizures predict hospital course and long-term seizure control after hemispherectomy. *Epilepsia* 2004; 45(5):527–533.
58. Cohen-Gadol AA, Ozduman K, Bronen RA, Kim JH, et al. Long-term outcome after epilepsy surgery for focal cortical dysplasia. *J Neurosurg* 2004; 101(1):55–65.
59. Mathern GW, Giza CC, Yudovin S, Vinters HV. Postoperative seizure control and antiepileptic drug use in pediatric epilepsy surgery patients: the UCLA experience, 1986–1997. *Epilepsia* 1999; 40(12):1740–1749.
60. Kun Lee S, Young Lee S, Kim DW, Soo Lee D, et al. Occipital lobe epilepsy: clinical characteristics, surgical outcome, and role of diagnostic modalities. *Epilepsia* 2005; 46(5):688–695.
61. Aykut-Bingol C, Bronen RA, Kim JH, Spencer DD, et al. Surgical outcome in occipital lobe epilepsy: implications for pathophysiology. *Ann Neurol* 1998; 44(1):60–69.
62. Kim DW, Lee SK, Yun CH, et al. Parietal lobe epilepsy: the semiology, yield of diagnostic workup, and surgical outcome. *Epilepsia* 2004; 45(6):641–649.
63. Sinclair DB, Wheatley M, Snyder T, Gross D, et al. Posterior resection for childhood epilepsy. *Pediatr Neurol* 2005; 32(4):257–263.
64. Yun CH, Lee SK, Lee SY, Kim KK, et al. Prognostic factors in neocortical epilepsy surgery: multivariate analysis. *Epilepsia* 2006; 47(3):574–579.
65. Dalmagro CL, Bianchin MM, Velasco TR. Clinical features of patients with posterior cortex epilepsies and predictors of surgical outcome. *Epilepsia* 2005; 46(9):1442–1449.
66. Tellez-Zenteno JF, Dhar R, Wiebe S. Long-term seizure outcomes following epilepsy surgery: a systematic review and meta-analysis. *Brain* 2005; 128(5):1188–1198.
67. Lachhwani DK, Pestana E, Gupta A, Kotagal P, et al. Identification of candidates for epilepsy surgery in patients with tuberous sclerosis. *Neurology* 2005; 64(9):1651–1654.
68. Koh S, Jayakar P, Dunoyer C, et al. Epilepsy surgery in children with tuberous sclerosis complex: presurgical evaluation and outcome. *Epilepsia* 2000; 41(9):1206–1213.
69. Weiner HL, Carlson C, Ridgway EB, Zaroff CM, et al. Epilepsy surgery in young children with tuberous sclerosis: results of a novel approach. *Pediatrics* 2006; 117(5): 1494–1502.
70. Jarrar RG, Buchhalter JR, Raffel C. Long-term outcome of epilepsy surgery in patients with tuberous sclerosis. *Neurology* 2004; 62:479–481.
71. Gonzalez-Martinez JA, Gupta A, Kotagal P, et al. Hemispherectomy for catastrophic epilepsy in infants. *Epilepsia* 2005; 46(9):1518–1525.
72. Carreno M, Wyllie E, Bingaman W, Kotagal P, et al. Seizure outcome after functional hemispherectomy for malformations of cortical development. *Neurology* 2001; 57(2):331–333.
73. Devlin AM, Cross JH, Harkness W, Chong WK, et al. Clinical outcomes of hemispherectomy for epilepsy in childhood and adolescence. *Brain* 2003; 126(Pt 3):556–566.
74. Jonas R, Nguyen S, Hu B, et al. Cerebral hemispherectomy: hospital course, seizure, developmental, language, and motor outcomes. *Neurology* 2004; 62(10):1712–1721.
75. Kossoff EH, Vining EP, Pillas DJ, et al. Hemispherectomy for intractable unihemispheric epilepsy etiology vs outcome. *Neurology* 2003; 61(7):887–890.
76. Van Oijen M, De Waal H, Van Rijen PC, Jennekens-Schinkel A, et al. Dutch Collaborative Epilepsy Surgery Program. Resective epilepsy surgery in childhood: the Dutch experience 1992–2002. *Eur J Paediatr Neurol* 2006; 10(3):114–123.
77. Sinclair DB, Aronyk K, Snyder T, et al. Extratemporal resection for childhood epilepsy. *Pediatr Neurol* 2004; 30(3):177–185.
78. Wyllie E, Comair YG, Kotagal P, Bulacio J, et al. Seizure outcome after epilepsy surgery in children and adolescents. *Ann Neurol* 1998; 44(5):740–748.
79. Schiller Y, Cascino GD, So EL, Marsh WR. Discontinuation of antiepileptic drugs after successful epilepsy surgery. *Neurology* 2000; 54(2):346–349.
80. Schmidt D, Baumgartner C, Loscher W. Seizure recurrence after planned discontinuation of antiepileptic drugs in seizure-free patients after epilepsy surgery: a review of current clinical experience. *Epilepsia* 2004; 45(2):179–186.
81. Berg AT, Vickrey BG, Langfitt JT, et al; Multicenter Study of Epilepsy Surgery. Reduction of AEDs in postsurgical patients who attain remission. *Epilepsia* 2006; 47(1):64–71.
82. Hoppe C, Poepel A, Sassen R, Elger CE. Discontinuation of anticonvulsant medication after epilepsy surgery in children. *Epilepsia* 2006; 47(3):580–583.
83. Camfield P, Camfield C. The frequency of intractable seizures after stopping AEDs in seizure-free children with epilepsy. *Neurology* 2005; 64(6):973–975.
84. Gilliam F, Wyllie E, Kashden J, et al. Epilepsy surgery outcome: comprehensive assessment in children. *Neurology* 1997; 48(5):1368–1374.
85. Turanli G, Yalnizoglu D, Genc-Acikgoz D, Akalan N, et al. Outcome and long term follow-up after corpus callosotomy in childhood onset intractable epilepsy. *Childs Nerv Syst* 2006; 22(10):1322–1327.
86. Kawai K, Shimizu H, Yagishita A, Maehara T, et al. Clinical outcomes after corpus callosotomy in patients with bihemispheric malformations of cortical development. *J Neurosurgery* 2004; 101(Pediatrics 1):7–15.
87. Wong TT, Kwan SY, Chang KP, et al. Corpus callosotomy in children. *Childs Nerv Syst* 2006; 22(8):999–1011.
88. Benifla M, Otsubo H, Ochi A, Snead OC 3rd, et al. Multiple subpial transections in pediatric epilepsy: indications and outcomes. *Childs Nerv Syst* 2006; 22(8):992–998.
89. Blount JP, Langburt W, Otsubo H, et al. Multiple subpial transections in the treatment of pediatric epilepsy. *J Neurosurg* 2004; 100:118–124.
90. Vickrey BG, Hays RD, Rausch R, et al. Outcomes in 248 patients who had diagnostic evaluations for epilepsy surgery. *Lancet* 1995; 346:1445–1449.
91. Selwa LM, Schmidt SL, Malow BA, Beydoun A. Long-term outcome of nonsurgical candidates with medically refractory localization-related epilepsy. *Epilepsia* 2003; 44(12):1568–1572.
92. Bien CG, Schulze-Bonhage A, Soeder BM, Schramm J, et al. Assessment of the long-term effects of epilepsy surgery with three different reference groups. *Epilepsia* 2006; 47(11):1865–1869.
93. Sperling MR, Harris A, Nei M, Liporace JD, et al. Mortality after epilepsy surgery. *Epilepsia* 2005; 46 Suppl 11:49–53.
94. Hirsch E, Schmitz B, Carreno M. Epilepsy, antiepileptic drugs (AEDs) and cognition. *Acta Neurol Scand Suppl* 2003; 180:23–32.
95. Oguni H, Mukahira K, Tanaka T, Awaya Y, et al. Surgical indication for refractory childhood epilepsy. *Epilepsia* 2000; 41 Suppl 9:21–25.
96. Vargha-Khadem F, Isaacs E, van der Werf S, Robb S, et al. Development of intelligence and memory in children with hemiplegic cerebral palsy. The deleterious consequences of early seizures. *Brain* 1992; 115 Pt 1:315–329.
97. Vargha-Khadem F, Polkey CE. A review of cognitive outcome after hemidecortication in humans. *Adv Exp Med Biol* 1992; 325:137–151.
98. Duchowny M, Jayakar P, Resnick T, et al. Epilepsy surgery in the first three years of life. *Epilepsia* 1998; 39(7):737–743.
99. Freitag H, Tuxhorn I. Cognitive function in preschool children after epilepsy surgery: rationale for early intervention. *Epilepsia* 2005; 46(4):561–567.
100. Battaglia D, Chieffo D, Lettori D, Perrino F, et al. Cognitive assessment in epilepsy surgery of children. *Childs Nerv Syst* 2006; 22(8):744–759.
101. Caplan R, Siddarth P, Mathern G, et al. Developmental outcome with and without successful intervention. *Int Rev Neurobiol* 2002; 49:269–284.
102. Jonas R, Asarnow RF, LoPresti C, et al. Surgery for symptomatic infant-onset epileptic encephalopathy with and without infantile spasms. *Neurology* 2005; 64(4):746–750.
103. Westerveld M, Sass KJ, Chelune GJ, et al. Temporal lobectomy in children: cognitive outcome. *J Neurosurg* 2000; 92(1):24–30.
104. Lah S, Joy P, Bakker K, Miller L. Verbal memory and IQ in children who undergo focal resection for intractable epilepsy: a clinical review. *Brain Impairment* 2002; 3:114–121.
105. Szabo CA, Wyllie E, Stanford LD, et al. Neuropsychological effect of temporal lobe resection in preadolescent children with epilepsy. *Epilepsia* 1998; 39(8):814–819.
106. Gleissner U, Sassen R, Lendt M, Clusmann H, et al. Pre and postoperative verbal memory in pediatric patients with temporal lobe epilepsy. *Epilepsy Res* 2002; 51:287–296.
107. Adams CBT, Beardsworth ED, Oxbury SM, Oxbury JM, et al. Temporal lobectomy in 44 children: outcome and neuropsychological follow-up. *J Epilepsy* 1990; 3(Supp 1):157–168.
108. Lou Smith M, Elliott IM, Lach L. Memory outcome after pediatric epilepsy surgery: objective and subjective perspectives. *Child Neuropsychol* 2006; 12(3):151–164.
109. Gleissner U, Sassen R, Schramm J, Elger CE, et al. Greater functional recovery after temporal lobe epilepsy surgery in children. *Brain* 2005; 128(12):2822–2829.

110. Vaz SA. Nonverbal memory functioning following right anterior temporal lobectomy: a meta-analytic review. Seizure. 2004 Oct; 13(7):446-52.
111. Lendt M, Helmstaedter C, Elger CE. Pre and postoperative neuropsychological profiles in children and adolescents with temporal lobe epilepsy. *Epilepsia* 1999; 40:1543–1550.
112. Lendt M, Gleissner U, Helmstaedter C, Sassen R, et al. Neuropsychological outcome in children after frontal lobe epilepsy surgery. *Epilepsy Behav* 2002; 3(1):51–59.
113. Helmstaedter C, Gleissner U, Zentner J, Elger CE. Neuropsychological consequences of epilepsy surgery in frontal lobe epilepsy. *Neuropsychologia* 1998; 36(7):681–689.
114. Lah S. Neuropsychological outcome following focal cortical removal for intractable epilepsy in children. *Epilepsy Behav* 2004; 5(6):804–817.
115. Lassonde M, Sauerwein HC, Jambaque I, Smith ML, et al. Neuropsychology of childhood epilepsy: pre- and postsurgical assessment. *Epileptic Disord* 2000; 2(1):3–13.
116. Helmstaedter C, Lendt M. Neuropsychological outcome of temporal and extratemporal lobe resection in children. In: Jambaque I, Lassonde M, Dulac O, eds. *Neuropsychology of Childhood Epilepsy*. New York: Kluwer Academic Plenum Publishers, 2001; 215–227.
117. Luerding R, Boesebeck F, Ebner A. Cognitive changes after epilepsy surgery in the posterior cortex. *J Neurol Neurosurg Psychiatry* 2004; 75(4):583–587.
118. Kuehn SM, Keene DL, Richards PM, Ventureyra EC. Are there changes in intelligence and memory functioning following surgery for the treatment of refractory epilepsy in childhood? *Childs Nerv Syst* 2002; 18(6–7):306–310.
119. Mabbott DJ, Smith ML. Memory in children with temporal or extra-temporal excisions. *Neuropsychologia* 2003; 41(8):995–1007.
120. Vigevano F, Bertini E, Boldrini R, Bosman C, et al. Hemimegalencephaly and intractable epilepsy: benefits of hemispherectomy. *Epilepsia* 1989; 30(6):833–843.
121. Wyllie E. Surgery for catastrophic localization-related epilepsy in infants. *Epilepsia* 1996; 37 Suppl 1:S22–S25.
122. Wyllie E, Comair YG, Kotagal P, Raja S, et al. Epilepsy surgery in infants. *Epilepsia* 1996; 37(7):625–637.
123. Sugimoto T, Otsubo H, Hwang PA, Hoffman HJ, et al. Outcome of epilepsy surgery in the first three years of life. *Epilepsia* 1999; 40(5):560–565.
124. Pulsifer MB, Brandt J, Salorio CF, Vining EP, et al. The cognitive outcome of hemispherectomy in 71 children. *Epilepsia* 2004; 45(3):243–254.
125. Vasconcellos E, Wyllie E, Sullivan S, et al. Mental retardation in pediatric candidates for epilepsy surgery: the role of early seizure onset. *Epilepsia* 2001; 42(2): 268–274.
126. Asarnow RF, LoPresti C, Guthrie D, et al. Developmental outcomes in children receiving resection surgery for medically intractable infantile spasms. *Dev Med Child Neurol* 1997; 39:430–440.
127. Tellez-Zenteno JF, Dhar R, Hernandez-Ronquillo L, Wiebe S. Long-term outcomes in epilepsy surgery: antiepileptic drugs, mortality, cognitive and psychosocial aspects. *Brain* 2007; 130:334–345.
128. Klein B, Levin BE, Duchowny MS, Llabre MM. Cognitive outcome of children with epilepsy and malformations of cortical development. *Neurology* 2000; 55(2):230–235.
129. Kolb B. Synaptic plasticity and the organization of behaviour after early and late brain injury. *Can J Exp Psychol* 1999; 53(1):62–76.
130. Seidenberg M, Hermann BP, Schoenfeld J, Davies K, et al. Reorganization of verbal memory function in early onset left temporal lobe epilepsy. *Brain Cogn* 1997; 35(1):132–148.
131. Stiles J. The effects of early focal brain injury on lateralization of linguistic and cognitive function. *Curr Dir Psychol Sci* 1998; 7:21–26.
132. Akshoomoff NA, Feroleto CC, Doyle RE, Stiles J. The impact of early unilateral brain injury on perceptual organization and visual memory. *Neuropsychologia* 2002; 40(5):539–561.
133. Curtiss S, de Bode S, Mathern GW. Spoken language outcomes after hemispherectomy: factoring in etiology. *Brain Lang* 2001; 79(3):379–396.
134. Boatman D, Freeman J, Vining E, et al. Language recovery after left hemispherectomy in children with late-onset seizures. *Ann Neurol* 1999; 46(4):579–586.
135. Dlugos DJ, Moss EM, Duhaime AC, Brooks-Kayal AR. Language-related cognitive declines after left temporal lobectomy in children. *Pediatr Neurol* 1999; 21(1):444–449.
136. de Bode S, Firestine A, Mathern GW, Dobkin B. Residual motor control and cortical representations of function following hemispherectomy: effects of etiology. *J Child Neurol* 2005; 20(1):64–75.
137. van Empelen R, Jennekens-Schinkel A, Buskens E, Helders PJ, et al; Dutch Collaborative Epilepsy Surgery Programme. Functional consequences of hemispherectomy. *Brain* 2004; 127(Pt 9):2071–2079.
138. Rutter M, Tizard J, Yule W, Graham P, et al. Research report: Isle of Wight Studies, 1964–1974. *Psychol Med* 1976; 6(2):313–332.
139. Davies S, Heyman I, Goodman R. A population survey of mental health problems in children with epilepsy. *Dev Med Child Neurol* 2003; 45(5):292–295.
140. Danielsson S, Rydenhag B, Uvebrant P, Nordborg C, et al. Temporal lobe resections in children with epilepsy: neuropsychiatric status in relation to neuropathology and seizure outcome. *Epilepsy Behav* 2002; 3(1):76–81.
141. Szabo CA, Wyllie E, Dolske M, et al. Epilepsy surgery in children with pervasive developmental disorder. *Pediatr Neurol* 1999; 20(5):349–353.
142. Wilson P. Cerebral hemispherectomy for infantile hemiplegia. A report of 50 cases. *Brain* 1970; 93(1):147–180.
143. White HH. Cerebral hemispherectomy in treatment of infantile hemiplegia. *Confin Neurol* 1961; 25:1–50.
144. Neville BG, Harkness WF, Cross JH, et al. Surgical treatment of severe autistic regression in childhood epilepsy. *Pediatr Neurol* 1997; 16(2):137–140.
145. Lendt M, Helmstaedter C, Kuczaty S, Schramm J, Elger CE. Behavioural disorders in children with epilepsy: early improvement after surgery. *J Neurol Neurosurg Psychiatry* 2000; 69(6):739–744.

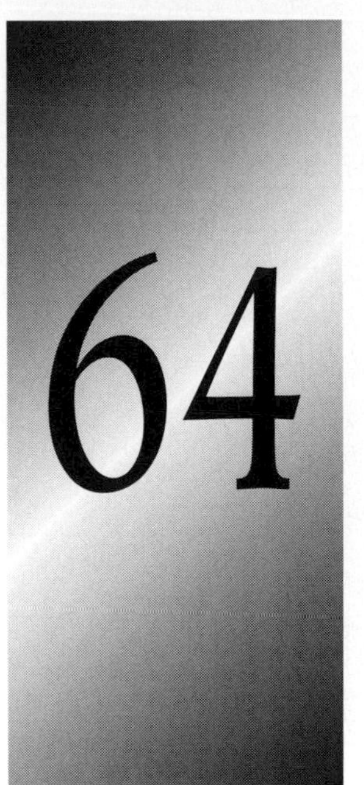

64 Vagus Nerve Stimulation Therapy in Pediatric Patients: Use and Effectiveness

James W. Wheless

Childhood epilepsies are often characterized by a wide range of seizure types and accompanying comorbidities such as mental retardation or developmental delay (MR/DD), autism, and language disorders, often making treatment difficult. However, advances in our understanding of the underlying mechanisms that result in seizures and epilepsy syndromes have also led to advances in epilepsy treatments. Traditionally, the two primary treatment modalities used to control seizures have been mono- and polytherapy with antiepileptic drugs (AEDs) and epilepsy surgery. Among pediatric patients, the ketogenic diet is used among a small number of children.

In 1997, however, the United States (U.S.) Food and Drug Administration (FDA) approved a new, nonpharmacologic treatment—vagus nerve stimulation (VNS) therapy—for adjunctive use among patients aged 12 years and older with partial-onset seizures refractory to standard therapies. Although VNS therapy is not currently approved in the United States for children younger than age 12 years, studies indicate that success with VNS therapy can be achieved independent of patient age and seizure type or syndrome. Reports indicate that VNS therapy may have unique benefits for pediatric patients (aged less than 18 years), including improvements in quality of life resulting from the lack of pharmacologic interactions known to impair development, and success at reducing seizure frequency and severity among patients with age-related and difficult-to-control syndromes such as Lennox-Gastaut syndrome (LGS). This chapter outlines both the safety and effectiveness of VNS therapy among pediatric patients with epilepsy, as discerned from current treatment practices and reports in the literature.

THE VAGUS NERVE STIMULATION THERAPY SYSTEM

Vagus nerve stimulation (VNS) was the first nonpharmacologic therapy approved by the FDA for the treatment of seizures. The treatment, which attenuates seizure frequency, severity, and duration by chronic intermittent stimulation of the vagus nerve, is intended for use as an adjunctive treatment with AED therapies. As of March 2006, more than 35,000 patients with epilepsy have been implanted with the VNS therapy system worldwide, with approximately 30% of those patients being younger than age 18 at the time of their first implant. Approximately one-third of patients receiving VNS therapy experience at least a 50% reduction in seizure frequency with no adverse cognitive or systemic effects (1, 2). Moreover, clinical findings indicate that the effectiveness of VNS therapy continues to improve over time (2–8), independent of changes in AEDs or stimulation parameters (9). Also notable is the fact that tolerance, which is often accompanied by a reduction in efficacy for many treatments, does not appear to be a factor with VNS therapy, even after extended (>10 years) periods of time (2). Response to VNS therapy may be delayed for some patients (8, 10). As a result, the long-term safety and effectiveness seen with this treatment have made VNS therapy a mainstream treatment option for a broad range of epilepsy patients, including children and adolescents. VNS therapy is second only to AED therapy as a treatment category for childhood epilepsy in the United States.

The VNS therapy system consists of the implantable pulse generator and bipolar VNS therapy lead, a programming wand with software, a tunneling tool, and a hand-held magnet. The original systems consisted of the Model 100 and Model 101. However, in June 2002, Cyberonics, Inc. (Houston, Texas), introduced a new generator model, the Model 102 system, which is thinner (6.9 mm), lighter (25 g), and has less volume (52.2 mm in diameter) than the previous models (11). The smaller size of the Model 102 offers children an improved cosmetic appearance and increased comfort. In addition, the Model 102 has a single- rather than a dual-pin lead, making it easier and faster to implant than the previous models. Both the Model 101 and Model 102 are currently being implanted. The average battery life for the generator (Model 101 or 102) is approximately 7 to 10 years with normal use (11). Increases in stimulation intensities or frequency will decrease battery life.

The magnet provided to patients as part of the VNS therapy system allows for on-demand stimulation, which has the potential to abort seizures, either consistently or occasionally, among some patients or caregivers who are able to anticipate the onset of their seizures (12–14). The additional stimulus train that results when the magnet is held over the generator is typically stronger than the programmed stimulus parameters. This added ability of on-demand stimulation provides a greater sense of control for patients and their caregivers over their disorder, which can help improve how they perceive their quality of life. The magnet also allows temporary interruption of stimulation if needed, particularly when singing or playing wind instruments or during speaking engagements. However, stopping the stimulus should be done sparingly and with care, as doing so creates the potential risk of breakthrough seizures.

Implantation Procedure

The implant surgery is most often performed under general anesthesia and typically lasts about 1 hour (4). The pacemaker-like generator device is generally implanted in the subcutaneous tissues of the upper left pectoral region, with a lead then run from the generator device to the left vagus nerve in the neck, where it is attached by a coiled electrode (Figures 64-1, 64-2) (15, 16). Two incisions are made during the procedure: one in the chest to create the generator pocket, and the other along a fold in the neck to expose the vagus nerve for placement of the electrode (Figures 64-3, 64-4). A loop of lead wire is coiled beside the generator to allow for strain relief and patient growth.

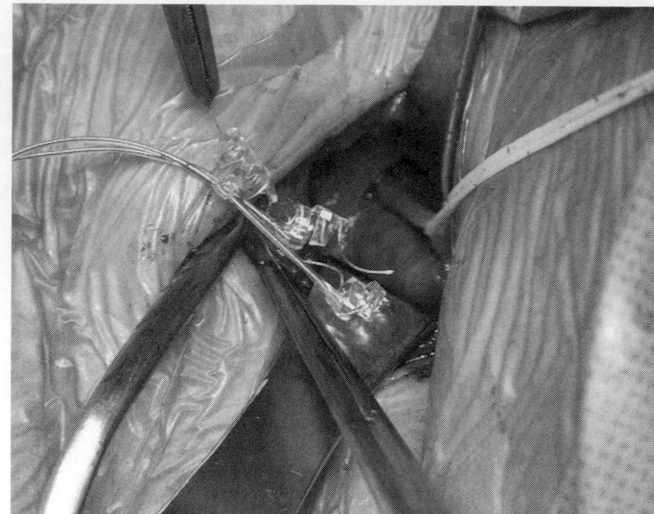

FIGURE 64-1

VNS lead wire prior to placement on the left vagus nerve. Cathode electrode (green suture) placed proximal (right side of picture), then anode electrode (white suture), then anchor tether (green suture; caudal; left side of picture).

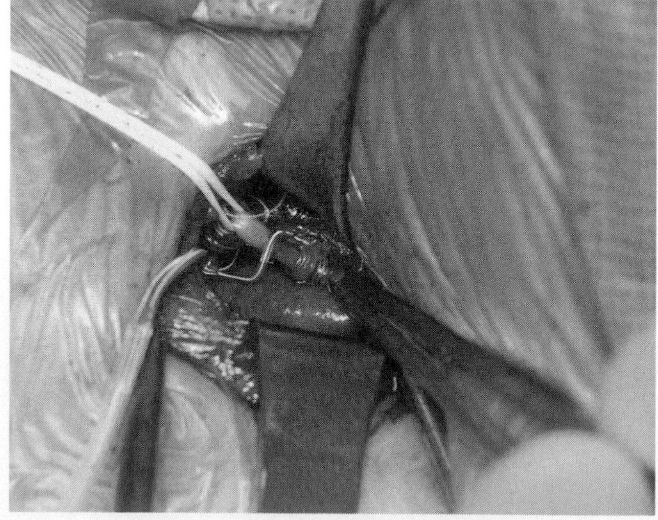

FIGURE 64-2

Lead wire starting to be placed on the left vagus nerve.

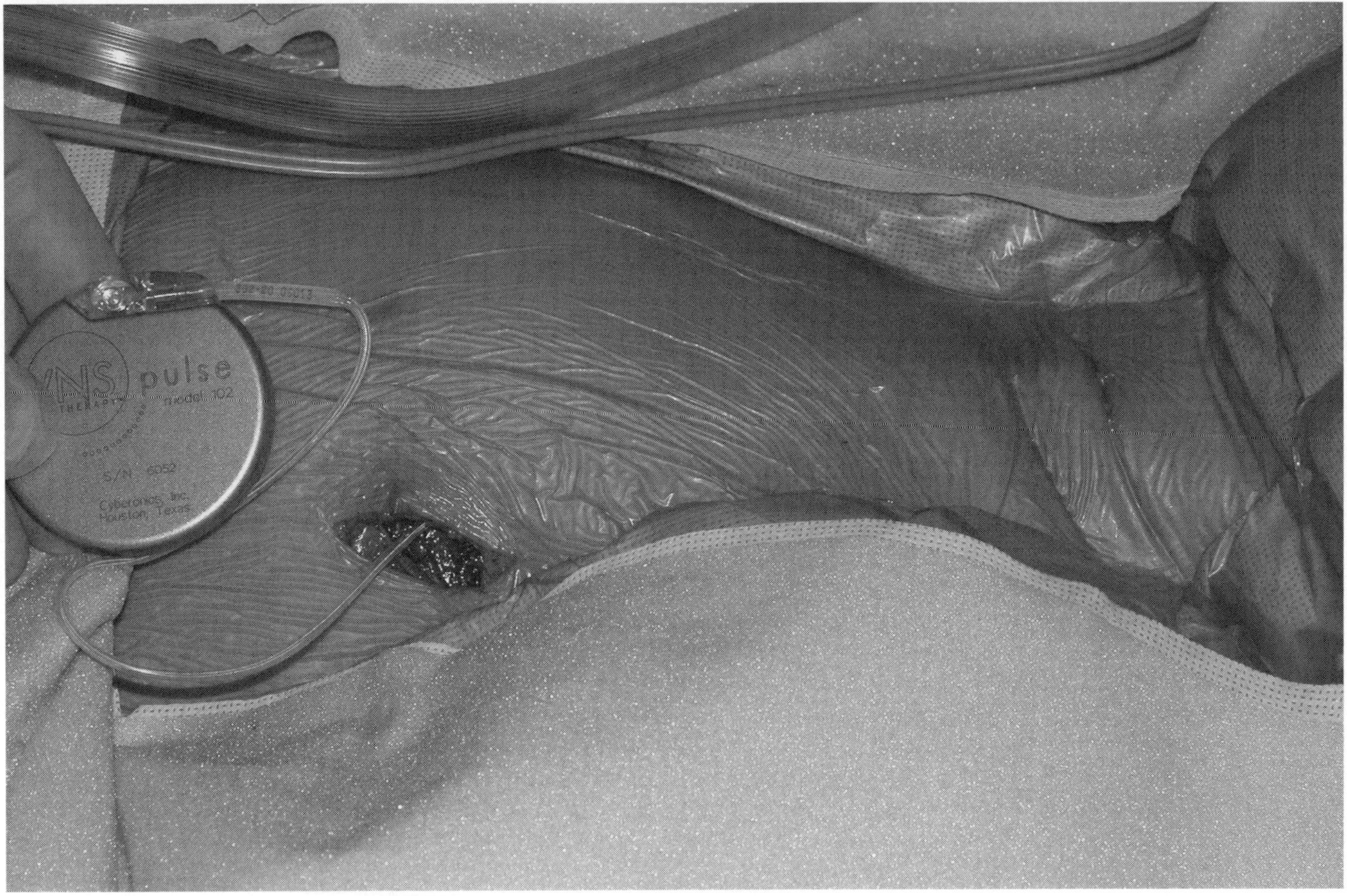

FIGURE 64-3

Implantation of the Model 102.

The procedure is well tolerated in both children and adults (17, 18) and is usually performed as outpatient surgery; however, in some cases, patients may be kept in the hospital overnight for observation. The device is often turned on in the operating room or in the office immediately after surgery, generally with a low initial setting of 0.25 mA (Figure 64-5) (19). The programming wand (Figure 64-6) is used at follow-up visits to check and fine-tune the stimulation settings according to patient comfort and level of seizure control. Instructions concerning care of the incision sites, magnet use, and necessary follow-up visits are given to patients and their families before the patient leaves the hospital.

The length of battery life for the VNS generator is dependent on the device model implanted and the stimulation parameters used (20). Often an increase in seizure frequency or intensity suggests clinical end of service (20). Other indications of battery failure include a sudden stop in sensing stimulation or unexpected changes in stimulation. Once a generator reaches end of service, another surgery is required to replace the generator. The entire generator is replaced rather than just the battery so as to prevent opening the hermetically sealed titanium case of the generator, which could lead to a rejection reaction (21). The generator-replacement surgery typically lasts approximately 10 to 15 minutes and is performed on an outpatient basis. Because the leads remain untouched during a generator replacement, only one incision is needed. Generator replacement is recommended and preferred by patients before the battery is completely depleted so as to prevent an interruption in treatment (20). A 12-year follow-up study showed that multiple device replacement surgeries are well tolerated (2). Often, however, tolerated device currents are lower after reimplantation but are not equated with a reduction in benefit from VNS therapy, which suggests improved battery strength in the newer models of VNS generators; parameter settings other than current are generally the same as with the initial device (20). For patients not obtaining a substantial level of benefit from VNS, it has been suggested that stimulation parameters be tapered down over an extended period of time before end of service to allow for explantation of

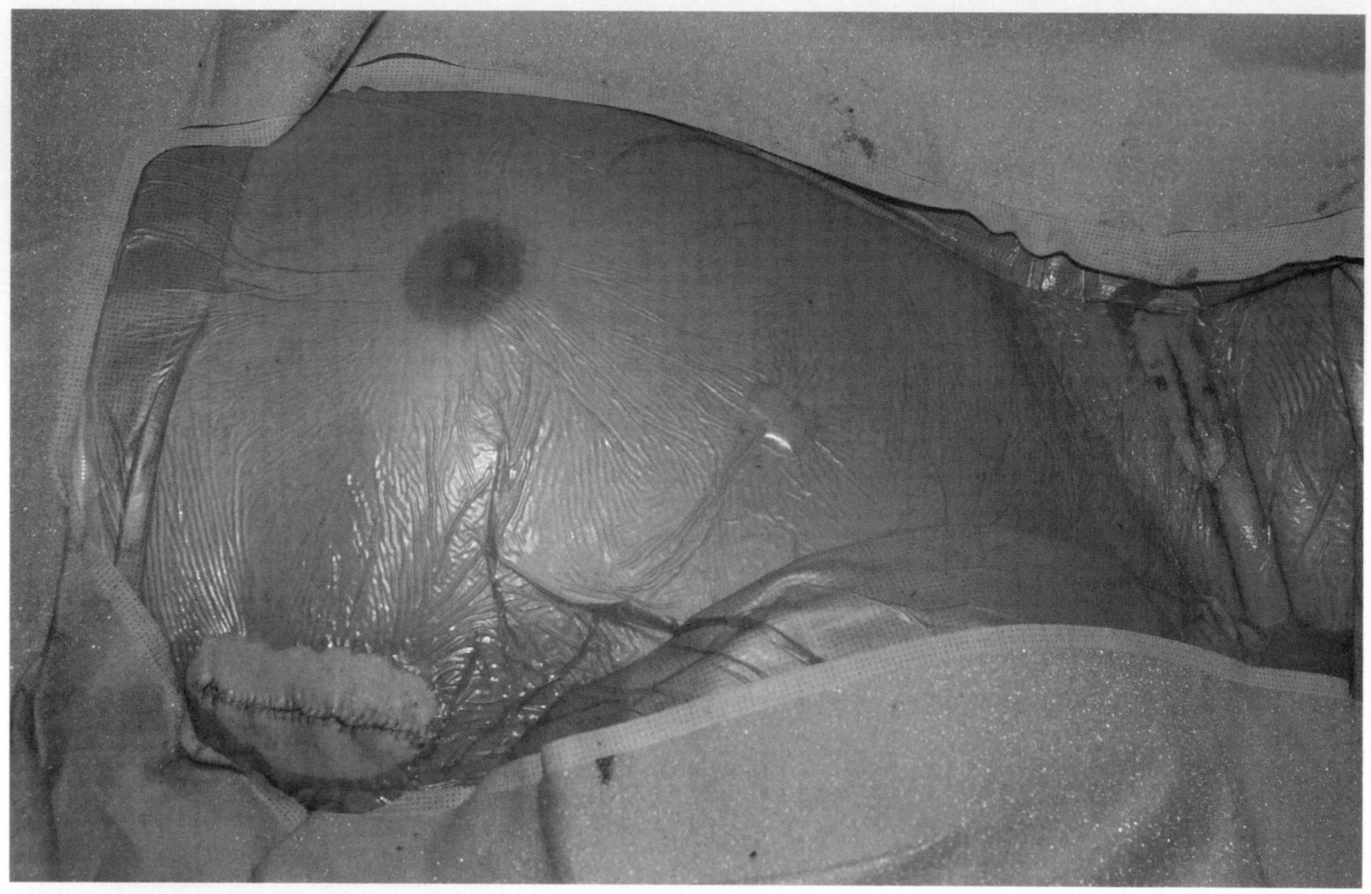

FIGURE 64-4

Neck incision (right) after final closure with Durabond; chest incision after final closure (bottom left).

the device before clinical signs of generator dysfunction become evident (20).

Potential Complications. Although the implant surgery is a relatively simple procedure that is safe and well tolerated by the vast majority of VNS therapy patients, complications can arise. One possible risk resulting from the implant surgery is an infection at the implant site. This risk may be increased in the pediatric population because young children or patients with neurocognitive disorders may tamper with the wound before the incision has had time to heal properly (22–24). Such infections can be treated with antibiotics but typically lead to explantation of the device if antibiotic treatment is not effective or if tampering continues (25, 26). Stimulator pocket infections among the pediatric population have been relatively uncommon, however (25, 27). No infections were observed in a recent study of 36 children aged younger than 18 years who were followed up for an average of 30 months (27).

The routine lead test performed during surgery also has resulted in reports of bradycardia and asystole in a small number of patients (~0.1%) (28–31). Neither of these cardiac events, however, has occurred after surgery during day-to-day treatment with VNS therapy or in children; these events are usually transient and self-limiting and are rarely of clinical significance (28–31). Vocal cord paresis, although rare, can be caused by manipulation of the vagus nerve during the implant procedure, but such paresis is most often transient (32). On the whole, the surgery required with VNS therapy is much less invasive and generally better tolerated than other traditional epilepsy surgeries. Although side effects associated with the surgery cannot be avoided completely, they can be minimized with a correct technical procedure (27). In addition, the implant surgery is not associated with any performance or cognitive impairments and can be reversed if the treatment is not effective.

Alternative Generator Placements. Depending on the circumstances of the patient, alternative generator placements have been reported with successful results. Le et al (22) successfully used an interscapular placement of the generator to reduce the risk of wound tamper-

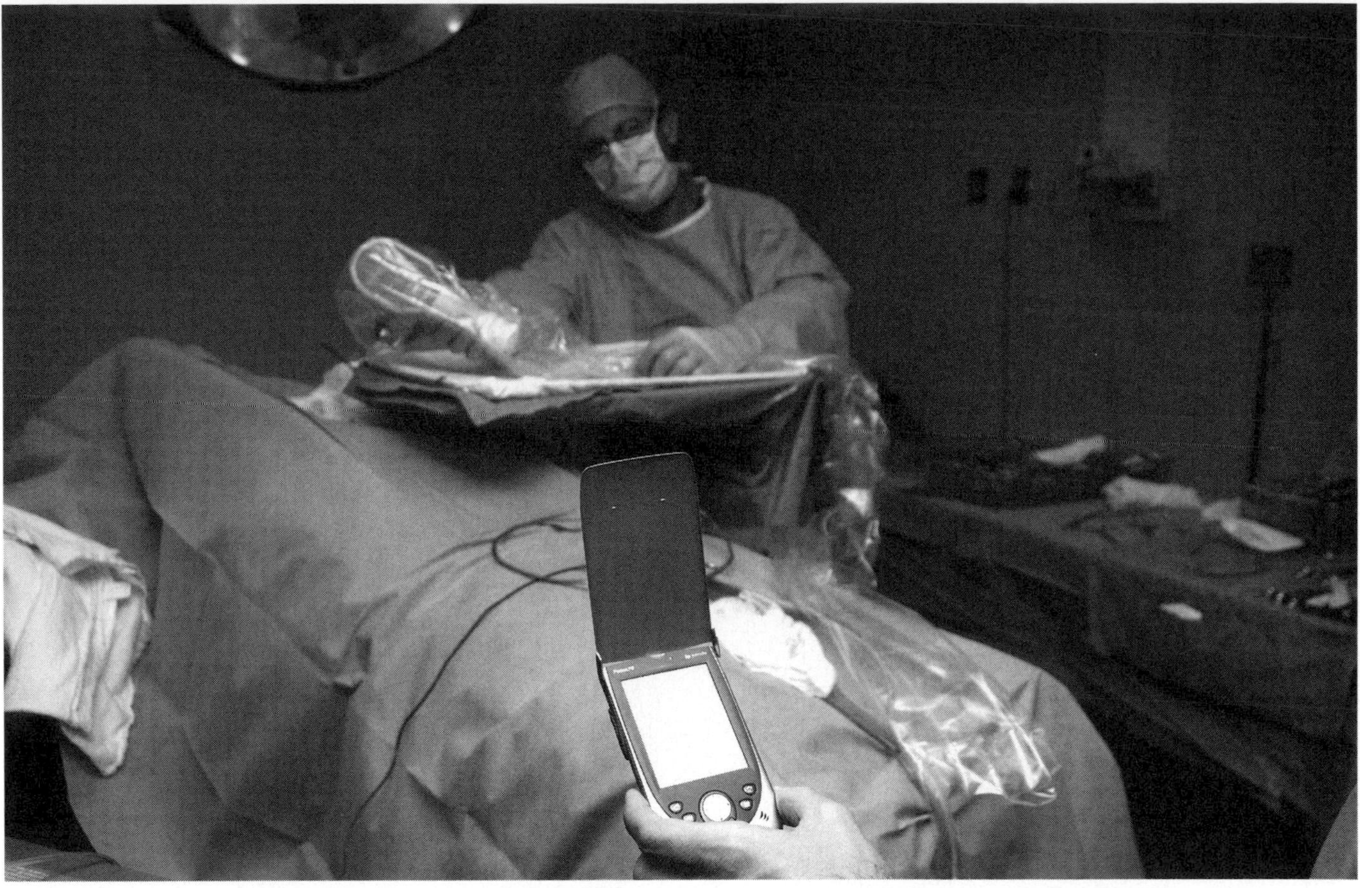

FIGURE 64-5

Intraoperative use of the handheld computer and programming wand to initiate stimulation.

ing among pediatric patients with cognitive delay who may be prone to tampering with the wound. Of the nine patients with an interscapular generator placement, none required explant; no discomfort or changes in daily routine (e.g., sleeping positions) were reported; and the effects of VNS therapy on seizure reduction and quality of life were consistent with the results seen with the traditional generator placement. An infraclavicular placement also has been used for developmentally delayed children, as well as for young women and children with small muscular mass (33, 34). Three children have had a device reimplanted on the right side rather than the left after undergoing explantation of a VNS device owing to infection (35). All three patients had been deriving benefit from the left-sided implant, but reimplantation of another device on the left side was not pursued because of the potential of inflicting nerve damage. The right-sided implantations were effective in once again reducing seizure frequencies, but a difference was noted in the level of seizure control achieved between the right- and left-sided implants. Although right-sided implantations are not recommended by the device manufacturer because of possible cardiac side effects, no cardiac events presented among these three children; however, two of the three children did experience transient respiratory events.

Stimulation Parameters

VNS therapy "dosing" is defined by five interrelated stimulation parameters (Figure 64-7): output current (measured in mA), signal frequency (Hz), pulse width (μs), signal On time (s), and signal Off time (s/min). The output current, signal frequency, and pulse width define how much energy is delivered to the patient, with the combination of settings for these three parameters being analogous to the size or dose of a pill. The signal On and Off times constitute the duty cycle (i.e., how often the energy is delivered) and are analogous to the dosing schedule for drug therapy. An optimal dose-response relationship for VNS therapy, however, is elusive, in part because of the interindividual variability between patients and in part because of the number of parameters involved in regulating the dose.

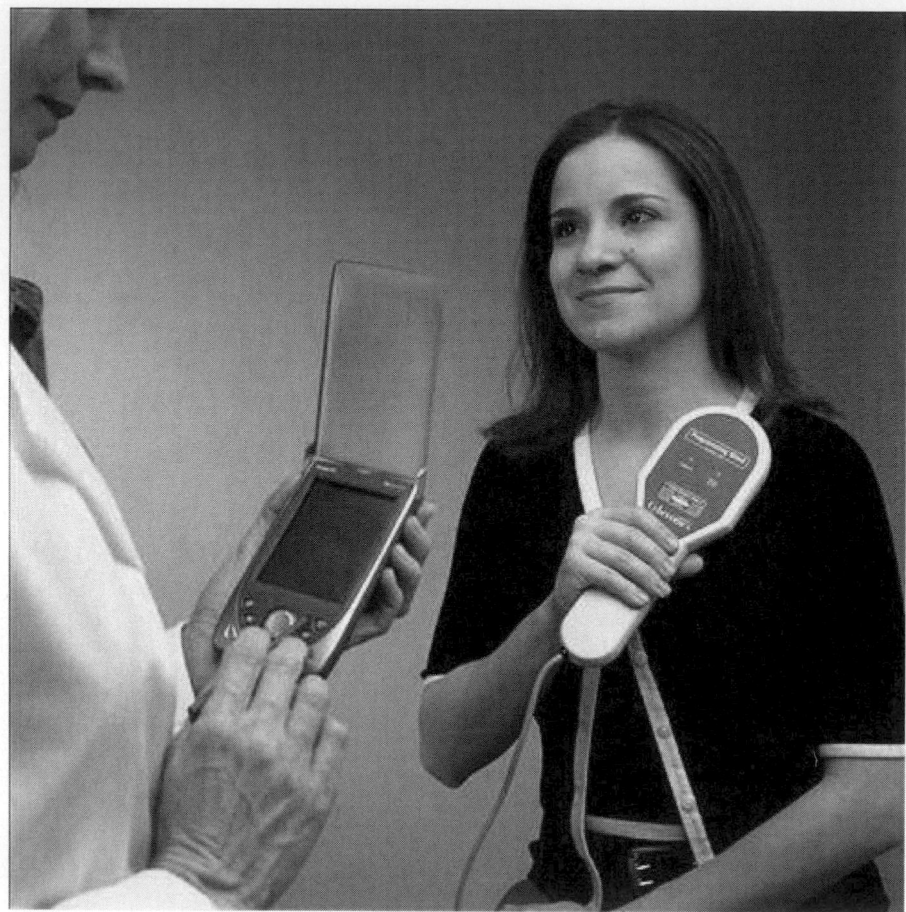

FIGURE 64-6

A programming wand is held by the patient over the device while a physician checks and/or adjusts stimulation parameters using a handheld computer.

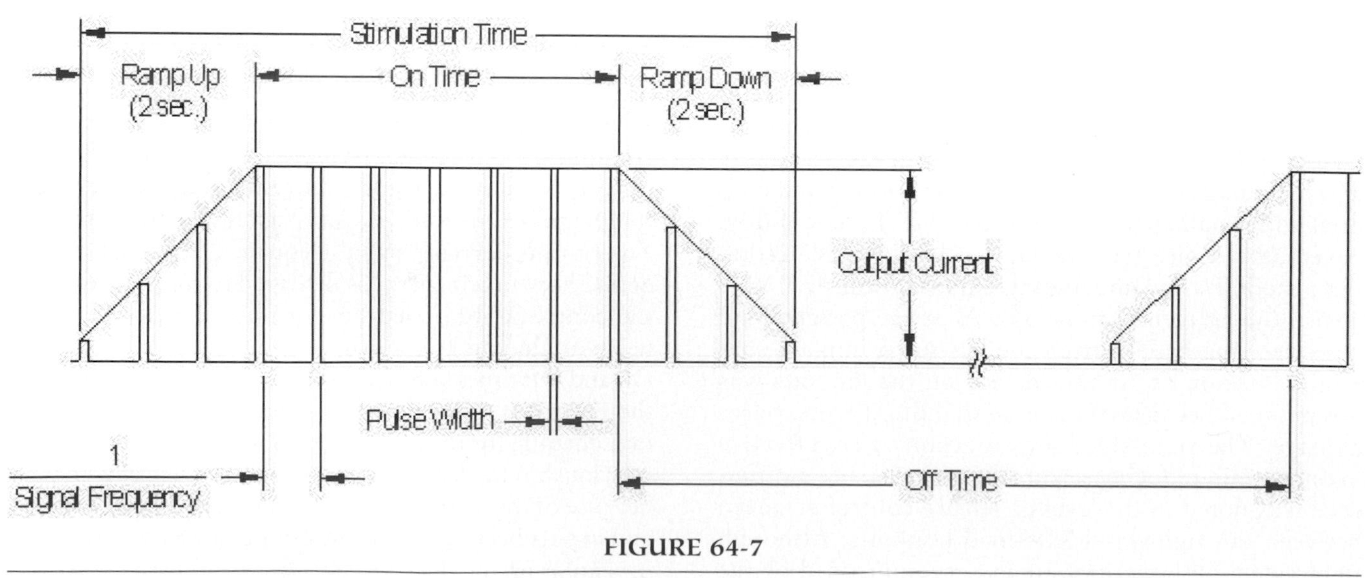

FIGURE 64-7

Stimulation parameters (all duty cycles except low output [≤10 Hz]).

TABLE 64-1
Stimulation Parameter Setting Ranges

		Median Settings			
		Pediatric (n = 743)		Adult (n = 1,486)	
Parameter	Typical Range	3 Months	12 Months	3 Months	12 Months
Output current	0.25–3.5 mA	1.25 mA	1.75 mA	1.00 mA	1.50 mA
Signal frequency	20–30 Hz	30 Hz	30 Hz	30 Hz	30 Hz
Pulse width	250–500 μs	500 μs	500 μs	500 μs	250 μs
Signal on time	7–270 s	30 s	30 s	30 s	30 s
Signal off time	12 s–180 min	5 min	3 min	5 min	3 min

*No standard settings have been defined on the basis of patient age or seizure type. The median settings shown here are taken from the VNS therapy patient outcome registry (Cyberonics, Inc; Houston, Texas).

Standard parameter settings, as determined from the clinical trials and outlined by Heck et al (36), range from 20 to 30 Hz at a pulse width of 250 to 500 ms and an output current of 0.25 to 3.5 mA for 30 s On time and 5 min Off time (Table 64-1). Initial stimulation is set at the low end of these ranges and slowly adjusted over time and within the safety limits (Figure 64-8) on the basis of patient tolerance and response. Patients should be closely monitored during the dose adjustment phase of VNS therapy, typically every 2 to 4 weeks for the first 2 to 8 weeks following generator implantation. Once a patient responds to a tolerated dose, further parameter adjustments are performed only as clinically necessary. However, routine assessment of lead-wire integrity and generator function should be performed.

Response to VNS therapy has been shown to be age dependent and therefore VNS stimulus parameters may need to be adjusted differently for the pediat-

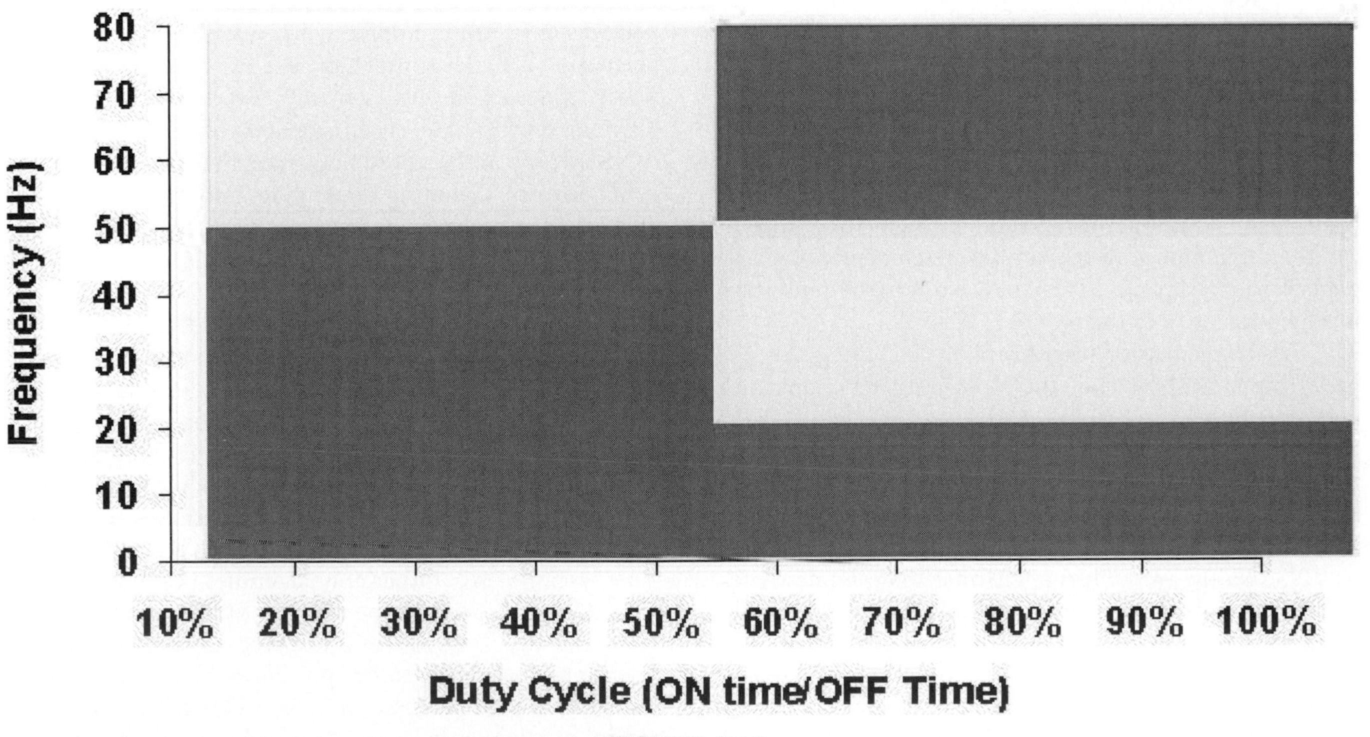

FIGURE 64-8

Safety ranges for VNS therapy stimulation parameters.

ric patient (37). Several studies indicate that pediatric patients may require higher output currents (Table 64-1) than those used in adult patients to reach a therapeutic dose (2.0 to 2.5 mA compared with 1.0 to 1.75 mA, respectively), particularly when lower (≤250 μs) pulse durations are used (33, 36, 38). Additional reports indicate clinically significant responses with low stimulation intensities (1.25 to 1.50 mA) (2, 5, 17). A multicenter, randomized trial looking at device parameter efficacy showed that various duty cycles were equally effective (39). Some reports among children with severe epileptic syndromes showed an increase in seizure frequency and severity at higher output currents (10, 40). Functional magnetic resonance imaging (fMRI) in humans also suggests that pulse width is an important variable in producing brain effects (41). Optimal parameter settings for specific ages and seizure types or syndromes, if they exist, have yet to be defined.

Mechanisms of Action

The mechanisms of action of VNS therapy are not fully understood, but they are believed to be manifold, owing to the diffuse distribution of vagal afferents throughout the central nervous system, and are distinct from those of traditional AED therapy (42, 43). Studies suggest that altered vagal afferent (not efferent) activities resulting from VNS are responsible for mediating seizures (43, 44). Such altered activities have been recorded in both cerebral hemispheres. Rat studies indicate that VNS activation of the locus coeruleus may be a significant factor for the attenuation of seizures (45–47). Human imaging studies also implicate the thalamus in having an important role in regulating seizure activity (48, 49). The exact antiseizure role of the thalamus is likely to be complex, however, because of the diffuse connections of the thalamus throughout the brain (48). Additionally, the reticular activating system, central autonomic network, limbic system, and noradrenergic projection system all may play a role in the antiseizure mechanisms of VNS therapy (43, 50–53).

Positron emission tomography (PET) imaging studies in humans show that the VNS-induced changes in cerebral blood flow (CBF) and synaptic activity vary over time (53). Widespread alterations in CBF activation during acute VNS was much more restricted after prolonged VNS, indicating that those sites of persisting VNS-induced changes may reflect the antiseizure actions of VNS therapy (53). During chronic VNS, no new sites of CBF alterations that were not also affected acutely were observed (53). Additional human imaging studies using various methods, including functional magnetic resonance imaging (fMRI) and single-photon emission computed tomographic (SPECT) techniques, have produced similar findings in both acute and chronic studies (53). These imaging findings, coupled with the clinical findings that the effectiveness of VNS therapy continues to improve over time, seem to indicate that rapidly occurring subcortical effects rather than rapidly occurring cortical effects may be more important in the VNS antiseizure mechanism (53). It is believed that rapidly altered intrathalamic synaptic activities as well as other mechanisms likely occurring independently of thalamic activation constitute the therapeutic mechanisms of VNS (53). Electroencephalogram (EEG) observations also suggest that unilateral rather than bilateral abnormalities may show more benefit from VNS (2). Other human studies show that some antiepileptic mechanisms affected by VNS are either modulated by or are the reflection of EEG changes, although the effect of VNS on the EEG background remains uncertain (54). Finally, gamma-aminobutyric acid (GABA) receptor ($GABA_A$) plasticity may contribute to the ability of VNS to modulate the cortical excitability of brain areas associated with epileptogenesis (55). Like medications, many different actions probably contribute to the efficacy of VNS therapy; therefore, determining whether there is a single mechanism that is most important may not be possible.

Animal Trials

VNS therapy was developed on the basis of early findings of neuroinhibition in the regulation of emesis, and changes in EEG activity resulting from vagal stimulation (56–58). Studies among animals showed that VNS therapy worked both acutely to abort seizures and chronically to control seizures (59, 60). In addition, VNS was effective beyond the period of active stimulation and across a wide range of seizure types and severities, thereby indicating the potential for long-term, phase-dependent seizure control. Tests of VNS therapy in the traditional animal models used to test AED efficacy, including rat, canine, and monkey models (60–64), further indicated that VNS therapy, like AEDs, may be effective for multiple seizure types. The clinical trials that followed proved the safety and efficacy of VNS therapy for controlling seizures, with few and mild side effects that were generally related to stimulation intensities.

A more recent PET imaging study in rats revealed differences between acute and chronic changes in glucose metabolism during VNS, which may reflect cerebral adaptation to VNS (65). These findings are in line with clinical findings and other animal and human studies that show improvements in seizure control and changes in CBF over time (3–5, 65, 66). Other animal studies also have shown that VNS may facilitate the recovery of function following brain damage, both in the rate of recovery and in the final level of performance reached postinjury, as well as enhance memory storage processes (67, 68). This enhancement of neural plasticity is believed to occur by the ability of VNS to enhance norepinephrine release throughout the neuraxis, but further studies are needed to explore the mechanisms behind these effects more fully (68, 69). Improvements in behavior among rats with induced brain damage also are suggestive of a neuroprotective effect of VNS, which may also help to reduce the behavioral deficits associated with seizures among humans receiving VNS therapy as part of their antiepileptic treatment (67).

SEIZURE EFFICACY

Clinical Trials

A series of acute-phase studies with long-term follow-up data proved the safety and efficacy of VNS therapy for the treatment of refractory epilepsy and thereby led to its approval by the FDA in 1997. Results from two randomized, placebo-controlled, double-blind trials (E03 and E05) were pivotal in demonstrating the antiseizure effect of VNS therapy. Patients in the 14-week acute E03 study (n = 113) who received therapeutic doses of stimulation (high; 30 Hz, 500 μs, up to 3.5 mA for 30 s every 5 min) showed a significantly higher median decrease in seizure frequency of 24.5% compared with only a 6.1% median decrease among patients receiving nontherapeutic levels of stimulation (low; 1 Hz, 130 μs, ≤3.5 mA for 30 s every 90 min; $p = 0.01$) (70).

Seizure frequency reductions of at least 50% were reported for 31% of patients in the high-stimulation group and for 13% in the low-stimulation group ($p = 0.02$). In the acute E05 study, the median reduction in seizure frequency was 27.9% for the 94 patients in the high-stimulation group and 15.2% for the 102 patients in the low-stimulation group at 3 months ($p = 0.04$) (71).

Long-term follow-up of patients in the acute E03 and E05 studies showed that the effectiveness of VNS therapy was cumulative. After the acute phase of these studies, patients receiving low stimulation had their stimulation levels titrated to therapeutic (high) settings, and all patients were then followed for an additional 12 months of treatment. For the 100 patients in the E03 open-label extension study treated for the additional 12 months, the median reduction in seizure frequency increased to 32% at 12 months from only 20% at 3 months (5). For the 196 patients with evaluable seizure data in the E05 trial, the median reduction in seizure frequency was 45% after an additional 12 months of treatment in the prospective, long-term extension study (4). At this same time point, 35% of patients had at least a 50% reduction in seizure frequency, and 20% had at least a 75% reduction. These seizure frequency reductions were sustained over time.

Pediatric Outcomes

Although the controlled clinical trials did not focus specifically on the pediatric patient, the children and adolescents included in one of the five clinical studies (E04) responded at least as favorably as the adults (14, 72). Of the 60 pediatric patients included in the E04 open, prospective study, 16 were younger than age 12 (mean age, 13.5 years). At 3 months, the median reduction in seizure frequency was 23% (n = 60); for the 46 patients with follow-up data available at 18 months, the median reduction was 42%. The results, although in a much smaller group, were similar for the patients aged 11 years and younger, indicating that age does not seem to be a factor in the effectiveness of VNS therapy to control seizures. Moreover, data from other pediatric study experiences with VNS therapy indicate that younger patients may have a higher tolerance and more effective response than adult patients (14, 17, 72–75).

The largest study to date to evaluate the effectiveness, tolerability, and safety of VNS therapy among pediatric patients was a six-center, retrospective study of 125 patients aged 18 years or younger (41 patients aged less than 12 years) (19). This study showed greater reductions in seizure frequency than those found in the pediatric subgroup of the E04 clinical trial, with a median reduction in seizure frequency at 3 months of 51.5% (range, −100% to +312%; n = 95) and 51.0% at 6 months (range, −99.9% to +100.0%; n = 56). A similar response was reported at 6 months for children aged less than 12 years (median seizure frequency reduction of 51%; n = 20). These reductions did not differ between patients with different seizure types.

Special Patient Populations

Although few prospective or controlled trials have been performed among pediatric epilepsy patients, the number of young patients receiving VNS therapy across the United States and Europe is growing. Observations of pediatric patients with age-related or specialized syndromes receiving VNS therapy indicate that this treatment is safe and effective across a broad range of seizure types and syndromes, independent of age. Table 64-2 (2–5, 7–9, 14, 16, 18, 19, 24, 38, 70–74, 76–85) shows the epilepsy syndromes, seizure types, and associated conditions in which VNS therapy may be helpful. Additionally, VNS therapy also seems to be a palliative treatment option for patients who have failed cranial surgery (Figure 64-9) (83, 86).

Lennox-Gastaut Syndrome, Infantile Spasms, and Ring Chromosome 20 Syndrome

Lennox-Gastaut syndrome (LGS) and infantile spasms are rare but difficult-to-treat epileptic disorders. These conditions are also accompanied by neurologic comorbidities that can be exacerbated by the cognitive adverse side effects typically associated with drug therapy. Although

TABLE 64-2
Epilepsy Syndromes, Seizure Types, and Associated Conditions in which VNS Therapy May Be Helpful

Epilepsy Syndrome, Seizure Type, and/or Associated Condition	References
Simple partial seizures Simple partial seizures progressing to complex partial seizures or secondary generalization	(2–5, 7–9, 14, 16, 18, 70–72, 74)
Complex partial seizures with or without secondary generalization	
Symptomatic generalized tonic-clonic seizures	(14, 19, 24, 72, 74, 76)
Drop attacks in Lennox-Gastaut syndrome	(19, 38, 73, 77)
Primary generalized epilepsy (JME)	(76, 78–80)
Tuberous sclerosis complex with complex partial or generalized tonic-clonic seizures	(81)
Autism with symptomatic epilepsy	(82)
Status epilepticus	(83–85)

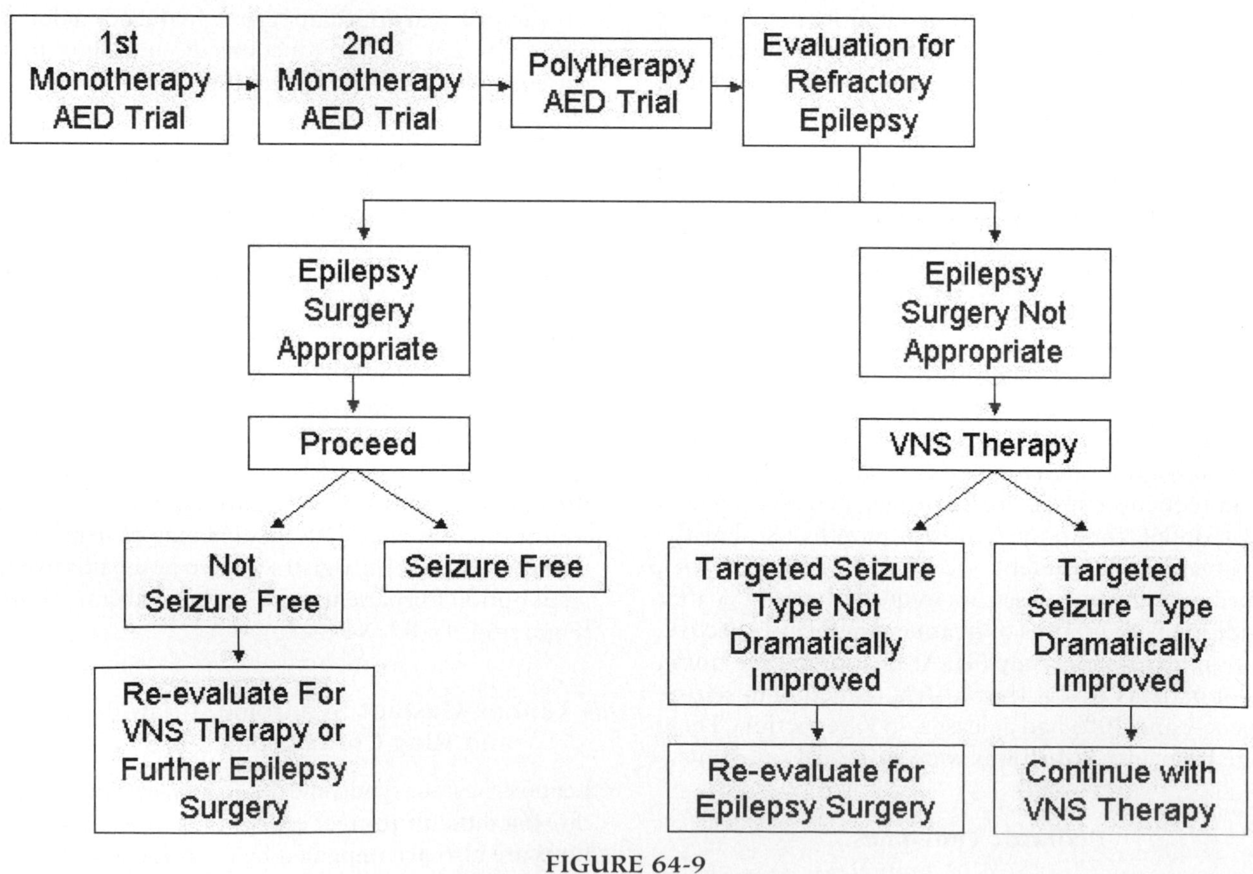

FIGURE 64-9

Suggested treatment sequence flowchart for patients with epilepsy.

limited data are available for children receiving VNS therapy for the treatment of infantile spasms (87), recent retrospective studies of the efficacy of VNS therapy among patients with LGS have shown some success in reducing seizure frequency without adverse side effects (10, 34, 38, 73, 779).

The largest retrospective study of LGS patients receiving VNS therapy was done by Frost et al (73) on 50 patients from six centers (median age at implant was 13 years; range, 5 to 27 years). This study showed that median reductions in seizure frequency at 1, 3, and 6 months of VNS therapy were 42%, 58.2%, and 57.9%, respectively ($n = 46$ who had complete seizure data available). Seizure reductions at 6 months by type showed an 88% decrease in drop attacks and an 81% decrease in atypical absence seizures. At 3 months, a 23% decrease was seen in complex partial seizures. In addition, improvements in quality of life with minimal and tolerable side effects from both the surgery and therapy were reported for this patient population. The most notable change in quality of life was an increase in alertness reported for more than half of the patients. Previous corpus callosotomy was not a contraindication for VNS therapy among this patient population, with the five patients who had undergone such surgery showing a 69% reduction in seizure frequency at 6 months. However, the one patient with a previous lobectomy surgery did not show a change in seizure frequency with VNS therapy. Age also was not a contraindication, because those patients aged less than 12 years showed similar response rates to the group as a whole.

A smaller, longer-term study on the behavior of 19 patients with LGS receiving VNS therapy showed no deterioration from baseline in either quality of life or cognitive measures after 24 months of treatment (88). In addition, a positive increase in cognitive measures indicated a gain in mental age of 4.2 months at follow-up. These findings were independent of seizure response to VNS therapy, indicating a potential additional treatment benefit from VNS therapy to patients with LGS. Two-year follow up of 19 children (aged 7 to 18 years) with LGS or Lennox-like types of epilepsy, mental retardation, and multiple seizure types, along with a high seizure frequency, showed that four patients had a seizure frequency reduction of at least 50% (34). One patient remained seizure free 2 years postimplantation. Atypical absence seizures responded better to VNS than other seizure types; moreover, higher baseline seizure frequency, the lowest quantity of interictal epileptic activity, and the highest baseline mental level seemed to predict a higher response rate. A mild improvement in mental age, though modest, and a positive effect on behavior that was independent of seizure control were seen over time. However, unlike some studies that show increased effectiveness over time with VNS therapy, the duration of treatment in this small study did not appear to increase VNS efficacy among this group of patients.

A case study by Buoni et al (10), however, indicated that the ability of VNS to reduce seizure frequency among patients with LGS may require extended periods of treatment before positive outcomes are observed. A 22-year-old man with LGS reported no reductions in seizure frequency for 1 year of VNS therapy, although improvements in alertness and appetite were achieved. But by 3 years, the patient's seizures abruptly disappeared, and his EEG was borderline normal without any changes in drug therapies or stimulation parameters.

Three separate cases of the use of VNS therapy among patients with ring chromosome 20 have been reported in the literature (40, 89, 90). In 2002, the first report of a girl aged 6 years indicated that VNS may be successfully used to treat the medically refractory generalized clonic epilepsy characteristic of this disorder, which also is marked by developmental delay (90). After receiving VNS therapy, the child became free of seizures and remained seizure free 9 months postimplantation. Moreover, the child was reported to have an increased level of alertness and less lethargy, and, after 4 months of VNS treatment, spontaneous vocalization was reported. The achievement of new developmental milestones after the initiation of VNS therapy was encouraging. A second report of a male implanted with a VNS device at the age of 8 years also showed a good response to VNS therapy (40). Seizures began at the age of 5 years, and the patient was experiencing numerous absence and nocturnal tonic-clonic seizures as well as nonconvulsive status epilepticus at the time of VNS implantation. Following initiation of VNS, seizure frequencies were eventually reduced to only occasional nocturnal episodes and some previously lost skills were reacquired, including ambulation, eye contact, social smiling, and improved mood. The third report was a 14-year-old male with ring chromosome 20 syndrome who was also diagnosed with LGS and experiencing a range of seizure types and severe impairment of cognitive functions. However, he did not show similar results to those reported previously (90). Following implantation of the VNS device at the age of 11 years, the child experienced a 50% reduction in seizure frequency. However, tonic seizures during sleep and secondary generalized seizures continued at a rate of 1 to 3 seizures per day. At age 13 years, a corpus callosotomy was performed with no additional benefit in terms of seizure frequency reduction, but some reduction in seizure severity was achieved. An increase in behavioral problems, fear attacks, and visual hallucinations began after callosotomy. These case reports suggest, therefore, that earlier use of VNS therapy among patients with ring chromosome 20 syndrome may be more beneficial.

Mental Retardation/Developmental Delay

Mental retardation or developmental delay (MR/DD) often co-occur among patients with epilepsy, and the causal relationship between these disorders is complex (91). Both the seizures caused by the epilepsy and the AEDs used to treat the epilepsy are, however, known to potentially exacerbate delays in development, which can complicate treatment among this patient population. The likelihood of additional behavioral and psychiatric disorders, which are estimated to be about sevenfold higher among this population, also further complicates the treatment regimen (91). Moreover, the increased use of polytherapy among this population is indicative of the large number of patients with MR/DD experiencing refractory seizures (92, 93). Therefore, VNS therapy may be an attractive treatment option among patients with developmental and behavioral comorbidities in addition to epilepsy, because VNS therapy may reduce the frequency of seizures without the pharmacologic side effects or interactions of additional drug therapy. Another potential benefit is the fact that VNS therapy is delivered automatically, meaning that compliance and caregiver reliance for treatment are minimized, which is particularly attractive for this patient population because many are unable to care for themselves.

Studies of the effects of VNS therapy among patients with MR/DD show success with VNS therapy (24, 93, 94). A retrospective study by Andriola and Vitale (24) of 21 mildly to severely affected MR/DD patients (age range, 3 to 56 years; 5 patients <16 years) with a range of seizure types and etiologies showed VNS therapy to be both effective and well tolerated. Seventy-one percent (15 of 21) saw some degree of change for the better in seizure frequency or severity. Of the 16 patients who had known pre- and postoperative seizure data available, all of them had some degree of seizure reduction reported, with 11 (68%) having at least a 50% reduction. One patient with secondary generalized seizures became seizure free and remained that way at 3 years postimplant. Improvements also were reported by caregivers for many areas of the patients' functional status, including alertness, mood, and daily task participation. In addition, such improvements were not always associated with decreases in either seizures or AEDs.

Similar findings were found by Gates et al (94) in a retrospective study comparing outcomes of patients receiving VNS therapy living in residential treatment facilities (RTFs) with those not living in RTFs. Despite numerous statistical differences in the demographics and medical histories found between the 86 RTF (age range, 7 to 59 years) and 690 non-RTF (age range, 2 to 79) patients, the 12-month responder rates (≥50% reduction in seizure frequency) for the two groups were similar at 55% and 56%, respectively. Patients in both groups were reported to have some degree of improvement in alertness, verbal communication, memory, achievement at school or work, mood, postictal period, and seizure clustering, with more improvements reported at 12 months than at 3 months, thereby indicating a cumulative effect of VNS therapy.

A more recent, prospective study among 40 patients institutionalized with MR/DD and followed for 2 years of VNS therapy confirmed that VNS was an effective treatment option for this population (93). Most patients (34 of 40) had some reduction in seizure frequency. More notable, however, is the fact that this group experienced fewer epilepsy-related hospitalizations after receiving VNS therapy, and postictal recovery periods were reduced among 75% of the patients. Furthermore, the quality of life for these patients was improved by significant improvements at both 1 and 2 years in attention span, word usage, clarity of speech, standing balance, ability to wash dishes, and ability to perform household chores. Other areas of improvement included an increase in their ability to dress themselves, interact with their peers, express themselves nonverbally, and perceive auditory and visual stimuli.

All of these studies to date indicate that VNS therapy was well tolerated and did not introduce the central nervous system or cognitive side effects that commonly occur when a new AED is added to a treatment regimen (24, 93, 94). Reported side effects were minimal and manageable with changes in stimulus parameters. In addition, the surgery was less invasive and thereby more tolerable than other epilepsy surgeries. However, wound tampering can be a potential problem with this patient population. One patient in the Andriola et al (24) study was explanted as a consequence of self-inflicted wound infection. This patient was reimplanted and extra measures (extensive bandages over the implant site and additional barriers) were taken to prevent wound tampering until after the implant incisions had healed. As discussed earlier, a second option to prevent wound tampering would be an interscapular placement of the generator (22).

Tuberous Sclerosis Complex, Autism, and Landau-Kleffner Syndrome

A retrospective, multicenter, open-label study of 10 patients (mean age of 13 years) with tuberous sclerosis complex (TSC) receiving at least 6 months of VNS therapy (with a mean of 22 months) found a high response rate to VNS therapy, with 9 out of 10 patients experiencing at least a 50% reduction in seizure frequency (81). More notably, 5 of the 10 patients experienced a more than 90% reduction in seizure frequency. In addition, three patients were reported to be more alert by their parents and teachers, two were reported to have briefer seizures, and one was reported to have less-intense seizures in addition to the reduction in seizure frequency. A patient diagnosed with an autism spectrum disorder in addition to TSC also was reported to have an 80% reduction in injurious behavior after the start of VNS therapy. These results were not countered by any major complications or side effects. In addition, the high response rate of patients with TSC receiving VNS therapy, compared with patients of similar age and seizure frequencies who were also receiving VNS therapy but did not have TSC, indicated that this patient population may be more responsive to VNS therapy. However, the small number of patients involved in this study was not enough to determine any statistical significance between responses among the TSC and non-TSC groups.

Preliminary data also suggest that VNS therapy may be effective among patients with epilepsy and either autism or Landau-Kleffner syndrome (LKS), which are both childhood disorders known to co-occur with epilepsy (82). Among 6 patients with LKS, 3 experienced a reduction in seizure frequency of at least 50% at 6 months of VNS therapy. Of 59 patients with autism, 58% experienced at least a 50% reduction in seizure frequency at 12 months. More notable, however, were the reported improvements in quality of life, particularly in the area of alertness; 4 of 6 children with LKS and 76% of the children with autism were reported more alert at 6 and 12 months, respectively. Therefore, the benefit of VNS therapy for patients with such disorders may extend beyond or be independent from seizure frequency reductions.

Hypothalamic Hamartomas

A small study of six pediatric patients (≤16 years) with hypothalamic hamartomas and refractory epilepsy indicates that VNS therapy may have the ability to independently improve behavior and, to a lesser extent, decrease seizure frequency or severity in this patient population (95). Three of the six patients experienced some degree of seizure control. However, the immediate and notable improvements in behavior among four of the patients characterized as having severe behavioral problems are of particular interest. Such behavioral improvements were seen independent of seizure control and were dependent on ongoing stimulation. One patient who had the generator turned off for a 2-week period for stereotactic surgery had the injurious and antisocial behavior return in the absence of VNS therapy. Those behaviors once again subsided when stimulation was restarted.

Status Epilepticus

Four pediatric patients (83, 84) and one adult patient (85) have seen a complete cessation of status epilepticus upon initiation of VNS therapy. As reported in a case report by Winston et al (83), a 13-year-old boy was implanted with the vagus nerve stimulator 15 days after being admitted to the hospital for pharmacoresistant generalized convulsive status epilepticus. While he was hospitalized, his condition continued to deteriorate despite numerous pharmacologic treatments. The patient also had previously undergone a 90% anterior corpus callosotomy, which had been followed by the return of seizures up to 80% of the preoperative frequency. Immediately following the initiation of stimulation in the operating room, the child's refractory status epilepticus ceased. Over the next year and half, the status epilepticus never reappeared, the rate and severity of seizures significantly decreased with little or no postictal phase, and the patient's neurologic condition, nutritional state, and quality of life all improved.

Another case series presented by Malik et al (94) reports on three children (aged 14 months to 10 years) who also presented with pharmacoresistant status epilepticus and who were emergently implanted with the VNS device. All three children experienced complete resolution of the status epilepticus and continued to have a marked reduction in seizure frequency at their 8-week follow-up visit. The seizure types varied for each of these three patients, with one experiencing atonic, hypomotor, and partial seizures; another atonic, general tonic-clonic, and myoclonic seizures; and the third, multifocal-onset seizures. A 30-year-old man who presented with pharmacoresistant status epilepticus and was placed in a pentobarbital coma also experienced a cessation of seizures and remained seizure free 19 days postimplantation. These preliminary case reports suggest that VNS therapy should be considered as a nonpharmacologic treatment option among children with pharmacoresistant status epilepticus independently of seizure type.

SAFETY

Adverse Events

Adverse events reported with VNS therapy are generally transient and mild, and are often related to the duration and intensity of stimulation. Serious adverse events have not been reported with standard therapy, and no patients have died or had a higher mortality risk as a result of VNS therapy (96). The most common adverse events reported during the clinical trials were mild hoarseness or voice alterations, coughing, and paresthesia (primarily at the implant site and decreasing over time) and were not considered clinically significant (4, 18, 70, 71). Other adverse events reported less frequently during these studies include dyspnea, pain, headache, pharyngitis, dyspepsia, nausea, vomiting, fever, infection, depression, and accidental injury (4, 70, 71). Not all of these events were related to VNS therapy. Outside of the clinical trials, occasional reports of additional adverse events such as shortness of breath (3) and vocal cord paresis (97) have been reported, but did not result in discontinuation of therapy. Many of the side effects initially reported with VNS therapy, such as lower facial weakness and lead breaks, have been resolved. Adverse events associated with the implant surgery are discussed earlier in the chapter in the description of the implantation procedure.

Generally, the side effects associated with VNS therapy are well tolerated and not prohibitive to patients receiving this adjunctive treatment (28). Moreover, many of the side effects tend to diminish or disappear altogether, as patients adjust to the stimulation therapy. If side effects persist or are bothersome to the patient, reductions in stimulation intensity or frequency oftentimes alleviate the side effects, most of which occur only during active stimulation (98). Overall, the mechanisms of action of VNS therapy are different from those of traditional AED therapy and, therefore, produce a unique side effect profile that does not cause the cognitive, sedative, visual, affective, or coordination side effects typically associated with AEDs.

Pediatric Safety

Pediatric patients seem to have a higher tolerance for the treatment. Technical complications (99) and pain at the implant site (17) have been reported among some pediatric patients. However, the smaller and lighter design of the current Model 102 generator has reduced some of these types of complications. Increased salivation (19, 73, 100) and increased hyperactivity (19) have been reported for pediatric patients. Zamponi et al (17) also reported increased salivation and asthenia in one pediatric patient who was switched to rapid-cycling stimulation parameters; these events ceased once standard cycling was resumed. Lundgren et al (100) reported swallowing difficulties among two severely impaired pediatric patients with a history of swallowing difficulties. However, a study of eight patients without a history of swallowing difficulties by Schallert et al (101) showed that VNS therapy did not put patients at an increased risk of aspiration. Overall, the side effects reported for pediatric patients are often mild and transient, and not a contraindication to VNS therapy for this patient population.

Device Safety

Safety features are built into the VNS therapy system to protect patients from stimulation-related nerve injury. The primary safety feature is the "off switch" effect of the magnet. If a patient begins to experience continuous stimulation or uncomfortable side effects as a result of VNS therapy, the magnet can be held or taped over the generator to stop stimulation until the patient can visit the physician. A watchdog timer also is programmed into the device to monitor the number of pulses a patient receives. If a certain number of pulses is delivered without an Off time, the device will turn itself off to prevent excess stimulation from potentially causing nerve injury.

Procedures such as diathermy and full-body MRI scans, which have the potential to heat the device leads around the vagus nerve and thereby result in either temporary or permanent tissue and nerve damage, are contraindicated among patients receiving VNS therapy. Patients requiring an MRI should have the procedure performed with a head coil, which has been done successfully in VNS therapy patients (102). Of 27 MRI scans performed among 25 patients across 12 centers, 24 scans were performed with the VNS device turned off as recommended by the manufacturer. No stimulation was induced either during these scans or during the three scans performed with the device remaining in the on position. One child (age 11) reported chest pain while experiencing severe claustrophobia during the scan, and one patient had a mild objective voice change lasting several minutes (102). A successful body-coil MRI with the use of an ice pack over the area of the device leads was reported for three patients receiving VNS therapy, but is not recommended by the manufacturer (103). As recommended by the FDA, any instructions for MRI imaging that may be in the labeling for the implant should be followed exactly, and information on the types and/or strengths of MRI equipment that may have been previously tested for interaction with the implanted device should be noted (104). And because leads or portions of leads are sometimes left in the body among patients who have had the pulse generator explanted, it is important to get information regarding previously implanted devices, as the remaining leads could possibly become heated and damage the surrounding tissue (104). A bench study also supported anecdotal evidence that the VNS therapy magnet may inadvertently adjust the settings of programmable shunt valves commonly used to treat hydrocephalus (105). Therefore, physicians should be aware of the possibility of potential device interactions as the development and use of other implantable devices continues to evolve (105).

CANDIDATE SELECTION

Because the mechanisms of action are not well defined, the selection of patients for VNS therapy does not follow a clear set of guidelines. In addition, the clinical trials for VNS therapy could not distinguish any correlation between patient response and seizure type or etiology, age, sex, frequency of seizures, or frequency of interictal spikes on EEG (106) from which to generate any obvious candidate selection criteria. The number of coadministered AEDs or seizure types (78–80) or the type of coadministered AEDs (107) are not predictors of response, either. Therefore, as with AED therapy, there are currently no markers to predict the success of VNS therapy on a case-by-case basis. The safety and effectiveness of this treatment, achieved without the common adverse side effects associated with traditional AED therapy, and the fact that VNS therapy is reversible if a patient does not respond, make VNS therapy an attractive adjunctive treatment option for patients with refractory epilepsy who are not surgical candidates. VNS therapy is particularly attractive for the pediatric population, given the added benefit of the freedom from compliance issues associated with this therapy (108). Figure 64-9 shows a suggested treatment sequence flowchart that can be helpful in determining which palliative surgical procedures to chose when patients are experiencing refractory seizures.

Patients of any age should be considered for VNS therapy if they experience seizures refractory to other therapies, including AEDs, the ketogenic diet, and epilepsy surgery. Preliminary data suggest that patients treated with VNS therapy earlier in the course of their epilepsy (i.e., when seizures fail to respond to treatment with two or three AEDs within 2 years of epilepsy onset) may have a higher response rate to treatment (109). Early use of VNS therapy in treatment-resistant children would further allow physicians to decrease the negative side effects associated with AED therapy, which are compounded after long-term use and known to hinder development in this population (89, 110). Earlier use may also improve response to VNS therapy among the pediatric population because of a higher degree of neuronal plasticity at an early age that has the potential for permanent damage from long-term epilepsy (78). Earlier use of VNS therapy during the course of pharmacoresistant epilepsy (<6 years) also has been shown to be twice as likely to eliminate seizures than when VNS was initiated among patients who had been experiencing for 6 or more years, which reinforces the view that lesser cumulative seizure loads may improve patients' chances for recovery (111).

Precautions should be taken with patients predisposed to cardiac dysfunction and obstructive sleep apnea (OSA), because stimulation may increase apneic events, and chronic obstructive pulmonary disease may increase the risk of dyspnea (112, 113). A study by Nagarajan et al showed that seven of eight children (aged 4 to 16 years) receiving VNS therapy had respiratory pattern changes during sleep, but these changes were not associated with significant hypoxia or hypercapnia (114). Also, no apnea or hypopnea indexes were in the abnormal range. Although the changes in respiratory patterns during sleep appear to be mild, care should be taken when using VNS therapy among those with sleep apnea syndromes or compromised respiratory function, because vagal afferents influence respiratory control centers (113, 114). Lowering the stimulus frequency or increasing the Off time may prevent exacerbation (112, 114). It is not known whether the effects of VNS on sleep-related breathing diminish over time (113). The daytime effects of the altered nighttime breathing patterns also are not clear, because VNS has been shown both to facilitate and to inhibit REM sleep (115). A case report by Holmes et al (116) showed that an adult patient began experiencing sleep apneas and arousals associated with the intermittent VNS stimulation patterns, which led to the development of excessive daytime sleepiness. However, reports by Rizzo et al (115, 117) on a broader sample of 10 patients show that sleep modifications induced by VNS therapy among patients with refractory epilepsy actually enhance sleep EEG power, reduce rapid eye movement sleep, and improve daytime alertness. A study by Malow et al (112) among 16 patients receiving VNS therapy also showed an improvement in daytime sleepiness independent of seizure frequency control.

Patients who have undergone a bilateral or left cervical vagotomy are not considered candidates for VNS therapy (11). Evaluation by a cardiologist is recommended for patients with a personal or family history of cardiac dysfunction. If clinically indicated, Holter monitoring and electrocardiograms also should be done before implant.

COST EFFECTIVENESS

Previous cost analyses for VNS therapy indicate that the initial costs of VNS are offset over time by reductions in health care costs and hospital admissions following implantation (118–121). The reductions in economic burden for both patients and society were seen even among patients with less than a 25% reduction in seizures, indicating that even those without a substantial benefit in terms of seizure frequency reductions receive some benefit from the device (118). Although the efficacy of VNS therapy has been shown to increase over time, a cost analysis study calculated from 18 months before to 18 months after VNS device implantation showed that intensive care unit and ward admissions decreased from the very start of treatment with VNS (118). From a financial standpoint, the economic argument against VNS therapy is weak, particularly considering the potential for meaningful reductions in seizure frequency among patients with refractory epilepsy and the fact that efficacy remains and possibly increases over the long-term (119, 121). Therefore, the decision as to whether to proceed with VNS therapy for a patient population with few options should be made on the basis of clinical judgment rather than short-term costs (119).

CONCLUSION

VNS is emerging at the forefront of epilepsy treatments as a well-tolerated adjunctive therapy. With its minimal adverse side effects, lack of pharmacokinetic interactions with drug therapies, negligible compliance issues, residual improvement in quality of life, and improved efficacy over time, VNS therapy may be particularly effective among special patient populations, including pediatric patients and patients with comorbid conditions. Use of VNS therapy, however, must be balanced against the necessity of surgery, although VNS therapy surgery is well tolerated. As our understanding of what characterizes refractory epilepsy continues to evolve, adjunctive treatments such as VNS therapy will play an increasingly larger role in improving the lives of patients with epilepsy.

References

1. Buchhalter JR, Jarrar RG. Therapeutics in pediatric epilepsy, Part 2: Epilepsy surgery and vagus nerve stimulation. *Mayo Clin Proc* 2003; 78:371–378.
2. Uthman BM, Reichl AM, Dean JC, et al. Effectiveness of vagus nerve stimulation in epilepsy patients: a 12-year observation. *Neurology* 2004; 63:1124–1126.
3. Morris GL 3rd, Mueller WM. Long-term treatment with vagus nerve stimulation in patients with refractory epilepsy. The Vagus Nerve Stimulation Study Group E01-E05. *Neurology* 1999; 53:1731–1735.
4. DeGiorgio CM, Schachter SC, Handforth A, et al. Prospective long-term study of vagus nerve stimulation for the treatment of refractory seizures. *Epilepsia* 2000; 41:1195–1200.
5. Salinsky MC, Uthman BM, Ristanovic RK, Wernicke JF, et al. Vagus nerve stimulation for the treatment of medically intractable seizures. Results of a 1-year open-extension trial. Vagus Nerve Stimulation Study Group. *Arch Neurol* 1996; 53:1176–1180.
6. Schachter SC. Vagus nerve stimulation: where are we? *Curr Opin Neurol* 2002; 15: 201–206.
7. Amar AP, Levy ML, McComb JG, Apuzzo ML. Vagus nerve stimulation for control of intractable seizures in childhood. *Pediatr Neurosurg* 2001; 34:218–223.
8. Spanaki MV, Allen LS, Mueller WM, Morris GL 3rd. Vagus nerve stimulation therapy: 5-year or greater outcome at a university-based epilepsy center. *Seizure* 2004; 13:587–590.
9. Labar D. Vagus nerve stimulation for 1 year in 269 patients on unchanged antiepileptic drugs. *Seizure* 2004; 13:392–398.
10. Buoni S, Zannolli R, Macucci F, et al. Delayed response of seizures with vagus nerve stimulation in Lennox-Gastaut syndrome. *Neurology* 2004; 63:1539–1540.
11. Cyberonics, Inc. Physician's manual. VNS Therapy™ Pulse Model 102 Generator and VNS Therapy (TM) Pulse Duo Model 102R Generator. Cyberonics, 2003. http://www.vnstherapy.com/Epilepsy/forvnstherapypatients/manuals.aspx (accessed April 7, 2006).
12. Boon P, Vonck K, Van Walleghem P, et al. Programmed and magnet-induced vagus nerve stimulation for refractory epilepsy. *J Clin Neurophysiol* 2001; 18:402–407.
13. Morris GL 3rd. A retrospective analysis of the effects of magnet-activated stimulation in conjunction with vagus nerve stimulation therapy. *Epilepsy Behav* 2003; 4:740–745.
14. Murphy JV, Torkelson R, Dowler I, Simon S, et al. Vagal nerve stimulation in refractory epilepsy: the first 100 patients receiving vagal nerve stimulation at a pediatric epilepsy center. *Arch Pediatr Adolesc Med* 2003; 157:560–564.
15. Reid SA. Surgical technique for implantation of the neurocybernetic prosthesis. *Epilepsia* 1990; 31 Suppl 2:S38–S39.
16. Amar AP, Heck CN, Levy ML, et al. An institutional experience with cervical vagus nerve trunk stimulation for medically refractory epilepsy: rationale, technique, and outcome. *Neurosurgery* 1998; 43:1265–1276; discussion 1276–1280.
17. Zamponi N, Rychlicki F, Cardinali C, Luchetti A, et al. Intermittent vagal nerve stimulation in paediatric patients: 1-year follow-up. *Childs Nerv Syst* 2002; 18:61–66.
18. Ramsay RE, Uthman BM, Augustinsson LE, et al. Vagus nerve stimulation for treatment of partial seizures: 2. Safety, side effects, and tolerability. First International Vagus Nerve Stimulation Study Group. *Epilepsia* 1994; 35:627–636.
19. Helmers SL, Wheless JW, Frost M, et al. Vagus nerve stimulation therapy in pediatric patients with refractory epilepsy: retrospective study. *J Child Neurol* 2001; 16: 843–848.
20. Tatum WO 4th, Ferreira JA, Benbadis SR, et al. Vagus nerve stimulation for pharmacoresistant epilepsy: clinical symptoms with end of service. *Epilepsy Behav* 2004; 5:128–132.
21. Vonck K, Dedeurwaerdere S, Groote LD, et al. Generator replacement in epilepsy patients treated with vagus nerve stimulation. *Seizure* 2005; 14:89–99.
22. Le H, Chico M, Hecox K, Frim D. Interscapular placement of a vagal nerve stimulator pulse generator for prevention of wound tampering. Technical note. *Pediatr Neurosurg* 2002; 36:164–166.
23. Farooqui S, Boswell W, Hemphill JM, Pearlman E. Vagus nerve stimulation in pediatric patients with intractable epilepsy: case series and operative technique. *Am Surg* 2001; 67:119–121.
24. Andriola MR, Vitale SA. Vagus nerve stimulation in the developmentally disabled. *Epilepsy Behav* 2001; 2:129–134.
25. Patel NC, Edwards MS. Vagal nerve stimulator pocket infections. *Pediatr Infect Dis J* 2004; 23:681–683.
26. Smyth MD, Tubbs RS, Bebin EM, Grabb PA, et al. Complications of chronic vagus nerve stimulation for epilepsy in children. *J Neurosurg* 2003; 99:500–503.
27. Rychlicki F, Zamponi N, Cesaroni E, et al. Complications of vagal nerve stimulation for epilepsy in children. *Neurosurg Rev* 2006; 29:103–107.
28. Ben-Menachem E. Vagus nerve stimulation, side effects, and long-term safety. *J Clin Neurophysiol* 2001; 18:415–418.
29. Asconape JJ, Moore DD, Zipes DP, Hartman LM, et al. Bradycardia and asystole with the use of vagus nerve stimulation for the treatment of epilepsy: a rare complication of intraoperative device testing. *Epilepsia* 1999; 40:1452–1454.
30. Tatum WO 4th, Moore DB, Stecker MM, et al. Ventricular asystole during vagus nerve stimulation for epilepsy in humans. *Neurology* 1999; 52:1267–1269.
31. Ali II, Pirzada NA, Kanjwal Y, et al. Complete heart block with ventricular asystole during left vagus nerve stimulation for epilepsy. *Epilepsy Behav* 2004; 5:768–771.
32. Zalvan C, Sulica L, Wolf S, Cohen J, et al. Laryngopharyngeal dysfunction from the implant vagal nerve stimulator. *Laryngoscope* 2003; 113:221–225.
33. Crumrine PK. Vagal nerve stimulation in children. *Semin Pediatr Neurol* 2000; 7:216–223.
34. Majoie HJ, Berfelo MW, Aldenkamp AP, Renier WO, et al. Vagus nerve stimulation in patients with catastrophic childhood epilepsy, a 2-year follow-up study. *Seizure* 2005; 14:10–18.
35. McGregor A, Wheless J, Baumgartner J, Bettis D. Right-sided vagus nerve stimulation as a treatment for refractory epilepsy in humans. *Epilepsia* 2005; 46:91–96.
36. Heck C, Helmers SL, DeGiorgio CM. Vagus nerve stimulation therapy, epilepsy, and device parameters: scientific basis and recommendations for use. *Neurology* 2002; 59: S31–S37.
37. Koo B, Ham SD, Sood S, Tarver B. Human vagus nerve electrophysiology: a guide to vagus nerve stimulation parameters. *J Clin Neurophysiol* 2001; 18:429–433.
38. Majoie HJ, Berfelo MW, Aldenkamp AP, Evers SM, et al. Vagus nerve stimulation in children with therapy-resistant epilepsy diagnosed as Lennox-Gastaut syndrome: clinical results, neuropsychological effects, and cost-effectiveness. *J Clin Neurophysiol* 2001; 18:419–428.
39. DeGiorgio C, Heck C, Bunch S, et al. Vagus nerve stimulation for epilepsy: randomized comparison of three stimulation paradigms. *Neurology* 2005; 65:317–319.
40. Parr JR, Pang K, Mollett A, et al. Epilepsy responds to vagus nerve stimulation in ring chromosome 20 syndrome. *Dev Med Child Neurol* 2006; 48:80; author reply 80.
41. Mu Q, Bohning DE, Nahas Z, et al. Acute vagus nerve stimulation using different pulse widths produces varying brain effects. *Biol Psychiatry* 2004; 55:816–825.
42. Schachter SC, Saper CB. Vagus nerve stimulation. *Epilepsia* 1998; 39:677–686.
43. Henry TR. Therapeutic mechanisms of vagus nerve stimulation. *Neurology* 2002; 59: S3–S14.
44. Rutecki P. Anatomical, physiological, and theoretical basis for the antiepileptic effect of vagus nerve stimulation. *Epilepsia* 1990; 31 Suppl 2:S1–S6.
45. Groves DA, Bowman EM, Brown VJ. Recordings from the rat locus coeruleus during acute vagal nerve stimulation in the anaesthetised rat. *Neurosci Lett* 2005; 379:174–179.
46. Krahl SE, Clark KB, Smith DC, Browning RA. Locus coeruleus lesions suppress the seizure-attenuating effects of vagus nerve stimulation. *Epilepsia* 1998; 39:709–714.
47. Jimenez-Rivera C, Voltura A, Weiss GK. Effect of locus ceruleus stimulation on the development of kindled seizures. *Exp Neurol* 1987; 95:13–20.
48. Petrucci M, Hoh C, Alksne JF. Thalamic hypometabolism in a patient undergoing vagal nerve stimulation seen on F-18 FDG PET imaging. *Clin Nucl Med* 2003; 28:784–785.
49. Liu WC, Mosier K, Kalnin AJ, Marks D. BOLD fMRI activation induced by vagus nerve stimulation in seizure patients. *J Neurol Neurosurg Psychiatry* 2003; 74:811–813.
50. Henry TR, Votaw JR, Pennell PB, et al. Acute blood flow changes and efficacy of vagus nerve stimulation in partial epilepsy. *Neurology* 1999; 52:1166–1173.
51. Henry TR, Bakay RA, Votaw JR, et al. Brain blood flow alterations induced by therapeutic vagus nerve stimulation in partial epilepsy: I. Acute effects at high and low levels of stimulation. *Epilepsia* 1998; 39:983–990.
52. Henry TR, Votaw JR, Bakay RAE, et al. Vagus nerve stimulation-indcued cerebral blood flow changes differ in acute and chornic therapy of complex partial seizures. *Epilepsia* 1998; 39:92.
53. Henry TR, Bakay RA, Pennell PB, Epstein CM, et al. Brain blood-flow alterations induced by therapeutic vagus nerve stimulation in partial epilepsy: II. Prolonged effects at high and low levels of stimulation. *Epilepsia* 2004; 45:1064–1070.
54. Marrosu F, Santoni F, Puligheddu M, et al. Increase in 20–50Hz (gamma frequencies) power spectrum and synchronization after chronic vagal nerve stimulation. *Clin Neurophysiol* 2005; 116:2026–2036.
55. Marrosu F, Serra A, Maleci A, Puligheddu M, et al. Correlation between GABA(A) receptor density and vagus nerve stimulation in individuals with drug-resistant partial epilepsy. *Epilepsy Res* 2003; 55:59–70.
56. Lesser RP. Unexpected places: how did vagus nerve stimulation become a treatment for epilepsy? *Neurology* 1999; 52:1117–1118.
57. Zabara J. Neuroinhibition in the regulation of emesis. In: Bianchi AL, Grelot L, Miller AD, King GL, eds. *Mechanisms and Control of Emesis*. Colloque INSERM/John Libbey Eurotext Ltd, 1992:285–295.

58. Zabara J, Chaffee RB Jr, Tansy MF. Neuroinhibition in the regulation of emesis. *Space Life Sciences* 1972; 3:282–292.
59. Zabara J. Peripheral control of hypersynchronous discharge in epilepsy. *Electroencephelogr Clin Neurophysiol* 1985; 61:P26.05.
60. Zabara J. Time course of seizure control to brief, repetitive stimuli. *Epilepsia* 1985; 26:518.
61. Woodbury JW, Woodbury DM. Vagal stimulation reduces the severity of maximal electroshock seizures in intact rats: use of a cuff electrode for stimulating and recording. *Pacing Clin Electrophysiol* 1991; 14:94–107.
62. Woodbury DM, Woodbury JW. Effects of vagal stimulation on experimentally induced seizures in rats. *Epilepsia* 1990; 31 Suppl 2:S7–S19.
63. Lockard JS, Congdon WC, DuCharme LL. Feasibility and safety of vagal stimulation in monkey model. *Epilepsia* 1990; 31 Suppl 2:S20–S26.
64. Lockard JS, Congdon WC. Effects of vagal stimulation on seizure rate in monkey model. *Epilepsia* 1986; 27:626 (abstract).
65. Dedeurwaerdere S, Cornelissen B, Van Laere K, et al. Small animal positron emission tomography during vagus nerve stimulation in rats: a pilot study. *Epilepsy Res* 2005; 67:133–141.
66. Dedeurwaerdere S, Vonck K, Claeys P, et al. Acute vagus nerve stimulation does not suppress spike and wave discharges in genetic absence epilepsy rats from Strasbourg. *Epilepsy Res* 2004; 59:191–198.
67. Clark KB, Smith DC, Hassert DL, Browning RA, et al. Posttraining electrical stimulation of vagal afferents with concomitant vagal efferent inactivation enhances memory storage processes in the rat. *Neurobiol Learn Mem* 1998; 70:364–373.
68. Smith DC, Modglin AA, Roosevelt RW, et al. Electrical stimulation of the vagus nerve enhances cognitive and motor recovery following moderate fluid percussion injury in the rat. *J Neurotrauma* 2005; 22:1485–1502.
69. Hassert DL, Miyashita T, Williams CL. The effects of peripheral vagal nerve stimulation at a memory-modulating intensity on norepinephrine output in the basolateral amygdala. *Behav Neurosci* 2004; 118:79–88.
70. A randomized controlled trial of chronic vagus nerve stimulation for treatment of medically intractable seizures. The Vagus Nerve Stimulation Study Group. *Neurology* 1995; 45:224–230.
71. Handforth A, DeGiorgio CM, Schachter SC, et al. Vagus nerve stimulation therapy for partial-onset seizures: a randomized active-control trial. *Neurology* 1998; 51:48–55.
72. Murphy JV. Left vagal nerve stimulation in children with medically refractory epilepsy. The Pediatric VNS Study Group. *J Pediatr* 1999; 134:563–566.
73. Frost M, Gates J, Helmers SL, et al. Vagus nerve stimulation in children with refractory seizures associated with Lennox-Gastaut syndrome. *Epilepsia* 2001; 42:1148–1152.
74. Hornig GW, Murphy JV, Schallert G, Tilton C. Left vagus nerve stimulation in children with refractory epilepsy: an update. *South Med J* 1997; 90:484–488.
75. Tanganelli P, Ferrero S, Colotto P, Regesta G. Vagus nerve stimulation for treatment of medically intractable seizures. Evaluation of long-term outcome. *Clin Neurol Neurosurg* 2002; 105:9–13.
76. Labar D, Nikolov B, Tarver B, Fraser R. Vagus nerve stimulation for symptomatic generalized epilepsy: a pilot study. *Epilepsia* 1998; 39:201–205.
77. Hosain S, Nikalov B, Harden C, Li M, et al. Vagus nerve stimulation treatment for Lennox-Gastaut syndrome. *J Child Neurol* 2000; 15:509–512.
78. Labar D, Murphy J, Tecoma E. Vagus nerve stimulation for medication-resistant generalized epilepsy. E04 VNS Study Group. *Neurology* 1999; 52:1510–1512.
79. Ng M, Devinsky O. Vagus nerve stimulation for refractory idiopathic generalized epilepsy. *Seizure* 2004; 13:176–178.
80. Holmes MD, Silbergeld DL, Drouhard D, Wilensky AJ, et al. Effect of vagus nerve stimulation on adults with pharmacoresistant generalized epilepsy syndromes. *Seizure* 2004; 13:340–345.
81. Parain D, Penniello MJ, Berquen P, Delangre T, et al. Vagal nerve stimulation in tuberous sclerosis complex patients. *Pediatr Neurol* 2001; 25:213–216.
82. Park YD. The effects of vagus nerve stimulation therapy on patients with intractable seizures and either Landau-Kleffner syndrome or autism. *Epilepsy Behav* 2003; 4: 286–290.
83. Winston KR, Levisohn P, Miller BR, Freeman J. Vagal nerve stimulation for status epilepticus. *Pediatr Neurosurg* 2001; 34:190–192.
84 Malik SI, Hernandez AW. Intermittent vagus nerve stimulation in pediatric patients with pharmacoresistant status epilepticus. *Epilepsia* 2004; 45(suppl 7):155–156.
85. Patwardhan RV, Dellabadia J Jr, Rashidi M, Grier L, et al. Control of refractory status epilepticus precipitated by anticonvulsant withdrawal using left vagal nerve stimulation: a case report. *Surg Neurol* 2005, 64:170–173.
86. Amar AP, Apuzzo ML, Liu CY. Vagus nerve stimulation therapy after failed cranial surgery for intractable epilepsy: results from the vagus nerve stimulation therapy patient outcome registry. *Neurosurgery* 2004; 55:1086–1093.
87. Fohlen MJ, Jalin C, Pinard JM, Delalande OR. Results of vagus nerve stimulation in 10 children with refractory infantile spasms. *Epilepsia* 1998; 39(suppl 6):170.
88. Aldenkamp AP, Majoie HJM, Berfelo MW, et al. Long-term effects of 24-month treatment with vagus nerve stimulation on behaviour in children with Lennox-Gastaut syndrome. *Epilepsy Behav* 2002; 3:475–479.
89. Chawla J, Sucholeiki R, Jones C, Silver K. Intractable epilepsy with ring chromosome 20 syndrome treated with vagal nerve stimulation: case report and review of the literature. *J Child Neurol* 2002; 17:778–780.
90. Alpman A, Serdaroglu G, Cogulu O, Tekgul H, et al. Ring chromosome 20 syndrome with intractable epilepsy. *Dev Med Child Neurol* 2005; 47:343–346.
91. Devinsky O. What do you do when they grow up? Approaches to seizures in developmentally delayed adults. *Epilepsia* 2002; 43 Suppl 3:71–79.
92. Pellock JM, Hunt PA. A decade of modern epilepsy therapy in institutionalized mentally retarded patients. *Epilepsy Res* 1996; 25:263–268.
93. Huf RL, Mamelak A, Kneedy-Cayem K. Vagus nerve stimulation therapy: 2-year prospective open-label study of 40 subjects with refractory epilepsy and low IQ who are living in long-term care facilities. *Epilepsy Behav* 2005; 6:417–423.
94. Gates J, Huf R, Frost M. Vagus nerve stimulation for patients in residential treatment facilities. *Epilepsy Behav* 2001; 2:563–567.
95. Murphy JV, Wheless JW, Schmoll CM. Left vagal nerve stimulation in six patients with hypothalamic hamartomas. *Pediatr Neurol* 2000; 23:167–168.
96. Annegers JF, Coan SP, Hauser WA, Leestma J, et al. Epilepsy, vagal nerve stimulation by the NCP system, mortality, and sudden, unexpected, unexplained death. *Epilepsia* 1998; 39:206–212.
97. Ben-Menachem E, Hellstrom K, Waldton C, Augustinsson LE. Evaluation of refractory epilepsy treated with vagus nerve stimulation for up to 5 years. *Neurology* 1999; 52:1265–1267.
98. Liporace J, Hucko D, Morrow R, et al. Vagal nerve stimulation: adjustments to reduce painful side effects. *Neurology* 2001; 57:885–886.
99. Murphy JV, Hornig GW, Schallert GS, Tilton CL. Adverse events in children receiving intermittent left vagal nerve stimulation. *Pediatr Neurol* 1998; 19:42–44.
100. Lundgren J, Amark P, Blennow G, Stromblad LG, et al. Vagus nerve stimulation in 16 children with refractory epilepsy. *Epilepsia* 1998; 39:809–813.
101. Schallert G, Foster J, Lindquist N, Murphy JV. Chronic stimulation of the left vagal nerve in children: effect on swallowing. *Epilepsia* 1998; 39:1113–1114.
102. Benbadis SR, Nyhenhuis J, Tatum WO 4th, Murtagh FR, et al. MRI of the brain is safe in patients implanted with the vagus nerve stimulator. *Seizure* 2001; 10:512–515.
103. Wilfong AA. Body MRI and vagus nerve stimulation. *Epilepsia* 2002; 43,347.
104. Schultz DG. FDA Public Health Notification: MRI-caused injuries in patients with implanted neurological stimulators. Published May 10, 2005. http://www.fda.gov/cdrh/safety.html (accessed March 14, 2006).
105. Jandial R, Aryan HE, Hughes SA, Levy ML. Effect of vagus nerve stimulator magnet on programmable shunt settings. *Neurosurgery* 2004; 55:627–629; discussion 629–630.
106. Wheless JW, Baumgartner J, Ghanbari C. Vagus nerve stimulation and the ketogenic diet. *Neurol Clin* 2001; 19:371–407.
107. Labar DR. Antiepileptic drug use during the first 12 months of vagus nerve stimulation therapy: a registry study. *Neurology* 2002; 59:S38–S43.
108. Wheless JW, Venkataraman V, Helmers S, et al. Vagus nerve stimulation (VNS) in children: efficacy. *Epilepsia* 1999; 40:120–121.
109. Renfroe JB, Wheless JW. Earlier use of adjunctive vagus nerve stimulation therapy for refractory epilepsy. *Neurology* 2002; 59:S26–S30.
110. Scherrmann J, Hoppe C, Kral T, Schramm J, et al. Vagus nerve stimulation: clinical experience in a large patient series. *J Clin Neurophysiol* 2001; 18:408–414.
111. Helmers SL, Griesemer DA, Dean JC, Sanchez JD, et al. Observations on the use of vagus nerve stimulation earlier in the course of pharmacoresistant epilepsy: patients with seizures for six years or less. *Neurologist* 2003; 9:160–164.
112. Malow BA, Edwards J, Marzec M, Sagher O, et al. Vagus nerve stimulation reduces daytime sleepiness in epilepsy patients. *Neurology* 2001; 57:879–884.
113. Marzec M, Edwards J, Sagher O, Fromes G, et al. Effects of vagus nerve stimulation on sleep-related breathing in epilepsy patients. *Epilepsia* 2003; 44:930–935.
114. Nagarajan L, Walsh P, Gregory P, Stick S, et al. Respiratory pattern changes in sleep in children on vagal nerve stimulation for refractory epilepsy. *Can J Neurol Sci* 2003; 30:224–227.
115. Rizzo P, Beelke M, De Carli F, et al. Chronic vagus nerve stimulation improves alertness and reduces rapid eye movement sleep in patients affected by refractory epilepsy. *Sleep* 2003; 26:607–611.
116. Holmes MD, Chang M, Kapur V. Sleep apnea and excessive daytime somnolence induced by vagal nerve stimulation. *Neurology* 2003; 61:1126–1129.
117. Rizzo P, Beelke M, De Carli F, et al. Modifications of sleep EEG induced by chronic vagus nerve stimulation in patients affected by refractory epilepsy. *Clin Neurophysiol* 2004; 115:658–664.
118. Ben-Menachem E, Hellstrom K, Verstappen D. Analysis of direct hospital costs before and 18 months after treatment with vagus nerve stimulation therapy in 43 patients. *Neurology* 2002; 59:S44–S47.
119 Forbes RB, Macdonald S, Eljamel S, Roberts RC. Cost-utility analysis of vagus nerve stimulators for adults with medically refractory epilepsy. *Seizure* 2003; 12:249–256.
120. Boon P, Vonck K, D'Have M, O'Connor S, et al. Cost-benefit of vagus nerve stimulation for refractory epilepsy. *Acta Neurol Belg* 1999; 99:275–280.
121. Boon P, Vonck K, Vandekerckhove T, et al. Vagus nerve stimulation for medically refractory epilepsy; efficacy and cost-benefit analysis. *Acta Neurochir (Wien)* 1999; 141:447–452; discussion 453.

VII

PSYCHOSOCIAL ASPECTS

65 Economics of Pediatric Epilepsy

Charles E. Begley

The economic aspects of epilepsy have received considerable attention in recent years. This interest has been generated by the need to contain the cost of medical care, allocate scarce research funds, and justify new therapies and health care services. There are two fundamental types of research on the economics of epilepsy: cost-of-illness and cost-benefit studies.

Cost-of-illness studies attempt to measure the economic burden of epilepsy to society (1). They are used by advocacy groups to promote research and fund services, and by planning and policymaking groups to allocate resources. Such studies measure the amount and distribution of direct cost associated with medical care and social service items, such as drug costs and counseling, and indirect costs from the disability and premature mortality effects of epilepsy, such as lost earnings and productivity. Cost-of-illness studies may also examine the distribution of cost among patients with different types of epilepsy, such as intractable epilepsy versus remitting epilepsy, and in different stages of illness, such as new cases versus prevalent cases.

COST OF ILLNESS STUDIES

In cost-of-illness studies, direct cost includes three broad categories:

1. The cost of medical care, including professional services, laboratory tests, medications, hospital care, medical supplies, and equipment
2. Nonmedical direct cost, including social services and resources related to special education, transportation, and modifications to the residence
3. Imputed costs of patients' and caregivers' time devoted to accessing care or providing care

Indirect costs of illness include the following:

1. Loss of earnings associated with reduced employment
2. Reduced earnings because of illness or reduced productivity on the job
3. The lost value of household production when people are unable to conduct household work
4. The lost earnings because of productive years of life lost from increased mortality attributable to epilepsy; productive years are usually defined as ages 18 through 64; although the pediatric ages are not included, childhood-onset epilepsy may have an impact on the productive years of life as adults

Cost-of-illness studies vary in time perspective. Cross-sectional studies present annual costs for prevalent cases. Longitudinal studies estimate the cost borne throughout the lifespan for incident cases that occur in a given year. The longitudinal perspective is used to evaluate the long-term effects of a new treatment. For example, to evaluate the economic effects of a new drug, one should estimate the lifetime impact on direct and indirect costs related to relapse seizures, side effects, future employment, and mortality. The cross-sectional perspective is useful for understanding the impact of a change in the healthcare delivery system. For example, the economic impact of managing patients with primary care or specialty physicians can be assessed by comparing the direct and indirect costs of patients in different treatment settings.

COST-BENEFIT STUDIES

In contrast to cost-of-illness studies, which measure the total burden of disease in economic terms, cost-benefit studies are used to evaluate the economic impact of specific interventions in prevention, diagnosis and treatment, or rehabilitation (2). The main objective of cost-benefit studies is to compare specific therapies or systems of health care delivery in terms of their relative benefits and costs. Cost-benefit studies depend on a thorough understanding of the detailed costs of an intervention. In addition, they require data on the outcomes of interventions. The following are examples of cost-benefit questions:

1. A new drug or device is introduced with additional costs, more or less adverse side effects, more or less need for monitoring, but some gain in efficacy. What are the costs and benefits of the new therapy versus the old therapy?
2. In a health care delivery system or network, what is the benefit of a neurologist versus a general practitioner evaluating and treating first-seizure patients and at what additional cost? The cost-benefit evaluation would apply to the accuracy of the diagnostic procedures and resulting patient outcomes, including seizure control and adverse drug affects.
3. What are the costs and benefits of specific tests such as magnetic resonance imaging (MRI) versus computed tomography (CT) scans in improving the accuracy of diagnoses in patients with epilepsy?

Economic studies of epilepsy are methodologically challenging. Cost-of-illness studies face unresolved issues regarding case definition, attribution of costs, and estimation of nonmedical direct and indirect costs. There are standardized methods for conducting cost-benefit studies (3), but data limitations often prevent researchers from following all the recommended procedures. In epilepsy cost-benefit studies lack standardized measures of treatment outcomes.

HOW THE COST OF EPILEPSY IS MEASURED

Because the total direct and indirect costs of illness include many components, one must combine data from several sources to estimate these costs. Direct medical cost typically is determined either from utilization and billing records of patients (4, 5), patient or population surveys (6), or simulated from a disease prognosis models (7, 8). Data collection studies may be prospective or retrospective. Nonmedical direct cost is more difficult to measure but can be obtained for pediatric epilepsy through interviews with caregivers of a representative sample of patients and families. Indirect cost is measured by comparing unemployment rates, lost work due to sick days, reduced productivity at home and at work, and lost work and household production due to premature mortality for people with epilepsy compared with the general population. National age- and sex-specific earnings data, available from the U.S. Bureau of the Census and the Bureau of Labor Statistics, are used to estimate lost earnings. The indirect costs related to differences in employment and wages may have to be inferred from information about the educational achievement of children. Age-specific person years of productive life lost can be determined from studies that measure the excess mortality in individuals with epilepsy.

CASE DEFINITION FOR PEDIATRIC COST STUDIES

Cost-of-illness estimates are strongly influenced by the case definition used. If cases of epilepsy are restricted to patients with recurrent unprovoked seizures that typically are seen in referral centers, then only 1 percent of children will be affected by their eighteenth birthday. However, should single unprovoked seizures, which occur in approximately 0.3 percent of children per year, be included in cost of epilepsy studies? The first seizure, if the patient is identified at that time, is when the major diagnostic workup occurs, and it is a significant direct medical cost. However, many of these children never receive a diagnosis of epilepsy. For this reason, a practical definition would include all cost from the second recognized seizure in the general population.

Cost related to the diagnosis and treatment of febrile convulsions have not been included in the cost of epilepsy. Even though the direct and indirect cost per febrile seizure case usually are low, the large number, four percent of all children, who have such seizures, would greatly increase the pediatric cost of epilepsy if febrile convulsions were included. Approximately 0.5% of all children experience acute symptomatic seizures—seizures related to transient central nervous system insults, the most common of which in children are traumatic brain injury, encephalitis, and perinatal insults. The cost of these seizures is not included in the cost of epilepsy studies and is more appropriately considered part of the cost of the underlying causes. In addition to children found to have had epilepsy or seizures, there are many who have symptoms suggestive of seizures and incur direct medical cost as a result. Cost of epilepsy studies tend to exclude this sizable population as well.

SEPARATING THE COST OF EPILEPSY FROM THAT OF OTHER ILLNESSES

Some pediatric epilepsy patients have severe comorbidities, especially cerebral palsy and mental retardation, that contribute to their direct medical and indirect cost because of potential unemployment and excess mortality. If the cost of epilepsy is to be separated from that of other illnesses, one must determine what proportion should be reasonably attributed to epilepsy. In cases of severe neurologic deficits, presumably present from birth (i.e., preceding the epilepsy), only the cost related to the seizure disorder should be attributed to epilepsy. If all the direct and indirect costs in children with severe neurologic deficits and epilepsy are attributed to epilepsy, the total cost of pediatric epilepsy is greatly inflated in the portion of cost incurred by children with neurologic deficit (6). To avoid this problem, only the direct cost related to the management of seizures in these children should be attributed to epilepsy. Likewise, in cases of postnatal acquired epilepsy—mainly traumatic brain injury, central nervous system infections, and intracranial tumors in children—only those components of direct cost related to seizures should be included. There is a small but, in terms of cost, very important group of children with catastrophic epilepsy of childhood in whom the other disabilities may be a product of epilepsy.

STUDIES OF THE COST OF EPILEPSY

A number of recent studies have estimated the direct medical care cost of epilepsy in people of all ages (5, 9–12). One study in Italy provided separate cost estimates for children. Table 65-1 indicates a range for annual direct medical care cost of $126 to almost $2,000 per person for inactive cases and $800 to over $3,000 per year for active cases. The range reflects variation in medical care prices and treatment patterns in epilepsy as well as methodological differences used in the studies. Because of data limitations, most studies do not address the non-medical direct or indirect costs of epilepsy.

Estimates of incidence-based cost come from three studies (13–15) (Table 65-2) and indicate first-year

TABLE 65-1
Prevalence-Based Estimates of the Annual Cost of Epilepsy

STUDY	TETTO ET AL, 2002 (9)	GUERRINI ET AL, 2000 (10)	JACOBY ET AL, 1998 (11)	COCKERELL ET AL, 994 (NES) (5)	VAN HOUT ET AL, 1997 (12)
Country	Italy	Italy	UK	UK	France, Germany, UK
Population	525 all ages	189 youth (age 0–18)	785 all ages	1,628 all ages	300 adults (age 18–65)
Case selection	Referral patients	Referral patients	General population	General population	Referral population
Study design	Prospective	Prospective	Retrospective	Retrospective	Retrospective
Direct cost per person per year	$420 inactive	$851 inactive	$243 inactive	$126 inactive	$1,748 inactive
	$1,657 active non drug-resistant	$1,104 active non-drug-resistant	$1,238 active <1 seiz\mo	$803 active (at least one seizure in prev two yrs)	$3,208 active (ranging from <1\mo to >1\day)
	$2,240 active drug-resistant cases	$3,256 active drug-resistant	$2,288 active >1 seiz\mo		

Reproduced from Begley and Beghi (1).

TABLE 65-2
Incidence-Based Estimates of the Annual Cost of Epilepsy

Study	Cockerell et al, 1997 (NGPSE) (13)	De Zelicourt et al, 1996 (14)	Begley et al, 2000 (15)
Country	UK	France	US
Population	602 all ages	1,942 all ages	500 all ages
Case selection	General	General	General
Study design	Prospective	Prospective	Retrospective
Direct cost per person per year	$917 in year 1	$2,432 in year 1	$3,157 in year 1
	$282 in year 4	$640 in year 2	$702 in year 2
	$254 in year 8		$471 in year 3
			$411 in year 4

medical costs ranging from $917 to over $3,000 per person and subsequent-year costs 60–70% below first-year cost, reflecting the large number of cases that achieve remission and the lower level of cost for maintenance therapy compared to initial therapy at onset. The most significant cost-driving factor in epilepsy is severity, expressed as seizure frequency. Costs do not appear to vary significantly among different epilepsy syndromes, nor across age groups or by gender.

THE TOTAL COST OF EPILEPSY

A study was conducted to estimate the total cost of epilepsy in the United States in 1995 (16). A model was constructed that considered the annual number of cases, the variable prognosis of epilepsy for three different groups, the variation in the use of services and medications by prognostic group and time from the diagnosis, and per case estimates of direct cost and indirect cost. The estimated U.S. lifetime cost, based on 1995 incidence cases, was $11.1 billion; the total annual cost, based on 2.3 million prevalent cases, was $12.5 billion. Indirect costs account for 85% of the total and concentrated in people with intractable epilepsy.

The distribution of direct costs of prevalent cases by age and type of epilepsy is presented in Table 65-3 in 1995 dollars. These include the cost of emergency services, inpatient hospitalizations, outpatient visits, diagnostic procedures, laboratory tests, antiepileptic drugs (AEDs), and surgery. The largest direct cost item was AEDs, which accounted for almost 31% of the cost of epilepsy. Hospital admissions were second, accounting for 24% of total costs, and outpatient physician visits were third, with 8% of costs.

COST-BENEFIT STUDIES OF ANTIEPILEPTIC DRUGS

AED therapy, either monotherapy or polytherapy, is the mainstay of treatment for people with epilepsy. Approximately 60% to 70% of people with epileptic seizures are able to control their seizures quite well with drug therapy. Since 1993, there has been a dramatic increase in the number of new AEDs available in the United States,

TABLE 65-3
Annual Direct Costs for 1995 by Age and Type of Epilepsy

	Age 0–14 yr	Age 15–64 yr	Age 65+ yr	All Ages
Prognostic Group				
Inactive	165,287 (9.8)	532,967 (31.6)	252,991 (15.0)	951,245 (56.3)
Active	64,091 (3.8)	526,221(31.2)	146,735 (8.7)	737,047 (43.7)
	229,378 (13.6)	1,059,118 (62.7)	399,726 (23.7)	1,688,292 (100.0)

Source: Begley et al 2000 (16).

TABLE 65-4
Acquisition Costs of First- and Second-Generation AEDs

AEDs	Common Maintenance Dosage (mg/day)	2003 Acquisition Cost/Month	2004 Acquisition Cost/Month
Second-Generation AEDs			
Zonisamide	100–600	63–375	65–387
Oxcarbazepine	600–2,400	102–192	105–198
Tiagabine	36–64	111–195	115–201
Levetiracetam	1,000–3,000	118–348	122–359
Felbamate	1,800–3,600	144–287	149–296
Gabapentin	900–3,600	155–195	160–201
Lamotrigine	300–500	174–262	180–271
Topiramate	200–400	206–267	213–276
Pregabalin	NA	NA	NA
First-Generation AEDs			
Phenobarbital	60–240	<5–32	<5–33
Phenytoin	300	28	29
Ethosuximide	500–1,500	62–185	64–191
Carbamazepine	800–1,600	68–136	70–140
Valproate	750–2,250	90–159	93–164
Primidone	750–1,500	NA	NA

Source: Begley 2005 (17).

including felbamate, gabapentin, lamotrigine, levetiracetam, oxcarbazepine, pregabalin, tiagabine, topiramate, and zonisamide.

All second-generation AEDs have been approved as add on therapy for patients with partial epileptic seizures, and three of them have been approved as add-on therapy for patients having generalized epileptic seizures. Most of the second-generation AEDs have been approved for children as well as adults, and four (felbamate, lamotrigine, oxcarbazepine, and topiramate) are approved for monotherapy. Because the new-generation drugs are much more expensive than earlier drugs, the cost-benefit ratio of these agents is a topic of ongoing debate (17) (Table 65-4).

A cost-benefit framework has been applied to evaluate the economic impact of the second-generation AEDs (2). The cost-benefit analysis compares the cost of treatment with one therapy type compared with another intervention, such as a first-generation AED versus a second-generation AED. It then compares the effects, expressed in a clinically relevant outcome measure or patient-based outcome measure, reflecting the benefit of the therapy. To carry out the study in the cost-benefit framework, several versions of analysis can be performed: cost-minimization analysis, cost-effectiveness analysis, and cost-utility analysis. These approaches differ slightly in terms of the data required to perform the economic evaluation of the new therapies.

Cost-benefit studies have compared the first- and second-generation AEDs in monotherapy. These studies indicate that the overall treatment costs for new patients with epilepsy are relatively low compared to the costs of other major chronic diseases. To date, the data also indicate that the first-generation AEDs are more likely to be cost-effective in monotherapy for new patients, but the results are uncertain. The acquisition costs for first-generation AEDs are significantly cheaper, but the cost differences, when considering rates and severity of adverse effects and tolerability, narrow the gap, indicating that payors should take into consideration these treatment cost differences as well as acquisition cost differences (2, 17).

Cost-benefit studies comparing first- and second-generaltion AEDs as adjunctive therapy illustrate that epilepsy is indeed a costly disorder for people with refractory seizures. They also illustrate that the second-generation AEDs are generally both more effective and more costly as adjunctive therapy—that is, they add cost, but they improve outcomes for refractory patients. Therefore, balancing of the additional cost versus the additional gain or additional benefit of newer AEDs becomes complicated. Patients have fewer adverse effects and drug interactions from the second-generation AEDs, which can significantly lower adverse-effects treatments. Last, second-generation AEDs appeared to be cost effective at a threshold level of about $40,000 per quality-adjusted life year, which is under the $50,000 gold standard (17).

Additionally, second-generation AEDs as add-on therapy may be no more expensive than first-generation AEDs as add-on therapy and appear to be cost effective in the long term. This is particularly true when considering the possible reduction in surgical evaluation and surgery. Some second-generation AEDs may be more cost effective than others, and although there are several studies comparing them, the studies are limited and the results are inconclusive (2, 17).

CONCLUSIONS

The total direct cost of all pediatric epilepsy and unprovoked seizure cases in the United States in 1995 was estimated to be approximately $230 million, representing 14% of total direct costs for all ages. The cost per case was $726, but this reflects the cost of cases with inactive as well as active epilepsy. Compared with other cross-sectional prevalence-based studies, these estimates appear to be conservative. Presumably, this difference is largely due to the inclusion of only those direct costs that can reasonably be attributed to epilepsy rather than comorbidities.

Although the second-generation AEDs tend to be more costly, they also potentially offer cost savings if patients become seizure free, experience fewer adverse effects from their drugs, or require less monitoring of the newer drugs. It appears from the preliminary studies that the second-generation AEDs have most economic value as add-on therapy in refractory patients and therefore need to be carefully evaluated to determine their value as monotherapy in new patients.

ACKNOWLEDGMENT

The author acknowledges Tom Reynolds and Sharon Coan for their assistance in preparation of this chapter.

References

1. Begley CE, Beghi E. The economic cost of epilepsy: a review of the literature. *Epilepsia* 2002; 43(Suppl 4):3–9.
2. Heaney DC, Begley CE. Economic evaluation of epilepsy treatment: a review of the literature. *Epilepsia* 2002; 43(Suppl 4):10–16.
3. Gold MR, Siegel JE, Russell LB, Weinstein MC. Cost-effectiveness in health and medicine. New York: Oxford University Press, 1996.
4. Banks GK, Regan KJ, Beran RG. The prevalence and direct costs of epilepsy in Australia. In: Beran RG, Pachlatko C, eds. *Cost of Epilepsy: Proceedings of the 20th International Epilepsy Congress*. Baden, Germany: Ciba-Geigy Verlag, 1995:39–48.
5. Cockerell OC, Hart YM, Sander JW, Shorvon SD. The cost of epilepsy in the United Kingdom: an estimation based on the results of two population-based studies. *Epilepsy Res* 1994; 18:249–260.
6. Commission for the Control of Epilepsy and Its Consequences, Economic Cost of Epilepsy. *Plan for Nationwide Action on Epilepsy, Vol. IV.* DHEW Publication No. 78-279. Washington, DC (NIH): 1978; 117–148.
7. Begley CE, Annegers JF, Lairson DR, Reynolds TF, et al. Cost of epilepsy in the United States: a model based on incidence and prognosis. *Epilepsia* 1994; 35:1230–1243.
8. Murray MI, Halpern MT, Leppik IE. Cost of refractory epilepsy in adults in the USA. *Epilepsy Res* 1996; 23:139–48.
9. Tetto A, Manzoni P, Millul A, Beghi E, et al. A prospective cost-of-illness study in referral patients with disease of different severity. *Epilepsy Research* 2002; 48:207–216.
10. Guerrini R, Battini R, Ferrari AR, Veggiotti P, et al, and the Epilepsy Collaborative Study Group. The costs of childhood epilepsy in Italy. Comparative findings from three health care settings. *Epilepsia* 2001; 42: 641–646.
11. Jacoby A, Buck D, Baker G, McNamee P, et al. Uptake and costs of care for epilepsy: findings from a U.K. regional study. *Epilepsia* 1998; 39:776–786.
12. van Hout B, Gagnon D, Souetre E, Ried S, Remy C, et al. Relationship between seizure frequency and costs and quality of life of outpatients with partial epilepsy in France, Germany, and United Kingdom. *Epilepsia* 1997; 38:1221–1226.
13. Cockerell OC, Johnson AL, Sander JWAS, Shorvon SD. Prognosis of epilepsy: a review and further analysis of the first nine years of the British National General Practice Study of Epilepsy, a prospective population-based study. *Epilepsia* 1997; 38: 31–46.
14. De Zelicourt M, Buteau L, Fagnani F, Jallon P. The contributing factors to medical cost of epilepsy: an estimation based on a French prospective cohort study of patients with newly diagnosed epileptic seizures (the CAROLE study). *Seizure* 2000; 9:88–95.
15. Begley CE, Lairson DR, Reynolds TF, Coan S. Early treatment cost in epilepsy and how it varies with seizure type and frequency. *Epilepsy Res* 2001; 47:205–215.
16. Begley CE, Famulari M, Annegers JF, Lairson DR, et al. The cost of epilepsy in the United States: an estimate from population-based clinical and survey data. *Epilepsia* 2000; 41:342–352.
17. Begley CE. Costs of care: first- and second-generation antiepileptic drugs. *Managed Care Consultant* 2005; 4:11–20.

Quality of Life in Children with Epilepsy

Joan K. Austin
Nancy Santilli

Recent changes in health care have led to an increased emphasis on documenting outcomes of care. In childhood epilepsy, the goal of care has traditionally been optimal seizure control. Recently, however, with the increased recognition of the importance of quality-of-life outcomes in the treatment of chronically ill children (1), there has been an impetus to assess the quality of life in children with epilepsy. This chapter provides a general introduction to health-related quality of life (HRQOL) in children and adolescents with epilepsy.

Although references to HRQOL per se are relatively new in the field of pediatric epilepsy, there has been longstanding interest in issues relevant to the quality of life of the child with epilepsy. For example, the emotional, learning, and social problems experienced by children with epilepsy have been a concern to clinicians, and these problems are related to quality of life in these children. Moreover, a clinician's asking "How are you doing?" can be viewed as an attempt, albeit unrefined, to assess quality of life in the clinical setting (2). The recent emphasis on quality-of-life outcomes, however, has led to a need for more formal or systematic approaches to the assessment and treatment of the quality of life of children with epilepsy. A relatively formal approach to HRQOL is the focus in this chapter. Major areas addressed are core domains, quality-of-life problems, measurement of quality of life in the clinical setting, and clinical interventions.

HEALTH-RELATED QUALITY OF LIFE

Core Domains

Although definitions of health-related quality of life in the literature are inconsistent (3), there is general agreement that it refers to a patient's (and sometimes his or her caregiver's) perceptions of the patient's state of functioning and well-being across multiple areas of concern (4, 5). In children these domains most commonly include those related to physical, psychologic, and social functioning and well-being (4). There also is general consensus that, in the measurement of HRQOL, information should be included that is disease specific or relevant to the child's particular condition and that addresses both the impact of the condition and the effects of treatment. Finally, there is a growing agreement that both subjective perceptions and objective data related to the child's quality of life are important (3, 4). Most studies investigating quality of life in children with epilepsy are consistent with these recommendations in that a multidomainal approach is used and information specific to epilepsy is included. For example, Austin and colleagues (6, 7) conceptualized quality of life around four domains: physical, psychologicl, social, and school. Information on seizure frequency was included in their measurement of the physical domain (6). In the process of developing a quality-of-life questionnaire for children with epilepsy, Ronen et al used focus groups to identify components of quality of life (8). They conceptualized quality of life in five domains: the epilepsy experience (e.g., how seizures feel), life fulfillment (regular activities), social issues (e.g., stigma), impact of epilepsy (e.g., psychologic), and "attribution" (concerns specific to epilepsy). In a final study Wildrick and colleagues (9) conceptualized quality of life in children with epilepsy in five domains: self-concept, home life (e.g., family relationships), school life, social activities, and medication (e.g., compliance).

For the purposes of this chapter, five domains relevant to health-related quality of life in children with epilepsy are presented in Table 66-1 and described in the next section. The domains presented here are based on the literature on quality of life in epilepsy as well as in other chronic conditions and, although independent, are highly interrelated. The core domains represent a broad-based conceptualization of HRQOL in pediatric epilepsy. The first four domains focus on aspects of child functioning and well-being. Because the family environment is integral to child well-being, the final domain focuses on family adjustment related to the child's epilepsy.

TABLE 66-1
Quality of Life Domains for Pediatric Epilepsy

Epilepsy and Treatment
Neurologic functioning
Cognitive functioning
Attention, memory, abstract reasoning, psychomotor functioning
Epilepsy syndrome
Seizure type, seizure frequency
Antiepilepsy medication effects
Physical, cognitive, and behavioral side effects
Psychologic
Emotional status
Happiness and satisfaction
Anxiety, depression, behavioral problems, and psychiatric disturbance
Self-esteem
Feelings about epilepsy
Concerns and fears
Attitude toward having epilepsy
Perceptions of stigma
Social
Completion of age-appropriate psychosocial developmental tasks
Satisfaction with family relationships
Peer relationships
Engagement in activities
Sports, clubs, hobbies, teams, organizations
School
Academic achievement
Learning problems
Adaptive characteristics
Works hard, behaves appropriately
Family
Seizure-management skills
Psychologic adjustment to epilepsy
Concerns and fears
Attitude toward epilepsy in child
Perceptions of stigma
Supervision of child's activities
Leisure activity participation

Epilepsy and Treatment

Assessment in this domain addresses epilepsy-specific information, including neurologic and cognitive functioning and information on the nature of the epilepsy as well as effects of treatment. Information on physical functioning is not generally included in the assessment of quality of life because children with epilepsy should not have physical limitations as a result of their seizure condition. Much of the epilepsy-specific data would be routinely obtained in a clinical setting as a core component of medical care. Assessments made in establishing a diagnosis generally include a complete neurologic examination that provides information about possible neurologic deficits. Moreover, in diagnosing and classifying epileptic syndromes, information on the nature of patients' seizures is collected. Once medications are prescribed, side effects also are regularly assessed. Thus, in the domain of epilepsy and treatment, only the information related to cognitive functioning, such as attention, memory, abstract reasoning, and psychomotor functioning, may not be routinely assessed in all children with epilepsy.

Psychologic

Two areas are covered in this assessment domain: emotional status and feelings about epilepsy. Emotional status includes common behavioral problems experienced by children who have any chronic physical condition and problems specific to epilepsy. Children with chronic neurologic conditions, such as epilepsy, are more likely to experience emotional problems than are children with non-brain-related physical chronic conditions (10, 11). Therefore, it is critical that this domain include anxiety, depression, behavioral problems, and psychiatric disturbances. Based on Ware's (12) recommendation that the full range of the health state be included in an assessment of quality of life, positive aspects of psychologic well-being (e.g., happiness, satisfaction, and self-esteem) should also be assessed. The second area of this domain relates to the feelings associated with having epilepsy. To what extent are children concerned and fearful about having epilepsy? Do they have negative feelings or a negative attitude about having epilepsy? Do they perceive a stigma associated with epilepsy to the point that it negatively affects their behavior?

Social

Assessment of social functioning and well-being is included because children with neurologic conditions have poorer social competence than children with other chronic conditions (6, 7, 13). An important component of social functioning is the accomplishment of developmental tasks. Because children with epilepsy manifest problems in areas of social competence (14), their assessment is included in this domain. Information on social functioning in both family relationships and peer relationships also is included. The last area included in this domain relates to the child's engagement in age-appropriate activities, including participation in sports, clubs, hobbies, teams, and organizations.

School

Success at school is important precursor of successful employment in adulthood. Functioning at school is especially important to measure in children with epilepsy because they have high rates of learning problems (15), which in some cases predate the onset of epilepsy (16). In addition, these children have poorer academic achievement than would be expected based on intelligence (17) and disproportionately high rates of school failure (18). Because success at school is partially dependent on behaviors such as working hard, school-adaptive characteristics also are included in this domain.

Family

Assessment of the family is important for two major reasons. First, it is the persons in the child's immediate environment who are in a position to exert the most influence on the child's quality of life (19). The family's adjustment to the epilepsy and the child's psychologic functioning are closely linked. Second, a chronic condition in a child negatively affects the adjustment of other family members, especially the mother (20). Also included in the family domain are factors related to the parents' ability to manage the epilepsy and their psychologic adjustment to the epilepsy. Do parents feel competent in their ability to handle future seizures? Are parents overly concerned and fearful about their child's condition? Are siblings unduly worried? Do family members have an optimistic attitude toward the epilepsy? Are family members unduly concerned about a stigma being associated with epilepsy? Is parents' supervision of the child's activities appropriate for the child's age? Finally, information on the participation of the family in leisure activity is included in this domain because of the importance of such participation in relation to family interaction and cohesion (21). Are family activities being overly restricted because of the epilepsy?

QUALITY-OF-LIFE PROBLEMS

Although a large number of studies have investigated a particular domain of function or well-being in children with epilepsy, far fewer studies have measured multiple quality-of-life domains in this population (22). Austin and colleagues (6) compared differences in four domains of quality of life (physical, psychologic, social, and school) between 136 children with epilepsy and 134 children with asthma age 8 to 13 years. Compared to children with asthma, the children with epilepsy had better functioning in the physical domain and poorer functioning and well-being in the psychologic, social, and school domains. A 4-year follow-up study again comparing quality of life in these same two groups indicated that those with epilepsy were still experiencing a poorer quality of life than those with asthma, even though substantially more of the children with epilepsy had inactive conditions. When the group with epilepsy was grouped by severity (inactive, low severity, and high severity), those with the most severe seizures were faring the worst, especially in the social domain. In the psychologic domain, girls had more anxiety, less happiness, and more negative feelings about having epilepsy than boys did (7). In a Japanese study of the quality of life of children (23), investigators studied quality of life in two environments: home and school. They included the assessment of problems as perceived by the children themselves, by their families, and by their schoolteachers. The children's main concerns were related to medication and seizures. Parents were most concerned about their child's future, their seizures, and their child's school performance. The most common problems the children experienced at school were keeping up with academic work and developing peer friendships.

A review of the literature indicates that functioning in one domain is often related to functioning in other domains. Because information on epilepsy, cognitive, and psychiatric comorbidities is covered in other chapters in this book, the focus here is on the psychologic, social, school, and family quality-of-life domains.

Psychologic

There is strong evidence that children with epilepsy are at risk for poor psychologic functioning and well-being. Epidemiologic studies indicate that children with epilepsy are up to 4.8 times more likely to have mental health problems than children from the general population (11, 24, 25). Children with epilepsy differ most from normative controls in the areas of internalizing problems (e.g., anxiety or depression), attention problems, and somatic complaints (26). The psychologic problems found in children with epilepsy do not appear to be solely from having a chronic illness, however, because the prevalence rate of problems is higher in children with epilepsy than in children with other chronic conditions (11, 24). For example, Davies et al (25) found that the prevalence of psychiatric disorders among children with uncomplicated epilepsy was approximately 2.5 times higher than among children with diabetes.

Few studies have focused on children's perceptions and coping responses related to having epilepsy. One study investigating the relationship between coping responses and mental health outcomes in youth with epilepsy found that coping responses of competence, optimism, compliance, and seeking support were associated with fewer behavioral problems and a positive self-concept. In contrast, coping responses of irritability, feeling different, and social withdrawal were related to more behavioral problems and a poorer self-concept (27). Austin and Huberty (28) found children's negative attitudes toward epilepsy to be related to poor self-concept and behavioral problems. In another study, children's attitudes or feelings about having epilepsy, an unknown locus of control, and low satisfaction with family relationships were associated with symptoms of depression in youth with epilepsy (29).

Some have hypothesized that mental health problems are caused by underlying neurologic dysfunction that causes both the seizures and the behavioral problems, a hypothesis with some empirical support. Children with epilepsy who also have deficits in neurologic functioning appear to be at an increased risk for mental health problems (30–33). Moreover, the relatively higher rates of psychiatric disorders found in children with chronic conditions involving the brain (10, 11) also provide support for this hypothesis. In addition, studies of children with new-onset seizures found relatively higher rates of behavior problems before the onset of their seizures (34, 35). For example, in a study of 224 children with a first recognized seizure, approximately 32% of children were in the clinical or at-risk range for behavior problems on a standardized scale (35).

Social

For optimal social development, children need an environment in which they can develop autonomy and initiative (36). Children with epilepsy have problems with developing independence. For example, Hoare (37) studied child dependency on the mother in four groups: children with newly diagnosed epilepsy, children with chronic epilepsy, children with newly diagnosed diabetes, and children with chronic epilepsy. Comparison of these groups with population-based norms indicated that children with either newly diagnosed or chronic epilepsy were more dependent on their mothers in three of four areas. In contrast, no differences were found between the control subjects and children with newly diagnosed diabetes. Finally, children with chronic diabetes differed from norms in only one dependency area.

Studies investigating seizure variables related to social functioning have led to inconsistent results. Austin and colleagues (7) found youth with the most severe epilepsy to be faring the worst socially. In contrast, Camfield and colleagues (18) did not find epilepsy-related variables (e.g., age of onset, seizure type) to be related to social functioning. Furthermore, in that study remission of epilepsy did not predict social functioning.

There is some support in the literature that the social functioning in children might be influenced by parenting behaviors. In an early descriptive study of 12 families, Mulder and Suurmeijer (38) found a relationship between parental control and dependency in children with epilepsy. Long and Moore (39) hypothesized that parents might have different expectations for a child with epilepsy than for a healthy sibling, which might lead to more restrictive parenting practices and subsequently more adaptation problems in the child with epilepsy. In a study of 19 families, Long and Moore (39) found that parents had different expectations for their children with epilepsy than for their healthy children. For example, they expected children with epilepsy to have more emotional problems, to be more unpredictable, and to be more "high-strung" than their siblings. Moreover, in this study parents perceived themselves as being more restrictive in parenting their children with epilepsy than their healthy brothers and sisters. Lothman et al (40) studied parenting behaviors of children with epilepsy through observing mother-child interactions and found praise to be related to child competence and positive affect. In contrast, intrusive and overcontrolling parenting behaviors were related to less autonomy and confidence in these children.

School

School problems are overrepresented in children with epilepsy. Research comparing academic achievement across different chronic childhood conditions consistently indicates that children with epilepsy are one of the most vulnerable groups. For example, an early comparison study of 270 children with 11 different conditions showed that children with epilepsy, sickle cell disease, or spina bifida were doing the poorest (41). Academic performance in children with epilepsy has consistently been found to be poorer than would be expected by intellectual ability (17). In one study children with uncomplicated epilepsy were, on average, about 1 year delayed in overall reading ability and that approximately 20% demonstrated severe deficits (42). In another study among children with epilepsy and normal intelligence, 39.7% had repeated at least one grade in school (43). When academic achievement on school-administered tests was compared between children with epilepsy and those with asthma, children with epilepsy had significantly lower scores in reading, mathematics, language, and vocabulary (44). In this study boys with the most severe epilepsy fared worst.

The relationship between seizures and academic functioning is unclear. Some studies have found that seizure type and frequency are related to academic achievement (45). In addition, Westbrook and colleagues (46) found that adolescents with mild idiopathic epilepsy had more problems with academic functioning than would be expected. In another study, however, academic underachievement was not related to seizure variables or to medication variables (47). Moreover, newly diagnosed youth with epilepsy who had not been treated already had academic problems, a finding noted by other investigators (16).

Neurologic dysfunction is another potential cause of academic problems in children with epilepsy. It is hypothesized that neurologic deficits lead to cognitive impairments, which in turn lead to academic problems. Even though broad intellectual abilities are stable and normal in the majority of children with epilepsy, these same children often perform below expected levels in the classroom. Although cognitive impairments are related to academic problems, it appears that the family environment can moderate this relationship. For example, cognitive deficits had less of a negative impact on achievement in supportive and organized families than in children with cognitive deficits who lived in unsupportive and disorganized homes (48).

Family

Few studies have investigated the adjustment of family members of children with epilepsy. Hoare's study of the prevalence of psychiatric disorder in parents and school-aged siblings of children with either newly diagnosed or chronic epilepsy found that children with newly diagnosed epilepsy were more disturbed than their siblings (49). The siblings' scores, however, did not differ from population norms. In contrast, the siblings of the children with chronic epilepsy were more disturbed than both siblings of children newly diagnosed with epilepsy and population norms. In this study psychiatric disturbance in the child with chronic epilepsy was associated with psychiatric disturbance in their mothers, a relationship that was not present when the child's epilepsy was newly diagnosed. Hoare proposes that chronic epilepsy can lead to stress that can negatively affect the mental health of other family members (49).

Two studies have addressed the concerns of parents whose children have seizures. Ward and Bower (50) studied the parents of 81 children with epilepsy, 30 of whom were newly diagnosed. These parents reported many concerns and fears related to the nature of the seizure, effects of medications, causes of seizures, injury, effects of seizures on intelligence, brain damage, mental health problems, and social problems. Austin and colleagues (51) studied 100 parents of children within 4 months of their first recognized seizure to identify concerns and fears. Concerns and fears focused on two broad areas: epilepsy and treatment (e.g., effect of seizures on the brain, on the child's mental health, and on the child's future life) and management of the epilepsy (e.g., handling future seizures, negative responses of others, lifestyle changes, and preventing mental health problems).

As might be expected based on the high rates of fear, parents have high levels of need for information and help with handling their children's seizure disorder. In a study of the psychosocial care needs of parents of children with seizures, Shore et al (52) found that approximately two-thirds of the mothers still wanted information about their child's seizure condition 6 months after seizure onset. In addition, at the same time 70% still felt the need to discuss their fears about seizures.

It appears that teaching parents about epilepsy can help them parent their children with epilepsy. For example, Suurmeijer (53) found that families imposed fewer restrictions on their child with epilepsy when the parents perceived that the information given to them about their child's condition was adequate. The same investigator reported that parents also indicated that they would more easily accept, be less frightened about, and know better how to deal with the epilepsy if they received adequate information about the condition.

Families of children with epilepsy consistently fare worse than control families in relation to parent-child interaction, maternal negative mood, and overprotection (54). Although fewer studies have explored the relationship between family environment variables and quality-of-life problems in children with epilepsy, most support a relationship between them, and the most consistent finding is between parent psychologic control and child behavior problems (54). Families of children with epilepsy experience relatively more stress, which has been found to be related to child behavior problems. For example, Pianta and Lothman (55) found family stress to be associated with child behavioral problems even after epilepsy factors and child characteristics were controlled statistically. Finally, the few studies that have explored relationships between family variables and child functioning over time also support a relationship between parenting behaviors and child behavior problems. For example, in a 2-year prospective study an increase in parental emotional support to the child was associated with a decrease in internalizing behavior problems (19).

MEASURING HEALTH-RELATED QUALITY OF LIFE

Measurement of HRQOL has received less attention in children and adolescents than in adults. One of the reasons instrument development has lagged behind in pediatrics is the changing frame of reference that results from child development and maturation. In deciding how to assess quality of life in children with epilepsy, much depends on the purpose of the assessment. If the goal is research related, measurements should be made that will answer the research questions in the most valid and reliable manner. In a clinical trial, measurement would be targeted to the specific quality-of-life domains most likely to be affected by the treatment under study.

When HRQOL is assessed in the clinical setting, the goal is to select the method that provides the best data to guide treatment decisions. It is these decisions that are the focus of the issues addressed here. The two most common methods used in the clinical setting are structured interview and self-report questionnaire. Advantages of the interview are that the interviewer is available to explain things that are not clear, to answer questions, and to make sure that all questions are answered. Interviews can be conducted either in person or by telephone. Information on quality of life can also be part of the clinician's history taking. Advantages of using self-report questionnaires are scheduling flexibility because an interviewer is not needed. Disadvantages include questions being skipped and the lack of opportunity for children and families to ask questions when something is unclear.

The information that follows focuses on issues related to the use of self-report questionnaires in the clinical setting. When using any instrument, it is important that it be in the respondent's native tongue and be culturally relevant. Criteria for evaluating instruments, practical considerations, selection of respondents, and selection of scales are addressed.

Selecting Instruments

Criteria for selecting instruments to measure quality of life depend on the conceptualization of health-related quality of life as well the quality of the scale. A good instrument would be conceptually strong in that it would have a sound theoretical underpinning (56) and the domains measured would be consistent with the purpose for doing the assessment. A good instrument should also have robust psychometric properties and meet clinical standards.

Two important psychometric properties are reliability and validity. Reliability refers to the consistency or the extent to which a measuring instrument yields similar results over repeated administrations. Stability reliability is consistency over time, and internal consistency reliability refers to the homogeneity of the items measuring the concept. Validity, which is the extent to which an instrument measures what it is supposed to measure, is commonly of three types: content validity, criterion validity, and construct validity. Content validity answers the question "Do the items measure what they are supposed to?" Criterion validity refers to the extent that the score on an instrument is systematically related to some external criterion. Construct validity refers to the extent that scores on an instrument are logically related to other measures.

An instrument that meets clinical standards differentiates between different levels of severity within the condition. Recently, there has been an emphasis on the extent to which a scale is sensitive or responsive to change. The term *responsiveness* refers to the instrument's ability to detect clinical change over time (57). An instrument must be able to detect even small improvements in a condition if it is going to be used to show effects of treatment.

Practical Considerations

There also are practical considerations when selecting instruments. Length of time that is required for collecting information must be considered, because time is especially important in the clinical setting. Are the instruments easily administered in the clinical setting? Are there norms based on age and gender? Because of the large differences that occur at various ages, one must use well-developed scales with norms based on age of the child. In addition, because of the different trajectories of boys and girls at different ages, the scales must have norms based on gender.

The complexity of the scoring also is an important practical consideration. Clinical staff may need to assist children and families to complete the instruments. The staff must use instruments that are easily scored and interpreted so the information can be used immediately. Unfortunately, most scales that can be used for a wide age range because they have norms for age and gender also have complex scoring; however, most of these scales have computer scoring programs that are easy to use.

Staff cooperation and training and an infrastructure for collecting data, scoring instruments, and incorporating the information into treatment are necessary. The assessment must take place in a manner that best fits with the clinical practice. Will children and families be asked to complete instruments before, during, or after clinical visits? More time is available for completion of scales if they are done outside the clinical setting before the clinic visit. The instrument can be sent out with an appointment reminder for the family to bring to the visit. When there is only a short period of time available for measurement or completing a questionnaire (e.g., while in the waiting room), decisions must be made whether to do a comprehensive assessment on a few HRQOL areas or screen in all areas, or a combination of the two. Other questions that must be considered relate to frequency and timing of assessment. Will all children be screened at every visit? Will more complete assessments be carried out on new patients? Will children who show problems have additional testing? Will different domains be targeted for different age groups? An assessment of HRQOL could also be triggered by critical events that occur in the child's life such as age-related changes (e.g., beginning school, transition into adolescence), health-related changes (e.g., seizures increase, medication change), and social changes (e.g., new school, parent divorce, new sibling).

Selection of Respondent

An important decision focuses on who should provide the data. Generally, it is ideal to obtain data from multiple sources (e.g., parents, children, and teachers). According to Landfraf and Abetz (57), children as young as 5 years can provide reliable information on very concrete concepts such as pain. Austin and colleagues have

TABLE 66-2
Sample Instruments to Measure Quality of Life in Childhood Epilepsy

Generic Scales	
Child Health Questionnaire (61)	A generic scale for children ages 5 and older. There are three parent-completed versions of differing lengths that measure 14 concepts and one child-completed version with 12 concepts. The scale has good psychometric properties and norms.
PedsQL™ (62)	A generic scale for children ages 2–18 years. There are child self-report and parent-completed versions that measure physical, mental, social, and school domains. It has a family impact module. The scale showed responsiveness to clinical change over time.
Epilepsy Scales	
Quality of Life in Epilepsy—Adolescent (63)	A general epilepsy scale for adolescents 11 to 17 years. The scale has 48 items that measure effects of epilepsy and medicine, stigma, feelings about self, and general HRQOL concepts of family, friends, activities, mood, cognition, and memory.
Health-Related Quality of Life (HRQOL) in Children with Epilepsy (64)	A general epilepsy scale for children ages 8–15 years. There are child-report and parent-completed versions. The 25-item scale evaluates five child domains (social, worries, emotional, secrecy, and normality) and five parent domains (Interpersonal/social, future worries, recent worries, and intrapersonal/emotional, secrecy).

TABLE 66-3
Questions to Assess HRQOL in the Clinical Setting

Assessment Questions for Parents

Epilepsy and treatment

What concerns do you have about your child's seizure condition or treatment?
What concerns do you have about handling your child's seizures?

Psychologic

What concerns do you have about your child's ability to cope with seizures?
Do you think your child is unduly worried or sad about having seizures?

Social

Compared to other children, how well does your child get along with others?
Compared to other children, how involved in activities is your child?

School

What concerns do you have about handling your child's seizures at school?
Is your child having any learning problems with school?

Family

Are any members of your family having problems coping with the seizures?
Is your family avoiding doing any leisure activities because of the seizures?

Assessment Questions for Older Children and Adolescents

Epilepsy and treatment

What questions do you have about your seizure condition?
What questions do you have about your medication?

Psychologic

Have you been feeling sad or down in the dumps about having seizures?
What kinds of things worry you about having seizures?

Social

How well do you get along with other kids your age?
What things are you not doing because of worry about seizures?

School

Do you feel you have to work harder on school work than other kids?
Are you having any trouble paying attention in school?

Family

Do your brothers and sisters treat you differently because of the seizures?
Do your parents treat you differently because of the seizures?

HRQOL, Health-related quality of life.

obtained reliable information on abstract concepts from children with epilepsy as young as 8 years of age (27, 28). As a general rule, parents should provide most of the information when the children are younger than 7 years old. Even for older children, the decision about who should provide information is not an easy one. Cognitive development and the ability to understand abstract concepts must be considered. Children who have had seizures from a very young age may not be able conceptualize what life would be without epilepsy and would have trouble answering questions about their life compared with the best possible life.

When data are collected from different categories of respondents, a number of factors must be considered when interpreting results. For example, mothers tend to report more problems in children than do fathers (57). Moreover, children's ratings of certain areas consistently differ from those of their parents. There tends to be more agreement on concepts related to physical functioning (e.g., activities and chores) and less agreement on behavioral or mental health functioning. For example, adolescents with epilepsy rated themselves to have fewer behavioral problems than their mothers, fathers, and teachers did (58). Parents' reports on children's mental health problems are more valid than children's reports (59). However, the fact that parents, children, and teachers rate things differently does not mean that one viewpoint is better than the other, just that they provide different perspectives. Some information is available only from the child. It also is important to consider that only children can report their emotional feelings, so if this information is desired, it must be obtained from children.

Selection of Scales

In a comprehensive assessment of HRQOL done for research purposes, it is important to use both general and disease-specific scales (60). General scales allow comparisons across samples, although a disadvantage of using these scales is that they often contain questions irrelevant for epilepsy. Disease-specific scales generate data that can be compared with other samples of children with epilepsy. In the clinical setting, instruments should be selected that will provide the best data to guide treatment decisions. Foremost, the clinician must consider what to do with the information once it has been collected. For example, a screening survey could be administered first and then followed with more specific information on areas in which problems are identified.

CLINICAL APPLICATION OF HRQOL ASSESSMENT

Incorporating HRQOL information into the clinical care of children with epilepsy can improve the quality of care provided. Therefore, it is critical that a strategy for HRQOL assessment be developed that can be incorporated into the office routine efficiently. Assessments can identify children who are at risk for problems so that interventions can be initiated at the earliest opportunity. Assessments also can improve clinical decision making by increasing the clinician's understanding of the quality-of-life problems experienced by children with epilepsy and their families. Finally, information from assessment of HRQOL over time can be used to document treatment outcomes (61–64). Table 66-2 describes a few of the available instruments that could be used to measure quality of life.

An alternative to using a formal HRQOL assessment instrument is to ask patients open-ended questions about their care. Table 66-3 includes questions that help to elicit information about quality-of-life issues in the clinical setting.

In the treatment of a chronic condition such as childhood epilepsy, the clinician must be concerned not only about controlling seizures but also about preventing adverse consequences of the condition and optimizing the child's functioning and well-being. When the outcome is narrowly conceptualized to be optimal seizure control, care is based on assessment of seizures and treatment to reduce seizures. When the outcome is conceptualized to include the child's quality of life, it will result in comprehensive care and improved quality-of-life outcomes in the child.

References

1. Drotar D, Levi R, Palermo TM, et al. Clinical applications of health-related quality of life assessment for children and adolescents. In: Drotar D, ed. *Measuring Health-Related Quality of Life in Children and Adolescents*. Mahwah, NJ: Lawrence Erlbaum, 1998.
2. Hoffman LG, Rouse MW, Brin BN. Quality of life: a review. *Journal of the American Optometric Association* 1995; 66:281–289.
3. Rapley M. Quality of life research. Thousand Oaks, CA: Sage Publications, 2003.
4. Koot HM. The study of quality of life: concepts and methods. In: Koot HM, Wallander JL, eds. *Quality of Life in Child and Adolescent Illness: Concepts, Methods, and Findings*. East Sussex, UK: Brunner-Routledge, 2001.
5. Wallander JL. Theoretical and developmental issues in quality of life for children and adolescents. In: Koot HM, Wallander JL, eds. *Quality of Life in Child and Adolescent Illness: Concepts, Methods, and Findings*. East Sussex, UK: Brunner-Routledge, 2001.
6. Austin JK, Smith MS, Risinger MW, McNelis AM. Childhood epilepsy and asthma: comparison of quality of life. *Epilepsia* 1994; 35:608–615.
7. Austin JK, Huster GA, Dunn DW, Risinger MW. Adolescents with active or inactive epilepsy or asthma: a comparison of quality of life. *Epilepsia* 1996; 37:1228–1238.
8. Ronen GM, Rosenbaum P, Law M, Streiner DL. Health-related quality of life in childhood epilepsy: the results of children's participation in identifying the components. *Dev Med Child Neurol* 1999; 41:554–559.
9. Wildrick D, Parker-Fisher S, Morales A. Quality of life in children with well-controlled epilepsy. *J Neurosci Nurs* 1996; 28:192–198.
10. Howe GW, Feinstein C, Reiss D, Molock S, Berger K. Adolescent adjustment to chronic physical disorders—I. Comparing neurological and non-neurological conditions. *J Child Psychol Psychiatry* 1993; 34:1153–1171.
11. Rutter M, Graham P, Yule W. A neuropsychiatric study in childhood. Philadelphia: JB Lippincott, 1970.
12. Ware JE. Evaluating measures of general health concepts for use in clinical trials. *Quality of Life Assessment* 1990; 6:51–63.

13. Nassau JH, Drotar D. Social competence among children with central nervous system-related chronic health conditions: a review. *J Pediatr Psychol* 1997; 22:771–793.
14. Caplan R, Sagun J, Siddarth P, et al. Social competence in pediatric epilepsy: insights into underlying mechanisms. *Epilepsy Behav* 2005; 6:218–228.
15. Fastenau PS, Shen J, Dunn DW, Austin JK. Academic underachievement among children with epilepsy: proportion exceeding psychometric criteria for learning disability and associated risk factors. *J Learn Disabil* in press.
16. Berg AT, Smith SN, Frobish D, et al. Special education needs of children with newly diagnosed epilepsy. *Dev Med Child Neurol* 2005; 47:749–753.
17. Seidenberg M, Berent S. Childhood epilepsy and the role of psychology. *Am Psychol* 1992; 47:1130–1133.
18. Camfield C, Camfield P, Smith B, Gordon K, et al. Biological factors as predictors of social outcomes of epilepsy in intellectually normal children: a population-based study. *J Pediatr* 1993; 122:869–873.
19. Austin JK, Dunn DW, Johnson CS, Perkins SM. Behavioral issues involving children and adolescents with epilepsy and the impact of their families: recent research data. *Epilepsy Behav* 2004; 5:S33–S41.
20. Eiser C. Psychological effects of chronic disease. *J Child Psychol Psychiatry* 1990; 31:85–98.
21. Orthner DK, Mancini JA. Leisure impacts on family interaction and cohesion. *J Leisure Res* 1990; 22:125–137.
22. Hanai T. Quality of life in children with epilepsy. *Epilepsia* 1996; 37 Suppl 3:28–32.
23. McDermott S, Mani S, Krishnaswami S. A population-based analysis of specific behavior problems associated with childhood seizures. *J Epilepsy* 1995; 8:110–118.
24. Austin JK, Dunn DW. Children with epilepsy: quality of life and psychosocial needs. *Annu Rev Nurs Res* 2000; 18:26–47.
25. Davies S, Heyman I, Goodman R. A population survey of mental health problems in children with epilepsy. *Dev Med Child Neurol* 2003; 45:292–295.
26. Rodenburg R, Stams GJ, Meijer AM, Aldenkamp AP, et al. Psychopathology in children with epilepsy: a meta-analysis. *Pediatr Psychol* 2005; 30:453–468.
27. Austin JK, Patterson JM, Huberty TJ. Development of the coping health inventory for children. *J Pediatr Nurs* 1991; 6:166–174.
28. Austin JK, Huberty TJ. Development of the child attitude toward illness scale. *J Pediatr Psychol* 1993; 18:467–480.
29. Dunn DW, Austin JK, Huster GA. Symptoms of depression in children with epilepsy. *J Child Adolesc Psychiatry* 1999; 38:1132–1138.
30. Hermann BP. Deficits in neuropsychological functioning and psychopathology in persons with epilepsy: a rejected hypothesis revisited. *Epilepsia* 1981; 22:161–167.
31. Hermann BP. Neurological functioning and psychopathology in children with epilepsy. *Epilepsia* 1982; 22:703–710.
32. Papero PH, Howe GW, Reiss D. Neuropsychological function and psychosocial deficit in adolescents with chronic neurological impairment. *J Dev Phys Disabil* 1992; 4(4):317–340.
33. Schoenfeld J, Seidenberg M, Woodard A, et al. Neuropsychological and behavioral status of children with complex partial seizures. *Dev Med Child Neurol* 1999; 41:724–731.
34. Dunn DW, Austin JK, Huster GA. Behaviour problems in children with new-onset epilepsy. *Seizure* 1997; 6:283–287.
35. Austin JK, Harezlak J, Dunn DW, et al. Behavior problems in children before first recognized seizures. *Pediatrics* 2001; 107(1):115–122.
36. Ziegler RG, Erba G, Holden L, Dennison H. The coordinated psychosocial and neurologic care of children with seizures and their families. *Epilepsia* 2000; 41(6):732–743.
37. Hoare P. Does illness foster dependency? A study of epileptic and diabetic children. *Dev Med Child Neurol* 1984; 26:20–24.
38. Mulder HC, Suurmeijer TPBM. Families with a child with epilepsy: a sociological contribution. *J Biosoc Sci* 1977; 9:13–24.
39. Long CG, Moore JR. Parental perceptions for their epileptic children. *J Child Psychol Psychiatry* 1979; 20:299–312.
40. Lothman DJ, Pianta RC, Clarson SM. Mother-child interaction in children with epilepsy: relations with child competence. *J Epilepsy* 1990; 3:157–163.
41. Fowler MG, Johnson MP, Atkinson SS. School achievement and absence in children with chronic health conditions. *J Pediatr* 1985; 106:683–687.
42. Yule W. Educational achievement. In: Kulig BM, Meinardi H, Stores C, eds. *Epilepsy and Behavior*. Lisse, The Netherlands: Swets and Zeitlinger, 1980.
43. Huberty TJ, Austin JK, Risinger MW, McNelis AM. Relationship of selected seizure variables in children with epilepsy to performance on school-administered achievement tests. *J Epilepsy* 1992; 5:10–16.
44. Austin JK, Huberty TJ, Huster GA, Dunn DW. Academic achievement in children with epilepsy or asthma. *Dev Med Child Neurol* 1998; 40:248–255.
45. Seidenberg M. Academic achievement and school performance of children with epilepsy. In: Hermann BP, Seidenberg M, eds. *Childhood Epilepsies: Neuropsychological, Psychosocial and Intervention Aspects*. Chichester, UK: John Wiley & Sons, 1989.
46. Westbrook LE, Silver EJ, Coupey SM, Shinnar S. Social characteristics of adolescents with idiopathic epilepsy: a comparison to chronically ill and nonchronically ill peers. *J Epilepsy* 1991; 4:87–94.
47. Mitchell WG, Chavez JM, Lee H, Guzman BL. Academic underachievement in children with epilepsy. *J Child Neurol* 1991; 6:65–72.
48. Fastenau PS, Shen J, Dunn DW, et al. Neuropsychological predictors of academic underachievement in pediatric epilepsy: moderating roles of demographic, seizure, and psychosocial variables. *Epilepsia* 2004; 45(10):1261–1272.
49. Hoare P. Psychiatric disturbance in the families of epileptic children. *Dev Med Child Neurol* 1984; 26:14–19.
50. Ward F, Bower BD. A study of certain social aspects of epilepsy in childhood. *Dev Med Child Neurol* 1978; 20:1–50.
51. Austin JK, Oruche UM, Dunn DW, Levstek DA. New-onset childhood seizures: parents' concerns and needs. *Clinical Nursing Practice in Epilepsy* 1995; Winter:8–10.
52. Shore C, Austin J, Musick B, Dunn DW, et al. Psychosocial care needs of parents of children with new-onset seizures. *J Neurosci Nurs* 1998; 30(3):169–174.
53. Suurmeijer PBM. Quality of care and quality of life from the perspective of patients and parents. *Int J Adolesc Med Health* 1994; 7:290–302.
54. Rodenburg R, Meijer AM, Dekovic M, Aldenkamp AP. Family factors and psychopathology in children with epilepsy: a literature review. *Epilepsy Behav* 2005; 6:488–503.
55. Pianta RC, Lothman DJ. Predicting behavior problems in children with epilepsy: child factors, disease factors, family stress, and child-parent interaction. *Child Dev* 1994; 65:1415–1428.
56. Davis E, Waters E, Mackinnon A, et al. Paediatric quality of life instruments: a review of the impact of the conceptual framework on outcomes. *Dev Med Child Neurol* 2006; 48:311–318.
57. Landgraf JM, Abetz LN. Measuring health outcomes in pediatric populations: issues in psychometrics and application. In: Spilker B, ed. *Quality of Life and Pharmacoeconomics in Clinical Trials*. Philadelphia: Lippincott-Raven, 1996.
58. Huberty TJ, Austin JK, Harezlak J, et al. Informant agreement in behavior ratings for children with epilepsy. *Epilepsy Behav* 2000; 1:427–435.
59. Dadds MR. Families, children, and the development of dysfunction. Thousand Oaks, CA: Sage Publications, 1995.
60. Shumaker SA, Moinpour CM, Aaronson NK, et al. Design and implementation issues. *Quality of Life Assessment* 1990; 5:27–46.
61. Landgraf JM, Abetz L, Ware JE. Child health questionnaire (CHQ): a user's manual. Boston: The Health Institute, New England Medical Center, 1996.
62. Varni JW, Seid M, Knight TS, et al. The PedsQL™ 4.0 generic core scales: sensitivity, responsiveness, and impact on clinical decision-making. *J Behav Med* 2002; 25(2): 175–193.
63. Cramer J, Westbrook L, Devinsky O, et al. Development of the quality of life in epilepsy inventory for adolescents: the QOLIE-AD-48. *Epilepsia* 1999; 8:1114–1121.
64. Ronen GM, Streiner DL, Rosenbaum, the Canadian Pediatric Epilepsy Network. Health-related quality of life in children with epilepsy: development and validation of self-report and parent proxy measures. *Epilepsia* 2003; 44(4):598–612.

67 Epilepsy, Cerebral Palsy, and IQ

W. Edwin Dodson

In all cultures children with epilepsy exhibit a disproportionately high share of problems with learning and behavior and are at risk to have poor social outcomes (1–10). As a group, children with epilepsy have an average IQ that is 10 points below normal, resulting in a threefold increased risk of mental retardation (2, 11) (Figure 67-1). Even those children who are not retarded are at increased risk for academic underachievement or school failure and maladjustment in later life (3, 8, 12–14). In one study of Finnish children with epilepsy there was a more than 20-fold increased risk of mental retardation or other handicap (15). Pazzaglia and Frank-Pazzaglia (16) found that among children with epilepsy in Cesena, Italy, only half had normal scholastic records, one-third were in special classes, and 17% were one or more grades behind. Behaviorally, children with epilepsy have an increased risk of psychopathology (10, 17, 18). They also are at risk of being described as fidgety, restless, irritable, inattentive, not liked, worrisome, solitary, disobedient, fussy, or destructive, and they are more likely to tell lies and fight with other children (19). They are also more likely to have temper tantrums, tics, sleep difficulties, poor appetite, loss of bowel control, lisping, stuttering, and headaches.

The specific components of cognitive function that account for the problems of patients with epilepsy are multiple and not well defined. Studies in children with epilepsy who were not taking medications suggest that perceptual problems and attention are major factors that antedate the onset of both seizures and treatment (20–22). In adults with intractable seizures, verbal and comprehension problems contribute more to variability in their IQs than attention or perceptual issues (23).

Academic underachievement is more prevalent in boys than in girls, a trend that persists among children with epilepsy. In the study summarized in Table 67-1, boys did worse in spelling than girls. Many factors were associated with underachievement in arithmetic. These included older age, generalized versus partial seizures, an earlier age of onset, and more seizures.

It is often difficult to determine the cause when children with epilepsy have academic or behavioral complaints. Parents and teachers tend to blame the epilepsy or the medication for the child's every imperfection. Isolating a cause is always complicated because numerous factors affect learning and behavior simultaneously. These factors include temperament, intrinsic developmental capability, associated brain disease, parent-child interactions, socioeconomic level, seizures, and medication-induced side effects. Some investigators have emphasized the importance of epilepsy or uncontrolled seizures, whereas others have highlighted the importance of other factors, especially drug therapy (24, 25)

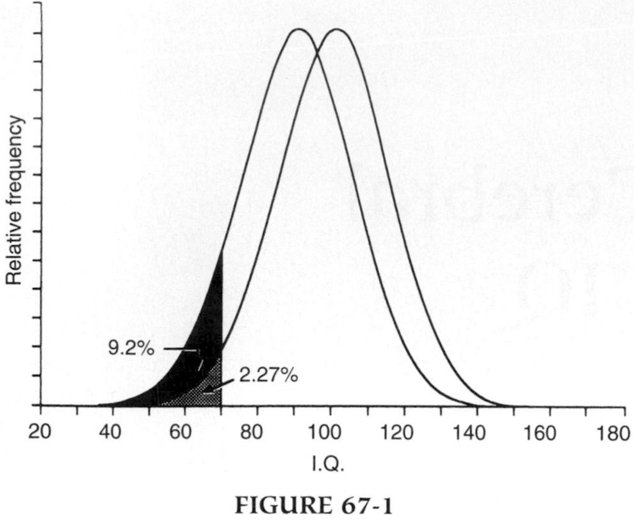

FIGURE 67-1

Frequency distribution of IQ in normal children and children with epilepsy. Adapted from Ellenberg et al (11).

(see Chapter 69). Relatively few studies have considered the confounding effects of socioeconomic level. Among the many factors that influence academic achievement in the population overall, socioeconomic status has the most pervasive influence (26, 27). Low socioeconomic status has also been linked to an increased incidence of medical conditions such as cerebral palsy and psychiatric disorders (28, 29).

Do seizures and epilepsy impair global intellectual ability? Usually they do not, but there are rare instances in which high seizure frequency is clearly linked to the stagnation of development and cognitive decline (30–33). Furthermore, children seem to be more vulnerable than adults to developing this consequence (34). A majority of children with epilepsy develop normally and enjoy normal cognitive ability. Aside from immediate ictal and postictal interruptions of awareness, seizures usually do not impair cognition permanently. Relationships between seizures, motor handicap, and intellectual impairment can, however, be complex. Overall etiology has the most powerful effect on intellectual outcome, but other seizure-related variables are influential as well. And, there are conditions in which childhood epilepsy and cognitive impairment progress simultaneously to result in permanent encephalopathy.

In exploring the relationship between epilepsy and cognitive function, a sequential approach helps to clarify the issues. First, factors that are not related to epilepsy are considered. Next, epilepsy-related factors such as etiology, comorbid conditions, seizure type, frequency, age of onset, and duration are discussed. Not discussed here are degenerative disorders in which neurologic deterioration is the primary feature and cognitive effects of drug treatment. Throughout this chapter it helps to remember that seizures, like mental retardation and cerebral palsy, are symptoms of abnormal brain function.

TABLE 67-1
Academic Achievement Among Children with Epilepsy

	Percent Underachieving	
WRAT Subtest	Boys	Girls
Word recognition	10.5	10.1
Spelling	33.3	15.9
Arithmetic	28.1	31.9
Reading comprehension	22.8	13.0

WRAT = Wide Range Achievement Test.
Adapted from Seidenberg et al (13).

TERMINOLOGY AND DEFINITIONS

The intelligence quotient (IQ) has been defined as an individual's mental age divided by chronological age times 100. In determining the IQ, many tests such as the Wechsler Adult Intelligence Scale (WAIS) do not require the actual calculation of a mental age but instead determine IQ based on standardized scale scores. The IQ is normally distributed in the general population with a mean of 100 and a standard deviation of 15 (Figure 67-2). Thus by definition, approximately 2.3% of the population has an IQ that is equal to or less than 70, the IQ value that is 2 standard deviations (SD) below the mean.

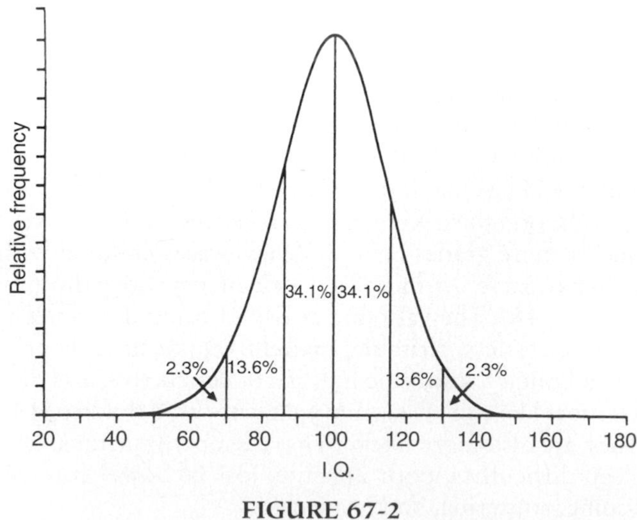

FIGURE 67-2

The distribution of IQ scores showing standard deviations and percent of the population in each group.

Most investigators who have studied the relationship between epilepsy and IQ report IQ values as group means and standard deviations. In these situations it is important to translate these values into terms that allow one to discern the magnitude of increased risk of mental retardation that is shared by group members. For example, if a particular group has an IQ of 90 with a standard deviation of 20, 16.5% of those groups are expected to have an IQ of 70 or less. In this example, even though most group members have normal intellect, the risk of mental retardation is increased sevenfold among group members. Although groups of patients with epilepsy who have been studied with IQ measurements do not necessarily have normally distributed values, for purposes of comparison in this chapter I have assumed that all group values are distributed normally.

The term *mental retardation* implies that an individual's global intellect and adaptation to the problems of living are defective and that these abnormalities have been present during development. Note that this definition encompasses more than an IQ criterion. However, the IQ score is one dimension of adaptive ability that is measured objectively, and it predicts academic performance. The IQ score also carries heavy weight in the diagnosis of mental retardation. Thus, for purposes of this chapter, an IQ score of 70 or less is considered to indicate mental retardation. Although this simplified approach has been adopted here for heuristic purposes, other dysfunctions such as learning disabilities, attention disorders, and disorders of language and communication all can have major adverse effects on learning, development, and socialization (35, 36).

Developmental disabilities are legally defined on a state-by-state basis. Nonetheless, federal legislation defined the condition as functional limitation in three or more major life activities. The major categories of activities include self-care, understanding and use of language, learning, mobility, self-direction, and capacity for independent living (37). The diagnosis of being developmentally disabled has important consequences because it may qualify the child for important educational and rehabilitative benefits. Although disabled children between the ages of 3 and 20 years have federal guarantees of access to educational and rehabilitative services, the authority to determine eligibility and the responsibility for providing services is vested in the states. Disability determinations are not categorical by diagnosis but rather depend on the child's functional ability (see Chapter 68). Thus, seizures may or may not be handicapping depending on their frequency, severity, and time of occurrence.

Cerebral palsy is a group of nonprogressive motor impairment syndromes secondary to lesions or brain abnormalities that arise early in development. The prevalence is 1.5–2.5 per 1,000 live births. The most common forms of cerebral palsy include hemiplegia (right side twice as frequent as left), spastic diplegia, and spastic quadriplegia. Less common forms include ataxic and athetoid disorders. Cerebral palsy, mental retardation, and epilepsy are often simultaneous manifestations of diffuse brain lesions that were acquired prenatally. The prevalence of various clinical patterns of cerebral palsy has changed, with more cases of spastic diplegia and fewer cases of spastic tetraplegia (quadriplegia). As a result of improvements in obstetrical and neonatal medicine, fewer full-term newborns suffer hypoxic ischemic encephalopathy, and more extremely low-birth-weight premature newborns survive hypoxic ischemic injury. If the latter children develop motor and other neurologic consequences of their encephalopathy, they generally have spastic diplegia and mental retardation, but they are less likely to have epilepsy than are full-term newborns who develop tetraplegia (38, 39).

Definitions of learning disability vary depending on the source, but generally the term implies that an individual's actual performance on measures of academic skills such as reading or arithmetic is substantially inferior to what would be predicted from that individual's global cognitive ability measured by the IQ. Most investigators designate an individual as learning disabled when that individual's IQ and measured academic skills differ by 1 SD or more. School systems in the United States have more complex definitions of learning disability, such that individuals with lower IQ scores require less statistical discrepancy between IQ and measures of scholastic skills to qualify for special remedial help than do individuals with normal or above-average IQ scores.

Studies of learning disabilities are more difficult to compare than studies of global cognitive ability because of the many issues that are involved in learning disabilities, including inconsistent definitions of the condition (40, 41). In studying learning disabilities, various investigators have different theoretical orientations and use different technical approaches. Although the role of factors such as strategic orientation, cognitive style, and motivation have been emphasized in the past, current theory points to defective auditory processing as the seminal abnormality in dyslexia, the most common learning disability (42).

In this chapter the focus will be on IQ scores. Similarly, cognitive functioning is emphasized more than behavior here, because the studies are more homogeneous and allow conclusions to be drawn.

NON-EPILEPSY-RELATED VARIABLES

Associated disease and social class are important background factors that interact with epilepsy and with antiepileptic therapy to influence behavior and cognitive ability (26, 27). Although many variables affect IQ, most of the determinants of IQ cannot be defined in large-scale investigations. In these types of studies, the largest determinant of IQ is socioeconomic class.

Socioeconomic Status

The National Collaborative Perinatal Project (NCPP) evaluated the relationship between various health-related and social factors and IQ measured at age 7 years. Overall, the strongest determinants of intellect were socioeconomic class and related variables such as maternal education. However, considering all predictor variables, the investigators could account for only 25% to 28% of the variance in IQ among whites and 15% to 17% among blacks (43). The highest correlation ($r = 0.38$) was found between socioeconomic index and IQ. This value yields a coefficient of determination of approximately 8%—indicating that 8% of the variability in IQ is linked to socioeconomic class. The correlation between the mother's nonverbal IQ and the child's IQ was lower ($r = 0.28$). The effects of socioeconomic factors are manifest in various ways. For example, 20.2% of children from families in the lowest socioeconomic class failed a test of language comprehension at age 8 years, compared to only a 2% failure rate for those from the highest social class (43).

Studies of epilepsy and IQ from diverse cultures that considered socioeconomic variables have confirmed that the influence of socioeconomic class on IQ is universal (44). Socioeconomic factors also influence many of the determinants and etiologies of epilepsy, cerebral palsy, and mental handicap, with children from the lowest socioeconomic groups faring worst in every outcome (15, 28, 29). Furthermore, sociocultural context plays a major role in the attitudes and behaviors about epilepsy (29, 45) and in the accessibility of educational and treatment opportunities for children challenged by handicaps (46).

The nature and quality of the parent-child interaction is also an important contributor to the child's cognitive development and behavior. Whereas seizure-related variables heavily influence medical outcome, sociocultural differences and the quality of the parent-child interactions exert enduring and pervasive effects on the child's behavioral outcome and statistically have a more far-reaching influence than disease-related factors (45, 47). Furthermore, even after seizures are controlled, flawed early psychosocial development can continue to thwart the maturation of skills necessary for productive, independent functioning (48). Having a child with epilepsy in the family increases the risk of maternal depression, lowers quality of the parent-child relationship, and promotes dissatisfaction with family relationships (18, 46).

Epilepsy-Related Variables and IQ

The most fundamental elements of neurologic diagnosis are etiologic and anatomic. Where is the lesion, and what caused it? Thus, it is not surprising that the etiology of a child's epilepsy predicts cognitive functioning best. Unfortunately, in a majority of children with epilepsy the etiology cannot be identified. As a result, the best diagnosis that can be made is usually descriptive, descriptive in terms of the child's seizure type(s) or type of epilepsy or epileptic syndrome. When the diagnosis is predominantly rooted in descriptive phenotypic features of the condition—that is, by seizure type or by epileptic syndrome—the relationship between epileptic variables and IQ is less predictable. Classification by seizure type is the least informative level of descriptive diagnosis. Diagnosis by type of epilepsy or epileptic syndromes provides a more complete description of the disorder and relationships between epileptic variables and IQ are more predictable. In fact, encephalopathy is a criterion for some syndromic categorizations.

SPECIFIC ETIOLOGIES

When the etiology is identified, the relationship between the epilepsy and intellect is usually clear cut. Among all epilepsy-related variables, the etiology of the epilepsy has the most pervasive effect on cognitive ability (Table 67-2).

TABLE 67-2
Examples of Etiologies of Symptomatic Epilepsy that also Affect Global Cognitive Function

- Perinatal asphyxia
- Symptomatic neonatal hypoglycemia
- Neurocutaneous disorders
  - Tuberous sclerosis
  - Neurofibromatosis
  - Hypomelanosis of Ito
- Chromosomal disorders
  - Down syndrome
  - Fragile X syndrome
  - Microdeletion syndromes
    - Angelman's syndrome
    - Prader-Willi syndrome
  - Inborn errors of metabolism (untreated)
- Ion channel disorders
  - Severe myloclonic epilepsy of infancy (SCNA1 channelopathy)
  - Rett's syndrome
- Progressive myoclonus epilepsies
  - Unverricht-Lundborg disease
  - Lafora body disease
  - Northern epilepsy syndrome
- CNS infections
  - Meningitis
  - Encephalitis
  - Human immunodeficiency virus
  - Subacute sclerosing panencephalitis (SSPE)

TABLE 67-3
Effect of Epilepsy on IQ at Age 7 years from the National Collaborative Perinatal Project (11)

	Epilepsy			Controls		
	n	IQ		*n*	IQ	
All children	368	90.0	(13)	NA	102.9	(13)
Sibling comparison	98	91.5	(20.9)	98	95.3	(15.1)
Normal early evaluation	59	99.8	(14.9)	59	98.0	(13)

Values shown are means and standard deviations.

In most cases where people with epilepsy are impaired intellectually or behaviorally, underlying brain disease, not recurrent seizures, is the major contributor to the difficulties.

Studies from the NCPP and from many other sources indicate that associated brain disease, not seizures, is the most important contributor to subnormal intellect among children with epilepsy (20). In population-based studies of epilepsy and IQ there is no evidence that epilepsy causes intellectual deficit. Rather, the antecedent conditions that cause epilepsy are associated with lowered group IQ. Among youngsters who began to have seizures between the ages of 4 and 7 years, the group IQ was similar to that of well-matched controls (11) (Table 67-3). By and large, the appearance of seizures in otherwise normal children does not predict reduced IQ.

In comparison to patients with idiopathic epilepsy, patients with symptomatic epilepsy have lower IQs. For example, in a prospective study of children with new-onset epilepsy, the mean IQ for the symptomatic group was 89.1 (SD 29.6) compared to 102.5 (SD 16.1) for the idiopathic group (45) (Figure 67-3). Differences of this magnitude lead to approximately a 10-fold increased chance of mental retardation among children with symptomatic epilepsy (25.8% vs. 2.3%).

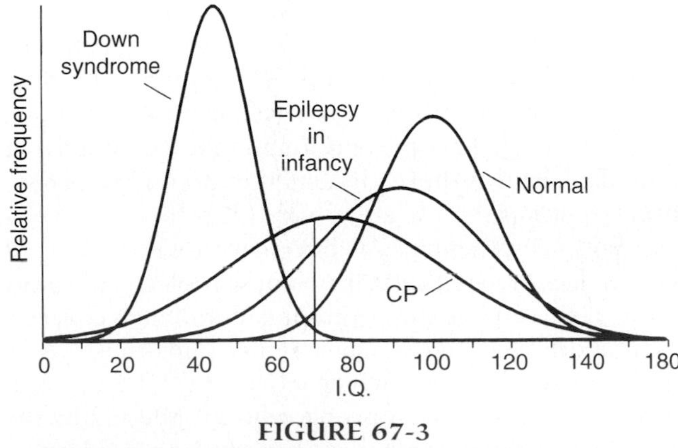

FIGURE 67-3

IQ distributions for people affected by disorders associated with epilepsy. Developed from information in the publication by Broman et al (43).

Symptomatic epilepsy due to a cerebral lesion heightens the chance of cognitive impairment even when the cause or precise extent of the lesion is unknown (49, 50). In a sample where 70% of children had symptomatic or presumed symptomatic (cryptogenic) epilepsy, 76% experienced learning problems including more than half of those with normal IQs. Factors that were linked to mental retardation were cerebral palsy, seizure onset before age 6 years, and lack of response to early drug treatment (51). Furthermore, the impact of structural brain abnormalities varies with the location of the lesion and the timing of its intrusion on brain circuitry as well as the intensity and frequency of the seizures that the lesion causes.

Brain malformations are prone to cause both epilepsy and mental impairment. Malformations range from being subtle and localized in the case of focal cortical dysplasia to pervasive and dramatic in the case of lissencephaly. Recently recognized cerebral malformations such as double cortex, frontal opercular syndrome, and congenital bilateral perisylvian syndrome have variably severe adverse effects on cognition (52–54). Despite improvements in imaging, specific brain malformations such as bilateral parasagittal polymicrogyria can still be difficult to detect on imaging tests and can cause a spectrum of cognitive problems plus epilepsy that begins early in life (55). The range of cognitive impairments linked to bilateral parasagittal polymicrogyria extends from normal functioning to mild retardation and includes subtle problems such as normal intelligence with slow mental processing.

In recent years, the proportion of epilepsy that is recognized as symptomatic of brain lesions has increased as a result of vast improvements in imaging techniques. These advances have allowed visualization of subtle, previously inconspicuous brain abnormalities such as heterotopias, areas of abnormal cerebral lamination, or small areas of atrophy (as in mesial temporal sclerosis) that can produce severe epilepsy and cognitive impairment (56). Whereas contemporary high-resolution magnetic resonance imaging (MRI) techniques allow visualization of mesial temporal lobe and other brain structures that previously were obscure, variations in these structures increasingly are being linked to cognitive differences among people with epilepsy. For example, Strauss et al found that among a group of people with epilepsy, the size of the posterior corpus callosum correlated positively with IQ (57). Similar observations have been made in children who were born prematurely with extremely low birth weights (58) and among mentally retarded men with fragile X syndrome (59). As more neurons connect to each other via the corpus callosum, the corpus callosum enlarges.

Chromosomal disorders illustrate how a particular etiology can produce both seizures and mental retardation independently. Among patients with Down syndrome the average IQ is 43.5 (SD 10.1), resulting in a 99% chance that patients with this disorder will be mentally retarded, independent of epilepsy (60). Angelman ("happy puppet") syndrome and Prader-Willi syndrome are both caused by a microdeletion of a portion of the long arm of chromosome 15 (61). Seizures are an invariable component of Angelman syndrome but occur in only 20% of children with Prader-Willi syndrome. However, subnormal intellect is a major feature of both disorders.

X-linked mental retardation is the most common inherited cause of mental subnormality. Associated with fragile X chromosome in 25% to 50% of cases, mental handicap is a uniform feature of this disorder. Although seizures occur in 20% of patients, they have a negligible relationship to intellect (62, 63).

In some instances of symptomatic seizures, both the etiology and the actual occurrence of seizures affect the cognitive outcome. The various causes of neonatal seizures help to illustrate how these relationships operate. Certain etiologies of neonatal seizures are benign, whereas others have grave consequences for intellectual outcome.

For example, hypocalcemia in the context of late neonatal tetany can cause dramatic and numerous seizures, but it does not increase the risk of mental retardation unless there are additional complications. On the other hand, neonatal hypoglycemia that causes seizures approximately doubles the risk of mental handicap compared to symptomatic neonatal hypoglycemia that does not cause seizures (64). Asymptomatic hypoglycemia only slightly increases the risk of subsequent cognitive impairment. Thus etiology can influence the cognitive consequences of the seizures. Furthermore, in certain etiologies such as hypoglycemia, the actual occurrence of seizures contributes a critical element in the pathogenesis of the adverse intellectual outcome.

In pyridoxine dependency, the number and duration of seizures contributes to the adverse cognitive outcome in children who otherwise would be normal if treated with vitamin B_6. Mental retardation occurs mainly in those individuals who have numerous seizures caused by pyridoxine dependency, but usually not in those who have only a few (43, 45, 47, 65). And pyridoxine dependency can be difficult to identify. Initially it was believed that pyridoxine dependency caused only neonatal seizures and neonatal status epilepticus. Subsequently, it was discovered that pyridoxine dependency could cause other types of seizures, including epileptic syndromes that are associated with cognitive decline. Those patients who experience the worst seizures in terms of seizure types, seizure frequency, and the duration of epilepsy have a high risk of irreversible cognitive impairment. And to make the condition all the more difficult to diagnose, the seizures due to pyridoxine dependency are partially responsive to antiepileptic drugs, like other forms of epilepsy.

The symptomatic etiology of epilepsy perinatal asphyxia causes a distinctive combination of cerebral palsy, mental retardation, and epilepsy. Findings from the NCPP revealed that when perinatal asphyxia in full-term newborns caused later epilepsy, it also caused cerebral palsy (60, 66). In the absence of cerebral palsy, no relationship was found between various measures of perinatal asphyxia and the occurrence of epilepsy in later childhood (66), a finding confirmed in a subsequent investigation (67). Among 87 newborns who had Apgar scores of 0–3 at 10 minutes and who did not develop cerebral palsy, none developed epilepsy during the 7-year follow-up period (68).

Similar to the relationship between etiology and cognitive impairment, underlying brain disease, more so than seizure-related variables, increases the risk of behavior disorders. Beran and Flanagan (68) compared adults who had posttraumatic versus idiopathic epilepsy of comparable severity using the Washington Psychosocial Seizure Inventory. There were differences across eight measures that indicated that the extent of brain dysfunction correlated with psychosocial dysfunction more than the severity of the epilepsy. Corbett et al concluded that among children with epilepsy, brain damage and dysfunction were of greater importance in causing behavior problems than medication (69). Deb studied the relationship between epilepsy and psychopathology among mentally retarded people and found that the underlying brain damage was more influential in producing behavioral symptoms than seizures were (70).

Etiology of epilepsy is intertwined with nearly all other epilepsy-related variables because etiology influences seizure type, response to medication, duration of epilepsy, and comorbidities, including cognitive impairment. As a result, etiology has far-reaching impact on global achievements and adjustment of people who are affected by the condition. Symptomatic etiology has adverse consequences for the chance of cessation of seizures, for educational and vocational achievement, for social adaptation, for driving, for employability and for other outcomes (9).

TABLE 67-4
*Thirty-Year Outcome of Childhood Onset Epilepsy from a Population of Children 70% of Whom Had Cryptogenic or Symptomatic Epilepsy**

Outcome	Epilepsy	Controls
Primary education only	49%	23%
No vocational training	69%	52%
Unpartnered	35%	10%
Childless	51%	16%
No driver's license	39%	16%
Unemployed	31%	8%

*Ongoing recurrent seizures that could not be prevented with medication were linked to the worst social outcomes (9).

Sillanpaa and colleagues reported the long term outcomes of 245 Finnish children with epilepsy that began before age 16 years. This group differed from most other population-based groups in which approximately 80% of cases are idiopathic epilepsy, because among the Finnish children with epilepsy only 28% of cases were idiopathic whereas 72% were either cryptogenic or symptomatic. When followed up after 30 years the adverse outcomes linked to symptomatic etiology and ongoing seizures were dramatic (Table 67-4).

ASSOCIATED NEUROLOGIC SYMPTOMS—COMORBIDITIES

The linkage between mental retardation, epilepsy, and cerebral palsy is well established. Historically one-third of children with cerebral palsy also have epilepsy. However, as obstetrical and perinatal medical care has improved, the distribution of different forms of cerebral palsy has changed and the incidence of epilepsy in cerebral palsy has changed, too (71). In various series, epilepsy has been most likely to occur in hypotonic, spastic hemiplegic, and tetraplegic forms of cerebral palsy (72, 73), in which the risk of epilepsy is approximately 50% (38, 74). Similarly, the risk of mental retardation is higher in patients with tetraplegia than in patients with spastic diplegia, especially when children with milder degrees of motor dysfunction are considered (75). For example, in one study of children with these disorders, the likelihood of mental retardation (IQ < 70) was 50% lower among children with diplegia than among those with tetraplegia (39). It is less common with spastic diplegia (73), even when the diplegia resulted from the most severe degree of intraventricular hemorrhage, which renders more than 70% of survivors mentally retarded (76). Cerebral palsy has also been linked to the onset of epilepsy in the first year of life, to neonatal seizures, and to a high incidence of mental retardation (74). In the NCPP, infants with hypotonia that was not further characterized had a mean IQ of 80 (SD 24.9), which translates into a 34.6% risk of mental retardation. In the same study among children with cerebral palsy, the mean IQ was 74.8 (SD 27.2), resulting in a 43.5% risk of mental retardation (43). Among young children, cerebral palsy is the most important single risk factor for severe epilepsy (77, 78).

For newborns with extremely low birth weight, the risk of cognitive and motor impairment is high and increases with increasing degrees of prematurity, with declining birth weight, with shorter gestation, and with more severe degrees of intraventricular hemorrhage when it is present (58, 79, 80). In the presence of periventricular leukomalacia and cognitive impairment, performance IQ was affected worse than verbal IQ. Thinning of the posterior corpus callosum correlated with reduced full-scale and performance IQ but not verbal IQ (58).

In the presence of mental retardation the risk of epilepsy increases with the severity of the mental handicap (Table 67-5). The lower the IQ, the more likely the child will also have epilepsy and the less likely that the seizures will respond to treatment (81). If the IQ is normal and the child has spastic diplegia, the child is more likely to have had a single seizure or to have responded to monotherapy (74). Conversely, among children who are mentally retarded, those who also have epilepsy tend to be more severely affected (82). Chelune et al reported that among people with IQ of 75 or less, the chance that surgical treatment would fail to cure epilepsy was fourfold greater than when the IQ was higher (83). The concurrence of multiple neurologic handicaps has an adverse compounding effect on the child's overall functionality, with the combined deficits having multiplicative rather than additive impact on the child's functioning (84).

A majority of severely retarded children have definable brain abnormalities that are known to heighten the risk of epilepsy. For example, in one series the causes of severe retardation (IQ < 50) included the following: 36%, chromosomal abnormalities; 20%, congenital

TABLE 67-5
Occurrence of Epilepsy Among Various Intellectual Categories

Intellectual Category	Prevalence of Epilepsy
Normal IQ	1%
Mild mental retardation (IQ 50–70)	15%
Severe mental retardation (IQ <50)	47%

Adapted from data in Susser et al (60).

malformations; 12%, perinatal complications or infections; and 7%, single-locus genetic diseases. Only 3% had postnatal causes, and the unknown/other category accounted for 22% (60).

Studies conducted since the completion of the NCPP have provided more refined information about the interrelationship between epilepsy, mental retardation, and cerebral palsy (85). Ignoring whether the mental retardation is associated with cerebral palsy, the overall risk of epilepsy among mentally retarded people is 15%. Among mentally retarded children without cerebral palsy, the risk of developing epilepsy by age 22 years is substantially lower, 5.2%. Mental retardation plus cerebral palsy increases the risk of developing epilepsy by age 22 approximately sixfold to 38%. Mental retardation that has been acquired as a result of postnatal causes carries an even higher risk of also developing epilepsy, 66%.

Other manifestations of brain disease and epilepsy are interrelated in children who are neurologically abnormal (Table 67-6). In young infants coincidental congenital disorders that do not seem to affect the nervous system directly nonetheless can be adversely related to IQ. For example, congenital heart disease is associated with a 10-point reduction in mean IQ from 100 to 90.4 (SD 23.5), resulting in a 19.8% risk of having an IQ below 70 (60). The mechanisms by which associated conditions such as this reduce IQ are undefined. Most of these patients have static, nonprogressive intellectual deficits unless additional insults to brain occur.

Thus, among youngsters with congenital neurologic abnormalities, the symptoms of mental retardation, motor disability, and epilepsy are tightly intertwined. These associations notwithstanding, the etiology of the brain dysfunction remains the principal determinant of IQ.

EPILEPTIC SYNDROMES (TYPES OF EPILEPSY)

A descriptive diagnosis by type of epilepsy or epileptic syndrome provides a more complete picture about the patient's epileptic condition than a diagnosis by seizure type does. Syndromes are nonspecific in regard to etiology and are defined by groups of symptoms that occur together. Several clinical elements define the various syndromes. These include seizure type(s), precipitating factors, electroencephalographic (EEG) patterns (both ictal and interictal), response to various medications, age on onset, natural history, and associated clinical features such as whether the patient has encephalopathy including motor deficits or mental handicap (86). The last two features, natural history, and the presence or absence of encephalopathy are central to this discussion because syndromic groupings usually imply an intellectual prognosis. For example, the encephalopathic epilepsies, such as West syndrome, Lennox-Gastaut syndrome, and Doose syndrome, are regularly associated with cognitive impairment. In other syndromes, such as childhood absence epilepsy, the prognosis is benign including the intellectual outcome (Table 67-7). Some syndromic phenotypes can

TABLE 67-6
Associations of Comorbid Neurologic Handicaps in Children from the National Collaborative Perinatal Project (NCPP)

Independent Variable	Dependent Variable			
	CP	SZ	MMR	SMR
CP		33.9%	30%	30%
CP and MR		38%		
Hemiplegia		50%		
Quadriplegia		27%		75%
SZ	19%		27%	
MR	20%	13–22%		
Postnatal MR		66%		
SMR	20%	47%		
Autism		25%		

CP = cerebral palsy; SZ = seizures; MMR = mild mental retardation; SMR = severe mental retardation.
Independent variables are listed in the leftmost column (60, 85, 153, 154).

TABLE 67-7
Examples of Epileptic Syndromes and Prognosis for Cognitive Function

Unfavorable Cognitive Development
- West syndrome (infantile spasms)
- Severe myoclonic epilepsy of Infancy
- Lennox-Gastaut syndrome
- Doose syndrome
- Landau-Kleffner syndrome
- Rett syndrome

Favorable Cognitive Development
- Febrile seizures
- Childhood absence epilepsy (petit mal, pyknolepsy)
- Benign partial epilepsy of childhood (rolandic epilepsy)
- Juvenile myoclonic epilepsy

evolve as the child grows older and as a result of other influences. Examples include the evolution of West syndrome to Lennox-Gastaut syndrome and the emergence of severe myoclonic epilepsy of infancy following febrile seizures.

Some syndromes evolve over time and most have indistinct boundaries (87, 88). A given syndrome can result from many causes and be either symptomatic or be idiopathic (primary). In most instances the idiopathic cases have the better prognosis for control with medication, for eventual remission and for intellectual outcome. Approximately 50% of children who have epilepsy can be categorized into one of the epileptic syndromes.

Encephalopathic Epilepsies

Epileptic encephalopathy (or encephalopathic epilepsy) is a term that has been used to describe the development of mental impairment that is often associated with a high frequency of seizures that are resistant to medication (89). The usual progression of events is stagnation of development, which causes the affected child to be left behind developmentally by his peers. Less often the child actually regresses developmentally through the loss of previously acquired skills and knowledge.

The mechanisms by which certain epilepsies lead to progressive encephalopathy are poorly understood (90). The major ones—West syndrome, Lennox-Gastaut syndrome, and severe myoclonic epilepsy of infancy (SMEI)—are characterized by early childhood onset, high frequencies of seizure, and multiple types of seizures. Others such as Landau-Kleffner syndrome and the syndrome of electrical status epilepticus during sleep (ESES, also called the syndrome of continuous spikes and waves during slow wave sleep, CSWS) have a low frequency of seizures or, in some cases, no seizures (91). The central elements of these disorders are severe encephalopathy manifested by language impairment. West syndrome and Lennox-Gastaut syndrome are interrelated in that approximately half of the infants who develop infantile spasms later evolve into the clinical pattern of Lennox-Gastaut syndrome (92). West syndrome consists of infantile spasms, an EEG pattern of hypsarrhythmia, and developmental arrest. Lennox-Gastaut syndrome includes multiple seizure types, especially tonic, astatic, partial, and atypical absence seizures, developmental arrest, and a slow spike wave pattern on EEG. In an epidemiological study that did not include mental retardation as a diagnostic criterion, 91% of affected children had IQs of 70 or less (93). Doose syndrome is the idiopathic version of Lennox-Gastaut syndrome. Normal intellect can be preserved if seizures can be controlled in Doose syndrome, but mental impairment accrues if seizures rage on. Although labeled as a syndrome, Rett syndrome is actually an etiologic entity. It is a genetic, progressive, relentlessly degenerative condition that has its onset in girls in the first or second year of life (94, 95).

Seizure Type

The ictal behavior that occurs during a seizure determines the seizure type and depends on the area(s) of brain in which the abnormal neuronal discharges are occurring. Any specific type of seizure can have a multiplicity of causes. As a result seizure type is generally a feeble correlate of other aspects of the epileptic condition. Furthermore there is a high rate of error in the clinical diagnosis of seizure types, especially when the behavior in question is epileptic staring.

Generalized seizures and generalized epileptiform patterns on the EEG have been linked to greater degrees of cognitive impairment than partial seizures, but these types of relationships are inconsistent. One comparison of neuropsychologic test results from people with partial seizures to those with partial secondarily generalized seizures found that those with secondarily generalization perform less well on tests of concentration and mental flexibility (96). Moreover, these differences were present before drug therapy was initiated. In another study that looked at the effects of partial versus partial secondary generalized seizures, patients with only partial seizures did better than those with secondary generalization on subtests of arithmetic, digit span, digit symbol, block design, and object assembly (97). Wilkus and Dodrill found that on 11 of 15 Halstead-Reitan measures patients with generalized EEG discharges performed worst, patients with focal EEG discharges had intermediate performances, and patients with no epileptiform EEG discharges performed best (98).

Data from Farwell et al (3) (Table 67-8) and from Bourgeois et al (1) (Figure 67-4) illustrate how the patients' predominant seizure types correlate with IQ overall. For example, generalized absence seizures are a

TABLE 67-8
Seizure Types and Average IQ Among Children 6–15 Years Old (3)

Seizure Type	Group Average IQ
Minor motor	70
Atypical absence	74
Partial and generalized	96
Partial only	98
Generalized tonic-clonic	99
Classical absence and generalized tonic-clonic	106

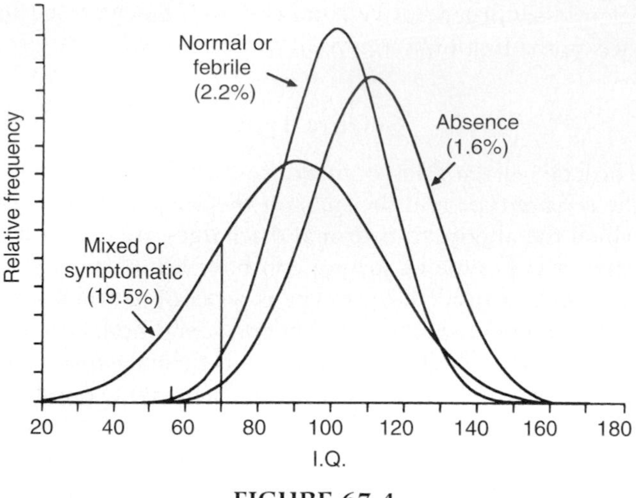

FIGURE 67-4

Frequency distributions of IQ scores among children with various seizure types. The percentage values shown in parentheses indicate the proportion of the group that is expected to have an IQ of 70 or less. The average and standard deviations (SD) for the groups are febrile 100.7 (SD 24.0), mixed 91.2 (SD 22.7), and generalized absence 109.7 (SD 16.4).

feature of many epileptic syndromes, some benign and some ominous. Absence seizures that occur in petit mal epilepsy bear a substantially better prognosis than atypical absence seizures that are coupled with other types of generalized seizures such as astatic seizures or drop attacks. Atypical absence seizures and astatic or drop seizures have been labeled collectively as minor motor seizures; these have a poor prognosis for mental development and functioning. Groups of children with classic absence seizures have a mean IQ that is above average. These youngsters probably have childhood absence epilepsy (petit mal epilepsy, pyknolepsy), whereas those patients with classic absence plus generalized tonic-clonic seizures most likely have juvenile myoclonic epilepsy, both of which are genetically determined and are linked to normal or superior intellect. However, absence seizures, especially atypical absence seizures, are linked to some of the worst cognitive outcomes when they occur in children with encephalopathic epilepsy such as infantile spasms or Lennox-Gastaut syndrome. Consistent with these relationships, hospital-based studies of children have found that nonconvulsive absence seizures are associated with lower cognitive scores than convulsive seizures (20).

The major drawback with trying to relate seizure type to intellectual outcome is that the classification of seizure types provides only limited information (99). Seizure types are ictal behavioral phenotypes. Although they provide clues as to the anatomical origin of the epileptic discharges, they are nonspecific in relation to either etiology or epileptic syndrome. Whereas individual seizure types have many causes and occur in many different syndromes, attempts to correlate seizure types with cognitive ability usually fall short.

Localization of Partial Seizures

Along with seizure type, seizure frequency, and epileptic syndrome, the localization of partial seizures is sometimes related to cognitive difficulty (20, 50, 100, 101). Fixed cerebral lesions and neurologic deficits produce more consistent clinical pictures than interictal EEG epileptic foci, which tend to wander over time in conditions such as benign partial epilepsy of childhood (BPEC), also known as benign rolandic epilepsy. Compared to children with the transient condition BPEC, children with chronic temporal lobe epilepsy scored lower on reading comprehension and reading speed. Notably, both groups were affected, but children with temporal lobe epilepsy were affected more so (102). Moreover, the types of abnormality found in repeated recordings from the same individuals can fluctuate over time, switching from focal to generalized epileptiform patterns and vice versa (103). Localized discharges also vary in their distant effects on other brain regions that play key roles in cognition. Positron emission tomography (PET) scans have demonstrated depressed cerebral metabolic activity in areas that are remote from EEG-defined epileptic foci (104, 105). These mechanisms of distant neuronal suppression appear to impair cognitive processing more so than memory.

Nonetheless, many investigators have found relationships between the cerebral localization of focal seizures and cognitive and/or behavioral outcomes. The results of this line of research generally support the theory that left-sided abnormalities are prone to interfere with verbal cognitive functions (106). High frequency of seizures has been linked to inattention (107, 108).

Although children with BPEC have normal IQs (109, 110), there are reports of heterogeneous patterns of difficulties with fine motor control, visual learning, and attention (109). No single cognitive profile has been identified, but some investigators have found that school difficulties and transiently weak scores improved after the EEG abnormalities abated (111). Other investigators found spike frequency to have greater impact on cognition than spike localization (112). Among 40 children with benign rolandic epilepsy (BRE), deficits in IQ were linked to spike frequency but not seizure frequency, lateralization of focus, and duration since spike focus was first identified. Perisylvian discharges were linked to learning difficulties at school and with language dysfunction affecting reading, spelling, auditory verbal learning, expressive grammar, and auditory discrimination (113).

Some investigators have drawn attention to the transient adverse effects of nocturnal EEG discharges in BPEC (113). Frequent subclinical nocturnal EEG discharges were linked to a heterogeneous group of educational, language, and behavioral impairments that, in themselves, were another mixed bag of disorders (114). After epileptic discharges in sleep stopped (remission of interictal discharges), IQ scores improved, as did performances on several subtests including visuomotor coordination attention and picture naming (115). Children with dyslexia and EEG trait of BPEC had attention impairment comparable to those with dyslexia but no BPEC (116). The occurrence of seizures during sleep is a noteworthy feature of the severe epileptic encephalopathies including Lennox-Gastaut syndrome, Doose syndrome, Landau-Kleffner syndrome, and ESES.

In a group of eight children with frontal lobe seizures who were studied in detail, IQ was spared but performance varied with lateralization, frequency, and age of onset (107). Left-sided EEG localization affected verbal long-term memory and visuospatial analysis. Hendriks and colleagues (108) identified verbal memory problems with temporal lobe epilepsy, but deficits also were intensified by high frequency of seizures, early age of onset, and long duration. Compared to children with generalized absence epilepsy or with temporal lobe epilepsy, children with frontal lobe seizures had reduced performance speed and were more distractible (117). Children with idiopathic occipital lobe epilepsy scored lower on attention and memory problems than nonepileptic controls (118).

Early onset of temporal lobe epilepsy can cause speech and language functions to relocate to nontypical cortical regions. These changes may be linked to reduced performance on subtests, but overall measures of intelligence are usually within the range of normal (119). Children with BPEC may relocate language away from the site of originally recorded spike focus (119, 120). Children who have left-sided brain abnormalities and shift language to either extratremporal bilateral or right brain language localization also show so-called crowding effects with nonverbal memory deficits.

Muszkat et al compared test results from 26 children with partial epilepsy to those from 61 control children who did not have epilepsy (121). Overall the children with epilepsy did less well than the control group. Furthermore, right-hemisphere EEG spike lateralization was linked to lower scores on measures of spatial ability and nonverbal attention. Left-hemisphere spike lateralization was linked to low scores on only digit span. Mitchell et al found that children with epilepsy tended to have slower reaction time, more variable performance, and make more errors of omission, but not commission, than normal control children (22). In another study of eight children with frontal lobe epilepsy, left-sided EEG localization affected verbal long-term memory and visuospatial analysis, whereas high frequency of seizures was linked to attention deficit (108).

Left hippocampal atrophy on MRI has been linked to problems with verbal memory (122). Among patients with left versus right mesial temporal sclerosis, those with left hippocampal atrophy had inferior general memory, verbal memory and verbal fluency, and naming (122, 123). Hermann et al compared patients with left versus right temporal lobe EEG foci (124). Subjects with left EEG foci did worse than either patients with right temporal foci or control subjects on verbal learning ability, immediate memory, and retrieval of verbal material from memory. Patients with left temporal lobe foci also had more problems with semantic organization, whereas the group with right temporal abnormalities did as well as controls. In another study, adult patients with left, but not right, temporal lobe EEG foci had reduced recognition of symbols presented tachistoscopically in their right visual fields. However, epileptic patients as a group had worse retention (memory) for the symbols than controls (125). In yet other studies left-sided lateralization of the epileptic focus was linked to loss of verbal abilities, whereas right-sided lateralization was linked to loss of nonverbal cognitive functions (126). Verbal-manual tasks used to assess cerebral organization for language indicate those children with left, but not right, hemisphere EEG foci have atypical patterns of cerebral dominance such as bihemispheric dominance (127). Right-sided temporal lobe epileptiform activity due to BPEC was accompanied by deficits in recognition memory (108, 119, 128). Billingsly and Smith reported lowered performance on both verbal and nonverbal IQ subtests by children with atypical cortical representation of speech (119).

Whereas linkages between cognitive difficulties and the laterality of EEG foci tend to be inconsistent, structural hemispheric lesions that produce hemiplegia have more dependable relationships to cognitive outcome. Sussova et al reported that among children with hemiplegic cerebral palsy, 80% had paroxysmal EEG features, although less than half actually had seizures (129). In these children the presence of epilepsy, not simply EEG abnormalities, was linked to lower IQ scores, an observation that was confirmed subsequently by others (130). Interestingly, in this particular study, right hemisphere lesions were more often linked to low IQ than left hemisphere lesions. In a different study, left hemispheric dysfunction producing right hemiplegia and epilepsy was linked to reduced IQ scores (26).

In children with tuberous sclerosis, the higher the number of lesions on MRI, the lower the IQ, the worse the behavior and the more severe the epilepsy (131). There are also relationships between the age of onset and cognitive outcome in tuberous sclerosis.

Epileptic foci in the left hemisphere have been linked to behavior disturbances, too. Corbett et al found that patients whose seizures originated in the left hemisphere were more likely to have behavior problems including

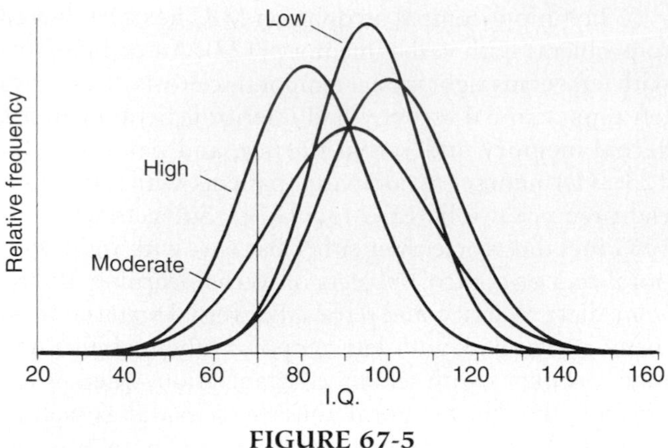

FIGURE 67-5

Effect of seizure frequency on full-scale IQ among people having seizure frequencies that were low (3 or fewer seizures per year), moderate (4–12 seizures per year), or high (12 or more seizures per year). Data are from Dikmen et al (133).

destruction of property, worrying, irritability, fussiness, and being resentful and aggressive (69).

Overall, however, in comparisons of the influence of various epilepsy-related variables on cognitive outcome, laterality of the epileptic seizure has been a less powerful covariable than age of onset (132).

Interrelationships of Epilepsy-Related Variables

Epilepsy-related variables that are linked to cognitive ability tend to be interrelated and often occur simultaneously. As will be seen in the sections that follow, age of onset and duration of epilepsy are closely intertwined. Collectively, these variables relate loosely to the overall intensity of the epileptic disorder. Dikman and colleagues evaluated 14 measures from the Halstead-Reitan Battery in adults who were categorized on the basis of seizure frequency, age of onset, and duration of epilepsy (133). Seizure frequency was directly related to reductions on 7 of 14 measures. Specifically, the average full-scale IQ declined from 95 to 81 as seizure frequency increased from 3 or fewer per year to more than 12 per year (Figure 67-5). When these investigators combined all three risk factors and compared the 12 patients with lowest risk to the 12 who had the highest risk, most cognitive measures were worse in the highest risk group—those patients who had the earliest onset, longest duration, and highest frequency of seizures. Similar findings have been reported by others (134).

Age of Onset of Epilepsy

Many investigations have found relationships between the age of onset of seizures and IQ (1, 3, 133, 135). In the study by Farwell et al the correlation between age of onset and full-scale IQ was 0.30: the older the age of onset, the higher the IQ 3. Overall, the onset of epilepsy in the first year of life has an ominous prognosis (136, 137). A long-term prospective study of 133 children whose epilepsy began in the first year found that 11% died before reaching age 7 years, 40% were severely retarded, and only 40% had an IQ of greater than 70 (138). The prognosis was the same no matter whether the child had infantile spasms or another type of epilepsy.

In the NCPP, epilepsy in the first year of life was associated with an average IQ of 91.8 (SD 22.0), which would result in 16.7% of this group being mentally retarded (11). In clinic-based studies the variables of age of onset and duration of epilepsy are usually interrelated. For example, Dikmen et al found that among adults with persistent epilepsy that began in childhood, the average group IQ declines in relation to the age of onset, the younger the age of onset the lower the IQ score (133) (Table 67-9). In addition, the early-onset group did worse

TABLE 67-9
Age of Seizure Onset and IQ Among Adults who Had Childhood Onset of Epilepsy that Lasted for 4 or More Years

	Age of Onset			
	Early (0–5 Years)		Late (10–15 Years)	
Number of subjects	22		22	
Duration (years)	22.28	(10.4)	23.6	(9.68)
Verbal IQ	81.04	(13.45)	91.00	(17.37)*
Performance IQ	78.14	(15.25)	88.41	(16.22)*
Full-scale IQ	78.5	(14.1)	89.36	(17.22)*
Fraction retarded	28.5%		13.7%	

*$P < 0.01$.
Values in parentheses are standard deviations.
Adapted from Dikmen et al (133).

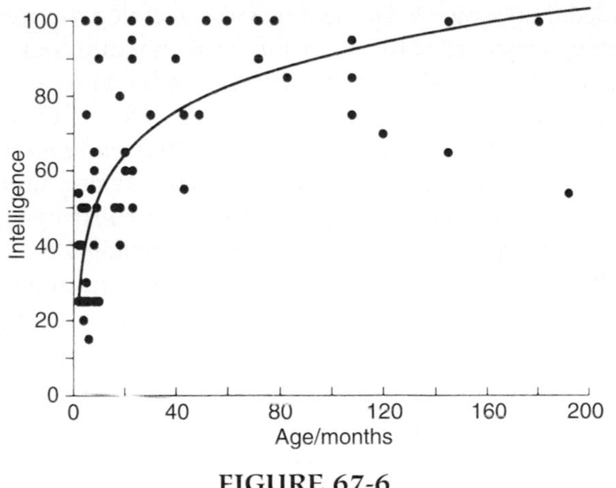

FIGURE 67-6

Relationship of age onset of seizures to IQ scores in children with tuberous sclerosis. Reproduced from Gomez (135) with permission.

on all 10 WAIS subtests, with statistically significant differences occurring on information, comprehension, arithmetic, and object assembly.

Seizure-related variables can interact simultaneously with etiology and the location of cerebral lesions to contribute to the child's cognitive capabilities. For example, in tuberous sclerosis the age of onset of seizures correlates with IQ: the earlier the onset of seizures, the lower the IQ (135) (Figure 67-6). Whereas most people with tuberous sclerosis are mentally retarded, virtually all mentally retarded patients with tuberous sclerosis have epilepsy, too. Finally, the location, number, and extent of cerebral lesions in tuberous sclerosis play central roles in shaping the overall clinical picture (131).

Seizure Frequency

Seizure control usually results in improved cognitive function (138–141) (Table 67-10.). Farwell et al found that among children whose seizures were controlled, the mean IQ was 99.6 compared to 87.0 for the group with continuing seizures (3). Among those patients whose seizure frequency declined there were overall improvements in IQ plus improvements on 8 of 11 subtests. By contrast, only the performance IQ and object assembly score improved on repeated testing among those whose seizure frequency remained the same or increased.

TABLE 67-10
Effect of Improved Seizure Control Among Young Adults with Epilepsy

	Test		Retest	
Verbal IQ	91.96	(12.51)	95.55	(12.02)
Performance IQ	86.09	(12.51)	96.32	(16.41)
Full-scale IQ	88.78	(12.12)	95.64	(13.76)

Values shown are means and standard deviations.
Adapted from Seidenberg et al (153).

Although the severity of the epilepsy has been linked to the degree of mental handicap, severe mental handicap does not preclude good seizure control (141).

In BPEC spike frequency, not seizure frequency or lateralization of the focus, has been linked to reduced IQ and other measures of cognition (112). Compared to control children, children with rolandic spikes tended to suffer from impaired IQ, defective visual perception, short-term memory disturbance, plus deteriorated psychiatric status and fine motor performance. However, after rolandic epilepsy remits, the cognitive impediments usually resolve (142).

Intuitively, seizure frequency would seem to be associated with cognitive impairment because of the extremely high frequency of seizures among children with encephalopathic epilepsies. In practice this association has proven difficult to document, especially when the seizure frequency is moderate to low. For example, among children with febrile seizures, neither the number of seizures nor the duration of individual seizures was associated with a reduction in IQ among patients compared to siblings. In the NCPP, among 36 children who had three or more febrile seizures, the full-scale IQ was 95.9 (SD 10.8) versus 95.9 (SD 11.6) in control siblings (143).

Duration of Epilepsy

In most studies the duration of epilepsy is related to the age on onset in that an early age of onset tends to be followed by a prolonged duration of the disorder. Thus, both of these factors are associated with reductions in group IQ scores. In some studies the duration of epilepsy has been inversely correlated with IQ in children with a correlation coefficient of −0.40 (3). When adjusted for duration of seizure-free years, the correlation has been even stronger, −0.62.

Factors that predict persistent seizures are also linked to adverse cognitive outcomes for children with epilepsy. These include frequent seizures, an early age of onset, secondary generalization, symptomatic epilepsy due to structural brain lesions, and abnormal neurologic status (143). When clinic-based groups of children who have partial seizures have been followed for long periods of time, those who have these features are at high risk for cognitive and social morbidity plus seizure-related death (144, 145). Among children with epilepsy due to Sturge-Weber syndrome, those with lower IQs had longer duration of epilepsy and more seizures (105).

Although population-based studies do not provide evidence that cognitive decline occurs in people with epilepsy, studies from institutions and from referral centers indicate that severe epilepsy is occasionally followed by declining IQ scores. Whereas these changes materialize insidiously over years to decades, repeated evaluations over long periods of time are needed to identify when this is occurring (9). Corbett et al found that 15.7% of patients at Lingfield Hospital experienced a reduction in IQ of 15 or more points (69). Factors that were associated with decreased IQ included higher levels of primidone and phenytoin and lower folate levels, but not the severity of EEG abnormalities or the seizure frequency. In a prospective clinic-based study of children with epilepsy, decreasing IQ scores were associated with earlier age of onset, more difficult-to-control seizures, having drug levels in toxic range, and having more drugs that caused toxicity (1). However, the mean IQ for the group as a whole did not decline. Although IQ scores declined in 11.1%, they increased in 16.7%.

Long-term follow-up of children with temporal lobe epilepsy indicates that a high percentage encounter academic failure if seizures continue unabated for years. In the series reported by Lindsay et al, there were 4 seizure-related deaths before age 16 years. A total of 10 of 58 children who were candidates for epilepsy surgery died. Among those whose seizures persisted and who were not treated surgically, only 25 of 45 completed regular school and 16 of 45 experienced early cognitive deterioration (144). Only 4 of the 45 members of this group were employable, and only 6 obtained driver's licenses. In another study (134), compared to healthy controls, people with prolonged temporal lobe epilepsy had reduced performance on tests of intelligence, language, motor speed, and executive function with longer duration associated with declining mental capability. As noted previously, symptomatic etiology can be linked to long-duration epilepsy and poor social adjustment in adult life (9).

Epilepsy and Neuropsychiatric Adaption

Although adults with epilepsy have a greater risk of neuropsychiatric problems, the nature and extent of these problems is difficult to characterize. In the Veterans Administration Collaborative Study 118, patients were compared to normal controls before therapy (146). Patients with epilepsy had significantly worse scores on 14 of 18 neuropsychologic measures before medication was started. However, the risk of neuropsychologic compromise among adult patients with epilepsy seems to be the same as among patients with other chronic neurologic ailments. Hermann et al found no differences due to seizure type or age of onset on Minnesota Multiphasic Personality Inventory (MMPI) measures of psychopathology, but epilepsy per se was associated with a greater risk of problems (147). After an extensive analysis of MMPI profiles from the literature, other investigators have concluded that compared to people without epilepsy, patients with epilepsy are at higher risk for psychopathology, but the risk associated with epilepsy is similar to that associated with chronic disease in general (148). In a later report, Dodrill and Batzel reiterated that patients with epilepsy are at greater risk than normal, but they argued that the risk of psychopathology for people with epilepsy is the same as for people with other neurologic disease; both of the neurologic disease groups, epileptic and nonepileptic, have higher risk than patients with chronic, non-neurologic diseases (149). The excess of psychopathology among people with neurologic disease is manifest primarily as a high prevalence of psychotic MMPI profiles for both epileptic and other neurologic groups.

Studies in adults that relate seizure type to distinctive personality profiles are controversial. Although some investigators have suggested that adults with temporal lobe epilepsy have distinctive personalities, others have been unable to confirm it (148, 149). Thus a majority of investigators conclude that temporal lobe epilepsy is no worse than any other type of epilepsy in this regard. Dodrill and Batzel, in reviewing this issue, also criticized the item content of the MMPI as being inappropriate for patients with epilepsy (149). In general, when adults with epilepsy have psychopathology, it tends to be severe (148). Depression is a particularly common problem (150).

Psychological tests in teenagers do correlate with overall adjustment later in adulthood. Dodrill and Clemmons followed up patients with epilepsy 5.9 (SD 1.86) years after their original evaluations during adolescence. The patients were rated on vocational adjustment (unemployed to full-time employment in four categories) and on daily life functioning (fully dependent to independent in three categories) (151). The MMPI did not predict either vocational or life functioning. Predictive measures of being fully functional (adequate in both vocational and independence measures) included the Halstead Impairment Index, Seashore Rhythm, Aphasia Screening (total errors), and verbal, performance, and full-scale IQ. Discriminant function analysis indicated that vocational adjustment related best to the Halstead Impairment Index, whereas independence in living was predicted by Seashore Rhythm and thematic perception test (TPT) (memory). Language skills were especially important. In a separate study, marital adjustment among adults with epilepsy was more related to emotional adjustment, whereas living independently was related to mental ability (152).

CONCLUSIONS

Although most children with epilepsy are developmentally and behaviorally normal, children with epilepsy as a group have an average IQ that is approximately 10 points lower than in children without epilepsy. Learning disabilities are also more prevalent among children with epilepsy. Boys are at higher risk than girls. The lower IQ found among groups of epileptic children is largely a consequence of antecedent, etiologically specific neurologic abnormalities rather than a consequence of seizures or antiepileptic drug therapy.

Although seizures do not cause i\ntellectual decline in most cases, certain exceptional encephalopathic epileptic syndromes are associated with abnormal development and intellectual decline. These severe epilepsies are so rare that they are not encountered to a meaningful extent in most population-based studies. Among all epileptic syndromes, childhood absence epilepsy (pyknolepsy or petit mal epilepsy) alone is associated with an above average IQ.

Among all epilepsy-associated variables, etiology plus the location and extent of cerebral lesion(s) best predict cognitive abilities in children with epilepsy. The risk of associated mental retardation in patients with epilepsy is increased when there is associated motor impairment, when epilepsy begins at an early age, when the duration of epilepsy is prolonged, when there are multiple seizure types—especially minor motor seizures—and when multiple drugs in high doses are required. Childhood epilepsy with uncontrolled seizures that persists into adulthood can cause dramatic and pervasive disruption of the acquisition of adult social and cognitive skills.

References

1. Bourgeois BF, Prensky AL, Palkes HS, et al. Intelligence in epilepsy: a prospective study in children. *Ann Neurol* 1983; 14(4):438–444.
2. Addy DP. Cognitive function in children with epilepsy. *Dev Med Child Neurol* 1987; 29(3):394–397.
3. Farwell JR, Dodrill CB, Batzel LW. Neuropsychological abilities of children with epilepsy. *Epilepsia* 1985; 26(5):395–400.
4. Ellenberg JH, Hirtz DG, Nelson KB. Do seizures in children cause intellectual deterioration? *N Engl J Med* 1986; 314(17):1085–1088.
5. Nelson KB, Ellenberg JH. Antecedents of seizure disorders in early childhood. *Am J Dis Child* 1986; 140(10):1053–1061.
6. Nelson KB, Ellenberg JH. Antecedents of cerebral palsy. Multivariate analysis of risk. *N Engl J Med* 1986; 315(2):81–86.
7. Sturniolo MG, Galletti F. Idiopathic epilepsy and school achievement. *Arch Dis Child* 1994; 70(5):424–428.
8. Jalava M, Sillanpaa M, Camfield C, Camfield P. Social adjustment and competence 35 years after onset of childhood epilepsy: a prospective controlled study. *Epilepsia* 1997; 38(6):708–715.
9. Sillanpaa M, Jalava M, Kaleva O, Shinnar S. Long-term prognosis of seizures with onset in childhood [see comment]. *N Engl J Med* 1998; 338(24):1715–1722.
10. Rodenburg R, Stams GJ, Meijer AM, et al. Psychopathology in children with epilepsy: a meta-analysis. *J Pediatr Psychol* 2005; 30(6):453–468.
11. Ellenberg JH, Hirtz DG, Nelson KB. Do seizures in children cause intellectual deterioration? *N Engl J Med* 1986; 314(17):1085–1088.
12. Epir S, Renda Y, Baser N. Cognitive and behavioural characteristics of children with idiopathic epilepsy in a low-income area of Ankara, Turkey. *Dev Med Child Neurol* 1984; 26(2):200–207.
13. Seidenberg M, Beck N, Geisser M, et al. Academic achievement of children with epilepsy. *Epilepsia* 1986; 27(6):753–759.
14. Jennekens-Schinkel A, Linschooten-Duikersloot EM, Bouma PA, et al. Spelling errors made by children with mild epilepsy: writing-to-dictation. *Epilepsia* 1987; 28(5):555–563.
15. Sillanpaa M. Epilepsy in children: prevalence, disability, and handicap. *Epilepsia* 1992; 33(3):444–449.
16. Pazzaglia P, Frank-Pazzaglia L. Record in grade school of pupils with epilepsy: an epidemiological study. *Epilepsia* 1976; 17(4):361–366.
17. Caplan R, Siddarth P, Gurbani S, et al. Psychopathology and pediatric complex partial seizures: seizure-related, cognitive, and linguistic variables. *Epilepsia* 2004; 45(10): 1273–1281.
18. Rodenburg R, Meijer AM, Dekovic M, Aldenkamp AP. Family factors and psychopathology in children with epilepsy: a literature review. *Epilepsy Behav* 2005; 6(4):488–503.
19. Kurokawa T, Matsuo M, Yoshida K, et al. Behavioral disorders in Japanese epileptic children. *Folia Psychiatr Neurol Jpn* 1983; 37(3):259–265.
20. Mandelbaum DE, Burack GD. The effect of seizure type and medication on cognitive and behavioral functioning in children with idiopathic epilepsy. *Dev Med Child Neurol* 1997; 39(11):731–735.
21. Caplan R, Sagun J, Siddarth P, et al. Social competence in pediatric epilepsy: insights into underlying mechanisms. *Epilepsy Behav* 2005; 6(2):218–228.
22. Mitchell WG, Zhou Y, Chavez JM, Guzman BL. Reaction time, attention, and impulsivity in epilepsy. *Pediatr Neurol* 1992; 8(1):19–24.
23. Bornstein RA, Drake ME Jr, Pakalnis A. WAIS-R factor structure in epileptic patients. *Epilepsia* 1988; 29(1):14–18.
24. Aldenkamp AP, Weber B, Overweg-Plandsoen WC, et al. Educational underachievement in children with epilepsy: a model to predict the effects of epilepsy on educational achievement. *J Child Neurol* 2005; 20(3):175–180.
25. Aldenkamp AP, Arends J, Verspeek S, Berting M. The cognitive impact of epileptiform EEG-discharges; relationship with type of cognitive task. *Child Neuropsychol* 2004; 10(4):297–305.
26. Glosser G, Cole LC, French JA, et al. Predictors of intellectual performance in adults with intractable temporal lobe epilepsy. *J Int Neuropsychol Soc* 1997; 3(3):252–259.
27. Mitchell WG, Chavez JM, Lee H, Guzman BL. Academic underachievement in children with epilepsy. *J Child Neurol* 1991; 6(1):65–72.
28. Odding E, Roebroeck ME, Stam HJ. The epidemiology of cerebral palsy: incidence, impairments and risk factors. *Disabil Rehabil* 2006; 28(4):183–191.
29. Caplan R, Arbelle S, Magharious W, et al. Psychopathology in pediatric complex partial and primary generalized epilepsy. *Dev Med Child Neurol* 1998; 40(12):805–811.
30. Boel MJ. Behavioural and neuropsychological problems in refractory paediatric epilepsies. *Eur J Paediatr Neurol* 2004; 8(6):291–297.
31. Hrdlicka M, Komarek V, Propper L, et al. Not EEG abnormalities but epilepsy is associated with autistic regression and mental functioning in childhood autism. *Eur Child Adolesc Psychiatry* 2004; 13(4):209–213.
32. Oguni H, Hayashi K, Osawa M. Long-term prognosis of Lennox-Gastaut syndrome. *Epilepsia* 1996; 37 Suppl 3:44–47.
33. Korkman M, Granstrom ML, Kantola-Sorsa E, et al. Two-year follow-up of intelligence after pediatric epilepsy surgery. *Pediatr Neurol* 2005; 33(3):173–178.
34. Bjornaes H, Stabell K, Henriksen O, Loyning Y. The effects of refractory epilepsy on intellectual functioning in children and adults. A longitudinal study. *Seizure* 2001; 10(4):250–259.
35. Aylward GP. Cognitive and neuropsychological outcomes: more than IQ scores. *Ment Retard Dev Disabil Res Rev* 2002; 8(4):234–240.
36. Caplan R, Guthrie D, Komo S, et al. Social communication in children with epilepsy. *J Child Psychol Psychiatry* 2002; 43(2):245–253.
37. Hauser W, Hesdorffer D. Epilepsy frequency, causes and consequences. New York: Demos, 1990.
38. Peduzzi M, Defontaine E, Misson JP. Epilepsie chez des enfants infirmes moteurs-cerebraux. *Rev Med Liege* 2006; 61(4):237–239.
39. Pleacher MD, Vohr BR, Katz KH, et al. An evidence-based approach to predicting low IQ in very preterm infants from the neurological examination: outcome data from the Indomethacin Intraventricular Hemorrhage Prevention Trial. *Pediatrics* 2004; 113(2):416–419.
40. Feagans L. A current view of learning disabilities. *J Pediatr* 1983; 102(4):487–493.
41. Hammill DD. On defining learning disabilities: an emerging consensus. *J Learn Disabil* 1990; 23(2):74–84.
42. Shaywitz BA, Fletcher JM, Shaywitz SE. Defining and classifying learning disabilities and attention-deficit/hyperactivity disorder. *J Child Neurol* 1995; 10 Suppl 1:S50–S57.
43. Broman S, Nichols P, Kennedy W. Preschool IQ prenatal and early developmental correlates. Hillsdale, NJ: Lawrence Erlbaum Associates, 1975.
44. Singhi PD, Bansal U, Singhi S, Pershad D. Determinants of IQ profile in children with idiopathic generalized epilepsy. *Epilepsia* 1992; 33(6):1106–1114.
45. Mitchell WG, Scheier LM, Baker SA. Psychosocial, behavioral, and medical outcomes in children with epilepsy: a developmental risk factor model using longitudinal data. *Pediatrics* 1994; 94 4 Pt 1:471–477.
46. Hammal D, Jarvis SN, Colver AF. Participation of children with cerebral palsy is influenced by where they live [see comment]. *Dev Med Child Neurol* 2004; 46(5):292–298.
47. Pianta RC, Lothman DJ. Predicting behavior problems in children with epilepsy: child factors, disease factors, family stress, and child-mother interaction. *Child Dev* 1994; 65(5):1415–1428.
48. Chovaz CJ, McLachlan RS, Derry PA, Cummings AL. Psychosocial function following temporal lobectomy: influence of seizure control and learned helplessness. *Seizure* 1994; 3(3):171–176.
49. Nolan MA, Redoblado MA, Lah S, et al. Intelligence in childhood epilepsy syndromes. *Epilepsy Res* 2003; 53(1-2):139–150.
50. Bulteau C, Jambaque I, Viguier D, et al. Epileptic syndromes, cognitive assessment and school placement: a study of 251 children. *Dev Med Child Neurol* 2000; 42(5):319–327.

51. Sillanpaa M. Learning disability: occurrence and long-term consequences in childhood-onset epilepsy. *Epilepsy Behav* 2004; 5(6):937–944.
52. Kuzniecky R, Andermann F. The congenital bilateral perisylvian syndrome: imaging findings in a multicenter study. CBPS Study Group. *AJNR Am J Neuroradiol* 1994; 15(1):139–144.
53. Ono J, Mano T, Andermann E, et al. Band heterotopia or double cortex in a male: bridging structures suggest abnormality of the radial glial guide system. *Neurology* 1997; 48(6):1701–1703.
54. Gleeson JG, Allen KM, Fox JW, et al. Doublecortin, a brain-specific gene mutated in human X-linked lissencephaly and double cortex syndrome, encodes a putative signaling protein. *Cell* 1998; 92(1):63–72.
55. Guerrini R, Dubeau F, Dulac O, et al. Bilateral parasagittal parietooccipital polymicrogyria and epilepsy. *Ann Neurol* 1997; 41(1):65–73.
56. Guerrini R, Sicca F, Parmeggiani L. Epilepsy and malformations of the cerebral cortex. *Epileptic Disord* 2003; 5 Suppl 2:S9–S26.
57. Strauss E, Wada J, Hunter M. Callosal morphology and performance on intelligence tests. *J Clin Exp Neuropsychol* 1994; 16(1):79–83.
58. Fedrizzi E, Inverno M, Bruzzone MG, et al. MRI features of cerebral lesions and cognitive functions in preterm spastic diplegic children. *Pediatric Neurol* 1996; 15(3):207–212.
59. Stromme P, Sundet K, Mork C, et al. X linked mental retardation and infantile spasms in a family: new clinical data and linkage to Xp11.4-Xp22.11. *J Med Genet* 1999; 36(5):374–378.
60. Susser M, Hauser W, Kiely J, et al. Quantitative estimates of prenatal and perinatal risk factors for perinatal mortality, cerebral palsy, mental retardation, and epilepsy. NIH Publ. No. 85-1149. Bethesda, MD: National Institutes of Health, 1985.
61. Schinzel A. Microdeletion syndromes, balanced translocations, and gene mapping. *J Med Genet* 1988; 25(7):454–462.
62. Wisniewski KE, French JH, Fernando S, et al. Fragile X syndrome: associated neurological abnormalities and developmental disabilities. *Ann Neurol* 1985; 18(6):665–669.
63. Hagerman RJ. Fragile X syndrome. *Curr Prob Pediatr* 1987; 17(11):621–674.
64. Fluge G. Neurological findings at follow-up in neonatal hypoglycaemia. *Acta Paediatr Scand* 1975; 64(4):629–634.
65. Singhi PD, Bansal U, Singhi S, Pershad D. Determinants of IQ profile in children with idiopathic generalized epilepsy. *Epilepsia* 1992; 33(6):1106–1114.
66. Nelson KB, Ellenberg JH. An epidemiological approach to the problems of cerebral palsy. In: Maekawa K, Yamaguchi K, eds. *International Congress Series No. 579: Child Neurology*. Ámsterdam: Excerpta Medica, 1981:341–350.
67. Funayama CA, de Moura-Ribeiro MV, Goncalves AL. Encefalopatia hipoxico-isquemica em recem-nascidos a termo. Aspectos da fase aguda e evolucao. *Arq Neuropsiquiatr* 1997; 55(4):771–779.
68. Beran RG, Flanagan PJ. Psychosocial sequelae of epilepsy: the role of associated cerebral pathology. *Epilepsia* 1987; 28(2):107–110.
69. Corbett JA, Trimble MR, Nichol TC. Behavioral and cognitive impairments in children with epilepsy: the long-term effects of anticonvulsant therapy. *J Am Acad Child Psychiatry* 1985; 24(1):17–23.
70. Deb S. Mental disorder in adults with mental retardation and epilepsy. *Compr Psychiatry* 1997; 38(3):179–184.
71. Hagberg B, Hagberg G, Olow I, van Wendt L. The changing panorama of cerebral palsy in Sweden. VII. Prevalence and origin in the birth year period 1987–90. *Acta Paediatr* 1996; 85(8):954–960.
72. Kaushik A, Agarwal RP, Sadhna. Association of cerebral palsy with epilepsy. *J Indian Med Assoc* 1997; 95(10):552–554, 565.
73. Hadjipanayis A, Hadjichristodoulou C, Youroukos S. Epilepsy in patients with cerebral palsy. *Dev Med Child Neurol* 1997; 39(10):659–663.
74. Kwong KL, Wong SN, So KT. Epilepsy in children with cerebral palsy. *Pediatr Neurol* 1998; 19(1):31–36.
75. Kulak W, Sobaniec W, Smigielska-Kuzia J, et al. A comparison of spastic diplegic and tetraplegic cerebral palsy. *Pediatr Neurol* 2005; 32(5):311–317.
76. Futagi Y, Toribe Y, Ogawa K, Suzuki Y. Neurodevelopmental outcome in children with intraventricular hemorrhage. *Pediatr Neurol* 2006; 34(3):219–224.
77. Aksu F. Nature and prognosis of seizures in patients with cerebral palsy. *Dev Med Child Neurol* 1990; 32(8):661–668.
78. Eriksson K, Erila T, Kivimaki T, Koivikko M. Evolution of epilepsy in children with mental retardation: five-year experience in 78 cases. *Am J Ment Retard* 1998; 102(5):464–472.
79. Mikkola K, Ritari N, Tommiska V, et al. Neurodevelopmental outcome at 5 years of age of a national cohort of extremely low birth weight infants who were born in 1996–1997. *Pediatrics* 2005; 116(6):1391–1400.
80. Doyle LW, Casalaz D, Victorian Infant Collaborative Study G. Outcome at 14 years of extremely low birthweight infants: a regional study. *Arch Dis Child Fetal Neonatal Ed* 2001; 85(3):F159–F164.
81. Eriksson K, Erila T, Kivimaki T, Koivikko M. Evolution of epilepsy in children with mental retardation: five-year experience in 78 cases. *Am J Ment Retard* 1998; 102(5):464–472.
82. Forsgren L, Edvinsson SO, Blomquist HK, et al. Epilepsy in a population of mentally retarded children and adults. *Epilepsy Res* 1990; 6(3):234–248.
83. Chelune GJ, Naugle RI, Hermann BP, et al. Does presurgical IQ predict seizure outcome after temporal lobectomy? Evidence from the Bozeman Epilepsy Consortium. *Epilepsia* 1998; 39(3):314–318.
84. Beckung E, Uvebrant P. Motor and sensory impairments in children with intractable epilepsy. *Epilepsia* 1993; 34(5):924–929.
85. Goulden KJ, Shinnar S, Koller H, et al. Epilepsy in children with mental retardation: a cohort study. *Epilepsia* 1991; 32(5):690–697.
86. Roger J, Dravet C, Bureau M, et al. Epileptic syndromes in infancy, childhood, and adolescence. London: John Libbey and Company, 1985.
87. Korff CM, Nordli DR Jr. Epilepsy syndromes in infancy. *Pediatr Neurol* 2006; 34(4):253–263.
88. Dulac O. Benign epilepsies of childhood—distinct syndromes and overlap. *Epileptic Disord* 2000; 2 Suppl 1:S41–S43.
89. Shields WD. Catastrophic epilepsy in childhood. *Epilepsia* 2000; 41 Suppl 2:S2–S6.
90. Rho JM. Basic science behind the catastrophic epilepsies. *Epilepsia* 2004; 45 Suppl 5:5–11.
91. Smith MC, Hoeppner TJ. Epileptic encephalopathy of late childhood: Landau-Kleffner syndrome and the syndrome of continuous spikes and waves during slow-wave sleep. *J Clin Neurophysiol* 2003; 20(6):462–472.
92. Trevathan E, Murphy CC, Yeargin-Allsopp M. The descriptive epidemiology of infantile spasms among Atlanta children. *Epilepsia* 1999; 40(6):748–751.
93. Trevathan E, Murphy CC, Yeargin-Allsopp M. Prevalence and descriptive epidemiology of Lennox-Gastaut syndrome among Atlanta children. *Epilepsia* 1997; 38(12):1283–1288.
94. Moretti P, Zoghbi HY. MeCP2 dysfunction in Rett syndrome and related disorders. *Curr Opin Genet Dev* 2006; 16(3):276–281.
95. Bradbury J. Advance made in understanding Rett's syndrome. *Lancet Neurol* 2005; 4(2):83.
96. Prevey ML, Delaney RC, Cramer JA, Mattson RH. Complex partial and secondarily generalized seizure patients: cognitive functioning prior to treatment with antiepileptic medication. VA Epilepsy Cooperative Study 264 Group. *Epilepsy Res* 1998; 30(1):1–9.
97. Giordani B, Sackellares JC, Miller S, et al. Improvement in neuropsychological performance in patients with refractory seizures after intensive diagnostic and therapeutic intervention. *Neurology* 1983; 33(4):489–493.
98. Wilkus RJ, Dodrill CB. Neuropsychological correlates of the electroencephalogram in epileptics: I. Topographic distribution and average rate of epileptiform activity. *Epilepsia* 1976; 17(1):89–100.
99. Anonymous. Proposal for revised clinical and electroencephalographic classification of epileptic seizures. From the Commission on Classification and Terminology of the International League Against Epilepsy. *Epilepsia* 1981; 22(4):489–501.
100. Berent S, Giordani B, Sackellares JC, et al. Cerebrally lateralized epileptogenic foci and performance on a verbal and visual-graphic learning task. *Percept Mot Skills* 1983; 56(3):991–1001.
101. Mungas D, Ehlers C, Walton N, McCutchen CB. Verbal learning differences in epileptic patients with left and right temporal lobe foci. *Epilepsia* 1985; 26(4):340–345.
102. Chaix Y, Laguitton V, Lauwers-Cances V, et al. Reading abilities and cognitive functions of children with epilepsy: influence of epileptic syndrome. *Brain Dev* 2006; 28(2):122–130.
103. Camfield P, Gordon K, Camfield C, et al. EEG results are rarely the same if repeated within six months in childhood epilepsy. *Can J Neurol Sci* 1995; 22(4):297–300.
104. Jokeit H, Seitz RJ, Markowitsch HJ, et al. Prefrontal asymmetric interictal glucose hypometabolism and cognitive impairment in patients with temporal lobe epilepsy. *Brain* 1997; 120 Pt 12:2283–2294.
105. Lee JS, Asano E, Muzik O, et al. Sturge-Weber syndrome: correlation between clinical course and FDG PET findings. *Neurology* 2001; 57(2):189–195.
106. Trimble MR, Thompson PJ. Neuropsychological and behavioral sequelae of spontaneous seizures. *Ann N Y Acad Sci* 1986; 462:284–292.
107. Riva D, Saletti V, Nichelli F, Bulgheroni S. Neuropsychologic effects of frontal lobe epilepsy in children. *J Child Neurol* 2002; 17(9):661–667.
108. Hendriks MP, Aldenkamp AP, Alpherts WC, et al. Relationships between epilepsy-related factors and memory impairment. *Acta Neurol Scand* 2004; 110(5):291–300.
109. Giordani B, Caveney AF, Laughrin D, et al. Cognition and behavior in children with benign epilepsy with centrotemporal spikes (BECTS). *Epilepsy Res* 2006; 70(1):89–94.
110. Staden U, Isaacs E, Boyd SG, et al. Language dysfunction in children with Rolandic epilepsy. *Neuropediatrics* 1998; 29(5):242–248.
111. Deonna T, Zesiger P, Davidoff V, et al. Benign partial epilepsy of childhood: a longitudinal neuropsychological and EEG study of cognitive function. *Dev Med Child Neurol* 2000; 42(9):595–603.
112. Weglage J, Demsky A, Pietsch M, Kurlemann G. Neuropsychological, intellectual, and behavioral findings in patients with centrotemporal spikes with and without seizures. *Dev Med Child Neurol* 1997; 39(10):646–651.
113. Nicolai J, Aldenkamp AP, Arends J, et al. Cognitive and behavioral effects of nocturnal epileptiform discharges in children with benign childhood epilepsy with centrotemporal spikes. *Epilepsy Behav* 2006; 8(1):56–70.
114. Pinton F, Ducot B, Motte J, et al. Cognitive functions in children with benign childhood epilepsy with centrotemporal spikes (BECTS). *Epileptic Disord* 2006; 8(1):11–23.
115. Baglietto MG, Battaglia FM, Nobili L, et al. Neuropsychological disorders related to interictal epileptic discharges during sleep in benign epilepsy of childhood with centrotemporal or Rolandic spikes. *Dev Med Child Neurol* 2001; 43(6):407–412.
116. Carlsson G, Igelbrink-Schulze N, Neubauer BA, Stephani U. Neuropsychological long-term outcome of rolandic EEG traits. *Epileptic Disord* 2000; 2 Suppl 1:S63–S66.
117. Hernandez MT, Sauerwein HC, Jambaque I, et al. Attention, memory, and behavioral adjustment in children with frontal lobe epilepsy. *Epilepsy Behav* 2003; 4(5):522–536.
118. Gulgonen S, Demirbilek V, Korkmaz B, et al. Neuropsychological functions in idiopathic occipital lobe epilepsy. *Epilepsia* 2000; 41(4):405–411.
119. Billingsley R, Smith ML. Intelligence profiles in children and adolescents with left temporal lobe epilepsy: relationship to language laterality. *Brain Cogn* 2000; 43(1–3):44–49.
120. Hommet C, Billard C, Motte J, et al. Cognitive function in adolescents and young adults in complete remission from benign childhood epilepsy with centro-temporal spikes. *Epileptic Disord* 2001; 3(4):207–216.

121. Muszkat M, De Vincenzo NS, Masuko A, et al. Analise da assimetria funcional hemisferica de criancas com epilepsia parcial e QI normal pelo desempenho nos subtestes do WISC. *Arq Neuropsiquiatr* 1991; 49(4):392–398.
122. Alessio A, Damasceno BP, Camargo CH, et al. Differences in memory performance and other clinical characteristics in patients with mesial temporal lobe epilepsy with and without hippocampal atrophy. *Epilepsy Behav* 2004; 5(1):22–27.
123. Alessio A, Bonilha L, Rorden C, et al. Memory and language impairments and their relationships to hippocampal and perirhinal cortex damage in patients with medial temporal lobe epilepsy. *Epilepsy Behav* 2006; 8(3):593–600.
124. Hermann BP, Wyler AR, Richey ET, Rea JM. Memory function and verbal learning ability in patients with complex partial seizures of temporal lobe origin. *Epilepsia* 1987; 28(5):547–554.
125. Masui K, Niwa S, Anzai N, et al. Verbal memory disturbances in left temporal lobe epileptics. *Cortex* 1984; 20(3):361–368.
126. Gadian DG, Isaacs EB, Cross JH, et al. Lateralization of brain function in childhood revealed by magnetic resonance spectroscopy. *Neurology* 1996; 46(4):974–977.
127. Piccirilli M, D'Alessandro P, Tiacci C, Ferroni A. Language lateralization in children with benign partial epilepsy. *Epilepsia* 1988; 29(1):19–25.
128. Gleissner U, Kurthen M, Sassen R, et al. Clinical and neuropsychological characteristics of pediatric epilepsy patients with atypical language dominance. *Epilepsy Behav* 2003; 4(6):746–752.
129. Sussova J, Seidl Z, Faber J. Hemiparetic forms of cerebral palsy in relation to epilepsy and mental retardation. *Dev Med Child Neurol* 1990; 32(9):792–795.
130. Muter V, Taylor S, Vargha-Khadem F. A longitudinal study of early intellectual development in hemiplegic children. *Neuropsychologia* 1997; 35(3):289–298.
131. Jambaque I, Cusmai R, Curatolo P, et al. Neuropsychological aspects of tuberous sclerosis in relation to epilepsy and MRI findings. *Dev Med Child Neurol* 1991; 33(8):698–705.
132. Strauss E, Loring D, Chelune G, et al. Predicting cognitive impairment in epilepsy: findings from the Bozeman epilepsy consortium. *J Clin Exp Neuropsychol* 1995; 17(6):909–917.
133. Dikmen S, Matthews CG, Harley JP. Effect of early versus late onset of major motor epilepsy on cognitive-intellectual performance: further considerations. *Epilepsia* 1977; 18(1):31–36.
134. Oyegbile TO, Dow C, Jones J, et al. The nature and course of neuropsychological morbidity in chronic temporal lobe epilepsy. *Neurology* 2004; 62(10):1736–1742.
135. Gomez M. Tuberous sclerosis. 2nd ed. New York: Raven Press, 1988.
136. Chevrie JJ, Aicardi J. Convulsive disorders in the first year of life: neurological and mental outcome and mortality. *Epilepsia* 1978; 19(1):67–74.
137. Chevrie JJ, Aicardi J. Convulsive disorders in the first year of life: persistence of epileptic seizures. *Epilepsia* 1979; 20(6):643–649.
138. Czochanska J, Langner-Tyszka B, Losiowski Z, Schmidt-Sidor B. Children who develop epilepsy in the first year of life: a prospective study. *Dev Med Child Neurol* 1994; 36(4):345–350.
139. Gilliam F, Wyllie E, Kashden J, et al. Epilepsy surgery outcome: comprehensive assessment in children. *Neurology* 1997; 48(5):1368–1374.
140. Gordon K, Bawden H, Camfield P, et al. Valproic acid treatment of learning disorder and severely epileptiform EEG without clinical seizures. *J Child Neurol* 1996; 11(1):41–43.
141. Marcus JC. Control of epilepsy in a mentally retarded population: lack of correlation with IQ, neurological status, and electroencephalogram. *Am J Ment Retard* 1993; 98 Suppl:47–51.
142. D'Alessandro P, Piccirilli M, Tiacci C, et al. Neuropsychological features of benign partial epilepsy in children. *Ital J Neurol Sci* 1990; 11(3):265–269.
143. Duchowny M, Levin B, Jayakar P, et al. Temporal lobectomy in early childhood. *Epilepsia* 1992; 33(2):298–303.
144. Lindsay J, Glaser G, Richards P, Ounsted C. Developmental aspects of focal epilepsies of childhood treated by neurosurgery. *Dev Med Child Neurol* 1984; 26(5):574–587.
145. Lindsay J, Ounsted C, Richards P. Long-term outcome in children with temporal lobe seizures. IV: Genetic factors, febrile convulsions and the remission of seizures. *Dev Med Child Neurol* 1980; 22(4):429–439.
146. Prevey ML, Delaney RC, Cramer JA, Mattson RH. Complex partial and secondarily generalized seizure patients: cognitive functioning prior to treatment with antiepileptic medication. VA Epilepsy Cooperative Study 264 Group. *Epilepsy Res* 1998; 30(1):1–9.
147. Hermann BP, Schwartz MS, Karnes WE, Vahdat P. Psychopathology in epilepsy: relationship of seizure type to age at onset. *Epilepsia* 1980; 21(1):15–23.
148. Whitman S, Hermann BP, Gordon AC. Psychopathology in epilepsy: how great is the risk? *Biol Psychiatry* 1984; 19(2):213–236.
149. Dodrill CB, Batzel LW. Interictal behavioral features of patients with epilepsy. *Epilepsia* 1986; 27 Suppl 2:S64–S76.
150. Robertson MM, Trimble MR, Townsend HR. Phenomenology of depression in epilepsy. *Epilepsia* 1987; 28(4):364–372.
151. Dodrill CB, Clemmons D. Use of neuropsychological tests to identify high school students with epilepsy who later demonstrate inadequate performances in life. *J Consult Clin Psychol* 1984; 52(4):520–527.
152. Batzel LW, Dodrill CB. Neuropsychological and emotional correlates of marital status and ability to live independently in individuals with epilepsy. *Epilepsia* 1984; 25(5):594–598.
153. Seidenberg M, O'Leary DS, Berent S, Boll T. Changes in seizure frequency and test-retest scores on the Wechsler Adult Intelligence Scale. *Epilepsia* 1981; 22(1):75–83.

68 Academic Deficits and Interventions in Pediatric Epilepsy

Caroline E. Bailey
Rochelle Caplan

In this chapter, we address issues of academic achievement and educational intervention for children with epilepsy. We approach this discussion on two levels. First, we highlight common educational concerns for children with epilepsy. We then review research on educational interventions and teacher attitudes toward epilepsy and discuss the impact this has on classroom education. Likewise, we discuss specific academic deficits in the areas of reading and language that are associated with pediatric epilepsy. We explain what is known about the underlying cognitive correlates of these difficulties, both in epilepsy and in other neurobehavioral disorders with similar symptom profiles. We discuss empirically supported interventions used to treat these academic deficits in other populations and examine their applicability to the pediatric epilepsy population. At the end of the chapter, we address this issue clinically using our experiences as practitioners and advocates working with patients and families. We provide guidelines on how to design an appropriate intervention for a specific child. We discuss the importance of teacher awareness and parent-teacher-student communication and make suggestions for obtaining special education services for children with epilepsy. In conclusion, we stress the importance of the role of the clinician as an educational advocate, and advocate for empirical investigations of academic interventions for children with epilepsy.

ACADEMIC DEFICITS IN PEDIATRIC EPILEPSY

Academic achievement difficulties are well documented in children with epilepsy (1–7). Yet, comparatively few investigations have examined these deficits in terms of the underlying cognitive and illness-related variables contributing to specific areas of academic weakness. In the linguistic domain, these areas of academic concern include reading and spelling (2, 4, 6, 8), spoken language, vocabulary development, rapid naming, verbal memory, and higher-level discourse deficits (2, 3, 9–11). Whereas important environmental factors such as family support and socioeconomic status affect academic achievement (3, 4), identifying the cognitive and linguistic correlates associated with academic failures in children with epilepsy is a key component in the process of understanding the academic needs of this population. This is particularly germane to the important task of determining appropriate educational interventions for children with epilepsy. Although educational interventions for children with learning disabilities have been well researched, educational interventions for the academic deficits associated with pediatric epilepsy remain grossly unstudied, in contrast to other conditions such as dyslexia, language impairment, and autism. At this point in time, empirically supported educational interventions for children with epilepsy are sorely lacking, in contrast to the large number of academic interventions geared toward other populations with learning difficulties. Few academic intervention studies have been conducted among children with epilepsy, largely because empirical groundwork is still being laid in terms of identifying the underlying mechanisms associated with academic failure in these patients. From the perspective of the advocate (a role often filled by the pediatric specialist), it is not sufficient to simply identify academic deficits in children with epilepsy without understanding their underlying cognitive mechanisms. Hence, it is timely and appropriate for educational issues in pediatric epilepsy to be addressed.

EDUCATIONAL CONCERNS

Many parents of children with epilepsy are concerned about finding appropriate school placements for their children. Given that children with epilepsy are at risk for academic failure and poor vocational outcome (12) and have been shown to manifest social, cognitive, and academic difficulties (2, 13), this concern is important and well founded. Of particular importance to parents are issues of special education and access to appropriate educational services. Although savvy parents are able to advocate for the immediate health needs of their children with epilepsy, many caregivers have difficulty accessing appropriate educational interventions. Likewise, some school districts may be hesitant to recognize that children with epilepsy may experience learning difficulties in conjunction with their medical illness. Given the lack of well-controlled studies investigating specific academic interventions with the pediatric epilepsy population, parents and educators are often unable to identify appropriate classroom options. In many cases, educational professionals lack sufficient knowledge of epilepsy to provide expert guidance. When this occurs, the clinician familiar with pediatric epilepsy plays a vital role as an educational advocate.

TEACHER AWARENESS OF AND ATTITUDES TOWARD EPILEPSY

Teachers report a lack of knowledge of the academic challenges associated with epilepsy (14). Despite evidence that children with pediatric epilepsy use special education services both before and after diagnosis of epilepsy (15), teachers appear unaware of their special education needs. A recent community-based study of 613 children with newly diagnosed epilepsy indicates that 58% received special education services 5 years after diagnosis (15). Although children with remote symptomatic epilepsies were most likely to be identified for services, approximately 50% of the children in the sample with cryptogenic and idiopathic epilepsy also used special education services.

A common misconception among educators is that academic deficits in children with epilepsy are a result of medication and other illness-related variables and therefore cannot be treated with educational strategies and interventions. However, it is well documented that many children with epilepsy have already begun receiving special education before seizure onset, illustrating that behavioral and neurocognitive processing deficits precede the onset of seizures in many cases (15–17). Given the broad effect of epilepsy-related academic deficits, learning disabilities associated with pediatric epilepsy constitute a unique area of clinical concern, ripe for awareness and development of sound educational interventions.

Historically, in the United States, teachers' attitudes toward students with epilepsy have been negative, in part because of knowledge gaps about epilepsy (14). However, as more information about epilepsy has been disseminated, attitudes have improved, and once commonly held misconceptions such as that "children with epilepsy are insane or prone to criminal activity" have decreased among educators (18). Bishop and Boag found that as a group, teachers hold positive attitudes toward students with epilepsy (14), but teachers' attitudes are influenced by teacher-related factors including their age, level of education, and classroom experience. Happily, teachers with experience working with students with epilepsy demonstrated the most positive attitudes toward epilepsy, supporting the notion that education about epilepsy helps create positive attitudes about the condition. Despite these positive findings, teachers still hold misconceptions and biases such as that "students with epilepsy are more accident prone" and "families of children with epilepsy should not be provided additional social support services"—suggesting that more teacher education is needed.

Teachers generally are aware that they are undereducated about the needs of children with epilepsy. Despite their positive attitudes toward students with epilepsy, as a group teachers report that they lack their knowledge of epilepsy and educational strategies appropriate for teaching children with epilepsy. In the Bishop and Boag study, approximately 70% of teachers reported having below-average knowledge of life circumstances and conditions of students living with epilepsy (14). Teachers felt unprepared to teach students with epilepsy because of lack of knowledge of the disease and its impact on classroom learning. This is in part because the education curriculum for teachers does not address the learning needs of children with epilepsy. Moreover, the lack of controlled studies of educational intervention for these students is likely a further contributor to educators' unfamiliarity with the learning needs of pediatric epilepsy patients. To date, only one published study has addressed this issue (19). Nonetheless, a majority of teachers want to learn more about management of epilepsy in the classroom.

CURRENT EDUCATIONAL INTERVENTIONS FOR CHILDREN WITH EPILEPSY

In an important step toward implementing evidence-based instruction methods for children with epilepsy and prominent learning disabilities, Humphries et al conducted a pilot study examining the effectiveness of Direct Instruction on a group of 55 students with intractable epilepsy and severe learning difficulties (19). Based on the principles of teacher-directed lessons, Direct Instruction techniques feature highly sequenced and scripted teaching geared toward teaching students to accomplish salient, individualized tasks. Students received instruction in a small classroom setting 3 to 4.5 days per week for up to 16 weeks. At pretest, students were underachieving in both reading and mathematics. At posttest, after the intervention, gains occurred in all areas except word identification. Treatment gains were related to IQ, not to seizure-related variables.

Children with severe epilepsy are receptive to highly structured, sequential learning tasks targeting specific academic areas (19). Given that more severely ill children do well with these techniques, it is likely that structured intervention techniques may benefit less severely affected children, too. Furthermore, many current interventions for learning disabilities usze a similar structured approach (20, 21). Although no controlled studies have evaluated specific techniques, these remediation methods merit further clinical research.

COGNITIVE AND ACADEMIC DEFICITS ASSOCIATED WITH PEDIATRIC EPILEPSY

Language and reading deficits are frequently associated with childhood epilepsy. Research on educational interventions used in children with and without epilepsy who demonstrate similar learning deficits provide clinicians with information about options for educational interventions. Although these treatments have not been specifically studied in the pediatric epilepsy population, there is good evidence that they are efficacious in children demonstrating similar language-based learning difficulties (22, 23).

Language Skill Deficits

How many times have clinicians heard parents report that their child with epilepsy "just doesn't listen," "won't follow directions," or "doesn't express himself well verbally or on paper"? Although comorbid attention deficit hyperactivity disorder (24) and illness-based reasons for difficulty with spoken and written language, such as high frequency of seizures or medication intoxication, should not be overlooked, language disorder is a common problem among children with epilepsy (11, 25). In a recent study 42% of children with epilepsy had some degree of language difficulty. Furthermore, children with focal epilepsies were 30% more likely manifest language disorder than those with other varieties of epilepsy (26).

Many children with complex partial seizures (CPS) have delayed verbal language skills (11, 27, 28). Schoenfeld et al compared a group of children with CPS to a sibling control group and found that the patients had expressive language deficits in the areas of oral vocabulary, oral fluency, and category fluency (27). Fastenau and colleagues found below-average performance on the Stroop naming tasks, suggesting underdeveloped confrontation naming skills and slowed verbal retrieval (3). Caplan et al found deficits in how children with CPS use language to formulate their thoughts. In conversations with CPS children, listeners often experience difficulty following who and what the child is talking about (10). Children with CPS have deficits in expressive language skills and phonological processing (28).

Basic language deficits in children with CPS are related to seizure frequency, to number of antiepileptic drugs (11), and to age of onset (27), suggesting a correlation between the degree of language impairment and the severity of epilepsy. Higher-level discourse skills are associated with verbal IQ, gender, seizure frequency, and age in these children (29). However, in children with intractable epilepsy who were surgical candidates as well as in children who were treated medically, cognitive functioning falls below age expectations across a wide variety of areas including language skill (30). Thus, seizure-related variables account for some but not all of the language difficulty in children with CPS.

Language difficulties are also present in children with benign childhood epilepsy with centrotemporal spikes (BECTS) including problems such as poor articulation, stuttering, and word-finding difficulties (31). Children with active BECTS and those in remission experience difficulty with expressive language, particularly in grammar (32). However, language deficits in these children appear to be strongly associated with atypical seizure characteristics (33).

Research on language skill in other forms of childhood epilepsy indicates problems that are less well documented. Compared to normal peers, children with generalized tonic-clonic seizures and children with absence seizures exhibit different patterns of brain activity when performing semantic processing and phonological tasks (34). Likewise, Caplan et al found that children with absence seizures and children with CPS have similar deficits in their abilities to use language to formulate thoughts (10). In contrast, Pavone et al suggested that language skills in patients with childhood absence epilepsy were relatively intact (35). In yet another study of children with absence seizures, communication deficits were related to duration of illness, male gender, and seizure frequency (36).

In summary, it is clear that many children with pediatric epilepsy struggle with expressive language skills. These skills are an integral to gaining access to their educational curriculum and to scholastic achievement. Although at this time, there are no language interventions designed specifically for children with epilepsy, there are several intervention methods that have been studied in other populations.

Language Interventions—Important Considerations

There are many options for language intervention for children with epilepsy. However, before committing to a specific intervention, parents who suspect their child is experiencing language difficulties should consult with a certified speech and language pathologist and request an assessment. This assessment is designed to identify the child's specific strengths and weaknesses across speech and language domains including vocabulary, phonetics, grammar, pragmatic language, articulation, listening, and comprehension. This information is critical to tailoring interventions to the individual child's needs.

In most areas, a request for a speech and language assessment can be made through the public schools. However, it has been our experience that, even in cases where children are receiving special education services on the basis of their medical illness, parents must ask the school authorities to conduct this testing, rather than relying on the authorities to refer their child for services spontaneously. In cases where school-based assessment is not available (i.e., where a child is attending a private school), many reputable and talented practitioners in private practice are licensed to provide this service. Physicians must make caregivers aware of these resources and must be willing to make referrals themselves to speech and language pathologists.

Wallach recently reviewed important ideas to consider when seeking speech and language intervention (37). Most importantly, interventions should be relevant to the curriculum and should focus on the question "What interventions will facilitate this child's academic success?" Language disorders present on a continuum, resulting in wide variability in symptom profiles. In most cases spoken language difficulties are related to written language difficulties. As such, written language skill is an important area for assessment. Likewise, reading is a language-based process. Children with language difficulty are prone to developing reading difficulties, a finding that has been supported by a large body of work (21). Hence, assessment must be comprehensive and focus on deeper linguistic skills and language-related difficulties, rather than addressing isolated symptoms.

Specific Language Intervention Strategies

Although there are no treatments that have been studied specifically for application to language disorder in children with epilepsy, there is a great deal of information regarding interventions for children with specific language impairment (SLI). Although these interventions may not have been customized with children with epilepsy in mind, we argue that information from the SLI treatment literature can serve as an important reference when considering treatment for language disability in children with epilepsy. Some of these interventions are described in the following paragraphs.

Verbal and nonverbal deficits in children with specific language impairment not only result in decreased school achievement but also can lead to behavioral problems in school (38). In many cases, grammatical knowledge presents a distinct difficulty for children with SLI. Fey and colleagues listed 10 principles that are fundamental to grammatical intervention in children with SLI (38). Generally speaking, interventions must be developmentally appropriate, with specific goals that are designed to increase the child's fluent use of grammar in conversational language. Furthermore, interventions should take place in environments where social and linguistic context is stressed and where a systematic approach highlights morphological and phonological information.

The narrative-based language intervention has been evaluated as an approach to helping children with SLI improve their conversational skills (39). Poverty of speech content is a problem that plagues children with SLI. This intervention was designed to assist children in developing richer story content, as well as good story form and sentence form. The narrative-based language intervention has enhanced the quality and detail of children's narratives but not grammatically based elements of storytelling.

Fast ForWord® (a product of the Scientific Learning Corporation) is a computerized program designed to assist children with specific language impairment or other expressive language disorders in developing fundamentals of oral language. It offers a variety of programs geared toward developing auditory discrimination, vocabulary, and phonological skills. One appealing component of this program is that it can be implemented both at home and in an educational setting, providing children with access to resources outside of school. Additionally, Fast ForWord offers a variety of programs geared toward children of different skill levels and ages. It targets both oral language skills and reading development.

Evaluations of the efficacy of Fast ForWord have produced mixed results. Troia and Whitney reported that children with poor expressive oral language improved significantly on a standardized oral language measure after intervention with Fast ForWord in comparison to an untreated control group (40). However, there were no differences between the experimental and control groups on measures of reading and phonological processing skill. Additional studies indicate that Fast ForWord produced gains for children with auditory temporal processing difficulties (41, 42). Cohen et al performed a larger randomized, controlled trial of the effects of Fast ForWord (43). When the Fast ForWord group was compared to two control groups, consisting of a group receiving commercially available language-based computer programs and a no-treatment group, all groups were found to improve, and over time there were no between-group differences. Likewise, in another study that compared the effectiveness of Fast ForWord, Earobics, and LiPS in children with reading and language deficits, no effects on language or reading performance were found (44). Thus, Fast ForWord is neither more nor less effective than other commercially available school-based interventions.

In regard to developing phonological skills, Patricia and Charles Lindamood's Auditory Discrimination in Depth program has been proven to generate both long-term and short-term gains in both phonological awareness and articulation skills in children with reading disability and in children with language disabilities (20). This structured, multisensory phonics approach teaches students core principles of articulation of speech sounds and discrimination of speech sounds. Systematic phonics instruction methods such as the Auditory Discrimination in Depth program help children to master the phonological processing skills required in single-word decoding more effectively than other unstructured methods (45).

Reading Skill Deficits in Pediatric Epilepsy

Literacy is fundamental to academic achievement. Reading skill is defined broadly by an amalgam of orthographic, phonological, and semantics skills that culminate in fluent single-word decoding and reading comprehension (46). Hence, children need phonological, orthographic, and semantic skills to become fluent, accurate readers (47). Failure to master any one of these key components can result in a disabled reading profile (46, 47). Understanding the specific nature of reading impairment allows for tailored interventions. Despite evidence of reading difficulties in pediatric epilepsy patients, few studies have examined cognitive correlates of reading disability in epilepsy patients (5, 8, 48). The information we do have regarding reading in children with epilepsy comes largely from patients with partial epilepsies (5, 8, 48).

Children with CPS experienced more reading problems, in particular problems with phonological skill and slow reading rate, than age-matched normal peers after controlling for differences in IQ (49). Children with left-sided CPS had more difficulty reading and experienced a greater degree of delays in phonological decoding, reading comprehension, and word recognition than those with right-sided CPS. Phoneme sequencing was particularly impaired among the left CPS group in comparison to both normal children and those with a right-sided epileptic focus. Children with right-sided CPS demonstrated visual-spatial but not language-based difficulties.

Reading deficits have been reported in children with temporal lobe epilepsy (TLE) (8). Children with TLE performed less well than those with idiopathic generalized epilepsy and those with BECTS on measures of reading speed and comprehension. However, these findings were affected by seizure-related variables, suggesting a relationship between illness severity and decreased reading skills. In the TLE group, children with left-sided epileptic activity (LTLE) demonstrated more reading difficulties than those with right-sided foci (RTLE). Phonological and semantic problems were prominent in the LTLE group compared to the RTLE group, suggesting that phonological processing difficulties may be sensitive to the lateralization of an epileptic focus.

In a study of French-speaking children with epilepsy, children with TLE, frontal lobe epilepsy, and childhood absence epilepsy (CAE) had reading deficits compared to healthy peers (48). Although children with TLE performed significantly less well than control subjects on overall reading ability, they did not demonstrate phonological deficits, as did children with frontal lobe epilepsy. Children with CAE showed deficits only in phonemic segmentation, implying a milder phonological delay. As a group, children with epilepsy did not differ from controls on language tasks, suggesting that reading deficits do not stem from underlying language problems. Children in the epilepsy groups did not differ on seizure frequency, age of onset, or duration of illness. No effect was found for monotherapy versus polytherapy with antiepileptic medications. The authors suggest the difficulty that the frontal lobe epilepsy patients had with single-word decoding may have resulted from decreased attention or reduced executive functioning.

In a study comparing written language skills of Greek-speaking children with benign rolandic epilepsy to normal peers, children with acute symptoms performed worse than controls on reading comprehension, reading aloud, and spelling (5). The Greek version of the Bangor

Dyslexia Test produced significant differences between children with epilepsy and controls.

Reading Interventions—Important Considerations

The majority of research on intervention in reading disability, in particular developmental dyslexia, has been focused around the idea that dyslexic readers have core deficits in phonological processing (21). This phonological deficit limits the individual's ability to manipulate speech sounds within words, to learn spelling to sound correspondences, and to decode single words accurately (50–52). However, phonological deficits can manifest themselves in many ways and are not limited to deficits in single-word decoding. Dyslexics of all reading levels have been shown to perform poorly in comparison to same-age normal control subjects on tasks of phoneme deletion, position analysis, speech perception, letter naming, spelling, lexical access, verbal working memory, and auditory processing of fast temporal stimuli (53–57). The phonological core deficit hypothesis proposes that dyslexics' reading difficulties are related to specific deficits in the representation and use of phonological information (21, 55, 58). Whereas reading deficits such as poor comprehension may not necessarily be phonologically based, the majority of poor readers do demonstrate some degree of phonological impairment (47). This being said, a savvy advocate for a child with epilepsy will want to investigate the variety of phonics-based interventions available.

There are a variety of structured, multisensory phonics programs that emphasize teaching students to understand grapheme-phoneme correspondences and single-word decoding strategies. As mentioned earlier, structured, systematic phonics approaches to instruction are the most effective with poor readers (45). Key components of successful systematic phonics interventions involve intensity of teaching and frequency of instruction (20). Likewise, early phoneme awareness intervention in kindergarten reduces the incidence of reading disability in at-risk children in both short-term and long-term follow-up (58). Moreover, the practitioner must be qualified to administer the intervention. In most cases, teachers must obtain specialized training that results in certification to be able to provide this instruction (i.e., Orton-Gillingham, Slingerland, Wilson Reading). In selecting a teacher or learning specialist it is important to ascertain whether that person is certified in these approaches. Overviews of some of these methods are provided herein.

Specific Reading Intervention Strategies

Orton-Gillingham is a multisensory phonics intervention designed to be delivered on an individualized basis (59). This program uses auditory, visual, and kinesthetic sensory input to create a total language approach that first emphasizes grapheme-phoneme correspondence rules (e.g., "A" says /a/ as in apple) and moves on to teach phonograms, vowel patterns, and syllable patterns. Written instruction, including letter formation, is taught along with phonological instruction to reinforce multisensory connections and teach spelling patterns. Reading whole words is introduced when the child has mastered simple vowel patterns and phonograms. Later, Beth Slingerland adapted this approach to be used in a classroom setting. Hence, the Slingerland method is the classroom adaptation of Orton-Gillingham and follows the same pedagogical principles (60).

Wilson Reading is also a structured, multisensory approach to reading designed originally for one-to-one instruction and is based on the Orton-Gillingham model (61). Originally designed for adolescents and adult poor readers, this 12-step, sequential program emphasizes awareness of individual speech sounds as well as six syllable types. From a teacher's perspective this system is very accessible because it comes with many premade instruction materials and can be adapted to work in a small group setting.

As described previously, Auditory Discrimination in Depth (20) is an effective method of teaching phonological awareness to children. Since its inception Patricia Lindamood has collaborated with Nancy Bell to form what is now called the Lindamood-Bell approach. Similar in content to Auditory Discrimination in Depth, Lindamood-Bell also incorporates training in orthographic knowledge and reading fluency (62).

Project Read is a school-based approach to reading remediation aimed at delivering phonics instruction to children falling in the lower quartile in reading and spelling skills (63). The curriculum, which is used frequently in school settings, is composed of the following three phases: (1) multisensory phonics instruction using Orton-Gillingham-like techniques, (2) reading comprehension and vocabulary skills, and (3) written language skills (spelling and sentence structure). This program is quite cost-effective and can be administered in a small-group setting. Another strength of the program is that it is designed for any child who is a poor reader, not just for dyslexic children. Hence, this intervention is quite broadly based and may be more suited to "garden variety" poor readers.

SUMMARY AND IMPLICATIONS

Language-based learning disabilities are associated with various types of pediatric epilepsy and often occur independently of epilepsy-related variables. Given that many academic problems such as reading, spelling, and language disabilities have specific underlying cognitive mechanisms (i.e., phonological deficits in the case of reading impairments), the key to intervention lies in pinpointing the cognitive processing mechanisms interfering with optimal learning. Efficacious intervention is best conducted by implementing appropriate, valid educational methods. Using tools such as a comprehensive neuropsychologic evaluation, we are able to identify a particular child's cognitive strengths and weaknesses and to tailor an appropriate educational strategy. If one considers learning disability as a presenting symptom, following it to its underlying cause facilitates proper treatment. Although no educational interventions are specific for children with epilepsy, much can be learned from existing methods of remediation for reading and language deficits for children with similar learning problems.

Clinical Implications

Although each child is an individual requiring a tailored educational approach, in our experience there are fundamental areas of concern that affect many children with epilepsy. Based on this, we offer the following guidelines in choosing an appropriate educational intervention.

First, we recommend a comprehensive, psychoeducational or neuropsychologic testing assessing for learning disabilities. Although it is often difficult to ascertain which symptoms (i.e., psychomotor slowing) are illness related and which indicate learning disorder, simply identifying the child's specific cognitive strengths and weaknesses is essential to developing an educational plan. This assessment is highly specialized and should be conducted by a licensed educational psychologist, pediatric neuropsychologist, or clinical psychologist with appropriate training.

Second, close communication between parents, students, and teachers is essential. Developing open lines of communication with the child's primary instructor is crucial to academic success. Knowing that many teachers do not have adequate knowledge of epilepsy, we encourage parents to provide teachers with this information. Succinct resource guides are often quite effective because most busy teachers prefer concise sources of information. Teaching children good coping skills, such as becoming their own advocates how to discuss their illness with peers and adults is also a key factor in academic success (64). One way to do this is to perform role playing exercises with the child, teaching him or her how to explain his or her special needs to an adult.

Third, after specific learning difficulties have been identified, parents should work with educational therapists and school psychologists to develop an intervention strategy. This should be a collaborative effort between caregivers and educators. In discussing this plan with educational professionals, it is essential to set measurable and appropriate academic goals for the child. These goals should be documented and revisited appropriately. Due to a lack of evidence, we cannot recommend specific educational intervention strategies. However, we encourage parents whose children have reading and language disabilities to explore the array of available methods. Examples of these methods include Lindamood-Bell, Wilson, and Orton-Gillingham for reading difficulties and Fast ForWord for language problems.

Last, we encourage health care professionals to advocate for parents attempting to obtain services from their child's school. Often, parents are unsure of the specific steps necessary to qualify their child for special education services. By becoming familiar with the steps required in the local community, health care professionals can guide parents through this process. This process typically requires submitting to the school district a written request for a special education evaluation and following a predetermined protocol. Frequently, parents will ask their treating physician to document their child's illness and the ways in which it impacts the child's learning. Providing supporting documentation with clearly outlined requests for specific educational services greatly increases the patient's chances of obtaining an optimal educational intervention. It is imperative to request all reasonable academic accommodations and assessments to ensure that proper resources are allocated to the child.

Depending on circumstances, the process of obtaining special education services for a child can be time consuming and frustrating. Parents should be encouraged to be both patient and persistent in their pursuit. Many school districts are not aware that children with epilepsy have both illness-related educational needs and specialized learning needs. Therefore, educational administrators have little knowledge of the sorts of academic accommodations that children with epilepsy and associated learning difficulties require. Educating school professionals about the needs of pediatric epilepsy patients is essential, as is encouraging continued research regarding educational interventions for children with epilepsy. However, what is paramount is supporting our patients in the process of securing appropriate educational interventions and helping them to understand that just learning differently does not mean that they cannot learn.

References

1. Aldenkamp A, Arends J. The relative influence of epileptic EEG discharges, short nonconvulsive seizures and type of epilepsy on cognitive function. *Epilepsia* 2004; 45(1):54–63.
2. Austin JK, Huberty TJ, Huster GA, Dunn DW. Does academic achievement in children with epilepsy change over time? *Dev Med Child Neurol* 1999; 41:473–479.
3. Fastenau P, Shen J, Dunn DW, Perkins SM, et al,. Neuropsychological predictors of academic underachievement in pediatric epilepsy; moderating roles of demographic, seizure and psychosocial variables. *Epilepsia* 2004; 45(10):1261–1272.
4. Mitchell WG, Chavez JM, Lee H., Guzman BL. Academic underachievement in children with Epilepsy. *J Child Neurol* 1991; 6:65–72.
5. Papavasiliou A, Mattheou D, Kotsalis C, Paraskevoulakos E. Written language skills in children with benign childhood epilepsy with centrotemporal spikes. *Epilepsy Behav* 2005; 6:50–58.
6. Seidenberg M, Beck N, Geisser M, O'Leary DS, et al. Neuropsychological correlates of academic achievement of children with epilepsy. *J Epilepsy* 1988; 1:23–29.

7. Williams J, Phillips T, Griebel ML, Sharp GB, et al. Factors associated with academic achievement in children with controlled epilepsy. *Epilepsy Behav* 2001; 2:217–223.
8. ChaixY, Laguitton V, Lauwers-Cances V, Daquin G, et al. Reading abilities and cognitive functions of children with epilepsy: influence of epileptic syndrome. *Brain Dev.* in press.
9. Caplan R, Guthrie D, Komo S, Shields WD, et al. Conversational repair in pediatric epilepsy. *Brain Lang* 2001; 78(1):82–93.
10. Caplan R, Gutherie D, Komo S, Siddarth P, et al. Social communication in children with epilepsy. *J Psychol Psychiatry* 2002; 43(2):245–253.
11. Caplan R, Siddarth P, Gurbani S, Ott D, et al. Psychopathology and pediatric complex partial seizures: seizure-related, cognitive and linguistic variables. *Epilepsia* 2004; 45(10):1273–1281.
12. Sillanpaa M. Learning disability: occurrence and long-term consequences in childhood-onset epilepsy. *Epilepsy Behav* 2004; 5:937–944.
13. Wirrell EC, Camfield CS, Camfield PR, Dooley JM, et al. Long-term psychosocial outcome in typical absence epilepsy. Sometimes a wolf in sheeps' clothing. *Arch Pediatr Adolesc Med* 1997; 151(2):152–158.
14. Bishop M, Boag EM. Teachers' knowledge about epilepsy and attidues toward students with epilepsy: results of a national survey. *Epilepsy Behav* 2006; 8(2):397–405.
15. Berg AT, Smith SN, Frobish D, Levy SR, et al. Special educational needs of children with newly diagnosed epilepsy. *Dev Med Child Neurol* 2005; 47(11):749–753.
16. Oostrom KJ, van Teeseling H, Smeets-Schouten A, Peters AC, et al; Dutch Study of Epilepsy in Childhood (DuSECh). Three to four years after diagnosis: cognition and behaviour in children with "epilepsy only." A prospective, controlled study. *Brain* 2005; 128 Pt 7:1546–1555.
17. Schouten A, Oostrom KJ, Pestman WR, Peters AC, et al; Dutch Study Group of Epilepsy in Childhood. Learning and memory of school children with epilepsy: a prospective controlled longitudinal study. *Dev Med Child Neurol* 2002; 44(12):803–811.
18. Bauman RJ, Wilson JF, Wiese HJ. Kentuckians' attitudes toward children with epilepsy. *Epilepsia* 1995; 36(10):1003–1008.
19. Humphries T, Neufeld M, Johnson C, Engels K, et al. A pilot study of the effect of Direct Instruction programming on the academic performance of students with intractable epilepsy. *Epilepsy Behav* 2005; 6(3):405–412.
20. Torgeson JK. Instructional interventions for children with reading disabilities. In: Shapiro BK, Accardo PJ, Capute AJ, eds. *Specific Reading Disability*. Timonium, MD: York Press, 1998:197–220.
21. Lyon GR. Toward a definition of dyslexia. *Ann Dyslexia* 1995; 45(3):3–27.
22. Olson RK, Wise B, Ring J, Johnson M. (Computer based remedial training in phoneme awareness and phonological decoding. Effects on the post-training development of word recognition. *Scientific Studies of Reading* 1997; 1(13):235–253.
23. Snowling M. Dyslexia. Oxford: Basil Blackwell, 2000.
24. Dunn DW, Austin JK, Harezlak J, Ambrosius WT. ADHD and epilepsy in childhood. *Dev Med Child Neurol* 2003; 45(1):50–54.
25. Siddarth P, Gurbani S, Lanphier E, Bailey C, et al. Language deficits in pediatric epilepsy. Annual Meeting of the International League Against Epilepsy, Singapore, July 2007.
26. Parkinson GM. High incidence of language disorder in children with focal epilepsies. *Dev Med Child Neurol* 2002; 44(8):533–537.
47. Antonello JL. Epilepsy and reading in children. *Dissertation Abstracts International* 1999; 60(3,a), 644.
27. Schoenfeld J, Seidenberg M, Woodard A, Hecox K, et al. Neuropsychological and behavioral status of children with complex partial seizures. *Dev Med Child Neurol* 1999; 41:724–731.
28. Kolk A, Beilmann A, Tomberg T, Napa A, et al. Neurocognitive development of children with congenital unilateral brain lesion and epilepsy. *Brain Dev,* 2001; 23:88–96.
29. Caplan R, Siddarth P, Bailey CE, Lanphier EK, et al. Thought disorder : a developmental disability in pediatric epilepsy. *Epilepsy Behav* 2006; 8(4):726–735.
30. Smith ML, Elliot IM, Lach L. Cognitive skills in children with intractable epilepsy: comparison of surgical and non-surgical candidates. *Epilepsia* 2002; 43(6):631–637.
31. Deonna T. Rolandic epilepsy: neuropsychology of the active epilepsy phase. *Epileptic Disord* 2000; 2(1):S59–S61.
32. Monjauze C, Tuller L, Hommet C, Barthez MA, et al. Language in benign childhood epilepsy with centro-temporal spikes abbreviated form: rolandic epilepsy and language. *Brain Lang* 2005; 92(3):300–308.
33. Vinayan KP, Biji V, Thomas SV. Educational problems with underlying neuropsychological impairment are common in children with benign epilepsy of childhood with centotemporal spikes (BECTS). *Seizure* 2005; 14(3):207–212.
34. Henkin Y, Kishon-Rabin L, Pratt H, Kivity S, et al. Linguistic processing in idiopathic generalized epilepsy; an auditory event-related potential study. *Epilepsia* 2003; 44(9): 1207–1217.
35. Pavone P, Bianchini R, Trifiletti RR, Incorpora G, et al. Neuropsychological assessment in children with absence epilepsy. *Neurology* 2001; 56(8):1047–1051.
36. Caplan R, Sagun J, Siddarth P, Gurbani S, et al. Social comptenece in pediatric epilepsy: insights into underlying mechanisms. *Epilepsy Behav* 2005; 6(2):218–228.
37. Wallach GP. A conceptual framework in language learning disabilities, school aged language disorders. *Topics in Language Disorders* 2005; 25(4):292–301.
38. Fey ME, Long SH, Finestack LH. Ten principles of grammar facilitation for children with specific language impairments. *Am J Speech Lang Pathol* 2003; 12(1):3–15.
39. Swanson LA, Fey ME, Mills CE, Hood LS. Use of narrative-based language intervention with children who have specific language impairment. *Am J Speech Lang Pathol* 2005; 14(2):131–143.
40. Troia GA, Whittney SD. A close look at the efficacy of Fast ForWord language for children with academic weaknesses. *Contemporary Educational Psychology* 2003; 28(4):465–494.
41. Gillam RB. Treatment for temporal processing deficits: computer-assisted language intervention using Fast ForWord: theoretical and empirical considerations for clinical decision making. *Language, Speech and Hearing Services in Schools* 1999; 30(4):363–370.
42. Gillam RB, Crofford JA, Gale MA. Language change following computer-assisted instruction with Fast ForWord or Laureate Learning Systems Software. *Am J Speech Lang Pathol* 2001; 10(3):258–268.
43. Cohen W, Hodson A, O'Hare A, Boyle J, et al. Effects of computer-based intervention through acoustically modified speech (Fast ForWord) in severe mixed receptive-expressive language impairment: outcomes from a randomized controlled trial. *Journal of Speech, Language and Hearing Research* 2005; 48(3):715–729.
44. Pokorni JL, Worthington CK, Jamison PJ. Phonological awareness intervention: comparison of Fast ForWord, Earobics, and LiPS. *The Journal of Education Research* 2004; 97(3):147–157.
45. Ehri LC, Nunes SR, Stahl SA. Systematic phinics instruction helps students learn to read: evidence from the National Reading Panel's meta-analysis. *Review of Educational Research* 2001; 71(3):393–447.
46. Harm MW, Seidenberg MS. Phonology, reading and dyslexia. Insights from connectionist models. *Psychol Rev* 1999; 106 (3):491–528.
47. Adams MJ. Beginning to read: thinking and learning about print. Cambridge, MA: MIT Press, 1994.
48. Vanasse CM, Beland R, Carmant L, Lassonde M. Impact of childhood epilepsy on reading and phonological processing abilities. *Epilepsy Behav* 2005; 7(2):288–296.
49. Antonello JL. Epilepsy and reading in children. *Dissertation Abstracts International* 1999; 60(3,a):644.
50. Liberman IY, Shankweiler D. Phonology and the problems of learning to read and write. *Remed Spec Educ* 1985; 6(6):8–17.
51. Stanovich KE. Explaining differences between the dyslexic and the garden-variety poor reader: the phonological-core variable-difference model. *J Learn Disabil* 1988; 21:590–612.
52. Manis FR, Seidenberg MS, Doi LM, McBride-Chang C, et al. On the basis of two subtypes of developmental dyslexia. *Cognition* 1996; 58:157–195.
53. Castles A, Coltheart M. Varieties of developmental dyslexia. *Cognition* 1993; 47: 149–180.
54. Wagner RK, Torgesen JK. The nature of phonological processing and its causal role in the acquisition of reading skills. *Psychol Bull* 1987; 101:192–212.
55. Vellutino F. Dyslexia. In: Wang William, S-Y, ed. The emergence of language: development and evolution: readings from "Scientific American" magazine. NewYork: H.W. Freeman, Times Book, Henry Holt & Co., 1991.
56. Joanisse MF, Manis FR, Seidenberg MS, Keating P. Language deficits in dyslexic children: Speech perception, phonology, and morphology. *J Exp Child Psychol* 2000; 77(1):30–60.
57. Bruck M. Persistence of dyslexics' phonological awareness deficits. *Dev Psychol* 1992; 28(5):874–886.
58. Elbro C, Petersen DK. Long-term effects of phoneme awareness and letter sound training: an intervention study with children at risk for dyslexia. *Journal of Educational Psychology* 2004; 96(4):660–670.
59. McNelis AM, Johnson CS, Huberty TJ, Austin JK. Factors associated with academic achievement in children with recent-onset seizures. *Seizure* 2005; 14(5):331-339.
60. Slingerland BH. *Book 1, A Multi-Sensory Approach to Language Arts for Specific Language Disability Children: A Guide for Primary Teachers.* Cambridge, MA: Educators Publishing Service, 1996.
61. Gillingham A, Stillman BW. *The Gillingham Manual: Remedial Training for Students with Specific Disability in Reading, Spelling and Penmanship*, 8th ed. Boston, MA: Educators Publishing Service, 1997.
62. Wilson B. *Matching student needs to instruction in learning disabilities, literacy and adult education.* In: Reder S, Vogel SA, eds. Learning Disabilities, Literacy, and Adult Education. Baltimore, MD: Brookes Publishing, 1998.
63. Calfee R, Wadleigh C. How Project Read builds inquiring schools. Educational Leadership, 1992; (50):28–32.
64. Eden, GF, Jones KM, Cappell K, Gareau L, et al. Neural changes following remediation in adult developmental dyslexia. *Neuron* 2004; 44(3):411–22.

69 Cognitive Side Effects of Antiepileptic Drugs

David E. Mandelbaum
Christine L. Trask

Cognitive side effects have emerged as a key consideration when an antiepileptic drug (AED) is being selected for the treatment of childhood seizure disorders. In years past, despite concerns about side effects, when the choice of antiepileptic medication was limited to phenobarbital and phenytoin, their adverse effects were accepted as a "necessary evil." After the Perinatal Collaborative Project demonstrated the generally benign course of recurrent febrile seizures (1), thinking shifted to the view that it might be best to avoid phenobarbital in the treatment of febrile seizures because it appeared that "the cure was worse than the disease" given concerns about adverse cognitive and behavioral effects of phenobarbital. In the early 1970s the emergence of carbamazepine as an alternative to phenytoin for partial seizures generated interest in the cognitive side effects of medications and stimulated debates as to whether carbamazepine had a side effect profile that was preferable to those of phenytoin and phenobarbital. Since then there has been a remarkable increase in options for the pharmacological management of seizures. As treatment options have increased there has been a commensurate increase in the interest in the side effect profiles of these drugs. For the most part, phase III trials reveal that there is little, if any, difference in efficacy among the different drugs. Thus, although the choice of an AED is driven, in part, by seizure type or epilepsy syndrome, in the final analysis the selection of an AED for a particular patient is heavily influenced by the side effect profile.

When drugs are brought to market, relatively little is known about their cognitive and behavioral side effects. Unfortunately, formal psychometric testing has not routinely been included in the studies done as part of the Food and Drug Administration (FDA) approval process. As a result, the information available regarding cognitive and behavioral side effects is limited and incomplete. Although some phase II and III trials have included quality of life assessments, these are not a substitute for objective, standardized, and quantifiable psychometric measures of the impact of these medications on cognition.

The epilepsy itself is an important confounding factor in assessing the cognitive effects of AEDs. Epilepsy can be associated with cognitive problems by virtue of the intrinsic neuropathology underlying both the mental impairment and the epilepsy. Cognition can also be affected by the seizures themselves, interictal electroencephalographic (EEG) activity, psychosocial problems, familial factors, and, of course, the effects of the AEDs (2).When AEDs suppress epileptiform discharges and decrease seizure frequency, they can improve cognitive function (3). However, the mechanisms by which AEDs suppress seizures may also affect normal neuronal mechanisms such as ion channel permeability, receptors, neurotransmitter kinetics, and second messengers and interfere with cognitive function. The mechanisms of action of the various anticonvulsant drugs are reviewed in Chapter 30 of this textbook.

Many of the studies assessing the cognitive side effects of AEDs in adults and children suffer from major methodological flaws, limiting the information that can be gleaned. Before reviewing these studies, it is advisable to review these methodological issues.

The first issue in the study of AEDs relates to who is being studied. Studies vary by patient selection criteria, including type of seizures, age of subjects, and duration of exposure to medication. In examining the influence of AEDs on cognition in patients with epilepsy, many studies include patients with any type of epilepsy. This can be problematic because, compared to patients with idiopathic epilepsy, patients with symptomatic epilepsy are more likely to have associated or underlying neurological disorders that directly impair neurological function, including cognition, attention, mood, and behavior (4). People with symptomatic epilepsy may also be more sensitive to the neurological adverse effects of AEDs.

Even within the category of idiopathic epilepsy, different seizure types are associated with varying cognitive impairments. For example, in a study of 43 children with new-onset idiopathic seizures, Mandelbaum and Burack (5) found that cognitive functioning was worse in children with generalized versus partial seizures, and nonconvulsive versus convulsive seizures, a difference that also may have an impact on adverse responses to AEDs.

Another methodological issue in studying the effect of AEDs on cognition is the composition of control groups. Studies may use either an "active" control (e.g., people receiving another medication, or with another medical disorder) or a "healthy" control. In some studies AEDs have been administered to normal adult volunteers. Although these studies have the virtue of isolating the effects of the AEDs from the effects of epilepsy or other medications, they have disadvantages as well. Most of them are limited to a short-term period of observation. None of them could detect a beneficial interaction between the AED and the epileptic brain. Furthermore, there are important differences between the mature, adult brain and the developing child's brain, which limit the applicability of studies in normal adult volunteers to children.

The use of a medical control group has the potential advantage of controlling for the socioemotional effects of dealing with a health condition. These types of control subjects may include children with other neurological or systemic illnesses. For example, in a study comparing children with newly diagnosed diabetes to children with newly diagnosed seizures before and 6 months after initiation of treatment, Williams and colleagues (6) found no differences over time between the groups on measures of cognitive or behavioral functioning. In contrast, Seidel et al (7) found that in a repeated-measures design, 14 children with untreated migraine headaches exhibited higher verbal memory scores in comparison to 10 children with benign rolandic epilepsy treated with carbamazepine. In a study by Bourgeois and others (4), the IQ score of the sibling controls of children with symptomatic epilepsy was much lower than the IQ score of the sibling controls of children with idiopathic epilepsy, illustrating the importance of socioeconomically (and, perhaps, genetically) matched controls.

Controlling for practice effects is important when studies follow children over time, with testing done before and after treatment. For this reason a separate control group is of considerable importance to interpreting the significance of changes in scores over time. Normal individuals who undergo repeated cognitive assessment as long as 4 years apart, much longer than is traditionally associated with a test-retest effect, show notable increases in test scores during repeated administrations (8). This raises the possibility that a lack of practice effect, that is, stable scores over time, indicates an adverse effect on learning.

Comparison of different studies is thwarted by significant variability in the measures used by individual researchers. Cochrane and colleagues (9) reviewed 40 randomized, controlled trials and noted a lack of uniform approach to neuropsychological assessment with approximately 87 different measures being used. The most commonly identified measures were the Stroop Color Word and Finger Tapping Test. Nevertheless, these tests were not used or reported uniformly, a lack of consistency that creates significant obstacles for integrating information across different studies. Furthermore, the decision of what is and is not included in the test battery can significantly affect the results. A drug may "look good" or "look bad" depending on the type of testing that was done. For example, in some of the early testing with carbamazepine it was demonstrated that carbamazepine enhanced sitting behavior, yet other studies showed adverse effects on motor tasks.

When reporting test results, it is essential that the nature of the data being used (e.g., raw scores, standardized scores based on manual-provided information, or specific reference to independent normative samples) be identified. Table 69-1 represents a battery of well-developed and widely available measures. This battery is proposed as a more uniform approach to studies of the cognitive effects of AEDs. In this battery the Stroop color word phenomenon is assessed as part of the Delis-Kaplan Executive Function System (D-KEFS), Color Word (10). Completion of comprehensive neuropsychological testing has practical limitations and choices must be made about which tests to administer. For example, the test battery listed in Table 69-1 would take 5 to 6 hours to

TABLE 69-1
Proposed Psychometric Battery

Intellect

WISC-IV (11): Block Design, Matrix Reasoning, Similarities, Vocabulary

Attention

WISC-IV – Integrated (12): Digit Span, Letter-Number Sequencing, Spatial Span, Cancellation

Continuous Performance Test, such as the CPT-II (13)

Simple and complex reaction time

Executive

D-KEFS (10): Number-letter switching, Category switching, Color Word Inhibition, Tower

WCST (14)

WISC-IV (11): Processing speed—Coding, Symbol Search

Language

WISC-IV (11): Vocabulary

PPVT-III (15)

EOWPVT-R (16)

D-KEFS (13): Letter fluency, category fluency

Visual-spatial

WISC-IV (11): Block Design

VMI, Beery VMI Developmental Test of Visual Perception (17)

Rey Complex Figure–Copy trial (18)

NEPSY: Arrows (19)

Memory

WRAML2—immediate, delayed, and recognition (20)

Rey Complex Figure (18)

Sensory-Motor

Grooved pegboard (21)

Finger tapping (22)

Grip strength (22)

Sensory exam

Academic

WJ-III (23)

TOWL-3 (24)

Socioemotional/behavioral

Parent report: BASC (25)

Child report: Beck Youth Inventories–II (26)

BASC (25)

administer and another 1 or 2 hours to score. The cost of doing such studies becomes immediately apparent, not to mention the challenge of assuring compliance with serial measures.

Research investigating the cognitive effects of AEDs must control for other potentially confounding variables, including parental intellectual level, family dynamics (e.g., level of disorganization, level of negative affect), and other stressors, including financial limitations. Socioeconomic status is one of the strongest predictors of intelligence in children with epilepsy (27). Oostrom and colleagues (28) found that cognitive and behavioral outcomes in 42 children with idiopathic or cryptogenic, newly diagnosed epilepsy followed over 3.5 years were related to the child's prediagnostic learning history, as well as to the parents' ability to cope effectively with their child's epilepsy. Children from disorganized and unsupportive homes were also more likely to have a poorer academic outcome (29, 30).

As a result of selection bias when subjects are chosen, results from studies of AEDs on cognition may not be generalizable to the population at large. For example, the majority of research in pediatric epilepsy has been conducted at epilepsy centers, where patients are more likely to have associated handicaps and severe forms of epilepsy (31).

There are differences of opinion on how the data on cognitive aspects of AEDs should be collected. A major research design question is whether to use cross-sectional versus prospective approaches. Cross-sectional studies are useful in that they help identify variables that show relationships with the identified area of interest by providing a snapshot of that relationship. Prospective, randomized studies are essential to establish the causal aspect of a relationship. Ideally, an initial neuropsychological assessment should be completed when epilepsy is diagnosed and before initiation of medication, with serial measures after treatment is initiated.

Other factors can also influence cognition among children with epilepsy. Subclinical or subtle seizures can affect test results. Thus, it is optimal to have EEG monitoring done at the time of testing, or at least in close proximity to the time of testing. The effect of AEDs on test performance may be influenced by drug concentrations (32), including whether testing is done at the time of peak or trough levels. Whereas drug concentrations fluctuate throughout the day, testing at a consistent time of day can minimize the confounding influence of this variable.

Finally, in any study comparing two groups, the null hypothesis—that is, that there is no difference between the two groups (treatment vs. placebo, drug A vs. drug B)—has to be disproved to a degree of statistical probability. Usually a two-tailed test with the P value set to <0.05 is used when a single outcome is being evaluated. A poorly designed or executed study or a study with

TABLE 69-2
Methodological Issues

Subject Selection	Control Groups	Environmental Factors	Outcome Variables	Analyses
Idiopathic vs. symptomatic	"Active control" e.g., headaches, diabetes	SES/Parental functioning	Different measures in different studies	Sample size
Focal vs. generalized	Siblings	Investigator and parental bias	Subjective vs. objective measures	Cross-sectional vs. longitudinal studies
Healthy adults	"Internal controls" (practice effect)	Peak vs. trough levels		

SES = socioeconomic status

inadequate power (as with a sample size that is too small) can fail to detect important differences. Many studies on this topic are single-center studies that have a small sample size that may miss important differences between study conditions. Likewise, when many outcomes are considered simultaneously, such as multiple subtest scores in a psychometric test battery, the probability value used to reject the null hypothesis must be made more stringent. If the P value is set at 0.05 and 20 dependent variables are evaluated, one or more dependent variables is likely to attain a level of significant difference by chance alone. Setting the P value at 0.01 or 0.001 is required to avoid this pitfall in data analysis.

The limitations of the literature notwithstanding (Table 69-2), representative studies that have looked at the question of cognitive effects of AEDs will now be reviewed. The reader is also directed to a supplement of the *Journal of Child Neurology* that was devoted to this topic (33).

PHENOBARBITAL

Because phenobarbital is the drug that has been used longest to treat epilepsy, there is a fairly extensive body of literature regarding its adverse effects. Phenobarbital is widely considered to have substantial adverse side effects, particularly as it relates to cognition. However, in a comprehensive review of the literature on phenobarbital, Pal stated, "The overall design quality and statistical methodology of clinical trials in this area is poor, especially for those trials conducted in the 1970's and 1980's" (34). Pal reported that blinded studies of childhood epilepsy did not show significant differences of behavioral or cognitive side effects when phenobarbital was compared to other AEDs, in contrast to studies in which the investigators were unblinded, hence subject to observer bias. In his review of the literature, there was one double-blinded, randomized, placebo-controlled study of phenobarbital for febrile seizures that showed an adverse effect of phenobarbital on IQ after 2 years of treatment that persisted for 6 months after discontinuation of therapy (35). However, this study had several confounding features including the following: Among 638 children eligible to enroll 421 declined, mostly because of parental reluctance to have the child take phenobarbital. The lowest-IQ group showed the greatest decrease in IQ compared to placebo, and it was the low-IQ phenobarbital group that had the greatest number of dropouts, with only 11 of 24 available for testing at 2 years and 13 of 24 at 2.5 years. Furthermore, although the analysis was done on the basis of intention to treat, because of breakthrough seizures and side effects, many participants did not complete the study. For example, approximately 25% of children assigned to placebo were taking phenobarbital by the end of the study, and only about half of the children assigned to phenobarbital were still taking phenobarbital at the end of the study. It is impossible to know how these factors impacted on the outcomes reported, but statistical assumptions had to be made to analyze the results.

Concerns have been raised about behavioral problems from phenobarbital (36). But, as pointed out by Pal, these data represent parental report in an unblinded, nonrandomized, uncontrolled study. A study comparing the efficacy of phenobarbital, valproate, and intermittent rectal diazepam, in which subjects were randomly assigned to treatment group, found that the parents of 8 of 41 children taking phenobarbital discontinued it because of side effects. In contrast, only 3 of 50 parents discontinued valproate (37).

In an effort to use surrogate neurophysiological data to assess the effect of phenobarbital on central nervous system (CNS) function, Chen et al (38) noted a prolongation of P-300 latencies in auditory evoked potentials in children treated with phenobarbital and not in those treated with carbamazepine or valproate monotherapy.

PHENYTOIN

Aman and colleagues in 1994 (39) investigated the cognitive impact of phenytoin by assessing children at both trough and peak levels and found no effect on cognitive performance, although the drug concentrations studied were rather low. A study of phenytoin compared to placebo in healthy adults found impaired memory, concentration, and mental and motor speed while taking phenytoin (40). An open-label study of cognitive function in children with epilepsy treated with either phenytoin, carbamazepine, or valproate monotherapy found that the phenytoin group did worse than the valproate group on a single measure of processing speed after 1 month, but not after 6 or 12 months of treatment (41).

CARBAMAZEPINE

Carbamazepine, approved for epilepsy in 1974, provided the first major alternative to phenobarbital and phenytoin for localization-related epilepsies. Studies of the cognitive impact of carbamazepine have shown both beneficial and adverse effects on cognition. Aman and colleagues (42) studied 50 children on carbamazepine monotherapy at trough and peak concentrations and found that the children performed significantly better at peak carbamazepine concentrations on measures of activity, attention span, motor steadiness, and task-specific response times. In a study by Forsythe and colleagues (41), 64 children with newly diagnosed epilepsy were randomly assigned to carbamazepine, phenytoin, or valproate. Cognitive testing was done before initiation of treatment and three times over the first year of treatment. The authors concluded that carbamazepine in moderate doses adversely effected memory, whereas valproate and phenytoin did not. A study by Stores and colleagues (43) compared 63 newly diagnosed children randomly assigned to either carbamazepine or valproate with 47 matched controls. Cognitive testing done before initiation of treatment and at intervals over 1 year revealed modest effects of both carbamazepine and valproate on cognitive abilities. There were no effects on behavioral measures, and there was no difference between carbamazepine and valproate. A study by Berg and colleagues (44) evaluated 64 children newly diagnosed with epilepsy who were randomly assigned to carbamazepine, phenytoin, or valproate. Behavioral measures were done before medication and after 1 and 6 months of treatment. The authors found that carbamazepine and valproate were associated with minor behavioral difficulties after 1 month, but these problems were not present at 6 months. In another study of children with both generalized and focal epilepsy, carbamazepine resulted in impaired reaction time variability that persisted over 12 months of treatment (45). In this group of patients there were attention problems at baseline, before medication was started. In most measures of cognitive functioning there were no adverse effects after initiating treatment with anticonvulsants.

VALPROIC ACID

Valproic acid, approved in the United States 4 years after carbamazepine, is useful in localization-related, generalized, convulsive, and nonconvulsive epilepsies. A study of children randomly assigned to valproic acid, carbamazepine, or phenytoin showed valproate to have fewer negative effects than carbamazepine or phenytoin (41). One study of children with newly diagnosed epilepsy found that scores on 4 tests of a total of 30 administered over a 12-month period were significantly worse in the children treated with valproate than in controls; a similar result was found for the carbamazepine group (43). However, it is worth noting that valproate has been used successfully to treat children with explosive temper and mood lability (46).

NEWER DRUGS

There is less information about the newer AEDs introduced since 1992. Among these drugs, topiramate appears to have more adverse cognitive effects than lamotrigine, oxcarbazepine, and levetiracetam. (47)

Lamotrigine

Among the newer AEDs, one of the better studied drugs is lamotrigine. Lamotrigine administered to normal adult volunteers caused no adverse effect on cognitive function compared to controls (48, 49); nor did lamotrigine result in any adverse effects in adults with epilepsy (50, 51). A study by Meador et al (52) comparing treatment with lamotrigine and carbamazepine in a double-blinded, randomized, crossover design demonstrated lamotrigine to have a side effect profile preferable to that of carbamazepine. Studies in children have suggested positive effects such as behavioral improvement and increased alertness, even in the absence of seizure reduction (53, 54).

Gabapentin

Gabapentin has been associated with behavioral problems in children. In a double-blind, placebo-controlled, add-on study among children with refractory partial-onset seizures, gabapentin was associated with an increased incidence of somnolence, hostility, emotional lability, and hyperkinesias compared to placebo (55). Other reports indicate that children with mental retardation are at greater risk than children with normal IQ for developing aggressive behavior while taking gabapentin (56). Studies in adult volunteers have shown no adverse effect of gabapentin at doses of 2,400 mg/day (57, 58). In the study by Meador et al, of 31 variables assessed there were 6 in which the subjects taking no drug did better than they did while taking gabapentin, as opposed to 15 variables in which the no-drug group did better than those taking carbamazepine. On 8 variables performance while taking gabapentin was superior to that while taking carbamazepine. Carbamazepine was not superior to gabapentin on any variables in this study. Note, however, that although this was a blinded study and the subjects were studied while not taking and while taking the two drugs, there was no placebo group.

Tiagabine

Tiagabine, which acts by increasing the effect of gamma-aminobutyric acid (a mechanism shared by barbiturates), variably causes disturbances in mood and behavior. In placebo-controlled studies, tiagabine, as either monotherapy or add-on in 162 subjects with epilepsy, was reported to cause no adverse cognitive effects (59). However, an open-label study of tiagabine as adjunctive therapy in children with refractory, complex partial seizures reported complaints of somnolence, headache, dizziness, and nervousness. These complaints diminished over time and were less frequent when the drug was used as monotherapy (60).

Vigabatrin

In an open label, randomized study comparing vigabatrin and carbamazepine monotherapy in adults with newly diagnosed epilepsy, there were no adverse effects of vigabatrin on cognitive functions, thus demonstrating a better adverse effect profile than carbamazepine (61). A similar, open label, randomized trial comparing vigabatrin to carbamazepine in children found that 6 of 38 children taking vigabatrin were described as having excessive irritability and excitability, whereas 6 of 32 children taking carbamazepine were excessively sedated (62). Vigabatrin, which is not FDA approved for sale in the United States, is largely limited to treatment of children with infantile spasms, particularly those with tuberous sclerosis. Little data are available on cognitive effects in this severely involved group of patients. Although vigabatrin has been shown to have significant neurotoxic effect in animal models, consisting of intramyelinic edema with microvacuoles in the optic tracts, cerebellum, hippocampus, and columns of the fornix in rodents and dogs (63), no effects on white matter have been found on magnetic resonance imaging (MRI) studies of humans who took vigabatrin. However, vigabatrin causes irreversible visual field constriction in what appears to be an at least partially dose- or duration-dependent fashion. Of note, in most cases these visual field defects were not overtly symptomatic (64).

Topiramate

Topiramate has been linked to difficulties with word finding and coding on psychometric tests. Meador and colleagues (65) compared the cognitive effects of topiramate to those of valproate or carbamazepine in adults with partial epilepsy. On the symbol-digit modalities test, 20% of the patients taking topiramate had a worsening in their performance of greater than 1 standard deviation, as opposed to none of the patients taking valproate. On a controlled word-association task, about 25% of the topiramate group performed more than 1 standard deviation below their baseline scores compared with about 10% in the valproate group. A double-blind, randomized, placebo-controlled study of topiramate as add-on therapy for children with intractable partial seizures noted increased incidences of emotional lability, fatigue, attention and concentration problems, and forgetfulness, compared to placebo; and this was despite improved seizure control (66). In another study of 42 patients with juvenile myoclonic epilepsy treated with valproate (62%) or topiramate (38%) monotherapy, among 27 items in the psychometric battery, the topiramate group performed significantly worse in 3. Two of the three were measures of memory, attention, and speed processing, and one a measure of verbal fluency (67).

Oxcarbazepine

In general, oxcarbazepine has not been linked to adverse cognitive effects. A study of the cognitive effects of oxcarbazepine, carbamazepine, and valproic acid in adults with newly diagnosed epilepsy showed no deterioration of cognitive function in patients in any of the treatment groups. In fact, there was improvement in learning and memory tests in the oxcarbazepine and carbamazepine groups, but not the valproate group. The patients who were treated with valproate showed improvement in attention and psychomotor speed (68). In studies on healthy volunteers, oxcarbazepine improved attention and writing speed and had no effect on long-term memory (69). One add-on study of oxcarbazepine in children with intractable epilepsy reported a 35% incidence of somnolence in children taking oxcarbazepine compared to a 14% incidence of somnolence in the placebo group (70).

Levetiracetam

Levetiracetam, although chemically related to piracetam, a drug with cognitive enhancing effects including improvement in learning and memory, has not been shown to have the same nootropic effect (71). A review of the adult literature comparing the behavioral effects of levetiracetam in adults with epilepsy versus adults with cognitive or anxiety disorders showed a greater incidence of depression, nervousness, hostility, anxiety, and emotional lability in epileptic patients treated with levetiracetam compared to placebo (72). A study of the cognitive and neurophysiologic measures in healthy volunteers treated with carbamazepine, oxcarbazepine, and levetriracetam found motor slowing in the volunteers treated with carbamazepine and oxcarbazepine, but not levetiracetam. Attention span increased from baseline levels with all three drugs. Carbamazepine and oxcarbazepine induced changes in some components of the visual evoked potential responses, whereas levetiracetam did not. Similarly, oxcarbazepine and carbamazepine, but not levetiracetam, resulted in slowing of the EEG (73). An open-label, retrospective study of levetiracetam as add-on therapy in children with intractable seizures found that among 41 of 59 children still taking levetiracetam at 12 months, 28% had adverse behavioral effects and 24% were lethargic in a non-dose-dependent fashion (74).

Zonisamide

Zonisamide, approved in the United States in 2000, was not studied in children before its release. Clinical experience, particularly in Japan, indicates that it is effective in a wide range of seizure types in children and adults (75). An open-label study of cognitive functioning in adults treated with zonisamide as add-on therapy showed effects on the acquisition and consolidation of new information with no effect on previously learned material or psychomotor performance. Verbal learning was affected, whereas visual-perceptual learning was not. There was a correlation between the impairment of cognitive function and the plasma concentration. There was also evidence of the development of tolerance to the adverse effects over time (76). In a retrospective review of their experience with children with intractable epilepsy treated with zonisamide as add-on therapy, Mandelbaum and colleagues (77) reported that at 12 months, among the 19 of 35 children still taking zonisamide, 7 (37%) were described as lethargic, 3 had behavior problems, and 3 had decreased appetite in a non-dose dependent manner.

Pregabalin

A study of pregabalin administered to healthy adult volunteers demonstrated an effect of pregabalin on a subset of psychometric tests; specifically, of a total of seven psychometric tests, there was an adverse effect in three and an improvement in one, compared to placebo. Functions adversely affected included arousal and reaction time, both of which were affected transiently. The test on which there was an improvement on pregabalin was also an assessment of reaction time. The third test in which pregabalin treatment was associated with a worse score was a subjective report of sedation. (78). No studies of children have been reported.

Clobazam

A drug that has not been approved for sale in the United States, clobazam is one of the few AEDs that have been studied in children using formal psychometric measures. A study comparing clobazam to carbamazepine or phenytoin found that the scores on performance IQ and memory tests were inversely related to clobazam serum concentrations. Whereas practice effects were evident in children on carbamazepine and phenytoin tested after a year of treatment, the children taking clobazam did not have a practice effect (79). As discussed previously, the absence of a practice effect likely indicates impairment of cognitive function (8).

VAGUS NERVE STIMULATION

A study by Clark et al (80) compared 10 patients with vagus nerve stimulation (VNS) to a control group of patients with sham stimulation and found that VNS stimulation of 0.5 milliamperes administered after reading a paragraph enhanced word recognition; there was no improvement with stimulation intensities of 0.75 to 1.5 mA and no improvement if the stimulation was done before reading the paragraph.

CONCLUSION

The nature of the data available, coupled with individual variability in response to the various AEDs, make it difficult to predict how an individual child will respond to a specific drug. The newer AEDs have the advantage of requiring less monitoring for medically serious adverse effects such as bone marrow suppression or hepatic dysfunction. For absence seizures, ethosuximide is a safe, effective drug with little in the way of adverse effects (81). For partial seizures and generalized convulsive seizures there are some clues as to which drugs are more or less likely to be problematic (Table 69-3). When administered prudently, lamotrigine, tiagabine, oxcarbazepine, levetiracetam, and zonisamide are effective, safe, and have favorable cognitive side-effect profiles. Topiramate and clobazam appear be more likely to cause cognitive side effects, and gabapentin has been linked to adverse behavioral effects. It is of interest that a critical review of the

TABLE 69-3
Summary of Predominant Adverse Cognitive and Behavioral Effects

Drug	Behavioral/Cognitive Effects	References
Phenobarbital	IQ effects, irritability	34, 35, 36, 37
Phenytoin	Processing speed	39, 40, 41
Carbamazepine	Memory, behavior	41, 42, 43
Valproic acid	(cognitive teratogenic effects)	41, 42
Lamotrigine		53, 54
Gabapentin	Behavior	55, 56
Tiagabine	Somnolence, nervousness	59, 60
Vigabatrin	Irritability, excitability	62
Topiramate	Cognitive	66, 67
Oxcarbazepine	Somnolence	70
Levetiracetam	Behavior	72, 74
Zonisamide	Cognitive, behavior	77
Pregabalin	No childhood studies	
Clobazam	IQ and memory	79

literature on phenobarbital suggests that its reputation for adverse cognitive and behavioral side effects is not fully documented. Hopefully, multicenter, blinded, head-to-head studies of different AEDs using a uniform battery of formal psychometric measures will be done to address these questions more conclusively. Pharmaceutical company–sponsored studies of new drugs should include objective, quantifiable psychometric testing in addition to the subjective, qualitative adverse effect reports that are currently the norm.

References

1. Nelson KB, Ellenberg JH. Prognosis in children with febrile seizures. *Pediatrics* 1978; 61:720–727.
2. Lennox WG. Brain injury, drugs and environment as causes of mental decay in epilepsy. *Am J Psychiatry* 1942; 99:174–180.
3. Mayor-Dubois C, Gianella D, Chaves-Vischer V, Haenggeli CA, et al. Speech delay due to a prelinguistic regression of epileptic origin. *Neuropediatrics* 2004; 35:50–53.
4. Bourgeois BFD, Prensky AL, Palkes HS, et al. Intelligence in epilepsy: a prospective study in children. *Ann Neurol* 1983; 14:438–444.
5. Mandelbaum DE, Burack GD. The effect of seizure type and medication on cognitive and behavioral functioning in children with idiopathic epilepsy. *Dev Med Child Neurol* 1997; 39:731–735.
6. Williams J, Bates S, Griebl ML, et al. Does short term anti-epileptic in children result in cognitive or behavioral changes? *Epilepsia* 1998; 39:1064–1069.
7. Seidel WT, Mitchell WG, et al. Cognitive and behavioral effect of carbamazipine in children: data from benign rolandic epilepsy. *J Child Neurol* 1999; 14:716–723.
8. Hermann BP, Seidenberg M, Schoenfeld J, et al. Empirical techniques for determining the reliability, magnitude and pattern of neuropsychological change after epilepy surgery. *Epilepsia* 1996; 37:942–950.
9. Cochrane HC, Marson AG, Baker GA, Chadwick DW. Neuropsychological outcomes in randomised controlled trials of antiepileptic drugs: a systematic review of methodology and reporting standards. *Epilepsia* 1998; 39:1088–1097.
10. Delis DC, Kaplan E, Kramer JH. Delis-Kaplan executive function system (D-KEFS). San Antonio, TX: Psychological Corporation, 2001.
11. Wechsler D. WISC-IV technical and interpretive manual. San Antonio, TX: Psychological Corporation, 2003.
12. Wechsler D, Kaplan E, Fein D, et al. WISC-IV: integrated. San Antonio, TX: Psychological Corporation, 2004.
13. Conners CK. Conners' Continuous Performance Test II (CPT II). North Tonawanda, NY: MHS, 2000.
14. Heaton RK, Chelune GJ, Talley JL, et al. Wisconsin card sorting test manual, revised and expanded. Odessa, FL: Psychological Assessment Resources, 1993.
15. Dunn LM, Dunn LM. Peabody picture vocabulary test. 3rd ed. Circle Pines, MN: American Guidance Service, 1997.
16. Gardner MF. Expressive one-word picture vocabulary test—revised manual. Novato, CA: Academic Therapy Publications, 1990.
17. Beery KE, Beery NA. The Beery-Buktenica developmental test of visual-motor integration VMI. 5th ed. Minneapolis, MN: NCS Pearson, 2004.
18. Meyers JE, Meyers KR. Rey complex figure test and recognition trial manual. Odessa, FL: Psychological Assessment Resources, Inc., 1995.
19. Korkman M, Kirk U, Kemp S. NEPSY: a developmental neuropsychological assessment. San Antonio, TX: Psychological Corporation, 1998.
20. Sheslow D, Adams W. Wide Range assessment of memory and learning. 2nd ed. Wilmington, DE: Wide Range Inc., 2003.
21. Klove H. Clinical neuropsychology. In: Forster FM, ed. *The Medical Clinics of North America*. New York: Saunders, 1963:1647–1658.
22. Reitan RM, Wolfson D. The Halstead-Reitan neuropsychological test battery: theory and clinical interpretation. Tucson, AZ: Neuropsychology Press, 1993.
23. Woodcock R, McGrew K, Mather N. Woodcock-Johnson III tests of achievement. Itasca, IL: Riverside Publishing, 2001.
24. Hammill D, Larsen S. Test of written language (TOWL). 3rd ed. Austin, TX: Pro-ed, 1996.
25. Reynolds CR, Kamphaus RW. Behavior assessment system for children—second edition (BASC-2). Circle Pines, MN: American Guidance Service, 2004.
26. Beck JS, Beck AT, Jolly JB, et al. Manual for Beck youth inventories—second edition. San Antonio, TX: Harcourt, 2005.
27. Singhi PD, Bansal U., Singhi S, et al. Determinants of IQ profile in children with idiopathic generalized epilepsy. *Epilepsia* 1992; 33:1106–1114.
28. Oostrom KJ, van-Teeseling H, Smeets-Schouten A, et al. Three to four years after diagnosis: Cognition and behaviour in children with "epilepsy only." A prospective, controlled study. *Brain* 2005; 128:1546–1555.
29. Fastenau PS, Shen J, Dunn DW, et al. Neuropsychological predictors of academic underachievement in pediatric epilepsy: moderating roles of demographic, seizure, and psychosocial variables. *Epilepsia* 2004; 45:1261–1272.
30. Adewuya AO, Oseni SB, Okeniyi JA. School performance of Nigerian adolescents with epilepsy. *Epilepsia* 2006; 47:415–420.
31. Hermann BP, Whitman S. Behavioral and personality correlates of epilepsy: a review, methodological critique, and conceptual mode. *Psychol Bull* 1984; 95:451–497.
32. Dodrill CB, Troupin AS. Neuropsychological effects of carbamazepine and phenytoin: a reanalysis. *Neurology* 1991; 41:141–143.
33. Pellock JM, ed. Behavioral and cognitive disorders in pediatric epilepsy. *J Child Neurol* 2004; 19 Suppl 1.
34. Pal DK. Phenobarbital for childhood epilepsy: systematic review. *Paediatric and Perinatal Drug Therapy* 2006; 7: 31–42.
35. Farwell JR, Lee YJ, Hirtz DG, et al. Phenobarbital for febrile seizures-effects on intelligence and seizure recurrence. *N Engl J Med* 1990; 322:364–369.

36. Wolfe SM, Forsythe A. Behavior disturbance, phenobarbital and febrile seizures. *Pediatrics* 1978; 61:728–731.
37. McKinlay I, Newton R. Intention to treat febrile convulsions with rectal diazepam, valproate or phenobarbitone. *Dev Med Child Neurol* 1989; 31:617–625.
38. Chen Y, Chi Chow J, Lee I, et al. Comparison of the cognitive effect of antiepileptic drugs in seizure-free children with epilepsy before and after drug withdrawal. *Epilepsy Res* 2001; 44:65–70.
39. Aman MG, Werry JS, Paxton JW, Turbott SH. Effect of phenytoin on cognitive-motor performance in children as a function of drug concentration, seizure type and time of medication. *Epilepsia* 1994; 35:172–180.
40. Thompson P, Huppert FA, Trimble M. Phenytoin and cognitive function: effects on normal volunteers and implications for epilepsy. *Br J Clin Psychol* 1981; 20:155–162.
41. Forsythe I, Butler R, Berg I, McGuire R. cognitive impairment in new cases of epilepsy randomly assigned to carbamazepine, phenytoin and sodium valproate. *Dev Med Child Neurol* 1991; 33:524–534.
42. Aman MG, Werry JS, Paxton JW, et al. Effect of carbamazepine on psychomotor performance in children as a function of drug concentration, seizure type, and time of medication. *Epilepsia* 1990; 31:51–60.
43. Stores P, Williams PL, Styles E, et al. Psychological effects of sodium valproate and carbamazepine in epilepsy. *Arch Dis Child* 1992; 67:1330–1337.
44. Berg I, Butler A, Ellis M, Foster J. Psychiatric aspects of epilepsy in childhood treated with carbamazepine, phenytoin or sodium valproate: a randomized trial. *Dev Med Child Neurol* 1993; 35:149–157.
45. Mandelbaum DE, Burack G, Bhise V. Assessment of cognition and atttention before and after anticonvulsant therapy in children with new-onset idiopathic epilepsy: a prospective study. *Neurology* 2005; 64:A117.
46. Donovan SJ, Stewart JW, Nunes EV, et al. Divalproex treatment for youth with explosive temper and mood lability; a double-blind, placebo-controlled crossover design. *Am J Psychiatry* 2000; 157:818–820.
47. Aldenkamp AP, De Krom M, Reijs R. Newer antiepileptic drugs and cognitive issues. *Epilepsia* 2003; 44 Suppl 4:21–29.
48. Cohen AF, Ashby L, Crowley D, et al. Lamotrigine (BW430C), a potential anti-convulsant. effects on the central nervous system in comparison with phenytoin and diazapam. *Br J Clin Pharmacol* 1985; 20:619–629.
49. Smith D, Baker G, Davies G, et al. Outcomes of add-on treatment with lamotrigine in partial epilepsy. *Epilepsia* 1993; 34:312–322.
50. Marciani MG, Stanzione P, Mattia D, et al. Lamotrigine add-on therapy in focal epilepsy: electroencephalographic and neuro-psychological evaluation. *Clin Neuropharmacol* 1998; 21:41–47.
51. Aldenkamp AP, Mulder OG, Overweg J, et al. Cognitive effects of lamotrigine in patients with localization-related (partial) epilepsy. *J Epilepsy* 1997; 10:117–121.
52. Meador KJ, Loring DW, Ray PG, et al. Differential cognitive and behavioral effects of carbamazepine and lamotrigine. *Neurology* 2001; 56:1177–1182.
53. Eriksson AS, Knutsson E, Nergardh A, et al. The effect of lamotrigine on epileptiform discharges in young patients with drug-resistant epilepsy. *Epilepsia* 2001; 42:230–236.
54. Uvebrant P, Bauziene R. Intractable epilepsy in children: the efficacy of lamotrigine treatment, including non-seizure-related benefits. *Neuropediatrics* 1994; 25:284–289.
55. Appleton R, Fichtner K, Lameroux L et al; the Gabapentin Paediatric Study Group. Gabapentin as add-on therapy with children with refractory partial seizures: a 12 week, multicentre, double blind, placebo controlled study. *Epilepsia* 1999; 40:1147–1154.
56. Tallian KB, Nahatamc, Low W, Tsaocy, et al. Gabapentin associated with aggressive behavior in pediatric patients with seizures. *Epilepsia* 1996; 37:501–502.
57. Martin R, Kuzniecky R, Ho S, et al. Cognitive effects of topiramate, gabapentin and lamotrigine in healthy young adults. *Neurology* 1999; 52:321–327.
58. Meador KJ, Loring DW, Ray PG, et al. Differential cognitive effects of carbamazepine and gabepentin. *Epilepsia* 1999; 40:1279–1285.
59. Dodrill CB, Arnett JL, Sommerville, KW, Shu V, et al. Cognitive and quality of life effects of differing doses of tiagabine in epilepsy. *Neurology* 1997; 48:1025–1031.
60. Pellock JM, et al. Tiagabine (Gabatril) experience in children. *Epilepsia* 2001; 42 Suppl 3:49–51.
61. Kalviainen R, Aikia M, Saukkonenam, et al. Vigabatrin versus carbamazepine monotherapy in patients with newly diagnosed epilepsy in a randomized controlled study. *Arch Neurol* 1995; 52:989–996.
62. Zamponi N, Cesare Cardinali C. Open comparative long-term study of vigabatrin vs carbamazepine in newly diagnosed partial seizures in children. *Arch Neurol* 1999; 56:605–607.
63. Graham D. Neuropathology of vigabatrin. *Br J Clin Pharmacol* 1989; 27 Suppl 1: 43S–45S.
64. Malmgren K, Ben-Menachem, V, Frisen L. Vigabatrin visual toxicity: evolution and dose dependence. *Epilepsia* 2001; 42:609–615.
65. Meador KJ, Loring DW, Hulihan JF, et al; the CAPSS-027 Study Group. Differential cognitive and behavioral effects of topiramate and valproate. *Epilepsia* 2003; 60:1483–1488.
66. Elterman RD, Glauser TA, Wyllie E, et al. A double-blind, randomized trial of topiramate as adjunctive therapy for partial-onset seizures in children. *Neurology* 1999; 52:1338–1344.
67. De Araujo Filho GM, Pascalicchio TF, Lin K, et al. Neuropsychiatric profiles of patients with juvenile myoclonic epilepsy treated with valproate or topiramate. *Epilepsy Behav* 2006; 8:606–609.
68. Sabers A, Moller, A, Dam M, et al. Cognitive function in anti-convulsant therapy: effective monotherapy in epilepsy. *Acta Neurol Scand* 1995; 92:19–27.
69. Curran HV, Java R. Memory and psycho-motor effect of oxcarbazepine in healthy human volunteers. *Eur J Clin Pharmacol* 1993; 44:529–533.
70. Glauser TA, Nigro M, Sachdeo R, et al; the Oxcarbazepine Pediatric Study Group. Adjunctive therapy with oxcarbazepine in children with partial seizures. *Neurology* 2000; 54:2237–2244.
71. Gentin P, Van Vleymen B. Piracetam and levetiracetam: close structural similarities but different pharmacological and clinical profiles. *Epileptic Disord* 2000; 2:199–105.
72. Kramer JA, DeRue K, Divinski O, et al. A systematic review of the behavioral effects of levetiracetam in adults with epilepsy, cognitive disorders, or anxiety aduring clinical trials. *Epilepsy Behav* 2003; 4:124–132.
73. Mecarelli O, Vicenzini E, Pulitano P, et al. clinical, cognitive, and neurophysiologic correlates of short-term treatment with carbamazepine, oxcarbazepine, and levetiracetam in healthy volunteers. *Ann Pharmacother* 2004; 38:1816–1822.
74. Mandelbaum DE, Bunch M, Kugler SL, et al. Efficacy of levetiracetam at 12 months in children classified by seizure type, cognitive status, and previous anticonvulsant drug use. *J Child Neurol* 2005; 20:590–594.
75. Glauser TA. Zonisamide in pediatric epilepsy: review of the Japanese experience. *J Child Neurol* 2002; 17:87–96.
76. Berent S, Sackelleres JC, Giordani V, et al. Zonisamide (CI-192) and cognition; results from a preliminary study. *Epilepsia* 1987; 28:61–67.
77. Mandelbaum DE, Bunch M, Kugler SL, et al. Broad spectrum efficacy of zonisamide at twelve months in children with intractable epilepsy. *J Child Neurol* 2005; 20:594–597.
78. Hindmarch I, Trick L, Ridoug F. A double blind placebo and positive internal controlled investigation of the cognitive and psychomotor profile of pregabalin in healthy volunteers. *Psychopharmacology* 2005; 183; 133–143.
79. Bawden HN, Camfield CS, Camfield PR, et al. The cognitive and behavioural effects of clobazam and standard monotherapy are comparable. Canadian study for childhood epilepsy. *Epilepsy Res* 1999; 33:133–143.
80. Clark KB, Naritoku DK, Smith DC. Enhanced recognition memory following vagus nerve stimulation in human subjects. *Nat Neurosci* 1999; 2:94–98.
81. Trimble MR, Reynolds EH. Anticonvulsant drugs and mental symptoms: a review. *Psychol Med* 1976; 6:169–178.

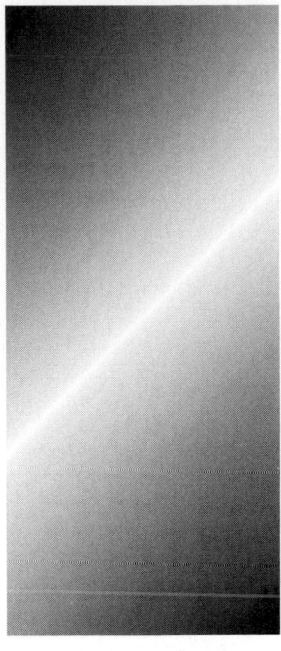

Index

Page numbers followed by f indicate figures; t, tables; b, boxes.